Surgery of the Chest

Surgery of the Chest

Volume **I**

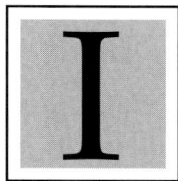

SIXTH EDITION

David C. Sabiston, Jr., M.D.

James B. Duke Professor of Surgery
Duke University School of Medicine
Chief of Staff
Duke University Medical Center
Durham, North Carolina

Frank C. Spencer, M.D.

George David Stewart Professor
Chairman, Department of Surgery
New York University School of Medicine
New York, New York

W.B. SAUNDERS COMPANY
A Division of Harcourt Brace & Company
Philadelphia   London   Toronto   Montreal   Sydney   Tokyo

W.B. SAUNDERS COMPANY
A Division of Harcourt Brace & Company

The Curtis Center
Independence Square West
Philadelphia, Pennsylvania 19106

Library of Congress Cataloging-in-Publication Data

Surgery of the chest / [edited by] David C. Sabiston, Jr., Frank C.
Spencer.—6th ed.
        p. cm.

    Includes bibliographical references and index.

    ISBN 0–7216–5271–9

    1. Chest—Surgery.   I. Sabiston, David C.
II. Spencer, Frank Cole.
        [DNLM: 1. Thoracic Surgery. WF 980 S961 1995]

RD536.G48   1995

617.5′4059—dc20

DNLM/DLC   94–22780

SURGERY OF THE CHEST   ISBN 0–7216–5271–9

Last digit is the print number: 9   8   7   6   5   4   3   2   1

Contributors

Alon S. Aharon, M.D.
Department of Surgery Resident, Cardiothoracic Division, University of California at Los Angeles Medical Center, Los Angeles, California
Congenital Malformations of the Mitral Valve

Robert W. Anderson, M.D.
The David C. Sabiston Professor and Chairman, Department of Surgery, Duke University Medical Center; Duke University Hospital, Durham, North Carolina
Shock and Circulatory Collapse

Mark P. Anstadt, M.D.
Resident in Chief in General Surgery, Duke University Medical Center, Durham, North Carolina
Assisted Circulation

Erle H. Austin III, M.D.
Professor of Surgery, University of Louisiana, Department of Surgery; Chief, Pediatric Cardiac Surgery, Kosair Children's Hospital, Louisville, Kentucky
Pulmonary Atresia with Intact Ventricular Septum; Univentricular Heart

John A. Bartlett, M.D.
Assistant Professor of Medicine, Duke University Medical Center, Durham, North Carolina
Thoracic Disorders in the Immunocompromised Host

Thomas M. Bashore, M.D.
Professor of Medicine; Director, Fellowship Training Program, Associate Director, Duke Heart Center, Duke University Medical Center, Durham, North Carolina
Cardiac Catheterization, Angiography, and Interventional Techniques in Valvular and Congenital Heart Disease; Coronary Arteriography

Harvey W. Bender, Jr., M.D.
Professor of Surgery, Vanderbilt University, School of Medicine; Chairman, Department of Cardiac and Thoracic Surgery, Vanderbilt University Medical Center, Nashville, Tennessee
Major Anomalies of Pulmonary and Thoracic Systemic Veins

Arthur D. Boyd, M.D.
Professor of Surgery, New York University School of Medicine; Attending Surgeon, Tisch Hospital of the New York University Medical Center; Attending Surgeon, Bellevue Hospital Center; Attending Surgeon, Manhattan Veterans Administration Center, New York, New York
Endoscopy: Bronchoscopy and Esophagoscopy; Tracheal Intubation and Mechanical Ventilation: The Surgeon's Viewpoint

Robert M. Califf, M.D.

Associate Professor of Medicine, Duke University; Director, Coronary Care Unit; Director, Clinical Epidemiology and Biostatistics, Duke University Medical Center, Durham, North Carolina
Fibrinolytic Therapy in the Management of Acute Myocardial Infarction

David N. Campbell, M.D.

Associate Professor of Surgery, University of Colorado, Health Services Center, Denver, Colorado
Thrombosis and Thromboembolism of Prosthetic Cardiac Valves and Extracardiac Prostheses

Aldo R. Castañeda, M.D., Ph.D.

Director, The Aldo Castañeda Institute for Congenital Heart Disease, Clinique de Genolier, Genolier, Switzerland
Anatomic Correction of Transposition of the Great Arteries at the Arterial Level

Jessie Chai, M.D.

Brigham and Women's Hospital, Boston, Massachusetts
Role of Computed Tomographic Scans in Cardiovascular Diagnosis

Robbin G. Cohen, M.D.

Assistant Professor of Surgery, Division of Cardiothoracic Surgery, Department of Surgery, University of Southern California School of Medicine; University of Southern California University Hospital; University of Southern California—Kenneth Norris Jr. Cancer Hospital; LAC University of Southern California Hospital, Los Angeles, California
The Pleura

Lawrence H. Cohn, M.D.

Professor of Surgery, Harvard Medical School; Chief, Division of Cardiac Surgery, Brigham and Women's Hospital, Boston, Massachusetts
Thoracic Aortic Aneurysms and Aortic Dissection

Stephen B. Colvin, M.D.

Associate Professor of Surgery, New York University Medical School; Director, Cardiac Surgical Residency and Pediatric Cardiac Surgery, New York Medical Center, New York, New York
Atrial Septal Defects, Atrioventricular Canal Defects, and Total Anomalous Pulmonary Venous Return; Acquired Disease of the Mitral Valve; Bypass Grafting for Coronary Artery Disease

Joel D. Cooper, M.D.

Joseph C. Bancroft Professor of Surgery; Head, Section of General Thoracic Surgery, Division of Cardiothoracic Surgery, Washington University School of Medicine, Barnes Hospital, St. Louis, Missouri
Lung Transplantation

James L. Cox, M.D.

Evarts A. Graham Professor of Surgery, Washington University School of Medicine; Professor of Surgery, Chief, Division of Cardiothoracic Surgery, Barnes Hospital at Washington University School of Medicine, St. Louis, Missouri
The Surgical Management of Cardiac Arrhythmias

Fred A. Crawford, Jr., M.D.

Professor and Chairman, Department of Surgery, Medical University of South Carolina, Charleston, South Carolina
Thoracic Incisions

Ronald D. Curran, M.D.
Fellow, Cardiovascular and Thoracic Surgery, Northwestern University Medical School, Chicago, Illinois
Shock and Circulatory Collapse

Thomas A. D'Amico, M.D.
Fellow in Cardiothoracic Surgery, Duke University Medical Center, Durham, North Carolina
Carcinoma of the Lung; Benign Tumors of the Lung and Bronchial Adenomas; Immunology and Immunotherapy of Carcinoma of the Lung; Surgical Management of Pulmonary Metastases; Kawasaki's Disease

Gordon K. Danielson, M.D.
Roberts Professor of Surgery, Mayo Medical School and Graduate School of Medicine; Consultant, Cardiothoracic Surgery, Mayo Clinic/Foundation, Rochester, Minnesota
Atrioventricular Canal; Ebstein's Anomaly

Charles J. Davidson, M.D.
Associate Professor of Medicine, Northwestern University Medical School; Chief, Cardiac Catheterization Laboratories, Northwestern Memorial Hospital, Chicago, Illinois
Cardiac Catheterization, Angiography, and Interventional Techniques in Valvular and Congenital Heart Disease; Coronary Arteriography

R. Duane Davis, Jr., M.D.
Assistant Professor of Surgery, Duke University School of Medicine, Durham, North Carolina
The Mediastinum

Tom R. DeMeester, M.D.
Professor and Chairman, Department of Surgery, University of Southern California School of Medicine, Los Angeles, California
The Pleura

Roberto M. Di Donato, M.D.
Professor of Clinical Surgery, Professor of Clinical Pediatrics, University of Medicine and Dentistry of New Jersey; Director, Division of Pediatric Cardiothoracic Surgery, Children's Hospital of New Jersey, United Hospitals Medical Center, Newark, New Jersey
Anatomic Correction of Transposition of the Great Arteries at the Arterial Level

J. Michael DiMaio, M.D.
Chief Resident in Surgery, Duke University Medical Center, Durham, North Carolina
Thoracic Disorders in the Immunocompromised Host

James M. Douglas, Jr., M.D.
Director of Cardiovascular Surgery, St. Joseph Hospital, Bellingham, Washington
The Pericardium; Thoracoscopic Surgery

John J. Downes, M.D.
Professor of Anesthesia and Pediatrics at the University of Pennsylvania; Department of Anesthesia and Critical Care Medicine, Children's Hospital of Philadelphia, Philadelphia, Pennsylvania
Respiratory Support in Infants

André Duranceau, M.D.
Professor of Surgery, Faculté de Médecine, Université de Montreal; Division of Thoracic Surgery, Hôtel-Dieu de Montréal, Montréal, Québec, Canada
Disorders of the Esophagus in the Adult

L. Henry Edmunds, Jr., M.D.
Julian Johnson Professor of Cardiothoracic Surgery, University of Pennsylvania; Staff, Division of Cardiothoracic Surgery, Hospital of the University of Pennsylvania, Philadelphia, Pennsylvania
Respiratory Support in Infants

T. Bruce Ferguson, Jr., M.D.
Associate Professor of Surgery, Division of Cardiothoracic Surgery, Washington University School of Medicine; Associate Surgeon, Barnes Hospital, St. Louis, Missouri
Congenital Lesions of the Lung and Emphysema

Thomas B. Ferguson, M.D.
Emeritus Professor of Surgery, Washington University School of Medicine at Barnes Hospital, St. Louis, Missouri
Congenital Lesions of the Lung and Emphysema

Gregory P. Fontana, M.D.
Assistant Clinical Professor, University of California at Los Angeles School of Medicine, Division of Cardiothoracic Surgery, Department of Surgery; Attending Cardiothoracic Surgeon, Cedars-Sinai Medical Center, Department of Cardiothoracic Surgery, Los Angeles, California
Acute Pulmonary Embolism

Robert M. Freedom, M.D., F.R.C.P.(C.), F.A.C.C.
Professor of Paediatrics (Cardiology) and Pathology, University of Toronto, Faculty of Medicine; Head, Division of Cardiology, The Hospital for Sick Children, Toronto, Ontario, Canada
The Mustard Procedure

David A. Fullerton, M.D.
Assistant Professor, Department of Surgery, University of Colorado; Chief, Cardiothoracic Surgery, Veterans Administration Medical Center; Surgeon, Denver Children's Hospital, Denver, Colorado
Prosthetic Valve Endocarditis

Aubrey C. Galloway, M.D.
Associate Professor of Surgery, New York University Medical School; Director of Surgical Research, New York University Medical Center, New York, New York
Atrial Septal Defects, Atrioventricular Canal Defects, and Total Anomalous Pulmonary Venous Return; Acquired Disease of the Mitral Valve; Bypass Grafting for Coronary Artery Disease

William A. Gay, Jr., M.D.
Professor, Department of Surgery, Washington University School of Medicine; Attending Surgeon, Cardiothoracic Surgery, Barnes Hospital, St. Louis, Missouri
Cardiac Transplantation

J. William Gaynor, M.D.
Assistant Professor of Surgery, Pediatric Cardiothoracic Surgery, Children's Hospital of Philadelphia, Philadelphia, Pennsylvania
Patent Ductus Arteriosus, Coarctation of the Aorta, Aortopulmonary Window, and Anomalies of the Aortic Arch; Pulmonary Atresia or Stenosis with Intact Ventricular Septum

Brian Ginsberg, M.D., B.Ch.
Assistant Professor of Anesthesiology, Duke University Medical Center, Durham, North Carolina
Acute Pain Management After Surgical Procedures

Donald D. Glower, Jr., M.D.

Associate Professor of Surgery, Duke University, Durham, North Carolina
Acquired Aortic Valve Disease

William J. Greeley, M.D.

Division Chief, Division of Pediatric Anesthesia and Critical Care Medicine; Associate Professor of Anesthesiology; Associate Professor of Pediatrics, Duke University Medical Center, Durham, North Carolina
Anesthesia and Supportive Care for Cardiothoracic Surgery

Katherine Grichnik, M.D.

Assistant Professor of Anesthesiology, Duke University Medical School; Assistant Professor of Anesthesiology, Duke University Medical Center, Durham, North Carolina
Anesthesia and Supportive Care for Cardiothoracic Surgery; Acute Pain Management After Surgical Procedures

Hermes C. Grillo, A.B., M.D.

Professor of Surgery, Harvard Medical School; Visiting Surgeon, Thoracic Surgery, Massachusetts General Hospital, Boston, Massachusetts
Congenital Lesions, Neoplasms, Inflammation, Infections, Injuries, and Other Lesions of the Trachea

Michael A. Grosso, M.D.

Assistant Professor of Cardiothoracic Surgery, University of Medicine and Dentistry of New Jersey, Cooper Hospital/University Medical Center, Camden, New Jersey
Left Ventricular Aneurysm

Frederick L. Grover, M.D.

Professor of Surgery; Head, Division of Cardiothoracic Surgery, University of Colorado Health Sciences Center; Chief, Surgical Service, Veterans Administration Medical Center, Denver, Colorado
Prosthetic Valve Endocarditis; Thrombosis and Thromboembolism of Prosthetic Cardiac Valves and Extracardiac Prostheses

John R. Guyton, M.D.

Associate Professor of Medicine; Assistant Professor of Pathology, Duke University Medical Center, Durham, North Carolina
Dietary and Pharmacologic Management of Atherosclerosis

John W. Hammon, Jr., M.D.

Professor of Cardiothoracic Surgery, Bowman Gray School of Medicine of Wake Forest University; Attending Cardiothoracic Surgeon, Medical Center of Bowman Gray School of Medicine and North Carolina Baptist Hospital, Winston-Salem, North Carolina
Major Anomalies of Pulmonary and Thoracic Systemic Veins

John R. Handy, Jr., M.D.

Assistant Professor of Surgery, Medical University of South Carolina College of Medicine, Charleston, North Carolina
Tricuspid Atresia

Alden H. Harken, M.D.

Staff Surgeon, Veterans Administration Hospital; Professor and Chairman, Department of Surgery; Staff Surgeon, Cardiovascular Surgery, University of Colorado; Staff Surgeon, Rose Medical Center, Denver, Colorado
Left Ventricular Aneurysm

J. Kevin Harrison, M.D.
Assistant Professor of Medicine; Assistant Director, Diagnostic and Interventional Catheterization Laboratories, Duke University Medical Center, Durham, North Carolina
Cardiac Catheterization, Angiography, and Interventional Techniques in Valvular and Congenital Heart Disease; Coronary Arteriography

Lucius D. Hill, M.D.
Clinical Professor of Surgery, University of Washington, Seattle, Washington
The Nissen Fundoplication; The Hill Repair; Paraesophageal Hernia

William L. Holman, M.D.
Associate Professor in Surgery, University of Alabama at Birmingham; Associate Professor in Surgery, Veterans Administration Medical Center, Birmingham, Alabama
Aneurysms of the Sinuses of Valsalva

O. Wayne Isom, M.D.
Professor of Cardiothoracic Surgery, Cornell University Medical College; Cardiothoracic Surgeon-in-Chief, The New Hospital, New York, New York
Aortic Grafts and Prostheses; Occlusive Disease of Branches of the Aorta

Robert H. Jones, M.D.
Mary and Deryl Hart Professor of Surgery; Associate Professor of Radiology, Duke University School of Medicine; Duke University Medical Center, Durham, North Carolina
Radionuclide Imaging in Cardiac Surgery

Allen B. Kaiser, M.D.
Professor of Medicine, Vanderbilt University School of Medicine; Vice-Chairman, Department of Medicine, Vanderbilt University Medical Center, Nashville, Tennessee
Use of Antibiotics in Cardiac and Thoracic Surgery

Robert B. Karp, M.D.
Professor of Surgery, University of Chicago, Chicago, Illinois
Acquired Disease of the Tricuspid Valve

James K. Kirklin, M.D.
Professor of Surgery, University of Alabama at Birmingham, School of Medicine; Professor and Surgeon, University of Alabama at Birmingham, Hospitals and Clinics, Birmingham, Alabama
Cardiopulmonary Bypass for Cardiac Surgery; Surgical Treatment of Ventricular Septal Defect

Joseph A. Kisslo, M.D.
Professor, Division of Cardiology, Department of Medicine; Director, Echocardiography, Duke University Medical Center, Durham, North Carolina
Ultrasound Applications in Cardiac Surgery: Echocardiography

John M. Kratz, M.D.
Professor of Surgery, Medical University of South Carolina, Charleston, South Carolina
Thoracic Incisions

Marino Labinaz, M.D., F.R.C.P.(C.)
Assistant Professor of Medicine (Cardiology), University of Ottawa, Heart Institute, Ottawa, Ontario, Canada
Percutaneous Transluminal Coronary Angioplasty

Edwin Lafontaine, M.D., F.R.C.S.(C.)
Assistant Professor of Surgery, Department of Surgery, University of Montreal; Attending Surgeon, Department of Surgery, Hospital Hôtel-Dieu, Montreal, Quebec, Canada
The Pleura

Hillel Laks, M.D.
Professor and Chief, Cardiothoracic Surgery Department, University of California at Los Angeles Medical Center, Los Angeles, California
Congenital Malformations of the Mitral Valve

Kevin P. Landolfo, M.D.
Assistant Professor of Surgery, Duke University Medical Center, Durham, North Carolina
Postoperative Care in Cardiac Surgery; Congenital Deformities of the Chest Wall; Postinfarction Rupture of the Papillary Muscles and Ischemic Mitral Insufficiency

Bruce Leone, M.D.
Associate Professor of Anesthesiology; Assistant Professor of Medicine; Chairman, Duke University Animal Care and Use Committee; Director, Anesthesiology Cardiopulmonary Research Laboratory, Duke University Medical Center, Durham, North Carolina
Anesthesia and Supportive Care for Cardiothoracic Surgery

John Leslie, M.D.
Clinical Professor of Anesthesiology, Duke University Medical School; Staff Attending, Duke University Medical Center; Staff Anesthesiologist, The Duke Heart Center, Durham, North Carolina
Anesthesia and Supportive Care for Cardiothoracic Surgery

Gary K. Lofland, M.D.
Clinical Professor of Surgery, Georgetown University, Washington, District of Columbia; Director, Columbia/HCA Congenital Heart Center; HCA Henrico Doctors' Hospital, Richmond, Virginia
Truncus Arteriosus

Floyd D. Loop, M.D.
Chairman, Board of Governors and Executive Vice President, The Cleveland Clinic Foundation, Cleveland, Ohio
Repeat Coronary Artery Bypass Grafting for Myocardial Ischemia

James E. Lowe, M.D.
Professor of Surgery; Associate Professor of Pathology, Attending Surgeon, Cardiothoracic Surgery, Duke University Medical Center, Durham, North Carolina
Bronchoplastic Techniques in the Surgical Management of Benign and Malignant Pulmonary Lesions; Cardiac Pacemakers and Implantable Cardioverter-Defibrillators; Congenital Malformations of the Coronary Circulation; Prinzmetal's Variant Angina and Other Syndromes Associated with Coronary Artery Spasm; Assisted Circulation

Philip D. Lumb, M.B.B.S., F.C.C.M.
Professor of Anesthesiology; Professor of Surgery; Chairman, Department of Anesthesiology, Albany Medical College; Anesthesiologist-in-Chief, Co-Director, Surgical Intensive Care Unit, Albany Medical Center Hospital, Albany, New York
Perioperative Pulmonary Physiology

H. Kim Lyerly, M.D.
Associate Professor of Surgery; Assistant Professor of Pathology, Duke University Medical Center, Durham, North Carolina
Thoracic Disorders in the Immunocompromised Host; Pulmonary Arteriovenous Fistulas

Neil R. MacIntyre, M.D.
Associate Professor of Medicine; Medical Director, Respiratory Care Services, Duke University Medical Center, Durham, North Carolina
Tracheal Intubation and Assisted Ventilation: The Anesthesiologist's Viewpoint

David C. McGiffin, M.D.
Associate Professor of Surgery, University of Alabama at Birmingham, Birmingham, Alabama
Cardiopulmonary Bypass for Cardiac Surgery

Eli Milgalter, M.D.
Division of Cardiothoracic Surgery, Hadassah Hospital, Jerusalem, Israel
Congenital Malformations of the Mitral Valve

Jon F. Moran, M.D.
Division of Cardiac Surgery, Department of Surgery, School of Medicine, East Carolina University, Greenville, North Carolina
Surgical Treatment of Pulmonary Tuberculosis

James J. Morris, M.D.
Associate Professor of Surgery, Mayo Medical School; Consultant, Cardiovascular Surgery, Mayo Clinic; Associate, Department of Physiology, Mayo Graduate School of Medicine, Mayo Clinic, Rochester, Minnesota
Utilization of Autologous Arterial Grafts for Coronary Artery Bypass

Kurt D. Newman, M.D.
Associate Professor of Surgery and Pediatrics, George Washington University School of Medicine; Senior Attending Surgeon, Children's National Medical Center, Washington, District of Columbia
Surgery of the Esophagus in Infants and Children

William I. Norwood, M.D., Ph.D.
The Aldo Castañeda Institute, Chief of Surgery, Clinique de Genolier, Genolier, Switzerland
Hypoplastic Left Heart Syndrome

H. Newland Oldham, Jr., M.D.
Professor of Surgery, Duke University Medical School; Professor of Surgery, Duke University Medical Center, Durham, North Carolina
The Mediastinum

Mark B. Orringer, M.D.
Professor and Head, Section of Thoracic Surgery, University of Michigan Medical School, Ann Arbor, Michigan
Short Esophagus and Reflux Stricture

A. D. Pacifico, M.D.
John W. Kirklin Professor of Surgery, University of Alabama at Birmingham, School of Medicine; Director, Division of Cardiothoracic Surgery, Vice Chairman, Department of Surgery, University of Alabama at Birmingham, Hospitals and Clinics, Birmingham, Alabama
Surgical Treatment of Ventricular Septal Defect; The Senning Procedure for Transposition of the Great Vessels

Peter C. Pairolero, M.D.
Chair, Department of Surgery; Professor, Mayo Medical School, Mayo Graduate School of Medicine, Rochester, Minnesota
Surgical Management of Neoplasms of the Chest Wall

G. Alexander Patterson, M.D.

Professor of Cardiothoracic Surgery, Department of Surgery, Washington University School of Medicine, St. Louis, Missouri
Lung Transplantation

Robert B. Peyton, M.D.

Carolina Cardiovascular Surgical Associates, P.A., Wake Heart Center, Rex Hospital, Raleigh, North Carolina
Aortic Grafts and Prostheses; Occlusive Disease of Branches of the Aorta

Harry R. Phillips III, M.D.

Associate Professor, Division of Cardiology, Department of Medicine; Co-Director, Interventional Cardiovascular Program, Duke University Medical Center, Durham, North Carolina
Percutaneous Transluminal Coronary Angioplasty

William S. Pierce, M.D.

College of Medicine, The Pennsylvania State University; Professor of Surgery, University Hospital, The Milton S. Hershey Medical Center, Hershey, Pennsylvania
The Artificial Heart

Francisco J. Puga, M.D., F.A.C.S., F.A.C.C.

Professor of Surgery, Mayo Medical School and Graduate School of Medicine; Consultant, Cardiothoracic Surgery, Mayo Clinic/Mayo Foundation, Rochester, Minnesota
Atrioventricular Canal

Judson Randolph, M.D.

Professor of Surgery, Meharry Medical College; Attending Surgeon, Metropolitan Nashville General Hospital, Nashville, Tennessee
Surgery of the Esophagus in Infants and Children

J. Scott Rankin, M.D.

Clinical Associate Professor, Department of Cardiac and Thoracic Surgery, Vanderbilt University Medical Center; Attending Surgeon, St. Thomas Hospital, Nashville, Tennessee
Cardiopulmonary Resuscitation; Physiology of Coronary Blood Flow, Myocardial Function, and Intraoperative Myocardial Protection; Utilization of Autologous Arterial Grafts for Coronary Artery Bypass; Postinfarction Ventricular Septal Defect

Russell C. Raphaely, M.D.

Professor of Anesthesia and Pediatrics, University of Pennsylvania School of Medicine; Associate Director, Department of Anesthesiology and Critical Care Medicine; Director, Division of Critical Care Medicine, Children's Hospital of Philadelphia, Philadelphia, Pennsylvania
Respiratory Support in Infants

Maruf A. Razzuk, B.Sc., M.D.

Professor in Thoracic and Cardiovascular Surgery, University of Texas Southwestern Medical School; Baylor University Medical Center, Dallas, Texas
Thoracic Outlet Syndrome

Bruce A. Reitz, M.D.

Professor and Chairman, Department of Cardiothoracic Surgery, Stanford University School of Medicine, Stanford; Chief of the Pediatric Cardiac Surgical Services, Lucile Salter Packard Children's Hospital at Stanford; Chief of the Cardiac Surgical Service, Stanford Health Services, Palo Alto, California
Clinical Heart-Lung Transplantation

J. G. Reves, M.D.
Professor and Chairman, Department of Anesthesiology; Director, The Duke Heart Center, Duke University Medical Center, Durham, North Carolina
Anesthesia and Supportive Care for Cardiothoracic Surgery

Greg H. Ribakove, M.D.
Assistant Professor of Surgery; Attending Cardiac Surgeon, New York University Medical Center, New York, New York
Tracheal Intubation and Mechanical Ventilation: The Surgeon's Viewpoint

William C. Roberts, M.D.
Executive Director, Baylor Cardiovascular Institute; Dean, A. Webb Roberts Center for Continuing Education, Baylor University Medical Center, Dallas, Texas
Pathology of Coronary Atherosclerosis

Bradley M. Rodgers, M.D.
Professor of Surgery and Pediatrics; Chief, Pediatric Surgery, University of Virginia Health Sciences Center, Charlottesville, Virginia
Management of Infants and Children Undergoing Thoracic Surgery

David C. Sabiston, Jr., M.D.
James B. Duke Professor of Surgery, Duke University School of Medicine; Chief of Staff, Duke University Medical Center, Durham, North Carolina
Congenital Deformities of the Chest Wall; The Mediastinum; Carcinoma of the Lung; Bronchoplastic Techniques in the Surgical Management of Benign and Malignant Pulmonary Lesions; Benign Tumors of the Lung and Bronchial Adenomas; Immunology and Immunotherapy of Carcinoma of the Lung; Surgical Management of Pulmonary Metastases; Acute Pulmonary Embolism; Chronic Pulmonary Embolism; Pulmonary Arteriovenous Fistulas; Patent Ductus Arteriosus, Coarctation of the Aorta, Aortopulmonary Window, and Anomalies of the Aortic Arch; Physiology of Coronary Blood Flow, Myocardial Function, and Intraoperative Myocardial Protection; Congenital Malformations of the Coronary Circulation; Tumors of the Heart

Robert M. Sade, M.D.
Professor of Surgery, Medical University of South Carolina, Charleston, South Carolina
Tricuspid Atresia

Mark W. Sebastian, M.D.
Department of Surgery, Duke University Medical Center, Durham, North Carolina
Chronic Pulmonary Embolism; Benign and Malignant Tumors of the Esophagus

David B. Skinner, M.D.
Professor of Surgery, Cornell University Medical College; Attending Surgeon, President/Chief Executive Officer, The Society of the New York Hospital, New York, New York
The Condition: Clinical Manifestations and Diagnosis; The Belsey Mark IV Antireflux Repair

Robert N. Sladen, M.B., Ch.B., M.R.C.P.(U.K.), F.R.C.P.(C.)
Associate Professor of Anesthesiology, Associate Professor of Surgery, Assistant Professor of Cell Biology, Duke University School of Medicine; Vice-Chair, Department of Anesthesiology, Co-Director, Surgical Intensive Care Unit, Duke University Medical Center, Durham, North Carolina
Tracheal Intubation and Mechanical Ventilation: The Anesthesiologist's Viewpoint

Peter K. Smith, A.B., B.M.E, M.D.
Professor of Surgery; Associate Professor of Biomedical Engineering, Duke University Medical Center; Division Chief, Thoracic and Cardiovascular Surgery; Medical Direc-

tor, Cardiac Acute Care Unit; Director, Core Cardiac Physiology Laboratory, Duke University Medical Center, Durham, North Carolina
Preoperative Assessment of Pulmonary Function: Quantitative Evaluation of Ventilation and Blood Gas Exchange; Postoperative Care in Cardiac Surgery; Computer Applications in Cardiothoracic Surgery; Ultrasound Applications in Cardiac Surgery: Echocardiography

Peter Snopkowski, M.D.

Resident in Surgery, Ryan Hill Research Foundation, Seattle, Washington
The Hill Repair

Robert J. Sparaco, B.S., J.D., R.R.T.

Associate Professor, Department of Allied Health Sciences, Nassau Community College, Garden City; Educational Coordinator, Respiratory Care Department, Tisch Hospital of New York University Medical Center, New York, New York
Tracheal Intubation and Mechanical Ventilation: The Surgeon's Viewpoint

Frank C. Spencer, M.D.

George David Stewart Professor and Chairman, Department of Surgery, New York University Medical Center, New York, New York
Atrial Septal Defects, Atrioventricular Canal Defects, and Total Anomalous Pulmonary Venous Return; Acquired Disease of the Mitral Valve; Bypass Grafting for Coronary Artery Disease

Charles E. Spritzer, M.D.

Associate Professor; Director, Body Magnetic Resonance Section; Co-Director, Magnetic Resonance Imaging, Duke University Medical Center, Durham, North Carolina
Role of Computed Tomographic Scans in Cardiovascular Diagnosis; Role of Magnetic Resonance Imaging in Cardiovascular Diagnosis

Richard S. Stack, M.D., F.A.C.C.

Associate Professor of Medicine; Director, Interventional Cardiovascular Program, Duke University Medical Center, Durham, North Carolina
Percutaneous Transluminal Coronary Angioplasty

James M. Steven, M.D.

Assistant Professor of Anesthesia and Pediatrics, University of Pennsylvania School of Medicine; Associate Anesthesiologist, Children's Hospital of Philadelphia, Philadelphia, Pennsylvania
Respiratory Support in Infants

John H. Stevens, M.D.

Chief Resident, Department of Cardiothoracic Surgery, Stanford University School of Medicine, Stanford, California
Clinical Heart-Lung Transplantation

Bret W. Stolp, M.D., Ph.D.

Assistant Professor, Department of Anesthesiology; Associate, Department of Cell Biology, Duke University Medical Center, Durham, North Carolina
Tracheal Intubation and Assisted Ventilation: The Anesthesiologist's Viewpoint

Mark Tedder, M.D.

Cardiothoracic Surgery Fellow, Duke University Medical Center, Durham, North Carolina
Bronchoplastic Techniques in the Surgical Management of Benign and Malignant Pulmonary Lesions

George A. Trusler, M.D., F.R.C.S.(C.)
Professor Emeritus, Department of Surgery, University of Toronto; Senior Surgeon, Cardiovascular Surgery Division, Hospital for Sick Children, Toronto, Ontario, Canada
The Mustard Procedure

Ross M. Ungerleider, M.D.
Professor of General and Thoracic Surgery; Associate Professor of Pediatrics; Chief, Pediatric Cardiac Surgery, Duke University Medical Center, Durham, North Carolina
Tetralogy of Fallot; Pulmonary Atresia or Stenosis with Intact Ventricular Septum; Congenital Aortic Stenosis

Harold C. Urschel, Jr., A.B., M.D.
Professor of Thoracic and Cardiovascular Surgery, University of Texas Health Science Center at Dallas (Southwestern Medical School); Baylor University Medical Center, Dallas, Texas
Thoracic Outlet Syndrome

Peter Van Trigt III, M.D.
Professor of Surgery, Surgical Director, Cardiopulmonary Transplantation, Duke University Medical Center, Durham, North Carolina
Lung Infections and Diffuse Interstitial Lung Disease; Diaphragm and Diaphragmatic Pacing; Tumors of the Heart

Andrew S. Wechsler, M.D.
Stuart McGuire Professor and Chairman, Department of Surgery; Professor of Physiology, Virginia Commonwealth University Medical College of Virginia; Chairman of Surgery, Medical College of Virginia Hospitals, Richmond, Virginia
Surgical Management of Myasthenia Gravis

J. Marcus Wharton, M.D.
Associate Professor of Medicine; Director, Clinical Cardiac Electrophysiology, Duke University Medical Center, Durham, North Carolina
Cardiac Pacemakers and Implantable Cardioverter-Defibrillators

David H. Wisner, M.D.
Associate Professor, Department of Surgery, University of California at Davis, Sacramento, California
Trauma to the Chest

Walter G. Wolfe, M.D.
Attending Cardiothoracic Surgeon; Professor of Surgery, Duke University Medical Center, Durham, North Carolina
Preoperative Assessment of Pulmonary Function: Quantitative Evaluation of Ventilation and Blood Gas Exchange; Benign and Malignant Tumors of the Esophagus

Preface

It is astonishing to reflect on the wide number of advances made in cardiac and thoracic surgery since the last edition of *Surgery of the Chest* was published in 1990. Many changes have occurred that have led to improved diagnostic techniques and therapeutic procedures for a host of disorders.

As advances occur, it is important to add new subjects and contributors to this work. In the Sixth Edition of *Surgery of the Chest*, there are 40 new authors and additional subjects. Drs. Robert N. Sladen, Bret Stolp, and Neil R. MacIntyre have added a completely new chapter on "Tracheal Intubation and Assisted Ventilation: The Anesthesiologist's Viewpoint" and a new co-author, Dr. Greg H. Ribakove, has been added to the chapter on "Tracheal Intubation and Mechanical Ventilation: The Surgeon's Viewpoint." Drs. Katherine Grichnik and Bruce Leone are new authors of the chapter on "Anesthesia and Supportive Care for Cardiothoracic Surgery." Drs. Brian Ginsberg and Katherine Grichnik have contributed a new chapter on "Acute Pain Management After Surgical Procedures." Dr. Ronald D. Curran is also a new author with Dr. Robert W. Anderson of an extensively revised and updated chapter on "Shock and Circulatory Collapse." Dr. Kevin P. Landolfo has been added as an author of "Postoperative Care in Cardiac Surgery" and Dr. James M. Steven for the chapter on "Respiratory Support in Infants." The chapter on "Trauma to the Chest" has been completely rewritten by Dr. David H. Wisner, and Dr. Kevin P. Landolfo has been added to the authorship of "Congenital Deformities of the Chest Wall," as has Dr. Robbin G. Cohen to the chapter on "The Pleura." Dr. Thomas A. D'Amico is a new author for the chapter on "Carcinoma of the Lung" and Dr. Mark Tedder on the chapter "Bronchoplastic Techniques in the Surgical Management of Benign and Malignant Pulmonary Lesions." Drs. Thomas A. D'Amico and David C. Sabiston, Jr., have completely rewritten the chapters on "Benign Tumors of the Lung and Bronchial Adenomas," "Immunology and Immunotherapy of Carcinoma of the Lung," and "Surgical Management of Pulmonary Metastases." Dr. J. Michael DiMaio has been added as one of the authors of "Thoracic Disorders in the Immunocompromised Host." Dr. Gregory P. Fontana is a new co-author of the chapter "Pulmonary Embolism," and Dr. Mark W. Sebastian is a co-author of the chapter on "Chronic Pulmonary Embolism." The chapter on "Benign and Malignant Tumors of the Esophagus" has been completely rewritten by Drs. Walter G. Wolfe and Mark W. Sebastian, as has the chapter on "Disorders of the Esophagus in the Adult" by Dr. André Duranceau. Dr. Lucius D. Hill has rewritten the chapter on "The Nissen Fundoplication" and, with Dr. Peter Snopkowski, has redone "The Hill Repair." Dr. J. Kevin Harrison has been added as an author of "Cardiac Catheterization, Angiography, and Interventional Techniques in Valvular and Congenital Heart Disease." New authors for the chapter on "Percutaneous Transluminal Coronary Angioplasty" are Drs. Marino Labinaz and Harry R. Phillips.

Many advances have been made in "Fibrinolytic Therapy in the Management of Acute Myocardial Infarction" and this chapter has been completely revised by Dr. Robert M. Califf. Similarly, the chapters on the "Role of Computed Tomographic Scans in Cardiovascular Diagnosis" and the "Role of Magnetic Resonance Imaging in Cardiovascular Diagnosis" have been completely rewritten by a new author, Dr. Charles E. Spritzer. Dr. David C. McGiffin has been added as an author to the chapter on "Cardiopulmonary Bypass for Cardiac Surgery." The chapter on "The Pericardium" has been rewritten by Dr. James M. Douglas, Jr., and Drs. Aubrey C. Galloway and Stephen B. Colvin have been added as authors of the chapter on "Atrial Septal Defects, Atrioventricular Canal Defects, and Total Anomalous Pulmonary Venous Return." A completely new chapter, "Pulmonary Atresia or Stenosis with Intact Ventricular Septum," has been written by Drs. Ross M. Ungerleider and J. William Gaynor. Dr. Alon S. Aharon is a new co-author of the chapter on "Congenital Malformations of the Mitral Valve." Completely new chapters have been written by Dr. Erle H. Austin III on "Pulmonary Atresia with Intact Ventricular Septum" and "Univentricular Heart." Dr. John R. Handy, Jr., has been added as an author of the chapter on "Tricuspid Atresia" and Drs. Aubrey C. Galloway and Stephen B. Colvin have been added as co-authors of the chapter on "Acquired Disease of the Mitral Valve." Totally new chapters have been written on "Prosthetic Valve Endocarditis" by Drs. David A. Fullerton and Frederick L. Grover and on "Thrombosis and Thromboembolism of Prosthetic Cardiac Valves and Extracardiac Prostheses" by Drs. David N. Campbell and Frederick L. Grover. Dr. Donald G. Glower is the new author of "Acquired Aortic Valve Disease." Dr. J. Marcus Wharton is the new co-author of "Cardiac Pacemakers and Implantable Cardioverter-Defibrillators." In the chapter on "Coronary Arteriography," Dr. J. Kevin Harrison has been added as a co-author, and Drs. Aubrey C. Galloway and Stephen B. Colvin are additional authors on "Bypass Grafting for Coronary Artery Disease." An additional author, Dr. James J. Morris, has been added on "Utilization of Autologous Arterial Grafts for Coronary Artery Bypass." Dr. Michael A. Grosso has been added as a co-author of the chapter on "Left Ventricular Aneurysm," and Dr. Kevin P. Landolfo has written a new chapter on "Postinfarction Rupture of the Papillary Muscles and Ischemic Mitral Insufficiency." Dr. J. Scott Rankin has added a new chapter on "Postinfarction Ventricular Septal Defect," and Drs. Mark P. Anstadt and James E. Lowe have written the new chapter on "Assisted Circulation."

Since the last edition, the role of "Dietary and Pharmacologic Management of Atherosclerosis" has received increasing attention, especially in relationship to reducing the severity of atherosclerosis. This subject chapter has been completely rewritten by Dr. John R. Guyton. For the chapter on "Lung Transplantation," Dr. Joel D. Cooper has added his colleague Dr. G. Alexander Patterson as a co-author, and Dr. John H. Stevens is the new co-author of "Clinical Heart-Lung Transplantation."

For this edition of *Surgery of the Chest,* a companion *Atlas of Cardiothoracic Surgery* is now available in its first edition, published by W. B. Saunders. This atlas is a comprehensive text of cardiac and thoracic surgical procedures. Included are more than 700 illustrations of correction of congenital deformities of the sternum, tracheal and bronchial procedures, the thoracic outlet syndrome, and surgical procedures involving the mediastinum and diaphragm. Neoplasms of the chest wall and thoracic sympathectomy are covered and thoroughly illustrated. The text contains a host of pulmonary procedures for benign and malignant lesions. There is an extensive section on *thoracoscopic* surgery, which is increasingly utilized in a variety of thoracic procedures. Surgical procedures for acquired heart disease are covered in detail, and congenital lesions of the heart are illustrated with the various procedures indicated for their correction. An extensive chapter describes cardiac neoplasms and their surgical management, and cardiac and pulmonary transplantation are extensively illustrated. Coronary bypass procedures are illustrated by multiple drawings describing various alternative techniques that can be utilized. This *Atlas* is a comprehensive one, including all the surgical techniques currently used in cardiac and thoracic surgery.

This edition of *Surgery of the Chest* is viewed as an essentially unabridged work designed to be a reference resource for the pathogenesis, pathologic features, diagnosis, and treatment of all cardiac and thoracic disorders.

DAVID C. SABISTON, JR.
FRANK C. SPENCER

Contents

VOLUME I

VOLUME II

Surgery of
the
Chest

1

Preoperative Assessment of Pulmonary Function: Quantitative Evaluation of Ventilation and Blood Gas Exchange

Peter K. Smith and Walter G. Wolfe

INTERPRETATION OF PULMONARY FUNCTION STUDIES

He is fat and scant of breath.

Shakespeare, *Hamlet*, Act V

Pulmonary function studies should be evaluated carefully in the preoperative patient's work environment, personal history, and smoking history. Any history of pulmonary disease should be assessed carefully, as should any history of other chronic or debilitating diseases.

Pulmonary function must also be evaluated preoperatively in patients (1) undergoing thoracotomy for removal of pulmonary tissue, (2) undergoing thoracotomy without excision of tissue, (3) undergoing median sternotomy, (4) undergoing upper and lower abdominal procedures, and (5) under certain circumstances for procedures on the extremities or elsewhere. Each patient responds in a slightly different manner with regard to the effect of the operation and anesthesia on pulmonary function. Postoperative expectations and problems can be predicted on the basis of the magnitude of the surgical procedure and the postoperative complications that might be expected.

Irrespective of the procedure, every effort should be made to optimize postoperative pulmonary function as soon as possible and to return the functional residual capacity (FRC) to the preoperative level. Supplemental oxygen should be used when needed to prevent hypoxemia. Generally, if attention is given to these areas, ventilation-perfusion matching also returns to normal. These guidelines are important because all patients who have anesthesia and surgical procedures experience reduced pulmonary volume and reduced ventilation. If severe hypoxemia ensues, respiratory insufficiency and failure may progress rapidly.

Applied respiratory physiology has become increasingly important in evaluating pulmonary function. To accurately measure pulmonary ventilation and gas exchange under various clinical situations, physicians must become skilled in the interpretation of such data.

An understanding of all the factors that contribute to and alter pulmonary ventilation and gas exchange requires a detailed knowledge of pulmonary function at the alveolar level. *Ventilation* serves to replenish the gas in the lungs in order to maintain high oxygen and low carbon dioxide tension and to produce maximal gradients for diffusion. The mass movement of air into and out of the lung is effective only to the extent that it adequately replenishes the gas in the alveoli. *Distribution* is the delivery of ambient air to the separate gas exchange units through the successively bifurcating tracheobronchial tree. *Diffusion* is the transfer by random molecular motion of gas molecules across the alveolar membranes from a region of high concentration (partial pressure). The blood-air barrier of more than 90 M^2 in normal adult humans is condensed into a pulmonary volume of only 5 l, which is made possible by the small radius (150 M^2) and large number (300 million) of alveoli. *Perfusion* is the means by which the outflow of the right ventricle is brought into intimate contact with the alveolar capillary bed.

The physician must understand that no *single test* is available to evaluate pulmonary function. All too frequently, because of convenience or the appeal of simplicity, the physician may draw conclusions from simple tests that would not have been justified if more detailed laboratory techniques had been applied. The measurement of the static and dynamic pulmonary volumes, elastic properties of the tissue, forced expiratory volume, and efficiency of gas transfer as reflected by the carbon monoxide diffusion capacity and arterial blood gases can provide a more complete analysis of the overall pulmonary function. Right-sided catheterization of the heart may sometimes be necessary for a complete evaluation.

The necessity for measurement of pulmonary function is usually obvious clinically. Initially, the tests are done to determine whether actual functional impairment is present and to apply the information to the preoperative and postoperative care of the patient. The studies are valuable later in determining whether the patient's condition has improved, is unchanged, or has deteriorated after the illness or operation.

When the history and physical examination do not suggest any evidence of pulmonary disease, measurement of vital capacity (VC) and forced expiratory volume in 1 second (FEV$_1$), combined with a normal chest film and normal blood-gas determination, sufficiently screens the patient and supports the clinical impression that no significant underlying pulmonary disease is present. However, in patients with obvious or even suspected pulmonary disease, more detailed studies are necessary to completely elucidate the malfunction.

When tests of pulmonary function are requested, the interpretation of the examination must be combined with a complete clinical assessment. Laboratory technology must be competent and reliable, and the patient's cooperation during testing must be considered. Errors in mathematical interpretation should be uncommon because of the computerized techniques that allow tests to be done simply and conveniently. However, the people doing or interpreting these studies should be familiar with the mechanisms and basic measurements.

Blood for gas analysis should be drawn expertly and anaerobically. The patient's temperature must be noted because, with a raised temperature, the PaO$_2$ may not represent the true state of the patient's arterial partial pressure of oxygen. The time taken between the drawing and the measurement of the gases should be minimized. A test is only as good as the physician's ability to interpret the results. If the aforementioned errors have been eliminated, an objective evaluation of the patient's pulmonary function should result (Comroe and Nadel, 1970) (Table 1–1; Fig. 1–1).

PULMONARY VOLUME

Pulmonary volume is the oldest assessment of pulmonary function, and it dates back to 1800. There is a long and interesting history of enlightened investigation in the methods, measurement, and interpretation of pulmonary volumes that constitutes an essential foundation for the student of pulmonary physiology (Bates et al., 1971; Comroe et al., 1962; Cotes, 1968). In the measurement of pulmonary volumes, the gas volume is usually expressed at body temperature and pressure and is saturated (BTPS) with water vapor as it would exist within the lungs. However, the volume reflected in the spirometer is at ambient temperature and pressure saturated (ATPS) with water vapor at that temperature. The correction for pulmonary volumes from the temperature of the spirometer of 25°C to body temperature increases the volume approximately 7.5% at sea level. This correction also allows comparison of the measured pulmonary volumes with the volumes predicted in tables of normal values and corrects for changes that otherwise would falsely seem to occur at high altitude. One of the pulmonary volumes, the VC, permits the detection of small changes in individuals. Individual variation is so great that pulmonary volume is not a very sensitive method for detecting disease at one measurement, although it can be used to show improvement or deterioration in sequential measurements. The pulmonary volumes are important in training physicians to think physiologically, in giving an approximate index of the severity of some patterns of dysfunction, and in occasionally noting changes in the severity of the dysfunction.

Several terms were formerly applied to the various subdivisions of the lung, but the standardized terminology published in 1950 has resolved this confusion (Federation of American Societies for Experimental Biology, 1950).

Respiratory excursion (i.e., the amount of air inspired and expired) is called *tidal volume* (V$_T$). The amount of gas contained in the lung at the end of quiet expiration is called the FRC. The patient then makes a maximal inspiration and increases his pulmonary volume over the volume contained at the peak of V$_T$,

HEIGHT 73.   WEIGHT 188.   MALE   AGE   43.

DETERMINATION	ACTUAL	PRED	%PRED
VITAL CAPACITY,L (FVC)	5.73	5.16	111.
FORCED EXP VOL,L(FEV1)	4.23	4.07	104.
TIMED VC, %1SEC,(FEV1%)	74.	79.	94.
MAX MID FLOW, L/SEC	3.25	4.30	76.
PEAK FLOW, L/MIN	580.	513.	113.
MAX BR CAP,L/MIN (MVV)	218.7	171.9	127.
RESPIRATORY RATE (F)	25.		
VENTIL,L/MIN (VE)	14.44		
TIDAL VOL,ML (VT)	580.		
O2 UPT.,ML/MIN (VO2)	265.		
VENT EQUIV L/100ML	5.5	<2.5	
INSP CAPACITY,L (IC)	3.99		
EXP RESERVE,L (ERV)	1.36		
CALC VC, L	5.36	5.16	104.
FUNC RES VOL,L (FRC)	3.52		
TOT LUNG CAP,L (TLC)	7.51	6.74	111.
RESID VOL,L (RV)	2.15	1.62	133.
(RV/TLC) X 100,%	29.	24.	121.
HE MIX TIME,MIN	2.0	<3	

ARTERIAL BLOOD

pH	7.44
PaO2	77
PaCO2	36
O2 Sat	96%

FIGURE 1–1. A standard pulmonary function laboratory report. Initially, one should look at the static volumes to see whether they are normal, increased, or reduced. The residual volume and functional residual capacity are noted with respect to their fraction of the total lung capacity. Dynamic flow rates (FEV$_1$) indicate whether there is an obstruction or restriction. Arterial blood gas detects whether there is hypoxemia. The PCO$_2$ of 36 mm Hg is probably based on hyperventilation before the needle stick. If marked abnormalities are noted on these initial studies, determinations of carbon dioxide diffusing capacity, dead-space ventilation, compliance, and airway resistance should be obtained.

■ Table 1–1. TYPICAL VALUES IN PULMONARY FUNCTION TESTS

These values are for a healthy, resting, recumbent young man (1.7 M^2 surface area) breathing air at sea level, unless other conditions are specified. They are presented to give approximate figures. These values may change with position, age, size, sex, and altitude; there is variability among members of a homogeneous group under standard conditions.

Pulmonary Volumes

Inspiratory capacity, ml	3600
Expiratory reserve volume, ml	1200
Vital capacity, ml	4800
Residual volume (RV), ml	1200
Functional residual capacity, ml	2400
Thoracic gas volume, ml	2400
Total lung capacity (TLC), ml	6000
RV/TLC $\times$ 100, %	20

Ventilation

Tidal volume, ml	500
Frequency, respirations/min	12
Minute volume, ml/min	6000
Respiratory dead space, ml	150
Alveolar ventilation, ml/min	4200

Distribution of Inspired Gas

Single-breath test (% increase N_2 for 500 ml expired alveolar gas), % N_2	<1.5
Pulmonary nitrogen emptying rate (7 min test) % N_2	<2.5
Helium closed-circuit (mixing efficiency related to perfect mixing), %	76

Diffusion and Gas Exchange

O_2 consumption (STPD), ml/min	240
CO_2 output (STPD), ml/min	192
Respiratory exchange ratio, R (CO_2) output/O_2 uptake)	0.8
Diffusing capacity, O_2 (STPD) resting, ml/O_2/min/mm Hg	>15
Diffusing capacity, CO (steady state) (STPD) resting ml CO/min mm Hg	17
Diffusing capacity, CO (single-breath) (STPD) resting, ml CO/min/mm Hg	25
Diffusing capacity, CO (rebreathing) (STPD) resting ml CO/min/mm Hg	25

Alveolar Ventilation/Pulmonary Capillary Blood Flow

Alveolar ventilation (l/min) blood flow, l/min	0.8
Physiologic shunt/cardiac output $\times$ 100, %	<7
Physiologic dead space/tidal volume $\times$ 100, %	<30

Pulmonary Circulation

Pulmonary capillary blood flow, ml/min	5400
Pulmonary artery pressure, mm Hg	25/8
Pulmonary capillary blood volume, ml	75–100
Pulmonary "capillary" blood pressure (wedge), mm Hg	8

Alveolar Gas

Oxygen partial pressure, mm Hg	104
CO_2 partial pressure, mm Hg	40

Arterial Blood

O_2 saturation (% saturation of Hb with O_2), %	97.1
O_2 tension, mm Hg	100
CO_2 tension, mm Hg	40
Alveolar-arterial P_{O_2} difference (100% O_2), mm Hg	33
O saturation (100% O_2), %	100
O_2 tension (100% O_2) mm Hg	640
pH	7.4

Mechanics of Breathing

Maximal voluntary ventilation l/min	125–170
Forced expiratory volume, % in 1 sec	83
% in 3 sec	97
Maximal expiratory flow rate (for 1 l), l/min	400
Maximal inspiratory flow rate (for 1 l), l/min	300
Compliance of lungs and thoracic cage, l/cm H_2O	0.1
Compliance of lungs, l/cm H_2O	0.2
Airway resistance, cm H_2O/l/sec	1.6
Work of quiet breathing, kg-M/min	0.5
Maximal work of breathing, kg-M/breath	10
Maximal inspiratory and expiratory pressure, mm Hg	60–100

which is called the *inspiratory reserve volume* (IRV). He then forcibly expires and forces as much air as possible out of the lungs. The total volume expired from the maximal inspiration to the maximal expiration is the VC. The amount of air that remains in the lungs after maximal expiration is the *residual volume* (RV) (Fig. 1–2). All of the pulmonary volumes except the RV and the FRC may be measured directly. These two volumes, and as a result the total lung capacity (TLC), can be determined by one of three different methods: inert gas dilution or washout, whole-body plethysmography, or radiologic techniques (Ball et al., 1962; Bedell et al., 1956; DuBois et al., 1956).

The residual volume is calculated by subtracting

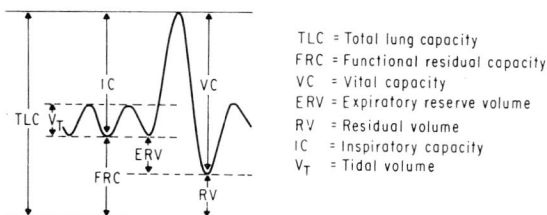

TLC = Total lung capacity
FRC = Functional residual capacity
VC = Vital capacity
ERV = Expiratory reserve volume
RV = Residual volume
IC = Inspiratory capacity
V_T = Tidal volume

FIGURE 1–2. Subdivisions of pulmonary volume.

expiratory reserve volume (ERV) from FRC, because the respiratory midposition may be reproduced more easily than the forced expiratory position. Three methods are used to measure the FRC. Two methods are based on measurements made with inert gases, and the third method is based on the application of Boyle's law. When FRC is measured by analysis of inert gas, either helium or nitrogen is used. When helium is used, the patient rebreathes a known concentration of helium until the concentration reaches a constant level (i.e., until it equilibrates within the lung and the spirometer). If a nitrogen washout is done to calculate FRC, the patient breathes 100% oxygen.

These two methods measure the RV of all alveolar units in communication with an airway. Poorly ventilated units are also included in the overall calculation if helium equilibration and nitrogen washout are maintained for sufficiently long periods. Although 7 minutes are typically used for nitrogen washout, more than 15 minutes may be necessary for patients with emphysema (Bedell et al., 1956).

The body plethysmographic method measures all gas in the lung and does not depend on the communication of the airway. The volume is properly called *thoracic gas volume* (TGV), and the difference between

TGV and FRC, measured by the dilution techniques, is an index of maldistribution of ventilation and indicates the presence of poorly ventilated pulmonary units. The discrepancy between TGV and FRC is particularly striking in patients with bullous disease. Body plethysmography is useful for measuring the FRC and airway resistance and also for constructing a pressure-volume curve for measuring compliance (Bedell et al., 1956; DuBois et al., 1956; Mead and Whittenberger, 1953).

Boyle's law states that the product of pressure and volume of the gas is constant for the same temperature. The patient is placed within a body plethysmograph, and the pressure within the plethysmograph and the mouth pressure are measured. Any change in the thoracic volume produces a reciprocal change in the plethysmographic volume, which in turn changes the plethysmographic pressure. Thus, an increase in thoracic volume reduces the plethysmographic volume and increases the plethysmographic pressure. At the end of quiet expiration, the airway is occluded by an electrically operated shutter, and the patient is asked to continue to pant against the obstructed airway. Because gas does not flow during the period of obstruction, mouth pressure is assumed to be equal to alveolar pressure. This increase in pressure is determined from the rise in plethysmographic pressure.

Maximal Breathing Capacity (MBC)

The MBC of an individual is defined as the largest volume of air that can be moved in and out of the chest in a minute. The maximal voluntary ventilation (MVV) indicates the maximal volume of gas breathed per unit under particular testing conditions (Bates et al., 1971).

The MVV is measured either by a closed-circuit system in which the patient rebreathes into a low-resistance spirometer or by an open-circuit system in which the patient breathes through a low-resistance two-way valve into a Douglas bag. The volume of the bag is measured in a Tissot spirometer or by a simple dry gas meter. The maximal value of three determinations is usually selected. This test appears to correlate well with the subjective symptom of dyspnea, and an index of the patient's ventilatory status may be obtained by comparing resting and maximal ventilation. An analysis of VC and MBC permits differentiation of the ventilatory abnormality into obstructive or restrictive disease, because MBC is reduced greatly in obstructive disease. The air velocity index is a ratio of the percentage of predicted MBC divided by the percentage of predicted VC. If the index is below 0.8, obstructive pulmonary disease is suspected, whereas if the index is more than 1.0, restrictive pulmonary disease is usually diagnosed.

Specific Abnormalities of Pulmonary Volume

In restrictive disease, the TLC and VC are small, whereas in obstructive diseases uncomplicated by fi-brosis, the RV is large. In emphysema, the FRC and TLC are large and the VC is normal or less than normal. Certain restrictive diseases have a small FRC, that is, muscular weakness, pulmonary granulomatosis, heart failure, and mixed restriction and obstruction. The patient with kyphoscoliosis, or the "jackknife" spine, typically has a small FRC. Some patients with obstructive diseases, such as moderate asthma and acute bronchitis, do not have a large FRC.

Patients with chronic emphysema and pulmonary cysts have an increased FRC. The ratio of RV to TLC is enlarged in emphysema and may increase in restrictive disease. Therefore, this ratio is not beneficial without simultaneous measurement of the absolute figures for RV and TLC.

Serial measurements of VC may be used to monitor the patient; however, the VC is reduced by so many different conditions that alone it has little value in a differential diagnosis. The VC may be useful in preoperative evaluation; thus, when the VC and the MBC are half of their normal value, the surgeon is usually reluctant to recommend thoracotomy or removal of more pulmonary tissue. Prognostically, when the VC is less than 1 l, the physician must consider that the patient is in danger of suffocation from insufficient ability to expand the lungs. Complications such as pneumonia, atelectasis, hydrothorax, or hypoventilation from any cause may be fatal.

DYNAMIC PROPERTIES OF THE LUNGS

Flow Rates

In patients with airway obstruction such as bronchitis or emphysema, more effort is required to produce airflow (Ayres and Grace, 1969; Hogg et al., 1968). The airflow that is produced even with maximal effort may be reduced. When the surgeon suspects that obstructive disease exists, the diagnosis can be confirmed usually by use of the spirometer. The patient inhales maximally and then exhales forcefully into a spirometer with a device that records the volume and the time. A common test of maximal expiratory airflow is the FEV_1. The FEV_1 is reduced in the presence of bronchial obstruction, but the values may also be reduced in restrictive pulmonary disease. Thus, the FEV_1 is usually related to the total exhaled VC. This ratio of FEV_1 to VC may be reduced in the presence of airway obstruction but is normal in restrictive pulmonary disease (Fig. 1–3).

Expiratory flow may be reduced in diseases of the airways, such as asthma and bronchitis, and in diseases associated with loss of pulmonary tissue, which is seen in patients with emphysema. In the presence of reduced expiratory flow rate, measurements of pulmonary compliance and diffusing capacity may help to differentiate among these diseases (Comroe, 1974; Comroe et al., 1962; Comroe and Nadel, 1970). A tangential line drawn at any point on the expiratory spirogram may be used to calculate the flow rate. Thus, the entire spirogram may be visualized as an

FIGURE 1–3. Changes in the forced expiratory volume (FEV) (1) in the normal patient, (2) in fibrosis or restrictive pulmonary disease, and (3) in obstruction. Because FEV$_1$ may sometimes be reduced in restrictive pulmonary disease, it should be related to the total exhaled vital capacity (VC). The ratio of FEV$_1$ to VC may be reduced in the presence of bronchial obstruction but is normal in restrictive disease.

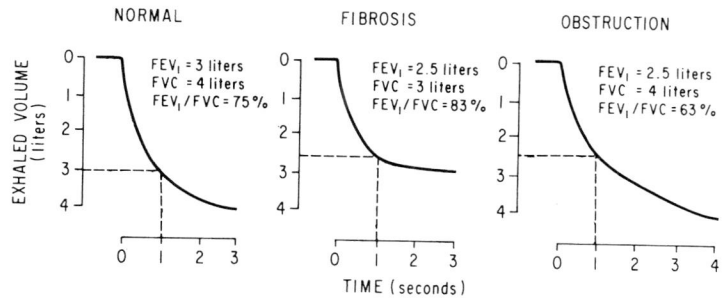

infinite series of instantaneous flow rates at a particular pulmonary volume. The slope of expiration has the units of flow because it represents volume change over time change.

Airway resistance is the pressure drop from the alveoli to the mouth divided by flow, which requires the measurement of flow with a flowmeter and measurement of alveolar pressure with a body plethysmograph. In normal lungs, most airway resistance is in airways larger than 2 mm in internal diameter, and changes in the dimensions of these airways, such as changes due to bronchospasm, may be detected with this technique. Measurement of airway resistance is useful to detect bronchial constriction and can be used to evaluate the efficiency of therapy in patients with increased airway resistance (DuBois et al., 1956; Mead and Whittenberger, 1953). Forced breathing with increased effort gives further important information about the properties of the lungs and is the basis of dynamic and spirometric tests to detect airway obstruction. The expiratory flow rate would be expected to increase with increased effort. Although this finding is true at or near total VC, midexpiratory flow no longer responds to increased expiratory effort because of the dynamic compression of intrathoracic airways. Over the lower two-thirds of expired VC, maximal flow occurs with submaximal effort; thus, flow measured at these pulmonary volumes reflects the properties of the lung and airways, can be reproduced, and is independent of effort by the patient.

Diffusion of Gas in the Lung

The physical definition of diffusion capacity is straightforward, but the details of its measurement and interpretation of the results obtained are not simple, particularly in clinical conditions in which no homogeneity of alveolar gas exists. Seven methods of measuring diffusion capacity with carbon monoxide have been described, excluding methods involving the use of radioactive carbon monoxide. Only the single-breath test is considered here (Bates et al., 1971; Comroe and Nadel, 1970).

Several factors affect diffusion in a single alveolus. The thickness of the alveolar lining membrane is important, as are the thickness of the protoplasm of the alveolar lining cell, the permeability of the capillary wall, and the thickness of the layer of plasma between the capillary wall and the red blood cell. Finally, the permeability of the red blood cell membrane to carbon monoxide or oxygen must be considered, as must the rate of reaction of hemoglobin with carbon monoxide or oxygen. In the single-breath carbon monoxide diffusion capacity, the presence of carbon monoxide–hemoglobin in the pulmonary arterial blood reduces the rate of carbon monoxide transfer.

A single-breath carbon monoxide diffusion capacity should be considered a screening test. The patient is required to inhale a low, nontoxic concentration of carbon monoxide, to hold the breath for 10 seconds, and to exhale. This test is rapid, simple, safe, and painless; however, it requires expensive equipment. The test can be done and the results can be calculated in approximately 10 minutes. It is useful particularly in patients with dyspnea who have a normal VC and normal maximal expiratory flow rates. A reduction in the pulmonary diffusion capacity (DL_{CO}) may be the earliest detectable abnormality in collagen disease, sarcoidosis, and industrial disease such as asbestosis. A reduced DL_{CO} is also found in patients with pulmonary emboli on a perfusion scan of the lung, and an arteriogram may be indicated to confirm this diagnosis (Wagner et al., 1964). It is increased in mitral stenosis, left-sided heart failure, or polycythemia. The test can be repeated frequently and thus is useful to evaluate the course of the disease in response to therapy.

Several factors affect a single-breath carbon monoxide diffusion capacity. As with the single-breath nitrogen washout, certain details of the procedure, such as inspiration and expiration time, should be controlled. Variations in values of each individual may be the result of differences in size. Results for a single subject vary with pulmonary volume during the breath-holding period when the measurement is being made. The subject's position is also important, because the diffusion capacity is greater in the supine position than in the sitting position.

Airway Resistance

The plethysmographic method for measurement of airway resistance (Comroe et al., 1962; DuBois et al., 1956) relies on Boyle's law for compression of gases. The patient sits inside a closed chamber that has either a sensitive pressure gauge or a lightweight spirometer attached to measure small changes in intrathoracic gas volume. As the patient breathes the air inside the box, the expired air expands or contracts slightly from changes in temperature and water vapor. These changes can be eliminated by shallow panting through a heated flowmeter or by rebreathing air in a warm, wet bag. The only remaining changes of gas volume that occur are changes caused by the expansion of alveolar air during expiratory gas flow. These alveolar volume changes produce changes in body volume that are measured with the pressure or volume gauge attached to the body plethysmograph, which are compared with the rate of airflow measured with the pneumotachygraph at the mouth. To calculate alveolar pressure changes, changes in body volume are converted to alveolar pressure changes by the use of Boyle's law, which states

$$\frac{P_1V_1}{T_1} = \frac{P_2V_2}{T_1}$$

The airway resistance is calculated in centimeters of water per liter per second, and normal values are from 0.6 to 2.4 cm $H_2O/l/sec$. Abnormal values in airway obstruction can rise to 10 times the average normal value. The airway resistance varies inversely with the pulmonary volume at which it is measured because of increased pulmonary tissue tension at greater pulmonary volume. Therefore, measurement of pulmonary volume may be used to predict the normal range of an individual's airway resistance. An alternative way in which the relationship between airway resistance and pulmonary volume may be expressed is by the use of airway conductance, which is the reciprocal of resistance. Conductance is directly proportional to the pulmonary volume. Conductance approaches zero as the airways close, which may occur at pulmonary volumes of 3 l in the patient with air trapping and explains why RV is so large.

Pulmonary Elasticity

In emphysema, the pulmonary compliance is often high, and therefore the FRC is large. Lungs that are in this condition show little elastic recoil at the measured FRC. As a result, the resting intrapleural pressure is not as negative as it would be in the normal person. This absence of negative intrapleural pressure allows the bronchi to collapse at a volume of only slightly less than FRC because the bronchi do not have either a negative pleural pressure around them or the outwardly pulling force of the pulmonary tissues surrounding them to keep them open. With collapsed bronchi, the patient with emphysema has difficulty in emptying the air from the lungs to reach a volume below the large FRC; therefore, the RV is enlarged (Bedell et al., 1956).

Measurement of dynamic pulmonary compliance provides only limited information regarding the elastic properties of the lungs (Fig. 1–4). Dynamic compliance is influenced by pulmonary volume history, by

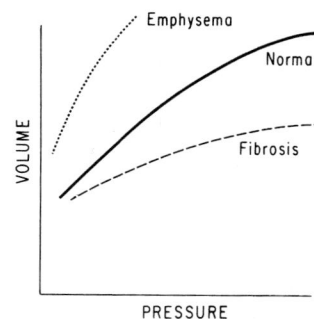

FIGURE 1–4. The pressure-volume curve. Compliance is equal to $1/E$ (E = elasticity). If there is increased elasticity of the lung, greater pressure is required to increase the volume, which is evident by the shifting of the curve down and to the right side in such diseases as fibrosis or sarcoidosis. In patients with emphysema or the loss of elastic recoil, a small increase in pressure causes a sharp increase in volume, which shifts the curve up and to the left side. A decrease in pulmonary compliance indicates to the physician that the patient's lowered vital capacity is due to stiff lungs. When pulmonary compliance is normal, the physician must look for another cause of reduced vital capacity. Patients with obstructive emphysema have increased compliance. The pressure-volume curve may help to differentiate patients with obstruction, because in patients with airway disease such as bronchitis the pulmonary compliance may be normal. Therefore, an evaluation of the changes in compliance depends on the knowledge of pulmonary volume (i.e., the changes in vital capacity and the dynamic expiratory flow rates).

whether a deep inspiration or full expiration has been made immediately before the measurement of compliance, by respiratory frequency, by the type of disease studied, and by time. Adequate assessment of the lung's elastic properties can be done only by measuring the static pressure-volume curve in which absolute transpulmonary pressure is related to absolute pulmonary volume over the whole VC during both inflation and deflation.

To correct for body size in patients with suspected pulmonary disease, static elastic recoil pressure may be plotted against a percentage of predicted TLC. In patients with emphysema, the curve is shifted upward to the left and indicates a noticeable loss of elastic recoil. Patients with pulmonary fibrosis have a downward shift of the curve to the right side, which indicates a sharp increase in elastic recoil at all pulmonary volumes. Many factors contribute to the shape and position of a static pressure-volume curve. Pulmonary volume history is an important factor. Another factor is age, because the elastic recoil decreases with age. The state of pulmonary tissue and the nature of the air-liquid interface of the lung are other important determinants. It is not yet clear how the recoil may change, which it apparently does in asthma, or exactly why aging of the lung should be associated with a loss of recoil that is disproportionate to any other changes.

Pressure-Volume Curve

The static elastic recoil pressure of the lung is caused mainly by surface tension at the alveoli-air interface. If the alveoli are filled with saline, the surface tension is abolished at a particular pulmonary volume, which effectively separates the elastic recoil of the lungs into two components—one component is attributed to the pulmonary tissue and the other component is attributed to the surface tension. The difference noted in pressure-volume curves and hysteresis loops between the air-filled and the liquid-filled interfaces is thus attributed to the surface tension at the alveolar level. The finding of the difference in the two pressure-volume loops led to the postulation that alveoli are not lined simply with proteins in water but instead with a watery solution containing lipoproteins, which, when compressed together, exert a surface pressure on each other. In a surface that consists of lipoproteins in water, the surface pressure of the lipoproteins may completely oppose the surface tension of the water and have no resultant net force. Substances recovered from the lungs by washing appear to contain a phospholipid combined with a type of protein. The phospholipid consists mainly of dipalmitoyl lecithin, which is a surfactant that could exert sufficient surface pressure to lower the surface tension to zero.

VENTILATION–PERFUSION ABNORMALITIES

Blood flow is wasted in an atelectatic lung, and ventilation is wasted when there is pulmonary vascular obstruction (Fig. 1–5). Impairment of gas exchange may be expressed in terms of wasted pulmonary blood flow, venous admixture, or right-to-left shunt. Venous admixture, or a mixture of venous blood and arterial blood, is by analogy the dead space of blood perfusion of the lungs, and except during pure oxygen breathing, the venous admixture is an expression of both true shunts and shunt-like effects. The former represent contributions to the arterial blood that has not been through ventilated areas of the lungs, and the latter are an expression of the effects of regions with a low ventilation-perfusion ratio. By giving the

patient pure oxygen, a true shunt can be distinguished from a low-ventilation-perfusion effect, because the arterial oxygen tension is the same in both the low and the high ventilation-perfusion regions. Therefore, if hypoxemia persists, a true shunt is the only cause of arterial hypoxemia (Comroe, 1974; Rahn and Farhi, 1964; Woodbury, 1973). However, arterial PO_2 rises appreciably in a patient with a true shunt when pure oxygen is breathed because the unshunted blood plasma absorbs more dissolved oxygen at a higher tension. In some instances, the arterial saturation of oxygen can be raised almost to 100% on pure oxygen, even in the presence of a true shunt; however, a widened alveolar-arterial oxygen tension difference still shows the existence of a shunt. A true shunt contains components from right-to-left intracardiac shunts, abnormal communications between pulmonary arteries and veins, and alveoli that are perfused but not ventilated. In healthy individuals at rest, the total shunt is less than 5% of the total cardiac output. The true shunt is approximately 1 to 2%. Normally, little blood flow is wasted (approximately 5%) compared with ventilation (approximately 30%) (Comroe, 1974; Rahn and Farhi, 1964).

Physiologic dead space (V_D) represents wasted ventilation (i.e., ventilation of nonperfused alveoli), and its magnitude can be used to express one aspect of impaired gas exchange (Wagner et al., 1964). The difference between anatomic dead space measured with an insoluble gas such as helium and V_D measured with an exchanging gas reflects the component of wasted ventilation. This space has been called alveolar dead space (Severinghaus and Stupfel, 1957) and is measured usually by substituting the arterial PCO_2 for the alveolar PCO_2 in the Bohr equation (Figs. 1–3 to 1–6). The V_D is often expressed in relation to the V_T. In normal young subjects, the V_D is on the average a little less than one-third of the V_T and tends to decrease during exercise. With advancing age, the V_D/V_T ratio increases. The ratio of V_D to the V_T is greater in newborn infants than in adults and indicates some nonuniformity of the ventilation-perfusion ratio or perhaps a small V_T in the lung immediately

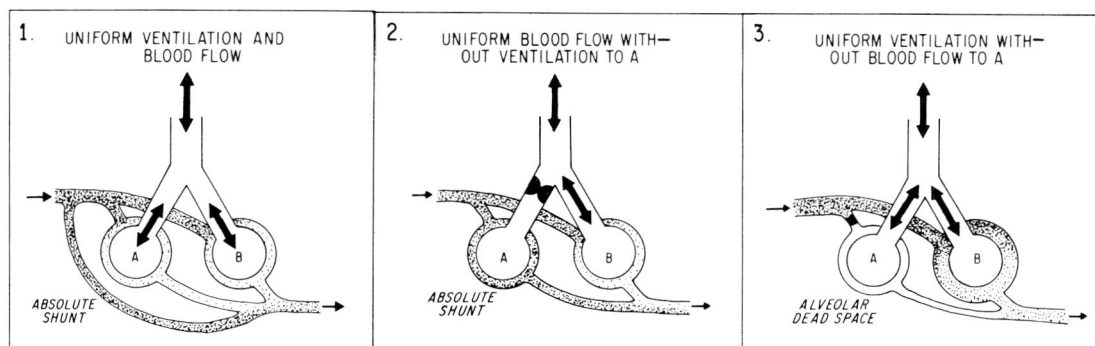

FIGURE 1–5. The problem of uneven ventilation and blood flow. 1, There is uniform ventilation and blood flow, but an absolute shunt or an anatomic shunt is present. 2, The problem seen with bronchial obstruction or atelectasis, in which there is continued uniform blood flow but absent ventilation, which produces a shunt. 3, Uniform ventilation but pulmonary vascular occlusion such as that seen with pulmonary emboli, in which dead space is increased. (Adapted from Comroe, J. H., Jr.: Physiology of Respiration. 2nd ed. Copyright © 1974 by Year Book Medical Publishers, Inc., Chicago. Reproduced by permission.)

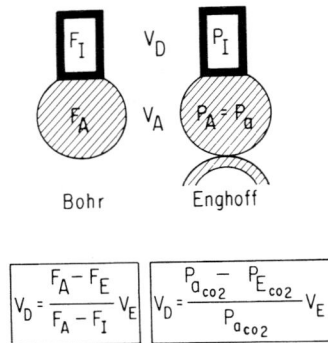

$$V_D = \frac{F_A - F_E}{F_A - F_I} V_E \qquad V_D = \frac{P_{a_{CO_2}} - P_{E_{CO_2}}}{P_{a_{CO_2}}} V_E$$

FIGURE 1–6. The measurement of dead space initially as described by Bohr. Dead space is obtained by measuring the fraction of carbon dioxide and the volume of expired gas. The Enghoff modification assumes that arterial carbon dioxide is equal to alveolar carbon dioxide. The measurement is done using partial pressure rather than a fraction. Using this more simplified measurement of dead space, the arterial carbon dioxide, expired carbon dioxide, and expired volume are the only measurements needed. If the assumption can be safely made that PA is equal to Pa, this method is an excellent and quick way to obtain the bedside measurement of dead-space ventilation.

after birth. However, by the age of 24 hours, the V_D/V_T ratio is of the same order as the ratio in adults.

Part of each breath is wasted because some inspired air never comes within diffusion distance of alveoli. This portion of wasted gas is called *anatomic dead space* and is equal to the volume of the tracheobronchial tree. The mouth and the pharynx contribute approximately 66 ml of dead space to an average total of 150 ml in normal humans. This value drops to 35 ml with depression of the jaw and flexion of the neck, whereas protrusion of the jaw increases the value to 105 ml. Anatomic dead space may be estimated in milliliters as being equal to an adult's ideal weight in pounds (Nunn et al., 1959).

The remaining portion of tidal air passes during inspiratory airflow beyond the tracheobronchial tree and into the remaining lung, where the gas mixes with gas that was previously present in the central regions. The gas then rapidly diffuses back and forth between central and peripheral regions of each lobule. This gas must span a distance of only about 0.05 mm, which is approximately the radius of a pulmonary lobule. The time for diffusion over such a short distance is less than 0.1 second. Using the formula for minute volume ventilation (minute volume = $V_T \times$ respiratory frequency) and dead space ventilation (dead space ventilation = volume of dead space × respiratory frequency), it is apparent that lobular and thus alveolar ventilation are equal to the minute volume minus the dead space ventilation.

Each inspiration brings some fresh air into the lobules and the alveoli. However, the alveolar air does not consist entirely of inspired fresh air, because the blood returning from the body tissues to the capillaries of the lung transports some carbon dioxide to the alveoli and also absorbs some oxygen. In the steady state, the carbon dioxide added to alveolar air by the blood is exactly equal to the carbon dioxide removed

from the body in the expired alveolar air. The amount of oxygen transferred from the alveolar air to the pulmonary blood is exactly equal to the amount of oxygen extracted from the inspired air. The expired alveolar air reflects this depletion of oxygen. Because slightly less carbon dioxide is excreted than oxygen is absorbed, there is a 1% reduction in the volume of expired alveolar air compared with inspired alveolar air and at the same time a corresponding concentration effect of 1% on all the gases in the alveolar air, which is called a respiratory quotient (RQ) effect.

The RQ is defined as a ratio of metabolic carbon dioxide output to oxygen uptake. The RQ varies with the composition of the food that is metabolized. If only carbohydrates are metabolized, the RQ is 1.0, because the number of oxygen equivalents in a carbohydrate molecule balances the number of hydrogen equivalents. However, when proteins are added to the diet, the RQ becomes 0.8, and if fat is added, the RQ falls to 0.7. The average person who fasts uses carbohydrate, protein, and fat in proportions that give a net RQ of approximately 0.81, which explains why slightly more oxygen is taken up from the inspired air than carbon dioxide is added to it (Bates et al., 1971; Comroe et al., 1962).

Measurement of Arterial Blood Gases

When liquid is in equilibrium with gas, the partial pressure of the gas dissolved in the liquid is proportional to the partial pressure of the gas in the gas phase. The gas partial pressure in the liquid is equal to the barometric pressure multiplied by the fractional gas concentration. Therefore, the gas mixture contains 50% oxygen, and the barometric pressure is 760 torr. The PO_2 is equal to 760 × 0.5, which is equal to 380 torr. This relationship is true for any liquid in equilibrium with any gas. The solubility of a gas in a simple solution is an expression of the volume of the liquid at some stated temperature and pressure. The relationship between the gas content of a simple solution such as distilled water and the gas tension of the fluid is linear at any particular temperature, but it is not linear if the solution contains a buffer or special methods of gas transport, which are contained within the red blood cell.

Oxyhemoglobin (HbO$_2$) Dissociation Curve

The unusual properties of the HbO_2 curve are shown in Figure 1–7 and are a result of the remarkable chemical substance, hemoglobin. Because the top of the HbO_2 dissociation curve is flat, oxygen tension may fall considerably at the top end of the curve with a relatively small change in oxygen content. A fall in the arterial PO_2 from 95 to 60 torr results in a reduction in oxygen content of less than 10%. Thus, hyperventilation with a consequent elevation of alveolar PO_2 results in only a small increase in the amount of oxygen taken up by the blood under normal circum-

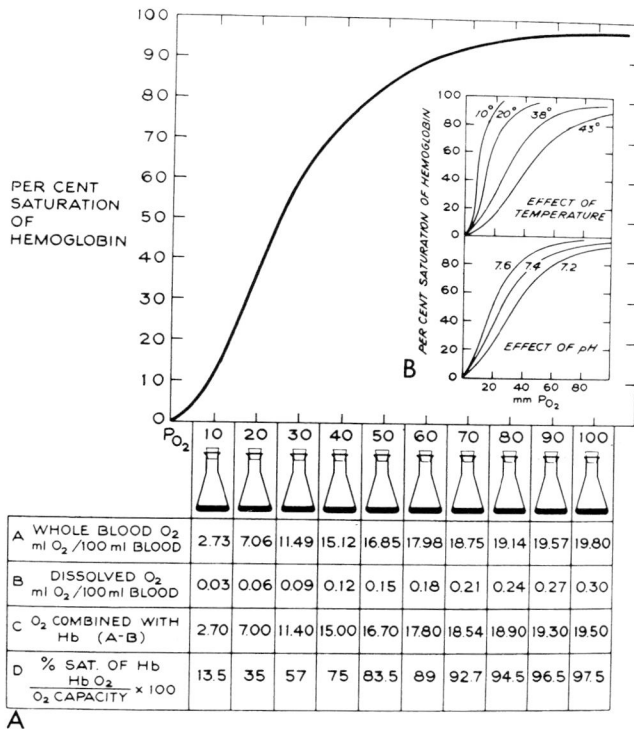

		10	20	30	40	50	60	70	80	90	100
A	WHOLE BLOOD O₂ ml O₂ /100 ml BLOOD	2.73	7.06	11.49	15.12	16.85	17.98	18.75	19.14	19.57	19.80
B	DISSOLVED O₂ ml O₂ /100ml BLOOD	0.03	0.06	0.09	0.12	0.15	0.18	0.21	0.24	0.27	0.30
C	O₂ COMBINED WITH Hb (A−B)	2.70	7.00	11.40	15.00	16.70	17.80	18.54	18.90	19.30	19.50
D	% SAT. OF Hb Hb O₂ / O₂ CAPACITY × 100	13.5	35	57	75	83.5	89	92.7	94.5	96.5	97.5

FIGURE 1–7. *A,* "Standard" HbO_2 dissociation (and association) curve. For a normal man with hemoglobin A; blood pH, 7.40; and body temperature, 37° C. P_{50} = blood Po_2 required for 50% saturation of hemoglobin with O_2 at 37° C and pH 7.40. *B,* Variations in the HbO_2 dissociation curve. Effect of changes in temperature. Effect of changes in blood pH. (*A,* Data from Severinghaus, J. W.: Blood gas calculator. J. Appl. Physiol. 21:1108, 1966; *B,* Reproduced with permission from Comroe, J. H.: Physiology of Respiration. 2nd ed. Copyright © 1974 by Year Book Medical Publishers, Inc., Chicago.)

stances. Therefore, hyperventilation of one part of the lung cannot compensate for reduced ventilation in other parts. The shape of the dissociation curve is altered by a change in blood pH, Pco_2, and temperature, and by the presence of carbon monoxide (see Fig. 1–7). As arterial blood enters the capillary of a working tissue and the carbon dioxide diffuses into the blood, the consequent fall in blood pH assists the unloading of oxygen into the tissue. A parallel process occurs at the other end of the capillary when hemoglobin increases the volume of the carbon dioxide that the blood can transport, thus assisting the removal of carbon dioxide from the metabolically active tissue. Furthermore, red blood cells contain the enzyme carbonic anhydrase, which enables carbon dioxide to be released quickly during the short passage of blood through the pulmonary capillary (Filley, 1971; Hills, 1973; Woodbury, 1973).

Oxygen

Oxygen equilibrated with blood exists in two forms: the first form is in simple physical solution, and the second form is in a reversible combination

with hemoglobin. Normal blood hemoglobin concentration is 15 g/100 ml blood, and the HbO_2 capacity is normally 1.34 ml/g × 15 g = 20.1 ml O_2 standard temperature and pressure, dry (STPD)/100 ml blood. Mixed venous blood is usually approximately 75% saturated at a venous Po_2 of 40 torr and pH of 7.37. Thus, mixed venous blood contains 1.34 ml/g × 15 g × 0.75 = 15.1 ml O_2 STPD/100 ml blood. The remainder has been delivered to the tissues, on average 20.1 − 15.1 = 5 ml O_2/100 ml blood flow. Additional oxygen can, therefore, be delivered under the same conditions only by lowering mixed venous saturation and thus the mixed venous Po_2.

The amount of oxygen combined with hemoglobin depends on the Po_2 dissolved in the blood; that is, the amount of dissolved oxygen is related linearly to the partial pressure. The amount of oxygen combined with hemoglobin is nonlinear and is described usually as a sigmoidal relationship (see Fig. 1–7). The principal messages of this curve are contained in three points (Fig. 1–8): (1) at a partial pressure of 100 torr, the arterial point, the saturation is 97.5%; (2) at a partial pressure of 50 torr, the saturation is approximately 84%; (3) at a Po_2 of 40 torr, the venous point, it is 75%. Between points 1 and 2, there is a 50-torr change in Po_2, but only a 13% change in saturation. However, in the steep portion of the curve, between points 2 and 3, there is essentially a linear relationship (i.e., for a 10-torr Po_2 change, there is a 10% saturation change), which provides important clinical information with reference to arterial hypoxemia. The range in which patients live or die is usually between 2 and 3. In this zone small changes in Po_2 can be translated to large changes in the percentage of saturation and significant changes in oxygen transport. However, between points 1 and 2 large changes in Po_2 result in small changes in the percentage of saturation and small changes in oxygen transport. As shown in Fig-

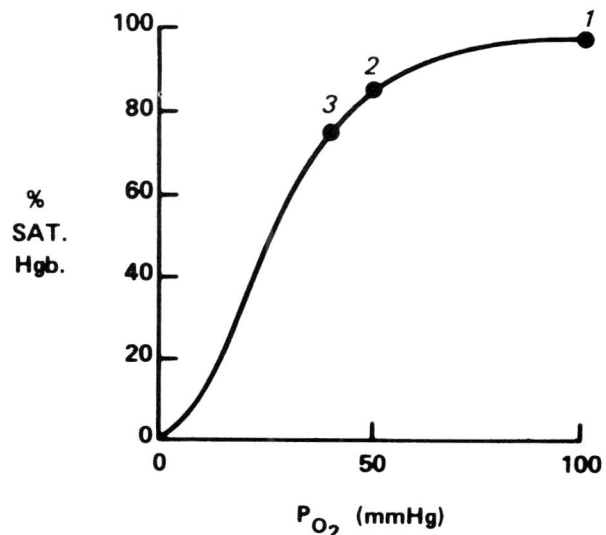

FIGURE 1–8. The oxyhemoglobin-dissociation curve. (From Tisi, G. M.: Pulmonary Physiology in Clinical Medicine. Copyright © 1980, The Williams & Wilkins Company, Baltimore. Used by permission.)

ure 1-7, the position of the oxygen-hemoglobin curve is not fixed; it is shifted by pH, P_{O_2}, and temperature. A shift to the right is produced by a fall in pH, a rise in P_{CO_2}, and an increase in temperature. Shifts to the left are produced by the opposite shades of each of these variables. Such shifts in the curve explain why certain patients with pneumonia look pinker than arterial oxygen would indicate. Patients with pneumonia tend to hyperventilate and have a low P_{CO_2}, which results in an increase in the pH. Thus, the curve is shifted to the left and results in a higher percentage of saturation. In such patients, the magnitude of pneumonia may be miscalculated owing to the absence of clinical cyanosis.

Carbon Dioxide

Carbon dioxide, like oxygen, also reacts with the blood. Unlike oxygen, most of the carbon dioxide is carried as a bicarbonate ion in the plasma. However, the hemoglobin buffers the hydrogen ions that are formed, and the carbon dioxide reacts with water to form ionized H_2CO_3, which then dissociates into H^+ and HCO_3^-. The red blood cells also have a role in that they contain carbonic anhydrase, which speeds up the conversion of CO_2 to H_2CO_3 and thus to bicarbonate. Also, hemoglobin combines as a protein directly with carbon dioxide. As venous blood enters the lung, carbon dioxide in physical solution begins to diffuse freely into the alveoli; the venous partial pressure of carbon dioxide is 46 torr, whereas the alveolar partial pressure of carbon dioxide is 40 torr. To replace the carbon dioxide that has left the blood, some H_2CO_3 dissociates to form carbon dioxide and water. This reaction is catalyzed by the carbonic anhydrase of the red blood cells to replace the H_2CO_3 that is dissociated in the red blood cells. Some hydrogen ions leave the hemoglobin in which they have been combined with bicarbonate ions in the red blood cells to form H_2CO_3. As a concentration of bicarbonate ions in the red blood cells decreases, the ions in the plasma diffuse through the red blood cell membrane into the red blood cells. In exchange, chloride ions diffuse from the red blood cells into the plasma. This entire process continues until the P_{CO_2} in the blood is equal to the P_{CO_2} in the alveolar air. The half-time for much of this process is approximately 0.2 second and is almost completed by the time that the blood has left the capillaries of the lung (transit time of 0.7 second).

Measurement of Oxygen and Carbon Dioxide Tension

Great advances have been made in these techniques in recent years. At present, the tension of oxygen and carbon dioxide in the blood can be determined in several ways, each of which has, in skilled hands, a standard deviation of approximately $\pm$ 2 torr. The first oxygen tension measurements became possible with the use of the polargraphic technique. The transi-

tion from the polargraphic method to electrodes based on the use of a membrane between blood and the platinum tip is very important clinically. The oxygen electrode, which was originally designed by Clark (1956) and described by Severinghaus and Bradley (1958), consists of a silver anode and a platinum cathode covered by a polyethylene membrane. Severinghaus and Bradley also described an electrode used for measuring carbon dioxide tension, which incorporates the Teflon membrane lying over a cellophane membrane that retains a solution of 0.01 M $NaHCO_3$ and 0.1 NaCl in front of the cathode, an arrangement that has produced satisfactory stability and accuracy of performance. Both oxygen and carbon dioxide electrodes require careful heat stabilization, meticulous maintenance, and routine calibration checks against blood or water of a known gas tension.

Measurements of oxygen and carbon dioxide tension have now shifted from the experimental and developmental stages into the clinical arena. Although one might think that the speed and accuracy of determination are the greatest assets, another major advantage lies in the fact that gas tensions of up to 600 torr for oxygen and up to 300 torr for carbon dioxide can be measured with the same facility as gas tensions at the lower end of the scale.

In the clinical management of patients, knowledge of Pa_{CO_2} alone is insufficient; therefore, the pH must also be determined. Until recently, accurate measurement of blood pH presented technical problems. Most of these problems have been solved, except for the difficulty of the glass electrode, which may become unstable with repeated use of blood because of blockage of the porcelain plug by plasma proteins. Careful routine standardization with freshly prepared buffer solutions ensures prompt detection of any error so that the electrode can be replaced.

The measurement of Pa_{CO_2} provides an immediate indication of the patient's alveolar ventilation. A Pa_{CO_2} of 40 torr is normal, and the range is from 34 to 46 torr. A Pa_{CO_2} of more than 46 torr means that there is alveolar hyperventilation, whereas a Pa_{CO_2} of less than 34 torr indicates that the patient has more alveolar ventilation than is required.

The measurement of arterial P_{O_2} is useful to evaluate the function of the lungs. An alveolar-arterial P_{O_2} difference ($P[A-a]O_2$) of approximately 10 torr is found customarily in young healthy adults, and a 20-torr difference is found in healthy older adults. Greater differences (i.e., an arterial P_{O_2} less than 80 torr in the absence of hypoventilation) require another explanation. The possibilities include a right-to-left shunt, a diffusion "barrier" (an incomplete diffusion equilibrium between alveolar gas and end-capillary blood), or uneven distribution of ventilation and blood flow. To test for a right-to-left shunt, when the patient is given 100% oxygen, the arterial blood P_{O_2} should increase to more than 600 torr. If the arterial P_{O_2} is less than predicted but more than 150 torr, then the percentage of right-to-left shunting can be calculated. This result represents the ratio for mixing between the venous and arterial streams:

$$\% \text{ shunt} = \frac{\dfrac{(673 - \text{Pa}_{O_2})\, 2.3}{760}}{\dfrac{673 - (\text{Pa}_{O_2})\, 2.3}{760} + 4.5} \times 100$$

assuming that 2.3 is the solubility of oxygen in plasma and 4.5 is the usual arteriovenous difference.

The normal shunt is 1 to 5%; in obese patients, the normal shunt may be up to 10%. Shunts more than 6% are usually abnormal. The pulmonary diffusion capacity is a test used to evaluate the presence of a diffusion "barrier" using carbon monoxide.

An oxygen difference can be caused by uneven distribution of ventilation and blood flow throughout the lung and is the remaining possible explanation for a $P(A-a)O_2$ when alveolar hypoventilation, right-to-left shunt, and diffusion "barrier" have been excluded.

Alveolar-Arterial Oxygen Gradient

There is a large pressure decrease in oxygen tension from atmospheric to cellular level (Fig. 1–9). The partial pressure of inspired oxygen, $P_{I_{O_2}}$, is approximately 159 torr. The alveolar oxygen tension is 110, and Pa_{CO_2} is normally 40 torr. The normal range for arterial oxygen tension is 80 to 100 torr. Oxygen tension of the mitochondrial level is approximately 1 torr. The difference in the oxygen tension between any two levels is referred to as a gradient. The gradient between alveolar and arterial levels, $P(A-a)O_2$, is basic to the understanding of arterial hypoxemia. The $P(A-a)O_2$ can be calculated by determining the Pa_{O_2} and the Pa_{CO_2} of arterial blood. Using the corrected formula, the PA_{O_2} is equal to $713 - F_{I_{O_2}} - Pa_{CO_2}$. This

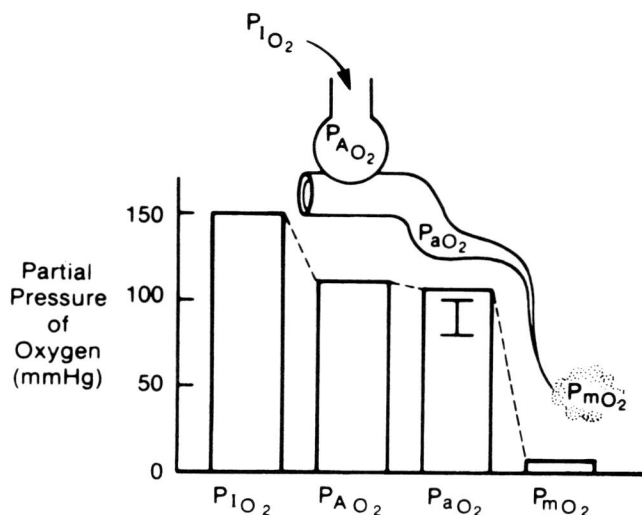

equation for PA_{O_2} is derived from the assumptions that the water-vapor pressure is 47 torr and the K, the correction factor that depends on $F_{I_{O_2}}$ and the respiratory quotient, can for clinical purposes be neglected. At sea level, where barometric changes are minimal, barometric pressure (PB) can be assumed to be 760 torr, and therefore, the derivation of the equation becomes $PA_{O_2} = 150 - Pa_{CO_2}$. Consequently, the only major value that must be determined is the Pa_{CO_2}. The Pa_{O_2} can then be subtracted from PA_{O_2} and the alveolar-arterial gradient is obtained. The normal $P(A-a)O_2$ at all ages is less than 25 torr.

Causes of Hypoxemia

The $P(A-a)O_2$ is an important measurement and provides one of the principal means for distinguishing the causes of arterial hypoxemia.

Central hypoventilation is defined as a reduction in the volume of air moving into and out of the mouth per minute or decreased minute ventilation. With central hypoventilation, there is hypoxemia and hypercapnia with a normal $P(A-a)O_2$. If the patient with central hypoventilation presents with an increased $P(A-a)O_2$, superimposed problems should be suspected (i.e., aspiration and atelectasis).

A reduced inspired oxygen tension is the second important cause of hypoxemia. It is important to be confident at sea level of the true measurement of $F_{I_{O_2}}$. Diffusion limitation has a minor role in arterial hypoxemia at sea level and for clinical purposes can be disregarded. Another important reason for arterial hypoxemia is right-to-left shunting. The arterial blood gas pattern for a shunt is hypoxemia with a greatly increased $P(A-a)O_2$, usually more than 60 torr, combined with a lack of response to supplemental oxygen.

Finally, with airway closure such as the closure that occurs with atelectasis, aspiration, and pneumonia, the resultant ventilation-perfusion mismatch is the most common cause for arterial hypoxemia. The regional pulmonary unit may be underventilated but is normally perfused. The most reliable way to define a reduction in ventilation-perfusion is to note the response to supplemental oxygen; the cause of the arterial hypoxemia most likely is abnormal ventilation-perfusion matching as opposed to a shunt.

EVALUATION OF ACID–BASE BALANCE

The acid-base status of the body has been characterized traditionally by the acid-base status of the blood because the blood is readily available for analysis. Blood does come into contact with all other organ systems of the body and presumably reflects their status. However, it accounts for only one-fourth of the buffering capacity of the entire body and under special conditions may not actually reflect changes in other areas (Filley, 1971).

FIGURE 1–9. The normal gradient in oxygen tension between atmospheric ($P_{I_{O_2}}$), alveolar (PA_{O_2}), arterial (Pa_{O_2}), and mitochondrial (Pm_{O_2}) levels. (From Tisi, G. M.: Pulmonary Physiology in Clinical Medicine. Copyright © 1980, The Williams & Wilkins Company, Baltimore. Used by permission.)

Physiologic Compensations

The principal buffering systems in the body are bicarbonate, phosphates, and cells. During acute changes, the extracellular bicarbonate and hemoglobin are the major buffers. In addition to chemical buffering, there are physiologic responses to alterations in acid-base status that are also critical in minimizing changes in pH for each of the four types of acid-base disturbances. The Henderson-Hasselbalch equation describes the bicarbonate/carbon dioxide buffering system, or the relationship among the pH, P_{CO_2}, and H_2CO_3

$$pH = pK + \log \frac{[H_2CO_3]}{[HCO_3^-]} \text{ or } pH = 6.1 + \log \frac{[HCO_3^-]}{0.03 \times P_{CO_2}}$$

where 6.1 = the pK_a of carbonic acid and 0.03 is the solubility of carbon dioxide in blood.

Wherever compensation occurs for primary respiratory acid-base disturbances, there must be a physiologically induced metabolic alteration that is usually renal. Primary metabolic disturbances are corrected initially by using a respiratory mechanism. The urinary excretion of acid, although starting rapidly, may take hours to days to complete; thus, renal adjustments in acid-base balance occur slowly. However, sudden loads of carbon dioxide can be eliminated almost completely in approximately 30 minutes, making this respiratory mechanism suitable for rapid adjustment in pH.

The interpretation of blood pH in terms of respiratory and metabolic acidosis becomes difficult if the blood samples are obtained after therapy has been initiated. With the availability of potent diuretics, rapid changes in blood pH by renal mechanism are possible without necessarily changing the intracellular pH. It is not uncommon to find normal arterial P_{CO_2}, which indicates good respiratory drive, in the presence of alkaline blood pH if the person has been treated with thiazide diuretics.

Respiratory Acidosis

Respiratory acidosis is compensated for by renal retention of bicarbonate or excretion of acid, which is a part of the same chemical process. Renal compensation begins immediately when respiratory acidosis develops but takes days to weeks to reach a maximum. This mechanism can return blood pH completely to normal, if there is sufficient time and if the steady-state Pa_{CO_2} is 60 to 65 torr or less. Above this level of hypercapnia, the kidney cannot increase its rate of reabsorption of bicarbonate to maintain normal pH, and the blood pH will fall. If the blood gases of the patient with hypercapnia show that the pH is normal because of a superimposed metabolic alkalosis rather than because of potassium secretion or loss of gastric juice, the indication is that respiratory acidosis is chronic, because hypercapnia must have been present for some days or weeks. If the pH is low and

the Pa_{CO_2} is below 60 torr, respiratory acidosis is likely to be acute or subacute. The range of normal values of plasma bicarbonate for a particular chronic elevation of Pa_{CO_2} has been determined. Bicarbonate concentrations are obviously higher than concentrations for acute elevations of Pa_{CO_2}, because chronic hypercapnia leads to bicarbonate retention.

The effect of respiratory acidosis on the sensorium is probably due to lowering of pH of the cerebrospinal fluid (CSF) with which blood carbon dioxide equilibrates rapidly. Because the CSF pH is corrected toward normal by accumulation of bicarbonate in CSF, within a few days of the onset of hypercapnia patients with chronic hypercapnia may have a clear sensorium at a level of Pa_{CO_2} that would cause coma if this condition developed acutely. Thus, clinical observation in the patient with known hypercapnia can often indicate whether hypercapnia is acute or chronic.

Respiratory Alkalosis

Controversy continues regarding compensation of the kidney in chronic respiratory alkalosis by excretion of bicarbonate and retention of acid. There is suggestive evidence that such compensation occurs, at least in chronic situations, but it is probably incomplete.

Metabolic Acidosis

Metabolic acidosis is corrected by inducing respiratory alkalosis. Chemoreceptors, both in the aortic-carotid areas and in the area on or near the floor of the fourth ventricle, account for at least half and possibly much more of the respiratory stimulation occurring during metabolic acidosis. The aortic-carotid area is affected rapidly by changes in the CSF pH. The maximal respiratory response to an acid load is delayed for some hours or days. For any particular blood pH during chronic metabolic acidosis, the Pa_{CO_2} is lowered appropriately. A Pa_{CO_2} that is inappropriately above or below the response to uncomplicated metabolic acidosis suggests the presence of a superimposed primary respiratory acidosis or alkalosis.

Metabolic Alkalosis

Metabolic alkalosis is compensated by the development of respiratory acidosis. However, under ordinary circumstances, Pa_{CO_2} does not increase above 50 torr despite the severity of the metabolic alkalosis. The usual minimal effect on Pa_{CO_2} appears to result from the fact that ventilation is linked to the rate of oxygen consumption or carbon dioxide production in some unknown manner. This link prevents the development of more severe hypercapnia by taking precedence over the compensatory mechanism.

CARDIOVASCULAR MANIFESTATIONS OF RESPIRATORY INSUFFICIENCY

One of the obvious cardiovascular manifestations of pulmonary insufficiency is cardiac enlargement on the chest film, which could be equated with primary heart disease. Complete knowledge of the patient is necessary to differentiate cardiomegaly secondary to respiratory insufficiency (Rao et al., 1968). Obstructive pulmonary disease, obesity, and chest-wall deformity may cause pulmonary insufficiency and cardiomegaly. In such primary processes, there is usually hypoxemia and an arterial oxygen saturation below 85%.

Pulmonary hypertension induced by hypoxemia and frequently accompanied by respiratory acidosis and tachycardia are factors that contribute to the problem of increased workload of the right ventricle. Pneumonia may occur as a complication of primary pulmonary disease that causes worsening of pulmonary function and the appearance of hypoxemia and respiratory acidosis in many patients. The chest film may show cardiomegaly and perihilar infiltrates and may make the physician believe that the problem is primarily left-sided heart failure. Digitalis and diuretics do not correct this situation, and they may induce cardiac arrhythmias. Attention to the airways, proper administration of oxygen therapy, antibiotics, and bronchodilators are necessary to reverse the situation.

It is not unusual to find pulmonary vascular congestion and Kerley B lines with severe obstructive airway disease associated with arterial hypoxemia and hypercapnia. Pulmonary edema may also be evident, with sharp anemia with hemoglobin less than 7 g/100 ml when associated with pneumonia, pulmonary emboli, neoplasia, or uremia. The low oxygen-carrying capacity of the blood results in peripheral tissue hypoxemia and stimulates an increase in cardiac output. Although the myocardial tissue is required to do more work, it also has less oxygen with which to accomplish its task.

Arrhythmias

Cardiac arrhythmias are a common accompaniment of abnormal gas exchange. As many as 77% of patients with chronic obstructive pulmonary disease and respiratory failure develop sinus tachycardia or arrhythmias, and major supraventricular arrhythmias may be present in as many as 50% of patients who are admitted in acute respiratory failure. Therefore, blood gases of patients on mechanical ventilators should be monitored carefully to prevent hypoxemia. Ventilation that is too vigorous can cause alkalosis with consequent arrhythmias (Flemma and Young, 1964; Hudson et al., 1973). Loss of chloride ion may increase serum bicarbonate in patients predisposed to alkaline pH values even without significant hypocapnia. In a study of patients who had thoracotomy and who were undergoing continuous online monitoring of respiratory and cardiovascular parameters, 50% of patients with respiratory difficulties also developed serious cardiac arrhythmias (Osborn et al., 1971). The latter could be corrected only by normalizing the blood gases. Usually, respiratory difficulty was suspected only after arrhythmia appeared.

Cardiac arrhythmias may be induced by beta-adrenergic stimulating drugs used to treat bronchospasm. Sinus tachycardia and ventricular ectopy may develop if excessive doses are administered systemically or absorbed across the mucous membranes. These drugs are invaluable in the treatment of airway obstruction and are administered to correctly minimize associated side effects in a patient who is already prone to arrhythmias. Those patients with respiratory insufficiency who are also receiving digitalis are prone to arrhythmias. Reduced potassium concentration in cells, common in patients with obstructive pulmonary disease, accounts for this predisposition. It must be kept in mind that hypertension and tachycardia are usually associated with hypoxemia. Acute carbon dioxide retention leads to respiratory acidosis and results in cerebral vasodilation and increased intracranial pressure. Cerebral edema and then systemic hypertension may follow. Therefore, hypertension concurrent with pulmonary insufficiency must be treated.

Pulmonary Insufficiency in Renal Failure

Edema in patients with chronic respiratory failure suggests that altered renal function accompanies the condition. However, when the patient is chronically hypoxemic, a considerable amount of subcutaneous fluid may accumulate in loose connective tissue. Many surgical patients who develop combined metabolic and respiratory acidosis may have virtual anuria. This finding is more common in obese patients in whom compensation for the acidosis may be difficult. A common finding of reduced output of urine may reflect respiratory insufficiency and hypoxemia, and when the patient's ventilation has improved, renal function returns completely. Generally, this renal failure is usually on a prerenal basis (Petty and Neff, 1971).

Respiratory depression during hemodialysis is not uncommon. The mechanism for this depression is explained on the basis that breathing before dialysis is under the control of carotid bodies that respond to hypoxemia and are potentiated by the acid pH. During dialysis, however, a patient may be made acutely alkalotic because accumulated acids are removed and bicarbonate is increased. This removes the acid stimulus to breathe, reduces the ventilatory drive, and makes the patient more hypoxemic. This problem is compounded when accompanied by pneumonia. Because severe hypoxemia depresses the natural respiratory control mechanism, it may induce apnea. Consequently, the patient who has a large pH increase during renal dialysis, when simultaneously hypoxemic because of pulmonary edema, uremia, or pneumonia, is at a high risk of respiratory arrest.

PULMONARY FUNCTION IN INFANTS AND CHILDREN

Almost every aspect of pulmonary function that has been measured in adults has also been measured in newborn infants and children (Avery et al., 1981; Cotes, 1968) (Table 1–2). The hemoglobin dissociation curve for oxygen in the fetus is to the left of the curve in the adult. This displacement facilitates the absorption of oxygen in the maternal blood. Before birth, the lung is not expanded, and there is a small blood supply. At birth, the situation alters dramatically with the termination of placental circulation and resultant expansion of the lung, which reduces the resistance to blood flow in the pulmonary bed and raises the resistance in systemic circulation. These changes in blood flow cause a pressure gradient to develop between the left atrium and the right atrium, which leads to the closure of the foramen ovale. At the same time, the ductus arteriosus is occluded by constriction of the muscle wall. This process diverts the entire cardiac output through the lung. The blood gases are probably the most useful single measurement for ventilatory adequacy at any age. Micromethods are available for determination of pH, Pa_{CO_2}, and Pa_{O_2}. Use of capillary blood may be inadequate in the distressed infant, and direct arterial sampling is necessary.

Hypoxemia at birth appears to be an unreliable stimulus for respiration and often exerts a depressant effect rather than a stimulatory effect. A more normal response develops after the first few days of life. At birth, the FRC becomes stabilized within the first few breaths, and thereafter the minute ventilation, alveolar ventilation, and work of breathing are comparable to those in adults, with allowance made for difference in metabolic rate. The FRC is smaller than expected and is associated with the relatively high frequency of breathing. In normal circumstances, the

respiratory apparatus of the infant adapts rapidly and completely to the conditions of extrauterine life, and in rare instances when it fails to do so, the condition called *respiratory distress of the newborn* is seen. Also, premature infants suffer from incompletely developed and weak respiratory muscles, which may compound this problem. The medullary respiratory center in the infant may be depressed because of drugs, anesthesia, or head trauma during birth (Comroe, 1974).

In the treatment of cardiac or pulmonary disease in the infant, the physician should be aware that an operation may increase the likelihood of respiratory distress and should be prepared to manage pulmonary insufficiency with increased positive end-expiratory pressure or continuous positive airway pressure (Gregory et al., 1971).

The lungs of children are smaller than the lungs of adults, and the muscles of respiration are less strong. The results of tests in which size and strength are important variables may be difficult to evaluate. The TLC and its subdivisions are smaller in children than in young adults. However, the proportion of pulmonary capacity that is accompanied by the RV is approximately the same, 24%. The airway resistance when measured at FRC is greater in children than in adults because the airways have a small diameter to match the small size of the lung. These differences result in a lower VC in children than in adults when a comparison is made in terms of MBC or forced air volume.

The differences in the mechanical properties of the lung between children and adults give rise to differences in respiratory frequency. Respiratory frequency is greatest in infancy and decreases progressively during childhood. The V_T is correspondingly small in children, and the proportion that is expended in ventilating the V_D is consequently larger. However, when the minute volume is standardized, the consumption of oxygen tends to be higher in children than in adults. By contrast, alveolar ventilation, when similarly standardized, is relatively independent of age.

The surface area of alveolar capillary membranes that is available for exchange of gas and the volume of alveolar capillaries are related to the size of the lung; they are, therefore, smaller in children than in adults. When the diffusing capacity is expressed per liter of pulmonary volume, higher values are obtained in children than in adults. This increase is caused apparently by the relatively larger volume of blood in the alveolar capillaries of children. The differences are probably a function of the relatively small size of the alveolar spaces and capillaries in children, but whether the walls of the alveoli contain a higher density of capillaries or the capillaries contain more red blood cells must still be determined. During childhood, the function of the lungs is similar for boys and girls of equal size. After puberty, the lines diverge, and throughout life, after age and size are taken into account, men have a greater pulmonary capacity than women. However, as men grow older their lungs

■ **Table 1–2.** APPROXIMATE VALUES FOR PULMONARY FUNCTION IN A 3-KG NEWBORN BABY

Vital capacity (vigorous cry)	120 ml
Functional residual capacity	80 ml
Total lung capacity	160 ml
Residual volume	40 ml
Tidal volume	16 ml
Anatomic dead space	7 ml
Frequency of breathing	40/min
Minute volume of breathing	640 ml/min
Alveolar ventilation	360 ml/min
Pulmonary compliance	0.006 l/cm H_2O
Pulmonary compliance/FRC	0.07 l/cm H_2O/l
Airway resistance	18 cm H_2O/l/sec
Arterial O_2 saturation*	88–100%
Arterial P_{CO_2}*	34–40 mm Hg
Arterial pH*	7.3–7.4 units
Arterial hemoglobin	17.6 g/100 ml

From Comroe, J. H., Jr.: Physiology of Respiration. 2nd ed. Copyright © 1974 by Year Book Medical Publishers, Inc., Chicago. Reproduced by permission.
*Varies during the first day of life, depending on time and completeness of closure of venous-to-arterial shunts (foramen ovale and ductus arteriosus) and opening of all alveoli.

deteriorate more than do the lungs of women, and the initial differences are reduced (Cotes, 1968).

EVALUATION OF THE RISK OF PULMONARY RESECTION

Effect of Surgical Procedures on Pulmonary Function

The degree of pulmonary dysfunction after operation is related directly to the type of procedure and the preoperative pulmonary function. For example, operations done on the extremities generally have little effect on pulmonary function (Tisi et al., 1983). Abdominal procedures can cause significant respiratory depression, especially when an upper midline incision is used (Latimer et al., 1971). Thoracic procedures, particularly procedures involving pulmonary resection, cause severe depression of respiratory function.

The TLC and all the subdivisions of pulmonary capacity are reduced after nonextremity procedures (Meyers et al., 1975; Smith et al., 1960). Thus, the surface area available is reduced for gas exchange and promotes airway closure because the FRC is reduced below the closing volume. The resultant atelectasis, either macroscopic or microscopic, can produce arterial hypoxemia. Atelectasis can also be due to retained secretions, the quality of which may be altered by anesthetic agents. The elimination of these secretions is hampered by diminished cough, which is caused by pain or administration of narcotics. There may be a dysfunction of ciliary activity and a clearance of microbial agents.

Airway closure is also due to postoperative splinting of the chest. The breathing pattern is altered characteristically to accomplish adequate minute ventilation with a lowered V_T at an increased respiratory rate. Sighing, a normal mechanism for opening the airways, is eliminated in the early postoperative period (Hyatt et al., 1975). Restriction of the patient to bed, primarily in the supine position, is also deleterious (Tucker et al., 1960). In addition, abnormal positioning of the patient during operation can result in pulmonary dysfunction and is evident particularly in the thoracic patient, for whom the lateral decubitus position can lead to dependent pulmonary consolidation (Lumb, 1983).

Increased age and a history of smoking increase the closing volume (Hyatt et al., 1975). Obesity diminishes the FRC and ERV, such that the end V_T is close to the closing volume. Patients with obstructive pulmonary disease have a reduced ERV. The additional effect of a postoperative reduction in FRC and ERV results in airway closure and atelectasis in patients with these characteristics.

Preoperative Evaluation of Risk

Obstructive pulmonary disease is the most important risk factor in surgical patients, and the degree of expiratory obstruction is related directly to the risk of postoperative complications (Stein et al., 1962). Restrictive pulmonary disease is usually tolerated more easily, despite the fact that pulmonary volumes are reduced postoperatively, owing to better maintenance of expiratory flow and clearing of secretion.

The use of preoperative pulmonary function testing has allowed an approximation of risk based on obstruction. Generally, an FEV_1 of more than 2 l is associated with minimal risk. Increased risk is associated with FEV_1 of from 1 to 2 l. When the FEV_1 is less than 0.8 l, there is a moderate risk of severe complications and the risk becomes prohibitive with an FEV_1 of less than 0.5 liters (Burrows et al., 1975). The 5-year survival rate of patients with an FEV_1 of less than 0.75 l may be as little as 10%, a factor that should be considered in elective surgical procedures (Burrows et al., 1969).

Thoracotomy and pulmonary resection are even less well tolerated (Burrows et al., 1975). The loss of functional pulmonary tissue and the more direct effects of thoracic incisions tend to depress postoperative pulmonary function more severely. The presence of pulmonary hypertension and hypercapnia ($P_{CO_2} > 45$) probably contraindicates pulmonary resection (Stein, 1962). If the FEV_1 is less than 2 l, the MVV is less than 50% of the predicted value, and the predicted postoperative FEV_1 is less than 0.8 l (Olsen et al., 1973, 1975), the patient is at increased risk with pulmonary resection and should probably not undergo pneumonectomy.

The use of standard pulmonary function tests to predict operability in patients who undergo pulmonary resection has been applied extensively (Table 1–3). Generally, these tests can identify patients who are at low risk with pulmonary resection (Gass, 1986; Mittman, 1961; Tisi, 1979), but do not function well as sole criteria for operability when significant abnormalities are present (Keagy et al., 1983; Lockwood, 1973; Peters, 1983).

More recently, various more specific approaches have been taken. The residual pulmonary function should be estimated for a patient before operation (Fig. 1–10) and requires accurate clinical staging as well as an evaluation of regional pulmonary function. Methods have been developed to predict postoperative pulmonary function by subsegmental analysis, which, combined with accurate clinical staging, can be used to predict the number of functional subsegments that must be removed to cure the patient. The remaining subsegments can be used to predict the postoperative FEV_1.

The postoperative FEV_1 has a significant relationship to complication rate for patients older than 65 years of age, and respiratory difficulties occur when the values are 52% of normal or less. Patients with predicted postoperative FEV_1 of 67% or more do not suffer complications. This analysis is less effective in patients younger than 65 years of age (Nakahara et al., 1985). This approach may be combined with radionuclide methods to determine regional perfusion and ventilation to further delineate predicted functional

■ **Table 1–3.** RISK OF PULMONARY RESECTION BY PULMONARY FUNCTION TESTING

Source	Operation	MVV*	FEV₁†	FEF₂₅₋₇₅‡	Mortality Rate
		%			%
Miller, 1993	Pneumonectomy	>55	>21	>1.61	4.97 (8/153)
Miller, 1993	Lobectomy	>40	>11	>0.61	0.39 (3/653)
Miller, 1993	Wedge or segmental	>35	>0.61	>0.61	0.21 (1/475)
Miller, 1987	Less than lobectomy	<40	≤1.01	≤0.61	0 (0/32)

*MVV = maximal voluntary ventilation.
†FEV_1 = forced expiratory volume at 1 second.
‡FEF_{25-75} = forced expiratory flow rate from 25–75% of vital capacity.

loss (Kristersson et al., 1972; Markos et al., 1989, Peters, 1983).

Analysis of exercise tolerance of patients undergoing thoracic procedures reveals information regarding the overall cardiopulmonary status of the patient. The measurement of *pulmonary vascular resistance (PVR) with exercise* has been found to correlate closely with postoperative survival. Five of eight patients who were unable to reduce pulmonary vascular resistance below 190 dyn/sec/cm^{-5} died postoperatively of pulmonary failure (Fee et al., 1978). In nine patients whose initial PVR was more than 190 at rest, but less than 190 with exercise, there were no deaths. In another study, 75 patients were exercised maximally, and patients who completed the tests successfully experienced no postoperative complications, whereas 57% of patients who could not complete the test experienced significant complications. These two groups could not be discriminated by routine pulmonary function testing (Reichel, 1972).

Although some researchers have been unable to show discrimination by exercise testing (Colman et al., 1982), others have used *maximal oxygen consumption* (MVO₂) and the development of measured lactic acidosis as predictors (Table 1–4). The anaerobic threshold and oxygen consumption can be determined conveniently during pulmonary function testing by analysis of expired gases (Whipp, 1987) and may show impending cardiopulmonary failure to provide adequate oxygen delivery to the tissues (Wasserman, 1987).

Eugene and associates maximally exercised 19 patients and determined the minute oxygen consumption. There were no deaths if oxygen consumption was more than 1 l/min, whereas there was a 75% mortality rate in patients who were unable to generate oxygen consumptions of 1 l/min or greater (Eugene et al., 1980). In another study, all patients with an oxygen consumption of less than 15 ml/kg/min had pulmonary complications, whereas only one in ten did when oxygen consumption was more than 20 ml/kg/min. In the intermediate range, 66% had complications (Smith et al., 1984). In a study of 33 patients subjected to incremental exercise testing until an arterial lactate level of 20 mg/dl was achieved, mortality was well predicted. This test, however, did not discriminate well for pulmonary complications (Miyoshi et al., 1987).

Bechard and co-workers assessed exercise oxygen consumption in 50 consecutive patients who had pulmonary function testing. Mortality rate was 29% and morbidity rate was 43% when the MVO₂ was less than 10 ml/kg/min. When the MVO₂ was between 10 and 20 ml/kg/min, there was a 10.7% morbidity and mortality rate. When the MVO₂ was more than 20 ml/kg/min, there was no morbidity or death (Bechard et al., 1987). The determination of oxygen consumption may be a valuable addition to the evaluation of patients who are marginal, but the lower limit of acceptability has not been defined.

The decision to operate on high-risk patients must be balanced against the alternatives available (Peters, 1987). With the advent of limited pulmonary resection as a potentially curative procedure for non-small-cell bronchogenic carcinoma, significant survival can still be obtained in high-risk patients. In one series, lim-

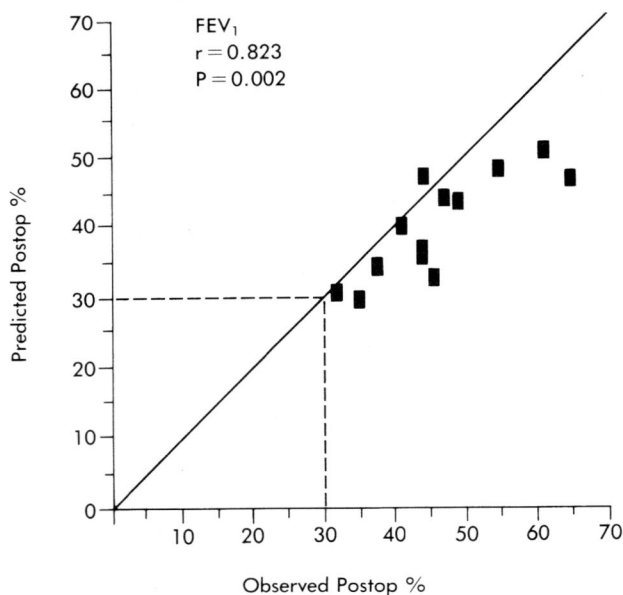

FIGURE 1–10. Plot of the relationship between FEV₁ as a percentage of normal as predicted before pneumonectomy and as observed postoperatively. A *line of identity* shows the excellent relationship obtained in this series of 13 patients, and the *dashed lines* represent the lower limit of patients accepted for pneumonectomy in this study. (From Gass, G. D., and Olsen, G. N.: Preoperative pulmonary function testing to predict postoperative morbidity and mortality. Chest *89*:127, 1986; normal values from Morris, J. F., Koski, A., and Johnson, L. C.: Spirometric standards for nonsmoking healthy adults. Am. Rev. Respir. Dis. *103*:57, 1971.)

■ **Table 1–4.** RISK OF PULMONARY RESECTION BY EXERCISE TESTING

Source	Operation	MVO$_2$*		Morbidity (%)	Mortality (%)
Eugene, 1980	More than lobectomy	>1	l/min	—	0 (0/15)
Eugene, 1980	More than lobectomy .	<1	l/min	—	75 (3/4)
Smith et al., 1984	Any resection	<15	ml/kg/min	100 (10/10)	17 (1/6)
Smith et al., 1984	Any resection	15–20	ml/kg/min	67 (4/6)	17 (1/6)
Smith et al., 1984	Any resection	>20	ml/kg/min	10 (1/10)	0 (0/10)
Bechard and Weststein, 1987	Any resection	<10	ml/kg/min	43 (3/7)	29 (2/7)
Bechard and Weststein, 1987	Any resection	10–20	ml/kg/min	10.7 (3/28)	0 (0/28)
Bechard and Weststein, 1987	Any resection	>20	ml/kg/min	0 (0/15)	0 (0/15)

*MVO$_2$ = maximal oxygen consumption with exercise.

ited resection has been applied to patients with MVV of less than 40% of predicted, FEV$_1$ of less than or equal to 1 l, and a forced expiratory flow rate of less than or equal to 0.6 l/sec. In this group, a 2-year survival rate of 84% and a 5-year survival rate of 31% were achieved without operative mortality (Miller et al., 1987). These findings tend to justify limited operations in high-risk patients (Miller et al., 1981; Martini et al., 1986).

With the advent of limited postoperative radiation as an adjunctive agent, the degree to which a successful pulmonary resection can be limited may result in even further strides than the strides achieved in the transition from the classic pneumonectomy to lobectomy initiated by Churchill (Churchill et al., 1950).

PERIOPERATIVE CARE

Preoperative Preparation

Every effort should be made to convince the patient to stop smoking preoperatively. Ideally, the patient should stop smoking at least 2 weeks before operation, although there is great benefit from cessation for as little as 1 week. The identification of other treatable preoperative conditions is essential. Sputum culture and the start of appropriate antibiotics are imperative in patients with a productive cough.

Education and training of patients are important parts of preoperative preparation. Breathing exercises strengthen the respiratory musculature. Instructions on coughing and deep breathing improve postoperative cooperation. Instruction in the use of narcotics, as needed, to allow coughing and deep breathing gives the physician a valuable ally in the titration of these drugs postoperatively. Chest percussion and postural drainage may be necessary in patients with copious pulmonary secretion.

Medical Management of Bronchospasm

A larger variety of therapeutic agents are now available to optimize pulmonary function. An organized approach in the use of these agents is important because there are many potential drug interactions and serious side effects that may limit therapy.

Adrenergic Agonists and Bronchodilator Aerosol Therapy

Beta-agonists are currently the most popular initial bronchodilating agents. The effect of adrenergic agonists is primarily due to direct effects on bronchial smooth muscle because there is no significant direct sympathetic innervation in humans. The beta-2 effects are bronchodilatory and anti-inflammatory by inhibition of mediator release. Mucociliary clearance is also improved.

The prototype sympathomimetic drug is epinephrine, but its use has been limited by adverse cardiac effects when given systemically and by poor bioavailability in oral forms. The development of metaproterenol and albuterol has allowed oral dosage and has minimized cardiac or beta-1 effects. Beta-2 selective agents, such as salbutamol, have been recently introduced (Pesenti et al., 1993).

The effects of adrenergic agents are dose-related and show no response plateau. Therapy can be limited by systemic side effects, which include tremor, nervousness, and cardiac arrhythmias. Aerosol administration allows greater effective dosing with fewer side effects. In acute bronchospasm, the aerosol route may not result in uniform airway distribution, and effectiveness can be delayed. The bronchodilatory effects of the adrenergic agents are probably additive when used in combination with theophylline (Shim, 1984).

Corticosteroids

Current trends in the management of reactive airway disease include the early employment of intravenous corticosteroids. Although steroids may adversely effect wound healing, their powerful anti-inflammatory action is of overriding importance, particularly in acute bronchospastic disorders. Intravenous administration is usually accompanied by beta-agonist therapy and a short course prescribed in the immediate perioperative period. Patients already receiving chronic steroid therapy for obstructive lung disease should be given perioperative steroids because of adrenal suppression.

The introduction of beclomethasone dipropionate has increased the therapeutic efficacy of steroid use because it is administered by inhalation. Adrenal suppressive effects are not seen with normal prescription. Long-term studies have not shown any adverse histologic effects on the bronchial mucosa (Brogden et al., 1984).

Anticholinergic, Antimuscarinic Bronchodilators

The primary efferent innervation of the lung is parasympathetic, cholinergic, and excitatory, so that there is a predominant vagal tone resulting in bronchoconstriction and increased mucous secretion. Atropine has long been recognized as a potent bronchodilator, but its use has been limited by its side effects. Even with aerosol administration, systemic levels are high, resulting in bladder outlet obstruction, meiosis, and tachycardia. The dangers of inspissation of viscid secretions with chronic anticholinergic therapy may be only a theoretical adverse effect.

The introduction of the quaternary ammonium congeners of atropine, atropine methonitrate, and ipratropium bromide has resulted in the clinical revival of the anticholinergic agents. These drugs are poorly absorbed after aerosol administration and thus have few systemic effects. They are very potent bronchodilators that act to remove tonic stimulation and interact synergistically with currently available agents. The most particular specific indication for these drugs is in the treatment of bronchospasm induced by beta-blockade (Gross et al., 1984). High-dose ipratropium bromide (8 to 12 puffs every 2 hours) is frequently used in patients with severe airway obstruction who are being mechanically ventilated.

Theophylline

Theophylline is a member of the xanthine family. Its mechanism of action is unclear at this time, but it is known to inhibit phosphodiesterase and to specifically antagonize adenosine. Although formerly the most popular initial therapeutic agent for airway obstruction, theophylline has now become less frequently used and has assumed an adjunctive role (Newhouse, 1990). The specific effects of theophylline preparations are:

1. Bronchodilatation.
2. Increase in respiratory drive.
3. Inhibition of mast cell mediator release.
4. Increase in mucociliary clearance.
5. Pulmonary arterial vasodilatation.
6. Increase in contractility and reduction in fatigability of the diaphragm (Aubier et al., 1981).

Bronchodilatation is dose-related over a relatively narrow therapeutic range (10 to 20 μg/ml). The maintenance of appropriate serum theophylline levels has been made possible by the development of a clinically available radioimmunoassay. Adverse gastrointestinal effects can be seen with levels greater than 15 μg/ml. Cardiac effects are also seen at higher levels, but no studies have demonstrated adverse effects in the therapeutic range.

Intravenous loading with 5.6 mg/kg is indicated in acute bronchospasm, followed by a continuous infusion at a rate dependent on age, smoking habits, and other medical conditions. Conversion to an oral preparation should be accomplished within 48 hours. Serum levels should be monitored throughout the initial period of use. The possibility that concomitant bronchodilatation and pulmonary arterial dilatation may be distributed in such a way as to worsen ventilation-perfusion matching, and thus lead to hypoxemia, should always be considered (Bukowskyj et al., 1984; Cummiskey et al., 1984).

Perioperative Management

Intraoperative measures to diminish splinting and therefore permit deeper breathing and improved ability to cough productively have been recognized to improve the patient's postoperative course. Thoracic neurectomy has been shown to significantly reduce postoperative pulmonary dysfunction as measured by FEV_1 (Smith et al., 1960). More practically, an intrathoracic intercostal nerve block has been shown to be equally effective in improving postoperative FEV_1 and FVC (Toledo-Pereyra et al., 1979; Deneuville et al., 1993; Richardson et al., 1993) and to permit a reduction in the overall narcotic requirement postoperatively. Continuous (El-Baz et al., 1986) and intermittent (Shulman et al., 1984; Yeager et al., 1987) epidural infusion of morphine has salutary effects. Selected patients may benefit from administering their own analgesics by an infusion pump.

Generally, if preoperative evaluation has been complete, postoperative management should be a continuation of preoperative therapy. Supplemental oxygen is administered to correct hypoxemia caused by central hypoventilation in the immediate postoperative period. Oxygen therapy is discontinued when it is no longer required, as documented by arterial blood gas determinations. The patient is placed in position with the head slightly elevated, if possible, and the position in bed is changed at frequent intervals. Inspiratory exercises, with the encouragement of deep breathing, are the most effective means of minimizing airway closure (Bartlett et al., 1973). Narcotics are administered to minimize postoperative pain and to allow effective coughing. When the cough is ineffective, endotracheal suctioning may be necessary.

Early ambulation has proved to be an effective means to prevent postoperative pulmonary complications. An upright sitting position and ambulation increase the FRC, lead to improvement in all pulmonary volumes, and counteract the changes induced by operation (Craig, 1981). The risk of a pulmonary embolism is also reduced.

SUMMARY

The role of the pulmonary function laboratory is to quantify the severity of derangement in pulmonary function. The physician must decide on the basis of the clinical manifestations what functional evaluations are pertinent in the management of the patient. The initial measurement of the blood gases with an arterial sample is most useful. The evaluations of pulmonary volumes and the VC are important and are measured easily if the patient is able to cooperate. Their use is limited in the very ill patient and is not feasible generally in children under 5 years of age. The use of the dynamic pulmonary volumes such as the timed VC, FEV_1, and MBC provides an index of obstructive airway disease. Other tests that may be important in the diagnosis of the patient's pulmonary disease are tests to determine the diffusion capacity, distribution of ventilation, FRC, compliance, and airway resistance. These tests require more elaborate instrumentation and experience and for practical purposes should be considered research and teaching approaches. Exercise testing, ventilation and perfusion lung scanning, angiography, and cardiac catheterization may contribute important information about the malfunction of the pulmonary system, and bronchoscopy and bronchography may help to localize abnormalities of the airways.

After years and thousands of spirometric studies, there is apparently no spirometric number, percentage, or category that absolutely separates patients who need operation from patients who should not have surgical therapy. The preoperative pulmonary function evaluation provides an estimation of the risk and guidelines but does not provide absolutes. In dealing with the risk of mortality, the physician should remember that although statistics apply to groups, they may not apply to an individual patient.

SELECTED BIBLIOGRAPHY

Avery, M. E., Fletcher, B. D., and Williams, R.: The Lung and Its Disorders in the Newborn Infant. 4th ed. Philadelphia, W. B. Saunders, 1981.

This volume is essential for any physician involved with the problem of respiratory insufficiency in infants and children. This work forms a solid background from which one can evaluate the constantly evolving methods for management of respiratory problems in newborns and infants.

Bates, D. V., Macklem, P. T., and Christie, R. V.: Respiratory Function in Disease. 2nd ed. Philadelphia, W. B. Saunders, 1971.

This outstanding text correlates respiratory physiology and pulmonary disease. It reviews the basic pulmonary function studies and discusses individual disease processes that alter pulmonary function and the types of alteration that may be encountered. It contains the most complete and current bibliography on this subject.

Churchill, E. D., Sweet, R. H., Soutter, L., and Scannell, J. G.: The surgical management of carcinoma of the lung. J. Thorac. Surg., 20:349, 1950.

A classic article that reviews the Massachusetts General Hospital experience in thoracic surgery from 1930 to 1950 in patients with clinical diagnosis of carcinoma of the lung. The authors show essentially equivalent 5-year survival for lobectomy and pneumonectomy at a time when pneumonectomy was the standard operation. This paper, and the discussion that follows it from its presentation at the 30th Annual Meeting of the American Association for Thoracic Surgery, contains many arguments that continue to be used in seeking more limited, yet still successful, pulmonary resection for carcinoma of the lung in high-risk patients. The article is required reading for any thoracic surgeon.

Comroe, J. H., Jr.: Physiology of Respiration. 2nd ed. Chicago, Year Book Medical, 1974.

This introductory monograph apprises the reader of what is known about respiratory physiology. Dr. Comroe states that this book "is intended for students of medicine—whether in medical school, residency training, or in the practice of medicine." This book is essential for a student of respiration.

Comroe, J. H., Jr., Forster, R. E., II, DuBois, A. B., et al.: The Lung. Chicago, Year Book Medical, 1962.

This classic text is written for physicians and medical students rather than for pulmonary physiologists and it explains in simple language with explicit diagrams those aspects of pulmonary physiology that are important to clinical medicine. The monograph also presents the rationale for treatment of acute and chronic respiratory pulmonary disorders.

Miller, J. I., Jr.: Physiologic evaluation of pulmonary function in the candidate for lung resection. J. Thorac. Cardiovasc. Surg., 105:347, 1993.

This is the most recent update of the surgical results in 2340 patients undergoing thoracotomy or pulmonary resection under the supervision of one staff surgeon. This report relates operative mortality and morbidity to detailed pulmonary function testing and is a useful reference for predicted mortality rates based on these studies. It is important to note that operation was denied to less than 1% of the patients considered for surgical resection.

Tisi, G. M.: Pulmonary Physiology in Clinical Medicine. Baltimore, Williams & Wilkins, 1980.

This current monograph is well illustrated and offers an excellent clinical approach to the physiologic interpretation of pulmonary function. It specifically covers clinical situations commonly encountered in practice in both medical and surgical disciplines.

BIBLIOGRAPHY

Ashbaugh, D. G., and Petty, T. C.: Positive end-expiratory pressure: Physiology, indications, and contraindications. J. Thorac. Cardiovasc. Surg., 65:165, 1973.

Aubier, M., DeTeroyer, A., Sampson, M., et al.: Aminophylline improves diaphragmatic contractility. N. Engl. J. Med., 305:249, 1981.

Avery, M. E., Fletcher, B. D., and Williams, R.: The Lung and Its Disorders in the Newborn Infant. 4th ed. Philadelphia, W. B. Saunders, 1981.

Ayres, S. M., and Grace, W. J.: Inappropriate ventilation and hypoxemia as causes of cardiac arrhythmias: The control of arrhythmias without antiarrhythmic drugs. Am. J. Med., 46:495, 1969.

Ayres, S. M., Kozam, R. L., and Lukas, D. S.: The effects of intermittent positive-pressure breathing on intrathoracic pressure, pulmonary mechanics, and the work of breathing. Am. Rev. Respir. Dis., 87:370, 1963.

Ball, W. C., Jr., Stewart, P. B., Newsham, L. G. S., and Bates, D. V.: Regional pulmonary function studies with xenon 133. J. Clin. Invest., 41:519, 1962.

Bartlett, R. H., Gazzaniga, A. B., and Geraghty, T.: Respiratory maneuvers to prevent postoperative pulmonary complications: A critical review. J. A. M. A., 224:1017, 1973.

Bates D. V., Macklem, P. T., and Christie, R. V.: Respiratory Function in Disease. 2nd ed. Philadelphia, W. B. Saunders, 1971.

Bechard, D., and Weststein, L.: Assessment of exercise oxygen consumption as preoperative criterion for lung resection. Ann. Thorac. Surg., 44:344, 1987.

Bedell, G. N., Marshall, R., DuBois, A. B., and Comroe, J. H., Jr.: Plethysmographic determination of the volume of gas trapped in the lungs. J. Clin. Invest., 35:664, 1956.

Bendixen, H. H., Egbert, L. D., Hedley-Whyte, J., et al.: Respiratory Care. St. Louis, C. V. Mosby, 1965.

Brogden, R. N., Heel, R. C., Speight, T. M., and Avery, G. S.: Beclomethasone dipropionate: A reappraisal of its pharmacodynamic properties and therapeutic efficacy after a decade of use in asthma and rhinitis. Drugs, 28:99, 1984.

Bukowskyj, M., Nakatsu, K., and Munt, P. W.: Theophylline reassessed. Ann. Intern. Med., 101:63, 1984.

Burrows, B., and Earle, R. H.: Course and prognosis of chronic obstructive lung disease. N. Engl. J. Med., 280:397, 1969.

Burrows, B., Knudson, R. J., and Kettel, L. J.: Respiratory Insufficiency. Chicago, Year Book Medical, 1975.

Churchill, E. D., Sweet, R. H., Soutter, L., et al.: The surgical management of carcinoma of the lung. J. Thorac. Surg., 20:349, 1950.

Clark, L. C., Jr.: Monitor and control of blood and tissue oxygen tensions. Trans. Am. Soc. Artif. Intern. Organs, 2:41, 1956.

Colman, N. C., Schraufnagel, D. E., Rivington, R. N., and Pardy, R. L.: Exercise testing in evaluation of patients for lung resection. Am. Rev. Respir. Dis., 125:604, 1982.

Comroe, J. H., Jr.: Physiology of Respiration. 2nd ed. Chicago, Year Book Medical, 1974.

Comroe, J. H., Jr., Forster, R. E., II, DuBois, A. B., et al.: The Lung: Clinical Physiology and Pulmonary Function Tests. 2nd ed. Chicago, Year Book Medical, 1962.

Comroe, J. H., Jr., and Nadel, J. A.: Current concepts: Screening tests of pulmonary function. N. Engl. J. Med., 282:1249, 1970.

Cotes, J. E.: Lung Function. Philadelphia, F. A. Davis, 1968.

Craig, D. B.: Postoperative recovery of pulmonary function. Anesth. Analg., 60:46, 1981.

Cummiskey, J. M., and Popa, V.: Theophyllines—A review. J. Asthma, 21:243, 1984.

Deneuville, M., Bisserier, A., Regnard, J. F., et al.: Continuous intercostal analgesia with 0.5% bupivacaine after thoracotomy: A randomized study. Ann. Thorac. Surg., 55:381, 1993.

DuBois, A. B., Botelho, S. Y., and Comroe, J. H., Jr.: A new method for measuring airway resistance in man using a body plethysmograph: Values in normal subjects and in patients with respiratory disease. J. Clin. Invest., 35:327, 1956.

El-Baz, N., and Ivankovich, A. D.: Management of postoperative thoracotomy pain: continuous epidural infusion of morphine. In Kittle, C. F. (ed): Current Controversies in Thoracic Surgery. Philadelphia, W. B. Saunders, 1986.

Eugene, J., Brown, S. E., Light, R. W., et al.: Maximum oxygen consumption: A physiologic guide to pulmonary resection. Surg. Forum, 33:260, 1980.

Federation of American Societies for Experimental Biology: Standardization of definitions and symbols in respiratory physiology. Fed. Proc., 9:602, 1950.

Fee, H. J., Holmes, E. C., Gewirtz, H. S., et al.: Role of pulmonary vascular resistance measurements in preoperative evaluation of candidates for pulmonary resection. J. Thorac. Cardiovasc. Surg., 75:519, 1978.

Filley, G. F.: Acid-Base and Blood Gas Regulation. Philadelphia, Lea & Febiger, 1971.

Flemma, R. J., and Young, W. G., Jr.: The metabolic effects of mechanical ventilation and respiratory alkalosis in postoperative patients. Surgery, 56:36, 1964.

Gregory, G. A., Kitterman, J. A., Phibbs, R. H., et al.: Treatment of the idopathic respiratory-distress syndrome with continuous positive airway pressure. N. Engl. J. Med., 284:1333, 1971.

Gross, N. J. and Skorodin, M. S.: Anticholinergic, antimuscarinic bronchodilators. Am. Rev. Respir. Dis., 129:856, 1984.

Hills, A. G.: Acid-Base Balance: Chemistry, Physiology, Patho-physiology. Baltimore, Williams & Wilkins, 1973.

Hogg, J. C., Macklem, P. T., and Thurlbeck, W. M.: Site and nature of airway obstruction in chronic obstructive pulmonary disease. N. Engl. J. Med., 278:1355, 1968.

Hudson, L. D., Kurt, T. L., Petty, T. L., and Genton, E.: Arrhythmias associated with acute respiratory failure in patients with chronic airway obstruction. Chest, 63:661, 1973.

Hyatt, R. E., and Rodarte, J. R.: Closing volume: One man's noise—Other men's experiment. Mayo Clin. Proc., 50:17, 1975.

Keagy, B. A., Schorlemmer, G. R., Murray, G. F., et al.: Correlation of preoperative pulmonary function testing with clinical course in patients after pneumonectomy. Ann. Thorac. Surg., 36:253, 1983.

Kristersson, S., Lindell, S., and Svanberg, L.: Prediction of pulmonary function loss due to pneumonectomy using ^{133}Xe-radiospirometry. Chest, 62:694, 1972.

Latimer, R. G., Dickman, M., Day, W. C., et al.: Ventilatory patterns and pulmonary complications after upper abdominal surgery determined by preoperative and postoperative computerized spirometry and blood gas analysis. Am. J. Surg., 122:622, 1971.

Lockwood, P.: Lung function test results and the risk of postthoracotomy complications. Respiration, 30:529, 1973.

Lumb, P. D.: Perioperative pulmonary physiology. In Sabiston, D. C., Jr., and Spencer, F. C. (eds): Gibbon's Surgery of the Chest. 4th ed. Philadelphia, W. B. Saunders, 1983.

Markos, J., Mullan, B. P., Hillman, D. R., et al.: Preoperative assess-

ment as a predictor of mortality and morbidity after lung resection. Am. Rev. Respir. Dis., 139:902, 1989.

Martini, N., McCaughan, B. C., McCormack, P. M., and Bains, M. S.: The extent of resection for localized lung cancer: Lobectomy. In Kittle, C. F. (ed): Current Controversies in Thoracic Surgery. Philadelphia, W. B. Saunders, 1986, pp. 171–175.

Mead, J., and Whittenberger, J. L.: Physical properties of human lungs measured during spontaneous respiration. J. Appl. Physiol., 5:779, 1953.

Meyers, J. R., Lembeck, L., O'Kane, H., and Baue, A. E.: Changes in functional residual capacity of the lung after operation. Arch. Surg., 110:576, 1975.

Miller, J. I., Grossman, G. D., and Hatcher, C. R.: Pulmonary function test criteria for operability and pulmonary resection. Surg. Gynecol. Obstet., 153:893, 1981.

Miller, J. I., and Hatcher, C. R., Jr.: Limited resection of bronchogenic carcinoma in the patient with marked impairment of pulmonary function. Ann. Thorac. Surg., 44:340, 1987.

Mittman, C.: Assessment of operative risk in thoracic surgery. 1960. Am. Rev. Respir. Dis., 84:197, 1961.

Miyoshi, S., Nakahara, K., Ohno, K., et al.: Exercise tolerance test in lung cancer patients: The relationship between exercise capacity and postthoracotomy hospital mortality. Ann. Thorac. Surg., 44:487, 1987.

Morris, J. F., Koski, A., and Johnson, L. C.: Spirometric standards for nonsmoking healthy adults. Am. Rev. Respir. Dis., 103:57, 1971.

Nakahara, K., Monden, Y., Ohno, K., et al.: A method for predicting postoperative lung function and its relation to postoperative complications in patients with lung cancer. Ann. Thorac. Surg., 39:260, 1985.

Newhouse, M. T.: Is theophylline obsolete? Chest, 96:1, 1990.

Nunn, J. F., Campbell, E. J. M., and Peckette, B. W.: Anatomical subdivisions of the volume of respiratory dead space and effect of position of the jaw. J. Appl. Physiol., 14:174, 1959.

Olsen, G. N., and Block, A. J.: Pulmonary function testing in evaluation for pneumonectomy. Hosp. Prac., September 1973, pp. 137–144.

Olsen, G. N., Block, A. J., Swenson, E. W., et al.: Pulmonary function evaluation of the lung resection candidate: A prospective study. Am. Rev. Respir. Dis., 111:379, 1975.

Osborn, J. J., Raison, J. C. A., Beaumont, J. O., et al.: Respiratory causes of "sudden unexplained arrhythmia" in postthoracotomy patients. Surgery, 69:24, 1971.

Pesenti, A., Pelosi, P., Rossi, N., et al.: Respiratory mechanics and bronchodilator responsiveness in patients with the adult respiratory distress syndrome. Crit. Care Med., 21:78, 1993.

Peters, R. M.: Pulmonary reserve in patients after pneumonectomy. Ann. Thorac. Surg., 36:245, 1983.

Peters, R. M.: How big and when? Ann. Thorac. Surg., 44:338, 1987.

Petty, T. L., and Neff, T. A.: Renal function in respiratory failure. J. A. M. A., 217:82, 1971.

Rahn, H., and Farhi, L. E.: Ventilation, perfusion, and gas exchange—The VAQ Concept. In American Physiological Society: Handbook of Physiology. Washington, D. C., American Physiological Society, 1964, pp. 735–766.

Rao, B. S., Cohn, K. E., Eldridge, F. L., and Hancock, E. W.: Left ventricular failure secondary to chronic pulmonary disease. Am. J. Med., 45:229, 1968.

Richardson, J., Sabanathan, S., Eng, J., et al.: Continuous intercostal nerve block versus epidural morphine for postthoracotomy analgesia. Ann. Thorac. Surg., 55:377, 1993.

Reichel, J.: Assessment of operative risk of pneumonectomy. Chest, 62:570, 1972.

Severinghaus, J. W., and Bradley, A. F.: Electrodes for blood Po_2 and Pco_2 determination. J. Appl. Physiol., 13:147, 1958.

Severinghaus, J. W., and Stupfel, M.: Alveolar dead space as an index of distribution of blood flow in pulmonary capillaries. J. Appl. Physiol., 10:335, 1957.

Shim, C.: Adrenergic agonists and bronchodilator aerosol therapy in asthma. Clin. Chest Med., 5:659, 1984.

Shulman, M., Sandler, A. N., Bradley, J. W., et al.: Postthoracotomy pain and pulmonary function following epidural and systemic morphine. Anesthesiology, 61:569, 1984.

Smith, T. C., Cook, F. D., DeKornfeld, T. J., and Siebecker, K. L.:

Pulmonary function in the immediate postoperative period. J. Thorac. Cardiovasc. Surg., *39*:788, 1960.

Smith, T. P., Kinasewitz, G. T., Tucker, W. Y., et al.: Exercise capacity as a predictor of post-thoracotomy morbidity. Am. Rev. Respir. Dis., *129*:730, 1984.

Stein, M., Koota, G. M., Simon, M., and Frank, H. A.: Pulmonary evaluation of surgical patients. J. A. M. A., *181*:765, 1962.

Tisi, G. M.: Preoperative evaluation of pulmonary function: Validity, indications, and benefits. Am. Rev. Respir. Dis., *119*:293, 1979.

Tisi, G. M.: Pulmonary Physiology in Clinical Medicine. 2nd ed. Baltimore, Williams & Wilkins, 1983.

Toledo-Pereyra, L. H., and DeMeester, T. R.: Prospective randomized evaluation of intrathoracic intercostal nerve block with bupivacaine on postoperative ventilatory function. Ann. Thorac. Surg., *27*:203, 1979.

Tucker, D. H., and Sieker, H. O.: The effect of change in body position on lung volumes and intrapulmonary gas mixing in patients with obesity, heart failure and emphysema. Am. Rev. Respir. Dis., *83*:787, 1960.

Wagner, H. N., Jr., Sabiston, D. C., Jr., McAfee, J. G., et al.: Diagnosis of massive pulmonary embolism in man by radio-isotope scanning. N. Engl. J. Med., *271*:377, 1964.

Wasserman, K: Determinants and detection of anaerobic threshold and consequences of exercise above it. Circulation, *76VI*:29, 1987.

West, J. B.: Ventilation/Blood Flow and Gas Exchange. Oxford, Blackwell Scientific, 1965.

Whipp, B. J.: Dynamics of pulmonary gas exchange. Circulation, *76VI*:18, 1987.

Woodbury, D. M.: Physiology of body fluids. *In* Ruch, T. C., and Patton, H. D. (eds): Physiology and Biophysics. 20th ed. Philadelphia, W. B. Saunders, 1973.

Yeager, M. P., Glass, D. D., Neff, R. K., and Brinck-Johnsen, T.: Epidural anesthesia and analgesia in high-risk surgical patients. Anesthesiology, *66*:729, 1987.

2

Perioperative Pulmonary Physiology

Philip D. Lumb

No longer is the operation the primary intervention with recovery assumed to be the responsibility of a "higher" authority. Rather, meticulous attention to all aspects of the patient's illness enables the practitioner to modify and control its outcome.

Norman Chevers
Guy's Hospital Report, 1842

Too frequently, the respiratory function is first noticed when a patient fails to breathe adequately following anesthesia and surgery. The incidence of postoperative respiratory complications is difficult to ascertain, with estimates ranging from almost nonexistent to as much as 40 to 75% of postsurgical morbidity. Despite this extreme difference of opinion, it is undoubted that pulmonary problems account for a substantial proportion of increased hospital costs and either unnecessary or inappropriate use of expensive support modalities (Conference on the Scientific Basis of In-Hospital Respiratory Therapy, 1974, 1979). In a critical review of 153 postoperative deaths, Chevers (1842) reported that 86 were caused by pneumonia, pleurisy, or other respiratory complications, for an incidence of 53%. Since this review, respiratory complications have ranked with hemorrhage and wound infection as the important triad of threats in the postoperative period. Therefore, not only is a thorough knowledge of ventilatory support necessary but also an understanding of pulmonary pathophysiology is required, which enables the clinician to predict which patients are likely to require postoperative respiratory care. This chapter discusses the development of respiratory physiology and ventilatory support and attempts to draw useful clinical correlations between scientific principles and patient care.

HISTORICAL REVIEW

The history of airway management is long, with the use of expired air and positive-pressure ventilation predominating in attempts to revive the apparently dead. Elijah is reported in the Bible to have "restored the son of the Shunammite woman to life, putting his mouth to his mouth" (Book 2 of Kings, Chapter IV). This is probably the first reference to positive-pressure ventilation, and this technique is still in first-line use for emergency airway management (CPR Guidelines, 1992). Tracheostomy was performed in the 12th and

13th centuries in the treatment of the drowned, and Paracelsus (1493–1541) introduced the use of a bellows to ventilate the lungs (Lee and Atkinson, 1973). In 1543, Vesalius passed a reed into the "rough artery" or trachea, and between 1760 and 1780 the physiologic roles of oxygen and carbon dioxide were elucidated. By 1796, a technical manual that incorporated all available techniques for the resuscitation of drowned persons had been published (Herholdt and Rafn, 1796), but widespread use of positive-pressure ventilation would not develop for another 150 years, when methods of intubation became well established.

Mechanics

The physiologic basis of respiratory support is over 300 years old and probably begins with clockmaker Robert Hooke's "The Theory of Springs" (Hooke, 1678), which provided the scientific background for subsequent studies of static compliance characteristics of the lungs and the distribution of gas within the thoracic cavity. Pulmonary dynamics were not appreciated until the period between 1923 and 1956, during which rapid progress was made. In 1933, Hermanssen first proposed the maximal voluntary ventilation test, and this, together with the earlier work of Hutchinson (1846), established the predictive role of pulmonary function tests.

Clinical respiratory physiology required the ability to match the theoretical advances in mechanical function of the lungs with knowledge of the effectiveness of air-blood exchange. Humans are, after all, aerobic creatures at the level of individual cellular metabolism, and no study of respiration is possible "without simultaneous analysis of both ventilation and blood flow" (Laver et al., 1981). The studies of Riley and Cournand (1949, 1951) and Rahn and Fenn (1955) and more recent investigations with radioactive gases (West and Jones, 1965; West, 1977; Laver et al., 1981) have led to the understanding of the relationships between ventilation and perfusion on which effective exchange and transport of oxygen depend. It is interesting to note that an apparent decrease in physiologic experimentation coincided with an increase in availability of ventilatory support modes that followed the Copenhagen poliomyelitis epidemic in 1952 and that heralded the modern development of intermittent positive-pressure ventilation and pulmonary management techniques.

Development of mechanical ventilation parallels the previously described review, and Vesalius can be credited with the first application of *intermittent positive-pressure ventilation* (IPPV) for thoracotomy in his description of an animal experiment in which the rhythmic inflation of the lungs was accomplished with bellows while the chest was open. Because of difficulty in connecting the trachea to dependable devices for inflating the lungs, interest in positive-pressure ventilation declined, and methods of ventilation that incorporated either passive positional changes or body-encircling negative-pressure devices were popular until the mid-1900s. Poliomyelitis epidemics in Los Angeles in 1948 and 1949 and in Copenhagen in 1952 (Grenvik et al., 1980) not only showed the cumbersome nature of negative-pressure devices but also proved that mortality could be decreased by application of intermittent positive-pressure devices. "Before 1955, negative pressure ventilation with a tank ventilator was associated with a 50 percent mortality in 48 patients, while 24 patients treated in 1960 using IPPV sustained a mortality of only 17 percent" (Grenvik et al., 1980).

In 1967, Ashbaugh and associates reported the use of positive end-expiratory pressure during exhalation in the treatment of respiratory failure; this marks the advent of the current varieties of ventilatory support devices that combine forms of positive-pressure lung insufflation with various means of providing end-expiratory pressure. Discussion of these techniques becomes clearer after one understands the mechanisms and requirements of pulmonary ventilation and perfusion.

Table 2–1 reviews the historical development of the physiologic and mechanical components of mechanical ventilation discussed in this section.

Webster (1975) defines respiration as

1: (a) The placing of air or dissolved gases in intimate contact with the circulating medium of a multicellular organism (as by breathing); (b) a single complete act of breathing. 2: The physical and chemical processes by which an organism supplies its cells and tissues with the oxygen needed for metabolism and relieves them of the carbon dioxide formed in energy-producing reactions. 3: Any of the various energy-yielding oxidative reactions in living matter.

Implicit in this set of statements is the knowledge that oxygen and carbon dioxide exchange at the alveolar-capillary junction must match the metabolic requirements of the organism. To perform this function, the distribution of blood flow within the lungs must match as closely as possible the tidal flow of gas into and out of the lung. The next sections deal with the matching of ventilation and perfusion, the distribution of gas and blood within the lungs, and the mechanics of gas movement.

DISTRIBUTION OF VENTILATION

Ultimately, distribution of ventilation depends on the shape of the structure into which gas is expected to flow. At thoracotomy, the exposed lung collapses to a small, airless mass unless kept inflated by the use of positive-pressure ventilation. Obviously, the relationship between the intact thorax and the lung parenchyma is essential in preserving the spatial relationships in which gas exchange occurs. Physiology classes concentrate too often on the smoked drum kymographic tracings produced by ventilation in a closed-system spirometer rather than on the reality of the underlying changes in pulmonary volume that support blood-gas exchange. The information that is generated by such devices and incorporated into more sophisticated pulmonary function apparatus unfortunately becomes divorced from the practicality of gas exchange. The pulmonary volumes that are

■ **Table 2–1.** HISTORICAL DEVELOPMENT OF MECHANICAL VENTILATION: PHYSIOLOGY AND EQUIPMENT

Physiology	Mechanical
Elijah—first practical application	
	1493–1541 Paracelsus; Bellows to inflate lungs
	1543 Vesalius: "Intubation"
1678 Hooke: The Theory of Springs	
1679 Borelli: Tidal volume	
1760–1780 Physiology of O_2 and CO_2 elucidated	
	1796 Life saving measures for drowning persons Negative-pressure devices
1843 Chevers: Postoperative pulmonary complications	
	1864 Jones: Described "iron lung"
	1876 Willey (Paris, France): Spirosphere—first working iron lung
1887 Orth: Distribution of blood flow in the lungs	*1904* Sauerbruch: Differential pressure ventilation
1910 Pasteur: Active lobar collapse	*1931* Emerson: The modern iron lung
	1938 Cranford: IPPV anesthesia
1949 Fowler: Single-breath nitrogen washout—closing volume determination	*1950s* Negative-pressure devices for long-term support
1941–1951 Riley and Cournand	*1960s* IPPV
1955 Rahn and Fenn — Distribution of ventilation and perfusion	*1967* Ashbaugh: PEEP
1965 West and Jones	*1972* Kirby: IMV
1970 West	*1975* Suter: "Best" PEEP
	1977 Sjostrand: High-frequency positive-pressure ventilation

produced remain as two-dimensional tracings rather than as actual volumes with clinical importance (Fig. 2–1).

A much simplified model of the lung, shown in Figure 2–2, demonstrates lung volumes and gas flows. Although it is an incomplete diagram and much individual variation exists in the quoted volumes, the concepts presented are useful in that initial assessments can be made about the ventilatory function of the lungs. In the awake individual, normal oxygen uptake and carbon dioxide elimination are maintained at a precise, metabolically determined respiratory exchange ratio by balancing the ventilation of all the air spaces with perfusion of those particular alveoli that are in intimate contact with circulating blood. This implies that a certain portion of ventilation and circulation is wasted, because conducting airways are not well perfused and some lung areas remain perfused without receiving the benefits of fresh gas flow. Commonly described deviations from the normal distribution are shown in Figure 2–3. The lung is represented as a two-alveoli system with appropriate blood supply to each unit. Deviations of oxygen and carbon dioxide homeostasis are demonstrated by changing the relative proportions of ventilation and perfusion at each unit.

The most common situations are as follows:

1. *Normal:* (a) well-matched ventilation and perfusion; (b) O_2 delivery approximately 250 ml/min; (c)

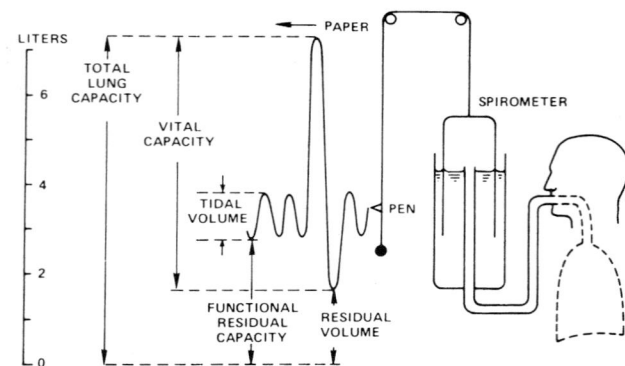

FIGURE 2–1. Pulmonary volumes determined by spirometry. Residual volume and functional residual capacity cannot be measured with the spirometer and require either washout or plethysmographic techniques for measurement. Exhalation is represented as a downward deflection on the chart. Normal values for such tests are

Tidal volume (VT): 500 ml = normal inhalation and exhalation

Vital capacity (VC): 6000 ml = maximal exhalation after maximal inhalation

Inspiratory reserve volume (IRV): 5000 ml = maximal inhalation from normal expiratory level

Residual volume (RV): 1600 ml = gas that remains in lung at end of maximal expiratory effort

Functional residual capacity (FRC): 2800 ml = gas in lungs after a normal expiration

Aging erodes the volume buffer between RV and FRC as small airways "close." Postoperative atelectasis also causes encroachment of RV on FRC, and it may lead to postoperative hypoxia secondary to increased intrapulmonary shunt. (From West, J. B.: Respiratory Physiology. 2nd ed. Copyright © 1979 by The Williams & Wilkins Company, Baltimore. Reproduced by permission.)

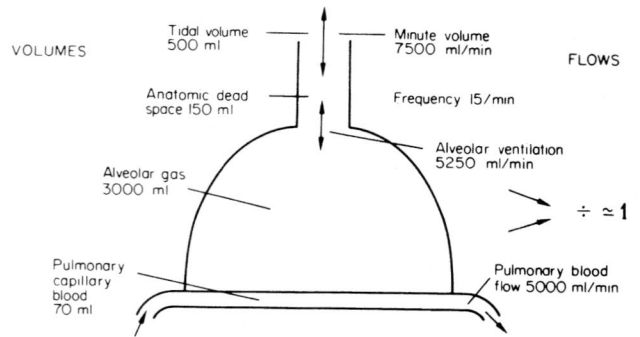

FIGURE 2–2. Simplified diagram of the lung and pulmonary circulation that shows typical gas volumes and blood flows in a resting subject. There is much individual variation around these values, and these numbers are intended only to approximate the normal situation. A simple rule aids in calculating dead space and alveolar and tidal ventilatory volume:

Body weight in lb × 1 = anatomic dead space
× 2 = alveolar ventilation/breath
× 3 = tidal volume

Therefore, if normal respiratory rate = 16 breaths per minute and the individual weighs 150 lb:

Alveolar ventilation = 16 × 300 = 4.8 l/min
Minute ventilation = 16 × 450 = 5.2 l/min

(From West, J. B.: Ventilation-Blood Flow and Gas Exchange. 4th ed. Oxford, Blackwell, 1985.)

CO_2 elimination approximately 200 ml/min; and (d) respiratory exchange ratio of 0.8.

2. *Ineffective O_2 exchange:* (a) shunt; (b) continued perfusion of a nonventilated unit; and (c) overperfusion of an underventilated unit may produce atelectasis.

3. *Ineffective CO_2 exchange:* (a) dead space; and (b) nonperfusion of a ventilated alveolus.

As Figure 2–3 shows, all blood-gas abnormalities can be seen as arising from a mismatch in normal ventilation-perfusion ratio. For ease of discussion, lung units are considered as either dead space (infinite ventilation without perfusion) or shunt (zero ventilation with continued perfusion) units.

These ideas can be unified in the following example:

A normal 70-kg man is expected to demonstrate:
1. Dead space (VD) = 150 ml (approximates the patient's weight in pounds)
2. Tidal volume (VT) = 450 ml (the dead space/tidal volume ratio, or VD/VT, is approximately 0.3, with a range of 0.2 to 0.4)
3. Alveolar ventilation ($\dot{V}A$)/breath = 300 ml ($\dot{V}A$ = VT − VD)
4. Respiratory rate (f) = 15 breaths/minute
5. Pa_{CO_2} = 40 torr − normal arterial P_{CO_2}
6. Respiratory exchange ratio = 0.8; i.e.,

$$\frac{\text{Carbon dioxide production (200 ml/min)}}{\text{Oxygen consumption (250 ml/min)}}$$

Therefore, the average man at rest requires a minute ventilation of 6.75 l to maintain oxygen and carbon dioxide homeostasis. Of this total volume, 4.5 l is the alveolar ventilation responsible for gas exchange, and approximately one-third of the minute ventilation

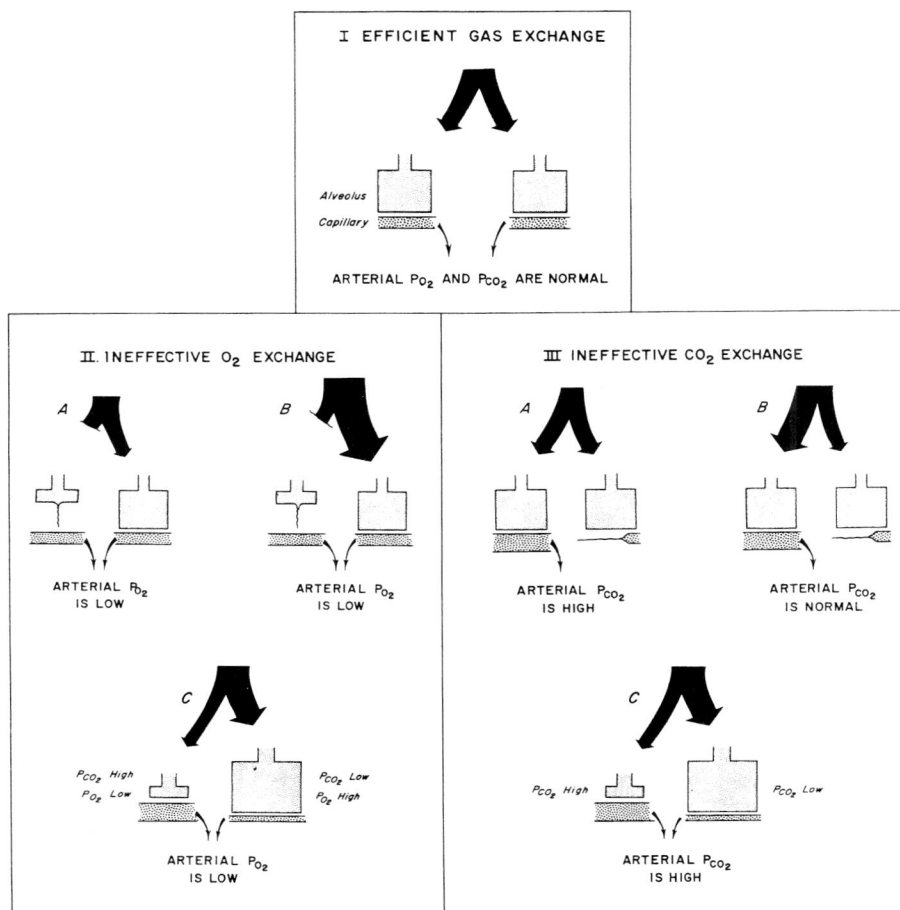

FIGURE 2–3. Variations in ventilation and perfusion that cause disturbances in exchange of oxygen and carbon dioxide. *I,* Adequate and well-matched ventilation and perfusion maintain normal arterial oxygenation and elimination of carbon dioxide. *IIA* and *B,* Collapse of terminal airway leads to arterial hypoxemia even if ventilation to unaffected areas increases. The reduction in P_{O_2} depends on the amount of blood that continues to flow through the collapsed pulmonary segments. Alveolar hypoxia invokes hypoxic pulmonary vasoconstriction, which tends to limit the amount of wasted perfusion or "shunt" blood flow. *C,* Marked maldistribution of ventilation and perfusion can also lead to hypoxia (i.e., if most of the perfusion goes to poorly ventilated areas, inefficient gas exchange results). This condition is seen in later examples as the patient's position or cardiac output is changed. *III,* Continued ventilation of a nonperfused alveolus results in wasted or dead-space ventilation. In addition, hypotension or reduced cardiac output can result in reduced perfusion of ventilated alveoli with similar effects. In the presence of dead-space units, an increase in total minute ventilation can accommodate rising carbon dioxide tension and return P_{CO_2} levels to normal limits. Therefore, it is important to look not only at blood gas results when assessing the respiratory status of a patient but also at the effort required to obtain the measured values. Dead space can obviously be seen to be of two types: (1) Anatomic dead space ($V_{D_{anat}}$)—areas of conducting airways in which no blood-gas exchange occurs; and (2) alveolar dead space ($V_{D_{alv}}$)—areas of lung parenchyma in which blood-gas exchange is expected but is decreased owing, for example, to pulmonary embolism or hypoperfusion. The total contribution of dead space is the sum of (1) and (2) and is called the physiologic dead space ($V_{D_{phys}}$).

will be wasted as dead space. This simple introduction will assume much greater importance in discussing mechanical ventilation of the lung, because all tests of respiratory function must be compared with the patient's predicted normal values. Efficiency of gas exchange and the response of patients to various therapies do not depend on making arterial blood-gas values fall within acceptable ranges, but rather permit comparison of the degrees of assistance required to produce acceptable values.

Modern ideas about ventilatory support have been developed following more complete understanding of the factors controlling distribution of ventilation and perfusion and the mechanism by which the lung matches these two to provide optimal gas exchange (Dolfuss et al., 1967; Milic-Emili et al., 1966; Minh et al., 1974). The lung is influenced by many forces, including the force of gravity, diaphragmatic tone and motion, and the presence of an intact, airtight chest wall. Problems encountered in mechanical ventilation and weaning of infants are in part different from those seen in adults because of compliance differences in the chest wall. Therefore, to appreciate fully the abnormalities in perioperative physiology, the normal situation must be understood first. The interaction of mechanical support superimposed on this normal balance also requires careful attention to normal detail.

In upright humans, lung function can be demonstrated by a model (Fig. 2–4*A*). A child's Slinky toy is

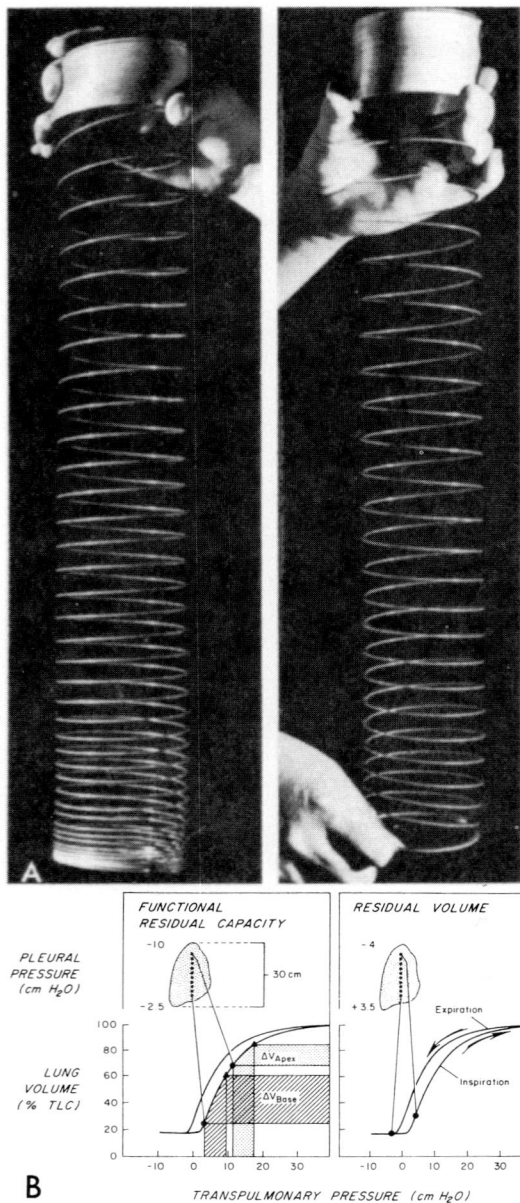

FIGURE 2–4. *A,* A child's Slinky spring held in midair and extended by its own weight represents alveolar size distribution in the lung at end-expiration. Inspiration is mimicked by stretching the spring with traction applied to the dependent end. As the spring is pulled, the lower spring coils (basal lung segments) are expanded more than the already stretched upper coils (apical segments). In the lung, basal alveoli can be shown to expand more during inspiration than the apical areas. Unlike the spring, pulmonary expansion is aided and equalized by pulmonary surfactant, which tends to equalize compliance of all areas of lung, irrespective of their relative size. *B,* Influence of end-expiratory volume on the distribution of gas during inspiration due to changes in pressure-volume relationships. In the *left panel,* pleural pressure becomes less negative from the apex of the lung to the base owing to the reduced influence of gravity and increased tissue volume in the base of the lung. Therefore, airway distending pressure (transpulmonary pressure) is less at the base than at the apex—this is measured at end-expiration with open glottis when atmospheric pressure is equal to alveolar pressure. In *both panels,* pulmonary volume changes are shown by the curves marked inspiration and expiration. The lack of identity between the two curves is called hysteresis and is due to pulmonary surfactant that lines the terminal pulmonary units in health. Inspiratory and expiratory curves are identical if these changes in volume are measured with a saline-filled lung.

If an inspiration is initiated from FRC (*left panel*), the changes in transpulmonary pressure are of equal magnitude in the apex and the base, but the alveolar expansion in the two areas is different because alveoli in these areas are on different portions of the pressure-volume curve. Expansion is greater in the basilar segments of the lung and gas flow during inspiration is preferentially to the bases of the lung. If, however, inspiration is initiated from pulmonary volumes less than FRC, basal alveoli remain collapsed during the early phase of inspiration and open only during the later portion of inspiration. The distribution of gas flow is directed preferentially to the apex of the lung in this situation. This may cause derangements in the relationship of ventilation and perfusion and lead to inequality of gas exchange with the possibility of increased dead space ventilation. (*A,* From Laver, M. B., and Austen, W. G.: Respiratory function: Physiologic considerations applicable to surgery. *In* Sabiston, D. C., Jr [ed]: Davis-Christopher Textbook of Surgery. 12th ed. Philadelphia, W. B. Saunders, 1981; *B,* Redrawn from Bates, D. V., Macklem, P. T., and Christie, R. V.: Respiratory Function in Disease. 2nd ed. Philadelphia, W. B. Saunders, 1971.)

an excellent model; as the Slinky hangs under its own weight, separation of the loops are markedly different at the two ends. Therefore, the areas encompassed by the loops are also different, with greater area at the nondependent portion of the spring. However, if stretch is increased by traction on the lower end of the spring, further separation is maximal in the dependent regions. The differing separation of spring loops determines each loop's specific compliance for a particular position of stretch, and further expansion of the loop depends on the deforming forces and the compliance of the loop. Therefore, a comparator must be chosen, at which point lung inflation characteristics can be determined. The logical and generally accepted lung volume against which increases or reductions are made is the position of the lung at rest following a normal expiration. This volume is called

the *functional residual capacity* (FRC) and is composed of the residual volume and the expiratory reserve volume (see Fig. 2–2).

In the normal lung, a spontaneous breath initiated at FRC alters the volume of basal and apical alveoli according to their respective compliance in a fashion analogous to movement of the spring coils. Therefore, because volume change has been seen to be nonuniform, gas movement also is nonuniform and parallels volume changes. Unlike the spring, the lung also has pleural pressure gradients acting across its surface that change in proportion to the relative height of the segment of lung concerned. This relationship is shown in Figure 2–4B, and it can be seen that the pleural pressure is less negative at the lung base. The source of the pleural pressure gradient is not certain, but there is agreement that in a breath initiated at normal FRC, the inspired volume is distributed preferentially to the lung bases. It is in this location that regional changes in gas volume are the greatest (Macklem, 1978; Minh et al., 1974).

In part, the gradient is caused by the characteristics of the isolated lungs and chest wall superimposed on one another. At FRC, the natural tendency of the thoracic cage is to expand, whereas the unsupported lungs would collapse to an airless mass of tissue. The lack of communication between atmosphere and pleural space causes these two forces to balance one another and helps keep the lungs inflated. This causes the pleural pressure to be subatmospheric. When the glottis is open, pressure throughout the alveoli is atmospheric, but there is still a subatmospheric pleural pressure, which is measured as the arithmetical difference between the pleural or esophageal pressure and the atmospheric pressure. As the lung expands with increasing thoracic volume, the recoil force of the lung increases, as does the transpulmonary pressure—that is, it becomes more negative. Obviously, this pressure is applied to all intrathoracic structures, and it is an important consideration when discussing the distribution of blood flow through the lungs and the effects of various modes of mechanical ventilatory assistance.

A decrease in FRC affects the compliance characteristics of the various lung segments and may change overall gas distribution when a breath is initiated from low lung volume. It is important to visualize the lung as a honeycomb of air spaces of differing sizes. The various lung volumes that are discussed and represented either as two-dimensional graphs or tracer gas distribution diagrams merely represent available areas for blood-gas exchange. If the volumes are reduced, some areas must have been closed and are no longer available. This alters significantly the

distribution of ventilation, which depends on the volume history of the previous exhalation (hysteresis) (Laver et al., 1976), and the compliance of the closed unit, which becomes more difficult to inflate. Each individual lung unit exists on a compliance curve that determines its ability to expand and contract. The actual changes in the alveolar shape during expansion and contraction are not well understood, but recent evidence suggests that alveolar infoldings play a part in the changing alveolar shape (Mazzone et al., 1978, 1980; Mazzone, 1981). The effect of end-expiratory lung volume and the subsequent distribution of gas flow is seen in Figure 2–5. It should be obvious why current concepts of postoperative patient management place such great emphasis on the preservation of the normal FRC, that is, the preservation of the individual's normal lung volume. The importance of this emphasis is coupled with the concept that certain areas of lung collapse if a certain alveolar volume is not maintained.

It has been shown that many of the abnormalities in respiratory function during anesthesia and following operation are due to the closure of small airways in the lung bases. This leads to decreased compliance in these areas, and segments of lung become airless (atelectatic) and difficult to reinflate; this contributes to decreased arterial oxygen saturation, because the blood that continues to perfuse the area is not oxygenated. If an individual exhales to residual volume, nitrogen concentration throughout the lung is relatively uniform, although alveolar size at the bases is smaller than at the apex, because lung volumes at the base are distorted by the weight of the lung. If a slow vital-capacity inspiration of 100% oxygen is taken, the alveoli throughout the lung become more uniformly sized, and the nitrogen concentration at the base has been more diluted than the apical concentration be-

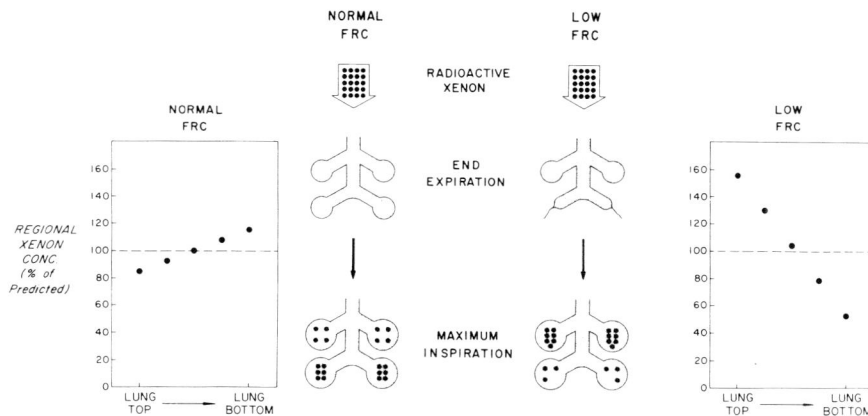

FIGURE 2–5. Effect of end-expiratory pulmonary volume on the distribution of an inspired breath. Radioactive xenon is breathed during inspiration, and the distribution of radioactivity is measured with external chest counters placed over different areas of the lung. An inspiration initiated at normal FRC is preferentially distributed to the bases of the lung. If these areas become closed during expiration (as may happen with increased age) or closed owing to low pulmonary volume (postoperative atelectasis), the nondependent areas receive most of the inspired gas. Because perfusion of the gravity-dependent areas is greater than the perfusion in the apices, a maldistribution of ventilation to perfusion results. Blood continues to flow through areas of poorly ventilated lung, which results in diminished oxygenation of arterial blood. This situation is also shown in Figure 2–3II. (From Pontoppidan, H., Laver, M. B., and Geffin, B.: Acute respiratory failure in the surgical patient. Adv. Surg., 4:163, 1970. Copyright © 1970 by Year Book Medical Publishers, Inc., Chicago. Redrawn from data of Milic-Emili, J., Henderson, J. A. M., Dolovich, M. B., et al.: Regional distribution of inspired gas in the lung. J. Appl. Physiol., 21:749, 1966.)

cause of the increased gas movement at the base. During a subsequent expiration, expired nitrogen content indicates the pattern of lung deflation and the distribution of gas flow. Initially, a short phase in which no nitrogen concentration is detected represents oxygen washout of the upper airways or dead-space zone of the lung. Subsequently, nitrogen concentration rises quickly as alveolar gas washes out and replaces the dead space component. A relatively constant nitrogen concentration is then reached, which represents uniform emptying of the alveoli of all lung segments. This concentration rises slowly for reasons that are not fully understood; perhaps there are some regions of lung that, because of poor ventilation, receive relatively small amounts of the oxygen breathed (West, 1979). Therefore, these regions have relatively high nitrogen concentrations and tend to empty last, which may account for the slow rise in phase 3 of the nitrogen concentration curve. Toward the end of this expiration, nitrogen concentration again rises as small airways in the lung bases close, because the higher apical concentration now preferentially affects the expired nitrogen concentration (Fig. 2–6). The volume of lung at which this change in concentration is measured is called the *closing volume.* The closing volume plus residual volume is known as the *closing capacity* and is expressed as a percentage of total lung capacity on respiratory function test reports.

The importance of this concept of gas distribution and flow relates to the ways in which age and disease affect the distribution of gas in the lung and the volumes at which alveolar closure occurs. Figure

2–7A shows the compliance changes in an exaggerated manner at two different times of life. Owing to an aging-dependent loss of compliance, basal alveoli in the elderly may close before end-expiration or FRC, even though the pleural pressure gradient is similar for the two ages. This phenomenon occurs in the young only if expiration is forcefully continued so that lung volume is decreased below FRC. The effect of aging on closing volume by using a radioactive xenon tracer technique is shown in Figure 2–7B. The higher incidence of postoperative pulmonary complications in the elderly population may be, in part, due to the encroachment of FRC by closing volume. This is represented in Figure 2–8, which shows the narrowing, ultimate elimination, and subsequent reversal of the buffer zone between FRC and airways closure. Other components affected by aging are reduced elastic recoil forces and decreased chest wall compliance.

Another interesting feature in the relationship between closing volume and FRC is the relative independence of the effect of posture on closing volume. FRC changes little with increasing age in the upright individual, but it decreases by approximately 20% in the supine position. Closing volume does not alter substantially with changes in posture; the supine reduction in FRC creates a situation in which closing volume begins to exceed FRC in 44-year-old patients on the operating table. This condition also exists in upright 65-year-olds (Laver et al., 1976).

Therefore, atelectasis in some lung segments is inevitable in situations in which closing volume exceeds FRC, and this is partially responsible for decreased oxygenating ability in the elderly. A question now

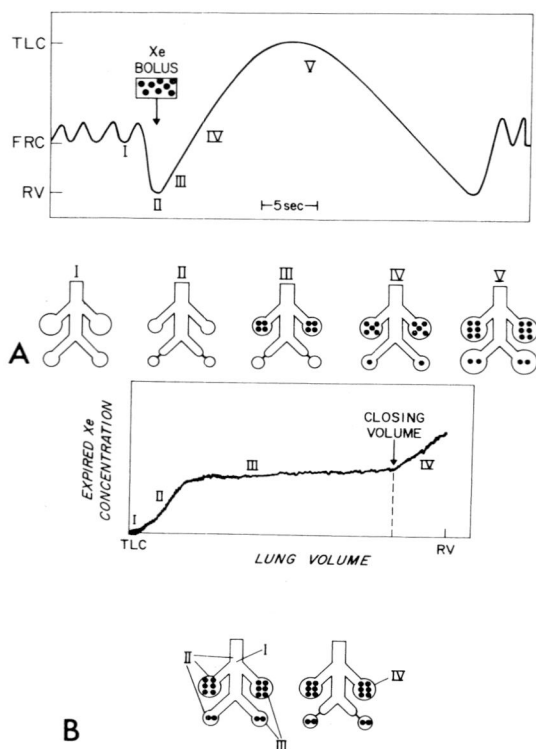

FIGURE 2–6. Patterns of gas distribution during measurement of closing volume—tracer gas technique. The text describes closing volume measurement using the resident gas method. Tracer gas determinations are also used to measure this value. The following example describes this method. *A, Inspiration.* A spirometer record and a four-alveoli lung model are represented. Spontaneous ventilation and gas distribution are represented in I. As an exhalation to residual volume is taken (II), basal alveolar closure occurs. At residual volume, a bolus of xenon tracer gas is injected at the mouthpiece, and a slow inspiration to total lung capacity (TLC) is taken. Initial and final distribution of gas and alveolar size are indicated in III, IV, and V. At TLC, all alveoli are of equal size, but the greater volume (and concentration) of inspired tracer gas is in the nondependent segments. *B, Expiration.* Concentration of helium in the expired gas is plotted against TLC-expired gas volume. During slow exhalation, four distinct zones are shown. Zone 1 (shown as I): No helium is detected. This represents pure dead-space gas. Zone 2: Rapid rise of xenon concentration; non-dead-space gas with differing contributions from all areas of the lung. Zone 3: "Alveolar plateau" represents the mean alveolar concentration of xenon in the alveoli. This portion of the curve rises slowly. This rise is probably due to unequal distribution of ventilation perhaps secondary to different time constants in various alveolar areas. Zone 4: Increase in tracer gas caused by closure of basal alveoli and the relative increase in tracer found in the apical alveoli, which were preferentially ventilated initially. The onset of Zone 4 is determined visually from the graph and is called the *closing volume.* This volume is expressed usually as a proportion of TLC and is called *closing capacity.* Irrespective of the techniques used for measurement, the implication that small airway closure occurs at reduced pulmonary volume emphasizes the importance of maintenance of optimal expansion of the lung at all times, especially postoperatively.

FIGURE 2–7. *A,* Effect of aging on regional compliance and distribution of ventilation. Owing to decreased proportion of elastic tissue in the elderly lung, recoil force and, therefore, transpulmonary pressure will be reduced. Basal alveoli lie on a portion of the pressure-volume curve that is below their closing volume. During early inspiration, transpulmonary pressure does not increase enough to exceed the critical alveolar opening pressure, and alveoli remain closed. Later in inspiration, the alveoli open as transpulmonary pressure increases, and gas distribution in the bases of the lung increases as the pulmonary volume increases. Thus, recruitment of basal alveoli by postoperative pulmonary exercises is a valuable adjunct in the elderly patient because it promotes increased expansion in the already compromised base of the lung. *B,* Effect of age on closing volume. Note that the FRC in both age groups is similar but that residual volume is significantly increased in the elderly. This is due to reduced elastic tissue and diminished recoil force that leads to a continuous state of relative hyperinflation of the lung. At TLC, the distribution of a radioactive tracer gas is similar in both age groups. However, during expiration, no change in gas distribution is detected in the young adult until the pulmonary volume is well below FRC. This distribution is altered in the elderly owing to the earlier closure of small airways, which occurs at pulmonary volumes greater than FRC. In elderly patients, airways at the bases of the lung close during normal tidal ventilation. The implication of this is obvious in the postoperative period when pulmonary volumes are significantly reduced—the elderly patient is at greater risk to develop small airway closure and resultant intrapulmonary shunting. Therefore, vigorous postoperative respiratory care is mandatory for these patients. Too often, inspiration is thought to be the key to good pulmonary function; however, the inability to expire and subsequent increase in residual volume have greater significance in elderly patients (see also Fig. 2–31). (*A,* From Pontoppidan, H., Laver, M. B., and Geffin, B.: Acute respiratory failure in the surgical patient. Adv. Surg., 4:163, 1970. Copyright © 1970 by Year Book Medical Publishers, Inc., Chicago; *B,* Redrawn from Milic-Emili, J., Macklem, P. T., Holland, J., et al.: Regional distribution of pulmonary ventilation and perfusion in elderly subjects. J. Clin. Invest., 47:81, 1968.)

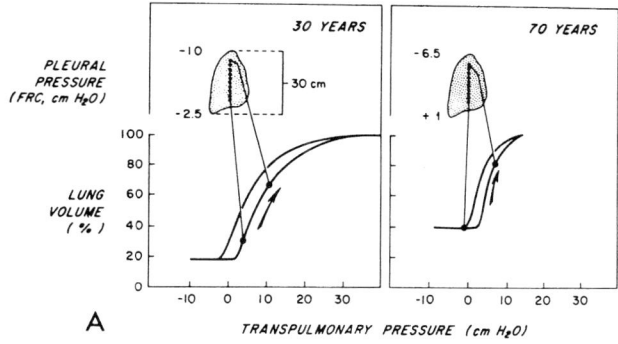

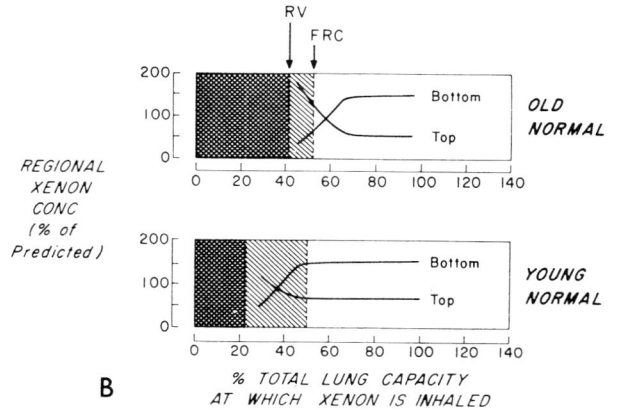

arises as to the fate of the gas volume trapped in closed alveoli. In part, this depends on the subsequent re-expansion of the alveoli, the composition of the gas, and its solubility in blood. It is absorption of the gas that leads to atelectasis in basilar lung segments. As the inspired oxygen concentration is increased, the higher alveolar oxygen tension favors increased solubility in blood and may be responsible for increases in intrapulmonary shunt when this value is measured on 100% inspired oxygen (Rehder et al., 1979): Gas washout from the alveoli exceeds entry, intra-alveolar nitrogen content is reduced, and the alveoli close, producing a shunt unit. It should be recognized that the intra-alveolar nitrogen concentration is an important alveolar stabilizing force. Nitrogen is a poorly diffusible gas and therefore acts to splint alveoli open.

Unfortunately, tests involving FRC and closing volume require patient cooperation and are difficult to perform. Therefore, in the clinical setting, more practical guidelines are required. The important point is that lung volume is a recruitable space that is capable of gas exchange and of being measured. Standard postoperative chest films are beneficial in estimating lung volume, because lung expansion to the eighth rib (counting posteriorly) is compatible with FRC in most situations. Therefore, lung expansion and recruitment can be estimated from serial radiographs. Changes in the appearance of lung expansion in acute

respiratory failure parallel increasing ventilatory support, usually with increasing levels of *positive end-expiratory pressure* (PEEP). All chest radiographs, including those taken with the patient receiving mechanical ventilatory assistance, are exposed at end-inspiration. This provides an optimal view of pulmonary expansion and, if compromised, the physiologic impact can be expected to be proportionately greater because during the respiratory cycle the lung is seldom operating at this peak surface area.

General anesthesia is known to impair pulmonary gas exchange in all patients (Dueck et al., 1980; Rehder et al., 1979) and postoperative respiratory compromise is the rule, not the exception (Craig, 1981). Respiratory impairment is unpredictable and is divided into two periods: an early phase, which is seen during the first 2 postoperative hours and may be due to anesthetic effects, and a delayed phase, due to mechanical abnormalities. Defects in gas exchange may persist for several weeks. FRC returns to normal values within 2 weeks, but vital capacity may require 3 weeks or longer to be reestablished. Arterial oxygen values may grossly underestimate the abnormality in ventilation and perfusion that exists in this situation because of routine use of supplemental inspired oxygen support postoperatively. Carbon dioxide retention at constant ventilation or an increasing respiratory rate may be a better guide and a measure of compromise. The recognition of the importance of

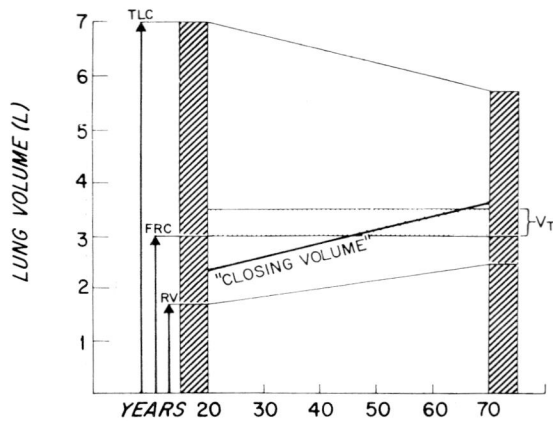

FIGURE 2–8. Effect of age on TLC, FRC, residual volume, and closing volume. These values are for a normal, supine adult. Note: In the fifth decade, the closing volume exceeds the FRC during normal tidal ventilation, (i.e., small airways close before end-expiration). This causes increasing ventilation-perfusion inequality with age and accounts for the normally seen arterial hypoxemia in elderly patients. It may also explain the increased incidence of acute respiratory failure in the elderly postoperative patient. (Modified and reproduced with permission from Pontoppidan, H., Geffin, B., and Lowenstein, E.: Acute Respiratory Failure in the Adult. Boston, Little, Brown, 1973.)

FRC as an essential lung volume may provide a physiologic end-point for goal-oriented respiratory therapy, and the long period over which respiratory function remains depressed should be an important reminder that adequate progress during the first 2 or 3 postoperative days should not indicate that the patient continues to do well.

The changing volume of the lung has been shown to alter the individual and overall compliance characteristics of the lung. Decreased lung volumes lead to decreased respiratory compliance; thus, increased breathing work is required to provide adequate gas exchange. Although airway closure can be documented physiologically (Engle et al., 1975) and histologically (Hughes et al., 1970), the concept must be viewed in terms of its functional rather than its morphologic importance. Airway closures leading to mechanical derangements in lung and chest wall function cause significant redistribution of gas flow and impairment of blood-gas exchange in the immediate and prolonged postoperative recovery period. If these changes are prevented or minimized, postoperative recovery may be accelerated.

DISTRIBUTION OF BLOOD FLOW

The concept that blood flow within the lung is not uniform and may be influenced by gravitational forces and the interaction of vascular and airway pressures is not new. In 1887, Johannes Orth, in *Aetiologisches und Anatomisches uber Lungenschwindsucht*, postulated that the weight of the column of blood in upright lungs might be sufficient to cause hypoperfusion or "anemia" of the apical zone. However, it has

been only with the advent of radioactive tracer gas techniques that this postulate has been studied. It has been demonstrated that, as with ventilation, lung perfusion depends on gravitational effects (West, 1977), the state and degree of lung inflation (Howell et al., 1961; Hughes et al., 1968), and pulmonary artery and venous perfusion pressures (Hughes et al., 1968; Permutt et al., 1962).

A model helps to clarify this situation (Fig. 2–9). Regardless of body position, the lung is subject to the effects of gravity, modified by mode of ventilation, degree of lung expansion, and pulmonary vascular pressures. In an erect human, with an open glottis, alveolar pressure is constant in all areas. As shown in Zone 1, with alveolar pressure greater than pulmonary arterial pressure, an area of no flow is created because the thin-walled, collapsible capillaries are exposed directly to alveolar pressure. Under normal conditions, Zone 1 probably does not exist, but conceptually it becomes important when one tries to interpret pressure data from indwelling pulmonary artery catheters in patients being mechanically ventilated. Zone 1 is not only the apical portion of lung;

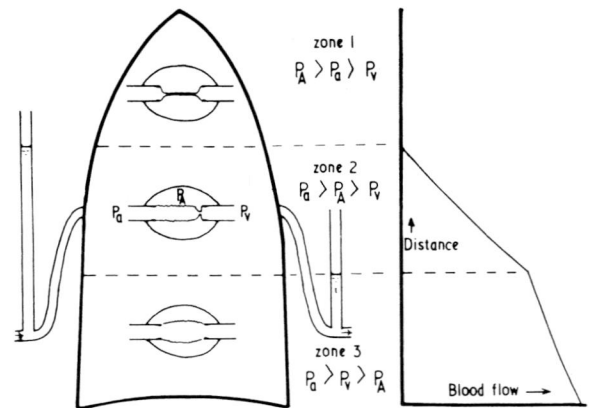

FIGURE 2–9. Diagram of blood flow in the isolated lung. Uneven distribution of blood flow in the lung is based on the relationship between perfusion pressure and the pressures affecting the capillaries within the lung. *Zone 1:* Alveolar pressure exceeds perfusion pressure in the apex of the lung, and theoretically, no flow occurs. This zone is unlikely to exist in healthy individuals. (Alveolar pressure > pulmonary arterial pressure > pulmonary venous pressure.) *Zone 2:* Pulmonary arterial pressure now exceeds alveolar pressure, but alveolar pressure is greater than pulmonary venous pressure. In this zone, the capillaries behave like Starling's resistors (see Fig. 2–10), and flow increases down the zone owing to the increasing hydrostatic pressure that is secondary to gravitational effects; i.e., flow is determined by the arterial-alveolar pressure difference, which is the "waterfall" area of the lung. *Zone 3:* In this area, pulmonary venous pressure exceeds alveolar pressure and flow is determined by the pulmonary arterial-venous pressure difference that remains constant throughout the region. As the base of the lung is approached, flow can be shown to decrease despite increasing hydrostatic pressure. This area, *Zone 4* (see text), is caused by constriction of arterioles due to the increased mass of tissue that is compressed owing to the effects of gravity. This area varies and depends on the degree of expansion. With reference to previous discussion, this area decreases with increased age. (From West, J. B., Dollery, C. T., and Naimark, A.: Distribution of blood flow in isolated lung; relation to vascular and alveolar pressures. J. Appl. Physiol., *19:*713, 1964.)

depending on patient position, it is also any lung area that is superior to the pressure reference point (phlebostatic axis) of the left atrium. Therefore, if a pulmonary artery catheter tip lies in a Zone 1 area, owing to either initial placement or subsequent change in patient position, the pressures obtained during mechanical ventilation are significantly higher than when the patient breathes spontaneously, because of the effect of changing alveolar pressure (Geer, 1977; Roy et al., 1977; Stanley et al., 1977). Clinically, this situation can be anticipated if it is noted that a wide fluctuation in pulmonary artery pressure occurs with each mechanical breath. Confirmation of catheter position may be obtained in a cross-body lateral chest film—the catheter tip is seen to lie superior to the left atrium. Therefore, it is always important to read pulmonary artery pressures at the time of end-expiration in an attempt to minimize the effects of increased airway pressure on pulmonary artery pressure. Also, clinicians must recognize that the more compliant the lung, the more likely it is that intrathoracic pressure is transmitted to the alveolar space. Paradoxically, in sick patients with "stiff" lungs, it is often easier to interpret invasive hemodynamic data than in patients with normal pulmonary compliance. This is detailed further during the discussion of mechanical ventilation and positive end-expiratory pressure.

In Zone 2, pulmonary arterial pressure is greater than alveolar pressure, but alveolar pressure is greater than pulmonary venous pressure. The vessels in this area of lung behave like the resistor in a Starling heart-lung model (Fig. 2–10): The vessel is represented as a collapsible tube surrounded by a pressure chamber. Blood flow through this area depends not on the gradient of pulmonary artery to pulmonary vein pressure but on the pulmonary artery-to-alveolar pressure difference. The reason is that the vessel itself offers no resistance to the collapsing pressure, so that the pressure inside and outside the tube is the same. Consequently, the perfusing pressure is determined by the gradient between pulmonary artery and alveolus. Because the alveolar pressure within the lung is uniform at all levels and the pulmonary artery pres-

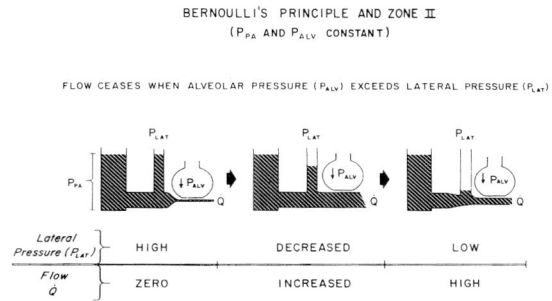

FIGURE 2–11. The control of blood flow through Zone 2 by the interaction between vascular and alveolar pressure. Left, The situation is identical to the conditions in Zone 1 with alveolar pressure exceeding intravascular or perfusion pressure; therefore, a state of zero flow exists. Center, As blood continues to enter the lung, increasing vascular and hydrostatic pressures are sufficient to overcome alveolar pressure, and flow begins. Right, As blood flow increases (increasing hydrostatic pressure down Zone 2 with alveolar and pulmonary artery pressures constant), the lateral vascular pressure decreases (Bernoulli's principle). With further increases in blood flow and in lateral pressure, a point is reached at which alveolar pressure exceeds lateral vascular pressure and flow again ceases. This condition probably accounts for decreased flow in the so-called Zone 4. The preceding situation is similar to the simple suction apparatus used in chemistry laboratories in which a vacuum is produced by a stream of water with a side port on the side of the spigot. As flow is initiated, air is entrained into the water stream, which creates a vacuum (decreases lateral vascular pressure). It can be appreciated, then, that in the crowded basal segments of the lung, geometric considerations may alter flow through the lung.

sure increases inferiorly in the lung because of a gravitational hydrostatic effect, blood flow increases as Zone 2 is traversed. This is reflected in the diagram. Zone 2 has also been described as the waterfall zone because, in a waterfall, flow across the brim is independent of the height of the waterfall above the collecting reservoir and is constant until reservoir height (pulmonary vein) exceeds the height of the waterfall (pulmonary artery perfusing pressure). Therefore, flow in this zone is independent of the gradient of alveolar to left atrial pressure. At times, intra-alveolar pressure exceeds intravascular pressure, and the blood vessels may intermittently close or "flutter," which leads to disturbances in lung parenchymal perfusion and alters ventilation-perfusion ratios. As is discussed, this deficit is probably temporary but may be partly responsible for the low specificity of defects seen in postoperative perfusion lung scans (Walker et al., 1981; Wagner, 1978). The intermittent nature of blood flow in Zone 2 is illustrated in Figure 2–11.

In Zone 3, both intravascular pressures exceed alveolar pressure, and the vessel is held open at all times. Flow is now determined by the arterial-venous pressure difference in the usual manner. As in Zone 2, an increase in flow down the lung is observed, which is at first difficult to explain, because the pulmonary arterial-venous pressure gradient is constant. However, the hydrostatic effect increases down the lung, causing pressure inside the small vessels to increase down the zone. The small vessels will distend slightly, thereby decreasing their resistance to flow. Any

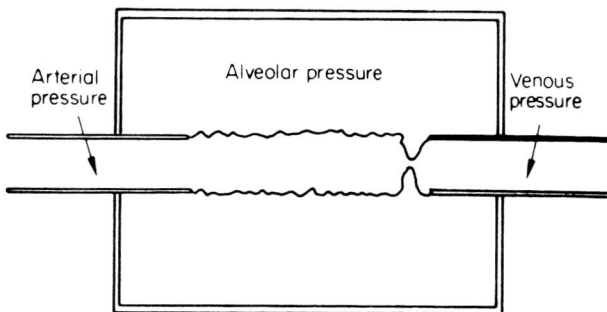

FIGURE 2–10. Diagram of a Starling resistor or flutter valve. The capillary network can be visualized as a collapsible tube within the alveolar pressure chamber. This model accounts for the increased blood flow down Zone 2 of the lung. (From West, J. B.: Ventilation-Blood Flow and Gas Exchange. 4th ed. Oxford, Blackwell, 1985.)

change in body position or vascular status that subjects large portions of the lung to conditions seen in Zone 3 will predispose to increased distention of pulmonary vasculature and ultimately will enhance the accumulation of interstitial pulmonary fluid, especially if left atrial pressure is abnormally high.

In patients receiving mechanical ventilatory assistance, it is possible to postulate the existence of another zone that may develop geographically within Zone 3 secondary to the high airway pressures necessary to ventilate patients with poor pulmonary compliance. Overdistention of alveoli results, which decreases pulmonary blood flow in the affected area and produces areas of dead-space ventilation. Some authorities have suggested that these areas should be called a Zone 4 condition. Effects of body position on the distribution of lung perfusion are illustrated in Figure 2–12.

The interaction of vascular and alveolar pressures is responsible for the distribution of pulmonary blood flow. Situations that alter normal perfusion pressure would be expected to change ventilation-perfusion characteristics and alter blood-gas exchange. Figure 2–13 demonstrates the effects of hypotension and left ventricular failure on the distribution of pulmonary vascular pressures. Implicit in this discussion of the pulmonary vasculature are some points that are often overlooked. The pulmonary artery receives 100% of the cardiac output and must, therefore, be able to adapt to a wide range of blood flows (ranges in normal adults may be from 5 to 56.6 l/min, or roughly 80 to 800 ml/sec) (Rerych et al., 1978, 1980). Heterogeneity of vascular distribution is essential for effective gas exchange, and the ability of the lungs to tolerate these fluctuations in flow is partly due to the fact that certain areas of lung are not perfused some of the time. In general, a rise in pulmonary artery pressure increases perfusion in nondependent lung areas and reduces the physiologic dead space. The mechanisms underlying the increase in perfusion are

either distention of already perfused vascular beds or recruitment of available but not perfused vascular channels.

In the extreme situation, the changes are responsible for the radiographic appearances of pulmonary edema, with initial perihilar fluffiness occurring secondary to distention of the pulmonary vessels; ultimately, cephalization of blood flow is seen as the normally underperfused apical vessels are recruited. It is interesting to note that the initial hilar congestion begins in the right lung, presumably because the right pulmonary vein is longer than the left and is influenced by distention of the right atrium, which is enlarged in cardiac failure. As left atrial pressure increases, the extent of Zones 1 and 2 will be decreased, and that of Zone 3 will be increased. This is reflected as a decrease in pulmonary vascular resistance, because a greater number of collapsible alveolar vessels is held open and the rate of blood flow depends on the pressure gradient between the pulmonary artery and the left atrium. However, the rate of fluid flow into the lung interstitium in Zone 3 areas is, in part, proportional to the pressure gradient between the left atrium and the alveolus ($P_{LA} - P_{ALV}$). This assumes that the alveolar-capillary membrane separating the two is osmotically competent and that the serum oncotic pressure is within normal limits. Regardless of other considerations, interstitial lung water will accumulate until left atrial pressure is lowered.

Hypotension and left ventricular failure are two causes of abnormal pulmonary blood flow distribution seen commonly in the perioperative period. In Figure 2–13, both situations are shown: The patient has been placed in the lateral position to emphasize the effects on blood-gas exchange. During thoracotomy, severe respiratory dysfunction may occur secondary to these effects as well as to the effects of anesthetic agents on the distribution of ventilation and perfusion. In the normal situation, the upper lung is ventilated preferentially and perfused poorly

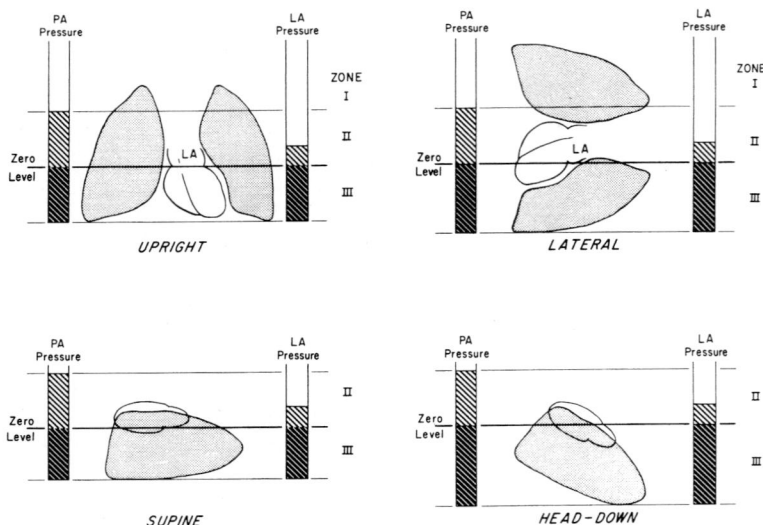

FIGURE 2–12. Effect of body position on the distribution of pulmonary perfusion. The normal distribution is shown in the *upper left diagram.* All other positions are noted to cause an increase in Zone 3 (shown as Zone III) areas, either uniformly in both lungs (*bottom panels*) or almost exclusively in one lung (as in the lateral position). The supine position increases Zone 3 primarily in the posterior segments of the lung from apex to base, and the Trendelenburg position causes the most significant increase in Zone 3 areas. Pulmonary edema tends to form most easily in Zone 3 areas. Therefore, good postoperative pulmonary care will include frequent position changes and early ambulation. (From Laver, M. B., Hallowell, P., and Goldblatt, A.: Pulmonary dysfunction secondary to heart disease: Aspects relevant to anesthesia and surgery. Anesthesiology, 33:161, 1970.)

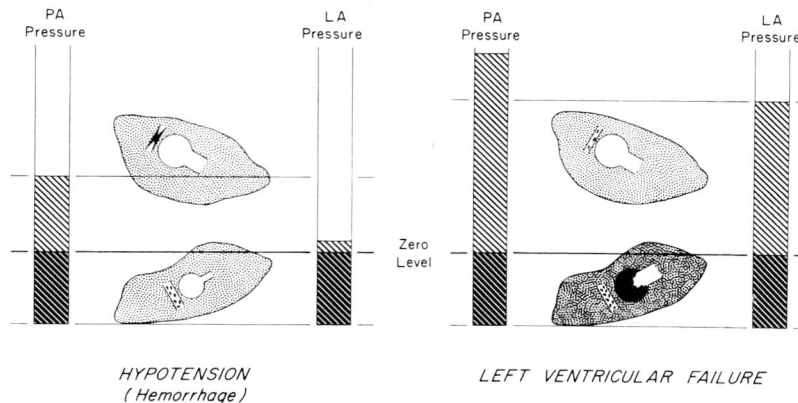

FIGURE 2–13. Effect of hypotension and left ventricular failure on the distribution of vascular pressures (see also Fig. 2–12). The patient is placed in the lateral position to simplify the zone changes and to emphasize the possible derangements in blood-gas exchange. Decreased blood pressure causes a reduction in blood flow to the nondependent lung, which results in a ventilated but not perfused lung segment (dead space). Conversely, increased left atrial pressure seen in congestive cardiac failure leads to increased perfusion of nondependent zones of the lung. However, the increased hydrostatic effects in the dependent lung lead to the formation of pulmonary edema with resultant collapse of terminal airways. This region allows continued perfusion of nonventilated alveoli (shunt effect) and increases the likelihood of arterial hypoxemia. The effective pressure in the dependent and nondependent lung is measured as the total of left atrial pressure (zero reference height is at the level of the mitral annulus) and the hydrostatic pressure within the column of blood below it. From this relationship, the possibility of dead-space pulmonary units is shown. (From Laver, M. B., and Austen, W. G.: Respiratory function: Physiologic considerations applicable to surgery. In Sabiston, D. C., Jr. [ed]: Davis-Christopher Textbook of Surgery. 12th ed. Philadelphia, W. B. Saunders, 1981.)

because of gravitational effects. During operation, collapse of the operated lung leads to alveolar hypoxia in the atelectic segments. This hypoxia normally causes a reflex pulmonary vasoconstriction, which decreases blood flow to the hypoxic areas and thereby minimizes venous admixture or shunt. The *hypoxic pulmonary vasoconstrictor reflex* (HPVR) may be diminished by use of inhalational anesthetic agents (halothane, enflurane, isoflurane), which are commonly used for one-lung anesthesia during thoracotomy. These potent agents permit the use of high inspired oxygen concentrations, which may be required if the patient becomes hypoxic. High-dose narcotic anesthetic techniques, which may be beneficial because of theoretic preservation of the HPVR and subsequent decreased pulmonary-venous admixture, may be contraindicated owing to an unacceptable incidence of patient recall of intraoperative events or prolonged recovery times. The use of a continuous infusion of ketamine has been shown to diminish intrapulmonary shunting during one-lung anesthesia and to preserve the HPVR (Lumb et al., 1979; Silvay et al., 1980) and is an acceptable alternative anesthetic technique. Balanced anesthetic techniques using narcotics (fentanyl, sufentanil, alfentanil) and hypnotics (diazepam, midazolam, lorazepam) have become the main agents used in thoracic surgical procedures. The recent introduction of propofol into anesthetic practice provides an agent with useful characteristics for thoracic anesthesia. It will likely gain in acceptance and be used more frequently for these procedures.

Of practical consideration, the treatment of hypoxia during one-lung anesthesia may be managed by altering the ventilation-perfusion mismatch caused by surgical manipulation, lung collapse, and diminished HPVR. Commonly employed techniques require either complete deflation of partially collapsed lung segments in order to maximize HPV or gradual reexpansion of lung segments to provide an increased gas exchange area. The latter is accomplished by applying a continuous, low distending pressure (*continuous positive airway pressure* [CPAP]) to the collapsed lung. In either approach, the physiologic endpoint is more appropriate matching of available ventilation and perfusion, producing improved oxygenation. Cooperation between the anesthesiologist and the operating surgeon is of paramount importance to ensure success because, ultimately, each must recognize the physiologic goals and constraints placed upon the other.

Other factors that contribute to deranged pulmonary function during thoracotomy (or during any procedure that requires the lateral position for long periods) are the increase in Zone 3 areas due to hydrostatic pressure gradients in the dependent lung and an increase in Zone 1 areas in the nondependent lung. This situation produces gross mismatch of ventilation and perfusion, with dead-space effects in the nondependent lung requiring increased minute ventilation to control carbon dioxide retention. In the dependent lung, accumulation of interstitial pulmonary fluid is increased, which leads to defective alveolar gas transport and the appearance of shunt units secondary to airway collapse and atelectasis. It is not surprising that the lateral position is tolerated poorly by patients who initially have poor myocardial reserve (Fig. 2–14).

The problems of distribution of ventilation and perfusion are increased significantly during mechanical ventilation because of intrathoracic pressure reversal and altered diaphragmatic activity. This is discussed further in the section dealing specifically with me-

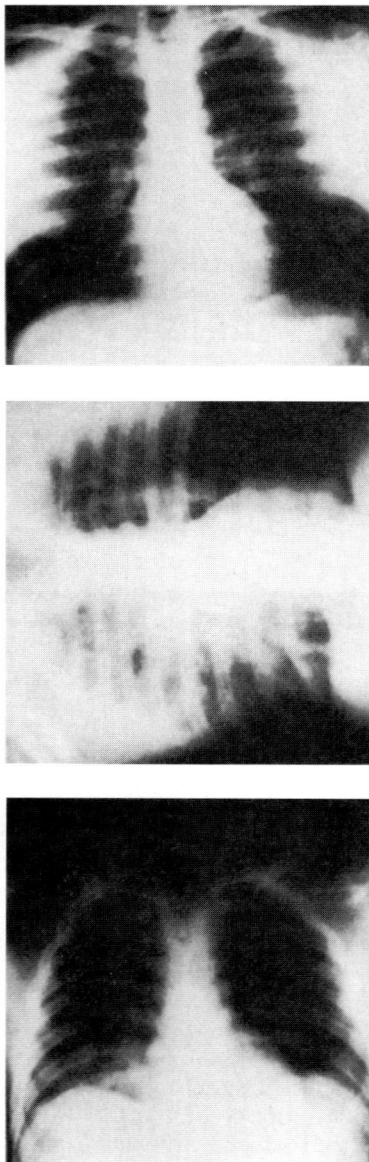

FIGURE 2-14. The practical consequence of prolonged operation in the lateral position in a patient with congestive heart failure. The operation, left hip arthroplasty, lasted for 5 hours. One hour postoperatively, the patient developed all the clinical signs of severe pulmonary edema. The chest film at the *top* was taken preoperatively, the film in the *center* (obtained with the patient in an upright position), taken at the time of pulmonary edema (1 hour postoperatively), is placed on its side, similar to the position maintained by the patient during operation. The film at the *bottom* was taken 48 hours later, after pulmonary edema had resolved. The most prominent congestive changes appeared in the dependent (right) lung. (From Laver, M. B., and Austen, W. G.: Respiratory function: Physiologic considerations applicable to surgery. *In* Sabiston, J. C., Jr. [ed]: Davis-Christopher Textbook of Surgery. 12th ed. Philadelphia, W. B. Saunders, 1981).

chanical ventilation and the regulation of ventilation and perfusion. First, further consideration must be given to the distribution of blood flow in the upright lung during inspiration and expiration. Analysis of blood flow in the upright lung during spontaneous breathing suggests that there are two separate vessel systems that respond differently to lung expansion, and they have been classified as intra-alveolar and extra-alveolar vessels (Howell et al., 1961; Hughes et al., 1968). During inspiration, the small, intra-alveolar capillaries are most affected by the rise in airway pressure, and flow through this region decreases proportionally to the increase in transmural pressure (Laver et al., 1981). On the other hand, the extra-alveolar vessels are surrounded by a negative pressure that depends on the state of lung inflation (West, 1977). At high lung volumes, these larger vessels are tethered open and their vascular resistance is decreased. At FRC, when the lung parenchyma at the base is poorly expanded, the extra-alveolar vessels are collapsed, which increases their resistance, and blood flow is decreased. The diagram in Figure 2-15 emphasizes the difference between alveolar and extra-alveolar vessels. Figure 2-16 shows a composite of the factors that influence the distribution of perfusion in the upright lung.

It should be clear that alterations in the geometry of the airways alter the cross-sectional area of the extra-alveolar blood vessels and vice versa. These relationships interact to produce a good but incomplete method of adjusting ventilation to perfusion, which will be discussed in the next section. However, the understanding that lung volume changes are reflected also as changes in the compliance of the respiratory system should alert the clinician that preserving postoperative lung volume is a priority. Basal airways collapse because of thoracic or abdominal splinting or raised intra-abdominal pressure, and lung compliance in this area decreases, which decreases blood flow in these areas. This leads to a quantity of blood flowing past nonventilated airways, which effectively adds nonoxygenated blood to the systemic circulation. Ultimately, arterial hypoxemia ensues. These changes are accentuated in obese patients, who have all the disadvantages of the postoperative condition in addition to a markedly reduced FRC due to the increased abdominal and chest wall

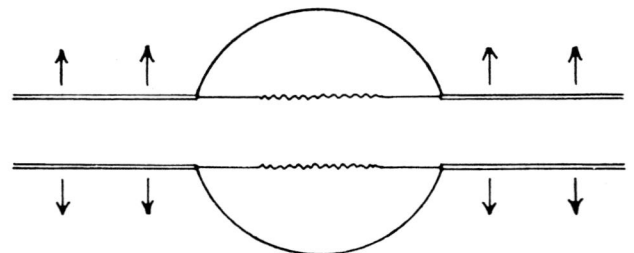

FIGURE 2-15. Extra-alveolar vessels that are more than 100 μ in diameter and include arteries, veins, and vessels in alveolar-septal junctions are expanded during pulmonary expansion. Alveolar capillaries are constricted during increases in transmural pressure. However, equalization of flow is seen at times of constant pulmonary volume when intra-alveolar pressure equalizes to atmosphere. Thus, pressure recordings of intraparenchymal vessels are taken at a constant position of end-expiration with an open glottis. (From West, J. B.: Respiratory Physiology. 2nd ed. Copyright © 1979 by The Williams & Wilkins Company, Baltimore. Reproduced by permission.)

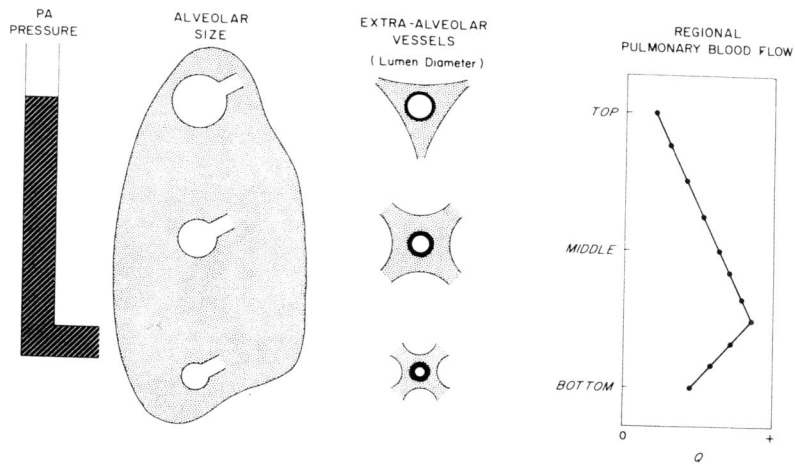

FIGURE 2–16. Factors influencing pulmonary blood flow in the upright lung. The effects of alveolar shape, effective perfusion pressure, and gravity are shown. Perfusion pressure at the apex of the lung is lowest, but anatomic and gravitational factors combine to increase alveolar size (see also Fig. 2–4). Traction on extra-alveolar vessels also increases the size of the lumen in this region. As the lung is traversed from apex to base, increasing effective perfusion pressure tends to increase blood flow; this is counterbalanced by increasing distortion to the blood vessel architecture by pressure due to the relative increase in weight of the lung and reduced alveolar size. Perfusion is greatest just above the bases of the lung, at which point the increased perfusion pressure is least affected by reductions in extra-alveolar size. The occurrence of Zone 4 is less abrupt than shown in this diagram. (From Laver, M. B., and Austen, W. G.: Respiratory function: Physiologic considerations applicable to surgery. *In* Sabiston, D. C., Jr. [ed]: Davis-Christopher Textbook of Surgery. 12th ed. Philadelphia, W. B. Saunders, 1981).

weight that functionally erodes lung volume. Figure 2–17 demonstrates this situation.

THE VENTILATION–PERFUSION RELATIONSHIP

Although the preceding two sections have attempted to deal with ventilation and perfusion as isolated entities, it has been impossible to separate the discussions. Not only are the anatomic relationships between airway and vessel diameters and resistances close but also the ultimate function of the lungs and circulation is to support aerobic metabolism. Therefore, blood-gas exchange efficiency is really the clinical correlate, and methods of assessing this efficiency are the basis of this section. Although disorders of arterial oxygenation are often the most urgent of the problems of blood-gas exchange, chronic disorders of ventilation and perfusion are no longer the exception in patients presenting for elective surgery, and the perioperative management of chronic lung disease poses a major problem. Throughout the following discussion, oxygen transport and extraction are stressed, rather than a more traditional approach that highlights arterial oxygen tension as being an adequate reflection of satisfactory aerobic metabolism.

Oxygen Transport

Oxygen is transported in the blood in two forms: dissolved and in combination with hemoglobin (West, 1979).

Dissolved Oxygen

The amount of oxygen dissolved in blood follows Henry's law, which states that the amount dissolved is proportional to the partial pressure of oxygen (Fig. 2–18). For each millimeter of mercury of P_{O_2}, there is 0.0031 ml of oxygen dissolved in 100 ml of blood. Therefore, in normal arterial blood with a P_{O_2} of 100 mm Hg, 0.3 ml of O_2 will be transported in each 100 ml of blood. This method of oxygen transport is shown to be inadequate in the following example (West, 1979).

Assume that O_2 consumption during strenuous exercise is 3000 ml/min and that there is total extraction of oxygen from the blood by peripheral tissues. The Fick principle states that the oxygen consumption per minute ($\dot{V}_{O_2}$) is equal to the amount of oxygen taken up by the blood in the lungs per minute. Because the oxygen content difference between the arterial and the venous blood equals the oxygen uptake, and because the minute volume of uptake is dependent on cardiac output, this relationship can be expressed as Cardiac output = Oxygen consumption/Arterial-mixed venous oxygen content difference, or

$$Q = \frac{\dot{V}_{O_2}}{A\text{-}V_{O_2}}$$

then

$$Q = \frac{3000}{0.003} \text{ where } Ca_{O_2} = 0.003 \text{ ml } O_2/\text{ml blood}$$
$$= 1{,}000{,}000 \text{ ml/min, or } 1000 \text{ l/min}$$

Because the highest recorded cardiac output in a trained athlete is approximately 56 l/min (Rerych et al., 1978, 1980), an additional method of transporting

UPRIGHT LUNG

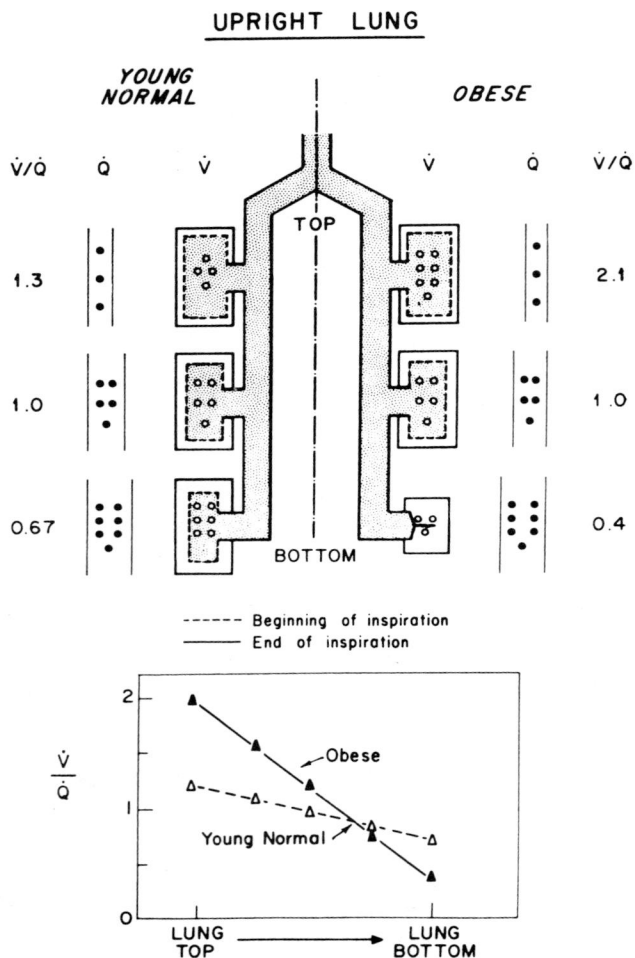

FIGURE 2–17. A comparison of the distribution of ventilation and perfusion in young normal and obese individuals. A sharp increase in abdominal and chest wall weight leads to an increase in the Zone 3 area at the base of the lung. In the supine position, basal alveolar collapse is marked, and relative hypoxemia results. The distribution of ventilation and perfusion in the upper zones of the lung is reversed, and severe respiratory dysfunction may be present in the normal state. The *open* and *closed circles* represent units of ventilation and perfusion, respectively. In the normal lung, the ratio of ventilation to perfusion ($\dot{V}/\dot{Q}$) is highest although perfusion and gas flow are greatest at the bases of the lungs in absolute terms. This high ratio is due to the relative lack of perfusion at the apex of the lung and is reduced as perfusion increases down the lung.

In the obese patient, the changes in $\dot{V}/\dot{Q}$ are more marked and more rapidly progressive down the lung, which leads to increased areas of wasted perfusion and ultimately arterial hypoxia (*bottom graph*). The reason for this change is that the distribution of gas flow is reversed from the normal situation owing to intermittent basal alveolar closure and redistribution of gas flow during inspiration. These considerations emphasize the importance in obese patients of early postoperative mobilization.

The situation is analogous to that of the plunger within the barrel of a syringe. The chest wall is represented as the syringe barrel and the diaphragm as the plunger. The normal situation is that the plunger moves freely within the syringe and appropriately changes the volume of enclosed gas or fluid. However, in obese patients, because of the increased hydrostatic pressure of abdominal contents that press upward on the diaphragm, free motion is prevented and the patient attempts to move the chest wall on the diaphragm (or move the syringe while keeping the plunger fixed). This situation is poorly tolerated and may lead to significant postoperative morbidity in these patients. (From Pontoppidan, H., Laver, M. B., and Geffin, B.: Acute respiratory failure in the surgical patient. Adv. Surg., 4:163–254, 1970. Redrawn with permission from data of Holley, H. S., Milic-Emili, J., Becklake, M. R., et al.: Regional distribution of pulmonary ventilation and perfusion in obesity. J. Clin. Invest., 46:475, 1967.)

oxygen is needed. It should be remembered that the measurements of $P_{A_{O_2}}$ obtained clinically in the blood-gas laboratory reflect only the amount of oxygen dissolved in plasma. The amount of oxygen dissolved in blood changes markedly in hyperbaric conditions, and by raising the inspired P_{O_2} to 3 atmospheres, the amount of dissolved oxygen in arterial blood can be increased to about 6 ml/100 ml of blood (see Fig. 2–18). In this situation, all the metabolic needs of the resting individual can be met with dissolved oxygen alone. However, this condition clinically is not feasible for prolonged treatment, and oxygen combined with hemoglobin provides the bulk of clinically significant oxygen transport.

Oxygen in Combination with Hemoglobin

The maximal amount of oxygen that can be combined with hemoglobin is called the oxygen capacity. It is measured by tonometry of blood at a very high P_{O_2} and subtraction of the dissolved oxygen. One gram of hemoglobin can combine with 1.39 ml of oxygen, although this figure is variably reported as either 1.34 or 1.36 ml. This discrepancy occurs because under normal conditions some of the hemoglobin is in forms such as methemoglobin and thus is not

available for combination with oxygen. However, most blood-gas calculators use 1.39 ml O_2/g hemoglobin in logic circuitry; therefore, this value is used for the remainder of this discussion. In addition, it is now common for modern blood-gas analyzers to separately measure the concentrations of carboxyhemoglobin and methemoglobin, and their influences on oxygen transport can be quantitated. Therefore, in a situation in which the hemoglobin concentration is 15 g/100 ml of blood and hemoglobin is fully saturated, the oxygen capacity is about 20.8 ml of oxygen/100 ml of blood. Figure 2–18 illustrates the oxygen-hemoglobin dissociation curve drawn at a temperature of 37° C and a pH of 7.4. As can be appreciated, oxygen delivery to the tissues is enhanced, as shown by the shape of the descending portion of the curve. The upper flat portion of the curve demonstrates the ineffectiveness of using high inspired oxygen concentrations to increase oxygen loading.

More important to the oxygen capacity of blood in the most favorable state is the carriage of oxygen by hemoglobin in the clinical context. The oxygen saturation of hemoglobin is expressed as:

$$\frac{\text{Oxygen combined with hemoglobin}}{O_2 \text{ capacity}} \times 100$$

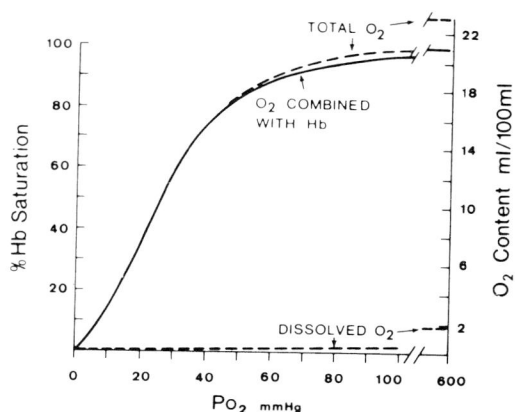

FIGURE 2–18. The oxygen dissociation curve is drawn for a hemoglobin concentration of 15 g/100 ml of blood at pH of 7.4 and P_{CO_2} of 40 mm Hg at 37° C. Dissolved oxygen content is represented by the *dotted line* at the base of the graph and is obviously inadequate for normal aerobic metabolism. Dissolved oxygen is shown at normal Pa_{O_2} and at 1 atmosphere of oxygen pressure. An initial increase in dissolved oxygen from 0.0031 ml/100 ml of blood to almost 2 ml/100 ml of blood is obtained by breathing 100% oxygen. It can be inferred that at 3 atmospheres of pressure, dissolved oxygen would increase to 6 ml/100 ml of blood and for normal aerobic metabolism, hemoglobin would become unnecessary. (From West, J. B.: Respiratory Physiology. 2nd ed. Copyright © 1979 by The Williams & Wilkins Company, Baltimore. Reproduced by permission.)

The oxygen saturation of arterial blood with a P_{O_2} of 100 mm Hg is about 97.5%, and that of desaturated venous blood with a P_{O_2} of 40 mm Hg is about 75%. With this information, it is possible to determine the oxygen content of arterial and venous blood. This has previously been shown to be an important link in the calculation of oxygen delivery and cardiac output, and it depends on the amount of oxygen combined with hemoglobin plus the oxygen dissolved in plasma. This can be expressed as:

$$\text{Oxygen content} = \text{Hb} \times \% \text{ saturation} \times 1.39 + 0.0031 \times P_{A_{O_2}}$$

The relationships between P_{O_2}, oxygen saturation, oxygen content, and hemoglobin are shown in Figure 2–19. For example, a patient at normal temperature and pH, with normal lungs and a hemoglobin of 15 g/100 ml and $P_{A_{O_2}}$ of 100 mm Hg has an arterial oxygen content ($C_{A_{O_2}}$) of $15 \times 97.5 \times 1.39 + 0.0031 \times 100$.

Situation 1:
$$C_{A_{O_2}} = 20.32 + 0.31 = 20.63 \text{ ml}/100 \text{ ml}$$

Compare this content with the same physiologic parameters after blood loss with a resultant hemoglobin of 13 g/100 ml:

Situation 2:
$$C_{A_{O_2}} = 13 \times 0.975 \times 1.39 + 0.0031 \times 100$$
$$= 17.62 + 0.31 = 17.93 \text{ ml}/100 \text{ ml}$$

If metabolic demands remain constant and the mixed

venous oxygen saturation does not change, the following becomes evident:

$$\text{Oxygen consumption} = \text{cardiac output} \times \text{A-V}_{O_2}$$

In Situation 1:

Arterial oxygen content ($C_{A_{O_2}}$) = 20.63 ml/100 ml
Mixed venous oxygen content ($C\bar{V}_{O_2}$) = 15.94 ml/100 ml
Therefore $\dot{V}_{O_2} = Q \times 4.69$.

In Situation 2:
$$C_{A_{O_2}} = 17.93 \text{ ml}/100 \text{ ml}$$
$$C\bar{V}_{O_2} = 13.86 \text{ ml}/100 \text{ ml}$$
Therefore $\dot{V}_{O_2} = Q \times 4.07$.

If oxygen consumption is to remain constant, one of two compensatory changes must occur: Either the arterial blood must be more thoroughly depleted of oxygen in the peripheral tissues, which decreases the mixed venous saturation, or the cardiac output must increase. Both situations occur and are well tolerated in health. With illness, especially in patients with increased metabolic needs (sepsis, burns, the postoperative state); with previous respiratory disease, which decreases the efficiency of arterial oxygenation; or with cardiac disease, which decreases the ability to increase cardiac output without danger of myocardial ischemia, compensation may be more difficult, and dangerous tissue hypoxia associated with anaerobiasis and metabolic acidosis may result. Therefore, the clinician is faced with the problem of juggling all of these factors in an attempt to maximize oxygen delivery to meet tissue metabolic demands without jeopardizing individual organ function. Pulmonary artery catheters with an indwelling fiberoptic bundle

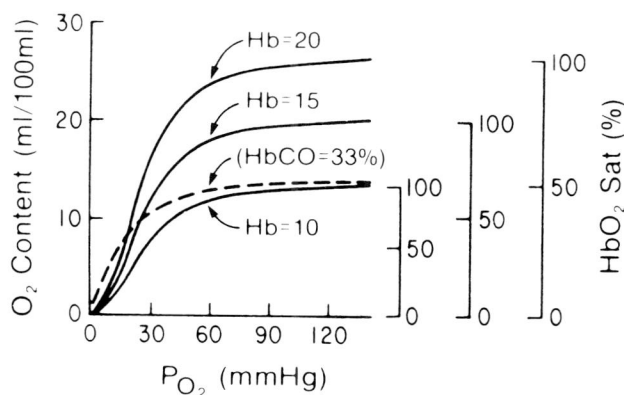

FIGURE 2–19. Effects of anemia and polycythemia on oxygen content and saturation. The effects of carbon monoxide binding to hemoglobin are shown by the *dashed line*. Note that oxygen saturation that depends on oxygen dissolved in plasma is unaffected by hemoglobin concentration, but that the oxygen content is greatly reduced as red blood cells are lost. All aspects of oxygen delivery must be assessed when interpreting arterial blood gas results. Oxygen delivery is expressed as: $\dot{Q} \times Ca_{O_2}$, where $Ca_{O_2} = \text{Hb} \times 1.39 \times$ arterial saturation $+ Pa_{O_2} \times 0.0031$. (From West, J. B.: Respiratory Physiology. 2nd ed. Copyright © 1979 by The Williams & Wilkins Company, Baltimore. Reproduced by permission.)

are used to monitor mixed venous oxygen saturation, continuously using the principle of reflectance spectrophotometry. This capability may be useful in optimizing hemodynamic parameters in patients with compromised cardiovascular function (Shoemaker, 1992).

Oxygen delivery to peripheral tissues now can be calculated easily from the following equation:

$$\text{Oxygen delivery} = \text{cardiac output} \times \text{arterial oxygen content}$$

$$DO_2 = Q \times CA_{O_2}$$

$$CA_{O_2} = Hb \times 1.39 \times \% \text{ saturation} + 0.0031 \times PA_{O_2}$$

$$\text{Oxygen consumption} = \text{cardiac output} \times \text{arterial-venous oxygen content difference}$$

$$\dot{V}O_2 = Q \times A\text{-}V_{O_2}$$

A useful combination of oxygen delivery and consumption data is expressed as the oxygen extraction ratio:

$$O_{2ER} = \frac{O_2 \text{ consumption}}{O_2 \text{ delivery}}$$

In health, this is less than 0.25. Concern should be evident if the O_{2ER} becomes greater than 0.3.

The following example demonstrates this value using the previously calculated data, assuming a cardiac output of 5.5 l/min.

Situation 1:
$\dot{V}O_2 = 5.5 \times 4.69 = 258$ ml O_2/min
O_2 delivery $= 5.5 \times 20.63 = 1135$ ml O_2/min
$O_{2ER} = 0.223$

However, to achieve this constancy, the overall oxygen consumption in Situation 2 was reduced. Physiologically, this is impossible below certain levels (except in states of hibernation and hypothermia), and in order to maintain oxygen consumption, the extraction has to increase if cardiac output remains fixed.

Situation 2:
O_2 delivery $= 986$ ml O_2/min
$\dot{V}O_2$ fixed $= 258$ ml O_2/min
$O_{2ER} = 0.26$

It is possible to backtrack and calculate the increase in venous desaturation that is required to maintain oxygen consumption (venous saturation = 67%), but more important is the understanding of possible dangers inherent in extracting excessive amounts of oxygen from the venous blood: The tissue anaerobic threshold is approached more rapidly, and acidosis is likely to result.

The decreasing partial pressure of oxygen from atmospheric to tissue concentrations is shown in Figure 2–20. Here the implication is that oxygen flows down a concentration gradient at each stage of its transfer

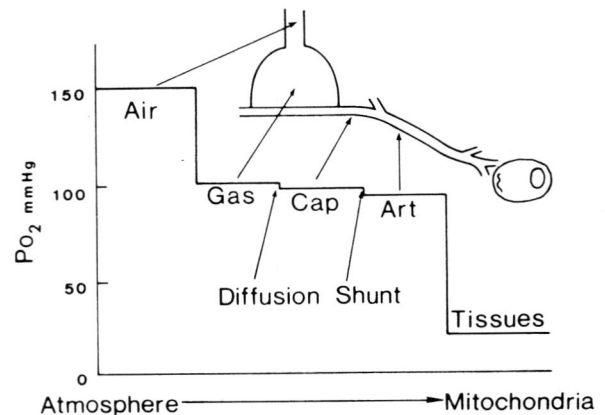

FIGURE 2–20. Oxygen partial pressure gradients from room air to mitochondria. Room air PO_2 at sea level is (760) (0.21) or 160 mm Hg. This is reduced rapidly in the alveoli by humidification and the mixing of metabolic carbon dioxide. Alveolar PO_2 (PA_{O_2}) is expressed in the simplified alveolar gas equation as (West, 1979):

$$PA_{O_2} = PI_{CO_2} - \frac{Pa_{CO_2}}{R} + F$$

$$\text{and } PI_{O_2} = (760 - 47) \times 0.21 + 2 = 152$$

$$\text{Therefore, } PA_{O_2} = 152 - \frac{40}{0.8} = 102 \text{ mm Hg}$$

Diffusion effects at the alveolar-capillary membrane and intrapulmonary shunt abnormalities cause a further reduction in PO_2 to a normal arterial tension of 95 mm Hg. A rapid desaturation in the tissues enables adequate aerobic metabolism, and the oxygen partial pressure of mixed venous blood after normal tissue oxygen extraction is approximately 40 mm Hg. (Modified from West, J. B.: Ventilation-Blood Flow and Gas Exchange. 4th ed. Oxford, Blackwell, 1985.)

from air to mitochondria. The arterial oxygen partial pressure is considered the driving force of oxygen out of the blood into the tissues, but it is the venous oxygen tension that reflects the reserves present in the metabolic situation. In the clinical context, the venous blood that reflects most accurately the overall oxygen extraction is that obtained from the pulmonary artery just prior to the location of alveolar oxygenation. This "mixed venous" blood is fully desaturated and does not reflect regional oxygen extraction, which occurs when blood is sampled from the superior or inferior vena cava. In addition, oxygen contents of coronary veins and the thebesian circulation are represented in samples taken from the pulmonary artery. However, this is a composite sample and does not reflect oxygen extraction in specific organs—for example, blood drawn from the coronary sinus is the most highly desaturated blood found. Therefore, the normal mixed venous oxygen tension ($P\bar{v}_{O_2}$) of 40 mm Hg with a saturation of 75% may be viewed as a measure of the blood oxygen reserves.

Some investigators have tried to determine the mixed venous saturation compatible with acceptable oxygenation of all tissue mitochondria. Obviously, this is a theoretical and difficult number to derive, but Bryan-Brown and others have stated that a partial pressure of 20 mm Hg in mixed venous blood is minimally acceptable to ensure adequate oxygenation of the peripheral tissues (Bryan-Brown, 1976). Therefore, the mixed venous oxygen can be regarded as a reflection of the minimally acceptable measurable oxygen partial pressure compatible with adequate aerobic tissue metabolism. Also, changes in mixed venous oxygenation may reflect metabolic derangements and, in sepsis, peripheral shunting may cause an inappropriately elevated saturation that, if not understood in the context of the disease process, creates a false sense of security with respect to patient well-being. PA_{O_2} and $P\bar{v}_{O_2}$ are physiologically interdependent, and the two values must be considered together. The PA_{O_2} determines the concentration gradient that will cause oxygen to move into the cells. Because oxygen delivery to peripheral tissues depends on the shape and position of the oxygen-hemoglobin dissociation curve, the oxygen partial pressure at 50% hemoglobin saturation (P_{50}) may need to be determined in critically ill patients in order to assess peripheral oxygenation. The mixed venous saturation is a more accurate indication of the P_{50} than $P\bar{v}_{O_2}$ is. Therefore, in patients with a low $P\bar{v}_{O_2}$, the mixed venous oxygen saturation should also be determined, and the P_{50} should be calculated (Coetzee and Rossouw, 1980). If the position of the oxygen-hemoglobin curve is determined to be unfavorable for oxygen unloading in peripheral tissues, as reflected by the calculated or measured P_{50} value, therapeutic measures may be undertaken to alter the position of the curve. This changes the affinity of hemoglobin for oxygen and may permit better oxygenation of peripheral tissues in unfavorable situations.

It is necessary to return to a discussion of the mechanisms through which the distribution of alveolar ventilation and perfusion is responsible for affecting overall gas exchange and, ultimately, oxygen transport.

Oxygenation

As previously stated, oxygenation of the arterial blood is accomplished by means of a series of decreasing partial pressure gradients between room air and the tissues, as seen in Figure 2–20. This is shown in simplified form in Figure 2–21.

In the alveolus, the P_{O_2} is further reduced to approximately 100 mm Hg, because the P_{O_2} of alveolar gas is governed by two processes: the removal of oxygen by the pulmonary capillary blood (oxygen transport) and its continued replenishment by alveolar ventilation. The rate of removal of oxygen from the lung is governed by the metabolic rate of the tissues and changes little under resting conditions. The other gases present in the alveolus are the waste product of metabolism, carbon dioxide, and atmospheric nitrogen, which is important in maintaining the stability of the alveolus. When systemic blood reaches the tissue capillaries, further oxygen extraction occurs, as previously described, and in some cells, the P_{O_2} is as low as 1 mm Hg. Therefore, the

ultimate partial pressure gradient between atmospheric oxygen and the tissue is 150/1, and the lung is the essential link in this process. It must be remembered that the lung is a passive link, in that the amount of oxygen removed from the alveoli by the blood and the amount of carbon dioxide added to the alveolar gas by the blood are predetermined for the lung by the body's metabolic demands. The response of the blood-gas exchange system must be adequate to meet these demands. The relationships are diagrammed in the preceding figure (see Fig. 2–20).

In practice, the difference between the partial pressure of oxygen in the alveolus and in the arterial blood $P(A-a)_{O_2}$ provides a measure of the efficiency of the gas exchange system. Alveolar oxygen tension can be calculated from the alveolar gas equation, which allows calculation of the ideal alveolar P_{O_2} if the composition of the inspired gas, the respiratory exchange ratio (R), and the ideal alveolar carbon dioxide concentration (assumed to be equal to the arterial P_{CO_2}) are known (West, 1977):

$$R = \dot{V}_{CO_2}/\dot{V}_{O_2}$$

and

$$PALV_{O_2} = PI_{O_2} - \frac{P_{CO_2}}{R} + PALV_{CO_2} \times FI_{O_2} \times \frac{1 - R}{R}$$

Formerly, it was recommended that a patient be placed on 100% inspired oxygen in order to simplify calculation of $PALV_{O_2}$. The equation becomes $PALV_{O_2} = PB - (PA_{CO_2} + PH_2O)$. However, breathing 100% oxygen causes an absorption atelectasis in some lung areas, which may increase the disparity between alveolar and arterial oxygen partial pressures by creating lung units that are perfused but not ventilated. Therefore, this does not reflect accurately the situation at the patient's resting inspired oxygen concentration (Dantzker et al., 1979; Nunn et al., 1978; Tonnesen et al., 1977; Wagner et al., 1974). Practically any inspired oxygen concentration greater than room air allows the following approximation to be made:

$$PALV_{O_2} = FI_{O_2} (PB - PH_2O) - PA_{CO_2}$$

The alveolar-arterial oxygen tension gradient reflects the degree of mixing of well-oxygenated and poorly oxygenated blood. As previously noted in the section on oxygen transport, changes in cardiac output affect the degree of mixing, and a more sophisticated approach is necessary to derive the degree of mixing in the clinical setting.

The common deviations from ideal gas exchange seen during the perioperative period have been discussed (see Fig. 2–3). Efficient gas exchange requires that the cardiac output be directed past well-ventilated alveoli. Although gas exchange continues and physiologic homeostasis is maintained, decreased efficiency is noted in two instances: First, ventilation occurs in the absence or excess of perfusion, leading to wasted ventilation. This is reflected as alveolar

Po$_2$ 159 mm Hg

Humidification

Po$_2$ 149 mm Hg

Po$_2$ 109 mm Hg

O$_2$ extraction

(Arterial Po$_2$~100 mm Hg)

CO$_2$ addition

(Arterial Pco$_2$~40 mm Hg)

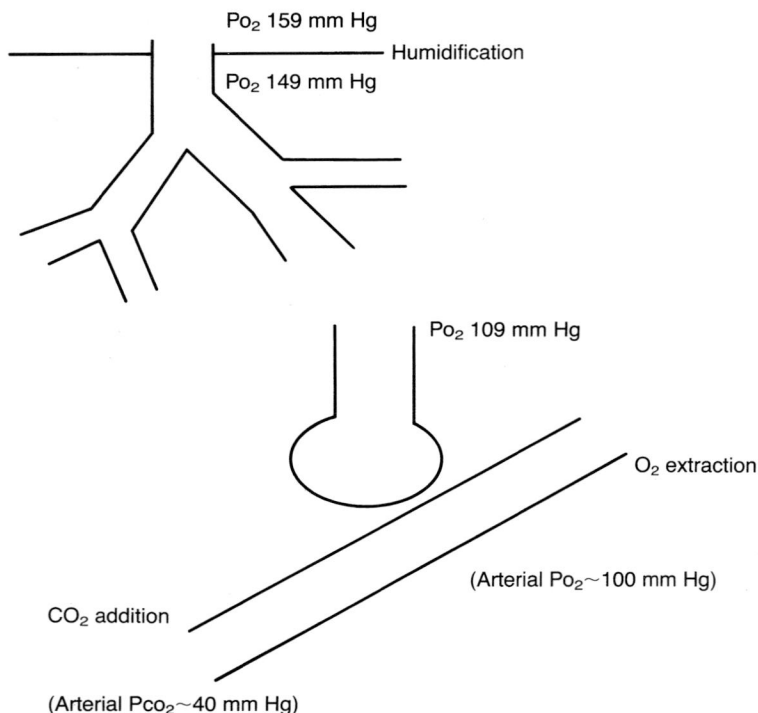

FIGURE 2–21. Simplified view of oxygenation of arterial blood by a series of decreasing partial pressure gradients between room air and the tissues.

Atmospheric pressure (P$_B$) at
sea level = 760 mm Hg

Inspired oxygen percentage
(F$_{IO_2}$) room air = 20.9%

Therefore, room air Po$_2$ = 760 × 0.209 = 159 mm Hg

However, as the air is inhaled, it becomes saturated with water vapor at body temperature, so that a correction factor must be applied to account for the partial pressure of water vapor. At 37° C, this is 47 mm Hg. The Po$_2$ of moist, inspired gas is therefore 0.209 × (760 − 47) = 149 mm Hg.

dead space, because carbon dioxide levels will rise unless minute alveolar ventilation is increased. Second, perfusion occurs in the absence or excess of gas exchange, leading to wasted perfusion. In this situation, blood that has had its oxygen extracted is allowed to return to the circulation, where it mixes with well-oxygenated blood. This mixing causes an overall decrease in the total oxygenation of the arterial blood and, if severe, may cause hypoxemia. It is obvious that of these two situations, the second is more hazardous to the patient, because the administration of increased amounts of oxygen to the alveoli does not provide proportionate increases of oxygen in the circulation. This occurs because the "shunted" blood does not contact the alveoli, and the oxygenated blood already is almost fully saturated. Therefore, an increased F$_{IO_2}$ can only increase the oxygen-carrying capacity of already oxygenated blood on the upper, flat portion of the oxygen-hemoglobin dissociation curve (see Fig. 2–19). The additional oxygen gained by this maneuver is small. But a rise in alveolar dead space characterized by an elevated carbon dioxide tension can be tolerated well if a small increase in inspired oxygen concentration is made. In this case, arterial oxygen tension is well maintained because of the absence of shunt.

The calculation of intrapulmonary shunt is a useful index of the degree of severity of respiratory insufficiency and has been used as an end-point of treatment (Gallagher et al., 1978; Jardin et al., 1979). The calculation is based on the following assumptions:

1. The total amount of oxygen transported in the blood per unit of time is a function of the cardiac output and the arterial oxygen content.

2. The total amount of oxygen in the pulmonary venous system (i.e., blood that is fully oxygenated) is the total blood flow ($\dot{Q}_T$) multiplied by the oxygen concentration in the arterial blood (C$_{AO_2}$), or $\dot{Q}_T$ × C$_{AO_2}$.

3. $\dot{Q}_T$ × C$_{AO_2}$ must equal the sum of oxygen in normally circulated blood that has become oxygenated in the pulmonary capillary beds and the amount of oxygen in the shunted blood ($\dot{Q}_S$).

4. The amount of oxygen in end-capillary blood can be represented as total oxygen content minus shunted content, or Cc'_{O_2} × ($\dot{Q}_T$ − $\dot{Q}_S$).

5. The amount of oxygen in shunted blood is expressed as $\dot{Q}_S$ × C$\bar{v}_{O_2}$, or shunt blood flow × the oxygen content of the mixed venous (desaturated) blood.

6. These expressions can be assembled as follows:

$$\dot{Q}_T \times C_{AO_2} = (\dot{Q}_S \times C\bar{v}_{O_2}) + (\dot{Q}_T - \dot{Q}_S) \times Cc'_{O_2}$$

7. This can be rearranged to produce the familiar "shunt" equation:

$$\dot{Q}_S/\dot{Q}_T = \frac{Cc'_{O_2} - C_{AO_2}}{Cc'_{O_2} - C\bar{v}_{O_2}}$$

A clinical problem in obtaining this value lies in the fact that direct measurement of end-capillary oxygen content is impossible. Therefore, calculations based on the alveolar Po$_2$ and the oxygen-hemoglobin dissociation curve are usually employed. This, in turn, causes further difficulty, because the respiratory exchange ratio is not measured commonly, and to assume a normal ratio of 0.8 in sick patients who are receiving supplemental oxygen is probably not

justified. In addition, measurements of end-capillary oxygen saturation that do not consider the effects of the dyshemoglobins (carboxy-, met-, and sulf-) on apparent shunt calculation are inaccurate and underestimate the true value (Cane et al., 1980; Cohn and Engler, 1979). End-capillary oxygen content is calculated correctly in the following manner (Maffėo et al., 1981):

$$Cc'_{O_2} = 1.39 \times Hb \times [1 - (\% \text{ Met Hb} + \% \text{ COHb})] + PA_{O_2} \times 0.0031$$

However, despite these described difficulties, shunt calculations are frequently performed in automated physiologic profiles (Shabot et al., 1977), and if consistency is used within the patient population, useful trends can be obtained that may aid patient management. It is important for the clinician to understand the mathematical package used in the monitoring program if true comparisons are to be made between measurements and to reported values. Before the ready availability of pulmonary artery catheterization, clinical approximation of shunt required the inspired oxygen concentration to be raised in order to ensure maximal hemoglobin saturation. All of these clinical approximations, however, used assumptions regarding the respiratory exchange ratio that were probably unjustified. The preceding discussion is represented diagrammatically in Figure 2–22.

It is crucial to understand the importance of atmospheric nitrogen as a buffer of alveolar integrity. Figure 2–23 shows the effect of alveolar nitrogen on the alveolar-arterial P_{O_2} gradient and the integrity of terminal air units in a two-alveoli model. Thus, a poorly ventilated alveolus may have an oxygen inflow that potentially is less than the amount of oxygen transferred from the alveolus into the blood per unit of time. Nitrogen is taken up poorly by the blood, so that it remains within the alveolus following oxygen extraction. If 100% oxygen is breathed in an attempt to alleviate hypoxia, the nitrogen eventually is eliminated from the alveolus, but the increased oxygen supply may not exceed the potential transfer of oxygen out of the alveolus. Therefore, as oxygen is extracted, no gas remains within the alveolus as a structural support, and the alveolus becomes unstable and collapses. This creates a shunt area. Figure 2–24 further highlights this situation. The importance of the prediction of intrapulmonary shunt from $P_{ALV_{O_2}}$ or the calculation of the alveolar-arterial gradient is not necessarily that documentation of the degree of gas exchange inefficiency aids in patient management, but that an appreciation of the magnitude of the problem helps to estimate the degree of illness. Too often, acceptable blood-gas values are noted on a patient's flow sheet, and the degree of ventilatory support necessary to produce adequate oxygenation or pH is forgotten. Therefore, calculations of shunt and $P(A-a)_{O_2}$ are useful tools in comparing the severity of illness between patients and in following a single patient's progress during the course of respira-

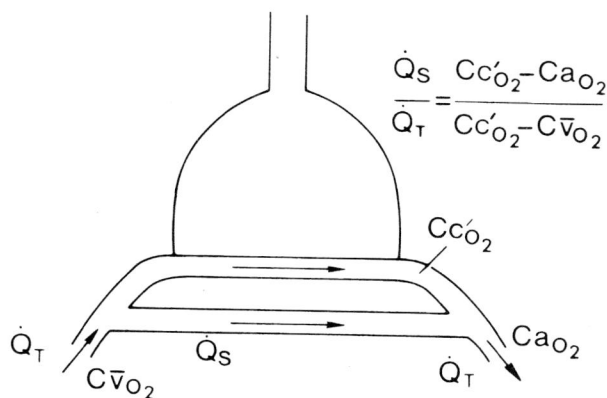

FIGURE 2–22. Calculation and measurement of intrapulmonary shunt. The oxygen carried in the arterial blood is equal to the sum of the oxygen carried in the capillary blood and that in the shunted blood or

$$\dot{Q}_T \times Ca_{O_2} = (\dot{Q}_S \times C\bar{v}_{O_2}) \times (\dot{Q}_t - \dot{Q}_s) \times Cc'_{O_2}$$

The major problem encountered in shunt measurement is the calculation of end-capillary oxygen content (Cc'_{O_2}). However, this situation has been remedied with common availability of oxy-, carboxy-, and met-hemoglobin measurements. Calculation of intrapulmonary shunt in a normal individual breathing room air would be accomplished as follows:

Hb – 15 g O_2 satn—98% carboxy Hb—1.5% met Hb—0.5%
$\dot{Q}$ – 5.5 l/min Pa_{O_2} – 98 mm Hg $P\bar{v}_{O_2}$ – 40 mm Hg mixed venous satn—70%

then: $\quad\quad\quad\quad Pa_{CO_2}$ – 40 mm Hg

$$Ca_{O_2} = 15 \times 1.39 \times 0.98 + 0.0031 \times 98 = 20.63 \text{ ml/100 ml}$$

$$Cv_{O_2} = 15 \times 1.39 \times 0.70 + 0.0031 \times 40 = 14.72$$

Cc'_{O_2}—The problem in this calculation is to assess the alveolar oxygen saturation and the alveolar P_{O_2}. Ultimately, assumptions need to be made, but the saturation can best be approximated as 1— (carboxy Hb + met Hb) (Hoyt, 1981 ASA Abstracts). PA_{O_2} is calculated from the alveolar gas equation (see Fig. 2–20) with the assumption that the respiratory exchange ratio on an oxygen-enriched inspired gas concentration is 1. For purposes of this example in a normal individual, this value is taken as 0.8.

Therefore,

$$Cc'_{O_2} = 15 \times 1.39 \times 1 - (1.5 + 0.5) + PA_{O_2} \times 0.0031,$$

$$\text{where } PA_{O_2} = FI_{O_2} \times (760 - 47) - \frac{Pa_{CO_2}}{R} + F$$

$$= 0.21 (713) - \frac{40}{0.8} + 2$$
$$= 149.7 - 50 + 2$$
$$= 101.7$$
$$= 20.43 + 101.7 \times 0.0031$$
$$= 20.43 + 0.32$$
$$= 20.75$$

Therefore,

$$\dot{Q}_S/\dot{Q}_T = \frac{20.75 - 20.63}{20.75 - 14.72} = \frac{0.12}{6.03} \times 100 = 1.99 \text{ or } 2\%$$

(From West, J. B.: Respiratory Physiology. 2nd ed. Copyright © 1979 by The Williams & Wilkins Company, Baltimore. Reproduced by permission.)

tory dysfunction. Other techniques of indexing the degree of respiratory support are listed below:

1. The mixed expired oxygen level of each breath reflects rapid changes in the ventilation-perfusion re-

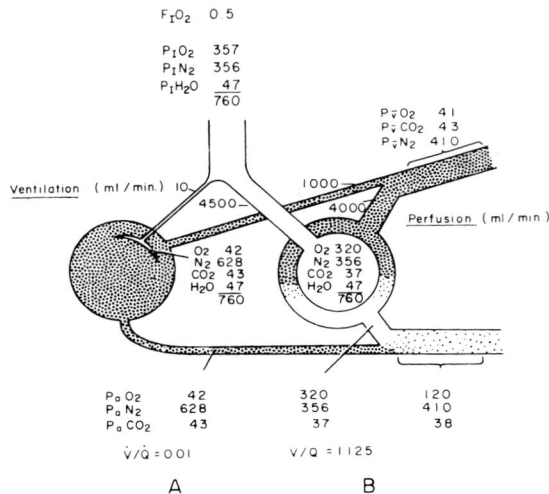

FIGURE 2–23. Effect of nitrogen on the alveolar-arterial P_{O_2} gradient and on the geometric integrity of terminal alveoli. For purposes of clarity, $\dot{V}/\dot{Q}$ maldistribution is exaggerated in a two-alveoli model on an $F_{I_{O_2}}$ of 0.5:

Alveolus A receives: 10 ml gas/min ($\dot{V}$)   } Therefore
                      1000 ml blood/min ($\dot{Q}$) } $\dot{V}/\dot{Q}$ = 0.01
                      5 ml O_2/min
                      5 ml N_2/min   ($F_{I_{O_2}}$ = 0.5)

Alveolus B receives: 4500 ml gas/min ($\dot{V}$)   } Therefore
                      400 ml blood/min ($\dot{Q}$)   } $\dot{V}/\dot{Q}$ = 1.125
                      2250 ml O_2/min
                      2250 ml N_2/min

The amount of oxygen absorbed into 100 ml of blood from alveolus A raises the end-capillary Pa_{O_2} from 41 mm Hg to 42 mm Hg, as seen in the diagram. This is obviously inadequate for full arterial saturation owing to the sharp inequality between ventilation and perfusion. Alveolus A also receives 5 ml/min of nitrogen. Solubility of nitrogen in blood is approximately half that of oxygen, so that nitrogen content is approximately 0.0015 ml/mm Hg/100 ml of whole blood. At a blood flow of 100 ml/min to alveolus A, the rise from pulmonary venous to end-capillary nitrogen (410–628 mm Hg) is associated with a nitrogen content uptake of 1000 × (628 − 410) × 0.0015/100 = 3.3 ml N_2/min. Therefore, in the example thus stated, gas delivery to alveolus A provides an excess of nitrogen in the face of inadequate oxygen.

If the inspired oxygen concentration is increased to 100% alveolus A receives 10 ml of O_2/min. If a normal arterial − mixed venous oxygen content difference $C(a − \bar{v})_{O_2}$ is assured, then to fully saturate 100 ml of blood, 400 ml O_2/min is needed. Clearly, 40 ml O_2/min delivered is inadequate to meet this demand. In the absence of small amounts of alveolar nitrogen, alveolus A collapses in this situation; that is, demand exceeds supply. Without structural nitrogen buttressing, the alveolus closes. (From Pontoppidan, H.: The black box illuminated. Anesthesiology, 37:1, 1972.)

lationship or in cardiac output. The changes produce temporary situations in which more or less oxygen will be taken up from each breath by the pulmonary blood flow until equilibrium between cellular oxygen consumption and oxygen delivery is re-established (Zinn et al., 1980).

2. The respiratory index or $(A-a)D_{O_2}/PA_{O_2}$ has been used as a comparator between various therapeutic trials within similar patient populations (Hegyi and Hiatt, 1981).

3. The a/A P_{O_2} ratio is useful for predicting the effects of a change in $F_{I_{O_2}}$ on subsequent arterial oxygenation at constant oxygenation with unchanged al-

veolar ventilation. The formula used is (Gross and Israel, 1981):

$$\frac{\text{old } Pa_{O_2}}{\text{old } PA_{O_2}} = \frac{\text{new } Pa_{O_2}}{\text{new } PA_{O_2}}$$

when

$$PA_{O_2} = (P_B − 47)(F_{I_{O_2}}) − \frac{Pa_{CO_2}}{R}$$

and

$$\text{new } F_{I_{O_2}} = \frac{(\text{new } Pa_{O_2})(\text{old } F_{I_{O_2}})}{\text{old } Pa_{O_2}}$$

$$+ \frac{\text{old } Pa_{CO_2}[1 − \text{new } Pa_{O_2}]}{R(P_B − 47)} \quad \text{old } Pa_{O_2}$$

4. Intrapulmonary shunt can be predicted from various tables given the arterial P_{O_2} and assuming constant pH, hemoglobin concentration, and oxygen consumption. An example of this is shown in Figure 2–25 (Benatar et al., 1973; Fournier and Major, 1981).

Oxygenation of arterial blood is a function of ade-

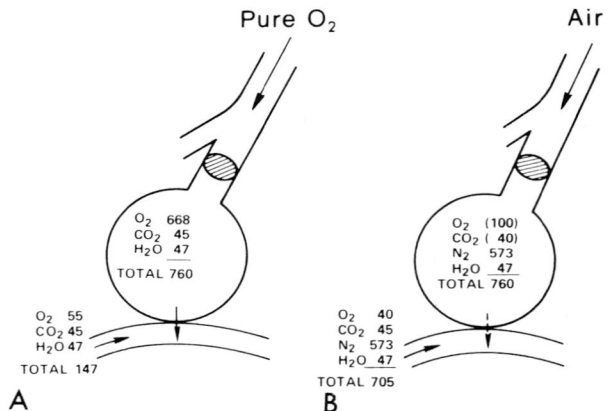

FIGURE 2–24. Absorption atelectasis—a comparison of oxygen and air breathing. In this example, a mucous plug produces a low $\dot{V}/\dot{Q}$ unit. Because the total pressure of the alveolar gas is 760 mm Hg, and if 100% O_2 is replaced as the inspired gas, the partial gas pressures of O_2, CO_2, and H_2O are as indicated. The sum of the gas partial pressures in mixed venous blood is much lower, because even if 100% O_2 is breathed, mixed venous oxygen tension does not increase significantly. Therefore, because there is a large partial pressure gradient between alveolus and pulmonary artery blood, absorption of gas from the alveolus is rapid. If gas inflow is inadequate to meet metabolic demand, the alveolus empties and collapse is inevitable. If the patient breathes air, although nitrogen is only half as soluble as oxygen in blood, eventually an equilibrium is reached, which leads to a much lower partial pressure gradient between alveolus and pulmonary artery blood. Therefore, the speed of gas absorption is slower and is dependent on the absorption of nitrogen. Nitrogen is a buffer against absorption atelectasis, although, unless the $\dot{V}/\dot{Q}$ ratio changes, alveolar collapse is inevitable ultimately. In B, O_2 and CO_2 values are shown in parentheses because they change with time. (A and B, From West, J. B.: Respiratory Physiology. 2nd ed. Copyright © 1979 by The Williams & Wilkins Company, Baltimore. Reproduced by permission.)

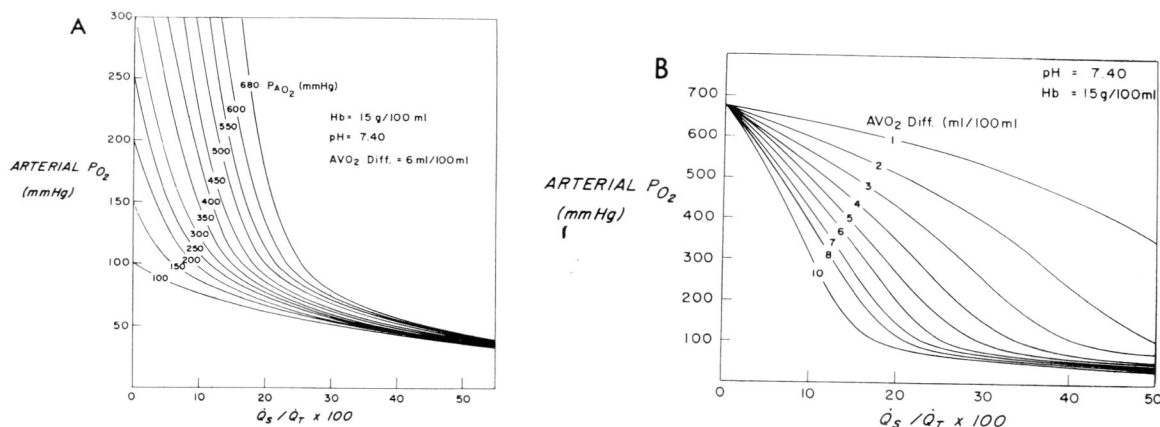

FIGURE 2-25. *A*, Relation between arterial P_{O_2} (Pa_{O_2}) and intrapulmonary right-to-left shunt at different levels of alveolar P_{O_2} (PA_{O_2}) or arteriovenous oxygen content differences (AVO_2 diff.). PA_{O_2} varies according to the inspired oxygen concentration. The curves were calculated on the basis of a standard oxyhemoglobin dissociation curve (i.e., P_{O_2} at 50% saturation = 26.6 mm Hg), a pH of 7.4, and a hemoglobin concentration of 15 g/100 ml. Note the convergence of arterial P_{O_2} values as $\dot{Q}_S/\dot{Q}_T \times 100$ rises. *B*, Effect of a change in the arterial minus mixed venous oxygen content (AVO_2 diff.) (secondary to an alteration in cardiac output or oxygen consumption) on arterial P_{O_2}. Note the sharp rise in arterial P_{O_2} as AVO_2 falls at moderate levels of right-to-left shunt (i.e., $\dot{Q}_S/\dot{Q}_T \times 100$, range of 10 to 20%). If $\dot{Q}_S/\dot{Q}_T \times 100 = 30\%$ and $AVO_2 = 8$ ml/100 ml, arterial P_{O_2} can be raised from approximately 80 to 400 mm Hg by a fourfold rise in cardiac output. (*A* and *B*, From Pontoppidan, H., Laver, M. B., and Geffin, B.: Acute respiratory failure in the surgical patient. Adv. Surg., 4:163–254, 1970. Graphs kindly prepared by Dr. M. A. Duvelleroy.)

quate matching of ventilation and perfusion. Gross changes in distribution or volume of gas flow, cardiac output, or regional perfusion affect oxygenation. This change is reflected in the $P(A-a)_{O_2}$, as can be seen in Table 2–2, or in the measured intrapulmonary shunt. It must be remembered that increased cardiac output at constant ventilation can produce an increased intrapulmonary shunt (Dantzker et al., 1980; Jardin et al., 1979; Siegel et al., 1979). This is seen by reconsidering the Fick equation, which provides that:

$$Q = \dot{V}_{O_2}/CA_{O_2} - C\overline{V}_{O_2}$$

Thus, at constant oxygen consumption, the arterial-venous oxygen content difference must increase as

■ **Table 2–2.** FACTORS THAT INFLUENCE THE ALVEOLAR-ARTERIAL OXYGEN TENSION DIFFERENCE $P(A-a)_{O_2}$*

1. Right-to-left shunt ($\dot{Q}_S/\dot{Q}_T \times 100$), i.e., percentage of cardiac output ($\dot{Q}_T$) flowing past nonventilated alveoli ($\dot{Q}_S$).
2. Arteriovenous oxygen content difference $C(a-\overline{v})_{O_2}$.
3. Oxygen consumption ($\dot{V}_{O_2}$) $\dot{Q}_T = \dot{V}_{O_2}/C(a-\overline{v})_{O_2}$.
4. Cardiac output ($\dot{Q}_T$)
   A. Secondary to change in $C[a - q\ \overline{v}_{DO_2}]$ when oxygen consumption ($\dot{V}_{O_2}$) remains constant $\dot{Q}_T = \dot{V}_{O_2}/C(a-\overline{v})_{O_2}$.
   B. Secondary to redistribution of pulmonary blood flow.
5. Inspired oxygen concentration (uneven distribution plays a greater role when less than 100% oxygen is inspired).
6. Position of the hemoglobin-oxygen dissociation curve (pH, body temperature, red blood cell 2,3-disphosphoglyceric acid concentration).
7. Position of the arterial point (PA_{O_2}) on the oxygen-hemoglobin dissociation curve; i.e, above or below full saturation.

From Laver, M. B., and Austen, W. G.: Respiratory function: Physiologic considerations applicable to surgery. *In* Sabiston, D. C., Jr. (ed): Davis-Christopher Textbook of Surgery. 12th ed. Philadelphia, W. B. Saunders, 1981.

*Not included is the influence of a change in distribution of ventilation or body position as discussed in the text.

cardiac output decreases, which is reflected as increased pulmonary efficiency, although the practical aspects of this situation are opposite. Therefore, following the level of the shunt fraction may create a false sense of security if the ultimate objective of tissue oxygen delivery is not remembered.

There are more sophisticated methods for measuring ventilation-perfusion relationships in the acutely diseased lung. They involve the infusion of several gases with different blood solubility coefficients into the pulmonary venous circulation and the measurement of the expired concentrations of these gases. Calculation of $\dot{V}_A/Q$ is made according to the quantities retained when these gases pass through the lung into the arterial circulation (Rehder et al., 1979; West, 1979).

Carbon Dioxide Removal

As previously stated, an imbalance between ventilation and perfusion may alter the removal of carbon dioxide. At one extreme, this is seen as the continued ventilation of a nonperfused alveolus, which produces wasted ventilation and has the same effect as adding dead-space tubing to a ventilator circuit or rebreathing into a closed paper bag.

The amount of carbon dioxide expired with each breath depends on the respiratory exchange ratio and thus on total carbon dioxide production ($\dot{V}_{CO_2}$). It consists of the volume of CO_2 in the gas from ventilated and perfused alveoli, which can be expressed as $\dot{V}_A \times PA_{CO_2}$. A proportion of expired gas comes from the anatomic dead space (V_{Danat}) and from areas of unstable ventilation/perfusion ratios, which help form the variable physiologic dead space (V_{Dphys}). This concept can be expressed as $\dot{V}_D = V_{Dphys} +$

VD_{anat}, and the contribution of CO_2 from dead-space areas is $VD \times PD_{CO_2}$. Then, $VD \times PD_{CO_2} + \dot{V}A \times PA_{CO_2}$ equals the total volume of exhaled gas (VE) times the mixed expired carbon dioxide concentration ($P\bar{E}_{CO_2}$), or

$$VE \times P\bar{E}_{CO_2} = VD \times PD_{CO_2} + \dot{V}A \times PA_{CO_2}$$

We can assume that $PA_{CO_2} = Pa_{CO_2}$, that VD_{CO_2} is zero, and that $\dot{V}A = VE - VD$; then

$$VT \times P\bar{E}_{CO_2} = (VT - VD) \times Pa_{CO_2}$$

This equation may be rewritten as:

$$VD/VT = \frac{Pa_{CO_2} - P\bar{E}_{CO_2}}{Pa_{CO_2}} = 1 - \frac{P\bar{E}_{CO_2}}{Pa_{CO_2}}$$

An increase in the calculated VD/VT ratio implies a decreased efficiency of carbon dioxide removal and requires an increase in either tidal volume or ventilatory rate if Pa_{CO_2} is to remain constant. The normal ratio of dead space to tidal volume is 0.2 to 0.35 during resting breathing (West, 1979). Potential sources of increased physiologic dead space in the perioperative period are diagrammed in Figure 2–26. The most common causes of continued ventilation of a nonperfused segment of lung are pulmonary embolism, hypotension, and a decreased cardiac output. In chronic obstructive lung disease, high $\dot{V}/\dot{Q}$ areas are probably due to the capillary obstruction found in emphysema, so that areas are still ventilated but receive little perfusion. Absence of shunt and low $\dot{V}/\dot{Q}$ areas in the face of severe obstruction probably reflect lack of sputum and good collateral ventilation. It is interesting to note that when patients with chronic obstructive lung disease are given 100% oxygen to breathe, the arterial PO_2 fails to increase as expected, probably because of a slow nitrogen washout rate, which delays the rise in PA_{O_2}. Therefore, arterial PO_2 does not distinguish between shunt and $\dot{V}/\dot{Q}$ anomaly in these patients, and shunt is greatly overestimated. In patients with advanced, generalized interstitial lung disease, two populations of lung units can be recognized: units able to maintain normal $\dot{V}/\dot{Q}$ ratios in spite of severe disease and essentially destroyed units associated with near-zero ventilation but some continued perfusion. There is a striking absence of units with intermediate to low $\dot{V}/\dot{Q}$ ratios, which is currently not understood (Wagner, 1978).

Other important considerations in the immediate postoperative period are temperature changes and the effect of shivering with its coincident increase in carbon dioxide production. This may be associated with respiratory depression following the use of narcotic analgesics and may cause significant respiratory acidosis during recovery from anesthesia. The patient with a low postoperative core temperature, who paradoxically may be vasodilated peripherally secondary to the use of a volatile anesthetic agent, is at risk for carbon dioxide retention in the recovery period. This is accentuated if the patient begins to shiver and increases his metabolic demands. For this reason, prophylactic oxygen is administered by face mask or T tube to any patient in the postoperative recovery area who has received a general anesthetic. All such patients have depressed ventilatory drive. Unlike the hypoxemia secondary to intrapulmonary shunt, the hypoxia and attendant hypercarbia of hypoventilation are easily eliminated with small quantities of supplemental oxygen. The following example should clarify this point: $Pa_{O_2} = 55$; $Pa_{CO_2} = 60$; $pH = 7.24$; $FI_{O_2} = 0.21$. Although the degree of acidosis and hypercarbia may require treatment, administration of 40% inspired oxygen by mask provides the following change: At 40% inspired O_2, what will the predicted Pa_{O_2} be, assuming constant ventilation?

$$Pa_{O_2} \, 40\% = \frac{Pa_{O_2} \, 21\%}{PA_2 \, 21\%} \times PA_{O_2} \, 40\%$$

$$= \frac{55}{90} \times 225 = 137$$

Therefore, although problems of acidosis may be significant, arterial hypoxemia secondary to pure hypoventilation can be prevented easily with an increase in inspired oxygen concentration.

Another easily avoided situation that may lead to unacceptable carbon dioxide retention is an improperly set or functioning mechanical ventilator. The system must include all airway connections and the endotracheal tube cuff seal. Alveolar ventilation is proportional to carbon dioxide production and inversely proportional to alveolar carbon dioxide pressure. This relationship is expressed as:

$$\dot{V}A = \frac{0.863 \times \dot{V}_{CO_2}}{PA_{CO_2}}$$

where 0.863 is a conversion factor required to change units from standard temperature and pressure, dry gas phase (STPD), which is used in the calculation of $\dot{V}_{CO_2}$, to body temperature and atmospheric pressure, saturated gas phase, which is used for measurement of $\dot{V}A$. By following end-expired carbon dioxide partial pressure, insight into the adequacy of mechanical ventilation can be assessed, and conjectures about the distribution of ventilation can be made also. These concepts will be discussed in the section on mechanical ventilation.

All the equations relating to cardiac output and physiologic shunt previously solved using oxygen as a monitor can also be computed using carbon dioxide production and excretion as the monitor. For example, an increase in cardiac output at constant alveolar ventilation decreases dead space–to–expired tidal volume ratio, and carbon dioxide removal is enhanced. The parallel for oxygen is that this situation is reflected as an increase in shunt fraction due to perfusion of nonventilated alveoli.

Table 2–3 shows the effect of aging on arterial PO_2 and PCO_2 at rest during ambient-air breathing. It is always useful to compare a patient's values with the

SOURCES OF MIXED ARTERIAL TO MEAN ALVEOLAR CO$_2$ GRADIENTS

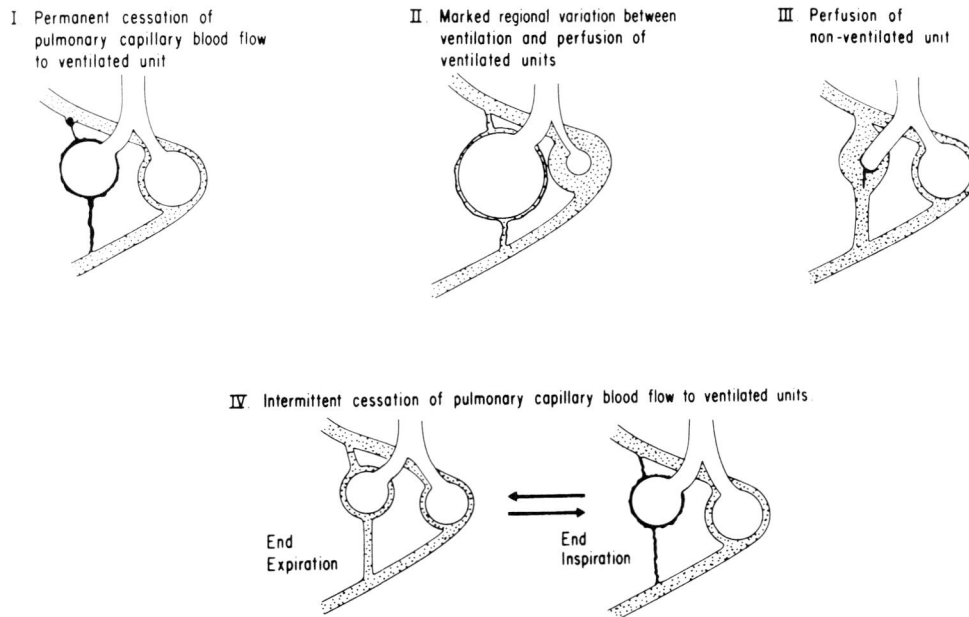

I. Permanent cessation of pulmonary capillary blood flow to ventilated unit

II. Marked regional variation between ventilation and perfusion of ventilated units

III. Perfusion of non-ventilated unit

IV. Intermittent cessation of pulmonary capillary blood flow to ventilated units

End Expiration

End Inspiration

FIGURE 2–26. Increased postoperative physiologic dead space secondary to abnormal $\dot{V}/\dot{Q}$. *Zone 1 (shown as I):* Permanent or transient cessation of pulmonary artery flow to a continuously ventilated unit results in wasted ventilation. This condition is seen in hypotension, postural changes, and pulmonary embolism (see Fig. 2–13). *Zone 2:* Marked regional difference in ventilation and perfusion is seen during thoracotomy (see Figs. 2–12 and 2–14) and in patients with chronic obstructive lung disease (COLD). Changes seen in COLD are presumably secondary to the variable emptying time constants of individual units of the lung. *Zone 3:* Perfusion of a nonventilated unit (shunt) not only causes hypoxemia, but also increases arterial P_{CO_2}. This occurs in a manner analogous to the reduction in oxygenation seen with desaturated blood entering the pulmonary vein; i.e., blood with a high carbon dioxide level that comes from these units enters pulmonary venous blood and elevates in CO_2 content. This is a "pseudo" dead-space effect. *Zone 4:* Intermittent cessation of pulmonary capillary blood flow to ventilated units occurs in Zone 4 regions of the lung previously described. These areas increase in patients suffering from acute respiratory failure, who require high airway pressures to provide adequate ventilation. In these patients, the lungs are variably noncompliant, and overdistention of the more compliant alveoli rather than recruitment of collapsed segments compress interalveolar blood vessels and cause an increase in apparent dead space (i.e., areas of ventilation without adequate perfusion). (From Laver, M. B., and Austen, W. G.: Respiratory function: Physiologic considerations applicable to surgery. *In* Sabiston, D. C., Jr. [ed]: Davis-Christopher Textbook of Surgery. 12th ed. Philadelphia, W. B. Saunders, 1981.)

expected normal values at a given age. Carbon dioxide exchange is well maintained with increased age, whereas arterial oxygenation decreases, perhaps owing to the decrease in elastic properties of the lungs. These features are discussed in the next section, which considers the diffusion of gas between atmospheric air and the capillary blood.

GAS DIFFUSION INSPIRED AIR AND PULMONARY CAPILLARY BLOOD

Oxygenation of pulmonary capillary blood occurs secondary to the large partial pressure gradient of oxygen between inspired air and mixed venous blood. Consumption of oxygen by tissue metabolism is responsible for the desaturation of mixed venous blood. At the same time, aerobic metabolism produces the waste product carbon dioxide, which is transported in venous blood in three forms (dissolved, as bicarbonate, and in combination with proteins) and excreted in the lungs. The overall concentration gradient for carbon dioxide is far less than that for oxygen,

and the relative importance of ventilation versus perfusion can be seen by studying blood-gas changes in apnea. During apnea for periods as long as 55 minutes with the endotracheal tube attached to a reservoir of oxygen, blood flowing through the lung continues to take up oxygen, and arterial saturation remains high. Tissue metabolism appears to be unaffected during this procedure. The partial pressure of oxygen in the reservoir is almost atmospheric, whereas that in the mixed venous blood is approximately 40 mm Hg. This gradient (greater than 700 mm Hg if 100% oxygen is placed in the reservoir) is sufficient for oxygen to be supplied almost as fast as it is removed by blood flow. Conversely, the carbon dioxide gradient is significantly less (mixed venous P_{CO_2} is 45 to 55 mm Hg, and P_{CO_2} in the upper airway is almost zero) in the region of 50 mm Hg. This gradient is insufficient to allow adequate removal of carbon dioxide solely by diffusion. The rate of rise of carbon dioxide in the steady state is readily predictable, and values of 3 to 4 mm Hg/min of apnea are seen clinically (Loeschke et al., 1953; Frumin et al., 1959; Eger and Severinghaus, 1961).

■ **Table 2–3.** EFFECT OF AGE ON ARTERIAL P_{O_2} AND P_{CO_2} WHILE BREATHING AMBIENT AIR AT REST

Age Group (in Years)	No. Obs.	$P_{A_{O_2}}$ Mean	± SD (mm Hg)	$P_{A_{CO_2}}$ Mean	± SD (mm Hg)
< 30 (median = 23)	38	94.2	3.31	39.0	1.8
31–40 (median = 36)	30	87.2	3.47	38.5	2.0
41–50 (median = 46)	30	83.9	4.07	39.6	2.4
51–60 (median = 55)	30	81.2	3.74	39.0	1.9
> 60 (median = 71)	24	74.3	4.43	39.8	2.1

From Sorbini, C. A., Grassi, V., Solinas, E., and Muiesan, G.: Arterial oxygen tension in relation to age in healthy subjects. Respiration, 25:3, 1968.

Diffusion through tissues is described by Fick's law of diffusion, which states that the rate of transfer of a gas through a tissue sheet is (1) proportional to the tissue area and the difference in gas partial pressure between the two sides and (2) inversely proportional to the tissue thickness. In the lung, the surface area of the blood-gas barrier is large, and the thickness of the alveolar-capillary membrane is negligible. Therefore, the barrier dimensions are ideally suited for gas diffusion. In addition, the rate of transfer is proportional to a diffusion constant, which is proportional to the solubility of the gas and inversely proportional to the square root of the molecular weight. These relationships are illustrated in Figure 2–27. Practically, this means that oxygen diffuses slightly more rapidly than carbon dioxide in air, but that carbon dioxide is approximately 20 times more rapid than oxygen in diffusing through tissue sheets because it has a much higher solubility. The implication of gas solubility in

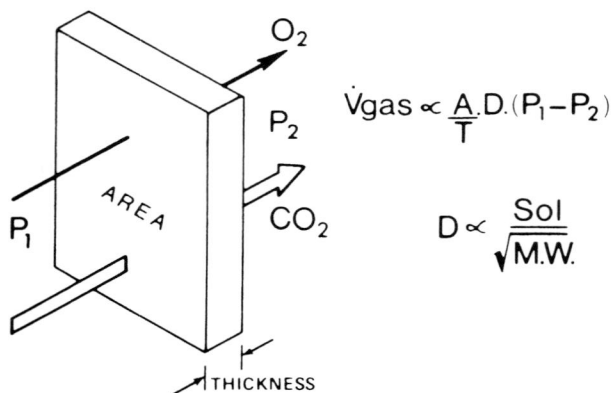

FIGURE 2–27. Fick's law of diffusion through a tissue sheet. The amount of gas transferred per unit time ($\dot{V}$ gas) is proportional to the tissue surface area (A), a diffusion constant (D), and the partial pressure difference across the sheet ($P_1 - P_2$). Initially, the relationship was stated for the concentration difference across the sheet, but partial pressure is clinically more applicable. $\dot{V}$ gas is inversely proportional to the thickness of the tissue sheet. D is proportional to the solubility of the gas, but inversely proportional to the square root of its molecular weight.

Because the surface area of the lung blood gas barrier is approximately 50 to 100 m^2 and its thickness is less than 0.5 μm, the barrier characteristics are ideally suited for diffusion. In comparing O_2 and CO_2 despite their similar molecular weights, it is seen that CO_2 diffuses across the barrier about 20 times more rapidly than O_2 because it has a higher solubility. (From West, J. B.: Respiratory Physiology. 2nd ed. Copyright © 1979 by The Williams & Wilkins Company, Baltimore. Reproduced by permission.)

blood raises an important consideration that is of practical importance in pulmonary function testing and in general anesthesia. A gas that binds to the hemoglobin molecule within the red cell is taken up with almost no increase in partial pressure of the gas across the alveolar-capillary membrane. Therefore, the gas continues to move rapidly across the alveolar wall. The quantity of this gas that will pass across the alveolar wall is limited, not by the amount of blood flowing through the capillary bed, but rather by the diffusion characteristics of the blood-gas barrier. Carbon monoxide binds rapidly to hemoglobin, and the partial pressure within the blood rises quickly. This in turn causes a significant back pressure of gas across the alveolar wall, and diffusion will cease until more gas can be removed by a fresh inflow of blood. A corollary can be drawn to explain the slower onset of action of an inhalation anesthetic with a low blood-gas partition coefficient (low solubility in blood) in patients with decreased cardiac output—that is, transfer of the agent depends on cardiac output. Low cardiac output states thus delay the necessary rise in brain partial pressure of the agent necessary to produce anesthesia. An example of an agent with low blood solubility is nitrous oxide. Nitrous oxide transfer is therefore said to be perfusion-limited. Halothane, enflurane, and isoflurane, however, are much more soluble in blood and provide a more rapid onset of anesthesia as long as minute ventilation is well maintained. The depression of cardiac output that accompanies use of these drugs does not usually delay the induction of anesthesia.

There are two major barriers to the transfer of a gas from the alveolus to the red cell. The first is the alveolar-capillary membrane (M), and the second is the rate of reaction (O) between the hemoglobin molecule and the gas (carbon monoxide is the tracer gas used in testing diffusion capacity). As previously stated, the amount of gas transferred across a sheet of tissue by diffusion is expressed as:

$$\dot{V}_{gas} = \frac{A}{T} \times D \times (P_1 - P_2)$$

For the lung, the thickness of the barrier cannot be measured, and the preceding equation is rewritten using the concept of the lung diffusing capacity as:

$$\dot{V}_{gas} = D_L \times (P_1 - P_2)$$

For carbon monoxide, the diffusing capacity is expressed as:

$$D_L = \frac{\dot{V}_{CO}}{P_1 - P_2}$$

However, the partial pressure of carbon monoxide in capillary blood is negligible. Therefore, this can be rewritten as:

$$D_L = \frac{\dot{V}_{CO}}{P_{A_{CO}}}$$

Thus, the diffusing capacity of the lung for carbon monoxide is the volume of carbon monoxide transferred in milliliters per minute per millimeter of mercury of alveolar partial pressure.

To combine the reaction rate of combination of carbon monoxide with hemoglobin (the second barrier to gas transfer) with the membrane diffusion barrier described earlier, an analogue of electrical resistance can be used by taking the inverse of D_L. The combination of reaction rate and diffusion barrier can now be expressed as:

$$\frac{1}{D_L} = \frac{1}{D_M} + \frac{1}{O \times V_C}$$

where V_C is the volume of capillary blood and gives the effective diffusing capacity of the rate of gas combination with hemoglobin. In practice, the resistances offered by the membrane and blood components are approximately equal. This concept is diagrammed in Figure 2–28. Figure 2–29 shows the time course for oxygen in the pulmonary capillary for normal and abnormal diffusion states. The time course for oxygen

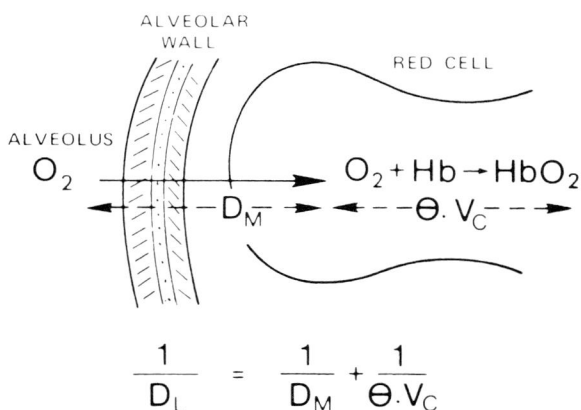

FIGURE 2–28. The two components that make up the diffusing capacity of the lung (D_L). The first component is that previously described in Figure 2–27; i.e., that due to the diffusion process. The other consideration concerns the time taken for oxygen (or any tracer gas such as carbon dioxide used in the clinical measurement of D_L) to react with hemoglobin ($\theta \cdot V_C$). Carbon dioxide is used in clinical practice because of its high affinity for hemoglobin. (From West, J. B.: Respiratory Physiology. 2nd ed. Copyright © 1979 by The Williams & Wilkins Company, Baltimore. Reproduced by permission.)

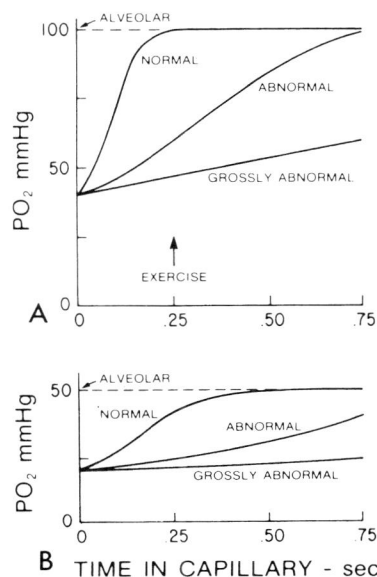

FIGURE 2–29. Oxygen time courses in the pulmonary capillary for normal and abnormal diffusion states. A, Time course for normal alveolar P_{O_2}. B, Slower time for oxygenation when alveolar P_{O_2} is low. Exercise decreases the time available for oxygenation in both states. Normally, a red blood cell takes approximately 0.75 second to pass through a capillary. Therefore, in most instances adequate oxygenation occurs. However, in disease states such as sepsis in which alveolar-capillary membrane dysfunction occurs coincident with increased metabolic demands (i.e., the organism is exposed to stresses similar to those seen in exercise), oxygenation may become inadequate and arterial hypoxia develops. (A and B, From West, J. B.: Respiratory Physiology. 2nd ed. Copyright © 1979 by The Williams & Wilkins Company, Baltimore. Reproduced by permission.)

transfer lies between that of carbon monoxide and nitrous oxide. Unlike nitrous oxide, oxygen combines with hemoglobin, but far less avidly and rapidly than carbon monoxide does. Under normal conditions, oxygen transfer across the capillary membrane is supported by enormous diffusion reserves. However, this situation changes if either $P_{A_{O_2}}$ is decreased (e.g., by breathing a hypoxic gas mixture or breathing at altitude) or the membrane becomes less diffusible to the oxygen molecule.

The two respiratory gases of concern are carbon dioxide and oxygen, both of which are adequately transferred under normal conditions in the lung. Carbon dioxide requires more time to achieve equilibrium because of the associated carbonic anhydrase reaction and shift of chloride from plasma into erythrocyte to maintain electrical neutrality. An exposure time of 150 msec is required if pulmonary venous blood is to be in equilibrium with alveolar gas. In conditions of severe pulmonary dysfunction in which both membrane permeability and contact time are altered, changes in oxygen and carbon dioxide homeostasis are common.

ACID–BASE BALANCE

A comprehensive review of acid-base balance cannot be presented within the limits of a chapter on respiratory physiology. However, a brief description of the common abnormalities observed in the perioperative period complements the preceding discussions concerning ventilation-perfusion ratios. Although an apparent mystique has grown up around the subject of acid-base balance, it is important to state that the core of the problem is not discovery of an amount of "buffer base" or "fixed cation" but rather maintenance of the hydrogen ion concentration of the extracellular fluid. Dietary proteins contain sulfate and phosphate groups that, when protein is metabolized, remain as H_2SO_4 and H_3PO_4. The hydrogen ion load from this source is approximately 150 mEq/day. The carbon dioxide formed by metabolism in the tissue is in large part hydrated to H_2CO_3, and the total hydrogen ion source from this load is over 12,500 mEq/day. Most of the CO_2 is excreted in the lungs, and only small quantities of the hydrogen ion from this source are excreted by the kidneys.

Common sources of extra acid loads are strenuous exercise or tissue hypoperfusion (lactic acid), dietetic ketosis (acetoacetic and β-hydroxybutyric acid), and ingestion of acidifying salts such as ammonium and calcium chloride, which, in effect, add hydrochloric acid to the body. Failure of diseased kidneys to excrete the normal acid load is also a cause of acidosis. Fruits are the main dietary source of alkali. They contain sodium and potassium salts of weak organic acids, and the anions of these salts are metabolized to carbon dioxide, leaving $NaHCO_3$ and $KHCO_3$ in the body. A common source of alkalosis is loss of acid from the body due to vomiting of gastric juice rich in hydrochloric acid. A more insidious alkalosis occurs following diuretic administration in which sodium and potassium excretion are artificially elevated and adequate replacement of these electrolytes is neglected. This leads to an excessive kaliuresis, and potassium is replaced by hydrogen ion to maintain electrical charge neutrality in the urine. This, in turn, leads to severe depletion of hydrogen and potassium ions, with resultant metabolic alkalosis, which may prolong the weaning period from mechanical ventilatory assistance (Gallagher, 1979).

Historically, the development of knowledge of acid-base balance can be outlined as follows:

The law of mass action states that the ratio of the product of the ionized components to that of the unionized components of a solution at equilibrium is equal to a constant, or:

$$K = \frac{[H^+][A^-]}{[HA]} \quad (1)$$

and that the dissociation of an acid can be expressed as:

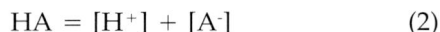

$$HA = [H^+] + [A^-] \quad (2)$$

1908: Henderson rearranged (1) for blood buffers:

$$H = K\frac{[HA]}{[A^-]} = \frac{[H_2CO_3]}{[HCO_3]} \quad (3)$$

1912: Sorensen established "puissance hydrogen" (the power of hydrogen), or pH, as the negative logarithm of the hydrogen ion concentration.

1916: Hasselbalch stated (3) in negative logarithmic form:

$$pH = pK + \log\frac{[H_2CO_3]}{[HCO_3]}$$

This can be simplified to:

$$pH = 6.1 + \log[HCO_3] \text{ or } 0.03 \times P_{CO_2}\frac{kidney}{lung}$$

where 6.1 = the pKA of carbonic acid and 0.03 is the solubility of CO_2 gas dissolved in blood.

Most of the buffering action occurs within 1 pH unit of the pK of the buffering system. The most important intravascular buffering system is the carbonic acid–bicarbonate buffer pair, or:

$$pH = 6.1 + \log[HCO_3] \text{ or } [H^+] = \frac{24\ P_{CO_2}}{[HCO_3]}$$

where 24 equals the numerical value of the Bunsen coefficient of $CO_2 \times KH_2CO_3$. Because its pK is 6.2, its buffering capacity at a pH of 7.4 is poor. The division of buffering between (H_2CO_3) and P_{CO_2} leads to the commonly named metabolic and respiratory components of acid-base balance:

$$P_{CO_2}\ (lungs)$$
$$\downarrow$$
$$CO_2 + H_2O = H_2CO_3 = H^+ + HCO_3$$
$$\downarrow$$
$$kidney$$

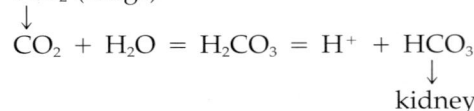

1920: van Slyke described a manometric method for the measurement of CO_2 content.

1922: Hughes described the operation of a glass electrode for the measurement of pH based on Sorenson's work in the early 1900s, noting a voltage differential between two sides of a thin glass membrane placed in fermenting beer and yeast cultures.

1923: Bronsted defined an acid as a molecule capable of giving off a hydrogen ion and a base as one capable of taking up a hydrogen ion. Stadie developed a functional electron tube voltmeter necessary for measurement of voltage changes across the glass membranes of the electrodes.

1948: Hastings and Singer defined "buffer base."

1950s: Astrup, Siggard-Anderson, Engle, and Jorgensen defined and described base excess and standard bicarbonate.

1956: Clark developed the oxygen electrode.

By the late 1950s, theory, experimentation, and technology had coalesced. This enabled clinicians to obtain acid-base determinations and to ascertain the state of arterial oxygenation of their patients as routine test procedures. Today, major surgical operations of all kinds, especially thoracic and thoracoabdominal procedures, are performed with an indwelling arterial cannula. This is useful, not only for monitoring blood pressure on a continuous basis, but also for immediate access to arterial blood samples for determination of a wide range of variables. Soon, optodes will be available for continuous invasive blood gas measurement. In the absence of this invasive technology, however, noninvasive pulse oximetry and capnography are routinely used in all anesthetizing locations and aid greatly in the management of any patient with abnormalities of cardiac or respiratory function. The most commonly used values with direct bearing on the subject matter of this chapter are P_{O_2}, pH, P_{CO_2}, bicarbonate, base excess, oxygen saturation, carboxyhemoglobin saturation, methemoglobin saturation, reduced hemoglobin, and total oxygen content. The blood-gas analyzers in clinical use base all measurements at a temperature of 37° C, which is maintained carefully within the sample chamber. For this reason, correction of measured blood-gas values to the patient temperature has been considered a clinical necessity. The P_{O_2}, P_{CO_2}, and pH of a sample of blood are temperature-dependent, and correction of P_{O_2} to patient temperature has been well described (Nunn, 1970).

However, controversy has arisen about whether or not pH and P_{CO_2} values should be temperature-corrected (Ream et al., 1982). Hemoglobin saturation is temperature-independent; direct measurement of this variable (e.g., with a CO-oximeter) will give maximal information about oxygen transport. In those cases in which saturation is not measured, P_{O_2} values can be temperature-corrected with reference to a standard nomogram (Nunn, 1977). However, the clinician independently should decide whether or not to correct measured values for pH and P_{CO_2} also (Williams and Marshall, 1982). In addition, the clinician must realize that some of the aforementioned values are measured directly, and others are calculated. The directly measured parameters in a blood-gas analyzer are pH, P_{O_2}, and P_{CO_2}, from which is calculated the bicarbonate value. Specific concerns about adequate oxygen transport are raised during cardiopulmonary bypass at greatly reduced temperatures. The solubility of carbon dioxide in blood increases when blood with a constant oxygen content is cooled. This forces more carbon dioxide into solution, reducing the gaseous form. In turn, this causes a temperature-dependent decrease in P_{CO_2} and an increase in pH. During cardiopulmonary bypass and in the immediate postoperative period when marked temperature gradients exist, gross differences in pH and P_{CO_2} measurements may be noted. With "alpha-stat" management, the blood gases are measured at 37° C and reported directly. In "pH-stat" management, the blood gases are measured in the same fashion, remembering that the analyzers maintain 37° C internally within tight limits, but then the values are "corrected" to the patient's temperature at the time of sampling using standard nomograms.

There is no universal agreement on measurement standardization or management technique. However, the clinician must be aware of the norms used in his or her institution in order to understand the results and their impact upon patient management. For example, at the reduced temperatures used during cardiopulmonary bypass, maintenance of a temperature-corrected P_{CO_2} of 40 mm Hg may cause excessive amounts of dissolved carbon dioxide in the blood. In turn, this causes cerebral hyperperfusion through the mechanism of hypercarbic dilatation of the central vasculature (Smith, 1992).

The CO-oximeter measures hemoglobin by a colorimetric method that depends on analysis of the red cells with a zero buffer reference solution. Reduced hemoglobin is then measured specifically, and this value is used subsequently in the calculation of base excess. Specific wavelengths also measure oxyhemoglobin, carboxyhemoglobin, and methemoglobin saturation. Total oxygen content is calculated from oxyhemoglobin saturation and the measured hemoglobin concentration. It is important to realize the interrelationship between measured and calculated values, because significant mistakes can be made if therapeutic decisions are made on data that are biologically inappropriate.

Primary derangements in acid-base balance in the perioperative period are seen secondary to alterations in carbon dioxide production or removal, low cardiac output and peripheral hypoperfusion, and electrolyte imbalance.

During thoracotomy and major abdominal procedures, large tissue areas are exposed. Evaporation and diffusion of body fluids may lead to profound temperature loss. In the recovery area, temperatures as low as 32 to 33° C are not uncommon. As patients are rewarmed, several problems may develop that affect acid-base homeostasis. Initially, peripheral vasoconstriction and poor peripheral perfusion may promote anaerobiasis and lactic acid production, which produces a metabolic acidosis (i.e., an acid pH with normal P_{CO_2} and base deficit more negative than -2). Subsequently, the forced vasodilation or rewarming may exacerbate the metabolic acidosis unless adequate volume infusion is maintained to support circulating blood volume as an increased number of vascular beds are recruited. Also, if the patient begins to shiver during this period, carbon dioxide production increases and adequacy of minute alveolar ventilation requires reassessment by frequent referral to arterial blood-gas values or, in appropriate cases, capnography data.

Metabolic alkalosis in association with electrolyte imbalance is a common finding in the postoperative period. The condition may follow large infusions of *acid citrate dextrose* (ACD) blood or inappropriate continuation of Ringer's lactate solution following resuscitation. Following cardiopulmonary bypass, patients frequently receive large doses of loop diuretics in an attempt to decrease the extravascular crystalloid load received during the pump run. This iatrogenic, electrolyte-losing (especially potassium ion) diuresis promotes hydrogen ion loss at the nephron. In turn, despite continuous potassium replacement, this often leads to a metabolic alkalosis, which compounds the respiratory acidosis commonly seen following anesthesia and analgesic administration in the postoperative period. Metabolic alkalosis has been shown to prolong weaning time from mechanical ventilatory assistance (Gallagher, 1979). Chronic diuretic therapy creates a situation of total body potassium deficit, and intracellular potassium deficiencies are common despite normal serum potassium values (Schimert et al., 1966). Carbon dioxide homeostasis and its relationship to mechanical ventilation are discussed later.

The ready availability of arterial blood-gas determinations with measured base deficit has made the routine correction of metabolic acidosis by administration of sodium bicarbonate a common clinical practice. Until recently, bicarbonate administration during cardiopulmonary resuscitation was recommended based on the time course of the cardiac arrest according to the following formula (CPR Guidelines, 1980):

$$\text{Required } (HCO_3) \text{ mEq/l} = \text{Measured base excess} \times 0.2 \text{ (body weight)}$$

The body weight is measured in kilograms, and 0.2 is the factor used to approximate the value of the extracellular space. Common practice called for administration of one-half to one-third of the calculated value, because full therapeutic correction may cause profound metabolic alkalosis if resuscitation has been rapid. However, more recent evidence supports the association of bicarbonate use during resuscitation with the production of paradoxic intracellular acidosis, and this has led the American Heart Association to alter recommendations for bicarbonate administration during resuscitation (1987). New standards support the use of sodium bicarbonate only after other definitive interventions, such as endotracheal intubation with appropriate ventilation, chest compressions to produce an effective circulation, and early defibrillation, have been initiated. This change is based on the fact that acidosis, per se, may be less detrimental to cardiac function than the elevated levels of carbon dioxide (respiratory acidosis) seen with inadequate ventilation. Even modest respiratory compensation of metabolic acidosis can prevent intracellular acidosis (Adler et al., 1965), whereas administration of sodium bicarbonate causes the rapid generation of carbon dioxide, which is a potent negative inotrope. Myocardial function is closely related to the carbon dioxide tension; newer recommendations suggest minimizing the role of sodium bicarbonate and using other methods to ensure adequate correction of the mixed metabolic and respiratory acidosis attendant upon cardiac arrest. The use of end-tidal CO_2 monitors during ventilation in an arrest situation is gaining popularity (Weil, 1988). Additionally, new research into the differences between arterial and mixed venous pH levels may improve insight into the most appropriate resuscitation techniques. In summary, rapid restoration of pH to normal values with bicarbonate infusion based

on arterial blood gas analysis can no longer be recommended for routine practice.

Respiratory acidosis secondary to accumulation of carbon dioxide is a well-recognized postoperative problem following all surgical procedures in which narcotic analgesics are employed. However, with the advent of intermittent ventilatory modes, it is becoming more common to follow changes in arterial pH and not Pco_2. Many patients show a high normal pH with high Pco_2 secondary to previously mentioned metabolic changes. Although Pco_2 can be lowered by mechanical ventilation, the underlying metabolic alkalosis will be worsened, and weaning will be prolonged. Vigorous correction of serum potassium deficits, use of acetazolamide (Diamox) to decrease bicarbonate concentration by promoting an alkaline diuresis, and judicious infusion of dilute solutions of hydrochloric acid or ingestion of ammonium chloride may ameliorate this complex situation, which prolongs the requirement of mechanical ventilatory assistance.

PREOPERATIVE EVALUATION OF PULMONARY FUNCTION

In animals where there is no circulation there can be no lungs; for lungs are an apparatus for the air and blood to meet, and can only accord with motion of blood in vessels.
. . . As the lungs are to expose the blood to the air, they are so constructed as to answer this purpose exactly with the blood being brought to them, and so disposed in them as to go hand in hand.

John Hunter
(*Philosophical Transactions*, 66:412, 1776)

The purpose of respiration is to carry off the putrid effluvium or to discharge that phlogiston which had been taken into the system with the aliment.

Joseph Priestley
(*Philosophical Transactions*, 66:226, 1776)

These two statements reflect the long interest in and concern about the interrelated functions of the heart and lungs. Not only is the expert performance of surgery and anesthesia mandatory for the successful outcome of major thoracic and cardiac procedures, but also, as techniques of prolonged life support have become more sophisticated, accurate prediction of the long-term effect of operation on pulmonary function has become mandatory. An operation would be contraindicated if the result required lifelong mechanical ventilatory support for adequate pulmonary function. Of greater importance, accurate prediction of preoperative risk factors that could be modified in the perioperative period might be expected to decrease postoperative pulmonary morbidity. Unfortunately, although a highly sophisticated testing apparatus is now available, the ability to predict outcome or to prevent complications is still inexact and depends to a great extent on the desire and motivation of the patient.

The goal of pulmonary function testing is to identify low- and high-risk surgical patients so that preoperative and postoperative measures can be attempted to decrease morbidity. Unfortunately, "the assessment of risk is based on statistics, which, although they apply to groups, need not and often do not apply to individual patients" (Tisi, 1979). Therefore, the clinician is faced with two basic questions: Should pulmonary function testing be performed; and, if so, on which patients? How should the results of such tests be viewed?

Obviously, the wide acceptance of pulmonary function testing indicates that the answer to the first part of the first question is affirmative, but the selection of patients is confusing. The value of testing is in the identification and prevention of pulmonary morbidity. Therefore, patients in whom perioperative clinical and laboratory examination indicates that normal postoperative pulmonary derangements will be tolerated poorly require testing to see whether or not prophylactic measures can be undertaken to improve pulmonary function prior to operation and to prepare the patient in such a way as to improve her postoperative course. This may involve breathing exercises and the use of expiratory loading measures before surgery (Gothe and Cherniack, 1980; Pardy et al., 1981).

Postoperative pulmonary changes are most marked in the following areas:

Lung Volumes. Total lung capacity and all subdivisions decrease postoperatively following abdominal and thoracic procedures but not following procedures on the extremity (Anscombe and Buxton, 1958; Beecher, 1933; Churchill and McNeil, 1927; Diament and Palmer, 1966, 1967). The decrease is greater for upper abdominal and thoracic surgery. The importance of these volume losses is that available surface area for blood-gas exchange decreases. Of extreme importance are decreases in expiratory reserve volume, which promote small airway closure and subsequent atelectasis. Pasteur (1910) was the first to describe massive collapse of the lung, and although he treated this complication with "spirits," it is also noteworthy that the resultant coughing was probably as beneficial as our conventional "stir-up regimens" and endotracheal suctioning. Atelectasis is still of primary concern because, although initially a noninfective complication, continued blood flow through the collapsed lung segments leads to direct right-to-left intrapulmonary shunting and the development of arterial hypoxemia. The most common causes of atelectasis are retained secretions, decrease in expiratory reserve volume, and changes in respiratory pattern (e.g., decreased frequency of spontaneous sighs).

Postoperative atelectasis is seen not just in patients with thick tracheobronchial secretions; indeed, many patients with normal lungs and minimal secretions develop atelectasis. However, the likely cause of atelectasis in the presence of secretions is that perfusion to an occluded segment initially continues in excess of the available ventilation. Absorption of gas continues from the occluded alveolus, and depending on the contained gas and its rate of absorption into blood,

the alveolar segments gradually become airless and collapse. Nitrogen acts as an alveolar support because it is absorbed slowly, and breathing room air produces the slowest development of atelectasis. This theory was submitted when higher oxygen concentrations were studied (Coryllos and Birnbaum, 1932; Dale and Rahn, 1953), and has been implicated in the studies showing that an inspired oxygen fraction of 100% increases absorption atelectasis, which in turn increases the measured intrapulmonary shunt (Carlon et al., 1980; Douglas et al., 1976; Oliven and Burstein, 1980; Reines and Civetta, 1979; Tonnesen et al., 1977). Therefore, although retained secretions are only partially responsible for postoperative atelectasis, attention to circulating blood volume (hydration) and adequate humidification of inspired gases with use of low levels of inspired oxygen concentration should minimize the influence of secretions on deranged pulmonary function.

Decreased lung volume causes two other major derangements in ventilation. At normal end-expiration, recoil lung forces and expansile chest wall forces are balanced at a point of optimal compliance for each individual. If this relationship is altered by decreased total lung volume, the lungs become less compliant, more difficult to expand. This, in conjunction with the pain of the operative procedure and the automatic abdominal splinting that protects the patient from further incisional pain, produces rapid, shallow respirations. Although this is abnormal, initially oxygenation is well supported because alveolar PO_2 is increased, and the rapid rate allows for adequate carbon dioxide elimination. Ultimately, however, small airways closure and subsequent intrapulmonary shunting will eventually cause arterial hypoxemia and deranged pulmonary function. The largest proportion of postoperative decreased lung volume is a consequence of small airways closure secondary to decreases in the tidal volume and sigh excursions, mentioned previously. This decrease in expiratory reserve volume—the volume of gas that must be exhaled prior to the initiation of a large inspiration—has been related to the lung volume at which airways close. In normal people, the point at which small airways close is above residual volume and below the end-tidal point of each breath. If closing volume is smaller than expiratory reserve volume, it will lie below the end-tidal point, and closure is avoided. However, the closing volume has been noted to increase with age, is greater in those people with a history of smoking, and is an early predictor of small airways disease. Figure 2–30 shows these relationships.

Gas Exchange. Arterial hypoxemia develops secondary to changes previously described.

Defense Mechanisms. The cough mechanism can be thought of as having two aims: to clear large airways of secretions and to place small particles in distal airways in proximity to the pulmonary macrophage system with ultimate elimination by pulmonary lymphatic drainage. "The clearance of inhaled particles postoperatively is affected to the extent to

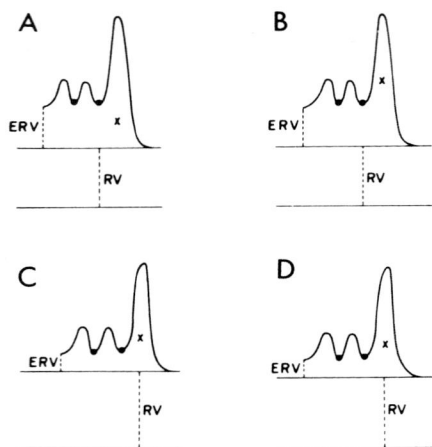

FIGURE 2–30. Relationship between closing volume (CV) and expiratory reserve volume (ERV). The closed circle (•) represents the end-tidal point of spontaneous breathing, and x is the CV. *A,* Normal. CV is less than ERV and is below the end-tidal point (i.e., collapse of alveoli does not occur during normal breathing). *B,* Smoker. VC is increased and is greater than the ERV and occurs above the end-tidal point. Therefore, even during normal breathing, some alveoli close on expiration and may increase postoperative morbidity. *C,* Obesity. ERV is reduced and CV occurs above the end-tidal point (see Fig. 2–17). *D,* Postoperative normal. ERV is reduced, and CV occurs above the end-tidal point. Therefore, a comparison of this and changes seen in *B* and *C* implies that even more severe abnormalities in blood-gas exchange can be expected in obese patients and in smokers. Also, the importance of postoperative exercise designed to recruit FRC is shown in these diagrams. ERV recruitment by early mobilization and "stir up" regimens is beneficial. (RV = residual volume.) (*A–D,* From Tisi, G. M.: Preoperative evaluation of pulmonary function. Am. Rev. Respir. Dis., *119:293, 1979.)

which normal ciliary function is decreased, and the extent to which the complex mixture of secretions that comprise mucus is altered. The clearance of microbial agents is decreased by arterial hypoxemia, one of the pulmonary changes that may develop postoperatively" (Tisi, 1979).

Pulmonary complications are accentuated normal postoperative changes. Postoperative pulmonary morbidity can be characterized as follows: atelectasis, infectious complications, and prolonged mechanical ventilatory requirement. Therefore, the benefits of patient testing and identification will be that the inoperable patient is identified and immediate postoperative mortality avoided, and prophylaxis in high-risk patients may be begun as early as possible.

Table 2–4 identifies the pulmonary function guidelines that indicate high perioperative risk. Table 2–5 indicates those patients who should be considered for preoperative pulmonary function testing. These guidelines are only relative, because certain individuals show marked postoperative improvement despite poor preoperative values. For example, preoperative hypoxemia may be a poor indicator of risk if the defect is due to increased intrapulmonary blood flow to an atelectatic lung segment that is obstructed by an intrabronchial lesion. Theoretically, removal of the affected lung segment diminishes the blood flow through the nonventilated segment, thereby decreas-

■ **Table 2–4.** PULMONARY FUNCTION GUIDELINES THAT INDICATE HIGH RISK OF MORBIDITY AND MORTALITY

Spirometric
1. Maximal breathing capacity <50% predicted (Gaensler et al., 1955; Didolkar et al., 1974; Mittman, 1961)
2. Forced expiratory volume in 1 second < 2 l (Boushy et al., 1971; Lockwood, 1973)

Arterial Blood Gases
1. Arterial PCO_2 > 45 mm Hg (Bjork and Hilty, 1953; Burrows and Earle, 1969; Diener and Burrows, 1975; Segall and Butterworth, 1966)
2. Hypoxemia is unreliable

Pulmonary Vasculature
1. Pulmonary arterial pressure during temporary unilateral occlusion of left or right main pulmonary artery > 30 mm Hg (Laros and Swierenga, 1967)

Modified from Tisi, G. M.: Preoperative evaluation of pulmonary function. Am. Rev. Respir. Dis., *119:302, 1979.

ing inappropriate and wasteful perfusion and improving pulmonary function overall.

The commonly available pulmonary function tests are:

1. *Spirometry.* This was one of the earliest methods available and still is probably one of the most valuable of all tests. It enables measurement of all lung volumes and of maximal breathing capacity or maximal voluntary ventilation. This test is exceptionally valuable because not only are assessments of individual physiologic variation performed, but also the patient's stamina, motivation, and ability to cooperate with respiratory support personnel can be estimated.

2. *Arterial blood gases.* The baseline, resting Pa_{CO_2} is especially useful. Increased postoperative morbidity has been shown for patients with Pa_{CO_2} values greater than 45 mm Hg, and preoperative bronchodilator therapy with breathing exercises and antibiotics (if indicated) may greatly reduce postoperative risk (see Table 2–4).

3. *Ventilation and perfusion studies.* These may indicate specific preoperative lesions. However, although Wagner (1978) has provided an excellent review of this subject, usefulness of this test in the postoperative

■ **Table 2–5.** POSSIBLE CANDIDATES FOR PREOPERATIVE EVALUATION OF PULMONARY FUNCTION

1. Patients scheduled for thoracic surgery (Boushy et al., 1971; Gaensler et al., 1955; Karliner et al., 1968; Lockwood, 1973; Mittman, 1961)
2. Patients with a history of heavy smoking and cough (Latimer et al., 1971; Morton and Camb, 1944)
3. Obese patients (Putman et al., 1974)
4. Patients older than 70 years of age (Klug and McPherson, 1959; Zeffren and Hartford, 1972)
5. Patients with preoperative pulmonary disease (Gaensler et al., 1955; Miller et al., 1956; Mittman, 1961)
6. Patients scheduled for upper abdominal surgery (Anscombe and Buxton, 1958; Beecher, 1933; Diament and Palmer, 1966)

Modified from Tisi, G. M.: Preoperative evaluation of pulmonary function. Am. Rev. Respir. Dis., *119:303, 1979.

period has been criticized by Walker and associates (1981) because of its low specificity. The defects seen on lung scan are often nonspecific and may be seen in healthy individuals who have no evidence of pulmonary embolism by pulmonary angiography. In fact, 25% of patients with a postoperative complaint of chest pain can be expected to yield abnormal lung-ventilation scan results whether or not a pulmonary embolus is present.

4. *Balloon occlusion of the pulmonary artery.* This test is indicated in patients with pulmonary artery hypertension who are being considered for pulmonary resection. In these patients, the rise in pulmonary artery pressure following unilateral pulmonary artery occlusion may indicate whether or not the remaining pulmonary vascular bed is adequate following the procedure.

5. *Individual lung spirometry.* Each lung can be isolated by passage of a special double-lumen endotracheal tube. This enables the contribution of each lung to the total blood-gas exchange mechanism to be measured. From these data, patients with significant pulmonary disease about to undergo pneumonectomy or lung resection may be spared an operation that would lead to a postoperative inability of the remaining lung to support the metabolic requirements of the individual.

These last two tests are always described, but they are rarely performed. Clinically, decisions to proceed with pulmonary resection are based on many variables, and no single function test can be considered diagnostic. Unfortunately, no "gold standard" exists against which these tests can be evaluated.

Although much has been learned about the likelihood of an individual patient's developing postoperative pulmonary complications, no data predict accurately the danger of postoperative mortality. The guidelines outlined here may be suggestive, but no absolute predictions can be made. Therefore, the current success of major abdominal and especially thoracic surgery must, in part, be viewed as the increased awareness of the value of preoperative and postoperative pulmonary prophylaxis. This includes:

1. *Discontinuation of smoking for as long as possible preoperatively.* Even a 12-hour abstention may increase the effectiveness of the mucociliary transport mechanisms for evacuation of upper airway debris.

2. *Patient education.* The patient must be aware of the importance of postoperative coughing and deep breathing maneuvers. Incentive spirometric devices may aid the patient in these exercises.

3. *Judicious analgesia.* Although postoperative narcotic administration may cause retention of carbon dioxide and respiratory acidosis secondary to depression of the respiratory center, the careful use of analgesia enables the patient to cooperate more fully with postoperative pulmonary exercises. It has been found that epidural narcotics or continuous low-dose narcotic infusions may be an important adjunct to the care of the severe pulmonary cripple in the postoperative period. Additionally, *patient-controlled analgesia*

(PCA) devices are an alternative method to traditional narcotic administration and may be very useful in the postoperative care of these patients. Also, the importance of various local anesthetic blocks that may provide excellent analgesia should not be discounted, and installation of local anesthetic solutions into the pleural cavity is gaining wide acceptance as an effective method of postoperative pain management.

4. *Preoperative antibiotic and bronchodilator therapy* may be extremely beneficial for patients who suffer from chronic bronchitis and obstructive pulmonary disease. Also, elective scheduling of procedures during the summer months may minimize the incidence of postoperative respiratory infections in susceptible patients.

5. *Long-term goals may involve changes in the patient's habitus and life-style.* Weight reduction and exercise programs may benefit greatly some patients with severe pulmonary limitations. The recommended prophylaxis for preventing postoperative respiratory morbidity is shown in Table 2–6.

Distinguishing among life-saving operations—necessary, elective, and irresponsible—is crucial in justifying the risks of any procedure to the patient and, increasingly important, to a society reluctant to commit costly resources to salvage inappropriate therapy. The goal of preoperative pulmonary function testing is to predict the likelihood of a bad postoperative pulmonary outcome so that it can be changed or eliminated. Therefore, predictors, rather than descriptors, of the potential complications must be identified. Unfortunately, although the literature is replete with many proposed tests, their specificity, individually and collectively, remains poor. Preoperative hypercarbia appears to correlate positively with a number of studies indicating prolonged postoperative respiratory recovery in thoracic and abdominal procedures. Indeed, and as would be expected, site of incision also relates to the severity of complications.

Forced expiratory volume in one second (FEV_1) is a test that has been postulated to predict postoperative pulmonary morbidity, and when results are reason-

■ **Table 2–6.** PROPHYLACTIC MEASURES RECOMMENDED TO REDUCE POSTOPERATIVE COMPLICATIONS

Preoperatively: Education of patients to ensure optimal postoperative compliance and performance; cessation of smoking; training in proper breathing (incentive spirometry); bronchodilatation and control of infection and secretions when indicated; and weight reduction when appropriate

Intraoperatively: Reduction in time under anesthesia; control of secretions; prevention of aspiration; maintenance of optimal bronchodilatation; and intermittent hyperinflations

Postoperatively: Continuation of preoperative measure with particular attention to hyperinflation, mobilization of secretions, early ambulation, encouragement to cough, and control of pain, with attention to the effects of analgesia on the pattern of breathing

From Tisi, G. M.: Preoperative evaluation of pulmonary function. Am. Rev. Respir. Dis. *119*:303, 1979.

ably normal (FEV$_1$ > 70% predicted), spirometry is appropriately reassuring. However, if FEV$_1$ results are abnormal, further pulmonary evaluation should be undertaken. Preoperative spirometry may help predict postoperative respiratory complications statistically within populations, but it is not particularly helpful individually. As noted above, a number of preoperative interventions make physiologic sense and can be demonstrated on pulmonary function testing, such as preoperative bronchodilator use, smoking cessation, and treatment of pulmonary infections. Other aspects of pulmonary procedures, such as the surgical site and amount of tissue to be resected, remain unchanged by any preoperative preparation. In general, if a patient at risk elects a procedure and shows hypercarbia and an FEV$_1$ of less than 40% predicted on preoperative testing, it is wise to reassess the necessity of the procedure, because the likelihood of postoperative complications is, not surprisingly, high.

Modern surgical, anesthetic, and perioperative support techniques have decreased the morbidity of thoracic surgical procedures, but the reality remains that, for some patients scheduled for operation and resection, postoperative pulmonary function proves inadequate. Although this situation can be minimized, the risk always exists, so it is important not to allow patients to succumb to the readily reversible defects in pulmonary function that occur in all patients following operations. "To put it shortly, there is a sporting element in the speciality; it is a game of skill in which chance also figures to some degree" (Barton, 1920).

ADULT RESPIRATORY DISTRESS SYNDROME OR ACUTE RESPIRATORY FAILURE

Adult respiratory distress syndrome (ARDS) describes many acute, diffuse infiltrative lung lesions of diverse etiologies when they are accompanied by severe arterial hypoxemia. The term was chosen because of several clinical and pathologic similarities between such acute illnesses in adults and the neonatal respiratory distress syndrome. However, in the neonatal form, immaturity of alveolar surfactant production and a highly compliant chest wall are primarily involved in the pathophysiology, whereas in the adult form, alveolar surfactant changes are secondary to the primary process, and the chest wall is not compliant. ARDS develops in approximately 150,000 patients per year (Murray, 1975), most of whom are young and usually previously healthy. The mortality rate from ARDS was soon found to be higher than initially reported with the publication of the results of the extracorporeal membrane oxygenator (ECMO) project supported by the National Heart, Lung, and Blood Institute. This was an 18-month collaborative study at nine American medical centers in which 686 patients aged 12 years and older were admitted into the perfusion group if they required intubation, mechanical ventilation for 24 hours or more, or an inspired oxygen concentration of 50% or greater.

The mortality rate in isolated respiratory failure in the 12- to 65-year-old age group was 41% and rose to 68% in patients over 65 years old. If complications from other organ systems developed, the mortality rate was higher, and only 15% of patients in the 12- to 65-year-old age group with respiratory and renal failure survived (Pontoppidan, 1979). The intervening years have provided significant improvements in the pharmacology, technology, and nutritional support available to the critical care teams caring for these patients, but the mortality rate of the disease has remained virtually unchanged.

Although the etiologic possibilities are numerous, and include diffuse pulmonary infections, aspiration of gastric content, inhalation of toxins and irritants, narcotic-overdose pulmonary edema, non-narcotic drug effects, immunologic response to host antigens, effects of nonthoracic trauma with hypotension, association with systemic reactions to processes initiated outside the lung, and postcardiopulmonary bypass, the clinical characteristics, respiratory pathophysiologic derangement, and current techniques for management of these acute abnormalities are remarkably similar. Obviously, the conditions listed do not always lead to respiratory failure, and the treatment of the underlying diseases will be different; however, seeing the pathologic similarities of the response of the lungs to trauma may make it possible to derive a logical plan on which this discussion can focus.

The pathologic changes observed in the lung in respiratory failure are mostly secondary to the physiologic disturbances that precede them. The clinical syndrome is characterized by hypovolemic shock and a gradual rise in the respiratory rate to compensate for a fall in the tidal volume. The PA$_{O_2}$ falls progressively during the first 12 hours, and the patients become increasingly cyanosed and hypocapnic. The cyanosis is unrelieved by oxygen therapy and is caused mainly by shunting blood through the unaerated lung. Post-traumatic respiratory insufficiency was divided by Moore (1969) into the following four clinical stages:

Stage I   Period of shock
            Spontaneous hyperventilation/
               hypocapnia
Stage II Early respiratory distress
            Hypoxia—shunt 10 to 20% of cardiac
               output
            Hyperventilation/hypocapnia
Stage III Gross hypoxia
            Requires mechanical ventilatory
               assistance
            Chest film—shock lung
Stage IV Terminal anoxemia
            Finally, hypercapnia

At postmortem examination, the following conditions are apparent (Spencer, 1977; Ingram, 1980):

Interstitial and intra-alveolar edema: 85%

Intra-alveolar hemorrhage: 55%
Interstitial hemorrhage: 25%
Patchy atelectasis: 70%
Fat embolism: 65%
Bronchopneumonia: 25%

Pathophysiology

Regardless of the initiating process, ARDS is invariably associated with an increase in lung water. Thus, it is a form of pulmonary edema; yet it is distinct from cardiogenic pulmonary edema because pulmonary capillary hydrostatic pressures are not raised. Initially, there is injury to the alveolar-capillary membrane that causes leakage of liquid, macromolecules, and cellular components from the blood vessels into the interstitial space and, with increasing severity, into the alveoli. Alveolar collapse occurs secondary to the effect of the intra-alveolar liquid, especially its fibrinogen, that interferes with normal surfactant activity and because of possible impairment to further surfactant production by injury to the granular pneumocytes. The lungs become less compliant (i.e., they stiffen because of interstitial edema, alveolar collapse, and increase in surface forces). Because of the decreased compliance, large inspiratory pressures must be generated by the respiratory muscles in order to support oxygenation so that the work of breathing is increased. Both hypoxemia and the stimulation of receptors in the stiff lung parenchyma cause an increase in respiratory frequency, a decrease in tidal volume, and deterioration of gas exchange.

Pathology

In the absence of demonstrable specific pathogens, the pathology is remarkably similar among the various conditions causing ARDS, because the lung has a limited number of ways in which it reacts to an almost limitless number of injuries. Grossly, the lungs are heavy, edematous, and almost airless, with regions of hemorrhage, atelectasis, and consolidation. Light microscopy shows edema and cellular infiltration of interalveolar septa and interstitial spaces surrounding airways and blood vessels, atelectasis and hyaline membranes in many regions, engorgement of vessels with red blood cells, and aggregates of platelets along with interstitial and alveolar hemorrhage. In addition, both hyperplasia and dysplasia of the granular pneumocytes are often present.

To return to the simplified, morphologic classification presented previously, changes seen early in ARDS can be summarized as follows (Pontoppidan, 1979):

1. Intra-alveolar and interstitial high-protein-content pulmonary edema and hemorrhage
2. Hyaline membrane formation
3. Necrosis of the alveolar lining epithelium (Type 1 pneumocyte) and endothelial cells

4. Appearance of microthrombi in the small vessels

The pathologic changes at this time do not suggest major alterations in the underlying lung architecture. The basic normal pattern of alveolar space and interstitial matrix has been retained, recruitable air space and vasculature are still present in most cases, and reversibility of morphologic changes would seem possible if effective therapeutic measures were available.

If the illness is prolonged (longer than 10 days), there is often a surprising amount of fibrosis in addition to the acute changes. In patients who recover and subsequently die from another cause, significant interstitial fibrosis and emphysematous changes may be found in the previously affected lungs. However, a significant number of patients recover completely if vigorous supportive measures are instituted rapidly. The late changes in severe ARDS that take place over days or weeks can be summarized as follows (Pontoppidan, 1979):

1. Vasculature
   a. Thrombi in small and medium arteries
   b. Intact megakaryocytes prominent in small vessels
   c. Endothelial cell necrosis; no neovascularization
   d. Extensive vessel loss in respiratory lung regions
2. Alveolar lining and spaces
   a. Hyperplasia of Type II cells—evidenced by multilayered cuboidal epithelium
      i. Intra-alveoloar hyaline membrane
      ii. Intra-alveoloar fibrosis
3. Interstitium
   a. Increase in connective tissue matrix, especially collagen; total lung collagen may increase two to three times normal
   b. Decrease in lung elastic tissue
   c. Disruption of lung architecture

Although pulmonary morphologic changes are frequently described as being diffuse, they have a distinct focal distribution, with areas of well-preserved lung interspersed between areas of severe destruction of normal architecture. This therefore alters the normal ventilation and perfusion relationships, which are determined by gravity and alveolar pressure; rather, mini-zones of unknown $\dot{V}/\dot{Q}$ are the new determinants of ultimate gas exchange.

A patient suffering from shock often develops a series of structural changes in the lungs. These are important, because even if the patient survives the disturbances elsewhere in the body, the lung changes may still cause gross functional impairment of gas exchange and even death. However, death due to primary respiratory insufficiency is becoming less common because of better understanding of the physiology of ventilatory support modes.

Treatment

All the major treatment modalities available can be classified as supportive rather than primary therapeutic measures. In large measure, the treatment plan is confounded by an apparently irrational approach to the problem of a patient with increased lung water. Traditionally, pulmonary edema is controlled by fluid restriction, use of diuretic therapy, and, in the recent past, by phlebotomy, rotating tourniquets, and vasodilator therapy. However, in ARDS the edema may form secondary to an impairment in capillary osmotic properties that allows protein-rich fluid to leak from the intravascular space. Capillary leak is, a priori, almost impossible to document, so a high index of suspicion must accompany the initial diagnosis of pulmonary edema in the surgical or trauma patient.

Radiographic changes consistent with ARDS were described by Greene (1979): diffuse lung consolidation, air bronchograms, and low lung volumes.

An association with any of the mentioned etiologies should alert the care team to the immediate possibility that major pulmonary damage has occurred and that the normal function of the alveolar capillary membrane has been compromised. After this, a progressive increase in pulmonary interstitial water occurs in the following manner: extra-alveolar interstitial connective tissue compartment around large blood vessels and airways, alveolar wall thickening, and alveolar filling, which only follows interstitial overload.

There is no correlation between positive water balance and pulmonary extravascular water, and the extravasation of water is neither cardiogenic nor osmotic, at least in the early stages of the process. At the turn of the century, Starling (1896) discussed the mechanics of fluid passage across semipermeable membranes, and the ideal situation in which application of his principles might be expected to be useful has been questioned recently. Therefore, in an abnormal situation in which the barrier is no longer selectively permeable (rather, the barrier has no flow-restrictive properties), fluid pools within the lung interstitium and eventually leads to progressive alveolar flooding and the clinical picture of fulminant pulmonary edema.

Treatment of ARDS is logically divided into three stages: resuscitation, prolonged support, and weaning from all support modalities. Regardless of etiology, all forms of ARDS are associated with increased interstitial pulmonary water. Many patients present with hemodynamic instability reflected as hypotension, tachycardia, and oliguria. It is of prime importance during this period to provide optimal volume loading in an attempt to restore normal hemodynamics while supporting respiratory function.

The patient suffering from ARDS has interstitial edema, atelectasis, and decreased lung parenchymal compliance. Therefore, increased work of breathing is extremely detrimental, and ventilatory support modes must accomplish the following: stabilization of lung function; recruitment of additional alveolar surface area; control of arterial pH and, secondly, PCO_2; minimal depression of cardiac output; and overall decrease in work of breathing.

Cardiovascular stability is provided initially by volume resuscitation until adequate filling pressure is obtained. Preload and afterload management in addition to specific inotropic agents subsequently may become an essential consideration. An important concern surrounding these decisions is that myocardial oxygen consumption increases least with respect to increased output (sometimes measured as the *rate pressure product* [RPP]) if preload augmentation is used rather than inotropic support. A controversy continues over the correct choice between crystalloid and colloid resuscitation. Arguments are persuasive for use of either fluid type, but other considerations are probably equally important. Patients require blood and blood products (e.g., fresh frozen plasma, platelets, granulocytes) in large quantities for specific reasons. The mistake often made with colloid use is to think that it will clear pulmonary and peripheral capillary dysfunction. This is not true, and instead of intravascular recruitment of peripheral edema fluid, leakage of albumin into the interstitium may occur. In most tissues, this is not a significant problem. However, if leakage occurs in either the lungs or the kidneys, significant deficits in oxygen saturation or renal function become apparent.

It appears reasonable to propose resuscitation in the following manner: Transfuse with packed red cells to a stable hematocrit of 30 to 35%; use fresh frozen plasma to correct clotting factors; administer platelets as indicated; and use isotonic crystalloid solutions to maintain hemodynamic stability and adequate renal function. Patient weight gain may be considerable during this time, and respiratory support is an important treatment adjunct. Optimal values for hematocrit will continue to be controversial as long as the blood supply remains at risk from varieties of hepatitis, HIV, and other related transfusion conditions. Public awareness is high on this point, and the popularity of self-donation programs continues to rise.

Resuscitation and support stages blend into one another, and in most instances, accurate monitoring is necessary for accurate therapy. The most common monitoring priorities are as follows (Lumb, 1981):

1. *Arterial blood gases:* Assess saturation, oxygen transport; determine FI_{O_2} and positive end-expiratory pressure (PEEP).
2. *Mixed venous blood gases:* Assess peripheral oxygen consumption and cardiac output; determine volume loading, inotropic support, acceptable oxygenation levels.
3. *Cardiac output:* Estimate cardiac work.
4. *Pulmonary compliance:* Grossly estimate recruited lung volume or functional residual capacity.
5. *Renal function:* Monitor urine quality as well as quantity. Standard investigation should include (a) serum chemistry: BUN, creatinine, glucose, osmolarity; (b) urine: electrolytes (Na^+, K^+), timed creatinine, osmolarity, presence of glucose or ketones, specific gravity; and (c) derived: creatinine clearance, osmolar clearance, free water clearance.

Virgilio and associates (1979) stated that the primary goal of fluid resuscitation in shock and trauma is to protect major organ function by the rapid and safe restoration of hemodynamic stability. This is a reasonable and generally acceptable desire; the question now centers on the most satisfactory manner in which this can be accomplished. During the past several years, noninvasive methods for assessing blood pressure, cardiac output, arterial oxygen saturation, and end-tidal carbon dioxide concentration have become available and reliable in the clinical setting. Already, more efficient weaning techniques from mechanical ventilatory support have been reported using noninvasive measurements (Sharer and Sladen, 1988), and it is likely that these techniques will become standard for the management of all postoperative and critically ill patients. Assessment of intrapulmonary shunt can be made continuously by using continuous arterial and mixed venous oxygen saturation data, which may improve the rapidity of controlling pulmonary complications in mechanically ventilated patients. However, as with the use of any new technology, the clinician must be aware of inherent inaccuracies in any of the devices used. Just as direct pulmonary artery pressure measurements in patients on mechanical ventilators can produce errors in interpretation, the noninvasive devices are open to errors in sampling and interpretation: The pulse oximeter, although now used widely in a variety of clinical settings, has demonstrable inaccuracies in a variety of clinical situations (Eisenkraft, 1988).

End-points of volume resuscitation can be formulated. Invasive monitoring, despite undoubted potential for complication, is the most complete and reproducible source of data currently available. Various indices of ventricular performance can be calculated, and the trends in a patient's progress during hemodynamic manipulation may lead to optimal volume replacement plus or minus inotropic support in most cases. Pulmonary artery monitoring also permits speculation on the overall metabolic state of the patients. The human body is, after all, an aerobic, oxidative mechanism, and support of mitochondrial oxygenation is the ultimate therapeutic goal.

MECHANICAL VENTILATORY SUPPORT

Current concepts in mechanical ventilation separate the need for ventilation from the need for maintenance of lung volume or FRC. The mode of ventilation that provides minimum cardiac depression coincident with adequate alveolar gas exchange appears to be *intermittent mandatory ventilation* (IMV). Recruitment of functional residual capacity is provided by increasing amounts of PEEP. Mechanical support of ventilation has two primary purposes: control of Pa_{O_2} and maintenance of pH.

Patients requiring mechanical ventilatory assistance will present management problems associated with the two preceding categories. These problems include hypoxemia, respiratory acidosis, and respiratory alkalosis.

Hypoxemia. This condition is often due to increased interstitial lung water secondary to vigorous volume resuscitation with either crystalloid or colloid solutions. It may also occur following cardiac surgery and the large crystalloid volume infused with the pump prime. Hypoxemia is exacerbated by ventilation-perfusion abnormalities and atelectasis of variably located alveolar segments. Although this deficit often can be alleviated with large tidal volume ventilation and increased inspired oxygen concentration, PEEP provides a more rational means of support. The increase in FRC associated with the application of PEEP provides a greater gas-exchange surface area (FRC) and enables optimal ventilatory support at relatively low mean intrathoracic pressures. Recent practice supports the concept that pulmonary damage secondary to ventilator-induced barotrauma may be as much a function of excessive volume expansion as applied positive pressure. Therefore, clinicians should consider the conflicting goals of ventilator therapy (alveolar expansion, applied pressure, and cyclical airflow) when they prescribe volume, flow, and rate parameters.

Respiratory Acidosis. Often this is due to residual muscle weakness from intraoperative muscle relaxation or continued postoperative anesthetic depression. Usually both of these situations respond to pharmacologic antagonism. More insidious is respiratory acidosis secondary to progressive neurologic disorders (e.g., Guillain-Barré disease) or to errors in management of patients with chronic pulmonary disorders that alter normal respiratory drive mechanisms (e.g., inappropriate provision of supplemental oxygenation), which may lead to respiratory depression by reducing a normal hypoxic ventilatory stimulus.

Respiratory Alkalosis. Respiratory alkalosis may be seen following resuscitation in which excessive amounts of sodium bicarbonate have been administered; it also occurs in patients with pre-existing potassium or chloride depletion and in those with considerable induced diuresis. The presence of a large base excess and alkalosis has been associated with an increase in the time necessary for weaning from mechanical ventilatory assistance (Gallagher, 1979). As intermittent mandatory ventilation has gained popularity, control of pH has become more important than the more traditional control of P_{CO_2}. P_{CO_2} levels in the 50 to 55 mm Hg range are now accepted during weaning as long as arterial oxygen saturation and pH are within normal limits. This is also important with newer management techniques for postoperative pain management, such as PCA devices and epidural or intrathecal narcotic administration.

Mechanical ventilatory assistance, therefore, should provide support that does not alter the normal physiologic state but that provides adequate support of arterial oxygen saturation and pH with minimal effect on cardiac output and hemodynamic stability. Of the currently available ventilatory modes, intermittent mandatory ventilation appears to afford the best compromise, allowing for a gradual return from complete apnea to full spontaneous ventilatory effort without the paradoxic movement that often accompanies controlled positive-pressure ventilation or an improperly adjusted assist-controller. IMV also reduces the commonly observed alveolar hyperventilation that accompanies return of cognitive function on assist-control modes. However, increasing availability of pressure support (PS) and augmented minute ventilatory (AMV) or mandatory minute ventilatory (MMV) modes has already modified the premier position of IMV. Whatever the mechanical support chosen, the approach in the postsurgical patient should be to stimulate voluntary ventilatory effort, support FRC, and cause minimal deviation from the patient's preoperative homeostatic levels. The effort should not be directed at "normalizing" numbers. Rather, the patient's native pulmonary function should be supported and returned to baseline as rapidly as possible. This is even more important when weaning patients who have been ventilator-dependent for a considerable time. In these difficult patients, PS is becoming increasingly popular and successful. The following is a synopsis of the available ventilatory modes in common use.

Control Ventilation

In this method of mechanical ventilation, a preset tidal volume is delivered to the patient under positive pressure at regular, preset intervals and at a constant rate. During times of ventilator inactivity, no gas is available to the patient, even though he may be making respiratory efforts. This leads to paradoxic movement of the chest wall, and the patient appears to "fight" the ventilator. This is the most commonly used mode of ventilation in anesthesia ventilators and for paralyzed patients in the intensive care unit.

Assist-Control Ventilation (ACV)

In this mode, characteristics of gas flow do not change from those used in controlled ventilation, but the patient may initiate delivery of a breath by her own inspiratory efforts. The machine is designed to sense either negative pressure (Bennett MA-1, MA-2, Bird) or movement of gas (Bourns Bear II, V, Siemens) caused by the patient's inspiratory effort. Once the operator-set delivery threshold is reached, the machine delivers a preset tidal volume in response to the patient's inspiratory effort. The threshold can be adjusted so that increasing effort will be required to initiate a breath. This has been thought to aid in weaning the patient from the ventilator. However, because each breath delivers a full tidal volume, an agitated patient may hyperventilate inappropriately.

Intermittent Mandatory Ventilation (IMV)

This mode functions as a controller in the apneic patient. However, as the patient begins to make inspiratory efforts, a circuit modification enables the pa-

tient to receive humidified gas at the constant, prescribed inspired oxygen concentration in volumes that depend on inspiratory effort with minimal resistance to gas flow. Therefore, the patient does not make a paradoxic effort and does not receive a preset tidal volume for each effort. This decreases the incidence of discomfort for the patient and the likelihood of inappropriate hyperventilation. Unfortunately, even in the most carefully designed systems, the inspired and expired work of breathing imposed by demand valves, high gas flows, and resistors is significant and may frustrate efforts to wean weakened, chronically debilitated patients.

Intermittent Positive-Pressure Breathing (IPPB)

Traditionally, this has been a respiratory therapy treatment mode rather than one used for therapeutic, long-term support. It is delivered by a pressure-limited device that delivers a continuous flow of gas until a preset inflation pressure is reached. Gas flow is initiated by negative inspiratory pressure. Initially, this was believed to be beneficial postoperatively as a method of maintaining good lung expansion. There is no evidence to support its routine use (Conference on the Scientific Basis of Respiratory Therapy, 1974), and after early enthusiastic use, IPPB was replaced by incentive spirometry and other techniques to invoke patient participation. However, patients with tracheostomies (who have no control over glottic closure) and selected patients who present difficult weaning problems may benefit from IPPB treatments every 4 hours with the addition of nebulized bronchodilators. It is important to ensure that the patient receives a mechanical breath of adequate volume to expand the lung to FRC and beyond (12 to 15 ml/kg) for this therapy to be effective. Too frequently, the breath is curtailed by the preset pressure limit of the device before the patient has received an augmented tidal volume. In this setting, failure of the technique is guaranteed. Additionally, pressure-limited and reverse-ratio ventilation are being used effectively in a number of patients in whom the peak inflation pressures reached by conventional settings are not tolerated.

Mandatory Minute Ventilation (MMV)

This technique is becoming more commonly used in the United States and is enthusiastically supported in Europe. Designed to guarantee a minimal minute ventilation, the machine quantitates the patient's exhaled volume and supplements this with additional breaths if necessary. The ventilator adds breaths only if the patient's own exhaled volume falls below the selected minimum value. Back-up support modes can be established to prevent the patient from maintaining the minimum minute ventilation with a large number of low-volume breaths. Theoretically, rapid postoperative weaning should be possible with this ventilator, because after the initial set-up, the patient should gradually take over from the machine without further intervention. This method creates physiologic weaning, rather than weaning that relies on the clock or appropriate blood-gas values before ventilatory changes are made. Further safety can be ensured with this technique by monitoring end-tidal CO_2 levels and continuous arterial oxygen saturation, both of which are performed noninvasively. Unfortunately, in practice the technique has failed to meet its promise, and further work is necessary to define the role of this technique in the intensive care unit (ICU) and postoperative settings.

High-Frequency (Positive-Pressure) Ventilation (HF[PP]V)

HFV is defined by ventilatory rates greater than 50 breaths/minute and a tidal volume at or below dead space (Arndt, 1992). Although it was first described by Oberg and Sjostrand during experiments on the carotid sinus reflex, its most commonly intraoperative use today is a derivative of injector techniques used during bronchoscopy and laryngeal surgery. The technology is advanced, and several varieties of "airway vibrators"* are available. Interest in this ventilatory pattern is now high because of several potential advantages, including low mean intrathoracic pressure, minimal cardiovascular compromise coincident with use, excellent blood-gas exchange, good vibratory properties for removal of secretions, and specific advantages during thoracotomy and in situations of cardiac tamponade. The place of this ventilatory mode in routine practice remains to be elucidated. However, specific uses in one-lung anesthetic techniques and lung transplantation are becoming more common. Also, it is increasingly employed for patients with bronchopleural fistulas which are difficult to control. In practice, in the postoperative/ICU setting, HFV offers no advantages over conventional techniques, and technical considerations (humidification of inspired gases) limit its use.

Airway Pressure Release Ventilation (APRV)

This experimental technique developed by Downs and Stock employs a high-flow CPAP system to improve lung compliance and arterial oxygenation. However, it differs from a conventional CPAP circuit by mechanically ventilating the lungs by interrupting the positive pressure and briefly allowing system pressure to fall to ambient pressure. In this manner, the lungs are allowed to exhale passively, and they reinflate with resumption of the basal level of CPAP. By the nature of the circuit, time-cycled and pressure-limited, the inspiratory time is long and the I/E ratio

*The first vibrator patent was filed by the J. H. Emerson Company of Boston, MA, in March 1955.

may be reversed. Although this is an interesting development, it is important to study its impact when more information about its efficacy is available, especially in more complex management situations. "APRV produces lower peak and mean airway pressures, normalizes mean interpleural pressure, and may decrease barotrauma" (Arndt, 1992).

The ventilatory modes discussed above are useful primarily in the control of arterial pH and subsequent P_{CO_2}. Current treatment of hypoxia is directed toward recruiting additional lung units by the addition of positive end-expiratory pressure to the ventilator circuit. The following discussion focuses on the concepts and hemodynamic consequences of the institution of PEEP therapy.

Positive End-Expiratory Pressure (PEEP)

In 1967, Ashbaugh and associates reported the use of positive end-expiratory pressure to treat hypoxemia associated with acute respiratory failure. PEEP increases alveolar surface area for gas exchange, which is reflected as an increase in FRC. This has been shown to increase arterial oxygen tension. Since this time, PEEP has become used increasingly as a therapeutic tool. However, studies in both animals (Prewitt and Wood, 1979; Summer et al., 1979) and patients (Cournand et al., 1948; Powers et al., 1973) have shown that PEEP decreases cardiac output. Qvist and colleagues (1975) reported that changes in cardiac index were related solely to changes in filling pressures and not to changes in contractility. The reported effects of PEEP were as follows: (1) A reduction in ventricular filling pressure causes the decrease in cardiac index and stroke index observed when ventilation is altered by the addition of PEEP to mechanical ventilation. (2) Once such a decrease has occurred, it persists for prolonged periods without evidence of return to baseline levels. (3) Augmentation of blood volume by transfusion reverses these changes. (4) The hemodynamic consequences of relative hypervolemia will become evident once PEEP is discontinued.

This last point is echoed in work by Annest and co-workers (1980), who stated that endotracheal intubation should be accompanied by low levels of end-expiratory pressure and that end-expiratory pressure should not be discontinued before extubation. The detrimental effect of PEEP removal is cited as a decrease in mean expiratory airway pressure, which is reversed at the time of extubation when the patient regains the glottic mechanism. Prophylactic use of PEEP may also prevent respiratory insufficiency, according to some authors (Schmidt et al., 1976; Valdes et al., 1979).

More recently, attention has been focused on the effects of PEEP and left ventricular geometry. Cassidy and associates (1979) noted that as end-diastolic right ventricular septal-to-lateral wall dimensions increased with PEEP, end-diastolic left ventricular septal-to-lateral free wall dimensions decreased. They also questioned whether or not the use of PEEP led to increased extravascular lung water. Jardin and colleagues (1981) noted that increasing levels of PEEP are associated with a gradual increase in the radius of septal curvature at both end-diastole and end-systole; a progressive decrease in end-diastolic and end-systolic left ventricular dimension; equalization of right and left ventricular transmural end-diastolic pressures; and unaltered or slightly increased myocardial contractility. They showed that the hemodynamic effects of PEEP are mediated by ventricular interaction; hence, volume loading to reverse depression of cardiac output is of limited value at high levels of PEEP. At these levels, a relatively large increase in transmural filling pressure is associated with further flattening of the septum and only a slight increase in left ventricular dimensions.

Other investigators have disagreed with the finding that contractility is unaltered during PEEP, and some have suggested the presence of a circulating, humoral myocardial depressant factor in patients treated with PEEP (Manny et al., 1978). In addition, depression of cardiac output secondary to a reflex depression of cardiac function due to overdistention of the lungs with stimulation of pulmonary stretch receptors has been shown (Cassidy et al., 1978). Haynes and co-workers (1980) tried to encompass most of these ideas when they observed the relationship between PEEP and left ventricular diastolic pressure-area curves. They found that PEEP altered pressure-volume relationships, and they postulated intrinsic and extrinsic left ventricular myocardial effects:

1. Intrinsic factors
   a. Incomplete ventricular relaxation
   b. Coronary vascular engorgement
   c. Altered viscoelastic properties secondary to rapid ventricular filling
2. Extrinsic myocardial constraints
   a. Right and left ventricular diastolic pressure-volume characteristics depend on the degree of right ventricular distention, possibly owing to mutually shared circumferential fibers. Therefore, increased right ventricular volume may distend the right ventricle and subsequently alter left ventricular characteristics.
   b. The pericardium may augment the effects of increased volume by causing a correspondingly greater pressure increase in the right ventricle with possible septal shift and geometric alteration of the left ventricle and encroachment on the left ventricular outflow tract.

All of the various mechanisms responsible for the decreased cardiac output associated with the application of PEEP involve a potential decrease in ventricular activity that is related to an increase in mean intrathoracic pressure. An important feature of this fact is that ventilatory modes that increase intrathoracic pressure decrease cardiac output. However, modern practice uses IMV to control arterial pH and uses PEEP to recruit diffusible membrane area (FRC).

It is important to decide how to begin the weaning from ventilatory assistance. Each spontaneous breath initiated by the patient decreases the mean intrathoracic pressure from baseline end-expiratory values. Conversely, each machine-initiated (positive-pressure) breath raises the mean intrathoracic pressure and further depresses cardiac output. Therefore, the appropriate practice is to decrease the rate of mechanical ventilation before decreasing PEEP in order to maximize the expansion of the lung while minimizing depression of cardiac output. At this juncture, another common ventilatory mode must be discussed. *Continuous positive airway pressure* (CPAP) causes some confusion whenever it is mentioned, and this review will oversimplify the terminology in current use. (For a full discussion of this subject, see Grenvik et al., 1980; Kirby and Graybar, 1980.)

In the apneic patient, PEEP produces a constant end-expiratory plateau that is maintained until the next breath is administered. PEEP is produced by a mechanical valve or water column situated in the exhalation limb of the ventilator circuit. Therefore, back pressure is generated within the system. If the patient begins to breathe spontaneously, a significant increase in the work of breathing results unless the back pressure within the system is flow-compensated or mechanically compensated. Gas flow must occur as soon as inspiration is initiated. For this purpose, CPAP circuits were developed. These circuits provide a pressurized reservoir that allows continuous gas flow through the ventilator system at all times except during ventilator inspiration. This mechanism decreases the inspiratory work required of the patient. Other advantages of CPAP systems are that they do not require intubation, and CPAP has been shown to minimize surfactant consumption, improve the pattern and regularity of respiration, improve oxygenation, and retard the progress of respiratory distress (Hegyi and Hiatt, 1981). However, in spite of these theoretical advantages, the systems also demonstrate significant disadvantages. Inefficient resistors may increase the expiratory work of breathing significantly and cause significant patient morbidity. Inappropriate application of uncompensated end-expiratory pressure devices on spontaneously breathing patients may lead to weaning difficulties, as shown in the following example.

The patient was a 13-year-old male who had just undergone repair of a pectus excavatum deformity. He was placed on a Bear II ventilator in the recovery room on an IMV rate of 8 breaths at 700 ml tidal volume (patient's weight was 60 kg). Initial blood-gas values were acceptable, and as the patient began to awaken, an IMV circuit was added to the system. The patient continued to do well clinically, and arterial blood-gas values remained good. The decision to add PEEP to the system to prevent basilar atelectasis was made, and 5 cm of H_2O pressure was added to the expiratory limb. No consideration was given to the increased work of breathing imposed by the ventilator at these settings due to the flow characteristics of the pressurized circuit and the postoperative instability of the patient's chest wall. The resultant increased work of breathing for the patient and his subsequent course are detailed in Table 2–7.

The discrepancy between an abdominal count of respiration and that determined by auscultation reflects the inability of this patient to overcome the resistance to breathing imposed by an uncompensated PEEP device. This example merely underscores the importance of understanding the full implications of the various devices currently available for respiratory support and provides an introduction for the next topic to be discussed, pressure support ventilation (PSV).

Pressure Support Ventilation (PSV)

The goals of mechanical ventilatory assistance are to support adequate oxygenation through restoration and preservation of FRC, to ensure appropriate ventilation as determined by pH and P_{CO_2} homeostasis, to provide subjective relief of dyspnea, and to begin the process of reconditioning the respiratory muscles so that unaided ventilation will be resumed as soon as possible. These goals have been met by using the wide range of assist devices described earlier. A new technique has evolved that attempts to integrate many support philosophies into a coherent package. The stated problems associated with conventional positive pressure support modes include myocardial depression due to mechanical and humoral events; discoordinate assistance provided by the machine, in some circumstances actually increasing oxygen consumption during mechanical ventilation (Harpin et al., 1987); increased expiratory work of breathing associated with some mechanical PEEP valves (Manni et al., 1985); prolonged weaning times due to chronic dependence on mechanical ventilatory assistance (Browne, 1984); and confusion among physicians as to the appropriate support mode for an individual patient, although intermittent mandatory ventilation has been established as the most common form of mechanical ventilation in the United States (Venus et al., 1987). Additionally, although modern ventilators have become extremely sophisticated, and intelligent integration of ventilation to patient is possible, complications may arise from the complexity of the machines themselves, and inappropriate patient outcomes have been reported with AMV (Bagley et al., 1987).

PS has been introduced to supplement conventional positive-pressure and continuous-flow machines to overcome mechanical inefficiencies and is available with most ICU ventilators. PS supports a patient's native respiratory efforts. The clinician selects a positive airway pressure at which the machine supports the patient's inspiratory effort. Selection of the level of PS depends either on controlling the patient's tidal volume or respiratory rate or on providing a theoretic level of support that overcomes the mechanical resistance of the ventilator and circuit and minimizes external work of breathing. In practice, PS selection is relatively easy, and clinical bias supports the use of this mode in patients who are not expected to wean easily by more conventional methods. As determined by MacIntyre (1986), "PSV was a reasonable form of mechanical ventilatory support in patients with spontaneous ventilatory drives. It improves patient comfort, reduces the patient's ventilatory work, and provides a more balanced pressure and volume change form of muscle work to the patient. The clinical significance of these properties during the weaning remains to be determined." As is often the case with new techniques, PSV has become accepted widely and uncritically. However, it does seem to offer advantages in the management of patients who do not wean rapidly, who are nutritionally compromised, and in whom other methods have failed. PSV also allows for a more normal variation in tidal volume than do other forms of mechanical ventilation, and, because of flow characteristics of the ventilator circuit, less expiratory work of breathing is demanded of the patient, which appears to be extremely beneficial to weaning. Certainly, the roles of PSV and AMV remain to be determined. Undoubtedly, they will prove to be valuable additions to the support modes required for successful weaning of complex, ventilator-dependent patients.

"Ideal" Ventilatory Support

The ultimate goal of mechanical ventilatory support is to provide the most physiologic support possible for compromised pulmonary function. By the very nature of positive-pressure ventilation, normal intrathoracic pressure relationships are reversed, and cardiac depression is assured. In addition, passive displacement of the diaphragm is associated with a greater degree of ventilation-perfusion mismatch than is active contraction (Froese and Bryan, 1974) (Fig. 2–31). Therefore, maintenance of spontaneous ventilation is beneficial, because more normal distribution of

■ **Table 2–7.** INAPPROPRIATE PEEP APPLICATION AND INCREASED WORK OF BREATHING

	Before PEEP	PEEP	T Tube	Extubated
Pulse (beats/min)	100	144	120	106
Resp. rate—abdominal count (resp/min)	18	36	24	22
Resp. rate—auscultation (resp/min)	18	8	24	22
P_{O_2} (mm Hg)	202	200	179	160
P_{CO_2} (mm Hg)	36	52	38	38
pH	7.39	7.3	7.4	7.39

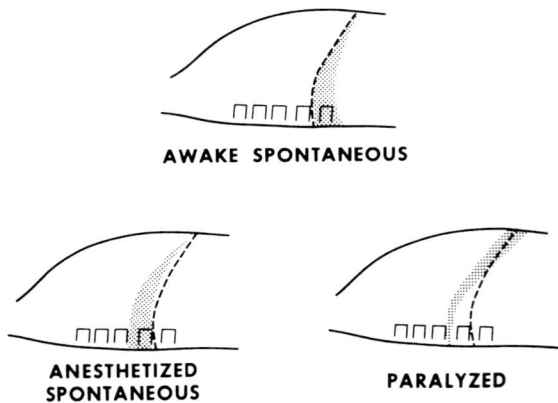

AWAKE SPONTANEOUS

ANESTHETIZED SPONTANEOUS   **PARALYZED**

FIGURE 2–31. These three examples show the benefits of spontaneous ventilation over mechanical ventilation in a paralyzed patient. In an awake, supine patient, active diaphragmatic contraction causes more volume increase in the posterior basal segments of the lung. Under anesthesia, the distribution of ventilation does not change, but an erosion of total pulmonary volume is seen. This occurs at the expense of the expiratory reserve volume, although ventilation-perfusion ratios are not altered initially. In paralyzed humans, greater changes are seen as ventilation-perfusion ratios throughout the lung are altered. The reasons for these changes are: (1) Approximately a 25 cm H_2O gradient exists between the anterior abdominal wall and the back owing to weight of the abdominal contents pressing against the inferior diaphragmatic surface. (2) Diaphragmatic displacement is governed by the law of La Place, which provides that: pressure = tension/radius. Therefore, in the anterior diaphragmatic segments with a larger radius of curvature, diaphragmatic tension is less and displacement per unit pressure greater. Therefore, anterior segments move more freely and lead to the large change in volume distribution seen in the diagram. (3) Positive-pressure breathing reduces venous return to the right side of the heart and may reduce cardiac output, further reducing perfusion in anterior lung segments. (From Froese, A. B., and Bryan, A. C.: Effects of anesthesia and paralysis on diaphragmatic mechanics in man. Anesthesiology, *41*:242, 1974.)

ventilation is obtained, which diminishes ventilation-perfusion mismatch; mean intrathoracic pressure is minimized owing to spontaneously generated negative inspiratory effort, regardless of the end-expiratory pressure; maintenance of a negative (or relatively negative) inspiratory effort theoretically supports venous return to the right heart and improves cardiac output; patients appear more comfortable and require less sedation while receiving ventilatory support; and higher PEEP levels are tolerated more readily with decreased requirement for inotropic or volume support of the circulation. Spontaneous breathing decreases mean intrathoracic pressure and promotes venous return to the right heart. Even when associated with PEEP, overall mean intrathoracic pressure is lowered by spontaneous breaths.

From the time of inception of mechanical ventilation assistance, a therapeutic priority will be weaning and extubation. Therefore, a rational physiologic progression to extubation should include the following:

1. Initiation of IMV ventilation with 5 to 15 cm H_2O PEEP as determined by arterial saturation with an $F_{I_{O_2}}$ of 0.4 and ventilation supported mechanically to preserve a pH of 7.35.

2. Rapid progression to decrease ventilatory support is supported by the following observations:
   a. If there is no dyspnea or paradoxic respiratory movement, the patient is considered an acceptable weaning candidate.
   b. If respiratory paradox is apparent, consider either sedation, if discomfort is a problem, or more vigorous ventilatory support, if blood gases are unacceptable.
   c. A possible weaning formula includes the following:
      i. Maintain Pa_{O_2} between 80 and 100 mm Hg; increase PEEP as indicated.
      ii. Maintain pH at 7.35 or higher.
      iii. Maintain Pa_{CO_2} below 55 mm Hg; increase IMV as necessary.
      iv. Check ventilatory status hourly or half-hourly, as indicated.
      v. Consider IMV of 2 breaths and PEEP of 6 cm H_2O as indicating readiness for extubation if adequate respiratory mechanics are documented.
      vi. Extubate from low-rate IMV and CPAP. Patients do not require to be placed routinely on a T tube.
      vii. Consider initial diuretic therapy in patients who continue to hypoventilate in the face of a rising Pa_{CO_2} with metabolic alkalosis and normal serum potassium with 250 to 500 mg acetazolamide (Diamox), administered intravenously. This dose may be repeated two or three times as indicated to maintain normal bicarbonate levels.

Pulmonary support is directed toward recruiting lung volume to increase the available aveolar exchange area and to provide a regulated, enriched inspired oxygen concentration. The goal of respiration is the optimal oxygenation of individual mitochondria, but the most common measurement of respiration is the arterial blood gas. Because of the nature of the oxyhemoglobin dissociation curve, guidelines can be established that relate unacceptable peripheral oxygenation to varying arterial saturations. Indeed, estimation of pulmonary venous admixture (shunt) can be made accurately from arterial blood-gas values alone (Benatar et al., 1973). Mechanical ventilation should be tailored to respond to specific abnormalities while causing minimal derangements in normal pulmonary function. For this reason, support of FRC has been separated from regulation of pH.

With carefully applied PEEP and IMV, most patients can be supported successfully on a nontoxic concentration of inspired oxygen until safe weaning is feasible. Every effort should be made to allow the patient to do as much work as possible and to diminish ventilator dependence. Mechanical ventilation is not a benign intervention, and careful assessment of hemodynamic and renal function is essential in all ventilated patients. In some instances, exemplary blood gases are unobtainable, and it is important that the patient's condition not be allowed to suffer during the search for ideal ventilator settings.

Weaning from Mechanical Ventilation

Although appropriate matching of patient to machine is an appropriate goal, the most important goal of mechanical ventilatory assistance is to separate the patient from all support. For this reason, it is important to consider the parameters against which a patient's unaided performance is compared with various extubation criteria. Additionally, it becomes apparent that although some criteria are appropriate for patients who require ventilation for comparatively short periods, other indices may be necessary to successfully manage chronic patients (duration of ventilatory support in excess of 30 days) (Morganroth et al., 1984). In most cases, especially those seen following routine operations, the following criteria predict accurately the patient who can be weaned and extubated:

1. Negative inspiratory force greater than (more negative than) -25 mm Hg
2. Minute ventilation less than 10 l/min
3. Vital capacity of greater than 10 to 15 ml/kg
4. Tidal volume of 5 to 8 ml/kg
5. Resting respiratory rate less than 25 breaths per minute (Tobin et al., 1986)

Additionally, in the immediate postoperative period, restoration of core temperature to greater than 36° C aids in the ability of a recently anesthetized patient to maintain ventilatory homeostasis. If extubated while cold, many narcotized patients have an inadequate ventilatory response to the metabolic demands of rewarming and shivering. Hypercapnia and associated respiratory acidosis may develop.

It is appropriate to decrease mechanical support with the following hierarchy:

1. Decrease $F_{I_{O_2}}$ to 40% or less to support a stable arterial oxygen saturation of 90% or more.
2. Decrease IMV rate so that the patient is supporting more than 80% of the calculated required alveolar ventilation.
3. Wean PEEP or CPAP commensurate with maintenance of adequate oxygenation at a stable $F_{I_{O_2}}$ (Borman et al., 1986).

In general, patients should not be discontinued from PEEP before extubation, and most patients tolerate weaning from 5 to 8 cm H_2O PEEP. In fact, patients who have been receiving mechanical support with PEEP and who are placed on a T tube before extubation may develop atelectasis and a worsened intrapulmonary shunt, which may delay extubation.

PSV was developed not as an improved ventilatory support mode but as a buffer to the increased work of breathing imposed by most commercial ventilator demand valves and circuits. Therefore, it is in the realm of weaning patients that the technique has gained widespread, if uncritical, popularity. Theoretically similar to IPPB, "PSV systems work by maintaining a constant pressure during a plateau phase of spontaneous inspiration" (Arndt, 1992). The machines are servo-controlled and maintain a constant airway pressure by controlling inspiratory flow, thereby establishing the mechanism through which a patient's inspiratory effort is sensed. Flow is constant at the preset pressure for the duration of spontaneous inspiration, and it is terminated when sensed flow falls below a threshold of either 5 l/min or 25% of the peak inspiratory flow, depending on the equipment. The patient's subjective response to this modality has been positive, and of all newly introduced techniques in respiratory care, this one has probably gained the most general acceptance. PSV can be regarded as an adjunct to most forms of ventilatory support and should be used in patients who have adequate respiratory drive but who are unable to "drive" conventional devices. Clinicians familiar with the technique attempt to eliminate the ventilator as a work source for the patient. In this manner, PSV is used as a weaning adjunct and not as a primary means of ventilatory support.

SUMMARY

The relationship between pulmonary ventilation and perfusion is important. The lungs are unique because they receive the entire cardiac output, except for blood involved in direct right-to-left intracardiac shunts. The function of the lungs is to provide adequate oxygenation of the arterial blood with the concomitant elimination of carbon dioxide, the volatile acid waste product of aerobic metabolism. Within this framework, the requirements of the perioperative period have been discussed, and the detrimental effects of mechanical ventilation and muscle relaxation on the distribution of perfusion have been explored. A physiologic framework on which mechanical ventilatory support can be prescribed has been presented. At all times, the relationships between ventilation and cardiac performance must be remembered. Robotham (1981) summarizes the cardiac effects of spontaneous ventilation as follows:

During spontaneous respiration with each inspiratory decrease in pleural pressure, the right ventricle distends because of an increased venous return and an increased right heart afterload. This causes the left ventricle to be effectively stiffer, increasing the left ventricular diastolic pressure, decreasing pulmonary venous return, and hence, the left ventricular stroke volume. This phenomenon interacts with the increase in left ventricular afterload created by the decrease in pleural pressure, further increasing left ventricular diastolic pressure and decreasing left ventricular stroke volume.

Obviously, these changes gain significance in patients for whom the pleural pressure gradients are increased (e.g., in respiratory insufficiency). It is therefore imperative that the clinician view the total mechanism of pulmonary gas exchange rather than focus on either the head or the lungs. This is emphasized in the choice of mechanical ventilatory support modes required in the operating room and in the ICU. Intermittent mandatory ventilation, although originally viewed as a means of more rapid patient weaning (Downs et al., 1971), has become the mainstay of ventilatory support for the conscious patient. Advantages of this technique include:

1. Respiratory muscle conditioning during spontaneous respiratory efforts, with relaxation of these areas during mechanical inspiration, thereby reducing the risk of muscle fatigue (Muller et al., 1979)

2. Maintenance of spontaneous distribution of ventilation interspersed with mechanical breaths, preventing atelectasis and ventilation-perfusion mismatch (Froese and Bryan, 1974)

3. Improvement of systemic venous return with each spontaneous inspiration (Morgan et al., 1966)

PEEP has been presented as a means of preserving or augmenting the available surface area for gas diffusion. Adequate perfusion of this surface area (FRC) requires continual balancing of the necessities of increased circulating blood volume with the potential for developing pulmonary venous congestion with increased pulmonary vascular pressures and decreased gas diffusion.

At no time can the discussion of pulmonary physiology escape the need to combine ventilation (the lung) and perfusion (the circulation). Pulmonary function is diminished following all abdominal and thoracic surgical procedures. Anesthetic agents are all negative inotropes. This combination can produce significant postoperative morbidity. Careful attention to the derangement, careful physiologic preparation, and adjustment of commonly measured variables may diminish the complications and relegate them to the status of interesting benignities.

SELECTED BIBLIOGRAPHY

Physiology

Nunn, J. F.: Applied Respiratory Physiology. 2nd ed. London, Butterworth, 1977.

Although now an old text, this book provides an excellent review of pulmonary physiology for the interested investigator. All chapters are extremely well written and have good references. The sections on mechanisms of pulmonary ventilation, distribution of inspired gas, and the pulmonary circulation are exceptionally good, not only for the detailed and understandable discussion, but also for the completeness of the review from a historical as well as a scientific point of view. This volume is useful for serious research into the physiologic mechanisms of pulmonary function, and it provides in-depth information on all important aspects of respiratory physiology.

West, J. B.: Ventilation-Blood Flow and Gas Exchange. 3rd ed. Philadelphia, J. B. Lippincott, 1977.
West, J. B.: Respiratory Physiology: The Essentials. 2nd ed. Baltimore, Williams & Wilkins, 1979.
West, J. B.: Pulmonary Pathophysiology: The Essentials. Baltimore, Williams & Wilkins, 1977.

These three textbooks, taken as a unit, provide an excellent basis for the understanding of ventilation-perfusion characteristics of the lung, methods of physiologic measurement, and derangements in pulmonary function in common disease states. The approach to pulmonary physiology is logical and very well presented, and it is designed to equip the reader with the fundamentals necessary for understanding clinical application of respiratory physiology and mechanical ventilation support. A good basis on which to follow pulmonary function testing is provided, and all three books have useful references in the appendices. These volumes have been a mainstay in teaching pulmonary physiology since they were first published, and they deservedly enjoy this high reputation.

Preoperative Pulmonary Testing

Gass, G. D., and Olsen, G. N.: Preoperative pulmonary function testing to predict postoperative morbidity and mortality. Chest, 89:127–135, 1986.
Markos, J.: Preoperative assessment as a predictor of mortality and morbidity after lung resection. Am. Rev. Respir. Dis., 139:902–910, 1989.
Olsen, G. N.: The evolving role of exercise testing prior to lung resection. Chest, 95:218–225, 1989.
Tisi, G. M.: Preoperative evaluation of pulmonary function. Am. Rev. Respir. Dis., 119:293–310, 1979.

These references delineate the current approaches to pulmonary function testing and preoperative prophylaxis. Oxygen consumption ($\dot{V}O_2$) studies at rest and at exercise are discussed and may help predict the reserves of the cardiopulmonary-muscular axis. Critical evaluation of $\dot{V}O_2$ measurements may improve the reliability of pulmonary function tests in current use and improve risk stratification in lung resection operations. [133]Xe radiospirometry and ventilation scans are discussed in relation to other conventional tests, and although the sophistication and cost of the preoperative evaluation has increased, reliable outcome prediction has not.

Mechanical Ventilation

Eklund, J., Jarnberg, P. O., Norlander, O., and Santesson, J.: Opsscula Medica 1981 Supplementum LIII. Intensive Care IV. New Aspects on Artificial Ventilation. Stockholm, Sweden, 1981 (OPMSA7 53–1981).

This short, intelligent discussion of the physiology and mechanical interrelationships between circulation and ventilation. Sections on overall physiology, the pulmonary circulation, $\dot{V}/\dot{Q}$ relationships, and PEEP, as well as articles on techniques of ventilation, are well presented. A brief description of HFPPV is included, and the entire article is well referenced for further study.

Kirby, R. R., and Graybar, G. B. (eds): Intermittent mandatory ventilation. Int. Anesthesiol. Clin., 18:1, 1980.

This is an excellent review of modern techniques of mechanical ventilation. Common misconceptions in definition and application are explored, and a realistic attempt to explain the "alphabet soup" of ventilator jargon is made. The authors are all experts in the field, and the text extends from a good historical introduction to the most up-to-date types of mechanical ventilatory equipment. This is a good book for individuals who are seriously interested in understanding ventilatory support. It is an almost indispensable volume for people involved in full-time intensive care medicine.

MacIntyre, N. R.: Respiratory function during pressure support ventilation. Chest, 89:667, 1986.

This insightful article by a recognized expert on mechanical ventilatory support provides a good introduction to the use of and technical considerations supporting pressure support ventilation. The article provides some of the first clinical information available documenting potential benefits of the mode, and interested readers will find the text carefully written, the illustrations concise and helpful, and the references excellent.

Pathology

Ingram, R. H., Jr.: Adult respiratory syndrome. In Isselbacher, K. J., Adams, R. D., Braunwald, E., et al. (eds): Harrison's Principles of Internal Medicine. 9th ed. New York, McGraw-Hill, 1980, pp. 1276–1278.
Donald, K. J., Iverson, O. H., and Whimster, W. F.: Pathology of the respiratory system. 2nd ed. In Iverson, O. H. (ed): IPALS. Oslo, Universitats forlaget, 1978, pp. 22–33.
Spencer, H.: Pathology of the Lung. 3rd ed. New York, Pergamon Press, 1977, pp. 503–504.

Taken as a group, these references provide a good description of normal lung development and the pathology that is most frequently encountered in the postoperative period. Specific lesions are not addressed, but the overall situation that causes acute respiratory failure is well covered. The possible responses of the lung to trauma are described, and specific reference is made to the changes in lung architecture that are consistent with noncardiogenic pulmonary edema. Mechanisms of pulmonary edema are described, and the quoted references are valuable for further research.

Acute Respiratory Failure

Ashbaugh, D. G., Bigelow, D. B., and Petty, T. L.: Acute respiratory distress in adults. Lancet, 2:319, 1967.

Ayres, S. M.: The structural basis of pulmonary function. *In* Shoemaker, W. C., and Thompson, W. L. (eds): Critical Care—State of the Art. Soc. Crit. Care Med., *2*(A):1, 1981.

Bone, R. C.: Treatment of severe hypoxemia due to the adult respiratory distress syndrome. Arch. Intern. Med., *140*:85, 1980.

Kirby, R. R., Downs, J. B., Civetta, J. M., et al.: High level positive end expiratory pressure (PEEP) in acute respiratory insufficiency. Chest, *67*:156, 1975.

Murray, J. F.: Mechanisms of acute respiratory failure. Am. Rev. Respir. Dis., *107*:115, 1977.

Pontoppidan, H.: Mechanisms of acute respiratory failure. Presented at 30th Annual Refresher Course Lectures, American Society of Anesthesiologists, October 20–24, 1979, p. 223.

Staub, N. C.: Pulmonary edema. Physiol. Rev., *54*:678, 1974.

Each of the preceding articles or chapters provides insight into specific aspects of acute respiratory failure. Taken in sequence, they yield an up-to-date view of the current concepts used in managing patients who are classified as having noncardiogenic pulmonary edema and respiratory failure. The articles also provide a historical perspective on the development of modern therapeutic and mechanical ventilatory support modes. The references are well balanced, and the more recent articles will afford an excellent basis on which to pursue specific points of interest.

All selected references have been chosen because they provide a combination of historical insight and practical clinical approach that is based on an excellent physiologic foundation. References are pertinent and extensive. The interested reader should be able to research fully the topics covered in this chapter. Clinical applications of these physiologic principles often follow technologic initiative; therefore, the student is advised that source references are often more important than the latest treatise describing the therapeutic fashion of the moment.

BIBLIOGRAPHY

American Cardiac Life Support. Chicago, American Heart Association, 1987, 1992, p. 132.

Annest, S. J., Gottlieb, M., Paloski, W. H., et al.: Detrimental effects of removing end-expiratory pressure prior to endotracheal extubation. Ann. Surg., *191*:539, 1980.

Anscombe, A. R., and Buxton, R.: Effect of abdominal operations on total lung capacity and its subdivisions. Br. Med. J., *2*:84, 1958.

Arndt, G. A., and Stock, M. C.: Mechanical ventilation in postoperative period. Probl. Urol., *6*:102–115, 1992.

Ashbaugh, D. G., Bigelow, D. B., Petty, T. L., and Levine, B. E.: Acute respiratory in adults. Lancet, *2*:319, 1967.

Ayres, S. M.: The structural basis of pulmonary function. *In* Shoemaker, W. C., and Thompson, W. L. (eds): Critical Care—State of the Art. Soc. Crit. Care Med., *2*(A):1, 1981.

Bartel, L. P., Bazik, J. R., and Powner, D. J.: Compression volume during mechanical ventilation: Comparison of ventilators and tubing circuits. Crit. Care Med., *13*:710–713, 851, 1985.

Barton, G. A. H.: Backwaters of Lethe: Some Anesthetic Notions. New York, Paul B. Hoeber, 1920.

Beecher, H. K.: Effect of laparotomy on lung volume: Demonstration of a new type of pulmonary collapse. J. Clin. Invest., *12*:651, 1933.

Beecher, H. K.: The measured effect of laparotomy on the respiration. J. Clin. Invest., *12*:639, 1933.

Benatar, S. R., Hewlett, A. M., and Nunn, J. F.: The use of iso-shunt lines for control of oxygen therapy. Br. J. Anaesth., *45*:711, 1973.

Bjork, V. O., and Hilty, H. J.: The arterial oxygen and carbon dioxide tension during the post operative period in cases of pulmonary resections and thoracoplasties. Surgery, *27*:455, 1953.

Bone, R. C.: Treatment of severe hypoxemia due to the adult respiratory distress syndrome. Arch. Intern. Med., *140*:85, 1980.

Borman, K. R., Weigelt, J. A., and Aurbakken, C. M.: Guidelines for weaning from positive end-expiratory pressure in ventilated patients. Am. J. Surg., *152*:687–690, 1986.

Boushy, S. F., Billeq, D. M., North, L. B., and Helgason, A. H.: Clinical course related to preoperative and postoperative pulmonary function in patients with bronchogenic carcinoma. Chest, *59*:383, 1971.

Bryan-Brown, C. W.: Oxygen transport and the oxyhemoglobin dissociation curve. *In* Berk, J. L., Sampliner, J. E., Artz, J. S.,

and Vinocur, B. (eds): Handbook of Critical Care. Boston, Little Brown, 1976.

Browne, R. G.: Weaning patients from mechanical ventilation. Intensive Care Med., *10*:55–58, 1984.

Burrows, B., and Earle, R. H.: Prediction of survival in patients with chronic airway obstruction. Am. Rev. Respir. Dis., *99*:865, 1969.

Cane, R. D., Shapiro, B. A., Harrison, R. A., et al.: Minimizing errors in intrapulmonary shunt calculations. Crit. Care Med., *8*:294, 1980.

Carlon, G. C., Howland, W. S., Turnbull, A. D., and Kahn, R. C.: Pulmonary venous admixture during mechanical ventilation with varying $F_{I_{O_2}}$ and PEEP. Crit. Care Med., *8*:616, 1980.

Cassidy, S. S., Eschenbacher, W. L., Robertson, C. H., Jr., et al.: Cardiovascular effects of positive-pressure ventilation in normal subjects. J. Appl. Physiol., *47*:453, 1979.

Cassidy, S. S., Robertson, C. H., Jr., Pierce, A. K., et al.: Cardiovascular effects of positive end-expiratory pressure in dogs. J. Appl. Physiol., *44*:743, 1978.

Chevers, N.: Observations on the diseases of the orifice and valves of the aorta. Guy's Hospital Report, *7*:387, 1842.

Churchill, E. D., and McNeil, D.: The reduction in vital capacity following operation. Surg. Gynecol. Obstet., *44*:483, 1927.

Coetzee, A., and Rossouw, J.: [Letter to the editor]. S. Afr. Med. J., *5*:377, 1981.

Cohn, J. D., and Engler, P. E.: Shunt effect of carboxyhemoglobin. Crit. Care Med., *7*:54, 1979.

Conference on the Scientific Basis of Respiratory Therapy, Philadelphia, May 2–4, 1974.

Conference on the Scientific Basis of In-Hospital Respiratory Therapy, Atlanta, November 14–16, 1979.

Coryllos, P. N., and Birnbaum, G. I.: Studies in pulmonary gas absorption in bronchial obstruction: Behavior and absorption times of oxygen, carbon dioxide, nitrogen, hydrogen, helium, ethylene, nitrous oxide, ethyl chloride and ether in the lung. Am. J. Med. Sci., *183*:347, 1932.

Cournand, A., Motley, M. L., Werko, L., and Richards, D. W.: Physiological studies on the effect of intermittent positive-pressure breathing on cardiac output in man. Am. J. Physiol., *152*:162, 1948.

CPR guidelines. JAMA, *244*:453, 1980.

Craig, D. B.: Postoperative recovery of pulmonary function. Anesth. Analg., *60*:46, 1981.

Dale, W. A., and Rahn, H.: Rate of gas absorption during atelectasis. Am. J. Physiol., *170*:606, 1953.

Dantzker, D. R., Brook, C. J., Dehart, P., et al.: Ventilation-perfusion distributions in the adult respiratory distress syndrome. Am. Rev. Respir. Dis., *120*:1039, 1979.

Dantzker, D. R., Lynch, J. P., and Weg, J. G.: Depression of cardiac output is a mechanism of shunt reduction in the therapy of acute respiratory failure. Chest, *77*:636, 1980.

Diament, M. L., and Palmer, K. N. V.: Postoperative changes in gas tensions of arterial blood and in ventilatory function. Lancet, *2*:180, 1966.

Diament, M. L., and Palmer, K. N. V.: Spirometry for preoperative assessment of airways resistance. Lancet, *1*:1251, 1967.

Didolkar, M. S., Moore, R. H., and Takita, H.: Evaluation of the risk in pulmonary resection for bronchogenic carcinoma. Am. J. Surg., *127*:700, 1974.

Diener, C. F., and Burrows, G.: Further observations on the course and prognosis of chronic obstructive lung disease. Am. Rev. Respir. Dis., *111*:719, 1975.

Dolfuss, R. E., Milic-Emili, J., and Bates, D. V.: Regional ventilation of the lung studied with boluses of xenon. Respir. Physiol., *2*:234, 1967.

Donald, K. J., Iverson, O. H., and Whimster, W. F.: Pathology of the respiratory system. 2nd ed. *In* Iverson, O. H. (ed): IPALS. Oslo, Universitats Forlaget, 1978, pp. 22–33.

Douglas, M. E., Downs, J. B., Dannemiller, F. J., et al.: Change in pulmonary venous admixture with varying inspired oxygen. Anesth. Analg., *55*:688, 1976.

Downs, J. B., Klein, E. F., Desautels, D., et al.: Intermittent mandatory ventilation. A new approach to weaning patients from mechanical ventilators. Chest, *64*:331, 1973.

Dueck, R., Young, I., Clausen, J., and Wagner, P. D.: Altered distribution of pulmonary ventilation and blood flow following induction of inhalational anesthesia. Anesthesiology, 52:113, 1980.

Eger, E. I. O., and Severinghaus, J. W.: The rate of rise of $P_{A_{CO_2}}$ in the apneic anesthetized patient. Anesthesiology, 22:419, 1961.

Eklund, J., Jarnberg, P. O., Norlander, O., and Santesson, J.: Opsscula Medica 1981 Supplementum LIII. Intensive Care IV. New Aspects on Artificial Ventilation. Stockholm, 1981 (OMPSA7 53-1981).

Engel, L. A., Grassino, A. E., and Anthonisen, N. R.: Demonstration of airway closure in man. J. Appl. Physiol., 38:1117, 1975.

Fournier, L., and Major, D.: Comparison between a clinical short-cut method and a precise laboratory estimation of intrapulmonary shunt and A-aDo_2. Can. Anaesth. Soc. J., 28:263, 1981.

Froese, A. B., and Bryan, A. C.: Effects of anesthesia and paralysis on diaphragmatic mechanics in man. Anesthesiology, 41:242, 1974.

Frumin, M. J., Epstein, R. M., and Cohen, G.: Apneic oxygenation in man. Anesthesiology, 20:789, 1959.

Gaensler, E. A., Cugell, D. W., Lingren, I., et al.: The role of pulmonary insufficiency in mortality and invalidism following surgery for pulmonary tuberculosis. J. Thorac. Surg., 29:163, 1955.

Gallagher, T. J.: Metabolic alkalosis complicating weaning from mechanical ventilation. South. Med. J., 72:786, 1979.

Gallagher, T. J., and Civetta, J. M.: Goal-directed therapy of acute respiratory failure. Anesth. Analg., 59:831, 1980.

Gallagher, T. J., Civetta, J. M., and Kirby, R. R.: Terminology update: Optimal PEEP. Crit. Care Med., 6:323, 1978.

Geer, R. T.: Interpretation of pulmonary-artery wedge pressure when PEEP is used. Anesthesiology, 46:383, 1977.

Gothe, B., and Cherniack, N. S.: Effects of expiratory loading on respiration in humans. J. Appl. Physiol., 49:601, 1980.

Greene, R.: Diagnostic radiology in intensive care. Presented at ASA 30th Annual Refresher Course Lectures, San Francisco, October 22–24, 1979.

Grenvik, A., Eross, B., and Powner, D.: Historical survey of mechanical ventilation. Int. Anesthesiol. Clin., 18:1, 1980.

Grindlinger, G. A., Mauney, J., Justice, R., et al.: Presence of negative inotropic agents in canine plasma during positive end-expiratory pressure. Circ. Res., 45:460, 1979.

Gross, R., and Israel, R. H.: A graphic approach for prediction of arterial oxygen tension at different concentrations of inspired oxygen. Chest, 79:311, 1981.

Harpin, R. P., Baker, J. P., Bowner, J. P., et al.: Correlation of the oxygen cost of breathing and length of weaning from mechanical ventilation. Crit. Care Med., 15:807–812, 1987.

Haynes, J. B., Carson, S. D., Whitney, W. P., et al.: Positive end-expiratory pressure shifts in left ventricular diastolic pressure-area curves. J. Appl. Physiol., 48:670, 1980.

Hegyi, T., and Hiatt, I. M.: The effect of continuous positive airway pressure on the course of respiratory distress syndrome: The benefits of early initiation. Crit. Care Med., 9:38, 1981.

Herholdt, J. D., and Rafn, C. G.: Life Saving Measures for Drowning Persons. Copenhagen, 1796. Reprinted by the Scandinavian Society of Anesthesiology, 1960.

Hermannsen, J.: Untersuchungen uber die maximale Ventilationsgrosse (Ateingrenzwert). Ztschr. Ges. Exper. Med., 90:130, 1933.

Hooke, R.: The Theory of Springs. De Potential Restitutive, 1678.

Howell, J. B., Permutt, S., Proctor, D. F., and Riley, R. L.: Effect of inflation of the lung on different parts of the pulmonary vascular bed. J. Appl. Physiol., 16:71, 1961.

Hughes, J. M. B., Glazier, J. B., Maloney, J. E., and West, J. B.: Effect of extra-alveolar vessels on distribution of blood flow in the dog lung. J. Appl. Physiol., 25:701, 1968.

Hughes, J. M. B., Glazier, J. B., Maloney, J. E., and West, J. B.: Effect of lung volume on the distribution of pulmonary blood flow in man. Respir. Physiol., 4:58, 1968.

Hughes, J. M. B., Rosenzweig, D. Y., and Kivitz, P. B.: Site of airway closure in excised dog lungs: histolic demonstration. J. Appl. Physiol., 29:340, 1970.

Hunter, J.: Philosophical Transactions, 66:412, 1776.

Hutchinson, J.: On the capacity of the lungs, and on the respiratory functions, with a view of establishing a precise and easy method of detecting disease by the spirometer. Med. Chir. Trans., 29:137, 1846.

Ingram, R. H., Jr.: Adult respiratory distress syndrome. In Isselbacher, K. J., Adams, R. D., Braunwald, E., et al. (eds): Harrison's Principles of Internal Medicine. 9th ed. New York, McGraw-Hill, 1980.

Jacob, H. S.: Damaging role of activated complement in myocardial infarction and shock lung: Ramifications for rational therapy. In Shoemaker, W. C., and Thompson, W. L. (eds): Critical Care—State of the Art. Soc. Crit. Care Med., 1:(L):1, 1980.

Jardin, F., Gurdjian, F., Desfonds, P., and Margairaz, A. P.: Effect of dopamine on intrapulmonary shunt fraction and oxygen transport in severe sepsis with circulatory and respiratory failure. Crit. Care Med., 7:273, 1979.

Jardin, F., Farcot, J. C., Boisante, L., et al.: Influence of positive end-expiratory pressure on left ventricular performance. N. Engl. J. Med., 304:387, 1981.

Karliner, J. S., Coomaiaswamy, R., and Williams, M. H.: Relationship between preoperative pulmonary function studies and prognosis of patients undergoing pneumonectomy for carcinoma of the lung. Dis. Chest, 54:32, 1968.

Kirby, R. R., and Graybar, G. B. (eds): Intermittent Mandatory Ventilation. Int. Anesthesiol. Clin., 18:1, 1980.

Kirby, R. R., Downs, J. B., Civetta, J. M., et al.: High level positive end expiratory pressure (PEEP) in acute respiratory insufficiency. Chest, 67:156, 1975.

Klug, T. J., and McPherson, R. C.: Postoperative complications in the elderly surgical patients. Am. J. Surg., 97:713, 1959.

Laros, C. D., and Swierenga, J.: Temporary unilateral pulmonary artery occlusion in the preoperative evaluation of patients with bronchial carcinoma. Med. Thorac., 24:269, 1967.

Latimer, G., Dickman, M., Clinton Day, W., et al.: Ventilatory patterns and pulmonary complications after upper abdominal surgery determined by preoperative and postoperative computerized spirometry and blood gas analysis. Am. J. Surg., 122:622, 1971.

Laver, M. B., and Austen, W. G.: Respiratory function: Physiologic considerations applicable to surgery. In Sabiston, D. C., Jr. (ed): Davis-Christopher Textbook of Surgery. 12th ed. Philadelphia, W. B. Saunders, 1981.

Laver, M. B., Austen, W. G., and Wilson, R. S.: Blood-gas exchange and hemodynamic performance. In Sabiston, D. C., Jr., and Spencer, F. C., (eds): Gibbon's Surgery of the Chest. 3rd ed. Philadelphia, W. B. Saunders, 1976.

Laver, M. B., Hallowell, P., and Goldblatt, A.: Pulmonary dysfunction secondary to heart disease: Aspects relevant to anesthesia and surgery. Anesthesiology, 33:161, 1970.

Lee, J. A., and Atkinson, R. S.: Resuscitation. In Lee, J. A., and Atkinson, R. S. (eds): A Synopsis of Anaesthesia. 7th ed. Bristol, John Wright, 1973.

Lockwood, P.: The principles of predicting risk of post-thoracotomy function-related complications in bronchogenic carcinoma. Respiration, 30:329, 1973.

Loeschcke, H. H., Sweel, A., Kough, R. H., and Lambertsen, C. J.: The effect of morphine and meperedine (Dilantin, Demerol) upon the respiratory response of normal men to low concentrations of inspired carbon dioxide. J. Pharmacol. Exp. Ther., 108:376, 1953.

Lumb, P. D.: The use and abuse of diuretics. Mt. Sinai J. Med., 48:381, 1981.

Lumb, P. D., Silvay, G., Weinreich, A. I., and Shiang, H.: A comparison of the effects of continuous ketamine infusion and halothane on oxygenation during one-lung anesthesia in dogs. Can. Anaesth. Soc. J., 26:394, 1979.

MacIntyre, N. R.: Respiratory function during pressure support ventilation. Chest, 89:5, 677, 1986.

Macklem, P. T.: Respiratory mechanics. Ann. Rev. Physiol., 40:157, 1978.

Maffeo, C. J., Hoyt, J. W., and Swain, R. F.: Venous admixture: Efforts and clinical decisions. Anesthesiology, 55:A80, 1981.

Manny, J., Patten, M. T., Liebman, P. R., and Hechtman, H. B.: The association of lung distension, PEEP and biventricular failure. Ann. Surg., 187:151, 1978.

Marini, J. J., Culver, B. H., and Kirk, W.: Flow resistance of exhalation valves and positive end-expiratory pressure devices used in mechanical ventilation. Am. Rev. Respir. Dis., 131:850, 1985.

Matthay, R. A., and Wood, L. D.: Cardiovascular function in respiratory failure. I. Introduction: The functionally integrated cardiovascular-pulmonary unit. Am. J. Cardiol., 47:683, 1981.

Mauney, J., Grindlinger, G., Mathe, A. A., and Hechtman, H. B.: Positive end-expiratory pressure, lung stretch, and decreased myocardial contractility. Surgery, 84:201, 1978.

Mazzone, R. W.: Influence of pulmonary edema on capillary morphology. Presented at Fed. Proc. Abstracts. 65th Annual Meeting, Atlanta, Georgia, 1981.

Mazzone, R. W., Durand, C. M., and West, J. B.: Electron microscopy of lung rapidly frozen under controlled physiological conditions. J. Appl. Physiol., 45:325, 1978.

Mazzone, R. W., Kornblau, S., and Durand, C. M.: Shrinkage of lung after chemical fixation for analysis of pulmonary structure-function relations. J. Appl. Physiol., 48:382, 1980.

Milic-Emili, J., Henderson, J. A. M., Dolovich, M. B., et al.: Regional distribution of inspired gas in the lung. J. Appl. Physiol., 21:749, 1966.

Miller, W. F., Wu, N., and Johnson, R. L., Jr.: Convenient method of evaluating pulmonary ventilatory function with a single breath test. Anesthesiology, 17:480, 1956.

Minh, V. D., Kurihara, N., Friedman, P. J., and Moser, K. M.: Reversal of pleural pressure gradient during electrophrenic stimulation. J. Appl. Physiol., 37:496, 1974.

Mittman, C.: Assessment of operative risk in thoracic surgery. Am. Rev. Respir. Dis., 84:197, 1961.

Moore, F. D.: A critical analysis of causes and treatment of surgical types of shock. J. Trauma, 9:143, 1969.

Morgan, B. C., Martin, W. E., Hornbein, T. F., et al.: Hemodynamic effects of intermittent positive pressure respiration. Anesthesiology, 27:584, 1966.

Morganroth, M. L., Morganroth, J. L., Nett, L. M., and Petty, T. L.: Criteria for weaning from prolonged mechanical ventilation. Arch. Intern. Med., 144:1012–1016, 1984.

Morton, H. J. V., and Camb, D. A.: Tobacco smoking and pulmonary complications after operation. Lancet, 1:368, 1944.

Muller, N., Gulston, G., Cade, D., et al.: Diaphragmatic muscle fatigue in the newborn. J. Appl. Physiol., 46:688, 1979.

Muller, N., Volgyesi, G., Becker, L., et al.: Diaphragmatic muscle tone. J. Appl. Physiol., 47:279, 1979.

Murray, J. F.: ARDS—May it rest in peace. Am. Rev. Respir. Dis., 111:716, 1975.

Murray, J. F.: Mechanisms of acute respiratory failure. Am. Rev. Respir. Dis., 107:115, 1977.

Murray, J. F.: The Normal Lung. Philadelphia, W. B. Saunders, 1976.

Nunn, J. F.: Applied Respiratory Physiology. 2nd ed. London, Butterworth, 1977.

Nunn, J. F.: Carriage of oxygen in the blood. In Nunn, J. F. (ed): Applied Respiratory Physiology. 2nd ed. London, Butterworth, 1977, p. 405.

Nunn, J. F.: The distribution of inspired gas during thoracic surgery. Ann. R. Coll. Surg. Engl., 28:223, 1961.

Nunn, J. F., Williams, L. P., and Jones, J. G.: Detection and reversal of pulmonary absorption collapse. Br. J. Anaesth., 50:91, 1978.

Oliven, A. A. E., and Burstein, S.: The influences of varying inspired oxygen tensions on the pulmonary venous admixture (shunt) of mechanically ventilated patients. Crit. Care Med., 8:99, 1980.

Orth, J.: Distribution of Blood Flow in Lungs. Aetiologisches und Anatomisches uber Lungenschwindsucht, Berlin, 1887, Breitkreuz 8.1M.

Pardy, R. L., Rivington, R. N., Depas, P. D., and Macklem, P. T.: The effects of inspiratory muscle training on exercise performance in chronic airflow limitation. Am. Rev. Respir. Dis., 123:426, 1981.

Pasteur, W.: Active lobar collapse of the lung after abdominal operations: A contribution to the study of postoperative lung complications. Lancet, October 1910, pp. 1080–1082.

Patten, M. T., Liebman, P. R., Manny, J., et al.: Humorally mediated alterations in cardiac performance as a consequence of positive end-expiratory pressure. Surgery, 84:201, 1978.

Permutt, S.: Effect of interstitial pressure of the lung on pulmonary circulation. Med. Thorac., 22:118, 1965.

Permutt, S., Bromberger-Barnea, B., and Bane, H. N.: Alveolar pressure, pulmonary venous pressure, and the vascular waterfall. Med. Thorac., 19:239, 1962.

Pontoppidan, H.: The black box illuminated. Anesthesiology, 37:1, 1972.

Pontoppidan, H.: Mechanisms of injury and natural history of acute respiratory failure. Presented at ASA 30th Annual Refresher Course Lectures, San Francisco, October 22–24, 1979, p. 223.

Pontoppidan, H., Geffin, B., and Lowenstein, E.: Acute Respiratory Failure in the Adult. Boston, Little Brown, 1973.

Pontoppidan, H., Laver, M. B., and Geffin, B.: Acute respiratory failure in the surgical patient. Adv. Surg., 4:163, 1970.

Powers, S. R., Manual, R., Neclino, M., et al.: Physiologic consequences of positive end-expiratory pressure (PEEP) ventilation. Ann. Surg., 178:265, 1973.

Prewitt, R. M., and Wood, L. D. H.: Effect of positive end-expiratory pressure on ventricular function in dogs. Am. J. Physiol., 236:H534, 1979.

Priestley, J.: Philosophical Transactions, 66:412, 1776.

Putnam, L., Jennicek, J. A., Cellan, C. A., and Wilson, R. D.: Anesthesia in the morbidly obese. South. Med. J., 67:1411, 1974.

Qvist, J., Pontoppidan, H., Wilson, R. S., et al.: Hemodynamic responses to mechanical ventilation with PEEP: The effect of hypervolemia. Anesthesiology, 42:45, 1975.

Rahn, H., and Fenn, W. O.: A Graphical Analysis of the Respiratory Gas Exchange. Washington, D. C., American Physiological Society, 1955.

Ream, A. K., Reitz, B. A., and Silverberg, G.: Temperature correction of P_{CO_2} and pH in estimating acid-base status: An example of the emperor's new clothes? Anesthesiology, 56:41, 1982.

Rehder, K., Knopp, T. J., Sessler, A. D., and Didier, E. P.: Ventilation-perfusion relationship in young, healthy, awake and anesthetized-paralyzed man. J. Appl. Physiol., 47:745, 1979.

Reines, M. D., and Civetta, J. M.: The inaccuracy of using 100% oxygen to determine intrapulmonary shunt fraction in spite of PEEP. Crit. Care Med., 7:301, 1979.

Rerych, S. K., Scholz, P. M., Newman, G. E., et al.: Cardiac function at rest and during exercise in normals and in patients with coronary heart disease: Evaluated by radionuclide angiocardiography. Ann. Surg., 187:449, 1978.

Rerych, S. K., Scholz, P. M., Sabiston, D. C., Jr., et al.: Effects of training on left ventricular function in normal subjects: A longitudinal study. Am. J. Cardiol., 45:244, 1980.

Riley, R. L., and Cournand, A.: Analysis of factors affecting partial pressures of oxygen and carbon dioxide in gas and blood of lungs: Theory. J. Appl. Physiol., 4:77, 1951.

Riley, R. L., and Cournand, A.: "Ideal" alveolar air and the analysis of ventilation-perfusion relationships in the lungs. J. Appl. Physiol., 1:825, 1949.

Robotham, J. L.: Cardiovascular disturbances in chronic respiratory insufficiency. Am. J. Cardiol., 47:941, 1981.

Roy, R., Powers, S. R., Jr., Feustel, P. J., et al.: Pulmonary wedge catheterization during positive end-expiratory pressure ventilation in the dog. Anesthesiology, 46:385, 1977.

Sabiston, D. C., Jr. (ed): Davis-Christopher Textbook of Surgery. 12th ed. Philadelphia, W. B. Saunders, 1981.

Salzano, J. V.: Lecture Notes in Physiology—Respiratory. Durham, NC, Dept. of Physiology, Duke University Medical Center, 1979.

Schimert, G., Hunt, O. R., Lillenstein, M., et al.: Sodium/potassium ratios in papillary muscle biopsies obtained during mitral valve replacement. J. Thorac. Cardiovasc. Surg., 52:152, 1966.

Schmidt, G. B., O'Neill, W. W., Kotb, K., et al.: Continuous positive airway pressure in the prophylaxis of the adult respiratory distress syndrome. Surg. Gynecol. Obstet., 143:613, 1976.

Segall, J. J., and Butterworth, A.: Ventilatory capacity in chronic bronchitis in relation to carbon dioxide retention. Scand. J. Respir. Dis., 47:215, 1966.

Shabot, M. M., Shoemaker, W. C., and State, D.: Rapid bedside computation of cardio-respiratory variables with a programmable calculator. Crit. Care Med., 5:105, 1977.

Sharer, K., and Sladen, R.: Evaluation of perioperative ischemia by ST segment analysis in patients with coronary artery disease undergoing noncardiac surgery. Abstract of paper presented at the Society of Cardiovascular Anesthesiologists 10th Annual Meeting, New Orleans, April 10–13, 1988.

Siegel, J. H., Giovannini, I., and Coleman, B.: Ventilation:perfusion maldistribution secondary to the hyperdynamic cardiovascular state as the major cause of increased pulmonary shunting in human sepsis. J. Trauma, 19:432, 1979.

Silvay, G., Weinreich, A. I., Lumb, P. D., and Shiang, D. V. M.: Continuous infusion of ketamine for thoracic surgery using one-lung ventilation. *In* Aldrete, J. A., and Stanley, T. H. (eds): Trends in Intravenous Anesthesia. Miami, Symposia Specialists, 1980.

Smith, H., and Lumb, P. D.: Acid-Base Balance in Clinical Anesthesia. 2nd ed. Philadelphia, J. B. Lippincott, 1992, pp. 237–250.

Sorbini, C. A., Grassi, V., Solinas, E., and Muiesan, G.: Arterial oxygen tension in relation to age in healthy subjects. Respiration, *25*:3, 1968.

Spencer, H.: Pathology of the Lung. 3rd ed. New York, Pergamon Press, 1977.

Stanley, T. H., Liu, W. S., and Gentry, S.: Effects of ventilatory techniques during cardiopulmonary bypass on post-bypass and postoperative compliance and shunt. Anesthesiology, *46*:391, 1977.

Starling, E. H.: On the absorption of fluids from the connective tissue spaces. J. Physiol., *19*:312, 1896.

Staub, N. C.: Pulmonary edema. Physiol. Rev., *54*:678, 1974.

Summer, W. R., Permutt, S., Sagawa, K., et al.: Effects of spontaneous respiration on canine left ventricular function. Circ. Res., *45*:719, 1979.

Sykes, M. K., Adams, A. O., Finlay, W. E. I., et al.: The effects of variations in end-expiratory inflation pressure on cardiorespiratory function in normo-hypervolemic dogs. Br. J. Anaesth., *42*:669, 1970.

Tisi, G. M.: Preoperative evaluation of pulmonary function. Am. Rev. Respir. Dis., *119*:293, 1979.

Tobin, M. J., Perez, W., Guenther, S. M., et al.: The pattern of breathing during successful and unsuccessful trials of weaning from mechanical ventilation. Am. Rev. Respir. Dis., *134*:1111–1118, 1986.

Tonnesen, A. S., Gabel, J. C., Guidry, O. F., et al.: Lack of effect of 100% O_2 breathing on shunt. Abstracts of scientific papers, ASA Annual Meeting, New Orleans, 1977, pp. 13–14.

Valdes, M. E., Powers, S. R., Shah, D. M., et al.: Continuous positive airway pressure in the prophylaxis of the adult respiratory distress syndrome (ARDS) in trauma patients. Surg. Forum, *29*:187, 1979.

Venus, B., Smith, R. A., and Mathru, M.: National survey of methods and criteria used for weaning from mechanical ventilation. Crit. Care Med., *15*:530, 1987.

Vesalius, A.: De Humani Corporis Fabrica Libri Septem. 2nd ed. Basel, Oporinus, 1555, p. 818.

Virgilio, R. W., Rice, C. L., Smith, D. E., et al.: Crystalloid vs. colloid resuscitation: Is one better? Surgery, *85*:129, 1979.

Wagner, P. D.: Measurement of the distribution of ventilation-perfusion ratios. *In* Davis, D. G., and Barnes, C. D. (eds): Regulation of Ventilation and Gas Exchange. New York, Academic Press, 1978.

Wagner, P. D., Lavoroso, R. B., Uhl, R. R., et al.: Continuous distribution of ventilation-perfusion ratios in normal subjects breathing air and 100% oxygen. J. Clin. Invest., *54*:54, 1974.

Wagner, P. D., Dantzker, D. R., Dueck, R., et al.: Ventilation-perfusion inequality in chronic obstructive pulmonary disease. J. Clin. Invest., *59*:203, 1977.

Walker, I., Aukland, P., Hirsch, J., et al.: The low specificity of postoperative perfusion lung scan defects. CMA J., *124*:153, 1981.

Webster's New Collegiate Dictionary: Springfield, MA, G. & C. Merriam, 1975.

West, J. B.: Pulmonary Pathophysiology. Baltimore, Williams & Wilkins, 1977.

West, J. B.: Respiratory Physiology. 2nd ed. Baltimore, Williams & Wilkins, 1979.

West, J. B.: Ventilation-Blood Flow and Gas Exchange. 3rd ed. Philadelphia, J. B. Lippincott, 1977.

West, J. B., and Jones, N. L.: Effect of changes in topographical distribution of lung blood flow on gas exchange. J. Appl. Physiol., *20*:825, 1965.

Williams, J. J., and Marshall, B. E.: A fresh look at an old question. Anesthesiology, *56*:1, 1982.

Zeffren, S. E., and Hartford, C. E.: Comparative mortality for various surgical operations in older versus younger age groups. J. Am. Geriatr. Soc., *20*:185, 1972.

Zinn, S. E., Ozanne, G. M., and Fairley, H. B.: Mixed expired gas transients as a noninvasive index of the effect of PEEP. Anesthesiology, *52*:261, 1980.

3

Endoscopy: Bronchoscopy and Esophagoscopy

Arthur D. Boyd

Because endoscopy provides direct access to the tracheobronchial tree and esophagus, it plays an essential role in the diagnosis and treatment of patients with chest diseases. Although attempts to visualize the tracheobronchial tree and esophagus were made early in the 19th century, real progress began when instruments with incandescent lighting became available. Endoscopy as an art and science reached a peak in what may be called the Philadelphia School of Bronchoesophagology founded by Chevalier Jackson. During his long, productive career as a clinical investigator and teacher, Chevalier Jackson made bronchoesophagology a specialized subject and attracted students from all over the world. He trained such leaders as Clerf, Tucker, C. L. Jackson, and Hollinger, who devoted their full energies to establishing the principles of endoscopy and to increasing the information about chest diseases. Hollinger, for example, made a significant contribution to the teaching of endoscopy by producing a series of films that show most of the lesions that are encountered in an active endoscopic clinic.

During the 1980s, the scope and use of endoscopy of the respiratory tract and esophagus have increased dramatically. The Hopkins rod-lens optical system, developed for use in rigid open-tube endoscopes and flexible fiberoptic endoscopes, has introduced exciting new dimensions to endoscopy. These instruments allow better visualization and more precise biopsy of lesions than was previously possible. The introduction of updated endoscopes, with greater visual and operative capabilities, lasers, and endoscopic instruments, such as more refined biopsy forceps, brushes, dilators, and endoluminal prostheses, and more sophisticated techniques for obtaining and processing specimens contribute significantly and increasingly to the care of patients with chest diseases.

BRONCHOSCOPY

Bronchoscopy is performed for both diagnostic and therapeutic reasons in patients with pulmonary pathology. Diagnostic bronchoscopy includes not only the direct inspection and observation of the larynx, trachea, and bronchi, but also the removal of tissue, secretions, brushings, and washings for histologic, bacteriologic, viral, protozoal, chemical, antibody, and cytologic study. Therapeutic bronchoscopy, although done less frequently than diagnostic procedures, is still very important. Removal of secretions and foreign bodies, control of massive bleeding, and opening of narrowed tracheal and bronchial segments can be accomplished by an experienced bronchoscopist.

Before bronchoscopy is attempted, a complete clinical examination should be performed and chest films should be taken. During the bronchoscopy, the patient must be relaxed and cooperative. The surgeon must be skillful and gentle, particularly when he introduces a straight rigid bronchoscope into the naturally angulated air passages. Similar skill and gentleness are also required with the flexible fiberoptic bronchoscope, although its introduction is easier than the introduction of the rigid scope.

Indications

The numerous indications for bronchoscopy, both diagnostic and therapeutic, are shown in Table 3–1. The most common indication for the performance of a diagnostic bronchoscopy is the suspicion of bronchogenic carcinoma. Radiographic findings that suggest the presence of a pulmonary tumor or bronchial obstruction, as well as cough, hemoptysis, or wheezing, are all indications for bronchoscopy.

Frequently, pulmonary infections (bacterial, fungal, tuberculous, viral, and protozoal) require bronchoscopic examination, especially when these infections occur in patients who are immunocompromised from the use of chemotherapeutic agents and steroids, as well as in patients with acquired immunodeficiency syndrome (AIDS). Interstitial pulmonary disease is often investigated by bronchoscopy and transbronchial biopsy of the lung. Bronchoscopy must be performed by the operating surgeon before thoracotomy on all patients in whom a pulmonary resection is contemplated. Bronchoscopy is also useful diagnostically to monitor the course of chest diseases and to evaluate the larynx, trachea, and bronchi of patients who have had trauma to these structures or who have had prolonged endotracheal intubation.

Therapeutic bronchoscopy is performed to remove secretions and foreign bodies, to control massive bleeding, and to open narrowed tracheal or bronchial segments.

■ **Table 3–1.** DIAGNOSTIC AND THERAPEUTIC INDICATIONS FOR BRONCHOSCOPY

Diagnostic bronchoscopy
  Abnormal thoracic radiogram, localized lesion
  Unresolving lobar or segmental pneumonia
  Lung biopsy for diffuse parenchymal lung disease
  Bronchoalveolar lavage
  Hemoptysis
  New or unexplained cough
  Stridor or localized wheezing
  Suspected bronchiectasis
  Suspected foreign body
  Suspected broncholithiasis
  Malignant pleural effusion
  Neoplasm suggested by cytologic examination of
    sputum
  Immunocompromised patient with new pulmonary
    infiltrate
  Major thoracic trauma
  Upper esophageal lesions
Therapeutic bronchoscopy
  Postoperative atelectasis
  Retained sections or mucus plugs
  Removal of a foreign body
  Localized management of tumors with phototherapy,
    laser cautery, or cryotherapy
  Brachytherapy
  Management of life-threatening bleeding

From Brutinel, W. M., and Sanderson, D. R.: Bronchoscopy. *In* Practice of Surgery. Vol. 5, Chap. 4, Sect. 1. Philadelphia, Harper & Row, 1985, pp. 1–8. By permission of the publisher.

Specific Indications

Cough. A chronic persistent cough of unexplained origin with or without expectoration may be the only symptom of a neoplasm in an adult or of a foreign body in a child. Bronchoscopy may be the only method to determine the presence of these conditions. Cough may precede any other evidence of pulmonary disease, and therefore should not be dismissed lightly as being due to smoking or chronic bronchitis. All too often the serious mistake of withholding bronchoscopy is made in these circumstances because the procedure is considered too distressing to the patient.

Hemoptysis. Hemoptysis is a common clinical event and an important indication of pulmonary disease. Hemoptysis in association with an abnormal chest film is an indication for prompt bronchoscopy. With a normal chest film, intermittent hemoptysis of more than 1 week's duration, especially in patients at risk for lung cancer, is also an indication for prompt

bronchoscopy (Snider, 1979; Weaver et al., 1979). Mild, limited hemoptysis in association with acute bronchitis occasionally may be observed (Shure, 1987). Because the risk and degree of discomfort of bronchoscopy with the flexible fiberoptic bronchoscope are so small, it is preferable to pursue bronchoscopy aggressively rather than not to do this procedure. Hemoptysis has many causes, among which pulmonary neoplasms are the most common. Bronchiectasis, tuberculosis, aspergillosis, and mitral stenosis are other causes. Bronchoscopy is usually necessary to establish the etiology of hemoptysis and, if possible, should be performed when bleeding is subsiding. The bleeding thus does not interfere with visualization and can be traced to the lesion or to the segmental bronchus from which it arises.

In one series of patients with hemoptysis and normal chest films, 16% had endobronchial tumors at bronchoscopy (Zavala, 1975). In another series of patients with abnormal chest films, the site of bleeding was frequently found to be in an area other than the abnormal area on the chest film (Smiddy and Elliott, 1973). In 8 to 10% of patients, the site of bleeding could not be established, even after a complete diagnostic survey that included bronchoscopy and bronchography.

Wheezing and Bronchial Obstruction. Wheezing, particularly when restricted to one area of the chest, is an important finding because it may signify partial obstruction of a bronchus. Bronchial obstruction is also indicated by films that show either atelectasis or localized emphysema. The causes of bronchial obstruction are either intrinsic lesions, such as neoplasms, foreign bodies, or strictures (Fig. 3–1), or extrinsic lesions, such as enlarged nodes, neoplasms, and vascular abnormalities, that compress a bronchus (Fig. 3–2).

Diagnostic Bronchoscopy

Bronchoscopic Procedure

RIGID BRONCHOSCOPE

Instruments. A complete set of endoscopic instruments is essential. The correctly sized bronchoscope is one that enters the larynx without causing trauma and yet provides good visibility and working space.

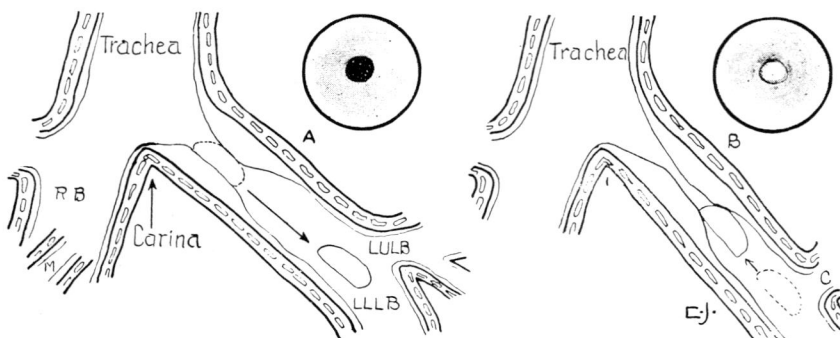

FIGURE 3–1. Mechanism of ball-valve obstructive emphysema. A foreign body lodged in the bronchus moves downward with inspiration and allows air to pass into the lung, as shown in *A*. On expiration, the lumen becomes blocked by the impacted foreign body in contact with the swollen mucous membrane, as shown in *B*, and forms an effective cork. Air is trapped in the distal lung. (*A* and *B*, From Jackson, C., and Jackson, C. L.: Bronchoesophagology. Philadelphia, W. B. Saunders, 1950.)

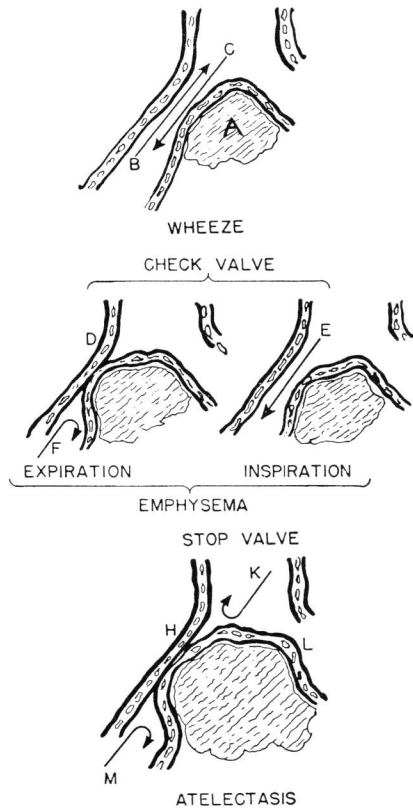

FIGURE 3–2. Changes produced by a compressing extrabronchial lesion. As the mass increases in size the bronchial stenosis progresses to (1) partial obstruction, (2) obstructive emphysema, and (3) complete obstruction with atelectasis. (From Jackson, C., and Jackson, C. L.: Diseases of the Nose, Throat and Ear. 2nd ed. Philadelphia, W. B. Saunders, 1959.)

■ **Table 3–2.** GAUGE OF BRONCHOSCOPE IN RELATION TO AGE OF PATIENT*

Age	Bronchoscope
Adult	8 mm × 40 cm
Adolescent	7 mm × 40 cm
6–12 yr	6 mm × 35 cm
2–5 yr	5 mm × 30 cm
12–24 mo	4 mm × 30 cm
6–12 mo	3.5 mm × 25 cm
Under 6 mo	3 mm × 25 cm

*Gauges and ages are averages, and the gradation of the instrument may have to be altered according to the size rather than the age of the patient.

In infants and children, the selection of the correct size is especially important because the subglottic space is narrow and its tissues tend to swell. The sizes of the bronchoscopes that are appropriate for each age group are shown in Table 3–2.

Recent technical developments have improved bronchoscopic observation and have extended its range (Marsh, 1978). Fiberoptic light carriers have improved illumination, and telescopic attachments at the proximal end of bronchoscopes provide a magnified image for more detailed viewing (Fig. 3–3). Metallurgic advances have made it possible to produce thin-walled bronchoscopes with the same outside diameter but with larger lumens (Berci, 1978). The Hop-kins rod-lens optical system, however, has provided the most significant breakthrough in rigid open-tube bronchoscopy (Hopkins, 1976). This system provides increased light transmission, brighter images, better resolution, greater depth of field, and a wider viewing angle than did previously available lens systems (Fig. 3–4). The rod-lens system can also be miniaturized for use in pediatric bronchoscopes; and by incorporating biopsy forceps with the telescope (optical biopsy forceps), more precise biopsies can be obtained with unobstructed vision of the lesion (Fig. 3–5). Zero-degree straight, 30-degree forward oblique, and 90-degree lateral telescopes with approximately 70-degree viewing angles are available; and they have dramatically improved the diagnostic capabilities of the rigid open-tube bronchoscope (Fig. 3–6). Flexible-tip aspirating and biopsy forceps make it possible to obtain secretions and tissue specimens from the upper lobe bronchi beyond the range of visibility of the rigid bronchoscope (Fig. 3–7). The flexible fiberoptic bronchoscope is superior to the rigid bronchoscope for these purposes.

For examining patients under general anesthesia, ventilating bronchoscopes are available with an observation window that closes the proximal end of the bronchoscope and with a side arm that attaches to anesthesia equipment. Thus, a closed circuit for ventilating is established. The observation window can be removed to introduce aspirators and biopsy forceps. Perforated diaphragms, which cover the proximal end of the bronchoscope and through which telescopes and optical biopsy forceps can be inserted, as well as Sanders-Venturi ventilating systems (Fig. 3–8), also permit positive-pressure ventilation (Sanders, 1967). One model of ventilating bronchoscope has the extra convenience of batteries contained in its handle,

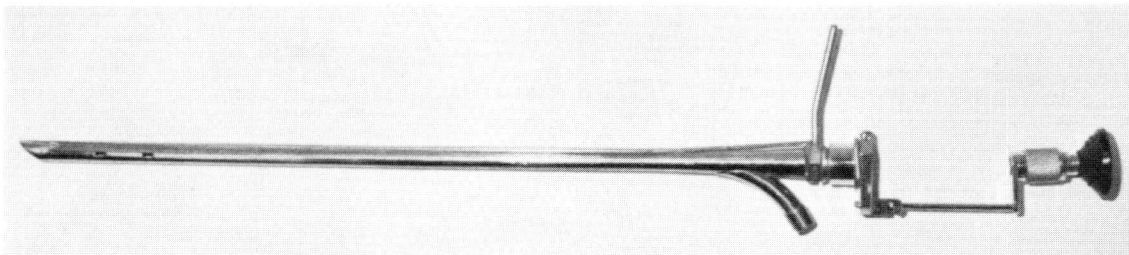

FIGURE 3–3. Bronchoscope with telescopic attachment.

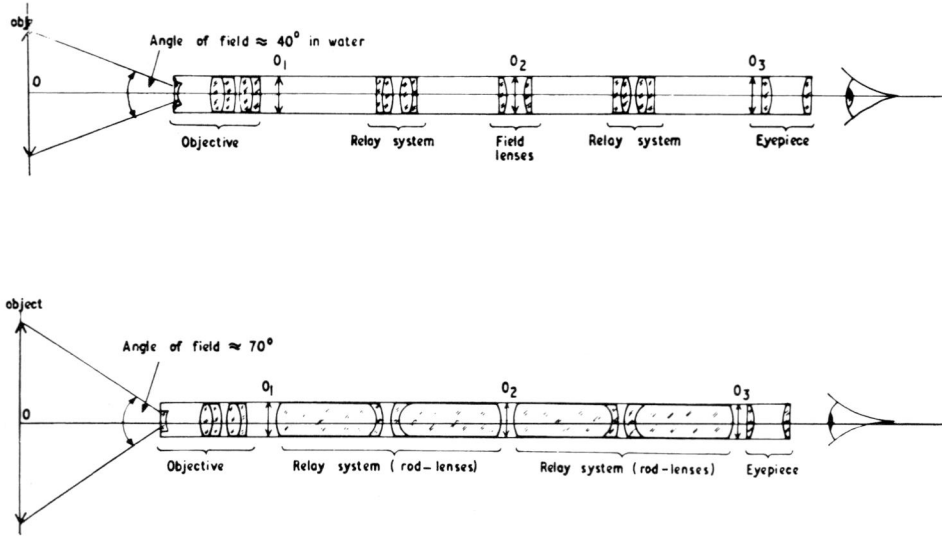

FIGURE 3–4. *Top,* Diagram of standard telescopic lens. A significant portion of light is absorbed by the air columns situated between the lenses. *Bottom,* Hopkins' rod-lens system. Glass rods are used instead of air columns. Lenses are cemented to the ends of the glass rods. Light transmission is significantly increased. Angle of field is wider. (From Hopkins, H. H.: Optical principles of the endoscope. *In* Berci, G. [ed]: Endoscopy. New York, Appleton & Lange, 1976.)

FIGURE 3–5. Optical biopsy forceps. *A,* Telescope and biopsy forceps. *B,* Close-up of tip of telescope and biopsy forceps. *C,* Jaws do not obscure view through the telescope. (*A–C,* From Berci, G.: Chevalier Jackson Lecture: Analysis of new optical systems in bronchoesophagology. Ann. Otol. Rhinol. Laryngol., *87:*451, 1978.)

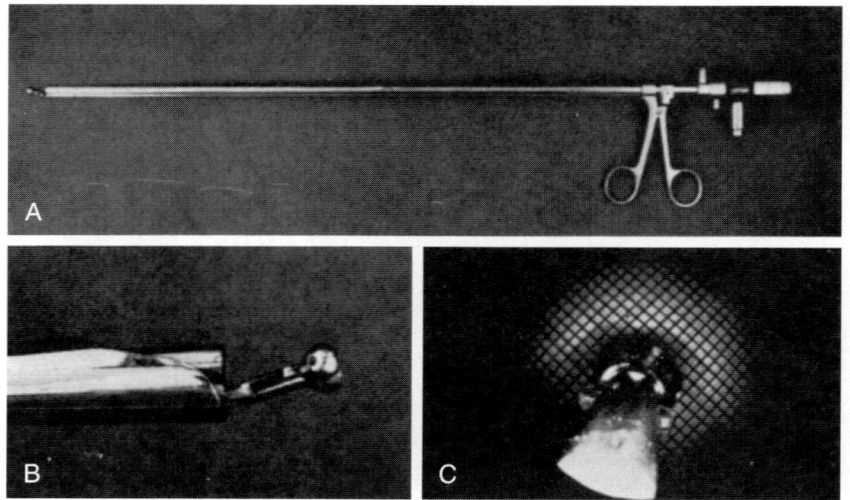

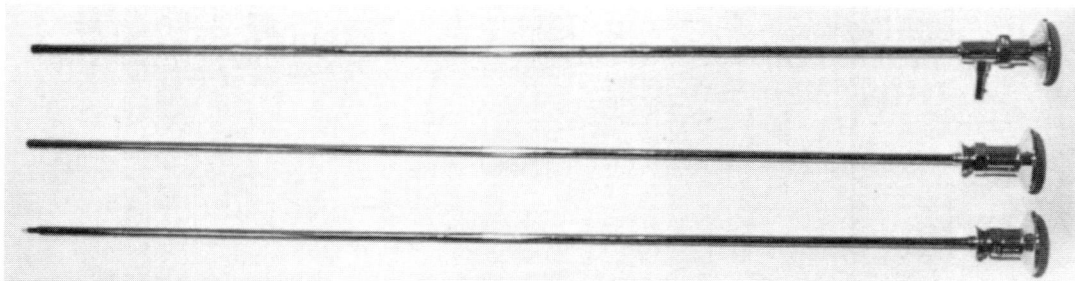

FIGURE 3–6. Telescopic inserts. *Top,* Right-angle fiberoptic telescope. *Middle,* Right-angle incandescent telescope. *Bottom,* Forward oblique incandescent telescope.

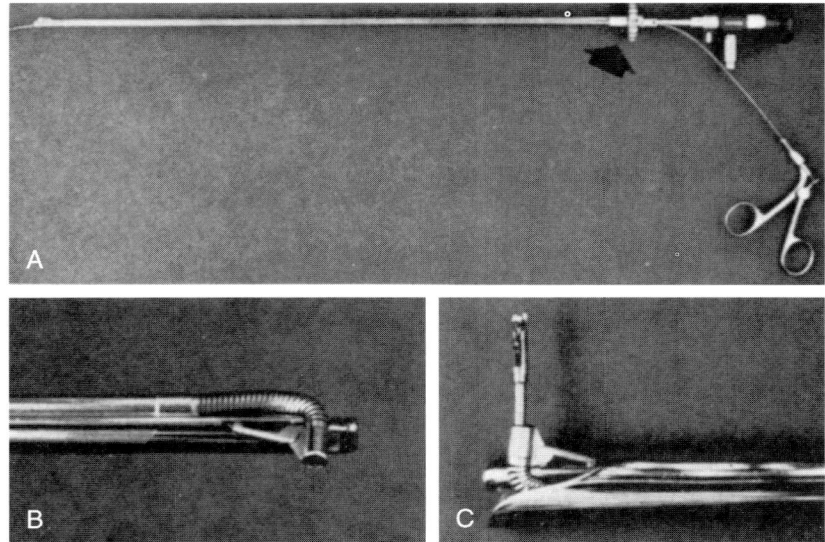

FIGURE 3–7. Lateral telescope with biopsy forceps deflector. *A,* Wheel that activates the bending mechanism. *B,* Close-up of the distal end of the bending mechanism. *C,* Forceps advanced through the bending mechanism. (*A–C,* From Berci, G.: Chevalier Jackson Lecture: Analysis of new optical systems in bronchoesophagology. Ann. Otol. Rhinol. Laryngol., *87:*451, 1978.)

which makes it portable and ready for immediate use (Fig. 3–9). Although bronchoscopic procedures can be performed under various circumstances—at the patient's bedside, in an operating room, or in an outpatient department—it is highly desirable to have a specially equipped endoscopic room that is staffed with trained personnel, particularly when the number of bronchoscopies justifies it.

Preparation of the Patient. Bronchoscopy in the adult may be performed under local anesthesia, with the patient awake and cooperating. Food and liquid are restricted for 6 hours before the examination. The patient is given sufficient premedication to relieve anxiety and to ensure relaxation during the procedure. Medication and dosage should be based on the age, body size, and general condition of the patient. In adults, pentobarbital sodium, up to 200 mg, may be given with up to 100 mg of meperidine (Demerol) 1 hour before the examination. Atropine sulfate is not given routinely because the drug has a drying effect on secretions. If, however, secretions are copious and become a problem during the application of topical anesthesia, atropine sulfate, 0.6 mg, may be given intravenously. If the physician takes some time to explain the procedure to the patient, she or he will gain the patient's confidence and cooperation during the bronchoscopy.

Topical Anesthesia. Careful monitoring of the patient is indicated while topical anesthesia is being applied and during the bronchoscopic examination. Continuous monitoring of the patient's electrocardiogram (ECG) is essential, and oxygen saturation should be observed continuously if a pulse oximeter is available. Before bronchoscopy, dental plates are removed and loose teeth are extracted. The oral pharynx is sprayed with lidocaine hydrochloride (Xylocaine 2%). Cotton pledgets soaked in lidocaine hydrochloride are applied to the piriform sinuses. With the aid of a laryngeal mirror, this solution is applied to the epiglottis and vocal cords from a laryngeal syringe while the patient is phonating. The trachea and bronchi are then anesthetized by placing lidocaine hydrochloride between the cords. The agent reaches the carina and enters the right main bronchus. The solution can be made to enter the left main bronchus by having the patient lean to the left. The tracheobronchial tree may also be anesthetized by transtracheal injections. The anesthetic agent is introduced into the trachea through a needle inserted into the midline between the tracheal cartilages or through the cricothyroid membrane. Another method is to ask the patient to breathe the vaporized anesthetic solution from a nebulizer that is held in the mouth.

Other topical agents that are used to anesthetize

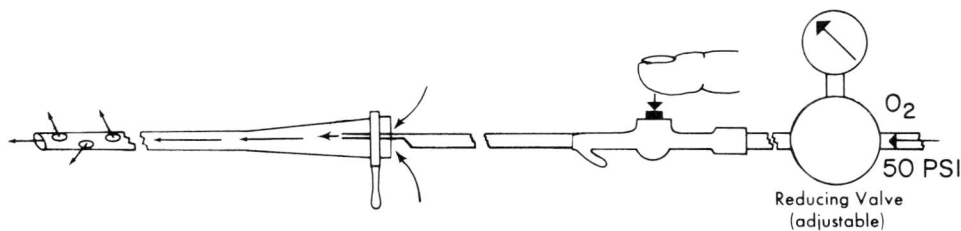

FIGURE 3–8. A schematic representation of the Sanders-Venturi ventilation system showing from right to left: oxygen at 50 psi entering an adjustable reducing valve, passing from there through a manually operated flow controller, and then coming out of the jet into the bronchoscope, causing entrainment of air. (From Carden, E.: Recent improvements in techniques for general anesthesia for bronchoscopy. Chest, *73*[Suppl.]:697, 1978.)

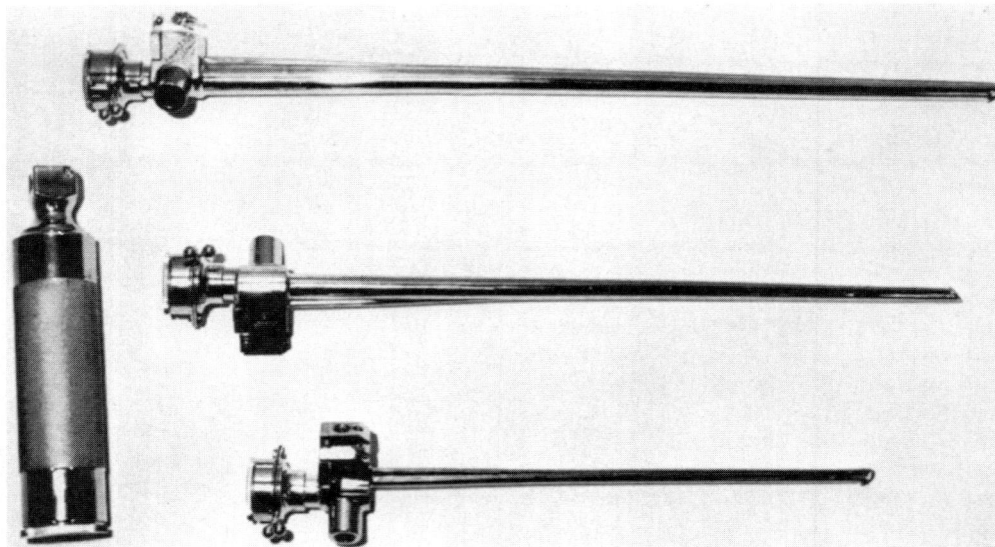

FIGURE 3–9. Ventilating bronchoscopes and battery handle.

the tracheobronchial tree are cocaine hydrochloride in either a 4% or a 10% solution, tetracaine hydrochloride (Pontocaine) in a 0.5% solution and hexylcaine hydrochloride (Cyclaine) in a 5% solution. Tetracaine hydrochloride is four times as toxic as cocaine hydrochloride and should be used carefully because fatal reactions to this drug have been reported. The dose of lidocaine hydrochloride as a 2% solution should not exceed 20 ml (400 mg). Ten to 15 drops of 10% cocaine hydrochloride are adequate to anesthetize the larynx and tracheobronchial tree. An additional brief spray of 4% cocaine hydrochloride may be necessary when the bronchoscope enters the left main bronchus. Because toxic reactions can occur with any local anesthetic that is applied topically, only a measured quantity of these drugs should be used. As an additional precaution, administration of these agents should be fractionated over a 20-minute period. For control of convulsive reactions to these drugs, an ampule of thiopental sodium (Pentothal sodium) should be available in addition to equipment for resuscitation.

General Anesthesia. Jackson strongly advocated that all endoscopic examinations should be performed with the patient under topical anesthesia, and he warned against the hazards of general anesthesia (Jackson and Jackson, 1950). There is a growing preference, however, for general anesthesia (Carden, 1978), especially when a skilled anesthesiologist and a ventilating bronchoscope are available.

Moribund or generally debilitated patients or patients with limited cardiopulmonary reserve due to pooling of secretions, massive atelectasis, or cardiac failure who do not require premedication and who need little topical anesthesia are better managed under local anesthesia than under general anesthesia. In infants, children, and some adults, general anesthesia is desirable and is often necessary, especially if a long procedure is anticipated. The technique varies with and depends on the judgment and experience of the anesthesiologist. Thiopental sodium, given intravenously in combination with a muscle relaxant, is preferred by many anesthesiologists. With this method, oxygen can be given throughout the procedure through the side arm of the bronchoscope. The patient's ECG, blood pressure, and oxygen saturation should be monitored carefully throughout the procedure.

Position of the Patient. The patient is placed in the dorsal recumbent position with the shoulders flat at the edge of the table and the head elevated and extended. An assistant to the physician can help the patient achieve this position by supporting the patient's occiput with his left hand and by moving the patient upward on the table until the edge of the table is at the midscapular level. The head is then raised 15 degrees and is extended so that the oral cavity and larynx are aligned (Fig. 3–10). Bronchoscopy also can be performed with the patient sitting in a straight-backed chair or in bed with the head of the bed raised. The bronchoscope is introduced into the right side of the mouth. As the bronchoscope is advanced, it raises the base of the tongue, and the rim of the epiglottis is seen. The tip of the bronchoscope lifts the epiglottis as it advances and brings the vocal cords and glottis into view. A soft epiglottis may curl in front of the advancing bronchoscope and thus may obscure the view of the vestibule. In this situation, the bronchoscope is withdrawn to the point where the rim of the epiglottis is again identified, the midline position of the bronchoscope is confirmed, and the maneuver is repeated. With the handle of the bronchoscope up and the glottis clearly in view, the bronchoscope is advanced between the vocal cords. Alternatively, the handle may be turned to the right and, with the left cord clearly in view, the tip of the bronchoscope will then be in the midline position and will pass readily between the cords. In some patients, it may be necessary to first expose the larynx with

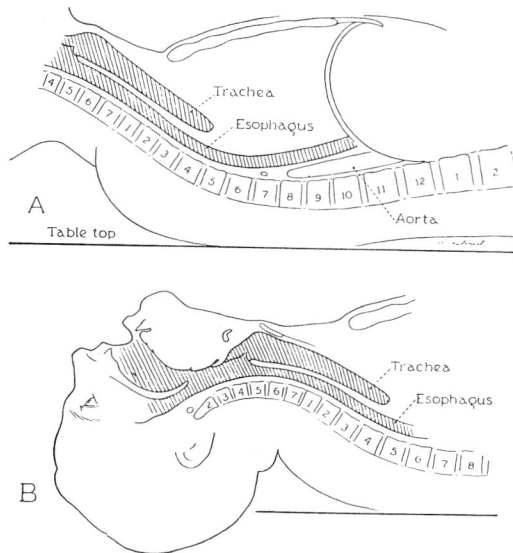

FIGURE 3–10. *A,* The correct position for the introduction of endoscopic instruments with the head elevated and the shoulders flat on the table. After the bronchoscope is passed through the larynx or the esophagoscope passes the cricopharyngeus, the head is lowered and extended as in *B. (A* and *B,* From Jackson, C., and Jackson, C. L.: Bronchoesophagology. Philadelphia, W. B. Saunders, 1950.)

a laryngoscope and to introduce the bronchoscope through the laryngoscope into the trachea. The laryngoscope is subsequently disengaged by removing its slot.

Inspection of the larynx and tracheobronchial tree is performed systematically, beginning with the epiglottis, ventricular bands, vocal cords, trachea, carina, right and left main bronchi, and orifices of the lobar bronchi. The scope is then withdrawn to the carina, and the Hopkins rod-lens telescopes are used to examine the tracheobronchial tree in detail (Fig. 3–11). The right upper lobe bronchus is inspected by turning the handle of the bronchoscope to the left and by carrying the head toward the left shoulder. The right-angle telescope is used to inspect the right upper lobe bronchus. The orifices of its three segmental branches can be seen through the telescope. The lower lobe bronchus and the orifices of its segmental branches can be seen with the zero-degree straight telescope. Because the right middle lobe approaches the anterior wall of the intermediate bronchus, the head is lowered to bring the middle lobe orifice into view. A 30-degree forward oblique telescope helps for detailed viewing of the middle lobe bronchus and its two segmental orifices. The superior segmental bronchus is examined with a 90-degree right-angle telescope. The bronchoscope is withdrawn to the carina, the head is carried to the right shoulder, and the bronchoscope is advanced into the left main bronchus. The orifice of the left upper lobe is seen on the lateral wall with the 90-degree telescope. The orifice of the superior segmental bronchus of the left lower lobe is seen on the posterior wall with the 90-degree tele-

scope. The basilar segmental orifices are seen with the zero-degree straight telescope. The 30-degree forward oblique telescope is used to examine the lingular bronchi. The tracheobronchial tree is inspected and a notation is made of any widening or fixation of the carina, the appearance of the bronchial mucosa, movement of the bronchi with respiration and heartbeat, compression or fixation of the bronchial wall, and the presence and location of any secretions, bleeding, foreign bodies, or pathologic lesions. Secretions are collected for bacteriologic and cytologic studies. Because these studies so often prove to have unexpected value, specimens should be obtained routinely when every bronchoscopy is done. Biopsies are taken as the last step in the procedure because bleeding may obscure further inspection.

Ball-tip or cup forceps are best suited for removing specimens of tissue. Punch biopsy forceps that may bite through a bronchial wall are unsafe because they may initiate an uncontrollable hemorrhage. Biting through the spur of a bronchial orifice is particularly dangerous because of the proximity of large vessels. Fatal hemorrhage has resulted when the spur of the left lower lobe bronchus has been biopsied. A superficial biopsy at the bronchial bifurcation proximal to a gross tumor should be obtained to define the upper extent of the tumor and the proper site of resection. The carina should be biopsied in all patients with tumors that involve a mainstem bronchus or the right upper lobe bronchus.

FLEXIBLE FIBERBRONCHOSCOPE

With the introduction of the flexible fiberbronchoscope by Ikeda in 1967 (Ikeda, 1970), the bronchoscopist gained a valuable new diagnostic instrument (Fig. 3–12). Various models of fiberoptic bronchoscopes are produced by several manufacturers, and each model has particular advantages and limitations. These models differ in outer diameter from less than 4 mm to more than 6 mm and also in arc of bending from 60 to 180 degrees. Viewing angles vary from 66 to 100 degrees, and side-channel diameters range from 1.2 to 3.2 mm. Ultrathin fiberoptic bronchoscopes (1.8 to 2.2 mm) are also now available, but their usefulness is still under evaluation.

Besides a standard model, every endoscopy suite should have several other models available—that is, a thin bronchoscope with a wide, bending angle for examination and biopsy of upper lobe bronchi and a model with a large side channel so that generous biopsies can be obtained and thick secretions can be aspirated. Facilities for still photography to document bronchoscopic findings and for video imaging for teaching purposes should also be available in well-equipped endoscopy suites.

The indications for bronchoscopy with the flexible fiberoptic bronchoscope are similar to the indications given for the rigid open scope. The flexible scope is particularly useful in patients with peripheral and upper-lobe lesions; however, its use is limited in the presence of copious, thick secretions or large amounts

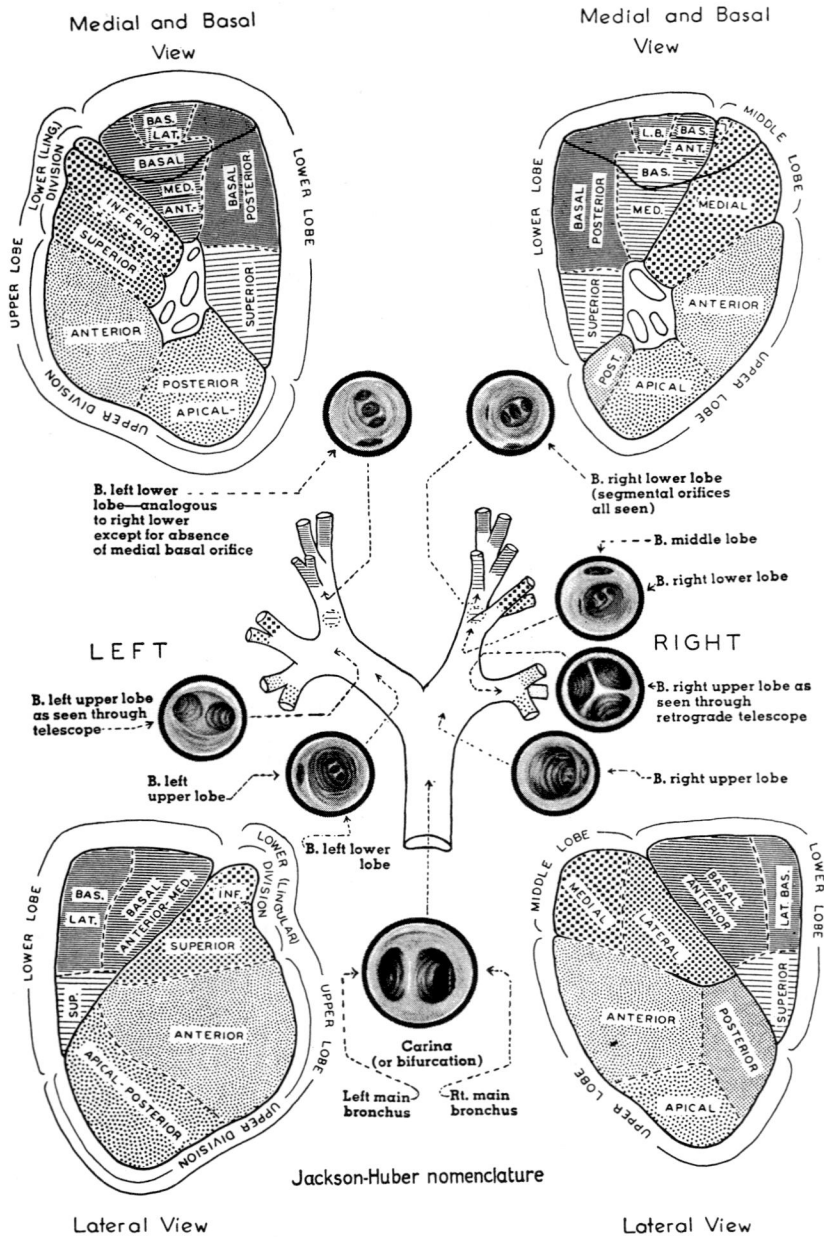

FIGURE 3–11. Drawings showing the pulmonary segments and the lobar bronchi and their segmental branches. The inset circles show the schematic representation of the landmarks seen endoscopically at the various points. The bronchial tree is shown "upside down," because it is desired to represent the structures in the same relations observed by the bronchoscopist when the patient is examined in the usual position of dorsal recumbency. (From Jackson, C., and Jackson, C. L.: Bronchoesophagology. Philadelphia, W. B. Saunders, 1950.)

of blood. The ease of introduction has made this instrument appealing and widely accepted.

Preoperative preparation of the patient is similar to that described for the rigid bronchoscope, and the procedure may be performed with the patient under either local or general anesthesia. The scope may be inserted through the nose or mouth under direct vision or through a standard rigid bronchoscope or endotracheal tube of sufficient size (8 mm or larger) to provide an adequate airway around the fiberoptic scope. If general anesthesia is to be used, an adapter (Fig. 3–13) on the end of the endotracheal tube or rigid bronchoscope provides a closed system and permits the maintenance of adequate ventilation. A Sanders-Venturi adapter can also be used to provide ventilation through an open rigid bronchoscope or

endotracheal tube through which the flexible scope is passed. After the scope has been inserted, care must be taken to visualize the entire tracheobronchial tree systematically. This procedure is accomplished through rotation of the instrument and flexion of its tip. This instrument provides unparalleled views of the entire tracheobronchial tree, especially the upper lobes and superior segments, and often extends to the third or fourth bronchial subdivisions.

The side channel of these scopes accepts flexible biopsy forceps, transbronchial biopsy needles, brushes, and curettes (Fig. 3–14). Placing the tip of the flexible scope into the appropriate segmental or subsegmental bronchus allows these instruments to be inserted precisely and directed fluoroscopically into position for biopsying, needling, brushing, or

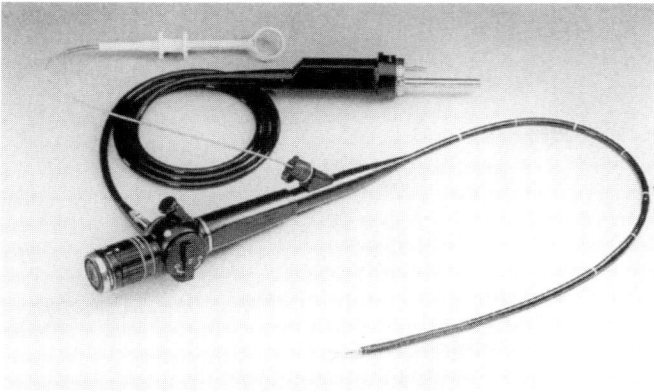

FIGURE 3–12. Flexible fiberoptic bronchoscope (Olympus OES Bronchoscope, Model BF–XT20D) with biopsy forceps in position. (Courtesy of Olympus America, Inc., Melville, NY.)

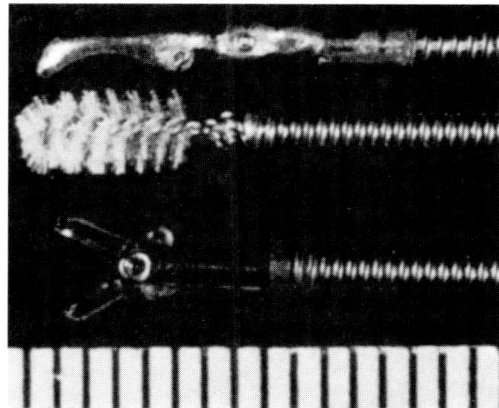

FIGURE 3–14. Biopsy forceps, brush, and curette. (From Marsh, B. R.: Advances in bronchoscopy. Otolaryngol. Clin. North Am., 11:371, 1978.)

curetting discrete or diffuse peripheral pulmonary lesions. The relation of the instrument tip to the pulmonary lesion must be confirmed in two planes by biplane fluorography, by a C-arm fluoroscope, or by rotation of the patient during fluoroscopy. When the instrument is in position, samples are taken from the lesion, and the material is then sent for appropriate examinations.

The ability to wedge the tip of a flexible bronchoscope into a segmental or a subsegmental bronchus also permits bronchoalveolar lavage, a diagnostic technique that is being widely investigated. The tip

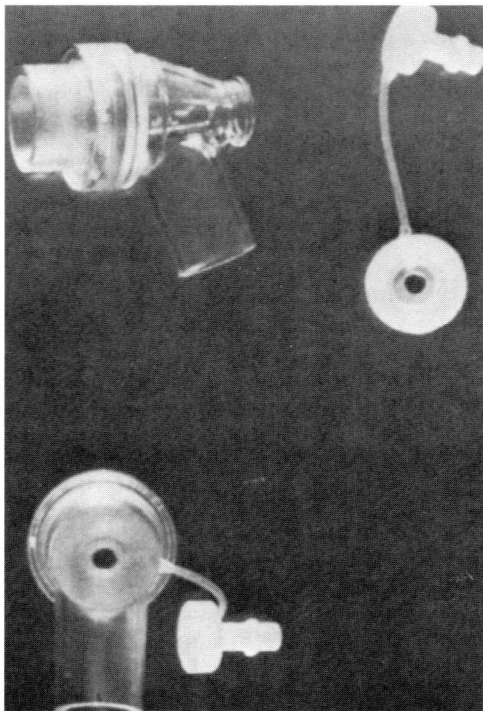

FIGURE 3–13. Two special adapters, cap removed and plug out, above (shown from the side) and cap in place with plug out, below (shown from above). (From Carden, E.: Recent improvements in techniques for general anesthesia for bronchoscopy. Chest, 73[Suppl.]:697, 1978.)

of the fiberoptic bronchoscope is placed in position in the segmental orifice that leads to the involved area of the lung. Aliquots of 20 ml of isotonic saline and then 10 ml of air are injected slowly into the bronchus and are then removed with low suction. The amount that is usually injected is 100 ml of saline, of which 40 to 60 ml is generally retrieved. This fluid is then centrifuged. Differential cell counting is done on the cells that are removed and various biochemical analyses are done on the fluid. The usefulness of the information obtained through bronchoalveolar lavage is controversial and still evolving (Reynolds, 1987; Turner-Warwick and Haslam, 1987).

The advantages of the flexible fiberoptic bronchoscope are numerous: This bronchoscope can be readily passed with little discomfort to the patient; it provides unparalleled visualization of the segmental bronchi, especially of the upper lobes; and it is ideal for use in patients with cervical arthritis or other conditions that prevent hyperextension of the neck. This bronchoscope has helped greatly in difficult tracheal intubations and in placing double-lumen endobronchial tubes in proper position. Its principal disadvantages are partial obstruction of the airway owing to the presence of the scope in the trachea, difficulty in removing thick secretions and blood, and the small size of the material obtained at biopsy, which may be insufficient for pathologic diagnosis.

Some experts have suggested that the flexible bronchoscope will supplant the rigid bronchoscope. This viewpoint is unfortunate because these two instruments with their different capabilities complement rather than compete with each other. Bronchoscopy with both the rigid and the flexible scopes can be done easily as a single procedure. A bronchoscopist should be adept with both the rigid and the flexible bronchoscopes so that the most complete diagnostic and therapeutic bronchoscopy can be performed in every patient.

Bronchoscopy in Specific Conditions

BRONCHOGENIC CARCINOMA

The suspicion of bronchogenic carcinoma is the most common indication for bronchoscopy. Bronchoscopy has an important role not only in the diagnosis of cancer of the lung but also in the staging of this disease. Because of the ease of insertion and the relative comfort for the patient during the procedure, the flexible fiberoptic bronchoscope is the preferred instrument for most patients.

Diagnosis. Shure (1987) has described five ways in which cancer involving the lung can present, each of which can be diagnosed at bronchoscopy: endobronchial masses that can be seen directly through the bronchoscope; submucosal or peribronchial involvement; peripheral masses (primary or metastatic carcinomas); diffuse metastatic disease; and occult carcinomas.

Endobronchial Masses. Endobronchial masses, even masses that arise in an upper lobe or superior segment, can usually be easily seen, and a biopsy can be performed through the flexible fiberoptic bronchoscope. These tumors present as friable, red or white necrotic lesions. Direct biopsy provides diagnostic material in almost 100% of these lesions (Kvale et al., 1976; Shure and Astarita, 1983; Zavala, 1975). Four biopsies of an endobronchial tumor are usually sufficient (Popovich et al., 1982). Although some experts believe that the size of the biopsy forceps does not influence the diagnostic yield (Shure, 1987), this author has not had this experience, and has resorted occasionally to the rigid open-tube bronchoscope with its larger biopsy forceps to obtain diagnostic tissue from necrotic endobronchial lesions. If the biopsy forceps tend to detach from an endobronchial lesion, a spear forceps (Fig. 3–15) or a curette is used to obtain tissue for making a diagnosis. Bronchial washings and brushings that yield positive cytologic findings in approximately 80% of patients with endobronchial lesions improve the diagnostic yield somewhat over direct biopsy alone. The addition of bronchial brushing, which is the most effective of the two, however, is probably sufficient (Richardson et al., 1974; Funahashi et al., 1979).

Bronchoscopy is important in reevaluating patients with endobronchial small-cell carcinomas (Ihde et al., 1978). In 35 to 60% of patients studied by Bye and associates (1980) and Ihde and co-workers (1978), the bronchoscopic findings differed from the radiographic assessment after chemotherapy. Thus, bronchoscopy is the most accurate method to use in evaluating the results of chemotherapy in patients with endobronchial small-cell carcinomas of the lung.

Submucosal and Peribronchial Involvement. Direct biopsy of an involved bronchial wall is difficult, and it frequently fails to obtain diagnostic material. Needle aspiration of submucosal or peribronchial areas, however, is more often productive. In one series of 31 patients, 55% of the lesions were diagnosed by biopsy alone; 71% were diagnosed by needle aspiration; and the combination of the two procedures produced positive diagnoses in 78% of the patients. Bronchial washings and brushings presented for cytologic evaluation raised the diagnostic yield to 97% in this study (Shure and Fedullo, 1985).

To biopsy a submucosal mass by needle aspiration, the needle (Fig. 3–16) is inserted into the mass at an

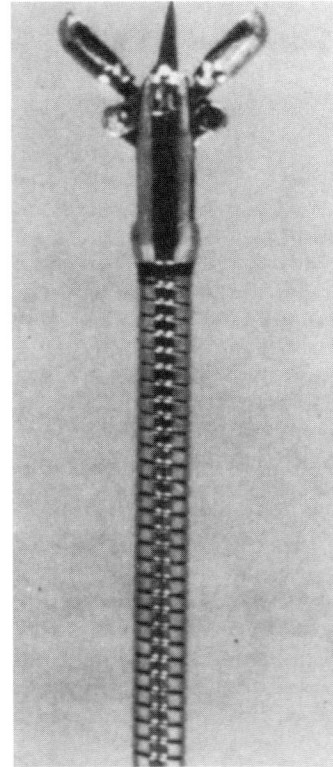

FIGURE 3–15. Spear forceps. (Courtesy of Olympus Corporation, Lake Success, NY.)

oblique angle, whereas when peribronchial tissue is sought, the needle is inserted perpendicularly between cartilaginous rings (Shure and Fedullo, 1985). In both cases, suction is applied to the needle, which is then agitated for 10 seconds and removed. After gentle release of the suction, the specimen is sent for cytologic examination.

Peripheral Masses. At present, it appears that a peripheral nodule is the most common presentation of bronchogenic carcinoma. Transbronchial biopsy and brushings done under fluoroscopic control have been reported to diagnose these lesions in 30 to 90% of patients, or 60% on average (Fletcher and Levin, 1983; Hanson et al., 1976; Popovich et al., 1982; Tierstein et al., 1978; Zavala, 1975; Zavala et al., 1973). Lesions in the lower half of the lung, away from the hilum, which can be reached more directly than lesions in the upper lung, and lesions that are larger than 3 cm and are supplied by three or more bronchi are the most likely to be diagnosed (Cortese and McDougall, 1979; Dougherty, 1984; Fletcher and Levin, 1983; Radke et al., 1979). Smaller lesions that have only one or two bronchi entering them are less likely to be located by the biopsy forceps or brush (Tsuboi et al., 1967). Although some endoscopists advocate obtaining six biopsies from peripheral nodules (Popovich at al., 1982), Shure and Astarita (1983) believe that four biopsies are sufficient. At the time of transbronchial biopsy, bronchial washings and brushings should also be obtained because pathologic and

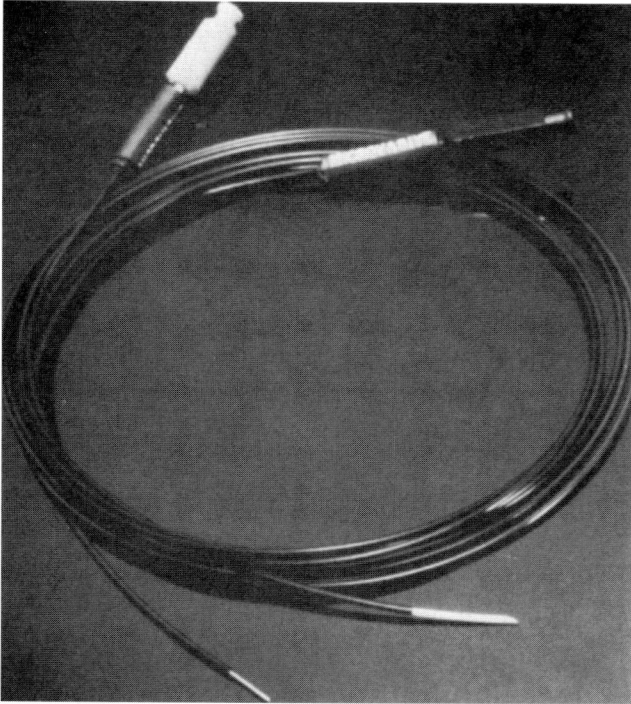

FIGURE 3–16. Transbronchial and transcarinal aspiration needles. Sofcor plastic needle *(top)* and Stifcor stainless-steel needle *(bottom).* (Courtesy of MicroVasive, Milford, MA.)

cytologic analyses of these specimens increase the diagnostic yield over transbronchial biopsy alone (Arroliga and Matthay, 1993; Shure and Fedullo, 1983).

Transthoracic needle aspiration (TTNA), a nonbronchoscopic technique, is proving to be very helpful in diagnosing peripheral lung lesions. Wallace and Deutsch (1982) found the diagnostic yield of TTNA to be twice that of flexible fiberoptic bronchoscopy. Currently, we favor TTNA for upper lung lesions and lesions smaller than 3 cm in diameter.

In instances where the biopsy forceps cannot be manipulated into a peripheral nodule, a transbronchial aspiration needle has helped to obtain a diagnostic specimen (Shure and Fedullo, 1983; Wang et al., 1984). In one report, needle aspiration was diagnostic in 33% of nodules smaller than 2 cm in diameter and in almost 80% of lesions 2 cm or more in diameter (Shure and Fedullo, 1983). Needle aspiration is useful particularly when the transbronchial biopsy forceps can be passed to the edge of a nodule but not into it. The transbronchial needle often can be passed into the mass, suction can be applied, and the needle can be moved in and out and finally withdrawn (see Fig. 3–16). A core of tissue and cytologic sample from the mass are obtained occasionally in this manner (Shure, 1987). Wang and Britt (1991) reported on the use of a needle brush (Mill-Ross Laboratory, Mentor, OH). They suggest that the needle brush is more productive than the standard brush, but more experience with this instrument is required.

Metastatic Nodules. The diagnostic yield of transbronchial biopsy in peripheral metastatic deposits,

generally reported to be less than 50% (Cortese and McDougall, 1981; Zavala, 1975), is lower than that in primary lung tumors, probably as a result of the vascular origin of the metastatic lesion as opposed to the bronchial origin of a primary tumor. As bronchoscopists gain greater skill in using the transbronchial aspiration needle, the success in obtaining tissue from metastatic nodules should improve and the diagnostic yield should consequently increase. A TTNA should also be considered when a metastatic nodule is suspected (Salazar and Westcott, 1993).

Diffuse Metastatic Disease. Metastatic cancer to the lung can present as an endobronchial mass, as a peripheral nodule, or as diffuse lymphangitic involvement. Endobronchial metastases, usually from the breast, kidney, or colon, can be diagnosed by direct biopsy. Diffuse lymphangitic spread of carcinoma can also be diagnosed by random transbronchial biopsy of the lung in more than 90% of patients (Shure, 1987).

Occult Carcinomas. Occult lung cancers are cancers that present with positive findings on sputum cytology but that have negative x-rays. Because the positive cytologic findings may be the result of upper airway tumors, a thorough examination of the nose, mouth, and pharynx should be performed. If no abnormality is found in these areas, a careful bronchoscopic examination should be done. Most frequently, the positive cytologic findings arise from a centrally located squamous cell carcinoma (Woolner et al., 1984). Sixty to 70% of these tumors are detected on the first routine bronchoscopic examination (Shure, 1987). If, however, the site of the tumor is not readily apparent, then repeated, selective segmental brushings and washings should be done at 3-month intervals in an attempt to localize the tumor.

Photodynamic detection of small or occult carcinomas of the lung is done in only a few centers. A hematoporphyrin derivative (HPD), which is given intravenously, is absorbed and retained by malignant cells. The tumor that contains HPD fluoresces when exposed to a special blue-violet light (405 nm), which permits the identification and biopsy of the cancer at a subsequent bronchoscopy (Sanderson, 1986).

Staging. Bronchoscopy also has a significant role in the staging of bronchogenic carcinoma by permitting an evaluation of the extent of bronchial involvement and the status of peritracheal, subcarinal, and parabronchial lymph nodes. An evaluation by biopsy of the bifurcation of the tracheobronchial tree just proximal to an endobronchial tumor permits the surgeon to determine whether that level is a suitable site at which to divide the bronchus at the time of a pulmonary resection. A tumor that involves the right upper lobe bronchus may not be amenable to simple right upper lobectomy. A biopsy of the right upper lobe origin should be taken, and if the result is positive, a pneumonectomy, sleeve resection, or bronchoplastic procedure is required. The main carina should also be biopsied in all patients with tumors that involve a main bronchus or the origin of the right upper lobe. If the mucosa of the carina is red and thick, biopsies have been reported to be positive in 40% of patients

(Shure et al., 1985). Routine carinal biopsies in patients with endobronchial tumors have been shown to be positive approximately 5% of the time (Robbins et al., 1979; Shure et al., 1985). Because carinal involvement usually indicates inoperability, careful carinal evaluation is essential in all patients with central lesions. Bronchogenic tumors are reported to be multicentric in 9 to 15% of patients (Marsh et al., 1978; Woolner et al., 1984). Although these figures are at variance with the author's experience, the incidence of multicentricity is sufficiently high to warrant a thorough bronchoscopic search for second areas of involvement in all patients with bronchogenic tumors.

The presence of subcarinal and paratracheal lymph node involvement with carcinoma contraindicates surgical resection. A course of neoadjuvant chemotherapy should be given and the patient reevaluated (Martini et al., 1993). The presence of a widened, fixed carina, compression of the trachea, or demonstration of enlarged subcarinal or paratracheal lymph nodes on computed tomography (CT) scans are indications for transtracheal, transcarinal, or transbronchial needle aspiration. The three areas on the carina in which biopsies are usually done are shown in Figure 3–17. The metal aspiration needle (see Fig. 3–16), longer than 1 cm, must clearly puncture the carinal wall. As previously described, suction is applied to the needle and the needle is removed. Because of the problem with inserting the needle laterally through the tracheal wall, aspiration of paratracheal nodes is more difficult than aspiration of subcarinal nodes. In one series in which the CT scan of the chest was used for guidance, the sensitivity of paratracheal nodal aspiration was 50%, with a specificity of 96% (Schenk et al., 1986). Shure (1987) found that aspiration of a widened, fixed carina yielded a positive result in 40% of patients, whereas the results of subcarinal aspiration were positive in 25% of patients with central endobronchial tumors. The author's current position is to do paratracheal and carinal aspiration on all patients with widened and fixed carinas, with enlarged subcarinal nodes, or with paratracheal lymph node masses that indent the tracheal wall.

False-positive results in these studies are unusual, and complications are infrequent (Schenk et al., 1986; Shure and Fedullo, 1984; Versteegh and Swierenga, 1963) and occur at a rate of only 1.4% (Wang et al., 1984b). No significant bleeding has been described, but pneumothorax and pneumomediastinum have been encountered. Aspiration of mediastinal cysts has been described (Schwartz et al., 1985) but has not been widely used because of the potential hazards from infection.

PULMONARY INFECTIONS

Since the early 1980s, the use of bronchoscopy in the diagnosis of pulmonary infections has increased significantly, particularly with the proliferation of patients with AIDS and the increased number of patients who receive chemotherapy and steroids.

Bacterial Infection. Contamination by upper airway flora may complicate an accurate identification of the infectious organism in patients with bacterial pneumonia. To aid in obtaining an uncontaminated specimen for culture, a protected specimen brush is needed (Bordelon et al., 1983; Chastre et al., 1984; Joshi et al., 1982). Quantitative culturing of the obtained specimen is advisable because small numbers of colonies of multiple organisms suggest contamination of the specimen, whereas large numbers of a single or a few organisms are more likely to be an accurate representation of the cause of the pneumonia.

Tuberculous and Fungal Infections. Bronchoscopy helps particularly to diagnose sputum-smear-negative tuberculosis. Thirty to 50% of patients can be diagnosed by staining the bronchoscopic specimens (Danek and Bower, 1979; Sarkar et al., 1980; So et al., 1982; Suratt et al., 1977; Uddenfeldt and Lundgren, 1981), whereas a significant number of the remainder can be diagnosed by culturing these specimens (Danek and Bower, 1979).

The diagnosis of fungal infections is more difficult to achieve than that of bacterial infections. Finding characteristic thick brown plugs that contain fungi at bronchoscopy permits the diagnosis of allergic bronchopulmonary aspergillosis. In cases of invasive aspergillosis, however, even an open lung biopsy may not be diagnostic (Albelda et al., 1984; McCabe et al., 1985). Of patients with coccidioidomycosal fungal infections, 50% can be diagnosed by bronchoscopy (Wallace et al., 1981).

Immunocompromised Host. Opportunistic infections that present as diffuse pulmonary infiltrates, such as *Pneumocystis carinii* and cytomegalovirus infections, are common in the immunocompromised host. Bronchoalveolar lavage and transbronchial biopsy have frequently been successful in diagnosing such lesions. Bronchoalveolar lavage alone is also frequently diagnostic and is indicated in patients with clotting abnormalities. The diagnostic yield in diffuse

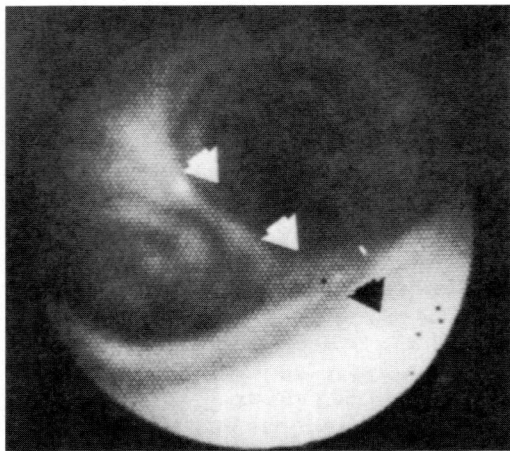

FIGURE 3–17. Transcarinal aspirates are done at anterior, mid, and posterior points *(arrows)* along the carina. (From Shure, D.: Fiberoptic bronchoscopy—Diagnostic applications. Clin. Chest Med., *8:*1, 1987.)

infiltrates, such as in immunocompromised patients, is greater (Broaddus et al., 1985; Ognibene et al., 1984; Stover et al., 1984) than that in patients who have received chemotherapeutic agents and who are likely to have drug-related pulmonary changes and fibrosis (Jaffe and Maki, 1981). If bronchoscopic specimens are inadequate for diagnosis, open lung biopsy must be considered (Toledo-Pereya et al., 1980).

Interstitial Pulmonary Disease. The role of bronchoscopy in noninfectious, non-neoplastic diffuse interstitial pulmonary disease is unsettled (Zavala, 1978b). Bronchoscopy is effective in the diagnosis of sarcoidosis (Koerner et al., 1975). Gilman and Wang (1980) report that a histologic diagnosis can be made in 90% of patients with sarcoidosis if four random biopsies are taken. Endobronchial biopsies also often show granulomas (Pauli et al., 1984). Pulmonary alveolar proteinosis can be diagnosed by finding the characteristic periodic acid–Schiff (PAS)–positive material in specimens from bronchoalveolar lavage and transbronchial biopsies (Daniele et al., 1985). Other conditions such as hypersensitivity pneumonitis, vasculitis, and idiopathic pulmonary fibrosis are diagnosed infrequently (Shure, 1987).

Therapeutic Bronchoscopy

Foreign Bodies. Most foreign bodies that are aspirated into the tracheobronchial tree can be removed by bronchoscopy. Although the rigid open bronchoscope is chosen most often for removal of foreign bodies (Holinger, 1978), the recent development of several foreign body forceps (Fig. 3–18) for use with

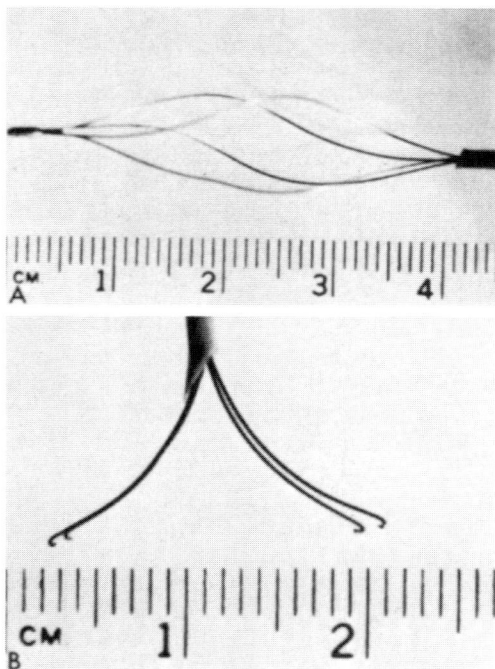

FIGURE 3–18. Foreign body forceps. A, Basket type. B, Grasping type. (A and B, From Marsh, B. R.: Advances in bronchoscopy. Otolaryngol. Clin. North Am., 11:371, 1978.)

the flexible fiberoptic bronchoscope provides an alternative instrument that has been used successfully (Cunanan, 1978). A history of cough, wheezing, and fever in a young child should always suggest the possibility of aspiration. Because, in children as well as in adults, the aspiration episode may not have been observed by others or may have been forgotten, a diagnosis of aspiration of a foreign body should always be considered in the differential diagnosis of chest disease. Clinical chest findings may vary because of shifting of a foreign body in the bronchi, even from one side of the chest to the other. If the foreign body is not opaque, its presence may be indicated only by lobar or segmental collapse or by obstructive emphysema. Chest films should be obtained in both inspiration and expiration to detect localized emphysema or mediastinal shift (Fig. 3–19).

Removal of a foreign body is not usually an emergency, and adequate preparation should be made so that the first attempt at removal is successful. The type of scope used depends on the patient and the skill and experience of the bronchoscopist. An anesthesiologist should be available, and in children and many adults, general anesthesia greatly facilitates removal. Vital signs should be monitored carefully because obstruction of the airways, arrhythmias, and even cardiac arrest may occur during the procedure. Appropriate instruments for grasping the foreign body must be available. The use of the balloon-tip catheter (Fogarty catheter) for the removal of foreign bodies has become popular (Bonfils-Roberts and Nealon, 1975; Saw et al., 1979). A duplicate of the foreign body should be obtained if possible, and some practice trials should be made at grasping it.

A foreign body must be seen clearly so that it can be grasped securely with the foreign-body forceps (Fig. 3–20). When the forceps have a secure grasp, the bronchoscope is advanced until contact is made with the foreign body. The bronchoscope, forceps, and foreign body are then withdrawn as a unit. Passage through the larynx is facilitated by maintaining the foreign body in contact with the end of the bronchoscope and by rotating the foreign body into the axis of the glottis. Hopkins' rod-lens optical grasping forceps offers the clearest unobstructed view of a foreign body and permits secure application of the forceps. Foreign bodies beyond the range of visibility of a rigid bronchoscopete can often be removed by a flexible scope either under direct vision or with a biplane or single-plane fluoroscope that guides the endoscopist. A balloon-tip catheter often can be advanced beyond a foreign body, the balloon can be distended, and the catheter can be withdrawn. The foreign body is thus displaced into a more proximal bronchus, where it can be grasped and removed. Removal of a foreign body by surgical intervention should only rarely be required.

If the first attempt at removal of a foreign body from a child is unsuccessful, it is better not to persist for more than 15 minutes because the incidence of complications increases with time. A second attempt can be made after 2 to 3 days.

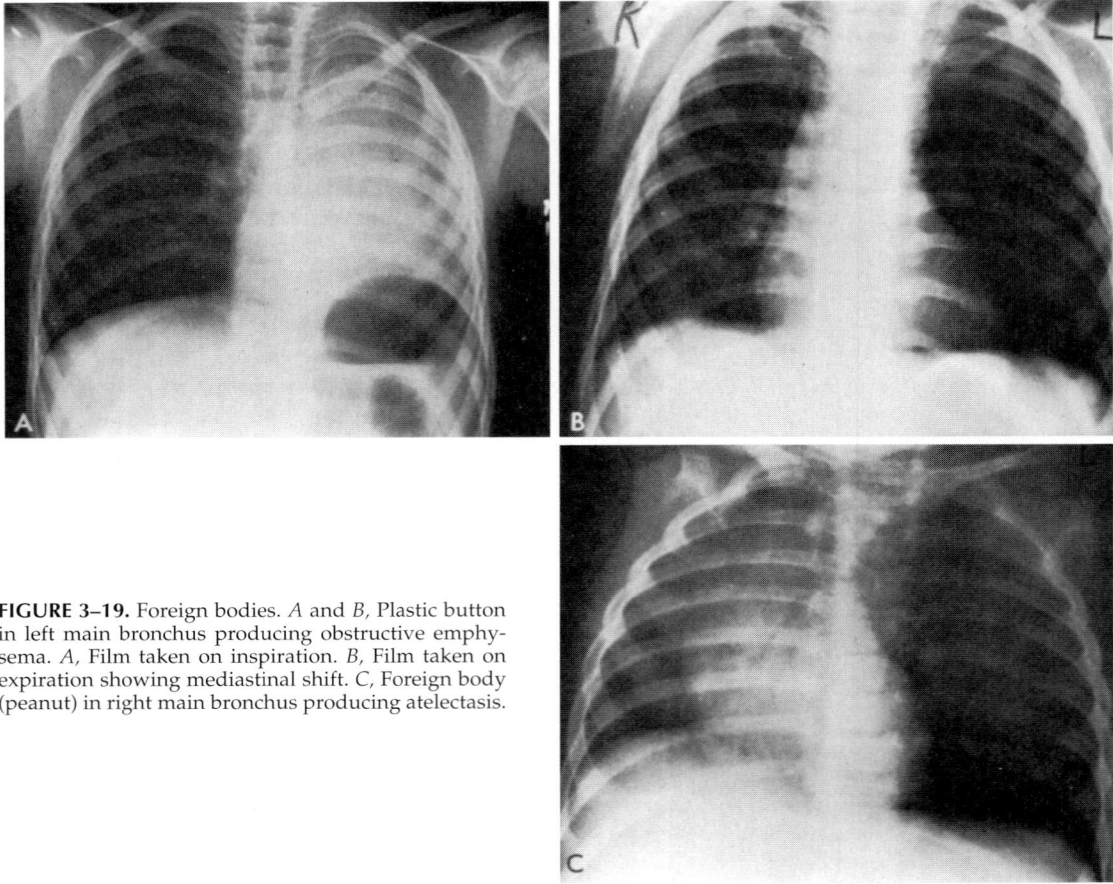

FIGURE 3–19. Foreign bodies. *A* and *B*, Plastic button in left main bronchus producing obstructive emphysema. *A*, Film taken on inspiration. *B*, Film taken on expiration showing mediastinal shift. *C*, Foreign body (peanut) in right main bronchus producing atelectasis.

Retained Secretions. Bronchoscopy is often required to remove thick, tenacious secretions when nasotracheal suctioning is unsuccessful. A flexible fiberoptic bronchoscope with a large side channel (2.6 mm) is usually adequate to remove the secretions. If suctioning through the flexible scope is unsuccessful, a rigid bronchoscope may be needed. Bronchoscopy is also useful in pulmonary suppuration, bronchiolitis, fibrocystic disease, asthma, and childhood tuberculosis in which rupture of a caseous lymph node may occlude a bronchus.

Endobronchial Tumors. Palliative treatment of endobronchial tumors and some benign conditions has become popular. Mechanical removal of tumor tissue through an open-tube ventilating rigid bronchoscope is possible, but the risk of a serious hemorrhage is real. Cryotherapy has been used to coagulate tumors that subsequently shrink, alleviating obstruction (Sanderson et al., 1981).

Laser therapy, often in association with radiation and chemotherapy, is, however, the most popular method used to treat unresectable, obstructing, and

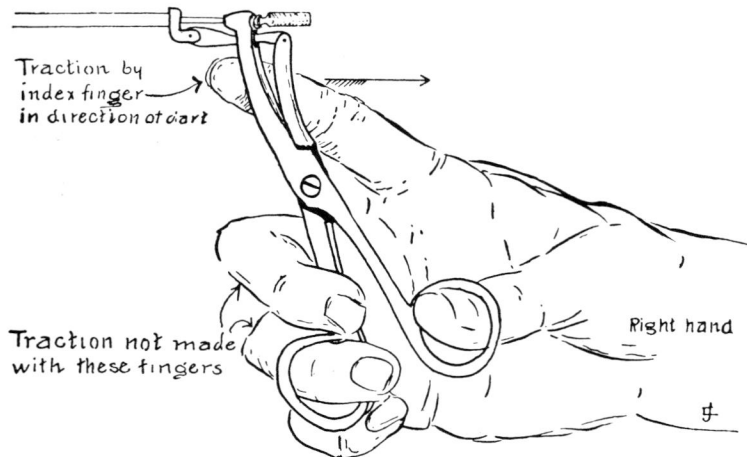

Traction by index finger in direction of dart

Traction not made with these fingers

Right hand

FIGURE 3–20. Proper method of grasping the forceps. The thumb and ring finger are inserted into the rings for opening and closing the forceps, the middle finger steadies the handle, and traction is exerted solely by the index finger along the shaft of the forceps. (From Jackson, C., and Jackson, C. L.: Bronchoesophagology. Philadelphia, W. B. Saunders, 1950.)

bleeding lesions of the tracheobronchial tree. Initially, the carbon dioxide laser was used, but because it requires a system of mirrors and an open rigid bronchoscope, it is unwieldy. More recently, the neodymium:yttrium-aluminum-garnet (Nd:YAG) laser (Fig. 3–21) has become available. The Nd:YAG laser causes coagulation necrosis of the tumor, which allows the mechanical removal of the obstructing tissue. Hemorrhage is unlikely to occur after the removal of the coagulated tissue, and good palliation is generally achieved in patients who have been properly selected (e.g., patients with endobronchial tumors with an adequate distal lumen) (Cavaliere et al., 1988). The Nd:YAG laser is preferred for use in the tracheobronchial tree to control bleeding and to remove obstructing tumor tissue because it is more easily used and is more hemostatic than the carbon dioxide laser.

Brachytherapy. The positioning of an ionizing radiation source in proximity to the target tissue has also helped treat obstructing lesions of the tracheobronchial tree. Afterloading catheters placed through such lesions with subsequent insertion of ^{192}Ir beads have proved to be beneficial (Sanderson, 1986).

Phototherapy. HPD phototherapy is used in some centers as an investigative technique to treat tumors

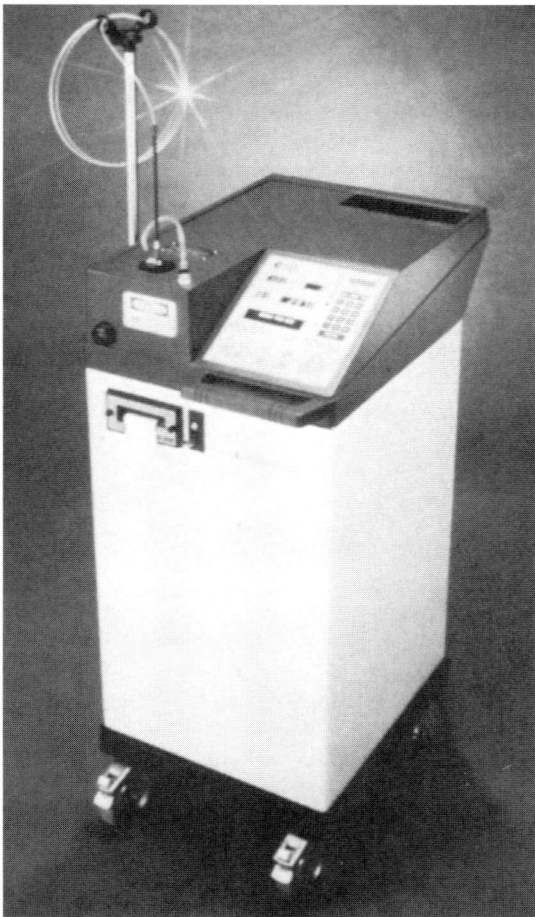

FIGURE 3–21. Neodymium:yttrium-aluminum-garnet (Nd:YAG) laser (Sharplan 2100). (Courtesy of Sharplan Laser, Inc., Allendale, NJ.)

of the respiratory tract in patients who are not candidates for operation. The HPD is picked up by tumor cells. A 630-nm light, which is produced by an argon-pumped dye laser, is introduced through the bronchoscope. The light activates the HPD that is concentrated in the tumor tissue and causes a photoreaction that releases toxic oxygen free radicals that kill malignant cells. Patients treated with HPD phototherapy become sensitive to the sun and must avoid exposure for 2 weeks after the treatment. They may also develop bronchial obstruction from the formation of eschar and edema (Sanderson, 1986).

Pediatric Bronchoscopy. Bronchoscopy in infants and children presents a special challenge because of the small caliber of the tracheobronchial trees. History, physical findings, and radiographic findings that suggest the presence of a foreign body are frequent indications for bronchoscopy in this age group. Persistent infections, compression, and deformity of the tracheobronchial tree in children with cardiovascular abnormalities and the presence of congenital bronchopulmonary stenosis can also be evaluated by bronchoscopy. In an H-type tracheoesophageal fistula, tracheoscopy using a forward-viewing pediatric telescope has been successful in locating the opening of the fistula in the posterior wall of the trachea. This information particularly helps the surgeon choose a cervical or thoracic approach when films do not show the level of the fistula (Killian, 1964). Bronchoscopy is also the only reliable method of establishing a diagnosis of endobronchial tuberculosis in its childhood form as well as its adult form (Daly, 1958).

Open-tube ventilating bronchoscopes are generally used in pediatric patients. Flexible bronchoscopes, some of which are as small as 2.7 mm in diameter (Wood and Fink, 1978), may help to make a rapid initial evaluation. Thus, the examiner who performs bronchoscopy on pediatric patients should be adept at both rigid and flexible bronchoscopy (Sanderson, 1986).

Complications. Pneumothorax, bleeding, hypoxia, and bronchospasm are the most common complications encountered during and after bronchoscopy (Shure, 1987). Preparation for managing severe bleeding and a significant pneumothorax must be made before bronchoscopy. A pneumothorax kit (Fig. 3–22), a balloon-occlusion catheter (Fig. 3–23), equipment for tracheal intubation, and resuscitative equipment should be available immediately wherever bronchoscopies are done.

Through the use of fluoroscopy, the incidence of pneumothorax, which is occasionally seen after transbronchial biopsy, has decreased significantly (Simpson et al., 1986). A pneumothorax, when it occurs, is usually small and requires only observation. A chest tube must be inserted occasionally to evacuate a large pneumothorax or to relieve a tension pneumothorax. A pneumothorax kit (Cook, Inc., Bloomington, IN) that is compact and can be stored conveniently on a bronchoscopy cart is easy to use and is effective for controlling a pneumothorax caused by a small pleural leak.

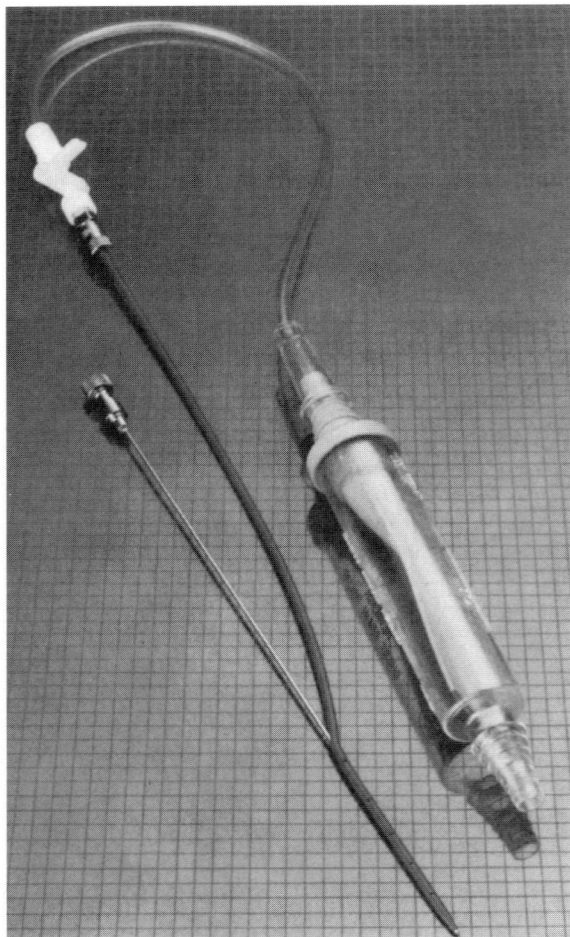

FIGURE 3–22. Pneumothorax set (C–TPT–100). (Courtesy of Cook, Inc., Bloomington, IN.)

Severe bleeding after bronchoscopy, although uncommon, does occur. If the bronchoscope is wedged in the segmental bronchus from which the bleeding is coming, the bleeding is usually localized, clotting occurs, and the bleeding stops (Zavala, 1978a). This maneuver occasionally is unsuccessful, and a balloon-

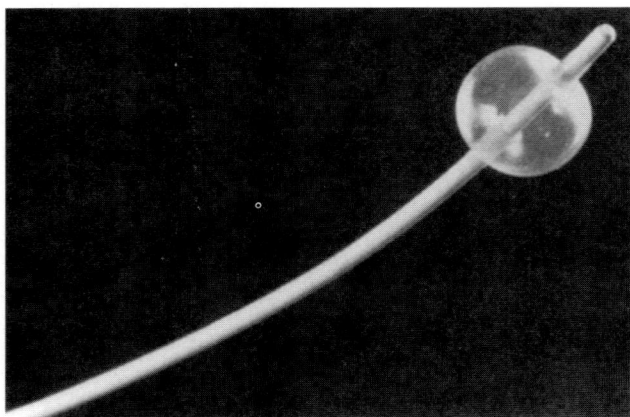

FIGURE 3–23. Balloon-occlusion catheter for controlling bleeding from the bronchial tree. (Courtesy of MicroVasive, Milford, MA.)

occlusion catheter that can block the bronchus from which the blood is coming must be inserted. The balloon is distended and the catheter is left in place until the bleeding stops (Sanderson, 1986).

The incidence of bronchospasm, which is often encountered in asthmatic patients, has been reduced by proper preoperative preparation (Belen et al., 1981). Fever, which often occurs after bronchoscopy, is rarely caused by bacterial infections of the lung (Suratt et al., 1977). Hypoxia, also frequently encountered during and after bronchoscopy, has been reduced by administering supplemental oxygen before, during, and for several hours after bronchoscopy (Albertini et al., 1974; Karetzky et al., 1974). The administration of oxygen also reduces the occurrence of cardiac arrhythmias during and after bronchoscopy (Lakshminarayan and Shrader, 1978). Reduced pulmonary volumes and hypoxia are associated with bronchoalveolar lavage and may last up to 24 hours. The administration of supplemental oxygen during the first day after the procedure has been recommended for all patients who have bronchoalveolar lavage (Burns et al., 1983; Tilles et al., 1986).

The reported operative morbidity for fiberoptic bronchoscopy varies from 0.08 to 0.15%, and the mortality varies from 0.01 to 0.4% (Credle et al., 1974; Simpson et al., 1986; Suratt et al., 1976). Morbidity and mortality increase when a transbronchial biopsy of the lung is performed. Simpson and colleagues (1986) have reported that the morbidity and mortality is 2.7 and 0.12% when a biopsy was performed, compared with 0.12 and 0.04% when no biopsy was taken. Although complications occur with bronchoscopy, particularly when a transbronchial biopsy is done, morbidity and mortality are sufficiently low and the information obtained is so helpful that bronchoscopy continues to be used extensively.

ESOPHAGOSCOPY

Esophagoscopy is technically more difficult to do than bronchoscopy, and it carries with it a risk of serious complications, even when performed by an experienced endoscopist (Anderson and Higgins, 1978). The esophagus is a flexible, thin-walled tube that is easily perforated, especially at its upper cervical constriction and just above the diaphragm (Fig. 3–24). Both rigid open esophagoscopes and flexible fiber gastroscopes are used widely. Another recent addition to the endoscopist's armamentarium is video endoscopy (Classen and Phillip, 1984). Its efficacy is still being determined.

Indications

Symptoms of dysphagia, regurgitation of food, hematemesis, retrosternal burning, or a history of swallowing a foreign body or caustic substance are all indications for esophagoscopy. Esophagoscopy is

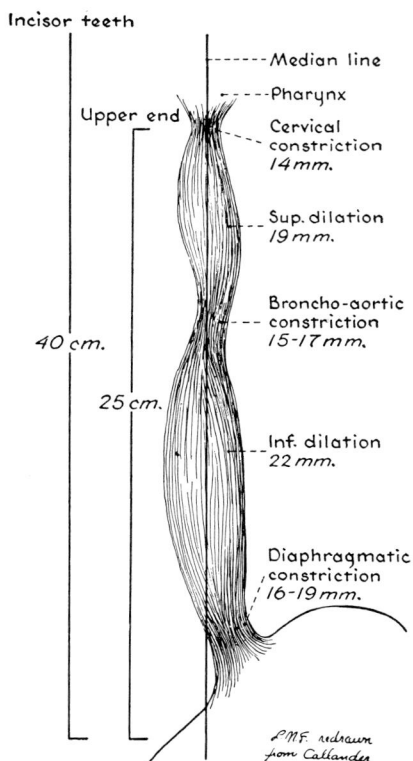

FIGURE 3–24. Sites of narrowing in the esophagus. (From Boies, L. R., Hilger, J. A., and Priest, R. E.: Fundamentals of Otolaryngology. 4th ed. Philadelphia, W. B. Saunders, 1964.)

also useful in locating the site of traumatic tears (Carter and Hinshaw, 1965).

Important diagnostic information is obtained from esophagograms and fluoroscopic studies of the swallowing mechanism. These studies should generally precede esophagoscopy because they localize and characterize the type of pathology that is encountered by the endoscopist.

Contraindications to esophagoscopy are few. Patients with aortic aneurysms have always been considered unsuitable for esophagoscopy because of the potential risk of rupture of the aneurysm. However, when the procedure is definitely indicated, it can be performed carefully with a fibergastroscope, and pressure on the wall of the aneurysm can be avoided. A sharp deformity of the cervical spine due to arthritis or sharp kyphosis may make esophagoscopy impossible or may limit the extent of the examination. In certain situations, a flexible scope can sometimes be inserted where a rigid scope cannot. A flexible scope, however, is passed blindly through the area of the cricopharyngeal muscle and the upper esophagus. The presence of pathology in this area makes passage of a flexible scope hazardous.

Technique

Rigid Open-ended Esophagoscope

The rigid open-ended esophagoscope is used widely because it can be passed under direct vision and it provides a large working space and sharp, clear visualization of the esophagus. The 9-mm × 45-cm esophagoscope is generally used for adults. Smaller-caliber esophagoscopes are available for use in children Table 3–3). An examination of the lower esophagus and cardia in patients with long chest walls is possible with a 9-mm × 53-cm esophagoscope. Recently, esophagoscopes fitted with a channel for injecting air to inflate the esophagus, Hopkins' rod-lens telescopes, and rigid high-quality optical biopsy forceps and foreign-body forceps have become available. These instruments have also been miniaturized for pediatric use (Fig. 3–25). The high-quality optics and stability of the current rigid open-ended esophagoscopes have greatly improved the esophagoscopist's ability to visualize and to perform a biopsy of the esophagus and also to grasp foreign bodies. Consequently, there has been a resurgence in the use of the rigid esophagoscope.

ANESTHESIA

Esophagoscopy may be done with the patient under topical anesthesia, as described for bronchoscopy, or under general anesthesia. The author prefers to use general anesthesia because it provides relaxation that permits the esophagoscope to be passed with greater ease and thus with less danger of perforation.

POSITION OF THE PATIENT

The patient is placed in the dorsal recumbent position with the head and shoulders over the edge of the table. In this position, the assistant can move the head in any direction. The neck is flexed and the head is extended on the atlanto-occipital joint to bring the pharynx and upper esophagus in line with the thoracic inlet.

With the handle up, the esophagoscope is introduced into the right side of the mouth. The shaft of the instrument rests on the thumb of the esophagoscopist's left hand, the fingers of which are placed on the patient's teeth or alveolar ridge (Fig. 3–26). A gauze pad protects the upper teeth. As the esophagoscope is advanced, the base of the tongue and the epiglottis are raised. The right arytenoid cartilage is

■ Table 3–3. GAUGE OF ESOPHAGOSCOPE IN RELATION TO AGE OF PATIENT*

Age	Esophagoscope
Adult	9 mm × 45 cm
	or
	9 mm × 53 cm
Adolescent	8 mm × 45 cm
6–12 yr	7 mm × 45 cm
2–5 yr	6 mm × 35 cm
12–24 mo	5 mm × 35 cm
6–12 mo	4 mm × 30 cm
Under 6 mo	4 mm × 30 cm

*Gauges and ages are averages, and the gradation of the instrument may have to be altered according to the size rather than the age of the patient.

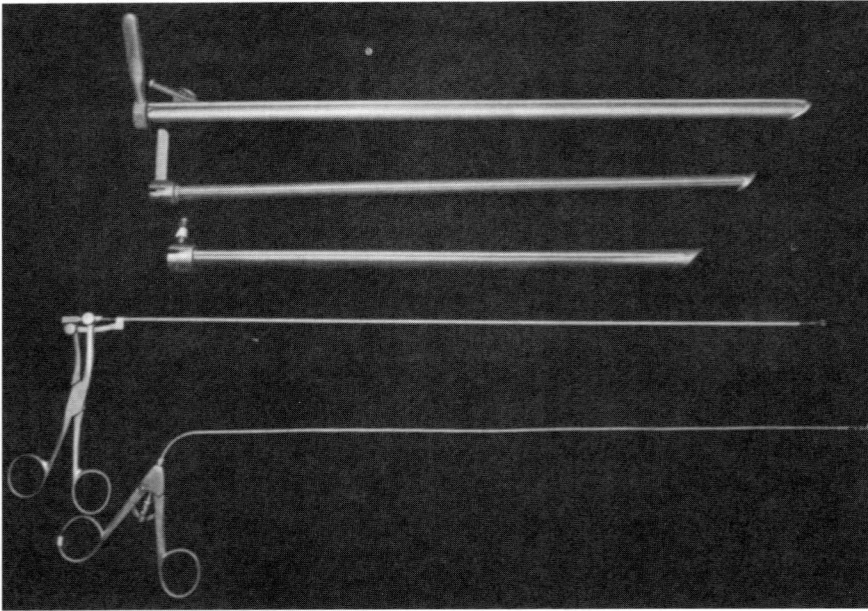

FIGURE 3–25. Pediatric esophagoscopes and forceps. *Top to bottom,* Jackson, Roberts, and Jesberg types of esophagoscope; globular object-grasping and tissue forceps (Jackson type) and right-angle cup forceps (center-action type).

identified and the lip of the instrument is passed behind it into the right piriform fossa. The esophagoscope is advanced slowly by a lifting motion of the left thumb. As the cricopharyngeal muscle is approached, the walls of the piriform sinus converge until a faint horizontal line is observed. The position of the esophagoscope must be maintained in line with the sternal notch. With steady downward pressure, the tip of the esophagoscope is advanced by the left thumb. Gentle pressure is placed on the cricopharyngeal muscle (Fig. 3–27). If the sphincter does not relax, a small bougie is inserted to locate the lumen. This is the most critical point in the procedure. Force must not be used with the tip of the esophagoscope or with the bougie. Once the bougie has passed through the esophageal opening, it serves as a guide and the instrument is advanced over it under direct vision. As the esophagoscope passes the cricopharyngeal muscle, the patient's head is lowered gradually. As the lower end of the esophagus is reached, the head must be depressed farther and must be carried to the right so that the esophagoscope may pass through the diaphragmatic hiatus. If difficulty is experienced in finding the opening at the cardia, a small bougie is inserted to aid in identification. The gastroesophageal junction is identified by the abrupt change from pale esophageal mucosa to the bright red gastric mucosa. A thorough examination of the esophageal wall is made with the Hopkins rod-lens telescope while the instrument is withdrawn. Retrograde inspection of the esophagus is important because a lesion or foreign body may be hidden by a fold of mucosa pushed in front of the advancing scope.

Flexible Fibergastroscope

Hirschowitz and associates (1958) introduced a flexible fiberscope for examination of the upper gastrointestinal tract. Subsequently, the fibergastroscope (Fig. 3–28) has been modified and provided with greatly improved optics. Several manufacturers produce these instruments, which vary in diameter from 7.9 to 12.6 mm and have tips that can be flexed in wide arcs. These instruments also have side channels through which air and fluid can be injected, suction applied, and biopsy forceps or cytology brushes inserted. Two-channel models suitable for therapeutic esophagoscopy are also available. The biopsy forceps for these scopes are small and the tissue obtained is occasionally insufficient for a pathologic diagnosis. The flexible fiberoptic gastroscopes, however, are excellent instruments for diagnostic esophagoscopy. Foreign-body removal through the flexible fibergastroscope has become possible with the development of grasping forceps and baskets similar to those used with the flexible bronchoscope (see Fig. 3–18).

Before the examination, the patient fasts for 6 hours. Topical anesthesia with supplemental sedation, if necessary, is generally adequate. The left lateral position is used, and the scope is generally inserted easily and comfortably through the mouth and into the esophagus with gentle pressure while the patient swallows. Introduction of air distends the esophagus and complete visualization of the esophageal wall is possible. The scope is passed under direct vision into the stomach and the upper stomach is examined. The esophagus is again visualized during withdrawal of the instrument. The passage of the flexible scope through the cricopharyngeal muscle and upper esophagus is done blindly, which makes insertion hazardous in patients with Zenker's diverticulum, cervical arthritis, or lesions of the upper third of the esophagus. When such pathology is suspected, the use of a rigid open esophagoscope is preferred because it is inserted under direct vision.

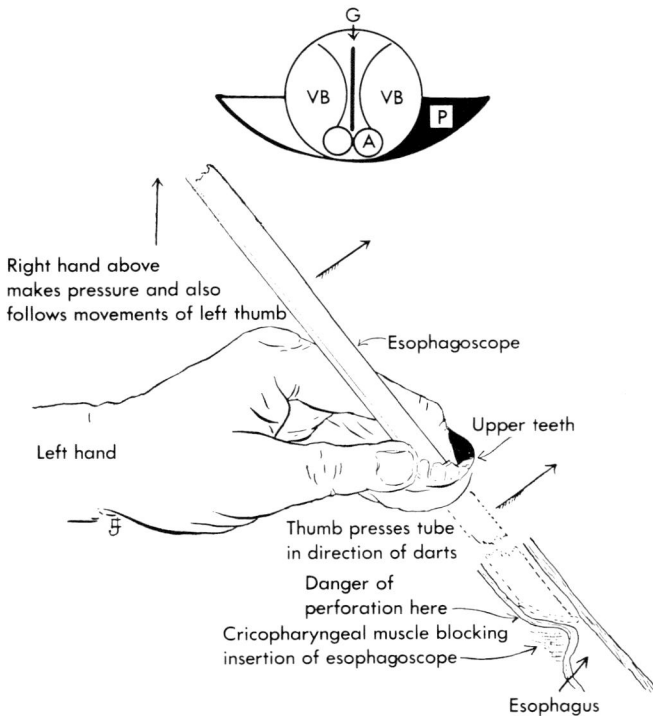

FIGURE 3–26. The *upper illustration* shows schematically the method of finding the pyriform sinus in the method of esophagoscopy. The large circle represents the cricoid cartilage. The pyriform sinuses are the normal food passages. G = glottic chink, spasmodically closed; VB = ventricular band; A = right arytenoid eminence; P = right pyriform sinus, through which the tube is passed in the recumbent patient.

The *lower illustration* shows the movements necessary for passing the cricopharyngeus. It also shows how the esophagoscope may at any time be fixed against the upper teeth, as, for example, when a foreign body is presented. The sketch represents the patient in a *dorsally recumbent* position; unless this is understood the illustration will be confusing. The "handle" of the esophagoscope is, and should be, vertical, to place the slanted distal end in proper position to override the cricopharyngeal mounding. (From Jackson, C., and Jackson, C. L.: Bronchoesophagology. Philadelphia, W. B. Saunders, 1950.)

Complications

The most common and serious complication of esophagoscopy is perforation of the esophagus, which can occur even when the flexible fiberscope is inserted carefully and gently. Perforation occurs most frequently at the upper opening of the esophagus and is due to forceful pressure against the weak posterior wall used in attempting to overcome a tightly closed cricopharyngeal sphincter (Fig. 3–29). The esophagus may also be perforated at the diaphragmatic hiatus by forceful pressure of the esophagoscope against its wall or during removal of a foreign body. Perforation may also result from a deep biopsy or bougienage and forceful dilatation of a stricture. Chest pain immediately after esophagoscopy or subcutaneous emphysema of the neck is a clinical indication of perforation. Films of the chest and neck should be obtained immediately. The treatment of a perforation is discussed elsewhere (see Chapter 27). At the New York Univer-

sity Medical Center, in more than 12,000 endoscopies, the incidence of esophageal perforation with the flexible scope has been lower than 0.1%. This experience compares favorably with the incidence of perforation of 0.25% reported with the rigid open esophagoscope by Palmer and Wirts (1957).

Esophagoscopic Findings in Diseases of the Esophagus

Films and CT scans of the chest and neck and esophagrams and fluoroscopic studies of the swallowing function provide most of the information needed for diagnosis of esophageal diseases. Radiographic studies thus define the esophageal problem and indicate what additional information must be sought at esophagoscopy.

Reflux Esophagitis. The precise biopsy technique possible with the rigid open esophagoscope and optical biopsy forceps makes possible a close correlation between the endoscopic and the pathologic changes that occur with reflux esophagitis. The initial pathologic lesion is a localized area of epithelial erosion and granulocytic infiltration of the lamina propria. Endoscopically, this lesion is seen as localized, supravestibular erythematous spots, some of which are

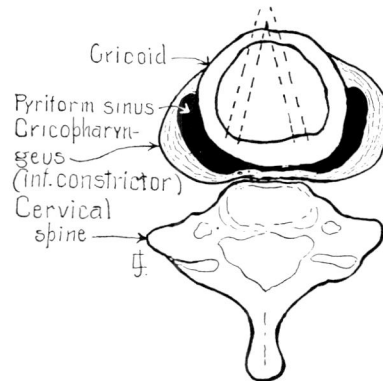

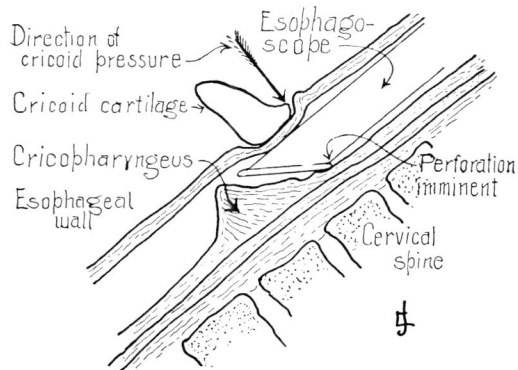

FIGURE 3–27. Anatomic relation of the cricoid cartilage and the cricopharyngeus that closes the esophageal opening like a pinchcock and forms the basis for difficulty in introduction of the esophagoscope through this area. (From Jackson, C., and Jackson, C. L.: Diseases of the Nose, Throat and Ear. 2nd ed. Philadelphia, W. B. Saunders, 1959.)

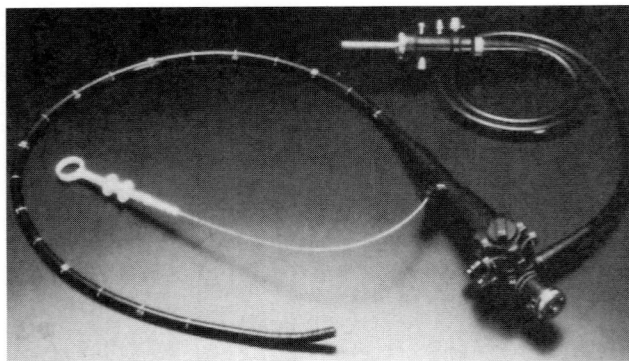

FIGURE 3–28. Flexible fibergastroscope (Olympus OES Gastroscope Model 61F–Q20) with biopsy forceps in position. (Courtesy of Olympus Corporation, Lake Success, NY.)

covered with an exudate (Stage I). When red areas become confluent, but do not involve the entire circumference of the esophagus, Stage II of reflux esophagitis has been reached. When the entire circumference is involved, Stage III is present. The typical appearance is an edematous, red mucosa, often with flat ulcerations covered by a thin, fibrous membrane that bleeds readily when touched by an instrument. Stage IV esophagitis consists of complications such as deep ulcers, stenotic lesions, and columnar epithelial metaplasia (Barrett's esophagus) (Savary and Miller, 1978).

Barrett's Esophagus. Stratified squamous epithelium of the lower esophagus may be destroyed by chronic reflux of gastric secretions. The esophagus responds to this insult by replacing the destroyed mucosa with columnar epithelium (metaplasia). This columnar-lined esophagus (Barrett, 1950) may become the site of a stricture or a discrete ulcer—"Barrett's ulcer." These ulcers have a deep, punched-out appearance with rounded edges. A biopsy should

be taken of the lesion to distinguish it from a malignant ulceration. The endoscopist should also try to determine whether normal esophageal mucosa separates the ulcerated area from gastric mucosa or whether the ulcer is in gastric mucosa that has been drawn up above the diaphragm (Allison and Johnstone, 1953).

Because the risk of developing cancer in patients with Barrett's esophagus is 75 times that in the normal population, yearly endoscopic biopsies seem to be an effective technique of surveillance. If high-grade dysplagia or carcinoma is found, surgical resection should be performed immediately (Streitz et al., 1993).

Stenosis. In congenital stenosis, the upper portion of the esophagus is moderately dilated. The stenosis is usually firm and is covered with normal mucosa. It is frequently associated with a congenitally short esophagus. The term *congenitally short esophagus* is used widely, but may be misleading. The recognition that hiatal hernia and gastric reflux occur frequently in infants suggests that the short esophagus is *acquired* rather than *congenital*. The diagnostic findings of the congenitally short esophagus are the transition to gastric mucosa at the stenosis and the presence of a portion of the stomach above the diaphragm. The stenosis is usually tight and does not permit the passage of the esophagoscope. Acquired stenosis is usually associated with esophagitis, esophageal ulcer, or esophagitis and hiatal hernia.

Corrosive Esophagitis. Corrosive esophagitis due to the ingestion of strong alkalis or acids usually causes scarring that results in stenosis, irregular strictures, and pockets. During the acute phase (Table 3–4), the burned area is covered with a grayish slough (Noirclerc et al., 1987). The esophageal walls become edematous and the lumen becomes narrow. Because the esophageal walls are edematous and friable, the risk of perforation by the passage of an esophagoscope is great. To avoid perforation, the examination

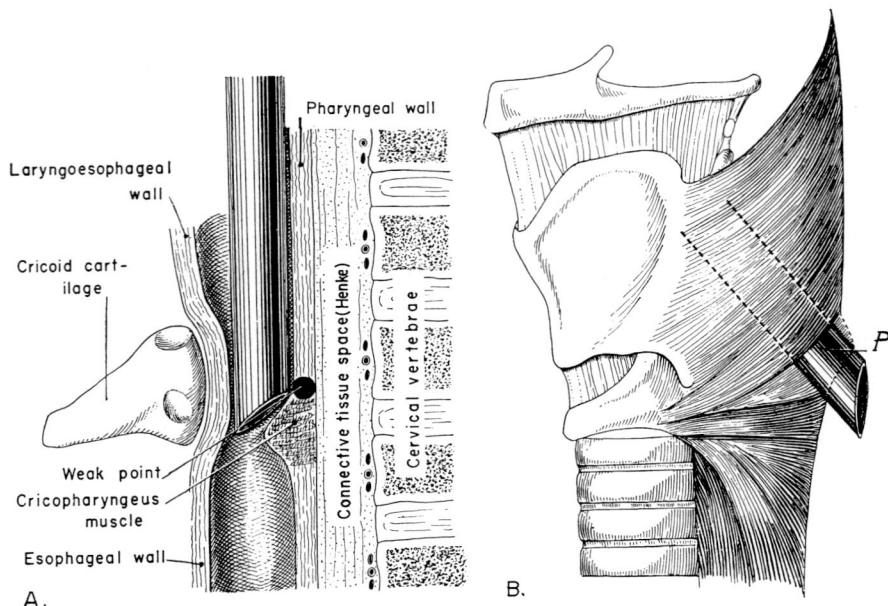

FIGURE 3–29. Schematic illustration of the anatomic basis for high instrumental perforation of the esophagus. The cricopharyngeal muscle closes the esophageal opening tightly by pulling the cricoid cartilage backward toward the cervical spine. Relaxation of the cricopharyngeal pinchcock, as in swallowing, is necessary to pass this area, and force is never exerted. *A*, The end of the instrument is resting on the weak spot. Pressure exerted on the weak spot as shown in *B* causes the tube to perforate this area. (*A* and *B*, From Terracol, J., and Sweet, R. H.: Diseases of the Esophagus. Philadelphia, W. B. Saunders, 1958.)

■ Table 3–4. ENDOSCOPIC STAGES

Stage		Characteristics
I		Inflammation of the mucosa
II		
	A	Ulceration, little hemorrhage
	B	Limited or circular necrosis
III		Extensive necrosis involving the whole organ and massive hemorrhage
IV		Characteristics of Stage III and intravascular disseminated coagulopathy and metabolic acidosis

Reproduced by permission from Noirclerc, M. J., DiCostanzo, J., Sastre, B., et al.: Surgical management of caustic injuries to the upper gastrointestinal tract. *In* DeMeester, T. R., and Matthews, H. R. (eds): International Trends in General Thoracic Surgery: Benign Esophageal Disease. Vol. 3, Chap. 18. St. Louis, C. V. Mosby, 1987.

should be concluded when the first burned area is encountered.

Diverticulum. In diverticulum of the esophagus, esophagoscopy is used to inspect the walls of the diverticulum to exclude ulceration and possible associated neoplasm. In pharyngoesophageal diverticulum, no difficulty is experienced in finding the diverticulum because the esophagoscope passes directly into the mouth of the diverticulum. It is difficult, however, to find the opening into the esophagus because it is closed tightly by the cricopharyngeal muscle. Esophagoscopy has been used to help the surgeon locate the diverticulum and then, by inserting the esophagoscope into the esophagus, to define the lumen of the esophagus while the neck of the diverticulum is being amputated.

Varices. Esophagoscopy is more successful in diagnosing esophageal varices than is roentgenography because small varices may be missed by the latter. The typical appearance is a bluish, longitudinal elevation at the lower end of the esophagus. Varices differ greatly in appearance from small elevations to very dilated veins that fill the lumen of the esophagus. The examination can be performed with little risk to the patient during the active phase of bleeding to distinguish esophageal from gastric bleeding.

Hiatal Hernia. Only the true hiatal hernia and the hernia with a short esophagus have characteristic findings. In the short esophagus, the gastroesophageal junction is located above the diaphragm and is narrow, and the lower end of the esophagus is ulcerated. In a true hiatal hernia, in which the gastroesophageal junction and stomach are above the diaphragm, the lower esophagus has redundant folds and, as the esophagoscope passes into the stomach, the firm support of the leaves of the diaphragm is not encountered. The paraesophageal sliding hernia has no characteristic findings.

Achalasia. The characteristic esophagoscopic findings of achalasia are wide dilatation of the esophagus and retention of food and secretions in the presence of a gastroesophageal sphincter of normal tone. In an advanced stage, the esophagus becomes enormously dilated and elongated and rests on the right leaf of the diaphragm. The walls are greatly thickened, leathery, and chronically inflamed by infection and by

irritation of decomposing food. At this stage, it may be impossible to find the lumen at the hiatus without the help of a swallowed thread. A small lead shot on the end of a thread helps the thread enter the stomach and also makes it possible to determine when the thread is anchored in the intestinal tract. The thread can then be used to guide dilators into position. Lavage and emptying of the esophagus with a wide-bore stomach tube should be done before esophagoscopy.

Neoplasm. Esophagoscopy is indicated whenever a neoplasm is suspected on clinical or roentgenographic evidence. Areas of reduced motility in the esophageal wall, as seen fluoroscopically, should be examined with the esophagoscope.

Carcinoma. Intraepithelial or microinvasive esophageal carcinomas are conditions that are now firmly established. They present as surface irregularities with a light discoloration of the mucosa (leukoplakia, erythroplakia, or leukoerythroplakia). A raised leukoplakia-type lesion is easily recognized and biopsied, whereas recognition and diagnosis of the more common flat erythroplakia-type lesion requires a rigid high-performance optical biopsy system. Vital staining of early esophageal carcinomas (with Lugol's solution or toluidine blue) has also improved the endoscopist's ability to diagnose these lesions by localizing and defining their limits (Monnier and Savary, 1987).

The typical finding in esophageal carcinoma is a large fungating lesion that bleeds with the slightest manipulation. The lesion presents occasionally as a smooth stenosis covered by edematous mucosa. The ulceration is beyond the vision of the esophagoscope, but specimens of tissue can be obtained by inserting biopsy forceps and a brush through the stenotic opening. These two methods give a positive diagnosis in more than 90% of carcinomas of the esophagus (Halter et al., 1977). A malignant tumor of the cardia not infrequently infiltrates the lower end of the esophagus and produces a stenosis covered with normal mucosa.

Benign Neoplasms. Benign neoplasms of the esophagus are uncommon, and leiomyomas are the most frequently seen. Fibromas and lipomas of the esophagus may develop long pedicles that may be regurgitated into the pharynx or even the mouth. These lesions are usually covered by normal esophageal mucosa. Operative removal is preferred to attempts made through the esophagoscope.

Endoscopic Ultrasonography

Endoscopic ultrasonography has made the evaluation of some esophageal lesions even more precise than has been possible using endoscopic and radiographic inspection, particularly in the definition of benign and malignant esophageal tumors and esophageal varices (Caletti et al., 1986; Strohm and Classen, 1986; Tio et al., 1986; Tio and Tytgat, 1984, 1986; Yasuda et al., 1986). Some tumors have characteristic echo densities. Leiomyomas, for example, have been found to be discrete masses of low echo density (Fig. 3–30), whereas esophageal carcinomas are indistinct echo-poor lesions. A site of origin of some tumors in the muscularis mucosa or muscularis propria can be recognized. The extent of esophageal wall involvement, extension into periesophageal structures, and lymph node involvement can also be evaluated with ultrasonography. In some cases, ultrasonography has been found to be superior to CT scanning for an evaluation of operability of carcinomas of the esophagus (Monnier and Savary, 1987).

Esophageal varices—periesophageal, submucosal, and deep intramural—in transverse section can be recognized as round, echo-poor structures. Ultrasonography has also proved useful in evaluating patients for sclerotherapy (Monnier and Savary, 1987).

Therapeutic Esophagoscopy

Removal of Foreign Bodies. Most esophageal foreign bodies can be removed endoscopically. A rigid optical foreign-body forceps incorporating a Hopkins rod-lens telescope passed through a rigid esophagoscope is the best instrument for visualizing, grasping, and removing foreign bodies. The flexible gastroscope also provides good visualization of foreign bodies, and the availability of grasping forceps and baskets for use through the flexible scope makes the removal of a foreign body feasible. Coins, fish and chicken bones, a bolus of meat, safety pins, and dentures are common objects that are swallowed inadvertently and become lodged in the esophagus (Fig. 3–31). The most common sites are the cervical esophagus just below the level of the cricopharyngeal muscle and the lower

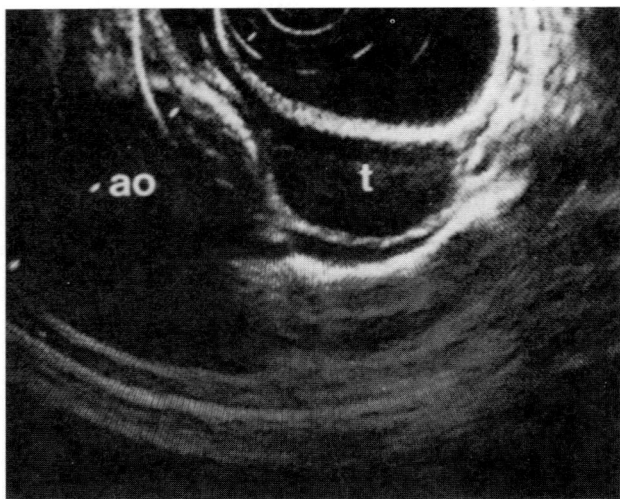

FIGURE 3–30. Endoscopic ultrasonographic image compatible with a leiomyoma. Endoscopic ultrasonography shows an ellipsoid hypoechogenic homogeneous echo pattern with sharply demarcated borders (t) beyond normal mucosa adjacent to the descending aorta (ao). (From Tio T. L., and Tytgat, G. N. J.: Atlas of Transintestinal Endosonography. Aalsmeer, The Netherlands, Drukkerij Mur-Kostverloren, 1986.)

esophagus at the level of the diaphragm. Objects with sharp points that become embedded in the wall of the esophagus present a special problem because of the danger of perforation. An open safety pin or a dental plate with sharp clips or points is particularly dangerous. The safest method of removing an open safety pin is to grasp the spring with a rotating forceps and to carry the pin with its point trailing into the stomach. With fluoroscopic guidance, version of the pin is accomplished and the pin is withdrawn with the point trailing. Other methods, such as sheathing the point with the esophagoscope, closure, and dangling, are more difficult to accomplish.

Dilatation of Esophageal Strictures. Strictures of the esophagus may be dilated through the rigid esophagoscope with Jackson's woven bougies. This method of bougienage is valuable in the initial assessment of a stricture, but the caliber of the esophagoscope places a limit on the size of the bougie that can be used. Passage of metal olive-tipped bougies (Eder-Puestow) over a swallowed string or wire has been widely used (Smith, 1986), especially when strictures are multiple and the esophageal lumen is irregular (Fig. 3–32). The incidence of perforation with these techniques has unfortunately been high (Earlam and Cunha-Melo, 1981; Luna, 1983; Tulman and Boyce, 1981).

The introduction of Savary-Gilliard bougies has reduced the incidence of iatrogenic perforation greatly and has also increased the effectiveness of dilatation (Monnier et al., 1985; Monnier and Savary, 1987). The Savary dilators are made of polyvinyl chloride; they measure 100 cm in length, and they have a central lumen through which a guidewire can pass. They are smooth and noncompressible, but flexible in the longitudinal axis. The proximal tip consists of a narrow straight 8-cm segment that is followed by a dilator cone (Fig. 3–33). The metal guidewire over which the dilators are inserted is passed endoscopically through the stricture. The tip of the metal guidewire is made of a flexible coil that resists perforating the esophagus even if the tip is placed perpendicularly against the esophageal wall. The endoscopist's method of dilating an esophageal stricture with these dilators has proved to be safe and effective. Three medical centers have reported more than 1000 dilatations without a perforation using these dilators, and thus confirm their safety (Dumon et al., 1984).

When a gastrostomy is in position, retrograde dilatation using Tucker's rubber dilators is a safe and effective method (see Fig. 3–32). A string must be passed from above into the stomach and is brought out through the gastrostomy opening, which allows the dilators to be drawn retrograde up through the esophagus. A string is maintained in the lumen of the esophagus between dilatations. Dilatation of esophageal strictures with flexible fiberscopes is now possible using balloon dilators that can be passed through these instruments. Balloon dilators are effective, but no more so than other dilators, and strictures seem to recur more quickly after balloon dilatation (Cox et al., 1985).

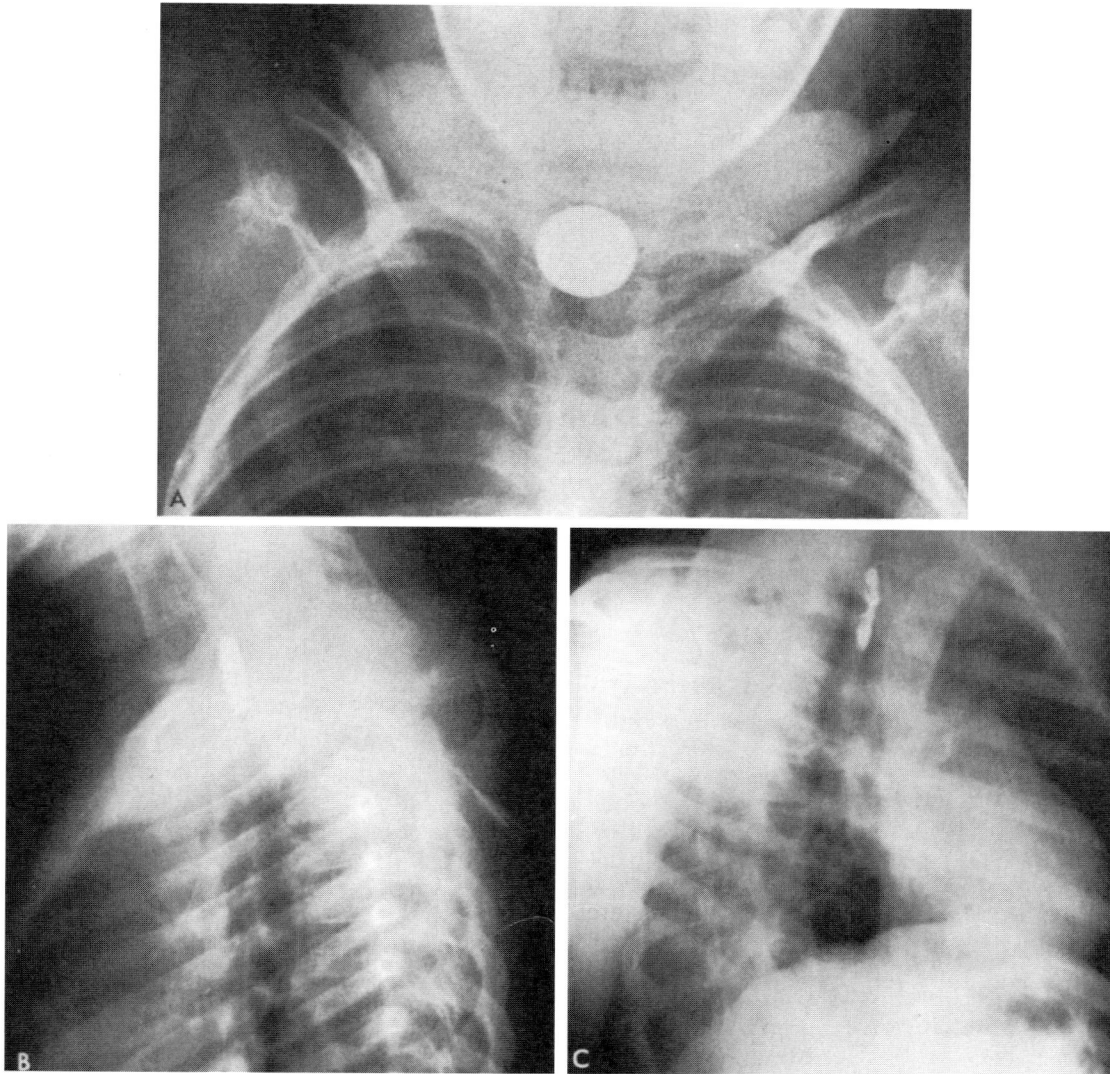

FIGURE 3–31. *A,* A coin in the cricopharyngeal sphincter of a 2-year-old child. *B,* The typical position of a coin in the cricopharyngeal sphincter is in the coronal plane. The lateral film shows an on-end view. *C,* Denture in the upper third of the esophagus. Sharp clasps were shielded during the removal to avoid tearing the esophagus.

Judgment and experience dictate the number and frequency of dilatations performed. When the esophagus has been dilated to a point at which the patient can maintain her weight, she is taught to swallow a Hurst mercury-weighted bougie to maintain the esophageal lumen (see Fig. 3–32).

Corrosive Esophagitis. After ingestion of caustic materials, the esophagus undergoes a necrotic phase followed by a healing phase (see Table 3–4). If the injury does not involve the submucosa (Stage II), healing usually is complete in 20 to 30 days. Burns that involve the submucosa (Stage III) require 90 to 120 days to heal (Noirclerc et al., 1987).

Historically, prophylactic dilatations that begin 3 to 4 days after injury were advocated to prevent strictures (Fig. 3–34A). This treatment was successful in 80% of patients (Salzer, 1920).

Since the early 1970s, the author's routine has been to perform esophagoscopy to confirm the presence of

a burn and to be careful not to pass the esophagoscope beyond the first burned area. A polyethylene nasogastric tube is introduced for nutritional support and nothing is allowed by mouth. Prophylactic bougienage is not used. The patient is maintained on a regimen of antibiotics and prednisone for 3 to 4 weeks, or until the esophagus heals, recognizing that the use of these agents is controversial (Fig. 3–34B–C). This regime has been successful in preventing strictures in 90% of patients. Five per cent of patients developed strictures that were treated successfully by dilatation from above with olive-tipped bougies passed over a string or guidewire. More recently, Savary's dilators have been used successfully. The remaining 5% of patients were lost to follow-up (Daly, 1968).

Carcinoma. Palliation of inoperable carcinoma of the esophagus can be accomplished by dilatation, laser resection, insertion of prosthetic tubes, and

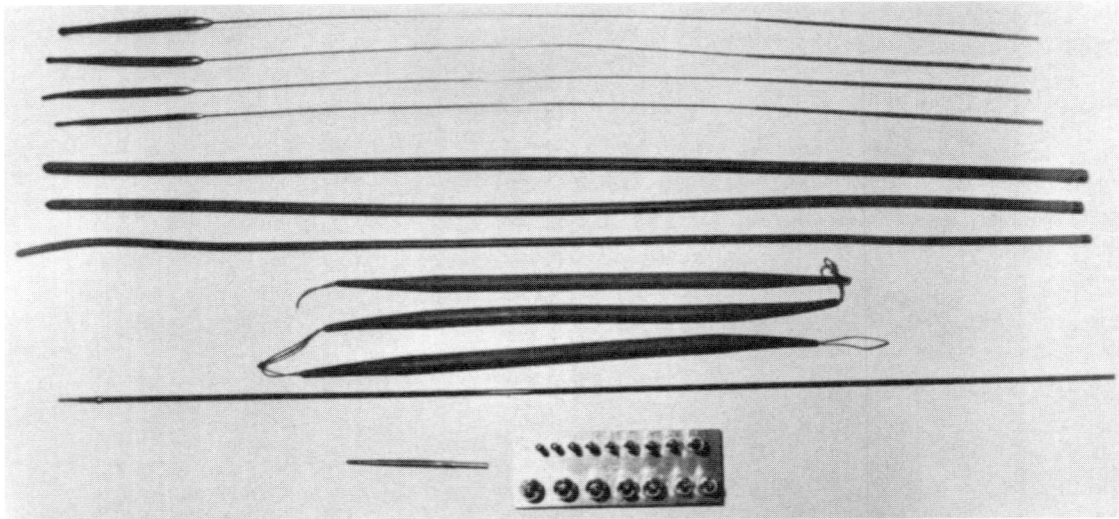

FIGURE 3–32. Bougies for esophageal dilatation. *Top,* Jackson woven bougies. *Middle,* Hurst bougies for dilatation from above. *Bottom,* Tucker bougies for retrograde dilatation over a swallowed thread.

brachytherapy. Palliation by dilatation is usually not effective for any prolonged period, and must be followed by laser resection or insertion of a prosthesis in most patients. Among the numerous prosthetic tubes currently available, plastic tubes (Mackler's, Celestin's, and Fell's types), metal spring tubes (Souttar's), and most recently, the Dumon-Gilliard prosthesis (Fig. 3–35) have been used extensively. Prosthetic tubes have been helpful particularly in managing patients with tracheoesophageal fistulas (Angorn and Haffejee, 1988).

The initial use of the Nd:YAG laser to control bleeding in the upper gastrointestinal tract has evolved into its use for widening the lumen through carcinomas of the esophagus (McElvein, 1988; Overholt, 1985). Most authors have reported using the laser from above downward. This method often requires several sessions to obtain complete opening of a passage through the tumor. More recently, reports of using the laser from below upward after dilatation have appeared (McElvein, 1988; Overholt, 1985). This approach seems effective and can often be done in a single sitting.

The Nd:YAG laser with its hemostatic properties is effective in coring a passage through esophageal carcinomas and permitting relatively normal swallowing. There is also one report of increased longevity in patients treated with the laser (Karlin et al., 1987). Although these palliative measures have helped in some situations, surgical excision or bypassing an esophageal carcinoma continues to be the best methods of palliation for this dreadful disease.

Brachytherapy. Brachytherapy is radiation therapy in which the ionizing source is placed in position close to the tissue that is to be treated. Several centers have reported their experience with this therapy. In

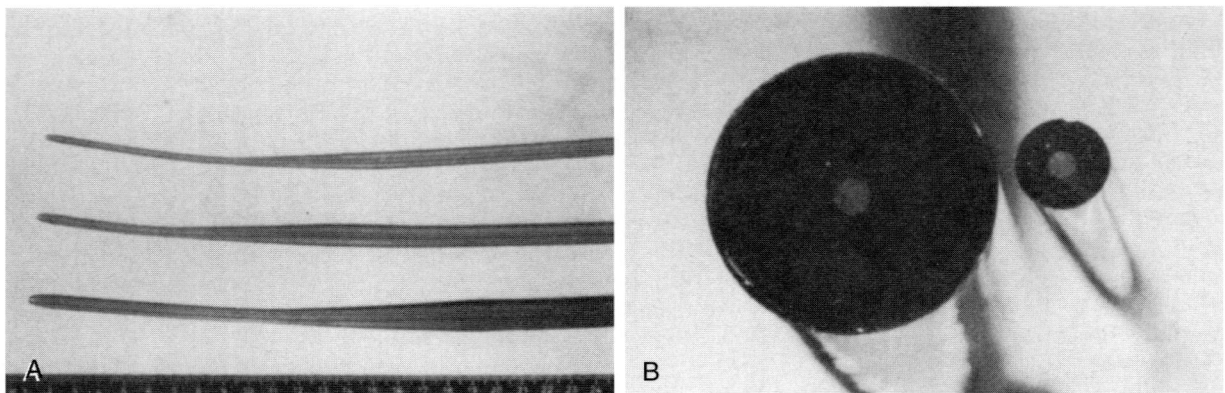

FIGURE 3–33. Savary-Gilliard dilatation bougies. *A,* The dilatation cone is extremely profiled. It follows an 8-cm straight segment and stays in a constant 4- or 5-degree angle, depending on the caliber of the bougie. Because of this construction, dilatation is gentle and progressive and causes minimal mucosal trauma. *B,* The bougies have a hollow core, 1.8 mm in diameter, which allows them to be advanced on a guidewire. (*A* and *B,* Reproduced by permission from Monnier, P., and Savary, M.: New endoscopic techniques. *In* DeMeester, T. R., and Matthews, H. R. [eds]: International Trends in General Thoracic Surgery: Benign Esophageal Disease. Vol. 3, Chap. 5. St. Louis, C. V. Mosby, 1987.)

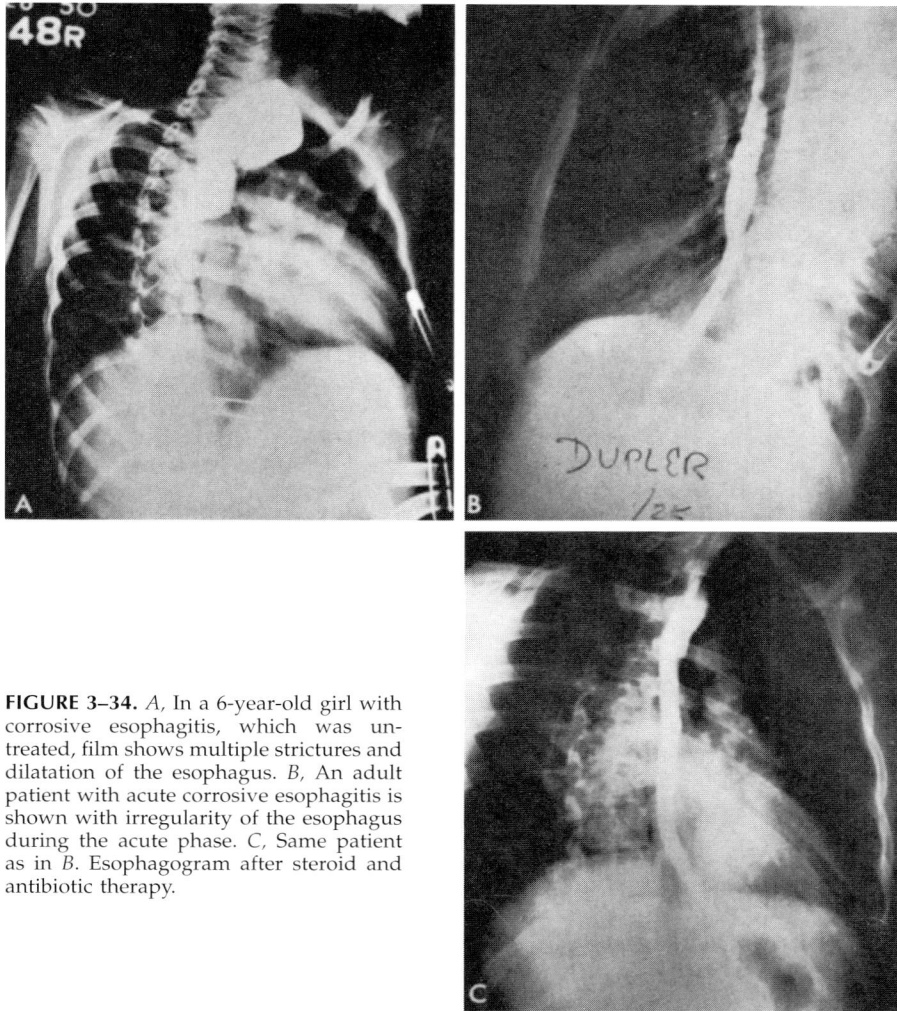

FIGURE 3–34. *A*, In a 6-year-old girl with corrosive esophagitis, which was untreated, film shows multiple strictures and dilatation of the esophagus. *B*, An adult patient with acute corrosive esophagitis is shown with irregularity of the esophagus during the acute phase. *C*, Same patient as in *B*. Esophagogram after steroid and antibiotic therapy.

one report by Pagliero and Rowland (1988), intracavitary irradiation in 72 patients with inoperable carcinoma of the esophagus was presented. They used ^{137}Cs applied through an afterloading applicator. The tumor was evaluated and dilated at esophagoscopy. A guidewire was advanced through the carcinoma, and the applicator was placed in position at the appropriate level in the esophagus. In a shielded environment, the radioactive isotope was inserted and approximately 3500 cGy was administered at the surface of the tumor, which took approximately 75 minutes. The procedure was well tolerated and had few side effects. Survival appeared to be better than survival with intubation. Fewer than half the patients, however, were alive after 6 months, but some patients did survive for 1 year. The exact role for brachytherapy in the treatment of inoperable carcinoma of the esophagus is still evolving (Pagliero and Rowland, 1988).

Photodetection and Photodynamic Therapy of Early Carcinomas of the Esophagus. Although still in an experimental stage, HpD has been used to detect and treat early carcinomas of the esophagus. HpD accumulates in malignant tumors and fluoresces when exposed to a 405-nm light, which permits tumor recognition. Exposure to another wavelength (630 nm) causes a photochemical reaction that releases oxygen free radicals that theoretically destroy carcinoma cells. The usefulness of these currently evolving techniques holds promise for the future (Dougherty, 1984; Hayata et al., 1985; Kessel, 1984; McCaughan and Williams, 1988; Monnier and Savary, 1987).

Dilatation of Achalasia. In most institutions, a surgical myotomy (Heller's procedure) is performed as the primary therapy for achalasia unless contraindications to thoracotomy exist. Symptomatic relief can be obtained in 70 to 80% of patients with achalasia by dilatation of the gastroesophageal junction. The dilatation consists of a submucosal avulsion of the muscle fibers of the sphincter. Either a hydrostatic or an aerostatic bag is introduced, with fluoroscopic guidance, over a string to the junction between the esophagus and the stomach. When the bag is in the proper position, pressure is raised to the point of tolerance or to 15 mm Hg, and is maintained at this pressure for 10 minutes (Fig. 3–36). Several dilatations performed at 3- to 6-month intervals are usually necessary. If symptoms are not relieved after three dilata-

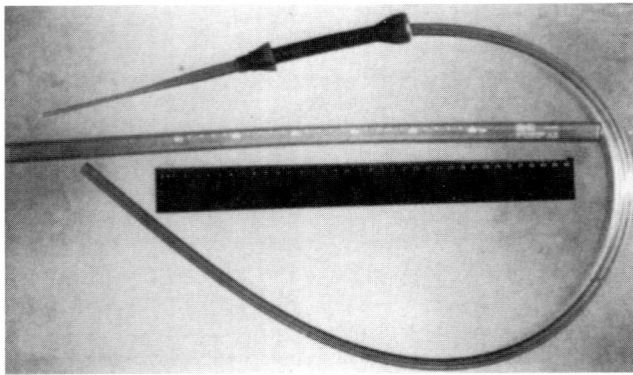

FIGURE 3–35. Dumon-Gilliard prosthesis introducer. This system is composed of a Savary bougie measuring 10.5 mm in diameter and 100 cm in length. The prosthesis introducer is passed through the cuff of the prosthesis and is attached to the proximal end by means of a conical ring. The bougie prosthesis/prosthesis introducer system is a single unit that allows easy introduction. (Reproduced by permission from Monnier, P., and Savary, M.: New endoscopic techniques. *In* DeMeester, T. R., and Matthews, H. R. [eds]: International Trends in General Thoracic Surgery: Benign Esophageal Disease. Vol. 3, Chap. 5. St. Louis, C. V. Mosby, 1987.)

tions, the procedure should be considered unsuccessful and a surgical myotomy should be done. Perforations due to mucosal tears during dilatation are a definite risk. Abdominal or chest pain or splinting of the upper abdomen is an indication that a perforation may have occurred.

Variceal Bleeding. Variceal bleeding is a serious complication of portal hypertension with a high mortality (Joffe, 1984). The use of the Ng:YAG laser to control bleeding has been reported. Sclerotherapy and electrocautery also have been used. The data on electrocautery are incomplete, and laser photocoagulation is unlikely to prevent rebleeding because only sealing of the varix is accomplished, not obliteration (Jensen et al., 1983). Sclerotherapy, although successful in many patients, is followed by rebleeding in 40% (Geenen, 1982). Endoscopic variceal ligation has been

used in patients in whom sclerotherapy has failed (Saeed et al., 1990). Further evaluation of these techniques for the treatment of esophageal varices is needed.

A basic endoscopic set includes the following instruments:

1 Laryngoscope, adult size
1 Laryngoscope, child size
1 Laryngoscope, infant size
1 Bronchoscope, 8 mm × 40 cm
1 Bronchoscope, 7 mm × 40 cm
1 Bronchoscope, 6 mm × 35 cm
1 Bronchoscope, 4 mm × 30 cm
1 Bronchoscope, 3.5 mm × 25 cm
1 Bronchoscope, 3 mm × 25 cm
3 Flexible fiberbronchoscopes (different models including a pediatric bronchoscope)
1 Esophagoscope, 9 mm × 45 cm
1 Esophagoscope, 9 mm × 53 cm
1 Esophagoscope, 7 mm × 45 cm
1 Esophagoscope, 6 mm × 35 cm
1 Esophagoscope, 4 mm × 30 cm
1 Esophagoscope, 9 mm × 45 cm (full lumen)
2 Flexible fibergastroscopes (diagnostic and therapeutic models)
1 Forceps, ball, 60 cm
1 Forceps, right-angle, rotation, 50 cm
1 Forceps, cupped, forward-grasping, 50 cm
1 Forceps, ball, 50 cm
1 Forceps, peanut, 40 cm
10 Bougies (esophageal nos. 8 to 28F)
Savary-Gilliard Bougies (complete set with metallic guidewire)
3 Aspirating tubes, velvet-eye 20, 50, 60 cm
3 Bronchial aspirating tubes, spiral, flexible (2 straight and 1 curved)
2 Aspirating tubes for infant scope
Sponge carriers, specimen collectors, and atomizers
Hopkins' rod-lens telescopes and optical biopsy and grasping forceps for use with both

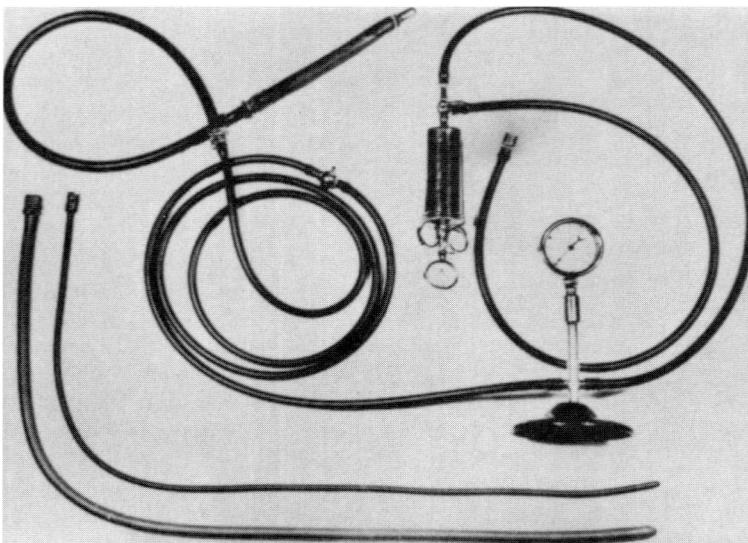

FIGURE 3–36. Hydrostatic dilator with gauge and hand pump. *Below and to the left,* Hurst mercury-filled bougies.

bronchoscopes and esophagoscopes (zero-degree straight, 30-degree forward oblique, and 90-degree lateral)

Biopsy and grasping forceps for use with the flexible bronchoscope and esophagoscope

SELECTED BIBLIOGRAPHY

Arroliga, A., and Matthay, R.: The role of bronchoscopy in lung cancer. Clin. Chest Med., *14*:87, 1993.

The current role of bronchoscopy in the diagnosis and staging of lung cancer is discussed. The techniques used in both central and peripheral lesions are included.

Berci, G.: Chevalier Jackson lecture: Analysis of new optical systems in bronchoesophagology. Ann. Otol. Rhinol. Laryngol., *87*:451, 1978.

A lucid description of the Hopkins rod-lens and flexible endoscope optical system is presented. Optical biopsy forceps and miniature endoscopes are also discussed.

Monnier, P., and Savary, M.: New endoscopic techniques. *In* De-Meester, T. R., and Matthews, H. R. (eds): International Trends in General Thoracic Surgery: Benign Esophageal Diseases. Vol. 3, Chap. 5. St. Louis, C. V. Mosby, 1987.

The most current diagnostic and therapeutic aspects of esophagoscopy are discussed. Emphasis is placed particularly on the advances made possible by the superb optical qualities and precise biopsy capabilities of the rigid open-tube esophagoscope.

Salazar, A., and Westcott, J.: The role of transthoracic needle biopsy for the diagnosis and staging of lung cancer. Clin. Chest Med., *14*:99, 1993.

This report is an up-to-date, concise, and thorough review of the role of transthoracic needle biopsy in the diagnosing and staging of lung cancer.

Sanderson, D. R.: Bronchoscopy. Br. Med. Bull., *42*:244, 1986.

This article presents a comprehensive overview of the approach made by the Mayo Clinic to both diagnostic and therapeutic bronchoscopy.

Shure, D.: Fiberoptic bronchoscopy—Diagnostic applications. Clin. Chest Med., *8*:1, 1987.

The diagnostic applications of fiberoptic bronchoscopy are discussed in detail in this review article. The various techniques that are applicable to the fiberoptic bronchoscope and their rationales are presented.

BIBLIOGRAPHY

Albelda, S. M., Talbot, G. H., Gerson, S. L., et al.: Role of fiberoptic bronchoscopy in the diagnosis of invasive pulmonary aspergillosis in patients with leukemia. Am. J. Med., *76*:1027, 1984.

Albertini, R. E., Harrell, J. H., Kurihara, N., et al.: Arterial hypoxemia induced by fiberoptic bronchoscopy. J. A. M. A., *230*:1666, 1974.

Allison, P. R., and Johnstone, A. S.: The oesophagus lined with gastric mucosa membrane. Thorax, 8:87, 1953.

Anderson, H. A., and Higgins, J. A.: Current status of esophagoscopy. Otolaryngol. Clin. North Am., *111*:391, 1978.

Angorn, I. B., and Haffejee, A. A.: Endoesophageal intubation for palliation in obstructing esophageal carcinoma. *In* Delarue, N. C., Wilkins, E. W., Jr., and Wong, J. (eds): International Trends in General Thoracic Surgery: Esophageal Cancer. Vol. 4, Chap. 51 St. Louis, C. V. Mosby, 1988.

Arroliga, A. C., and Matthay, R. A.: The role of bronchoscopy in lung cancer. Clin. Chest Med., *14*:87, 1993.

Barrett, N. R.: Chronic peptic ulcer of the oesophagus and oesophagitis. Br. J. Surg., *38*:175, 1950.

Belen, J., Neuhaus, A., Markowitz, D., et al.: Modification of the effect of fiberoptic bronchoscopy on pulmonary mechanics. Chest, *79*:516, 1981.

Berci, G.: Chevalier Jackson Lecture: Analysis of new optical systems in bronchoesophagology. Ann. Otol. Rhinol. Laryngol., *87*:451, 1978.

Bonfils-Roberts, E. A., and Nealon, T. F., Jr.: Balloon catheter for

endoscopic removal of foreign bodies. Ann. Thorac. Surg., *19*:196, 1975.

Bordelon, J. Y., Jr., Legrand, P., Gewin, W. C., and Sanders, C. V.: The telescoping plugged catheter in suspected anaerobic infections: A controlled series. Am. Rev. Respir. Dis., *128*:465, 1983.

Broaddus, C., Dake, M. D., Stulbarg, M. S., et al.: Bronchoalveolar lavage and transbronchial biopsy for the diagnosis of pulmonary infections in the acquired immunodeficiency syndrome. Ann. Intern. Med., *102*:747, 1985.

Burns, D. M., Shure, D., Francoz, R., et al.: The physiologic consequences of saline lobar lavage in healthy human adults. Am. Rev. Respir. Dis., *127*:696, 1983.

Bye, P. T. P., Harvey, H. P. B., Woolcock, A. J., et al.: Fiberoptic bronchoscopy in small cell lung cancer: Findings pre and post chemotherapy. Aust. N. Z. J. Med., *10*:397, 1980.

Caletti, G. C., Bolondi, L., Zani, L., et al.: Detection of portal hypertension and esophageal varices by means of endoscopic ultrasonography. Scand. J. Gastroenterol., *21*(Suppl. 123):74, 1986.

Carden, E.: Recent improvements in techniques in general anesthesia for bronchoscopy. Chest, *73*(Suppl.):697, 1978.

Carter, R., and Hinshaw, D. B.: Use of the esophagoscope in the diagnosis of rupture of the esophagus. Surg. Gynecol. Obstet., *120*:1304, 1965.

Cavaliere, S., Foccoli, P., and Farina, P. L.: Nd:YAG laser bronchoscopy: A five-year experience with 1396 applications in 1000 patients. Chest, *94*:15, 1988.

Chastre, J., Viau, F., Brun, P., et al.: Prospective evaluation of the protected specimen brush for the diagnosis of pulmonary infections in ventilated patients. Am. Rev. Respir. Dis., *130*:924, 1984.

Classen, M., and Phillip, J.: Electronic endoscopy of the gastrointestinal tract: Initial experience with a new type of endoscope that has no fiberoptic bundle for imaging. Endoscopy, *16*:16, 1984.

Cortese, D. A., and McDougall, J. C.: Biopsy and brushing of peripheral lung cancer with fluoroscopic guidance. Chest, *75*:141, 1979.

Cortese, D. A., and McDougall, J. C.: Bronchoscopic biopsy and brushing with fluoroscopic guidance in nodular metastatic lung cancer. Chest, *79*:610, 1981.

Cox, J. C., Winter, R. K., Jones, R., et al.: Balloons against bougies for dilatation of benign oesophageal stricture—A randomised prospective trial. Gut, *26*:A1136, 1985.

Credle, W. F., Smiddy, J. F., and Elliott, R. C.: Complications of fiberoptic bronchoscopy. Am. Rev. Respir. Dis., *109*:67, 1974.

Cunanan, O. S.: The flexible fiberoptic bronchoscope in foreign body removal. Chest, *73*:725, 1978.

Daly, J. F.: Corrosive esophagitis. Otolaryngol. Clin. North Am., *1*:119, 1968.

Daly, J. F.: Endoscopic aspects of primary tuberculosis in children. Ann. Otol. Rhinol. Laryngol., *67*:1089, 1958.

Danek, S. J., and Bower, J. S.: Diagnosis of pulmonary tuberculosis by flexible fiberoptic bronchoscopy. Am. Rev. Respir. Dis., *119*:677, 1979.

Daniele, R. P., Elias, J. A., Epstein, P. E., et al.: Bronchoalveolar lavage: Role in the pathogenesis, diagnosis and management of interstitial lung disease. Ann. Intern. Med., *102*:93, 1985.

Dougherty, T. J.: Photodynamic therapy (PDT) of malignant tumors. Crit. Rev. Oncol. Hematol., *2*:83, 1984.

Dumon, J. F., Castro, R., Merrick, B., et al.: Experience of 1100 esophageal dilatations. *In* Book of Abstracts. 4th ed. Symposium Internationale D'endoscopie Digestive, Paris, May 1984.

Earlam, R., and Cunha-Melo, J. R.: Benign esophageal strictures: Historical and technical aspects of dilatation. Br. J. Surg., *68*:829, 1981.

Fletcher, E. C., and Levin, D. C.: Flexible fiberoptic bronchoscopy and fluoroscopically guided transbronchial biopsy in the management of solitary pulmonary nodules. West J. Med., *138*:364, 1983.

Funahashi, A., Browne, T. K., Houser, W. C., et al.: Diagnostic value of bronchial aspirate and post bronchoscopic sputum in fiberoptic bronchoscopy. Chest, *76*:514, 1979.

Geenen, J. E.: New diagnostic and treatment modalities involving endoscopic retrograde cholangiopancreatography and esophagogastroduodenoscopy. Scand. J. Gastroenterol., 77(Suppl.):94, 1982.

Gilman, M. J., and Wang, K. P.: Transbronchial lung biopsy in sarcoidosis: An approach to determine the optimal number of biopsies. Am. Rev. Respir. Dis., 122:721, 1980.

Halter, F., Witzel, L., Grétillat, P. A., et al.: Diagnostic value of biopsy-guided lavage and brush cytology in esophagogastroscopy. Am. J. Dig. Dis., 22:129, 1977.

Hanson, R. R., Zavala, D. C., Rhodes, M. L., et al.: Transbronchial biopsy via flexible fiberoptic bronchoscope: Results in 164 patients. Am. Rev. Respir. Dis., 114:67, 1976.

Hayata, Y., Kato, H., Okitsu, H., et al.: Photodynamic therapy with hematoporphyrin derivative in cancer of the upper gastrointestinal tract. Semin. Surg. Oncol., 1:1, 1985.

Hirschowitz, B. I., Curtiss, L. E., Peters, C. W., and Pollard, H. M.: Demonstration of a new gastroscope, the fiberscope. Gastroenterology, 35:50, 1958.

Holinger, P. H.: Use of the open-tube bronchoscope in the extraction of foreign bodies. Chest, 73:721, 1978.

Hopkins, H. H.: Optical principles of the endoscope. In Berci, G. (ed): Endoscopy. New York, Appleton-Century-Crofts, 1976, pp. 3, 26.

Ihde, D. C., Cohen, M. H., Bernath, A. M., et al.: Serial fiberoptic bronchoscopy during chemotherapy for small cell carcinoma of the lung: Early detection of patients at high risk of relapse. Chest, 74:531, 1978.

Ikeda, A.: Flexible bronchofiberscope. Ann. Otol. Rhinol. Laryngol., 79:916, 1970.

Jackson, C., and Jackson, C. L.: Bronchoesophagology. Philadelphia, W. B. Saunders, 1950.

Jaffe, J. P., and Maki, D. G.: Lung biopsy in immunocompromised patients: One institution's experience and an approach to management of pulmonary disease in the compromised host. Cancer, 48:1144, 1981.

Jensen, A. M., Silpe, M. L., Jorge, T. I., et al.: Comparison of different methods of endoscopic hemostasis of bleeding canine esophageal varices. Gastroenterology, 84:1455, 1983.

Joffe, S. N.: Nonoperative management of variceal bleeding. Br. J. Surg., 71:85, 1984.

Joshi, J. H., Wang, K. P., de Jongh, C. A., et al.: A comparative evaluation of two fiberoptic bronchoscopy catheters: The plugged telescoping catheter versus the single-sheathed nonplugged catheter. Am. Rev. Respir. Dis., 126:860, 1982.

Karetzky, M. D., Garvey, J. W., and Brandstetter, R. D.: Effect of fiberoptic bronchoscopy on arterial oxygen tension. N. Y. State J. Med., 74:62, 1974.

Karlin, D. A., Fisher, R. S., and Krevsky, B.: Prolonged survival and effective palliation in patients with squamous cell carcinoma of the esophagus following endoscopic laser therapy. Cancer, 5:1969, 1987.

Kessel, D.: Hematoporphyrin and HPD: Photophysics, photochemistry and phototherapy. Photochem. Photobiol., 39:851, 1984.

Killian, D. A.: Endoscopic catheterization of H-type tracheoesophageal fistula. Surgery, 55:317, 1964.

Koerner, S. K., Sakowitz, A. J., Appelman, R. I., et al.: Transbronchial lung biopsy for the diagnosis of sarcoidosis. N. Engl. J. Med., 293:268, 1975.

Kvale, P. A., Bode, F. R., and Kini, S.: Diagnostic accuracy in lung cancer: Comparison of techniques used in association with flexible fiberoptic bronchoscopy. Chest, 69:752, 1976.

Lakshminarayan, S., and Shrader, D. L.: The effect of fiberoptic bronchoscopy on cardiac rhythm. Chest, 73:821, 1978.

Luna, L. L.: Endoscopic treatment of esophageal strictures. Endoscopy, 15:203, 1983.

Marsh, B. R.: Advances in bronchoscopy. Otolaryngol. Clin. North Am., 11:371, 1978.

Marsh, B. R., Frost, J. K., Erozan, Y. S., and Carter, D.: Diagnosis of early bronchogenic carcinoma. Chest 73:716, 1978.

Martini, N., Kris, M. G., Flehinger, B. J., et al.: Preoperative chemotherapy for stage IIIa (N2) lung cancer: The Sloan-Kettering experience with 136 patients. Ann. Thorac. Surg., 55:1365, 1993.

McCabe, R. E., Brooks, R. G., and Mark, J. B. D.: Open lung biopsy in patients with acute leukemia. Am. J. Med., 78:609, 1985.

McCaughan, J. S., and Williams, T. E., Jr.: Palliation of esophageal malignancy with photodynamic therapy. In Delarue, N. C.,

Wilkins, E. W., Jr., and Wong, J. (eds): International Trends in General Thoracic Surgery: Esophageal Cancer. Vol. 4, Chap. 50. St. Louis, C. V. Mosby, 1988.

McElvein, R. B.: Laser therapy as palliation for advanced nonresectable carcinoma. In Delarue, N. C., Wilkins, E. W. Jr., and Wong, J. (eds): International Trends in General Thoracic Surgery: Esophageal Cancer. Vol. 4, Chap. 49. St. Louis, C. V. Mosby, 1988.

Monnier, P., Hsieh, V., and Savary, M.: Endoscopic treatment of esophageal stenosis using Savary-Gilliard bougies: Technical innovations. Acta Endoscopia, 15:119, 1985.

Monnier, P., and Savary, M.: New endoscopic techniques. In DeMeester, T. R., and Matthews, H. R. (eds): International Trends in General Thoracic Surgery: Benign Esophageal Diseases. Vol. 3., Chap. 5. St. Louis, C. V. Mosby, 1987.

Noirclerc, M. J., DiCostanzo, J., Sastre, B., et al.: Surgical management of caustic injuries to the upper gastrointestinal tract. In DeMeester, T. R., and Matthews, H. R. (eds): International Trends in General Thoracic Surgery: Benign Esophageal Diseases. Vol. 3, Chap. 18. St. Louis, C. V. Mosby, 1987.

Ognibene, F. P., Shelhamer, J., Gill, V., et al.: The diagnosis of Pneumocystis carinii pneumonia in patients with the acquired immunodeficiency syndrome using subsegmental bronchoalveolar lavage. Am. Rev. Respir. Dis., 129:929, 1984.

Overholt, B. F.: Laser treatment of esophageal cancer. Am. J. Gastroenterol., 80:719, 1985.

Pagliero, K. M., and Rowland, C. G.: Brachytherapy for inoperable cancer of the esophagus and cardia. In Delarue, N. C., Wilkins, E. W., Jr., and Wong, J. (eds): International Trends in General Thoracic Surgery: Esophageal Cancer. Vol. 4, Chap. 45. St. Louis, C.V. Mosby, 1988.

Palmer, E. D., and Wirts, C. W.: Survey of gastroscopic and esophagoscopic accidents. J. A. M. A., 164:2012, 1957.

Pauli, G., Pelletier, A., Bohner, C., et al.: Transbronchial needle aspiration in the diagnosis of sarcoidosis. Chest, 85:482, 1984.

Popovich, J., Jr., Kvale, P. A., Eichenhorn, M. S., et al.: Diagnostic accuracy of multiple biopsies from flexible fiberoptic bronchoscopy: A comparison of central versus peripheral carcinoma. Am. Rev. Respir. Dis., 125:521, 1982.

Radke, J. R., Conway, W. A., Eyler, W. R., and Kvale, P. A.: Diagnostic accuracy in peripheral lung lesions: Factors predicting success with flexible fiberoptic bronchoscopy. Chest, 76:176, 1979.

Reynolds, H. Y.: Bronchoalveolar lavage: State of art. Am. Rev. Respir. Dis., 135:250, 1987.

Richardson, R. H., Zavala, D. C., Mukerjee, P. K., et al.: The use of fiberoptic bronchoscopy and brush biopsy in the diagnosis of suspected pulmonary malignancy. Am. Rev. Respir. Dis., 109:63, 1974.

Robbins, H. M., Morrison, D. A., Sweet, M. E., et al.: Biopsy of the main carina—Staging lung cancer using the fiberoptic bronchoscope. Chest, 75:484, 1979.

Saeed, Z. A., Michaletz, P. A., Winchester, C. B., et al.: Endoscopic variceal ligation in patients who have failed endoscopic sclerotherapy. Gastrointest. Endosc., 36:572, 1990.

Salazar, A.M. and Westcott, J. L.: The role of transthoracic needle biopsy for the diagnosis and staging of lung cancer. Clin. Chest Med., 14:99, 1993.

Salzer, H.: Early treatment of corrosive esophagitis. Wien. Klin. Wochenschr., 33:307, 1920.

Sanders, R. A.: Two ventilating attachments for bronchoscopy. Del. Med. J., 39:170, 1967.

Sanderson, D. R.: Bronchoscopy. Br. Med. Bull., 42:244, 1986.

Sanderson, D. R., Neel, H. B., III, and Fontana, R. S.: Bronchoscopic cryotherapy. Ann. Otol. Rhinol. Laryngol., 90:354, 1981.

Sarkar, S. K., Sharma, G. S., and Gupta, P. R.: Fiberoptic bronchoscopy in the diagnosis of pulmonary tuberculosis. Tubercle, 61:97, 1980.

Savary, M. and Miller, G.: The Esophagus. Handbook and Atlas of Endoscopy. Solothurn, Switzerland: Gassman, 1978.

Saw, H. S., Ganendran, A., and Somasundaram, K.: Fogarty catheter extraction of foreign bodies from tracheobronchial trees of small children. J. Thorac. Cardiovasc. Surg., 77:240, 1979.

Schenk, D. A., Bower, J. H., Bryan, C. L., et al.: Transbronchial needle aspiration staging of bronchogenic carcinoma. Am. Rev. Respir. Dis., 134:146, 1986.

Schwartz, D. B., Beals, T. F., Wimbish, K. J., et al.: Transbronchial fine needle aspiration of bronchogenic cysts. Chest, 88:573, 1985.

Shure, D.: Fiberoptic bronchoscopy—Diagnostic applications. Clin. Chest Med., 8:1, 1987.

Shure, D., and Astarita, R. W.: Bronchogenic carcinoma presenting as an endobronchial mass: Optimal number of biopsy specimens for diagnosis. Chest, 83:865, 1983.

Shure, D., and Fedullo, P. F.: The role of transcarinal needle aspiration in the staging of bronchogenic carcinoma. Chest, 86:693, 1984.

Shure, D., and Fedullo, P. F.: Transbronchial needle aspiration in the diagnosis of submucosal and peribronchial bronchogenic carcinoma. Chest, 88:49, 1985.

Shure, D., and Fedullo, P. F.: Transbronchial needle aspiration of peripheral masses. Am. Rev. Respir. Dis., 128:1090, 1983.

Shure, D., Fedullo, P. F., and Plummer, M.: Carinal forceps biopsy via the fiberoptic bronchoscope in the routine staging of lung cancer. West. J. Med., 142:511, 1985.

Simpson, F. G., Arnold, A. G., Purvis, A., et al.: Postal survey of bronchoscopic practice by physicians in the United Kingdom. Thorax, 41:311, 1986.

Smiddy, J. F., and Elliott, R. C.: The evaluation of hemoptysis with fiberoptic bronchoscopy. Chest, 64:158, 1973.

Smith, P. M.: Therapeutic endoscopy of the upper gastrointestinal tract. Br. Med. Bull., 42:249, 1986.

Snider, G. L.: When not to use the bronchoscope for hemoptysis. Chest, 76:1, 1979.

So, S. Y., Lam, W. K., and Yu, D. Y.: Rapid diagnosis of suspected pulmonary tuberculosis by fiberoptic bronchoscopy. Tubercle, 63:195, 1982.

Stover, D. E., Zaman, M. B., Hajdu, S. I., et al.: Bronchoalveolar lavage in the diagnosis of diffuse pulmonary infiltrates in the immunosuppressed host. Ann. Intern. Med., 101:1, 1984.

Streitz, J. M., Andrews, C. W., Jr., Ellis, F. H., Jr.: Endoscopic surveillance of Barrett's esophagus. Does it help? J. Thorac. Cardiovasc. Surg., 105:383, 1993.

Strohm, W. D., and Classen, M.: Benign lesions of the upper GI tract by means of endoscopic ultrasonography. Scand. J. Gastroenterol., 21(Suppl. 123):41, 1986.

Suratt, P. M., Gruber, B., Wellons, H. A., et al.: Absence of clinical pneumonia following bronchoscopy with contaminated and clean bronchofiberscopes. Chest, 71:52, 1977.

Suratt, P. M., Smiddy, J. F., and Gruber, B.: Deaths and complications associated with fiberoptic bronchoscopy. Chest, 69:747, 1976.

Teirstein, A. S., Chuang, M. T., Choy, A. R., et al.: Flexible bronchoscopy in nonvisualized carcinoma of the lung. Ann. Otol., Rhinol. Laryngol., 87:318, 1978.

Tilles, D. S., Goldenheim, P. D., Ginns, L. C., et al.: Pulmonary function in normal subjects and patients with sarcoidosis after bronchoalveolar lavage. Chest, 89:244, 1986.

Tio, T. L., Den Hartog Jager, F. C. A., and Tytgat, G. N. J.: The role of endoscopic ultrasonography in assessing local resectability of oesophagogastric malignancies. Scand. J. Gastroenterol., 21:78, 1986.

Tio, T.L. and Tytgat, G. N. J.: Atlas of Transintestinal Ultrasonography. Aalsmeer, The Netherlands, Smith Kline and French, Drukkerij Mur-Kostverloren B. V., 1986.

Tio, T. L., and Tytgat, G. N. J.: Endoscopic ultrasonography in the assessment intra- and transmural infiltration of tumours in the oesophagus, stomach and papilla of Vater and in the detection of extra-oesophageal lesions. Endoscopy, 16:203, 1984.

Toledo-Pereya, L. H., DeMeester, T. R., Kinealey, A. L., et al.: The benefits of open lung biopsy in patients with previously nondiagnostic transbronchial lung biopsy. Chest, 77:647, 1980.

Tsuboi, E., Ikeda, S., Tajima, M., et al.: Transbronchial smear for diagnosis of peripheral pulmonary carcinomas. Cancer, 20:687, 1967.

Tulman, A. B., and Boyce, H. E.: Complications of esophageal dilatation and guidelines for their prevention. Gastrointest. Endosc., 27:229, 1981.

Turner-Warwick, M., and Haslam, P. L.: Clinical applications of bronchoalveolar lavage. Clin. Chest Med., 8:15, 1987.

Uddenfeldt, M., and Lundgren, R.: Flexible fiberoptic bronchoscopy in the diagnosis of pulmonary tuberculosis. Tubercle, 62:197, 1981.

Versteegh, R. M., and Swierenga, J.: Bronchoscopic evaluation of the operability of pulmonary carcinoma. Acta Otolaryngol., 56:603, 1963.

Wallace, J. M., Cantanzaro, A., Moser, K. M., et al.: Flexible fiberoptic bronchoscopy for diagnosing pulmonary coccidioidomycosis. Am. Rev. Respir. Dis., 123:286, 1981.

Wallace, J. M., and Deutsch, A. L.: Flexible fiberoptic bronchoscopy and percutaneous needle lung aspiration for evaluating the solitary pulmonary nodule. Chest, 81:665, 1982.

Wang, K. P., and Britt, E. J.: Needle brush in the diagnosis of lung mass or nodule through flexible bronchoscope. Chest, 100:1148, 1991.

Wang, K. P., Haponik, E. F., Britt, E. J., et al.: Transbronchial needle aspiration of peripheral pulmonary nodules. Chest, 86:819, 1984a.

Wang, K. P., Haponik, E. F., Gupta, P. K., et al.: Flexible transbronchial needle aspiration: Technical considerations. Ann. Otol. Rhinol. Laryngol., 93:233, 1984b.

Weaver, L. J., Solliday, N., and Cugell, D. W.: Selection of patients with hemoptysis for fiberoptic bronchoscopy. Chest, 76:7, 1979.

Wood, R. E., and Fink, R. J.: Applications of flexible fiberoptic bronchoscopes in infants and children. Chest, 73:737, 1978.

Woolner, L. B., Fontana, R. S., Cortese, D. A., et al.: Roentgenographically occult lung cancer: Pathologic findings and frequency of multicentricity during a 10-year period. Mayo Clin. Proc., 59:453, 1984.

Yasuda, K., Nakajima, M., and Kawai, K.: Endoscopic ultrasonography in the diagnosis of submucosal tumor of the upper digestive tract. Scand. J. Gastroenterol., 21(Suppl. 123): 59, 1986.

Zavala, D. C.: Diagnostic fiberoptic bronchoscopy: Techniques and results of biopsy in 600 patients. Chest, 68:12, 1975.

Zavala, D. C.: Flexible Fiberoptic Bronchoscopy: A Training Handbook. Iowa City, University of Iowa Press, 1978a.

Zavala, D. C.: Transbronchial biopsy in diffuse lung disease. Chest, 73(Suppl.):727, 1978b.

Zavala, D. C., Richardson, R. H., Mukerjee, P. K., et al.: Use of the bronchofiberscope for bronchial brush biopsy: Diagnostic results and comparison with other brushing techniques. Chest, 63:889, 1973.

4 Use of Antibiotics in Cardiac and Thoracic Surgery

Allen B. Kaiser

Infection has long been the bane of the surgeon's trade. Before the antiseptic and antibiotic revolution, surgeons, despite their skill, were accustomed to seeing gains made at the time of operation lost with the onset of pyogenic infection within the surgical wound. Infection was so common through the end of the 19th century that surgeons were trained to expect, and even hope for, the development of "laudable pus" during the early postoperative period. However, the modern era of surgery began with the advent of Joseph Lister's *antiseptic surgery* in 1867, which caused a dramatic reduction in the incidence of devastating infection (Kaiser, 1991). Major surgical procedures could now be devised. The antibiotic revolution of the 1930s and 1940s further established the concept that infection-free surgical procedures were not only possible but also expected. The use of perioperative antisepsis and antibiotics and the availability of potent antibiotics to treat postoperative infections when they did occur created an environment in which complicated major procedures involving tissue trauma and implantable devices could be contemplated. The greatest effect of the "antibiotic revolution," in fact, may lie in its influence on the evolution of modern surgical procedures (McDermott and Rogers, 1982). It would be difficult to imagine cardiac and thoracic surgery as we know it today in an environment in which infection was common or untreatable. The next major breakthrough in this surgical subspecialty (e.g., transplantation surgery or implantation of the artificial heart) will probably await further advances in the prevention and management of infectious complications (Rice and Karchmer, 1988). Antisepsis and antibiotics have been the foundation of the development of modern cardiac and thoracic surgery.

HISTORICAL BACKGROUND

The chronology of the American surgeon's approach to the use of antimicrobials must be viewed from two perspectives: *therapy* and *prophylaxis*. The history of the use of antimicrobials for the *therapy* of established infection has been characterized by steady, data-driven advancements. Meleney's (1956) approach to the management of wound infections in the early antibiotic era is a paradigm of clinical medicine. Armed with only a handful of antimicrobials for systemic use (penicillin, streptomycin, bacitracin,

polymyxin, chloramphenicol, and tetracycline), Meleney outlined the appropriate use of Gram's stain and culture combined with an estimate of the depth of infection and the extent of the inflammatory process in designing the antimicrobial regimen. Whereas new antimicrobials and new diagnostic procedures have become available, the concept of correlating clinical observations with laboratory data to determine the most appropriate antimicrobial regimen to use in treating established infection has remained unimproved since its inception.

In contrast, the history of the use of antimicrobial for the *prophylaxis* of infection has been, at best, uneven. Early proponents of prophylactic antibiotics cited anecdotal benefits of perioperative prophylaxis. Perhaps influenced by Lister's early recommendations for aseptic surgery, which included spraying carbolic acid in and around the operative site, enthusiasts used available antibiotics in an excessive assortment of combinations and durations. In response, widespread opposition to the use of prophylactic antimicrobials in surgical procedures became firmly established during the early 1960s. Opponents noted both the lack of controlled studies supporting the efficacy of prophylactic antibiotics and the potential for the selection of antimicrobial-resistant pathogens. In fact, the first prospective, randomized, placebo-controlled study of prophylactic antibiotics, by Sanchez-Ubeda and colleagues (1958), showed no benefit of the prophylactic antibiotics. Moreover, these authors voiced concern over the in-hospital use of antibiotics for unproven indications, recalling the previously noted association of the widespread use of penicillin for therapeutic purposes and the dramatic rise in the incidence of nosocomial infection due to penicillin-resistant *Staphylococcus aureus*. The resolution of the controversy awaited a systematic and scholarly evaluation of the pathophysiology of surgical wound infection and its prevention.

BASIC CONCEPTS OF ANTIMICROBIAL PROPHYLAXIS

Between 1961 and 1963, two critical findings were identified and reported. First, investigators noted that, despite the most careful adherence to the principles of aseptic technique, pathogenic bacteria could almost always be isolated from the operative field during the procedure. The second critical finding demonstrated the importance of the timing of antibiotic administration relative to the contamination of the surgical wound.

Bacterial Contamination of the Surgical Field

By 1960, most authorities had conceded that prophylactic antibiotics had a role in surgical procedures involving contaminated and infected surgical fields, but the use of aseptic technique in clean surgical environments was thought to preclude the need for any additional prophylactic measures. However, between 1961 and 1963, three prospective, carefully conducted studies of bacterial contamination of clean surgical incisions performed in Cincinnati and Boston were published, clearly demonstrating that microbial contamination of the clean surgical incision was inevitable (Burke, 1963; Culbertson et al., 1961; Howe and Marston, 1962). The concept that aseptic techniques would guarantee a bacteria-free surgical incision was now understood to be incorrect. The benefits of aseptic operations were related to a reduction, not an elimination, of bacterial contamination of the wound. More recent careful studies by Whyte and co-workers (1982) and Whyte and associates (1991) have confirmed the universality of wound contamination, even under laminar flow conditions (Table 4–1). Therefore, the potential exists for prophylactic antibiotics to influence the outcome of clean operative procedures.

The sources of the pathogens, usually *S. aureus*, were never conclusively delineated by these early investigations. Today, however, with the availability of sophisticated epidemiologic investigational techniques such as plasmid fingerprinting, restriction-endonuclease-digestion analysis, ribotyping, and high-performance liquid chromatography, infecting pathogens have been traced with remarkable precision. The hands of an operative surgeon (Boyce et al., 1990), the skin and nares of a circulating nurse (Richet et al., 1991), and the tap water from the sink in the cardiac surgery recovery room (Lowry et al., 1991) have all been identified as the source or route of contamination. As experience is gained with these

tools, more insight into the epidemiology of surgical wound infection can be expected.

For *prosthetic valve endocarditis* (PVE), the time when bacteria are most likely to seed the newly implanted valve remains unknown, but the intraoperative, early postoperative, and late postoperative periods have all been implicated. All intravascular devices are vulnerable to seeding at any time after they have been inserted within the host. The demonstrated differences in the spectrum of pathogens between early and late PVE support the concept that different routes of infection exist, but the relative importance of the various routes of contamination has not been identified.

Similarly, for modern sternotomy incisions, opinions differ as to the importance of the various routes of contamination and subsequent infection. The weight of evidence suggests that bacterial seeding of the sternal incision is most likely to occur in the intraoperative period. As noted by earlier studies, careful preparation of the skin of patients and personnel prior to operation can at best eliminate only the superficial colonizing staphylococcal flora. Although face masks markedly decrease the chance for dissemination of upper respiratory pathogens, their use does not eliminate this possibility. The potential for intraoperative seeding of the incision is considerable, and the risk of contamination probably increases with the length of the procedure. Outbreaks of infection that have been traced to breaks in intraoperative aseptic technique reinforce the concept that modern asepsis can decrease, but never eliminate, bacterial contamination of the operative field.

The primarily closed median sternotomy incision may also be vulnerable to contamination and subsequent infection during the postoperative period. Stoney and colleagues (1978) noted a high incidence of infections of the median sternotomy associated with inadequate sternal stabilization, and speculated that an unstable sternum might behave like a bellows and suck contaminating bacteria into the incision during the postoperative period. This author has treated an unreported case of a deep pneumococcal abscess of the sternum occurring 3 months after uncomplicated coronary artery bypass surgery, which strongly suggests that late postoperative seeding of the sternal wound had occurred. More recently, Lowry and co-workers (1991) traced a cluster of postoperative sternal wound infections to the use of contaminated tap water for bathing postoperative patients in the cardiac surgery recovery room. Whatever the relative importance of the various routes of contamination, optimal management of the patient during the perioperative period awaits the results of carefully managed prospective studies and a better understanding of the pathophysiology of infection.

■ **Table 4–1.** MEDIAN BACTERIAL COUNTS DURING SURGERY

Patient's skin at incision*	980/100 cm²
Viseral surface at close*	15/100 cm² [360 cm²]
Wound wall at close*	60/100 cm² [240 cm²]
Conventional air†	413/m³ (105)
Laminar air†	4/m³ (3)

*Cholecystectomy procedures with sterile bile; brackets indicate estimated total surface area. Data from Whyte, W., Hambraeus, A., Laurell, G., and Hoborn, J.: The relative importance of routes and sources of wound contamination during general surgery. I. Non-airborne. J. Hosp. Infect., 18:93, 1991.
†Hip and knee replacement procedures; parentheses represent numbers of bacteria recovered from wound washouts. Data from Whyte W., Hodgson, R., and Tinkler, J.: The importance of airborne bacterial contamination of wounds. J. Hosp. Infect., 3:123, 1982.

Timing of Antibiotic Prophylaxis

The second critical finding in understanding the basic tenets of antimicrobial prophylaxis of surgical wound infection is related to the *timing of administration of the prophylactic antibiotic*. In 1946, Howes, working with a rabbit model of wound infection, noted a correlation between the amelioration of infection and the interval between the contamination of the wounds and the administration of antibiotics. In the early 1960s, Burke refined the concept in a guinea pig model of wound infection (Burke, 1961). He demonstrated that once tissues have been exposed to bacterial pathogens, a relatively narrow period of time is available for effective antibiotic prophylaxis. Specifically, antibiotics given slightly before or at the time of bacterial inoculation of an intradermal lesion with *S. aureus* significantly limited the size of the subsequent area of induration. In contrast, delaying the administration of the antibiotics by only 3 or 4 hours after bacterial inoculation virtually eliminated any benefits of prophylaxis. This finding helped explain why early clinical trials, such as Sanchez-Ubeda and colleagues' (1958) study of postoperative prophylaxis in general and orthopedic surgery, detected no benefit of prophylaxis. The crucial importance of the timing of the administration of prophylactic antibiotics has been noted recently by other investigators using different animal models, pathogens, and antibiotics. These studies led to the conclusion that antimicrobial prophylaxis can be effective in a wide variety of surgical procedures, but only if the antibiotics are in the tissues at the time of bacterial contamination.

The demonstration of an association between the timing of administration of prophylactic antibiotics and the magnitude of the subsequent wound infection implied that the delay of antibiotic administration allows the contaminating bacteria a 4- to 6-hour "head start" in establishing a wound infection. This information suggested that there are substantive differences in *bacterial contamination* of a wound versus *bacterial infection* of a wound, introducing, in effect, the concept of an *incubation period* between the contamination and the infection of a surgical wound.

Extensive research into the pathophysiology of other infectious processes (e.g., bacterial endocarditis, meningitis, gastroenteritis) suggests that the process of surgical wound infection also progresses through orderly stages of pathogen-host interactions (Table 4–2). The elucidation of this complex process could have profound implications for antibiotic prophylaxis of surgical wound infection. For example, attachment

of the bacteria to host tissues has been shown to be either enhanced or inhibited by subinhibitory concentrations of certain antibiotics (Alkan and Beachey, 1978; Beachey et al., 1982). Exposure of bacteria to antibiotics early in the infecting process has also been shown to enhance both phagocytosis of certain bacteria and intracellular killing of bacteria (Root et al., 1981). Chuard and associates (1993) focused attention on the importance of the rate of bacterial growth and the susceptibility of bacteria to antimicrobials. Through elegant studies designed primarily to explore the importance of the attachment of bacteria to surface structures (e.g., fibronectin), they demonstrated that once *S. aureus* have entered a static growth phase (achieved after 2 hours of growth), they are virtually unaffected by brief (i.e., <2 hour) exposure to a variety of antibiotics (Table 4–3). If these data are applied to the concept of antimicrobial prophylaxis of surgical wound infection, the "static phase" of bacterial growth is likely to represent the condition of potential pathogens 2 to 3 hours after implantation in an operative or traumatic wound. It would not be surprising, therefore, to find that antibiotics administered several hours after the contamination of the wound would have little to no effect. Whatever the essential features of the incubation period of bacterial infection of surgical wounds, future refinement in the use of prophylactic antibiotics in surgical procedures awaits the results of scholarly investigation of the pathophysiology of surgical wound infection.

CONTEMPORARY PROPHYLAXIS IN CARDIAC AND THORACIC SURGERY

Among clean operative procedures, none have been so actively evaluated for efficacy of antibiotic prophylaxis as the procedures associated with cardiac and thoracic surgery. Beginning with a placebo-controlled study of antibiotic prophylaxis in 71 patients undergoing valve replacement surgery in 1968, through studies of antimicrobial prophylaxis of median sternotomy infections involving more than 500 patients per study, the merits and limitations of prophylactic antibiotics have been addressed in more than 30 prospective studies. Numerous additional studies of infection risk factors and antimicrobial pharmacokinetics have been published. Although faults with the design or execution can be found in almost all of these clinical trials, important principles for the use of prophylaxis in cardiac and thoracic surgery have emerged.

Role of Antibiotics in Cardiac and Thoracic Surgery

The fulminant course of pneumococcal prosthetic valve endocarditis among placebo recipients in a prospective study of antimicrobial prophylaxis precluded any additional evaluation of placebo prophylaxis when prosthetic valves are at risk for infection (Good-

■ **Table 4–2.** THE INCUBATION PERIOD* OF BACTERIAL INFECTION OF SURGICAL WOUNDS

Attachment (mediated by nonspecific adherence of bacteria or by specific adherence of bacteria to receptors on host tissues)
Penetration (possibly mediated by microbial enzymes that disrupt connective enzymes)
Evasion of host defenses
  Avoidance or inactivation of phagocytic cells
  Avoidance of humoral immunity (antibody, complement)
  Avoidance of cell-mediated immunity
Tissue localization and multiplication
Toxin production

*Internal, between colonization and established infection.

■ **Table 4–3.** REDUCTION IN LOG COUNTS AT FOUR TIMES MINIMAL BACTERICIDAL CONCENTRATION OF FIBRONECTIN-ATTACHED *STAPHYLOCOCCUS AUREUS*

Phase	Oxacillin	Vancomycin	Fleroxacin	Gentamicin
Active growth [2 hr]	1.42 (2 hr)*	1.10 (2 hr)	2.53 (1 hr)	4.3 (½ hr)
Stationary phase [4 hr]	<0.5 (2 hr)	<0.5 (2 hr)	1.95 (1 hr)	1.06 (½ hr)
Active growth [2 hr]	>3.0 (24 hr)	>3.0 (24 hr)	>3.5 (24 hr)	>3.5 (24 hr)
Stationary phase [4 hr]	>3.0 (24 hr)	>3.0 (24 hr)	>3.5 (24 hr)	1.05 (24 hr)

Adapted from Chuard, C., Vaudaux, P., Waldvogel, F. A., and Lew, D.P.: Susceptibility of *Staphylococcus aureus* growing on fibronectin-coated surfaces to bactericidal antibiotics. Antimicrob. Agents Chemother., 37:625, 1993. Parallel fluid phase studies yielded similar results for all antibiotics except gentamicin.
*Parentheses indicate duration of organism exposure to antibiotic.

man et al., 1968) (Table 4–4*A*). Subsequently, in cardiac surgical procedures involving a median sternotomy incision but not valve replacement (e.g., coronary artery bypass surgery), placebo recipients have also had an unacceptable rate of postoperative infection. Two of the three placebo-controlled studies were modified early in the course of the evaluation because of an unacceptably high median sternotomy infection rate among the placebo recipients. The three placebo-controlled studies experienced a 21%, a 55%, and a 44% incidence of sternal wound infection in placebo recipients, respectively—an infection rate that would not be tolerated in cardiac surgery today (Table 4–4*B*). Accordingly, the use of prophylactic antibiotics should be considered a standard of care in any cardiothoracic procedure that involves a median sternotomy

■ **Table 4–4.** DEVELOPMENT OF PRINCIPLES OF ANTIMICROBIAL PROPHYLAXIS IN CARDIAC SURGERY

	Key Findings of Investigation	Implications
A	In prosthetic valve implantation, early onset (<5 days) of fulminant pneumococcal endocarditis among 2 of 15 placebo recipients led to the termination of the placebo arm of the study (Goodman et al., 1968)	*Role of antibiotics:* Because of the high morbidity and mortality of postoperative prosthetic valve endocarditis, no additional placebo-controlled trials of antibiotic prophylaxis in prosthetic valve implantation have been contemplated
B	A sternal wound infection rate of 21.3% was observed among patients randomized to receive placebo versus 0% for methicillin recipients ($p<.01$) (Fong et al., 1979)	*Role of antibiotics:* Antimicrobial prophylaxis is indicated in all patients undergoing a median sternotomy incision irrespective of valve replacement
	A sternal wound infection rate of 55% was observed among patients randomized to receive placebo versus 6.3% for cephradine recipients ($p<.002$) (Penketh et al., 1985), leading to termination of the study	
	Surgical wound infection occurred in 4 out of 9 placebo recipients versus 0 out of 6 cephalothin recipients, resulting in early termination of the placebo arm of the study ($p = .10$) (Austin et al., 1980)	
C	Wound infection developed in 3 of 11 patients with no cephalothin serum levels detectable at the close of surgery versus 2 of 175 patients with detectable levels ($p <.002$) (Goldmann et al., 1977)	*Pharmacokinetics:* Adequate antibiotic levels must be maintained throughout the bypass procedure
	Wound infections and sepsis were significantly more likely to occur in patients with low versus high antibiotic levels in atrial appendage tissue ($p<.05$) (Platt et al., 1984)	
D	Cephalothin was significantly more effective than methicillin in preventing sepsis and prosthetic valve endocarditis, 0 of 132 versus 11 of 129, respectively ($p<.001$) (Myerowitz et al., 1977)	*Differential efficacy:* Antibiotics may exhibit significant differences in efficacy as prophylactic agents in cardiac surgery. In general, cephalosporins are preferred to semisynthetic penicillins. Cephalosporins with low minimum inhibitory concentrations to staphylococci and high stability to staphylococcus beta-lactamase may provide improved prophylaxis. The differences in efficacy may be related in part to variations in pharmacokinetics, minimal inhibitory concentrations, and staphylococcal beta-lactamase stability
	Cefamandole was significantly more effective than cefazolin in preventing infection in both the sternal (1.8 versus 0.4%, respectively, $p < .05$) and donor site (1.3 versus 0%, respectively, $p < .02$) (Kaiser et al., 1987)	
	Cefamandole was significantly more effective than cefonicid in preventing chest wound and donor site infections and prosthetic valve endocarditis (2.2% vs. 6.3%, $p = 0.05$) (Gelfand et al., 1990)	
	Differences in deep sternal wound infection rates between cefamandole and cephalothin did not achieve significance (0% vs. 2.2%, respectively, $p=.06$) (Miedzinski et al., 1990)	
	Differences in infection rates of deep sternum or mediastinum between cefamandole and cefuroxime did not achieve significance (0.3% vs. 1.5%, respectively, $p = .06$) (Townsend et al., 1993)	

incision, regardless of whether cardiac valve reconstruction or replacement occurs during the procedure.

Pharmacokinetics of Perioperative Antibiotics

Investigators have also addressed the importance of providing adequate serum and tissue levels of antibiotics throughout the operative procedure (Table 4–4C). Goldmann and colleagues (1977) noted that wound infections were significantly increased in patients in whom serum levels were unmeasurable at the close of operation. Similarly, Platt and co-workers (1984) noted an increased incidence of wound infection and sepsis when atrial tissue levels of cephalothin were low. Because the low-to-absent antibiotic levels may be related to excessive durations of operative procedures, it is not possible in these studies to determine whether the increased infections were related primarily to the antibiotic levels or to other factors associated with prolonged surgical procedures. However, two large prospective studies of antimicrobial prophylaxis in cardiac surgery, each involving over 1000 patients, did not detect an association between the duration of the operation and the infection rate (Kaiser et al., 1987; Nagachinta et al., 1987). Given the current information, intraoperative redosing of prophylactic antibiotics should be routine and

based on the length of the surgical procedure and the pharmacokinetics of the antibiotics used in prophylaxis. It should also be remembered that the pharmacokinetics of antibiotics varies during the procedure, depending on whether the cardiopulmonary bypass pump is in use. In general, the half-life of the cephalosporins lengthens significantly during the period of cardiopulmonary bypass.

Differential Efficacy of Antibiotics Used in Prophylaxis

Cephalosporins alone have been compared in more than 20 prospective studies (Table 4–5). Nevertheless, a clear consensus regarding the most effective agent has not emerged. Cefazolin, for example, has been found to be superior, inferior, or equivalent in prophylactic efficacy to second-generation cephalosporins such as cefamandole and cefuroxime. Unfortunately, most studies have lacked adequate size to detect differences that may have existed. However, of prime importance is the fact that, with rare exceptions, these studies have failed to address adequately the important issue of pharmacokinetics and the duration of the surgical procedure. In only 5 studies are the pharmacokinetics of the comparative agents similar or have the study designs provided for redosing of antibiotics with relatively short half-lives dur-

■ **Table 4–5.** PROSPECTIVE COMPARATIVE STUDIES OF CEPHALOSPORIN PROPHYLAXIS OF WOUND INFECTIONS IN CARDIAC SURGERY

Date	First Author	Comparative Agents	Prophylaxis Efficacy*	No. of Patients	Intraoperative Redosing
1978	Archer	Cephalothin/cefamandole	(No infections)	30	No
1978	Kini	Cefazolin/cephalothin	Equivalent	99	No
1982	Parr	Cefamandole/cephalothin	Equivalent	178	No†
1983	Karney	Cephalothin/ceforanide	Equivalent	85	Yes
1983	Bryan	Cefamandole/cefazolin	(No infections)	34	No
1984	Beam	Ceftriaxone/cefazolin	Equivalent	104	Yes
1984	Platt	Ceforanide/cephalothin	Ceforanide > cephalothin	220	Yes‡
1985	Geroulanos	Cefuroxime/ceftriaxone	Equivalent	418	No
1986	Geroulanos	Cefuroxime/cefazolin	Equivalent	566	No
1986	Meszaros	Cefamandole /cephalothin	Equivalent	80	No
1986	Slama	Cefamandole/cefazolin/ cefuroxime	Cefuroxime/cefamandole > cefazolin	337	No
1987	Sexton	Cefuroxime/cefamandole	Equivalent	221	No
1988	Conklin	Cefuroxime/cefazolin	Equivalent	100	No
1987	Kaiser	Cefazolin/ cefamandole [Note: Gentamicin included in randomization]	Cefamandole > cefazolin	1030	Yes
1988	Gentry	Cefamandole/cefuroxime/cefazolin [Postoperative wound infections were not categorized; patients were not randomized]	Equivalent	620	No
1990	Doebbeling	Cefazolin/cefuroxime [Note ?Adequacy of cefuroxime redosing; 9% cefuroxime sternal wound infection rate]	Cefazolin > cefuroxime	213	No
1990	Gelfand	Cefamandole/cefonicid	Cefamandole > cefonicid	400	Yes
1990	Miedzinski	Cefamandole/cephalothin	Equivalent	448	No
1992	Maki	Cefazolin/cefamandole /vancomycin	Vancomycin > cefazolin	248	No
1993	Townsend	Cefamandole/cefazolin /cefuroxime	Equivalent	1641	Yes§

*p <.05
†Cephalosporins redosed at 6 hours
‡Protocol violations in 22% of patients
§Intraoperative redosing schedule did not predictably provide adequate levels for prolonged procedures.

ing prolonged procedures (Table 4–4D). Myerowitz and associates (1977) and Ghoneim and colleagues (1982) observed an impressive superiority of cephalosporins over semisynthetic penicillins. The increased efficacy of cephalothin noted by Myerowitz and associates may have been related to its broader spectrum of antimicrobial activity, particularly against non-staphylococcal pathogens. However, the significant advantage of cefamandole in Ghoneim and colleagues' study was apparently unrelated to its increased spectrum of antibiotic activity, as all cloxacillin failures were due to S. aureus. These data, in addition to the frequent history of penicillin allergy among hospitalized patients, have persuaded most cardiac surgeons to choose a cephalosporin for routine prophylaxis. However, conflicting results regarding the relative efficacy of cefazolin versus cefuroxime or cefamandole remain unresolved. The study by Kaiser and co-workers (1987) indicating a superiority of cefamandole is the largest prospective study to date in which multiple intraoperative doses of the cephalosporins were administered. Further investigations have suggested that the instability of cefazolin to staphylococcal beta-lactamase accounted for its inferior performance in this study (Kernodle and Kaiser, 1987). However, the study is complicated by the fact that, in addition to the randomization of cefamandole and cefazolin, patients were also randomized to receive or not receive gentamicin. Significant differences in infection rates were not observed when the gentamicin/nongentamicin groups were separated. Additional studies reveal that cefamandole's superiority over cefonicid, cephalothin, and cefuroxime is modest at best (see Table 4–4D), and a single additional infection in one arm or the other would strongly influence any conclusions regarding differences among these investigations. Given the fact that, with current preventative measures, wound infection rates following cardiac surgery are already extremely low, clinical trials with more than 1000 patients would be required to resolve these issues. Thus, although true differences in efficacy of cephalosporins may exist, they are certainly small and may be undetectable through the use of prospective clinical trials. Further advances in the understanding of prophylaxis in cardiac surgery will require a return to sophisticated in vitro and in vivo investigations.

GUIDELINES FOR ANTIMICROBIAL PROPHYLAXIS IN CARDIAC AND THORACIC SURGERY

Given the limitations of clinical studies and the paucity of in vivo studies of prophylactic efficacy, there are no "right" approaches to the choice, dose, and duration of antimicrobial prophylaxis in cardiac and thoracic surgery. Moreover, marked variations in the spectrum of infecting pathogens occur between institutions and within a given institution over time. Given these limitations, general guidelines to the pro-

phylaxis of infection in cardiac and thoracic surgery can be outlined (Table 4–6).

Median Sternotomy

The prophylactic regimen of choice for prevention of wound infection following elective median sternotomy remains controversial. Kreter and Woods (1992) performed a meta-analysis of 28 prospective comparative trials and determined that cefamandole and cefuroxime performed better than cefazolin. Nevertheless, as noted earlier, differences in efficacy are usually quite small. Accordingly, in hospital settings where risk factors are such that the deep sternal wound infection rate is less than 2% with an extant prophylactic regimen, it would be difficult to justify a change. Cefazolin is usually chosen in this setting because of its lower cost and longer half-life (see Table 4–6). Conversely, when deep sternal wound infection rates approach or exceed 2% and methicillin-sensitive S. aureus (MSSA) accounts for most of the infections, the weight of the literature would support changing to a second-generation cephalosporin for prophylaxis. In this regard, the trends of improved efficacy would support the use of cefamandole. Clearly, however, when methicillin-resistant S. aureus (MRSA) or methicillin-resistant coagulase-negative staphylococci (MRCNS) become important pathogens, vancomycin in addition to a cephalosporin regimen should be employed. Although the recommendation to continue to include a cephalosporin is largely theoretical, it is based on the demonstrated infection potential of gram-negative bacilli (Table 4–7) and the fact that cephalosporins offer a reasonable spectrum of activity against these pathogens.

Pacemaker Implantation

Infection rates following the insertion of permanent pacemakers have been uniformly low. Siddons and Nowak (1975) have argued against the routine use of prophylactic antibiotics, recommending that perioperative prophylactic antibiotics be reserved for high-risk patients (those with previous infections, operative contamination, or diabetes). However, prospective trials have indicated a benefit of prophylactic antibiotics (Muers et al., 1981). In general, if infection rates without the use of prophylaxis exceed 1% or 2%, consideration should be given to using routine antistaphylococcal prophylaxis (see Table 4–6).

Noncardiac Thoracic Surgery

For elective thoracic procedures not involving the heart, such as lobectomy and pneumonectomy, cephalothin has shown to be effective as a perioperative antibiotic (Ilves et al., 1981). Following penetrating thoracic trauma, patients randomized to receive antibiotics (specifically clindamycin, 300 mg every 6 hours for approximately 5 days) early in the course

■ **Table 4–6.** GUIDELINES FOR ANTIMICROBIAL PROPHYLAXIS IN CARDIAC AND THORACIC SURGERY

Surgical Procedure/Special Considerations	Prophylactic Regimen and Perioperative Considerations
Median sternotomy/deep sternal wound infection rate is low (i.e., <2%)	A. Cefazolin, 1 g IV initially, followed by 1 g IV q 6 hr intraoperatively, followed by 1 g IV q 6–8 hr postoperatively *or* B. Cefuroxime, 1.5 g IV initially, followed by 750 mg q 4 hr intraoperatively, followed by 750 mg q 6 hr postoperatively *or* C. Cefamandole, 2 g IV initially, followed by 1 g IV q 2 hr intraoperatively, followed by 1 g IV q 6 hr postoperatively
Median sternotomy/deep sternal wound infection rate is >2% and methicillin-sensitive *Staphylococcus aureus* accounts for a major portion of infections	D. Consider using cefamandole as outlined in C. Value, if any, of extending postoperative prophylaxis to 48 or 72 hr is not known
Median sternotomy/deep sternal wound infection rate is >2% and methicillin-resistant *S. aureus* (MRSA) accounts for a major portion of infections	E. Vancomycin, 15 mg/kg IV initial dose, followed by 10 mg/kg after coming off cardiopulmonary bypass, followed by 500 mg q 6 hr postoperatively (MRSA usually represents nosocomial colonization of the patient or environment. Careful attention to the perioperative environment [e.g., use of preoperative showering with antiseptic soaps, shortened preoperative hospital stay, avoidance of preoperative antibiotic use] may permit the continued use of cephalosporin prophylaxis) *In addition:* a cephalosporin as outlined (regimen A, B, or C) should be employed for continued prophylaxis against gram-negative enteric pathogens
Median sternotomy/deep sternal wound infection rate is >2% and methicillin-resistant coagulase-negative staphylococci (MRCNS) accounts for a major portion of infections	F. Vancomycin, as outlined in E. Based on in vitro data, consideration should also be given to using high-dose (see C) cefamandole in prophylaxis. *In addition:* a cephalosporin as outlined (regimen A, B, or C) should be employed for continued prophylaxis of gram-negative enteric pathogens
Prosthetic valvular surgery/early (<6 mo) prosthetic valve endocarditis (PVE) rates <2%	G. Cephalosporin regimens as outlined in A, B, and C. Longer postoperative prophylaxis (48 to 72 hr) has been recommended for valvular surgery, but without proof of efficacy
Prosthetic valve surgery/early PVE rates of >2%	H. Consider vancomycin and/or modifying perioperative environment as outlined in E. If MRCNS accounts for a major portion of infections, based on in vitro data, consideration should be given to using high-dose cefamandole in prophylaxis as outlined in C. There is, however, no clinical evidence that cefamandole provides enhanced efficacy in preventing PVE due to MRCNS
Pacemaker insertion/wound infection rate <2%	I. No proven benefit of antimicrobial prophylaxis
Pacemaker insertion/wound infection rate >2%	J. Cephalosporin prophylaxis as outlined in A, B, and C
Noncardiac thoracic surgery/elective, nontrauma	K. Cephalosporin prophylaxis as outlined in A, B, and C
Noncardiac thoracic surgery/trauma	L. Clindamycin, 300 mg IV q 6 hr for 5 days or until chest tubes are removed

of hospitalization experienced less clinical empyema than placebo recipients (p = .06, Fisher's exact test) (Grover et al., 1977). Antibiotics used in this way may actually represent therapy rather than prophylaxis. Additional studies are needed to determine the optimal choice and duration of antibiotic prophylaxis or therapy in trauma patients (see Table 4–6).

UNRESOLVED ISSUES

Role of Topical Antibiotics

Some surgeons routinely employ topical antibiotics, usually an aminoglycoside, as an adjunct to systemic antibiotic prophylaxis in cardiac and thoracic surgery. The usefulness of this practice is unproved. Although irrigating the wound at the time of closure with antibiotic-containing solutions has proved effective in prophylaxis of abdominal surgical procedures in which gross bacterial contamination may have occurred (e.g., appendectomy), the value of this practice in clean elective cardiac surgery is less obvious. In a nonrandomized study, Sutherland and associates (1977) reported that prophylaxis with topical antibiot-

ics alone (neomycin or cephalothin, administered in an irrigating solution) was not enhanced by the addition of systemic antibiotics (penicillin plus methicillin or cephalothin). However, topically applied cephalothin is readily absorbed in this setting and may have provided serum and tissue levels of antibiotic that are similar to those achieved with parenteral administration. Intravenous administration of prophylactic antibiotics would appear to be a more reliable method of administering readily absorbable antibiotics during cardiac and thoracic surgery.

For antimicrobials that are poorly absorbed from tissue surfaces, and in particular for the aminoglycosides for which excessive serum levels are associated with predictable toxicity, one could argue that topical antimicrobial irrigation would produce high antimicrobial concentrations at the site of bacterial contamination while avoiding any risk of toxicity. However, as appealing as this concept may be, there are absolutely no data on the efficacy of aminoglycosides when used in this way. On the other hand, Vander Salm and colleagues (1989) reported a reduction in sternal infection rates in patients in whom topical vancomycin was applied to the sternal edges at closure. Given the problems of vancomycin toxicity

■ **Table 4–7.** BACTERIAL ETIOLOGY OF STERNAL WOUND INFECTION AND MEDIASTINITIS*

Prophylactic Regimen	First Author (Date)	Wound Infection Rate	Total Reported Infections	Number of Pathogens Isolated					
				Staphylococcus aureus	*Coagulase-negative Staphylococci*	*Gram-negative Bacilli*	*Enterococci*	*Yeast*	*Other*
Placebo	Fong (1979)	21.3%†	10	7	1	1	—	—	1
	Penketh (1985)	54.5%	12	8	—	—	—	—	—
Total (% of total pathogens)			22	15 (83)	1 (6)	1 (5)			1 (6)
Beta-lactams‡	Sanfelippo (1972)	8.2%†	12	1	2	8	—	2	1
	Stoney (1978)	0.44%†	20	2	8	10	—	—	—
	Bor (1983)	3.4%†	21	5	6	11	—	—	2
	Grossi (1985)	0.97%†	77	35	12	14	9	9	17§
	Cheung (1985)	1.4%†	36	6	6	9	—	—	27§
	Dawson (1985)	0.98%	125	38	31	18	14	4	20
	Miholic (1985)	4.5%†	11	1	5	1	2	—	2
	Farrington (1985)	5.4%	10	5	7	1	—	—	2
	Sutherland (1985)	1.4%	34	21	2	4	1	—	6§
	Nagachinta (1987)	6.8%†	69	22	22	16	13	—	—
Total (% of total pathogens)			459	136 (30)	101 (22)	92 (20)	39 (9)	15 (4)	77 (19)
Beta-lactams‡ plus aminoglycosides‖									
	Engleman (1973)	1.6%†	27	6	—	15	1	4	—
	Culliford (1976)	1.5%†	39	[—18—]		—	16	—	5	—
	Wells (1983)	7.5%	13	3	—	11	—	—	—
	Rutledge (1985)	1.4%†	29	8	6	8	2	3	—
	Kaiser (1987)	1.1%†	11	4	3	3	—	2	—
Total (% of total pathogens)			119	21 (26) [—48 (40)—]	9 (11)	55 (46)	2 (2)	14 (18)	

*Studies of sternal wound infection and mediastinitis are included if 10 or more infections were reported in the referenced article.
†When sufficient information is given, only deep wound infections and associated pathogens are reported.
‡A variety of beta-lactam antibiotics were used including penicillin, cloxacillin, oxacillin, methicillin, cephalothin, cefazolin, or cefamandole.
§Infections yielding multiple pathogens that were not further delineated by the author are included as "Other" infections.
‖Includes those studies in which some or all patients received parenterally administered aminoglycoside (gentamicin or streptomycin).

when administered parenterally, this approach deserves further study.

Duration of Perioperative Prophylaxis

As established conclusively by the Burke animal model and numerous prospective clinical studies, prophylactic antibiotics need not be administered parenterally until the onset of the surgical procedure. The induction of anesthesia represents a convenient time to begin intravenous antibiotic administration. Beginning prophylactic antibiotics a day or even hours before operation is archaic and subjects the patient to all of the potential side effects of antibiotics at a time when there is no gain from their use.

Intraoperatively, every effort should be extended to ensure that adequate levels (i.e., serum levels greater than the *minimal inhibitory concentration* [MIC] of potential pathogens) are maintained throughout the operative procedure. Logistical support should be established to ensure redosing of antibiotics with short half-lives, or of any antibiotic, should unexpected prolongations in the operative procedure occur.

The continuation of the perioperative antimicrobial regimen into the postoperative period raises genuine concerns about excessive cost and theoretical concerns about the inducement of resistance among potential pathogens. Considerable controversy exists regarding this topic, however. Antibiotics begun preoperatively are commonly continued through the third or even the fifth postoperative day. Several reports in cardiac and thoracic surgery have documented that routine prolongation of prophylaxis beyond the first postoperative day provides no additional protection. However, these reports invariably have involved small numbers of patients with few documented infections. On the other hand, surgeons have been concerned that patients may remain at high risk for infection following cardiac surgery, particularly during the period of time when they are being monitored with intravascular devices. As early as 1961, Culbertson and co-workers suggested that hematogenous seeding of wounds might occur in the early postoperative period, and in 1983, Krieger and associates reported a 2.3% incidence of wound infections that appeared to be secondary to urinary tract infections that had developed postoperatively. In short, the relative risk and benefits of prolonged postoperative antibiotic prophylaxis have not been adequately studied and definitive recommendations cannot be made.

Complications Associated with Antimicrobial Prophylaxis

Side effects are to be expected with the use of any drug, and antibiotics are no exception. Various allergic and toxic reactions have been reported, and the issue of emergence or acquisition of resistant pathogens following antibiotic use continues to cause concern. Fortunately, in prophylaxis, toxic side effects have rarely been reported. For example, nephrotoxicity and ototoxicity, which occur with regularity during prolonged gentamicin therapy, have not been recognized as a complication of prophylaxis. This lack of toxicity in prophylaxis undoubtedly is related to the fact that a brief perioperative course of antibiotics provides maximal prophylactic efficacy while exposing the patient to only moderate amounts of drug.

However, several side effects of antibiotics that have been noted during prophylaxis deserve mention. The most frequently reported complication is pseudomembranous colitis. This complication has been reported with a wide variety of both orally and parenterally administered antibiotics. Ampicillin, clindamycin, and the cephalosporins remain the most common offending antibiotics. One institution reported a 6% incidence of pseudomembranous colitis associated with perioperative cefoxitin administration (Block et al., 1986). However, since published reports have been infrequent, pseudomembranous colitis would appear to be an unusual complication of prophylactic therapy.

A side effect of note associated with prophylaxis is a bleeding disorder. Certain beta-lactam antibiotics (penicillins and cephalosporins) possess the potential to induce bleeding, even after a brief perioperative exposure associated with prophylaxis. Hypoprothrombinemia may occur with therapeutic doses of cephalosporins possessing a methylthiotetrazole substitution in the beta-lactam molecule. Cefamandole, moxalactam, and cefoperazone possess this side chain, and the use of cefamandole in surgical wound prophylaxis was associated with an increased sensitivity to warfarin therapy in one retrospective study (Angaran et al., 1983). However, in cardiac and thoracic surgery, where considerable attention is given to the bleeding parameters of perioperative patients, major bleeding complications have not been associated with cefamandole prophylaxis. Moreover, a recent prospective evaluation of the bleeding tendencies associated with the use of cefamandole, cefuroxime, and cefazolin in perioperative prophylaxis in cardiac surgery did not reveal any differences among these agents (Townsend et al., 1993). It would be reasonable, however, to routinely check prothrombin times in patients receiving any of the cephalosporins in therapy or prophylaxis, especially in malnourished or severely ill patients. Other beta-lactam antibiotics (moxalactam, carbenicillin, and ticarcillin) have also been shown to impair platelet function. This complication has been associated with an alpha-carboxyl substitution on the beta-lactam ring. Bleeding times may be markedly prolonged in patients receiving these antibiotics, but because they have had a less prominent use in prophylaxis, the risk of bleeding in this setting is unknown.

A third side effect of importance in prophylaxis is the *red man syndrome*, which may occur with the intravenous administration of vancomycin. This syndrome is associated with vancomycin-inducement of histamine release, an idiosyncratic reaction that cannot be anticipated in any given patient. Investigators have suggested that this syndrome is related to the rapid intravenous infusion of the drug and recommend administering each dose over 60 minutes. However, the syndrome has occurred despite careful attention to the rate of infusion. Three studies of vancomycin use in prophylaxis were terminated because of an unacceptable incidence of reactions (Miedzinski et al., 1990; Nagachinta et al., 1987; Slama et al., 1986). A 7% incidence of reaction was noted in one study in which infusion rates were carefully controlled and administered over 1 hour (Maki et al., 1992). However, prophylaxis was able to be continued in five of eight patients by treatment with diphenhydramine and further slowing of the infusion rate.

There is little doubt that the widespread use of any antibiotic can be associated with the emergence of pathogens resistant to that antibiotic. The resistant pathogens can become established within the environment of a hospital, placing newly admitted patients at risk of acquiring these strains. Equally important, under the selective pressure of antibiotic use, resistant subpopulations of bacteria may emerge in an individual patient, dominating normal colonizing flora. In prophylactic use, for example, widespread use of gentamicin in cardiac surgery has been associated with the emergence of gentamicin-resistant gram-negative rods within the hospital environment (Roberts and Douglas, 1978). Similarly, even brief perioperative use of cephalosporins is associated with both the emergence and the acquisition of antibiotic-resistant *coagulase-negative staphylococci* (CNS) in patients undergoing cardiac surgery (Kernodle et al., 1988). Given the proven efficacy of antibiotics for use in prophylaxis of infection in cardiac and thoracic surgery, the use of "no prophylaxis" is not an option. However, several authorities have emphasized the importance of minimizing the amount and duration of perioperative prophylaxis. Some data suggest that prolonged (4 days) postoperative prophylaxis is associated with more antimicrobial resistance among infecting pathogens (Conte et al., 1972). However, as noted previously, there are theoretical advantages to continuing perioperative prophylaxis in cardiac surgery through the second or even third hospital day. Further data are needed to resolve the relative risks and benefits of continuing perioperative prophylaxis into the postoperative period in cardiac and thoracic surgery.

SPECTRUM OF PATHOGENS ENCOUNTERED IN CARDIAC AND THORACIC SURGERY

Epidemiology

Median Sternotomy Infection

Reported sternal wound infection rates vary greatly from institution to institution (see Table 4–7). Some of this variation can be explained by differences in methodology of reporting (e.g., including or excluding superficial wound infections and variations in length of follow-up). However, it is likely that true differences in infection rates exist, related possibly to the severity of underlying illness within patient populations, differences in environmental conditions, or surgical technique. Staphylococci, coagulase-positive (*S. aureus*) and coagulase-negative, account for most of the reported sternal wound infections and mediastinitis, but gram-negative bacilli occasionally dominate the pathogenetic spectrum (see Table 4–7). Because institutions differ markedly in their spectrum of pathogens isolated from infections and because significant changes occur within institutions over time, cardiothoracic surgeons must adopt their prophylactic and therapeutic strategies to their immediate circumstances. Prophylactic regimens undoubtedly have played a dominant role in shaping the bacterial patterns of postoperative infection. For example, in placebo-controlled studies, *S. aureus* was the dominant pathogen among placebo recipients compared with patients receiving antistaphylococcal prophylaxis (83% versus 29%, respectively; $p < .001$, Chi Square; see Table 4–7). Similarly, in institutions where aminoglycoside antibiotics are routinely included in the prophylactic armamentarium, gram-negative bacilli are isolated much more often than in institutions not using systemic aminoglycosides (46% versus 20%, $p < .0001$). Cause and effect are less evident in evaluating the impact of aminoglycoside antibiotics because the use of aminoglycosides may in fact represent only the response of investigators to a high prevalence of gram-negative bacillary infection in their environment.

Aside from the overall trends in pathogen distribution in sternal wound infections and mediastinitis over the past several years, numerous focal outbreaks of unexpected or unusual pathogens have also been reported. *Enterobacter, Serratia,* and *Mycobacterium fortuitum* are examples of pathogens that have dominated postoperative infections in cardiac surgery as a result of a break in standard aseptic technique. Close surveillance of pathogens and their susceptibility to antibiotics is an essential part of cardiac and thoracic surgery. Cardiothoracic surgeons must be prepared to carefully evaluate their operating environment when unusual pathogens appear and must be willing to modify their prophylactic regimens when persisting shifts occur in the antimicrobial susceptibility of infecting bacteria.

Donor Site Infections

Pathogens isolated from donor sites also vary widely from institution to institution. However, in general, cultures of donor site infections yield the same range of pathogens as those from sternal wound infections. There is also some association between the incidence with which gram-negative bacilli are isolated from infected donor site wounds and the inclusion of aminoglycosides in the prophylactic regimen (44% of pathogens in institutions not using systemic aminoglycosides versus 68% in those that do). As with sternal infections, this information does not in and of itself prove a cause-and-effect relationship. However, systemic gentamicin was administered randomly to half the patients in the study by Kaiser and co-workers (1987), and pathogens resistant to gentamicin occurred only among the gentamicin recipients.

Several patients with late-onset donor site infection due to streptococci were noted by Baddour and Bisno (1982). Such infections have been managed successfully with penicillin therapy, but recurrent infections are common.

Pacemaker

Following elective pacemaker insertion, pathogens isolated from infected sites are almost always coagulase-positive or coagulase-negative staphylococci. Patients hospitalized for several days before pacemaker implantation may be vulnerable to infection from the broader range of pathogens usually found in a hospital environment.

Noncardiac Thoracic Surgery

Ilves and colleagues (1981) noted that whether or not cephalothin prophylaxis was employed, *S. aureus* was the most common pathogen isolated from infections of wounds following noncardiac thoracic surgery. Pulmonary infections were more likely due to *Haemophilus influenzae*, pneumococcus, and *S. aureus*, in that order. Again, the use of cephalothin prophylaxis did not appear to influence the pathogen selection in pulmonary infections, although there was an associated decrease in infection rate.

Prosthetic Valve Endocarditis

Infecting pathogens of PVE have been well described. As noted elsewhere, CNS are the primary cause of infection in the early postoperative period (i.e., <6 months) and second only to alpha-streptococci as a cause of infection in the late-occurring cases.

Individual Pathogens

Coagulase-negative Staphylococci

The CNS are represented by a number of gram-positive coccal species, most frequently *Staphylococcus epidermidis*. These organisms are normal inhabitants of the skin flora and possess less virulence than *S. aureus*. CNS play a prominent role in infections in cardiac and thoracic surgery, related perhaps to the ability of these organisms to withstand prophylaxis or therapy with the semisynthetic penicillins or cephalosporins. Despite the fact that clinical laboratories often identify CNS as methicillin-sensitive or methicillin-resistant or even cephalosporin-sensitive or cephalosporin-resistant, the true susceptibility of these organisms to the beta-lactam antibiotics is difficult to determine. A major problem with the sensitivity testing of CNS is that they display heterogeneous resistance in that only a small percentage of a given population actually exhibits resistance in vitro. Thus, routine in vitro testing may miss the fact that, in vivo, under the pressure of antibiotic therapy, the resistant subpopulation can survive and lead to therapeutic failure. Specialized in vitro assays such as the use of salt-supplemented media and high inocula are required to recognize the presence of resistant strains. Prophylaxis and therapy are further complicated by the fact that differences exist among the cephalosporins in their ability to contain CNS in vitro. Cefamandole, for example, appears to be more effective against CNS than other cephalosporins (Woods et al., 1987).

This difficulty in characterizing the susceptibility of CNS has led most authorities to recommend that neither semisynthetic penicillins nor cephalosporins be used to treat established infection with MRCNS, no matter what the results of testing to cephalosporins may be. Infection due to methicillin-sensitive CNS (MSCNS) usually responds to therapy with semisynthetic penicillins or cephalosporins. However, as noted earlier, unless sophisticated testing procedures are employed, many authorities prefer avoiding the beta-lactam antibiotics altogether and using vancomycin in therapy, especially when treating life-threatening infection.

The difficulties in beta-lactam-susceptibility testing of CNS also have implications for the use of the cephalosporins in prophylaxis when CNS are frequently encountered. However, infection rates with these organisms in cardiac and thoracic surgery simply have been too low for controlled studies to identify any advantage of one antibiotic over the other.

The role of CNS in surgical wound infection versus PVE is somewhat paradoxical. The organisms are the dominant pathogen in early PVE, an infection associated with considerable morbidity and mortality. On the other hand, although they clearly can cause deep sternal wound infection and mediastinitis, CNS are more likely to be associated with superficial infections of the chest wall and donor sites.

Staphylococcus aureus

S. aureus is the single most common pathogen in cardiac and thoracic surgery, accounting for over 20% of all pathogens in present-day practice in which antistaphylococcal prophylaxis is routinely employed. The likely source of the organism is the patient's own flora or airborne contamination from nasal carriage or skin flora of the operating room personnel. S. aureus isolated from cardiac and thoracic infections are rarely susceptible to penicillin, but semisynthetic penicillins and cephalosporins are usually effective in treating established infection. Long-standing concern with the vulnerability of cefazolin to certain S. aureus beta-lactamases has led some authorities to avoid cefazolin

in therapy, but recent studies have yielded conflicting conclusions regarding its relative efficacy when used prophylactically in cardiac and thoracic surgery (see Table 4–5).

Although controversy regarding the relative efficacy of the various cephalosporins in prophylaxis has dominated the issue of prophylactic antibiotic use in cardiac and thoracic surgery for over a decade, the increasing prevalence of MRSA has sharply shifted the focus of these debates. MRSA now account for 15% of nosocomial S. aureus isolates (Panlilio et al., 1992). Although some differences exist among the various cephalosporins in antimicrobial activity against MRSA, this organism possesses true or *intrinsic* resistance to methicillin and all other penicillins and cephalosporins. The cell-wall target sites (known as *penicillin-binding proteins* [PBPs]) for the killing activity of these antibiotics has been altered in MRSA so that they are unaffected by the presence of these antibiotics. Significantly, there is no apparent loss of virulence. In some hospital settings, MRSA have become the most common form of staphylococcal infection. These organisms often resist other antibiotics such as clindamycin or erythromycin. The quinolone class of antibiotics once held promise as alternative therapies. However, MRSA have been found to acquire resistance to ciprofloxacin within months of this agent's introduction into a hospital environment, rendering it almost useless for therapy or prophylaxis of MRSA infection. Whether other quinolones with a higher tissue level/MIC ratio will perform satisfactorily remains to be seen.

Vancomycin is currently the only agent that can be administered via the intravenous route that possesses predictable in vitro activity against MRSA. It is for this reason that surgical prophylaxis currently accounts for 35% of intravenous vancomycin use (Ena et al., 1993). Although several studies have demonstrated that vancomycin is superior to placebo in surgical procedures, only one study to date has prospectively compared vancomycin with commonly used cephalosporins (Maki et al., 1992). However, excess infections due to S. aureus did not occur among any of the prophylactic regimens in this study. Accordingly, there are no clinical data that clearly document vancomycin to be superior to other agents in preventing MRSA infection.

Of more concern, however, is the question of the relative effectiveness of vancomycin versus cephalosporins in preventing infections due to MSSA. Recent data suggest that vancomycin may be inferior to beta-lactams for therapy of severe S. aureus infection. Levine and co-workers (1991) reported that patients with MRSA endocarditis who were treated with vancomycin remained febrile and bacteremic for a median of 7 days whereas the median duration of bacteremia with MSSA endocarditis, treated with nafcillin, is only 3 days. The slowness of the clinical response to vancomycin and uncertainties about its efficacy compared with beta-lactams have led some to caution against the use of vancomycin in patients with severe MSSA infections (Karchmer, 1991). Regarding prophylaxis of

MSSA infection, the relative efficacy of vancomycin versus the cephalosporins is simply unknown. However, Kernodle and Kaiser (1993) demonstrated in a guinea pig model of clean wound infection due to *S. aureus* that vancomycin is superior to cefazolin in preventing intramuscular infection by either MSSA or MRSA. As noted, there are no clinical data to collaborate these in vivo findings.

Gram-negative Bacilli

Various gram-negative bacilli that cause infection in cardiac and thoracic surgery have been reported, and recent trends suggest a rising prevalence of these organisms. Gram-negative bacilli can be isolated from almost any moist area within the environment. The gastrointestinal tract is normally populated with gram-negative bacilli, and the prevalence of these organisms increases in association with antibiotic use. Skin surfaces can also become colonized, especially within skin folds such as in the axilla and groin. Outbreaks of gram-negative bacillary infections have been reported in association with cardiac surgery. Such outbreaks are often related to contaminated environmental sources such as cardioplegic solutions. The antibiotic susceptibility of gram-negative bacilli varies widely, and therapy must be determined following in vitro susceptibility testing.

Enterococci

Enterococci are pathogens infrequently encountered in infections of deep sternal wounds and prosthetic valves. When encountered in wound infections, these organisms are usually found in association with other infecting pathogens, leaving some doubt as to the importance of enterococci as surgical wound pathogens. There is ample evidence, however, that enterococci may occasionally be the only pathogen isolated from a devastating deep sternal wound infection or PVE. These organisms are present in low numbers as a part of the normal human colon. However, with use of antibiotics and prolonged exposure to the hospital environment, the colonization and subsequent infection rates increase. Although vancomycin-resistant enterococcal strains are becoming increasingly prevalent in hospital environments, vancomycin remains the drug of choice for treating suspected enterococcal infection, pending culture and sensitivity results. If antimicrobial sensitivity tests indicate the organism to be susceptible to ampicillin, this antibiotic can be used successfully in therapy. Gentamicin is synergistic with both ampicillin and vancomycin in treating enterococcal infections, but because of the associated risk of renal toxicity with prolonged gentamicin use, most authorities have attempted to minimize its use in synergistic therapy.

Fungi

Fungal infections often occur as superinfections during or following antibiotic treatment of major in-fections caused by bacterial pathogens. Various fungal organisms, most often *Candida* species, have been isolated from deep sternal, mediastinal, and valvular infections following cardiac and thoracic surgery. Because the isolation of fungi from superficially cultured surfaces often represents colonization, not infection, most authorities require repeated isolations of fungal organisms from infected lesions or a single deep culture with positive Gram's stains from a deep, aseptically obtained culture before assuming that an established fungal infection is present. Conversely, hematogenous dissemination of candidal species, usually *Candida albicans*, often occurs despite persistently negative blood cultures. In this situation, the primary site of contamination/infection is often an in-dwelling intravascular line, surgical wound, urinary tract infection, or even the uninfected gastrointestinal tract. Such infections usually occur in debilitated or severely ill hosts, and the presence of established fungal infection is a poor prognostic sign. Newer antifungal agents such as fluconazole are being successfully employed in therapy of superficial and deep infections, but amphotericin B is often indicated in therapy of established deep or disseminated infection.

Anaerobic Bacteria

Scattered reports of mediastinitis due to anaerobic bacteria have been noted. However, the relatively low virulence of these organisms and the relatively low colonization rates in the skin of the chest make it unlikely that anaerobic bacteria are a dominant pathogen in cardiac and thoracic surgery.

Therapy of Established Infection

It is probably useful to classify sternal wound infection by the severity of the process (Table 4–8 and Fig. 4–1). Class I or superficial infections of the sternum involve the skin and superficial areas of subcutaneous

■ **Table 4–8.** CLASSIFICATION OF SEVERITY OF INFECTION* FOLLOWING MEDIAN STERNOTOMY

Category	Depth	Description
Class I	Superficial	Purulence involving the superficial subcutaneous tissues; such infections do not prolong hospitalization or require altered outpatient management
Class II	Deep	Purulence involving the deep subcutaneous tissues; ordinarily, such infections require surgical débridement and/or prolonged hospitalization and/or altered posthospitalization management
Class III	Deep	Sternal osteomyelitis
Class IV	Deep	Purulence extends into posterior mediastinal tissue planes

*Infection is identified by the presence of polymorphonuclear leukocytes (either grossly as pus or microscopically) within wound exudates or tissues. Results of bacterial cultures of tissues or exudates are not important in determining whether the wound is infected.

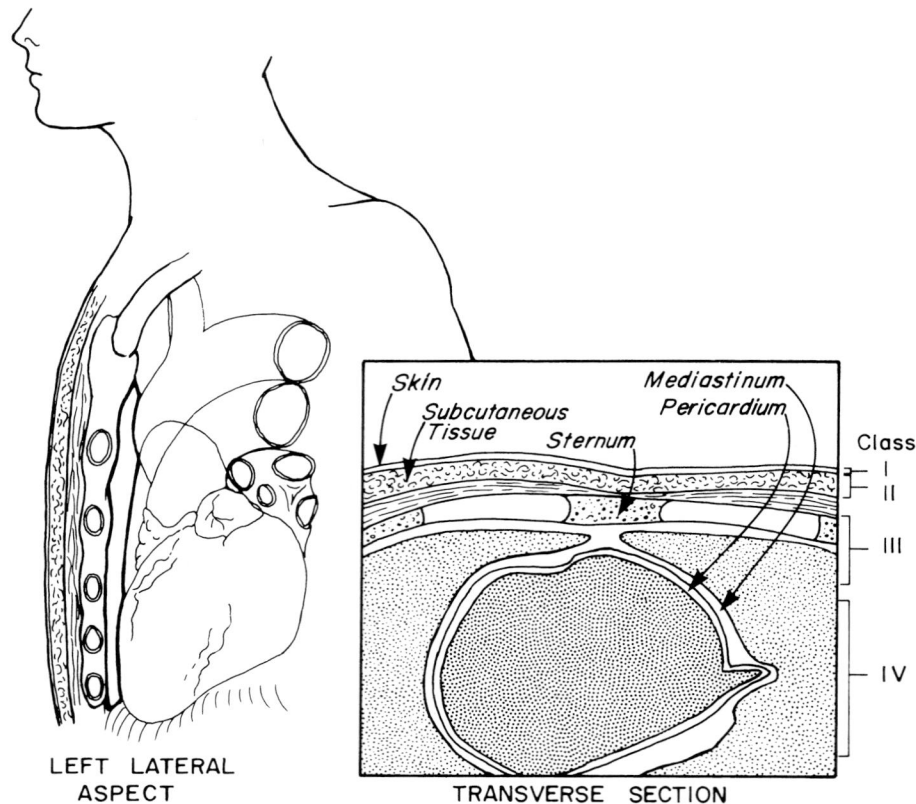

FIGURE 4–1. Schematic of the mediastinum and classification of the severity and depth of infection following a surgical procedure involving a median sternotomy incision. The morbidity, mortality, and cost related to infection increase substantially as the depth (of class) of infection increases. (From Kaiser, A. B.: Postoperative infections and antimicrobial prophylaxis. *In* Mandell, D. L., Douglas, R. D., Jr., and Bennett, J. E. (eds): Principles and Practice of Infectious Diseases. 3rd ed. Churchill Livingstone, New York, 1990, p. 2253.)

tissues. An increased frequency of CNS has been isolated in these infections, reflecting the fact that these infections most likely arise from late operative or early postoperative contamination of the superficial subcutaneous tissues with skin flora. Such infections often respond without therapy or with simple lancing of a stitch abscess. Antibiotic therapy, if needed, is usually successful with cloxacillin or erythromycin.

Class II infections involve deep subcutaneous tissues and often are defined retrospectively as those subcutaneous infections that require incision and drainage and antibiotic therapy for proper management. Gram's stain and culture and sensitivity testing should always be obtained in such cases before instituting antibiotic therapy. However, one should not wait for a positive culture report to begin antibiotic therapy. The demonstration of purulence within a deep subcutaneous lesion is evidence enough to begin empiric antibiotic therapy. Gram's stain can often differentiate among gram-positive, gram-negative, and fungal pathogens. As a rule of thumb, an antibiotic that has been used in prophylaxis should never be continued as empiric therapy of postoperative infection. Vancomycin should be employed after cultures are obtained or pending cultures have been reported. Gentamicin should be added if gram-negative rods are known to be common in a given institution. Once

culture and sensitivity reports are available, antibiotics should be changed to the least toxic and, if possible, least costly regimen that shows in vitro effectiveness. If signs and symptoms of infection persist, reevaluation of the diagnosis is indicated (e.g., is sternal involvement present?), as is repeated aspiration with culture and sensitivity testing of deep tissue sites.

Class III infections of the median sternotomy incision involve the sternum and are often associated with some sternal instability. When there is infection of the skin and subcutaneous tissue overlying a sternal incision, and the sternum is unstable to palpation, then the sternum is presumed to be involved in the infectious process. However, the subcutaneous tissues may not be involved in early sternal infections, and fever and a painful sternum may be the only signs or symptoms. Routine chest x-rays are not helpful. Radioisotope bone scans, indium-III leukocyte scans, and computed tomography of the thorax with careful attention to the sternum may occasionally identify focal areas of infection. Repeated needle aspiration of suspicious areas may yield evidence of infection. Occasionally, however, in patients with persistent pain, fever, and other nonspecific evidences of infection, the sternum must be explored. Most authorities have recommended that the infected sternum, once diagnosed, be débrided with reapproximation of the sternal edges (i.e., primary closure of the wound). Extensively involved tissues may require that a muscle flap be turned for proper wound healing and control of infection. Topical antibiotic irrigation of the freshly débrided wound via implanted subcutaneous catheters is commonly employed. Various antibiotics have been used, such as aminoglycosides, vancomycin, and beta-lactams. However, the value of topical antibiotic irrigation as an adjunct to parenterally administered antibiotics is unknown. Choice of parenteral antibiotics is identical to that for Class II sternal wound infection. Because some institutions have noted an increasing incidence of fungal involvement of the sternum, Gram's stain or culture of sternal fragments should be carefully evaluated for the presence of *Candida* or other fungi. If fungi are present, aggressive therapy with amphotericin B, fluconazole, or other potent antifungal agent is warranted.

Class IV infections indicate that extensive mediastinal involvement has occurred. Patients with such infections are readily identified, since most exhibit extreme prostration, with x-ray and physical findings suggestive of mediastinitis. Mediastinal exploration and drainage are indicated in the management of such patients. Antibiotic therapy is similar to that outlined for Class II and Class III infections.

Antibiotic Use in Prophylaxis and Therapy of Cardiac and Thoracic Surgery

Penicillin

Although the earliest trials of antibiotic use in prophylaxis of wound infection in cardiac surgery employed penicillin-G or beta-lactamase–resistant penicillins (e.g., methicillin) in the prophylactic regimen, most cardiac surgeons have discontinued using the penicillin analogues in prophylaxis. The beta-lactamase–resistant, semisynthetic penicillins possess outstanding activity against MSSA, but most lack significant activity against gram-negative bacilli, pathogens that are isolated from as many as one-half of wound infections following cardiac surgery (see Table 4–6). An exception is the ampicillin-sulbactam combination. The addition of the beta-lactamase inhibitor sulbactam confers both antistaphylococcal activity and an extended gram-negative spectrum. This agent has a relatively short half-life, however, and careful redosing (every 2 to 4 hours) during the intraoperative period is required.

It has been not a question of efficacy but one of safety that has minimized the use of penicillins in prophylaxis in cardiac surgery. Between 5 and 10% of the adult population have a history of penicillin allergy. In contrast, allergies to cephalosporins are unusual, and cephalosporins have been administered safely to patients with a history of mild reactions (e.g., rash) to penicillin. However, it should be noted that a history of penicillin and cephalosporin allergy should be sought in every patient before the use of prophylactic antibiotics. Cephalosporins should be avoided in patients with a history of an immediate or accelerated reaction (hypotension, bronchospasm, or urticaria, or a combination) to any of the penicillins as well as the cephalosporins.

The penicillins, especially the semisynthetic, penicillinase-resistant penicillins (nafcillin, oxacillin, methicillin), are important antibiotics for therapy of established infections secondary to MSSA. In addition, if sensitivity testing procedures are adequate, these antibiotics are also useful in therapy of MSCNS infection. Prolonged therapy (>4 weeks) with these agents for severe infections such as endocarditis has been associated with rare complications of reversible bone marrow suppression and interstitial nephritis. The latter is a syndrome characterized by decreasing renal function and eosinophilia. The syndrome is usually reversible with discontinuation of the therapy. Such complications may be less common with nafcillin therapy. So-called third-generation penicillins such as ticarcillin and piperacillin possess broad activity against hospital-acquired gram-negative rods and have an important role in treating serious infection that may arise following cardiac and thoracic surgery.

Cephalosporins

A low incidence of toxicity and side effects and a broad antibiotic spectrum have made the cephalosporins popular antibiotics for prophylaxis in clean surgical procedures. However, with changes in the spectrum of pathogens and the availability of newer antibiotics, it is uncertain whether this class of antibiotics will remain dominant as the prophylactic antibiotic of choice for cardiac and thoracic surgery.

FIRST-GENERATION CEPHALOSPORINS

Numerous clinical studies have verified the utility of the first-generation cephalosporins in cardiac surgery. Because of competitive pricing and its relatively long half-life, cefazolin has emerged as the predominant choice. One gram every 6 hours provides adequate serum and tissue levels throughout the perioperative period. However, two clinical trials noted that cefazolin failed to provide predictable protection from *S. aureus* infection of the sternal and donor sites (Kaiser et al., 1987; Slama et al., 1986). It is likely that cefazolin's susceptibility to staphylococcal beta-lactamase accounts for these observed failures (Kernodle and Kaiser, 1987). It was first noted in 1975 that the beta-lactamase of certain penicillinase-producing *S. aureus* (i.e., penicillin-resistant but MSSA) can more readily hydrolyze cefazolin than other cephalosporins (Regamey et al., 1975). Currently, clinical microbiology laboratories cannot reliably identify the staphylococci that produce beta-lactamases that are highly effective in hydrolyzing cefazolin. The clinical importance of staphylococcal beta-lactamases vis-à-vis *S. aureus* has been questioned by some, and the full implications of the differences in stability of the various cephalosporins to staphylococcal beta-lactamases in prophylaxis and therapy have yet to be elucidated fully. Indeed, recent comparative studies have detected no loss of prophylactic efficacy with cefazolin compared with second-generation cephalosporins (see Table 4–4). Nevertheless, the use of cefazolin in routine prophylaxis of cardiac and thoracic surgery should be evaluated carefully. In settings of cefazolin use where unexpected or persistent MSSA infections are noted, a change to another cephalosporin or another class of antibiotics should be considered.

Cephalothin, an older first-generation cephalosporin, has appeal as a prophylactic agent, primarily because of its enhanced stability against staphylococcal beta-lactamase. However, cephalothin has a relatively short half-life and frequent redosing (every 2 to 4 hours) is required to maintain adequate levels throughout the surgical procedure. Of equal concern has been the finding that human tissues contain enzymes that may inactivate (desacetylate) cephalothin in situ. It has been postulated that the desacetylating enzymes account for the observed failure of cephalothin to reliably treat bacterial meningitis. Whether this phenomenon has implications for the use of cephalothin as a prophylactic agent in operative procedures is unknown. Nevertheless, these factors should discourage a return to this antibiotic as a prophylactic choice in clean operations. Other first-generation cephalosporins have been evaluated as prophylactic agents in cardiac and thoracic surgery. In general, however, uncertainties over their beta-lactamase stability, variations in their MIC to S. aureus, and their relatively short half-lives have dissuaded interest in these antibiotics as prophylactic agents.

Therapeutically, first-generation cephalosporins have only limited usefulness in cardiac and thoracic surgery. These antibiotics should be avoided, if possible, in treating established S. aureus infection, and a semisynthetic penicillin or vancomycin should be used instead. Cephalothin with its resistance to S. aureus beta-lactamase and proven efficacy in clinical trials may be useful in settings of penicillin allergy. Sensitivity testing of CNS may indicate sensitivity to the cephalosporins, and if such organisms also test sensitive to methicillin, therapy of such infections with a first-generation cephalosporin may be considered. However, if organisms test resistant to methicillin, vancomycin should be used to treat any life-threatening infection due to CNS, no matter what the results of in vitro sensitivity testing to the cephalosporins (Karchmer et al., 1983).

SECOND-GENERATION CEPHALOSPORINS

Second-generation cephalosporins with modest extension of antibiotic spectrum were released for general use in the mid-1970s, and two deserve comment in the context of cardiac and thoracic surgery. Two studies found cefamandole to be superior to cefazolin as a prophylactic agent (Kaiser et al., 1987; Slama et al., 1986), and three other studies noted trends of improved efficacy with cefamandole versus other cephalosporins (see Table 4–4D). Cefamandole's enhanced stability to hydrolysis by certain staphylococcal beta-lactamases or improved binding to staphylococcal PBPs may account for its improved performance. This agent's MICs against CNS are among the lowest of any antibiotic, providing an advantage, unproved as yet, in preventing infection due to CNS. Its primary disadvantage is related to its relatively short half-life, demanding frequent redosing during operation. Use every 2 hours during operation was required to provide reliable serum levels throughout the perioperative period in one study (Ghoneim et al., 1982). The cefamandole molecule also possesses a methylthiotetrazole side chain, which has been associated with prolonged prothrombin times. An increased sensitivity to warfarin anticoagulation therapy has been noted in patients receiving cefamandole prophylaxis in cardiac surgery (Angaran et al., 1983). This remains a theoretical concern in prophylaxis, as no major bleeding problems have been noted associated with cefamandole prophylaxis.

Cefuroxime has emerged as an important prophylactic agent in cardiac and thoracic surgery. Like cefamandole, it possesses a good spectrum of activity against pathogens frequently associated with infection in cardiac surgery. MICs to CNS are higher than those of cefamandole. However, it possesses excellent stability against the common beta-lactamases of S. aureus. Unfortunately, compared with cefazolin, it has proved to be both a better and a worse prophylactic agent in cardiac surgery than cefazolin (Doebbeling et al., 1990; Slama et al., 1986). Although it possesses a somewhat longer half-life than cefamandole and has approval for use in prophylaxis with infrequent dosing, the half-life of cefuroxime is shorter than that of cefazolin. During the important intraoperative period, frequent dosing, every 4 to 6 hours, may be required to maintain reliable levels of antibiotic (see Table 4–6).

In therapy, the second-generation cephalosporins offer little advantage over other available antibiotics. Although some in vitro advantages may be noted with certain organisms, most authorities would be unwilling to treat established infection due to any of the staphylococci with the second-generation cephalosporins. These antibiotics have extended activity against gram-negative bacilli and may find a limited role in treating such infection if so indicated by sensitivity testing.

THIRD-GENERATION CEPHALOSPORINS

The third-generation cephalosporins are the most recently developed and marketed cephalosporins. In general, these agents possess an exceptionally broad spectrum of antibiotic activity. Many have extensive half-lives, allowing dosing every 12 or even 24 hours. Their extended gram-negative spectrum of activity may prove valuable in preventing infection at the median sternotomy site when a high prevalence of gram-negative bacilli is noted. However, although these agents have proved effective in treating staphylococcal infection, their MICs against S. aureus are higher than those of most of the first-generation and many of the second-generation cephalosporins. The implications of this finding in prophylaxis are unknown, but careful monitoring of prophylactic efficacy, particularly of *S. aureus* infection, is required if these agents are chosen for routine prophylaxis. Although the third-generation cephalosporins are, in general, much more expensive than either the first-generation or the second-generation compounds, their cost may be partially offset by their requirement for infrequent dosing. Some of these agents, specifically moxalactam and cefoperazone, tend to prolong the prothrombin time, but as with cefamandole, the short use of these agents in the perioperative period usually precludes the development of significant bleeding (Sattler et al., 1986). The third-generation cephalosporins deserve careful consideration for prophylaxis in cardiac and thoracic surgery, but careful monitoring of prophylactic efficacy is required before an endorsement of these agents can be offered.

The extended spectrum of activity against gram-negative bacilli has led to an important role for third-generation cephalosporins in the therapy of established infections. Nosocomially acquired gram-negative bacilli vary considerably in their susceptibility to the cephalosporins, so careful evaluation of sensitivity testing of infecting pathogens is warranted.

Aminoglycosides

Aminoglycosides have been used extensively in prophylaxis in cardiac and thoracic surgery, both systemically as streptomycin, gentamicin, kanamycin, tobramycin, and topically as kanamycin, neomycin, or gentamicin. These antibiotics possess a reasonable spectrum of antibiotic activity, since staphylococci and many gram-negative rods are predictably susceptible to these agents. Direct proof of efficacy in prophylaxis is lacking, however. Sutherland and co-workers (1985) reported very low infection rates involving cardiac surgery using topical neomycin as the prophylactic agent at the time of wound closure. Others have employed systemic gentamicin in high-risk settings such as emergency reexploration of the mediastinum. More important, results from at least two studies suggest that systemic gentamicin may actually be contraindicated as a prophylactic antibiotic in cardiac surgery. Roberts and Douglas (1978) reported that gentamicin resistance among *Pseudomonas* and *Serratia* isolates rose from 4 to 28% in their hospital following the institution of systemic gentamicin in routine perioperative prophylaxis in open heart surgery. Similarly, an increased incidence of gentamicin-resistant infection was encountered among gentamicin recipients in a prospective randomized study of antibiotic prophylaxis in cardiac surgery (Kaiser et al., 1987). Standard dosing of gentamicin (1–2 mg/kg/8 hr) predictably produces several hours of low (<2 mg/ml) gentamicin serum levels between doses. It may be that this interval of subtherapeutic gentamicin encourages the emergence of resistant subpopulations. Whatever the mechanism of emergence of resistance, pending further data to the contrary, systemic aminoglycosides should be avoided as a prophylactic agent in cardiac surgery or used under conditions where patterns of gentamicin resistance can be closely monitored.

Therapeutically, the aminoglycosides provide valuable assistance in managing existing infections due to gram-negative rods. They are also useful in synergy with semisynthetic penicillins or vancomycin in treating deep infections due to *S. aureus*. Their recognized ototoxicity and nephrotoxicity demand that gentamicin serum levels be monitored closely, taking care to keep nadir serum levels less than 2 mcg or 2 μg. Recent studies suggest that once-daily dosing of gentamicin (4 mg/kg) is as effective as traditional three-times-daily dosing, but with lower nephrotoxicity (Prins et al., 1993).

Vancomycin

Vancomycin offers predictable activity against all aerobic gram-positive cocci: coagulase-negative and coagulase-positive staphylococci and all streptococcal pathogens including enterococci. The antibiotic has proved effective as a prophylactic agent, and cross-allergy to the beta-lactams does not occur. Several programs have turned to vancomycin for routine prophylaxis, particularly in centers where MRSA wound infections or MRCNS prosthetic valve endocarditis is endemic.

However, numerous problems are associated with routine vancomycin prophylaxis. The most obvious concerns the critical role this antibiotic offers in therapy of established methicillin-resistant infection. The theoretical risk is that the widespread use of this agent leads to the emergence of vancomycin-resistant pathogens. The second problem with routine vancomycin prophylaxis concerns its toxicity. In addition to ototoxicity, seen with high serum doses, and frequent incidence of phlebitis, intravenous administration of vancomycin is associated with the *red man syndrome*, a peculiar reaction to the drug manifested by intense peripheral vasodilatation and, rarely, hypotension (Slight et al., 1985). As noted earlier, this reaction is less likely to occur if a 1-g dose is infused over 1 hour, and predosing with antihistamines may minimize the symptoms (see "Differential Efficacy of Antimicrobials Used in Prophylaxis," earlier in this chapter). The final problems with the use of vancomycin as a prophylactic agent concern its narrow antibiotic spectrum. The antibiotic has no activity against gram-negative bacilli, pathogens that account for up to 40% of infections in the sternum and donor sites. Concurrent use of other antibiotics may be necessary for adequate prophylaxis. In addition, the drug is expensive: a 24-hour prophylactic regimen may be several times the cost of a comparable cefazolin regimen. Farber and associates (1983) recommended an initial dose of 15 mg/kg followed by 10 mg/kg at the end of cardiopulmonary bypass. Dosage recommendations are not available for prolonged operative procedures.

Vancomycin used therapeutically should be administered 500 mg every 6 hours or 1 g every 12 hours. Doses should be modified considerably for patients who have impaired renal function.

Quinolones

The quinolone antibiotics have recently been introduced as broad-spectrum agents available both orally and parenterally. The first of this class, ciprofloxacin, offered promise in therapy and prophylaxis of both MSSA and MRSA. Enthusiasm has been tempered, however, by the rapid emergence of ciprofloxacin-resistance among MRSA isolates once this agent has been introduced into a hospital environment. Newer quinolones that offer higher MICs against *S. aureus* are in final stages of evaluation and may prove to provide long-term efficacy against staphylococci. Because the quinolones also possess an excellent spectrum of activity against gram-negative bacilli and, in general, have few side effects, they hold promise for the future. However, given the experience with ciprofloxacin, these agents must be used with caution and with careful monitoring, whether used in prophylaxis or in therapy. Side effects with the quinolones have been unusual, and the main contraindications concern its potential for impairing bone and cartilage growth. The antibiotic should be avoided in adolescents, children, and pregnant patients.

Rifampin

Rifampin shows bactericidal activity against a wide range of microorganisms. However, rapid emergence of resistance to rifampin develops during in vitro and in vivo use. In therapy of life-threatening staphylococcal infections, rifampin may have a role. Evidence shows that rifampin provides important synergistic activity with vancomycin against MRCNS and with nafcillin or vancomycin against MSSA and MRSA. However, in vitro and in vivo antagonism has also been noted with rifampin combinations, and careful microbiologic confirmation of efficacy should be sought before using this antibiotic in synergistic therapy of life-threatening staphylococcal infections.

SELECTED BIBLIOGRAPHY

Beam, T. R., Jr.: Perioperative prevention of infection in cardiac surgery. Antibiot. Chemother., 33:114, 1985.

The epidemiology of postoperative infectious complications of cardiac surgery is reviewed. A rationale for preventive measures that involve operating room personnel and the environment is presented, and a review of pathogens responsible for infections in cardiac surgery and antibiotics used in prophylaxis is provided.

Kaiser, A. B., Petracek, M. R., Lea, J. W., IV, et al.: Efficacy of cefazolin, cefamandole and gentamicin as prophylactic agents in cardiac surgery. Ann. Surg., 206:791, 1987.

A large (1030-patient) prospective randomized study of antibiotic prophylaxis in cardiac surgery. Information on risk factors, pathogens, and cost is provided. Cefazolin was found to be significantly less effective in the prevention of *Staphylococcus aureus* infection than cefamandole. The other important finding in the study was the higher incidence of gentamicin-resistant pathogens among patients randomized to receive gentamicin.

Nagachinta, T., Stephens, M., and Reitz, B.: Risk factors for surgical wound infections following cardiac surgery. J. Infect. Dis., 156:967, 1987.

This study involves more than 1000 patients who had elective cardiac surgery. An extensive evaluation of risk factors for infection is provided. After logistic regression analysis, four variables were found to persist as independent predictors of sternal wound infection: obesity, diabetes mellitus, length of preoperative stay in hospital, and cigarette smoking.

Rutledge, R., Applebaum, R. E., and Kim, B. J.: Mediastinal infection after open heart surgery. Surgery, 97:88, 1985.

An extensive retrospective review of 2031 patients who had median sternotomy at the National Heart Lung and Blood Institute between 1956 and 1981. A detailed analysis of the experience in the management of mediastinal infection is provided.

BIBLIOGRAPHY

Alkan, M. L., and Beachey, E. H.: Excretion of lipoteichoic acid by group A streptococci: Influence of penicillin on excretion and loss of ability to adhere to human oral epithelial cells. J. Clin. Invest., 61:671, 1978.

Angaran, D. M., Dias, V. C., Arom, K. V., et al.: The influence of prophylactic antibiotics on the warfarin anticoagulation response in the postoperative prosthetic cardiac valve patient. Ann. Surg., 199:107, 1983.

Archer, G. L., Polk, R. E., Duma, R. J., and Lower, R.: Comparison of cephalothin and cefamandole prophylaxis during insertion of prosthetic heart valves. Antimicrob. Agents Chemother., 13:924, 1978.

Austin, T. W., Coles, J. C., Burnett, R., and Goldbach, M.: Aortocoronary bypass procedures and sternotomy infections: A study of antistaphylococcal prophylaxis. Can. J. Surg., 23:483, 1980.

Baddour, L. M., and Bisno, A. L.: Recurrent cellulitis after saphenous venectomy for coronary bypass surgery. Ann. Intern. Med., 97:493, 1982.

Beachey, E. H., Eisenstein, B. I., and Ofek, I.: Adherence of bacteria: Prevention of the adhesion of bacteria to mucosal surfaces: Influence of antimicrobial agents. *In* Eickenberg, H. V., Hahn, H., and Opferkuch, W. (eds): The Influence of Antibiotics on the Host Parasite Relationship. Munich, Springer-Verlag, 1982, p. 171.

Beam, T. R., Raab, T. A., Spooner, J. A., et al.: Comparison of ceftriaxone and cefazolin prophylaxis against infection in open heart surgery. Am. J. Surg., 148:8, 1984.

Block, B. S., Mercer, L. J., Ismail, M. A., and Moawad, A. H.: *Clostridium difficile*–associated diarrhea follows perioperative prophylaxis with cefoxitin. Am. J. Obstet. Gynecol., 153:835, 1986.

Bor, D. H., Rose, R. M., Modlin, J. F., et al.: Mediastinitis after cardiovascular surgery. Rev. Infect. Dis., 5:885, 1983.

Boyce, J. M., Potter-Bynoe, G., Opal, S. M., et al.: A common-source outbreak of *Staphylococcus epidermidis* infections among patients undergoing cardiac surgery. J. Infect. Dis., 161:493, 1990.

Bryan, C. S., Smith, C. W., Sutton, J. P., et al.: Comparison of cefamandole and cefazolin during cardiopulmonary bypass. J. Thorac. Cardiovasc. Surg., 85:222, 1983.

Burke, J. F.: The effective period of preventive antibiotic action in experimental incisions and dermal lesions. Surgery, 50:161, 1961.

Burke, J. F.: Identification of the sources of staphylococci contaminating the surgical wound during operation. Ann. Surg., 158:898, 1963.

Cheung, E. H., Craver, J. M., Jones, E. L., et al.: Mediastinitis after cardiac valve operations: Impact upon survival. J. Thorac. Cardiovasc. Surg., 90:517, 1985.

Chuard, C., Vaudaux, P., Waldvogel, F. A., and Lew, D. P.: Susceptibility of *Staphylococcus aureus* growing on fibronectin-coated surfaces to bactericidal antibiotics. Antimicrob. Agents Chemother., 37:625, 1993.

Conklin, C. M., Gray, R. J., Neilson, D., et al.: Determinants of wound infection incidence after isolated coronary artery bypass surgery in patients randomized to receive prophylactic cefuroxime or cefazolin. Ann. Thorac. Surg., 46:172, 1988.

Conte, J. E., Jr., Cohen, S. N., Roe, B. B., and Elashoff, R. M.:

Antibiotic prophylaxis and cardiac surgery: A prospective double-blind comparison of single-dose versus multiple-dose regimens. Ann. Intern. Med., 76:943, 1972.

Culbertson, W. R., Altemeier, W. A., Gonzalez, L. L., and Hill, E. O.: Studies on the epidemiology of postoperative infection of clean operative wounds. Ann. Surg., 154:599, 1961.

Culliford, A. T., Cunningham, J. N., Jr., Zeff, R. H., et al.: Sternal and costochondral infections following open heart surgery: A review of 2594 cases. J. Thorac. Cardiovasc. Surg., 72:714, 1976.

Dawson, M. S., Keys, T. F., and Gill, C. C.: Sternal wound infections complicating median sternotomy (Abstract no. 488). Twenty-fifth Interscience Conference on Antimicrobial Agents and Chemotherapy. Minneapolis, American Society for Microbiology, 1985.

Doebbeling, N., Pfaller, M. A., Kuhns, K. R., et al.: Cardiovascular surgery prophylaxis. A randomized controlled comparison of cefazolin and cefuroxime. J. Thorac. Cardiovasc. Surg., 99:981, 1990.

Ena, J., Dick, R. W., Jones, R. N., and Wenzel, R. P.: The epidemiology of intravenous vancomycin usage in a university hospital. A 10-year study. J. A. M. A., 269:598, 1993.

Engelman, R. M., Williams, C. D., Gouge, T. H., et al.: Mediastinitis following open heart surgery. Arch. Surg., 107:772, 1973.

Farber, B. F., Karchmer, A. W., Buckley, M. J., and Moellering, R. C.: Vancomycin prophylaxis in cardiac operations: Determination of an optimal dosage regimen. J. Thorac. Cardiovasc. Surg., 85:933, 1983.

Farrington, M., Webster, M., Fenn, A., and Phillips, I.: Cardiothoracic wound infection at St. Thomas' Hospital. Br. J. Surg., 72:759, 1985.

Fong, I. W., Baker, C. B., and McKee, D. C.: The value of prophylactic antibiotics in aorta-coronary bypass operations: A double-blind randomized trial. J. Thorac. Cardiovasc. Surg., 78:908, 1979.

Gelfand, M. S., Simmons, B. P., Schoettle, P., et al.: Cefamandole versus cefonicid prophylaxis in cardiovascular surgery: A prospective study. Ann. Thorac. Surg., 49:435, 1990.

Gentry, L. O., Zeluff, B. J., and Cooley, D. A.: Antibiotic prophylaxis in open heart surgery: A comparison of cefamandole, cefuroxime, and cefazolin. Ann. Thorac. Surg., 46:167, 1988.

Geroulanos, S., Donfried, B., Schumacher, F., and Turina, M.: Cefuroxime versus ceftriaxone prophylaxis in cardiovascular surgery. Drugs Exp. Clin. Res., 11:201, 1985.

Geroulanos, S., Oxelbark, S., and Turina, M.: Preoperative antimicrobial prophylaxis in cardiovascular surgery. A prospective randomized trial comparing two-day cefuroxime prophylaxis with four-day cefazolin prophylaxis. J. Cardiovasc. Surg., 27:300, 1986.

Ghoneim, A. T. M., Tandom, A. P., and Ionescu, M. I.: Comparative study of cefamandole versus ampicillin plus cloxacillin: Prophylactic antibiotics in cardiac surgery. Ann. Thorac. Surg., 33:152, 1982.

Goldmann, D. A., Hopkins, C. C., Karchmer, A. W., et al.: Cephalothin prophylaxis in cardiac valve surgery: A prospective, double-blind comparison of two-day and six-day regimens. J. Thorac. Cardiovasc. Surg., 73:470, 1977.

Goodman, J. S., Schaffner, W., Collins, H. A., et al.: Infection after cardiovascular surgery: Clinical study including examination of antimicrobial prophylaxis. N. Engl. J. Med., 278:117, 1968.

Grossi, E. A., Culliford, A. T., Krieger, K. H., et al.: A survey of 77 major infectious complications of median sternotomy: A review of 7949 consecutive operative procedures. Ann. Thorac. Surg., 40:214, 1985.

Grover, F. L., Richardson, J. D., Fewel, J. G., et al.: Prophylactic antibiotics in the treatment of penetrating chest wounds. A prospective double-blind study. J. Thorac. Cardiovasc. Surg., 74:528, 1977.

Howe, C. W., and Marston, A. T.: A study on sources of postoperative staphylococcal infection. Surg. Gynecol. Obstet., 115:266, 1962.

Howes, E. L.: Prevention of wound infection by the injection of nontoxic antibacterial substances. Ann. Surg., 124:268, 1946.

Ilves, R., Cooper, J. D., Todd, T. R. J., and Pearson, F.: Prospective, randomized, double-blind study using prophylactic cephalothin for major, elective, general thoracic operations. J. Thorac. Cardiovasc. Surg., 81:813, 1981.

Kaiser, A. B.: Surgical wound infection. N. Engl. J. Med., 324:123, 1991.

Kaiser, A. B., Petracek, M. R., Lea, J. W., IV, et al.: Efficacy of cefazolin, cefamandole, and gentamicin as prophylactic agents in cardiac surgery. Ann. Surg., 206:791, 1987.

Karchmer, A. W.: Staphylococcus aureus and vancomycin: The sequel. Ann. Intern. Med., 115:739, 1991.

Karchmer, A. W., Archer, G. L., and Dismukes, W. E.: Staphylococcus epidermidis causing prosthetic valve endocarditis: Microbiologic and clinical observations as guides to therapy. Ann. Intern. Med., 98:447, 1983.

Karney, W., Correa-Coronas, R., Zajtchuk, R., et al.: Comparison of cephalothin and ceforanide prophylaxis in cardiac surgery with cardiopulmonary bypass. Antimicrob. Agents Chemother., 24:85, 1983.

Kernodle, D. S., Barg, N. L., and Kaiser, A. B.: Low-level colonization of hospitalized patients with methicillin-resistant coagulase-negative staphylococci and their emergence during surgical antimicrobial prophylaxis. Antimicrob. Agents Chemother., 32:202, 1988.

Kernodle, D. S., and Kaiser, A. B.: Comparative prophylactic efficacy of cefazolin and vancomycin in a guinea pig model of Staphylococcus aureus wound infection. J. Infect. Dis., 168:152, 1993.

Kernodle, D. S., and Kaiser, A. B.: Staphylococcus aureus infections failing cefazolin or cefamandole prophylaxis in cardiac surgery: Clinical relevance of beta-lactamase production (Abstract no. 87). Twenty-seventh Interscience Conference on Antimicrobial Agents and Chemotherapy. New York, American Society of Microbiology, 1987.

Kini, P. M., Fernandez, J., Causay, R. S., and Lemole, G. M.: Double-blind comparison of cefazolin and cephalothin in open heart surgery. J. Thorac. Cardiovasc. Surg., 76:506, 1978.

Kreter, B., and Woods, M.: Antibiotic prophylaxis for cardiothoracic operations. J. Thorac. Cardiovasc. Surg., 104:593, 1992.

Krieger, J. N., Kaiser, D. L., and Wenzel, R. P.: Nosocomial urinary tract infections cause wound infections postoperatively in surgical patients. Surg. Gynecol. Obstet., 156:313, 1983.

Levine, D. P., Fromm, B. S., and Reddy, B. R.: Slow response to vancomycin or vancomycin plus rifampin in methicillin-resistant Staphylococcus aureus endocarditis. Ann. Intern. Med., 115:674, 1991.

Lowry, P. W., Blankenship, R. J., Gridley, W., et al.: A cluster of Legionella sternal wound infections due to postoperative topical exposure to contaminated tap water. N. Engl. J. Med., 324:104, 1991.

Maki, D. G., Bohn, M. J., Stolz, S. M., et al.: Comparative study of cefazolin, cefamandole, and vancomycin for surgical prophylaxis in cardiac and vascular operations. A double-blind randomized trial. J. Thorac. Cardiovasc. Surg., 104:1423, 1992.

McDermott, W., and Rogers, D. E.: Social ramifications of control of microbial disease. Johns Hopkins Med. J., 151:302, 1982.

Meleney, F. L.: The present status of antibiotics in surgery. Surg. Clin. North Am., 36:273, 1956.

Meszaros, R., Windisch, M., Koltai, C., and Lukacs, L.: Comparative study of cefamandole versus cephalothin as antibiotic prophylaxis for open heart surgery. Cor Vasa, 28:61, 1986.

Miedzinski, L. J., Callaghan, J. C., Fanning, E. A., et al.: Antimicrobial prophylaxis for open heart operations. Ann. Thorac. Surg., 50:800, 1990.

Miholic, J., Hudec, M., Domanig, E., et al.: Risk factors for severe bacterial infections after valve replacement and aortocoronary bypass operations: Analysis of 246 cases by logistic regression. Ann. Thorac. Surg., 40:224, 1985.

Muers, M. F., Arnold, A. G., and Sleight, P.: Prophylactic antibiotics for cardiac pacemaker implantation: A prospective trial. Br. Heart J., 46:539, 1981.

Myerowitz, P. D., Caswell, K., Lindsay, W. G., and Nicoloff, D. M.: Antibiotic prophylaxis for open heart surgery. J. Thorac. Cardiovasc. Surg., 73:625, 1977.

Nagachinta, T., Stephens, M., and Reitz, B.: Risk factors for surgical wound infection following cardiac surgery. J. Infect. Dis., 156:967, 1987.

Panlilio, A. L., Culver, D. H., Gaynes, R. P., et al.: Methicillin-resistant Staphylococcus aureus in U.S. Hospitals, 1975–1991. Infect. Control Hosp. Epidemiol., 13:582, 1992.

Parr, G. V. S., and Aber, R. C.: Comparative efficacy and tolerance of cefamandole and cephalothin as prophylaxis for open heart surgery: A randomized double-blind study. J. Cardiovasc. Surg., 23:305, 1982.

Penketh, A. R. L., Wansbrough-Jones, M. H., Wright, E., et al.: Antibiotic prophylaxis for coronary artery bypass graft surgery. Lancet, 1:1500, 1985.

Platt, R., Munoz, A., Stella, J., et al.: Antibiotic prophylaxis for cardiovascular surgery: Efficacy with coronary artery bypass. Ann. Intern. Med. 101:770, 1984.

Prins, J. M., Buller, H. R., Kuijper, E. J., and Tange, R. A.: Once- versus thrice-daily gentamicin in patients with serious infections. Lancet, 341:335, 1993.

Regamey, C., Libke, R. D., Engelking, E. R., et al.: Inactivation of cefazolin, cephaloridine, and cephalothin by methicillin-sensitive and methicillin-resistant strains of *Staphylococcus aureus*. J. Infect. Dis., 132:291, 1975.

Rice, L. B., and Karchmer, A. W.: Artificial heart implantation: What limitations are imposed by infectious complications? J. A. M. A., 259:894, 1988.

Roberts, N. J., Jr., and Douglas, R. G., Jr.: Gentamicin use and *Pseudomonas* and *Serratia* resistance: Effect of a surgical prophylaxis regimen. Antimicrob. Agents Chemother., 13:214, 1978.

Root, R. K., Isturiz, R., Molavi, A., et al.: Interactions between antibiotics and human neutrophils in the killing of staphylococci. J. Clin. Invest., 67:247, 1981.

Richet, H. M., Craven, P. C., Brown, J. M., et al.: A cluster of *Rhodococcus (Gordona) bronchialis* sternal wound infections after coronary artery bypass surgery. N. Engl. J. Med., 324:109, 1991.

Rutledge, R., Applebaum, R. E., and Kim, B. J: Mediastinal infection after open heart surgery. Surgery, 97:88, 1985.

Sanchez-Ubeda, R., Fernand, E., and Rousselot, L. M.: Complication rate in general surgical cases: The value of penicillin and streptomycin as postoperative prophylaxis—A study of 511 cases. N. Engl. J. Med., 259:1045, 1958.

Sanfelippo, P. M., and Danielson, G. K.: Complications associated with median sternotomy. J. Thorac. Cardiovasc. Surg., 63:419, 1972.

Sattler, F. R., Weitekamp, M. R., and Ballard, J. O.: Potential for bleeding with the new beta-lactam antibiotics. Ann. Intern. Med., 105:924, 1986.

Sexton, D. J., Wlodaver, C., Smith, D. L , et al.: Antibiotic prophylaxis in cardiovascular surgery: Cefuroxime and cefamandole. Infect. Med., December 1987, p. 445.

Siddons, H., and Nowak, K.: Surgical complications of implanting pacemakers. Br. J. Surg., 62:929, 1975.

Slama, T. G., Sklar, S. J., Misinski, J., and Fess, S. W.: Randomized comparison of cefamandole, cefazolin, and cefuroxime prophylaxis in open heart surgery. Antimicrob. Agents Chemother., 29:744, 1986.

Slight, P. H., Gundling, K., Plotkin, S. A., et al.: A trial of vancomycin for prophylaxis of infections after neurosurgical shunts. N. Engl. J. Med., 312:921, 1985.

Stoney, W. S., Alford, W. C., Jr., Burrus, G. R., et al.: Median sternotomy dehiscence. Ann. Thorac. Surg., 26:421, 1978.

Sutherland, R. D., Martinez, H. E., Guynes, W. A., and Marier, R. L.: Antibiotics and coronary artery bypass operations: An 11-year experience. Infect. Surg., 4:585, 1985.

Sutherland, R. D., Martinez, H. E., Guynes, W. A., and Miller, L.: Postoperative chest wound infections in patients requiring coronary bypass: A controlled study evaluating prophylactic antibiotics. J. Thorac. Cardiovasc. Surg., 73:944, 1977.

Townsend, T. R., Reitz, B. A., Bilker, W. B., and Bartlett, J. G.: A clinical trial of cefamandole, cefazolin, and cefuroxime for antibiotic prophylaxis in cardiac surgery. J. Thorac. Cardiovasc. Surg., 106:664, 1993.

Vander Salm, T. J., Okike, O. N., Pasque, M. K., et al.: Reduction of sternal infection by application of topical vancomycin. J. Thorac. Cardiovasc. Surg., 98:618, 1989.

Wells, F. C., Newsom, S. W. B., and Rowlands, C.: Wound infection in cardiothoracic surgery. Lancet, 1:1209, 1983.

Whyte, W., Hambraeus, A., Laurell, G., and Hoborn, J.: The relative importance of routes and sources of wound contamination during general surgery. I. Non-airborne. J. Hosp. Infect., 18:93, 1991.

Whyte, W., Hodgson, R., and Tinkler, J.: The importance of airborne bacterial contamination of wounds. J. Hosp. Infect., 3:123, 1982.

Wood, G. L., Knapp, C. C., and Washington, J. A., II: Relationship between cefamandole and cefuroxime activity against oxacillin-resistant *Staphylococcus epidermidis* and oxacillin-resistant phenotype. Antimicrob. Agents Chemother., 31:1332, 1987.

5 Anesthesia

■ I Anesthesia and Supportive Care for Cardiothoracic Surgery

J. G. Reves, William J. Greeley, Katherine Grichnik,
John Leslie, and Bruce Leone

HISTORY

Although humankind had long seen the need for anesthesia to facilitate surgery, it was not until 1842 that Crawford Long used ether for a dental surgical procedure and 1848 that William Morton demonstrated that ether could be used successfully for surgery. It is unlikely that the surgeon and anesthesiologist of the mid-19th century could have envisioned the events that would follow over the next century and a half. Although there were many medical achievements in that time (Fig. 5–1), only a few might be considered essential in the development of anesthesia for thoracic surgery (Benumof, 1978; Kaplan, 1987). The single most important advance in thoracic anesthesia was the use of intermittent positive pressure ventilation during open chest surgery. The importance of this development was noted by the tho-

racic surgeon Matas, who reported in 1899 that "the procedure that promises the most benefit in preventing pulmonary collapse in operations on the chest is the artificial respiration by a tube in the glottis directly connected with a bellows." Despite Matas' observation and the fact that physiologists had long used endotracheal ventilation in laboratory experiments, it was not until World War II and the 1940s that the use of a laryngoscope (developed by Kirstein in 1895), a cuffed endotracheal tube (designed by Tuffier in 1895), and the forerunner of a ventilator (the Fell bellows with O'Dwyer intubating cannula, introduced in 1893) finally found common use for ventilation and anesthesia during surgery of the chest. During the 1930s, Gale and Waters in the United States and Magill in the United Kingdom emphasized the value of this technique with endotracheal intubation (using the direct laryngoscope devel-

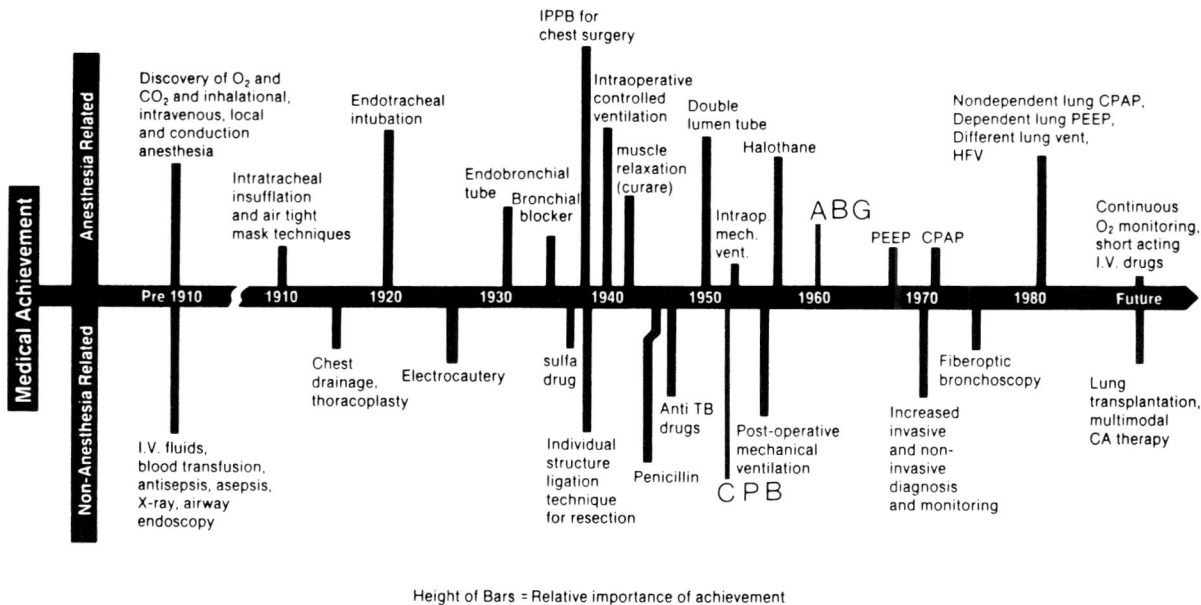

FIGURE 5–1. Evolution of modern anesthesia practice for cardiac and thoracic surgery. (ABG = arterial blood gas; CA = cancer; CPAP = continuous positive airway pressure; CPB = cardiopulmonary bypass; HFV = high-frequency ventilation; IPPB = intermittent positive-pressure breathing; I.V. = intravenous; PEEP = positive end-expiratory pressure; TB = tuberculosis.) (Modified from Benumof, J. L.: Anesthesia for Thoracic Surgery. Philadelphia, W. B. Saunders, 1987.)

117

oped by Jackson) and positive pressure ventilation, which permitted major thoracic surgical operations with an open pleural cavity.

Anesthesiologists are clinical physiologists and clinical pharmacologists; thus, progress in cardiothoracic anesthesia has been associated with the understanding of cardiopulmonary physiology and the introduction of potent new drugs. Two drugs were particularly important to the development of cardiothoracic anesthesia: curare in 1942 and halothane in 1956. With intravenous curare, anesthetists could paralyze the diaphragm, control respiration, and provide excellent operating conditions for surgeons—including the cessation of ventilation on the surgeon's request to facilitate delicate operative maneuvers. Halothane, a halogenated inhalation anesthetic, did not pose the same threat of hepatotoxicity as chloroform, nor was it explosive, as were ether and cyclopropane. Without toxicity and explosive hazards, longer and more complicated thoracic and cardiac operations could be planned, and electrocautery could be used with impunity.

Finally, important technologic advances have advanced cardiothoracic anesthesia. Among these is the ability to cannulate the radial artery and continuously monitor the systemic blood pressure as well as intermittently measure the arterial blood gases. The PO_2 electrode was developed by Clark in 1960 (Clark et al., 1960), and PO_2 measurement enabled the anesthesiologist to optimize methods of oxygenation, including such techniques as *continuous positive airway pressure* (CPAP), introduced by Gregory in 1971 (Gregory et al., 1971), and application of *positive end-expiratory pressure* (PEEP) in 1967 (Ashbaugh et al., 1967). The Severinghaus CO_2 electrode (1960) also permitted the anesthesiologist to assess the adequacy of ventilation by the direct measurement of PCO_2. The double-lumen tracheal tube devised by Carlens and Robertshaw, first used in the 1950s, permitted selective bronchial ventilation; this permitted isolation of each lung as well as deflation of a lung to facilitate surgery. The first mechanical ventilator for use during surgery was designed by Frenckner, a Swedish ear, nose, and throat surgeon, and was used initially in surgery by Crofoord in 1938. Use of postoperative ventilation was an outgrowth of the Copenhagen polio epidemic of 1952, which fostered the development of the Engstrom volume ventilator, first used for postoperative, poor-risk thoracic surgery patients in 1955 and popularized by John Gibbon in 1957. Gibbon had introduced the pump oxygenator in 1953. Although this machine revolutionized cardiac surgery, new anesthesia techniques were not required; however, electronic monitoring of the electrocardiogram (ECG) and display of cardiac and vascular pressures have greatly aided the operating team in assessing the cardiovascular status of the patient. The pulmonary artery catheter with thermodilution cardiac output capability, introduced by Swan and Ganz in 1971, gave the operating team accurate data regarding cardiac performance. These monitoring techniques permit the anesthesiologist to base selection and titration of appropriate anesthetic and vasoactive drugs for the cardiothoracic patient on physiologic and pharmacologic principles.

A critical step in the successful development of thoracic surgery has been the organization and implementation of the cardiothoracic surgical team. This concept assures the close cooperation of the various professionals required to produce optimal results. Members of this team are surgeons, anesthesiologists, perfusionists, and nurses who all work in concert, each doing his particular task, all with the common goal of superlative patient care. For the best results, each member of the team should be trained in those disciplines required of cardiothoracic subspecialists, and communication must be maintained always. The creation of heart centers, using the interdisciplinary work of subspecialists in the operating room as the model, extends this concept to improve all aspects of patient care, teaching, and research.

MONITORING

Assessment of Patients

Preoperative Evaluation

The preoperative visit and evaluation permit the surgeon and anesthesiologist to perform a thorough clinical assessment and to begin preparing the patient both physically and mentally. All patients need a current medical history and physical examination. These measures determine any pathologic or pathophysiologic conditions that may require perioperative therapy or that may alter the management plans. Not all the medical problems can be evaluated and corrected preoperatively; the surgeon and anesthesiologist must discuss the potential management problems and any need for further evaluation or interventions before beginning anesthesia or operative procedures.

From the anesthesiologist's view, patient care begins with the preoperative evaluation and preparation, follows the patient through anesthesia induction and maintenance, and continues into the postoperative period. By organizing the evaluation and management process with a specific care plan sequence, the clinician may estimate whether any of the pathologic conditions of the particular patient alter the care prescribed during the course of management. If so, appropriate interventions are made prior to the anticipated problem.

For example, a patient with severe chronic obstructive pulmonary disease and a history of congestive heart failure may require a detailed preoperative work-up of the cardiorespiratory system. The clinician is reminded to consider what preoperative tests (e.g., pulmonary function tests with and without bronchodilators, rest and exercise, multigated angiogram [MUGA] scan) or what preoperative interventions may be indicated (e.g., diuresis with potassium supplementation, antibiotics for chronic bronchitis).

The anesthesiologist also formulates treatment plans based on the need to perform tracheal intubation and extubation, positioning problems, muscle relaxation, or problems in using a particular anesthetic technique for a patient. Appropriate communication and cooperation between the anesthesiologist and surgeon will maximize patient care and facilitate expedient perioperative clinical management. The trend in more ambulatory surgery and same-day admission increases the need for coordinated evaluation and planning.

Preoperative therapy is intended to correct reversible disease processes that, if not treated, could lead to morbidity. The indicated assessments can be classified conveniently by the case-specific pathophysiology. Such an evaluation provides the clinician with a detailed assessment not only of the patient's current status but also, ideally, with an estimation of problems that may develop from pre-existing disease states or that may be complicated by the anesthetic and surgical interventions.

The best way to determine the extent of the preoperative work-up is a complete systems review. Maintenance antihypertensives, antiarrhythmics, antiseizure drugs, and antianginal medications should be continued preoperatively and reinstituted in the postoperative period. The routine prophylaxis for arrhythmias is controversial unless the patient's history confirms a high-risk situation. Many clinicians use prophylaxis for bronchospasm with continuous intravenous aminophylline infusions, but studies highlight potential problems with such therapy as well as the potential effectiveness of inhaled beta$_2$-agonists such as albuterol (Busse et al., 1986). Uncontrolled and untreated preoperative hypertension increases the amount of morbidity and mortality associated with anesthesia and operation.

Laboratory Studies

Preoperative laboratory assessment minimally requires a hemoglobin and hematocrit determination, serum creatinine and electrolytes, chest film, an ECG, and any other test necessary to provide an accurate and reasonably comprehensive assessment of the patient's disease state. If there is a history of bleeding problems or if the patient has been receiving anticoagulants or antiplatelet drugs, then further tests of the intrinsic and extrinsic coagulation cascade are needed. Abnormal values should not be dismissed as "laboratory error." An abnormality is not necessarily a reason to delay or cancel surgery unless the detected abnormality may affect patient safety and risk factors.

Airway Assessment

A significant level of anesthetic morbidity and mortality is related to airway management problems. These problems must be anticipated, and patients at risk must be identified. Thus, during the admission history and physical examination, the clinician should determine whether the patient may have a high-risk airway problem and alert the anesthesiologist so that she may perform any needed evaluations or make specific plans to manage anticipated problems. The major concerns with airway management include patients with obvious respiratory distress or obstruction requiring rapid assessment and intervention, patients with anticipated or obvious airway obstruction or respiratory distress, and patients in whom it may be difficult to place an endotracheal tube because of physiognomic or pathologic anomalies.

Airway management problems are present in patients with airway trauma, hypoxia, hypercarbia, unconsciousness, intercostal retractions, tracheal tug, significant agitation, dyspnea, or supraglottic lesions. A timely assessment of severity and appropriate therapy must be initiated. Stridor is a sign of partial airway obstruction. Dyspnea, for example, implies a markedly diminished respiratory reserve with a forced expiratory volume in 1 second (FEV$_1$) of less than 1500 ml.

The physical signs that suggest tracheal intubation problems include a short muscular neck, micrognathia, limited cervical spine or mandibular mobility, diminished distance from mandible to the thyroid notch (less than three finger breadths), protruding incisors, a high arched palate, or a narrow mouth. Mallampati described a classification to predict intubation difficulty by noting the visibility of intraoral structures when the patient maximally protrudes the tongue while in the erect position (Mallampati et al., 1985). These patients may require preoperative laryngoscopy, bronchoscopy, radiography, tomography, or pulmonary function studies.

Premedication

Sedative/anxiolytic drugs are administered to relieve anxiety and provide patients with the final preanesthetic doses of maintenance pharmacologic therapy for their underlying disease states. Anticholinergic drugs are excellent drying agents but may make patients very uncomfortable during the preoperative waiting period. The routine use of "heavy" premedication is controversial, and perhaps is best avoided by a thorough preoperative explanation designed to allay the patient's fears. An appropriate premedication is the foundation for an excellent anesthetic course.

Physiologic Monitoring

The monitoring used for a particular patient should depend on the condition of the patient and the type and extent of the surgical procedure. Modern anesthesia and surgical practice require routine monitoring of certain essential physiologic parameters, such as blood pressure, ECG, temperature, ventilation, inspired oxygen, and usually systemic arterial oxygen saturation (Barker and Tremper, 1985). Depending on the surgical procedure, these minimal monitoring requirements increase. For convenience, the various organ systems and monitoring techniques available are listed in (Fig. 5–2) and discussed later.

Neurologic System

The use of online recording of one or more channels of the electroencephalogram (EEG) is increasing. Numerous models of intraoperative EEG recorders, or cerebral function monitors, are commercially available and relatively simple to use. The proposed benefit of online continuous electroencephalographic monitoring is the early diagnosis of acute or potentially reversible brain ischemia or injury. The EEG also may be useful in detecting the level and depth of anesthesia. Loss of electroencephalographic activity should alert the clinician that an intervention is needed to prevent permanent and irreversible neurologic injury. The overall neurologic function of reflexes, pupillary size, diaphoresis, and spontaneous muscle movement may also signal *central nervous system* (CNS) activity or compromise.

Finally, specialized assessments of such variables as cerebral blood flow (CBF), cerebral blood oxygenation, near-infrared spectroscopy of intracranial hemoglobin saturation, jugular bulb oxygenation, or cerebral perfusion pressure may be used. Although such systems now are often limited to research protocols, the clinician may expect to use them online as the technology continues to improve. These growing improvements are of great importance, because neurologic problems are the last major area of morbidity associated with intrathoracic or cardiac surgery.

Cardiopulmonary System

An esophageal stethoscope provides information on the level and effectiveness of ventilation, heart sounds, and even early signs of cardiac rhythm changes. Temperature monitoring is important to detect malignant hyperthermia and to assess the effectiveness of cooling and rewarming during hypothermic cardiopulmonary bypass.

The potential for myocardial ischemia often is monitored by appropriate evaluation of ST-T wave seg-

Thoracic Surgery Perioperative Monitoring:
Instruments - Techniques - Variables

Neurologic System
Electroencephalogram
  • frequency, amplitude, spectral edge
Evoked potentials
  • auditory or visual
  • somatosensory
Routine examination
  • pupillary size/reactivity
  • diaphoresis
Specialized:
  • cerebral blood flow
  • carotid stump pressure
  • computerized tomography
  • retinal blood flow

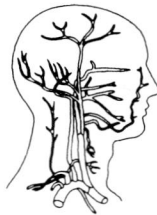

Cardiopulmonary Systems
Esophageal stethoscope
Electrocardiogram
  • ST-T wave segment analysis
  • esophageal ECG lead
Peripheral pulse oximeter
Arterial line catheter
  • blood pressure and gases
Ventilator parameters
Central venous catheter
Pulmonary artery catheter
  • pulmonary artery pressures
  • ventricular filling
  • cardiac output and venous oxygen
Transesophageal echocardiography

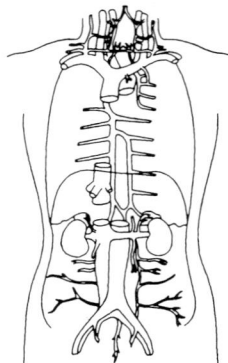

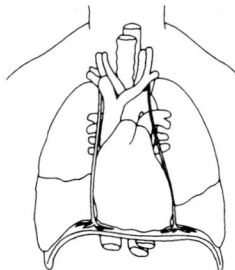

Other Organ Systems
Temperature
  • esophageal
  • rectal
  • blood
Foley catheter
  • urine output
  • osmolality/lytes
Coagulation
  • intrinsic system
  • extrinsic system
Peripheral nerve stimulator
Operative field losses
  • blood and fluids
  • nasogastric

JBL

FIGURE 5–2. The frequently used perioperative monitoring techniques are listed by the specific organ system monitored. The noninvasive and the more invasive techniques are included.

ments. This may require placement of a lateral precordial ECG lead, similar to V_5, before the sterile cleansing and draping of the patient. Because the familiar 12-lead ECG cannot be performed intraoperatively, it may be difficult to make electroencephalographic rhythm diagnoses without the aid of an esophageal lead (Greeley and Reves, 1988). This lead also may be used for temporary pacing.

The finger pulse oximeter is a simple device that provides beat-to-beat information on systemic arterial oxygen saturation, which is valuable on a real-time basis. This level of monitoring is indicated in all patients undergoing intrathoracic surgical procedures. It does not obviate the need for continuous intra-arterial pressure monitoring or for periodic arterial blood gas analysis.

Ventilation monitoring is important in thoracic surgery to provide information about abnormal physiology or to guide potential interventions to improve oxygenation. Changes in peak airway pressure, tidal volume, expiratory time, and minute ventilation may be early warnings of abnormal, but correctable, cardiopulmonary physiology. These variables, which usually are connected to pressure-sensing alarm systems during operations, may further warn of ventilation disconnection, endotracheal tube kinking, and partial or total obstruction.

The placement of a central venous catheter or a flow-directed pulmonary artery (PA) catheter is indicated for high-risk patients or for accurate assessment of the cardiovascular system during surgery. The recent incorporation of mixed venous oxygen saturation (MV_{O_2}) as an online variable also might be valuable. Normally, the mixed venous blood is 75% saturated, with a P_{O_2} of 40 to 50 mm Hg. Values below 60% saturation provide early detection of cardiac decompensation, acidosis, reduced oxygen-carrying capacity, light anesthesia or excessive "stress," and possible cellular injury. Excessively high levels of MV_{O_2} may warn of sepsis, physiologic or anatomic shunting, hypothermia, or a wedged catheter. Pulse oximeter and MV_{O_2} values also aid in determining the optimal level of PEEP and obviate the need for frequent blood-gas analysis during weaning from ventilatory support (Fahey and Harris, 1984). Not only do PA catheters provide the physiologic database listed in Figure 5–2, they also may be used perioperatively as temporary pacing catheters, provide a means of diagnosing physiologic or anatomic shunts, and help preload and afterload assessments.

Transesophageal or epicardial echocardiography may be used as an intraoperative monitor (deBruijn and Clements, 1987). Intraoperative echocardiography aids in evaluation of myocardial performance, valvular status, regional myocardial function, anatomic shunting, and intrachamber air or venting success. This minimally invasive technology is increasing in applicability, and may become an integral part of the monitoring of selected patients undergoing intrathoracic or major vascular surgery.

Other Organ Systems

As previously mentioned, the body temperature must be assessed continuously for numerous reasons.

The renal system also must be monitored, because the current mortality rate from perioperative renal failure in the surgical setting approaches 80%. Every effort must be made to assess renal function, and any alterations in renal function must be determined rapidly and treated, if possible. The coagulation system must be assessed preoperatively if there is historical evidence of potential abnormality or if the patient has been treated with anticoagulants. The various components of the intrinsic and extrinsic pathway are well known and will serve to direct the clinician's therapy.

Monitoring the Pediatric Patient

Standard monitoring for pediatric patients undergoing cardiac surgery is similar to that in adult patients. This includes a continuous ECG, an esophageal stethoscope, temperature measurement (usually of the esophagus and rectum), an automated blood pressure cuff, and pulse oximetry. Standard invasive monitoring usually includes direct arterial pressure monitoring from an arterial catheter, usually from a radial, ulnar, or femoral artery site. Also, a central venous pressure catheter is placed percutaneously into the internal or external jugular vein, providing central venous pressure measurement and a potential route for the continuous infusion of potent vasoactive substances. In general, the above-mentioned invasive and noninvasive monitoring is usually employed in most pediatric open heart cases, because the benefits clearly exceed the risks. The routine use of invasive monitoring in the pediatric patient is not as extensive as in the adult, because patient size is limited and placement can be risky. For example, the routine use of a pulmonary artery catheter is difficult in young patients because of the large catheter size. When indicated, transthoracic monitoring and infusion lines can be placed intraoperatively by the surgeon directly into the pulmonary artery and the atria, and they can be brought out the chest wall. As in any anesthetic plan, monitoring at its best takes into account the individual patient's condition, operative surgery, and planned postoperative management.

Newer monitoring techniques used in adults also are being applied in pediatric patients. These techniques include the use of an esophageal ECG lead for dysrhythmia analysis (Greeley and Reves, 1988), intraoperative echocardiography with color flow imaging assessing cardiac function and quality of repair (Ungerleider et al., 1987), the thromboelastogram for assessment of blood coagulation changes after bypass (Greeley et al., 1986), the use of continuous online processed EEG, and the measurement of CBF (Greeley et al., 1988). The usefulness of these new monitoring techniques and their effects on outcome have been demonstrated.

Complications

Invasive monitoring provides valuable and useful physiologic data that help the clinician provide minute-to-minute management of the patient, but these monitoring modalities have risks. Complications from arterial cannulation are usually related to low-flow states, chronic cannulation, or thrombogenesis. The size and type of catheter materials are important, as are frequent observations and the use of potential alternative arterial cannulation sites (Bedford, 1977). The most frequent complications from central venous or PA catheterization are vessel injury, pneumothorax, hemothorax, nerve injury, and hematoma. There are reports of fatal perforation of the pulmonary artery with these catheters, but complications should not dissuade the physician from using these monitoring modalities if the patient's condition warrants. Many complications can be prevented by careful attention to proper techniques during insertion of the catheter (Kaye, 1983; Matthay, 1983).

PHARMACOLOGY OF ANESTHETIC DRUGS

A variety of drugs may be used to provide anesthesia. Anesthesia groups include intravenous, inhalation, local, and muscle relaxants. With general anesthesia, the objective is to provide unconsciousness, analgesia, amnesia, and usually muscle relaxation.

Intravenous Anesthetic Drugs

Intravenous anesthetic drugs are used to induce and maintain general anesthesia, and some are employed postoperatively for sedation and analgesia. Many drugs are available. The anesthetist must know the pharmacology of these diverse compounds, whereas the surgeon should be familiar with some aspects of the pharmacology of these drugs. Knowledge of the primary CNS actions, the cardiovascular pharmacology, and the pharmacokinetics guides the selection of a drug in a particular patient. Because these drugs are given for particular actions, this section will group the drugs according to their primary indication.

Hypnosis (Unconsciousness)

Drugs that produce sleep are hypnotics. Among the most commonly used hypnotics in anesthesia are thiopental, midazolam, diazepam, etomidate, propofol, and ketamine. Except for ketamine, none of these drugs produce analgesia, so they must be given with other analgesic drugs to produce satisfactory anesthesia. They also are devoid of muscle paralysis properties, and therefore must be supplemented with neuromuscular blocking drugs if muscle relaxation is required. Benzodiazepines (diazepam, lorazepam, and midazolam) are very specific amnestic drugs: They produce dose-related amnesia, which can persist for many hours after administration. In general, hypnotics produce a dose-related effect on the CNS that reflects the plasma/brain equilibrium; however, there is wide interindividual variation in the dose-response

relationship. Benzodiazepines can be antagonized with flumazenil (Dunton et al., 1988).

Analgesia

Analgesic drugs block pain stimuli and thereby protect against the physiologic responses to noxious stimuli and other stresses. Opioids such as morphine, meperidine, fentanyl, sufentanil, alfentanil, and other similar compounds maintain analgesia during surgery and are used sometimes in cardiac surgery to induce anesthesia. As anesthetic drugs, the opioids are not reliable hypnotics or amnestics; therefore, they require supplementation with hypnotics or inhalation anesthetics. Like the hypnotics, there is a wide interindividual dose-response with opioids, as well as a ceiling effect in some patients (giving more drug does not produce greater analgesic effect).

Cardiovascular Pharmacology

Each drug has a particular cardiovascular profile. However, the hemodynamic effect of a drug depends on several factors: the drug per se, the patient's cardiovascular status (disease as well as condition), and concurrent pharmacologic therapy (Reves and Gelman, 1985). Table 5–1 lists the more relevant hemodynamic actions of commonly used intravenous anesthetic drugs. Thiopental is the most widely used hypnotic in the world, and in well-compensated patients with lung or cardiac disease, it is very safe. Its principal hemodynamic effect is a decrease in contractility, which is due to reduced availability of calcium to the myofibrils (Seltzer et al., 1980; Sonntag et al., 1975). To compensate for the slight decrease in blood pressure after thiopental, there is usually a small reflex increase in the heart rate. The benzodiazepines and opioids are not negative inotropes and are frequently used in patients with compromised cardiac function. Interestingly, when opioids and benzodiazepines are given together they can produce hypotension (Tomicheck et al., 1983), which does not occur when each is administered alone even in large doses (Lunn et al., 1979; Samuelson et al., 1981). Morphine was the first opioid to be used in high doses for cardiac anesthesia in patients with valvular heart disease (Lowenstein et al., 1969). Because of the histamine release and resultant hypotension, however, fentanyl replaced morphine as the most commonly used narcotic analgesia in cardiac anesthesia (Lunn et al., 1979). Ketamine is unique among these intravenous anesthetics, because it tends to produce a hyperdynamic hemodynamic response that is mediated by a sympathetic nervous system release of endogenous catecholamines (Zsigmond et al., 1974).

Pharmacokinetics and Drug Disposition

A drug is eliminated from the blood by redistribution and biotransformation. Major factors that are important in determining the pharmacokinetic fate of drugs are the tissue solubility of the drug and the

■ **Table 5–1.** HEMODYNAMIC EFFECTS OF ANESTHETIC DRUGS

Drug	Cardiac Index	Blood Pressure	Systemic Vascular Resistance	Heart Rate	Contractility
Diazepam	↔	↓	↓	↔	↔
Enflurane*	↓	↓	↓	↑	↓
Etomidate	↑	↔	↓	↑	↓
Fentanyl	↔	↔	↔	↓	↔
Halothane*	↓	↓	↔	↔	↓
Isoflurane*	↔	↓	↓	↑	↓
Ketamine	↑	↑	↑	↑	↔
Midazolam	↔	↓	↓	↔	↓
Morphine	↔	↓	↓	↔	↓
Propofol	↔	↓	↓	↔	↔↓
Sufentanil	↔	↔	↔	↓	↔
Thiopental	↓	↓	↑	↑	↓

Key: ↔ = no change; ↓ = decrease; ↑ = increase; ↔↓ = no change or decrease.
*Inhalation agents.

hepatic and renal metabolism (clearance) of the particular drug. The termination of an intravenous anesthetic drug action after a single bolus administration is due to the distribution of the drug from the blood and well-perfused tissues, such as the brain, to other less well-perfused tissues, such as muscle and fat (Brodie et al., 1950). Thus, 5 to 10 minutes after the administration of thiopental, a patient will begin to awaken if anesthesia is not maintained by repeated administration or with other anesthetic drugs. Drugs with high tissue solubility will disappear from the blood rapidly and have a short context-sensitive half-time (time for drug level to decrease by 50%) (Hughes et al., 1992). The context-sensitive half-time increases for each drug with the duration of infusion (Fig. 5–3). This information is necessary in choosing a drug as well as in anticipating the need for redosing and estimating awakening. Drugs with short half-times are used for short operations, whereas those with long half-times are more appropriate for longer surgical procedures or for prolonged sedation postoperatively. Pharmacokinetic data are also used to calculate continuous drug infusions either manually (Sprigge et al., 1982; Wagner, 1974) or by the simpler use of a computer-controlled infusion pump (Alvis et al., 1985; Jacobs, 1990; Theil et al., 1993). Intravenous anesthetic drugs should be given via continuous infusion during cardiac surgery to maintain adequate anesthetic depth (Theil et al., 1993).

Inhalation Drugs

Uptake and Distribution

The inhalation anesthetics rely on the respiratory tract for entry and elimination from the body. Although the precise mechanism for the action of inhalation agents is not completely understood, it is clear that the primary site of action is within the CNS (Eger, 1974). Thus, an adequate partial pressure of anesthetic in the brain is required for surgery. The brain and other tissues in the body tend to equilibrate with the partial pressure of the anesthetic drug delivered to them by arterial blood. The partial pressure of the inhalation drug in blood, in turn, is determined

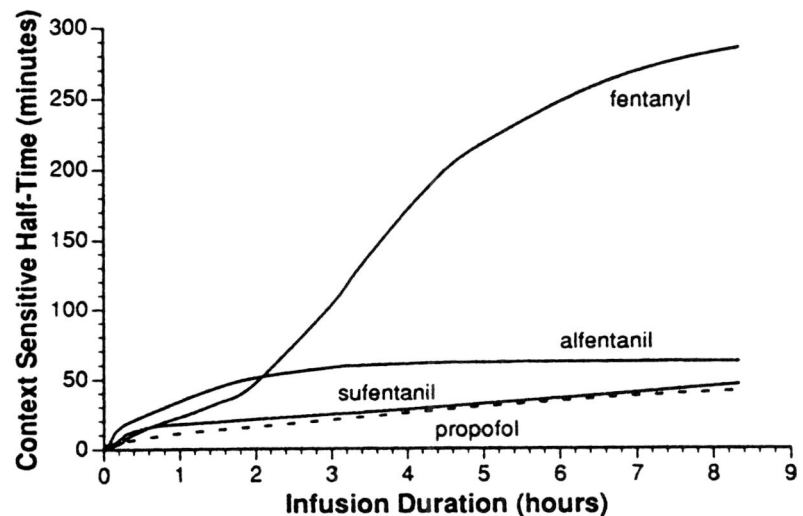

FIGURE 5–3. Context-sensitive half-times computed from simulation of three-compartment pharmacokinetic models for alfentanil, fentanyl, and sufentanil. Half-times for propofol are shown for comparison. (From Hughes, M., Jacobs, J., Glass, P.: Context sensitive half-time in multi-compartment pharmacokinetic models for intravenous anesthetic drugs. Anesthesiology, 76:334–341, 1992.)

by the alveolar partial pressure. Because the alveolar partial pressure governs the partial pressure of anesthetic in all body tissues, including the brain, the relationship between inspired and alveolar anesthetic partial pressures is an important first step in producing an anesthetic state (Eger, 1974).

Two factors determine the rate at which alveolar anesthetic tension rises toward the concentration of the anesthetic being inspired: First, increasing the inspired tension of the anesthetic will directly increase delivery of the drug and increase alveolar anesthetic tension; second, increasing the minute ventilation promotes increased alveolar anesthetic tension. Additional factors influence the level of alveolar anesthetic tension and, ultimately, general anesthesia. Decreased removal of anesthetic agent by the blood promotes an increase in alveolar anesthetic tension and a greater anesthetic effect. Decreased removal may derive from a decrease in cardiac output, a decrease in alveolar-venous anesthetic gradient, or a decrease in solubility of the specific anesthetic agent. Conversely, increased cardiac output, use of a very soluble agent, or a large alveolar-venous anesthetic gradient will promote increased removal of drug into the bloodstream, limiting the alveolar anesthetic tension buildup. Under the latter conditions, production of an anesthetic effect will be delayed.

The factors that govern the rate at which alveolar anesthetic concentration rises during the induction of anesthesia also affect the emergence from anesthesia. Recovery from anesthesia results from the elimination of the anesthetic from the brain by reversing the pressure gradient. The anesthetic agent is removed by the differential gradient from brain to blood to alveoli created by reducing the inspired concentration to zero. As ventilation reduces the concentration of anesthetic from alveoli, an anesthetic partial pressure gradient develops from the returning venous blood to the alveoli. This gradient drives the anesthetic into the alveoli, where it can be removed. Ultimately, this reversal of gradient decreases brain concentration of the anesthetic agent and permits recovery (Eger, 1974). The induction, maintenance, and recovery from inhalational anesthesia is, therefore, relatively rapidly controlled by alterations in the inspired concentration of the specific gas.

Pharmacodynamics

As with the intravenous anesthetic drugs, it is important to assess the anesthetic potency of the inhalation agents. The concept of *minimal alveolar concentration* (MAC) was developed as an index of anesthetic potency; this index facilitates the comparison of pharmacodynamic properties of all the inhalation anesthetic agents (Eger, 1974). MAC is the anesthetic concentration at 1 atmosphere of pressure that produces immobility to a noxious stimulus in 50% of subjects. This concept is analogous to the ED_{50}—the effective dose in 50% of subjects for any drug. Because MAC is measured at equilibrium between inspired and alveolar concentrations, the alveolar concentration and

brain partial pressures are assumed to be equal. Therefore, MAC represents the anesthetic concentration at the anesthetic site of action. Based on measurements of MAC, patient susceptibility to inhalation anesthetics is not altered significantly by gender, duration of anesthesia, metabolic alkalosis or acidosis, respiratory acidosis, anemia, or hypertension (Eger, 1974). However, increased susceptibility to anesthetic effects occurs with hypercarbia, hypoxemia, increasing age, decreasing body temperature, and exposure to other CNS depressants (Eger, 1974). Specifically, opioids, benzodiazepines, and the barbiturates decrease the amount of inhalation anesthetic required, because they have added depressant effects on the CNS. The ultimate clinical criterion for appropriate anesthetic depth is the patient's unique response to the balance between anesthetic-induced CNS depression and surgical stimulation.

Metabolism

All the potent inhalation anesthetic agents undergo some biotransformation in the liver by the microsomal enzymes (Cohen et al., 1970). However, unlike the intravenous anesthetics, the importance of metabolism to recovery from inhalation drugs is minimal. Under normal circumstances, the biotransformation of these agents is minimal and safe, because an oxidative reaction produces nontoxic, inert metabolites. However, the development of hepatic necrosis after the administration of halothane, enflurane, or isoflurane may depend on the chance combination of such events as genetic background, exposure to other drugs, reduced hepatic blood flow or hypoxia, the dose or molecular structure of the agent, and certain physiochemical properties promoting retention of anesthetic in tissues (Bunker et al., 1969).

Specific Inhalation Anesthetics

Contemporary inhalation anesthesia involves four drugs: the volatile liquids halothane, enflurane, and isoflurane, and the inert gas nitrous oxide (N_2O). Sevoflurane and desflurane are new volatile anesthetics, and their place in thoracic anesthesia is not established. The addition of fluoride to the aliphatic hydrocarbons has rendered the volatile liquids nonflammable. The physical properties of these anesthetic gases determine how they are supplied, influence the systems involved in their administration, and, most important, influence their uptake and distribution in the body. The laws of physics governing diffusion, solubility, differential partial pressures, and temperature are the basis for the differences in pharmacologic effects and clinical use of these anesthetics.

Cardiovascular Pharmacology

Each inhalation anesthetic has a specific cardiovascular profile (Table 5–1). As with the intravenous agents, their hemodynamic effects depend on the drug per se, the cardiovascular status of the patient, and concurrent pharmacologic therapy. Unlike the situation with intravenous drugs, cardiovascular effects of the inhalation agents are more similar to one another than they are different. The inhalation anesthetics often alter cardiac output and blood flow. All the inhalation agents exert a direct, dose-dependent negative inotropic effect on the myocardium (Brown and Crout, 1971; Merin, 1981; Price and Price, 1962). Between individual agents there are small differences in the degree of myocardial depression, as well as differences in the mechanism of myocardial contractility suppression. In general, halothane and enflurane reduce cardiac output to a greater degree than does isoflurane in healthy patients. The depressant effects of the volatile anesthetics on myocardial contractility in diseased states such as ischemic heart disease are additive (Mallow et al., 1976). Age, diseased myocardium, premedication, and adjuvant drugs also are important additive depressant factors. Halothane has minimal effect on the heart rate, whereas isoflurane and enflurane are associated with increased heart rate (Eger, 1981). Halothane, enflurane, and isoflurane produce relaxation of smooth muscle in the wall of blood vessels throughout the systemic vasculature (Venugopal et al., 1973). They influence the cerebral circulation both directly and indirectly. Halothane and enflurane cause cerebral vasodilation. Isoflurane also causes cerebral vasodilation (Eger, 1981), although this effect may be blunted by prior hyperventilation. Indirectly, these potent inhalation agents produce cerebral vasodilation by promoting increases in carbon dioxide secondary to hypoventilation. Isoflurane dilates coronary arteries to a greater extent than do enflurane and halothane. Isoflurane, halothane, and enflurane all reduce splanchnic and renal blood flow (Venugopal et al., 1973). The latter effects largely can explain the reductions in glomerular filtration rate that have been reported during anesthesia. Finally, all the potent anesthetic agents dilate skin and muscle blood vessels and reduce thermoregulatory control (Venugopal et al., 1973).

Muscle Relaxants

The clinical use of neuromuscular blocking drugs began in 1932 with the administration of D-tubocurarine to help control muscle spasms in patients with tetanus (West, 1932). Muscle relaxants now are administered to facilitate endotracheal intubation, to provide the surgeon with optimal working conditions during anesthesia, and to optimize mechanical ventilator support in some patients. Because the neuromuscular blockers do not produce analgesia, sedation, or amnesia, they cannot substitute for other supportive care in the potentially conscious patient. Muscle paralysis should not be performed without sedation or general anesthesia.

Mechanism of Action and Classification

The drugs are classified as either *depolarizing* or *nondepolarizing*, depending on their mechanism of blockade. A depolarizing neuromuscular blocker mimics the neural transmitter, acetylcholine, and produces sustained membrane permeability changes that prevent further depolarization of the postsynaptic membrane until the drug dissipates. Onset of muscle paralysis is very rapid. The nondepolarizing blockers compete with acetylcholine for the nicotinic cholinergic receptors; thus, nondepolarizing muscle relaxants are competitive antagonists that prevent acetylcholine binding and subsequent depolarization. Because of the relative excess of receptors, however, more than 70% of them must be blocked before there is clinically significant muscle weakness. The onset of nondepolarizers is slow compared with that of depolarizers, often requiring more than 5 minutes for the full paralyzing effect. These relaxants also exhibit characteristic responses to electrical nerve stimulation: diminished twitch response, fade during tetany, post-tetanic potentiation, and reversibility with anticholinesterases.

Administration Guidelines

Succinylcholine, the prototypic depolarizing neuromuscular blocker, is metabolized principally by plasma cholinesterase. The rate of metabolism of succinylcholine is reduced by a loss of effective hydrolysis enzyme in severe liver disease due to genetically atypical plasma cholinesterase. This may lead to unexpected prolongation in neuromuscular blockade. Because of this and other potential side effects (bradycardia, hypotension, dysrhythmias, hyperkalemia, postoperative myalgia, increased intracranial pressure, malignant hyperthermia), succinylcholine is not recommended for routine use except during anesthetic induction and in specific clinical situations.

The nondepolarizing blockers undergo hepatic and/or renal degradation leading to their elimination and the return of muscle function. Many factors can alter drug distribution, metabolism, and elimination, leading to potentially wide variability in dosing requirements and cautions. These include renal disease, hepatic disease, protein binding, age, temperature, and concomitant drugs. Table 5–2 lists commonly used relaxants and their frequently recommended doses.

Specific drugs may have advantages and/or disadvantages as relaxants when compared with each other. The major differences between the nondepolarizers relate to length of duration of blockade (intermediate vs. long-acting), the mechanism(s) of metabolism and clearance, and the autonomic side effects (tachycardia, hypotension, vagolytic). Pancuronium provides an excellent, long-acting state of muscle relaxation but may increase heart rate, especially if administered rapidly or in large doses. Atracurium has a unique mechanism of metabolism—Hoffman degradation—that occurs at a predictable in vivo rate

■ Table 5–2. NEUROMUSCULAR BLOCKING DRUG PHARMACOLOGY AND DOSING

Drug	Initial Dose (mg/kg)	Expected Duration (min)
Depolarizer		
Succinylcholine	1–1.5	3–5
Nondepolarizer		
D-Tubocurarine	0.5	60–90
Pancuronium	0.07–0.1	45–90
Atracurium	0.2–0.4	30–45
Vecuronium	0.1–0.2	30–45
Mivacurium	0.1–0.3	8–10
Pipecuronium	0.05–0.15	80 + *
Doxacurium	0.04–0.06	80 + *

*Follow neuromuscular blockade depth with twitch monitor.

such that clearance of the drug is unaltered even in the presence of severe hepatic or renal disease (Stenlake et al., 1983). Vecuronium has the lowest autonomic side effect profile and produces little hemodynamic alteration even with doses significantly larger than the recommended amounts (Morris et al., 1983). Atracurium and vecuronium may also be administered by continuous intravenous infusion (Shanks, 1986).

Neuromuscular Blocker Reversal

Depolarizing relaxants cannot be pharmacologically reversed. Patients with a genetic deficiency of plasma cholinesterase and others who experience a prolonged effect may improve with intravenous enzyme administration through a plasma transfusion. This is generally not recommended over appropriate sedation and support, including assisted ventilation, until the drug is metabolized by the postsynaptic membrane-bound enzyme.

The nondepolarizing relaxants can be reversed once the patient has recovered partial neuromuscular function. Anticholinesterase drugs (e.g., neostigmine, physostigmine, pyridostigmine, edrophonium) inhibit the acetylcholinesterase enzyme and permit accumulation of the acetylcholine at the postsynaptic junction. Acetylcholine competitively displaces residual nondepolarizing muscle relaxants. Potential problems in routine reversal of nondepolarizer drugs may complicate the clinical situation. Anticholinesterases also increase ganglionic neural transmission, thus necessitating the usual concomitant administration of an anticholinergic drug. The dose or duration of action of the competitive reversal agent may be shorter than the duration of the muscle relaxant, causing unexpected postreversal weakness and potential muscle paralysis. Properly administered and monitored, however, nondepolarizing relaxants and reversal agents can provide well-planned periods of optimal surgical relaxation (Shanks, 1986).

Local Anesthetics

Cocaine, the first drug used as a topical ophthalmic anesthetic, was administered by Koller in 1884. Halsted used cocaine to produce peripheral nerve blocks and spinal anesthesia for surgery. Procaine was the first synthetic local anesthesia, and lidocaine was synthesized in 1943. The local anesthetics are widely used to provide anesthesia for localized surgical procedures as well as to produce regional anesthesia (spinal, epidural, caudal, field block, intravenous, or Bier block). Their specific membrane-altering properties also make many drugs with local anesthetic properties useful for the treatment of cardiac dysrhythmias. Local anesthetics must be deposited near the neural conductive tissue to produce effective blockade of pain and/or motor and autonomic fibers. The drugs also have potentially lethal side effects if administered improperly or in excessive doses (Kendig, 1985).

Similar to the neuromuscular blocking drugs, local anesthetics interfere with neural transmission to produce their effects, though by different mechanisms. Local anesthetics reversibly block nerve conduction by decreasing the rate of depolarization. These drugs produce no permanent structural damage to neural tissue and can produce both sensory and motor block. Subsequent recovery of conduction occurs spontaneously. Onset of block requires diffusion across the lipid nerve membrane by the nonionized form of the drug. The local anesthetic's main site of action is within this lipid nerve membrane, where it inhibits transmission of nerve impulses by reducing sodium membrane permeability and the displacement of ionized calcium. Thus, the threshold potential for depolarization activation is not reached, and an action potential is not conducted. The duration of action of a local anesthetic is proportional to the time it is in direct contact with the nerve fiber.

All local anesthetics consist of a hydrophobic region (usually an aromatic ring) and a hydrophilic region (usually a tertiary amine), separated by an intermediate alkyl chain. The bond of the alkyl chain with the aromatic ring is either an ester (-CO-) or an amide bond (-NHC-). Thus, these drugs are classified as esters or amides depending on their linkage. Local anesthetics are themselves weak bases, which are poorly water-soluble and are therefore marketed as water-soluble, acidic, hydrochloride salts (pH 6). All local anesthetics except cocaine produce peripheral vasodilation by direct relaxation of vascular smooth muscle. Epinephrine (1:200,000) often is added to local anesthetic solutions (pH 4) to produce local vasoconstriction, reduce systemic drug absorption, and thus maintain a high drug concentration at the injection site. Carbonated local anesthetic solutions (pH 6.5) are preferred by some groups who believe that the onset of blockade with such solutions is more rapid and intense (Bromage et al., 1967). The properties of local anesthetics are determined by their lipid solubility (potency), pKa (onset time), and protein binding (duration) (Table 5–3).

There are important differences in the pathways of drug metabolism between the two classes of local anesthetics as well as differences in their potentials for producing allergic reactions and other side effects. Ester local anesthetics are metabolized by plasma cho-

■ **Table 5–3.** LOCAL ANESTHETIC PHARMACOLOGY AND DOSAGE

Drug (Generic)	Common Trade Name	Relative Potency	Duration (Minutes)	Maximal Single Dose (mg/kg)	pKa	Nonionized at pH 7.4 (%)	Protein Binding (%)
Esters							
Chloroprocaine	Nesacaine	4	30–60	10	8.7	5	(Unknown)
Procaine	Novocaine	1 (Standard)	45–60	7	8.9	3	6
Tetracaine	Pontocaine	16	120–480	2	8.5	7	76
Amides							
Bupivacaine	Marcaine	4	180–480	2	8.1	15	95
Ropivacaine*		<4	180–480	2.5	8	20	94
Etidocaine	Duranest	4	180–480	4	7.7	33	94
Lidocaine	Xylocaine	1 (Standard)	90–180	6	7.9	25	70
Mepivacaine	Carbocaine	1	90–180	5	7.6	39	77
Prilocaine	Citanest	1	90–180	5	7.9	24	55

Modified from Covino, B. G., and Vassallo, H. L.: Local Anesthetics: Mechanisms of Action and Clinical Use. New York, Grune & Stratton, 1976.
*Ropivacaine is a new local anesthetic—see text.

linesterase with *p*-amino benzoic acid as a metabolite. Esters therefore are more likely to produce allergic reactions than are amide local anesthetics. Amides are metabolized in the liver to multiple metabolites, none of which are particularly allergenic. However, preservative agents (e.g., methylparaben) may be added to ester or amide local anesthetics, which may cause allergic reactions. Allergy from local anesthetics generally remains a rare event.

Administration Guidelines

The onset of anesthesia after injection of a local anesthetic depends on site of injection, dose, concentration, characteristics of the drug, protein binding, and blood supply of the area (Covino and Vassallo, 1976). Acidosis at the site of injection causes a greater portion of the drug to become ionized and less diffusible across cell membranes. This is consistent with the observation of poor conduction analgesia produced in an area of infection and tissue acidosis.

Local anesthetic toxicity arises through a relative or absolute overdose of the drug resulting from inadvertent intravascular injection or from excessive intravascular absorption of local anesthetic from its injection site. Local anesthetic toxicity produces both CNS and cardiovascular system toxicity (Covino, 1992). Fortunately, the toxicity of local anesthetics is progressive, with CNS toxicity occurring well before cardiac toxicity. CNS toxicity is easier to treat and is usually without sequelae. Exceptions to this progression of events include the sedated patient in whom signs of CNS toxicity may be masked, and the use of bupivacaine, which has a very quick progression from CNS to CVS toxicity. The signs and symptoms of local anesthetic toxicity are shown in Table 5–4. CNS toxicity is manifested by lightheadedness, tinnitus, and circumoral numbness leading to seizures. Concurrently there may be signs of sympathetic nervous system activation as the result of increased cerebral activity.

With further increases in plasma local anesthetic concentration, signs of cardiovascular toxicity occur. Local anesthetics affect the cardiac electrical system, the myocardium, and the peripheral vascular smooth muscle. Cardiac electrical effects include increases in the ratio of the effective refractory period to the action potential duration, prolonged PR and QRS intervals, atrioventricular (AV)-nodal dysrhythmias, and, ultimately, sinus bradycardia and arrest. The mechanical effect of local anesthetics on cardiac muscle is negative inotropy, which is directly related to potency. Further, local anesthetics can cause arteriolar vasodilation. Bupivacaine is the local anesthetic most often associated with irreversible toxicity. Bupivacaine is a "fast-in, slow-out" drug that binds avidly to cardiac tissue. Bupivacaine toxicity causes an increased incidence of ventricular arrhythmias. Cardiopulmonary resuscitation from bupivacaine toxicity is extremely difficult; it may take supranormal doses of catecholamines and atropine or even cardiopulmonary bypass to treat it effectively. Ropivacaine is a new local anesthetic that is not yet clinically available. Ropivacaine is similar to bupivacaine but has less cardiac toxicity (Moller and Covino, 1990; Scott et al., 1989). The recommended doses of local anesthetics are given in Table 5–3. Dosages should be based on site of injection, use of vasoconstrictors, co-morbidity, and volume of drug necessary. Local anesthetic toxicity can be prevented by having a relatively alert patient who can report onset of symptoms, fractionating doses, aspirating for heme, and carefully placing the needle. Treatment of local anesthetic toxicity involves

■ **Table 5–4.** SIGNS AND SYMPTOMS OF LOCAL ANESTHETIC TOXICITY SYMPTOMS

Plasma Concentration	Mild	Severe
Low ↓ High	Lightheadedness Dizziness Tinnitus Circumoral numbness Disorientation Increased PR interval Decreased cardiac output Decreased blood pressure	Tremors Muscle twitching Unconsciousness Seizures Increased QRS interval Sinus bradycardia Severe hypotension Atrioventricular block Asystole

securing an airway and establishing ventilation. Seizures may be treated with benzodiazepines or barbiturates. Cardiovascular toxicity can be treated with catecholamines, atropine, and bretylium as necessary.

INTRAOPERATIVE MANAGEMENT OF SELECTED THORACIC PROCEDURES

The principles of intraoperative management of thoracic surgical procedures are based on an understanding of the pathophysiology of each disease process and the knowledge of the effects of various anesthetic and other pharmacologic interventions on the particular patient's condition.

Ischemic Heart Disease

Pathophysiology

The heart becomes ischemic and loses function when it is deprived of oxygen. Although ischemic heart disease has many causes, the most common is atherosclerosis, which diminishes oxygen supply over time. Acute ischemia from decreased or absent flow can be caused by local hyperreactivity of vascular smooth muscle (dynamic stenosis or spasm), thrombosis (platelet activation), plaque fissuring, and abnormal arachidonic acid metabolism (Brown et al., 1984; Conti and Mehta, 1987; Maseri et al., 1986). Ischemia can also result from increased oxygen demand in the presence of compromised supply. The primary determinants of myocardial oxygen consumption are heart rate, contractility, and wall tension (Sarnoff et al., 1958; Sonnenblick and Skelton, 1971). Oxygen supply depends primarily on adequate oxygen-carrying capacity of the blood and maintenance of coronary blood flow. When ischemia occurs, myocardial function is lost almost immediately; if not corrected, it can lead to worsened function, arrhythmias, infarction, and death. Intraoperatively, myocardial ischemia occurs very commonly in patients with coronary artery disease but is associated with hemodynamic perturbations in only about 50% of patients who manifest ST ischemia changes during operation (Slogoff and Keats, 1985, 1986). This suggests that factors other than a simple hemodynamic imbalance are responsible for ischemia. The single most useful predictor of ischemia is tachycardia (Slogoff and Keats, 1988), but the worst hemodynamic profile is hypotension with tachycardia (Mauney et al., 1970), because hypotension lowers the perfusion pressure and tachycardia increases oxygen consumption while reducing the time of coronary flow in diastole. Myocardial infarction occurs in about 8% of patients with ischemic heart disease who develop ST changes during cardiac (Slogoff and Keats, 1988) and noncardiac (Roy et al., 1979) procedures. *Perioperative myocardial infarction* (PMI) is a serious complication (London and Mangano, 1987), particularly in noncardiac operations, because it carries a high mortality rate, ranging from 28 to 68%.

Patient Assessment

Because of the significant implications of PMI, it is imperative that patients at risk for ischemia be identified, particularly for noncardiac surgical procedures in which myocardial revascularization will not be accomplished. Patients at greatest risk of acute ischemia and PMI are patients with advanced age, recent infarction, unstable angina, diabetes mellitus, ventricular arrhythmia, congestive heart failure, and thoracic surgery (Cheitlin, 1988; Eagle et al., 1987; Goldman et al., 1978; London and Mangano, 1987; Steen et al., 1978; Tarhan et al., 1972). In addition to the usual studies (such as 12-lead ECG), a relatively new nuclear cardiology test, the dipyridamole-thallium scan, seems to be useful in identifying which patients are at greatest risk of ischemia and might need coronary arteriography and/or some coronary revascularization procedure before operation. Patients who have undergone a previous coronary artery surgical bypass procedure and who require noncardiac operations are at less risk than those who have not undergone the surgical revascularization procedure (Mahar et al., 1978).

Intraoperative Management

Optimal anesthetic management of patients with ischemic heart disease maintains the appropriate oxygen supply-demand relationship. First, this involves maintaining patients on their preoperative antianginal therapy, which generally includes beta-adrenergic blockers, nitrates, and/or calcium entry blockers. These drugs should be administered in the usual dose on the day of operation. During anesthesia, care is taken to avoid anemia, hypoxia, hypotension, and tachycardia (Table 5–5). Choice of a particular anesthetic agent is less important when monitoring is appropriate and the physiologic guidelines are observed. If myocardial ischemia occurs during the operation, treatment is indicated immediately. Figure 5–4 depicts a treatment algorithm of myocardial ischemia. Treatment is based primarily on the hemodynamic setting, presuming that this reflects the underlying cause. These recommendations are based on pharmacologic studies demonstrating, for example, the vasodilating properties of nitroglycerin. Because anesthesia reduces the work of the heart while increasing oxygen-carrying capacity, it can be considered a myocardial protective strategy (Maccioli and Reves, 1988). However, the emergence from anesthesia and the immediate postoperative period are not safe times for patients because pain, fever, and other physiologic imbalances, which probably include a hypercoagulable state, create the setting in which myocardial ischemia and infarction are likely to occur. This is why most perioperative myocardial infarctions in noncardiac surgical patients occur not during surgery but during the first 3 postoperative days (London and Mangano, 1987; Tarhan et al., 1972).

◘ Table 5–5. PRINCIPLES OF INTRAOPERATIVE MANAGEMENT FOR ADULT CARDIAC DISEASE

	Heart Rate	Rhythm	Preload	Afterload	Contractility	Anesthetic Choice
Aortic insufficiency	Normal or slight increase	Sinus	Elevated usually (not a major)	Reduce	Maintain or increase	Balanced anesthesia with perhaps isoflurane or narcotic with pancuronium (avoid increases in afterload)
Aortic stenosis	Normal (70–80) (avoid tachycardia and bradycardia)	Sinus is essential	Increase or maintain	Maintain; do not decrease	Maintain	Any anesthesia that does not greatly alter heart rate, rhythm, and preload
Cardiac tamponade	Increased (80–100)	Sinus	Increase (avoid decreases)	Maintain	Increase	Ketamine, etomidate, narcotic (avoid dilators and depressants)
Coronary artery disease	Decreased (50–80)	Sinus	Normal	Normal	Decrease	Any anesthetic regimen that optimizes oxygen supply or demand to the heart
Dilated congestive cardiomyopathy	Increased (avoid tachycardia)	Sinus if possible	Maintain or increase	Decrease slightly	Increase	Ketamine, etomidate, midazolam, narcotic (avoid agents that decrease heart rate, contractility, and preload)
Hypertrophic cardiomyopathy	Normal (avoid tachycardia, bracycardia)	Sinus is essential	Maintain or increase	Maintain	Decrease	Thiopental, any of the inhalational drugs (carefully maintain preload)
Mitral insufficiency	Normal to slight increase	Usually atrial fibrillation (be sure digitalized)	Maintain	Reduce (will improve cardiac output)	Maintain or increase	Any anesthesia that avoids increases in afterload and profound myocardial depression
Mitral stenosis	Normal (avoid tachycardia)	Sinus, if possible; atrial fibrillation is frequent (be sure digitalized)	Maintain or increase	Maintain	Maintain	Any anesthetic drugs that keep heart rate and preload normal
Transplanted heart	Denervated (manipulation of heart rate requires pacing)	Sinus	Essential to maintain (avoid decreases)	Maintain or slightly decrease	Maintain or increase	Ketamine, etomidate, midazolam, or narcotic (avoid negative inotropic drugs; use vasodilators cautiously)

Cardiac Tamponade

Pathophysiology

There are many causes of cardiac tamponade, both acute (e.g., trauma or postoperative hemorrhage) and chronic (e.g., metabolic disorders). Blood or fluid accumulates in the pericardial sac in patients with pericardial tamponade. The pericardial sac is a nondistensible envelopment of the heart, and as pressure builds in it, ventricular diastolic pressure increases, thus decreasing the *atrioventricular* (AV) *valve* pressure gradient and causing a premature closure of the AV valve. This causes decreased ventricular filling and a decrease in *stroke volume* (SV). With a decrease in SV, a circular series of events begins: a decrease in cardiac output, hypotension with resultant myocardial hypoperfusion, and further decreased SV because of myocardial ischemia. If this series is not interrupted, death results.

Patient Assessment

The patient with significant cardiac tamponade has tachycardia, elevated jugular venous pressure, a narrow arterial pulse pressure ($\leq$ 30 mm Hg), and usually equalization of left and right atrial pressures. Often present are a paradoxic pulse, Kussmaul's sign, distant heart sounds, and a pericardial rub. In managing the patient, the clinician must ensure that intravenous access is adequate for administration of fluid. Findings of low blood pressure or shock require immediate intervention. Shock is a life-threatening emergency in patients with cardiac tamponade.

Intraoperative Management

The key to successful anesthetic management is to maintain the central venous pressure, SV, *heart rate* (HR), and myocardial contractility (see Table 5–5). In the presence of significant hypotension, pericardio-

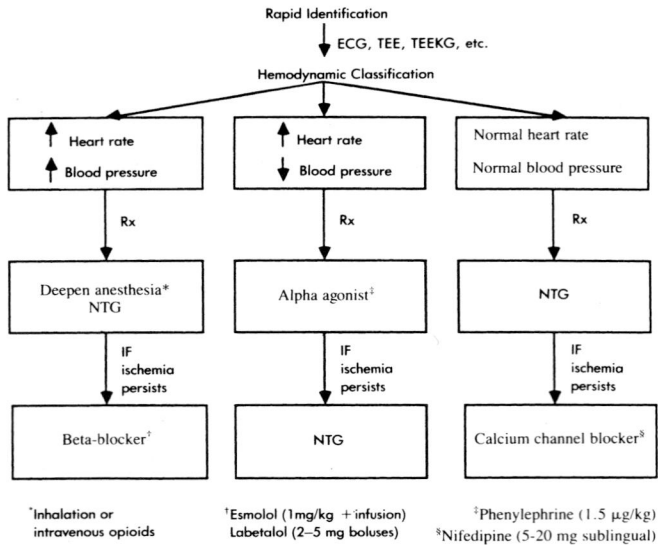

Rapid Identification
↓ ECG, TEE, TEEKG, etc.
Hemodynamic Classification

↑ Heart rate ↑ Blood pressure	↑ Heart rate ↓ Blood pressure	Normal heart rate Normal blood pressure
Rx	Rx	Rx
Deepen anesthesia* NTG	Alpha agonist‡	NTG
IF ischemia persists	IF ischemia persists	IF ischemia persists
Beta-blocker†	NTG	Calcium channel blocker§

*Inhalation or intravenous opioids

†Esmolol (1mg/kg + infusion) Labetalol (2–5 mg boluses)

‡Phenylephrine (1.5 μg/kg)
§Nifedipine (5-20 mg sublingual)

FIGURE 5–4. Treatment algorithm for myocardial ischemia based on the hemodynamic classification of the ischemia. Identification of ischemia is made by electrocardiography (ECG), transesophageal echocardiography (TEE), or transesophageal electrocardiography (TEEKG). (Rx = treatment; NTG = nitroglycerin.)

centesis should be performed before the induction of anesthesia. Ketamine or etomidate with pancuronium is useful; anesthesia may be maintained with any analgesics that do not reduce preload. Except in constrictive pericarditis, the cardiac output immediately improves with pericardiotomy, and any anesthetic technique may be employed at that time.

Aortic Stenosis

Pathophysiology

Aortic stenosis usually is either rheumatic or congenital bicuspid valve disease that progressively becomes calcific and obstructive. The primary pathology is obstruction to *left ventricular ejection*. An increased pressure overload of the left ventricle (LV) ensues, with an increase in left ventricular mass (concentric hypertrophy). This anatomic change reduces ventricular contractility and compliance. To maintain left ventricular diastolic filling and SV, the small thick-walled LV chamber depends on adequate blood volume and an effective and well-timed *left atrial contraction*. The hypertrophied LV is extremely vulnerable to ischemia because of increased myocardial oxygen consumption (greater pressure workload) as well as decreased coronary blood flow (increased left ventricular wall tension). If coronary artery disease is also present, as is frequently the case, ischemia is common. Late changes in aortic stenosis include decreased left ventricular contractility with dilation and, ultimately, a decrease in SV and *cardiac output* (CO).

Preoperative Evaluation

Typically the patient is about 50 years old, with recent onset of symptoms of fatigue and dyspnea on exertion. The triad of angina, syncope, and congestive heart failure signifies severe disease. Impaired renal and hepatic function indicate low CO. When evaluating the patient, the ECG should be examined carefully to note the rhythm and presence of junctional bradycardia, premature ventricular contractions (PVCs), and intraventricular conduction defects. The best indicator of severity of aortic stenosis is the calculated valve area that is obtained at cardiac catheterization (normal is 2.6 to 3.5 cm², and operative candidates usually are at < 0.75 cm²). The cardiac index, HR, and pressure measurements should also be examined in interpreting the valve area, because they influence the calculations. An ejection fraction of less than 50% indicates impairment of myocardial contractility. The LV-aorta gradient is not a very reliable measure of the severity of aortic stenosis, because ventricular function affects it (e.g., if a patient has poor left ventricular function, the LV-aortic gradient may be 20 to 30 mm Hg).

Intraoperative Management

HR of 70 to 80 bpm is optimal for patients with aortic stenosis (see Table 5–5). Faster HR may be desirable in maintaining CO, but tachycardia predisposes to ischemia because it increases myocardial oxygen consumption (MV$_{O2}$) and reduces the time of diastolic perfusion of the thick-walled LV. Sinus rhythm is essential because the hypertrophied LV obtains up to 40% of its diastolic filling from the atrial contribution (the atrial contribution to normal LV filling is only about 20%). Maintenance of preload is essential, because the noncompliant LV requires a high left ventricular pressure for adequate left ventricular volume. Hypotension can seriously jeopardize myocardial blood flow. After valve replacement, while the patient is still on cardiopulmonary bypass, maintenance of perfusion pressure is essential to reperfuse the thick-walled LV. Arrhythmias during reperfusion are common and are amenable to lidocaine and adequate (70 to 90 mm Hg) perfusion pressure. Postoperative hypertension is often a problem in patients with aortic stenosis.

Aortic Insufficiency

Pathophysiology

Aortic insufficiency, unlike stenosis, has multiple etiologies (aortic root disease, aortitis, intrinsic valve disease, and subvalvular causes). Chronic aortic insufficiency causes left ventricular volume overload with resultant increased myocardial fiber length and left ventricular volume. The CO is maintained at a relatively low MV$_{O2}$ (in contrast to the high MV$_{O2}$ used with aortic stenosis) early in the disease process. With time, the left ventricular wall tension increases, as does the mass, producing a noncompliant and less contractile LV and ultimately increased left atrial pressure, decreased SV, and a decrease in CO. The increased left ventricular volume and pressure create signs and symptoms of pulmonary venous hypertension. Acute aortic insufficiency is poorly tolerated compared with chronic aortic insufficiency. With acute aortic insufficiency, the pulmonary venous and arterial pressures are elevated, and the *right ventricle* (RV) cannot handle the sudden increase in work.

Preoperative Evaluation

Chronic aortic insufficiency can be tolerated well for years, but once failure occurs, the survival rate declines rapidly. It is important to distinguish chronic from acute aortic insufficiency. Cardiomegaly and a wide pulse pressure are commonly observed with chronic insufficiency, whereas signs and symptoms of pulmonary venous hypertension and a narrow pulse pressure are associated with acute insufficiency. In clinical assessment of the patient with aortic insufficiency, normal blood pressure may mean severe insufficiency and low CO. The severity of aortic insufficiency may be judged best by angiographic criteria. If 60% of SV is regurgitated back to the LV, then there is severe regurgitation. Other important data from the catheter are pulmonary artery wedge, *pulmonary arterial*, and *right atrial* pressures to determine the degree of right heart involvement. The patient with acute aortic regurgitation may need immediate operation.

Intraoperative Management

Maintaining HR in the normal range of 80 to 90 bpm reduces LV size and maintains SV (see Table 5–5). Bradycardia leads to left ventricular distention, increased wall tension, and MV_{O2} predisposing to ventricular arrhythmias and ischemic damage. Supraventricular arrhythmias are tolerated better by patients with aortic insufficiency than by those with aortic stenosis. Afterload is important in aortic insufficiency, and slightly decreasing afterload augments forward flow (CO). The LV in aortic insufficiency is very compliant compared with the noncompliant LV in aortic stenosis; therefore, when one measures filling pressures, relatively large changes in left ventricular volume may be reflected by small changes in mean left atrial or pulmonary arterial pressures. An anesthetic technique using perhaps isoflurane or a high-dose narcotic with pancuronium may be desirable in patients with aortic insufficiency. Avoidance of increases in afterload (hypertension) is the most important aspect of the anesthetic management. In acute aortic insufficiency, the failing RV often is the limiting factor in successful management.

Mitral Stenosis

Pathophysiology

Mitral stenosis (MS) usually results from rheumatic heart disease. The primary physiologic problem is obstruction of the mitral valve with impairment of left atrial emptying, which causes decreases in left ventricular filling. Increases in left atrial pressure also increase pulmonary venous pressure and cause perivascular edema and airway narrowing in the lungs with a decrease in pulmonary compliance and an increase in work of breathing. The pulmonary arterial pressure usually is elevated, and CO is decreased. End-stage mitral stenosis involves development of severe pulmonary arterial hypertension with an increase in pulmonary vascular resistance, which decreases after operation in many cases. In severe cases, right ventricular overload occurs, and there is low CO with left and right ventricular failure. In patients with long-standing mitral stenosis, intimal changes occur in pulmonary arteries and veins, so that pulmonary arterial resistance may remain elevated postoperatively.

Preoperative Evaluation

The optimal time for operation of mitral stenosis is before progressive debility occurs in the final two decades of life. Most patients are in *atrial fibrillation* (AF), and a rapid ventricular response to AF should be controlled throughout the perioperative period. As with aortic stenosis, valve pressure gradients may be deceptive and highly dependent on flow (cardiac function) and HR. The normal valve area is 4 to 6 cm^2, and valve areas less than or equal to 2.5 cm^2 produce symptoms that are severe at or below 1.0 cm^2. If the patient with MS is treated with excessive diuretic therapy, intraoperative volume replacement will be greater than anticipated. Signs and symptoms of pulmonary venous hypertension and right ventricular heart failure should be sought, because right ventricular function may be important in determining outcome.

Intraoperative Management

When SV is fixed, as it is with MS, CO is a function of HR. The optimal HR for patients with MS is 60 to 80 bpm, and because most are in AF, maintaining this HR depends on adequate digitalization (see Table 5–5). Intubation and other stresses during operation in inadequately digitalized patients increase HR. Ventricular response increases with intubation regardless of muscle relaxant; however, higher digoxin levels attenuate this response. Preload needs to be maintained or increased, but the left atrial pressure or pulmonary arterial wedge pressure do not reflect *left ventricular end-diastolic pressure* (LVEDP) in mitral stenosis. Because performance of the RV is important in MS, monitoring right atrial pressure and pulmonary arterial pressures is useful. The anesthetic of choice for patients with MS may be a high-dose narcotic or any other anesthetic technique that keeps HR and preload normal. Alpha-adrenergic agents should be avoided, because they may increase pulmonary vascular resistance and precipitate RV failure. After bypass, the pulmonary vascular resistance usually decreases, but when it does not, the RV may require inotropic support. Isoproterenol or dobutamine are of theoretical advantage, because they may decrease pulmonary arterial resistance. Avoid conditions that increase pulmonary vascular resistance, such as hypoxemia, hypercarbia, acidosis, hypothermia, and release of endogenous catecholamines.

Mitral Insufficiency

Pathophysiology

Mitral regurgitation, like aortic insufficiency, has multiple etiologies. Chronic regurgitation produces volume overloading of the LV and LA as in aortic insufficiency. Left ventricular and left atrial dilation occur rather than hypertrophy. The left atrial size and compliance dictate the level of pulmonary venous hypertension. If the process is chronic, left atrial and left ventricular enlargement is slow, and early in the course, right ventricular function may be maintained. However, with acute volume overloading (e.g., secondary to papillary muscle dysfunction or ruptured chordae tendineae), severe pulmonary arterial hypertension ensues with right ventricular failure.

Preoperative Evaluation

The optimal timing for operation of chronic mitral regurgitation usually follows decades of disease, but should take place before heart failure occurs, because such failure heralds a rapid decline in survival rate. With acute mitral regurgitation, immediate operation is usually warranted. Chronic mitral regurgitation should be differentiated from the acute kind. Chronic mitral regurgitation's signs and symptoms of pulmonary venous hypertension may not correlate with severity of disease. Acute mitral regurgitation often is associated with coronary artery disease and may be life-threatening, with low CO and pulmonary venous hypertension. Most patients have large central circulating blood volumes; preoperative assessment should center on the degree of pulmonary and right ventricular involvement. Patients with mitral regurgitation are generally in AF, so the adequacy of digitalization needs to be assessed. Assessment of left ventricular ejection fraction will identify those patients with chronic mitral regurgitation with a poorly compliant LV who are at high risk for anesthesia and operation. Assessment of the pulmonary arterial pressure and resistance will signify the degree of potential right heart stress, and an elevated right atrial pressure suggests right ventricular dysfunction.

Intraoperative Management

It is desirable to maintain a normal to slightly increased HR in the patient with mitral regurgitation (see Table 5–5). Afterload reduction is useful in improving CO in most patients. Preload should be maintained, as should contractility. Any anesthetic that avoids increases in afterload and profound myocardial depression is suitable for use in patients with mitral regurgitation. The LV may fail after bypass, because it is faced with significantly greater afterload (before mitral prosthesis placement, the LV was unloaded through the incompetent mitral valve). In such cases, therapy should be designed to reduce afterload and increase contractility, usually with vasodilators and positive inotropic drugs.

Hypertrophic Cardiomyopathy

Pathophysiology

Hypertrophic cardiomyopathy is also referred to as *idiopathic hypertrophic subaortic stenosis* (IHSS) or asymmetric septal hypertrophy. The incidence is not known, but many sudden deaths are attributed to IHSS among the young of both sexes. The major feature of IHSS is thickened and bizarrely arrayed muscle in the intraventricular septum and free wall of the LV. The result is decreased left ventricular compliance, diminished diastolic filling, obstruction to left ventricular outflow, and increased myocardial oxygen requirements. In symptomatic patients with obstructive IHSS, the LVEDP may increase with some left ventricular dilation. Ultimately, the LV may fail, or arrhythmias may occur.

Preoperative Evaluation

Clinical signs of failure, such as dyspnea or inadequate myocardial oxygenation reflected by angina, are important to elicit in the history. Other signs of severe disease are dizziness and arrhythmias. The degree of hydration is important to ascertain, as is what drugs the patient is taking, such as beta-adrenergic antagonists or calcium entry blockers. Catheterization data may not be particularly useful in documenting the severity of left ventricular obstruction, because IHSS is a "dynamic" disease, and LV-arterial gradients are variable. Severity of disease is much better documented by the symptoms listed earlier.

Intraoperative Management

Heavy sedation before induction prevents excitement and the release of endogenous catecholamines that may precipitate severe reduction in cardiac output. Anesthetic management is designed to avoid tachycardia, which limits left ventricular filling. Reductions in preload must be avoided. Anesthesia may be induced rapidly with thiopental and maintained with inhalation drugs in doses that do not decrease preload but do diminish contractility. It is important to maintain sinus rhythm, because the atrial contribution to ventricular filling is vital. If preload is reduced or tachycardia occurs during anesthesia, the obstruction will worsen, and SV will be severely reduced.

Dilated Congestive Cardiomyopathy

Pathophysiology

Dilated congestive cardiomyopathy is the most common form of cardiomyopathy. It occurs worldwide in persons of all races but predominates in men of middle age. That it is frequently called idiopathic indicates that the origin often is not known. The fundamental pathology is that both ventricles lose their contractile properties and dilate. The earliest compensatory response is an increase in ventricular volume and HR. HR increases are more effective in augmenting the reduced CO than are increases in preload. Ultimately, LVEDP and right ventricular end-diastolic pressure (RVEDP) rise with resultant increases in left atrial and right atrial pressures and signs of biventricular failure. The cardiac dilation that occurs increases wall tension; with further reduction of CO, the heart is unable to meet its increased metabolic requirement for oxygen, and it fails.

Preoperative Evaluation

Ejection fractions usually range from 10 to 20%. Symptoms of left and right heart failure are present. Right heart failure usually causes anasarca and passive hepatic congestion. Notation of liver function, including clotting abnormalities, is important. Medical therapy needs to be evaluated, especially the requirement for either positive inotropic or vasodilator drugs. These patients usually present for emergency cardiac transplantation surgery.

Intraoperative Management

Premedication should be light. Induction is accomplished best with an agent that does not decrease HR or contractility (e.g., ketamine or etomidate) and should be maintained with drugs that, besides maintaining HR and contractility, avoid decreases in preload. Inotropic and vasodilator drugs may be used to optimize CO; however, caution with vasodilators is required, because preload may be excessively decreased.

Transplanted Heart

The transplanted heart is a form of acquired heart disease. Usually, it is placed in a patient with a long history of cardiomyopathy. The unique feature of the transplanted heart is that it lacks sympathetic and parasympathetic innervation. The denervated heart relies on circulating catecholamines, as well as appropriate preload and afterload, to maintain CO. Whereas the normal heart adjusts HR to augment CO, this is impossible or delayed in the denervated heart. Management of the denervated heart consists of optimizing the preload and afterload to improve CO. It is desirable to pace the heart if epicardial or endocardial wires are present. Alternatively, exogenous catecholamines may be used to increase contractility and HR; apparently, the denervated heart is "suprasensitive" to catecholamines (Yusuf et al., 1987), so that greater response to beta-agonists may be expected. Transplant patients requiring anesthesia should receive anesthetic drugs that maintain contractility, HR, and preload. Pacing the heart at a desirable rate is a useful therapeutic modality but not always feasible.

Adult Thoracic Procedures

Pulmonary Resection

From the preoperative assessment of the patient, it is important to determine whether the patient has adequate pulmonary reserve to survive after the resection. Most patients undergoing pulmonary resections should undergo pulmonary function tests with and without bronchodilators, as well as arterial blood gas analysis. Any pulmonary, cardiac, nutritional, or other major system disorder that may be improved preoperatively must be treated appropriately. Patients who have undergone extensive pulmonary lobectomies or pneumonectomies require further testing (Banoub and Nugent, 1993). First, arterial blood gas (ABG) and routine pulmonary function tests need to be examined. High-risk results ($PA_{CO_2} > 45$, $FEV_1 < 2$ l, $FVC > 50\%$ predicted, FEV_1/FVC ratio $< 50\%$) require further testing with flow-volume loops and split-function tests. Flow-volume loops can help to differentiate intrathoracic from extrathoracic airway obstruction. Split-function tests allow one to determine the proportion of ventilation and perfusion to each lung. If the predicted postoperative FEV_1 (preoperative $FEV_1 \times$ percentage of perfusion to remaining postoperative lung) is less than 800 ml, then a third tier of pulmonary function tests is needed. A pulmonary artery catheterization and occlusion can mimic postoperative conditions and determine whether the patient will tolerate them. Predictors of a poor outcome include a rise in the mean pulmonary arterial pressure to greater than 40 mm Hg, a rise in the PA_{CO_2} to greater than 60 mm Hg, and a decrease in the PA_{O_2} to less than 40 mm Hg. The cardiovascular system also must be assessed for evidence of pulmonary hypertension, right ventricular hypertrophy, bundle branch block, and cor pulmonale.

Appropriate bronchodilators, including the inhaled beta$_2$-agonist albuterol, are often used perioperatively. Mucolytics, steroids, antibiotics, chest physiotherapy, diuretics, digitalis, and pulmonary vasodilators may be indicated for some patients preoperatively. The anesthetic technique and drug selection for the anesthesia should attempt to minimize ventilation-perfusion ($\dot{V}/\dot{Q}$) mismatching. A double-lumen tube used for one-lung anesthesia is common and recommended for most resections. (See "One-Lung Ventilation," later in this chapter).

The trachea should be extubated as soon as possible after the operation, ideally in the operating room. This will minimize the need for sedatives, minimize continued tracheal damage, permit better humidification, and avoid accidental higher peak airway pressures if the patient coughs as the ventilator is delivering peak flows. Further, positive pressure on the surgical suture lines is avoided. If postoperative ventilatory support is needed, the double-lumen tube should be changed to a standard single-lumen tube, unless it is appropriate to continue one-lung ventilation. This minimizes airway resistances, improves suctioning capabilities, and decreases airway trauma by the smaller mass tube. Beware of changing the endotracheal tube without a back-up plan; many patients who had normal airways at the beginning of an operation have abnormal airways after an operation secondary to swelling, positioning, and trauma.

Esophageal and Major Vascular Procedures

Esophageal and major vascular procedures in the thorax often require double-lumen endotracheal tube placement and one-lung ventilation. These are complicated procedures in patients with significant co-morbid disease. Such possible events as aortic clamping during thoracic aneurysm surgery and retraction of the heart during esophageal surgery must be anticipated and planned for. Further, our usual monitoring devices may not be appropriate, such as an esophageal stethoscope for esophageal surgery or a left radial arterial line for procedures near the aortic arch.

Thymectomy

The major anesthetic concerns relate to the loss of muscle strength and function as a result of myasthenia gravis. Despite preoperative anticholinesterase therapy and dialysis, the patient's pulmonary reserve is often critically low. Preoperative indications for postoperative ventilation include co-existing chronic obstructive pulmonary disease, pyridostigmine dose of greater than 750 mg/day, disease older than 6 years, and FVC of less than 2.9 l (Leventhal et al., 1980). It is debatable whether to treat a patient with anticholinergics on the morning of surgery. Many anesthesiologists advocate withholding medication and then using no neuromuscular blockade for the surgery. Alternatively, neuromuscular blockade agents can be used but should be titrated carefully, using starting doses as low as 10% of a normal dose. The patient usually is left intubated in the immediate postoperative period until the anesthesiologist, surgeon, and neurologist are confident that the patient will be able to maintain the needed pulmonary workload. Respiratory parameters and muscle strength must be assessed frequently even after the patient is extubated. Pulse oximetry and an intensive care setting may be continued for several days postoperatively as an early warning of a decline in arterial oxygenation.

Pacemaker Insertion

Many of these procedures do not require a general anesthetic. The term *anesthesia standby* is a misnomer.

The anesthesiologist is actively managing the patient and providing full anesthetic care, including monitoring, positioning, resuscitation, analgesia, and sedation. The patient is simply not medicated to the level classified as a general anesthetic, although the anesthesiologist is always prepared for this possibility. During pacemaker insertion, it is important to determine and document that the electrocardiographic tracings create an effective cardiac contraction and pulse pressure wave. This information may be detected by the finger pulse oximeter, palpation of the carotid pulse by the anesthesiologist, and blood pressure measurements. The careful recording of lead thresholds and maintenance of the patient during "nonpaced" periods also are important aspects of anesthesia for such procedures.

Lung Transplantation

With advances in techniques to avoid graft rejection and improved surgical technique, lung transplantation has become a viable alternative to death from end-stage chronic obstructive pulmonary disease (COPD), pulmonary fibrosis, cystic fibrosis, and many other pulmonary diseases. Lung transplantation requires coordination and cooperation among many professionals, including surgeons, anesthesiologists, pulmonologists, and intensivists. The anesthesia for a lung transplant is challenging, requiring a thorough knowledge of cardiopulmonary physiology. These patients are extremely ill and probably unsuitable for a general anesthetic used for any other surgical procedure. Because some patients with poor pulmonary reserve may not tolerate PA clamping, cardiopulmonary bypass must be available for emergency use. Transesophageal echocardiography (in addition to full invasive monitoring) may be useful to assess the function of the heart when the graft is in place. These patients often require complex manipulations of ventilation to prevent hypoxia and multiple vasoactive drugs to maintain systemic pressure with acceptable pulmonary artery pressures.

One-Lung Ventilation

The success and safety of the anesthetic one-lung ventilation technique have progressed significantly because of improvements in catheter design, the use of the bronchoscope, and elucidation of the physiologic changes in ventilation, pulmonary perfusion, and gas exchange that occur during one-lung ventilation. The original double-lumen endotracheal tube was designed by Carlens (Carlens, 1949) to insert into the left main stem bronchus. It has a carinal hook to aid in positioning the tube at the appropriate level. Problems in placement skills, trauma from the carinal hook, suctioning port size, and other difficulties led to the development of modern double-lumen catheters, which are easier to use and more efficient. These catheters bear the names of their developers: the White tube (a right-sided Carlens) and the Robertshaw tube (available either left- or right-sided without the carinal hooks). Figure 5–5A depicts the Carlens tube, and Figure 5–5B depicts a modern left-sided endobronchial catheter.

TECHNIQUE

The patient is often placed in the lateral decubitus position for many of the thoracic surgical procedures when one-lung ventilation is performed. This position places the nondependent lung in the operative field, and it becomes the nonventilated, collapsed, and atelectatic lung during the procedure. One-lung ventilation, therefore, is the delivery of ventilation only to the gravitationally dependent, downward lung ("down-lung"), which is not in the upper operative field. Because the nonventilated and atelectatic lung still receives pulmonary blood flow from the right ventricle, the initiation of one-lung ventilation produces an obligate right-to-left intrapulmonary shunt.

Three techniques can provide ventilation to only one lung. First, a conventional single-lumen endotracheal tube can be placed down either the left or right main stem bronchus by advancing the tube past the tracheal bifurcation. This positioning may be performed "blindly," with limited success in intubating the desired bronchus, or it may be performed with near 100% success by using the bronchoscope through the endotracheal tube. The major difficulties with routine use of this technique are occlusion and nonventilation of the right upper lobe bronchus by the tube cuff if inserted into the right main stem bronchus, the need to position the tube with bronchoscopy at a critical point in the operation with the patient positioned under the drapes, and the inability to suction the nonventilated lung, permitting cross-contamination when the tube is withdrawn. However, in an emergency, or if the need for one-lung ventilation develops intraoperatively, this technique may be the most expedient and practical.

The second technique uses specific endobronchial blockers or occluders to obstruct ventilation to one of the lungs. The bronchial blockers, Fogarty and similar catheters, are inserted with the bronchoscope and left in place, with a single-lumen endotracheal tube positioned in the standard midtracheal location. At the time of desired one-lung ventilation, the catheter balloon can be inflated to occlusion. The major problems have been malpositioning of the catheters, inability to suction the collapsed lung, and the significant time and skill required to place the catheters.

The third and most frequently practiced technique uses a specially designed double-lumen endotracheal tube, as depicted in Figure 5–5B. The two separate lumens permit isolated ventilation of each main bronchus, isolation of the lungs for suctioning, and even differential ventilation techniques (e.g., flow, gases, PEEP) for the two lungs at the same time. The modern disposable tubes have thinner walls, larger lumens, and special ports for maintaining right upper lobe ventilation with right-sided tube insertion.

Many physicians avoid potential obstruction or hypoventilation of the right upper lobe by using only left-sided tubes. During a left pneumonectomy, for example, the clinician simply pulls the tube back into the tracheal lumen immediately before cross-clamping the left main stem bronchus. The largest catheter that will pass easily through the larynx and vocal cords is usually inserted, thus maximizing suctioning catheter size and minimizing ventilation gas flow resistances. The catheter must be of the proper diameter so as not to damage the trachea or larynx. Of numerous techniques utilized to position the catheters properly, the most reliable is direct visualization with the ventilating bronchoscope. A pediatric bronchoscope (outer diameter, 4.5 mm) will pass down the lumen of modern double-lumen tubes (Nos. 41, 39, 37, and 35 French sizes). Proper tube placement requires sufficient air within the occluding cuffs but not enough to "herniate" over into the other bronchus and prevent proper ventilation of the other lung. If there is any concern about proper tube placement, occlusion by secretions, cuff inflation problems, or kinking, the clinician should withdraw the tube into the trachea to permit adequate bilateral ventilation and assess the situation with bronchoscopy.

CONTROL OF HYPOXIC PULMONARY VASOCONSTRICTION

The changes in the position of the patient and the necessity of anesthesia with paralysis can aggravate $\dot{V}/\dot{Q}$ mismatch (Benumof, 1983). With the patient in the supine position, there is a gradient of blood flow and ventilation from anterior to posterior, with the greatest ventilation and blood flow being relatively matched in the more dependent portions of the lung. With movement to the lateral decubitus position, the same principle applies, with the dependent lung (the nonoperative lung) receiving greater blood flow and ventilation, thus primarily preserving $\dot{V}/\dot{Q}$ matching in this position. With paralysis, anesthesia, and the onset of controlled ventilation, $\dot{V}/\dot{Q}$ mismatch is worsened because of multiple mechanisms. First, loss of diaphragmatic tone allows the diaphragm to displace abdominal contents toward the dependent lung. The mediastinal structures and positioning impinge on the dependent lung. The nondependent lung

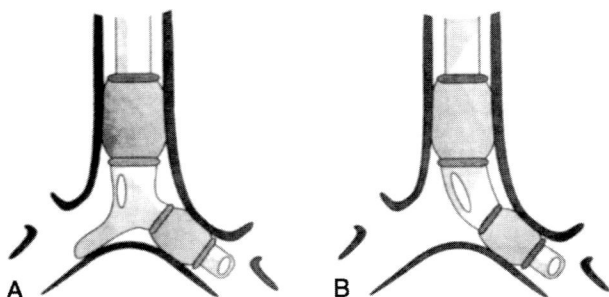

FIGURE 5–5. The proper endobronchial placement of both left- and right-sided endobronchial catheters. The early catheters were designed with carinal hooks to secure positioning at the bifurcation (A), whereas most modern catheters no longer have this hook (B), which may complicate safe and rapid placement or repositioning.

moves to a steeper portion of the compliance curve and thus receives a greater portion of the tidal volume than does the dependent lung. These factors lead to a significant $\dot{V}/\dot{Q}$ mismatch, with most of the perfusion going to the dependent lung and most of the ventilation going to the nondependent lung. Opening the chest again worsens mismatch, because the nondependent lung becomes even more compliant, and more of the ventilation is shunted to the nondependent lung. Furthermore, the diaphragmatic displacement of the dependent lung becomes maximal. When the nondependent lung is not ventilated under one-lung ventilation, an absolute shunt is created in which the portion of the pulmonary blood flow that goes to the nondependent lung is not exchanging oxygen. Control of oxygenation is achieved partially through hypoxic pulmonary vasoconstriction, with reduction in blood flow to the nondependent lung.

During one-lung anesthesia, the major reduction in blood flow to the nonventilated lung occurs as an active vasoconstrictive mechanism, *hypoxic pulmonary vasoconstriction* (HPV). The increase in pulmonary vascular resistance is a response to the atelectasis that results from nonventilation (Benumof, 1987). This selective decrease in blood flow to the nonventilated lung will decrease the pulmonary shunt fraction and potentially lessen the fall in arterial oxygenation that occurs with the initiation of one-lung ventilation. Thus, the usual measured shunt is only 25% of the CO, as opposed to the 40 to 50% expected in the absence of this reflex vasoconstriction.

INDICATIONS

There are several absolute indications for one-lung ventilation, thereby isolating the two lungs from each other. There are also other frequent indications for one-lung ventilation, and these are listed in Table 5–6. One absolute indication for one-lung isolation is to prevent spilling or cross-contamination from the diseased lung to the noninvolved lung as with an infection or from active or massive bleeding. One-lung ventilation also may be required to provide adequate ventilation in the presence of a large bronchopleural or bronchopleural cutaneous fistula and to perform unilateral lung lavage. Otherwise, all of the gas flow delivered into a standard single-lumen endotracheal tube would follow the path of minimal resistance and flow through the fistula.

The relative indications for the one-lung double-lumen tube involve improved surgical technique. Thus, the surgeon may expect better exposure for a procedure such as an upper lobectomy, a pneumonectomy, or a major thoracic aortic or esophageal surgical procedure with the nonventilated lung in the operative field. The other major benefit for the patient is that the procedure minimizes direct lung tissue trauma and further impairment of gas exchange, which will occur if the surgeon constantly must apply traction or manipulate the lung in the operative field (Anderson and Benumof, 1981). With modern double-lumen tubes, aids to placement such as fiberoptic bronchoscopy, and well-established methods to treat hypoxia, one-lung ventilation has become relatively efficacious and safe. Numerous thoracic surgical procedures benefit from one-lung ventilation.

TREATMENT OF HYPOXEMIA

The factors listed in Table 5–7 all contribute to $\dot{V}/\dot{Q}$ mismatching and an increased pulmonary shunt fraction, creating hypoxemia. All of the mechanical or position-related factors should be minimized to reduce the $\dot{V}/\dot{Q}$ mismatch problem. The inhibition of HPV occurs with the administration of systemic vasodilators such as nitroprusside, nitroglycerin, beta$_2$-agonists, and calcium channel blockers. Interestingly, vasoconstrictors increase the dependent ventilated lung pulmonary vascular resistance, and thus may increase the flow to the atelectatic lung. The remaining factors in Table 5–7 have also been shown to influence the shunt fraction but are not as significant as HPV itself.

If one-lung ventilation is initiated and the arterial oxygenation declines to an unsatisfactory level (PA_{O_2} < 70 mm Hg), the anesthesiologist must attempt to minimize the $\dot{V}/\dot{Q}$ abnormality. The inspired oxygen should be increased to 100% (FI_{O_2} 1.0), tube positioning should be confirmed (especially right upper lobe ventilation if appropriate), and the patency of the endobronchial tube lumen should be proven. The inspiratory tidal volume should be adjusted to approximately 10 ml/kg, the respiratory rate should maintain normocarbia, and the inspiratory/expiratory ratios should optimize flow and avoid high peak airway pressures. If needed, 5 to 10 cm H_2O of CPAP should be added selectively to the nonventilated lung. Then 5 to 10 cm H_2O of PEEP may be added to the ventilated lung and increased to 15 cm H_2O if needed. If oxygenation is still unacceptable, then the nondepen-

■ **Table 5–7.** FACTORS THAT AFFECT ONE-LUNG SHUNT FRACTION

Gravity	Vasoconstrictors
Position	Pulmonary vascular pressure
Cardiac output	Oxygen tension
Surgical manipulation/traction	Carbon dioxide tension
Preoperative $\dot{V}/\dot{Q}$ abnormalities	Airway pressures
	Infection
Anesthetic drugs	
Vasodilators	

■ **Table 5–6.** INDICATIONS FOR ONE-LUNG VENTILATION

Absolute	Relative
Pulmonary abscess	Thoracoscopy
Pulmonary hemorrhage	Pneumonectomy
Bronchopleural fistula	Upper lobectomy
Bronchopleural cutaneous fistula	Thoracic aortic surgery
Unilateral pulmonary cyst	Unilateral pulmonary emboli
Unilateral pulmonary lavage	Middle/lower lobectomy
	Esophageal surgery

dent lung must be ventilated intermittently or the one-lung ventilation technique must be discontinued. The other alternative may be to temporarily clamp the pulmonary artery of the nonventilated lung, thus eliminating most of the $\dot{V}/\dot{Q}$ mismatch. Use of the finger pulse oximeter is critical, as are frequent arterial blood gas determinations to document adequate $\dot{V}/\dot{Q}$ matching.

Pediatric Cardiac Care

Anesthetic management for pediatric cardiac surgery has improved significantly since the mid-1980s. These advances are due to a greater understanding of neonatal and pediatric medicine, better intravenous anesthetic agents and techniques, advances in monitoring, and extensive improvement in postoperative intensive care, especially respiratory therapy. The clinical and experimental data, generated primarily in pediatric intensive care units, have been especially invaluable in fostering the understanding of anesthetic management for children undergoing cardiac surgery.

The principles of anesthetic management in these patients are based on a firm understanding of the differences between adult and pediatric cardiovascular anesthesia. These differences are largely due to the immature physiologic processes of neonates and infants, the different disease states and functional consequences seen in congenital heart disease, and the complexity of surgical repair.

In general, the major organ systems of the young infant and child undergo continual developmental changes that affect physiologic function. During the first years of life, the major organ systems are immature and undergo rapid change. The cardiovascular system in the young infant differs in several developmental physiologic processes from that of the adult. In the newborn period, there is a dramatic change in blood flow patterns within the cardiovascular system (Rudolph, 1974). During fetal life, blood flow returning to the heart preferentially bypasses the collapsed, unventilated lung and uses the foramen ovale in the atrial septum and the *patent ductus arteriosus* (PDA) as bypass channels to provide for systemic flow. At the time of birth, closure of the PDA and patent foramen ovale bring about normal adult circulatory patterns, whereby all blood returning to the right atrium is diverted to the lung and all systemic blood flow is derived from the left ventricle. A congenital heart defect can disrupt this normal adaptation process, creating a transitional circulation whereby right-to-left shunting across the foramen ovale or ductus arteriosus may occur (Berman, 1985). Under some circumstances, continued presence of this transitional circulation leads to hemodynamic instability, which is poorly tolerated in the neonate. On the other hand, in treatment of a cyanotic congenital heart defect, the prolongation of transitional circulation is actually beneficial, allowing pulmonary blood flow and postnatal viability. An example of the latter

is pulmonary atresia with pulmonary blood flow coming from the PDA. Also worth noting is that the neonatal myocardium is less compliant than that of the normal adult, thereby limiting recruitable stroke volume with each heart beat (Friedman, 1972). As a consequence, these patients depend highly on heart rate and adequate circulating blood volume to maintain CO.

The infant respiratory system also differs from that of the adult, thus requiring a different approach to anesthetic management. First, infants have a higher rate of metabolism and therefore consume oxygen more rapidly and produce carbon dioxide in greater amounts (Wells et al., 1972). Infants rely heavily on the respiratory system to meet these increased metabolic needs. Specifically, they breathe at a faster rate and become hypoxemic more quickly than adults do during apnea. Second, lung-closing capacity is greater than functional residual capacity during normal tidal volume breathing. As a result, the oxygen reserve during apnea is greatly reduced, further placing infants at risk for hypoxemia. Finally, chest compliance, thoracic wall structure, and diaphragmatic function are different in young infants, placing them at risk for easy fatigability and hypoxemia.

The neonatal renal system is immature in the first months of life, with a reduced glomerular filtration rate. Therefore, young infants have a limited capacity to excrete excess water and salt loads and are at risk for fluid and salt overload during anesthesia. The liver also has an immature capacity for drug clearance during the first month of life. Specifically, pediatric patients demonstrate delayed drug clearance of certain narcotics and sedatives because of immature liver microenzyme systems and altered hepatic blood flow (Greeley and de Bruijn, 1988). Consequently, drug dosing in the young is complex and unpredictable. After 1 month of age, the pharmacokinetic processes of infants mature, and drug clearance and elimination become predictable. The CNS also is immature in young infants; this is especially evident in neonatal patterns of breathing. Some infants, especially premature ones, are periodic breathers, and others exhibit apnea. All infants hypoventilate in response to hypoxia. Neonates and small infants are very sensitive to the respiratory depressant effects of narcotics, and the abnormalities in breathing patterns are unmasked by their use. When narcotics are used in the young patient, mechanical ventilation should be available, and the patient should be closely observed in an intensive care unit or recovery area.

Congenital heart disease differs significantly from acquired adult cardiac disease and accounts for another major difference in approach between these two patient groups. Congenital heart defects often are complex and diverse, complicating any uniform approach to anesthetic management. The anesthesiologist must have complete knowledge of the defect and the intended operation. The spectrum of intracardiac shunts, valve stenoses, disrupted great artery connections, and the absence of one or more chambers of the heart preclude a uniform approach to these patients.

Moreover, myocardial changes can result from the hemodynamic stresses of these defects. The functional consequence of these changes is to place the myocardium at great risk for developing intraoperative ischemia and ventricular failure (Lee et al., 1973). Therefore, an understanding of the isolated defect and its treatment and associated developmental consequences is fundamental to the anesthetic management of these patients.

One final difference between adult and congenital heart surgery that influences anesthetic management is the nature of the surgical procedures themselves. There is a wide spectrum of operations for complex congenital heart disease. These repairs often require significant alterations in the operating conditions, such as the use of deep hypothermic cardiopulmonary bypass and circulatory arrest (Tharion et al., 1982). The immature physiologic systems of the young patient, coupled with a diverse group of complex heart defects and an often complex surgical operation, complicate the care of these patients in the operating room. These factors require that the anesthesiologist have an intimate knowledge of pediatric medicine, congenital heart disease, and surgical repair in addition to the fundamental knowledge and skills requisite for the clinical practice of anesthesia.

Preoperative Evaluation and Preparation

The preoperative visit allows the physician to evaluate the child and to prepare him for anesthesia and surgery. Preoperative evaluation should focus on the child's congenital heart defect and the functional capabilities of the cardiorespiratory system. Underlying medical diseases and therapy, prior anesthetic history, associated congenital anomalies, and recent intercurrent illnesses are also important to assess. The physical examination should include a complete assessment of the cardiopulmonary system. The ECG, complete blood count, electrolytes, blood urea nitrogen, creatinine, two-dimensional echocardiogram, and cardiac catheterization data all should be reviewed. Preoperative feeding should be tailored to each patient; one must consider the timing of the surgical procedure and the child's routine feeding schedule. In general, infants and children should not receive solids and nonclear liquids by mouth for 6 to 8 hours; clear liquids can be restricted for only 2 to 3 hours. Preoperative medications for the pediatric patient should also be tailored to the patient's need and institutional practices. Preoperative sedatives may be provided by an oral regime of a narcotic, sedative, and a minor tranquilizer such as meperidine, pentobarbital, and diazepam, or more conventionally by a short-acting benzodiazepine, midazolam. These premedications should be tailored to the individual patient and should be given prior to the induction of anesthesia. In some circumstances, a skillful preoperative visit with a cooperative patient may obviate the need for a premedication altogether.

General Principles of Anesthetic Management

The diverse array of congenital heart defects and surgical procedures makes an individualized anesthetic management plan essential. This plan takes into account the specific pathophysiologic process caused by the defect, the planned operative procedure, appropriate monitoring for the patient, and a working knowledge of the specific anesthetic agents to be used and their pharmacologic effects. The method of induction of anesthesia is determined primarily by the health of the child and cardiovascular reserve. In critically ill neonates and infants, an intravenous narcotic induction is best, because it preserves cardiovascular stability (Friesen and Lichtor, 1982). In infants, children, and adolescents with stable cardiovascular systems and some cardiac reserve, the choice of induction techniques is more flexible (Friesen and Lichtor, 1983; Hensley et al., 1985). Inhalation, intramuscular, rectal, and intravenous techniques have been used in this setting. The choice among these techniques depends on the age, hazard of regurgitation, and physical status of the patient. In young children and those who fear needles, mask induction is preferable. Once a child loses consciousness, an intravenous cannula is inserted, and maintenance intravenous anesthetics are administered. For the older child and adolescent, routine intravenous induction is used. In all circumstances, tracheal intubation is required, and ventilation is controlled under neuromuscular blockade, using one of the longer-acting muscle relaxants.

Maintenance of anesthesia in these patients depends on the age and condition of the patient, the nature of the surgical procedure, the duration of cardiopulmonary bypass, the development of complications, and the need for postoperative ventilation. For example, for infants who are critically ill in whom hemodynamic stability is essential or in patients in whom postoperative ventilation is required (e.g., pulmonary artery hypertension), a high-dose narcotic technique is desirable (Hickey et al., 1985). More important than the specific techniques and drugs is the skilled execution of the anesthetic plan, taking into account the anesthesiologist's experience, the patient's response to drug therapy, changes associated with direct and indirect surgical manipulation, and early recognition of intraoperative complications. For example, intraoperative hypotension may derive from a number of causes, including anesthetic effect, surgical manipulation of the aorta, and myocardial ischemia. Determining the specific etiology of the hypotension and appropriately adjusting the anesthetic plan are fundamentally more important than adhering strictly to a specific, inflexible anesthetic plan.

Cardiopulmonary Bypass

There are several management concerns during *cardiopulmonary bypass* (CPB). Of course, responsibilities are divided among the patient care team during this critical phase of the cardiac operation. The surgeon operates, the perfusionist maintains adequate perfusion, equipment, and technology, and the anesthesiologist maintains anesthesia and administers appropriate vasoactive drugs. All three must act in concert.

Blood Gas Management and Perfusion Pressure

The role of blood gas management has been clarified as it relates to whether or not temperature of blood gases should be corrected during hypothermic CPB (Schell et al., 1993). A blood gas management plan that employs temperature correction (pH stat) produces a relative hypercarbia compared to a non–temperature-corrected method (alpha stat). The pH stat method requires the addition of CO_2 to the oxygenator and is therefore more complex. Because the cerebral vasculature responds to CO_2 during CPB (Govier et al., 1984; Murkin et al., 1987; Prough et al., 1986), the pH stat method causes cerebral vasodilation, which appears to uncouple cerebral blood flow and metabolism (Murkin et al., 1987). Thus, a more physiologic approach to blood gas management is to use alpha stat (non–temperature-corrected methods) and maintain the arterial CO_2 near normal values. This approach matches CBF to metabolic requirements. Also, with this approach, the CBF and cerebral perfusion autoregulation remain intact (Govier et al., 1984; Murkin et al., 1987). Preserved pressure-flow autoregulation means that CBF remains constant over a very wide range of systemic pressures (30 to 100 mm Hg) in patients without known cerebral vascular disease (Govier et al., 1984). The single most important determinant of absolute CBF is temperature: Low temperatures cause cerebral vasoconstriction as cerebral metabolism decreases. The metabolic effect of temperature on cerebral metabolism can be defined as the change over 10° C, or Q10; the Q10 in anesthetized patients during cardiac surgery is 2.8, or a 2.8-fold change over 10° C (Croughwell et al., 1992). With normal pump flows ($\geq$ 1.6 l/min/m²), the systemic perfusion pressure can be maintained safely over the range of cerebral autoregulation (30 to 100 mm Hg). However, to adequately perfuse the heart and perhaps other organs that are known to have obstructive arterial lesions, perfusion pressures higher than 30 mm Hg may be required to prevent ischemia. The adequacy of perfusion is determined by assessing the urine output, the acid/base status, the evenness of cooling and warming at multiple temperature sites, and the measurement of mixed venous oxygen saturation.

Anticoagulation

The contact of blood with nonendothelial surfaces is a potent cause of blood coagulation. To prevent blood coagulation during cardiopulmonary bypass, the patient must be anticoagulated adequately. Heparin was introduced in 1938 as an effective anticoagulant and is currently the drug of choice to prevent coagulation during CPB. Heparin acts by binding to and activating antithrombin; because antithrombin in-

activates coagulation proteins throughout the entire coagulation cascade, heparin is an effective and nonspecific anticoagulant. There is, however, great interindividual variation in the dose response of heparin. Also, patients deficient in antithrombin are resistant to heparin, and a subset of patients, when maintained on prolonged heparin therapy, become heparin-resistant, presumably by depletion of antithrombin. The best method to monitor heparin effect is the *activated clotting time* (ACT), which was introduced as a quick, precise bedside coagulation test in 1966 (Hattersley, 1966). The normal ACT value is 107 seconds $\pm$ 13 seconds. Heparin administration will prolong the ACT in a dose-related manner (more heparin prolongs the ACT).

Adequate heparinization must be achieved before CPB begins. An original, individually quantitative method of anticoagulation using the ACT was introduced in 1975 (Bull et al., 1975). The method involves defining a dose-ACT effect in the patient, achieving a clearly defined (> 480 seconds) prolongation of the ACT, and reversal of the heparinization with a protamine dose (ratio of protamine to residual heparin ACT effect of 1.3:1). It is generally assumed that anticoagulation is achieved at ACT values of over 300 seconds, but animal data suggest that a value of at least 400 seconds is required (Young et al., 1978). Hypothermia will prolong this ACT, and care must be taken to be sure that the ACT is measured in a standardized fashion, including warming the sample. Use of commercial bedside instruments such as the Hemochron have improved the precision of the ACT measurement. There is, in general, a poor correlation between ACT and plasma heparin assays (Culliford et al., 1981), but it is the effect of heparin on coagulation, not the amount of plasma heparin, that is important when monitoring anticoagulation for CPB.

Stress Response and Anesthesia

The remarkably unphysiologic condition of CPB causes a stress response that has been well documented and characterized by the measurement of many markers of stress: catecholamines, cortisol, growth hormone, prostaglandins, complement, and many other substances. Causes of the elaboration of these substances include, but are not restricted to, contact of blood with foreign surfaces, hypotension, anemia, hypothermia, myocardial ischemia, and a nonpulsatile state. The production of stress-related substances coincides with conditions that reduce their metabolism and clearance: hypothermia, exclusion of the lungs and heart from circulation (organs responsible for metabolism of many of the substances), and reduced hepatic and renal blood flow. Usually, the stress response peaks during early rewarming in the course of customary cardiac operations (Reves et al., 1980). There is clear evidence that the stress response can be blunted by increasing the depth of anesthesia (Feldman et al., 1984; Flezzani et al., 1986; Samuelson et al., 1986) (Fig. 5–6). What is not clear is what, if any, significance there is to the high levels of stress-

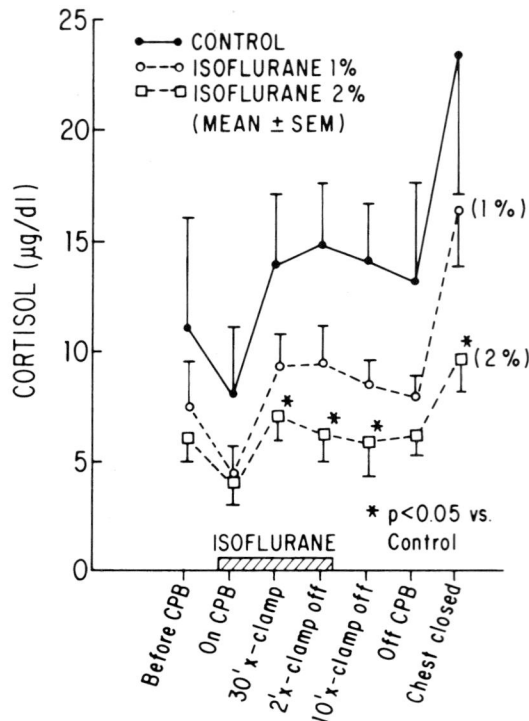

FIGURE 5–6. The stress response to cardiopulmonary bypass (CPB) and cardiac surgery is shown by cortisol plasma concentrations at various times during operation. These stress responses were attenuated in a dose-related manner by the increased concentration of anesthesia (isoflurane) during operation. The patients who were given 2% isoflurane had significantly lower cortisol values than patients who were anesthetized solely with fentanyl (control). (From Flezzani, P., Croughwell, N., McIntyre, R., and Reves, J.: Isoflurane decreases the cortisol response to cardiopulmonary bypass. Anesth. Analg., 65[11]:1117–1122, 1986.)

related substances. Many of the substances could mediate undesirable postoperative effects, such as myocardial damage (catecholamines), hypertension (catecholamines), pulmonary damage (complement), and graft closure (thromboxane), but except for hypertension (Wallach et al., 1980), none of these consequences has been proven. If depth of anesthesia is accomplished by the administration of excessively large doses of opioids (e.g., fentanyl or sufentanil), postoperative respiratory depression will result, and residual levels of inhalation anesthetic drugs (e.g., enflurane or isoflurane) can produce transient myocardial depression at the termination of CPB. It seems prudent to maintain a depth of anesthesia adequate to attenuate the stress response, but it may not be necessary to attempt to block the response altogether. Acceptable anesthesia is accomplished best by either the continuous administration of an inhalation anesthetic via the pump oxygenator or the continuous infusion of an opioid.

Management in Children

Management of CPB for congenital heart defects differs from CPB management for adults in the use of different perfusion techniques and in the extent of the inflammatory reaction to extracorporeal circulation (Greeley et al., 1988; Kirklin et al., 1983). A major cause of morbidity and mortality in the young patient has been the effects of CPB (Kirklin et al., 1981a, 1981b). Refinements in the technology of CPB as well as safer application of perfusion techniques have reduced these risks to an acceptable level.

In any patient, three externally controlled factors are managed during CPB: perfusion rate and pressure, temperature, and hemodilution. These factors are altered significantly more in children than in adults during CPB. Perfusion is regulated by adjusting the pump flow of the CPB circuit, which is maintained at a higher level in infants and children because of their higher metabolic rate. Because of the noncompliant cardiovascular system in children, this perfusion can be accomplished at very low mean perfusion pressures (15 to 30 mm Hg) (Kunkel et al., 1979). Usually, pump flow rate is adjusted to 2.4 to 2.6 l/min/m² in neonates and small infants and to 2.4 l/min/m² in older children at mild to moderate temperatures (28 to 30° C) so that repair is optimized. Flow rate can be reduced, because the temperature of the perfusate is reduced, allowing some flexibility and variation in CPB management.

Hemodilution can vary widely in small infants when they are exposed to the large priming volume of the CPB circuit. In neonates, the dilutional effects from the CPB circuit is 20 to 40 times greater than in adults. In children with polycythemia and in whom repair is going to take place at very cold temperatures, the hemodilution effects of the priming solution can be used to decrease blood viscosity (Milam et al., 1985). Ideally, during hypothermic CPB, the hematocrit should be maintained between 18 and 22%. This range of hematocrits will allow an adequate supply of oxygen to the body tissues and at the same time provide the optimal blood viscosity for cooler temperatures. To achieve this low hematocrit in neonates and young children, one must add packed red blood cells to the priming solution to avoid excessive hemodilution.

The temperature of the perfusate is reduced during CPB management in order to reduce the metabolic rate of the body. The resulting reduced flow optimizes surgical repair. Reducing the demand for oxygen reduces the need for its supply and minimizes tissue ischemia. Surgical repair of congenital heart defects takes place over a wide range of temperatures, varying in extremes of 18 to 20° C for repair of a ventricular septal defect in infancy to normothermia for repair of a small atrial septal defect. During the periods of cooling and rewarming, organs are at highest risk for ischemia because flow cannot meet the metabolic demands of tissue. Therefore, extraordinary vigilance is required during these phases of cooling and rewarming. Uneven cooling and rewarming of core and body surface temperatures suggest inadequate perfusion, and the cause must be readily identified and corrected. Preliminary studies suggest that despite the variation of perfusion pressure and low flow rates during hypothermia, organ perfusion, particularly CBF, appears to be maintained during these extreme variations in biologic conditions if bypass is executed in an exacting manner.

Neonates and small infants weighing less than 8 to 10 kg who require extensive repair of complex congenital heart defects may best be treated with deep hypothermic CPB with total circulatory arrest (Lamberti et al., 1978; Tharion et al., 1982). With this technique, surgical repair may be more exacting because of the bloodless, cannula-free field wherein CPB time is shortened and organ protection appears to be greater (Clarkson et al., 1980; Venugopal et al., 1973). Extensive clinical experience with this technique has shown that the duration of safe circulatory arrest periods is 50 to 60 minutes. Beyond this duration, the incidence of permanent and transient neurologic sequelae increases significantly (Dickinson and Sambrooks, 1979). These sequelae include seizures, choreoathetosis, subtle learning disabilities, and subtle intellectual deficits (Brunberg et al., 1974; Ehyai et al., 1984; Treasure et al., 1985; Wells et al., 1983; Wright et al., 1979). The "safe" period of total circulatory arrest still needs rigorous investigation, and the effects of this technique on the developing brain need to be determined.

Because of concern about neurologic dysfunction after total circulatory arrest, some institutions use low-flow bypass at deep hypothermic levels as an alternative technique. The potential of cerebral protection techniques such as barbiturates or calcium channel blockers is unknown (Artru and Michenfelder, 1981; Kass, 1984; Steen et al., 1985). No clinical studies have systematically examined the influence of these pharmacologic agents on outcome. Additionally, the effect of anesthetic agents and vasodilators should be investigated in terms of their potential protective effect.

Discontinuation of Cardiopulmonary Bypass

When weaning a patient from CPB, one can assess the requisite filling pressures by temporarily increasing preload prior to termination of CPB. Myocardial contractility is assessed by direct visualization and, more quantitatively, by intraoperative esophageal echocardiography (adults) or epicardial echocardiography (children). When specific concerns of left heart function are raised, the pulmonary arterial wedge pressure can be monitored or monitoring catheters can be placed in the left atrium by the surgeon. After adequate HR (by epicardial pacing if required) and rhythm, preload, contractility, warming, and acid/base status have been achieved, the patient can be weaned from bypass. This is accomplished best by slowly filling the heart by reducing venous return to the bypass machine and gradually reducing the arterial flow. In small patients, this can be accomplished by clamping the venous return cannula and turning off the arterial inflow immediately after adequate blood volume is achieved, thus abruptly terminating CPB. Thereafter, the slow infusion of residual pump perfusate or fluids can optimize blood pressure and perfusion. The cause of any difficulty in weaning a patient from CPB must be determined immediately. The primary cause in adults is poor pump function, either the left or the right ventricle, or both. The causes in children include poor surgical result needing re-repair, pulmonary artery hypertension, and right or left ventricular dysfunction or ischemia. Intraoperative echocardiography with color-flow imaging is very helpful in assessing and determining the specific cause in children (Ungerleider et al., 1987). Thereafter, drug therapy using vasodilators and inotropes, ventilation techniques, pacing, and other mechanical support can be specifically applied.

Blood Conservation During Cardiac Surgery

Early cardiac surgery involved routine use of blood products, particularly red blood cells, despite early opinions that priming solutions need not contain red blood cells (Panico and Neptune, 1959). Modern cardiac surgical procedures can be performed without use of blood products. Indeed, severe hemodilution to hematocrits as low as 7% can be tolerated well by young children without a significant increase in morbidity or mortality (Henling et al., 1985). Increased awareness of the risks of blood transfusions (Sazama, 1990), including hepatitis (Bove, 1987), human immunodeficiency virus (HIV) (Glück et al., 1990), and cytomegalovirus transmission (Adler, 1983), as well as potential immunosuppression (Murphy et al., 1991; Waymack et al., 1987), has led to further examination of the need for transfusion therapy. Thus, although screening techniques for donated blood have improved dramatically, the inherent risks of transfusion therapy dictate that blood products be given to reverse perioperative coagulopathies and to increase the hemoglobin (and oxygen-carrying capacity) to acceptable levels. Therefore, the management approach to blood conservation throughout the perioperative period should be comprehensive, with consideration of the anesthetic, surgical, and postoperative techniques used.

Perioperative blood conservation may begin with preoperative autologous blood donations. However, current recommendations exclude patients with significant cardiac disease (Consensus Conference, 1988). Although experimental evidence suggests that significant reductions in hemoglobin can be tolerated in the presence of severe coronary stenoses (Spahn et al., 1992, 1993), usually there is insufficient time between the diagnosis of severe coronary disease and surgical intervention to harvest sufficient autologous blood. The use of erythropoietin may increase the yield of autologous blood preoperatively, but this technique cannot decrease the time needed for autologous predonation. Thus, autologous predonation programs are not useful to cardiac surgery blood conservation management.

Acute normovolemic hemodilution has been employed successfully in cardiac and orthopedic surgery.

This technique involves harvesting of whole blood with crystalloid or colloid as volume replacement. One or two units of whole blood can be collected safely from a cardiac surgical patient prior to surgery; this blood is reinfused after the termination of CPB. Whether a patient is able to undergo acute normovolemic hemodilution depends on the preoperative hematocrit, the blood volume (and thus the weight of the patient), and the presence of co-existing diseases. As an example, although an elderly patient may have an adequate hematocrit, the presence of preoperative congestive heart failure, necessitating diuretic therapy, and preoperative unstable angina, necessitating bed rest, may contract the circulating blood volume and therefore artificially elevate the hematocrit. Acute normovolemic hemodilution is effective, and a preliminary report suggests that there may be some improvement in post-CPB coagulopathy with reinfusion of the perioperatively harvested whole blood (Whitten et al., 1992).

Although preoperative blood conservation techniques may help to conserve blood, by far the most blood product transfusions occur intraoperatively. Thus, surgical technique is critical to blood conservation. Use of adjuvant blood salvaging techniques, such as a cardiotomy reservoir for collecting operative blood loss after heparinization, will reduce blood loss from the surgical field. Other devices, such as blood-scavenging devices, can effectively salvage blood from the operative field in patients who do not need systemic heparinization. This technique is not associated with any clinically significant infections, although the reinfused blood is most often contaminated with skin commensurals such as coagulase-negative staphylococci (Bland et al., 1992). During CPB, volume can be manipulated with an ultrafiltration system that has a hollow fiber system of hemofiltration identical to that used during renal dialysis. This system can effectively remove excess volume, increasing the hematocrit during CPB, particularly during rewarming of the patient after hypothermia and cardioplegia. After discontinuation of CPB, the ultrafiltration system can be used to concentrate the remaining blood in the extracorporeal circuit during reinfusion into the patient. The cardiotomy system can be used further to collect the drainage from the chest for reinfusion; however, reinfusion of this blood is associated with transient, although clinically insignificant, mild coagulopathy (Fuller et al., 1991; Griffith et al., 1989).

Pharmacologic interventions have been used to decrease the extent of intraoperative and postoperative bleeding. Aprotinin and transaxemic acid are thought to inhibit serine protease, thus decreasing complement and platelet activation during extracorporeal circulation. Both of these agents have shown some benefit when administered before CPB (Harder et al., 1991). Aminocaproic acid, by inhibiting plasmin formation, is thought to decrease post-CPB bleeding by decreasing the formation of fibrin split products and other mediators of fibrinolysis. Aprotinin, transaxemic acid, and aminocaproic acid all may help to de-

crease the need for perioperative blood transfusions; further clinical studies are needed to determine the benefits and risks of these drugs.

Finally, although preoperative and perioperative whole blood harvesting, surgical technique, and pharmacologic interventions are important, postoperative management ultimately may determine whether transfusion therapy is necessary. Laboratory evidence suggests that, although most tolerance to normovolemic hemodilution is idiosyncratic as long as normovolemia is maintained, minimal transfusion therapy reverses myocardial dysfunction when it occurs (Spahn et al., 1993). However, clinical preliminary data have demonstrated that, postoperatively, patients experience more ischemia after peripheral vascular surgery when hematocrits are maintained below 29% (Christopherson et al., 1991). These patients experienced postoperative ischemia 24 to 72 hours after surgery; these ischemic episodes were associated with tachycardia, presumably during increasing ambulation of these patients. Thus, although significant normovolemic hemodilution may be tolerated well intraoperatively, postoperative optimal hematocrits may need to be higher because of the increased metabolic requirements associated with recovery and ambulation.

Perioperative blood conservation can effectively decrease or eliminate transfusion therapy during cardiac operations in a subset of cardiac surgical patients. The management of these patients should routinely incorporate blood conservation techniques, including preoperative and perioperative autologous donations (including the use of acute normovolemic hemodilution), meticulous surgical technique, pharmacologic interventions, scrupulous attention to maintenance of normovolemia, and judicious use of postoperative transfusion therapy tailored to individual patient needs.

PHARMACOLOGY AND USE OF VASOACTIVE DRUGS

Knowledge of adrenergic pharmacology and the cardiovascular pharmacology of other vasoactive drugs is essential for the understanding and appropriate use of the multitude of drugs available in the supportive care of patients undergoing cardiothoracic surgery (Reves, 1993). Three endogenous catecholamines (epinephrine, norepinephrine, and dopamine) are adrenergic agonists. The sympathetic nervous system has adrenoceptors in many tissues and various organs (Table 5–8).

Alpha- and Beta-Adrenergic Agonists

In 1906, Dale linked the actions of the sympathetic nervous system with the concept of a receptor-mediated phenomenon (Dale, 1906), and in 1948, Ahlquist classified the adrenergic receptors into alpha and beta subtypes (Ahlquist, 1948). Since the original descrip-

■ **Table 5–8.** PHYSIOLOGIC ADRENOCEPTOR EFFECTS

Tissue or Organ	Receptor Type Stimulated	Physiologic Response
Heart	Beta$_1$ (Beta$_2$)*	Increased rate
		Increased force of contraction
		Increased conduction
	(Alpha$_1$)	Increased force of contraction
Arteries	Alpha$_1$	Vasoconstriction
	Beta$_2$	Vasodilatation
Veins	Alpha	Vasoconstriction
Bronchial smooth muscle	Beta$_2$ (Beta$_1$)	Bronchodilatation relaxation
Liver	Beta$_2$	Glycogenolysis gluconeogenesis
Skeletal muscle	Beta$_2$	Glycogenolysis, lactate production
Pancreas	Alpha	Decreased insulin secretion
	Beta$_2$	Increased insulin and glucagon release
Kidney	Beta$_1$ (Beta$_2$)	Renin release

*Parentheses denote minor effect.

tion of alpha- and beta-receptor types, there now are two adrenoceptor subtypes that mediate important, different hemodynamic and physiologic effects. These subtypes have been reviewed (Hoffman and Lefkowitz, 1980; Vanhoutte, 1981). Understanding the adrenergic receptors and the very different alpha- and beta-agonist actions of drugs is fundamental to the rational use of these drugs and their antagonists. Although the endogenous catecholamines are both alpha- and beta-agonists, norepinephrine tends to activate alpha-adrenoceptors, and epinephrine the beta-receptors. Dopamine is close to epinephrine in relative proportion of alpha/beta activity, but it also stimulates dopaminergic receptors, which mediate renal arterial dilation (Goldberg, 1972). The spectral activity of catecholamines is illustrated in Figure 5–7: Methoxamine has primarily alpha-adrenergic activity, and isoproterenol has beta-adrenergic activity. These drugs have dose-related changes in position on this relative activity spectrum; for example, low doses of epinephrine tend to act more on beta-receptors, but higher doses have prominent alpha effects. There are also different receptor densities and levels of receptor responsiveness in patients of different ages and cardiovascular functional status; for example, beta$_1$-receptor responsiveness decreases with increasing age and in congestive heart failure (Feldman et al., 1984).

Knowledge of the adrenergic activity of catecholamines is used to select the appropriate drug and dose. Thus, if vasoconstriction is needed, a pure, or nearly pure, alpha$_1$-agonist, such as phenylephrine or norepinephrine, is used. Primary vasoconstriction is required when the systemic vascular resistance (SVR) is reduced, as with anesthetic or vasodilator drug therapy or during some forms of shock. Also, myocardial ischemia resulting from hypotension responds to increased perfusion pressure after intervention with a vasoconstrictor (often in conjunction with nitroglycerin). Table 5–9 lists commonly used vasoconstrictor drugs and recommended doses. If increased inotropic effect is desired, a beta-agonist such as isoproterenol or dobutamine would be selected. Many positive inotropic drugs are available (Table 5–10), and all catecholamines that have beta$_1$-adrenergic activity will increase myocardial contractility.

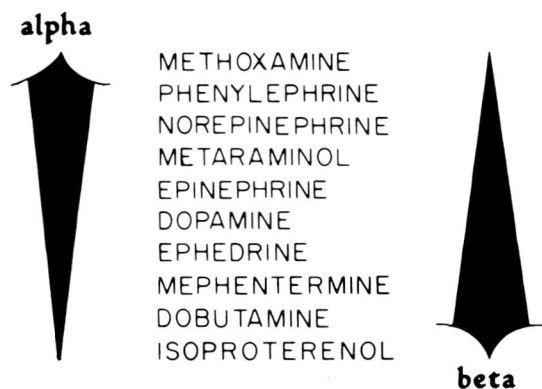

FIGURE 5–7. The spectrum of alpha- and beta-adrenergic activity among various pharmacologic agents. Methoxamine has the greatest alpha-adrenergic effect, and isoproterenol has the greatest beta-adrenergic effect. Positions of drugs along this spectrum can be alternated by the dose (i.e., higher doses tend to make pharmacologic agents such as epinephrine more alpha-adrenergic than lower doses). (From Reves, J.: Pharmacology of vasoactive drugs. *In* Thomas, S. [ed]: Manual of Cardiac Anesthesia. Churchill Livingstone, New York, 1993, pp. 315–335.)

Nonadrenergic Inotropic Drugs

Noncatecholamines (digoxin, glucoson, calcium chloride, and amrinone) increase contractility and have positive inotropic effects via nonadrenergic mechanisms. The common mechanism of increased myocardial contractility is enhanced intracellular calcium. Catecholamines stimulate the beta-receptor, increasing production of intramyocardial cyclic adenosine monophosphate (cAMP), which facilitates calcium entry into the cell. Digoxin increases calcium by inhibiting the sodium-potassium adenosine triphosphatase present on the cell membrane. This increases intracellular sodium, which limits transmembrane sodium-calcium exchange and causes a secondary rise

■ **Table 5–9.** PHARMACOLOGIC CHARACTERISTICS OF COMMONLY USED VASOCONSTRICTORS

Generic Name (Trade Name)	Alpha$_1$	Beta$_2$	Beta$_1$	Onset	Duration	Adult Intravenous Dose
Methoxamine (Vasoxyl)	+ + + +	0	0	1–2 min	5–8 min	0.2–0.5 mg bolus
Phenylephrine (Neosynephrine)	+ + + +	0	+	1–2 min	5 min	50–100 mg bolus
						0.10–0.5 mg/kg/min infusion
Norepinephrine (Levophed)	+ + + +	0	+ +	30 sec	2 min	0.05–0.15 mg/kg/min infusion
Ephedrine (Ephedrine)	+ + +	+	+ +	1 min	5–10 min	2.5–5 mg bolus

Note: The number of plus signs (+) denotes increasing activity or time, and 0 denotes no activity.

in intracellular calcium. Amrinone increases cAMP by inhibiting a phosphodiesterase isoenzyme (PDE III) and may secondarily interfere with the sodium-calcium membrane exchange. Amrinone, like the beta-agonists, produces systemic vasodilation as well as positive inotropic effect. Positive inotropes improve ventricular contractility but should be used only after preload and HR have been optimized. Selection of a particular inotrope is based primarily on the afterload, using a drug with vasodilation (beta-agonists or amrinone) when the SVR is high and a mixed alpha/beta-agonist when there is normal or reduced SVR. Figure 5–8 depicts the decision algorithm used in the selection of vasoactive drugs for low CO (cardiac index < 2.0 l/min/m^2).

Vasodilators

Vasodilators constitute a diverse pharmacologic group of drugs (see Table 5–11) used to lower blood pressure and to reduce afterload. The reduction of afterload can enhance SV of failing hearts and those with aortic and mitral valve insufficiency. There are several different mechanisms for the vasodilation: direct smooth muscle dilation (e.g., hydralazine, nitrates, calcium channel blockers), sympathetic ganglion blockers (e.g., trimethaphan), alpha$_1$-adrenergic antagonists (e.g., phentolamine, labetolol), and alpha$_2$-adrenergic agonists (e.g., clonidine). Indications for vasodilators include hypertension, low cardiac output (see Fig. 5–8), coronary artery spasm, and pulmonary hypertension. When vasodilators are given, care must be taken to maintain the preload.

Adrenergic Antagonists

The alpha- and beta-adrenoceptor blocking drugs in clinical use are competitive antagonists that inhibit the binding of the endogenous or other sympathomimetic neurotransmitters. Thus, competitive inhibition attenuates the activity of the baseline as well as the normal stress-induced increased activity of the sympathetic nervous system.

Competitive adrenergic antagonism causes a rightward shift in the dose-response curve for the agonist, but the slope remains the same. The antagonists produce pharmacologic responses according to their selective action at the various types of cell membrane receptors as expected from the known action of the receptor agonist. A sufficiently large dose of the appropriate agonist will reverse the blockade from a competitive antagonist. Thus, a beta$_1$-selective antagonist can be expected to produce negative chronotropic and inotropic effects, but it will not alter vascular resistances; it may induce bronchospasm or produce significant orthostatic hypotension.

Alpha-receptors have been subclassified as postsynaptic alpha$_1$ and presynaptic alpha$_2$. Alpha$_1$ blockade diminishes the vasoconstriction of alpha-agonists, whereas alpha$_2$ blockade permits increased presynaptic membrane release of norepinephrine. Alpha$_2$-agonists inhibit release of neurotransmitter. The beta-receptors are subclassified as either beta$_1$ or beta$_2$ and are further classified as to whether they possess any intrinsic sympathomimetic activity (ISA). Beta-blockers are similar in structure to isoproterenol. The specific physiologic effects of activation of these receptors will be the opposite of the agonist-induced changes listed.

■ **Table 5–10.** PHARMACOLOGIC CHARACTERISTICS OF POSITIVE INOTROPIC DRUGS

Generic Name	Receptor Activity: Vascular/Cardiac			Adult Intravenous Dose
	Alpha$_1$	Beta$_2$	Beta$_1$	
Epinephrine	+ + +	+	+ +	Infusion 0.05–0.15 mg/kg/min
Dopamine* (Intropin)	+ +	+	+ +	Infusion 1–10 μg/kg/min
Ephedrine (Ephedrine)	+ + +	+	+ +	Bolus 5–10 μg
Dobutamine (Dobutrex)	+	+	+ + +	Infusion 1–20 μg/kg/min
Isoproterenol (Isuprel)	0	+ + + +	+ + + +	Infusion 0.025–0.05 μg/kg/min
Calcium chloride (calcium)	0	0	0	Bolus 1–10 mg/kg
Digoxin (Lanoxin)	0	0	0	Bolus 0.125–0.25 mg
Amrinone (Inocor)	0	0	0	Bolus 0.5–2.0 mg/kg, then infusion 5–10 μg/kg/min

Note: The number of plus signs (+) denotes increasing activity or time, and 0 denotes no activity.
*Dopamine also stimulates dopaminergic receptors, which cause mild renal and splanchnic arterial dilatation.

Rapid Identification

↓

Thermodilution, SVO₂ ,
Calculate resistance

Hemodynamic Classification

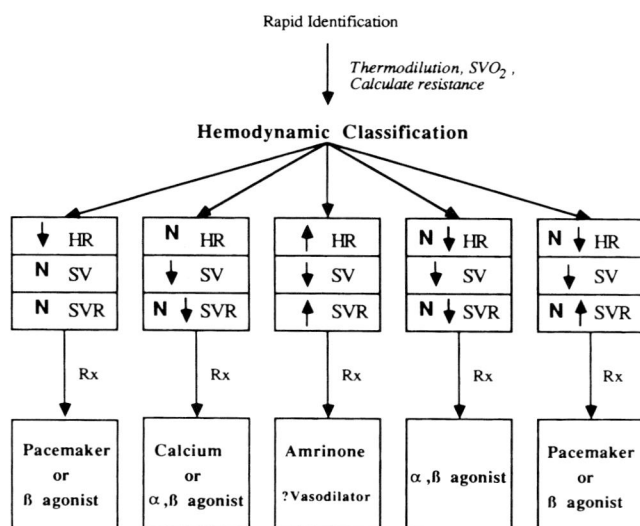

FIGURE 5–8. Treatment algorithm for low cardiac output (CO). Rapid identification is accomplished by measurement of CO by thermodilution or an alternative method. Also, observation of significantly reduced SVo₂ indicates low CO. Systemic resistance is calculated. After hemodynamic classification, therapy is indicated according to changes in heart rate (HR), stroke volume (SV), and systemic vascular resistance (SVR). Pharmacologic intervention is based on the need for alpha- or beta-agonist drugs or other positive inotropic drugs. (Rx = treatment; ↓ = decrease; ↑ = increase; N = normal.)

The various adrenergic blocking drugs, some basic pharmacology, and the usual drug dosing recommendations are listed in Table 5–12. Beta-adrenergic blockade should generally be maintained throughout the perioperative period to avoid the risk of rebound sympathetic hyperactivity and to maintain the desired effects of beta blockade (Boudoulas et al., 1977). Chronic administration of beta-adrenoceptor blockers increases the density of cell membrane beta-receptors (Maisel et al., 1987). The decrease in mortality produced by effective beta blockade in patients with ischemic heart disease is well known; furthermore, beta-blockers have been shown to decrease the incidence of perioperative myocardial ischemic events (Stone et al., 1988).

The currently recommended doses and routes of administration for the common alpha- and beta-adrenergic blockers are listed in Table 5–12. Drugs with

some intrinsic sympathomimetic activity generally are tolerated better by patients with poor left ventricular function, because these drugs produce less functional myocardial depression and bradycardia. The selectivity of the beta₁ drugs is lost at higher doses.

The alpha-antagonists may cause cardiac stimulation through an increase in reflex sympathetic activity. This may limit their effectiveness as single agents in patients with significant coronary artery disease, especially if tachycardia results. Orthostatic hypotension may be a problem, especially in the relatively hypovolemic patient. However, the effect of alpha-blockers on reducing the SVR can be valuable in many patients.

The selection among the various beta-blockers is often based on anticipated tolerance of potential side effects. Nonselective beta-antagonists should be avoided in patients with chronic lung disease or bronchospasm. Pure beta-antagonists limit exercise capacity and may produce other side effects, such as depression, cold extremities, impotence, and altered blood lipid profiles. Esmolol is a unique blocker with a half-life of only 9 minutes, permitting rapid titration of drug to the desired beta₁-antagonist effect by continuous infusion (Menkhaus et al., 1985). Labetalol is also unique in providing combined receptor blockade by providing vasodilation through alpha blockade and limiting reflex tachycardia by nonselective beta blockade. Labetalol has been used recently with success for the management of perioperative hypertension in a varied surgical patient population (Leslie et al., 1987).

POSTANESTHESIA MANAGEMENT

Immediate postoperative care of the patient who has undergone cardiothoracic surgery is important in the overall sequence of anesthetic and surgical management. Although the primary influence on outcome is the execution of the operation, postoperative care is the next most important factor. The postoperative period can be characterized by a series of physiologic and pharmacologic changes as the body convalesces from the abnormal biologic conditions of CPB and cardiac surgery toward a normal rehabilitative state (Kirklin et al., 1980; Kirklin and Archie, 1974).

■ **Table 5–11.** ANTIHYPERTENSIVE DRUG CLASSES

Arteriolar Dilator	Venodilator or Combined	Combined Beta and Alpha Blocker	Central Nervous System	ACE* Inhibitor	Angiotensin II Blocker
Hydralazine (Apresoline)	Nitroglycerine	Labetalol (Trandate)	Clonidine† (Catapres)	Captopril (Capoten)	Saralasin (Sarenin)
Diazoxide (Hyperstat)	Nitroprusside (Nipride)		Methyldopa (Aldomet)		
Minoxidil (Loniten)	Prazosin (Minipress)		Reserpine (Serpasil)		
	Nifedipine (Procardia)				

*ACE = Angiotensin converting enzyme.
†Alpha₂ agonist.

■ **Table 5–12.** ANDRENERGIC BLOCKING DRUG PHARMACOLOGY AND DOSES

Drug Generic (Trade)	Receptor(s) Blocked	Elimination Half-Life (Hours)	Adult Oral Dose (mg)	Adult Intravenous Dose (mg)
Propranolol (Inderal)	Beta$_1$, beta$_2$	2–6	40–1000	0.5–2*
Labetalol (Trandate)	Beta$_1$, beta$_2$, alpha$_2$	2–5	200–2400	2–20*
Nadolol (Corgard)	Beta$_1$, beta$_2$	20–24	40–640	NA
Pindolol (Visken)	Beta$_1$, beta$_2$	3–4	5–30	NA
Timolol (Blocadren)	Beta$_1$, beta$_2$	3–4	5–45	NA
Atenolol (Tenormin)	Beta$_1$	6–9	50–300	NA
Metoprolol (Lopressor)	Beta$_1$	3–4	50–400	1–5*
Esmolol (Brevibloc)	Beta$_1$	0.15	NA	100–300 µg/kg/min
Prazosin (Minipress)	Alpha$_1$	2–4	2–20	NA
Phentolamine (Regitine)	Alpha$_1$, alpha$_2$	0.5–1	NA	30–50 µg/kg
Phenoxybenzamine (Dibenzyline)	Alpha$_1$, alpha$_2$	18–24	10–100	NA

NA = Not available.
*May repeat if indicated.

During this postoperative period, the effects of the cardiac operation, the patient's underlying diseases, the effects of CPB, and special techniques such as profound hypothermia with circulatory arrest may create other special problems. In the immediate postoperative setting, abnormal convalescence and specialized problems must be recognized and managed appropriately. Fortunately, most patients are able to compensate for the surgical repair and CPB effects, with which morbidity and mortality rates remain low. Therefore, the guiding principle in managing the postoperative patient is understanding the distinction between normal convalescence after anesthesia and cardiac surgery, and abnormal convalescence, wherein specific complications are to be sought.

The immediate postoperative period is one of continuous physiologic changes for the patient because of the elimination of anesthetic agents and their pharmacologic effects and the ongoing physiologic changes secondary to surgical trauma and extracorporeal circulation. Anesthesia affects not only the patient's conscious state but also respiratory, renal, and hepatic function; fluid and electrolyte balance; and immunologic characteristics. In spite of all these changes, postoperative care should be simple for patients undergoing cardiac procedures.

In general, management in the cardiac patient takes several phases. First, during the transfer of the patient to the *intensive care unit* (ICU), the maintenance and continued monitoring of vital signs, ECG, blood pressure, ventilation, and oxygenation are very important. During this period, essential information pertinent to the patient's preoperative and intraoperative courses should be communicated to the ICU team, as should information about the anticipated residual anesthetic effects. Special regard should be given to the nature of the operation, the type of anesthesia, hemodynamic trends, plans for ventilation, recent hematocrit, electrolytes, arterial blood gas, urine output, temperature, cardiac output, and any intercurrent complications. During the second phase of postoperative management in the early ICU period, the patient goes through a transition, recovering from the residual effects of hypothermia to a rewarming phase. During

this time, SVR may drop, and hypovolemia is often evident. The third phase of ICU care in the uncomplicated patient is marked by hemodynamic and respiratory weaning. By the second postoperative day, the fourth and last phase of ICU care occurs, wherein fluids are mobilized.

The emergence from anesthesia in the immediate postsurgical period usually is uncomplicated, and the surgical outcome is obvious and expected. As long as hemostasis is adequate and major organ systems—including neurologic, cardiovascular, pulmonary, and renal systems—continue to recover function, invasive intervention and monitoring can be minimized, and postoperative care can be simplified. Although close physiologic monitoring, active pharmacologic therapy, and aggressive cardiopulmonary support are available to minimize or reverse adverse effects of anesthesia or surgery, these interventions usually are not necessary. Emergence from anesthesia should occur within the first few hours of the postoperative period when the patient regains consciousness and responds to simple commands. Major changes in neurologic function should not occur after uncomplicated cardiac and thoracic surgery. Transient abnormalities such as mental confusion, hallucination, and drowsiness may occur during "normal" convalescence and can be attributed to either residual anesthetic drug effect or the effects of CPB (Stewart et al., 1981). These symptoms usually subside within the first postoperative day or two, although cognitive dysfunction is reported in 35% of patients at time of discharge (Blumenthal et al., 1991; Newman et al., 1993).

Overt seizure activity, a focal neurologic examination, choreiform movements, or coma should be viewed as complications in patient management and immediately investigated. If a high-dose narcotic anesthetic technique is used intraoperatively, an extended period of patient unconsciousness lasting 8 to 16 hours may occur. Also, premedication rarely causes confusion in the patient postoperatively, especially in the elderly or the very young patient.

Under most circumstances, neuromuscular blocking agents are not reversed in the operating room if the patient is to be ventilated in the early postoperative period. Early postoperative immobility may be attributed to the neuromuscular blockade effects of these drugs. Within 4 to 6 hours, the effects of these drugs should not be present because of their metabolism by and elimination from the body. In patients in whom complete neuromuscular function is desirable immediately after the operation, reversal of muscle relaxants usually is accomplished in the operating room and is not a factor postoperatively. Shivering in the early postoperative period is a normal response to the CNS effects of certain anesthetic drugs and the temperature changes perioperatively. No treatment of shivering is necessary under most circumstances. If shivering produces serious reductions in Sv_{O_2}, it can be treated with small doses of a muscle relaxant (in anesthetized patients) or with meperidine in awaking patients.

In a convalescing patient without complications, a state of alertness is to be anticipated 2 to 4 hours postoperatively. Emergence from anesthesia also influences pulmonary function and ventilatory management. Under normal circumstances after CPB, tachypnea and mild pulmonary dysfunction are expected because of pulmonary water changes (Cleland et al., 1966; Cohn et al., 1971). Despite these changes, patients can be extubated early after cardiac surgery; this can be performed as soon as the effects of the anesthetic agents have worn off. This is usually accomplished in patients undergoing closed heart procedures, thoracotomies, and uncomplicated cardiac surgery (e.g., coronary artery bypass, grafting, or aortic valve replacement) or after repair of some congenital heart defects (e.g., atrial or ventricular septal defects). Such patients are extubated 2 to 6 hours after the operation, provided there are no ongoing complications, such as bleeding, pulmonary insufficiency, dysrhythmias, and neurologic dysfunction (Lell et al., 1979). In patients who are critically ill before surgery or who have undergone complex surgical procedures, extubation usually is not performed until the next morning or later. Under these circumstances, ventilatory management and appropriate sedation are continued in the postoperative period until extubation. Adult patients and children weighing more than 15 kg are managed best with a volume-cycled ventilator; children weighing less than 15 kg are managed best with a pressure-cycled ventilator. At the time of weaning, intermittent mandatory ventilation is gradually reduced to a level of 2 to 4 breaths per minute before extubation. While the patient is being mechanically ventilated, settings are minimized to achieve normal blood gases and to prevent barotrauma. Also, during mechanical ventilation, appropriate humidification and chest physiotherapy are performed to prevent pulmonary atelectasis.

Most important, the emergence from anesthesia effects the cardiovascular system in the postoperative period. The appropriate responses to withdrawal of anesthesia must be distinguished from inappropriate hemodynamic instability or behavior secondary to new physiologic process or complications related to the operation itself. This assessment of a patient's postoperative recovery involves defining an adequate scale of normal, uncomplicated convalescent cardiovascular recovery. For example, when a patient is recovering from the effects of anesthetic drugs, mental status is an indicator of adequate cerebral perfusion. In the somnolent, disoriented, or combative patient, one should consider that inadequate CBF may be due to low CO after ruling out residual anesthetic effects, hypoxia, and hypercarbia.

A normal, uncomplicated postoperative period occurs when CO meets organ perfusion and tissue metabolic needs (Kirklin and Archie, 1974). This assessment can be made by physical examination and quantitative measurement of CO. During normal convalescence from cardiac surgery, the physical examination in the early postoperative period should show normal blood pressure, good peripheral perfusion, normal body temperature, good color, adequate pulse strength, good capillary refill, alert mental status, good urine output, and an adequate arterial wave form on direct arterial measurement. When the physical examination is equivocal or decreased CO is suspected, quantitative measurement of cardiac output is warranted. However, most evaluations in patients during uncomplicated convalescence and assessment of the patient's cardiovascular status can be made without actually measuring CO. When cardiac index is above minimal levels, the patient can be said to be convalescing normally in terms of the cardiovascular system (Kirklin and Archie, 1974). When cardiac index is below acceptable values and a physical examination suggests low CO, pharmacologic support and more invasive measures are necessary to maintain circulation. The body's ability to maintain vigorous CO after a cardiac operation enhances the recovery from the damaging effects of CPB. Low CO syndrome can cause subsequent dysfunction of other organ systems, such as the pulmonary, central nervous, renal, and hematologic systems. Finally, residual anesthetic drug effects may persist in the postoperative period or be delayed because hepatic metabolism may be altered through the effects of CPB or reduced liver blood flow. Under such circumstances, drowsiness or somnolence may persist in the normal convalescing patient. Sedative drugs should be administered cautiously, because they may depress the patient further.

Coagulation abnormalities often appear in the postoperative cardiac patient who has no complications. Abnormal platelet count and function, prolongation of prothrombin and activated partial thromboplastin times, and decreased fibrinogen level often occur in these patients (Greeley et al., 1986). These changes stem from the exposure of nonendothelialized surfaces of the CPB circuitry and the dilutional effects on blood components. Usually, these coagulation abnormalities correct themselves within the first postoperative day and are not associated with excessive clinical bleeding. Therefore, routine correction of these abnormalities with the infusion of blood products is not warranted. The significant risk of infection associated with blood component therapy is an important reason for not administering blood products unless nonsurgical bleeding is significant (Bove, 1986; Miller et al., 1985). Intervention with blood products should not be made unless clinical evidence shows excessive bleeding.

One of the most important functions of the ICU team is to identify complications in the normal convalescent patient. These abnormalities often require closer observation, pharmacologic intervention, and increased cardiopulmonary technical support. Such complications include hypovolemia, decreased myocardial contractility, hyperdynamic circulation, pulmonary arterial hypertension, right ventricular failure, cardiac tamponade, dysrhythmias, cardiac arrest, oliguria, and CNS dysfunction (Kirklin et al., 1980; Kirklin and Archie, 1974). These special situations require specific therapy as discussed elsewhere in this book. It is critical to detect any departure from the normal convalescent course.

Postoperative complications specifically related to anesthesia have several etiologies. Failure to awaken usually is due to residual anesthetic effects, neuromuscular blockade, an intraoperative metabolic/electrolyte disorder, or a CNS event. Postoperative respiratory problems directly attributed to anesthetic effects include impaired ventilation due to upper airway obstruction, impaired respiratory drive due to residual narcotic or volatile anesthetic effect, altered ventilatory mechanisms due to residual neuromuscular blockade, or the effects of pain.

Under most circumstances, naloxone is not used to reverse residual narcotic effects. The release of catecholamines, the exacerbation of the stress response, and the resultant hypertension and tachycardia may cause hemodynamic instability and low CO due to myocardial ischemia after naloxone administration. Under such circumstances, it is best to continue ventilation rather than to reverse narcotic-induced respiratory depression. Reversal of muscle relaxants, if required, is facilitated by use of available neuromuscular blockade monitors. Flumazenil can be used to reverse the hypnotic, amnestic, and respiratory depressant effects of all benzodiazepines (Hughes et al., 1992).

The anesthesiologist also can contribute significantly to ablation of pain postoperatively. After thoracic and cardiovascular surgery, patients are especially prone to respiratory and cardiac complications, which may result from inadequate analgesia. Limiting the effects of inadequately managed pain can limit morbidity and possibly mortality after surgery. Adequately controlled pain can decrease physiologic responses to acute pain—including tachycardia, hypertension, splinting, tachypnea, and immobility—which may cause such complications as cardiac ischemia and acute respiratory failure. Further, the psychological aspects of acute pain can be allayed, increasing patient cooperation with procedures or pulmonary therapy. Multiple modes of pain management include passive cutaneous anaphylaxis, epidural analgesia, and peripheral nerve blocks. These modes are outlined in part II of this chapter, "Acute Pain Management After Surgical Procedures."

SUMMARY

The improvement in thoracic surgery that has occurred during the past decades has been accompanied by enormous progress in knowledge of anesthesia and supportive care. New drugs, better monitoring, greater physiologic understanding, new concepts of patient care, and creation of the specially trained cardiothoracic anesthesiologist as a member of the surgical team are factors responsible for the past and future success of the entire enterprise.

SELECTED BIBLIOGRAPHY

Benumof, J. L.: One-lung ventilation and hypoxic pulmonary vasoconstriction: Implications for anesthetic management. Anesth. Analg., 64:821–833, 1985.

This is a comprehensive review by a frequently quoted expert in the area of one-lung anesthesia. Numerous recent animal and human studies delineating the optimal anesthetic management techniques and methods of ventilation for one-lung anesthesia are presented. The potential indications for one-lung ventilation are discussed, and the physiology of one-lung ventilation and hypoxemia are reviewed in detail. A suggested sequence of treatment interventions for intraoperative hypoxemia is discussed, and a bibliography of 115 references is presented.

Bull, B. S., Huse, W. M., Brauer, F. S., and Korpman, R. A.: Heparin therapy during extracorporeal circulation. J. Thorac. Cardiovasc. Surg., 69:685–689, 1975.

This paper changed clinical practice. The concept of monitoring the effect of heparin with the activated clotting time (ACT) was advanced to ensure a standardized anticoagulant effect of heparin. The ACT is a simple, reliable bedside method of quantitating the anticoagulant effect of heparin. A method of determining the precise heparin and protamine dose in an individual patient is presented by constructing a heparin dose-response curve. Clinicians have used this new method to replace a very arbitrary method of heparin administration during cardiac surgery.

Govier, A. V., Reves, J. G., McKay, R. D., et al.: Factors and their influence on regional cerebral blood flow during nonpulsatile cardiopulmonary bypass. Ann. Thorac. Surg., 38:592–600, 1984.

This clinical study was the first to show that cerebral autoregulation was preserved during cardiopulmonary bypass (CPB) and that temperature and, to a lesser extent, CO_2 are the major determinants of cerebral blood flow during CPB. Cerebral blood flow is independent of mean arterial pressure (range 30 to 110 mm Hg) and pump flow (1.0 to 2.0 l/min/m²) in patients without known cerebrovascular disease during nonpulsatile CPB managed with alpha-stat pH strategy (non–temperature-corrected blood gas management).

Hughes, M., Jacobs, J., and Glass, P.: Context sensitive half-time in multi-compartment pharmacokinetic models for intravenous anesthetic drugs. Anesthesiology, 76:334–341, 1992.

This theoretical paper explains the choice of intravenous drug based on the disposition of the drug during the time (context) in which the drugs are used. The term context-sensitive half-time is explained and used to guide choice and method of intravenous drug delivery.

Kaye, W.: Invasive monitoring techniques: Arterial cannulation, bedside pulmonary artery catheterization, and arterial puncture. Heart Lung, 12:395–427, 1983.

An extensive review article outlining many of the principles of invasive hemodynamic monitoring and the basic techniques of insertion. Included are numerous representative waveform examples, a discussion of monitoring complications, and a suggested list of indications for the various levels of monitoring techniques. Numerous anatomic drawings are included to aid the description of the insertion techniques.

Slogoff, S., and Keats, A. S.: Does perioperative myocardial ischemia lead to postoperative myocardial infarction? Anesthesiology, 62:107–114, 1985.

This is a clinical study documenting the incidence of perioperative ischemia and relating the ischemia to outcome in 1023 elective coronary artery bypass surgery patients. Ischemia is common: 37% of patients had ischemia in the perioperative period. About half of the ischemic episodes were not associated with significant hemodynamic changes, but of the hemodynamic perturbations, tachycardia was most commonly associated with ischemia. Most ischemic episodes were benign and short-lived. Postoperative myocardial infarction (PMI) occurred in 6.9% of patients who had operative ischemia, whereas 93.1% of these patients did not have PMI. Significant predictors of PMI were ischemia before bypass, aortic cross-clamp time, and surgical rating of quality of the operation. Four per cent of all patients had PMI; of these, 12% died.

Stoelting, R. K.: Local anesthetics. *In* Stoelting, R. K. (ed): Pharmacology and Physiology in Anesthetic Practice. New York, J. B. Lippincott, 1987, pp. 148–168.

An excellent brief review of the potential mechanisms of action and overdose toxicity of local anesthetics. Included are the relevant pharmacokinetic parameters and points of comparison between the various local anesthetics. Several useful tables highlight drug selection for various regional blocks, drug metabolism and clearance mechanisms, and treatment of toxicity. The book also contains other valuable chapters detailing perioperative drug clinical pharmacology more practically than do most similar texts.

Tarhan, S., Moffitt, E. A., Taylor, W. F., and Giuliani, E. R.: Myocardial infarction after general anesthesia. J. A. M. A., *220*:1451–1454, 1972.

This is the first large outcome study to report the incidence of perioperative myocardial infarction (PMI) as a function of several perioperative descriptors of risk. The study encompassed 32,877 patients undergoing noncardiac surgery. Only 0.2% of this population had PMI, but it was determined that patients with previous myocardial infarction or undergoing thoracic surgery were 5 or 6 times, respectively, more likely to have PMI. PMI is more likely to occur on the third postoperative day and in patients with a history of a recent myocardial infarction. Mortality was very high (54%) in patients who did develop PMI. Type of anesthesia and duration of surgery were not predictors of PMI.

BIBLIOGRAPHY

Adler, S. P.: Transfusion-associated cytomegalovirus infections. Rev. Infect. Dis., *5*:977–993, 1983.

Ahlquist, R.: A study of the adrenotropic receptors. Am. J. Physiol., *153*:586–600, 1948.

Alvis, J. M., Reves, J. G., Govier, A. V., et al.: Computer-assisted continuous infusions of fentanyl during cardiac anesthesia: Comparison with a manual method. Anesthesiology, *63*:41–49, 1985.

Anderson, H., and Benumof, J.: Intrapulmonary shunting during one-lung ventilation and surgical manipulation. Anesthesiology, *55*:A377, 1981.

Artru, A., and Michenfelder, J.: Influence of hypothermia or hyperthermia alone or in combination with pentobarbital or phenytoin on survival time in hypoxic mice. Anesth. Analg., *60*:867, 1981.

Ashbaugh, D. G., Bigelow, D. B., Petty, T. L., et al.: Acute respiratory distress in adults. Lancet, *2*:319, 1967.

Banoub, M., and Nugent, M.: Thoracic anesthesia. *In* Rogers, M. (ed): Principles and Practice of Anesthesiology. St. Louis, Mosby Year Book, 1993.

Barker, S. J., and Tremper, K. K.: Transcutaneous oxygen tension: Physiological variable for monitoring oxygenation. J. Clin. Monit., *1*:130–134, 1985.

Bedford, R. F.: Radial arterial function following percutaneous cannulation with 18- and 20-gauge catheters. Anesthesiology, *47*:37–39, 1977.

Benumof, J. L.: History of anesthesia for thoracic surgery. *In* Benumof, J. (ed): Anesthesia for Thoracic Surgery. Philadelphia, W. B. Saunders, 1987.

Benumof, J. L.: Mechanism of decreased blood flow to atelectatic lung. J. Appl. Physiol., *46*:1047–1048, 1978.

Benumof, J. L.: Physiology of the open chest and one lung ventilation. *In* Kaplan, J. (ed): Thoracic Anesthesia. New York, Churchill-Livingstone, 1983.

Berman, W.: The hemodynamics of shunts in congenital heart disease. *In* Johansen, K., and Burggren, W. (eds): Cardiovascular Shunts: Phylogenetic, Ontogenetic, and Clinical Aspects. New York, Raven Press, 1985, pp. 399–410.

Bland, L. A., Villarino, M. E., Arduino, M. J., et al.: Bacteriologic and endotoxin analysis of salvaged blood used in autologous transfusions during cardiac operations. J. Thorac. Cardiovasc. Surg., *103*:582–588, 1992.

Blumenthal, J., Madden, D., Burker, E., et al.: A preliminary study of the effects of cardiac procedures on cognitive performance. Int. J. Psychosomat., *38*:13–16, 1991.

Boudoulas, H., Lewis, R., Kates, R., and Dalamangas, G.: Hypersensitivity to adrenergic stimulation after propranolol withdrawal in normal subjects. Ann. Intern. Med., *87*:433–436, 1977.

Bove, J. R.: Transfusion-associated hepatitis and AIDS. What is the risk? N. Engl. J. Med., *317*:242–245, 1987.

Brodie, B., Mark, L., and Papper, E.: The fate of thiopental in man and method for its estimation in biological material. J. Pharmacol. Exp. Ther., *98*:85, 1950.

Bromage, P., Burford, M., Crowell, D., and Traunt, A.: Quality of epidural blockade. III: Carbonated local anesthetic solutions. Br. J. Anaesth., *39*:197, 1967.

Brown, B., and Crout, R.: A comparative study of the effects of five general anesthetics on myocardial contractility. Anesthesiology, *34*:236, 1971.

Brown, B., Lee, A., Bolson, E., and Dodge, H.: Reflex constriction of significant coronary stenosis as a mechanism contributing to ischemic left ventricular dysfunction during isometric exercise. Circulation, *70*:18, 1984.

Brunberg, J., Doty, D., and Reilly, E.: Choreoathetosis in infants following cardiac surgery with deep hypothermia and circulatory arrest. J. Paediatr., *84*:232–235, 1974.

Bull, B., Huse, W., Brauer, F., and Korpman, R.: Heparin therapy during extracorporeal circulation. J. Thorac. Cardiovasc. Surg., *69*:685–689, 1975.

Bunker, J. P., Forrest, W. H., and Mosteller, F.: The National Halothane Study. A Study of Possible Association Between Halothane Anesthesia and Postoperative Hepatic Necrosis. Bethesda, MD, National Institute of General Medical Sciences, 1969.

Busse, W. W., Smith, A., and Bush, R. K.: The use of a single daily theophylline dose and metered-dose albuterol in asthma treatment. J. Allerg. Clin. Immunol., *78*:577–582, 1986.

Carlens, E.: A new flexible double-lumen catheter for bronchospirometry. J. Thorac. Surg., *18*:742–748, 1949.

Cheitlin, M. D.: Finding the high-risk patient with coronary artery disease. J. A. M. A., *259*:2271–2277, 1988.

Christopherson, R., Frank, S., Norris, E., et al.: Low postoperative hematocrit is associated with cardiac ischemia in high-risk patients [Abstract]. Anesthesiology, *75*:A99, 1991.

Clark, L. C., Jr., Bargeron, J. M., Jr., and Lyons, C.: Detection of right-to-left shunts with an arterial potentiometric electrode. Circulation, *22*:949, 1960.

Clarkson, P., MacArthur, B., and Barratt-Boyes, B.: Developmental progress after cardiac surgery in infancy using hypothermia and circulatory arrest. Circulation, *62*:855–861, 1980.

Cleland, J., Pluth, J., Tauxe, W., and Kirklin, J.: Blood volume and body fluid compartment changes soon after closed and open intracardiac surgery. J. Thorac. Cardiovasc. Surg., *52*:698, 1966.

Cohen, E. N., Trudell, J. R., and Edmunds, H. N.: Urinary metabolites of halothane in man. Anesthesiology, *43*:392, 1970.

Cohn, L., Angell, W., and Shumway, N.: Body fluid shifts after cardiopulmonary bypass I. Effects of congestive heart failure and hemodilution. J. Thorac. Cardiovasc. Surg., *62*:423, 1971.

Consensus Conference: Perioperative red blood cell transfusion. J. A. M. A., *260*:2700–2703, 1988.

Conti, C. R., and Mehta, J. L.: Acute myocardial ischemia: Role of artherosclerosis, thrombosis, platelet activation, coronary vasospasm, and altered arachidonic acid metabolism. Circulation, *75*:V84–V95, 1987.

Covino, B. G.: Clinical pharmacology of local anesthetic agents. *In* Cousins, M., and Bridenbaugh (ed): Neural Blockade. 2nd ed. Philadelphia, J. B. Lippincott, 1992, pp. 111–114.

Covino, B. G., and Vassallo, H. L.: Local Anesthetics: Mechanisms of Action and Clinical Use. New York, Grune & Stratton, 1976.

Croughwell, N., Smith, L., Quill, T., et al.: The effect of temperature on cerebral metabolism and blood flow in adults during cardiopulmonary bypass. J. Thorac. Cardiovasc. Surg., *103*:549–554, 1992.

Culliford, A., Gitel, S., and Starr, N.: Lack of correlation between activated clotting time and plasma heparin during cardiopulmonary bypass. Ann. Surg., *193*:105–111, 1981.

Dale, H.: On some physiological actions of ergot. J. Physiol. (Lond.), *34*:163, 1906.

deBruijn, N. P., and Clements, F. M.: Transesophageal Echocardiography. Boston, Martinus Nijhoff, 1987.

Dickinson, D., and Sambrooks, J.: Intellectual performance in children after circulatory arrest with profound hypothermia in infancy. Arch. Dis. Child., 54:1–6, 1979.

Dunton, A., Schwam, E., and Pitman, V.: Flumazenil: US clinical pharmacology studies. Eur. J. Anaesthesiol., 2:81, 1988.

Eagle, K. A., Singer, D. E., and Brewster, D. C.: Dipyridamole-thallium scanning in patients undergoing vascular surgery. J. A. M. A., 257:2185–2189, 1987.

Eger, E. I.: Isoflurane: A review. Anesthesiology, 55:559–576, 1981.

Eger, E. I. II: Anesthetic Uptake and Action. Baltimore, Williams & Wilkins, 1974.

Ehyai, A., Fenichel, G., and Bender, H.: Incidence and prognosis of seizures in infants after cardiac surgery with profound hypothermia and circulatory arrest. J. A. M. A., 252:3165–3167, 1984.

Fahey, P. J., and Harris, K.: Clinical experience with continuous monitoring of mixed venous oxygen saturation in respiratory failure. Chest, 86:748–756, 1984.

Feldman, R., Limbird, L., and Nadeau, J.: Alterations in leukocyte B-receptor affinity with aging. N. Engl. J. Med., 310:815–819, 1984.

Flezzani, P., Croughwell, N., McIntyre, R., and Reves, J.: Isoflurane decreases the cortisol response to cardiopulmonary bypass. Anesth. Analg., 65:1117–1122, 1986.

Friedman, W.: Intrinsic physiological properties of the developing heart. Prog. Cardiovasc. Dis., 15:87–111, 1972.

Friesen, R., and Lichtor, J.: Cardiovascular depression during halothane induction in infants: A study of three induction techniques. Anesth. Analg., 61:42–45, 1982.

Friesen, R., and Lichtor, J.: Cardiovascular effects of inhalation induction with isoflurane in infants. Anesth. Analg., 62:411–414, 1983.

Fuller, J. A., Buxton, B. F., Picken, J., et al.: Haematological effects of reinfused mediastinal blood after cardiac surgery. Med. J. Aust., 154:737–740, 1991.

Glück, D., Kubanek, B., Elbert, G., et al.: Risk of HIV infection from former blood donations of donors found to be HIV antibody-positive in blood bank routine testing. "Look-back" study in German Red Cross Blood Banks in the FRG. Infusionstherapie, 17:73–76, 1990.

Goldberg, L.: Cardiovascular and renal actions of dopamine: Potential clinical applications. Pharmacol. Rev., 24:1, 1972.

Goldman, L., Caldera, D. L., and Southwick, F. S.: Cardiac risk factors and complications in noncardiac surgery. Medicine, 57:357–370, 1978.

Govier, A., Reves, J., McKay, R., and Karp, R.: Factors and their influence on regional cerebral blood flow during nonpulsatile cardiopulmonary bypass. Ann. Thorac. Surg., 38:592–600, 1984.

Greeley, W., and deBruijn, N.: Changes in sufentanil pharmacokinetics within the neonatal period. Anesth. Analg., 67:86–90, 1988.

Greeley, W., Peterson, M., Kong, D., and Oldham, H.: Effects of cardiopulmonary bypass on eicosanoid metabolism during pediatric cardiovascular surgery. J. Thorac. Cardiovasc. Surg., 95:842–889, 1988.

Greeley, W. J., Quill, T. J., and Greenberg, C. S.: Blood coagulation and thromboelastogram changes during and after pediatric cardiovascular surgery. Proceedings of Society of Cardiovascular Anesthesiologists Meeting. Boston, Nijhoff, 1986.

Greeley, W. J., and Reves, J. G.: Transesophageal atrial pacing for the treatment of dysrhythmias in pediatric surgical patients. Anesthesiology, 68:282–285, 1988.

Greeley, W. J., Ungerleider, R. M., and Reves, J. G.: Deep hypothermic cardiopulmonary bypass with total circulatory arrest alters cerebral blood flow in infants. 14th Annual Meeting Western Thoracic Surgical Association, 1988.

Gregory, G. A., Kitterman, J. A., and Phibb, R. H.: Treatment of the idiopathic respiratory distress syndrome with continuous positive airway pressure. N. Engl. J. Med., 284:1333, 1971.

Griffith, L. D., Billman, G. F., Daily, P. O., and Lane, T. A.: Apparent coagulopathy caused by infusion of shed mediastinal blood and its prevention by washing of the infusate. Ann. Thorac. Surg., 47:400–406, 1989.

Harder, M. P., Eijsman, L., Roozendaal, K. J., et al.: Aprotinin reduces intraoperative and postoperative blood loss in membrane oxygenator cardiopulmonary bypass. Ann. Thorac. Surg., 51:936–941, 1991.

Hattersley, P.: Activated coagulation time of whole blood. J. A. M. A., 196:436–440, 1966.

Henling, C. E., Carmichael, M. J., Keats, A. S., and Cooley, D. A.: Cardiac operation for congenital heart disease in children of Jehovah's Witnesses. J. Thorac. Cardiovasc. Surg., 89:914–920, 1985.

Hensley, F., Larach, D., and Stauffer, R.: The effect of halothane/nitrous oxide/oxygen mask induction on arterial hemoglobin saturation in cyanotic congenital heart disease [Abstract]. Anesthesiology, 63:A3, 1985.

Hickey, P., Hansen, D., and Wessel, D.: Pulmonary and systemic responses to fentanyl in infants. Anesth. Analg., 64:483–486, 1985.

Hoffman, B., and Lefkowitz, R.: Alpha-adrenergic receptor subtypes. N. Engl. J. Med., 302:1390, 1980.

Hughes, M., Jacobs, J., and Glass, P.: Context sensitive half-time in multi-compartment pharmacokinetic models for intravenous anesthetic drugs. Anesthesiology, 76:334–341, 1992.

Jacobs, J.: Algorithm for optimal linear model-based control with application to pharmacokinetic model-driven drug delivery. IEEE Trans. Biomed. Eng., 37:107–109, 1990.

Kaplan, J. A.: Development of Thoracic Anesthesia. New York, Churchill Livingstone, 1987.

Kass, I.: Blocking CA^{++} entry protects against anoxic brain damage in vitro. Anesthesiology, 61:A367, 1984.

Kaye, W.: Invasive monitoring techniques: Arterial cannulation, bedside pulmonary artery catheterization, and arterial puncture. Heart Lung, 12:395–427, 1983.

Kendig, J. J.: Clinical implications of the modulated receptor hypothesis: Local anesthetics and the heart. Anesthesiology, 62:382–384, 1985.

Kirklin, J., and Archie, J.: The cardiovascular subsystem in surgical patients. Surg. Gynecol. Obstet., 139:17, 1974.

Kirklin, J., Blackstone, E., and Kirklin, J.: Intracardiac surgery in infants under age 3 months: Incremental risk factors for hospital mortality. Am. J. Cardiol., 48:500–506, 1981a.

Kirklin, J., Blackstone, E., and Kirklin, J.: Intracardiac surgery in infants under age 3 months: Predictors of postoperative in-hospital cardiac death. Am. J. Cardiol., 46:507–512, 1981b.

Kirklin, J., Daggett, W., and Lappas, D.: Postoperative care following cardiac surgery. In Johnson, R., Haber, E., and Austen, W. (eds): The Practice of Cardiology. Boston, Little Brown, 1980.

Kirklin, J., Westaby, S., Blackstone, E., and Kirklin, J.: Complement and the damaging effects of cardiopulmonary bypass. J. Thorac. Cardiovasc. Surg., 86:845, 1983.

Kunkel, R., Hagl, S., and Richter, J.: The effects of deep hypothermia and circulatory arrest on systemic metabolic state of infants undergoing corrective open heart surgery: A comparison of two methods. J. Thorac. Cardiovasc. Surg., 27:168–177, 1979.

Lamberti, J., Lin, C., and Cutiletta, A.: Surface cooling and circulatory arrest in infants undergoing cardiac surgery. Arch. Surg., 113:822–826, 1978.

Lee, J., Halloran, K., and Taylor, J.: Coronary flow and myocardial metabolism in newborn lambs: Effects of hypoxia and acidemia. Am. J. Physiol., 224:1381–1387, 1973.

Lell, W., Samuelson, P., Reves, J., and Strong, S.: Duration of intubation and ICU stay after open heart surgery. South. Med. J., 72:773, 1979.

Leslie, J., Kalayjian, R., and Sirgo, M.: Intravenous labetalol for treatment of postoperative hypertension. Anesthesiology, 67:413–416, 1987.

Leventhal, R., Orkin, F. K., and Hirsh, R. A.: Prediction of the need for postoperative mechanical ventilation in myasthenia gravis. Anesthesiology, 53:26, 1980.

London, M. J., and Mangano, D. T.: Assessment of perioperative cardiac risk. In Kirby R. R., and Brown, D. L. (eds): Problems in Anesthesia, Cardiovascular Anesthesia. Philadelphia, J. B. Lippincott, 1987.

Lowenstein, E., Hallowell, P., and Levine, F. H.: Cardiovascular response to large doses of intravenous morphine in man. N. Engl. J. Med., 281:1389–1393, 1969.

Lunn, J. K., Stanley, T. H., Eisele, J. H., et al.: High dose fentanyl anesthesia for coronary artery surgery: Plasma fentanyl concentrations and influence of nitrous oxide on cardiovascular responses. Anesth. Analg., 58:390–395, 1979.

Maccioli, G. A., and Reves, J. G.: Anesthesia: A method of protection in patients with ischemic heart disease. State of the Art Reviews: Cardiac Surgery, 2:145–154, 1988.

Mahar, L. J., Steen, P. A., Tinker, J. H., et al.: Perioperative myocardial infarction in patients with coronary artery disease with and without aorta-coronary artery bypass grafts. J. Thorac. Cardiovasc. Surg., 76:533–537, 1978.

Maisel, A., Motulsky, H., and Ansel, P.: Propranolol treatment externalizes beta-adrenergic receptors in pig myocardium and prevents further externalization by ischemia. Circ. Res., 60:108–112, 1987.

Mallampati, S. R., Gatt, S. P., Gugino, L. D., et al.: A clinical sign to predict difficult tracheal intubation: A prospective study. Can. Anaesth. Soc. J., 32:429–434, 1985.

Mallow, J. E., White, R. D., Cucchiara, R. F.: Hemodynamic effects of isoflurane and halothane in patients with coronary artery disease. Anesth. Analg., 55:135–138, 1976.

Maseri, A., Chierchia, S., and Davies, G.: Pathophysiology of coronary occlusion in acute infarction. Circulation, 73:233–239, 1986.

Matthay, M. A.: Invasive hemodynamic monitoring in critically ill patients. Clin. Chest. Med., 4:233–249, 1983.

Mauney, F. M., Ebert, P. A., and Sabiston, D. C.: Postoperative myocardial infarction: A study of predisposing factors, diagnosis and mortality in a high risk group of surgical patients. Ann. Surg., 172:497–503, 1970.

Menkhaus, P., Reves, J., and Kissin, I.: Cardiovascular effects of esmolol in anesthetized humans. Anesth. Analg., 64:327–334, 1985.

Merin, R. G.: Are the myocardial functional and metabolic effects of isoflurane really different from those of halothane and enflurane? Anesthesiology, 55:398–408, 1981.

Milam, J., Austin, S. F., and Nihill, M.: Use of sufficient hemodilution to prevent coagulopathies following surgical correction of cyanotic heart disease. J. Thorac. Cardiovasc. Surg., 89:623–629, 1985.

Miller, P., O'Connel, J., and Leipold, A.: Potential liability for transfusion-associated AIDS. J. A. M. A., 253:3419–3423, 1985.

Moller, R., and Covino, B. F.: Cardiac electrophysiologic properties of bupivacaine and lidocaine compared with those of ropivacaine, a new amide local anesthetic. Anesthesiology, 72:322–329, 1990.

Morris, R. B., Cahalan, M. K., Miller, R. D., et al.: The cardiovascular effects of vecuronium (ORG NC45) and pancuronium in patients undergoing coronary artery bypass grafting. Anesthesiology, 58:438–450, 1983.

Murkin, J., Farrar, J., Tweed, A., et al.: Cerebral autoregulation and flow/metabolism coupling during cardiopulmonary bypass. The influence of $P_{A_{CO_2}}$. Anesth. Analg., 66:825–832, 1987.

Murphy, P., Heal, J. M., and Blumberg, N.: Infection or suspected infection after hip replacement surgery with autologous or homologous blood transfusions. Transfusion, 31:212–217, 1991.

Newman, M., Schell, R., Croughwell, N., et al.: Pattern and time course of cognitive dysfunction following cardiopulmonary bypass. Anesth. Analg., 76:S294, 1993.

Panico, F. G., and Neptune, W. B.: A mechanism to eliminate the donor blood prime from the pump-oxygenator. Surg. Forum, 10:605–609, 1959.

Price, M. L., and Price, H. L.: Effect of general anesthetics on contractile response of rabbit aorta strips. Anesthesiology, 23:16–20, 1962.

Prough, D., Stump, D., and Roy, R.: Response of cerebral blood flow to changes in carbon dioxide tension during hypothermic cardiopulmonary bypass. Anesthesiology, 64:576–581, 1986.

Reves, J.: Pharmacology of vasoactive drugs. In Thomas, S. (ed): Manual of Cardiac Anesthesia. New York, Churchill Livingstone, 1993.

Reves, J., Karp, R., and Buttner, E.: Neuronal and adrenomedullary catecholamine release in response to cardiopulmonary bypass in man. Circulation, 66:49–55, 1980.

Reves, J. G., and Gelman, S.: Cardiovascular effects of intravenous

anesthetic drugs. In Covino, Fozzard, Rehder, and Strichartz (eds): Effects of Anesthesia. Bethesda, MD, American Physiological Society, 1985.

Roy, W. L., Edelilst, G., and Gilbert, B.: Myocardial ischemia during non-cardiac surgical procedures in patients with coronary artery disease. Anesthesiology, 51:393–397, 1979.

Rudolph, A. M.: Congenital Diseases of the Heart. Chicago, Year Book, 1974.

Samuelson, P., Reves, J., and Kirklin, J.: Comparison of sufentanil and enflurane-nitrous oxide anesthesia for myocardial revascularization. Anesth. Analg., 65:217–226, 1986.

Samuelson, P. N., Reves, J. G., Smith, L. R., and Kouchoukos, N. T.: Midazolam versus diazepam: Different effects on systemic vascular resistance: A randomized study utilizing cardiopulmonary bypass constant flow. Arzneim-Forsch. Drug Res., 31:2268–2269, 1981.

Sarnoff, S. J., Braunwald, E., Welch, J., and Case, R. B.: Hemodynamic determinants of oxygen consumption of the heart with special reference to the tension-time index. Am. J. Physiol., 192:148–156, 1958.

Sazama, K.: Reports of 355 transfusion-associated deaths: 1976 through 1985. Transfusion, 30:583–590, 1990.

Schell, R., Kern, F., Greeley, W., et al.: Cerebral blood flow and metabolism during cardiopulmonary bypass. Anesth. Analg., 76:849–865, 1993.

Scott, D. B., Lee, A., Fagan, D., et al.: Acute toxicity of ropivacaine compared with that of bupivacaine. Anesth. Analg., 69:563–569, 1989.

Seltzer, J. L., Gerson, J. L., and Allen, F. B.: Comparison of the cardiovascular effects of bolus v. incremetal administration of thippentone. Br. J. Anaesth., 52:527–530, 1980.

Shanks, C. A.: Pharmacokinetics of the nondepolarizing neuromuscular relaxants applied to calculation of bolus and infusion dosage regimens. Anesthesiology, 64:72–86, 1986.

Slogoff, S., and Keats, A. S.: Does chronic treatment with calcium entry blocking drugs reduce perioperative myocardial ischemia? Anesthesiology, 68:676–680, 1988.

Slogoff, S., and Keats, A. S.: Does perioperative myocardial ischemia lead to postoperative myocardial infarction? Anesthesiology, 62:107–114, 1985.

Slogoff, S., and Keats, A. S.: Further observations on perioperative myocardial ischemia. Anesthesiology, 65:539–542, 1986.

Sonnenblick, F. H., and Skelton, C. L.: Myocardial energetics: Basic principles in clinical implications. N. Engl. J. Med., 285:668–675, 1971.

Sonntag, H., Hellberg, K., and Schenk, H. D.: Effects of thiopental (trapanal) on coronary blood flow and myocardial metabolism in man. Acta. Anaesth. Scand., 19:69–78, 1975.

Spahn, D. R., Smith, L. R., McRae, R. L., and Leone, B. J.: Effects of acute isovolemic hemodilution and anesthesia on regional function in left ventricular myocardium with compromised coronary blood flow. Acta Anaesth. Scand., 36:628–636, 1992.

Spahn, D. R., Smith, L. R., Veronee, C. D., et al.: Acute isovolemic hemodilution and blood transfusion: Effects on regional function and metabolism in myocardium with compromised coronary blood flow. J. Thorac. Cardiovasc. Surg., 105:694–704, 1993.

Sprigge, J. S., Wynands, J. E., and Whalley, D. G.: Fentanyl infusion anesthesia for aortocoronary bypass surgery: Plasma levels and hemodynamic response. Anesth. Analg., 61:972–978, 1982.

Steen, P., Gisvold, S., and Milde, J.: Nimodipine improves outcome when given after complete cerebral ischemia in primates. Anesthesiology, 62:406–414, 1985.

Steen, P. A., Tinker, J. H., and Tarhan, S.: Myocardial reinfarction after anesthesia and surgery. J. A. M. A., 239:2566–2570, 1978.

Stenlake, J. B., Waigh, R. D., Urwin, J., et al.: Atracurium: Conception and inception. Br. J. Anaesth., 55:3S–10A, 1983.

Stewart, R., Blackstone, E., and Kirklin, J.: Neurological dysfunction after cardiac surgery. In Parenzan, L., Crupi, G., and Graham, G. (eds): Congenital Heart Disease in the First Three Months of Life: Medical and Surgical Aspects. Bologna, Italy, Patron Editore, 1981.

Stone, J., Foex, P., Sear, J., et al.: Myocardial ischemia in untreated hypertensive patients: Effect of a single small oral dose of a beta-adrenergic blocking agent. Anesthesiology, 68:495–500, 1988.

Tarhan, S., Moffitt, E. A., Taylor, W. F., and Giuliani, E. R.: Myocardial infarction after general anesthesia. J. A. M. A., 220:1451–1454, 1972.

Tharion, J., Johnsol, D., and Celemajer, J.: Profound hypothermia with circulatory arrest. J. Thorac. Cardiovasc. Surg., 84:66–73, 1982.

Theil, D., Stanley, T., White, W., et al.: Midazolam and fentanyl continuous infusion anesthesia for cardiac surgery: A comparison of computer-assisted versus manual infusion systems. J. Cardiothorac. Vasc. Anesth., 7:300–306, 1993.

Tomicheck, R. C., Rosow, C. E., and Philbin, D. M.: Diazepam-fentanyl interaction: Hemodynamic and hormonal effects in coronary artery surgery. Anesth. Analg., 62:881–884, 1983.

Treasure, T., Naftel, D., and Conger, K.: The effect of hypothermic circulatory arrest time on cerebral function, morphology, and biochemistry. J. Thorac. Cardiovasc. Surg., 86:761–770, 1985.

Vanhoutte, P.: Alpha- and beta-adrenergic receptors and the cardiovascular system. J. Cardiovasc. Pharmacol., 3:S1, 1981.

Venugopal, P., Olszowka, J., and Wagner, H.: Early correction of congenital heart disease with surface-induced deep hypothermia and circulatory arrest. J. Thorac. Cardiovasc. Surg., 66:375–385, 1973.

Wagner, J. D.: A safe method for rapidly achieving plasma concentration plateaus. Clin. Pharmacol. Ther., 16:691–700, 1974.

Wallach, R., Karp, R., Reves, J., and Oparil, S.: Pathogenesis of paroxysmal hypertension developing during and after coronary bypass surgery: A study of hemodynamic and humoral factors. Am. J. Cardiol., 46:559, 1980.

Waymack, J. P., Warden, G. D., Alexander, J. W., et al.: Effect of blood transfusion and anesthesia on resistance to bacterial peritonitis. J. Surg. Res., 42:528–535, 1987.

Wells, F., Coghill, F., and Caplan, H.: Duration of circulatory arrest does influence the psychological development of children after cardiac operation in early life. J. Thorac. Cardiovasc. Surg., 86:823–831, 1983.

Wells, R., Friedman, W., and Sobel, B.: Increased oxidative metabolism in the fetal and newborn lamb heart. Am. J. Physiol., 222:1488–1493, 1972.

West, R.: Curare in man. Proc. R. Soc. Med., 25:1107–1116, 1932.

Whitten, C., Allison, P., Latson, T., et al.: Autologous blood after cardiopulmonary bypass alters hemostatic and thromboelastographic parameters [Abstract]. Anesth. Analg., 74:S348, 1992.

Wright, J., Hicks, R., and Newman, D.: Deep hypothermic arrest: Observation on later development in children. J. Thorac. Cardiovasc. Surg., 77:466–468, 1979.

Young, J., Kisker, C., and Doty, D.: Adequate anticoagulation during cardiopulmonary bypass determined by activated clotting time and the appearance of fibrin monomer. Ann. Thorac. Surg., 26:231–240, 1978.

Yusuf, S., Theodoropoulos, S., Mathias, C. J., and Dhalla, N.: Increased sensitivity of the denervated transplanted human heart to isoprenaline both before and after β-adrenergic blockade. Circulation, 75:696–704, 1987.

Zsigmond, E. K., Kothary, S. P., and Matsuki, A.: Diazepam for prevention of the rise in plasma catecholamines caused by ketamine. Clin. Pharmacol. Ther., 15:223–224, 1974.

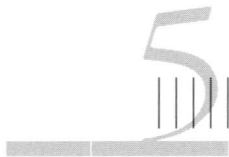

■ II Acute Pain Management After Surgical Procedures

Brian Ginsberg and Katherine Grichnik

Major progress has been made in the alleviation of acute pain. Since the mid-1980s, much attention has been focused on the concept of preemptive analgesia using opioids, nonsteroidal anti-inflammatory agents, and regional analgesia. Not only is the alleviation of pain a humanitarian need but numerous studies have documented that preventing and alleviating pain is associated with both reduced morbidity and reduced mortality (Cushieri et al., 1985; Wasylak et al., 1990; Yeager et al., 1987). Historically, pain management following surgery has relied on the *intramuscular* administration of opioids to relieve inevitable pain. However, this form of analgesia is far from ideal and has left many patients suffering from needless pain. Studies have reported an incidence of severe pain following surgery that has ranged from 35 to 75% (Marks and Sachar, 1973). The inadequacy of pain control has prompted the use of new techniques, drugs, and routes of administration. These techniques include patient-controlled analgesia, epidurally administered analgesics, transdermally administered opioids, transmucosally administered opioids, interpleural analgesia, and supplemental methods.

The gold standard of pain medication, intramuscularly administered opioids on a p.r.n. (pro re nata, as required) basis, has failed to provide adequate analgesia for a number of reasons: the amount and timing of the administered dose, the pharmacokinetics and pharmacodynamics of the opioids used, and the vast interindividual variability in the amount of opioid required by patients. In addition, the medical and nursing staff who are left to make the management decisions lack the confidence and skills to use the technique effectively.

The timing and amount of opioid to be administered intramuscularly are based on a prescription that indicates a range of doses and a variable frequency on a p.r.n. basis. A flexible dosing regimen should be ideal for the management of postoperative pain, because the amount of pain and the response to an analgesic vary. However, this flexibility results in patients receiving as little as 25% of the prescribed dose despite their reporting of inadequate pain relief (Marks and Sachar, 1973). The blame cannot rest entirely on the shoulders of the nursing staff, because the prescribing physicians tend to order inadequate amounts of opioids and fail to adjust the dosing regimen frequently enough to meet the patients' needs (Graves et al., 1983).

The intramuscular route of administration, although easy to use, increases the variability in response to the intramuscular medication. After intramuscular administration, the peak plasma level achieved varies by 5 times; the time taken to reach this peak level can vary by 15 times (Rigg et al., 1978). After intramuscularly administered opioids, the blood levels of the opioid will rise to a peak level and subsequently decline with time. This analgesic state is maintained until the waning plasma level falls below the threshold and pain is experienced. Because the frequency of the intramuscular dosing is restricted, larger doses than necessary are usually given, resulting in blood levels that exceed the analgesic threshold. Patients thus experience dose-related side effects of the opioids.

The plasma level of the opioid that provides analgesia, the *minimal effective analgesic concentration* (MEAC), varies with time and activity; there is up to a 5-fold difference among individuals in plasma levels that will provide analgesia (Dahlström et al., 1982; Tamsen et al., 1982). Unfortunately, except for age, little information helps to predict the analgesic requirements for any particular patient. Analgesic requirements decrease linearly with age. This marked interpatient variability in MEAC requires individualized pain management.

The aim of any analgesic regimen is an alert, pain-free patient with near-normal physiologic parameters who can cooperate with medical therapy. Before initiating therapy, physicians should consider the following:

1. The dose should maximize analgesia and minimize possible side effects.
2. The relationship between the plasma level and the antinociceptive effect of the analgesic should be simple (i.e., as the concentration increases, so will the analgesic efficacy).
3. The pharmacokinetics of the analgesic are altered by the effects of anesthesia and the surgical procedure.

Because the intramuscular route for giving pain medication is inadequate, other modes of analgesia have been developed. They include intravenous medication via patient-controlled analgesia (PCA), epidural analgesia, intrapleural analgesia, peripheral nerve block, transdermal and transmucosal analgesia, and adjuvant medications.

PATIENT–CONTROLLED ANALGESIA

PCA can individualize opioid dosing without extensive nursing intervention. However, to use PCA safely and effectively, one must understand the pharmacodynamics and pharmacokinetics of the drugs administered and the variables of the delivery system.

PCA is a device that allows patients to give themselves pain medication in a highly controlled manner. After analgesia has been established with a loading dose of opioid (usually in the recovery room), patients give themselves small doses of opioids to maintain their level of analgesia. Thus, patients do not have to wait for a third party to assess their pain, nor do they have to wait for an intramuscular opioid to work, sometimes with side effects secondary to the dose. Lock-out intervals and safe maximum doses are built into the program so that patients cannot give themselves too much.

Advantages

Patients intuitively perceive the theoretical advantages and disadvantages of PCA (Kluger and Owen, 1990). In a study before surgery, patients were asked to list the advantages and disadvantages of PCA. The major potential disadvantage was that the use of PCA would limit contact with the nursing staff. In addition, these patients were afraid that they could inadvertently administer an overdose. Inadequacy of analgesia and the possibility of becoming addicted to the opioid were other concerns. All of these fears can be allayed by adequate education of the patients and personnel. The major advantages of PCA as perceived by the patients were that they would not have to bother the nurse, the onset of analgesia would be rapid, and they would have control over their pain. This theoretical knowledge base has translated into adequate, effective use of PCA as demonstrated by a significant correlation between the amount of analgesic used and the objective pain level (Kluger and Owen, 1990).

When patients use PCA, they tend not to use the device to obtain complete analgesia. Most patients are satisfied with a level of "mild pain," 20 to 30 mm on a 100-mm VAS scale (a scale used to assess pain from 1 to 100 or from no pain to the worst pain imaginable) rather than complete analgesia. Patients keep their blood level of the opioid below the level that produces side effects. Even when patients titrated themselves to a level of analgesia that was not perfect, they still considered PCA superior to intramuscular analgesia (Bennett et al., 1982; Bollish et al., 1985).

PCA has been compared with many other forms to determine if PCA has any significant advantages. Compared with conventional intramuscular medication, PCA led patients to use less analgesia (Bennett et al., 1982; Bollish et al., 1985), suffer less sedation (Bennett et al., 1982), and ambulate earlier (Atwell et al., 1984). The period of ileus following bowel surgery was reduced in the group receiving PCA when compared with the group receiving conventional analgesia (Albert and Talbott, 1988). Patients on PCA have demonstrated a reduced incidence of postoperative fever as compared with intramuscularly medicated control subjects (Lange et al., 1988). Although PCA may improve the level of analgesia, this has not translated to a reduction in the catabolic response to operation (Moller et al., 1988). Further, these findings have not been universal. Some patients on PCA have required more analgesics and have had ileus longer than patients on conventional medication (Rogers et al., 1990).

When PCA was compared with intercostal block or intramuscularly administered morphine, more patients in the PCA group rated their analgesia as "good" (Rosenberg et al., 1984). The pain relief achieved with epidural opioids, however, was found to be superior to relief achieved with PCA (Eisenach et al., 1988; Harrison et al., 1988). Although the epidural opioids produced significantly lower visual analog pain scales than did PCA, the patients still preferred the analgesia that was achieved with PCA. The improved analgesia of PCA as compared with other modes was associated with earlier ambulation, diminished morbidity, and earlier discharge from the hospital following hysterectomy (Wasylak et al., 1990).

Initial concerns with the use of PCA included oversedation and use of the PCA in age extremes. With appropriate monitoring, these concerns should be no stronger than with conventional medications. In 83 elderly patients, PCA demonstrated superior analgesia to the control subjects receiving intramuscular medication (Egberts et al., 1990). Further, there was no increase in sedation or difference in oxygen saturation. PCA has also been used effectively to provide analgesia in children and adolescents (Berde et al., 1991). PCA also demonstrated its superiority over a constant-rate intravenous infusion in bone marrow transplant patients (Hill et al., 1990).

Clinical Use

When PCA is initiated, the following factors need to be considered:

- Loading dose
- Maintenance dose
- Lock-out interval
- Continuous infusion
- Opioid selection
- Monitoring protocols
- Complications of PCA
- Weaning from PCA

Loading Dose

An adequate loading dose given under the supervision of a doctor will enable patients to rapidly achieve a pain-free state. Postoperatively, a patient's level of awareness is reduced during the recovery period from anesthesia, limiting the ability to use PCA effectively (Dahlström et al., 1982). In addition, the pain level is highest during the immediate postoperative period. If the maintenance dose is used without the benefit of a loading dose, an analgesic state will not be prolonged.

The minimal effective analgesic concentration (MEAC) has been defined for a number of different opioids (Table 5–13). Because the MEAC is known for

■ **Table 5–13.** CHARACTERISTICS OF VARIOUS OPIOIDS

	Morphine	Meperidine	Dilaudid	Fentanyl
Octanol/H$_2$O at pH 7.4	1.4	39	8	813
MEAC (ng/ml)	16	455	4	1
T½ beta (minutes)	177	222	142	185

MEAC = minimal effective analgesic concentration.

the opioids, why not infuse the opioid to reach this plasma end-point using simple pharmacokinetics? The dose of the opioid in question could be determined by multiplying the MEAC (target concentration) by the volume of distribution of the opioid. Unfortunately, MEAC represents a range of plasma levels, not a specific value. The MEAC plasma level varies up to 5 times among individuals (Dahlström et al., 1982; Tamsen et al., 1982). The MEAC also varies with time and activity in a given patient. Because the MEAC varies so much, the loading dose is best titrated to effect. The total loading dose is usually broken into two or three equal doses repeated every 6 to 10 minutes until effective pain relief is achieved. Patients should not be discharged from the postanesthetic care unit before adequate pain control is achieved.

Most PCA units have a loading mode that will limit the need for any separate analgesics. This facility will also limit the amount of paperwork required to control opioids. If the PCA unit lacks a loading mode, an adequate loading dose must be given by the medical staff before maintenance therapy is initiated.

Maintenance Dose

PCA units use an intermittent bolus dose that is self-administered by the patient. Also called a PCA dose or a maintenance dose, it is usually administered intravenously. The maintenance dose can be administered by pressing and releasing a button that can either be on a hand-held pendant or attached to the PCA unit itself. When the button is released, some PCA units emit an audible signal. This audible tone is reassuring to patients who use PCA, and most patients appreciate this feature. Less anxiety and better pain control was reported when the signal was emitted after a successful request for PCA (Hecker and Albert, 1988).

The aim of the small, frequently injected dose in PCA is to safely maintain an analgesic blood level without producing sedation. The dose required to produce this effect is highly individualized, because pain tolerance and response to analgesics vary widely. (Dahlström et al., 1982). The analgesic requirement of patients decreases with age, is poorly related to height and weight, and may be related to gender (Bellville et al., 1971; Burns et al., 1989; Ginsberg et al., 1989). This poor correlation between PCA use and patient demographics is no different from the vast experience with intramuscularly administered opioids (Austin et al., 1980a).

It is important that the maintenance dose of PCA be optimized for each patient. If a small dose is selected in an attempt to minimize the risks of respiratory depression, inadequate analgesia can result. Some personnel assume that the patient will simply increase the number of demands to compensate for the small dose. However, patients cannot increase the number of demands sufficiently to compensate for an inadequate maintenance dose. Doses that are set too high can produce unacceptable side effects (Owen et al., 1989a).

The patient's weight is a useful guide in initiating PCA dosing, even though the ultimate correlation between analgesic requirements and weight is poor. Effectiveness of the dose selected must be appraised intermittently to ensure optimal analgesia and thus patient satisfaction. Patients are satisfied if they do not have to make too many repeated demands over too long a period. Clinically, we attempt to keep the average number of successful demands at approximately two to three per hour.

It is helpful to be able to obtain a history of the patient's demands and the machine's delivery from the PCA unit. Not only is the number of completed demands important, but valuable information can be obtained from the number of unsuccessful demands that are made. This demand-to-delivery ratio can be used as a guide to the patient's pain level, understanding of the PCA unit, and anxiety level. The doses that we generally administer for the commonly used opioids are summarized in Table 5–14. If patients demonstrate inadequate analgesia despite making sufficient demands, the dose is increased by 25 to 50%. This must not be automatic: The patient must be evaluated before the dose is increased to exclude an alteration in the patient's condition, such as a tight limb cast. Similarly, if the patient manifests signs of an overdose such as excessive sedation, the dose is reduced by 25 to 50%.

Lock-Out Interval

This is the period during which the PCA unit is refractory to further demands by the patient. The *lock-out interval* (LOI) is a needed safeguard to prevent patients from taking a further dose before they appreciate the full effect of the preceding dose. This will limit the potential for the patient to administer an inadvertent overdose.

The LOI should therefore take into account the speed of onset of the agent and the time during which adequate concentrations of the opioid are available (Mather and Owen, 1988). A shorter LOI would be required for an agent that has a rapid onset of action but that diffuses out of the effective compartment rapidly. The LOI will also be influenced by the size of the maintenance dose: with a larger maintenance dose, the LOI can be widened. The optimal LOI still has to be defined for the different analgesic agents in all settings. The manufacturers of PCA units allow a range of settings from 1 to 99 minutes. The average LOIs are depicted in Table 5–14.

Continuous Infusion

Most PCA units provide a number of options in addition to PCA that can be employed to provide analgesia. These options include constant-rate infusion and constant-rate infusion plus PCA.

Constant-Rate Infusion. Constant-rate infusion of opioids provides pain relief to patients after surgery. When an infusion is started, the plasma level of the opioid gradually increases until the rate of infusion matches the rate of elimination. The time taken for the analgesic to reach the plateau level will be dictated by the elimination half-life of the drug selected. Ninety-four per cent of the final concentration will be reached in four half-lives of the agent and 98% will be reached in six half-lives. The elimination half-lives of the commonly used agents are given in Table 5–13. With the use of a simple constant-rate infusion, the final level will be reached after 20 to 24 hours. Therefore, to reach the plateau level rapidly, either a loading dose or a variable infusion rate can be used.

Constant-rate infusion, although effective, cannot adapt to the marked variability among the analgesic requirements of different patients. Therefore, the rate of infusion must be continuously tailored to each patient. This requires constant adjustments in the infusion rate in both directions. In addition, the postoperative patient is assailed by at least two forms of pain. The first is the constant pain emanating from the wound, which can be adequately managed by a constant-rate infusion of analgesics. The second is the acute exacerbation of pain following movement induced by coughing, physiotherapy, or dressing changes. Constant-rate infusion adjusted by the nursing staff to the patient's pain level used more morphine than did continuous infusion of morphine supplemented with PCA (Zacharias et al., 1990).

Constant-Rate Infusion Plus PCA. A continuous or "background" infusion is often used to supplement intermittent bolus doses. The addition of a low-dose constant infusion should minimize the fluctuation in the plasma concentration of the analgesic and provide better analgesia. In addition, the continuous infusion theoretically reduces the number of demands and decreases the severe pain that many patients experience when awakening. If the infusion keeps the patient in or close to the MEAC, a small supplemental dose may be all that is required to provide complete

■ **Table 5–14.** DOSES OF OPIOIDS AND SETTINGS FOR PATIENT-CONTROLLED ANALGESIA

Drug	Dose (μg/kg)	Lock-Out Interval (minutes)	Loading Dose (μg/kg)
Morphine	20–30	8–12	50–100
Meperidine	200–250	8–12	500–750
Fentanyl	20–40	5–8	0.5–1
Hydromorphone	2–4	6–10	20–40
Sufentanil	0.01–0.02	5–8	0.1–0.2

analgesia. It has been demonstrated that only a small alteration in the plasma level of the opioid may be needed to relieve severe pain (Austin et al., 1980b).

Continuous infusion in addition to PCA has not been as beneficial as had been anticipated, but a study showed that the addition of a continuous infusion of 1.5 mg/hour to a PCA dose of 1 mg (LOI of 2 minutes) led to an increased use of morphine (73.8 ± 16.3 mg) when compared with PCA alone (33.9 ± 14.6 mg) with similar analgesic effectiveness (Owen et al., 1989b). Similarly, following abdominal surgery, the use of continuous infusion added to PCA increased morphine use (Hansen et al., 1991) with equal satisfaction. In a group of patients recovering from abdominal hysterectomy, the addition of a continuous infusion did not influence the quantity of morphine used or alter the time to recovery (Parker et al., 1989, 1991). Therefore, a continuous infusion should not be used routinely to manage acute pain even when combined with PCA, but should be reserved for specific indications.

Opioid Selection

The ideal PCA agent should have a rapid onset of action with a medium duration of action. There should be no ceiling to the analgesic effect, and the agent should not cause nausea, vomiting, respiratory depression, or impairment of bowel motility. Because no opioid is available with these properties, the agents selected for PCA represent a compromise. The use of the agonist-antagonist group of analgesics is limited by their ceiling effect on the level of analgesia that can be achieved. In addition, analgesics with very short or very long duration of action are inappropriate for PCA.

Morphine is one of the most commonly used analgesics for PCA. It has been used extensively with safety, is inexpensive, and is familiar to most medical personnel. The onset of action of morphine is slow compared with that of the more lipid-soluble opioids, but its duration of action is longer. In the first hour following surgery, a highly lipid-soluble opioid such as fentanyl more greatly reduced pain levels than did morphine even after an adequate loading dose (Ginsberg et al., 1989). After the initial 6 hours, the difference in opioids was no longer apparent, because the patients had compensated for the different properties of the opioid. Similarly, when morphine was compared with the more lipid-soluble meperidine and oxymorphone in PCA, the initial analgesia with morphine was not as good as with the other two agents (Sinatra et al., 1989). In addition, morphine also tends to cause more sedation than meperidine, oxymorphone, or sufentanil (Sinatra et al., 1989; Ved et al., 1989). Opioid use is characterized by wide interpatient variability in the amount of opioid used for similar procedures. Morphine, however, has a long efficacy and safety record.

Meperidine is the only opioid other than morphine that has been approved by the Food and Drug Administration (FDA) for PCA use. In a double-blind comparison of meperidine and morphine, no differences were found in the level of analgesia (at rest) or in side-effect profile (Bahar et al., 1985). The difference between the analgesics became apparent on deep breathing. Morphine provided superior analgesia with this physiologic stress. In patients who had undergone cesarean section, pain relief on movement also was inadequate with meperidine when compared with morphine or oxymorphone (Sinatra et al., 1989). A comparison of the total morphine and meperidine use over 72 hours of PCA for differing surgical procedures showed variation in the ratio of morphine to meperidine use. The ratio of meperidine to morphine use for this postoperative period was ±2:1 for abdominal procedures and ±3:1 for orthopedic procedures. These studies indicate a difference in the quality of analgesia among agents.

Although meperidine is an effective analgesic, its use is complicated by the possible accumulation of normeperidine, the principal metabolite of meperidine. Normoperidine causes dose-related central nervous system excitement manifesting as agitation, insomnia, and tremors that can culminate in seizures (Kaiko et al., 1983). Fifty-six per cent of the patients in this study experienced central nervous system excitation at doses that exceeded 250 mg of meperidine per day. Because normeperidine is renally excreted, the risks of potential toxicity are enhanced by renal failure.

Fentanyl has been used extensively to provide postoperative analgesia. Fentanyl has a more rapid onset than do less lipid-soluble drugs (Lehmann et al., 1986). The amount of fentanyl required with procedures ranging from hysterectomies to thoracotomies has varied from 0.4 to 2.55 μg/kg/hr, with a maintenance dose of 7.2 to 34.5 μg (Lehmann et al., 1988). Even when the type of surgery, anesthetic technique, and sex of the patient were standardized, they accounted for only a little of this variability (Lehmann et al., 1990). The hourly use of fentanyl in these studies has ranged from 0.68 ± 0.39 μg/hr for thoracotomy patients to 0.39 ± 0.31 μg/hr for abdominal surgery. Fentanyl is thus characterized by extremely varied interpatient requirements. Fentanyl is an excellent drug for intravenous use because it does not release histamine, as many opioids do, and it has few other side effects. In addition, the metabolites of fentanyl are not active.

Other opioids that have been used successfully for PCA include alfentanil, sufentanil, and hydromorphone. Use of alfentanil for PCA produced less sedation but equivalent levels of analgesia when compared with meperidine or fentanyl (Kay, 1981; Welchew and Hosking, 1985). However, patients using alfentanil experienced more pain in the first 6 hours of the study than did patients using meperidine, morphine, or sufentanil (Reedy et al., 1986; Welchew and Hosking, 1985). This could be a result of the brief duration of action of alfentanil. Sufentanil is an excellent agent for PCA because it is highly lipid-soluble and has an intermediate duration of action. In addition, sufentanil has been associated with less respiratory depression than fentanyl in healthy volunteers, regardless of dose (Bailey et al., 1990). In a study comparing sufentanil, alfentanil, and morphine, sufentanil provided a rapid onset of pain relief, less sedation, and less depression of oxygen saturation. Hydromorphone has also been used extensively in PCA and may be especially useful in patients with sickle cell anemia who are intolerant of other analgesics.

Butorphanol, nalbuphine, and buprenorphine are members of the mixed agonist-antagonist group of analgesics. Butorphanol is a fully synthetic morphine derivative that is 5 to 7 times as potent as morphine. It has been used to provide analgesia to patients following abdominal surgery via PCA without any ceiling effect to the level of analgesia (Reedy et al., 1986). Nalbuphine is as potent as morphine at low doses. Although it provided effective analgesia with PCA in one study, nalbuphine provided ineffective analgesia in another study, and its use always caused excessive sedation (Jaffe and Martin, 1985; Sprigge and Otton, 1983). Buprenorphine is highly lipid-soluble and is 25 to 30 times as potent as morphine. Buprenorphine use has been characterized by a high incidence of nausea (62%) (Gibbs et al., 1982).

Monitoring Protocols

Before a PCA service is initiated, protocols need to be established for the effective and safe use of this form of analgesia, including detailed instruction to the staff on the use of the PCA device, opioid control, and, most important, patient monitoring and care. The patient monitoring should include assessment at least every 4 hours of the patient's level of pain and sedation and respiratory rate. A simple verbal pain scale will track the patient's pain level and alert the staff if alterations in PCA settings are necessary. These parameters should be recorded on a flow sheet so that trends are apparent. Further, on every shift change, the PCA settings should be checked against the prescription to circumvent inadvertent programming errors.

Patient education will ensure optimal pain relief and should take place preoperatively. The teaching should include such topics as use of the PCA button often enough to keep pain at a minimum, rather than waiting until it is severe; use of the PCA device before painful activities such as movement or breathing exercises; reassurance of the unlikelihood of overdosage or addiction; reporting of side effects to nursing staff; and when to expect a change to oral medication. In addition, relatives and friends may be instructed to encourage the patient to use the PCA. However, relatives and friends may not be allowed to press the button for the patient. Currently, we attach a label to our PCA pumps warning relatives that the PCA pump is only safe if used by the patient.

Complications

The most feared complication of opioid use is respiratory depression. The onset of and recovery from respiratory depression will occur more rapidly with lipophilic opioids than with morphine. Respiratory rate and sedation scale checks are both used to detect the onset of respiratory depression. A decrease in respiratory rate is the classic sign of respiratory depression induced by opioids. However, in patients receiving a constant intravenous infusion of morphine, the oxygen saturation fell without a decrease in respiratory rate in postoperative patients (Catley et al., 1985). Constant infusion of an opioid and normal sleep depresses the ventilatory drive to CO_2 (Rigg et al., 1981). Therefore, CO_2 may accumulate and result in CO_2-induced narcosis. This can be detected by observing the patient's level of sedation at least every 4 hours (Table 5–15). A sedation scale rating of 3 or more indicates respiratory depression and warrants immediate therapy, including oxygen, naloxone, and discontinuation of the opioid.

Another manifestation of impaired ventilation is a decrease in oxygen saturation. PCA has caused periods of decreased oxygenation, although of less severity or less often than with epidurally or intramuscularly administered morphine following cesarean section (Brose and Cohen, 1989). Similarly, a comparison of PCA, epidurally administered diamorphine, and intramuscularly administered morphine demonstrated that the amount of time spent with a saturation level of less than 94% was statistically higher in the epidurally medicated group (Wheatley et al., 1990). Even in the elderly, the use of PCA when compared with intramuscularly administered morphine showed that the oxygen saturation did not differ from that of the intramuscularly medicated control subjects in the 3 days following abdominal surgery (Egberts et al., 1990). Although PCA depresses oxygenation, there is no indication for the routine use of pulse oximetry, because most desaturations are clinically insignificant (i.e., because O_2 saturation remains > 90%).

Anesthesia and surgery are associated with a high incidence of nausea and vomiting. Opioids contribute to the nausea and vomiting by directly stimulating the chemoreceptor trigger zone and sensitizing the vestibular apparatus to movement. It is not surprising that nausea and vomiting are the most common complaints of patients receiving PCA (Bollish et al., 1985; Dahl et al., 1987). The nausea and vomiting can be managed by adjusting the PCA dose, changing the analgesic, or using an antiemetic or a scopolamine patch.

■ **Table 5–15.** SEDATION SCALE USED TO MONITOR PATIENTS RECEIVING ANALGESIC THERAPY

Scale No.	Level	Description
1	None	Awake, alert, oriented
2	Mild	Sleepy but aroused by soft voice
3	Moderate	Requires physical stimulus to arouse, then oriented
4	Severe	Requires physical stimulus to arouse, not oriented

Opioids depress the peristaltic activity of the large and small intestine and increase the tone of the ileocecal and anal sphincters. All of these actions can promote ileus. In a 72-hour postoperative study, Albert and Talbott (1988) showed a decrease in the duration of ileus with PCA as compared with intramuscularly administered opioids. Clinical studies have yet to determine which opioid has the least severe effect on the gastrointestinal tract and whether a continuous infusion affects the length and/or severity of ileus. Although it might be anticipated that a drug such as nalbuphine, which is an antagonist at the μ-receptor and agonist at the κ-receptor, would improve bowel function, this has not been seen clinically.

Pruritus is a common complaint with the use of opiates via PCA, although it occurs less often with PCA than it does with epidurally administered morphine. Two separate studies reported that the incidence of pruritus ranged from 38 to 60% with morphine given via PCA compared with 72 to 85% with epidurally administered morphine (Eisenach et al., 1988; Harrison et al., 1988). The incidence of pruritus following intramuscularly administered morphine in the same two studies ranged from 17 to 35%. Mild itching can be treated with an antihistamine if necessary. In the event of more severe itching and urinary retention, the analgesic should be discontinued and an agent from a different chemical group substituted. Further, a low-dose infusion of naloxone may be able to relieve itching while preserving analgesia.

Weaning

PCA should continue until the recovering patient is able to take analgesics orally. This will only be possible when bowel function has returned. Because the patient must then be able to meet analgesic requirements with an oral agent, a knowledge of oral equivalence of the parenteral opioid is needed (Table 5–16).

EPIDURAL ANALGESIA

Epidural analgesia initially was limited to the use of local anesthetics for postoperative pain relief. The discovery that specific spinal receptors for opioids existed and that they modulated pain encouraged the use of both epidural and intrathecal opioids. Subsequently, epidural analgesia using opioid and local anesthetics has been used extensively to manage acute pain.

Mechanism of Action

Tissue damage or injury sets off a complex cascade of events that is eventually perceived as pain. This initial trauma stimulates nociceptive-sensitive nerve endings that transmit the impulse via peripheral nerve endings to the spinal cord. These peripheral nerve endings, or nociceptors, are found all over the body. A number of simultaneous reactions occur following tissue trauma, which alerts the body to the noxious stimulus (Fig. 5–9). The injured cell membranes release phospholipase, which ultimately forms prostaglandins and the leukotrienes. These prostanoids, although unable to stimulate nociception, potentiate the action of bradykinin, which is a potent pain-producing substance (Jensen et al., 1990). In addition, injury to the blood vessels activates clotting factors that activate kallikrein, which also releases bradykinin. Bradykinin can increase vasodilatation and vascular permeability, leading to further tissue injury.

Nerve fibers convey pain impulses from the periphery along A-delta and C fibers. Sharp, well-localized pain is conveyed along the poorly myelinated A-delta fibers, whereas the dull, poorly localized pain is conveyed along the C fibers. The A-delta and C fibers terminate in the gray matter of the dorsal horn of the

■ **Table 5–16.** EQUIANALGESIC OPIOID CONVERSIONS

Opioid	Equianalgesic Dose (mg)		Comments	Precautions
	Oral	*Intramuscular*		
Morphine	30–60	10	Gold standard Oral morphine sulfate q8–12hr	
Fentanyl	—	0.1	Transdermal route available; 25 μg/hr minimum dose	12-hr delay in onset and offset of transdermal patch, local heat and fever include rate of absorption
Meperidine	300	75	Oral administration not recommended	Toxic metabolite (normeperidine) causes seizures, especially doses > 600 mg/day; do not use with renal failure patients or those on monoamine oxidase inhibitors; caution patients with sickle cell anemia
Methadone	20	10	Long T½ (24–36 hr)	Accumulates; causes sedation after 2–3 days
Hydromorphone	7.5	1.5	Duration slightly shorter than that of morphine sulfate	
Oxycodone	15–30	—	Usually prepared with acetaminophen, 325–500 mg/tab	Acetaminophen dose not more than 4000 mg/day

Adapted from Principles of Analgesic Use in the Treatment of Acute and Cancer Pain. 3rd ed. American Pain Society, 1992.
Note: For all opioids, exercise caution in patients with sedation, marginal ventilation, asthma, increased intracranial pressure, liver failure, and renal failure.

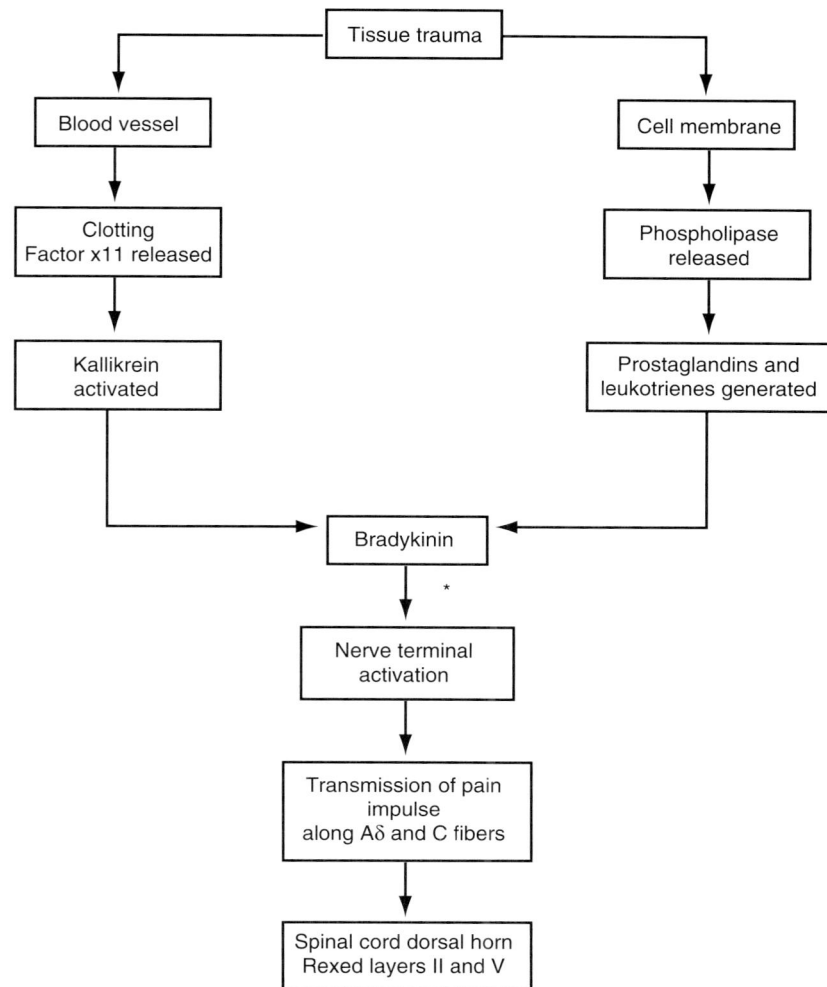

FIGURE 5–9. Cascade of events after tissue trauma.

Flowchart:

Tissue trauma → Blood vessel → Clotting Factor x11 released → Kallikrein activated → Bradykinin

Tissue trauma → Cell membrane → Phospholipase released → Prostaglandins and leukotrienes generated → Bradykinin

Bradykinin → * → Nerve terminal activation → Transmission of pain impulse along Aδ and C fibers → Spinal cord dorsal horn Rexed layers II and V

*Multiple factors are involved.

spinal cord in Rexed layer II or V of the spinal cord. These primary afferent nerve fibers release substance P as one of the many neurotransmitters responsible for further nociceptive transmission (Hamon et al., 1988). The nociceptive impulse is conveyed from the dorsal horn neurons via the contralateral spinothalamic tract for central integration. The dorsal horn neurons serve as a central modulating system that is influenced by fibers originating from higher centers and from the action of interneurons.

The mechanical action of epidural opioids has been inferred from radiolabeled binding studies and opioid receptor studies. Radiolabeled studies have shown that opioids bind in the substantia gelatinosa of the dorsal horn at Rexed layers II and V. Further, opioid receptors (mu, delta, and kappa) have been identified in the dorsal horn. Epidurally administered opioids diffuse to the spinal cord through multiple routes to act presynaptically and postsynaptically on second-order neurons, where the receptors are located (Jesse and Iversen, 1977; Lombard and Besson, 1989). It has been demonstrated that morphine inhibits the evoked release of substance P (Go and Yaksh, 1987). Morphine-induced analgesia does not affect other sensory modalities or motor functions.

Local anesthetics inhibit nerve impulses (including pain impulses) by inhibiting sodium channels along nerve fibers. Epidurally administered local anesthetics may act in this manner in a number of sites as the nerve fibers traverse the epidural space. The local anesthetics may act on the nerves in the intervertebral foramina or on the spinal roots in dural sleeves. In addition, the local anesthetics may act on the periphery of the spinal cord after penetrating the subarachnoid space. Local anesthetics affect multiple sensory modalities, including pain, sensation, and motor function. The degree of loss of sensory or motor function depends on the local anesthetic and the concentration of local anesthetic used.

Benefits

Epidural analgesia can relieve pain segmentally, so localized analgesia produces fewer systemic effects than intravenously administered analgesia does. Epidurally administered analgesia may be effected with opioids, local anesthetics, or a combination of the two.

Epidural opioid techniques, compared with many other forms of pain relief, have provided superb analgesia (Bromage et al., 1980). The percentage of patients reporting excellent pain relief was significantly higher following epidurally administered analgesia than following systemic narcotic administration with either PCA or intramuscularly administered opioids (Hamon et al., 1988).

Decreased sedation and more rapid recovery to presurgical levels of consciousness as compared with systemic narcotic administration are another benefit of epidurally administered analgesia (Berde, 1989; Berde et al., 1989). Because patients with epidurally administered analgesia have adequate pain control with less sedation, they are able to mobilize earlier and more effectively after operation. Patients are able to cooperate with respiratory therapy, mobilize secretions, and commence physical therapy earlier (Bromage, 1955; Craig, 1981; Simpson et al., 1961; Wahba et al., 1975), all of which decrease the incidence of pulmonary complications and venous thrombosis (Modig et al., 1980, 1983; White, 1982). Further, epidurally administered analgesia with local anesthetics may also improve graft flow in patients following vascular surgery through mild sympathetic blockade (Cousins and Wright, 1971). Earlier return of bowel function and a decreased stress response may also contribute to shorter hospitalizations and decreased morbidity (Breslow et al., 1989; Kehlet, 1979; Rawal et al., 1987; Rutberg et al., 1984, Scott and Kehlet, 1988). Some of these advantages have been documented in controlled prospective studies; overall decreased morbidity and mortality also has been demonstrated (Cuschieri et al., 1985; Eichorn, 1989; Ferrante et al., 1987; Yeager et al., 1987).

Indications

Epidurally administered analgesia has been effective in treating pain in the body below the upper thoracic level. Certain surgical procedures lend themselves well to epidurally administered anesthesia and analgesia: orthopedic, urologic, gynecologic, upper abdominal, and thoracic procedures (Cullen et al., 1985; Logas et al., 1987). Trauma victims especially can benefit from epidurally administered analgesia following a flail chest.

Epidural Analgesic Agents

The nociceptive pain impulse can be inhibited in the epidural space by local anesthetics, opioids, or the combination of local anesthetics and opioids (see Tables 5–17 through 5–19). Most of the drugs administered via the epidural route have not been approved by the FDA for epidural administration, so guidelines for such products are minimal. There appears to be a

■ **Table 5–17.** LOCAL ANESTHETIC CONCENTRATIONS FOR USE IN EPIDURAL ANALGESIA

Percentage as Fraction	Percentage as Decimal	Mg/ml
1/16%	0.0625%	0.625
1/8%	0.125%	1.25
1/4%	0.25%	2.5

general consensus in the United States that preservatives should not be administered epidurally, but a European study has refuted this claim (Wang et al., 1992). Case studies citing apparent neurologic damage from preservatives have been published, but clear-cut causality has not been determined (Sjoberg et al., 1992). Until these issues are resolved, it is prudent to administer drugs via the epidural route without preservatives. Currently, the only opioid approved for epidural administration is morphine. The antioxidants typically used with morphine for intravenous administration are sodium ethylene diaminetetracetic acid (EDTA) and sodium bisulfites. The products marketed for epidural administration are labeled "preservative-free" and do not contain any antioxidants. This standard, set by the United States Pharmacopeia (USP), only appears with these commercially available products or morphine intended for epidural administration. Whether products that contain antioxidants should be used for epidural administration is the subject of considerable disagreement.

Most of the products that have not received FDA approval will likely never do so because they are no longer under patent. It is legal and within good medical practice to administer opioids or other agents epidurally without FDA approval if the literature adequately documents both safety and efficacy for the product. It is especially important to note the studies documenting the drug's failure to cause direct nerve damage when administered via the epidural route. These studies require preliminary animal studies with proven models to evaluate the risk of direct nerve damage (Yaksh et al., 1987). The agents presented in this text have a long history of use and record of safety.

Local Anesthetics

Local anesthetic agents are often used to provide analgesia and anesthesia for patients undergoing

■ **Table 5–18.** COMMONLY USED EPIDURAL OPIOIDS

Drug	Bolus Dose (mg/kg)	Infusion Concentration (mg/ml)	Infusion Rates (ml/hr)
Fentanyl	0.001–0.002	0.0025–0.01	4–10
Morphine	0.03–0.10	0.1–0.2	1–5
Meperidine	0.35–0.7	1–2.5	4–10
Hydromorphone	0.01–0.02	0.05–0.1	1–5

■ **Table 5–19.** SUGGESTED EPIDURAL PROTOCOLS

I. Opioids Alone
   A. Morphine (preservative-free)
      1. *Bolus:* 0.07 mg/kg in total volume of 10 ml PFNS
         a. Can be given q8–12hr
   B. Demerol (preservative free)
      1. *Bolus:* 0.5–1.0 mg/kg in total volume of 10 ml PFNS
         a. Can be given q6–12hr
      2. *Infusion:* Demerol 0.15 mg/kg/hr
   C. Fentanyl
      1. *Bolus:* 0.001 mg/kg in total volume of 10 ml PFNS
         a. Can be given q3–4hr
      2. *Infusion:* Fentanyl 0.5 kg/hr
II. Local Anesthetics Alone
   A. Lidocaine—2%
      1. *Bolus:* 2 ml 2% lidocaine with or without epinephrine 1:200,000
         a. Can repeat 2 times, 5–10 min apart
      2. *Infusion:* not used as infusion
   B. Bupivacaine
      1. *Bolus:* 0.125%, 0.25%, or 0.5%, 2–4 ml
         a. Usually given without epinephrine
      2. *Infusion:* 0.125% or 0.25% at 4–6 ml/hr
III. Local Anesthetic and Opioid Combination
   A. Bupivacaine 0.125% and fentanyl 2–5 µg/ml, 4–6 ml/hr
      1. Useful for thoracotomy and for upper abdominal and orthopedic procedures (thoracic catheters are recommended)
   B. Bupivacaine 0.125% and demerol 2.5 mg/ml, 4–6 ml/hr
      1. Especially useful for abdominal procedures
   C. Bupivacaine 0.125% and morphine 0.01% at 4–6 ml/hr
      1. Especially useful for procedures with big incisions in which significant dermatomal spread is needed
   D. Bupivacaine 0.25% and fentanyl 2–5 µg/ml or demerol 2.5 mg/ml, 4–6 ml/hr
      1. Especially useful for lower-extremity orthopedic procedures

Data from Ferrante et al., 1987; Berde et al., 1987; Raj and Bridenbaugh, 1987.

PFNS = preservative-free normal saline.

Note: It is best to wait for some sign of recovery from motor blockade from epidural anesthesia before instituting an epidural infusion for postoperative analgesia, because prolonged motor blockade can result. Rates may be titrated to 10 ml/hr, but one must watch for side effects.

surgery. Selection of the most appropriate local anesthetic to use epidurally and the optimal delivery method depend on pharmacokinetics and pharmacodynamics. Lidocaine and bupivacaine are the agents most commonly used for postoperative epidural blockade. Although lidocaine has a higher safety index than the longer-acting bupivacaine, systemic accumulation is more marked with the shorter-acting local anesthetics (lidocaine), which increases risk of toxicity (Tucker et al., 1977). In general, lidocaine is limited to use in a bolus form to establish or rescue a block, whereas bupivacaine is used as an infusion or in bolus form. Bupivacaine has a long duration of action and has a differential between its sensory and its motor blockade. Analgesia can be provided with minimal muscle weakness when bupivacaine is used in appropriate concentrations.

It would be logical to assume that local anesthetics could be used to provide analgesia in the postoperative period. Local anesthetic can be administered epidurally either as a bolus or by continuous infusion. The effect of a bolus technique is short-lived, and the doses required to repeatedly reestablish the desired level of analgesia may precipitate physiologic alterations, a drop in blood pressure, or systemic toxicity. A continuous infusion of local anesthetic would circumvent these difficulties. However, constant-rate infusion of a local anesthetic through the epidural catheter may produce tachyphylaxis (Scott et al., 1989) characterized by a shrinking analgesic area with a fixed rate of infusion. This tachyphylaxis may represent an increase in the size of the pain field at the spinal cord level due to recruitment of more nociceptive endings, may be due to some pharmacologic alteration of the local anesthetic, or may represent an increase in blood flow within the epidural space that absorbs the local anesthetic more rapidly into the circulation (Morgenson et al., 1988). The development of tachyphylaxis has not been a universal phenomenon and is less likely at the extremes of age. In addition, tachyphylaxis may be circumvented, as when bupivacaine is administered in small, incremental boluses.

Another potential problem with the use of local anesthetic agents alone is accumulation of the local anesthetic agent in the systemic circulation. Systemic accumulation is more marked with the short-acting amides, such as lidocaine, than with the longer-acting amides (Tucker et al., 1977). The longer-acting agents bind more nonspecifically in the fat of the epidural space (Schweitzer and Morgan, 1987). Thus, although the potential for immediate systemic toxicity (secondary to intravascular injection) is higher with the longer-acting amides, the long-term results are more severe with the shorter-acting agents. The toxicity of the local anesthetics is less marked when the agents accumulate slowly, but there is an ever-present risk of central nervous system depression, convulsions, or cardiac arrest.

The concentration of local anesthetic will influence the analgesia and the profile of side effects. Constant-rate infusion of 0.5% bupivacaine may induce hypotension, muscle weakness, sensory block, and accumulation of toxic systemic levels (Scott et al., 1989). Plasma levels may be higher in the elderly and frail. Side effects may be attenuated by using lower concentrations of bupivacaine. The use of a low-dose constant-rate infusion of epidurally administered bupivacaine (0.1%) close to the dermatomal level desired for pain relief can significantly decrease the incidence of side effects inherent with the use of more concentrated solutions. Although a low concentration of bupivacaine is effective, it provides a lower level of analgesia than that of combining the bupivacaine with low concentrations of epidurally administered morphine or the use of morphine alone (Gregory et al., 1985; Rawal et al., 1981; Scott et al., 1989).

Opioids

Selection of the most appropriate opioid to use in the epidural space and optimal delivery method depends on understanding the pharmacokinetics and pharmacodynamics of the opioids used in the epidural space. Epidurally administered opioids must traverse the dura mater and the cerebrospinal fluid to reach the gray matter of the spinal cord. Only 2 to 3.6% of an epidurally administered dose of morphine crosses the dura (Sjostrom et al., 1987). The rate of transfer of opiates across the dura is proportional to the lipid solubility of the agent used (Chrubasik, 1988). The more lipid-soluble the opioid, the faster the onset of effect.

Once introduced into the epidural space, opioids can diffuse in a number of directions. The quantity of the opioid that is absorbed into the systemic circulation depends on the dose of the opioid used and the lipid solubility of the opioid. If the systemic level of the opioid exceeds the MEAC, this will contribute to the analgesia after epidural administration (Gourlay et al., 1986). However, the analgesia following epidurally administered morphine does not depend on the systemic levels. A 2-mg epidural dose of morphine provided adequate analgesia with plasma levels of only 5.1 ± 2 ng, well below the MEAC for morphine (Rawal et al., 1981). In addition, the duration of analgesia following epidural morphine administration exceeds the time during which morphine can be detected in significant amounts in the plasma. Thus, the major difference between epidurally and intramuscularly administered opiates is a higher, more sustained level of morphine in the cerebrospinal fluid (Kehlet, 1979).

Lipophilic opioids such as fentanyl have many potential advantages and disadvantages. The increased lipid solubility is reflected by rapid penetration across the dura and diffusion through the cerebrospinal fluid and to the opioid receptors. Further, the lipophilic opioid is quickly absorbed systemically, contributing to its analgesic effect. Just as these drugs have a rapid onset of action, they have a rapid elimination, which limits the duration of action of a bolus dose of a lipophilic agent. Repeated doses can cause systemic accumulation of the opioid with blood levels that can exceed its MEAC. This was demonstrated in a study comparing continuous epidural infusion of fentanyl with continuous intravenous infusion. The plasma levels of fentanyl were initially low in the epidurally medicated group and then reached a level that exceeded the MEAC of fentanyl after 18 hours (Loper et al., 1990). These levels were similar to that obtained with a continuous intravenous infusion of fentanyl. Maintaining systemic levels above the MEAC limits the theoretical value of maintaining an epidural catheter.

Opioid and Local Anesthetic Combination

An alternative method of providing pain relief is to infuse a combination of local anesthetics and opioids into the epidural space. Local anesthetics and opioids are thought to act synergistically (Fischer et al., 1988b; Gregg et al., 1988) to allow decreased concentrations and dosages of each agent to be used, thereby limiting the potential for side effects. This would provide the ideal form of analgesia. Bupivacaine has been used

most often in concentrations ranging from 0.1 to 0.25% with either morphine, fentanyl, or meperidine. The use of morphine and bupivacaine has produced effective analgesia in patients following thoracic, abdominal, and general surgery (Magora et al., 1980; Rawal et al., 1981; Rutberg et al., 1984; Scott et al., 1989). However, fentanyl combined with bupivacaine had a lower incidence of side effects when compared with the morphine-bupivacaine combination (Fischer et al., 1988b). In one comparative study of epidural fentanyl and fentanyl-bupivacaine, no differences in the level of pain relief, infusion rates, or resulting fentanyl levels were detected (Badner et al., 1991). Much further research is necessary to determine the best drug or combination of drugs for each procedure or situation.

Modes of Epidural Analgesia Delivery

Analgesia may be administered epidurally in multiple forms. Bolus administration is used with both opioids and local anesthetics (Chrubasik et al., 1988; DeCastro et al., 1991; Ferrante et al., 1991; Gregg et al., 1988; Yu et al., 1989). The duration of effect of the opioids or local anesthesia determines the interval dosing time. In general, morphine, meperidine, and dilaudid are used in bolus form because they last 6 to 12 hours. Fentanyl is rarely repeated in bolus form because its duration is 2 to 4 hours. Local anesthetics may be used for analgesia in bolus form, but this may cause side effects such as hypotension.

Analgesia may also be administered epidurally as a continuous infusion (Badner et al., 1991; El Baz et al., 1984; Ferrante et al., 1987; Hughes et al., 1986; Morgenson et al., 1988). The continuous infusion may consist of opioids, local anesthetics, or combinations of opioids and local anesthetics. Lidocaine generally is not used as a continuous infusion because of its potential for accumulation and toxicity. A third form of epidural analgesia is *patient-controlled epidural analgesia* (PCEA) (Chrubasik and Wiemers, 1985; Sjostrom et al., 1988). PCEA is similar to PCA using intravenously administered opioids. Small boluses of opioids and/or local anesthetics are available at defined intervals with defined maximum allowable dosages. A continuous background infusion of opioids and/or local anesthetics may be added to the patient-controlled intermittent mode (Chrubasik and Wiemers, 1985).

Pumps and Devices

Given the need to automate the delivery of opioids and other drugs to the epidural space, multiple pumps have been designed and marketed. Most of the pumps used for epidural administration were not specifically designed for it. Certain aspects of pump design are more important than others when choosing a pump. Table 5–20 lists several important criteria.

The ability to accurately deliver a small volume of

■ **Table 5–20.** IDEAL ANALGESIC PUMP CRITERIA

Accurate dose delivery over a wide range of doses
- Ability to dose in mg/μg/ml
- Simple to use and program

Alarms
- High pressure
- Prevention of free flow
- Device malfunction (low batteries)
- Low drug reservoir

Physical characteristics
- Small, portable, and lightweight
- Clear display of drug and doses
- Locks to prevent drug tampering
- Printer capability
- No infusion ports on connecting tubing
- Both battery and AC power

Adaptable (has many modes of delivery)

■ **Table 5–21.** TREATMENT OF SIDE EFFECTS FROM EPIDURAL OPIOIDS

Side Effect	Treatment	Dosage/70 kg
Respiratory depression	Naloxone IV	0.04–0.4 mg or infusion*
Urinary retention	Urinary catheter Naloxone IV	0.1–0.4 mg or infusion*
Pruritus	Antihistamine (less effective) Naloxone IV	0.1–0.4 mg or infusion*
Nausea and vomiting	Metaclopramide IV/IM Naloxone IV Droperidol IV	10 mg 0.1–0.4 mg or infusion* 1.25–2.5 mg
Constipation	Laxatives	—

Data from Bromage et al., 1982; De Castro et al., 1991; and Rawal and Wattwil, 1984.

Key: IV = Intravenous administration; IM = intramuscular administration.

*Infusion = 0.4–0.8 mg/hr; titrate to effect.

drug is extremely important. The volume of drug delivered via the epidural route varies from 0.5 to 15 ml/hr. Further, the pump should be able to dose in multiple formats, including milligrams, micrograms, and milliliters.

More institutions and home health care settings are turning to the PCEA method of administration, so the pump must be able to deliver both a continuous infusion and a patient-administered bolus on demand. This has led to adaptation of previously designed portable PCA pumps for PCEA use. The ability to obtain a history from the PCEA machine helps the pain team adjust therapy to meet the patient's needs.

Physical characteristics also influence the choice of a pump. The size and weight of the pump are important when ambulation is desired. In the recovering patient and the home-bound patient with epidural infusion or PCEA, a small, portable, easily managed pump is a necessity, as is a pump that uses nonrechargeable batteries instead of the heavier, rechargeable batteries found in the older models. Clear displays, locks, and tubing with no infusion ports to complement the pump are also useful.

Side Effects

Epidural analgesia administration does have side effects, including nausea, pruritus, and urinary retention (Bromage et al., 1982). The incidence of these side effects varies with the lipid solubility of the opioid used. These side effects can usually be treated with low-dose naloxone infusion (while retaining pain relief) or by altering the local anesthetic/opioid concentration (Berde et al., 1989) (Table 5–21). More serious complications include sedation and delayed respiratory depression. Delayed respiratory depression is thought to derive from the rostral spread of epidurally administered opioid to the brain stem with effects on the respiratory control centers in the floor of the fourth ventricle (Rawal and Wattwil, 1984). Bromage and associates, studying hypalgesia to cold and pin scratch after 10 mg of morphine was administered epidurally to volunteers, demonstrated that the effects of the morphine moved rostrally, reaching the trigeminal area in 9 hours in half of the subjects (Bromage et al., 1982). The rostral spread of morphine in the cerebrospinal fluid has been confirmed in both animal (Gregory et al., 1985) and human studies (Gourlay et al., 1987; Payne, 1987).

This rostral spread has been blamed for the emergence of delayed respiratory depression occurring 6 to 12 hours following the epidural administration of morphine. The incidence of respiratory depression ranges from 0.09 to 0.25 to 0.4% in two large retrospective studies (Gustaffoson et al., 1982 Rawal et al., 1987). The incidence of respiratory depression is highest in the elderly, patients given excessive amounts of concomitant sedatives, patients receiving thoracic epidural administration, and debilitated patients. The absolute rate of respiratory depression from epidurally administered analgesia needs to be defined better but may not appear significantly different from that of other forms of opioid therapy. This complication can be prevented by judicious opioid use and appropriate patient monitoring.

Epidural administration of local anesthetics may cause hypotension, motor block, or sensory loss in the dermatomal distribution of the catheter. Precautions should be taken to prevent and treat these complications, such as not allowing a patient with a lumbar catheter to ambulate because of motor weakness or loss of proprioception. These side effects can be managed further by changes in the local anesthetic concentration or by intravenous fluid infusion.

Subarachnoid migration of the catheter is an extremely rare complication that is manifested by increasing sensory and motor function loss. Agitation and seizures may also result from migration of the catheter to a blood vessel or from systemic absorption of local anesthetics. Again, appropriate monitoring of the patient allows early recognition and treatment of these complications.

Monitoring the Patient

Perhaps the most important aspect of epidural analgesia administration is to monitor the patient's safety.

To do so successfully, the primary care personnel should understand and recognize all the potential side effects of epidural neural blockade. In effect, monitoring regimens are set up to detect and treat side effects if they occur. Not only is detection important, but quick treatment may be life-saving. Therefore, all personnel caring for these patients should be adept at emergency treatment. Further, a physician from the pain treatment service should be immediately available to treat any adverse consequences of epidural analgesia administration.

Guidelines for monitoring epidurally administered analgesia have been established by many hospitals (Berde, 1987; Ferrante, 1987; Ready et al., 1988). Sensible protocols include the following: For every patient following or during an epidural administration, analgesia monitoring equipment and emergency drugs and equipment must be readily available. The patient's room should be equipped with at least oxygen, an air-mask-bag unit (AMBU), and a blood pressure cuff. Naloxone, 0.4 mg/ml, with a syringe should be present in a prominent position in each room (e.g., taped to the epidural pump or above the patient's bed). An emergency cart with full advanced cardiac life support capability should be immediately available on the floor.

Patients undergoing epidural analgesia administration should be assessed for respiratory rate and depth with a sedation scale once per hour. The purpose of the sedation scale is to detect respiratory depression that is not associated with the classic features of bradypnea. Epidurally administered opioids may depress the depth of ventilation without affecting the rate. This causes carbon dioxide retention, which manifests as sedation. For simplicity, we use a four-point sedation scale: 1—awake, alert, and oriented; 2—asleep but oriented when awakened with verbal stimulus; 3—as for 2 but physical stimulus is required; 4—disoriented when aroused. Shallow breathing, mild sedation, and decreased respiratory rate are some of the early signs of narcosis. Treatment is based on the amount of sedation and respiratory depression. It may range from simple stimulation to the administration of naloxone. The treatment of other side effects is given in Table 5–21. Absolutely no additional opioids or central nervous system depressant medication should be given without the approval of the pain treatment service.

Patients receiving a continuous infusion of local anesthetics or local anesthetics with opioids require an added level of monitoring. Vital signs should be assessed every 4 hours, including sensory level and the degree of motor block. Abnormal findings should be reported to the pain treatment service physician. Patients with epidurally administered analgesia should also be placed close to a nursing station so that they can be observed frequently.

Patients with lumbar or low thoracic epidural insertion points should not be allowed to ambulate. Although the patients may have adequate motor strength, they may lack the proprioception necessary to walk. Patients with higher thoracic catheters may ambulate with assistance.

The most important monitor, however, is good nursing personnel who regularly communicate with members of the pain treatment service or primary care physician. A member of the pain treatment service who is familiar with the patients should be available immediately to cope with problems and should be easily reachable to answer questions.

Guidelines for monitoring patients with epidurally administered analgesia are well established. Whether these monitoring guidelines are applied in an intensive care setting or on routine postoperative floors may be determined by the level of expertise and training of the team (anesthesiologist, surgeon, and nursing staff), by the resources available in the hospital, and by the individuals responsible for the epidural analgesia administration (Berde et al., 1989; Raj and Bridenbaugh, 1987; Rawal and Watwill, 1984; Ready, 1990).

How Epidural Catheters Are Placed

Epidural catheters may be used for acute postoperative pain management or for long-term chronic pain syndromes such as cancer. Epidural catheters used for immediate postoperative pain management are inserted subcutaneously using a loss-of-resistance technique and are threaded into the epidural space via a specially designed needle. The needle is removed, and the catheter is left in place before use. The catheter insertion site should be dressed with a clear sterile dressing so that the site may be visible for daily inspection. Epidural catheters may also be inserted at the time of surgery under direct vision. Of course, the type of surgery will determine the feasibility of the technique; lumbar laminectomy may yield the best exposure.

Patients receiving medications epidurally on a long-term basis (more than 1 to 2 weeks) usually undergo catheter implantation for several reasons (DuPen et al., 1987a). First, implanted catheters are sutured in place and are much less likely to be removed accidentally. Second, these catheters are designed to prevent infection via the exit site; a Dacron cuff helps prevent infection from tracking via the exit wound. Third, temporary catheters are hard for the patient to manipulate because they exit the skin from the back. Implanted catheters are tunneled to the lower chest, and the exit site is made easily accessible to the patient and/or caretaker. The catheter can then be externalized like venous access devices are or it can be made into a Mediport access site (wherein a needle is required to puncture the skin and access the catheter).

Conclusions

Epidural analgesia administration is an alternative to traditional pain therapy. It is extremely effective and safe if appropriate monitoring is employed. Epidural analgesia administration is uniquely useful for patients who undergo major thoracoabdominal, vascular, or orthopedic procedures; they benefit most from early mobility and return of pulmonary function. Trauma victims, especially those with a flail chest injury, also significantly benefit from epidural analgesia administration. Local anesthetics, opioids, or a combination of the two agents may be used to achieve analgesia. Side effects and complications are well described and are easily treated or avoided. Responses to epidural analgesia administration vary, so epidural analgesia administration regimens should be tailored to individual reactions.

INTRAPLEURAL ANALGESIA

In 1981, O'Kelley and Garry described an innovative technique of providing extensive analgesia to a patient with multiple rib fractures in whom conservative management with intramuscular meperidine (Demerol) had failed (O'Kelley et al., 1981). A 19-gauge needle was walked off the fifth rib, close to the angle of the rib and advanced into the intrapleural space with a loss-of-resistance technique. Twenty milliliters of plain bupivacaine, injected through the needle into the intrapleural space, provided 8 hours of pain relief accompanied by increased skin warmth in the analgesic area and improved respiratory function. Later, the procedure was repeated using a Tuouhy needle, through which an epidural catheter was passed. Intermittent injections of bupivacaine every 7 to 8 hours provided good analgesia for 6 days. After 4 days, the concentration of bupivacaine was decreased to 0.25%. The administration of a radiopaque contrast medium through the epidural catheter demonstrated the spread of the contrast over five interspaces on a chest film. A quantity of the dye was located in the paravertebral area, suggesting medial spread of the contrast medium. In 1984, a group of Norwegian anesthesiologists used this technique for postoperative pain relief in 81 surgical patients undergoing cholecystectomy via a subcostal incision, renal surgery, and unilateral breast surgery (Kvalheim and Reiestad, 1984). Effective and long-lasting analgesia was obtained in 90% of the patients with 20 ml of 0.5% bupivacaine with epinephrine. The duration of this analgesia ranged from 6 to 26 hours, with a mean duration of 10 hours. In this study, the intrapleural catheter was introduced at the end of surgery but while the patients were still anesthetized. Chest films were taken 2 hours after the completion of surgery and again 24 hours later, following removal of the catheter. No pneumothoraces were seen in any of the 81 patients studied.

Site of Action

Numerous theories describe the sites of action of the local anesthetics deposited in the intrapleural space. The principal site of action of intrapleural local

anesthetic agents is believed to be diffusion through the parietal pleura to anesthetize the intercostal nerves. The anatomic barriers between the local anesthetic inserted in the intrapleural space and the intercostal nerves vary along the course of the nerve. The intercostal nerves are separated from the parietal pleura by only a layer of fat in the paravertebral region. Lateral to this, a fascial layer, the posterior intercostal membrane, separates the nerves from the pleura. At the level of the angle of the ribs, the membrane is replaced by the fibers of the internal intercostal membrane. Local anesthetic deposited in the pleural space must diffuse through one of these layers to be effective.

The thoracic sympathetic chain runs along the ribs posterior to the parietal pleura. The close proximity of the thoracic chain indicates that the sympathetic nervous system could be involved following an intrapleural blockade. There have been no reports of significant alterations in any of the hemodynamic parameters measured in patients receiving intrapleural analgesia, probably because of the unilateral nature of these blocks. An increase in skin temperature has been noted over the affected dermatomes in many patients.

Technique of Insertion

The easiest and safest technique for inserting an intrapleural catheter is under direct vision by the surgeon at the time of a thoracotomy. A catheter is laid between the parietal and visceral pleura and then tunneled through the chest wall to exit laterally at the side of the chest. Different techniques have been used to identify the intrapleural space in patients whose chests are closed. Most studies have used a well-lubricated glass syringe attached to a Tuouhy needle, which is advanced immediately above the rib. In a spontaneously breathing patient, the intrapleural space is identified by the inward suction of the entire needle-syringe combination from negative pressure in the pleural space. The second technique has relied on the loss of resistance to pressure as the syringe advances through the pleural space. However, because the pleural space is limited in extent, lung damage may occur with vigorous advancement of the needle or catheter too far into the space (Kambam et al., 1987). When 18 intrapleural catheters were examined at the time of surgery after preoperative placement of the catheter, only 7 catheters were optimally positioned; 7 were in lung tissue, and a hemodynamically significant pneumothorax was created in one patient (Gomez et al., 1984). The hanging drop technique has also been used to indicate the negative pressure in the pleural space in a spontaneously breathing patient (Squier et al., 1989).

Drug Selection

Effective postoperative analgesia has been achieved for upper abdominal, flank, breast, and some thoracic procedures. The pain following an anterior thoracotomy is not relieved effectively with a unilateral intrapleural technique, because the nociceptive impulses are conveyed bilaterally (Kambam et al., 1987). The catheter must be positioned above and lateral to the incision to provide optimal analgesia (Chan et al., 1988). The intrapleural technique has also been used to manage patients suffering from chronic pain conditions.

Controversy exists regarding the optimal concentration and volume of local anesthetic agent to use with the intrapleural technique. Both bupivacaine and lidocaine have been used to provide analgesia with success. A 2% concentration of lidocaine produces a more rapid onset of analgesia than 0.5% lidocaine does (Kuhlman et al., 1988). The analgesia is equally effective, and duration was similar in these two groups, but the more concentrated solution resulted in a higher plasma level of lidocaine (without features of toxicity). Lidocaine, even in a 2% concentration, was not effective following a thoracotomy at a rate of 15 to 20 ml/hr with 1:200,000 epinephrine (El-Baz et al., 1988).

Effective analgesia has been obtained with concentrations of bupivacaine that have ranged from 0.25 to 0.75%, with volumes ranging from 8 to 30 ml. The 22 cholecystectomies (with subcostal incisions) in which patients received 20 ml of 0.25%, 0.375%, or 0.5% bupivacaine, only one patient in each of the lower-dose groups had inadequate pain relief from the initial bolus dose (Reiestad et al., 1986). The mean duration of analgesia ranged from 285 minutes in the low concentration to 500 minutes with 0.5% bupivacaine. Most studies have used 0.5% bupivacaine in volumes ranging from 20 to 30 ml.

Systemic absorption of the local anesthetic is a potential limitation to the use of a continuous infusion of local anesthetics into the pleural space. The use of 0.25% bupivacaine for a thoracotomy caused the serum level of bupivacaine to increase to a mean value of 1.64 μg/ml at 24 hours to 3.68 μg/ml at 48 hours, with a peak level of 4.24 μg/ml (Rosenberg et al., 1987). Adverse reactions were not apparent, probably because of either the slow rate at which the bupivacaine level rose or altered pharmacokinetics in the postoperative patient. An inflammatory response in the pleural space causes an increase in the speed of absorption. For example, 5 minutes after the injection of 30 ml of 0.5% bupivacaine into the intrapleural space from which straw-colored fluid was initially drained, a venous concentration of 4.9 μg/ml of bupivacaine was obtained. This was associated with a grand mal convulsion (Seltzer et al., 1987).

The degree of pain relief obtained from intrapleural analgesia has been compared with other forms of analgesia. When the intrapleural technique was compared with the use of saline in thoracotomy patients, the morphine requirements were significantly less in the intrapleurally medicated group (Symreng et al., 1989). The patients who received bupivacaine demonstrated a significant improvement in forced vital capacity, forced expiratory flow in 1 second, and peak flow. The analgesia obtained from a large dose (30 ml) of 0.5% bupivacaine has been compared with that of a continuous infusion of fentanyl via a thoracic epidural catheter (Seltzer et al., 1989). The level of analgesia obtained from the epidurally administered fentanyl was superior to that provided by the intrapleural administration of bupivacaine.

A contraindication to the use of intrapleural analgesia is fibrosis of the pleura because of the technical difficulty of isolating the pleural space. The presence of blood or fluid in the pleural space is also a contraindication because of the dilution of the local anesthetic and increased absorption of the local anesthetic from an inflamed pleura. Because tachycardia has been reported from the rapid absorption of an epinephrine-containing solution, a test dose would decrease the risk in injecting a larger amount of local anesthetic into the pleural space.

TRANSDERMAL OPIOIDS

Transdermally administered fentanyl has been approved for use in patients with cancer-induced pain. Many studies have explored the role of transdermal fentanyl administration in the management of postoperative pain. This technique may obviate the need for a functioning gastrointestinal tract or an intravenous or epidural catheter.

The major barrier to the absorption of the transdermally administered opioids is the stratum corneum of the intact skin. The permeability across the stratum corneum depends on the degree of lipophilicity of the agent (Roy and Flynn, 1989). Although the lipophilicity of the opioid increases, the rate of absorption does not increase in proportion to the lipophilicity but instead plateaus because of the aqueous barrier presented by the tissues. In addition, the opioid used must be potent enough to limit the area over which the agent has to be applied to be able to reach a therapeutic concentration. It has been estimated that to provide a 10-mg dose of morphine, the size of the patch would have to be 62,500 cm^2; to provide 150 mg of meperidine, the patch size would need to be 258 cm^2.

Fentanyl meets the criteria for use in a transdermal delivery system because it is both highly lipid-soluble and potent enough for transdermal use. The Transdermal Therapeutic System, or TTS (Alzo Corporation, Palo Alto, CA), is self-adhesive with a selectively permeable membrane, and it comes in different sizes to vary the rate of delivery. These patches provide the predicted amount of medication in the range of 25 to 100 μg/hr (Gourlay et al., 1989; Varrel et al., 1989).

Because the skin is not uniform, the rate of transfer varies with the site on which the patch is placed as well as the gender, age, blood flow, sweat gland activity, temperature, and pH of the skin. Therefore, to make the transdermal system predictable, the rate of transfer must be limited by the transdermal delivery system and must be less than the maximum rate of transfer of the opioid across the skin. The rate of transport thus will be set by the characteristics of the patch and will prevent excessive absorption in the patient who has more permeable skin.

There is a significant lag time before therapeutic levels of fentanyl are detected in the plasma. With a 75-μg/hr patch to relieve pain following orthopedic surgery, the median lag time following the application of fentanyl to detectable plasma levels was 2.25 hours (Plezia et al., 1989). Before appreciable plasma levels of fentanyl are obtained, a large number of rescue treatments are necessary at the beginning of therapy (Holley and Van Steennis, 1988). This can be circumvented by applying the patch early (Rowbotham et al., 1989). TTS fentanyl, 100 μg/hr, provides analgesia as effective as that of intravenous infusion of fentanyl, also at 100 μg/hr, provided that sufficient time is allowed for the fentanyl to be absorbed (Holley and Van Steennis, 1988).

The characteristic feature following the removal of the patch is a long elimination half-life. The elimination half-life has ranged from 17 to 22 hours following the removal of the patch (Holley and Van Steennis, 1988). Thus, the skin acts as both a reservoir for and a barrier to fentanyl. Therefore, analgesic requirements are reduced in the 24 hours following the removal of the patch. Fentanyl patches have been used for a total of 3 to 156 days and have provided excellent pain control with good correlation between the plasma fentanyl level and the predicted rate of delivery (Mier et al., 1989).

Fentanyl patches have been associated with some slowing in respiratory rate (Caplan et al., 1989; Latasch and Luders, 1989). This reduction in respiratory rate has not been accompanied by any statistically significant reduction in PA_{O_2} or increase in PA_{CO_2} when compared with a placebo patch. However, a 75-μg/ hr patch used in a smaller patient (50 kg) created higher plasma levels than predicted as well as respiratory impairment. The authors suggested that the size of the fentanyl patch used should be tailored to the patient's size to limit the incidence of respiratory depression. Even when the fentanyl patch sizes were varied according to anthropometric and psychological variables to provide analgesia following abdominal surgery, patch size had to be changed because of both inadequate analgesia and respiratory depression (Gourlay et al., 1989). This study demonstrated that these predictive measures did not help determine the optimal patch size and that the patches should be applied after the analgesic requirements are determined by other means. Fever or local heating, such as a heating pad, can increase the release of fentanyl and precipitate respiratory depression.

The other side effects inherent to the use of fentanyl include nausea and vomiting. The incidence of nausea reached 84%. However, when the transdermal patch was compared with intramuscularly administered morphine, 73% of patients with intramuscular medications suffered from vomiting as compared with 30% of those treated with the fentanyl patch (Caplan et al., 1989). The adhesive leaves only a transient period of redness when the patches are removed. Transder-

mally administered fentanyl provides effective analgesia but is difficult to titrate because of slow onset and prolonged elimination half-life.

TRANSMUCOSALLY ADMINISTERED OPIOIDS

With recent advances in technology, opioid administration has become available in a transmucosal delivery system. The mucosa of the mouth and nose has long been used for drug delivery (e.g., deamino-D-arginine-vasopressin [DDAVP], nifedipine). However, until recently, opioids have not been administered transmucosally.

To be effective transmucosally, a drug must be potent and nonirritating and have a high solubility. As anticipated, morphine was ineffective as an analgesic transmucosally (Fischer et al., 1988a). However, potent drugs with high solubility (such as buprenorphine, fentanyl, and methadone) have been absorbed significantly more than morphine sulfate has (Weinberg et al., 1988).

Transmucosal administration can take place in a number of sites, including the mouth (sublingual, buccal, and gingival), the nose, and the rectum. Each site presents advantages and disadvantages. The nose and mouth can yield swift absorption and onset of action with little first-pass metabolism. However, transmucosally administered medications given via the mouth (as compared with oral administration) may be diluted by saliva, and those given nasally may irritate. Rectal delivery may have advantages in uncooperative patients. However, absorption may be limited by bowel movements, mucosal irritation, and variable absorption, because the rectum has venous plexi drainage to the systemic and portal systems.

Advantages of a transmucosal drug delivery system are clear in the hospital and in outpatient settings: Patients without intravenous access may present in the emergency room; the drugs may be used for premedication before surgery; and in some patients, intravenous access has been discontinued or is difficult to obtain. For outpatients, opioids may be administered transmucosally as maintenance pain management therapy or as rescue therapy to treat breakthrough pain. Further, painful diagnostic procedures may be treated with transmucosally administered opioids (Streisand, 1992). Transmucosally administered opioids may be especially useful in treating cancer pain.

Current studies include the use of transmucosally administered opioids for premedication in children (Freisen and Lockhart, 1992), for treating cancer pain (Fine et al., 1991), and for treating acute postoperative pain in adults (Ashburn et al., 1993). Transmucosally administered opioids are not currently marketed but are in the investigative stage of development.

NONSTEROIDAL ANTI–INFLAMMATORY DRUGS

Nonsteroidal anti-inflammatory drugs (NSAIDs) may be used in the management of postsurgical pain. The

NSAIDs may be sufficient to relieve pain after simple procedures or may have additive (or synergistic) effects with other forms of analgesics (Dahl et al., 1990). NSAIDs may reduce the requirements for opioids. NSAIDs may be used before, during, or after a surgical procedure, and in this way they may limit the potential toxicity and side effects of other analgesic regimens. NSAIDs all produce antipyretic, analgesic, and anti-inflammatory effects, but the relative proportions of these effects vary with the different agents.

Rectally, intramuscularly, and intravenously administered NSAIDs have all demonstrated an opioid-sparing effect in patients following thoracotomy (Jones et al., 1985; Pavy et al., 1990; Rhodes et al., 1992). Ketorolac tromethamine is an NSAID that is FDA-approved for both intramuscular and oral administration. The use of ketorolac in this form improved respiratory function in elderly patients following abdominal surgery (Michaelides et al., 1992). Following major surgery with erratic gastric absorption, the systemic route is preferred. Although ketorolac is not yet approved by the FDA for intravenous administration, many studies have indicated that this form is as safe as using ketorolac intramuscularly. This agent is an effective analgesic with a paucity of side effects. However, as with other NSAIDs, there is always the possibility of enhanced postoperative or gastric bleeding. Ketorolac is contraindicated in patients with allergy to aspirin or in patients with nasal polyps, because there is the potential for an anaphylactic reaction. Further care should be taken in administering NSAIDs to patients with significant renal impairment.

After abdominal or orthopedic procedures, the intramuscular addition of ketorolac effectively reduced even the pain level (VAS < 1) achieved with intrathecally administered opioids (Gwirtz et al., 1992). In a study of patients who had undergone radical retropubic prostatectomy, ketorolac decreased epidural fentanyl use, decreased the time to recovery of gastrointestinal function, and produced less nausea on the third postoperative day (Grass et al., 1993). There was no difference in blood loss, hematocrit, or platelet count.

Ketorolac is absorbed rapidly and completely after oral and intramuscular administration (Mroszczak et al., 1990). The dose that is usually effective in young, healthy individuals is an intramuscularly administered loading dose of 60 mg followed by 30 mg every 6 hours. It is routinely recommended that the dose be reduced by 50% in patients under 65 years of age. In addition, it is recommended that ketorolac not be used for more than 5 consecutive days.

ACUTE PAIN MANAGEMENT: A TEAM APPROACH

The management of chronic pain is best controlled with a team approach. Development of an acute pain service in the hospital setting provides similar rewards for the treatment of acute pain (Ready et al.,

1988). The purpose of an acute pain service is to coordinate the skills and knowledge of all the personnel into a uniform plan to manage postoperative pain relief.

Several members are necessary in the postoperative setting to optimize the team approach to postoperative care. At most centers, each discipline is not involved on a full-time basis but can be assembled when necessary. Table 5–22 lists the disciplines that should be represented in some capacity for acute pain management.

A physician member is essential to provide the medical knowledge and direction for the team. All team functions are performed under the direction of the medical director of the service. Typically, the primary physician involved on these services is an anesthesiologist. The primary physician could also be from another discipline. Other physicians who should be in frequent contact with the acute pain service include the patient's primary care service and significant consultative services, such as oncology and radiology.

Nursing is an essential element of the team. Ideally, a full-time nurse provides continuity throughout the institution and is responsible for nursing inservices pertaining to pain management throughout the hospital. Nurses have the training and background necessary to provide excellent patient care in this setting and should never be excluded from this group. The nurse providing the day-to-day care of the patient has to work well with the acute pain team to provide adequate monitoring and feedback on the patient's progress.

A pharmacist should be a member of the acute pain service. This person (or persons) initially should be involved with decisions about products to be used, ranging from devices that provide epidural drug delivery to specialized drug products prepared by the pharmacy for specific applications. The pharmacist is also concerned with the stability and sterility of the products, as well as with direct patient evaluation, monitoring of side effects, and interactions with other drugs being administered.

Consultative membership in the acute pain service will be dictated by the patient's postoperative course. Other essential fields may include psychiatry/psychology, physical therapy, occupational therapy, social services, and pastoral services. These services typically are deeply involved with chronic pain services, but their roles may be much more limited in the acute setting. These team members may be especially useful when dealing with patients who may develop chronic pain or who have chronic pain syndromes and experi-

■ **Table 5–22.** ACUTE PAIN TEAM MEMBERS

1. Anesthesiologist	*Consultative:*
2. Nurse	Psychiatrist/psychologist
3. Pharmacist	Physical therapist
4. Physician—primary care	Occupational therapist
5. Surgeon	Social worker
	Pastor

ence acute pain through exacerbations or a new source.

The acute pain team must be able to respond to patients within minutes 24 hours a day, 7 days a week. The service should be managed by a physician who can respond quickly to patients' needs or provide other methods of responding quickly. The nurse is the most important link in any acute pain team and must communicate inadequate pain control or side effects to the acute pain team. The first 6 to 12 hours after operation typically constitute the period when it is most difficult to control the severity of pain and the potential for side effects of the pain or therapy.

BIBLIOGRAPHY

Albert, J. M., and Talbott, T. M.: Patient-controlled analgesia vs. conventional intramuscular analgesia following colon surgery. Dis. Colon Rectum, 31:83–86, 1988.

Ashburn, M. A., Lind, G. H., Gillie, M. H., et al.: Oral transmucosal fentanyl citrate (OTFC) for the treatment of postoperative pain. Anesth. Analg., 76:377–381, 1993.

Atwell, J. R., Flanigan, R. C., Bennet, R. L., et al.: The efficacy of patient controlled analgesia in patients recovering from flank incisions. J. Urol., 132:701–703, 1984.

Austin, K. L., Stapleton, J. V., and Mather, L. E.: Multiple intramuscular injections: A major source of variability in analgesic response to meperidine. Pain, 8:47–62, 1980a.

Austin, K. L., Stapleton, J. V., and Mather, L. E.: Relationship between blood meperidine concentrations and analgesic response: A preliminary report. Anesthesiology, 53:460–466, 1980b.

Badner, N. H., Reimer, E. J., Komar, W. E., and Moote, C. A.: Low-dose bupivacaine does not improve post-operative epidural fentanyl analgesia in orthopedic patients. Anesth. Analg., 72:337–341, 1991; Erratum Anesth. Analg., May 1991, p. 718.

Bailey, P. L., Streisand, J. B., East, K. A., et al.: Differences in magnitude and duration of respiratory depression and analgesia with fentanyl and sufentanil. Anesth. Analg., 70:8–15, 1990.

Bellville, J. W., Forrest, W. H., Miller, E., et al.: Influence of age on pain relief from analgesics: A study of postoperative patients. J. A. M. A., 217:1835–1841, 1971.

Bennett, R. L., Batenhorst, R. L., and Bivens, B. A.: Patient-controlled analgesia: A new concept of postoperative pain relief. Ann. Surg., 195:700–705, 1982.

Berde, C. B.: Children's Hospital Pain Treatment Service Protocols: Personal communication, 1987.

Berde, C. B.: Pediatric post-operative pain management. Pediatr. Clin. North Am., 36:921–940, 1989.

Berde, C. B., Lehn, B. M., Yee, J. D., et al.: Patient controlled analgesia in children and adolescents: A randomized, prospective comparison with intramuscular administration of morphine for postoperative analgesia. J. Pediatr., 118:460–466, 1991.

Berde, C. B., Sethna, N. F., Levin, L., et al.: Regional analgesia on pediatric medical and surgical wards. Intensive Care Med. J., 15:540–543, 1989.

Bollish, S. J., Collins, C. L., Kirking, D. M., et al.: Efficacy of patient controlled versus conventional analgesia for postoperative pain. Clin. Pharm., 4:48–52, 1985.

Breslow, M. J., Jordan, D. A., Christopherson, R., et al.: Epidural morphine decreases postoperative hypertension by attenuating sympathetic nervous system activity. J. A. M. A., 261:3577–3581, 1989.

Bromage, P. R.: Spirometry in assessment of analgesia after abdominal surgery. Br. J. Anaesth., 2:539–592, 1955.

Bromage, P. R., Camporesi, E., and Chestnut, D.: Epidural narcotics for postoperative pain relief. Anesth. Analg., 59:473–480, 1980.

Bromage, P. R., Camporesi, E. M., Durant, P. A., and Nielsen, C. H.: Non-respiratory effects of epidural morphine. Anesth. Analg., 61:490–495, 1982.

Brose, W. G., and Cohen, S. E.: Oxyhemoglobin saturation following cesarean section. Anesthesiology, 70:948–953, 1989.

Burns, J. W., Hodsman, N. B. A., McLintock, T. T. C., et al.: The influence of patient characteristics on the requirements for postoperative analgesia. Anaesthesia, 44:2–6, 1989.

Caplan, R. A., Ready, B. L., Oden, R. V., et al.: Transdermal fentanyl for postoperative pain management. J. A. M. A., 26:1036–1039, 1989.

Catley, D. M., Thornton, C., and Jordan, C.: Pronounced, episodic oxygen desaturation in the postoperative period: Its association with ventilatory pattern and analgesic regimen. Anesthesiology, 63:20–28, 1985.

Chan, V. W. S., Arthur, G. R., and Ferrante, M. F.: Intrapleural bupivacaine for pain relief following thoracotomy. Reg. Anesth., 13:25–70, 1988.

Chrubasik, J., and Wiemers, K.: Continuous-plus-on-demand epidural infusion of morphine for postoperative pain relief by means of a small, externally worn infusion device. Anesthesiology, 62:263–267, 1985.

Chrubasik, J., Wust, H., Schulte-Monting, J., et al.: Relative analgesia potency of epidural fentanyl, alfentanil and morphine in treatment of postoperative pain. Anesthesiology, 68:929–933, 1988.

Cousins, M. J., and Wright, C. J.: Graft muscle skin blood flow after epidural block in vascular surgical procedures. Surg. Gynecol. Obstet., 33:59–64, 1971.

Craig, D. B.: Post-operative recovery of pulmonary function. Anesth. Analg., 60:46–52, 1981.

Cullen, M. L., Staren, E. D., El-Ganzouri, A., et al.: Continuous epidural infusion for analgesia after major abdominal operations: A randomized, double-blind study. Surgery, 98:718–728, 1985.

Cuschieri, R. J., Morran, C. G., Howie, J. C., and McArdle, C. S.: Post-operative pain and pulmonary complications: Comparison of three analgesic regimens. Br. J. Surg., 72:495–498, 1985.

Dahl, J. B., Daugaard, J. J., Larsen, H. V., et al.: Patient-controlled analgesia: A controlled trial. Acta Anaesthesiol. Scand., 31:744–747, 1987.

Dahl, J. B., Rosenberg, J., Dirkes, W. E., et al.: Prevention of postoperative pain by balanced analgesia. Br. J. Anaesth., 64:518–520, 1990.

Dahlström, B., Tamsen, A., Paalzow, L., and Hartvig, P.: Patient controlled analgesic therapy. Part IV: Pharmacokinetics and analgesic plasma concentrations of morphine. Clin. Pharmacokinet., 7:266–279, 1982.

DeCastro, S., Meynadier, J., and Zenz, M. (eds): Regional Opioid Analgesia. Dordrecht, Kluwer Academic Press, 1991, pp. 80–109.

DuPen, S. L., Peterson, D. G., Bogosian, A. C., et al.: A new permanent exteriorized epidural catheter for narcotic self-administration to control cancer pain. Cancer, 59:986–993, 1987a.

DuPen, S. L., Ramsey, D., and Chin, S.: Chronic epidural morphine and preservative-induced injury. Anesthesiology, 67:987–988, 1987b.

Egberts, K. M., Parks, L. H., Short, L. M., and Burnett, M. L.: Randomized trial of postoperative patient controlled analgesia vs intramuscular narcotics in elderly men. Arch. Intern. Med., 150:1897–1903, 1990.

Eichorn, J. H.: Spinal anesthesia and anticoagulant therapy questions and answers. J. A. M. A., 262:411, 1989.

Eisenach, J. C., Grice, S. C., and Dewan, D. M.: Patient-controlled analgesia following cesarean section: A comparison with epidural and intramuscular narcotics. Anesthesiology, 68:444–448, 1988.

El-Baz, N., Faber, P. L., and Ivankovitch, A. D.: Intrapleural infusion of local anesthetic: A word of caution. Anesthesiology, 68:809–810, 1988.

El-Baz, N. M., Faber, P., and Jensik, R. J.: Continuous epidural infusion of morphine for treatment of pain after thoracic surgery: A new technique. Anesth. Analg., 63:757–764, 1984.

Ferrante, F. M.: Brigham and Women's Hospital Pain Treatment Service Protocols: Personal communication, 1987.

Ferrante, F. M., Lu, L., Jamison, S. B., et al.: Patient-controlled epidural analgesia: Demand dosing. Anesth. Analg., 73:547–552, 1991.

Fine, P. G., Marcus, M., Just DeBoer, A., and Van der Oord, B.: An open label study of oral transmucosal fentanyl citrate (OTFC) for the treatment of breakthrough cancer pain. Pain, 45:149, 1991.

Fischer, A. P., Fung, C., and Hanna, M.: Absorption of buccosal morphine, a comparison with slow release morphine. Anaesthesia, 43:552–553, 1988a.

Fischer, R., Lubenow, T. R., Liceaga, A., et al.: A comparison of continuous epidural infusion of fentanyl-bupivacaine and morphine-bupivacaine in management of post-operative pain. Anesth. Analg., 66:559–563, 1988b.

Friesen, R. H., and Lockhart, C. H.: Oral transmucosal fentanyl citrate for preanesthetic medication of pediatric day surgery patients with and without droperidol as a prophylactic antiemetic. Anesthesiology, 76:46–51, 1992.

Gibbs, J. M., Johnson, H. D., and Davis, F. M.: Patient administration of IV buprenorphine for postoperative pain relief using the "Cardiff" demand palliator. Br. J. Anaesth., 54:279–284, 1982.

Ginsberg, B., Cohen, N. A., Ossey, K. D., and Glass, P. S. A.: The use of PCA to assess the influence of demographic factors on analgesic requirements. Anesthesiology, 71:A688, 1989.

Go, V. L. W., and Yaksh, T. L.: Release of substance P from the rat spinal cord. J. Physiol., 39:1141–1167, 1987.

Gomez, M. N., Symreng, T., Johnson, B., et al.: Intrapleural bupivacaine for intraoperative analgesia: A dangerous technique. Anesth. Analg., 67:S266, 1984.

Gourlay, G. K., Cherry, D. A., and Cousins, M. J.: Cephalad migration of morphine in CSF following lumbar epidural administration in patients with cancer pain. Pain, 23:317–326, 1986.

Gourlay, G. K., Cherry, D. A., Plummer, J. L., et al.: The influence of drug polarity on the absorption of opioid drug into the CSF and subsequent cephalad migration following lumbar epidural administration: Application to morphine and pethidine. Pain, 31:297–305, 1987.

Gourlay, G. K., Kowalski, S. R., Plummer, J. L., et al.: The transdermal administration of fentanyl in the treatment of postoperative pain: Pharmacokinetics and pharmacodynamic effects. Pain 37:193–202, 1989.

Grass, J. A., Sakima, N. T., Valley, M., et al.: Assessment of ketorolac as an adjuvant to fentanyl patient-controlled analgesia after radical retropubic prostatectomy. Anesthesiology, 78:642–648, 1993.

Graves, D. A., Foster, T. S., Batenhorst, R. L., et al.: Patient controlled analgesia. Ann. Intern. Med., 99:360–366, 1983.

Gregg, R. V., Denson, D. D., Knarr, D. C., and Steubing, R. C.: Continuous epidural infusions of bupivacaine and morphine vs. systemic narcotic analgesics for post-operative pain relief. Anesthesiology, 69:A384, 1988.

Gregory, M. A., Brock-Utne, J. C., Bux, S., and Downing, J. W.: Morphine concentration in brain and spinal cord after subarachnoid morphine injection in baboons. Anesth. Analg., 64:929–932, 1985.

Gustaffoson, L. L., Schildt, B., Jackobsen, K. T., and Allvin, R.: Present state of extradural and intraspinal opiates: Report of a nationwide survey in Sweden. Br. J. Anaesth., 54:479–486, 1982.

Gwirtz, K. H., Helvie, J. E., Young, J. V., and Li, W.: Ketorolac enhances intrathecal analgesia after major abdominal surgery and orthopedic surgery. Reg. Anesth., 17:161, 1992.

Hamon, M., Bourgoin, S., and Lebars, D.: In vivo and in vitro release of central neurotransmitters in relation to pain and analgesia. Brain Res., 77:431–444, 1988.

Hansen, L. A., Noyes, M. A., and Lehman, M. E.: Evaluation of PCA versus PCA plus continuous infusion in postoperative cancer patients. Pain Symptom Management, 6:4–13, 1991.

Harrison, D. M., Sinatra, R., Morgenson, L., et al.: Epidural narcotic and patient-controlled analgesia for post-cesarean section pain relief. Anesthesiology, 68:454–457, 1988.

Hecker, B. R., and Albert, L.: Patient controlled analgesia: A randomized prospective comparison between two commercially available PCA pumps and conventional therapy for postoperative pain. Pain, 35:115, 1988.

Hill, H. F., Chapman, C. R., Kornell, J. A., et al.: Self-administration of morphine to bone marrow transplant patients reduces drug requirement. Pain, 40:121–129, 1990.

Holley, F. O., and Van Steennis, C.: Post operative analgesia with fentanyl: Pharmacokinetics and pharmacodynamics of con-stant-rate IV and transdermal fentanyl. Br. J. Anaesth., 60:806–813, 1988.

Hughes, S., Millar, W. L., and Reisner, L. S.: Clinical experience with continuous epidural fentanyl. Reg. Anesth., 11:44, 1986.

Jaffe, J. H., and Martin, W. R.: Opioid analgesics and antagonists. In Goodman, L. S., Gilman, A. Z., Rall, T. W., and Murad, F. (eds): The Pharmacological Basis of Therapeutics. New York, Pergamon Press, 1985.

Jensen, K., Tuxen, C., and Pedersen-Bjergaard, U.: Pain and tenderness in human temporal muscle induced by bradykinin and 5 hydroxytryptamine. Peptides, 11:1127–1132, 1990.

Jesse, T. M., and Iversen, L. L.: Opiate analgesics inhibit substance P release from the rat trigeminal nucleus. Nature, 268:549–551, 1977.

Jones, R. M., Cashman, J. N., Foster, J. M., et al.: Comparison of infusion of morphine and lysine acetyl salicylate for the relief of pain following thoracic surgery. Br. J. Anaesth., 57:259–263, 1985.

Kaiko, R. F., Foley, K. M., and Grabinski, P. Y.: Central nervous system excitatory effects of meperidine in cancer patients. Ann. Neurol., 13:180–185, 1983.

Kambam, J. R., Handte, R. E., Flanagan, J., et al.: Intrapleural analgesia for post thoracotomy pain relief. Anesth. Analg., 66:S287, 1987.

Kay, B.: Postoperative pain relief: Use of an on-demand analgesia computer (ODAC) and a comparison of the rate of use of fentanyl and alfentanil. Anaesthesia, 36:949–951, 1981.

Kehlet, H.: Influence of epidural analgesia on endocrine metabolic response to surgery. Acta Anesth. Scand. Suppl., 70:39–49, 1979.

Kluger, M. T., and Owen, H.: Patient expectations of patient controlled analgesia. Anaesthesia, 46:1072–1074, 1990.

Kuhlman, G., Vique, B., Duranteau, J., and Orhant, B.: Intrapleural lidocaine analgesia influence of volume and concentration [Abstract]. Anesthesiology, 71:A659, 1988.

Kvalheim, L., and Reiestad, F.: Interpleural analgesia in the management of postoperative pain [Abstract]. Anesthesiology, 61:A231, 1984.

Lange, P. M., Dahn, M. S., and Jacobs, L. A.: Patient-controlled analgesia versus intermittent analgesia dosing. Heart Lung, 17:495, 1988.

Latasch, L., and Luders, S.: Transdermal fentanyl against postoperative pain. Acta Anaesthesiol. Belg., 40:113–119, 1989.

Lehmann, K. A.: Patient controlled analgesia for postoperative pain. In Benedetti, C., Chapman, C. R., Giron, G. (eds): Advances in Pain Research and Therapy. New York, Raven Press, 1990, pp. 297–324.

Lehmann, K. A., Brund-Stavroulaki, A., and Dworzak, H.: The influence of demand and loading dose on the efficacy of postoperative patient controlled analgesia with Tamadol. Schmerz-Pain-Douleur, 7:146–152, 1986.

Lehmann, K. A., Heinrich, C., and van Heiss, R.: Balanced anesthesia and patient-controlled postoperative analgesia with fentanyl: Minimum effective concentrations, accumulation and acute tolerance. Acta Anaesthesiol. Belg., 39:11–22, 1988.

Logas, W. G., El-Baz, N., El-Ganzouri, A. et al.: Continuous thoracic epidural analgesia for postoperative pain relief following thoracotomy: A randomized prospective study. Anesthesiology, 67:787–791, 1987.

Lombard, M. C., and Besson, J. M.: Attempts to gauge the relative importance of pre and post synaptic effects of morphine on the transmission of noxious messages in the dorsal horn of the rat spinal cord. Pain, 37:335–345, 1989.

Loper, K. A., Ready, L. B., Downey, M., et al.: Epidural and intravenous fentanyl infusions are clinically equivalent after knee surgery. Anesth. Analg., 70:72–75, 1990.

Magora, F., Olshwang, D. L., Eimeri, D., et al.: Observation on extradural morphine analgesia in various pain conditions. Br. J. Anaesth., 52:247–252, 1980.

Marks, R. M., and Sachar, E. J.: Undertreatment of medical inpatients with narcotic analgesics. Ann. Intern. Med., 78:173–181, 1973.

Mather, L. E., and Owen, H.: The scientific basis for patient controlled analgesia. Anaesth. Intensive Care, 16:427–447, 1988.

Michaelides, S., Pappas, X., Pouliou, K., et al.: Comparative evaluation of the effects of morphine and ketorolac on gas exchange in elderly postoperative patients. Reg. Anesth., 17:154, 1992.

Mier, A. W., Narang, P. K., Dothage, J. A., et al.: Transdermal fentanyl for pain control in cancer patients. Pain, 37:15–21, 1989.

Modig, J., Borg, T., Karlstrom, G., et al.: Thromboembolism after total hip replacement: Role of epidural and general anesthesia. Anesth. Analg., 62:174–180, 1983.

Modig, J., Malbert, P., and Saldeen, T.: Comparative effects of epidural and general anesthesia on fibrinolysis function, lower limb rheology and thromboembolism after total hip replacement. Anesthesiology, 53:34–44, 1980.

Moller, I. W., Dinesen, K., Sondergard, S., et al.: Effect of patient controlled analgesia on plasma catecholamines, cortisol and glucose concentrations after cholecystectomy. Br. J. Anaesth., 61:160–164, 1988.

Morgenson, T., Hojaard, L., Scott, N. B., et al.: Epidural blood flow and the regression of sensory analgesia during continuous post-operative epidural infusion of bupivacaine. Anesthesiology, 67:809–813, 1988.

Mroszczak, E. J., Jung, D., Yee, J., et al.: Ketorolac tromethamine pharmacokinetics after intravenous, intramuscular, and oral administration in humans and animals. Pharmacotherapy, 10:33S–39S, 1990.

O'Kelley, E., and Gary, B.: Continuous pain relief for multiple fractured ribs. Br. J. Anaesth., 53:989–991, 1981.

Owen, H., Plummer, J. L., Armstrong, I., et al.: Variables of patient-controlled analgesia: Bolus size. Anaesthesia, 44:7–10, 1989a.

Owen, H., Szekely, S. M., Plummer, J. L., et al.: Variables of patient-controlled analgesia: Concurrent infusion. Anaesthesia, 44:11–13, 1989b.

Parker, R. K., Holtman, B., Woodring Brown, P., and White, P. F.: Effects of basal opioid infusion on postoperative analgesic requirements. Anesthesiology, 71:A763, 1989.

Parker, R. K., Holtman, B., Woodring Brown, P., and White PF: Patient controlled analgesia. Does a concurrent opioid infusion improve pain management after surgery? J. A. M. A., 266:1947–1952, 1991.

Pavy, T., Medley, C., and Murphy, D. F.: Effect of indomethacin on pain relief following thoracotomy. Br. J. Anaesth., 65:624–627, 1990.

Payne, R.: CSF distribution of opioids in animals and man. Acta Anaesth. Scand. Suppl., 85:38–46, 1987.

Plezia, P. M., Kramer, T. H., Linford, J., and Hameroff, S. R.: Transdermal fentanyl: Pharmacokinetics and preliminary clinical evaluation. Pharmacotherapy, 9:2–9, 1989.

Raj, P., and Bridenbaugh, L. D.: The experts opine: Should epidural narcotics be used for post-operative pain? Surv. Anesthesiol., 31:372–378, 1987.

Rawal, N., Arner, S., Gustafsson, L. L., and Allvin, R.: Present state of extradural and intrathecal opioid analgesia in Sweden. Br. J. Anaesth., 59:791–799, 1987.

Rawal, N., Sjostrand, U., and Dahlstrom, B.: Post operative pain relief by epidural morphine. Anesth. Analg., 60:726–731, 1981.

Rawal, N., and Wattwil, M.: Respiratory depression after epidural morphine: An experimental and clinical study. Anesth. Analg., 63:14, 1984.

Ready, L. B.: Issue Pro & Con: Are epidural narcotics safe for control of post-operative pain beyond the confines of the intensive care unit? ASRA NEWS, August 1990, pp. 3–4.

Ready, L. B., Oden, R., Chadwick, H. S., et al.: Development of an anesthesiology based post-operative pain management service. Anesthesiology, 68:100–106, 1988.

Reedy, M. E., Morris, L. E., Brown, D. I., et al.: Double blind comparison of butorphanol and morphine in patient controlled analgesia. Acute Care, 12(Suppl.):40–46, 1986.

Reiestad, F., Stromskag, K. E., and Holmqvist, E.: Intrapleural administration of bupivacaine in postoperative pain management [Abstract]. Anesthesiology, 65:A204, 1986.

Rhodes, M., Conacher, I., Morritt, G., and Hilton, C.: Nonsteroidal antiinflammatory drugs for post thoracotomy pain. A prospective controlled trial after lateral thoracotomy. J. Thorac. Cardiovasc. Surg., 103:17–20, 1992.

Rigg, J. R., Ilsley, A. H., and Vedig, A. E.: Relationship of ventilatory depression to steady-state blood pethidine concentrations. Br. J. Anaesth., 53:613–620, 1981.

Rigg, J. R. A., Browne, R. A., Davis, C., et al.: Variation in the disposition of morphine after i.m. administration in surgical patients. Br. J. Anaesth., 50:1125, 1978.

Rogers, D. A., Dingus, D., Stanfield, J., et al.: A prospective study of patient controlled analgesia. Am. Surg., 56:86–88, 1990.

Rosenberg, P. H., Heino, A., and Schein, B.: Comparison of intramuscular analgesia, intercostal block, epidural morphine and on demand IV fentanyl in the control of pain after abdominal surgery. Acta Anaesthiol. Scand., 28:603–607, 1984.

Rosenberg, P. H., Scheinin, B. M., Lepantalo, M. J., and Lindfors, O. L.: Continuous intrapleural infusion of bupivacaine for analgesia after thoracotomy. Anesthesiology, 67:811–813, 1987.

Rowbotham, D. J., Wyld, R., Peacock, J. E., et al.: Transdermal fentanyl for the relief of pain after upper abdominal surgery. Br. J. Anaesth., 63:56–59, 1989.

Roy, S. D., and Flynn, G. L.: Transdermal delivery of narcotic analgesics: Comparative permeability of narcotic analgesics through human cadaver skin. Pharm. Res., 6:825–832, 1989.

Rutberg, H., Hakanson, E., Anderberg, B., et al.: Effects of extradural administration of morphine or bupivacaine on the endocrine response to upper abdominal surgery. Br. J. Anaesth., 56:233–238, 1984.

Schweitzer, S. A., and Morgan, D. J.: Plasma bupivacaine concentrations during postoperative continuous epidural analgesia. Anaesth. Intensive Care, 15:425–430, 1987.

Scott, N. B., and Kehlet, H.: Regional anesthesia and surgical morbidity. Br. J. Surg., 75:299–304, 1988.

Scott, N. B., Morgenson, T., Big, D., et al.: Continuous thoracic extradural 0.05% bupivacaine with or without morphine: Effect on quality of blockade, lung function and the surgical stress response. Br. J. Anaesth., 62:253–257, 1989.

Seltzer, J. L., Bell, S. D., Moritz, H., and Cantillo, J.: A double-blind comparison of intrapleural bupivacaine and epidural fentanyl for post thoracotomy pain. Anesthesiology, 71:A665, 1989.

Seltzer, J. L., Larijajani, G. E., Goldberg, M. E., and Marr, A. E.: Intrapleural analgesia: A kinetic and dynamic evaluation. Anesthesiology, 67:798–800, 1987.

Simpson, B. P., Parkhouse, J., Marshall, R., et al.: Extradural analgesia and the prevention of post-operative respiratory complications. Br. J. Anaesth., 33:623–641, 1961.

Sinatra, R. S., Lodge, K., Sibert, K., et al.: A comparison of morphine, meperidine, and oxymorphone as utilized in patient-controlled analgesia following cesarean delivery. Anesthesiology, 70:585–589, 1989.

Sjoberg, M., Karlsson, P., Nordberg, C., et al.: Neuropathologic findings after long-term intrathecal infusion of morphine and bupivacaine for pain treatment in cancer patients. Anesthesiology, 76:173–186, 1992.

Sjostrom, S., Hartvig, P., Persson, M. P., and Tamsen, A.: Pharmacokinetics of epidural morphine and meperidine in humans. Anesthesiology, 67:877–888, 1987.

Sjostrom, S., Hartvig, P., and Tamsen, A.: Patient-controlled analgesia with extradural morphine or pethidine. Br. J. Anaesth., 60:358–366, 1988.

Sprigge, J. S., and Otton, P. E.: Nalbuphine versus meperidine for postoperative analgesia: A double-blind comparison using the patient controlled analgesic technique. Can. Anaesth. Soc. J., 30:517–521, 1983.

Squier, R. C., Morrow, J. S., and Roman, R.: Hanging drop technique for intrapleural analgesia. Anesthesiology, 70:882, 1989.

Streisand, J.: Controlled iontophoretic and transmucosal delivery of opioids. In Sinatra, R., Hord, A. H., Ginsberg, B., et al. (eds): Acute Pain: Mechanisms and Management. St. Louis, Mosby Year Book, 1992.

Symreng, T., Gomez, M. N., and Rossi, N.: Intrapleural bupivacaine vs saline after thoracotomy effects on pain and lung function: A double blind study. J. Cardiothorac. Anesth., 3:144–149, 1989.

Tamsen, A., Hartvig, P., Fagerland, C., et al.: Patient-controlled analgesic therapy. Part II: Individual analgesic demand and analgesic plasma concentrations of pethidine in postoperative pain. Clin. Pharmacokinet., 7:164–175, 1982.

Tucker, G. T., Cooper, S., Littlewood, D., and Buckley, S. P.: Observed and predicted accumulation of local anesthetics during continuous extradural analgesia. Br. J. Anaesth., 49:237, 1977.

Varvel, J. R., Shafer, S. L., Hwang, S. S., et al.: Absorption characteristics of transdermally administered fentanyl. Anesthesiology, 70:928–934, 1989.

Ved, S. A., Dubois, M., Carron, H., and Lea, D.: Sufentanil and alfentanil pattern of consumption during patient controlled analgesia: A comparison with morphine. Clin. J. Pain, 5:S63–S70, 1989.

Wahba, W. M., Don, H. R., and Craig, D. B.: Post-operative epidural analgesia: Effect on lung volumes. Can. Anesth. Soc. J., 22:519–527, 1975.

Wang, B. C., Budzilovich, G., Hiller, J. M., et al.: Are the preservatives sodium bisulfite and ethylene diaminetetracetate free from neurotoxic involvement? [Letter]. Anesthesiology, 77:602–603, 1992.

Wasylak, T. J., Abbott, F. V., English, M. J. M., and Jeans, M. E.: Reduction of postoperative morbidity following patient controlled analgesia. Can. J. Anaesth., 37:726–731, 1990.

Weinberg, D. S., Inturrisi, C. E., Beidenberg, B., et al.: Sublingual absorption of selected opioid analgesics. Clin. Pharmacol. Ther., 44:335–342, 1988.

Welchew, E. A., and Hosking, J.: Patient-controlled postoperative analgesia with alfentanil. Anaesthesia, 40:1172–1177, 1985.

Wheatley, R. G., Somerville, I. D., Sapsford, D. J., and Jones, J. G.: Postoperative hypoxemia: Comparison of extradural, IM and patient controlled opioid analgesia. Br. J. Anaesth., 64:267–275, 1990.

White, D. C.: The relief of post-operative pain. In Atkinson, R. S., and Hewer, C. L. (eds): Present Advances in Anesthesia and Analgesia. New York, Churchill Livingstone, 1982, pp. 121–139.

Yaksh, T. L., Durant, P. A. C., Gaumann, D. M., et al.: The use of receptor-selective agents as analgesics in the spinal cord: Trends and possibilities. J. Pain Symptom Management, 2:129–138, 1987.

Yeager, M. P., Glass, D. D., Nett, R. F., and Brinck-Johnson, T.: Epidural anesthesia and analgesia in high risk surgical patients. Anesthesiology, 66:729–736, 1987.

Yu, P. Y. H., Gamling, D. R., and McMorland, G. H.: A comparative study of patient-controlled epidural fentanyl and single dose epidural morphine for post-cesarean section analgesia. Can. J. Anaesth., 36:55–56, 1989.

Zacharias, M., Pfeifer, M. V., and Herbison, P.: Comparison of two methods of intravenous administration of morphine for postoperative pain. Anaesth. Intensive Care, 18:205–209, 1990.

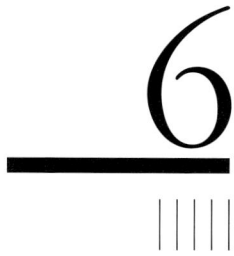

6 Shock and Circulatory Collapse

Ronald D. Curran and Robert W. Anderson

In fundamental terms, shock occurs when there is a failure of normal circulatory and metabolic homeostatic mechanisms that leads to cellular injury. Clinically, shock describes a wide spectrum of disease states and pathophysiology. Shock includes the physiologic response of the critically injured trauma victim with profound hypovolemia and vasoconstriction, but also encompasses the hyperdynamic pathologic response of the septic patient with low systemic vascular resistance and organ failure. Correspondingly, the shock state is associated with alterations in the function of virtually every organ system. The cause and severity of the shock state and the patient's baseline organ function determine the specific organ response. Hypovolemic shock may stimulate the kidney to appropriately reabsorb sodium and water; with more severe ischemia/reperfusion injury, it may lead to renal failure and the inability of the kidney to regulate fluid balance. The shock response to injury, whether it be the result of infection, pump failure, or tissue destruction, is the culmination of neural and humoral effects and the actions of cell-derived mediators. Increased sympathetic tone, release of the hormones glucagon, adrenocorticotropic hormone (ACTH), and growth hormone, as well as the production of cytokines such as tumor necrosis factor (TNF), interleukin-1 (IL-1), and interleukin-6 all act in concert to stimulate a variety of alterations in cellular metabolism. The specific cellular response to shock depends on the patient and the cause and severity of the shock state. Shock may stimulate the hepatocyte to synthesize an array of acute-phase proteins that protect the cells from proteolytic damage. In the more compromised patient, severe shock states may inhibit hepatocyte protein synthesis, which eventually leads to liver dysfunction. Shock affects a heterogeneous patient population presenting with a variety of organ responses and alterations in cellular metabolism.

Numerous attempts have been made to define the shock state. Initially, the term *shock* was used merely as a clinical description for the moribund patient with altered sensorium and signs of inadequate tissue perfusion. Recognition that there were consistent patterns in the shock response led to classification of shock according to the precipitating event or cause. However, this method of describing shock also has limitations, since multiple factors may act synergistically to induce the shock response. In addition, this static classification system does not reflect the multitude of events, such as nosocomial infections, stress-induced myocardial infarction, or gastrointestinal bleeding, that can complicate a patient's recovery from an episode of shock. Recent attempts to define shock have taken a more analytical approach, including physiologic and biochemical criteria. There are now a number of scoring systems, such as the Acute Physiology and Chronic Health Evaluation (APACHE), the Therapeutic Intervention Scoring System (TISS), and the Injury Severity Score (ISS), that use clinical, biochemical, and physiologic variables to precisely quantify a patient's status. These scoring systems have applications in directing patient care and can predict morbidity. Currently, an accurate description of a patient in shock should include both the cause or classification of the injury and the results of one of these numerical scoring systems. This information effectively separates the large diverse population of patients with shock into smaller, more homogeneous subgroups with similar injury severity and physiologic responses.

HISTORICAL ASPECTS

The nature of shock has been studied for approximately four centuries in attempts to formulate rational therapy in terms of the body's reaction to injury. Paré (1582) first described the syndrome following trauma on the battlefield as "petite mort," but it was not until the beginning of the 18th century that the word was first used medically in the English language in a translation of Henri François Le Dran's *A Treatise of Reflection Drawn from Experiences with Gunshot Wounds*. The development of theories on the cause and treatment of shock is the story of the development of medical thought in general. Early writings almost exclusively described patients who were examined on the battlefield and who had the clinical signs of circulatory failure. However, in 1831, Thomas Latta made a great contribution by recognizing the importance of hypovolemia in the treatment of patients who were critically ill with cholera. He reported (1832) infusion of intravenous saline solution to treat patients and showed dramatic clinical improvement in some of them. Since then, studies have been less concerned with clinical description and philosophic definitions than with clarifying the pathophysiology and developing types of therapy for managing shock.

The advent of experimental physiology and precise measurements focused the attention of early investigators on the determination of arterial blood pressure and its control by a vasomotor center, which acted by way of nerve pathways. Recognition of the interrelationship between cardiac function and vascular tone by way of the nervous system generated the concepts of vasomotor paralysis and cardiac failure that resulted from reflex vagal hyperactivity. The neurogenic theory of shock was summarized and advocated by Groenigen (1885), and because this hypothesis satisfied both those who believed in an overactive nervous system and those who believed that vasomotor exhaustion was the important factor in shock, the theory was widely accepted for several years.

At the end of the 19th century, Crile (1899) developed an experimental model of hemorrhagic shock in the dog and began to apply physiologic techniques to the study of shock. His reports helped to systematically define shock in the experimental animal, and he was the first to delineate the effects of hypovolemia on *central venous pressure* (CVP), the acceleration and deepening of respiration after hemorrhage, and the response of the animal in shock to an infusion of warm saline. Crile was impressed by the heart's ability to respond to an infusion of fluid in the late stages of shock, and he suggested early on that cardiac function remained unimpaired in the syndrome.

Because of the large number of traumatic injuries seen on the battlefield, war invariably stimulated interest in the definition and treatment of shock. The collaborative efforts of Cannon and Bayliss (1919) during World War I created an important precedent for future battlefield studies by investigative groups. These investigators did various physiologic and biochemical studies. Cannon (1918) first documented the correlation between low blood pressure and a reduction in alkaline reserve by the use of the Van Slyke apparatus. He surmised that the fall in alkaline reserve was due to the accumulation of fixed acids, such as lactic acid, and recognized that this was caused by impaired oxygen transport. He further identified acidosis as the secondary phenomenon and noted a striking improvement in patients in shock after the administration of sodium bicarbonate. Other studies were done by Keith (1919a, 1919b), who directly measured blood volume by means of the dye dilution method and showed clearly that the severity of shock correlated with the reduction in the blood volume. Many interesting observations were made concerning the nature of crush injuries among patients with war wounds. Numerous clinical descriptions were given of wounded soldiers who were in good condition with their limbs pinned under falling timbers. After the removal of these timbers, the soldiers' condition deteriorated rapidly into "traumatic shock," which led to death. It was also observed that when the limb was amputated before the timber was removed, the patient survived. This led to the concept of "traumatic toxemia" and stimulated Cannon and Bayliss to create an experimental model in the laboratory. Their experiments, interpreted in the light of the work of Dale and Richards (1918) on the toxic effects of histamine, suggested that the dominant factor in traumatic shock was the release of toxic materials into the systemic circulation. Substances such as histamine appeared to supply a basis for loss of vasomotor tone and to cause

the sequestration of blood and the failure of venous return to the heart. The concept of "traumatic toxemia" replaced the vasomotor paralysis theory, and the energies of many investigators were directed toward the isolation of toxic factors in experimental shock preparations.

Blalock (1930) and Parsons and Phemister (1930), working independently, challenged the concept of generalized vascular injury and traumatic toxemia when they showed in a series of classic experiments that a profound loss of blood and plasma occurred in crush injuries in and around the traumatized area, and blood and plasma infiltrated the tissue spaces beyond the area of local injury. This local loss of fluid caused systemic hypovolemia and shock. Their experiments demonstrated that hypovolemia, rather than mysterious toxic factors, in severe trauma continues to be the most important element in most clinical cases of shock.

World War II renewed interest in the study of shock, and the importance of volume restoration, secondary infection, and renal failure was stressed. Because new techniques had facilitated the study of the circulation, the pathophysiology of shock was expressed for the first time in hemodynamic terms that included not only blood pressure but also blood flow, resistance, and the effectiveness of perfusion. The clinical application of cardiac catheterization by Cournand and associates (1943) opened a new era in the investigation of shock. The reduction of cardiac output in relation to fluid loss was clearly confirmed by these investigators. Attention was then directed to the blood supply of certain organ systems such as the brain, lungs, liver, kidneys, and heart. The concept of microcirculatory transport was investigated for the first time, especially in relation to the "sludging" phenomenon that occurred during low-flow states by direct microcirculatory observation.

Information gained during the two World Wars was augmented by further studies conducted during both the Korean and the Vietnam wars. Rapid evacuation systems made it possible for casualties to be examined in resuscitation areas within 20 to 30 minutes after their injuries, and specialized groups were formed to study and to improve the care of casualties. The emphasis in Korea was on renal failure and hemodynamic changes, and in Vietnam on problems of pulmonary insufficiency and noncolloid methods of resuscitation. Between the Korean and the Vietnam wars, investigation of civilian shock was maintained and this led ultimately to the formation of the Shock Study Committee of the National Academy of Sciences. Under the impetus of this group, shock study units were developed and supported in the United States and provided extensive measurements of hemodynamic, biochemical, and clinical data in the various forms of civilian shock. Experience had clearly shown that none of the available experimental models precisely duplicated the situation in human clinical shock and that greater emphasis needed to be placed on the study of the critically ill patient rather than on the experimental animal.

Since 1940, a large volume of hemodynamic and metabolic data has been collected from patients with serious infections. During this period, septic shock has been recognized as a unique pathophysiologic entity, which differs from hypovolemic and cardiogenic shock in that, in many cases, a primary metabolic defect rather than a deficit in blood flow accounts for an overwhelming imbalance in homeostasis.

It was not until the mid-1960s, however, that it was clearly shown that shock associated with sepsis may present with either abnormally high or abnormally low cardiac output and that the high-output response to infection has a unique pathophysiology. In 1966, Clowes and colleagues reported a group of 25 surgical patients with peritonitis. Twelve of these patients recovered promptly from their infections, and all 12 patients had raised cardiac indices. Deaths occurred in patients who either never responded with increased cardiac output or could not sustain increased output confronted with intercurrent complications. MacLean and co-workers (1967) made similar observations in a study of 56 patients who had septic shock. Two distinct groups of patients were identified. Twenty-eight patients were categorized as presenting in "early" septic shock. Hemodynamically, the 24 survivors in this group had elevated CVP, increased cardiac output, reduced peripheral vascular resistance (PVR), and hypotension. A second group of patients presented initially with low CVP, decreased cardiac output, high PVR, and hypotension. If the patients in this second group were acidotic when studied initially, neither fluid nor vasopressors augmented their cardiac outputs, and most patients died.

Siegel and associates (1967) also distinguished two patterns of hemodynamic response to serious infection. In addition, this group made the critical observation that the patients with the highest cardiac output had abnormally high venous oxygen content and a narrow arterial-venous oxygen content difference (A-Vo$_2$). This finding suggested that the peripheral metabolic machinery of the septic patient does not respond appropriately to stress and that the high flows may be a response to a primary defect in aerobic metabolism. Studies by Siegel and colleagues (1971) showed that, in septic patients, increases in cardiac output and reductions in PVR can be correlated with the inability of the liver and skeletal muscle to use oxygen and substrate. At present, the primary lesion in high-output septic shock appears to be an abnormality in oxidative metabolism. The resultant metabolic deficits seem to induce an unbalanced circulatory response that may eventually exhaust cardiovascular reserves.

Since the mid-1980s, it has been recognized that, with the prompt treatment of trauma and infection and the expeditious correction of perfusion deficits, recovery can be expected in patients who were previously in good health. However, in patients in whom perfusion deficits are not immediately corrected and in whom infected or devitalized tissue is not completely débrided, an initial episode of shock may progress to a prolonged illness characterized by multiple organ dysfunction. In these patients, whether the initial stress was caused by hypovolemia, cardiac dysfunction, or infection, the final result appears much the same in terms of clinical presentation. Hepatic dysfunction and jaundice are early indicators of the development of this syndrome. Hyperglycemia and hypertriglyceridemia indicate the onset of a hypermetabolic state in which the lean body mass is rapidly catabolized. Serious renal and pulmonary dysfunctions are frequently the harbingers of a fatal outcome. A great deal of current research on shock focuses on this multiple organ failure syndrome and on its prevention. The exogenous and endogenous mediators that are responsible for this syndrome are now being investigated, and new developments in molecular biology may provide the means of interrupting the pathways that lead to its metabolic and hemodynamic sequelae. Research into the metabolic support of these critically ill patients may provide a method for postponing this syndrome until those factors that usually precipitate it (e.g., incomplete débridement of devitalized or infected tissues and persistent perfusion deficits) can be corrected.

CLASSIFICATION OF SHOCK

In 1934, Blalock (1934a, 1934b) summarized the physiologic studies done both by his group and by others and proposed a classification of circulatory failure from a physiologic standpoint. He indicated that the modern tendency was to classify all forms of acute circulatory failure that complicated operations and wounds, except organic heart failure, under the heading of shock. The terms that he used to designate the different types of shock were:

1. *Hematogenic:* The initial and most important circulatory change is the diminution in the blood volume.
2. *Neurogenic:* The primary alteration is vasodilatation, which depends on diminished constrictor tone as a result of influences acting through the nervous system.
3. *Vasogenic:* Vascular dilatation is brought on directly by agencies that act through the blood vessels.
4. *Cardiogenic:* Acute circulatory failure occurs as a result of a primary disturbance of the heart.

The current classification of shock outlined subsequently extends Blalock's original description by incorporating the work of Shires and co-workers (1973), and provides additional information on the factors that contribute to the development of shock in low-flow states.

A. Cardiogenic
  1. Primary myocardial dysfunction
    a. Myocardial infarction
    b. Cardiomyopathy
    c. Valvular heart disease
    d. Cardiac arrhythmia

    e. Myocardial depression from other causes
      (1) Trauma
      (2) Drug toxicity
  2. Extrinsic causes of impaired cardiac function
    a. Tension pneumothorax
    b. Vena caval obstruction
    c. Cardiac tamponade
    d. Pulmonary embolus
B. Hypovolemic
  1. Blood loss
    a. Trauma
    b. Gastrointestinal
    c. Ruptured aneurysm
    d. Spontaneous retroperitoneal hemorrhage
  2. Plasma loss
    a. Burns
    b. Pancreatitis
    c. Peritonitis
  3. Water loss
    a. Gastrointestinal
    b. Renal
  4. Any combination of these three items
C. Neurogenic: Brought about by central failure of the autonomic nervous system to maintain PVR
  1. Spinal anesthesia
  2. High spinal cord section
  3. Neurogenic reflexes, as in acute pain
D. Vasogenic: Resulting from decreased peripheral arterial resistance and increased central venous capacitance.
  1. Sepsis
    a. Infectious
    b. Noninfectious
    c. Either of these associated with multiple organ failure
  2. Anaphylaxis

In this classification system, patients are grouped according to the cause or pathogenesis of the shock episode. Clinically, the system is useful because patients within the same classification tend to exhibit similar physiologic responses to the shock state and in general share common treatment strategies. However, there are limitations to this classification system. In some cases, it will be difficult to classify a patient into one of these categories because multiple factors may combine to incite the shock state. Furthermore, this classification system fails to take into account secondary insults, which can complicate a patient's recovery from shock and often significantly affect the patient's outcome. The limitation of this classification system is most clearly illustrated in the case of a trauma victim with multiple injuries who is resuscitated from an initial episode of hypovolemic shock only to develop hyperdynamic sepsis with organ failure 3 to 5 days after injury. In this frequently encountered scenario, the patient's physiologic response to hypovolemic shock evolves directly into vasogenic shock, making it difficult to classify the patient into one category. Much of the overlap in this classification scheme of shock involves the category of sepsis with organ failure, since it frequently complicates an epi-

sode of shock or injury of different cause. Our understanding of septic shock and multiple organ failure is continuing to evolve, and it is now recognized that endogenously produced mediators such as cytokines, eicosanoids, and nitric oxide play an important role in the pathogenesis of this syndrome. In future classification schemes, when the pathogenesis of hyperdynamic sepsis and organ failure is even more clearly defined, it may be that sepsis resulting from noninfectious causes such as injury or inflammation will be considered no longer a category of shock but rather a physiologic response to shock of any cause.

Many other factors besides cause affect a patient's response to shock or injury. The patient's age, general condition, history of previous medical problems, and underlying organ dysfunction all profoundly influence the prognosis and treatment. In conjunction with these individual patient variables, the severity of the injury or physiologic derangement determines the severity of the shock episode. In the past, the physician had to combine information from a bedside evaluation of the patient with physiologic and biochemical data to generate an overall picture of the patient's condition, prognosis, and most appropriate course of therapeutic intervention. More recently, scoring systems have been proposed that quantify critical illness by assigning a numerical value to all the factors that influence prognosis. In 1985, Knaus and associates reported the revised Acute Physiology and Chronic Health Evaluations Score (APACHE II), which stratifies critically ill patients by physiologic variables, age, and chronic health status (Fig. 6–1). In this scoring system, 12 physiologic variables are objectively graded from 0 to 4 based on the most deranged reading during a patient's initial 24 hours in the intensive care unit. In addition, the patient receives points for chronologic age, the presence of chronic organ dysfunction or immunocompromised state, and whether he has undergone an emergency surgical procedure. A validation study of 5815 patients in intensive care units at 13 different hospitals found a direct relationship between APACHE II scores and observed hospital death rates. For each 5-point increase in an APACHE II score, there was a significant increase in death rate (Fig. 6–2). Obviously, use of this scoring system, or another like it, for patients with shock will more precisely describe the patient's clinical status. Thus, by combining a numerical score of critical illness with the previously described classification of shock, it will be possible to more accurately compare patient populations and treatment modalities.

MONITORING OF PATIENTS IN SHOCK STATES

Initial management of the patient in shock must include simultaneous evaluation and treatment. After assessing the patient's cardiopulmonary status, the physician must attempt to determine the cause of the shock episode as well as the severity of the physio-

THE APACHE II SEVERITY OF DISEASE CLASSIFICATION SYSTEM

PHYSIOLOGIC VARIABLE	HIGH ABNORMAL RANGE				0	LOW ABNORMAL RANGE			
	+4	+3	+2	+1	0	+1	+2	+3	+4
TEMPERATURE — rectal (°C)	≥41°	39°-40.9°		38.5°-38.9°	36°-38.4°	34°-35.9°	32°-33.9°	30°-31.9°	≤29.9°
MEAN ARTERIAL PRESSURE — mm Hg	≥160	130-159	110-129		70-109		50-69		≤49
HEART RATE (ventricular response)	≥180	140-179	110-139		70-109		55-69	40-54	≤39
RESPIRATORY RATE — (non-ventilated or ventilated)	≥50	35-49		25-34	12-24	10-11	6-9		≤5
OXYGENATION: A-aDO₂ or PaO₂ (mm Hg) a. FIO₂ ≥0.5 record A-aDO₂	≥500	350-499	200-349		<200				
b. FIO₂ <0.5 record only PaO₂					PO₂ >70	PO₂ 61-70		PO₂ 55-60	PO₂ <55
ARTERIAL pH	≥7.7	7.6-7.69		7.5-7.59	7.33-7.49		7.25-7.32	7.15-7.24	<7.15
SERUM SODIUM (mMol/L)	≥180	160-179	155-159	150-154	130-149		120-129	111-119	≤110
SERUM POTASSIUM (mMol/L)	≥7	6-6.9		5.5-5.9	3.5-5.4	3-3.4	2.5-2.9		<2.5
SERUM CREATININE (mg/100 ml) (Double point score for acute renal failure)	≥3.5	2-3.4	1.5-1.9		0.6-1.4		<0.6		
HEMATOCRIT (%)	≥60		50-59.9	46-49.9	30-45.9		20-29.9		<20
WHITE BLOOD COUNT (total/mm3) (in 1,000s)	≥40		20-39.9	15-19.9	3-14.9		1-2.9		<1
GLASGOW COMA SCORE (GCS): Score = 15 minus actual GCS									
A Total ACUTE PHYSIOLOGY SCORE (APS): Sum of the 12 individual variable points									
Serum HCO₃ (venous-mMol/L) [Not preferred, use if no ABGs]	≥52	41-51.9		32-40.9	22-31.9		18-21.9	15-17.9	<15

B AGE POINTS:
Assign points to age as follows

AGE(yrs)	Points
≤44	0
45-54	2
55-64	3
65-74	5
≥75	6

C CHRONIC HEALTH POINTS
If the patient has a history of severe organ system insufficiency or is immuno-compromised assign points as follows:
a. for nonoperative or emergency postoperative patients — 5 points
or
b. for elective postoperative patients — 2 points

DEFINITIONS
Organ insufficiency or immuno-compromised state must have been evident prior to this hospital admission and conform to the following criteria

LIVER: Biopsy proven cirrhosis and documented portal hypertension; episodes of past upper GI bleeding attributed to portal hypertension; or prior episodes of hepatic failure/encephalopathy/coma.

CARDIOVASCULAR: New York Heart Association Class IV.
RESPIRATORY: Chronic restrictive, obstructive, or vascular disease resulting in severe exercise restriction, i.e., unable to climb stairs or perform household duties; or documented chronic hypoxia, hypercapnia, secondary polycythemia, severe pulmonary hypertension (>40mmHg), or respirator dependency.
RENAL: Receiving chronic dialysis.
IMMUNO-COMPROMISED: The patient has received therapy that suppresses resistance to infection, e.g., immuno-suppression, chemotherapy, radiation, long term or recent high dose steroids, or has a disease that is sufficiently advanced to suppress resistance to infection, e.g., leukemia, lymphoma, AIDS.

APACHE II SCORE
Sum of A + B + C

A APS points

B Age points

C Chronic Health points

Total APACHE II

FIGURE 6–1. The revised Acute Physiology and Chronic Health Evaluation (APACHE II) severity of disease classification system. (From Knaus, W. A., Draper, E. A., Wagner, D.P., et al.: APACHE II: A severity of disease classification system. Crit. Care Med., 13:818–829, 1985.)

logic insult. Simultaneously, resuscitation of the shock victim must begin immediately, to halt any ongoing deterioration of the patient's cardiopulmonary status and to restore adequate perfusion before irreversible tissue injury occurs. Technical and methodologic advances now permit rapid hemodynamic monitoring of acutely ill patients. Numerous measurements of cardiovascular and pulmonary mechanics may be used to determine the efficacy of therapy. Selection of the most appropriate monitoring depends on many factors, such as the cause and severity of the shock episode, the patient's response to initial attempts at resuscitation, and individual patient characteristics. However, there are principles and standards of monitoring common to all shock victims. Experience has demonstrated that these critically ill patients are optimally managed in an intensive care unit, where highly trained nurses and clinicians, using sophisticated monitoring equipment, can detect and respond to changes in the patient's clinical status. In addition, some standards of monitoring are used for all patients with shock, regardless of cause.

1. Vital signs: Blood pressure, pulse rate, temperature, and respiratory rate
2. Electrocardiogram
3. Urine output and specific gravity
4. Hematocrit and electrolytes
5. Arterial blood gas analysis

Aside from these standards, decisions regarding additional cardiopulmonary monitoring should be individualized to each patient.

Analysis of cardiovascular function in the critically ill patient may require the assessment of both right and left ventricular function. Monitoring of right atrial pressure or CVP is an adequate estimate of the right ventricular end-diastolic pressure in the absence of tricuspid valvular disease. The estimation of left ventricular filling pressure requires a more sophisticated approach. Swan and colleagues (1970) described the clinical application of a flow-directed balloon-tip catheter that can be placed in the pulmonary artery without aid of fluoroscopy. The measurement of pulmonary capillary wedge pressure or pulmonary artery diastolic pressure is a reliable estimate of mean left-sided filling pressures in the absence of significant preexisting pulmonary parenchymal disease (Fig. 6–3). The level of left ventricular filling pressure is a determinant of cardiac performance because it affects diastolic ventricular stress. In the absence of mitral valve stenosis, there is a close correlation between mean left ventricular diastolic pressure and the pulmonary venous and pulmonary capillary pressures. If the left ventricular filling pressure is low, cardiac output may be inadequate. Conversely, if left ventricular filling pressure is raised, pulmonary congestion and edema, increasing respiratory and cardiac work, will occur. The presence of preexisting pulmonary artery disease imposes a severe limitation on the meaningfulness of recorded pulmonary artery pressures, and

APACHE II AND HOSPITAL DEATH
Nonoperative and Postoperative Patients

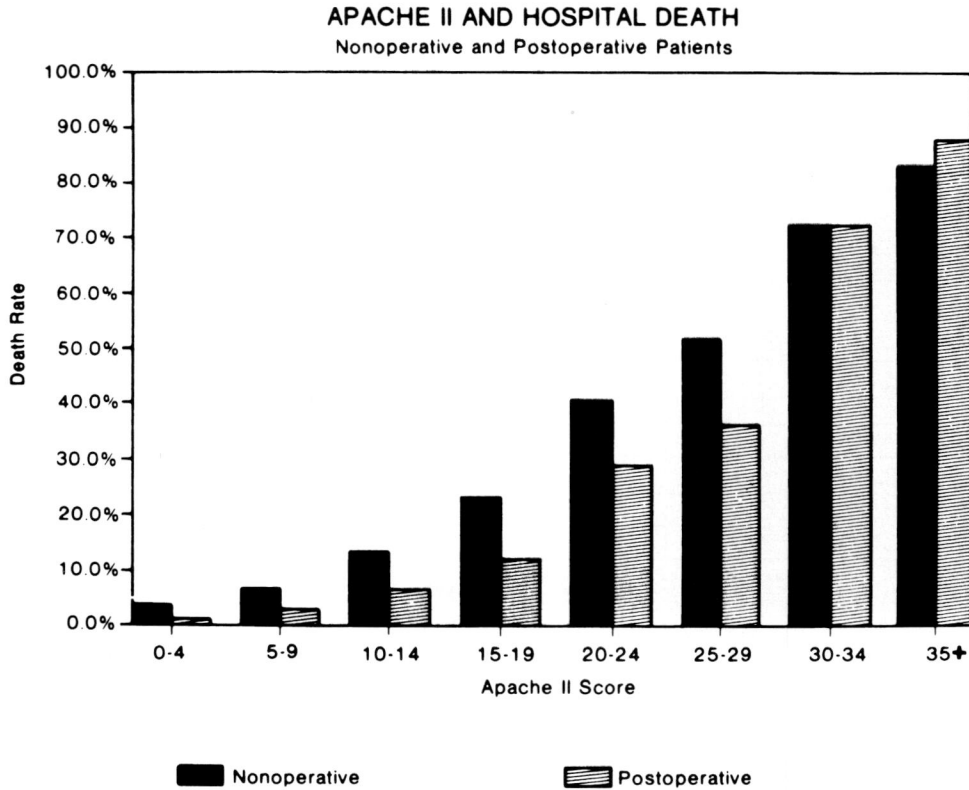

Nonoperative   **Postoperative**

FIGURE 6–2. The relationship between APACHE II scores and hospital mortality among 5815 intensive care unit (ICU) admissions for both postoperative and nonoperative patients. The data demonstrate that for each five-point increase in APACHE II score there is a significant increase in death rate. (From Knaus, W. A., Draper, E. A., Wagner, D. P., et al.: APACHE II: A severity of disease classification system. Crit. Care Med., *13*:818–829, 1985.)

occasionally a more direct assessment of ventricular function must be considered.

The measurement of CVP is an adequate system when dealing with patients who do not have evidence of left ventricular disease, but it has been observed on numerous occasions that patients with left ventricular dysfunction may have severely raised left atrial and left ventricular end-diastolic pressures in the presence of a normal or low CVP (Fig. 6–4). Therefore, the use of a pulmonary artery catheter to monitor left

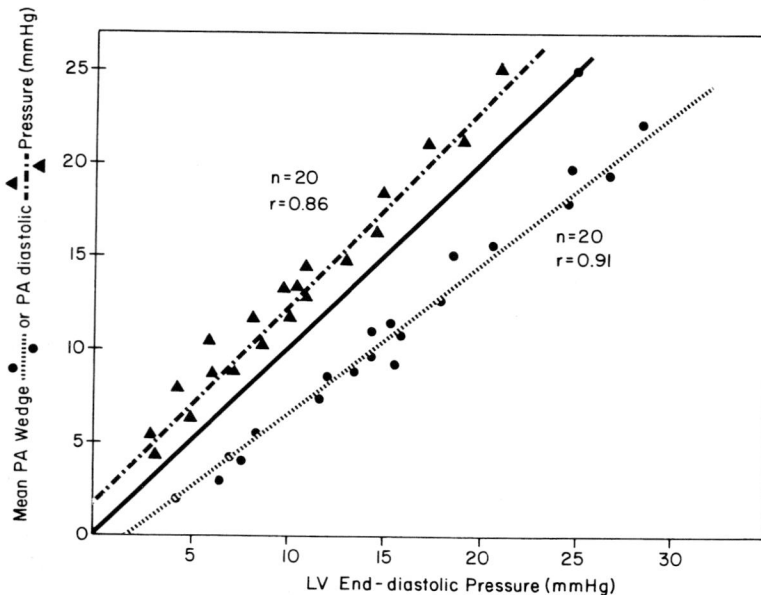

n = 20
r = 0.86

n = 20
r = 0.91

FIGURE 6–3. In 20 patients with coronary artery diseases and depressed ventricular function (ejection fraction less than 30%), good correlation was shown to exist between pulmonary capillary wedge pressure and pulmonary artery (PA) diastolic pressure and left ventricular (LV) end-diastolic pressure.

FIGURE 6–4. Thirty patients with coronary artery disease and depressed ventricular function (ejection fraction less than 30%) were studied postoperatively 4 hours after they returned to the recovery room. There was a very poor correlation in these patients between mean central venous pressure (CVP) as determined from a Swan-Ganz catheter. CVP almost invariably underestimates the left-sided filling pressure when left ventricular function is abnormal, which often causes overtransfusion and the development of pulmonary edema. PA = pulmonary artery.

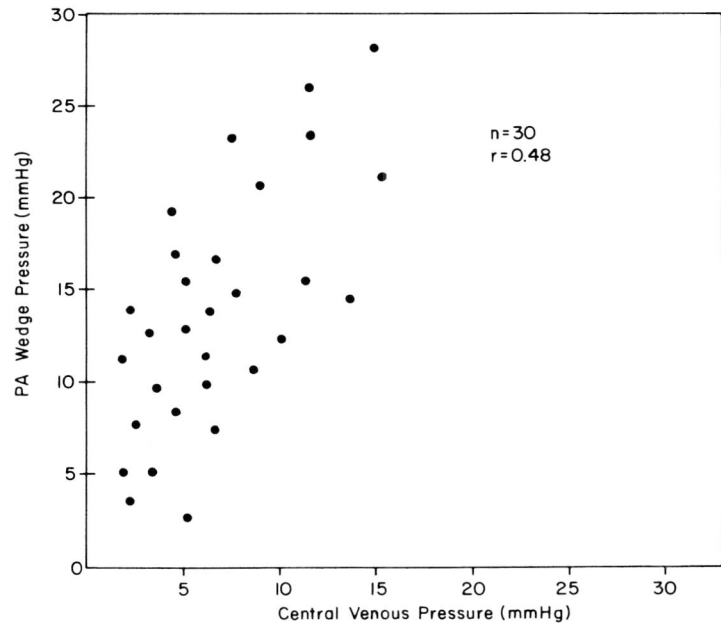

ventricular filling pressures is critical in the patient with compromised ventricular function, such as in the case of cardiogenic shock or shock of any other cause in an elderly patient with prior history of cardiac disease. In contrast, monitoring only the CVP is usually adequate in younger patients with hypovolemic shock in whom ventricular function should be normal.

Each of the various classes or causes of shock has a characteristic pattern of hemodynamic response. An additional advantage of the pulmonary artery catheter is that it permits the generation of an entire hemodynamic patient profile. Cardiac output can be determined by the thermal dilution technique, and then this value in conjunction with right and left ventricular filling pressures as well as systemic and pulmonary arterial pressures can be used to derive the patient's cardiac index, stroke volume, systemic and pulmonary vascular resistance, and ventricular stroke work. In some cases, the initial hemodynamic patient profile may be the first indication that a clinician has as to the cause or pathogenesis of the shock state. In addition, intermittent monitoring of the hemodynamic profile may be of assistance in following a patient's dynamic physiologic status and in evaluating the effectiveness of therapy.

In conjunction with the cardiac evaluation, it is necessary to assess the adequacy of tissue perfusion. A gross measure of tissue perfusion may be obtained by examining the temperature and color of the patient's extremities. Obviously, this is a very imprecise and subjective assessment. More objectively, arterial pH and serum lactate levels can be monitored, although these measures lack sensitivity and are only abnormal in more profound shock states. Careful monitoring of urine output, by indwelling catheter, is the most effective noninvasive method of evaluating tissue perfusion, providing an excellent overall guide

to the adequacy of circulation at the organ level. Both the volume and the specific gravity of the urine should be recorded frequently; further, the osmolarity and sodium and potassium concentration of the urine should be intermittently evaluated. Fixed osmolarity and an elevated urine sodium concentration suggest intrinsic renal injury associated with acute tubular necrosis from hypotension.

In contrast, a rising osmolarity and normal or low urine concentration of sodium in the presence of decreasing urine volume suggests decreased renal blood flow, usually secondary to a falling cardiac output.

The adequacy of tissue perfusion may also be evaluated by monitoring oxygen transport balance. This is an analytic method of comparing oxygen supply or delivery with oxygen demand or consumption. From the cardiac output, hemoglobin concentration, and arterial and venous blood gas analysis, it is possible to calculate the $A-V_{O_2}$, peripheral oxygen consumption, oxygen delivery, and oxygen utilization coefficient (Table 6–1). The $A-V_{O_2}$ defines the balance between oxygen consumption and cardiac output. An increase in the $A-V_{O_2}$ indicates that either blood flow and oxygen delivery are too low or oxygen consumption is too high. In critically ill patients, intermittent monitoring of these oxygen transport parameters detects imbalances in tissue perfusion, as manifested by imbalances in oxygen consumption versus oxygen delivery, long before clinical signs of shock or lactic acidosis develop. Normalization of oxygen supply and demand can also serve as a guide to adequate resuscitation of the shock victim.

One of the newer technologic advances in monitoring critically ill patients is the incorporation of fiberoptics into the pulmonary artery catheter, which allows continuous measurement of mixed venous oxygen saturation. The mixed venous oxygen saturation is a function of the cardiac output, arterial oxygen

■ **Table 6–1.** NORMAL RANGE, UNITS, AND DERIVATION FOR COMMON OXYGEN TRANSPORT TERMS*

Parameter	Normal Range	Units	Derivation
$C_{A_{O_2}}$	16–22	ml/dl	$(S_{A_{O_2}} \times Hgb \times 1.38) + P_{A_{O_2}} \times 0.0031$
$C_{V_{O_2}}$	12–17	ml/dl	$(S_{V_{O_2}} \times Hgb \times 1.38) + P_{V_{O_2}} \times 0.0031$
A-V_{O_2}	3.5–5.5	ml/dl	$C_{A_{O_2}} - C_{V_{O_2}}$
$\dot{V}_{O_2}$	180–280	ml/min	A-V_{O_2} $\times$ CO $\times$ 10
D_{O_2}	700–1400	ml/min	$C_{A_{O_2}} \times$ CO $\times$ 10
OUC	0.23–0.32	(fraction)	$\dot{V}_{O_2}/D_{O_2}$
$S_{V_{O_2}}$	0.68–0.77	(fraction)	Measured

*Normal ranges are approximate and may vary between laboratories. $C_{A_{O_2}}$ = arterial oxygen content; $S_{A_{O_2}}$ = arterial oxygen saturation; $P_{A_{O_2}}$ = arterial oxygen pressure; Hgb = hemoglobin; $S_{V_{O_2}}$ = mixed venous oxygen saturation; $C_{V_{O_2}}$ = mixed venous oxygen content; A-V_{O_2} = arterial-venous oxygen content difference; $\dot{V}_{O_2}$ = oxygen consumption; D_{O_2} = oxygen delivery; OUC = oxygen utilization coefficient (extraction ratio).

saturation, hemoglobin concentration, and oxygen consumption. Values within the normal range (0.68 to 0.77) suggest a balance between oxygen delivery and oxygen consumption, whereas an abrupt decrease in mixed venous oxygen saturation to below 0.65 indicates an oxygen transport imbalance secondary to a decrease in cardiac output, hemoglobin, or arterial oxygen saturation or an increase in oxygen consumption. Continuous measurement of mixed venous oxygen saturation may be a guide to resuscitation and the effectiveness of therapy of benefit in treating patients with shock. Additionally, continuous monitoring of mixed venous oxygen saturation provides an early warning system, alerting the clinician to untoward changes in the patient's hemodynamic status.

Siegel and Cerra and their associates revolutionized the monitoring of hemodynamic and metabolic data from critically ill patients by establishing a computerized database of measurements collected from patients in their intensive care units (Cerra et al., 1979b; Siegel et al., 1971). They have clearly shown the value of classifying the physiologic response to stress on the basis of multiple hemodynamic and metabolic variables. By following these variables over time, the physician can characterize a multidimensional trajectory of each patient's physiologic response to disease or trauma. The response can be quantified precisely and compared by statistical methods with well-characterized patterns of response to stress.

Arterial and central venous catheterization is necessary to monitor the variables that have been analyzed by Siegel's group. Those hemodynamic variables measured or calculated include cardiac index, right atrial pressure, ventricular ejection time, and total PVR. From the analysis of the cardiac output indicator dilution curves, a pulmonary dispersive volume (which correlates with pulmonary blood volume) and a cardiac mixing time (which correlates with ejection fraction) can be determined. These hemodynamic variables are used to characterize the determinants of cardiovascular performance: preload, afterload, and cardiac contractility. Venous and arterial blood gases are used to characterize the metabolic response to injury and disease. From blood-gas determinations, A-V_{O_2} and also an oxygen consumption index (the product of cardiac index and A-V_{O_2}) can be calculated.

Siegel's group compared the data that they col-

lected from critically ill patients with data that were previously collected from a group of nonstressed, preoperative general surgery patients who had fasted overnight. These patients constitute a reference (R) or control group. Each variable that is collected from critically ill patients is normalized in units of standard deviations from its mean value in the R group.

The data from patients with various diseases and trauma have been segregated to describe four patterns of response of stress: A, B, C, and D (Fig. 6–5). The A state represents a well-balanced and compensated response to stress. This response is characterized by a hyperdynamic cardiovascular response with increases in heart rate, cardiac output, and cardiac contractility. Pulmonary transit time, cardiac mixing time, and ventricular ejection time are all reduced. Arterial pressure is normal or increased, which indicates that there is an appropriate relationship between cardiac output and PVR. In the A state, the A-V_{O_2} difference is normal or slightly increased. The D state, at the opposite extreme of the physiologic spectrum, represents a response in which cardiac function is compromised. Cardiac output is low; PVR is high. The A-V_{O_2} difference is usually increased to compensate for deficits in blood flow, but oxygen consumption is reduced on the basis of poor perfusion.

The B state represents a state of unbalanced vascular tone, which is characterized by large increases in cardiac output and reductions in PVR. The reduction in resistance is disproportionate to the increase in flow and produces hypotension. Failure of the peripheral tissues to fully desaturate hemoglobin produces an inappropriately narrow A-V_{O_2} and an absolute reduction in oxygen consumption despite high flows. Some degree of metabolic acidosis is usually present. The B state is characteristic of patients with a high-output response to sepsis and of patients with multiple organ failure. Mortality is high if the metabolic derangements cannot be reversed. The C state is characterized by respiratory failure superimposed on the B state. The respiratory dysfunction usually cannot be corrected with ventilatory support. Profound metabolic and respiratory acidosis combined with intractable hypotension almost inevitably results in death.

If the appropriate hemodynamic and metabolic variables are followed in an individual patient, the data can be compared statistically with the mean data characterizing the five prototype states (R, A, B, C,

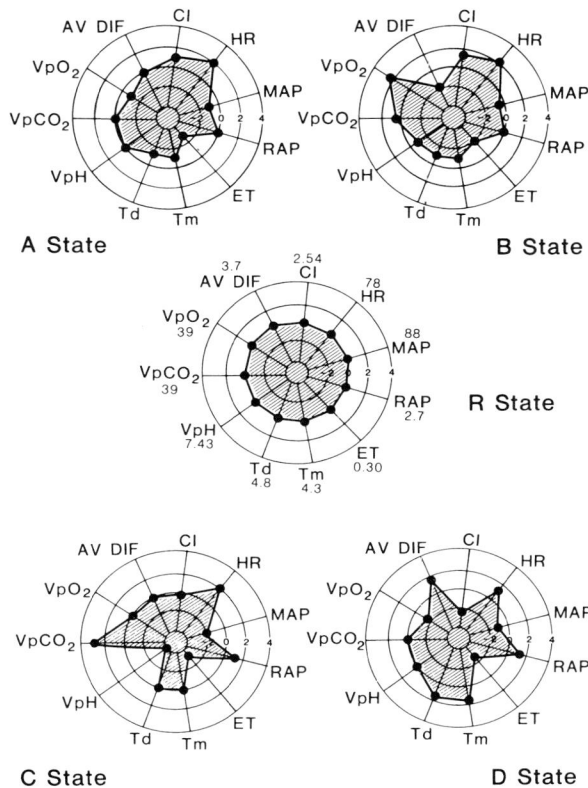

FIGURE 6–5. Physiologic patterns of response to stress: Siegel's patients have been segregated into five groups by statistical clustering techniques. The mean values of each physiologic parameter in the R state are shown in the central polar plot. In the four corners of the figure are the polar plots of the means of the parameters in states A, B, C, and D. For the purpose of these plots, each parameter has been normalized in terms of standard deviations from its mean value in the R state. CI = cardiac index (l/min/m²); HR = heart rate (beats per minute); MAP = mean arterial pressure (mm Hg); RAP = right atrial pressure (mm Hg); ET = cardiac ejection time (sec); Tm = cardiac mixing time (sec); Td = pulmonary dispersion time (sec); VpH = venous pH; VpCO₂ = venous carbon dioxide tension (mm Hg); VpO₂ = venous oxygen tension (mm Hg); AV DIF = A - VO₂ difference (volumes per cent).

and D). A patient's similarity or dissimilarity to each state can be measured in terms of a euclidian distance in multidimensions from each of these states. The existing physiologic state of the patient can then be characterized in terms of the prototype state to which the patient has the most resemblance at that moment. This pathophysiologic classification of acutely ill patients provides a useful method of monitoring their clinical course and the efficacy of types of therapy. The multivariate mapping of the patient's physiologic state increases the discriminatory power of analysis. Specific combinations of abnormalities (e.g., high cardiac output and narrow A-VO₂ in the B state) often signal early progression of pathophysiology that cannot be characterized by monitoring any one variable alone. By describing the patient's response to illness with comparisons to the five prototypic physiologic states, the clinician can monitor the patient's progress in much the same way an experienced navigator charts the course of a craft by distance from known beacons and potentially dangerous landmarks.

MULTIPLE ORGAN FAILURE

The syndrome of multiple organ failure was first observed by Tilney and co-workers (1973) in patients recovering from hemorrhagic shock after rupture of an abdominal aortic aneurysm. Since then it has become apparent that multiple organ failure may develop following all forms of shock, trauma, burns, pancreatitis, as well as infection. Regardless of the cause, the syndrome of multiple organ failure usually follows a predictable course. The organs that fail often are not directly involved in the primary disease process, and there is often a lag of several days between the initial inciting event and the development of distant organ failure. Characteristically, the organ dysfunction first becomes manifest in the lungs, and is then followed by hepatic, intestinal, and renal failure. The onset of central nervous system dysfunction, which can range from mild confusion to coma, may occur either early or late in the course of multiple organ failure, whereas hematologic and myocardial failure usually occur later. This characteristic sequential pattern of organ failure may be altered by the presence of preexisting organ dysfunction. For example, patients with underlying renal insufficiency are more likely to develop renal failure earlier in the course of multiple organ failure.

Despite intense clinical interest in the syndrome of multiple organ failure, the mortality ranges from 30 to 100%, depending on the number of organs involved, and has not significantly improved since the mid-1970s. The treatment remains essentially supportive because the precise cause and pathogenesis of multiple organ failure are not well understood. It has been hypothesized that the translocation of bacteria or endotoxin across the bowel wall into the portal circulation is critical to the pathogenesis of multiple organ failure. The translocation of bacteria induces organ dysfunction either by direct endotoxin injury to cells, such as hepatocytes, or by the activation of regulatory cells, which then secrete inflammatory mediators leading to tissue damage. The progressive atrophy of the intestinal mucosa with malnutrition and the overgrowth of aerobic gram-negative bacteria within the intestine from the use of antibiotics predispose the patient recovering from shock to bacterial translocation. It has also been proposed that excessive or prolonged stimulation of macrophages leading to uncontrolled cytokine secretion is critical in the pathogenesis of multiple organ failure. This hypothesis stems from the finding that the organs frequently involved in multiple organ failure syndrome contain large numbers of resident macrophages: Kupffer's cells within the liver, astrocytes within the central nervous system, mesangial cells in the kidney, and alveolar macrophages. Data from co-culture systems indicate that primary regulation of hepatocyte function and injury is mediated by the Kupffer cell. Cell-to-cell peptide mediators may be involved. West and associates (1985) and Keller and colleagues (1985) observed that hypoxemia presensitizes the Kupffer cell so that when endotoxin is then added, a severe reduction in hepatic protein synthesis is observed. This experimental observation correlates with the clinical observation that a perfusion deficit followed by an infection is a common clinical pathway that leads to the multiple organ failure syndrome. Macrophage modulation of muscle *adenosine triphosphate* (ATP) production under conditions of inflammation is another example of a paired cell-mediated change in metabolism as reported by Morris and co-workers (1985).

In most clinical series of patients with the multiple organ failure syndrome, the lung is the first organ to fail, which might suggest that the failure of this particular organ is important to the subsequent failure of other organs. However, hypoxia from respiratory failure usually does not cause further organ damage because adequate arterial oxygenation can usually be maintained with mechanical ventilation. Intense interstitial and intra-alveolar macrophage and neutrophil infiltration is seen characteristically in patients with respiratory dysfunction. The damaged lung may therefore act as a source of inflammatory mediators, which in turn causes distant organ damage. Richardson and associates (1982) noted that nosocomial pneumonia of various degrees is also evident in more than 50% of patients with *adult respiratory distress syndrome* (ARDS) and adds another source of bacteria and endotoxin for perpetuation of the systemic inflammatory response. The affected lungs may also fail metabolically and cause impaired clearance of vasodilator prostanoids and bradykinin and failed production of angiotensin II. More than 75% of patients dying of ARDS now die of multiple organ failure and systemic hemodynamic instability rather than of impaired gas exchange, according to Montgomery and colleagues (1985).

Progressive failure of liver function is also a critical factor in this syndrome. Initially, increased metabolic activity is necessary in the liver to clear the amino acid load that is generated by peripheral tissues and to increase glucose and acute-phase protein synthesis. Ultimately, there is progressive synthetic, metabolic, and phagocytic dysfunction. With metabolic failure, the liver can no longer balance the interorgan flow of substrate, and the plasma levels of glucose, triglyceride, lactate, ketones, and amino acids dramatically increase. Jones (1984) showed that hepatic secretion of IgA bile salts reduces the proliferation of gut bacteria and inhibits endotoxin detoxification. The hepatic reticuloendothelial system is important for protection of the lung and other organs from the bacteria and microemboli generated from a septic focus. Kupffer's cells, which constitute 70% of the total body macrophage content, are activated by inflammatory stimuli, bacteria, and endotoxin. They produce cytokines and other mediators that can have both local and systemic effects.

Renal dysfunction often follows lung and liver failure, even if volume loading and inotropic support have been initiated at an early stage. Lucas (1976) proposed that inadequate maintenance of perfusion pressure during the hyperdynamic state and redistri-

bution of blood flow away from the renal cortex are the mechanisms by which the kidney fails. The hepatorenal syndrome is another mechanism by which the kidney can be damaged. This phenomenon is still not well understood, but it may be caused by redistribution of intrarenal blood flow.

HYPOVOLEMIC SHOCK

Hypovolemia is the most common cause for shock in surgical patients. Hypovolemic shock results whenever blood, plasma, water, or a combination of body fluids is lost in sufficient degree to cause cardiovascular compromise. The exact intravascular volume deficit at which shock ensues depends on the rate, quantity, and nature of the fluid loss. Additionally, individual patient characteristics, such as age and the presence of preexisting cardiovascular disease, greatly influence the patient's ability to tolerate an episode of hypovolemia. Most patients with hypovolemic shock that the surgeon will care for are trauma victims. In these patients, the source of shock may be obvious, as with external hemorrhage. However, in some trauma patients, hypovolemic shock may result from occult fluid losses—for example, the blood and plasma sequestered into the tissue surrounding a fracture or the fluid lost by evaporation from a burn wound. Furthermore, these patients frequently have multiple injuries and their state of shock may be the result of numerous factors such as hemorrhage, tissue destruction, and intestinal perforation. Also, in some circumstances, the surgeon may encounter a patient in hypovolemic shock unrelated to trauma. Whether the hypovolemia is secondary to gastrointestinal hemorrhage, pancreatitis, or intestinal obstruction, the neurohumoral response to hypovolemic shock in these settings is essentially the same as that observed in trauma victims. Therefore, the initial management of the patient in hypovolemic shock is generally the same, regardless of the cause of the shock state.

The clinical signs and symptoms of hypovolemic shock reflect the severity of the intravascular volume deficit. Generally, a loss of 20% or less of the circulating blood volume is tolerated well by most patients and produces few symptoms (Table 6–2). As the circulating blood volume is reduced further, a graded increase in heart rate and decrease in blood pressure result. The arterial systolic, diastolic, and pulse pressure diminish and the pulse becomes thready and weak. Correspondingly, the patient exhibits changes in mental status, progressing from apprehension and anxiety to apathy and eventually to obtundation and coma. Cutaneous veins collapse and the skin appears pale, moist, and slightly cyanotic. Initially, the respiratory rate is rapid, but as the patient's mental status deteriorates, respirations slow and may become shallow or deep. The loss of intravascular volume eventually produces a characteristic hemodynamic profile of decreased right-sided and left-sided cardiac filling pressures, decreased cardiac output, increased sys-

■ **Table 6–2.** CLINICAL SIGNS AND SYMPTOMS OF HEMORRHAGIC SHOCK BASED ON THE SEVERITY OF BLOOD LOSS

Percent Loss of Circulating Blood Volume (For 70-kg man)	Pulse Rate	Systolic Blood Pressure	Pulse Pressure	Capillary Refill	Respirations	Central Nervous System	Urine Output
<15% (<750 ml)	<100	Normal	Normal	Normal	Normal	Normal	Normal
15–30% (750–1500 ml)	>100	Normal	Decreased (↑ diastolic blood pressure)	Delayed	Mild tachypnea	Anxious	20–30 ml/hr
30–40% (1500–2000 ml)	>120 Weak	Decreased	Decreased	Delayed	Marked tachypnea	Confused	<20 ml/hr
>40% (>2000 ml)	>140 Nonpalpable	Marked decrease	Marked decrease	Absent	Marked tachypnea	Lethargic	Negligible

temic vascular resistance, and decreased venous oxygen saturation.

The natural history of hypovolemic shock can be divided into three phases. Phase I begins with the onset of volume loss and ends when this loss has been contained. Phase II begins when the plasma volume has been restored to normal and the resulting perfusion deficit has been corrected. During Phase II, fluid is sequestered into the extracellular space; this phase ends when, as a result of this sequestration, the patient's weight gain is maximal. Fluid is translocated from the plasma volume into both the intracellular space and the interstitial fluid space. The duration and extent of this translocation depends on the volume loss incurred during Phase I. For example, in a patient who has been transfused with 10 to 20 units of blood during Phase I, Phase II will last an average of 24 to 36 hours, and the total body weight gain will be 10 to 15 kg. During Phase III, the plasma volume increases despite a reduction in the rate of fluid infused. Fluid is transfused into the plasma volume space from intracellular and interstitial fluid spaces. During this period, patients show a spontaneous diuresis and an improvement in oxygenation. If, during the initial phases of hypovolemic shock, fluid resuscitation has been incomplete and persistent regional perfusion deficits have permitted tissue devitalization or infection, the onset of Phase III, which heralds recovery, may be delayed indefinitely. In this case, multiple organ dysfunction becomes the basis of a prolonged critical illness.

Experimentation in humans and animals has defined the neurohumoral and cellular response to hypovolemia and, in particular, hemorrhagic shock. In response to a greater than 15% loss in circulating blood volume, certain homeostatic mechanisms are evoked, including baroreceptor reflexes, chemoreceptor reflexes, cerebral ischemic responses, reabsorption of tissue fluid, release of endogenous vasoconstrictor substances, and renal conservation of salt and water. The baroreceptor reflex, which is initiated at onset of hypovolemia, attempts to minimize the fall in arterial blood pressure (Fig. 6–6). Reductions in mean arterial pressure and pulse pressure during hypovolemia are detected by baroreceptors in the aortic arch and ca-

rotid sinus. In response to the decrease in blood pressure, the baroreceptors transmit less afferent stimuli to the vasomotor center in the medulla, which in turn enhances sympathetic neural output. The increase in sympathetic tone stimulates constriction of arterioles and capacitance veins, which in turn enhances systemic vascular resistance and venous blood return to the heart. The increased sympathetic discharge also produces an autotransfusion of blood into the circulation. In humans, the cutaneous, pulmonary, and hepatic vasculature are the principal reservoirs that provide this autotransfusion, whereas in dogs, blood is mobilized primarily by contraction of the spleen. In conjunction with the increase in sympathetic output, norepinephrine and epinephrine are released from adrenal medulla, producing tachycardia and a positive inotropic effect on atrial and ventricular myocardium. Therefore, the baroreceptor reflex, through generalized arteriolar vasoconstriction, increased venous blood return, and enhanced myocardial contractility, restores arterial blood pressure during hypovolemia. The baroreceptor response also redistributes blood flow. The arteriolar vasoconstriction is most intense in cutaneous, skeletal muscle, renal, and splanchnic vascular beds and is negligible or absent in the cerebral and coronary circulations. This nonuniform vasoconstrictor response is protective for the heart and brain, allowing these organs to receive a larger percentage of the available cardiac output and permitting them to continue to function during states of shock.

As hypovolemia and shock progress, peripheral chemoreceptors and cerebral ischemic responses are stimulated, further enhancing sympathetic neural output. With profound hypovolemia or hemorrhage, inadequate blood flow produces localized anoxia and chemoreceptor excitation. By further increasing sympathetic tone, chemoreceptor excitation augments the peripheral vasoconstrictor response initiated by the baroreceptor reflex. Maximal sympathetic discharge occurs in response to cerebral ischemia. When arterial blood pressure falls below 50 mm Hg, cerebral blood flow is diminished and the cerebral ischemic response is initiated. Cerebral ischemia maximally stimulates sympathetic output, causing even more intense vasoconstriction and myocardial contractility.

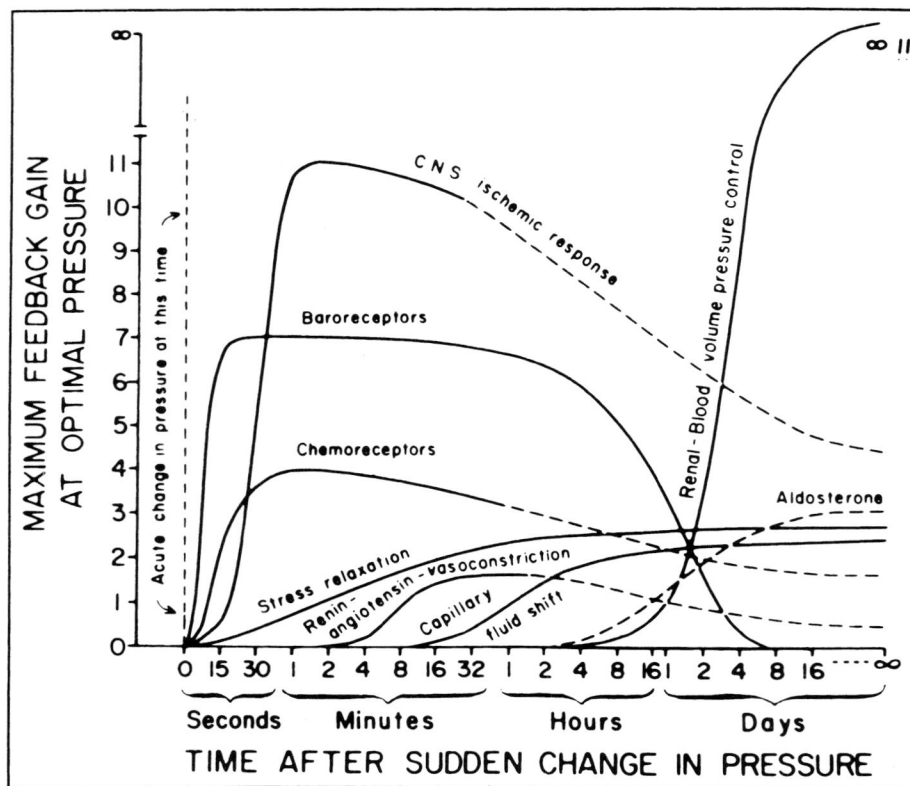

FIGURE 6–6. Neurohumoral responses to hypotension. The potency of various arterial pressure homeostatic mechanisms at different time intervals after the onset of hypotension is shown. Note the potential for infinite gain in the renal-body fluid pressure control mechanism that occurs after 2 days. CNS = central nervous system. (From Guyton, A. C.: Arterial Pressure and Hypertension. Philadelphia, W. B. Saunders, 1980.)

Hypovolemia and hemorrhage also initiate an array of humoral responses with increases in the plasma levels of ACTH, cortisol, glucagon, growth hormone, and catecholamines. The same stimuli that enhance sympathetic output induce the release of catecholamines from the adrenal medulla, which then reinforce the effects of the sympathetic nervous system. In response to hypovolemia, receptors in the left atrium and the carotid-aortic baroreceptors stimulate the posterior pituitary to release *antidiuretic hormone* (ADH). ADH induces vasoconstriction, particularly in the splanchnic circulation, and increases the reabsorption of water in the distal tubule of the kidney. Hypoperfusion of the juxtaglomerular apparatus of the kidney causes the secretion of renin and the formation of angiotensin. Angiotensin induces vasoconstriction as well as accelerates the release of aldosterone from the adrenal cortex, which in turn then stimulates the reabsorption of sodium in the renal tubules. Growth hormone promotes gluconeogenesis and lipolysis, and glucagon similarly opposes the effects of insulin by promoting gluconeogenesis, lipolysis, and glycogenolysis. The catecholamines epinephrine and norepinephrine also contribute to hyperglycemia by promoting gluconeogenesis and glycogenolysis and by inhibiting the release of insulin. Thus, glucagon, growth hormone, and catecholamines all combine to increase blood glucose and osmolarity, which promote the movement of fluid into the vascular bed and assist in maintaining intravascular volume. Therefore, the sympathetic cardiovascular response to hypovolemic shock is augmented by the stimulation of multiple endocrine pathways, all with the common end results of vasoconstriction, the conservation of water and electrolytes, and the ongoing supply of nutrients for the metabolic requirements of the heart and brain.

Further protection from an intravascular volume deficit involves the autoregulation of microcirculatory blood flow. In response to decreased mean arterial pressure, there is sympathetic mediated vasoconstriction of larger arterioles (90 to 150 μm in diameter) and reflex dilatation of smaller (20 to 50 μm) arterioles. This gradient in resistance from large to small arterioles produces lower capillary hydrostatic pressure and the net reabsorption of interstitial fluid into the vascular compartment. In conjunction with the fluid shift induced by hyperglycemia and increased osmolarity, autoregulation of capillary blood flow restores intravascular blood volume. The studies of human volunteers by Lister and co-workers (1963) and Moore and associates (1966) documented the importance of transcapillary refilling in the restoration of blood volume. Plasma refilling begins minutes after a 20% reduction in blood volume and proceeds at rates of 50 to 90 ml/hr during the first 2 hours. Total restoration of blood volume is accomplished in approximately 36 hours. Although transcapillary refilling restores total blood volume, plasma protein levels decrease, and thus the forces that maintain intravascular volume are reduced in accordance with Starling's law. The proteins within the interstitial fluid space are mobile and can be transported with extracellular fluid into the intravascular space via the lymphatic system. During hypovolemia, there is a flux of proteins out of the interstitial space as peptidoglycans in the interstitium alter their conformation, causing proteins to be excluded. Complete restoration of plasma proteins by synthesis and release from the liver is a more gradual process that occurs after the patient has recovered from shock.

Transcapillary refilling and the restoration of blood volume does not account for all of the reduction in the extracellular fluid volume observed during hypovolemic shock. Shires and co-workers (1973), using a triple isotope technique, demonstrated in a model of hemorrhagic shock that an extracellular fluid deficit persists even after all of the shed blood is returned. In further studies, these investigators demonstrated that the extracellular volume deficit was secondary to the uptake of interstitial fluid by injured cells. Thus, besides the neurohumoral and microcirculatory responses to hypovolemic shock, there are also well-defined alterations in cell structure and function. Much of the experimental work describing the cellular response to hypovolemic shock has used skeletal muscle, which accounts for 50% of the total body mass. In models of acute hemorrhagic shock, there is a progressive fall in skeletal muscle transmembrane potential. This alteration in membrane stability permits the influx of sodium, calcium, chloride, and water into the cell, causing isotonic cell swelling and mitochondrial dysfunction. The mechanism by which hypovolemic shock induces cell membrane instability is not known, although it has been suggested that it may be secondary to depletion of cellular ATP or hypoxia-induced dysfunction of the sodium-potassium exchange pump. More important, it has been demonstrated that these shock-induced alterations in cell function can be reversed by adequate volume resuscitation. Prompt and appropriate nonsanguinous volume resuscitation restores cell membrane integrity, allowing the water and electrolyte fluxes to return to normal.

In hypovolemic shock, the primary defect is a reduction in intravascular volume. Secondary physiologic alterations traceable to this low intravascular volume include reduced cardiac output, arterial pressure, CVP, left atrial pressure, and stroke index. In addition, there are increases in heart rate, PVR, and A-VO_2 difference. Protective vasoconstrictive reflexes that occur in the face of decreasing cardiac output due to hypovolemia maintain arterial blood pressure and perfusion of the heart and brain and play a vital protective role in the immediate response to hemorrhage. However, if blood loss continues, the compensatory mechanisms will be exceeded, and blood flow to the heart and brain will decrease. At this point, the patient loses consciousness and develops a profound metabolic acidosis, as blood flow to the liver falls below a critical level and lactic acid is no longer metabolized. A blood volume of 50% of normal cannot be tolerated for a long time, and even if hemorrhage is controlled, this degree of volume deficit will overwhelm the compensatory mechanisms. When this occurs, central aortic pressure falls below the level at which coronary perfusion can be maintained, and cardiac output decreases, causing a further fall in central aortic pressure. At this point, a vicious circle is initiated, with decreasing cardiac output producing a fall in coronary perfusion, and death rapidly ensues.

Treatment of Hypovolemic Shock

Many different clinical situations may lead to a deficit in intravascular volume and the development of hypovolemic shock. Intravascular volume depletion may result from a loss of whole blood, as seen with postoperative hemorrhage, gastrointestinal bleeding, and trauma. Burns, pancreatitis, and peritonitis may cause a significant loss of plasma and the depletion of intravascular volume. A total body water deficit leading to intravascular volume depletion may result from dehydration, loss of renal concentrating ability, and abnormal enteric losses such as vomiting, diarrhea, or a fistula. Despite their diverse causes, the therapeutic approach to these conditions is similar and relies on the replacement of the volume loss, control of the process that has produced the volume loss, and correction of any secondary or complicating events.

The hemodynamic and biochemical changes that occur after acute blood loss are determined by the rate, quantity, and duration of blood loss. Beecher (1952) emphasized that the loss of 50% of the blood volume in a young, healthy individual causes severe circulatory failure and the clinical manifestations of profound shock. With rapid blood loss, such as that observed with a ruptured abdominal aortic aneurysm, acute coronary insufficiency and myocardial failure occur early. In contrast, with gradual blood loss, compensatory reexpansion of the intravascular space by transcapillary refilling may prevent circulatory failure, and the only manifestation of blood loss will be a decrease in red blood cell mass, detected by a low hemoglobin or hematocrit value. The presence of an extracellular volume deficit from some dehydrating process reduces the tolerance for blood loss, so even a small hemorrhage may precipitate circulatory collapse. This occurs commonly in patients with prolonged illness requiring intravenous fluid replacement or in cardiac patients receiving chronic diuretic therapy. Furthermore, preexisting organ dysfunction complicates even minimal intravascular volume deficits, making them more refractory to appropriate therapy. An antecedent history of coronary atherosclerosis, chronic obstructive pulmonary disease, cirrhosis, or chronic renal insufficiency diminishes a patient's probability of recovery from an episode of hypovolemic shock.

The initial management of the patient in shock, regardless of the cause, must include an assessment of the patient's ventilatory status. It is optimal for the clinician to use an aggressive approach in the management of the patient's airway and breathing. Virtually all patients with severe shock and impending circulatory collapse require tracheal intubation and mechanical ventilatory support, even though acute respiratory failure may not yet have occurred. In patients with less severe episodes of shock, and especially in those who improve with initial resuscitation, decisions regarding mechanical ventilation should be based on the evaluation of the patient's gas exchange, work of breathing, and ability to maintain a patent airway. Important clinical signs that ventilatory support is necessary include severe tachypnea or bradypnea, use of accessory muscles, mental obtundation, and cyanosis. Auscultation of the chest may reveal rales, wheezing, or poor inspiratory air movement. Finally, arterial blood-gas analysis may reveal hypoxemia or inadequate respiratory compensation for a metabolic acidosis. The presence of any of these clinical signs, especially in combination with abnormal arterial blood-gas results, requires immediate consideration for intubation and ventilatory support. In the presence of shock, it is often necessary to reach a decision regarding intubation and mechanical ventilation even before the cause of the respiratory compromise is determined.

Additional therapeutic maneuvers used early in the management of hypovolemic shock include the Trendelenburg position and *military antishock trousers* (MAST). Theoretically, placing a patient in the headdown position should increase central blood volume, augmenting cardiac filling and stroke volume. However, recent studies of the Trendelenburg position have failed to demonstrate any significant effect on venous return or systemic vascular resistance in hypotensive patients. In fact, it has been suggested that the Trendelenburg position may actually be detrimental to the patient by compromising cerebral perfusion and pulmonary function. For these reasons, the Trendelenburg position should not be considered one of the standard initial therapeutic maneuvers for shock. There is also controversy surrounding the use of the MAST suit for shock. Initially, it was believed that the MAST suit augmented arterial blood pressure by returning blood from the periphery to the central circulation, in effect creating an autotransfusion. However, it is now known that the MAST suit enhances blood pressure primarily by increasing systemic vascular resistance and decreasing peripheral perfusion. In essence, the MAST suit further potentiates the neural and humeral redistribution of blood flow, increasing the possibility of ischemic injury in the cutaneous, skeletal muscle, renal, and splanchnic vascular beds. Even more important, use of the MAST suit has not enhanced survival in patients with shock, and numerous complications have been reported related to its improper use. Therefore, despite its positive effect on arterial blood pressure, equally important theoretical and practical disadvantages preclude the use of the MAST suit in the hospital care of the shock victim.

After adequate ventilation is assured, a quick assessment of the patient's circulatory status must be performed and then initial attempts at resuscitation instituted. At this point, the clinician must decide on the rate and volume of fluid replacement as well as the choice of fluid. Decisions regarding fluid resuscitation are based on the cause and severity of the shock episode, and also on the repeated monitoring of clinical, hemodynamic, and biochemical responses to resuscitation. The basic guide to fluid therapy in shock is the concept of titration according to the results of repeated clinical observations and hemodynamic measurements.

The clinician who treats shock, regardless of its origin, must be assured that cardiac filling pressures are adequate to produce an effective cardiac output and adequate peripheral circulation. In younger patients with hypovolemic shock, in whom left ventricular dysfunction is not suspected, CVP is an adequate indicator of circulatory status. CVP represents the filling pressure of the right ventricle and depends on the interrelationship of blood volume, venous tone, and right ventricular compliance. CVP should not be considered a static measurement, but should be evaluated in response to fluid challenges as an aid in assessing the patient's volume needs from a dynamic standpoint. CVP that rises in response to the 200-ml infusion of fluid suggests an adequate intravascular blood volume. In contrast, CVP that does not change with the rapid infusion of fluid suggests hypovolemia. In severe shock, such as in the patient with hypotension associated with hemorrhage and multiple injuries, a more aggressive approach to fluid resuscitation is indicated. In this situation, large volumes of fluid, 10 to 20 ml/kg, may be rapidly infused without the need for CVP monitoring. However, the response of the cardiac output and the cardiac filling pressures to a fluid challenge is the single most important measurement that can be made in a patient with hypovolemic shock. Arbitrary rules and flow diagrams guiding fluid replacement have limited utility, since the response to shock is dynamic, with changing venous capacitance, arterial vascular resistance, and myocardial contractility. For this reason, the routine monitoring of CVP as a guide to fluid resuscitation in hypovolemic shock is warranted. When the patient does not respond favorably to volume replacement as guided by the CVP measurement, a more direct measurement of left ventricular filling should be determined before additional fluid challenges are attempted. Similarly, in the elderly patient with hypovolemic shock, and in those patients in whom left ventricular dysfunction is suspected, monitoring the CVP is inadequate to evaluate the patient's volume status and response to fluid challenges. In these cases, the adequacy of left ventricular filling is best determined by measuring the filling pressure of the left side of the heart with a pulmonary artery catheter. Even with the use of a pulmonary artery catheter, the principles of fluid therapy in shock remain the same, with the titration of fluid volume according to the results of repeated clinical observations and hemodynamic measurements.

With the aforementioned guidelines to fluid replacement, the next question that must be addressed involves the selection of physiologic criteria to evaluate the adequacy or end-point of fluid resuscitation.

The conventionally accepted approach has been to administer fluid until the heart rate, blood pressure, urine output, and CVP have normalized. Blood pressure alone is an inadequate guide to resuscitation, since the homeostatic mechanisms previously described maintain systemic arterial blood pressure within the normal range, even when the circulating intravascular blood volume is reduced by 20 to 30%. Restoration of adequate tissue perfusion as evidenced by normal organ function is a more appropriate endpoint for volume resuscitation. Thus, a urine output of 0.5 to 1.0 ml/kg/hr, a normal heart rate, adequate capillary refill, and normal sensorium are all better indicators than blood pressure of adequate fluid resuscitation. Some authors favor a more aggressive approach to fluid resuscitation, advocating that the goal or end-point of volume replacement be a supranormal hemodynamic cardiac profile. They contend that the conventional physiologic criteria (heart rate, blood pressure, urine output, and CVP) correlate poorly with actual blood volume and that using these criteria to guide fluid replacement therapy allows for ongoing organ perfusion deficits (Fig. 6–7). In this state of incomplete resuscitation or compensated shock, the homeostatic mechanisms that redistribute blood flow place vulnerable organs such as the gut and kidney at further risk for oxygen debt and may lead to the development of multiple organ failure. Fleming and colleagues (1992) reported a prospective trial comparing supranormal hemodynamic resuscitation with conventional fluid replacement in patients with severe hemorrhagic shock secondary to trauma. They demonstrated significantly improved survival and a lower incidence of organ failure in patients resuscitated to supranormal values of oxygen delivery, oxygen consumption, and cardiac index within 24 hours of injury. These findings support the hypothesis that conventional fluid therapy in shock creates inadequate organ perfusion and the accumulation of an oxygen debt. Furthermore, this insult contributes to the development of organ failure unless resuscitation is directed toward maximizing oxygen delivery and tissue oxygen consumption. This approach to resuscitation requires further validation before it should be considered the standard of therapy. However, it is appropriate to monitor oxygen transport variables if the patient has a pulmonary artery catheter in place, to assure that fluid replacement has created a balance between oxygen delivery and consumption.

The choice of fluid for replacement in hypovolemic shock depends largely on the nature of the volume loss. Treatment of hemorrhagic shock continues to be adequate replacement with type-specific whole blood or packed red blood cells. Of the readily available fluids for resuscitation, only blood is able to restore oxygen-delivering capacity. Thus, extensive red blood cell loss or continuous or repeated blood loss must be treated at least in part with blood. Besides its oxygen-carrying capacity, blood supplies a relatively normal spectrum of plasma proteins and helps restore intravascular oncotic pressure. Furthermore, a transfusion

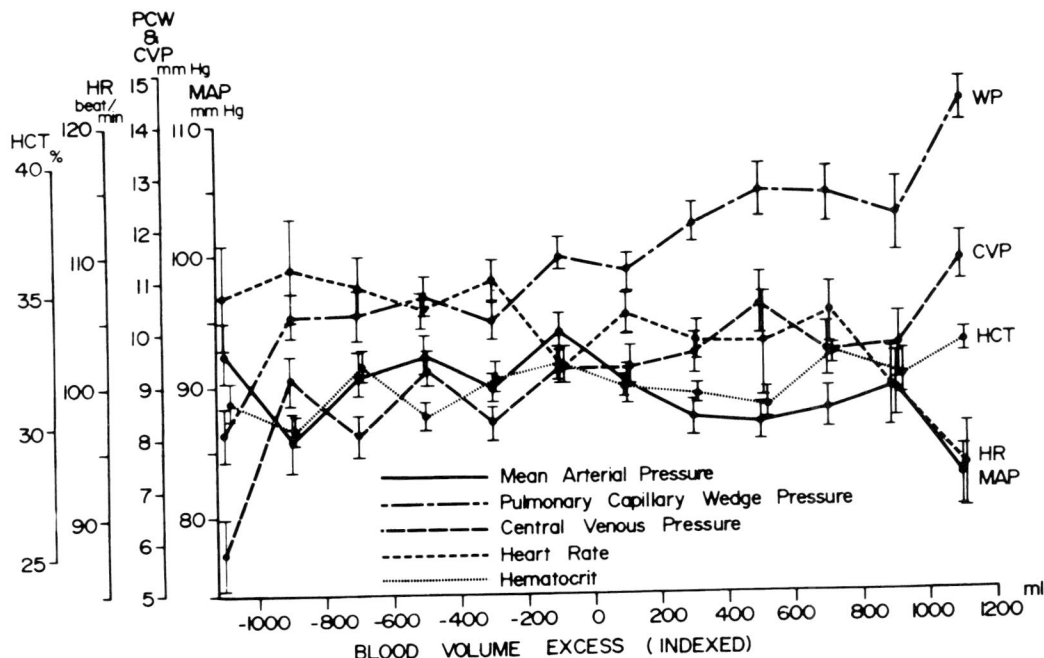

FIGURE 6–7. The relationship of blood volume to commonly monitored hemodynamic parameters. Mean ± SEM for the variables Hct, HR, CVP, WP, and MAP on the Y-axis plotted against the corresponding blood volume excess (+) or deficit (−) indexed. The data demonstrate that there is a high degree of variability in the hemodynamic parameters and overall a poor correlation throughout the range of blood volume. HCT = hematocrit; HR = heart rate; CVP = central venous pressure; PCW = pulmonary capillary wedge; MAP = mean arterial pressure; WP = wedge pressure. (From Shippy, C. R., Appel, P. L., and Shoemaker, W. C.: Reliability of clinical monitoring to assess blood volume in critically ill patients. Crit. Care Med., 12:107–112, 1984.)

of whole blood or packed red blood cells remains in the intravascular space for a significant period of time, effectively expanding the intravascular volume. Through the restoration of oxygen-carrying capacity and plasma oncotic pressure and the expansion of the intravascular compartment, blood provides the simplest and most expedient means of augmenting blood flow and the use of oxygen in states of shock. The optimal hemoglobin concentration and hematocrit in critically ill patients represent a compromise between oxygen-carrying capacity and plasma viscosity. For optimal oxygen transport, a hemoglobin concentration of 10 to 11.5 mg/dl or a hematocrit of 30 to 35% is recommended. However, a higher hemoglobin concentration and hematocrit will produce an increase in plasma viscosity and a resistance to blood flow. Therefore, to minimize the effect of hemoglobin on plasma viscosity and resistance to flow, it is better to maintain the hemoglobin concentration between 8 and 9 mg/dl. In most patients, cardiac output increases to compensate for these lower hemoglobin levels, and sufficient oxygen transport to the periphery is maintained.

The disadvantages of blood transfusion are well known and significant. Despite screening, there continues to be a small but measurable risk of transmitting diseases such as hepatitis and acquired immunodeficiency syndrome (AIDS). Exposure to blood may incite an immediate transfusion reaction or, over a longer time, induce a mild immunosuppressant effect. Blood procurement is difficult, and handling of blood and blood products requires extensive facilities and well-trained personnel. In addition, blood has a relatively short shelf life and it is expensive. The administration of large volumes of blood may lead to clotting factor deficiency, citrate toxicity, hyperkalemia, and hypocalcemia.

Fluid therapy for hemorrhagic shock must also include the administration of nonblood colloid or crystalloid solution. With an animal model of hemorrhagic shock, Shires and co-workers (1973) demonstrated that returning shed blood alone or shed blood plus plasma produced an 80% and 70% mortality, respectively. In contrast, returning the shed blood plus lactated Ringer's solution decreased the mortality to 30%. These results illustrate the importance of restoring extracellular fluid volume during resuscitation for hemorrhagic shock. As previously discussed, the extracellular fluid volume deficit occurs in part because of transcapillary refilling of the intravascular compartment and also the movement of fluid into the intracellular compartment, causing isotonic cell swelling. However, the exact mechanism for the extracellular fluid deficit is still of some debate; Anderson and co-workers (1969) failed to demonstrate the translocation of extracellular fluid in patients with shock from combat injuries. There are often more obvious sources of extracellular fluid loss. Most patients with hemorrhagic shock sequester significant amounts of fluid into areas of injury during the first several days after resuscitation. The volume of sequestered fluid is related to the degree of trauma and the seriousness

of the physical damage to tissues, and is increased by such complications as paralytic ileus or peritonitis. An additional benefit to the use of crystalloid solutions in resuscitation is the prevention of renal failure. The earlier that normal tissue perfusion is reestablished, the lower the incidence of subsequent renal failure. The institution of a saline diuresis appears to prevent the combined insults of hemorrhagic shock and trauma that otherwise tend to promote renal insufficiency. Crystalloid volume resuscitation and forced diuresis prevent the formation of concentrated urine, which is toxic to the renal tubules and also reduces the oxygen requirement of the tubules. All of these considerations favor the use of large volumes of both blood and crystalloid solution early in the resuscitation of hemorrhagic shock.

One of the great ongoing debates in surgical science involves the question of crystalloid versus colloid fluid therapy for hypovolemic shock. The theoretical advantage of albumin-containing colloid solutions is based on Starling's law, and assumes that albumin administration increases colloid osmotic pressure and allows movement of fluid from the interstitium into the intravascular compartment. The proponents for crystalloid fluid therapy are quick to point out that the use of colloid solutions for acute volume replacement or resuscitation has never been shown to alter patient outcome. They further justify their support for crystalloid fluid therapy by its lower cost and ability to restore extracellular fluid volume. In contrast, the use of colloid fluid resuscitation will further aggravate the extracellular fluid deficit by drawing fluid into the intravascular compartment. The use of colloid solutions for fluid resuscitation can also impair renal function, cause bleeding diathesis, and depress the function of the reticuloendothelial system. In fact, there is even debate about how much of the albumin in the colloid solution remains in the intravascular space. Numerous studies have demonstrated an increase in endothelial permeability to albumin during states of critical illness, including hypovolemic shock. Proponents of colloid fluid resuscitation argue that the albumin-containing solutions more efficiently restore plasma volume and more promptly improve cardiac hemodynamics. The use of colloid solutions during resuscitation is also advantageous because most of the fluid volume remains in the intravascular compartment, whereas the administration of crystalloid solutions creates a large increase in interstitial fluid volume. Therefore, the greatest benefit attributed to colloid fluid resuscitation in hypovolemic shock is the decrease in the accumulation of interstitial lung water and, consequently, better oxygenation and pulmonary mechanics.

New approaches to the design of replacement solutions with oxygen-carrying capacity have been tested throughout the late 1980s and early 1990s. The fluorocarbon solutions and stroma-free hemoglobin solutions have been the most widely used. Both of these products possess oxygen-carrying capacity as well as the ability to increase oncotic pressure. Unfortunately, both have limited half-lives in the circulation and have shown toxic side effects that restrict their use to carefully controlled investigative protocols.

REFRACTORY HEMORRHAGIC SHOCK

The reflex vasoconstriction in response to hemorrhage is acutely protective, but inevitably produces a relative ischemia by diminishing the blood supply to tissues such as skeletal muscle and the splanchnic bed. These regions suffer inadequate nutritional supply, which causes anaerobic metabolism, and if this period of relative ischemia is unduly prolonged, cell injury will eventually occur. With prolonged low blood flow and ischemia, the vasoconstriction response may diminish because of exhaustion of the vascular smooth muscle or depression of the autonomic nervous system, or because these are overcome by local metabolic vasodilatory influences. Eventually, a refractory form of hemorrhagic shock develops that does not respond to volume replacement. The clinician is rarely confronted with this most advanced form of hypovolemic shock, and much of our knowledge regarding the pathogenesis of this unusual problem has been derived from experimental studies. An irreversible refractory state of hemorrhagic shock can be created in a dog model by returning approximately 50% of the shed blood after a significant hemorrhage and interval of shock. The reinfusion of shed blood after a prolonged episode of shock induces a loss of vasomotor tone that is critical in the pathogenesis of the refractory shock state. It has been suggested that this loss of vasomotor tone is due either to the release of local mediators or to vasomotor paralysis. Mellander and Lewis (1963) suggested that prolonged hypoperfusion produces an irreversible alteration in the vasogenic and neurogenic mechanisms that normally control capillary transport and fluid balance, allowing for extravascular pooling even in the presence of an intravascular volume deficit. Although the clinical relevance of these experimental studies is not certain, they provide plausible mechanisms to explain the occasional occurrence of refractory hypovolemic shock.

It is difficult to determine whether the observed cardiac dysfunction during refractory hemorrhagic shock is a primary event or merely a consequence of circulatory collapse. The heart normally extracts virtually all of the available oxygen from its blood supply, leaving very little in reserve. Increased demands must be met by increases in coronary blood flow, and coronary blood flow depends on central aortic diastolic pressure as well as on the ability of the coronary vessels to dilate. During severe hypovolemic shock, the diastolic pressure falls, the work demands on the heart increase, and a high fraction of the cardiac cycle is spent in systole. These events place a critical demand on the coronary vessels to dilate, a demand that may not be obtainable in elderly patients with significant coronary atherosclerosis. Therefore, as hypotension and shock progress, the coronary blood flow falls below myocardial demand, causing ischemia and myocardial dysfunction. Some investigators contend that the myocardial dysfunction associated with prolonged episodes of hemorrhagic hypotension is mediated by a myocardial depressant factor released into the bloodstream. Although hypotheses regarding such a myocardial depressant factor have been proposed for years, the actual identification of such a mediator in hemorrhagic shock has been elusive. Recent studies have suggested that tumor necrosis factor (TNF) may be such a myocardial depressant factor. Alyono and associates (1978) demonstrated that diastolic properties of the canine left ventricle were adversely affected by prolonged hypotension. In their study, survival was determined by whether normal left ventricular diastolic mechanics could be restored after resuscitation. Again, whether these proposed mechanisms for myocardial dysfunction and refractory hemorrhagic shock are of clinical significance is not certain.

SEPTIC SHOCK

The fully developed clinical syndrome of septic shock is easily recognized: The patient presents with fever, tachycardia, hypotension, oliguria, and altered mental status. Similarly, septic shock has a characteristic hemodynamic pattern, consisting of elevated cardiac index, low systemic vascular resistance, and a low A-Vo$_2$. However, in other respects, septic shock is far more confusing than all of the other classes of shock. Within the medical community, disagreement exists about the definition of septic shock. Some clinicians propose that the term *septic shock* may include both hyperdynamic and hypodynamic cardiovascular responses, whereas others believe septic shock occurs only when the cardiac output fails to compensate for falling systemic vascular resistance, producing hypotension and inadequate organ perfusion. There is also debate regarding the cause of septic shock. Some clinicians believe that septic shock should include only infectious processes, and others feel that the term should also encompass noninfectious processes that produce a similar hemodynamic and metabolic response, such as pancreatitis and trauma. There is even confusion over appropriate terminology: Some investigators use the terms *sepsis, septicemia, septic shock,* and *hyperdynamic sepsis* interchangeably; others have attempted to separate these terms. Much of the confusion regarding the terminology and definition of septic shock results from the fact that the disease and the patient's response to it constitute a dynamic process. In early sepsis, it is not unusual for patients to present with increased cardiac index, decreased systemic vascular resistance, and hypotension. This hypotension, typically, is easily corrected with volume infusion, producing a further increase in cardiac index and development of a hyperdynamic state. Conversely, late in the course of sepsis, this hyperdynamic cardiovascular response decays into a hypodynamic state, associated with vasoconstriction, decreased cardiac index, and hypotension. These fluctuations in the patient's cardiovascular and metabolic response to septic shock occur as a continuum, making it impractical to attempt to separate these responses as different clinical entities. In this discussion, the term *septic shock* encompasses both hyperdynamic and hypodynamic cardiovascular responses secondary to infectious and noninfectious causes.

Septic shock is the most common cause of death in intensive care unit patients, and the 13th most common cause of death in the United States. Despite our increased understanding of the pathogenesis of this disease, the incidence of septic shock rises annually. Approximately half of the cases of septic shock are due to infection, most commonly of gram-negative bacterial origin. Finland and Jones (1959) demonstrated that the incidence of gram-negative bacteremia increased fivefold between 1935 and 1957 at the Boston City Hospital, and this trend has been confirmed at other centers. The rising incidence of gram-negative sepsis has been attributed to the widespread use of broad-spectrum antibiotics, with the development of a reservoir of virulent and resistent organisms. Furthermore, advances in the care of injured and critically ill patients, allowing them to survive the primary physiologic insult, have expanded the patient population at increased risk for developing septic shock. More extensive operations are being performed in generally older and sicker patients, also increasing the patient population at risk for gram-negative bacteremia. Finally, the use of steroids and other immunosuppressive agents has contributed to the rising incidence of septic shock.

The mortality rate of patients in septic shock ranges from 20 to 80%, depending on the cause of the septic episode and the patient population studied. Despite common physiologic responses, sepsis associated with urinary tract infection carries a considerably different prognosis than sepsis resulting from intestinal perforation and peritonitis. In addition, individual patient characteristics, such as their immune status and preexisting organ dysfunction, have a large impact on the prognosis in septic shock. Many factors may depress host defense mechanisms, including immunologic disorders, malignancy, cirrhosis, collagen vascular disease, chronic inflammatory diseases, burns, and traumatic injury. Preexisting organ dysfunction in the elderly, such as atherosclerotic coronary artery disease, chronic obstructive pulmonary disease, and chronic renal insufficiency, not only predisposes the patient to sepsis but also significantly worsens the prognosis. Freid and Vosti (1968), in a study of 270 patients with gram-negative bacteremia, documented mortality rates of 86% in patients with co-existing ultimately fatal medical diseases, compared with only 16% in patients who were otherwise in good health. Unfortunately, although many factors predispose the patient to develop sepsis, very little can be done to stop this physiologic response.

The gram-negative bacteria most commonly associated with septic shock are of intestinal origin or have colonized the hospital environment. *Escherichia coli*, *Klebsiella, Aerobacter, Pseudomonas, Proteus,* and *Bacte-*

roides are common pathogens, although the particular pattern of predominant organisms will vary depending on the site of infection and the hospital. Several genera of gram-positive bacteria are also associated with septic shock, most commonly *Staphylococcus, Streptococcus*, and pneumococcus. Less frequently, viral and fungal infections may cause septic shock, although their mechanism in producing this syndrome appears to be qualitatively different from that of bacterial organisms. Besides the particular organism, the site of infection is also of prognostic importance. The site of infection often dictates the size of the bacterial inoculum and the degree of host inflammatory response. In children, the primary sites of infection are the umbilical cord, burn wounds, and urinary tract; in adult patients, septic shock is most frequently associated with urinary tract infections, intestinal perforation, biliary tract disease, pneumonia, and burn wounds. Indwelling catheters and prosthetic devices are also common portals of entry for bacteria in both children and adults.

Not all septic-appearing patients have an underlying infection, and it is frequently impossible to differentiate clinically the patient with systemic infection from the patient who appears septic but does not have evidence of systemic infection. Devitalized or injured tissue appears to be able to replace bacteria as the stimulus for the septic response. Common noninfectious insults that may incite septic shock include pancreatitis, multiple trauma, resolving hematoma, burns, and multiple blood transfusions. That these diverse noninfectious processes as well as some infections create the same constellation of cardiovascular and metabolic responses obviously suggests that there are common mediators responsible for the expression of the septic shock syndrome. This finding is further strengthened by the observation that a septic response can be induced experimentally with exposure to endotoxin or cytokines, or both.

Clinical Patterns of Septic Shock

The onset of clinical septic shock is often heralded by a change in mental status, which may vary from mild confusion to delirium and should always alert the clinician to the possibility of this problem. Fever (ranging from 38 to 40° C) is usually present and often arouses suspicion of the correct diagnosis. Early in bacteremic shock, warm, moist skin and bounding pulses may be present, and transient hypotension and tachycardia may be the sole objective manifestations of a potentially lethal situation. The urine output may be satisfactory initially. With the development of low cardiac output and decreased perfusion, the patient becomes hypotensive and oliguric. The skin may become peripherally constricted and cold, and some degree of tachypnea without obvious ventilatory dysfunction is common. Blood cultures taken at this time are usually positive, and a profound leukocytosis is generally present. Clinical jaundice is often observed. In the hypotension associated with sepsis, there may be remarkable hyperventilation with arterial hypoxemia and hypocarbia. An initial respiratory alkalosis later proceeds toward a partially compensated metabolic acidosis as the hypoperfusion state persists and lactic acidemia develops. CVP is often reduced, and initial blood volume measurement in the untreated patient is often normal.

Since the mid-1970s, investigators in the field of septic shock have turned their attention to the study of patients, and a large volume of data has been recorded in the literature. Sepsis in humans appears able to cause several different patterns of hemodynamic abnormalities, and any attempts at instituting rational therapy require precise classification of the underlying pathophysiology in the individual patient. Patients may present in *hypodynamic septic shock* with a low arterial blood pressure, low cardiac index, and evidence of increased peripheral arterial resistance. Physiologic monitoring reveals a pattern characteristic of State D in Siegel's schema. The velocity of blood flow in the circulation is slow as measured by the mean transit time. The CVP and pulmonary capillary wedge pressure are often low initially, and the infusion of fluid sufficient to raise cardiac filling pressure often fails to raise the cardiac output and restore hemodynamic stability. There is evidence of organ hypoperfusion with decreased urine output, lactic acidemia, and a widened A-VO_2 resulting from normal or slightly increased oxygen consumption in the setting of decreased oxygen delivery. Pulmonary dysfunction and coagulation abnormalities are usually present. The physiologic defect in these patients appears to represent a combination of depressed myocardial function and an altered venous capacitance state with peripheral pooling of blood that does not respond completely to volume infusion. This *hypodynamic septic state* appears to represent a primary circulatory disturbance.

A second subset of patients presents with *hyperdynamic septic shock*. The hemodynamic pattern is characterized by Siegel's State B, with increased cardiac output and decreased PVR. The alteration in vascular tone and reduction in PVR often are so great that the hemodynamic response may become unbalanced and hypotension ensues. Because cardiac output dramatically increases, oxygen delivery far exceeds oxygen consumption, and the A-VO_2 and oxygen consumption index decrease. Lactic acidemia may initially be compensated for by respiratory effort, but eventually both arterial blood and venous blood become acidotic. These findings all suggest that the hyperdynamic form of septic shock may represent a primary metabolic derangement in which there is a failure of oxygen use by the cells of vital organs. The development of a hyperdynamic low-resistance circulatory state may be a compensatory mechanism to increase flow and oxygen supply to cells in the periphery that are unable to benefit from this response. Eventually, the compensatory cardiovascular response fails (Fig. 6–8). The persistence of the physiologic state may eventually exhaust both circulatory and metabolic reserves and evolve into a state in which perfusion deficits

become the primary pathophysiology. Patients with preexisting cardiovascular disease are most prone to this transition. Furthermore, when severe respiratory insufficiency is superimposed on the metabolic and circulatory demands of the hyperdynamic septic state, the physiologic derangements often cannot be reversed or supported with mechanical ventilation, and death inevitably follows. All forms of septic shock are associated with a high incidence of pulmonary dysfunction, and the results of treatment are dictated largely by the degree of preexisting illness and the secondary organ dysfunction that arises during the period of hypoperfusion.

The Pathophysiology of Septic Shock

The hemodynamic and metabolic responses of septic shock induced by gram-negative bacterial infection result from the release of endotoxin. Endotoxin is a phospholipopolysaccharide protein complex present in the cell wall of all gram-negative bacteria and released when the bacterium undergoes lysis. The lipopolysaccharide endotoxin is composed of three layers. In the outer layer are O-specific polysaccharides, which are repetitive units of sugars that convey the serologic specificity of the endotoxin. This O-specific region is linked to a core polysaccharide that is widely shared among gram-negative bacteria, so that antibodies generated against this region are broadly cross-reactive. Still within the outer region, the polysaccharide core is complexed to lipid A, which is the portion of the endotoxin responsible for inducing the septic response. The other layers of the lipopolysaccharide endotoxin consist of a middle mucopeptide and the inner cytoplasmic membrane. Although endotoxemia is usually associated with bacteremia, the presence of viable organisms in the blood is not necessary, and absorption of endotoxin from the intestinal tract or a septic focus such as the peritoneal cavity or genital urinary tract can cause shock. A major factor in the initiation of shock appears to be the quantity of endotoxin introduced into the bloodstream.

As with other types of shock, it is difficult to reproduce precisely all of the clinical features of septic shock in experimental models. Depending on the dose and the route of administration, injection of purified endotoxin into experimental animals may cause fever, leukopenia, skin reactions, Shwartzman's phenomenon, hemodynamic responses, disseminated intravascular coagulopathy, metabolic alterations, and ultimately death. Endotoxin preparations derived from one bacterial species may differ quantitatively in potency from preparations from other bacteria, but the effects produced by all endotoxins are qualitatively the same.

Endotoxin initiates the septic response through its actions on numerous cell types, inducing the secretion of a cascade of inflammatory mediators and cytokines. Most likely, in noninfectious septic shock, a similar group of mediators and sequence of responses

Post Op II (day 1)
A State Balanced _____

Post Op II (day 2)
B State Unbalanced _____

Post Op II (day 5)
D State Cardiogenic

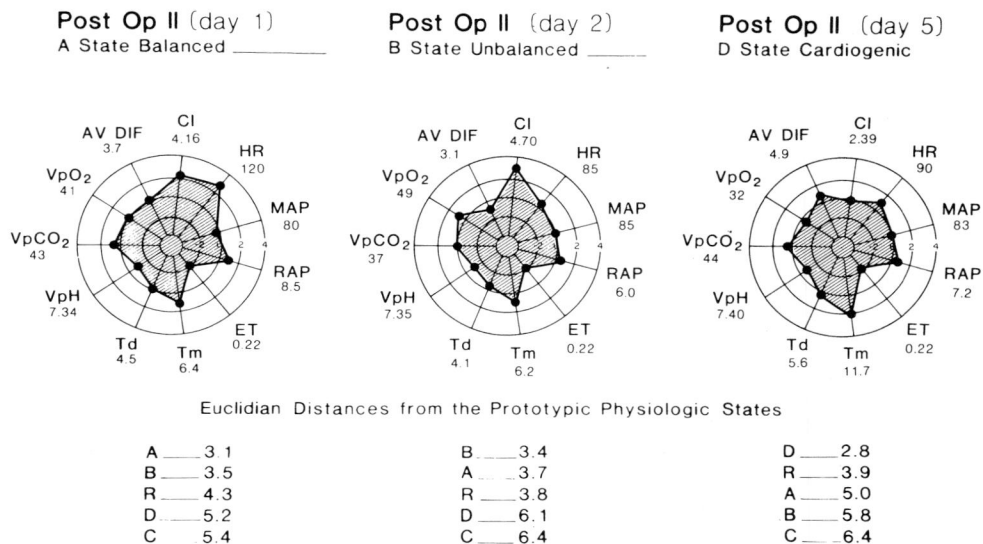

Euclidian Distances from the Prototypic Physiologic States

A	3.1	B	3.4	D	2.8
B	3.5	A	3.7	R	3.9
R	4.3	R	3.8	A	5.0
D	5.2	D	6.1	B	5.8
C	5.4	C	6.4	C	6.4

FIGURE 6–8. The postoperative course of a 62-year-old man who was operated on initially for small bowel infarction is illustrated in physiologic coordinates. Postoperative complications included peritonitis, sepsis, and abdominal wound dehiscence. During a second operative procedure (OP II), the patient underwent ileostomy, colostomy, tracheostomy, and repair of the dehiscence. The patient's changing physiologic pattern and the euclidean distances of each pattern of physiologic response from the prototypic states are shown. The patient progressed from a compensated A state response on day 1 to the B state of metabolic imbalance on day 2 and eventually to the D state of cardiac dysfunction on day 5. (For explanation of abbreviations and units, see Fig. 6–5.)

are initiated by either tissue destruction or an exaggerated inflammatory response. A vicious circle is entered, in which endotoxin-activated cells produce cytokines, causing inflammation that in turn stimulates the secretion of additional cytokines. Complicating this situation, injury or infection suppresses the host defense mechanisms, allowing bacterial translocation across the gastrointestinal tract, fueling the septic response even further. Furthermore, with this sequence of events, it is possible to remove the initial focus of infection or devitalized tissue without interrupting the septic response.

There is growing evidence that the primary defect in high-output septic shock is a metabolic or cellular abnormality that leads to circulatory insufficiency, rather than the converse. During sepsis, an alteration occurs in the use of oxygen and substrate at the cellular level, which is manifested by a reduction in the A-Vo$_2$ despite increased metabolic demand. The mediator or mediators responsible for this defect in cellular metabolism have yet to be identified. However, the net effect, if not reversed, is to cause gradual cardiovascular decompensation. The relationship between cardiac output and PVR becomes unbalanced, and hypotension results when decreases in resistance are disproportionate to increases in flow. Eventually, circulatory collapse occurs, either because of continued decreases in resistance and further hypotension or because the cardiac index falls as the patient's cardiovascular reserves fail. The following discussion considers the evidence for and against this point of view and describes the circulatory response to sepsis in terms of three primary targets of pathophysiology: the heart, the peripheral vascular beds, and the metabolic competence of the tissues.

The Heart

It is generally agreed that cardiac dysfunction is not the primary defect in septic shock, but experimental studies in humans and in animals during sepsis have demonstrated that ventricular function is abnormal. There is a decrease in the right and left ventricular ejection fractions, and an increase in the end-diastolic and end-systolic ventricular volumes. Controversy exists regarding the cause of this myocardial dysfunction, although depressed coronary blood flow, increased left ventricular afterload, direct endotoxin toxicity, and the presence of a circulating myocardial depressant factor have all been proposed as possible mechanisms. It is known that a history of preexisting cardiovascular disease predisposes the patient to cardiac failure during the course of a septic illness because of myocardial depression.

Hinshaw and associates (1972, 1973), in a canine model of endotoxemic shock, demonstrated left ventricular dysfunction as evidenced by depressed Starling's curves 3 to 6 hours after administration of endotoxin. In this model, which consisted of an isolated heart preparation supported by an intact animal, they showed that maintaining coronary perfusion pressure and flow alleviated the endotoxin-induced depression of left ventricular function. These findings suggest that myocardial ischemia caused by hypotension may contribute to circulatory collapse during the course of septic shock. In contrast, Cunnion and associates (1986) demonstrated that patients with septic shock had normal or increased coronary blood flow and extracted a similar amount of lactate from the circulation. These results argue against the hypothesis that global myocardial ischemia accounts for the myocardial depression in septic shock.

There is no evidence that endotoxin is able to directly alter the mechanical performance of the myocardium. However, for years, investigators have speculated about the presence of a circulating myocardial depressant factor. Lefer and Martin (1970), in a canine model of shock, demonstrated that a small polypeptide (myocardial depressant factor) contributed to the myocardial dysfunction observed following hemorrhagic or endotoxic shock. They showed that this factor was released from the splanchnic circulation of the dog after 3 to 4 hours of low flow or ischemia. Similar circulating myocardial depressant factors have been reported by other investigators, most originating within the splanchnic circulation in canine models of shock. However, endotoxin-induced intestinal ischemia observed in dogs is unique and does not appear to be present in septic shock in humans. Nonetheless, Parrillo and colleagues (1985) and Ellrodt and co-workers (1985) reported clinical studies of patients with septic shock that show reversible left ventricular dysfunction. The Parrillo group's study demonstrated that sera from septic patients, when incubated with myocardial cells in vitro, inhibited the extent and velocity of myocyte shortening, indicating that there was a depressant substance present within the sera. The exact identity of this myocardial depressant factor remains a mystery; however, recent studies suggest that TNF may be responsible. The administration of TNF to dogs depresses cardiovascular function in a manner that is temporally and qualitatively similar to that produced by administration of endotoxin or bacteria. Furthermore, TNF directly inhibits cardiac myocyte contractility in vitro.

Vascular Beds

The characteristic hemodynamic profile of septic shock includes increased cardiac output, decreased systemic vascular resistance, and a low A-Vo$_2$. This hyperdynamic state is difficult to reproduce in animal models of septic shock and requires a more indolent inflammatory process (e.g., septic hind-limb cellulitis, pericecal abscess, or septic cholecystitis), as opposed to the administration of a bolus of endotoxin. These experimental models of hyperdynamic sepsis have shown that regional vasodilatation does not simply serve the increased metabolic demands of the infected tissue. In the model of septic hind-limb cellulitis, increases in blood flow to the affected limb did not account for the observed 50% increase in cardiac output. There were equal or more significant increases in blood flow to the kidneys, splanchnic viscera, and the uninfected hind limb. Most significantly, the 50% increase in cardiac output was out of proportion to the 12% increase in oxygen consumption. Gump and associates (1970) made similar observations in patients with intra-abdominal infections. In patients who responded to their infections with increased cardiac output, mean splanchnic blood flow was almost double that of patients who responded with normal cardiac output. Forty-two per cent of the increase in cardiac output was accounted for by increases in

splanchnic flow. The available data suggest that regional blood flow is not directly related to the metabolic demands for oxygen substrate. The area of inflammation does command a greater share of the augmented cardiac output, but the intestines and liver often receive increased flow, even if intra-abdominal infection is not present. The extent to which this redistribution of blood flow is adaptive is unclear, but it does not appear that the vasodilatation and increased flow are merely a physiologic response to increased metabolic demands.

The decrease in A-Vo$_2$ during sepsis suggests that there is an alteration in oxygen use. This oxygen deficit may result from inadequate supply to the tissues, such as with arterial venous shunting or a maldistribution of capillary blood flow. In addition, this alteration in oxygen use could reflect a cellular abnormality in oxygen metabolism. Finley and colleagues (1975), using a xenon washout technique to study patients who responded to sepsis with increased cardiac output, found that capillary blood flow increased in parallel with cardiac output. These findings suggest that significant arterial-venous shunting does not occur in sepsis, at least not to a degree that would explain the alteration in oxygen use. Despite the increase in blood flow and the decrease in systemic vascular resistance, some investigators have proposed that the alteration in oxygen use may be the result of microvascular hypoperfusion.

Inflammatory mediators can cause local vasoconstriction and the aggregation of platelets and neutrophils, decreasing capillary blood flow. With the decrease in oxygen delivery, there is a shift from aerobic to anaerobic metabolism that leads to the accumulation of lactate as well as a decrease in the intracellular stores of high-energy phosphates. However, metabolic data collected by Cerra and associates (1979c) from severely ill septic patients indicate that the alterations in oxygen use do not result from inadequate microvascular perfusion. Although there are concomitant increases in both lactate and pyruvic levels in these patients, the pyruvate-lactate ratio (which falls dramatically in patients with lactic acidosis on the basis of low flow) is almost normal in septic patients if cardiac output is sustained. In addition, studies using phosphorus-31 nuclear magnetic resonance spectroscopy to evaluate cellular bioenergetics in experimental models of sepsis have demonstrated adequate levels of ATP and phosphocreatines in skeletal muscle, brain, and myocardium. These studies indicate that the altered oxygen use characteristic of hyperdynamic sepsis is not the result of a maldistribution of capillary blood flow, but instead appears to be secondary to abnormal cellular oxygen metabolism.

The vasoconstrictive response in septic shock develops in patients with preexisting cardiovascular disease and compromised ventricular function and also in patients whose cardiovascular reserves have been exhausted by a prolonged hyperdynamic state. The status of the peripheral vascular beds in this hypodynamic septic state resembles that observed during hypovolemic shock. Presumably, this response represents the final common pathway that is observed in all forms of irreversible circulatory insufficiency. It most likely represents the sympathetic and adrenal response to a prolonged imbalance between metabolic demands and circulatory performance.

Metabolic Characteristics of Septic Shock and Multiple Organ Failure

The characteristics of hypermetabolism in septic shock and multiple organ failure include increases in energy expenditure, oxygen consumption, cardiac output, and carbon dioxide production. Use of carbohydrates, fats, and amino acids as energy substrates is increased, and nitrogen in the urine is increasingly lost. The increase in resting energy expenditure is associated with a respiratory quotient in the 0.8 range, which is higher than that of starvation (0.7). This appears to indicate mixed fuel oxidation, with as much as 30% derived from the oxidation of amino acids, 40% from glucose, and 30% from fat, according to the data of Giovannini and co-workers (1983). This mixture persists until the late stage of organ failure, when the endogenous respiratory quotient exceeds 1.0, which indicates net lipogenesis that occurs predominantly in the liver.

The onset of the septic state is associated with progressive abnormalities in the substrate levels of glucose, fat, and many of the amino acids. One of the first observable metabolic derangements is the appearance of hyperglycemia that is refractory to the administration of exogenous insulin. The infusion of exogenous glucose can seriously aggravate this disorder and can induce a hyperosmotic state. The lactate-pyruvate ratio remains constant, which is strong evidence that the metabolic derangement is not the result of a perfusion-related deficit. Serum triglyceride levels also rise progressively, and the serum may become lipemic. A prolonged clearance time for administered triglyceride can be shown, and there is evidence of increased hepatic lipogenesis. Free fatty acid levels are raised, and initially there are large amounts of circulating ketone bodies. An enormous increase in muscle catabolism is characteristic of early untreated sepsis. The branched-chain amino acids are heavily used as the energy source in the peripheral tissues. However, as the septic state evolves, the peripheral tissues become less capable of catabolizing the branched-chain amino acids, and their levels in the bloodstream rise and are extremely high at the time of death. In patients who recover from the sepsis, the substrate levels eventually return to those appropriate for a person who fasts overnight. If sepsis is uncontrolled, the substrate levels continue to rise up to the time of death. The only exceptions are the plasma levels of ketone bodies and glucose, which tend to fall terminally and reach their lowest levels on the day of the patient's death.

The relationship between the hemodynamic abnormalities of sepsis (low PVR) and unbalanced metabolism can be best appreciated by doing a detailed analysis of one amino acid. Proline cannot be catabolized by muscle and must be processed by the liver. Proline levels in sepsis rise exponentially when the patient is dying. As proline levels rise, the PVR falls in a tight linear relationship (Fig. 6–9). This rise in proline is also associated with a fall in oxygen consumption index and progressive rises in both lactate and pyruvate levels.

The regulation of metabolism normally proceeds through a combination of local factors, with modulation, when necessary, by the neurohumoral systems. The result is a coordinated interorgan flow of substrate in accordance with demand. In patients with sepsis, there appears to be a progressive ineffectiveness of normal modulation and eventual failure of the metabolic machinery itself. Increased hepatic gluconeogenesis increases the mass flow of glucose to the periphery, where glucose oxidation is impaired. Burke and associates (1979) and Long and colleagues (1976) showed that this hepatic glucose production cannot be suppressed by the administration of exogenous glucose. Because glucose cannot be metabolized completely by the peripheral tissues, lactate, pyruvate, alanine, and glycerol are recycled back to the liver, which increases the substrate available for gluconeogenesis. Thus, although peripheral cellular uptake of glucose is normal, the mass flow of glucose is increased. The same ineffective recycling of substrate appears to occur also in fat cells, and the primary recycling occurs through glycerol. The increases in hepatic production of triglyceride that occur during sepsis coincide with reduced use of fats in the periphery.

The primary energy substrate in the body becomes muscle protein. The branched-chain amino acids appear to be preferentially used by the mitochondria in the peripheral tissues; but because the branched-chain

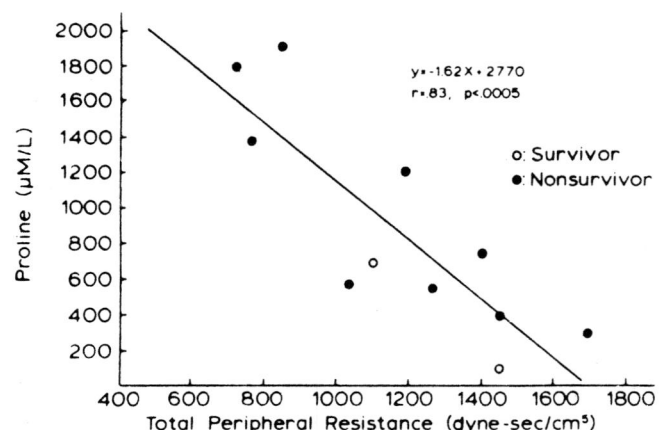

FIGURE 6–9. The data show the significant negative correlation between plasma proline levels and total peripheral resistance in septic patients. Falling peripheral resistance accompanied by hypotension is a hemodynamic hallmark of the B state response to a serious infection. Rising plasma proline levels are therefore a reliable predictor of metabolic and hemodynamic deterioration. (From Cerra, F. B., Caprioli, J., Siegel, J. H., et al.: Proline metabolism in sepsis, cirrhosis, and general surgery: The peripheral energy deficit. Ann. Surg., *190*:577, 1979.)

amino acids cannot be selectively removed from actin and myosin, all of the amino acids must be released from muscle. Some amino acids are converted to alanine and are transported back to the liver to make more glucose. Other amino acids that cannot be catabolized or interconverted by muscle are released into the bloodstream. The result is an increase in ureagenesis, ammonia production, creatinine release, and uric acid production, with all of these substances being excreted in increased quantities in the urine. The reduced level of total body protein synthesis can be supported by exogenous amino acids, but in much higher doses than are needed in uncomplicated starvation, as shown by Clowes and associates (1980) and by Cerra and co-workers (1980). Protein synthesis is increased in the liver to support the inflammatory process and the activation of immunologic mechanisms to combat infection. In patients in whom exogenous amino acids are unable to maintain protein synthesis, mortality is high, which is noted by Cerra and co-workers (1980).

As organ failure progresses, the liver eventually cannot properly metabolize the substrates that are recycled and transported to it, and hepatic protein synthesis begins to fail. At this point, exogenous amino acids appear only to increase an already accelerated rate of ureagenesis. The result of this process is a protein-energy-based economy with muscle wasting and a progressively unbalanced amino acid pattern. The fundamental manifestation of this multitude of metabolic derangements is malnutrition. If left unsupported, the lean body mass becomes rapidly depleted, and visceral protein mass soon follows. Moderate to severe malnutrition can occur in a few days, compared with a few weeks in uncomplicated starvation.

All the evidence suggests a primary defect in mitochondrial function that underlies these changes in substrate metabolism. There appears to be an energy deficit that is associated with a progressive fall in redox potential. This deficit may be related to an inability to regenerate nicotinamide-adenine dinucleotide (NAD) from NADH (the reduced form of NAD) with progressive failure of NAD-NADH-dependent systems. One of the most sensitive enzymes in this system is pyruvate dehydrogenase for the conversion of pyruvate to acetyl coenzyme A. Inhibition of pyruvate dehydrogenase would account for the abnormalities in levels of lactate, pyruvate, and glucose. Reduced use of fatty acids could be accounted for by an inhibition of fatty acid decarboxylase enzymes and subsequent reduced entry into the Krebs cycle through acetyl coenzyme A. The result is the progressive inability of substrate to enter the mitochondria for high-energy phosphate production.

Mediators of Septic Shock and Multiple Organ Failure

One focus of research in sepsis and multiple organ failure since the late 1980s has been to identify endogenous mediators and their interrelationships. The mediators of this syndrome can be divided into two broad categories: the mediators of the inflammatory response, which can have either local or systemic effects, and the neuroendocrine mediators. Bacteria, endotoxin, and injured or necrotic tissue can all activate the inflammatory response after trauma, infection, or an episode of shock. Activation of the complement cascade is an integral part of the inflammatory response to infection and tissue injury. Local tissue damage is the result of neutrophil attraction, margination, and activation with release of oxygen radicals and proteases. The role of the complement system is amplified at the local level by the production of oxygen radicals, which is shown by increased levels of circulating lipid peroxides and tissue lipid peroxidation. The anaphylatoxins (C3a and C5a) are the components of the complement cascade that can most readily affect the hemodynamic status of the host. They are released in soluble form, and therefore can exert systemic effects, including increases in vasodilatation, vascular permeability, neutrophil chemotaxis and aggregation, and mononuclear phagocyte chemotaxis. Their effects are amplified by the release of thromboxane from macrophages that are stimulated by C3a and the release of serotonin from platelets that are stimulated by C5a. The levels of the components of the complement cascade are known to be normal or to increase in the acute stages of clinical infection, but they are often decreased once systemic sepsis and septic shock have developed. Large increases in complement activation that occur in sepsis have been correlated with an ultimately poor prognosis.

Arachidonic acid, the parent compound of prostaglandins and leukotrienes, is produced when cell membrane phospholipids react with the enzyme phospholipase (Fig. 6–10). Cyclo-oxygenase and lipo-oxygenase determine whether arachidonic acid is further metabolized to the biologically active prostaglandins or leukotrienes. Prostaglandin H_2 (PGH$_2$) is the precursor of the five main prostaglandins: prostaglandin I_2 (PGI$_2$; prostacyclin), thromboxane A_2, prostaglandin D_2 (PGD$_2$), prostaglandin E_2 (PGE$_2$), and prostaglandin F_2 (PGF$_2$). The prostaglandins are metabolized quickly and therefore exert most of their effects locally, as shown by Bakhle (1983). Prostacyclin has vasodilator, bronchodilator, and membrane-stabilizing effects and is a potent antagonist to platelet aggregation. Its primary source appears to be the vascular endothelium. The effects of thromboxane A_2 are opposite those of prostacyclin. Thromboxane is a potent vasoconstrictor and bronchoconstrictor, has membrane-destabilizing properties, and promotes platelet aggregation. Numerous tissues have the capacity for prostaglandin synthesis, and it appears that a mixture of the five prostaglandins is synthesized by any given tissue. Some tissues, however, appear to elaborate a predominant type of prostaglandin. Vascular endothelium can secrete fairly substantial quantities of prostacyclin, whereas most thromboxane is produced by platelets. Under circumstances of confined tissue infection, the prostaglandins act as local inflammatory mediators. Thus, according to Whittle

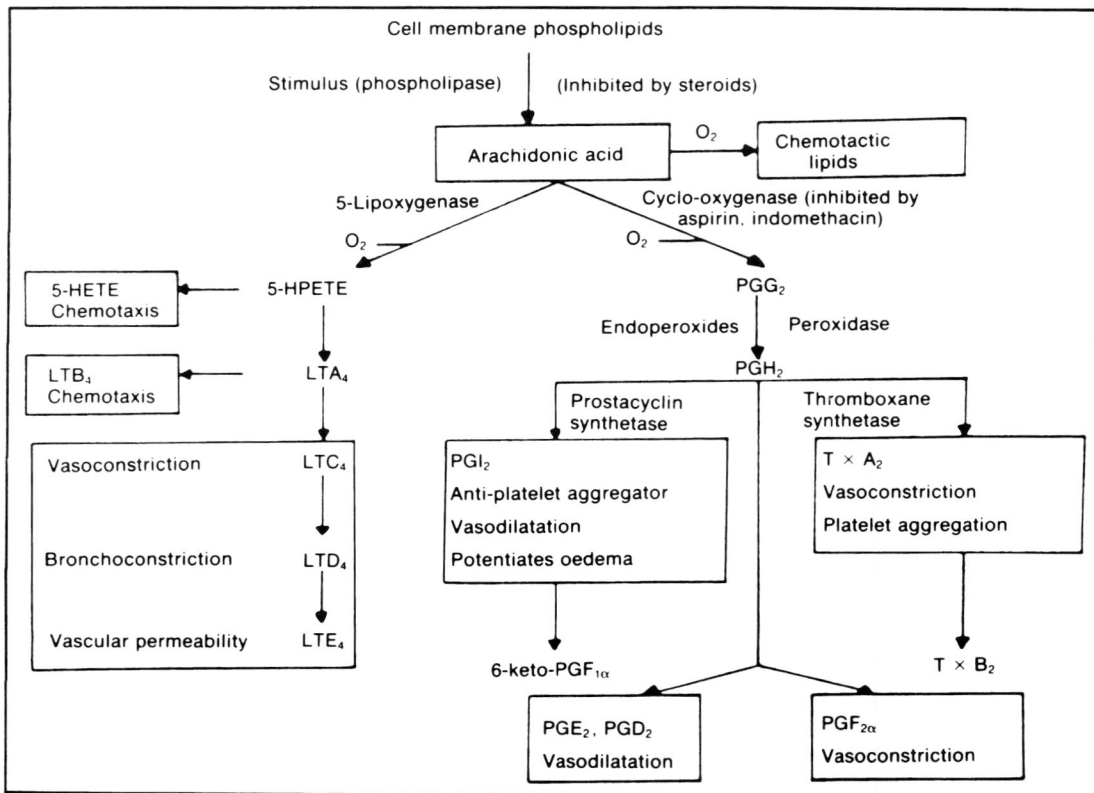

FIGURE 6–10. Arachidonic acid metabolites in inflammation. (From Ledingham, I. M., and MacKay, C. [eds]: Jamieson & Kay's Textbook of Surgical Physiology. 4th ed. Edinburgh, Churchill Livingstone, 1988, p. 479.)

and Moncada (1983), prostacyclin and thromboxane act to achieve the appropriate balance of vascular tone and tissue blood flow in the region of injury.

The role of the prostaglandins in the hemodynamic and metabolic changes that occur in systemic infection is less clear. The measurements of prostaglandin levels in the circulation have been confined primarily to the stable metabolites of prostacyclin (6-keto-PGF₁) and thromboxane A₂ (thromboxane B₂). Reines and associates (1982) showed that circulating levels of these substances under normal conditions are almost undetectable, but under circumstances of experimental and clinical sepsis, levels of both metabolites can be high. The agents that most clearly interfere with the synthetic pathways that produce prostaglandin are steroidal and nonsteroidal anti-inflammatory agents. The administration of prostaglandin inhibitors to animals rendered septic or endotoxemic has been revealing. In the dog, endotoxin creates a substantial fall in blood pressure and cardiac output. Changes in heart rate and PVR vary. The subsequent administration of a nonsteroidal anti-inflammatory agent increases blood pressure, cardiac output, and pH. Almquist's group (1984a, 1984b) and Fink and colleagues (1984), who studied a canine hyperdynamic sepsis model, found that the rises in cardiac output, heart rate, and temperature were partially reversed after an infusion of indomethacin. Almquist and co-workers (1984a, 1984b) have shown that survival can be prolonged in endotoxic dogs treated with ibupro-

fen. Although increases in the circulating levels of the metabolites of thromboxane and prostacyclin have been documented in clinical sepsis in humans, few well-controlled clinical studies investigate the role of prostaglandins. Although steroids block both prostaglandin and leukotriene synthesis by inhibition of arachidonic acid formation, their administration during sepsis has never produced a substantial immediate benefit or prolonged survival.

The leukotrienes represent an alternative pathway for arachidonic acid metabolism. These slow-reacting substances cause bronchoconstriction, white blood cell chemoattraction, and increases in vascular permeability. The vasoconstrictor leukotrienes C₄ and D₄ are believed to be involved in the early pulmonary changes of ARDS in addition to some of the acute hemodynamic abnormalities of sepsis, according to Demling (1982). Although investigation into their action is continuing, little is known about their role in infection and sepsis in animals or in humans.

The plasma kinins may also have an important role in septic shock. Hageman's factor (Factor XII) converts prekallikrein to kallikrein, which is the enzyme that cleaves the kinin precursors (the kininogens) to bradykinin and kallidin. The kinins are synthesized to a substantial degree only when the coagulation system is activated in response to inflammation or blood vessel injury. The most important effects of the kinins are potent vasodilatation, an increase in capillary permeability, and the local production of edema. They may also initiate prosta-glandin synthesis in particular tissues. During endo-toxemia, raised levels of circulating bradykinin have been found in both humans and nonhuman primates. The inability of investigators to find specific antago-nists for kinins has limited the extent to which these substances have been studied in sepsis. However, be-cause these substances have potent vasodilatory ef-fects, it has been assumed that they have some role in the hyperdynamic circulatory response.

Endogenous opioids are a family of peptide sub-stances produced in the pituitary gland and other neurologic tissues. The enkephalins and beta-endor-phins have been the most thoroughly characterized. The effects of these substances are believed to be mediated through the central nervous system. Experi-mental work on animals has shown them to exert potent respiratory depressant effects and to cause both hypotension and bradycardia. The opioid that is most often measured during stress and illness has been beta-endorphin. The studies of Rees and associ-ates (1983) and Oyama and colleagues (1983) show that levels of this substance are raised in animals during various stress and toxic states. Researchers have used the opioid antagonist naloxone to ascertain whether certain pathologic responses to sepsis can be ameliorated by the blockage of opioid receptors. Improvement in hemodynamic status subsequent to naloxone administration has been seen in numerous models of hemorrhagic and endotoxic shock, as re-ported by Gurll and co-workers (1981a, 1981b) and Reynolds and associates (1980). Clinically, opiate re-ceptor blockade has yielded equivocal results. Some patients respond with improvement in hemodynamic status according to Peters and colleagues (1981), but seldom with the consistency seen in animal studies. Thus, the ultimate role of the opiates in sepsis in humans is still being investigated.

Since the mid-1980s, considerable emphasis has been placed on the study of cytokines as mediators of the septic response. Cytokines are small peptide molecules secreted by numerous cell types, which serve as intercellular messengers, allowing cells of the immune system to interact. *Interleukin-1* (IL-1) is an important mediator in the response to tissue injury, inflammation, bacterial infection, and in the immune response. Two forms of IL-1 have been identified, IL-1β and IL-1α, with IL-1β predominating in humans. In response to infection or inflammation, IL-1 is se-creted by monocytes/macrophages, endothelial cells, keratinocytes, neutrophils, and B-lymphocytes. IL-1 induces fever, granulocytosis, and the hepatic acute-phase response. In sepsis and multiple organ failure, IL-1 promotes gluconeogenesis and proteolysis. Clowes and co-workers (1983, 1985) demonstrated that a proteolytic inducing factor, possibly a fragment of IL-1, was present in the circulation of patients with sepsis and after trauma, and was responsible for inducing skeletal muscle proteolysis. Zamir and co-workers (1992), in an experimental model of endo-toxic shock, showed that the administration of an IL-1 receptor antagonist inhibited skeletal muscle pro-

teolysis. These findings suggest that the increase in muscle protein breakdown during endotoxemia may be regulated, at least in part, by IL-1.

TNF shares many of the same biologic effects as IL-1, allowing these two cytokines to potentiate or am-plify one another. Similar to IL-1, TNF is secreted by cells of the monocyte/macrophage lineage, including astrocytes and Kupffer's cells, after exposure to endo-toxin, C5a, IL-1, and fungal or parasitic infection. The administration of TNF induces a constellation of physiologic responses virtually identical to that observed following exposure to endotoxin. De-pending on the concentration of TNF used, TNF may induce hypotension, lactic acidosis, disseminated in-travascular coagulation, and increased systemic and pulmonary vascular permeability. In addition, TNF exposure may cause organ dysfunction, affecting the heart, lungs, liver, kidneys, and gastrointestinal tract. Tracey and associates (1986) reported increased serum TNF levels in patients dying of septic shock. Michie and colleagues (1988) reported that endotoxin expo-sure in normal volunteers increased circulating levels of TNF. These findings, as well as other experimental and clinical evidence, suggest that TNF is the central mediator of septic shock and multiple organ failure. Although TNF is directly toxic to some cells, many of its damaging properties are due to TNF-stimulated release of other inflammatory mediators, such as platelet-activating factor and nitric oxide.

Nitric oxide (NO) is an important intercellular and intracellular messenger in such physiologic systems as the brain, kidney, gastrointestinal tract, and circula-tory systems. NO is produced by numerous cell types from the oxidation of a guanidino nitrogen of the amino acid L-arginine. Its major physiologic effect is to mediate vascular tone and vessel patency. Endo-thelial cells secrete NO when exposed to vasoactive substances, such as acetylcholine, bradykinin, and cal-cium ionophore. This endothelial-derived NO acti-vates guanylate cyclase in vascular smooth muscle cells, producing cyclic guanosine monophosphate (cGMP) and relaxing vascular smooth muscle. Through an identical cGMP-dependent pathway in platelets, endothelial-derived NO also maintains vas-cular integrity by inhibiting platelet aggregation and adherence. The in vivo administration of NO inhibi-tors increases systemic vascular resistance and mean arterial blood pressure, indicating that small amounts of endothelial NO are continuously produced and function to regulate basal vascular tone. It has also been proposed that excessive production of NO may be responsible for the decrease in systemic vascular resistance and hypotension observed in sepsis. Injection of endotoxin or cytokines such as TNF and interleukin-2 (IL-2) produces a sepsis-like syndrome. Concurrent with the endotoxin-induced or cytokine-induced decrease in vascular tone is an increase in NO production. Furthermore, in both experimental models of endotoxin-induced or cytokine-induced shock and in humans with septic shock, the adminis-tration of inhibitors of NO production have been shown to block the decrease in system vascular resistance and restore blood pressure. These findings suggest that NO may be the final common mediator in sepsis-induced hypotension.

Despite the deleterious effects that have been described, these inflammatory mediators also possess many beneficial biologic actions. In addition, there is considerable overlap in their effects, and during endotoxemia or septic shock, a cascade of mediators is secreted, each potentiating or further amplifying the inflammatory response. For these reasons, treatment strategies that attempt to neutralize only one of these mediators will most likely be unsuccessful.

It has been known for some time that the metabolic response to injury is associated with the release of hormones from the hypothalamic-pituitary axis as well as with an increase in outflow from the sympathetic nervous system. Stimulation of the hypothalamic nuclei can reproduce many of the metabolic responses, such as hyperglycemia and triglyceride mobilization. Increased autonomic tone can mobilize glycogen and stimulate glucose production as well as insulin output. Adrenal cortical hormones cause salt and water retention, proteolysis, and lipolysis. Growth hormone somatomedin output is reduced during sepsis and is associated with reduced protein synthesis. Glucagon and insulin levels are both increased, as is the glucagon-insulin ratio, which is associated with increased gluconeogenesis and lactate formation. Bessey and co-workers (1984) showed that catecholamine infusion induces glucose intolerance and insulin resistance and may reduce the activity of pyruvate dehydrogenase.

Treatment of Septic Shock

A wide range of microbial agents can cause profound cardiovascular alterations that lead to shock and death. Treatment of established septic shock is more controversial than that of either hypovolemic or cardiogenic shock, and the mortality remains greater than 50% in almost all reported series.

The prevention of septic shock in many patients is undoubtedly possible because an unfortunately high percentage of patients who develop septic shock do so on an iatrogenic basis. The indiscriminate use of prophylactic antibiotics, especially for prolonged periods, must be avoided. Attention to the overall nutrition of critically ill patients, meticulous care of indwelling lines and catheters, prompt correction of blood volume deficits, careful use of sterile techniques during pulmonary care procedures, avoidance of the indiscriminate use of corticosteroids and immunosuppressive agents, and an alert infection control committee in every hospital can do much to prevent the incidence of septic shock.

The most important factor in treating septic shock is prompt and early clinical recognition. The objective of the clinician must be to recognize those patients who are at high risk and to detect the shock syndrome in its early stages and, by means of supportive measures, to attempt to reverse the effects of inadequate perfusion of the tissues and organs. The unexplained appearance in any patient of hyperventilation, tachycardia, mental confusion, and fever must be interpreted as impending bacteremia and possible septic shock until proved otherwise. When these clinical findings are noted, appropriate monitoring and treatment must begin immediately. A careful examination of the patient for possible sources of bacteremia must be done, and cultures of blood, sputum, urine, wounds, and any other potential focus of infection must be obtained. The presence of an abscess or other surgical source of infection is an immediate indication for drainage or removal of intravenous lines.

Because the effects of bacteremia appear rapidly, it is urgent that antibiotics be started in all patients in whom there is a high clinical suspicion of infection as soon as appropriate cultures have been obtained. The choice of antibiotics must be dictated mainly by the site of the infection and local antibiotic resistance patterns for the most commonly involved organisms. In general, broad-spectrum antibiotic therapy against gram-positive and gram-negative aerobes and anaerobes should be instituted initially. Once the culture results are known, selection of appropriate, narrower antibiotic regimens can be guided by the antibiotic sensitivity pattern of the infecting pathogen.

Patients who develop septic shock often show evidence of pulmonary insufficiency. Administration of oxygen is invariably indicated, and in many cases, intubation and mechanical ventilation may be necessary. Blood gases and arterial pH should be monitored frequently, and urine output should be recorded carefully as soon as the diagnosis is suspected. Appropriate monitoring must be instituted to evaluate the patient's hemodynamic status. This should include a pulmonary artery catheter and an arterial catheter. Electrocardiographic monitoring is useful to detect arrhythmias.

The hemodynamic interventions instituted in septic shock should be aimed at augmenting cardiac output when demands for increased perfusion exist. When increases in cardiac output no longer augment oxygen consumption, additional increases in the delivery of oxygen and substrate are probably no longer helpful. The lactate-pyruvate ratio is a useful guide to the adequacy of cardiac output. When there is no excess of lactate relative to pyruvate, the delivery of oxygen to the capillary beds has probably been optimized. These concepts are predicated on the assumption that the oxygen content of the blood has been brought to a level that does not limit oxygen delivery.

To diagnose patients who present with either a low cardiac output or a cardiac output that has not been optimized to meet the demands for oxygen, the first consideration is whether intravascular volume is adequate. Care must be exercised in administering intravenous fluid to patients whose hemodynamic profiles suggest that they need it. Even transient volume overload in the presence of the pulmonary abnormalities that frequently accompany sepsis can cause pulmonary edema. Ventricular filling pressures should be monitored carefully, and frequent determinations of cardiac output should be made to ascertain when preload has been optimized.

When perfusion cannot be improved further by expanding the intravascular volume and by increasing preload, afterload reduction and inotropic interventions should be considered. Because intense vasoconstriction eventually causes ischemic injury to the viscera and peripheral tissues, vasodilators are a logical mode of therapy either alone or in combination with inotropic agents in the setting of abnormally increased peripheral resistance and low cardiac output. Anderson and associates (1967) have shown a favorable response to phenoxybenzamine. Cerra and colleagues (1978) proved the efficacy of augmenting cardiac output in septic patients with the application of topical nitroglycerin paste. Nitroprusside, a short-acting intravenous agent with direct effects on vascular smooth muscle, is now used to treat heart failure in many disease states. This agent reduces both preload and afterload while increasing cardiac output. Because nitroprusside is administered by continuous infusion, arterial blood pressure must be monitored with an arterial catheter. Often, a fall in arterial pressure occurs with the use of a vasodilator despite increases in cardiac output. Although this fall may be tolerated by otherwise healthy patients, patients with either severe coronary or cerebrovascular disease may be at substantial risk. Furthermore, the use of these drugs to augment cardiac output presupposes adequate inotropic reserves of the left ventricle. If these reserves are not present, profound hypotension may occur without an increase in cardiac output. Frequently, an inotropic agent must be administered at the same time that an afterload-reducing drug is instituted to offset this hypotension.

When afterload reduction fails to improve cardiac output, inotropic pharmacologic agents should be considered. The sympathomimetic drugs dopamine, dobutamine, and epinephrine can provide inotropic support with variable dose-related effects on the peripheral vasculature. Dopamine is uniquely advantageous because there seems to be a specific renal receptor for this drug, through which renal blood flow is augmented.

Patients with hyperdynamic septic shock pose an interesting dilemma in management because their cardiac outputs are usually more than sufficient to meet the demands for delivery of oxygen and substrate. The patient in this category is often refractory to pharmacologic interventions and, by sustaining very high flow, may eventually exhaust her cardiac reserves and progress to the hypodynamic state. Persistent hypotension in the face of high cardiac output may also pose a threat, especially to patients with preexisting cardiovascular disease. The use of vasoconstrictive agents may appear to be a logical choice in this setting, but this type of intervention may severely reduce cardiac output. Usually, if cardiac output with adequate arterial pressure cannot be sustained by manipulation of preload, contractility, and afterload, the clinical course is unaltered by the addition of vasoconstrictor drugs.

Metabolic Support in Septic Shock and Multiple Organ Failure

The treatment of the metabolic derangements that arise in prolonged sepsis and multiple organ failure is mainly investigational. Because this syndrome is well characterized by nutritional and metabolic abnormalities and because the severity of these abnormalities correlates with the outcome, nutritional and metabolic support has been the primary focus of this investigational work. Some experimental work has also examined the feasibility of counteracting the mediators that are activated in this syndrome.

Since clinical malnutrition and muscle protein catabolism are such prominent features of sepsis and organ failure, initial strategies for metabolic support focused on providing specific substrates in total parenteral nutrition. However, it was quickly discovered that the well-established regimens of hyperalimentation that had been successful in the treatment of starvation actually seemed to exacerbate organ dysfunction. Askanazi and co-workers (1980) demonstrated that caloric loads exceeding 50 kcal/kg increased carbon dioxide production and minute ventilation and predisposed the patient for ventilatory failure. In addition, a high caloric intake in sepsis may produce hyperglycemia, increased osmolarity, and hepatic steatosis. Many of these problems are solved when glucose loads and total caloric intake are reduced. The administration of 30 to 40 nonprotein cal/kg/day accomplishes most of the goals that can be attained by using total parenteral nutrition in these patients. With the availability of intravenous fat emulsions, a caloric mix can be provided that substitutes fat calories for carbohydrate calories, as shown by Nordenstrom and associates (1983) and Kirkpatrick and colleagues (1981). Without the administration of these fats, long-chain fat deficiency usually appears within 1 week. There has been some concern about the use of fat emulsions. Hepatic steatosis has been documented when the rate of administration exceeds 3 g/kg/day. Macrophages account for a large part of the emulsion clearance, and it has been suggested that bacterial and particulate clearance by the reticuloendothelial system may be impaired when these emulsions are administered. However, there is little evidence to support this hypothesis.

The general doses of amino acids used to treat starvation (1 g/kg/day) do not produce nitrogen balance or inhibit the redistribution of the lean body mass in multiple organ failure. Cerra and co-workers (1984) reported that in sepsis and multiple organ failure, nitrogen retention is directly proportional to the amino acid load at a constant administration rate of calories. Moyer and associates (1981) demonstrated that 2 to 3 g/kg/day of amino acids was necessary to achieve nitrogen balance during stress. As a guide to therapy, the ratio of nonprotein calories to grams of nitrogen administered as protein should be in the 100 : 1 range. To achieve better support for organ function, the amino acid composition in total parenteral nutrition has been altered to increase those amino acids for which there is an increased demand. The branched-chain amino acids can be oxidatively metabolized directly by skeletal muscle, so solutions rich in leucine, isoleucine, and valine have been advocated. At best, these solutions induce better nitrogen retention per gram of administered nitrogen and more hepatic protein synthesis. They do not reduce the catabolic rate or affect the redistribution of nitrogen in the body. Therefore, there is no demonstrable effect on hypermetabolism, although patients can be supported longer and more patients may recover instead of dying of malnutrition, as reported by Cerra and associates (1982) and Bower and colleagues (1986).

Since the mid-1980s, enteral nutrition has become more popular and is now the preferred route of alimentation. Various factors make enteral feeding more attractive than parenteral nutrition. There is a dramatic cost differential between the two therapies: parenteral nutrition is approximately five times more expensive than enteral feeding. Enteral alimentation also has physiologic advantages over parenteral nutrition. Enteral feeding stimulates gallbladder contraction, reducing the likelihood of bile stasis and gallstone formation. Enteral nutrition also maintains gut-associated lymphoid tissue and stimulates immune function. Enteral alimentation maintains the integrity of the gut, as evidenced by decreased risk of perforation, increased collagen deposition, and improved healing of surgical bowel anastomoses. In contrast, with parenteral nutrition, there is atrophy of the gut mucosa, loss of gut-associated lymphoid tissue, and increased gut permeability. It has been suggested that this promotes the translocation of bacteria across the intestinal wall into the systemic circulation and, furthermore, that the translocation of gut bacteria then stimulates the production of cytokines and other inflammatory mediators that lead to organ failure. Finally, enteral alimentation is associated with a lower risk of complications when compared with parenteral nutrition.

Concurrent with the increase in popularity of enteral feeding has been renewed enthusiasm to identify nutritional factors that stimulate the immune system, the so-called field of immunonutrition. Numerous nutritional additives, including arginine, RNA, glutamine, omega-3 fatty acids, and pectin, are beneficial. Arginine and RNA are immunostimulants that enhance T-lymphocyte production and function, including the secretion of interleukin-2. Traditionally, both parenteral and enteral feeding formulas provided fat in the form of omega-6 long-chain polyunsaturated fatty acids. Infusion of omega-6 fatty acids leads to the production of thromboxane A_2, PGE_2, and leukotriene B_4 (LTB_4). The culmination is a profound immunosuppressant effect. In contrast, omega-3 fatty acids, which are found in fish oils, generate a different variety of prostaglandins and leukotrienes that do not suppress the immune system. Therefore, replacing omega-6 fatty acids in enteral formulas with omega-3 fatty acids leads to enhanced cell-mediated immunity and a decrease in the production of inflammatory mediators. Glutamine and pectin exert a trophic effect

on the gut mucosa and in some studies have been shown to prevent bacterial translocation. Enteral formulas that combine all of these nutritional additives used in clinical trials of burn patients prevent infection, decrease length of hospital stay, and reduce mortality, as demonstrated by Alexander and Gottschlich (1990).

When critically ill patients are not fed enterally, the gastrointestinal tract becomes colonized with aerobic gram-negative bacteria. It is believed that this overgrowth of gram-negative bacteria in the gut promotes translocation and subsequently potentiates multiple organ failure. For this reason, selective decontamination of the intestinal tract has been advocated by McClelland and colleagues (1990) and Stoutenbeck and co-workers (1984) for patients who cannot receive enteral alimentation. The enteral administration of a combination of nonabsorbable antibiotics such as an aminoglycoside, polymyxin, and amphotericin B inhibits bacterial colonization and thus decreases the rate of nosocomial infections in intensive care unit patients. But although this therapy should theoretically eliminate the gut as the source of ongoing sepsis and organ failure, the use of gut decontamination has not improved the survival of critically ill patients.

Aggressive feeding regimens are not able to reverse the hypermetabolism associated with sepsis. Despite the intake of adequate calories and nutrients, patients with sepsis and organ failure exhibit increased energy expenditure, muscle protein catabolism, and negative nitrogen balance. Growth hormone is a potent anabolic hormone that stimulates the production of insulin-like growth factor-1 and insulin. Numerous studies have demonstrated that the administration of recombinant human growth hormone reduces the catabolic response to trauma and burns. Growth hormone therapy induces positive nitrogen balance, reduces protein oxidation, increases lipolysis, and appears to promote wound healing. The only side effects are hyperglycemia and increased sympathetic tone, as evidenced by tachycardia and increased body temperature. The role for growth hormone therapy in sepsis and organ failure has yet to be defined, but preliminary clinical trials are promising.

To date, most of the therapy for septic shock has been directed at supporting organ function. Recently, the focus has shifted to developing more aggressive therapeutic strategies to block or neutralize the mediators that initiate the septic response. Revhaug and associates (1988) reported that the nonsteroidal anti-inflammatory drug ibuprofen reduced the stress response in acute septic states. However, other attempts to nonspecifically inhibit the inflammatory response using corticosteroids have failed to demonstrate any survival benefit in the treatment of septic shock and multiple organ failure. It appears that the potential anti-inflammatory benefits of corticosteroids are offset by their deleterious side effects on immune function and wound healing. In an attempt to inhibit ischemia-reperfusion injury, Olson and colleagues (1987) administered oxygen radical scavengers to animals in septic shock and reversed the acute hemodynamic response. However, the greatest potential for the future treatment of septic shock rests with the development of monoclonal and polyclonal antibodies to endotoxin and other inflammatory cytokines. Ziegler and co-workers (1991), in a report from the HA-1A Sepsis Study Group, demonstrated in a multicenter trial of 543 patients with sepsis that treatment with a human monoclonal IgM antibody to endotoxin significantly improved the survival of patients with gram-negative bacteremia. Specifically, in patients with gram-negative septic shock, the mortality was 33% in those patients receiving the antiendotoxin antibody, compared with 57% in the control group. Despite these promising results, the use of this antibody to the lipid A component of endotoxin, and others like it, to treat septic shock is available only on an experimental basis. Similarly, monoclonal antibodies to TNF and IL-1 and their cell surface receptors are undergoing trials in the treatment of septic shock. Beutler and associates (1985) and Tracey and colleagues (1987) have demonstrated improved survival using a monoclonal antibody to TNF in experimental models of endotoxic and bacteremic shock.

Finally, many patients who develop a profound circulatory response to their infection die regardless of how this hemodynamic derangement is managed. If the infectious process remains uncontrolled, the function of the cardiovascular system as well as that of other organ systems deteriorates. Adherence to the principles of adequate surgical eradication of any foci of infection and effective antibiotic therapy based on systematic culturing of tissue and fluids remains fundamental in the treatment of the patient with septic shock.

CARDIOGENIC SHOCK

Shock may occur as a consequence of the heart's inability to maintain an adequate cardiac output in a variety of acute pathologic states. These states include myocardial infarction, myocarditis, pericardial tamponade, various arrhythmias, and acute mitral or aortic valvular insufficiency. The heart's inability to maintain adequate output of blood also causes shock in patients with massive pulmonary embolism, vena caval obstruction, or tension pneumothorax. After intracardiac procedures, a certain percentage of patients manifest a syndrome of ventricular dysfunction and low cardiac output, and this appears to be the most common cause of early postoperative death in these patients.

Cardiogenic Shock Due to Coronary Artery Disease

Cardiogenic shock occurs in approximately 10 to 15% of patients after acute myocardial infarction and is the primary cause of death of patients in the coronary care unit. Advances in hemodynamic monitoring, pharmacologic support, balloon counterpulsa-

tion, and thrombolytic therapy have not decreased the 80 to 100% mortality. Only recent reports of aggressive reperfusion of the infarct-related coronary vessel have demonstrated dramatic improvement in the outcome of cardiogenic shock from acute myocardial infarction.

The Myocardial Infarction Research Units supported by the National Heart and Lung Institute have adopted the following criteria for establishing the diagnosis of cardiogenic shock:

1. A systolic arterial pressure less than 80 mm Hg, or 30 mm Hg below the basal pressure, and a cardiac index less than 2 l/min/m² in the presence of adequate filling pressure.
2. Evidence of reduced blood flow, as indicated by low urine output (less than 20 ml/hr), impaired mental function, and signs of decreased peripheral perfusion.

Hypotension that is related to pain, drug reactions, rhythm disturbances, or hypovolemia is excluded from this definition. Factors such as heart rate abnormalities, hypovolemia, hypoxemia, or acidosis may precipitate the shock syndrome in patients who have an acute myocardial infarction; only when these factors have been corrected can the contribution of primary myocardial dysfunction to the shock syndrome be identified. If the patient continues to show symptoms of a low perfusion state after these other factors are corrected, then the diagnosis of cardiogenic shock is appropriate.

A number of widely differing clinical profiles may precede the development of a shock state after myocardial infarction. The nature, magnitude, and location of pathologic changes in the heart, the functional state of noninfarcted myocardium, compensatory mechanisms, and the presence of an increase in mechanical load are all involved. Many patients who have an acute total occlusion of the proximal portion of the coronary artery die immediately because of arrhythmias or because such a large portion of the left ventricle is suddenly rendered ischemic. Deaths due to cardiogenic shock in hospitalized patients appear to be associated with extensive three-vessel coronary artery disease, and there is often a documented history of previous myocardial infarction. The syndrome of cardiogenic shock after myocardial infarction is associated with more extensive loss of left ventricular musculature than is seen in patients without shock. This conclusion is based on total loss, both recent and old. In all cases in which shock was present, the nonviable portion of the ventricle exceeded 40%.

Theoretical considerations of left ventricular function as well as clinical and laboratory studies support the contention that left ventricular failure is related to the amount of left ventricular damage. Klein and co-workers (1967), in a theoretical analysis of nonfunctioning regions of left ventricular muscle, concluded that the Starling mechanism of functional compensation would fail when a region of akinesis approached

20 to 25% of the left ventricular surface areas. These observations support the concept that a vicious circle operates to produce the refractory course followed by most patients in cardiogenic shock (Fig. 6–11). It appears that a falling blood pressure increases depression of cardiac function through its influence on coronary perfusion and that a minimal amount of left ventricular muscle is necessary to maintain cardiac function. Once insufficient cardiac muscle remains, a deteriorating condition leading to death is inevitable because the remaining myocardium is unable to compensate for the akinetic areas and the continuing necrosis of myocardial cells that occur during the shock state.

The available evidence suggests that the important basic mechanical defect in humans during cardiogenic shock due to myocardial infarction is a reduction in myocardial strength subsequent to decreased coronary blood flow. The latter apparently destroys the myocardium's ability to contract normally, and the decrease in strength reduces stroke volume and thus decreases the minute output of the ventricle, which then produces a fall in arterial blood pressure and underperfusion of the peripheral tissues. After a variable delay, the fall in pressure causes reflex compensatory changes via the carotid sinus baroreceptor mechanisms, and the sympathetic nerves to the heart and blood vessels become more active. In addition, the adrenal medulla discharges catecholamines, producing tachycardia, stimulation of uninvolved ventricular musculature, and constriction of the capacitance bed, all of which tend to support the cardiac output. Total peripheral resistance tends to increase, although in some instances it has remained essentially normal, but the net result is a patient with a low cardiac output, low blood pressure, tachycardia, and evidence of peripheral hypoperfusion. Because of this tissue hypoperfusion, the secondary signs of altered mentation, decreasing urine output, and peripheral acidosis appear.

Since the mid-1980s, it has become increasingly clear from both experimental and clinical investigations that, after a coronary occlusion, there is an area of reversibly injured myocardium that surrounds the infarct zone. The severity of injury to this "stunned" myocardium depends on the duration and extent of blood-flow deprivation. Those areas that sustain the most severe reversible injury recover a portion of their preischemic level of function over several weeks. Less severely injured regions totally regain their preischemic level of function over a similar period. The prompt reperfusion of the infarct-related vessel is the most important factor in limiting the size of the infarcted zone and in accelerating the recovery of the reversibly injured myocardium. The most severely injured myocardium (with almost total loss of contractility during coronary occlusion) can be benefited only by prompt reperfusion (1 to 2 hours). Less severely injured myocardium may be benefited by reperfusion up to 3 to 6 hours. Reperfusion beyond 12 hours is unlikely to be beneficial.

Treatment of Cardiogenic Shock After Myocardial Infarction

The treatment of cardiogenic shock has changed dramatically since the early 1980s. The advent of bedside hemodynamic monitoring, inotropic support, thrombolysis, and ventricular assist devices provides the physician with a number of therapeutic options. All patients with cardiogenic shock should be monitored immediately and transferred to an area equipped and staffed for immediate resuscitation. Once the diagnosis of shock of cardiogenic origin is established, vital functions should be stabilized as quickly as possible. Particular attention should be paid to the cardiac rhythm and ventilatory status, and oxygen should be routinely administered. Assessment of ventricular filling pressures and the measurement of the cardiac output with the use of a pulmonary artery catheter is pivotal in the treatment of patients with cardiogenic shock. Continuous measurement of interarterial pressure is also strongly advised. If initial hemodynamic monitoring indicates that there is a degree of intravascular volume deficit (pulmonary capillary wedge pressure < 12 mm Hg), then fluid should be administered to raise left ventricular filling pressure to 15 to 20 mm Hg. If fluid administration creates hemodynamic improvement and the cardiac

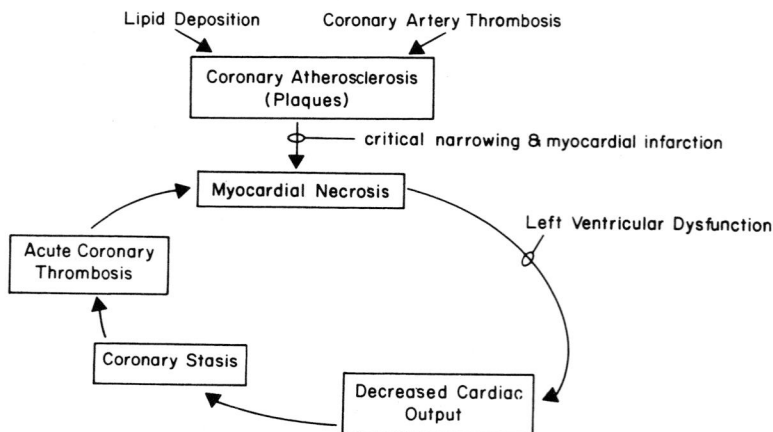

FIGURE 6–11. The incidence of acute coronary thrombosis is much higher in patients who die after an episode of cardiogenic shock than in patients who die with an arrhythmia after myocardial infarction. This finding supports the concept of a cycle of reduced coronary flow and stasis secondary to depressed left ventricular function and a depressed cardiac output. Interventions to reverse cardiogenic shock must be aimed at increasing cardiac output and preventing stasis with resultant myocardial necrosis that leads to additional left ventricular dysfunction.

index rises above 2 l/min/m², no further therapeutic interventions may be necessary. However, if no improvement occurs with volume expansion, or if ventricular filling pressures are initially high, the patient will require pharmacologic support until a more definitive therapeutic procedure to reperfuse the infarct-related coronary vessel can be performed.

The pharmacologic treatment of patients with shock after acute myocardial infarction who are not hypovolemic is directed toward hemodynamic improvement. Drugs that augment cardiac output either by direct (inotropic) stimulation of still-viable myocardium or by reduction of afterload (vasodilatation) are currently used. The sympathomimetic inotropic drugs commonly used include dopamine, dobutamine, and epinephrine. They produce their effects by stimulating one or a combination of specific adrenergic receptors: the cardiac inotropic and chronotropic effects are mediated via beta-1 adrenergic receptors, and the peripheral vascular effects are produced by stimulation of either alpha-1 receptors that cause vasoconstriction or the beta-2 receptors that lead to vasodilatation. Dopamine, dobutamine, and epinephrine all share similar pharmacokinetics, with half-lives of approximately 1.5 to 2.5 minutes, making them efficacious for use in the acute and often rapidly changing circumstances of shock. They are administered by continuous intravenous infusion and can be rapidly titrated to the individual patient's specific response.

Dopamine is the precursor of norepinephrine and epinephrine. It exerts its effects directly by stimulation of alpha-1, beta, and dopaminergic receptors, and indirectly by causing release of norepinephrine. At low doses (2 to 5 µg/kg/min), dopamine stimulates dopaminergic receptors, increasing renal and splanchnic blood flow. Doses in the range of 5 to 10 µg/kg/min stimulate beta-1 receptors and norepinephrine release, creating positive inotropic and chronotropic effects. At higher doses (10 to 20 µg/kg/min), dopamine stimulates alpha-1 receptors causing peripheral vasocontriction.

Dobutamine is a synthetic catecholamine that increases myocardial contractility by stimulating cardiac beta-1 receptors. In addition, dobutamine produces peripheral vasodilatation owing to beta-2 receptor stimulation. It does not stimulate the release of endogenous catecholamines and has no direct renal effects. Dobutamine improves diastolic function, increasing left ventricular compliance and causing a rightward shift in the pressure-volume curve that both lowers myocardial oxygen consumption and increases subendocardial perfusion. The net hemodynamic effect of dobutamine is to increase cardiac input, decrease pulmonary capillary wedge pressure, and decrease systemic vascular resistance. In comparison with dopamine, dobutamine is far less likely to induce tachyarrythmias, but its lack of vasopressor effect limits its use in the presence of hypotension.

Amrinone increases cardiac contractility by inhibiting cyclic adenosine monophosphate (cAMP)–specific phosphodiesterase activity. In addition, it exerts

a vasodilatory effect so that the net hemodynamic result is similar to that of dobutamine, with an increase in cardiac output, a fall in left ventricular filling pressure, and a decrease in systemic vascular resistance. It is given as a loading dose of 0.75 mg/kg followed by continuous infusion of 5 to 10 µg/kg/min. Its peak effect is observed within 10 to 15 minutes after administration, and the drug has a half-life of 3 to 6 hours.

The choice of inotropic agent depends on the degree of hypotension. In the setting of cardiogenic shock, with systolic arterial pressures less than 90 mm Hg, elevated left ventricular filling pressures greater than 18 mm Hg, and reduced cardiac index less than 2 l/min/m², initial treatment with dopamine is preferred. In this situation, dopamine increases both arterial pressure and cardiac output, although the increase in cardiac output is usually less than that obtained with dobutamine. If the patient's arterial pressure can be stabilized with dopamine, then dobutamine can be added to the regimen and the dopamine dose reduced.

The potential role for vasodilator drugs in the treatment of patients with cardiogenic shock is restricted to patients with clinical signs of shock, raised ventricular filling pressures, and normal or raised arterial pressure. Hemodynamic improvement in this limited subset of patients has been reported by many groups and appears to be related to a reduction in ventricular afterload. Increased cardiac output or reduced filling pressure suggests that ventricular function has been improved by reducing myocardial wall tension, perhaps by improving oxygenation of arterial blood secondary to a reduction in left atrial and pulmonary venous pressures. The vasodilator drugs most commonly employed in the treatment of cardiogenic shock are nitroprusside and nitroglycerin, which are administered by continuous intravenous infusion and can be titrated to the individual patient's hemodynamic response.

The ideal therapy for shock after myocardial infarction should reduce cardiac work while increasing coronary artery perfusion. The increase in coronary blood flow must be achieved by increasing coronary perfusion pressure, because flow through severely diseased vessels is pressure-dependent. Mechanical cardiac assist appears to be the only available intervention that fulfills these requirements. The pharmacologic agents that increase coronary perfusion pressure also increase cardiac work, whereas the pharmacologic agents that decrease cardiac work by lowering cardiac afterload and preload also decrease coronary perfusion pressure and blood flow in critical areas. The techniques advocated for cardiac assistance during cardiogenic shock have included total cardiopulmonary bypass, left atrial-arterial bypass, left ventricular-arterial bypass, and intra-aortic balloon pumping. At present, intra-aortic balloon pumping appears to be the easiest and safest method of providing mechanical cardiac assistance. This approach has been simplified by the development of the percutaneous method for insertion of the balloon catheter.

The intra-aortic balloon pump is a pulsatile, pneumatic device that inflates with gas during diastole and deflates during systole. The balloon pump decreases left ventricular afterload and increases coronary perfusion pressure, as well as decreasing myocardial oxygen consumption, which favorably alters the ratio of myocardial oxygen supply and demand. In normotensive patients with severe flow-limiting coronary atherosclerosis, the intra-aortic balloon pump most likely has little effect on coronary blood flow. However, in patients with moderate to severe hypotension and cardiogenic shock, the intra-aortic balloon pump appears to significantly increase coronary blood flow. Similarly, the hemodynamic effects of this device are variable and depend somewhat on the underlying cardiac function (Table 6–3). The cardiac output typically increases from 10 to 40%, and the pulmonary artery wedge pressure falls to between 10 and 20%.

When used early, the intra-aortic balloon pump can assist in myocardial recovery. It is effective in patients with acute myocardial infarction complicated by severe mitral insufficiency or ventricular septal defect. It also appears to benefit patients with acute myocardial infarction complicated by hemodynamically unstable refractory ventricular arrhythmias, presumably by improving the ratio of myocardial oxygen supply and demand. The intra-aortic balloon pump modestly decreases in-hospital mortality from cardiogenic shock in acute myocardial infarction, but in the long term, mortality and morbidity continue to be poor. When this device is used alone, without revascularization, the mortality is between 50 and 80%. Many of these patients become balloon-dependent unless timely revascularization or reperfusion of the infarct-related coronary vessel can be performed.

Trials using other forms of emergency mechanical cardiac-assist devices in the treatment of cardiac arrest or cardiogenic shock are ongoing. Percutaneous cardiopulmonary bypass, percutaneous left atrial–femoral artery circulatory support, and the continuous axial blood flow Hemopump all can be established rapidly and provide circulatory flow rates of approximately 3 l/min or more. Although these devices provide excellent systemic perfusion and hemodynamic support, their ability to provide myocardial protection is not known. These devices might even be detrimental to myocardial protection by inducing cardiac anaerobic metabolism.

The observations that pharmacologic therapy and mechanical circulatory assist generally produce only temporary hemodynamic improvement in cardiogenic shock and that long-term survival is not significantly affected stimulated the development of more definitive invasive cardiologic and surgical approaches. The two major goals of these invasive approaches are to increase coronary blood flow to ischemic but potentially viable myocardium and to correct mechanical defects that contribute to hemodynamic deterioration.

Reperfusion of the infarct-related coronary artery within the first 6 hours of the onset of chest pain in myocardial infarction can be rapidly and safely achieved by infusions of the thrombolytic agents tissue plasminogen-activating factor or streptokinase. Kennedy and associates (1983, 1988), the I.S.A.M. study group (1986), and G.I.S.S.I. trials (1987) have demonstrated an improvement in global left ventricular function and a reduction in mortality after prompt reperfusion with thrombolytic therapy in myocardial infarction. The institution of prompt reperfusion in the setting of coronary occlusion may prevent cardiogenic shock from complicating the myocardial infarction by limiting the area of necrosis and extent of reversible injury in the surrounding myocardium. However, if cardiogenic shock is already developed, the benefit of thrombolytic therapy is less certain. Theoretically, thrombolytic therapy that restores blood flow may be of benefit by improving myocardial function in reversibly injured ischemic areas. The contribution of these regions to cardiac contraction may be sufficient to reverse the shock state. However, in the G.I.S.S.I. study of 146 patients whose infarction was complicated by severe congestive heart failure (Killip class IV) the mortality rate with thrombolytic therapy was 70%, similar to the mortality rate for medical therapy alone.

Emergency coronary angioplasty has had the greatest effect on the survival from cardiogenic shock complicating acute myocardial infarction. According to Bates and Topol (1991) and Gacioch and associates (1992), in a review of the literature, the mortality rate for patients in cardiogenic shock after myocardial infarction treated with emergency coronary angioplasty ranges from 14 to 57%, averaging 44%. The patency rates for emergency angioplasty in acute myocardial infarction and cardiogenic shock are lower than in other patients with acute infarction. Successful reperfusion in those studies ranges from 62 to 100%, averaging 73%. This is a significant reduction in mortality when compared with the mortality rates reported for medical therapy alone in historical controls. Furthermore, in the 73% of patients who underwent successful reperfusion from coronary angioplasty, the mortality rate was lowered to 30%, whereas in patients who did not have successful angioplasty, the mortality rate remained 80%. These data demonstrate that emergency coronary angioplasty significantly improves the prognosis of pa-

■ **Table 6–3.** HEMODYNAMIC EFFECTS OF THE INTRA-AORTIC BALLOON PUMP

Effects	Change (%)
Peak systolic arterial pressure	5–15 decrease
Diastolic aortic pressure	70 increase
Left ventricular end-diastolic pressure	10–20 decrease
Pulmonary artery wedge pressure	10–20 decrease
Peak dp/dt*	10–20 decrease
Heart rate	5–10 decrease
Vmax	25 decrease
Cardiac output	10–40 increase

*dp/dt = ratio of change of ventricular pressure to change in time.

tients with cardiogenic shock complicating acute myocardial infarction. Other percutaneous interventional procedures, such as coronary atherectomy, laser angioplasty, and coronary stenting, should also be of benefit in producing coronary reperfusion in the setting of an acute myocardial infarction with cardiogenic shock.

The role of surgery in the treatment of cardiogenic shock after myocardial infarction is limited. Coronary artery bypass surgery effectively restores coronary artery blood flow provided there are adequate distal vessels for grafting and less than 60% of the left ventricle has been impaired. In addition, only patients in general good health without significant extracardiac disease, particularly of the pulmonary and renal systems, should be considered. A review of the literature since the mid-1980s indicates that, with proper selection of patients, coronary artery bypass in the setting of cardiogenic shock can be performed with a mortality of only approximately 30%. Furthermore, if surgical intervention is to be entertained, it is far more likely to be successful if performed early, less than 16 hours after the onset of infarction. Other indications for surgical intervention in the treatment of cardiogenic shock after myocardial infarction include the repair of a ventricular septal defect or rupture of the free wall and mitral valve repair or replacement for acute mitral insufficiency unresponsive to medical therapy and support with an intra-aortic balloon pump.

Optimal therapy for patients with acute myocardial infarction and cardiogenic shock includes pharmacologic or mechanical circulatory support and the early restoration of coronary blood flow to the infarct-related artery. Rapid and early restoration of coronary blood flow through thrombolytic therapy, percutaneous revascularization, or surgical intervention is most likely to improve ventricular function and survival. The ultimate success of these interventions depends on the time interval between the onset of infarction and the restoration of effective coronary blood flow. Although the role of intravenous thrombolytic therapy is not certain, these agents should probably be administered if there is to be a delay in performing emergent coronary angioplasty. Surgical intervention should be reserved for patients in whom percutaneous revascularization is unsuccessful or not feasible, provided they have adequate distal vessels and ventricular function. If myocardial damage is so extensive that it precludes surgical intervention in an otherwise healthy patient, the only possible treatment appears to be prolonged mechanical support and consideration of cardiac replacement on an emergency basis.

Postcardiotomy Cardiogenic Shock

The major causes of death and serious morbidity after intracardiac surgical procedures are pulmonary dysfunction and persistent low cardiac output. Left ventricular dysfunction, manifested by low cardiac output and raised left ventricular filling pressure, continues to be a major cause of morbidity and mortality after coronary artery bypass grafting, cardiac valve replacement, heart transplantation, left ventricular aneurysm repair, and congenital heart operation. Advances in postoperative care that allow the manipulation of preload and afterload have reduced the mortality of left ventricular dysfunction, but postcardiotomy cardiogenic shock still occurs in 2 to 6% of all patients undergoing myocardial revascularization or valvular heart operations.

In their excellent review, "Prevention of Myocardial Damage during Cardiac Operations," Kirklin and colleagues (1979) succinctly point out that death from acute cardiac failure soon after cardiac operation is most often related to new and often extensive perioperative myocardial necrosis. They further emphasize that this necrosis is also induced in patients who survive operation but in whom the long-term results are less than optimal. Almost all intracardiac procedures are associated with some laboratory evidence of myocardial damage. The functional significance of minor enzyme elevation during cardiac procedures remains obscure, but it is well documented that a strong correlation exists among enzyme elevation, histologically demonstrated myocardial necrosis, depressed left ventricular function, and surgical morbidity and mortality. Postoperative left ventricular dysfunction may be the result of preexisting deficits in myocardial performance, but all current techniques of intracardiac procedures cause transient and occasional permanent alterations in the performance of the left ventricle, despite modern methods of myocardial preservation.

Although one can suspect the presence of low cardiac output after operation by careful observation of the patient, the only way to evaluate cardiac output quantitatively is to measure it directly. The differential diagnosis between pericardial tamponade and intrinsic myocardial depression is frequently difficult to make and requires careful assessment by physical examination, hemodynamic monitoring, and assessment of chest films and drainage from mediastinal tubes.

Documentation of postoperative low cardiac output syndrome requires the initiation of a rational plan of therapy similar to the plan outlined in the treatment of cardiogenic shock due to myocardial infarction. Establishment of an optimal cardiac rate and rhythm and careful assessment of ventricular filling pressures should be the first and frequently the only steps that are necessary. Ventricular filling pressures in the left side should be raised to the maximal tolerable limit by the infusion of blood until the left atrial pressure reaches approximately 15 mm Hg. Adequate oxygenation must be assured and ventilatory adjustments must be made as necessary. If cardiac output remains dangerously low despite these initial measures, pharmacologic agents should be instituted. As with myocardial infarction, the drug used should be determined on the basis of the patient's hemodynamic profile. The presence of a low cardiac output and low arterial pressure warrants the use of an agent that will raise peripheral resistance and also have an inotropic effect on the heart. Dopamine, epinephrine, amrinone, and dobutamine, or combinations of these agents, are most commonly used. The presence of a low cardiac output with adequate arterial pressure can usually be treated successfully with dobutamine or dopamine and, in some cases, an agent to decrease afterload, usually nitroprusside or nitroglycerin.

Failure to respond to pharmacologic agents, with a deteriorating situation in the operating room, warrants consideration of mechanical support of the failing heart. In some cases, a brief period of support on total or partial cardiopulmonary bypass suffices and the myocardium recovers to the point at which cardiopulmonary bypass can be successfully terminated and adequate cardiac function can be maintained. If attempts at weaning the patient from cardiopulmonary bypass are unsuccessful, then mechanical support with an intra-aortic balloon pump should be instituted. Prompt institution of intra-aortic balloon counterpulsation, along with aggressive inotropic support, allows successful weaning from cardiopulmonary bypass in 75 to 85% of patients. Only approximately 0.2 to 1% of patients undergoing corrective cardiac surgery may need a more advanced circulatory assist device, such as a centrifugal or pneumatic ventricular assist device. The goal of mechanical circulatory assist in this group of patients is to provide adequate circulation and to diminish myocardial work, allowing for recovering of stunned myocardium.

In a report from the combined registry of the International Society for Heart Transplantation and the American Society for Artificial Internal Organs on 965 patients with ventricular assist devices for postcardiotomy cardiogenic shock, Pae and co-workers (1992) demonstrated that 44.9% of patients were successfully weaned from ventricular assistance and that, of these patients, 54.7% were discharged from the hospital, for an overall survival rate of 24.6%. The authors also demonstrated that there has been no significant improvement in the rates of weaning and survival since the late 1980s. The rate of weaning and successful hospital discharge were not related to the type of operative procedure performed or the type of mechanical assistance used. Patients requiring biventricular assistance had a slightly higher mortality. However, in the patients successfully weaned and discharged, the long-term outcome was good, with 86% of patients in New York Heart Association functional Class I or Class II. Although the overall rates of successful weaning from ventricular assistance and discharge from the hospital are low, the fact that 25% of the patients who otherwise would have died in the operating room were salvaged and ultimately went on to have functional lives is encouraging. Further detail regarding the use of these ventricular assist devices is discussed in other chapters.

RESPIRATORY INSUFFICIENCY IN SHOCK

As methods of treating the hemodynamic defects in critically ill patients have improved, a high inci-

dence of major respiratory impairments has appeared as a late complication. A spectrum of pulmonary insufficiency is observed in patients who are in shock. This insufficiency may include only the mild and transient hypoxemia observed after many injuries or surgical procedures, and may progress to the traditional postoperative complications of atelectasis and pneumonia. Occasionally, it may progress to post-traumatic pulmonary insufficiency or ARDS, which appears in a certain small percentage of patients and is characterized by increasing difficulties with oxygenation and ventilation without such obvious causes as pulmonary contusion, massive aspiration, end-stage chronic lung disease, or congestive heart failure. ARDS is an acute deterioration of pulmonary function, manifested by progressive hypoxemia and deleterious systemic effects. The progressive hypoxemia is the result of an alteration in the alveolar-capillary dynamics that causes a pulmonary venoarterial shunt. A rise in inspiratory pressure is observed, which produces a fall in pulmonary compliance and generally an increase in pulmonary vascular resistance and pulmonary arterial pressure. These changes are related to an increase in pulmonary capillary permeability, which appears to be secondary to the disruption of the pulmonary capillary endothelium and basement membrane in association with alveolar disruption, edema, hyaline membrane formation, and diffuse pneumonitis. A reduction in *functional residual capacity* (FRC) is observed, which impairs arterial blood oxygenation and carbon dioxide elimination.

Many elements contribute to the development of pulmonary dysfunction in critically ill patients. A single cause of post-traumatic pulmonary insufficiency or ARDS has not been described, and the exact role of shock, if any, is questionable. Although respiratory failure in association with shock has become a topic of great interest, it appears to have been described intermittently since the time of Laënnec (1819). The wide clinical application of blood-gas analysis has led to an increased awareness of the frequency and degree of hypoxemia in all seriously ill patients, and many shock units have reported a high incidence of major respiratory impairment. In fact, in some units, it has proved to be the leading cause of death. The overall incidence of ARDS in patients who have experienced an episode of shock is difficult to determine. Shires and co-workers (1973) reported that the incidence of pulmonary dysfunction in a group of 978 patients who were operated on for trauma was 2.1%, and "shock lung" was present in 1.4%. However, when these authors evaluated the incidence and degree of pulmonary dysfunction in a series of 49 of the most severely injured of these patients, they found that significant pulmonary dysfunction was present in 43% and the "shock lung" picture was present in 29%. Significant pulmonary dysfunction was defined as an arterial PO_2 below 60 mm Hg on room air or comparable hypoxemia on an increased inspired oxygen concentration. The syndrome of "shock lung" was defined as defective arterial oxygenation despite increased concentrations of inspired oxygen, plus evidence of "stiff lung" shown by a pattern of increasing inspired pressures to maintain tidal volume. The greatest incidence of all degrees of pulmonary dysfunction was found by these authors to occur in patients with sepsis, and there was no correlation between either the incidence or the severity of pulmonary dysfunction in septic patients and the demonstration of hypotension during their clinical course. These authors concluded that the initial impression of a causal relationship between hemorrhagic shock and the occurrence of post-traumatic pulmonary insufficiency was a questionable one, and that the presence of sepsis appeared to be a more important factor. Pepe and associates (1982) defined eight clinical conditions that were considered to be associated with the development of ARDS: septic shock; aspiration of gastric contents; pulmonary contusion; multiple emergency transfusions; multiple major fractures; near drowning; pancreatitis; and prolonged hypotension. They reviewed 136 consecutive patients with one of the eight conditions that predispose to ARDS and found that ARDS developed in 46 patients (34%). When only one of the eight conditions was present, 12 of the patients (25%) developed ARDS; when three conditions were present, 17 of the patients (42%) developed ARDS; and when three conditions were simultaneously present, the incidence of ARDS rose to 85%. Based on this study, Pepe and associates concluded that the significant risk factors for ARDS were septic shock, aspiration of gastric contents, multiple emergency transfusions, and pulmonary contusion.

Both mild pulmonary dysfunction and the more ominous ARDS are characterized by arterial hypoxemia that does not respond to elevated inspired oxygen concentrations in the presence of alveolar ventilation adequate to lower the carbon dioxide tension to levels below normal. The finding that was characteristically noted in these patients was a large alveolar-arterial difference or gradient in oxygen tensions. The increase in alveolar-arterial oxygen gradient may be the result of the interaction of three physiologic abnormalities: limited diffusion of oxygen across the blood-gas barrier; ventilation-perfusion inequalities in the lung that alter the normal balance between ventilation and perfusion of alveolar groups; and true venous shunting in the lungs through either anatomic or physiologic shunt channels. The early onset of ARDS is clinically evidenced by a patient who is hyperventilating and hypocarbic and who becomes clinically dyspneic. With time, the hypoxemia becomes more pronounced and less responsive to increased concentrations of inspired oxygen. Although these patients are frequently alkalotic and the arterial P_{CO_2} is low, it is ordinarily higher than would be expected in view of the patient's large tidal volumes, and this indicates an increase in dead-space ventilation because portions of the lung appear to be ventilated without adequate perfusion. With progression of the syndrome, an adequate arterial P_{O_2} becomes unobtainable, even with high inspired oxygen concentrations, and evidence of inadequate delivery of oxygen to tissues with increasing metabolic acidosis ap-

pears. In addition, dead-space problems become more prominent and arterial P_{CO_2} rises above normal. The clinical diagnosis of ARDS is based on: (1) the presence of hypoxemia that does not respond to increased inspired oxygen concentration, (2) decreasing pulmonary compliance, which requires increasing work to achieve adequate ventilation, and (3) a chest film showing an increase in extravascular water in the lungs, which is usually interpreted as interstitial pulmonary edema.

Many elements appear to contribute to the development of pulmonary dysfunction in patients who have had severe injury or illness often associated with a low perfusion state. Factors such as unsuspected aspiration of gastric contents, retained tracheobronchial secretions, narcotics and anesthetics, effects of surgical procedures, inability to clear secretions, and the ventilation-perfusion changes that occur with prolonged recumbency are factors that alter pulmonary mechanics and may contribute to altered ventilation states and to accumulation of pulmonary extravascular water in these patients. Fluid overload during resuscitation and left ventricular failure both increase pulmonary extravascular water and contribute to the development of compliance changes, and they may also alter ventilation-perfusion relationships and impair gas exchange. Fat embolization is undoubtedly an important factor in the development of post-traumatic pulmonary insufficiency in many patients with skeletal injuries, but the possible role of fat embolization in stress states is controversial. Prolonged exposure to high concentrations of oxygen causes changes in pulmonary tissue that are deleterious to pulmonary gas exchange and pulmonary circulatory function. Numerous studies have also shown that structural capillary damage, decreased compliance, and increased pulmonary resistance are the result of administration of endotoxin or living bacteria, so the role of sepsis in the development of ARDS must be stressed. Pneumonitis is a common complication and may be either a primary or a secondary event in the development of ARDS.

Blaisdell and colleagues (1970, 1977) and others have stressed the role of microaggregation and microembolization with associated intravascular clotting in the development of ARDS. Although significant clotting abnormalities occur in both hemorrhagic and septic shock in humans, the precise role of this mechanism in the development of problems in the lung in low perfusion states remains speculative. Although several studies have related hypoxemia after resuscitation to the amount of blood transfused and, by implication, to embolization from transfusion, Collins (1969) found that hypoxemia was related more closely to the type of injury. It is clear that particulate debris can be found in pulmonary capillaries after extensive transfusion in humans; therefore, the widespread use of effective filters during extensive transfusion certainly appears to be desirable. The "pump lung" picture that is occasionally thought to develop after open intracardiac surgical procedures has also been related to the infusion of microaggregates from the priming solution used in the extracorporeal circuit. The use of filters on the arterial side of the perfusion circuit appears to have significantly decreased the incidence of this complication. Patients who show significant pulmonary dysfunction after open heart operations almost invariably have an increased pulmonary extravascular water content on the basis of left ventricular dysfunction, which elevates the pulmonary capillary wedge pressure and interstitial pulmonary edema. Prolonged extracorporeal circulation and hemodialysis do cause alterations in blood, which includes activation of the complement system with the aggregation of white blood cells and platelets in the pulmonary capillary circulation.

Although many studies have recorded morphologic changes in experimental animals after episodes of hemorrhagic shock, there is little evidence that these changes have great functional significance after resuscitation. After resuscitation from complicated hemorrhagic shock, pulmonary function values appear to return to normal, and no permanent detrimental effects are noted. It has been speculated that pulmonary hypoperfusion causes ischemic injury to metabolic functions that normally occur in the lung. There is particular interest in studies that suggest that surfactant production decreases in the face of pulmonary hypoperfusion. Clements (1970), however, concluded that a primary defect of the surfactant system has never been shown conclusively to be the causative factor in the production of any pulmonary disease, including ARDS. Since the mid-1980s, several mediators have been suggested as being responsible for the pathophysiologic changes observed in ARDS. White blood cells are considered by many investigators to be major mediators of the acute injury to lungs in ARDS, and activated granulocytes are capable of injuring cellular systems in in vitro as well as in in vivo experimental models. These activated granulocytes injure tissues by releasing highly active oxygen-oxidant molecules, which include superoxide, hydrogen peroxide, and hydroxyl radicals.

In 1968, it was shown that mild hypoxemia occurred in patients who were placed on hemodialysis. This hypoxemia was related to activation of the complement cascade and an aggregation of neutrophils in the lung. An exaggerated version of these events was suggested as a possible cause of ARDS. Neutrophils are found in large numbers in the lungs of patients with ARDS, but their significance remains in doubt because patients with profound leukopenia can develop ARDS. This finding has cast serious doubt on the complement theory. Serotonin, thromboxane A_2, and the leukotrienes have all been suggested as important mediators of pulmonary damage in ARDS, but none has been confirmed to have a major role. There is at present no complete explanation of the pathophysiology of ARDS. In addition, no therapeutic methods have been proved based on the various pathogenetic mechanisms that have been proposed.

The development of ARDS in patients who have experienced an episode of shock appears to be the additive or synergistic result of many factors. Aspira-

tion, peritonitis, recumbency, pulmonary infection, fluid overload, fat embolization, left ventricular failure, prolonged mechanical ventilation, and oxygen toxicity all appear to be important factors. The precise role of shock is not known, but sepsis appears to be most important and is the most commonly identified factor in the development of ARDS when it occurs in patients who have no preexisting pulmonary dysfunction or left ventricular failure.

PRINCIPLES OF RESPIRATORY MANAGEMENT IN SHOCK PATIENTS

The treatment of pulmonary dysfunction in critically ill patients is a topic of considerable interest and concern. The recognition of ventilatory failure is now more common because of the widespread use of blood-gas analysis. Experience from intensive care units has documented that significant hypoxemia may exist in the absence of any clinical signs and that, only by routine serial blood-gas analysis, can the frequency and degree of hypoxia in patients with multiple system injuries be detected.

The patient who manifests a low-flow state or possibly sepsis should have routine arterial blood-gas analysis performed. The frequency of sampling should be determined by the status of the patient; it should be more frequent in the more seriously ill patients and in those with conditions that have an additional risk of pulmonary impairment, such as injuries that directly involve the chest wall or pulmonary parenchyma. Because oxygen itself is potentially damaging to the pulmonary parenchyma, oxygen therapy should not be used indiscriminately. Inspired oxygen tensions (FI_{O_2}) should be maintained at levels no higher than necessary for almost complete saturation of hemoglobin with oxygen. Because an arterial P_{O_2} of 70 mm Hg usually creates 90% hemoglobin saturation, there is little advantage in increasing the inspired oxygen concentration above levels necessary to achieve this arterial oxygen tension. Oxygen should be delivered with adequate humidification to prevent impairment in the clearing of bronchial secretions. Hypoxia itself is a common cause of hypoperfusion states in both postoperative and post-traumatic patients. Treatment of this condition requires methods that will ensure adequate ventilation, such as clearing obstructed airways of secretions, expansion of pulmonary tissue in the presence of a pneumothorax, stabilization of chest wall injuries, and institution of measures to prevent atelectasis. Many critically ill patients require only these measures to ensure an adequate airway and pulmonary ventilation to prevent the development of serious pulmonary dysfunction and ultimately ARDS.

Among patients who develop such serious pulmonary dysfunction that they may be classified as demonstrating ARDS, the broad objective of pulmonary support, regardless of cause of dysfunction, is to increase the number of functioning alveoli to restore balance between ventilation and perfusion and thus reestablish acceptable blood-gas exchange. Measures that are instituted must be designed both to improve pulmonary ventilation and gas exchange and to maintain an adequate oxygen transport to the periphery.

When a patient begins to develop evidence of severe pulmonary dysfunction, circulatory and respiratory monitoring is required to institute rational treatment. Monitoring of arterial, central venous, and pulmonary arterial pressure is essential both to obtain meaningful hemodynamic data and to serve as a source of blood for analysis. Intermittent measurements of cardiac output, the alveolar-arterial oxygen tension gradient, the degree of pulmonary shunting, and the pulmonary dead space, as well as measurements of the mechanics of the lung, allow additional decisions to be made in the care of these patients. Once it becomes clear that the respiratory workload is excessive, or that satisfactory gas exchange is not being achieved, ventilatory support through the use of a cuffed endotracheal tube and mechanical respirator should be instituted. The decision to proceed with tracheal intubation and artificial ventilation must be guided by pragmatic criteria.

The management of artificial ventilation in these critically ill patients, particularly if a low-flow state exists concomitantly, demands a high level of judgment and careful monitoring of the patients so that a proper choice of ventilation pattern and inspired oxygen concentration and a careful titration of fluids is maintained, which thus prevents the further progression of pulmonary complications.

In some patients, mechanical ventilation fails to achieve adequate oxygenation because a profound degree of pulmonary parenchymal disease exists. In this situation, additional measures must be taken to reduce pulmonary extravascular water and to increase alveolar ventilation. The judicious use of a diuretic may be beneficial in decreasing both interstitial and intra-alveolar edema. The most useful adjunct to conventional ventilatory therapy, however, appears to be the institution of positive end-expiratory pressure, which has shown benefits in improving oxygenation. Positive end-expiratory pressure recruits atelectatic areas for gas exchange and thus increases functional reserve capacity, compliance, and arterial oxygen tension. The institution of positive end-expiratory pressure, however, is not without hazards, and by overextending alveoli, it may reduce compliance and produce mechanical disruption and possibly pneumothorax. Experimental and clinical studies have shown the effects of increased airway pressure on cardiac hemodynamics and concluded that in the presence of hypovolemia, there may be profound depression of cardiac output as the result of excessive airway pressures.

In summary, pulmonary dysfunction is a common accompaniment of many shock states. ARDS occurs in some patients and appears to be due to various synergistic and additive factors, of which sepsis is the most prominent. The early recognition of this problem and prompt institution of appropriate therapy allow the salvage of many patients by correction of the increases in pulmonary extravascular water and the abnormal patterns of gas exchange that characterize the syndrome.

SELECTED BIBLIOGRAPHY

Barrett, J., and Nyhus, L. M. (eds): Treatment of Shock: Principles and Practice. 2nd ed. Philadelphia, Lea & Febiger, 1986.

This monograph on the management of the various forms of the shock state is written by experts in the field. As emphasized in the introduction, enormous strides have occurred in our understanding of the pathophysiology of the shock state since the mid-1970s. The microcirculation, volume replacement, monitoring, and the role of the central nervous system are reviewed. The specific effects of shock on the pathophysiology of the lung, brain, heart, kidney, and liver are covered in separate chapters. Special attention is given to the initial treatment of trauma, septic shock, and the immune response to shock. There is also a detailed account of pharmacologic therapy. This monograph is excellent for detailed reading.

Blalock, A.: Principles of Surgical Care, Shock, and Other Problems. St. Louis, C. V. Mosby, 1940.

This classic monograph summarizes the work by Dr. Blalock and many others up until 1940 and emphasizes the importance of hypovolemia in the traumatized patient. The problem is placed in historic perspective, and both experimental and clinical studies are used to show the principles of good surgical care.

BIBLIOGRAPHY

Alexander, J. W., and Gottschlich, M. M.: Nutritional immune modulation in burn patients. Crit. Care Med., 18:5149, 1990.

Almquist, P. M., Ekstrom, B., Kuenzig, M., et al.: Increased survival of endotoxin-injected dogs treated with methylprednisolone, naloxone, and ibuprofen. Circ. Shock, 14:129, 1984a.

Almquist, P. M., Kuenzig, M., and Schwartz, S. L.: Treatment of experimental endotoxin shock with ibuprofen, a cyclo-oxygenase inhibitor. Circ. Shock, 13:227, 1984b.

Alyono, D., Ring, W. S., and Anderson, R. W.: The effects of hemorrhagic shock on the diastolic properties of the left ventricle in the conscious dog. Surgery, 83:691, 1978.

Anderson, R. W., James, P. M., Bredenberg, C. E., and Hardaway, R. M.: Phenoxybenzamine in septic shock. Ann. Surg., 165:341, 1967.

Anderson, R. W., Simmons, R. L., Collins, J. A., et al.: Plasma volume and sulfate spaces in acute combat casualties. Surg. Gynecol. Obstet., 128:719, 1969.

Askanazi, J., Rosenbaums, H., Hyman, A., et al.: Respiratory changes induced by high glucose loads of total parenteral nutrition. J. A. M. A., 243:1444, 1980.

Bakhle, Y. S.: Synthesis and catabolism of cyclo-oxygenase products. Br. Med. Bull., 39:214, 1983.

Bates, E. R., and Topol, E. J.: Limitations of thrombolytic therapy for acute myocardial infarction complicated by congestive heart failure and cardiogenic shock. J. Am. Coll. Cardiol., 18:1077, 1991.

Beecher, H. K. (ed): Surgery and World War II: The Physiologic Effects of Wounds. Washington, DC, Office of the Surgeon General, Department of the Army, 1952.

Bessey, P., Waters, J., Soki, T., and Wilmore, D.: Combined hormone infusion simulates the metabolic response to injury. Ann. Surg., 200:264, 1984.

Beutler, B., Kilsark, J. A., and Cerami, A. C.: Passive immunization against cachectin/tumor necrosis factor prevents mice from lethal effect of endotoxin. Science, 229:869, 1985.

Blaisdell, F. W., and Lewis, F. R., Jr.: Respiratory Distress Syndrome of Shock and Trauma: Post-Traumatic Respiratory Failure. Philadelphia, W. B. Saunders, 1977.

Blaisdell, F. W., Lim, R. C., Jr., and Stallane, R. J.: The mechanism of pulmonary damage following traumatic shock. Surg. Gynecol. Obstet., 130:15, 1970.

Blalock, A.: Acute circulatory failure as exemplified by shock and hemorrhage. Surg. Gynecol. Obstet., 58:551, 1934a.

Blalock, A.: Experimental shock: Cause of low blood pressure produced by muscle injury. Arch. Surg., 22:959, 1930.

Blalock, A.: Shock: Further studies with particular reference to effects of hemorrhage. Arch. Surg., 29:837, 1934b.

Bower, R. H., Muggin-Sullam, M., Vallgren, S., and Fischer, J.: Branched chain amino acid–enriched solutions in the septic patient: A randomized, prospective trial. Ann. Surg., 203:13, 1986.

Burke, J. F., Wolfe, R., and Mullaney, J.: Glucose requirements and possible hepatic and respiratory abnormalities following excessive glucose intake. Ann. Surg., 190:274, 1979.

Cannon, W. B.: Acidosis in cases of shock, hemorrhage, and gas infection. J. A. M. A., 70:531, 1918.

Cannon, W. B., and Bayliss, W. M.: Notes on muscle injury in relation to shock. Special Report of the Medical Research Commission. No. 26, VIII:19, 1919.

Cerra, F. B., Caprioli, J., Siegel, J., and Border, J.: Proline metabolism in sepsis, cirrhosis, and general surgery: The peripheral energy deficit. Ann. Surg., 190:577, 1979a.

Cerra, F. B., Hasset, J., and Siegel, J. H.: Vasodilatory therapy clinical sepsis with low output syndrome. J. Surg. Res., 25:180, 1978.

Cerra, F. B., Mazuski, J., Chute, E., et al.: Branched-chain metabolic support. Ann. Surg., 199:286, 1984.

Cerra, F. B., Siegel, J. H., Border, J. R., et al.: Correlations between metabolic and cardiopulmonary measurements in patients after trauma, general surgery, and sepsis. J. Trauma, 19:621, 1979b.

Cerra, F. B., Siegel, J. H., Border, J. R., and Coleman, B.: The hepatic failure of sepsis: Cellular vs. substrate. Surgery, 86:409, 1979c.

Cerra, F. B., Siegel, J. H., Colman, B., et al.: Autocannibalism: A failure of exogenous nutritional support. Ann. Surg., 192:570, 1980.

Cerra, F. B., Upson, D., Angelico, R., et al.: Branched chains support postoperative synthesis. Surgery, 92:192, 1982.

Clements, J. A.: Pulmonary surfactant. Am. Rev. Respir. Dis., 101:984, 1970.

Clowes, G., George, B., and Villee, C.: Muscle proteolysis induced by a circulating peptide in patients with sepsis or trauma. N. Engl. J. Med., 308:545, 1983.

Clowes, G. H. A., Heidman, M., and Lindberg, B.: Effects of parenteral alimentation on amino acid metabolism in septic patients. Surgery, 8:532, 1980.

Clowes, G. H. A., Hirsch, E., George, B. C., et al.: Survival from sepsis: The significance of altered protein metabolism regulated by proteolysis-inducing factor, the circulating cleavage product of interleukin-1. Ann. Surg., 202:446, 1985.

Clowes, G. H. A., Jr., Vucinic, M., and Weidner, M. G.: Circulatory and metabolic alterations associated with survival or death in peritonitis: Clinical analysis of 25 cases. Ann. Surg., 163:866, 1966.

Collins, J. A.: The causes of progressive pulmonary insufficiency in surgical patients. J. Surg. Res., 9:685, 1969.

Cournand, A., Reilly, R. L., Bradley, S. E., et al.: Studies of circulation in clinical shock. Surgery, 13:964, 1943.

Crile, G. W.: An Experimental Research into Surgical Shock. Philadelphia, J. B. Lippincott, 1899.

Cunnion, R. E., Schaer, G. L., Parker, M. M., et al.: The coronary circulation in human septic shock. Circulation, 73:637, 1986.

Dale, H. H., and Richards, A. N.: Vasodilator actions of histamine and other substances, J. Physiol. (Lond.), 52:110, 1918.

Demling, R. H.: Role of prostaglandins in acute pulmonary microvascular injury. Ann. N. Y. Acad. Sci., 384:517, 1982.

Ellrodt, A. G., Riedinger, M. S., Kimchi, A., et al.: Left ventricular performance in septic shock: Reversible segmental and global abnormalities. Am. Heart J., 110:402, 1985.

Fink, M. P., MacVittie, T. J., and Casey, L. C.: Inhibition of prostaglandin synthesis restores normal hemodynamics in canine hyperdynamic sepsis. Ann. Surg., 200:619, 1984.

Finland, M., and Jones, W. F.: Occurrence of serious bacterial infections since introduction of antibacterial agents. J. A. M. A., 170:2188, 1959.

Finley, R. J., Duff, J. H., Holliday, R. L., et al.: Capillary muscle blood flow in human sepsis. Surgery, 78:87, 1975.

Fleming, A., Bishop, M., Shoemaker, W., et al.: Prospective trial of supranormal values as goals of resuscitation in severe trauma. Arch. Surg., 127:1175, 1992.

Freid, M. A., and Vosti, K. L.: The importance of underlying disease in patients with gram-negative bacteremia. Arch. Intern. Med., 121:418, 1968.

Gacioch, G. M., Ellis, S. G., Lee, L., et al.: Cardiogenic shock complicating acute myocardial infarction: The use of coronary angioplasty and the integration of the new support devices into patient management. J. Am. Coll. Cardiol., 19:647, 1992.

Giovannini, I., Boldrini, G., Castagnato, M., et al.: Respiratory quotient and patterns of substrate utilization in human sepsis and trauma. J. Parenter. Enter. Nutr., 7:226, 1983.

Groenigen, P.: Uber den Shock. Wiesbaden, 115:116, 1885.

G.I.S.S.I. (Gruppo Italiano per lo studio dello streptochi-nasi nell'infarto miocardico): Long-term effects of intravenous thrombolysis in acute myocardial infarction: Final report on the G.I.S.S.I. study. Lancet, 2:871, 1987.

Gump, F. E., Price, J. B., Jr., and Kinney, J. M.: Whole body and splanchnic blood flow and oxygen consumption measurements in patients with intraperitoneal infection. Ann. Surg., 171:321, 1970.

Gurll, N. J., Reynolds, D. G., and Vargish, T.: Primate endotoxemic shock reversed by opiate receptor blockade with naloxone. Physiology, 24:4, 1981a.

Gurll, N. J., Vargish, T., Reynolds, D. G., and Lechner, R. B.: Opiate receptors and endorphins in the pathophysiology of hemorrhagic shock. Surgery, 89:364, 1981b.

Hinshaw, L. B., Archer, L. T., Black, M. R., et al.: Prevention and reversal of myocardial failure in endotoxin shock. Surg. Gynecol. Obstet., 136:1, 1973.

Hinshaw, L. B., Greenfield, L. J., Owen, S. E., et al.: Precipitation of cardiac failure in endotoxin shock. Surg. Gynecol. Obstet., 135:39, 1972.

I.S.A.M. Study Group: A prospective trial of intravenous streptokinase in acute myocardial infarction (ISAM): Mortality, morbidity, and infarct size at 21 days. N. Engl. J. Med., 314:1465, 1986.

Jones, A. L.: The intestinal immune system. Gastroenterology, 87:236, 1984.

Keith, N. M.: Blood volume changes in wound shock and primary hemorrhage. Reports of the Special Investigations Committee on Surgical Shock and Allied Conditions, Vol. 9, 1919a.

Keith, N. M.: Report of Shock Committee. English Medical Research Committee, Vol. 27, March 1919b.

Keller, G., Barke, R., Harty, J., et al.: Decreased hepatic glutathione levels in septic shock: Predisposition of hepatocytes to oxidative stress. Ann. Surg., 120:941, 1985.

Kennedy, J. W., Martin, G. V., Davis, K. B., et al.: The Western Washington intravenous streptokinase in acute myocardial infarction randomized trial. Circulation, 77:345, 1988.

Kennedy, J. W., Ritchie, J. L., David, K. B., and Fritz, J. K.: Western Washington trial of intracoronary streptokinase in acute myocardial infarction. N. Engl. J. Med., 309:1477, 1983.

Killip, T., and Kimball, J. T.: Treatment of myocardial infarction in a coronary care unit: A two-year experience with 250 patients. Am. J. Cardiol., 20:457, 1967.

Kirklin, J. W., Conti, V. R., and Blackstone, E. H.: Prevention of myocardial damage during cardiac operations. N. Engl. J. Med., 301:135, 1979.

Kirkpatrick, J., Dann, M., and Haynes, M.: The therapeutic advantages of a balanced nutrition support system. Surgery, 89:370, 1981.

Klein, M. D., Herman, M. V., and Gorlin, R.: A hemodynamic study of left ventricular aneurysm. Circulation, 35:614, 1967.

Knaus, W. A., Draper, E. A., Wagner, D. P., and Zimmerman, J. E.: APACHE II: A severity of disease classification system. Crit. Care Med., 13:818, 1985.

Laënnec, R. T. H.: De l'auscultation mediate ou traité du diagnostic des maladies des poumons et du coeur, fondé principalement sur ce nouveau moyen d'exploration. Paris, 1819.

Latta, T.: Treatment of malignant cholera. Lancet, 2:1831, 1832.

Lefer, A. M., and Martin, J.: Origin of myocardial depressant factor in shock. Am. J. Physiol., 218:1423, 1970.

Lister, J., McNeil, I. F., Marshall, V. C., et al.: Transcapillary refilling and hemorrhage in normal man: Basal rates and volumes; effects of norepinephrine. Ann. Surg., 158:698, 1963.

Long, C., Kinney, J., and Geiger, J.: Nonsuppressibility of gluconeogenesis in septic patients. Metabolism, 25:193, 1976.

Lucas, E. E.: The renal response to acute injury and sepsis. Surg. Clin. North Am., *56:*953, 1976.

MacLean, L. D., Mulligan, W. G., McLean, A. P. H., and Duff, J. H.: Patterns of septic shock in man—A detailed study of 56 patients. Ann. Surg., *166:*543, 1967.

McClelland, P., Murray, A. E., Williams, P. S., et al.: Reducing sepsis in severe combined acute renal and respiratory failure by selective decontamination of the digestive tract. Crit. Care Med., *18:*935, 1990.

Mellander, S., and Lewis, D. H.: Effect of hemorrhagic shock on the reactivity of resistance and capacitance vessels and on capillary filtration transfer in cat skeletal muscles. Circ. Res., *13:*105, 1963.

Michie, H. R., Manogue, K. R., Spriggs, D. R., et al.: Detection of circulating tumor necrosis factor after endotoxin administration. N. Engl. J. Med., *318:*1481, 1988.

Montgomery, A., Stager, M., Carrico, J., et al.: Causes of mortality in patients with the adult respiratory distress syndrome. Am. Rev. Respir. Dis., *132:*485, 1985.

Moore, F. D., Dagher, F. J., Boyden, C. M., et al.: Hemorrhage in normal man. I: Distribution and dispersal of saline infusion following acute blood loss: Clinical kinetics of blood volume support. Ann. Surg., *163:*485, 1966.

Morris, A., Henry, W., Shearer, J., and Caldwell, M.: Macrophage interaction with skeletal muscle: A potential role of macrophages in determining the energy state of healing wounds. J. Trauma, 25:746, 1985.

Moyer, E. D., Border, J. R., McMenamy, R. H., and Caruana, J.: Multiple systems organ failure. V: Alterations in the plasma protein profile in septic trauma—Effects of intravenous amino acids. J. Trauma, 21:645, 1981.

Nordenstrom, J., Askanazi, J., Elwyn, D. H., and Kenney, J.: Nitrogen balance during total parenteral nutrition: Glucose vs. fat. Ann. Surg., *197:*27, 1983.

Olson, N. C., Grizzle, M. K., and Anderson, D. L.: Effect of polyethylene glycol–superoxide dismutase and catalase on endotoxemia in pigs. J. Appl. Physiol., *63:*1526, 1987.

Oyama, T., Yao, M., and Ishihara, H.: Effects of hemorrhagic shock and endotoxin shock on plasma levels of beta-endorphin and beta-lipotropin. Prog. Clin. Biol. Res., *111:*185, 1983.

Pae, W. E., Miller, C. A., Matthews, Y., et al.: Ventricular assist devices for postcardiotomy cardiogenic shock. J. Thorac. Cardiovasc. Surg., *104:*541, 1992.

Paré, A.: Les Oeuvres d'Ambroise Paré. Paris, Dupauye, 1582, p. 267.

Parrillo, J. E., Burch, C., Shelhamer, J. H., et al.: A circulating myocardial depressant substance in humans with septic shock: Septic shock patients with a reduced ejection fraction have a circulating factor that depresses in vitro myocardial cell performance. J. Clin. Invest., *76:*1539, 1985.

Parsons, E., and Phemister, D. B.: Hemorrhage and shock in traumatized limbs: Experimental study. Surg. Gynecol. Obstet., *50:*196, 1930.

Pepe, P. E., Potkin, R. T., Reus, D. H., et al.: Clinical predictors of the adult respiratory distress syndrome. Am. J. Surg., *144:*124, 1982.

Peters, W. P., Johnson, M. W., Friedman, P. A., and Mitch, W. E.: Pressor effect of naloxone in septic shock. Lancet, *1:*529, 1981.

Rees, M., Bowen, J. C., Payne, J. G., and Macphee, A. A.: Plasma beta-endorphin immunoreactivity in dogs during anesthesia, surgery, *E. coli* sepsis, and naloxone therapy. Surgery, *93:*386, 1983.

Reines, H. D., Halushka, P. V., and Cook, J. A.: Plasma thromboxane levels are elevated in patients dying with septic shock. Lancet, 2:174, 1982.

Revhaug, A., Michie, H., Manson, J., et al.: Inhibition of cyclooxygenase attenuates the metabolic response of endotoxin in humans. Arch. Surg., *123:*162, 1988.

Reynolds, D., Gurll, N. G., and Vargish, T.: Blockade of opiate receptors with naloxone improves survival and cardiac performance in canine endotoxin shock. Circ. Shock, 7:39, 1980.

Richardson, J. D., DeCamp, M. M., Garrison, R. N., et al.: Pulmonary infection complicating intra-abdominal sepsis: Clinical and experimental observations. Ann. Surg., *195:*732, 1982.

Shires, G. T., Carrico, C. J., and Canizaro, P. C.: Shock. Volume 13 of the series Major Problems in Clinical Surgery. Philadelphia, W. B. Saunders, 1973.

Siegel, J. H., Goldwyn, R. M., and Friedman, H. P.: Pattern and process in the evolution of human septic shock. Surgery, *70:*323, 1971.

Siegel, J. H., Greenspan, M., and Del Guercio, R. R. M.: Abnormal vascular tone, defective oxygen transport, and myocardial failure in human septic shock. Ann. Surg., *165:*504, 1967.

Stoutenbeck, C., Van Saene, H., Miranda, D., et al.: The effect of selective decontamination of the digestive tract on colonization and infection rate in multiple trauma patients. Intensive Care Med., *10:*185, 1984.

Swan, H. J. C., Forrester, J. S., Danzig, R., and Allen, H. N.: Power failure in acute myocardial infarction. Prog. Cardiovasc. Dis., *12:*568, 1970.

Tilney, N. L., Bailey, G. L., and Morgan, A. P.: Sequential system failure after rupture of abdominal aortic aneurysms: An unsolved problem in postoperative care. Ann. Surg., *178:*117, 1973.

Tracey, K. J., Fong, Y., Hesse, D. G., et al.: Anticachectin/TNF monoclonal antibodies prevent septic shock during lethal bacteremia. Nature, *330:*662, 1987.

Tracey, K. J., Lowry, S. F., Beutler, B., et al.: Cachectin/tumor necrosis factor participates in reduction of skeletal muscle plasma membrane potential: Evidence of bioactivity in plasma during critical illness. Surg. Forum, *37:*13, 1986.

West, M. A., Keller, G., Hyland, B., et al.: Hepatocyte function in sepsis: Kupffer cells mediate a biphasic protein synthesis response in hepatocytes after endotoxin and killed *E. coli.* Surgery, 98:388, 1985.

Whittle, B. J. R., and Moncada, S.: Pharmacologic interactions between prostacyclin and thromboxanes. Br. Med. Bull., *39:*232, 1983.

Zamir, A., Hasselgren, P. O., O'Brien, W., et al.: Muscle protein breakdown during endotoxemia in rats and after treatment with interleukin-1 receptor antagonist (IL-1ra). Ann. Surg., *216:*381, 1992.

Ziegler, E. J., Fisher, C. J., Sprung, C. L., et al.: Treatment of gram-negative bacteremia and septic shock with HA-1A human monoclonal antibody against endotoxin: A randomized, double-blind, placebo-controlled trial. N. Engl. J. Med., *324:*429, 1991.

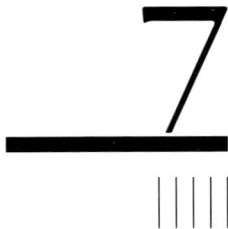

7 Thoracic Incisions

Fred A. Crawford, Jr., and John M. Kratz

HISTORY

Access to the mediastinum and the thoracic cavities has not been practical until modern times, because life-threatening pneumothorax prevented early surgeons from performing significant procedures within the thorax. The earliest attempts to treat intrathoracic disease were made approximately 2400 years ago, when Hippocrates described drainage of empyema. By the late 19th century, resection of the herniated lung or the lung firmly adherent to the chest wall had been accomplished. Routine operations within the thorax awaited the development of a negative pressure chamber by Sauerbruch in 1904 and the development of endotracheal anesthesia by Elsberg in 1911 (Meade, 1961).

In early thoracic surgical procedures, exposure was obtained by resection of the chest wall or flaps with division of at least two or three ribs. In 1892, Tuffier described the modern intercostal incision that was used to do the first successful resection for tuberculosis, and Meyer (1910) and Torek (1913) popularized the intercostal incision for access to the thoracic cavity. The median sternotomy was described by Milton in 1897 for exposure of mediastinal masses, and it was predicted at the time that this approach might well be used for cardiac surgery. Use of the median sternotomy was subsequently described by Holman and Willett (1949) for pericardiectomy and by Shumacker and Lurie (1953) for cardiac surgery. However, it was the report by Julian in 1957 that led to the widespread adaption of the sternotomy incision for all types of cardiac procedures.

Over the years, different approaches to organs within the thoracic cavity have varied in popularity. Some procedures may be satisfactorily done through several different incisions. For example, pulmonary resections are most commonly done through a posterolateral thoracotomy, but they can also be performed through a posterior or anterior thoracotomy and, more recently, through a median sternotomy. The choice of incision depends on the particular patient and the individual surgeon's experience, skill, and preference. The thoracic surgeon must have confidence and skill with each of the available incisions so that the most suitable operation for the anatomic and physiologic problems of the patient can be done.

INCISION AND CLOSURE

The key to successful thoracic surgical procedures is adequate and proper exposure. A well-chosen thoracic incision provides effortless and excellent exposure for almost any procedure. However, an ill-chosen or an improperly placed or performed incision often leads to a difficult and frustrating procedure with the danger of a failed operation.

Proper positioning of the patient on the operating table is essential to achieve a safe and satisfactory procedure. The patient must be positioned in a secure and stable manner. Plastic "bean bags" (Vacpac, Olympic Medical Co., Seattle, WA), which can be made firm by evacuating air after positioning, are helpful in maintaining position. Pressure points of nerves and vascular structures must be padded and protected to prevent injury during the operation. The electrocautery ground plate must be applied securely and must be kept dry when the skin is prepared. When positioning is satisfactory, the patient's respiratory and cardiovascular systems are easily accessed for monitoring and manipulation.

Several techniques are available for sterile preparation of the skin at the site of the incision. The surgeon must ensure that the area of operative exposure does not include any areas of ongoing sepsis, even to the most minor degree of skin scratches or irritation. Clipping is preferred to shaving hair as a method used to prevent injury to the skin. The area of skin prepared must be adequate for the primary incision as well as for vascular access, possible donor sites for vein grafts, or mobilization of gastrointestinal organs. The patient must then be draped to preserve the sterility of the wound throughout the surgical procedure. Current surgical practice demands a nonporous draping system to prevent contamination of the operative field through wet drapes and by bacterial migration. Large clear plastic adhesive drapes that are impregnated with iodine provide complete access to the operative site while ensuring a draping system that is impervious and resistant to displacement until the procedure is complete.

Before beginning the procedure, the surgeon should ensure that various peripheral support systems are in position and that these systems are functioning properly. Foley catheterization is usually indicated for long thoracic procedures. Arterial catheters should be easily accessed by the anesthesiologist, and intravenous access must be adequate. Placement of a double-lumen endotracheal tube prevents contamination of the opposite lung and enhances exposure for procedures such as correction of aneurysms, repair of a ruptured bronchus, and pulmonary resection through a median sternotomy. Correct positioning of this tube may be assisted by the use of a small bronchoscope that is inserted into the lumen of the tube.

The incision itself should be placed carefully so that it is located precisely where the operative procedure is to be done. Entry into an interspace that is higher or lower than intended may lead to unsatisfactory exposure. The incision should be long enough to provide complete exposure without too much tension on the tissues. Meticulous hemostasis throughout the operative procedure is essential; it should be obtained during the procedure and should not be postponed until later. Careful use of the electrocautery is essential to obtain satisfactory hemostasis during thoracic procedures and to ensure future healing.

Closure of thoracic incisions should provide for maximal stability and comfort in the postoperative period. Closure of all dead space in layers is essential. Chest tubes should be brought through the skin anteriorly enough to allow the patient to recline in the supine position comfortably without putting pressure on the tubes. Dressings that are applied to thoracic incisions should ensure adequate protection of the wound but should be as light as possible to ensure patient comfort.

RIB RESECTION

The technique of rib resection is particularly important because it is integral to many thoracic procedures. Resection of a rib may be the major part of the procedure itself (e.g., in rib resection for bone grafting or drainage of an empyema) or it may be necessary to improve exposure (e.g., in a posterolateral thoracotomy). For rib resection for bone graft harvesting, the patient is placed in a supine position on the operating table, and a slight roll is placed beneath the hip and the shoulder to rotate the side of the patient that is to undergo operation slightly upward. This position permits the choice of several different ribs if more than one is required and is adequate for most procedures. If extreme lengths of rib are required, the patient may be placed in a position similar to the one used for a standard posterolateral thoracotomy. When performing rib resection for drainage of an empyema, the site of empyema dictates the positioning so that exposure of the intended area is adequate. However, a standard lateral position similar to the position used in a posterolateral thoracotomy is generally indicated.

For drainage of an empyema, the site of incision must be selected carefully; the eighth rib is the area that is usually chosen for this procedure. Incisions at higher levels frequently do not provide adequate dependent drainage, whereas incisions at lower levels may be obstructed by the diaphragm. The incision is also placed in a position between the midaxillary and posterior axillary line, because incisions that are more anterior may not provide adequate drainage, and incisions that are more posterior cause discomfort for the patient while he is lying in the bed. The incision is made directly over the eighth rib, and sharp dissection is extended through the muscular layers to the

rib. Hemostasis must be complete while the muscular layers are being divided. Tissues are frequently inflamed, and hemostasis can be a problem without meticulous attention. Periosteal elevators are used to raise the periosteum from the surface of the rib (Fig. 7–1). A subperiosteal plane between the periosteum and rib is developed posteriorly. After the periosteum is excised completely from the rib, the rib is removed by using large bone shears. A large-bore needle is used to aspirate the underlying thoracic cavity to locate purulent material beneath the periosteal bed and thickened pleura. The bed of the periosteum is then incised, entering the empyema cavity, and the incision in the periosteum is extended for the full length of the rib resection. The cavity is irrigated and is emptied of its contents. Soft, large-bore rubber tubing is inserted, and careful attention is paid to the length to prevent undue pressure on the underlying pulmonary structures.

Subperiosteal resection of the rib is also indicated when bone graft material is being obtained or when increased exposure is necessary. If periosteum is removed with the rib for bone graft, the periosteum becomes necrotic and does not contribute to the graft. However, periosteum left within the site of rib resection usually regenerates a new rib. It is possible to obtain several portions of rib for grafting by alternating ribs that must be resected. A rib is left intact between each site of rib resection if considerable bone graft is required. Rib resection for donor bone graft

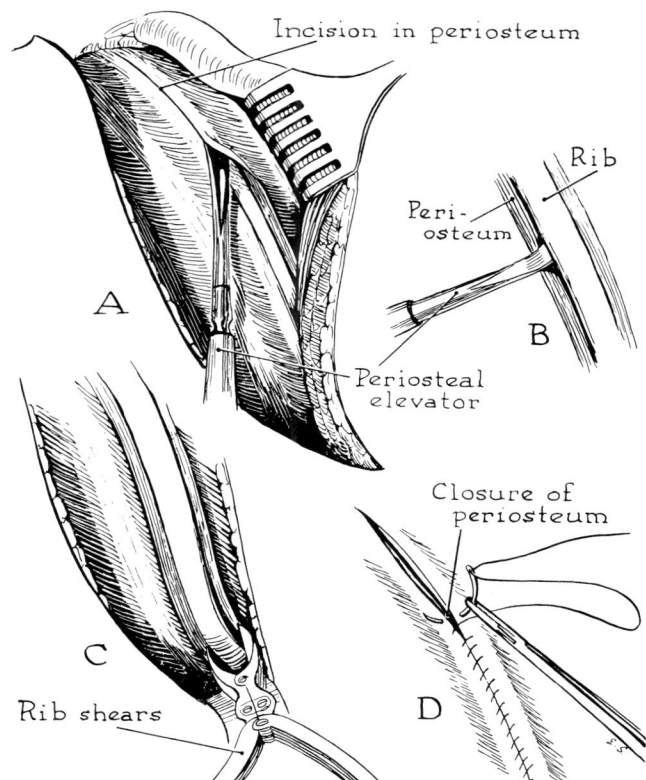

FIGURE 7–1. A–D, Technique of rib resection in posterolateral thoracotomy. Posteriorly, the rib is divided close to the transverse process.

may be closed with multiple layers of absorbable sutures, and the skin is closed according to preference.

POSTEROLATERAL THORACOTOMY

The posterolateral thoracotomy is one of the most frequently used incisions in thoracic surgery. Most pulmonary resections are easily performed with this approach, which also provides excellent access to the mediastinum for resection of mediastinal masses and esophageal procedures. Some cardiac procedures, such as coarctation repair, patent ductus arteriosus ligation, pulmonary artery banding, and thoracic aneurysm resection, may also be performed through this incision.

Positioning for posterolateral thoracotomy is important both to ensure patient stability during the procedure and to protect various neurovascular structures from injury by pressure. The patient is placed in a true lateral position on the operating table. A roll is placed beneath the axilla to protect the axillary contents from pressure during the procedure. The lower leg is flexed almost to a 90-degree angle, and the upper leg is extended straight after a pillow is

placed between the knees. The hips are stabilized with wide adhesive tape that extends from one side of the table to the other. The lower arm is supported with an armboard, and the upper arm is supported with pillows or an armboard. The upper arm should be fairly mobile during the procedure so that the shoulder girdle may be mobilized upward to allow access into higher interspaces. If access to the femoral vessels is necessary for cardiopulmonary bypass, the hips may be rotated more posteriorly.

The purpose of the initial incision is to mobilize the shoulder girdle to allow it to slide upward to expose the appropriate interspace for entry into the thoracic cavity. The incision in the skin extends from just below the nipple posteriorly to 1 inch below the tip of the scapula, and then the incision extends upward between the scapula and the spine (Fig. 7–2). Subcutaneous tissues are incised, after which the latissimus dorsi and the serratus anterior muscles are divided. Bleeding from these muscles during entry into the chest can be significant, and meticulous attention to hemostasis by cautery is essential. After the latissimus and serratus have been divided, the shoulder girdle glides upward and allows the scapula to retract away from the intended intercostal incision. The proper interspace may be found by counting ribs from the

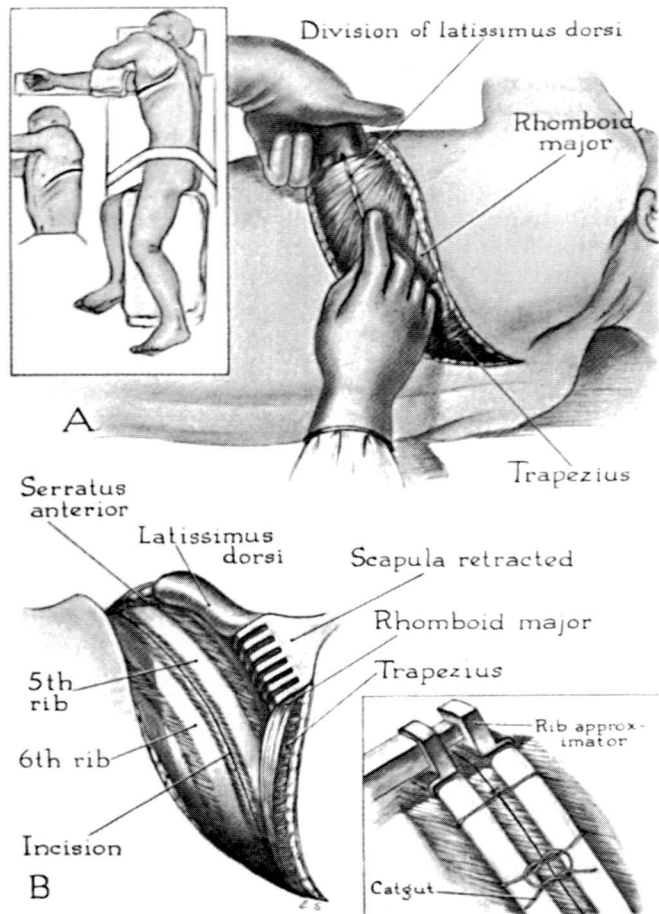

FIGURE 7–2. *A* and *B*, Posterolateral thoracotomy incision.

top of the ribs to the base of the ribs. The surgeon's hand is inserted beneath the scapula in a loose areolar plane and is moved upward. A moderately firm fascial layer usually prevents the surgeon's hand from reaching the first rib. The ribs are then counted downward from the second rib until the appropriate level is selected.

Operations that primarily require control of the hilum of the lung, such as pulmonary resection, are best done through the fifth intercostal space, whereas procedures such as ligation of a patent ductus arteriosus and coarctation repair are best done through the fourth intercostal space. The best approach for repair of hiatal hernia and Heller's esophagomyotomy is through the seventh or eighth intercostal space.

When the appropriate intercostal space has been selected, it is marked, and the intercostal muscles are divided for a short distance to obtain entry into the chest. Just prior to dividing the pleura, the surgeon must observe free motion of the lung beneath the pleural surface. If free motion is not observed, particular care must be taken to avoid inadvertent entry into the pulmonary parenchyma. Once the pleural cavity is entered, the lung is allowed to collapse and fall away from the chest wall. The intercostal muscle is divided for the length of the incision, and care is taken to avoid the intercostal artery by incising close to the lower rib. Care must also be taken posteriorly while the intercostal muscles are being divided, because transection of the intercostal artery and nerve may also occur easily at this site. A chest retractor is placed so as to spread the intercostal space and to retract the tip of the scapula from the operative field. The retractor should be opened gradually and gently so that rib fractures are avoided.

The first step in closure of the incision is placement of chest tubes within the thoracic cavity. A chest tube is placed anteriorly principally for evacuation of air, and a second tube is placed posteriorly for drainage of fluid and blood. These tubes leave the chest laterally through separate incisions. The ribs are approximated with a rib approximator, and five to six sutures of heavy absorbable material are used to restore the ribs to their normal position. Overzealous tightening of these sutures with collapse of the intercostal space should be avoided. Closure of the intercostal muscles is usually not required. The serratus anterior and latissimus dorsi are closed separately, and an accurate approximation of these muscles should be made carefully. The subcutaneous tissue and skin are then closed.

ANTEROLATERAL THORACOTOMY

The anterolateral thoracotomy and variations of this incision may be used for many thoracic procedures. The length of the incision may vary with the operative procedure. A short parasternal incision over the second or third intercostal space provides satisfactory exposure of the mediastinum and thoracic cavity for staging of carcinoma of the lung. This incision has been especially useful with lesions on the left side, which frequently metastasize to lymph nodes in the anterior mediastinum. A lengthened second or third intercostal anterior thoracotomy provides excellent exposure for limited pulmonary procedures such as bullectomy and open lung biopsy. Anterolateral thoracotomy in the fourth or fifth intercostal space affords adequate exposure for closure of atrial septal defects, mitral valve surgery, pacemaker insertion, some systemic pulmonary shunts, and ligation of patent ductus arteriosus.

The patient is placed in a supine position on the operating table. A pad is placed beneath the shoulder and the hip on the side that is to undergo operation to roll the patient approximately 20 degrees upward and to provide access to the lateral portion of the chest wall. Placing the hand of the operative side in the small of the back allows adequate exposure of the lateral chest wall and relaxes the muscles of the shoulder girdle. The incision is placed directly over the intended interspace, except in a woman, in which case the incision may be placed just below the breast. The pectoralis muscle is divided, and the chosen interspace is opened for the entire length of the incision. If the incision is extended to the sternum medially, the internal mammary artery and vein should be isolated and controlled. The intercostal space may be relaxed to allow further exposure by division of the intercostal muscles beyond the length of the incision from within the chest cavity. Closure is similar to closure for the posterolateral thoracotomy.

POSTERIOR THORACOTOMY

The posterior thoracotomy, which was popularized by Overholt and others, is described primarily for historical reasons. Although this incision has been used previously with excellent success for pulmonary procedures, it is now seldom used for this type of thoracotomy. The patient is placed in the prone position on a special table that not only allows the entire chest to be prepared but also adequately supports the patient. Entry is accomplished by a posterior intercostal incision. This incision provides the benefits of preventing accumulated blood or purulent material from the side undergoing the operation from draining into the lung that has not undergone operation, and it allows blood that has accumulated within the operative field to drain, thereby not obscuring exposure. Despite these advantages, the disadvantages of requiring a special table to support the patient and the difficulties in anesthetic management and observation of the patient have caused surgeons to choose other types of incision.

LATERAL MUSCLE–SPARING THORACOTOMY

Although it provides excellent exposure, the posterior lateral thoracotomy may be associated with severe postoperative pain and decreased pulmonary function. Late complications, including persistent incisional pain, frozen shoulder, pulmonary function impairment, and reduced arm strength, may also occur. With the advent of improved anesthesia using double-lumen tube ventilation, surgical stapling devices, and improved technical skills, surgeons have sought to use less extensive incisions in an attempt to avoid these complications. Many variations in the limited lateral muscle-sparing thoracotomy have been described. However, certain principles apply universally. The latissimus and serratus muscles are mobilized and retracted rather than divided, and rib retraction is limited with extensive division of the intercostal muscles to avoid fracture of a rib.

Most surgeons using these limited incisions feel that the benefits of *decreased pain* and *smoother recovery* are obvious in their patients. Three studies comparing the limited thoracotomy with the standard posterolateral thoracotomy have been performed. Lemmer and associates (1990) and Ponn and co-workers (1992) found improvement in pulmonary functions that require forced expiration in which accessory muscles of

the chest wall are used, such as forced vital capacity or 1-second expiratory volumes. Functions that measure capacity at rest, such as alveolar-arterial oxygen gradient, functional residual capacity, and total lung capacity, were not improved in any of the three studies. Lemmer and associates (1990) and Hazelrigg and co-workers (1991) found improvement in early muscle strength, perceived pain, and narcotic use in the group undergoing limited thoracotomy, but these advantages rapidly disappeared on longer follow-up. Most series have documented wound seromas in approximately 10% of patients as the result of extensive skin flap mobilization.

The patient is positioned just as for a posterolateral thoracotomy. The skin incision may be made either as a transverse incision from the submammary fold at the anterior axillary line to just below the scapular tip (Fig. 7–3A) or as a vertical incision beginning in the midaxillary line below the hairline and turning anteriorly to extend into the submammary fold. Subcutaneous skin flaps are developed to allow mobilization of the latissimus and serratus muscles (Fig. 7–3B). Once adequate skin flaps are developed, the anterior

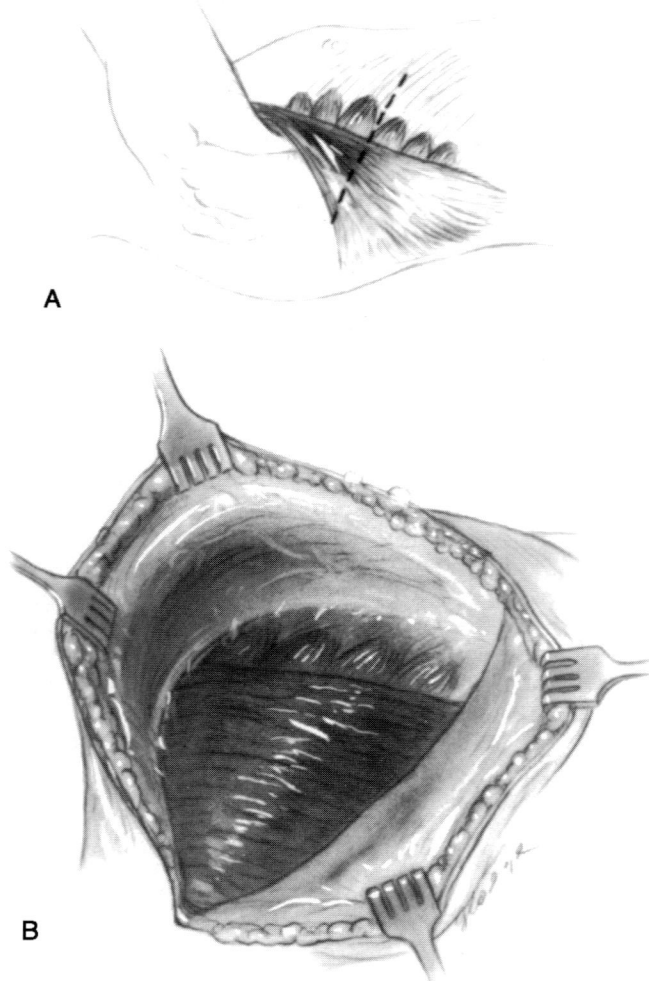

A

B

FIGURE 7–3. Muscle-sparing thoracotomy. *A,* Transverse incision. *B,* Subcutaneous flaps are developed over latissimus and serratus muscles.

Illustration continued on opposite page

border of the latissimus dorsi muscle is dissected. The entire latissimus is then developed bluntly, leaving its insertions intact (Fig. 7–3C). After the latissimus is mobilized and retracted posteriorly, the serratus anterior muscle is similarly dissected and mobilized, allowing it to be retracted anteriorly (Fig. 7–3D). The surgeon's hand is inserted beneath the muscles to determine the appropriate interspace for entry into the chest (Fig. 7–3E), the rib below the appropriate interspace for entry into the chest is scored (Fig. 7–3F), and the operator's finger is slipped beneath the serratus, and the muscle fibers overlying the level of intended entry are divided (Fig. 7–3G). Blunt dissection then divides the serratus muscle fibers over the interspace to be entered (Fig. 7–3H), the chest is entered in the appropriate interspace (Fig. 7–3I), and a Tuffier retractor is placed as the interspace is opened (Fig. 7–3J). After the chest is entered, the interspace is fully opened from the internal mammary artery anteriorly to the transverse processes posteriorly well past the extent of the skin and muscular opening (Fig. 7–3K). The ribs are spread with a single-bladed chest retractor, and a second retractor is placed at right angles to the first to retract the latissimus and serratus muscles (Fig. 7–3L). At the end of the procedure, the undivided muscles fall naturally into place without suture. Closed suction drains are placed beneath the skin flaps to prevent seroma formation (Fig. 7–3M).

THORACOABDOMINAL INCISION

Used less frequently than in the past, the thoracoabdominal incision is useful for increasing exposure to the upper abdomen, which may sometimes be needed for extended liver resections, removal of a massive enlarged spleen, total gastrectomy, and adrenalectomy or other retroperitoneal operations. It is also useful when simultaneous exposure of the upper abdomen and lower chest is needed (e.g., with tumors at the esophagogastric junction and for thoracoabdominal aortic aneurysms). The incision requires additional time for opening and closing and causes increased postoperative discomfort.

The patient's shoulders are placed in an almost lateral position, and the hips are rotated back toward

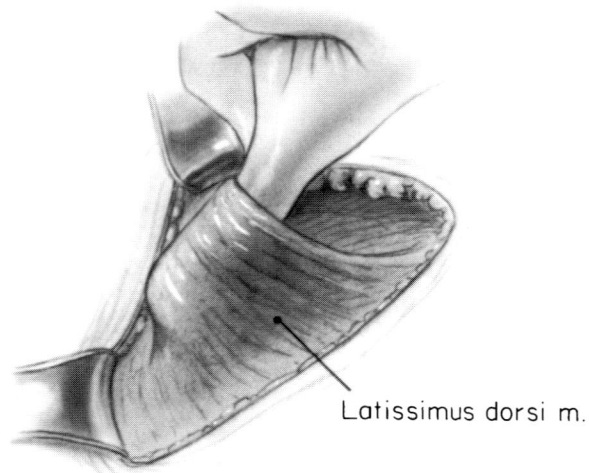

FIGURE 7–3 *Continued C,* The latissimus is developed bluntly. *D,* The serratus is similarly developed and retracted.

Illustration continued on following page

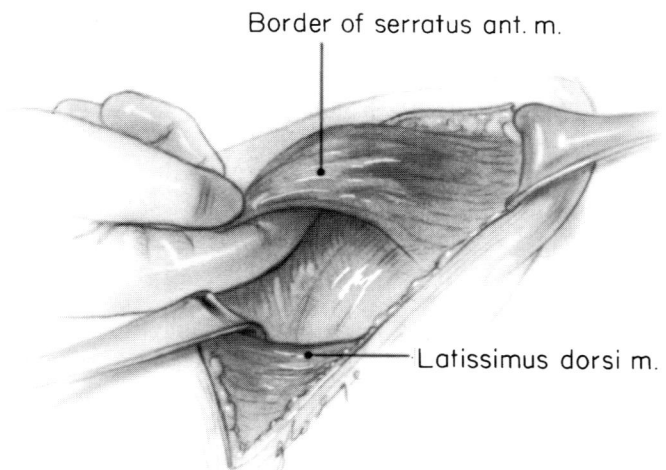

Latissimus dorsi m.

C

Border of serratus ant. m.

Latissimus dorsi m.

D

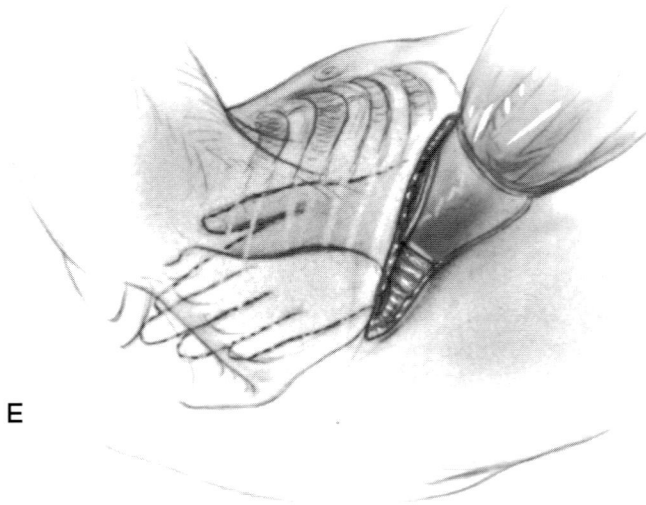

E

FIGURE 7–3 *Continued E,* Interspaces are counted from above downward. *F,* The appropriate interspace is marked with the cautery.

Illustration continued on opposite page

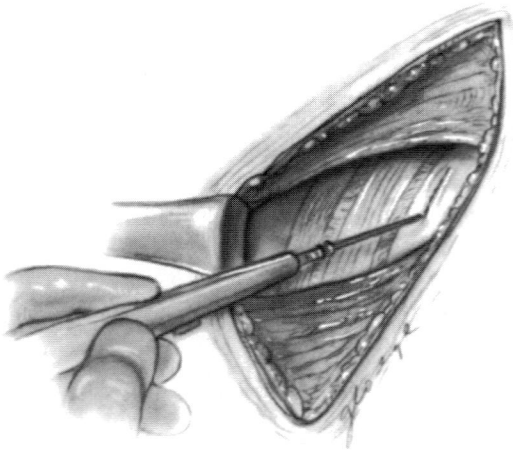

F

the supine position. The incision extends from the abdominal midline, midway between the xiphoid and umbilicus, up and across the costal margin and to the seventh or eighth intercostal space to the posterior axillary line (Fig. 7–4A). The serratus anterior and external oblique fibers are split in the line of the incision, the intercostal muscles are divided, and the pleural space is entered. The anterior rectus sheath, rectus muscle, and posterior rectus sheath are divided, and the peritoneal cavity is entered. The costal margin is divided sharply, and the diaphragm may be opened peripherally 3 to 4 cm from the costal margin or radially toward the esophageal hiatus. In either case, care must be taken to avoid direct or stretch injuries to the phrenic nerve and its branches. A second incision may be made in the fourth intercostal space when access to the upper thoracic cavity is required (Fig. 7–4B and C). Appropriate retractors are inserted, and the incision is opened. The extent of the incision into the chest wall and abdomen depends on the patient's size and the amount of exposure needed (Fig. 7–4D).

After the surgical procedure is completed, the diaphragm is repaired with interrupted nonabsorbable sutures. Several centimeters of costal cartilage may be removed to prevent friction between cut ends and to reduce postoperative pain. The thoracic and abdominal portions of the incisions are closed in layers.

RECONSTRUCTION OF THE CHEST WALL

Small resections of the chest wall are usually tolerated without requiring the reconstruction of the rigid thoracic cage. However, when large portions of the chest wall are resected, reconstruction of the chest wall may be necessary to preserve pulmonary and cardiac function.

In previous years, successful reconstruction of the chest wall was accomplished with fascia lata, polypropylene mesh, or stainless-steel mesh. Although these methods continue to suffice, they do not reconstitute a completely rigid chest wall, and some materials that are used are subject to fragmentation and deterioration later on. In 1981, McCormack and asso-

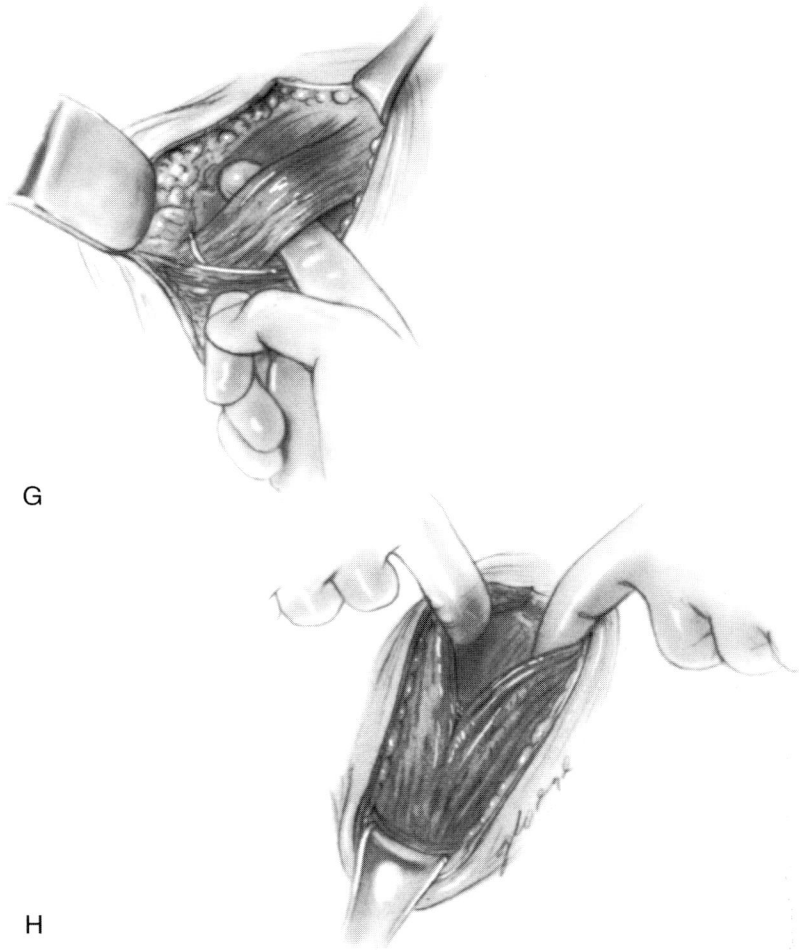

Illustration continued on following page

FIGURE 7–3 *Continued G,* The serratus muscle fibers over the chosen interspace are located. *H,* The identified muscle fibers are bluntly divided.

ciates described reconstruction of large chest wall defects with a sandwich of polypropylene mesh and methyl methacrylate glue. The sandwich may be constructed and allowed to solidify outside the body on the operating table and then sutured in place, or it may be formed within the defect to be reconstructed. Our preference is to suture a layer of polypropylene mesh to the parietal pleura. A moist laparotomy pad is placed beneath the mesh to protect the underlying organs, and methyl methacrylate glue is then mixed and applied to the mesh to fill the defect in the chest wall. A second layer of polypropylene mesh is then embedded within this layer of methyl methacrylate glue and is sutured to the chest wall. When this layer has hardened, a rigid shell takes shape, adheres to the chest wall, and replaces the excised segment of the chest wall. Methyl methacrylate glue undergoes an endothermic reaction while it is curing. Care must be taken to allow partial curing of the methyl methacrylate before applying it to the tissues. Underlying structures must be protected from the heat that is generated as a result of the endothermic reaction. In addition, the curing process, which is a chemical reaction, releases hydrogen ions and may cause systemic acidosis if the glue is exposed to raw tissue surfaces.

Large defects in the chest wall may also be repaired with muscular or myocutaneous flaps (Pairolero and Arnold, 1985). Three typical defects may require reconstruction. Large defects created as the result of removal of tumors in the chest wall or sternum may be closed by using muscular or myocutaneous flaps that are applied over the lung and heart or in conjunction with one of the aforementioned methods to make the chest wall rigid again. Muscles including the pectoralis major, serratus, latissimus dorsi, and rectus may be used. The defect may then be covered by skin grafting.

A second defect in which muscle transposition may be helpful is the post–pulmonary resection empyema space with or without bronchopleural fistula. The latissimus dorsi provides a bulky muscle to fill many defects, whereas the pectoralis major may fill the upper thorax, and the rectus may be used to fill the lower thorax. With larger defects such as the postpneumonectomy empyema, all of these muscles, with the possible addition of the serratus and omentum, may be required (Miller et al., 1984). Muscle transpo-

I

J

L

K

M

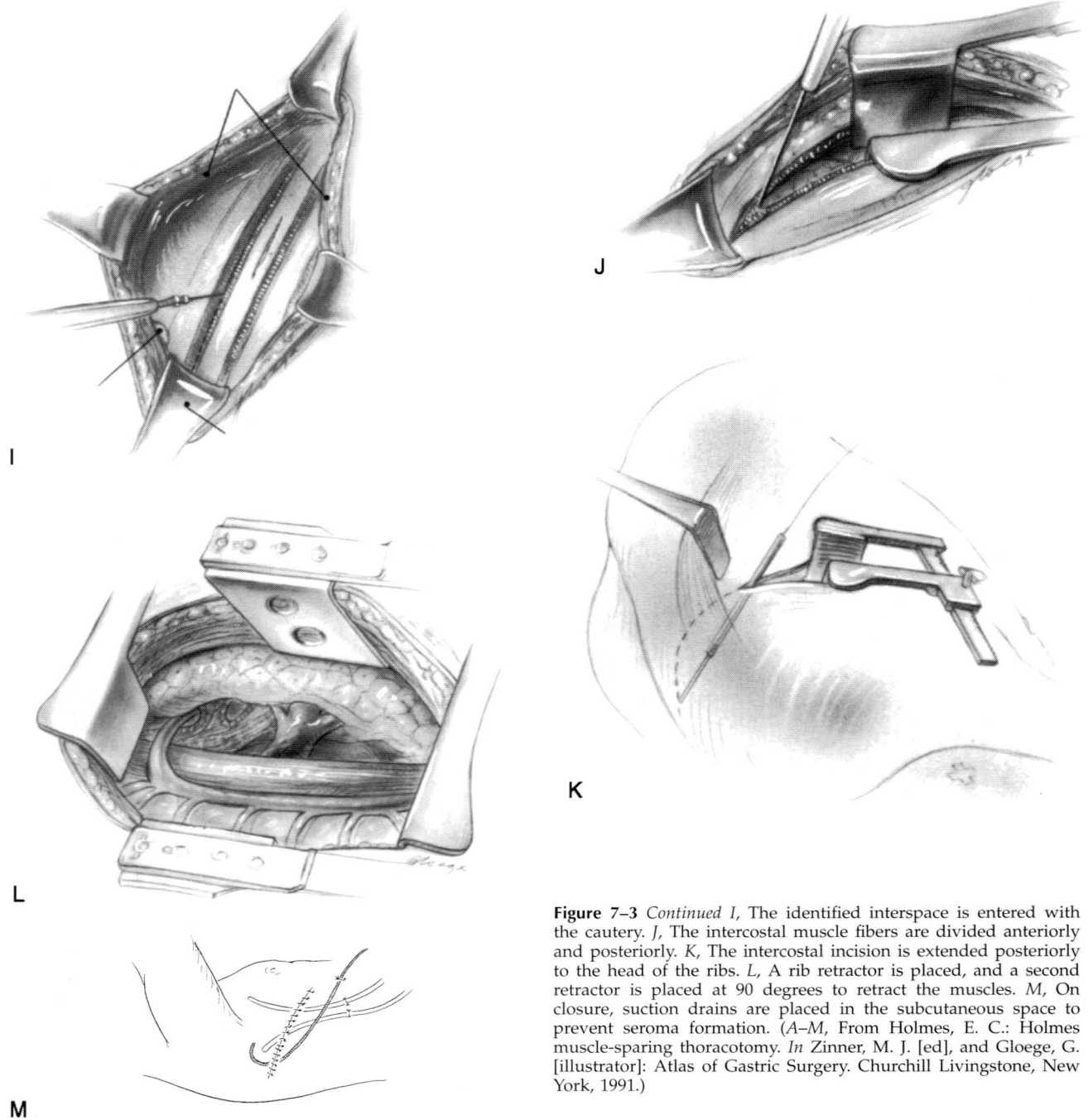

Figure 7–3 *Continued I,* The identified interspace is entered with the cautery. *J,* The intercostal muscle fibers are divided anteriorly and posteriorly. *K,* The intercostal incision is extended posteriorly to the head of the ribs. *L,* A rib retractor is placed, and a second retractor is placed at 90 degrees to retract the muscles. *M,* On closure, suction drains are placed in the subcutaneous space to prevent seroma formation. (*A–M,* From Holmes, E. C.: Holmes muscle-sparing thoracotomy. *In* Zinner, M. J. [ed], and Gloege, G. [illustrator]: Atlas of Gastric Surgery. Churchill Livingstone, New York, 1991.)

sition or a myocutaneous flap is also useful in the management of mediastinitis.

MEDIAN STERNOTOMY

Median sternotomy is now used for most cardiac operations as well as for other procedures that include thymectomy and resection of mediastinal tumors. Be-

cause of sternotomy's favorable characteristics, including familiarity, ease of performance, and simplicity, it has been suggested that various other common thoracic procedures may be performed as well via sternotomy as by the traditional thoracotomy approach. These procedures include bilateral simultaneous pleurodesis for recurrent pneumothorax (Kalnins et al., 1973), resection of multiple bilateral pulmonary metastases (Regal et al., 1985), and resection of bilateral bullous disease (Iwa et al., 1981). Urschel and

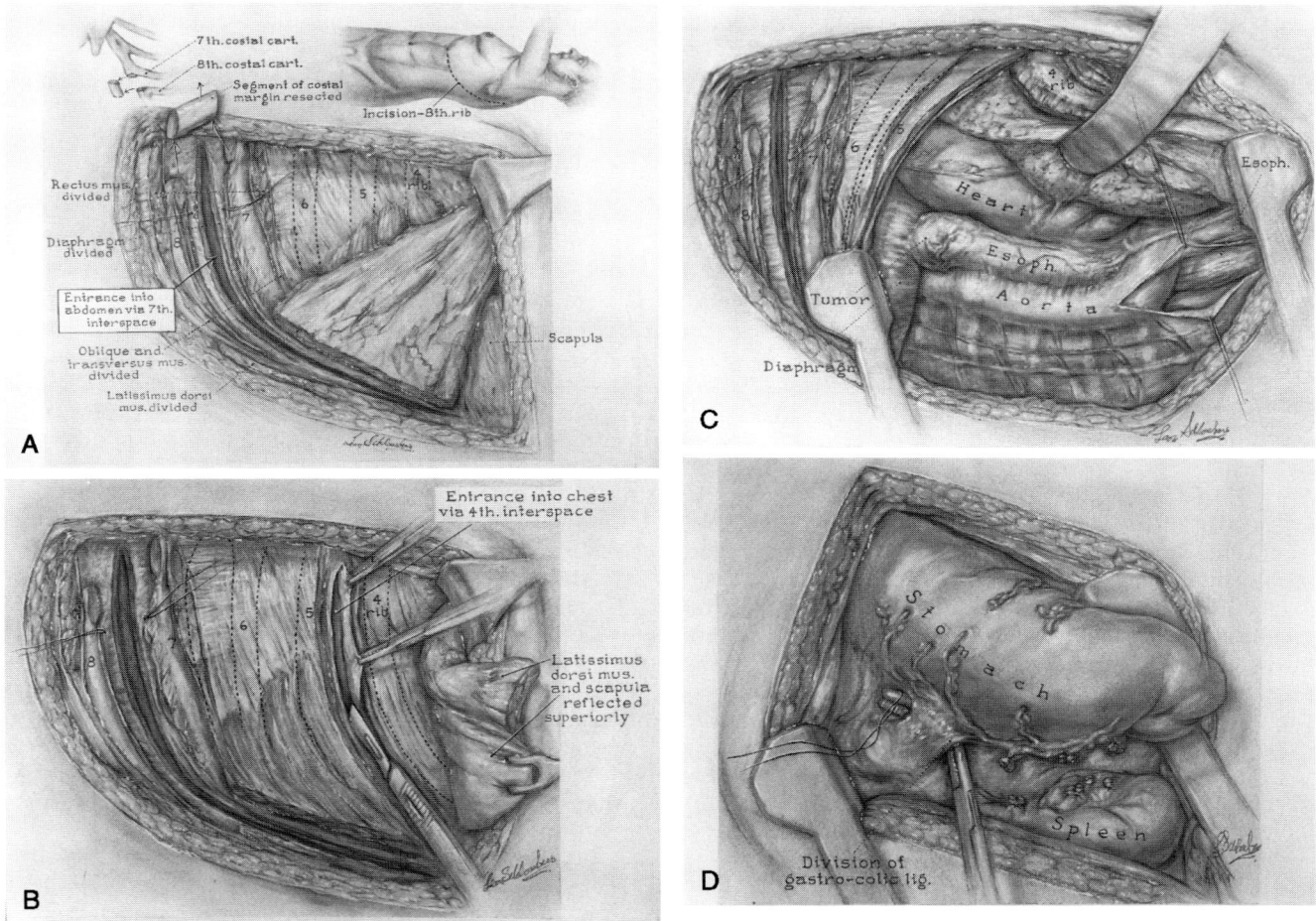

FIGURE 7–4. Thoracoabdominal incision. *A,* Patients are positioned as for a left thoracotomy. However, the hips are angled back to facilitate abdominal exposure. Also shown is the seventh interspace approach with the cut diaphragmatic edges marked with long silk sutures. *B,* Surgeon's view of exposed left quadrant. *C,* To perform a counterincision, the scapula is raised off the bony chest wall, and a second, higher interspace is entered. Seventh and fourth interspace incisions are shown here. *D,* Exposure of the supra-aortic esophagus through a separate fourth-interspace incision. (*A–D,* From Heitmiller, R. F.: The left thoracoabdominal incision. *46:*250–253, 1988. Reprinted with permission from the Society of Thoracic Surgeons [The Annals of Thoracic Surgery, 1988, Vol. 46, pp. 250–253].)

Razzuk (1986) reported a series of 174 patients who underwent pulmonary resection by median sternotomy. These included 23 pneumonectomies, 81 lobectomies, and 14 segmental resections. When compared with a similar group who underwent pulmonary resections with standard thoracotomy, the patients who had undergone sternotomy had a shorter time in operation, a shorter hospital stay, and less pain. Watanabe and associates (1988) confirmed these findings in a series of 73 patients.

The sternotomy incision is popular for cardiac procedures primarily because of the rapid and excellent exposure it provides of all parts of the heart. It also offers several advantages for pulmonary resection. The incision is quickly and easily made, which shortens operative time. Because no muscles are divided and the bone is stabilized after closure, most surgeons agree that this procedure is less painful than a standard thoracotomy incision. Perhaps because of this finding, many believe that pulmonary function is better and that atelectasis is reduced after sternotomy (Watanabe et al., 1988). Although vital capacity and

peak flow measurements were reduced after both sternotomy and thoracotomy, Cooper and associates (1978) showed that this reduction was significantly greater in patients who had undergone thoracotomy. In addition, recovery of function was faster after sternotomy.

The sternotomy incision is performed with the patient in the supine position. This alters the physiology of ventilation-perfusion less than the lateral thoracotomy incision does (in which the dependent lung provides most of the gas exchange). Because of the more normal physiology during operation and the improved pulmonary function postoperatively, it is reasonable to believe that patients with poor pulmonary function might be better surgical candidates if a sternotomy is used (Asaph and Keppel, 1984). Finally, some pulmonary problems are frequently bilateral (e.g., metastases and bullous disease). When these problems are approached through a sternotomy, both sides can be managed simultaneously, and the patient is spared the expense, pain, and loss of time necessitated by staged bilateral procedures.

The patient is placed in a supine position on the operating table, and the arms can be either extended or placed by the patient's side. Although most anesthesiologists prefer to have one or both of the patient's arms extended for access to arterial and intravenous lines, we have found that by careful positioning and padding of the arms, it is possible to routinely place both arms at the patient's sides, thus improving the comfort of the operating team. By placing a small pad between the patient's scapula and tilting the head slightly to one side, access to the upper end of the incision is improved, especially in obese patients.

The incision is made with a scalpel from just beneath the suprasternal notch to a point between the xiphoid and the umbilicus (Fig. 7–5). The incision is extended to the sternal periosteum and linea alba with either a scalpel or electrocautery. Excessive use of electrocautery may increase the incidence of postoperative sternal infection; accordingly, precise and discriminant use is recommended (Nishida et al., 1991). The periosteum is scored in the midline with electrocautery, the linea alba is divided at the xiphoid, and a plane is created behind the sternum at the suprasternal notch. It is unnecessary to dissect completely behind the sternum from the suprasternal notch to the xiphoid. The sternum is divided carefully in the midline using an electric sternal saw with a vertical oscillating blade. The sternal division is per-

formed equally well from the sternal notch to the xiphoid and in the opposite direction, depending on the surgeon's preference. Alternatively, the sternum can be divided using an oscillating saw or a Lebske knife, but both of these techniques are much less satisfactory. It is useful to have the anesthesiologist temporarily deflate the lungs as the sternum is divided. This may help prevent entering the pleural spaces, particularly in those patients with chronic obstructive pulmonary disease and hyperinflated lungs. Bleeding from the sternal periosteum is best controlled with electrocautery. In the past, bone wax was routinely used to control marrow bleeding, but its use has been abandoned on all but rare occasions because of the possibility of impaired wound healing and pulmonary complications related to the embolization of the wax to the lungs. Robicsek and associates (1981) demonstrated that postoperative bleeding does not increase when bone wax is not used. Accordingly, it is reserved for those patients who have refractory bleeding from sternal fractures, and even then, it should be used sparingly. A sternal retractor with broad blades is carefully positioned and opened slowly. The cross arm of the retractor may be positioned in either the upper or the lower end of the incision, depending on the surgeon's preference. By opening the retractor only a few turns at a time, one is usually able to avoid sternal fractures, especially in older patients with osteoporosis. The sternum should

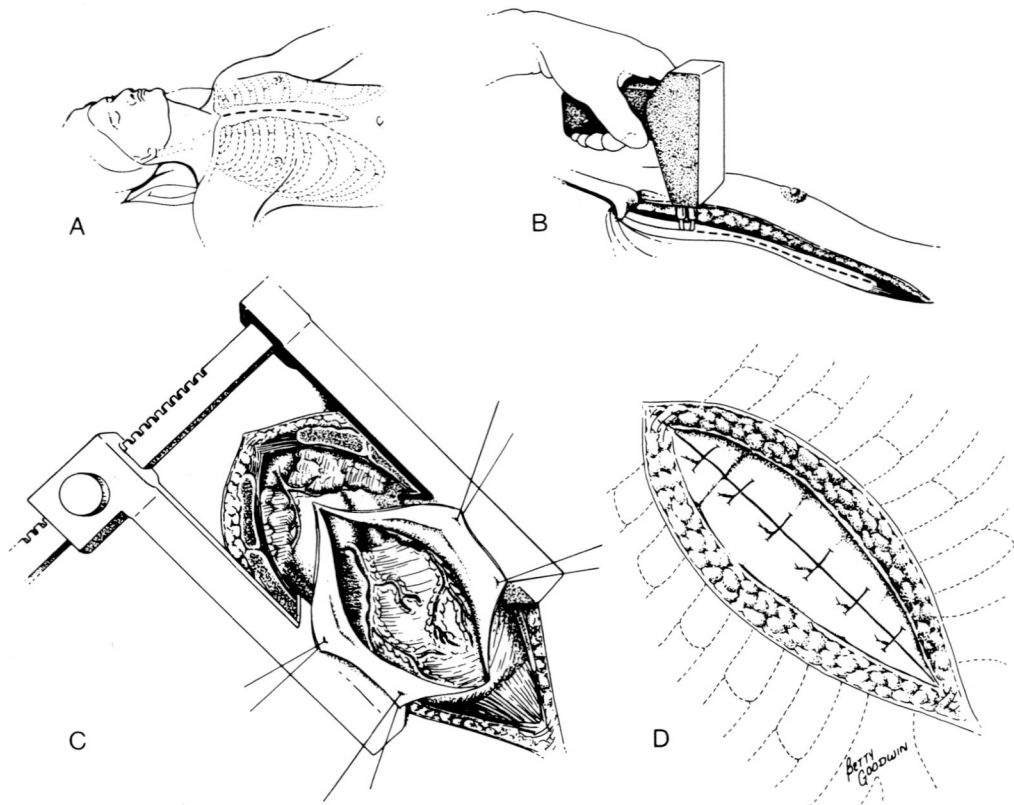

FIGURE 7–5. *A–D*, Median sternotomy. The illustration shows the use of a power-driven saw. In infants, the sternum can be divided with straight scissors.

be opened only as wide as is necessary to obtain adequate exposure. The planned operative procedure is then performed.

Once the operative procedure has been completed and hemostasis has been obtained, one or more large chest tubes are placed and led out through stab wounds at the lower end of the incision. The sternum is approximated with five to eight heavy stainless-steel wires passed through the sternum or, if one prefers or when the sternum is friable, around the sternum. If the wires are placed around the sternum, care must be taken to avoid injury to the internal mammary arteries. Traction is placed on these wires, and they are carefully tightened to achieve uniform approximation of the sternum. Care must be taken to avoid twisting the wires too tightly or they may cut through the sternum. Stainless-steel wire has been found to provide the most stable sternal closure when compared with other methods of closure including mersilene tape, stainless-steel bands, and plastic bands (Cheng et al., 1993). The twisted wires must be carefully turned down into the sternum so that they do not protrude externally and are not palpable, particularly in elderly thin patients or children. For these reasons and because sternal wires may break and protrude in the growing child, we have abandoned the use of wire for sternal closure in the pediatric patient. Instead, we have found that Maxon (Davis & Geck) provides equally secure sternotomy closure in the pediatric patient and thereby avoids any subsequent need to remove a painful or broken sternal wire. At the time of closure, care must be taken to avoid entrapment of pacing wires, pressure lines, and chest tubes. The linea alba is approximated with nonabsorbable sutures, as is the fascia. Subcutaneous tissue may be closed with either continuous or interrupted absorbable sutures. For skin closure, either staples or standard suture is satisfactory, but subcuticular skin closure with a continuous absorbable suture provides a superior cosmetic result and avoids the necessity of removing sutures, an especially important consideration in children. In addition, staples may hinder rapid reentry into the chest should this become necessary in the immediate postoperative period.

On rare occasions, closure of the sternum following long operative procedures compromises cardiac function. On these occasions, the sternum may be left open but protected by appropriate sterile drapes until cardiac function has improved, and delayed closure may be performed up to 2 weeks later. Although the incidence of infection is slightly increased in these patients, the technique is an acceptable alternative when primary closure is not possible (Furnary et al., 1992).

Although the median sternotomy offers many advantages, it has several disadvantages. One problem is that the incision is cosmetically unappealing, particularly in young females. In 1962, Brom proposed the use of a bilateral transverse submammary skin incision followed by the development of superior and inferior flaps and division of the sternum in the standard vertical manner (de la Riviere et al., 1981). This approach, which has been reported by others (Bedard et al., 1986; Bentz and Dunn, 1987), produces a better cosmetic result but requires additional operating time. Deutinger and Domanig (1992) reported no harm to breast development or lactation with this approach. Nandi and co-workers (1979) used a Y incision with the superior end placed much lower than the standard incision and also reported an improved cosmetic result. Tatebe and associates (1992) prefer to perform the standard sternotomy but through a very limited vertical skin incision; they claim improved cosmetic results without significant limitation in exposure. Wilson and co-workers (1992) described the use of a "partial" median sternotomy with a very limited skin incision in 182 infants and children undergoing correction of congenital heart defects; they indicate that this approach provides adequate exposure and superior cosmetic results.

Exposure of the great vessels, including the innominate, subclavian, and carotid arteries, may be improved by extending the sternotomy incision superiorly along the respective sternocleidomastoid muscle for the carotid and innominate vessels or to the supraclavicular fossa for exposure of the subclavian artery. Orringer (1984) has also utilized this approach for access to the upper thoracic esophagus. A "trap door" type of incision has been advocated for exposure of the great vessels. In these cases, the upper portion of the sternum is divided as usual, and the incision is then extended into the second or third intercostal space inferiorly and the supraclavicular fossa superiorly. Exposure of the subclavian artery may be enhanced by subperiosteal resection of the clavicle, which usually regenerates from the periosteum.

Brachial plexus injury has been reported to occur in a varied number of patients following sternotomy (Van der Salm et al., 1980) and is usually manifested by numbness in the fourth and fifth fingers. Initially, this was felt to be due to stretching of the brachial plexus from sternal retraction or from arm positioning. However, Van der Salm and associates demonstrated that this injury occurs with equal frequency regardless of the position of the arms and subsequently showed by radiographic and autopsy data that the injury is probably related to undetected first rib fractures producing direct brachial plexus injury. It was demonstrated that the incidence of fractures could be diminished by placing the blades of the retractor as far caudally as possible and by opening the sternum as little as possible. Others have confirmed these findings (Baisden et al., 1984).

Postoperative sternal wound complications are the other major problem with sternotomy incisions (Weber and Peters, 1986), and such complications have been reported to occur in 1 to 5% of patients undergoing sternotomy (Grossi et al., 1985; Nishida et al., 1991; Ottino et al., 1987). Wound problems include sterile serosanguinous drainage, unstable sternum, sternal dehiscence, superficial wound infection, and mediastinitis. The frequencies of such complications have been related to reoperative procedures; surgical technique, including the use of bilateral internal mammary arteries; reexploration for bleeding; patient-related factors such as diabetes mellitus; external cardiac massage; and prolonged mechanical ventilation with or without tracheostomy (Ottino et al., 1987).

Significant sternal instability even without obvious wound infection requires prompt reoperation in most patients. When the sternum is very friable, the technique of placing figure-of-eight sutures around the ribs, as described by Robicsek and associates (1977), is particularly useful in obtaining a secure closure (Fig. 7–6).

Sternal wound infections are usually manifested around the fifth to seventh postoperative day and may be heralded by pain, fever, leukocytosis, erythema, induration of the wound, or drainage from the wound. Superficial wound infections should be promptly opened and drained with cultures followed by administration of appropriate antibiotics. A midline radiolucent stripe on chest film may herald the development of sternal dehiscence (Escovitz et al., 1976). The development of frank mediastinitis is an ominous finding, because mortality may be high with this complication. Initial treatment for mediastinitis includes wide debridement of devitalized tissues, sternum, and mediastinum. Continuous mediastinal irrigation with a variety of solutions, including antibiotics and diluted povidone-iodine, has improved survival, but not uniformly. Molina (1993) described a different technique for irrigation with which there

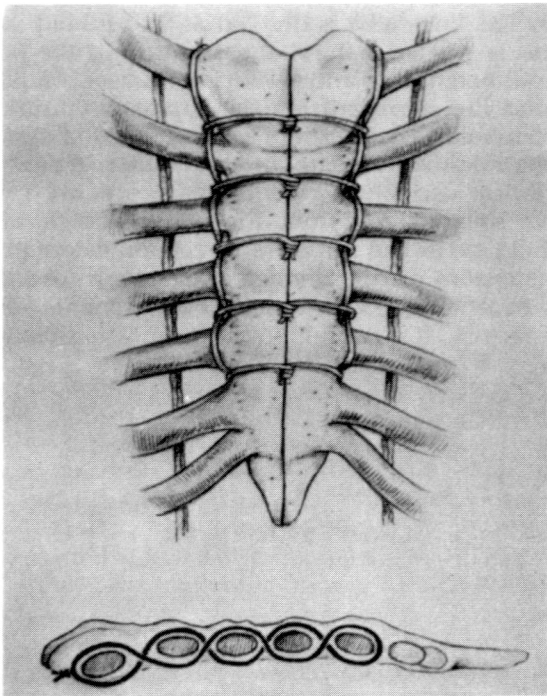

FIGURE 7–6. A method for prevention of sternal separation or correction of sternal separation if it has already occurred. (From Robicsek, F., Daughtery, H. K., and Cook, J. W.: The prevention and treatment of sternum separation following open heart surgery. J. Thorac. Cardiovasc. Surg., 273:267, 1977.)

were no failures, no deaths, and no recurrences in 16 patients followed for at least 8 years. Radical debridement of infected tissue including the sternum followed by placement of pedicled vascular flaps of pectoralis or rectus muscle into the mediastinum and skin closure over the flaps has improved survival rates (Grossi et al., 1985; Miller and Nahai, 1989; Pairolero and Arnold, 1984) (Fig. 7–7). Miller and Nahai described their technique in detail and reported 211 patients with an overall survival rate of 99.2%. Heath and Bagnato (1987) also reported improved results with omental transfer into the infected mediastinum.

Although mediastinitis remains a feared and life-threatening complication of median sternotomy incisions, these newer techniques of irrigation and flap closure of the infected wound offer much improved survival rates. Despite the improved survival rates, hospital stay length and hospital costs are markedly increased in this patient population, and it is clear that prevention of such complications is much preferred to treatment. Accordingly, meticulous surgical technique, appropriate use and harvesting of the internal mammary artery, discrete use of the electrocautery, meticulous hemostasis, use of systemic prophylactic antibiotics, and wound irrigation followed by careful wound closure minimizes the incidence of postoperative wound problems.

Subxiphoid hernia has been reported to occur in up to 4% of patients following median sternotomy incision and can be prevented by careful surgical technique (Davidson and Bailey, 1987).

Unfortunately, significant numbers of patients who have undergone successful cardiac surgery require reoperation at a later date. Occasionally, reoperation may be performed with a different approach, but it almost always requires reopening of the previous sternotomy incision. Repeat sternotomy requires meticulous technique to avoid an increased risk to the patient. The patient is placed in the supine position and prepared and draped so that the femoral vessels can be easily exposed. The perfusion team should be ready for immediate institution of cardiopulmonary bypass. The technique for reopening the sternum has been described in detail by Culliford and Spencer (1979) and includes sharp dissection of the retrosternal space with gradual division of the sternum under direct vision. Others have found the oscillating saw to be a safe method for dividing the sternum in patients who have undergone previous operations (Dobell and Jain, 1984). After the sternum is opened, further dissection allows identification and exposure of cardiac structures and preparation for cannulation and bypass. If significant bleeding is encountered at any point, the patient may be heparinized, cannulated via the femoral vessels, and placed on cardiopulmonary bypass with blood loss returned to the pump via cardiotomy suction. When these principles are followed, reoperation is possible without a significant increase in operative morbidity and mortality rates.

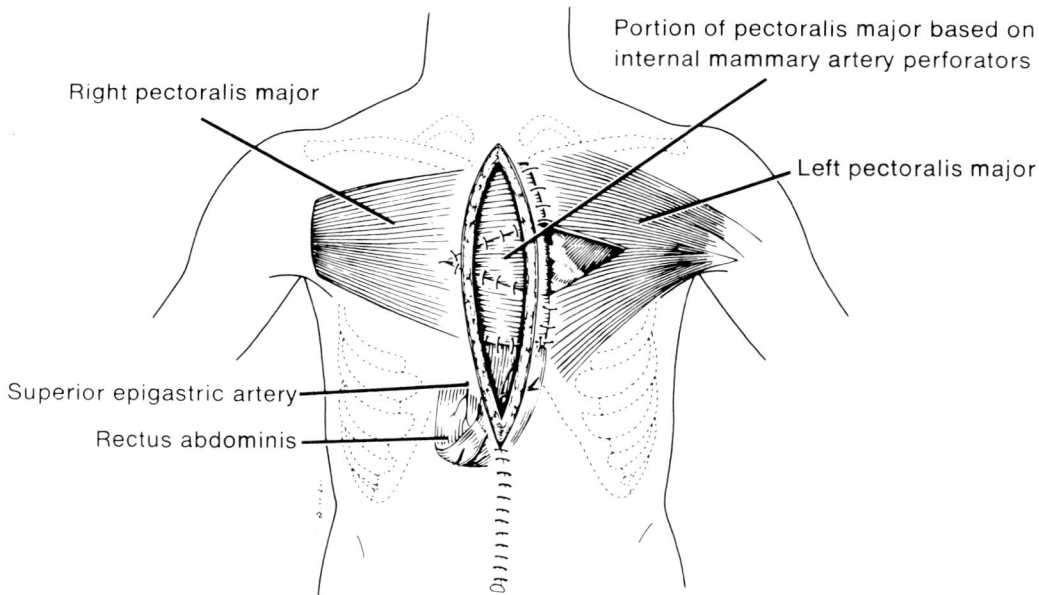

FIGURE 7–7. Multiple possible variations in reconstruction of sternal defect. A small portion of left pectoralis major muscle is transposed on its internal mammary perforating vessels and interdigitated with contralateral pectoralis major muscle based on its thoracoacromial vessel. A rectus abdominis flap is used to cover the inferior part of the defect. (From Fisher, J., Bone, D. K., and Nahai, F.: Reconstruction of the sternum. *In* Mathes, S. J., and Nahai, E. [eds]: Clinical Applications for Muscle and Musculocutaneous Flaps. St. Louis, C. V. Mosby, 1982.)

TRANS–STERNAL BILATERAL THORACOTOMY

This incision provides good exposure of the heart and anterior mediastinum. It was frequently used earlier but has been abandoned mainly because it is more time-consuming and more painful and causes more postoperative discomfort and pulmonary problems. Because a transverse skin incision is used, the scar may be more acceptable to women. Perhaps this incision is most frequently used today when it is necessary to extend either a right or left anterior thoracotomy across the midline position to improve exposure.

The patient is placed in the supine position, and the skin is prepared and draped as for a median sternotomy. A bilateral submammary incision is made that extends from the anterior axillary line on each side and crosses the sternum at the level of the fourth interspace. The pectoralis muscles are divided with a scalpel or electrocautery, as are the intercostal muscles in the fourth interspace, and the left and right pleural cavities are entered. The left and right internal mammary arteries and veins are carefully identified, ligated, and divided. The sternum may be divided with an electric saw or Gigli's saw. Appropriate retractors are inserted, and the incision is opened. When the operative procedure is completed, intercostal chest tubes are placed in each pleural space. The sternum must be approximated carefully and securely with several sutures of heavy-gauge stainless-steel wire so that no motion occurs at this point. The remainder of the incision is closed with the technique usually used for a thoracotomy incision.

THE AXILLARY APPROACH

This incision provides satisfactory exposure for first-rib resection, thoracic sympathectomy, and limited procedures within the thoracic cavity, and it requires the division of intercostal muscles only, without division of the major muscles of the chest wall. It is also small, hidden, and therefore cosmetically appealing.

The patient is placed in the lateral position with the chest rotated posteriorly approximately 20 degrees, and she is supported with sandbags. The chest, axilla, and forearm are prepared and draped. The arm is draped sterilely within the operative field so that its position may be changed by the assistant to improve exposure. A transverse incision is made in the axilla where the skin breaks from the chest wall. A slightly upward curved incision is made at each end from the pectoralis major anteriorly to the latissimus dorsi posteriorly (Fig. 7–8). The dissection is extended to the chest wall, and the lateral thoracic artery and thoracoepigastric vein are divided as they are encountered. On reaching the serratus anterior, one encounters a loose areolar plane just superficial to the muscle, and the axillary contents may be swept off the chest wall. The intercostal brachial nerve leaves the second intercostal space in the midportion and should be dissected free and protected during the operative procedure, when possible. Posterior dissection should be accomplished carefully to avoid injury to the long thoracic nerve (Roos, 1971).

If the procedure to be done is a cervical and thoracic sympathectomy, the second intercostal space is entered and opened through the extent of the incision.

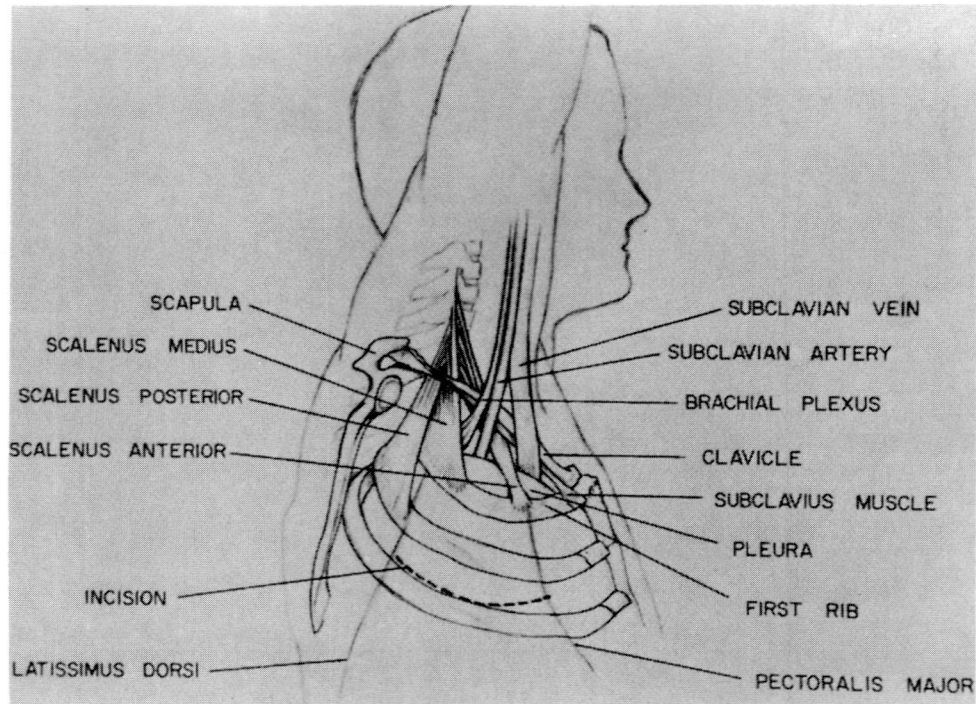

FIGURE 7–8. Anatomy of the right thoracic outlet from the axillary view with the upper extremity and shoulder elevated. (From Roos, D. B.: Experience with first rib resection for thoracic outlet syndrome. Ann. Surg., *173*:429, 1971.)

Exposure may be increased by lengthening the intercostal incision from within the chest to allow further retraction of the ribs. The apex of the lung is retracted with a malleable retractor, which exposes the stellate ganglion and the thoracic sympathetic chain that courses just below the parietal pleura.

If the procedure is a first-rib resection, further dissection is extended superiorly to the superior thoracic artery and vein, which are clamped and divided carefully to prevent them from being torn from the axillary vessels during the remainder of the operative procedure. A weak fascial layer, which interrupts the natural plane of dissection at this point and is attached to the lateral edge of the first rib, is divided sharply, allowing the surgeon's hand to enter the space that contains the axillary vessels. The subclavian vein and artery, as well as the scalenus anterior and medius muscles, may be visualized in their relationship to the first rib. In addition, portions of the brachial plexus may be identified and should be protected during the procedure. Adequate exposure of the axillary space for resection of the first rib depends on proper abduction and extension of the arm. The first rib may be excised, and the axillary contents should be duly protected.

If the thoracic cavity has been entered, a small chest tube may be brought out through a separate incision and left in position for underwater drainage or removed at the end of the closure of the incision if no untoward bleeding or air leakage is present. The ribs do not require approximation, and subcutaneous structures are closed in multiple layers.

SUBXIPHOID APPROACH

A subxiphoid approach provides adequate exposure for limited procedures on the heart and pericardium, which include attachment of pacing electrodes, drainage of pericardial fluid, and biopsy of the pericardium. This incision has the advantage of limited morbidity and may be easily extended to a median sternotomy if further exposure is required. A vertical midline incision is made from just over the xiphoid to 10 cm inferiorly. Dissection is extended to the midline abdominal fascia, and careful attention is paid to avoid entry into the peritoneum inferiorly. The xiphoid may be divided or removed as required for necessary exposure. Division of the lower 2 inches of sternum greatly improves exposure in difficult cases. The diaphragm is dissected from the pericardium, and the inferior pericardial surface is exposed. The pericardium is entered, and the incision is extended vertically to adequately expose the inferior surface of the heart and to access the contents of the pericardial cavity. This procedure allows pericardial biopsy, evacuation of pericardial fluid, exploration of the pericardial cavity for tumor involvement, and drainage of the pericardium. It also allows placement of myocardial electrodes for cardiac pacing and may be done under local anesthesia if indicated. If drainage is required, the tube should be brought out through a separate incision. The pericardium and diaphragm do not require closure, and the midline abdominal fascia is approximated with nonabsorbable sutures.

SUPRACLAVICULAR APPROACH

The supraclavicular approach may be used for biopsy of supraclavicular nodes in the staging of carcinoma of the lung; for exposure of the phrenic nerve, subclavian artery, and cervical ribs; and as a collar incision for thymectomy or tracheal reconstruction.

When excising supraclavicular lymph nodes for staging of lung cancer, a transverse incision of 3 to 4 cm is made following natural skin folds 2 cm above the clavicle. This incision extends laterally from the clavicular portion of the sternocleidomastoid muscle (Fig. 7–9). The platysma is divided and loose areolar tissue is dissected, exposing the lateral border of the sternocleidomastoid muscle and the omohyoid muscle. A fascial layer encountered overlying the supraclavicular fat pad is incised transversely, opening the contents of the fat pad. Dissection of the supraclavicular fat pad allows the identification of several lymph nodes for biopsy and examination. The medial limit of this space is defined by the internal jugular vein, and the subclavian artery defines the inferior limit of the supraclavicular space. The transverse cervical artery and vein are found coursing transversely in the depths of the supraclavicular fat pad. If the entire fat pad is dissected, the phrenic nerve may be seen coursing on the scalenus anterior muscle. Before closure, meticulous hemostasis must be ensured, because natural compression of bleeding does not occur in this space. The platysma is usually the deepest layer that requires closure.

Although most surgeons believe that a median sternotomy is the most appropriate incision for thymectomy for myasthenia gravis, some surgeons report satisfactory results with a supraclavicular col-lar incision (Cooper et al., 1988). The latter incision is made 2 cm above the sternal notch, and the strap muscles are divided in the midline position, exposing the cervical fascia that lies over the thymus. The fascia is opened, and the thymus is dissected by using a combination of traction with sharp and blunt dissection. Special care is indicated when crossing branches of the internal mammary that enter the thymus and where thymic veins enter the innominate vein.

Almost all strictures of the trachea may also be resected and reconstructed through a supraclavicular collar incision with the possible addition of a T into a limited upper median sternotomy. The trachea may be mobilized to the level of the carina by using blunt and sharp dissection while applying traction with a Penrose drain placed around the trachea at the level of stricture (Grillo, 1969).

INCISIONAL PAIN MANAGEMENT

Control of postoperative incisional pain after thoracotomy is of special importance. Rib-spreading incisions, such as posterolateral thoracotomies, frequently cause significant discomfort. This discomfort may lead to poor cough and inadequate inspired volumes, causing retained secretions and pulmonary collapse. Many solutions to this problem have been devised by thoracic surgeons. The previously described limited thoracotomies or median sternotomy incision may diminish pain experienced by the patient. The thoracic surgeon should be familiar with and skillful in the various techniques available, because a single approach may not always be appropriate. The pleura may be disrupted, preventing use of continuous inter-

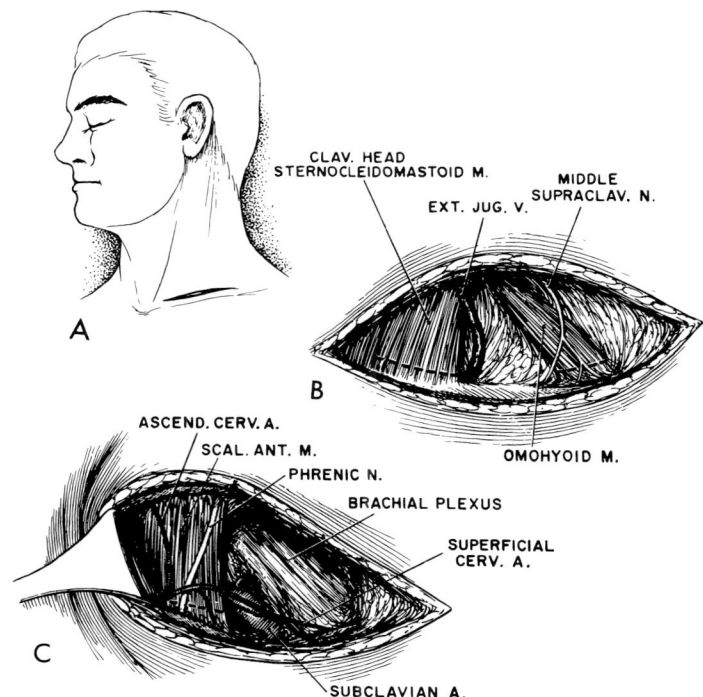

FIGURE 7–9. Supraclavicular (scalene) approach. For wider access to the supraclavicular fossa, the line of section of the sternocleidomastoid and omohyoid muscles is indicated in *B* and of the scalenus anterior muscle in *C*. (*A–C*, From Edwards, E. A., Malone, P. D., and Collins, J. J., Jr.: Superior aperture. *In* Operative Anatomy of the Thorax. Philadelphia, Lea & Febiger, 1972.)

costal infusion, or the patient may have a septic process, contraindicating the use of an epidural catheter.

Intermittent intramuscular narcotics have been traditionally used for pain relief. However, continuous intravenous infusion of narcotics with as-needed supplementation leads to smoother drug levels with a lessened chance of side effects. Patient control of additional bolus of drug is safe and provides more rapid response with decreased burden on the nursing staff.

Faber (1990) reported epidural catheter insertion at the beginning of the procedure with continuous infusion of morphine or fentanyl mixed with bupivacaine to provide good control of pain with few side effects. Morphine, being more hydrophilic, diffuses through the epidural space and may be used through a lumbar catheter. Fentanyl, being more lipophilic, diffuses less well and should be infused through a catheter placed at the level of the thoracic incision. However, side effects of sedation, pruritus, nausea, and respiratory depression are possible and must be anticipated and treated appropriately. Techniques such as continuous epidural anesthesia should be practiced with an experienced anesthesiology pain management team.

Sabanathan and associates (1988) described successful control of post-thoracotomy pain using continuous intercostal nerve block. At the time of thoracotomy, a multi-holed catheter of the type used for epidural anesthesia is inserted in the subpleural paravertebral area. Just prior to closing the chest, a 16-gauge Touhy needle is inserted through the skin into the chest just medial to the posterior end of the incision with entry at the angle of the rib. The catheter is advanced cranially in the extrapleural space. The pleura is closed over the catheter. Sabanathan then injects a methylene blue solution mixed with 10 ml of 0.5% bupivacaine through the catheter to check spread of the solution and to provide initial analgesia. Bupivacaine (0.5%) is infused at a rate of 5 ml/hr via constant infusion pump through the catheter. In a randomized trial comparing epidural anesthesia with continuous intercostal block, Richardson and co-workers (1993) found that both methods provided similarly adequate pain relief. However, the group receiving continuous intercostal block had far less nausea, vomiting, pruritus, and urinary retention.

SELECTED BIBLIOGRAPHY

Burch, B., and Miller, A.: Atlas of Pulmonary Resections. Springfield, IL, Charles C Thomas, 1965.

An atlas of noncardiac thoracic surgical procedures that demonstrates the technique of standard incisions and the approaches for exposure of intrathoracic structures in addition to demonstrating the technique for standard pulmonary resections. Demonstrated procedures will be of value to both the beginner and the experienced thoracic surgeon.

Meade, R.: A History of Thoracic Surgery. Springfield, IL, Charles C Thomas, 1961.

This text is an excellent review of the history of thoracic surgery, with several initial chapters describing the development of modern-day thoracic incisions. The reader will further appreciate the excellent exposure provided by currently available incisions after reading about their development.

Pairolero, P. C., and Arnold, P. G.: Management of recalcitrant

median sternotomy wounds. J. Thorac. Cardiovasc. Surg., 88:357, 1984.

This paper describes the Mayo Clinic experience with the use of muscle flaps for management of infected sternotomy incisions. The experience of others who have used the technique is reviewed in detail.

Urschel, H. C., and Razzuk, M. A.: Median sternotomy as a standard approach for pulmonary resection. Ann. Thorac. Surg., 41:130, 1986.

This paper reports one of the largest series of pulmonary resections utilizing the median sternotomy incision. Technical aspects are well described, and specific contraindications are discussed.

BIBLIOGRAPHY

Asaph, J. W., and Keppel, J. F.: Midline sternotomy for the treatment of primary pulmonary neoplasms. Am. J. Surg., 147:589, 1984.

Baisden, C. E., Greenwald, L. V., and Symbas, P. N.: Occult rib fractures and brachial plexus injury following median sternotomy for open-heart operations. Ann. Thorac. Surg., 38:192, 1984.

Bedard, P., Keon, W. J., Brais, M. P., and Goldstein, W.: Submammary skin incision as a cosmetic approach to median sternotomy. Ann. Thorac. Surg., 41:339, 1986.

Bentz, M. L., and Dunn, J. M.: The inframammary incision for median sternotomy in pediatrics. J. Cardiac Surg., 2:499, 1987.

Burch, B. H., and Miller, A. C.: Atlas of Pulmonary Resections. Springfield, IL, Charles C Thomas, 1965.

Cheng, W., Cameron, D., Warden, K., et al.: Biomechanical study of sternal closure techniques. Ann. Thorac. Surg., 55:737–740, 1993.

Cooper, J. D., Al-Jilaihawa, A. N., Pearson, F. G., et al.: An improved technique to facilitate transcervical thymectomy for myasthenia gravis. Ann. Thorac. Surg., 45:242, 1988.

Cooper, J. D., Nelems, J. M., and Pearson, F. G.: Extended indications for median sternotomy in patients requiring pulmonary resection. Ann. Thorac. Surg., 26:413, 1978.

Culliford, A. T., and Spencer, F. C.: Guidelines for safely opening a previous sternotomy incision. J. Thorac. Cardiovasc. Surg., 78:633, 1979.

Davidson, B. R., and Bailey, J. S.: Repair of incisional hernia after median sternotomy. Thorax, 42:549–550, 1987.

de la Riviere, A. B., Brom, G. H. M., and Brom, A. G.: Horizontal submammary skin incision for median sternotomy. Ann. Thorac. Surg., 32:101, 1981.

Deutinger, M., and Domanig, E.: Breast development and areola sensitivity after submammary skin incision for median sternotomy. Ann. Thorac. Surg., 53:1023–1024, 1992.

Dobell, A. R. C., and Jain, A. K.: Catastrophic hemorrhage during redo sternotomy. Ann. Thorac. Surg., 37:273, 1984.

Escovitz, E. S., Okulski, T. A., and Lapayowker, M. S.: The midsternal stripe: A sign of dehiscence following median sternotomy. Radiology, 121:521, 1976.

Faber, L. P.: Epidural analgesia: Different strokes for different folks. Ann. Thorac. Surg., 50:862–863, 1990.

Furnary, A., Magovern, J., Simpson, R., and Magovern, G.: Prolonged open sternotomy and delayed sternal closure after cardiac operations. Ann. Thorac. Surg., 54:233–239, 1992.

Grillo, H. C.: Surgical approaches to the trachea. Surg. Gynecol. Obstet., 129:347, 1969.

Grossi, E. A., Culliford, A. T., Krieger, R. H., et al.: A survey of 77 major infectious complications of median sternotomy: A review of 7,949 consecutive operative procedures. Ann. Thorac. Surg., 40:214, 1985.

Hazelrigg, S. R., Landreneau, J. L., Boley, T. M., et al.: The effect of muscle-sparing versus standard posterolateral thoracotomy on pulmonary function, muscle strength, and postoperative pain. J. Thorac. Cardiovasc. Surg., 101:394, 1991.

Heath, B. J., and Bagnato, V. J.: Poststernotomy mediastinitis treated by omental transfer without postoperative irrigation or drainage. J. Thorac. Cardiovasc. Surg., 94:355, 1987.

Holman, E., and Willett, F.: The surgical correction of constrictive pericarditis. Surg. Gynecol. Obstet., 89:129–144, 1949.

Iwa, T., Watanabe, Y., and Fukatani, G.: Simultaneous bilateral operations for bullous emphysema by median sternotomy. J. Thorac. Cardiovasc. Surg., 81:732, 1981.

Julian, O. C., Lopez-Belio, M., Dye, W. S., et al.: The median sternal incision in intracardiac surgery with extracorporeal circulation: A general evaluation of its use in heart surgery. Surgery, 42:753, 1957.

Kalnins, I., Torda, T. A., and Wright, J. S.: Bilateral simultaneous pleurodesis by median sternotomy for spontaneous pneumothorax. Ann. Thorac. Surg., 15:202, 1973.

Lemmer, J. L., Gomez, M. N., Symreng, T., et al.: Limited lateral thoracotomy: Improved postoperative pulmonary function. Arch. Surg., 125:873, 1990.

McCormack, P., Bains, M. S., Beattie, E. J., and Martini, N.: New trends in skeletal reconstruction after resection of chest wall tumors. Ann. Thorac. Surg., 31:45, 1981.

Meade, R. H.: A History of Thoracic Surgery. Springfield, IL, Charles C Thomas, 1961.

Meyer, W.: Some observations regarding thoracic surgery on human beings. Ann. Surg., 52:34, 1910.

Miller, J., and Nahai, F.: Repair of dehisced median sternotomy incision. Surg. Clin. North Am., 69:1091–1102, 1989.

Miller, J. I., Mansour, K. A., Nahai, F., et al.: Single stage complete muscle flap closure of the postpneumonectomy empyema space: A new method and possible solution to a disturbing complication. Ann. Thorac. Surg., 38:227, 1984.

Milton, H.: Mediastinal surgery. Lancet, 1:872, 1897.

Molina, E.: Primary closure for infected dehiscence of the sternum. Ann. Thorac. Surg., 55:459–463, 1993.

Nandi, P., Mok, C. K., and Ong, G. B.: Y incision for medial sternotomy. Aust. N. Z. J. Surg., 49:489, 1979.

Nishida, H., Grooters, R., Soltanzadeh, H., et al.: Discriminate use of electrocautery on the median sternotomy incision. J. Thorac. Cardiovasc. Surg., 101:488–494, 1991.

Orringer, M. B.: Partial median sternotomy: Anterior approach to the upper thoracic esophagus. J. Thorac. Cardiovasc. Surg., 87:124, 1984.

Ottino, G., De Paulis, R., Pansini, S., et al.: Major sternal wound infection after open-heart surgery: A multivariate analysis of risk factors in 2,579 consecutive operative procedures. Ann. Thorac. Surg., 44:173, 1987.

Pairolero, P. C., and Arnold, P. G.: Chest wall tumors. J. Thorac. Cardiovasc. Surg., 90:367, 1985.

Pairolero, P. C., and Arnold, P. G.: Management of recalcitrant median sternotomy wounds. J. Thorac. Cardiovasc. Surg., 88:357, 1984.

Ponn, R. B., Ferneini, A., D'Agostino, R. S., et al.: Comparison of

late pulmonary function after posterolateral and muscle-sparing thoracotomy. Ann. Thorac. Surg., 53:673, 1992.

Regal, A., Reese, P., Antkowiak, J., et al.: Median sternotomy for metastatic lung lesions in 131 patients. Cancer, 55:1334, 1985.

Richardson, J., Sabanathan, S., Engl., J., et al.: Continuous intercostal nerve block versus epidural morphine for post-thoracotomy. Ann. Thorac. Surg., 55:377, 1993.

Robicsek, F., Daugherty, H. K., and Cook, J. W.: The prevention and treatment of sternum separation following open heart surgery. J. Thorac. Cardiovasc. Surg., 73:267, 1977.

Robicsek, F., Masters, T. N., Littman, L., and Born, G. V. R.: The embolization of bone wax from sternotomy incision. Ann. Thorac. Surg., 31:357, 1981.

Roos, D. B.: Experience with first rib resection for thoracic outlet syndrome. Ann. Surg., 173:429, 1971.

Sabanathan, S., Smith, P. J. B., Pradhan, G. N., et al.: Continuous intercostal nerve block for pain relief after thoracotomy. Ann. Thorac. Surg., 46:425–426, 1988.

Sauerbruch, F.: Zur Pathologic des Offenen Pneumothorax und die Grudlagen Meines Verfahrens Zu seiner Ausschaltung, Mitt Grenzgeb. Med. Chir., 13:399, 1904.

Shumacker, H., and Lurie, P.: Pulmonary valvulotomy: Description of a new operative approach with comments about diagnostic characteristics of pulmonic valvular stenosis. J. Thorac. Surg., 25:173–186, 1953.

Tatebe, S., Eguchi, S., Miyamura, H., et al.: Limited vertical skin incision for median sternotomy. Ann. Thorac. Surg., 54:787–788, 1992.

Torek, F.: The first successful resection of the thoracic portion of the esophagus for carcinoma. J. A. M. A., 60:1533, 1913.

Tuffier, T.: Resection du Sommet du Poumon. Gaz. Hop. Toulouse, 6:257, 1892.

Urschel, H., and Razzuk, M.: Median sternotomy as the standard approach for pulmonary resection. Ann. Thorac. Surg., 41:130, 1986.

Van der Salm, T. J., Cereda, J. M., and Cutler, B. S.: Brachial plexus injury following median sternotomy. J. Thorac. Cardiovasc. Surg., 80:447, 1980.

Watanabe, Y., Ichihashi, T., and Iwa, T.: Median sternotomy as an approach for pulmonary surgery. Thorac. Cardiovasc. Surg., 36:227–231, 1988.

Weber, L. D., and Peters, R. W.: Delayed chest wall complications of median sternotomy. South. Med. J., 79:723, 1986.

Wilson, W., Ilbawi, M., DeLeon, S., et al.: Partial median sternotomy for repair of heart defects: A cosmetic approach. Ann. Thorac. Surg., 54:892–893, 1992.

8 Postoperative Care in Cardiac Surgery

Kevin Landolfo and Peter K. Smith

That the surgeon is primarily responsible for the patient is fundamental to the entire philosophy of surgery. . . . What is seriously debatable, however (and which we consider an intellectual myth), is that the science is so complex that only someone doing it full-time, an intensivist, can master it.

Spencer and Skinner, 1984

Critical care must be embraced as a branch of the tree of surgical knowledge that is practiced by fellow surgeons.

Weigelt, 1987

Postoperative care of the patient undergoing cardiothoracic surgery is particularly challenging and is directly affected by events that occur in the operating room. The surgeon's role as provider of postoperative care extends from the operative intervention. The postoperative course will be heavily influenced by the preoperative and intraoperative features of each patient. Postoperative care begins with the separation of the patient from *cardiopulmonary bypass* (CPB), and the central role of the surgeon remains paramount. The essence of this care consists of invasive monitoring and multisystem support to avoid, identify, and manage complications while permitting complete recovery of the patient.

INTENSIVE CARE UNIT

The initial postoperative environment, in virtually all cases, is an *intensive care unit* (ICU). A significant advantage accrues in ICU units that specialize in the care of cardiothoracic patients (Kron et al., 1984). Specific recommendations for ICU design and equipment have had a positive impact on patient outcome (Task Force on Guidelines, 1988). Specific monitoring should include the following:

- Continuous electrocardiogram (ECG)
- Intra-arterial blood pressure
- Pulmonary artery blood pressure and intermittent wedge pressures
- Central venous pressure

The following monitors are optional:

- Mixed venous oxygen saturation
- Left atrial pressure
- Pulse oximetry
- End-tidal CO_2

The following are experimental:

- Transcutaneous P_{O_2}
- Coronary sinus oxygen saturation

Most patients are ventilated for a minimum of 4 to 6 hours. This requires the frequent monitoring of arterial blood gases, pH, and ventilatory mechanics. Fluid balance must be logged hourly in the immediate postoperative period. Rapid changes in serum electrolytes, hematocrit, and the status of the coagulation system necessitate frequent laboratory testing.

Specialized nursing care is essential, with one nurse devoted to the care of each patient for the first several hours. The nurse also collates and maintains all the above-mentioned data on an intensive care flow sheet. The flow sheet shows data in an organized and time-oriented manner, allowing trend analysis and appropriate intervention. In many institutions, clerical aspects of nursing care have been delegated to a computer-based monitoring system, permitting nurses, house staff, and attending surgeons to focus attention on direct patient care (see Chapter 11).

The patient usually remains in the ICU for 24 to 48 hours, with a gradual reduction in care intensity and eventual transfer to a predischarge ward. The patient undergoes a transition from critical illness to relative wellness in a surprisingly short period. In the ICU, the avoidance of low-probability, potentially fatal events permits the performance of cardiothoracic surgery with low morbidity and mortality rates. The ICU setting allows rapid detection of physiologic change, which can be acted on before significant consequences occur. Any deterioration in the patient's status is identified by the ICU nurse specialist. The role of the nurse within the team effort required to manage these patients cannot be overemphasized.

GENERAL EVALUATION OF THE PATIENT

When the patient is admitted to the ICU, a complete evaluation is performed. This evaluation includes a review of the patient's history, the physical examination, the preoperative hospital course, and a comprehensive review of the conduct of the operation as reported by the surgical team.

After hemodynamic and respiratory function are deemed adequate, a physical examination is performed. Baseline neurologic evaluation is particularly important to recognize later abnormalities. Examination of the lungs may reveal unilateral absence of

230

breath sounds due to endotracheal tube malposition or pneumothorax. A midline trachea should be observed, and the pressure within the endotracheal tube cuff should be checked. Cardiac examination is of particular importance, especially in the patient with a prosthetic valve, although this examination may be difficult. Normal heart sounds, normal prosthetic valve sounds, and the absence of regurgitant or other murmurs should be documented. The abdominal examination reveals the presence or absence of bowel sounds and any signs of abnormal masses or distention, as well as location and character of the nasogastric tube drainage. The genitourinary examination should ascertain appropriate function of the indwelling catheter and the absence of phimosis or paraphimosis. A thorough inspection of the skin and extremities may reveal unrecognized intraoperative injuries, infiltration of intravenous infusions, absence of pulses, or signs of adverse drug or transfusion reactions.

The admission physical examination is completed by review of the patient's hemodynamic status and a notation of initial ventilatory parameters. Important hemodynamic parameters include the following:

- Blood pressure (BP) and arterial waveform (and correlation with noninvasive BP treatment)
- Pulmonary arterial catheter waveform
- Pulmonary arterial pressures
- Central venous pressure (CVP)
- Cardiac output
- Sv_{O_2}

Important ventilatory parameters include the following:

- Initial ventilator settings
- Peak airway pressures
- Pulse oximetry

The admission chest film is reviewed, with specific attention paid to the following:

1. Position of the endotracheal tube
2. Pneumothorax and mediastinal shift
3. Pleural and extrapleural fluid collections
4. Size of the mediastinal silhouette
5. Correct intravascular position of invasive lines and catheters
6. Normal position of radiopaque markers, sternal wires, and drainage tubes

An initial 12-lead ECG may be obtained and used as a baseline, but this is not imperative unless specific problems arise.

Following this assessment, admission orders are written. Particular attention must be paid to the patient's preoperative medical and drug history. Antianginal medications are not continued for patients who have undergone *coronary artery bypass grafting* (CABG). However, planned reinstitution of therapeutic agents such as digoxin, antiarrhythmic agents, thyroid supplementation, perioperative steroids, and perioperative antibiotics should be documented. Standard admission orders for cardiothoracic patients are

often used. Although this is efficient, it is important that each of these orders be reviewed and found appropriate using the same degree of thought as would be applied to the selection of a new medication or therapy.

MORBIDITY AND MORTALITY (RISK FACTORS IN CARDIAC SURGERY)

The mortality rate for isolated primary CABG has been reported to be as low as 0.8% (Cosgrove et al., 1984). Although much higher mortality rates have been reported both for CABG and for other cardiac operations, there is no consensus on a prohibitive mortality rate. Major morbidity and extended length of hospital stay are associated with advanced age (Roberts et al., 1985), significant preoperative renal and left ventricular dysfunction (Lahey et al., 1992), and valvular heart surgery (Katz et al., 1988). The following risk factors have been identified as independent predictors of mortality following coronary artery surgery (Gardner et al., 1985; Kouchoukos et al., 1980; Lytle et al., 1987; Naunheim et al., 1988; Roberts et al., 1985):

1. Advanced age
2. Reoperation
3. Impaired ventricular function
4. Emergency operation
5. Significant left main coronary artery disease
6. Incomplete revascularization

Gender was previously considered an independent risk factor; however, when data are adjusted for body surface area, small size, not gender, is associated with increased risk (Cosgrove, 1990; Grover et al., 1990).

The coupling of increasing age and increased medical problems has been associated with both increasing (Naunheim et al., 1988) and decreasing (Cosgrove et al., 1984) mortality rates. These data have been interpreted by some to suggest that high-risk candidates do not exist (Miller et al., 1983) and that patient selection is not a factor (Kouchoukos et al., 1980).

Cardiac dysfunction is becoming a less frequent cause of mortality, whereas morbidity from stroke, respiratory abnormalities, and renal dysfunction is increasing (Cosgrove et al., 1984, Hammermeister et al., 1990; Lahey et al., 1992) (Fig. 8–1). Multisystem organ failure as a cause of mortality increased from 7 to 21% in the period from 1974 to 1983 (Gardner et al., 1985).

The benefits of surgery are most apparent in higher-risk patients. Although patient selection may not be necessary to ensure beneficial results compared with medical therapy, its abandonment places a premium on the recognition and management of new and more prevalent postoperative complications.

CARDIOVASCULAR PHYSIOLOGY
Determinants of Cardiac Function

Cardiac function (cardiac output) is generally determined by the interrelation of preload, afterload, the

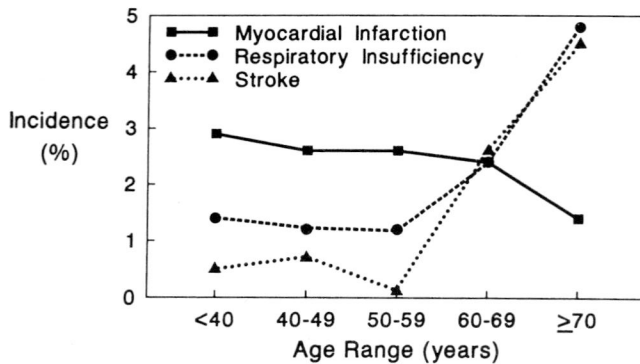

FIGURE 8–1. The incidence of myocardial infarction, respiratory insufficiency, and stroke as morbid events that follow primary myocardial revascularization. Data are grouped according to the decade of life and show an insignificant decrease in the incidence of myocardial infarction and a significant increase in the rate of both stroke and respiratory insufficiency with age. (Data from 24,672 patients analyzed by Cosgrove, D. M., Loop, F. D., Lytle, B. W., et al: Primary myocardial revascularization. J. Thorac. Cardiovasc. Surg., 88:673, 1984.)

inotropic state of each ventricle, and the heart rate. These factors are directly related to myocardial oxygen consumption (Sonnenblick and Skelton, 1971).

Normal and abnormal ventricular function can be expressed by the ventricular pressure-volume relationship, which is analogous to the force-length relationship in isolated heart muscle. Intraventricular pressure is graphed on the ordinate and intraventricular volume on the abscissa (Fig. 8–2). The pressure-volume relationship for an idealized cardiac cycle has four numbered phases: (1) passive ventricular filling during diastole (which is extended as a curvilinear dashed line to describe its behavior with different preload), (2) isovolumic systole (prior to aortic valve opening), (3) systolic ejection, associated with rapid intraventricular volume reduction and curvilinear pressure change, and (4) isovolumic relaxation, which is a rapid diminution in intraventricular pressure (aortic valve reclosure). The stroke volume for a particular cycle can be obtained by the arithmetical subtraction of the volume at end-systole from the volume

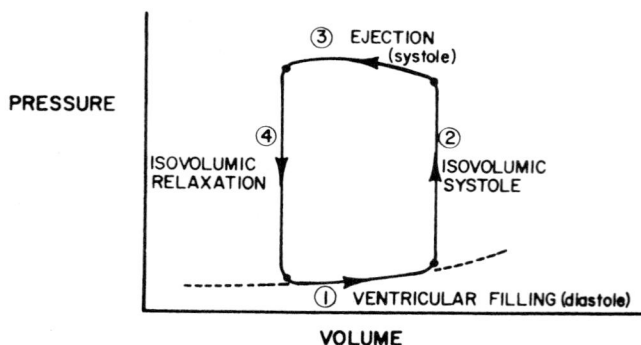

FIGURE 8–2. Idealized pressure-volume loop for the left ventricle representing a single cardiac cycle. (From Chatterjee, K., and Parmley, W. W.: The role of vasodilator therapy in heart failure. Prog. Cardiovasc. Dis., 19:301, 1977.)

at end-diastole. The ejection fraction can be determined by the fractional relationship between these two volumes.

The stroke work performed by the ventricle, excluding kinetic terms, is the area subtended by this idealized "work loop." Myocardial oxygen consumption is related to the amount of external work performed by each ventricle and is calculated as follows:

$$LVSWI = CI/HR \times MAP \times 0.0144$$
$$(\text{normal } 56 \pm 6 \text{ g-m/m}^2)$$

$$RVSWI = CI/HR \times MPAP \times 0.0144$$
$$(\text{normal } 8.8 \pm 0.9 \text{ g-m/m}^2)$$

where LVSWI = left ventricular stroke work index, CI = cardiac index, HR = heart rate, MAP = mean arterial pressure, RVSWI = right ventricular stroke work index, and MPAP = mean pulmonary artery pressure (Shoemaker et al., 1984a, p. 119). The minute work for either ventricle is obtained by multiplying stroke work by heart rate.

Clinically, intracavitary ventricular volume is not measured but rather assessed indirectly by pressure measurements obtained using a pulmonary arterial catheter. Ejection phase pressure is assumed to be equal to the systolic pulmonary artery pressure for the right ventricle and the peripheral arterial systolic pressure for the left ventricle in the absence of significant valvular, supravalvular, or subvalvular obstruction.

Diastolic-phase filling pressures are more indirectly determined. Central venous pressure in diastole closely reflects right ventricular diastolic pressure. Similarly, left atrial diastolic pressure closely reflects left ventricular diastolic pressure. In most patients, left atrial pressure is not measured directly, but rather is estimated by the pulmonary artery wedge pressure, which is in turn approximated by the pulmonary artery diastolic pressure. These three pressures are equal only under ideal circumstances. Generally, pulmonary arterial diastolic pressure exceeds pulmonary arterial wedge pressure, which exceeds mean left atrial pressure, the relationship being determined by gravitational effects related to pulmonary arterial catheter position and diastolic pressure gradients in the pulmonary vasculature. The latter can be significant in chronic obstructive pulmonary disease, acute respiratory distress syndrome (ARDS), left-sided valvular heart disease, and left ventricular failure. The relationship of pulmonary arterial diastolic pressure to left ventricular end-diastolic volume may also be altered in patients receiving positive airway pressure ventilation, whether positive end-expiratory pressure (PEEP) or continuous positive airway pressure (CPAP) (O'Quinn and Marini, 1983). Ideally, the flow-directed catheter should be placed in lung Zone 3 to determine accurate pulmonary wedge pressure (PWP) (Zone 3 defined as arterial pressure > venous pressure > alveolar pressure). Hypovolemia and PEEP/CPAP increase the proportion of Zones 1 and 2 relative to Zone 3 (Marini, 1991). If the catheter tip is located in Zone 1 or Zone 2, the pulmonary artery wedge pressure reading actually reflects alveolar pressure and not left atrial pressure. Pulmonary arterial catheters located below the level of the left atrium as viewed on lateral chest films usually reflect left atrial pressures accurately at all levels of PEEP/CPAP. In patients receiving PEEP/CPAP, pleural pressure is positive not only during mechanical inspiration but also during expiration. This pressure is transmitted to the intrathoracic vessels, elevating the measured PWP. Because transmural PWP most accurately reflects left ventricular end-diastolic pressure (LVEDP), a correction in patients with normal lung compliance can be made as follows (Jardin et al., 1981):

Transmural PWP = measured PWP − 0.5 × PEEP

Preload

Ventricular preload is the end-diastolic volume that is an estimation of average diastolic fiber length. The relationship between diastolic ventricular volume and pressure is curvilinear (see Fig. 8–2, *dashed line*) and depends on the passive viscoelastic properties of the heart. At high intraventricular volumes, the ventricle becomes stiffer, increasing end-diastolic pressure for equal added increments of volume. According to the Frank-Starling relationship, increases in preload cause increased stroke volume and stroke work. Beyond a certain point, preload augmentation of stroke work is lost, and left ventricular failure ensues. Clinically, the response to volume loading is the best test of preload adequacy. Following fluid challenge, measurements of systemic BP, CO, and PWP or pulmonary arterial diastolic pressure should be made. If a modest increase in pulmonary arterial diastolic pressure (< 3 to 4 mm Hg) is observed in association with an increase in systemic BP and CO, additional preload and higher pulmonary arterial diastolic pressures are desirable. If fluid challenge causes a large increase in pulmonary arterial diastolic pressure and minimal change in BP or CO, adequate preload should be assumed (O'Quinn and Marini, 1983). Low filling pressures imply low preload, whereas high filling pressures may be present with low, normal, or supranormal preloads.

Afterload

Afterload is a general term used to describe the hydraulic energetics at the ventricular outlet. Afterload is composed of forces tending to retard the ejection of blood and is primarily determined by the capacitive and resistive features of either the pulmonary or the systemic vasculature. These features interact with the quantity and quality of the ventricular ejection impulse to completely define the external work performed by the ventricle. An alternative concept is that afterload is the systolic ventricular wall stress (force per unit area) during ejection. Afterload is a dynamic measure that declines as ventricular volume and midwall radius decrease. The adverse

effect of ventricular dilatation is explained in part by this relationship.

In the systemic circulation, resistive features predominate because of the high systemic vascular resistance (SVR) and account for approximately 90% of external left ventricular work. SVR is calculated as follows:

$$SVR = MAP \ (mm \ Hg)/CO \ (l/min) \times 80$$

where the conversion factor of 80 is used to produce the units of SVR (dyn-sec/cm⁵). Strictly, MAP should be lessened by the CVP. The normal range for SVR is 900 to 1400 dyn-sec/cm⁵. The aorta and great vessels are relatively stiff, impeding ventricular ejection. Approximately 10% of the left ventricular work is expended in creating oscillations of pressure and flow about the mean.

The pulmonary circulation is characterized by low resistance and high compliance. Pulmonary vascular resistance (PVR) can be calculated as follows:

$$PVR = [MPAP − MLAP \ (mm \ Hg)]/CO \ (l/min) \times 80$$

where MPAP = mean pulmonary artery pressure, MLAP = mean left atrial pressure, and 80 is the conversion factor to express the result in dyn-sec/cm⁵. Normal PVR is 150 to 200 dyn-sec/cm⁵. Over 50% of the right ventricular external work is devoted to the creation of oscillations about the mean (this work properly viewed as being wasted).

The effect of afterload reduction is illustrated in the idealized pressure-volume loops of Figure 8–3. Two work loops are inscribed from equivalent end-diastolic pressure and volume. Work loop B shows systolic ejection against a higher pressure (afterload) than work loop A. A much larger stroke volume is evident in work loop A.

Inotropic State

The elusive inotropic state of the heart is a theoretical measure of intrinsic contractile ability. A direct measure of the inotropic state of the heart that is

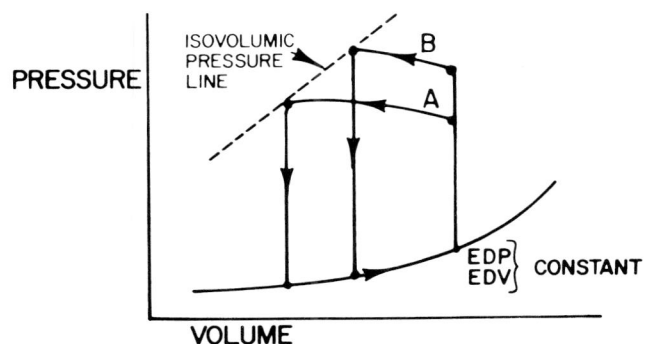

FIGURE 8–3. Two idealized pressure-volume loops at the same level of contractility and end-diastolic volume, but with a reduction in arterial pressure from loop B to loop A, which results in an increase in stroke volume. (From Chatterjee, K., and Parmley, W. W.: The role of vasodilator therapy in heart failure. Prog. Cardiovasc. Dis., *19*:301, 1977.)

independent of preload, afterload, and heart rate has been sought for many years. Two concepts for its approximation have emerged: preload recruitable stroke work and the systolic pressure-volume relationship.

Preload Recruitable Stroke Work. Although it is apparent that the relationship between stroke work and preload as determined by end-diastolic pressure is curvilinear (the Frank-Starling principle), it has long been suggested that the relationship between stroke work and end-diastolic volume might be linear (Sarnoff and Berglund, 1954). With improved methods of ventricular volume measurement, this relationship has been shown to be linear and minimally affected by afterload and heart rate (Fig. 8–4). The slope of the relationship between volumetric preload and stroke work appears to be a sensitive indicator of intrinsic myocardial performance, with measured increases following administration of inotropic agents (Glower et al., 1985) (Fig. 8–5).

Systolic Pressure-Volume Relationship. The evaluation of the entire pressure-volume relationship should be used to determine overall cardiac function in that it characterizes pump performance in both systole and diastole, and it offers information regarding the coupling between the ventricle and the vasculature (Kass and Maughan, 1988).

At a constant inotropic state, the end-systolic pressure-volume points create an isovolumic pressure line with varying preload and afterload conditions (Fig. 8–6). The slope of this line is the end-systolic elastance (E_{es}) of the ventricle (Sagawa et al., 1985). If cardiac contraction is viewed as a time-varying volume elastance, this elastance is maximal at end-systole and has been termed E_{max} (Sagawa et al., 1979). Neither of

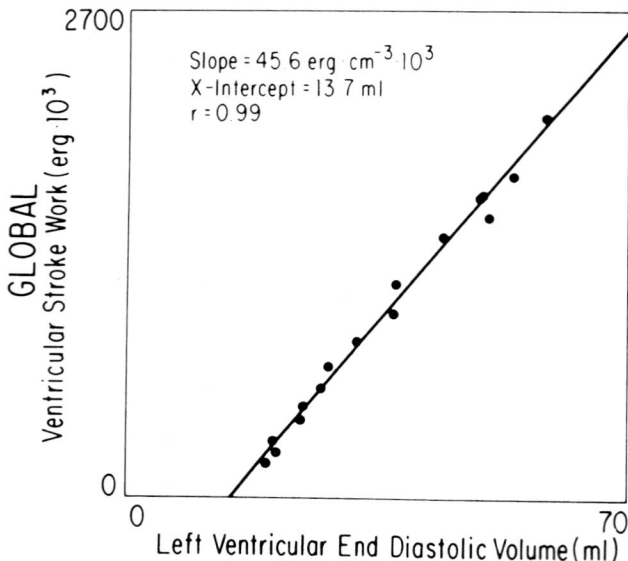

FIGURE 8–5. Linear relationship between left ventricular stroke work and left ventricular end-diastolic volume in the control state (*filled circles, solid line*) and after the infusion of calcium (*open circles, dashed line*), reflecting an increase in inotropic state under these conditions. (From Glower, D. D., Spratt, J. A., Snow, N. D., et al: Linearity of the Frank-Starling relationship in the intact heart: The concept of preload recruitable stroke work. Circulation, *71*:994, 1985. By permission of the American Heart Association, Inc.)

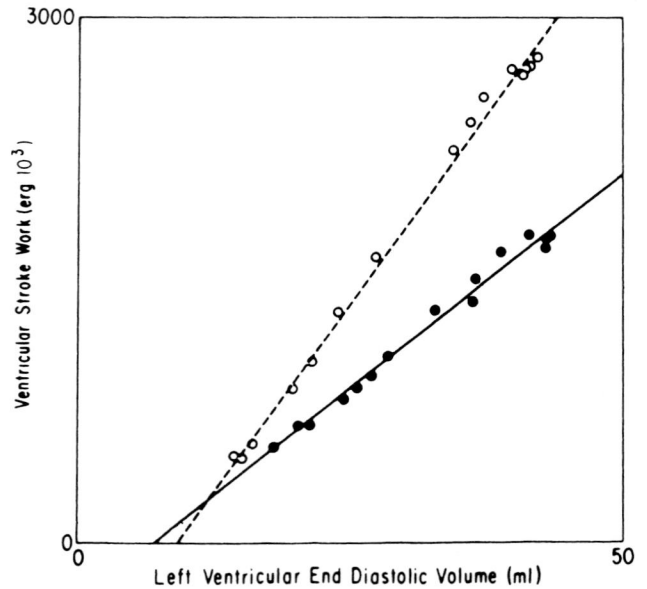

these relationships is strictly linear, particularly in relation to afterload. The end-systolic pressure-volume relationship is also sensitive to ventricular geometry, mass, and the characteristics of ejection (Kass and Maughan, 1988). Nonetheless, the slope and intercept of the isovolumic pressure line have yielded a good estimate of the inotropic state of the heart (Little et al., 1988) (Fig. 8–7).

Heart Rate

There is no simple relationship between heart rate and the other three determinants of cardiac function.

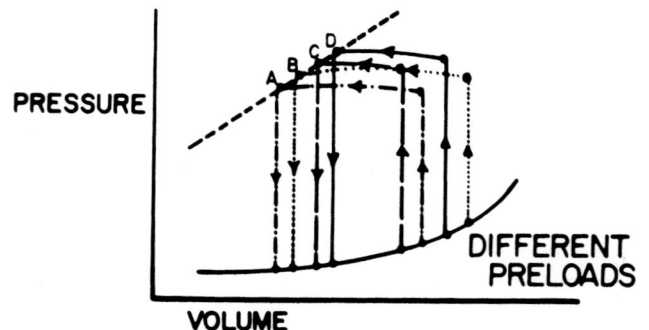

FIGURE 8–4. Representative linear relationship between global left ventricular stroke work and left ventricular end-diastolic volume. (From Glower, D. D., Spratt, J. A., Snow, N. D., et al: Linearity of the Frank-Starling relationship in the intact heart: The concept of preload recruitable stroke work. Circulation *71*:994, 1985. By permission of the American Heart Association, Inc.)

FIGURE 8–6. Series of idealized pressure-volume loops with alterations in end-diastolic volume and in arterial pressure. Despite these alterations, the end-points for contraction for each loop (A, B, C, D) fall on the dashed isovolumic pressure line. (From Chatterjee, K., and Parmley, W. W.: The role of vasodilator therapy in heart failure. Prog. Cardiovasc. Dis., *19*:301, 1977.)

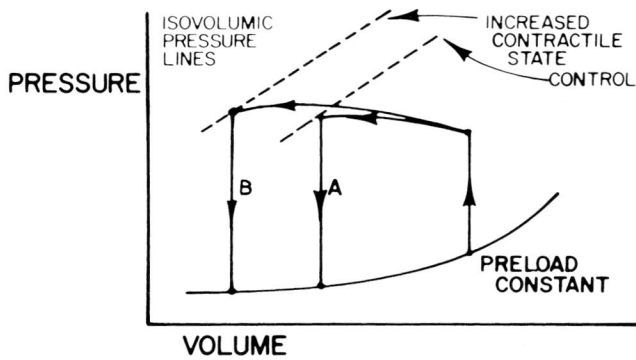

FIGURE 8–7. Pressure-volume loops inscribed under conditions of constant preload and afterload. An induced increase in inotropic state from loop A to loop B shifts the end-systolic pressure-volume relationship *(dashed lines)* and results in increased stroke volume in loop B. (From Chatterjee, K., and Parmley, W. W.: The role of vasodilator therapy in heart failure. Prog. Cardiovasc. Dis., *19*:301, 1977.)

Depending on other conditions, heart rates within the range of 50 to 130 beats per minute can generate adequate CO. Very low heart rates lead to a diminution in CO because of an inability to further increase stroke work volume through increased preload. At higher heart rates, an increase in contractility known as the Bowditch phenomenon is observed. This effect is probably mediated by sympathetic nerves (Higgins et al., 1973). At very high rates, a diminution in CO is observed, which is related to inadequate preload because of the shortened diastolic period (Strobeck and Sonnenblick, 1986). Although an optimal heart rate following cardiac surgery cannot be defined, it has been found that rates in the range of 90 to 110 beats per minute are usually satisfactory (Kouchoukos and Karp, 1976).

Myocardial Oxygen Supply-Demand Relationship

Increases in CO, afterload, inotropic state, and heart rate are all achieved at the expense of increased myocardial oxygen demand. Myocardial oxygen supply is determined by coronary blood flow (global and regional) and oxygen-carrying capacity. Arterial oxygen content is determined by the following parameters:

$$C_{A_{O_2}} = (S_{A_{O_2}} \times 1.39 \times Hb) + (P_{A_{O_2}} \times 0.0031)$$

where $C_{A_{O_2}}$ = arterial oxygen content, $S_{A_{O_2}}$ = oxygen saturation, and Hb = hemoglobin (mg/dl). Preserving both saturation and hemoglobin will maximize arterial oxygen content. The other aspect of myocardial oxygen supply is overall oxygen delivery. This can be calculated as follows:

$$\dot{D}_{O_2} = \text{arterial oxygen content} \times \text{cardiac index} \times 10 \ (ml/min/m^2)$$

where $\dot{D}_{O_2}$ = oxygen delivery.

In critically ill patients, attempts to increase oxygen delivery to supranormal levels with inotropic support have increased overall survival (Hayes et al., 1993; Shoemaker et al., 1973; Yu et al., 1993). This practice has not been translated to the routine postoperative cardiac surgical patient. In fact, inotropic support without overt cardiac failure may be deleterious in most patients (Lekven et al., 1988). In high-risk surgical patients, a significant postoperative increase in both $\dot{D}_{O_2}$ and oxygen consumption ($\dot{V}_{O_2}$) may occur and is predictive of increased survival. The explanation is that oxygen debt accrues during high-risk surgery and is then corrected in those patients who go on to recover uneventfully (Shoemaker et al., 1993).

The dominant feature of myocardial oxygen consumption is that oxygen extraction is virtually maximal at rest, so that increases in myocardial oxygen consumption can only be achieved by increased coronary blood flow. Most of the coronary flow occurs during diastole, because epicardial vessels are compressed during systole. Myocardial perfusion depends on the pressure gradient between the coronary arterial system and the left ventricle and the duration of diastole. Myocardial perfusion can be increased either by raising the arterial diastolic pressure or by lowering the LVEDP. Coronary perfusion pressure can be approximated from the difference between the diastolic arterial pressure and the pulmonary capillary wedge pressure. Pharmacologic interventions to improve ventricular performance must be chosen carefully. Nonselective increases in both diastolic arterial pressure and LVEDP do not improve coronary flow and do increase myocardial oxygen requirements (McGhie and Golstein, 1992). Tachycardia also adversely affects myocardial perfusion by shortening the length of diastole.

Low Cardiac Output Syndrome

Low CO after CPB historically has been recognized as a cause of sudden death (Boyd et al., 1959). Low CO resulting from ventricular dysfunction causes a series of adaptive neurohumoral responses as well as geometric changes (dilatation and hypertrophy) within the heart (LeJemtel and Sonnenblick, 1993). Acute losses of 20 to 25% of functioning myocardium (Swan et al., 1972) cause significant falls in CO and carry an extremely poor short-term (Kumon et al., 1986) and long-term prognosis (Massie and Conway, 1987).

The measurement and therapeutic manipulation of both CO and central filling pressures are critical to the postoperative care of cardiac surgical patients and predictive of survival (Appelbaum et al., 1976) (Fig. 8–8). Central pressures, CO, and venous saturation routinely are measured by means of a flow-directed pulmonary artery catheter. The cardiac index (CO expressed in l/min/m²) in 95% of normal range is from 2.1 to 4.9 l/min/m² (Reeves et al., 1961; Wade and Bishop, 1962). In adults, a cardiac index of at least 2.0 l/min/m² during the immediate postopera-

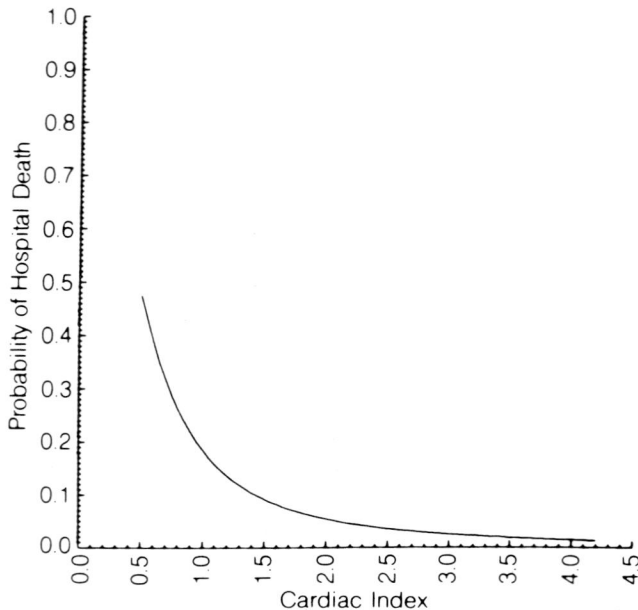

FIGURE 8–8. Relationship between postoperative cardiac index (l/min/m²) and probability of death for adults after mitral valve replacement. (From Kouchoukos, N. T. Detection and treatment of impaired cardiac performance following cardiac surgery. *In* Davila, J. C. [ed]: Henry Ford Hospital International Symposium on Cardiac Surgery. 2nd ed. New York, Appleton-Century-Crofts, 1977.)

tive period is required for normal convalescence (Appelbaum et al., 1976). Three patterns of low CO states have been identified:

1. Patients with high left ventricular filling pressures of greater than 18 mm Hg, low cardiac index (<2.0 l/min/m²), but a systolic arterial pressure of greater than 100 mm Hg
2. Patients with high left ventricular filling pressures (>18 mm Hg), reduced cardiac index (<2.0 l/min/m²), and low systolic arterial pressure (<90 mm Hg)
3. Patients with elevated right atrial and right ventricular diastolic pressures (>10 mm Hg), low cardiac index (<2.0 l/min/m²), and low systolic arterial pressure (<100 mm Hg) (i.e., significant right ventricular failure)

Shock is currently conceptualized as a clinical syndrome resulting from an imbalance of tissue oxygen demands and tissue oxygen supply. The general goals of postoperative care are to prevent shock and to provide adequate oxygen delivery. Oxygen delivery of less than 335 ml/min/m² has been associated with a decrease in oxygen consumption (Shibutani et al., 1983) and with the development of progressive lactic acidosis (Rashkin et al., 1985). Provision of supranormal oxygen delivery (>600 ml/min/m²) has been proposed to counteract the oxygen debt accumulated by patients in shock, although this approach in postoperative cardiac surgical patients has not been studied.

Lactic acidosis has been suggested as a metabolic monitor to correlate with total oxygen debt, the mag-

nitude of hyperperfusion, and the severity of shock (Broder and Weil, 1964; Mizock and Falk, 1992; Weil and Afifi, 1970). However, a direct relationship to total oxygen delivery has been disputed by others (Astiz et al., 1988). This discrepancy may be resolved by classifying patients with lactic acidosis (Cohen and Woods, 1976) into Type A (clinical evidence of tissue hypoxia) and Type B (no clinical evidence of tissue hypoxia). In Type A lactic acidosis, especially below the critical delivery threshold (the oxygen delivery level below which consumption and delivery become linearly related), lactate levels and oxygen delivery are closely related (Mizock and Falk, 1992).

Mixed venous oxygen saturation (MVO_2) is a useful index of the adequacy of circulation and reflects, to some extent, mean tissue oxygen level (Kirklin and Archie, 1974). MVO_2 is measured with specialized pulmonary artery catheters. Patients with a saturation of less than 60% or those who demonstrate a decrease of more than 5% suffer more frequent postoperative complications (Krauss et al., 1975). However, other authors have shown poor correlation between saturation, or trends in saturation, and outcome (Vaughn and Puri, 1988). Rapid changes in whole body oxygen consumption may reduce its overall predictive value.

Adequate regional oxygen delivery is even more difficult to determine. Organ requirements and hormonally activated reflex changes in regional blood supply may occur in the postoperative state (Fig. 8–9). For example, the kidney, skin, and resting muscles do not depend on the blood supply and maintain viability by increased oxygen extraction. The heart and brain, on the other hand, depend on the blood supply with near maximal oxygen extraction at rest. Sympathetically controlled reflexes compensate for these differences by a shift of blood flow from the skin and splanchnic region at low circulating volumes (Bryan-Brown, 1988). Increasingly, the effects of splanchnic hypoperfusion on postoperative complications and persistent acidosis are being recognized (Landow, 1993). Acute changes in regional blood supply may be mediated by differing degrees of sympathetic innervation to precapillary sphincters and arterioles (Mellander and Johansson, 1968).

Alterations in metabolic activity are common following heart surgery. These alterations can be monitored through capnography, which determines the partial pressure of CO_2 in expired gases (Chiara et al., 1987). Rewarming, with subsequent peripheral vasodilation, and shivering have been shown to increase metabolic and circulatory demands (Rodriguez et al., 1983) and can be eliminated with paralysis and sedation (see Chapter 5, part I). This promotes hemodynamic stability and decreases the need for inotropic support (Zwischenberger et al., 1987).

Thus, the actual definition of low CO syndrome must include evidence of inadequate oxygen delivery related to consumption. Clinical evidence of diminished peripheral perfusion and end-organ ischemia must be coupled with the measurement of metabolic parameters to establish this diagnosis.

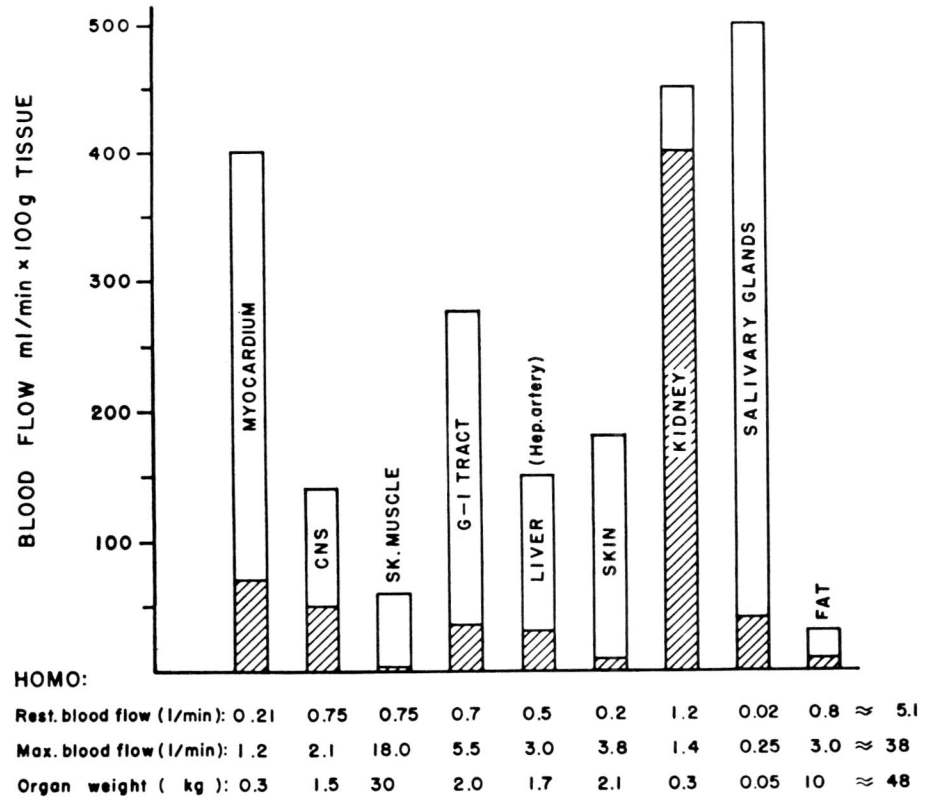

FIGURE 8–9. Approximate blood flows of various organs at maximal vasodilatation (*total areas*) and "at rest" (*hatched areas*) at a perfusion pressure of 100 mm Hg. Approximate figures for regional blood flows in a resting 70-kg man. (From Mellander, S., and Johansson, B.: Control of resistance, exchange, and capacitance functions in the peripheral circulation. Pharmacol. Rev., 20:117, 1968.)

HOMO:

Rest. blood flow (l/min):	0.21	0.75	0.75	0.7	0.5	0.2	1.2	0.02	0.8	≈ 5.1
Max. blood flow (l/min):	1.2	2.1	18.0	5.5	3.0	3.8	1.4	0.25	3.0	≈ 38
Organ weight (kg):	0.3	1.5	30	2.0	1.7	2.1	0.3	0.05	10	≈ 48

Management of Perioperative Cardiac Function

Preload

Maintenance of adequate preload is fundamental in the postoperative management of cardiac surgical patients. The optimal pulmonary capillary wedge pressure in postoperative cardiac surgical patients is unknown, but a range of 14 to 18 mm Hg has been suggested, with increases in extravascular lung water occurring above this level (Crexells et al., 1973). Preload correlates directly with the force of ventricular contraction, and the result is a ventricular volume change from end-diastole to end-systole determined by transmural pressure and compliance of the ventricular wall. Pericardial pressure is normally reflected by right atrial pressure. However, tight closure of the pericardium may adversely affect transmural pressure and decrease stroke volume (Angelini et al., 1990; Shabetai, 1988b; Tyberg et al., 1986). Pulmonary artery wedge pressures and the CVP, indicating left and right ventricular volumes, respectively, accurately reflect reduced filling pressures, whereas high filling pressures may be determined by changes in transmural pressure or myocardial compliance and may not accurately reflect preload. Most patients following cardiac surgery are relatively hypovolemic and have labile reactive vasculature (Hanson et al., 1976). In the immediate postoperative period, losses include large urine volumes, ongoing blood loss, and significant increase in vascular beds with rewarming.

The summation of these physiologic changes is a reduced preload, particularly to the left ventricle. This trend should be anticipated and managed with appropriate volume therapy to prevent precipitous hypotension and low CO. Immediate preload augmentation may be achieved with passive straight leg raising with a transient 8 to 10% increase in CO (Gaffney et al., 1982), although this should be viewed only as a temporizing measure and should be quickly supplanted by appropriate volume administration.

Afterload

Following a cardiac operation, afterload is often elevated. The incidence varies with cardiac pathology, operative procedure, and definition of the resulting hypertension. Following valve replacement, the reported incidence ranges between 8 and 12% (Estafanous et al., 1978). After myocardial revascularization, afterload is elevated in 8 to 61% of patients (Estafanous and Tarazi, 1980; Weinstein et al., 1987). Increased systemic vascular resistance at the arteriolar level appears to be the major determinant of arterial pressure after coronary artery surgery (Gall et al., 1982). The etiology of postoperative hypertension remains unclear, but contributing factors include decreased baroreceptor sensitivity (Fouad et al., 1979; Hanson et al., 1976) and elevated renin-angiotensin activity (Taylor et al., 1977, 1979), although this is disputed by others (Weinstein et al., 1987). Sympathetic stimulation and elevated levels of catechola-

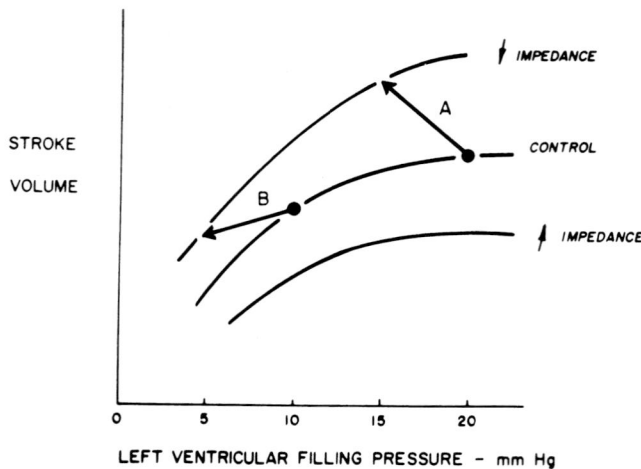

FIGURE 8–10. The Frank-Starling relationship is altered by afterload (impedance) modification. Decreased impedance shifts the relationship upward and to the left. A 5-mm Hg reduction in filling pressure induced by afterload reduction can result in an increase (A) or a decrease (B) in stroke volume, depending on filling pressure before intervention. (From Chatterjee, K., and Parmley, W. W.: The role of vasodilator therapy in heart failure. Prog. Cardiovasc. Dis., 19:301, 1977.)

mines also have been identified in the early postoperative period (Packer, 1988; Weinstein et al., 1987; Whelton et al., 1980). Further, postoperative pain may increase afterload and can be managed with the administration of morphine sulfate (Zelis et al., 1974).

Although pulmonary artery pressures are measured directly (right ventricular afterload), the ascending aortic pressure is inferred from measurements made at a peripheral artery (usually the radial). Systolic amplification may occur, thereby elevating the measured systolic radial artery pressure. However, mean pressures in the peripheral and central regions are similar, which should be considered when managing patients in the postoperative setting.

In the control of afterload, autoregulation at various sites should be considered. The central nervous system autoregulates between mean BPs of 50 to 150 mm Hg (Lassen, 1978), with a lower limit of 40 mm Hg for normal individuals. A reset lower limit for autoregulation may be higher (68 mm Hg in hypertensive patients) (Strandgaard et al., 1973). Renal autoregulation requires a mean BP of 70 mm Hg (Bryan-Brown, 1988). The heart with residual coronary disease also requires adequate mean arterial pressure (65 mm Hg),

as do patients with pathologic concentric myocardial hypertrophy (Marcus et al., 1987).

Acute afterload reduction in the postoperative period is frequently beneficial. Adequate preload must be achieved before the institution of vasodilating agents (Fig. 8–10). Afterload reduction with low filling pressures often produces a compensatory tachycardia, which may be deleterious. When afterload is reduced in patients with high filling pressures, there is usually no change or a slight reduction in heart rate. Additionally, experimental evidence suggests that afterload reduction, when applied to low or normally filled ventricles, may increase infarct size (Redwood et al., 1972). When applied in a setting of high preload, infarct size may be reduced (DaLuz et al., 1975; Watanabe et al., 1972). This may have implications for patients who have undergone incomplete myocardial revascularization.

The degree to which hemodynamic improvement can be obtained with afterload reduction is difficult to predict. Therapeutic results depend on the end-systolic pressure-volume relationship of each patient (Fig. 8–11). However, afterload reduction generally improves cardiovascular function and diminishes preload (Table 8–1). Preload augmentation coupled with afterload reduction has additional positive effects on overall cardiac function (Appelbaum et al., 1975; Stinson et al., 1977). Afterload reduction also improves forward ejection in patients with residual mitral regurgitation (Chatterjee et al., 1973; Chatterjee and Parmley, 1977) and aortic insufficiency (Bolen and Alderman, 1976).

Although various afterload-reducing agents are available, nitroglycerin and nitroprusside are the most frequently used agents in the immediate postoperative period. Nitroprusside may increase ST segment elevation in perioperative ischemia and cause significant shunt (Chiarello et al., 1976). However, it continues to be the agent of choice for the acute management of postoperative hypertension (Bixler et al., 1978; Chatterjee and Parmley, 1977; Franciosa et al., 1972). Nitroglycerin improves coronary collateral flow and may prevent coronary spasm, and it is frequently used for the first 12 to 24 hours following coronary revascularization (Chiarello et al., 1976; Goldstein et al., 1974).

The frequent use of nitroprusside mandates a knowledge of its adverse effects. The lethal dose is approximately 7 mg/kg (Davies et al., 1975). When high dosages are used (>7 µg/kg/min) for prolonged

■ Table 8–1. HEMODYNAMIC CHANGES AFTER ACUTE VASODILATOR THERAPY

Measurement	Nitroprusside	Nitroglycerin	Phentolamine	Prazosin
Mean aortic pressure	9% decrease	12% decrease	8% decrease	20% decrease
Pulmonary wedge pressure	45% decrease	60% decrease	39% decrease	41% decrease
Cardiac output	9% increase	No change	16% increase	42% increase
Venous resistance	48% decrease	53% decrease	23% decrease	69% decrease
Arterial resistance	44% decrease	No change	33% decrease	47% decrease

Modified from Ayres, S. M.: Ventricular function. In Shoemaker, W. C., Thompson, W. L., and Holbrook, P. R. (eds): Textbook of Critical Care. Chap. 49. Philadelphia, W. B. Saunders, 1984, p. 339.

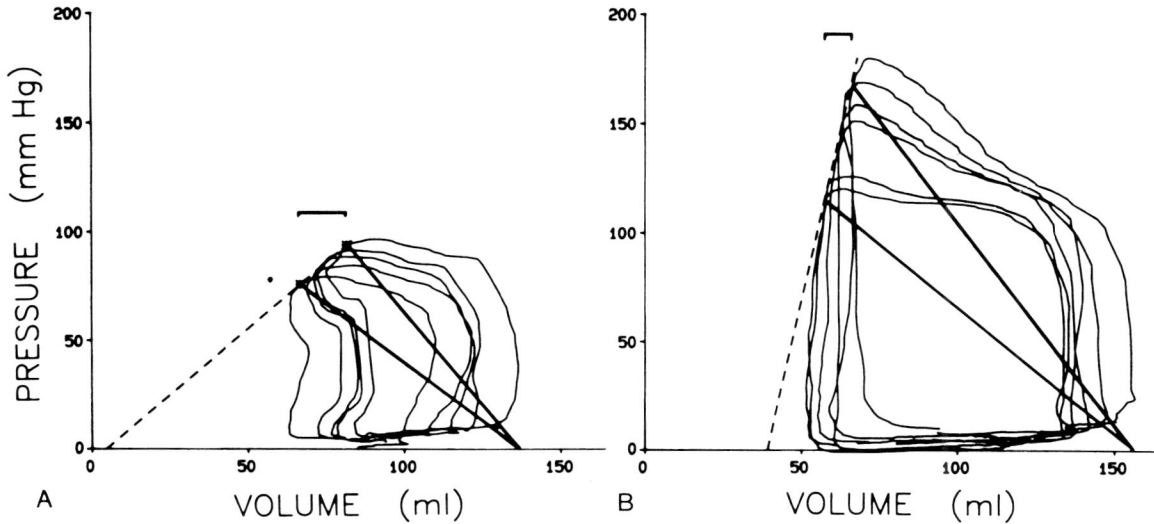

FIGURE 8–11. The pressure-volume relationship of two patients with dilated cardiomyopathy. *A*, The patient has a shallow end-systolic pressure-volume slope (*dashed line*) predicting a 30% increase in stroke volume (*brackets above loops*) after a 35% reduction in afterload (*solid lines*). *B*, A steep end-systolic pressure-volume relationship and similar afterload reduction predicts less than a 10% increase in stroke volume, with a greater effect on systolic pressure. (*A* and *B*, From Kass, D. A., and Maughan, W. L.: From "E$_{max}$" to pressure-volume relations: A broader view. Circulation, 77:1203, 1988. By permission of the American Heart Association, Inc.)

therapy, cyanogen, cyanide, and thiocyanate are potential toxic breakdown products. Signs of toxicity are subtle and include a narrowing of the arteriovenous oxygen difference and the development of metabolic acidosis (Michenfelder and Tinker, 1977). Thiocyanate levels may be measured under these circumstances; levels of 50 to 100 mg/l are associated with cyanate toxicity, and 200 mg/l may be lethal. Discontinuance and dialysis are the mainstays of treatment, although prophylactic infusion of hydroxocobalamin (25 mg/hr) has been shown to decrease cyanate concentration (Ram and Kaplan, 1984).

Alternative parenteral agents should be considered when high-dose nitroprusside therapy is necessary (Table 8–2). Hydralazine, although longer-acting, may also be effective (Sladen and Rosenthal, 1979). Phentolamine (Chatterjee and Parmley, 1977), trimethaphan (Stinson et al., 1975), and phenoxybenzamine (Buckberg et al., 1971), although effective, are not commonly used today. Sublingual nifedipine may also be employed and has the least depressive effect on myocardial performance of the calcium channel blockers (Mullen et al., 1988). Beta-blockers are also effective in the management of postoperative hypertension but should be used with caution in patients with left ventricular failure. Esmolol, a short-acting selective beta-blocker, may be particularly useful in this setting (see Chapter 5, part I).

Many patients require afterload reduction throughout their postoperative course. Patients with persistent hypertension and patients with reduced left ventricular function will benefit from long-term afterload reduction and should be switched to nonparenteral therapy (see Table 8–2). Chronic afterload reduction in patients with significant congestive heart failure has been shown to increase survival (Massie et al., 1981). In one large study of patients with symptomatic congestive heart failure (New York Heart Association [NYHA] Class II and Class III), long-term morbidity and mortality rates were reduced significantly in those treated with enalapril, an angiotensin-converting enzyme (ACE) inhibitor (Hood, 1993). Additional studies have confirmed that ACE inhibitors are particularly useful in the management of this problem (Davis et al., 1979; Konstam et al., 1990; Lotvin and Gorlin, 1993). Patients with asymptomatic left ventricular dysfunction (NYHA Class I and Class II) may benefit significantly from long-term therapy with ACE inhibitors. Although ACE inhibitor use yielded no significant difference in overall mortality when compared with placebo, they did lead to a 37% decrease in symptomatic congestive heart failure and a 36% decrease in hospital admission for congestive heart failure (Pitt, 1993). Although the mechanism of this positive impact has not been completely defined, two-dimensional echocardiographic studies in post-myocardial infarction patients have shown that ACE inhibitors attenuate left ventricular enlargement (St. John Sutton et al., 1994). Nitrates (Massie et al., 1981) and hydralazine (Cohn et al., 1986) have also been used; however, these agents are less effective than ACE inhibitors (Cohn et al., 1991).

■ **Table 8–2.** VASODILATOR DRUGS THAT HAVE PRODUCED BENEFICIAL HEMODYNAMIC EFFECTS

Parenteral	Nonparenteral
Sodium nitroprusside	Sublingual nitroglycerin
Nitroglycerin	Topical nitroglycerin
Hydralazine	Sublingual isosorbide dinitrate
Phentolamine	Oral isosorbide dinitrate
Trimethaphan	Hydralazine
Phenoxybenzamine	Captopril

Heart Rate

The postoperative control of heart rate is important and mandates standard application of temporary epicardial bipolar atrial and ventricular pacing wires in most patients (Harris et al., 1968; Hodam and Starr, 1969; Mills and Ochsner, 1973). Normal sinus rhythm, through synchronized end-diastolic preload augmentation, is responsible for approximately 25% of CO in the postoperative setting (Skinner et al., 1963) (Fig. 8–12).

Changes in heart rate are common following cardiac surgery and include sinus bradycardia, junctional rhythm, and first-degree, second-degree, or third-degree heart block. These phenomena are usually transitory and may be related to perioperative beta-blockade, intraoperative antiarrhythmics, or metabolic damage during cardioplegia administration (potassium or magnesium) (Ellis et al., 1980; Smith et al., 1983b). Inadequate myocardial protection may cause ischemia of the conduction system (Smith et al., 1983a, 1983c). However, permanent injury to the conduction system is most often due to direct surgical injury during intracardiac procedures.

Management of disturbances in heart rate must be individualized. Simple atrial pacing (in the range of 90 to 110 beats per minute) is optimal for sinus bradycardia or junctional arrhythmias. With atrial ventricular nodal blocks, which are often aggravated by quickened atrial pacing, the advantage of rate increase

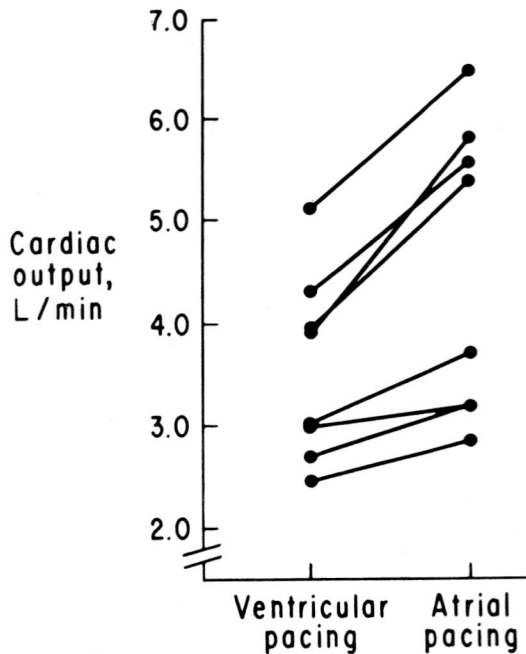

FIGURE 8–13. A comparison of atrioventricular (AV) sequential pacing and atrial pacing in patients with a prolonged postoperative PR interval (intrinsic and paced PR intervals are shown in milliseconds to the left for atrial pacing and to the right for AV sequential pacing). Note the uniform increase in cardiac output despite absolute differences in the shortening of the PR interval that is induced by pacing and overlap between paced PR intervals and intrinsic PR intervals between patients. (From Hartzler, G. O., Maloney, J. D., Curtis, J. J., and Barnhorst, D. A.: Hemodynamic benefits of atrioventricular sequential pacing after cardiac surgery. Am. J. Cardiol., 40:232, 1977.)

may be offset by the introduction of atrioventricular dyssynchrony. In this setting, atrioventricular pacing with an interval in the range of 150 to 175 msec is usually optimal (Guyton et al., 1976; Hartzler et al., 1977). The atrioventricular interval also depends on selected heart rate (Fig. 8–13). The normalization of atrioventricular synchrony by these means is associated with a loss of the normal ventricular activation sequence, depressing ventricular function at constant preload and afterload by approximately 10 to 15%. Optimal heart rate determination must be individualized with reference to measurements of CO.

When in place, temporary pacing wires constitute a *direct* current pathway to the heart and must be insulated when not in use. Caution should be practiced when connecting a rapid-pacing device to the wires ensuring atrial connection. The wires are removed on the fourth or fifth postoperative day. Temporary pacing wires may be left indefinitely, although high pacing thresholds are usually apparent within 2 weeks. When temporary pacing is not possible, bradyarrhythmias can be treated pharmacologically with atropine or isoproterenol. Alternatively, a pulmonary artery catheter with an additional pacing port may be used, or the Zoll transthoracic pacemaker may be employed (Zoll, 1952).

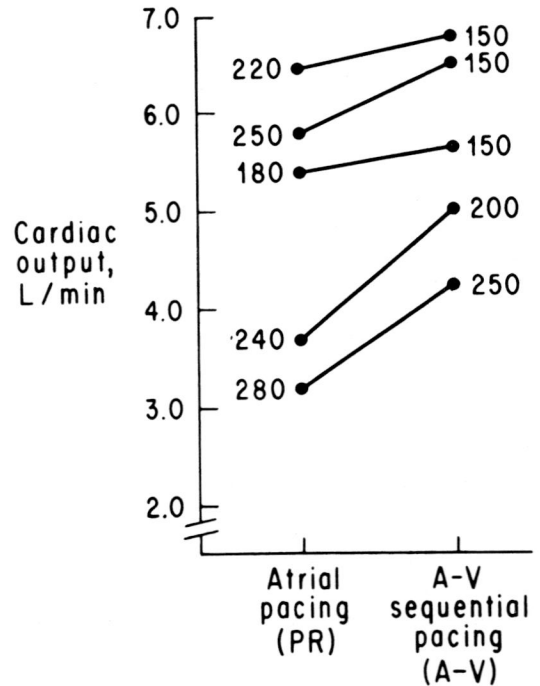

FIGURE 8–12. A comparison of cardiac output with ventricular pacing (without synchronous atrial systole) and with atrial pacing that shows an overall increase in cardiac output with atrial pacing of approximately 26% in patients after cardiac surgery. (From Hartzler, G. O., Maloney, J. D., Curtis, J. J., and Barnhorst, D. A.: Hemodynamic effects of atrioventricular sequential pacing after cardiac surgery. Am. J. Cardiol., 40:232, 1977.)

Inotropic State

Inotropic agents may be necessary to achieve cardiac function that adequately maintains peripheral oxygen delivery. Improvement in cardiac function by pharmacologic intervention is generally achieved at the expense of increased myocardial oxygen demand. Inotropic agents should be considered only after manipulations of heart rate, preload, and afterload have been maximized (Fig. 8–14). In general, myocardial function improves throughout the postoperative course, allowing weaning from inotropic support (Van Trigt et al., 1983).

Various inotropic agents are available, and all are administered by either intravenous bolus or continuous infusion. They should be administered through a central venous or pulmonary artery catheter whose intravascular position has been ascertained to prevent perivascular infiltration.

Most inotropic agents act through stimulation of adrenergic and dopaminergic receptors (see Tables 5–6 and 5–8). Most agents are adrenergic agonists whose actions are mediated through an increase in intracellular calcium concentration (Erdmann, 1988). Clinical experience using multiple inotropic agents has demonstrated synergism (Vernon et al., 1992) despite in vitro evidence that the maximal positive inotropic effect of one drug precludes augmentation by another (Brown, 1984). This may be due to alterations in the adenylate cyclase system in patients with heart failure (Erdmann, 1988) or to alterations in beta-adrenoreceptor density (Bristow et al., 1982; DiSesa, 1987; Erdmann, 1988; Fowler et al., 1986; Glaubiger and

Lefkowitz, 1977; Lefkowitz, 1979). Nonadrenergic inotropes include digoxin, calcium chloride, phosphodiasterase inhibitors (amrinone, milrinone, and enoximone), and triiodothyronine. The presence of metabolic acidosis may interfere with the effectiveness of inotropic agents (Kosugi and Tajimi, 1985; Tajimi et al., 1983).

Agents

Digoxin was first described for use by Withering in his classic monograph on the pharmacology of the leaves of the foxglove plant (*Digitalis purpurea*). Although the evidence is conflicting, there is support for the use of digoxin in patients with moderate to severe heart failure (NYHA Classes II, III, and IV) due to systolic ventricular dysfunction (Packer, 1993). An ongoing study from the Digitalis Investigators Group (DIG) sponsored by the National Heart, Lung, and Blood Institute of the National Institutes of Health has set out to determine whether routine prescription of a cardiac glycoside can be justified on the basis of improved survival.

Calcium is a positive inotropic agent only when used to normalize a low ionized calcium level. Calcium level should be checked upon admission of the patient to the ICU. Additional infusion in the setting of normal ionized calcium levels increases systemic vascular resistance (Drop and Scheidegger, 1980). Additionally, administration of calcium may blunt the patient's response to beta-adrenergic agonists (Zaloga et al., 1990). Administration is by bolus injection of 10 mg/kg. Calcium infusions may cause major disturbances in cardiac rhythm, including sinus arrhythmia, bradycardias, and atrioventricular dissociation (Drop, 1985).

Isoproterenol is a pure beta-adrenergic agonist. Its primary use is to increase heart rate and thus to increase CO with little effect on mean arterial BP (Lappas et al., 1977). It may also lower pulmonary vascular resistance.

Dopamine is an endogenous catecholamine and the immediate precursor of norepinephrine. Dopamine is a mixed alpha- and beta-adrenergic receptor agonist and causes release of norepinephrine from the myocardium. At low doses (2 to 4 μg/kg/min), a separate dopaminergic effect leading to renal, mesenteric, coronary, and cerebral arterial vasodilatation is seen without significant fall in peripheral vascular resistance (Goldberg and Rajfer, 1985; Lappas et al., 1977). The combination of dopamine and dobutamine may enhance cardiac function, especially in patients with significant right ventricular failure (Imai et al., 1992).

Dobutamine is a synthetic catecholamine and is an isoproterenol analogue (Sonnenblick et al., 1979). Improvements in CO of approximately 50% accompanied by a lowering of the PWP and variable decreases in both pulmonary and systemic vascular resistances have been noted (Orchard et al., 1982; Vernon et al., 1992). Significant tachycardia may result during administration. Dobutamine is particularly suitable for long-term administration because it undergoes less

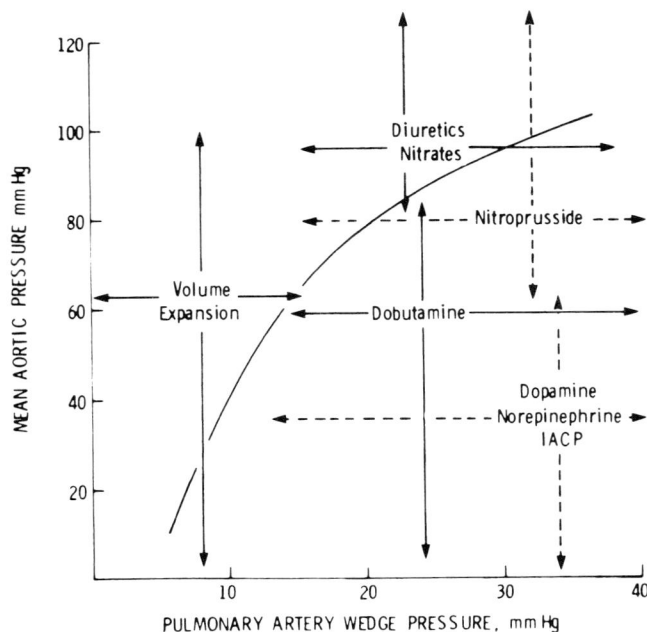

FIGURE 8–14. The hemodynamic indications for therapeutic interventions according to abnormalities of cardiac function described by the Frank-Starling relationship. (From Ayres, S. M.: Ventricular function. In Shoemaker, W. C., Thompson, W. L., and Holbrook, P. R. [eds]: Textbook of Critical Care. Philadelphia, W. B. Saunders, 1984.)

tachyphylaxis than is commonly seen with dopamine (MacCannell et al., 1983).

Epinephrine is a naturally occurring catecholamine that is a mixed alpha- and beta-adrenergic agonist (DiSesa, 1987; see Chapter 5, part I) and it significantly increases CO (by 40 to 60%) in the postoperative setting. Although epinephrine's effects are similar to those of other agents, it produces significant peripheral and splanchnic vasoconstriction, and may cause oliguria (Stephenson et al., 1976).

Norepinephrine is a naturally occurring catecholamine that is the neurotransmitter released at most sympathetic postganglionic fibers. Norepinephrine may be used at low doses (0.01 μg/kg/min) for profound hypertension. Higher doses may be used in instances of low CO that is unresponsive to other agents (Lollgen and Drexler, 1990).

Amrinone and *milrinone* inhibit cellular phosphodiasterase fraction 3 in both cardiac and smooth muscle. The benefit is an increase in intracellular concentrations of adenosine monophosphate (cAMP) (Alousi and Johnson, 1986; Endoh et al., 1986; Goldstein, 1986; Kaplan, 1989). Amrinone is the agent most frequently used in the postoperative setting. The effects of this class of agents include significant elevation in CO, a fall in pulmonary capillary wedge pressure and pulmonary artery pressure from both veno and arteriolar vasodilatation, and a significant fall in systemic vascular resistance (Kaplan, 1989, 1991; Kaplan and Levy, 1990). An important difference from adrenergic agonists is that with this class of agents, myocardial oxygen demand is not increased, and their use compares favorably with that of other inotropic agents in the postoperative setting (Dupuis et al., 1992). Major side effects are relatively rare, with an incidence of approximately 3%. Adequate preload often prevents significant hypotension. Other complications include gastrointestinal complaints and thrombocytopenia (3.4% and 2.4%, respectively) (Kaplan and Levy, 1990). In the postoperative setting, a higher loading dose of 1 to 3 mg/kg (over 5 to 10 minutes), followed by continuous infusion of 10 to 20 μg/kg/min, should be used (Kaplan, 1989).

Triiodothyronine (T3) has been reduced following CPB in both animal and clinical studies (Bremmer et al., 1979; Holland et al., 1991). In preliminary studies of patients undergoing myocardial revascularization, T3 significantly improved CO, decreased SVR, and reduced the need for postoperative inotropic support and cardiac assist devices (Novitzky et al., 1989, 1991). In animal models, CPB leads to a "sick euthyroid" state as manifested by decreased free T3, increased rT3, and slightly increased free thyroxine; this depresses myocardial function (Novitzky et al., 1989). One proposed mechanism of action for the observed effects of T3 on the myocardium is through cycling of intracellular sodium or calcium with resultant increases in free intracellular calcium and sodium channel current (Dyke et al., 1993). Evidence also exists for synergistic effects of T3 and ACE inhibitors (Pennock et al., 1993). Further elucidation of the role of T3 in the postoperative setting awaits the completion of ongoing prospectively randomized trials (Uppal et al., 1993).

Both the specific inotropic agent and its rate of administration are important considerations (Table 8–3). Increasing doses of agents with combined alpha- and beta-adrenergic properties, particularly dopamine and epinephrine, lead to a predominant alpha-adrenergic agonist effect at high doses, which may be deleterious (Feigl, 1987). Pure alpha-adrenergic effect is best obtained by using norepinephrine (Lappas et al., 1977) or other pure alpha-agonists (see Chapter 5, part I).

Dopamine and dobutamine are usually the agents of first choice, used alone or in combination. Low-dose dopamine may be used to improve renal perfusion (Davis et al., 1982). Dobutamine may be preferred in patients who require afterload and preload reduction, although the combination of dopamine and nitroprusside may allow easier titration (Table 8–4). Preload reserve may be obtained using a combination of an inotropic agent and afterload reduction (Miller et al., 1980).

Epinephrine and amrinone are usually reserved for patients with severe cardiac impairment. Epinephrine

■ **Table 8–3.** HEMODYNAMIC AND MYOCARDIAL METABOLIC RESPONSE OF SHOCK PATIENTS TO ADMINISTRATION OF FIVE AGENTS

Measurement	Isoproterenol	1-Norepinephrine	Dopamine	Dobutamine	IABP
Dosage	2–4 μg/min	2–8 μg/min	7 μg/kg/min	10 μg/kg/min	4–6 hours
Heart rate	27% increase	3% increase	10% increase	4% increase	13% decrease
Stroke index	27% increase	7% increase	54% increase	96% increase	54% increase
Cardiac index	63% increase	9% increase	59% increase	100% increase	39% increase
Mean arterial pressure	No change	38% increase	5% increase	5% increase	24% increase
Left ventricular systolic ejection resistance	33% decrease	28% increase	Decreased	Decreased	46% decrease
SVR	39% decrease	25% increase	38% decrease	44% decrease	11% decrease
Systolic ejection rate	49% increase	10% increase	29% increase	Increased	42% increase
Coronary blood flow	17% increase	39% increase	Decreased	—	34% increase
Arterial lactate	3% decrease	5% increase	Decreased	—	42% decrease
Myocardial oxygen extraction	7% decrease	3% decrease	4% increase	—	23% decrease

IABP = intra-aortic balloon counterpulsation; SVR = systemic vascular resistance.

Modified from Ayres, S. M.: Ventricular function. *In* Shoemaker, W. C., Thompson, W. L., and Holbrook, P. R. (eds): Textbook of Critical Care. Chap. 49. Philadelphia, W. B. Saunders, 1984, pp. 340 and 342. (Dobutamine data are from Mikulic et al., 1977; dopamine data from Stemple et al., 1978; and isoproterenol data from Mueller et al., 1970.)

■ Table 8–4. HEMODYNAMIC CHANGES AFTER ADMINISTRATION OF NITROPRUSSIDE, DOBUTAMINE, A COMBINATION OF THE TWO AGENTS, AND DOPAMINE WITH OR WITHOUT NITROPRUSSIDE

Measurement	Nitroprusside	Dobutamine	Nitroprusside + Dobutamine	Dopamine	Nitroprusside + Dopamine
Dosage	85 μg/min	10 μg/min		7 μg/kg/min	
Heart rate	7% decrease	7% decrease	3% decrease	10% increase	8% increase
Stroke index	40% increase	73% increase	120% increase	54% increase	82% increase
Pulmonary wedge pressure	48% decrease	32% decrease	56% decrease	3% increase	20% decrease
Systemic vascular resistance	32% decrease	35% decrease	69% decrease	38% decrease	55% decrease
Mean aortic pressure	12% decrease	2% decrease	14% decrease	5% increase	5% decrease

Modified from Ayres, S. M.: Ventricular function. *In* Shoemaker, W. C., Thompson, W. L., and Holbrook, P. R. (eds): Textbook of Critical Care. Chap. 49. Philadelphia, W. B. Saunders, 1984, p. 341. (Nitroprusside/dobutamine data are from Mikulic et al., 1977; nitroprusside/dopamine data are from Stemple et al., 1978.)

is usually the first drug weaned in a multi-inotropic agent environment because of its deleterious effect on peripheral and renal perfusion. Isoproterenol may be used in patients with pulmonary hypertension and right ventricular failure not controlled by other agents (DiSesa, 1987).

Mechanical Ventricular Assistance

Failure of conventional hemodynamic support can often be overcome with mechanical circulatory assist devices designed to provide circulatory support and to assist in myocardial recovery (Emery and Joyce, 1991; Miller, 1991). Following cardiac surgery, significant ventricular dysfunction requiring mechanical assist devices occurs in 2 to 10% of patients (Pennington et al., 1989). Most of these patients (60 to 90%) can be stabilized with an intra-aortic balloon pump (IABP); only a small percentage (0.2 to 1%) of patients require more advanced circulatory assist devices such as centrifugal or pneumatic ventricular assist devices (VADs) (Pennington et al., 1989). The objective for mechanical circulatory assist following cardiac surgery is to provide adequate circulation and to diminish myocardial work, allowing for recovery of stunned myocardium.

Intra-Aortic Balloon Counterpulsation (IABP). The IABP device is the simplest and most commonly used mechanical circulatory assistance device. Approximately 80,000 are inserted each year in the United States (Goldenberg, 1992). The device is a pulsatile pneumatic balloon that inflates with gas during diastole and deflates during systole. The result is a 70% increase in diastolic aortic pressure and a 10 to 40% increase in CO. As originally designed, the IABP device was introduced through an end-to-side Dacron graft placed in the common femoral artery. Percutaneous insertion techniques are now used routinely in most patients (Grayzel, 1982). Transthoracic insertion into the descending aorta (McGeehin et al., 1987) and insertion into the pulmonary artery (Moran et al., 1984; Skillington et al., 1991) have also been described in patients undergoing cardiac surgery. The complication rate of IABP has been as high as 30% (Goldberg et al., 1987). Complications are primarily vascular, including ischemia due to thrombosis or embolism, aortic dissection, aortic rupture, and bleeding, but

infection, hemolysis, thrombocytopenia, and gas leak also have been reported. Spinal cord ischemia causing paraplegia has also been observed in several patients (Harris et al., 1986; Rose et al., 1984; Tyras and Willman, 1978). Contraindications to IABP include significant aortic insufficiency and aortic aneurysm. Although percutaneous introduction of the IABP device is technically easier, the vascular complication rate with this method is slightly higher than with direct surgical insertion (Goldberg et al., 1987; Grayzel, 1982). However, improved percutaneous techniques allow safe insertion in most patients.

Proper balloon function requires synchronization using the ECG or monitored intra-arterial pressure. Interference and poor IABP augmentation may produce supraventricular or ventricular arrhythmias in patients. The complication rate is changed little by the duration of IABP assistance (Bolooki, 1986), and the mean duration of preoperative support is 2 to 3 days (McGee et al., 1980). One-to-one augmentation at a rate of 90 to 110 beats per minute and maximal balloon volume achieves full assistance capability. At higher heart rates, augmentation may fall because of balloon gas viscosity and incomplete systolic balloon collapse. Weaning from IABP is accomplished by gradual reduction in the rate of augmentation from 1:1 to 1:2 to 1:3. For every 24-hour period of IABP assistance, a 6-hour weaning time has been suggested (Bolooki, 1986). The removal of the IABP (percutaneous placement) is followed by 45 minutes of manual compression at the insertion site. Distal blood flow should be monitored with a transcutaneous Doppler device. Operatively placed IABP devices should be removed under direct vision.

Survival rates for IABP device insertion range from 27 to 63% in cardiac surgical patients who cannot be weaned from CPB (Bolooki, 1986; DiLello et al., 1988; Dowing et al., 1986); the rate is 53.4% when the device is inserted for preoperative cardiogenic shock (Pennington et al., 1983). Higher mortality rates are associated with postoperative insertion of IABP devices for perioperative myocardial infarction with associated cardiogenic shock (Golding et al., 1980).

Ventricular Assistance Devices. Assistance devices may be classified as left, right, or bi-ventricular assist devices. After IABP, centrifugal and roller pumps are the next most commonly used methods of mechanical assistance because of their commercial availability, low cost, and simplicity. These devices can provide univentricular or biventricular support. Three manufacturers produce centrifugal pumps: Biomedicus, Sarns, and Ares Medical. These devices can pump 5 to 6 l/min and therefore completely support the circulation. However, most centrifugal and roller pumps produce nonpulsatile flow (Rotello et al., 1992).

The Hemopump (Johnson & Johnson) is a continuous axial blood flow pump that propels blood from the left ventricle to the descending aorta. It is an intravascular pump using an Archimedean screw principle with rotations at approximately 20,000 RPM providing unidirectional nonpulsatile flow (Mooney et al., 1990).

External pulsatile VADs are still being investigated, and require Food and Drug Administration (FDA) approval. Examples include the Thoratec VAD and the Abiomed VVS support system.

Direct mechanical ventricular actuation is a biventricular support device requiring surgical application. Although it awaits further testing, this device, developed at Duke University Medical Center, does have the advantage of rapid application and does not require anticoagulation therapy (Anstadt et al., 1991; Lowe et al., 1991a).

Survival rates in patients requiring VADs following cardiac surgery approach 50% in patients with left-sided VAD and fall to 30% in patients requiring a biventricular assist device (Miller et al., 1990).

MANAGEMENT OF CARDIAC COMPLICATIONS

Perioperative Myocardial Infarction

The incidence of perioperative myocardial infarction has decreased with improvements in myocardial preservation and has been reported as low as 2.4% (Kouchoukos et al., 1980), with rates usually at about 6% (CASS, 1983). Reported perioperative infarction rates depend partially on the method used for diagnosis. Elevation of myocardial enzymes is associated with higher rates (Dixon et al., 1973; Gray et al., 1982; Moore et al., 1977) than are electrocardiographic indices (Alderman et al., 1973; Moore et al., 1977). The significance of perioperative myocardial infarction remains to be clearly defined. Perioperative myocardial infarction in patients with incomplete revascularization and in those with resulting depressed ejection fraction is associated with poor long-term survival compared with perioperative infarction in patients with well-preserved ventricular function (Force et al., 1990; Pennington et al., 1988). Perioperative myocardial infarction is often associated with bundle-branch block, particularly a new complete left bundle-branch block (Caspi et al., 1987), which makes the diagnosis difficult.

Intraoperative Injury and Graft Occlusion

Significant graft or coronary occlusion can have immediately perceptible hemodynamic effects (Fig. 8–15). Early graft failure is usually due to technical factors, although it may be produced by scarring and is seen more frequently in patients with inflammatory pericardial syndromes. Late graft failures are usually due to the development of new coronary lesions (47%) or the incorrect selection of anastomotic sites (23%) (Culliford et al., 1979). Graft survival is enhanced by the perioperative administration of antiplatelet agents. Initially, aspirin and dipyridamole were used (Chesebro et al., 1982). However, subsequent work suggests that low-dose aspirin alone (325 mg/day) is as effective as combination agents (Lorenz et al., 1984).

The simple occurrence of perioperative myocardial infarction has not been significantly related to graft patency, late survival, or cardiac status (Gray et al., 1982). Postoperative ventricular function and stress test performance are related to graft patency but not necessarily to the detection of myocardial injury in the perioperative period (Codd et al., 1978). Decreased survival has been noted by others (Namay et al., 1982), and the significance of perioperative myocardial infarction ultimately depends on postoperative ventricular function and completeness of revascularization.

The treatment of perioperative myocardial infarction consists primarily of supporting CO and treating coronary spasm. Early cardiac catheterization and graft revision should be considered when salvage of an occluded graft seems possible according to intraoperative findings (Lemmer and Kirsh, 1988). Supportive therapy with nitroglycerin (Flaherty et al., 1982) and afterload reduction with ACE inhibitors (SOLVD, 1990) can prevent recurrent hospitalization and improve long-term outcome (Cohn, 1993; Hood, 1993; Pitt, 1993; St. John Sutton et al., 1994). The effect of inotropic therapy on transmural blood flow distribution and on preformed collaterals should also be considered (Warltier et al., 1981).

The long-term treatment of patients suffering perioperative myocardial infarction may include beta-blockade, afterload reduction, and other drug therapy that has improved longevity in patients suffering from myocardial infarction (Beta-Blocker Heart Attack Trial Research Group, 1982; Norwegian Multicenter Study Group, 1981; Yusuf, 1987). Although significance of perioperative myocardial infarction has not been proved, exercise increase in ejection fraction months after surgery appears to be blunted in patients with perioperative myocardial infarction (Assad-Morrell et al., 1975).

Postoperative Coronary Spasm

The incidence of perioperative myocardial infarction caused by coronary spasm is as high as 1% (Lemmer and Kirsh, 1988). Spasm can occur in grafted vessels leading to ventricular fibrillation (Pichard et

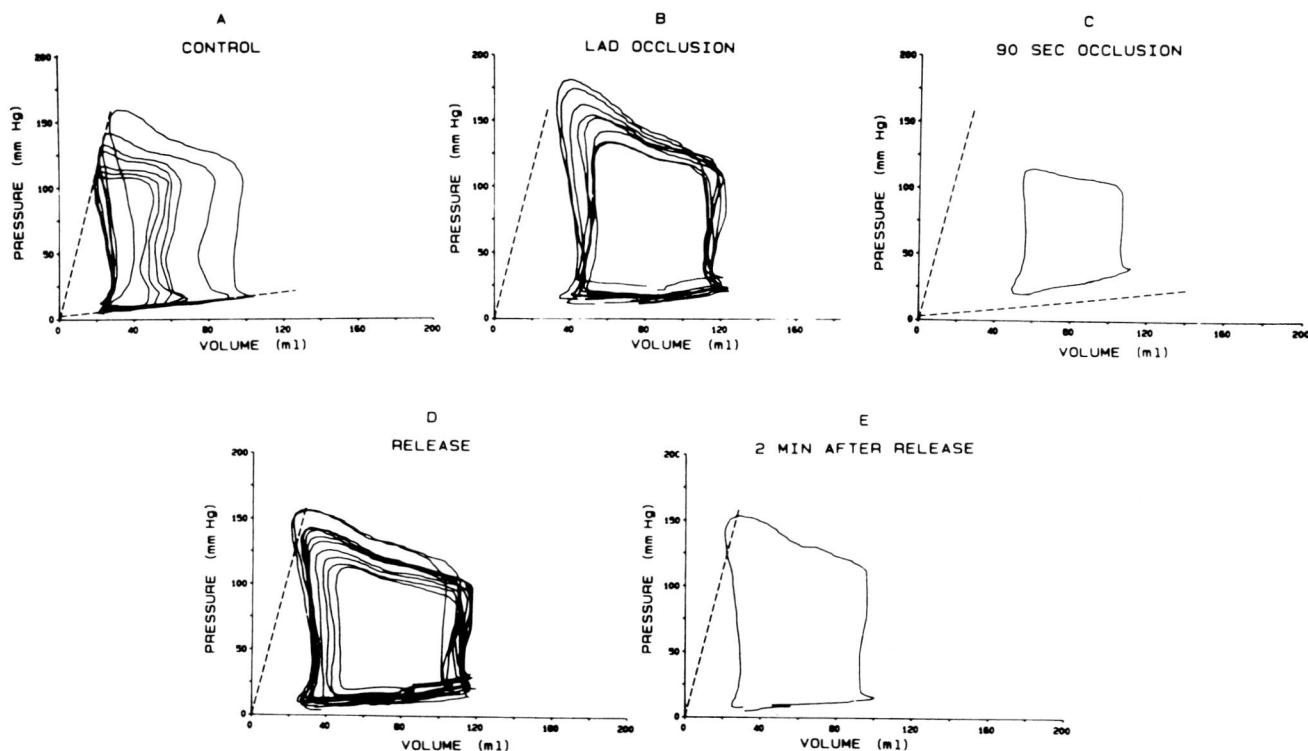

FIGURE 8–15. Pressure-volume relationship in the human heart during balloon occlusion of the left anterior descending (LAD) coronary artery. Ventricular volume was determined with a multielectrode conductance catheter. As can be seen in *B* and ultimately in *C*, sharp diminutions in inotropic state, stroke volume, and stroke work occur rapidly after coronary occlusion. *C*, A reduction in diastolic compliance is also noted. *D* and *E*, The reversibility of these changes is shown after momentary occlusion. (*A–E*, From Kass, D. A., and Maughan, W. L.: From "E_{max}" to pressure-volume relations: A broader view. Circulation, 77:1203, 1988. By permission of the American Heart Association, Inc.)

al., 1980). It may also occur in nongrafted vessels (Zeff et al., 1982), with a predilection for the right coronary artery (Buxton et al., 1981). In patients suffering perioperative myocardial infarction associated with a hyperdynamic state, elevated circulated catecholamine levels (Boudoulas et al., 1976) create an environment conducive to persistent coronary spasm. Perioperative coronary spasm should always be considered, and aggressive management with nitroglycerin and sublingual nifedipine should be instituted (Feldman, 1987). If pharmacologic therapy is unsuccessful, emergency cardiac catheterization and direct intracoronary injection of nitroglycerin or papaverine should be performed. In the unstable patient, re-exploration and direct injection into grafts has been used successfully (Lemmer and Kirsh, 1988). Long-term survival can be achieved with a low incidence of late postoperative spasm (Buxton et al., 1982).

Cardiac Tamponade

Cardiac tamponade results from occupation of the mediastinal space by fluid or clotted blood, which restricts the end-diastolic volume of both ventricles. It has been reported to occur acutely in 3.4 to 5.8% of cases (Craddock et al., 1968; Engelman et al., 1970; Nelson et al., 1969). The constellation of findings that is associated with acute postoperative cardiac tamponade includes the following:

1. Increased variation in blood pressure with respiration (pulsus paradoxus)
2. Equalization and elevation of the CVP, pulmonary artery diastolic pressure, and left atrial pressure or pulmonary artery wedge pressure (Weeks et al., 1976)
3. A fall in urine output (often an early finding)
4. Excessive chest tube drainage (or, paradoxically, minimal or no chest tube drainage, especially when heavy clots are noted within the chest tubes)
5. Mediastinal widening on chest film
6. Low CO (late)
7. Hypotension (late)

No single finding or combination of findings is sufficient to establish the diagnosis, and a high index of clinical suspicion should be maintained. Early postoperative tamponade is treated by reoperation, ideally in the operating room. However, patients in extremis may require reopening of their sternotomy in the ICU. Temporizing management consists of volume loading, reduction of airway pressure (removal of PEEP, anesthetizing agents, diminishing tidal volume with increasing ventilatory rate), and inotropic support.

Cardiac tamponade may be present with any amount

of retained blood or fluid, which in most cases is circumferential, but which may be loculated and may still adversely affect myocardial function (Fowler et al., 1988, Russo et al., 1993). In patients with decreased ventricular function, smaller amounts of space occupation are required to manifest tamponade physiology (Shabetai, 1988a). In patients with severe ventricular dysfunction, simple reapproximation of the sternum following cardiac surgery may not be possible. Delayed sternal closure may be necessary in 1 to 2% of high-risk patients, and subsequent closure is usually possible between the third and fourth days following initial operation (Furnary et al., 1992).

To a certain extent, the pleural and mediastinal spaces are continuous, and resulting intrathoracic pressure is distributed to affect the lungs and cardiac chambers simultaneously. An open pericardium and pleural space cannot prevent or minimize cardiac tamponade. Increases in airway pressure, which may result from changing lung compliance, application of PEEP, or a change in chest wall compliance, may be directly transmitted to the heart. Such increases in airway pressure cause additive space occupation and can bring about tamponade at lower volumes of retained fluid.

Although cardiac tamponade usually presents within the first 24 hours following surgery, there is a definite incidence of late presentation (Bortolotti et al., 1981; Ellison and Kirsh, 1974; Hardesty et al., 1978, Russo et al., 1993). Most cases occur in patients with large amounts of postoperative bleeding, patients who require anticoagulation, or patients with active inflammation (postpericardiotomy syndrome). Delayed diagnosis is attributed to the associated nonspecific symptoms of malaise, dyspnea, chest pain, and anorexia. Echocardiography serves as the mainstay in diagnosis (Fyke et al., 1985; Kronzon et al., 1983; Rifkin et al., 1987; Singh et al., 1984). As many as 85% of patients following cardiac surgery develop a pericardial effusion at some point in their postoperative course, without significant symptoms (Stevenson et al., 1984; Weitzman et al., 1984). In patients with circumferential pericardial effusions, echocardiography frequently reveals right ventricular diastolic collapse, right atrial collapse, and left atrial collapse, which are useful signs of cardiac tamponade (Spodick, 1983). These classic echocardiographic findings may be absent if the tamponade is caused by a regional pericardial effusion. Frequently, this effusion is localized posteriorly following surgery (Weitzman et al., 1984). Recent evidence suggests that early diastolic invagination of the left ventricular free wall, or left ventricular diastolic collapse, is a particularly useful echocardiographic finding in the postoperative patient (Chuttani et al., 1991). Occasionally, confirmation by right-sided catheterization is necessary to make a definitive diagnosis (Borkon et al., 1981; Hardesty et al., 1978).

Arrhythmias

Documented arrhythmias are frequent following cardiac surgery. Tachyarrhythmias occur in some form in up to 64% of patients (Michelson et al., 1979). Bradyarrhythmias and conduction system abnormalities also are common. Tachyarrhythmias are deleterious because of rapid rate, irregularity of a moderately increased rate, generation of an inefficient ventricular activation sequence, and loss of atrioventricular synchrony.

Supraventricular Arrhythmias

Sinus Tachycardia. Sinus tachycardia is usually a secondary phenomenon in response to other derangements. If inappropriate and deleterious, it may be treated with a beta-adrenergic antagonist.

Paroxysmal Atrial Tachycardia, Premature Atrial Contractions. Premature atrial contractions are common following cardiac surgery and frequently can be suppressed by maintaining the serum potassium concentration at the upper limit of normal (4.5 to 5.5 mEq/l) (Fisch et al., 1966). They may also be suppressed by overdrive atrial or atrioventricular pacing at a rate faster than the patient's spontaneous sinus rate. Paroxysmal atrial tachycardia may also be treated by rapid atrial pacing. Additional pharmacologic agents include beta-adrenergic antagonists and calcium and channel blockers. Adenosine appears to be as effective as calcium channel blockers for terminating paroxysmal supraventricular tachycardias.

Atrial Flutter. Postoperative atrial flutter is frequently difficult to treat (Wellens, 1991). Atrial flutter is generated by a macro–re-entrant phenomenon (Manolis and Estes, 1987) and can be treated rapidly and effectively with electrical stimulation. Although this arrhythmia may be interrupted by a single, appropriately timed, atrial extrasystole, it is most commonly interrupted by entrainment or by nonspecific rapid atrial stimulation (Waldo et al., 1977). The first method consists of determining the atrial rate and instituting atrial pacing at a slightly higher rate in order to capture the atria. Regularization of the ventricular response and an altered P-wave morphology are usually produced. Once accomplished, termination of pacing is ordinarily followed by normal sinus rhythm (Fig. 8–16).

Rapid atrial pacing is performed by introducing trains of atrial pacing at rates in the range of 450 to 600 beats per minute. Short trains (less than 1 second) effectively introduce single extra stimuli within the effective refractory period of the pacing site, thus interrupting atrial flutter and reinstating the normal sinus rhythm. If the train of rapid atrial pacing is too long, it may induce atrial fibrillation, which cannot be treated with these pacing techniques. However, in the atrial fibrillation that may ensue, the ventricular response is usually slower and thus better tolerated than that of atrial flutter (Lister et al., 1968). It is common for atrial fibrillation induced in this manner to spontaneously revert to normal sinus rhythm. Following acute treatment, superior long-term control of atrioventricular node conduction is usually obtained by digitalization. Digoxin is usually continued for 4 weeks postoperatively.

Pace Atria 350 beats/min—▶off

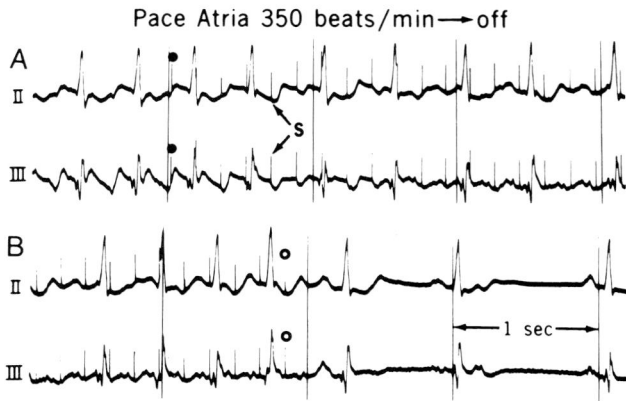

FIGURE 8–16. Electrocardiographic leads II and III show atrial flutter with 2:1 AV block. *A* and *B* are not continuous. At the *black dot* in *A,* atrial pacing at 350 beats/min is begun. Note that by the end of the tracing in *A,* the P-wave morphology has changed from negative to positive, which indicates entrainment. In *B,* after 30 seconds of pacing at 350 beats/min, atrial pacing is terminated (*open circle*). Sinus rhythm appears spontaneously. Time lines at 1-second intervals. (S = stimulus artifact.) (*A–B,* From Waldo, A. L., MacLean, W. A. H.: Diagnosis and Treatment of Cardiac Arrhythmias Following Open Heart Surgery. Mt. Kisco, NY, Futura Publishing, 1980.)

Atrial Fibrillation. Atrial fibrillation is the most common supraventricular arrhythmia following cardiac operation. The incidence has varied from 28 to 54% of patients undergoing cardiac operations (Lauer et al., 1989; Mills et al., 1983; Rubin et al., 1987; Silverman et al., 1982). The etiology is unknown, but has been postulated to be due to unprotected ischemia (Silverman et al., 1984; Smith et al., 1983c), multidose cardioplegic solution administration with high potassium concentration (Ellis et al., 1980), atrial dilatation or inadequate atrial protection (Cox, 1993; Podrid, 1992), or postoperative pericarditis (Page et al., 1986). The incidence of postoperative atrial fibrillation is higher in patients with echocardiographic evidence of pericardial effusion (Angelini et al., 1987). Certain patients may also have an inherent propensity to develop supraventricular arrhythmias related to the preoperative accumulation of catecholamines in intramyocardial axons (Kyosola et al., 1988). Additional risk factors predictive of an increased incidence of atrial fibrillation include advanced age, chronic obstructive pulmonary disease, and prolonged cross-clamp periods due to inadequate atrial protection (Creswell et al., 1993). Although this arrhythmia has not been shown to increase the 30-day mortality rate, it does prolong length of stay in patients undergoing CABG (Podrid, 1992). There is also an increased incidence of malignant ventricular rhythms (both ventricular tachycardia and ventricular fibrillation), as well as a significant increase in the postoperative stroke rate (Creswell et al., 1993). The risk of atrial fibrillation is increased in elderly patients, patients with chronic obstructive pulmonary disease, and patients in whom preoperative beta-adrenergic antagonists have been discontinued (Fuller et al., 1989; Podrid, 1992). Intraoperative identification of patients at risk

may be possible by determining the atrial threshold for induction of atrial fibrillation (Lowe et al., 1991b). Marked dispersion of the atrial refractory period (Cox, 1993) has been shown to lead to atrial fibrillation.

Treatment is aided by accurate diagnosis. Although various methods can be used, these have generally been supplanted by direct examination of atrial and ventricular bipolar ECGs (Waldo et al., 1977). The presence of chaotic and rapid atrial depolarization indicates atrial fibrillation, whereas regular rapid atrial depolarization with an organized ventricular response (usually 2:1 or 3:1) indicates atrial flutter (Fig. 8–17).

The therapeutic objectives in patients with atrial fibrillation are heart rate control, conversion to sinus rhythm, maintenance of sinus rhythm, and prevention of embolic complications. Heart rate control is the first objective for therapy of patients in atrial fibrillation. In general, heart rates controlled below 100 beats per minute maintain stroke volume in CO (Rawles, 1990). The drug of choice for controlling ventricular response is a calcium channel antagonist: either verapamil administered in 2.5- to 5-mg boluses to a total of 20 mg or diltiazem given as an intravenous load followed by a continuous infusion. These agents rapidly reduce the ventricular response by increasing atrioventricular block (Singh and Nademanee, 1987). The salutary effect of reduction in ventricular rate is usually more important than the negative inotropic effect of these drugs (Nayler and Szeto, 1972; Packer et al., 1987; Plumb et al., 1982). Adverse effects of calcium channel antagonists may be treated with calcium infusion (Perkins, 1978), glucagon (Linden and Aghababian, 1985), or inotropic agents (Singh and Williams, 1972). Alternatively, the use of beta-block-

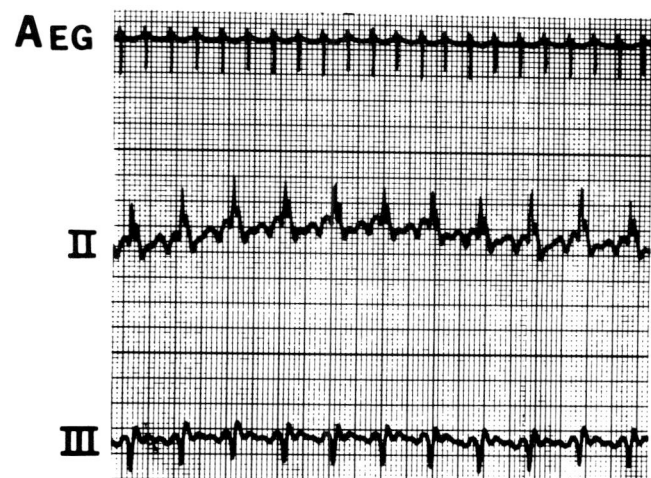

FIGURE 8–17. Bipolar atrial electrogram (AEG) is shown in the upper trace with simultaneous ECG leads II and III that show atrial flutter with 2:1 AV block. Recording speed, 25 mm/sec. (From Waldo, A. L., Cooper, T. B., and MacLean, W. A. H.: Cardiac pacing in the treatment of cardiac arrhythmias following open heart surgery: Use of temporarily placed atrial and ventricular wire electrodes. *In* Samet, P., and El-Sherif, N. [eds]: Cardiac Pacing. 2nd ed. Chap 24. New York, Grune & Stratton, 1980.)

ers, especially those with short action (esmolol), has been studied for the acute management of atrial fibrillation (Podrid, 1992). The response to beta-blockade varies considerably when it is used to treat atrial fibrillation following CABG. In addition, hypotension may be a significant side effect in as many as 20 to 40% of patients (Podrid, 1992). Digoxin has been similarly used, although immediate heart rate control is rarely achieved (Goldman et al., 1975).

Once heart rate control has been achieved, conversion and maintenance of sinus rhythm with a Class IA antiarrhythmic agent, either procainamide or quinidine, may be necessary (Morganroth et al., 1986). The Class IA agent should ordinarily be withheld until atrioventricular conduction has been controlled adequately, because it may enhance atrioventricular conduction and can convert atrial fibrillation into atrial flutter. This may cause deleterious hemodynamic effects. Intravenous beta-blockers are useful in controlling the atrioventricular node and thus the ventricular response, and they can induce normal sinus rhythm (Matloff et al., 1968). However, they have been largely supplanted by calcium channel antagonists, although this class of agents is ineffective in conversion to sinus rhythm (Heng et al., 1975). Multidrug combinations can be hazardous in patients without temporary pacing wires. The combination of digoxin, verapamil, and a beta-adrenergic antagonist can lead to complete heart block, whereas verapamil and a beta-adrenergic antagonist may lead to sinus arrest (Lee et al., 1986).

Rapid supraventricular arrhythmias causing significant hemodynamic compromise should be treated by cardioversion or defibrillation (see "Cardiopulmonary Resuscitation," later in this chapter).

There has been much interest in the prophylactic use of antiarrhythmic agents to diminish the incidence of supraventricular arrhythmias (atrial fibrillation in particular) following cardiac surgery. However, prophylactic use of antiarrhythmics in all patients may lead to unwanted side effects in patients who would otherwise convalesce normally. As attempts to identify perioperative risk factors continue, many cardiac surgeons prefer to treat arrhythmias only when they occur (Hashimoto et al., 1991). Numerous agents have been studied for prophylactic use in cardiac surgical patients. Digoxin has been found to be ineffective in this regard (Weiner et al., 1986), although it may blunt the initial ventricular response of supraventricular arrhythmias (Selzer and Walter, 1966). Prophylactic propranolol (10 mg given orally every 6 hours) can reduce the incidence by approximately 50% (Silverman et al., 1982; Stephenson et al., 1980) and can be administered safely in patients with acceptable left ventricular function within 24 hours of surgery (Boudoulas et al., 1978). Atenolol may also be given in doses of 25 mg every 8 hours with similar results. Prophylactic procainamide started intraoperatively has also been effective (Laub et al., 1993). The combination of digoxin and propranolol has been shown to reduce the incidence of arrhythmias from 30 to 3.4% (Mills et al., 1983) and yields the greatest reduction that may be achieved pharmacologically.

There is no clear consensus on perioperative management of cardiac surgical patients. As yet, no definitive preoperative factors predict the development of atrial fibrillation. Some surgeons treat all patients prophylactically to suppress atrial arrhythmias; many others, wishing to avoid unnecessary drug toxicities, treat only patients who develop postoperative arrhythmias.

Ventricular Arrhythmias

Perioperative ventricular tachyarrhythmias are potentially lethal. They may be heralded by premature ventricular contractions in as many as 29% of patients (Michelson et al., 1979), although arrhythmias such as ventricular fibrillation can occur spontaneously (Moran, 1984). These arrhythmias have numerous origins, including perioperative myocardial injury related to prolonged ischemia, incomplete myocardial revascularization, and graft occlusion. Treatable underlying causes include hypokalemia, acidosis, hypoxia, and irritation from malpositioned intracardiac catheters. In addition, hypomagnesemia (Boriss and Papa, 1988; Chernow et al., 1988; Dyckner and Wester, 1981; Iseri et al., 1983) and the use of catecholamines may promote ventricular irritability (Morady et al., 1988). However, ventricular escape rhythms may be physiologic in the setting of significant bradycardia.

The diagnosis is made principally by examination of continuous electrocardiographic monitoring and the 12-lead ECG. Ventricular tachycardia must be differentiated from sinus tachycardia with bundle-branch block and from supraventricular arrhythmia with aberrant conduction. Confirmation of ventricular origin requires demonstration of atrioventricular dissociation (Lown et al., 1973). A definitive diagnosis can usually be made from direct recording of atrial and ventricular bipolar electrodes (measured from the temporary epicardial pacing wires).

Treatment strategy includes simple observation, suppression with overdrive pacing (Beller et al., 1968; Mills and Ochsner, 1973), specialized pacing, and drug therapy. Conventional wisdom has been to assume a causal relationship between the presence of premature ventricular contractions (PVCs) and adverse outcome, which has led to the notion that suppression of PVCs should help these patients. The Cardiac Arrhythmia Suppression Trial (CAST), designed to test this hypothesis, revealed an increased mortality rate in patients whose PVCs were suppressed (CAST Investigators, 1989; Ruskin, 1989). No clear-cut relationship has been established between PVC frequency or morphology and the occurrence of life-threatening ventricular arrhythmias (Woosley, 1988). Similarly, it has never been demonstrated that nonsustained, ventricular tachycardia justifies drug therapy. The rationale for withholding drug therapy is related to the associated risk of adverse drug effects, including the well-documented proarrhythmic effect of most available agents (Bigger and Sahar, 1987; Dhein et al., 1983; Josephson, 1986; Prystowsky, 1988; Stanton et al., 1989; Vlay, 1985; Wellens, 1993; Woosley, 1988; Zipes, 1988). Supportive therapy with maintenance of normal serum electrolytes (particularly potassium and magnesium), the addition of overdrive suppression pacing, and the exclusion of hypoxia are always indicated. Most studies in this area relate to arrhythmias following acute myocardial infarction that occurs in the setting of additional coronary artery disease being managed medically. Thus, recommended therapy can be strictly applied only to less than 10% of patients undergoing cardiac operation (patients with incomplete revascularization who sustain perioperative infarction).

Premature Ventricular Contractions. Frequent PVCs (more than 6/min) or multifocal PVCs are commonly treated regardless of the presence or absence of symptoms or underlying ischemia. No definitive data support this practice, and such arrhythmias may accompany a benign postoperative recovery. Observation with continuous electrocardiographic monitoring and a predischarge 24-hour Holter monitor may suffice.

An alternative is to subject such patients to invasive electrophysiologic testing and PVC suppression by drugs identified during testing (ACC/AHA Task Force, 1989). Although mortality and morbidity may be increased in these patients, particularly if left ventricular function is depressed, the frequency and character of these arrhythmias have not been convincingly shown to be of *independent* predictive value (Califf et al., 1982; Surawicz, 1987). This approach has not been proved to affect morbidity and mortality in such asymptomatic patients.

PVCs associated with perioperative infarction should be treated with prophylactic beta-blockade. This has been effective in large trials of patients following myocardial infarction, although electrophysiologic end-points were not used. A rational plan would be to place such patients on beta-blockers either prophylactically or as a therapy for frequent PVCs. Continued monitoring and possible referral to an electrophysiologic consultant may be necessary.

Ventricular Tachycardia. Ventricular tachycardia is classified as nonsustained (3 beat runs) or sustained. Although certain forms of ventricular tachycardia may be hemodynamically tolerated, most lead to immediate hemodynamic compromise.

Ventricular tachycardia that is hemodynamically tolerated can be treated with drug therapy. Mechanical treatments such as a single precordial thump (which delivers a DC cardioversion of approximately 5 joules) may be effective and should be used. Ventricular tachycardia can also be abolished with a single induced extra stimulus or by entrainment, as outlined earlier for atrial flutter. Rapid ventricular pacing is contraindicated because it tends to induce ventricular fibrillation. Pacing therapy for ventricular tachycardia should be used only by those specifically trained in this area. Ventricular tachycardia leading to hemodynamic instability should be treated immediately with cardioversion.

Ventricular Fibrillation. This rhythm should be immediately treated with defibrillation (see following section).

Medical Therapy of Ventricular Arrhythmias. Antiarrhythmic agents can be divided into four groups (Table 8–5). In general, antiarrhythmic agents diminish ventricular automaticity and increase the effective refractory period of both conduction tissue and the myocardium (Singh et al., 1980). Class IB agents (lidocaine and tocainide) have a documented ability to increase the ventricular fibrillation threshold. Class I (all subgroups) and Class III agents all have documented effectiveness in reducing PVC frequency (37 to 86% reduction [Morganroth et al., 1986]). However, most agents have significant proarrhythmic features, and efficacy is related to therapeutic blood levels.

Clinically significant depression of sinus node function (disopyramide, flecainide, amiodarone, and bretylium) and atrioventricular conduction (disopyramide, flecainide, bretylium, encainide, and Class II and Class IV agents) should be considered when administering these drugs to patients with subclinical atrioventricular node injury or underlying disease of the conduction system (Morganroth et al., 1986). Procainamide may also elevate the epicardial pacing threshold in high doses.

Digoxin is a commonly prescribed medication, and understanding of its constellation of toxic effects is mandatory. Although almost any arrhythmia can be seen with toxicity, frequently encountered arrhythmias include atrial tachycardia with block, nonparoxysmal atrioventricular junctional tachycardia, bidirectional ventricular tachycardia (torsade de pointes), bigeminy, and multifocal PVCs (Bhatia and Smith, 1987). Measurement of serum digoxin level can be helpful in this diagnosis, although it is not definitive. Digoxin levels in the therapeutic range do not preclude toxicity, nor does an elevated digoxin level prove toxicity. The mean serum level in patients given nontoxic levels of digoxin whose left ventricular performance is improved is 1.4 ng/ml (Packer, 1993), whereas the mean serum level of patients with known toxic levels is approximately 2 to 3 times higher. Although the upper limit of normal is often stated to be 2 ng/ml, 10% of patients without toxicity will have higher levels, and 10% of patients with evidence of toxicity will have lower levels (Haber, 1985). The management of ventricular rate should be guided by adequate rate control rather than by serum levels of digoxin. Digoxin is not eliminated by CPB, is not dialyzable, and has a half-life of approximately 36 hours. Significant interactions with other drugs may cause toxicity. Initial therapy of toxicity-related arrhythmias includes lidocaine and dilantin. Hypokalemia should be aggressively managed because it exacerbates digitalis toxicity (Shapiro, 1978). Calcium is contraindicated, and cardioversion should be avoided. The definitive therapy for toxicity is the stoichiometric administration of digoxin-specific Fab fragments, which are effective within 30 minutes to 1 hour of their administration (Antman et al., 1990; Bhatia and Smith, 1987).

■ **Table 8–5.** CLASSIFICATION OF ANTIARRHYTHMIC DRUGS AND THERAPEUTIC BLOOD LEVELS*

Class I		Class II		Class III		Class IV	
IA							
Cibenzoline	(100–400 ng/ml)	Acebutolol	(1–2 µg/ml)	Amiodarone	(1–2.5 µg/ml)	Diltiazem	
Disopyramide	(2–4 µg/ml)	Atenolol		Bretylium		Verapamil	(100–400 ng/ml)
Pirmenol	(1–4 µg/ml)	Esmolol	(400–1200 ng/ml)	N-Acetylprocainamide	(<25 µg/ml)		
Procainamide	(4–10 µg/ml)	Metoprolol		Sotalol	(0.3–4.0 µg/ml)		
Quinidine	(1.5–4.0 µg/m)	Propranolol					
		Sotalol	(0.3–4.0 µg/ml)				
		Timolol					
IB							
Ethmozin	(0.2–1.5 µg/ml)						
Lidocaine	(2–5 µg/ml)						
Mexiletine	(0.5–2 µg/ml)						
Phenytoin	(10–20 µg/ml)						
Tocainide	(4–10 µg/ml)						
IC							
Encainide	(5–150 ng/ml)						
Flecainide	(0.2–1 µg/ml)						
Lorcainide	(150–500 ng/ml)						
Propafenone	(0.5–3.0 µg/ml)						

Modified from Morganroth, J., Frishman, W. H., Horowitz, L. N., et al. (eds): Cardiovascular Drug Therapy. Chicago, Year Book Medical, 1986; and Michelson, E. L., and Dreifus, L. S.: Newer antiarrhythmic drugs. Med. Clin. North Am., 72:275, 1988.
*Drugs are arranged alphabetically within each class. Therapeutic levels are in parentheses if available and potentially useful.

Cardiopulmonary Resuscitation

The loss of effective circulation following cardiac surgery can be sudden and unexpected. Long-term survival, however, is distinctly possible with appropriate therapeutic interventions. When this circulatory insufficiency occurs as part of progressive deterioration in patients requiring maximal pharmacologic support, survival is less likely (Fairman and Edmunds, 1981). Management of these patients requires an organized approach to deal with potential problems rapidly while supporting the circulation.

Diagnosis

Common causes of circulatory collapse include the following:

Arrhythmias. A common cause of circulatory collapse is malignant tachyarrhythmia, which should be recognized and treated with immediate cardioversion (see "Cardioversion or Defibrillation," below). Heart block, with resulting asystole or severe bradycardia, can be similarly recognized and treated by institution of temporary pacing or pharmacologic management with atropine and isoproterenol.

Alterations in Intrathoracic Pressure. A tension pneumothorax, which is shown on physical examination by a deviated trachea and a unilateral absence of breath sounds, may cause circulatory collapse. In the mechanically ventilated patient, observation of a sudden increase in peak inspiratory pressure can assist in the diagnosis. However, hemodynamic instability and increase in airway pressure may also be seen in severe cases of shivering and chest wall rigidity. Hemodynamic collapse is related to the magnitude of intrathoracic pressure rather than the size of the pneumothorax (Fig. 8–18). Although a chest film is

ideal for making the diagnosis, it may be necessary to rapidly decompress one or both hemithoraces with empirically positioned needles or blind tube thoracostomies. Additional respiratory causes of circulatory collapse include ventilator malfunction, endotracheal tube malposition, loss of endotracheal tube seal with rupture of the endotracheal cuff, and mucous plugging of a major airway. These causes may be ruled out by physical examination, endotracheal suctioning, and hand ventilation using an air-mask-bag unit (AMBU).

Bleeding. Sudden severe bleeding is usually evident on inspection of the mediastinal drainage tubes. Causes include a sudden disruption of a ligature, the opening of a vessel previously in spasm, and cardiac rupture (particularly following mitral valve replacement). Cardiac tamponade and the accompanying hypovolemia underlie this problem and are best treated with emergency reexploration in the ICU.

Specific Management

Cardioversion or Defibrillation. *Cardioversion* involves the synchronized delivery of a transthoracic electrical discharge that depolarizes a portion of the pathway of a re-entrant arrhythmia (DeSilva et al., 1980). Cardioversion is synchronized with the electrical impulse of the heart so that the electrical discharge is delivered during the R wave, thereby reducing the possibility of cardioversion-induced ventricular fibrillation (DeSilva et al., 1980). *Defibrillation* is an electrical transthoracic discharge applied in an unsynchronized mode and is intended to simultaneously depolarize most of the heart. It is applied primarily for ventricular fibrillation or pulseless ventricular tachycardia.

Complications (6 to 30%) resulting from cardiover-

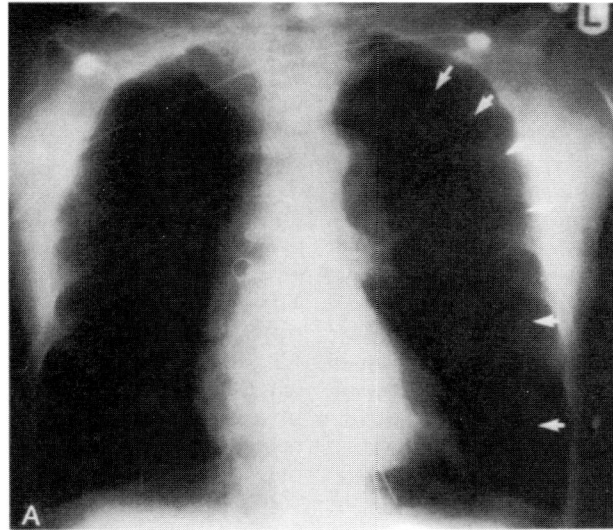

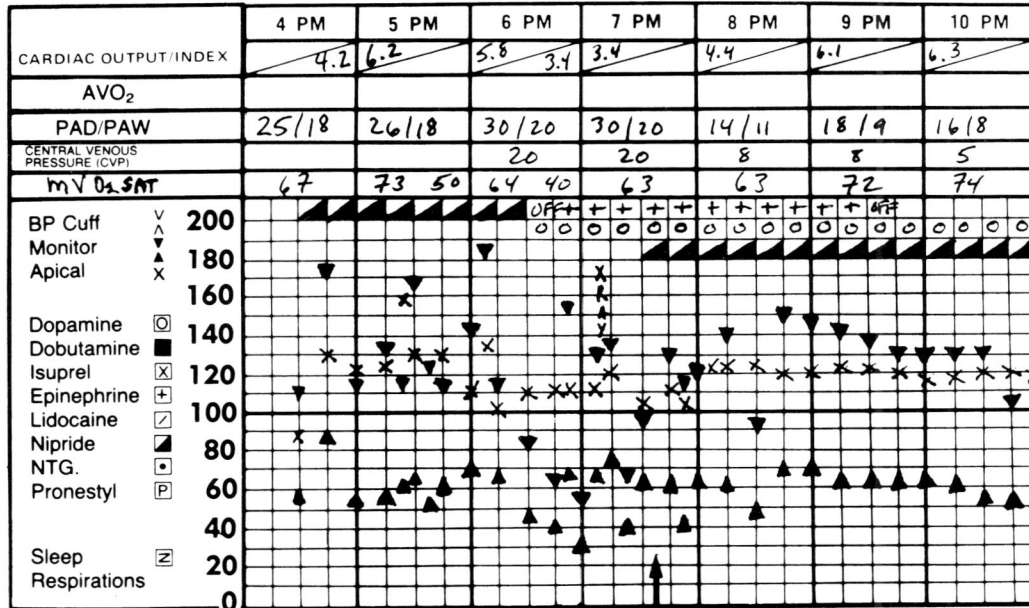

	4 PM	5 PM	6 PM	7 PM	8 PM	9 PM	10 PM
CARDIAC OUTPUT/INDEX	4.2	6.2	5.8 3.4	3.4	4.4	6.1	6.3
AVO$_2$							
PAD/PAW	25/18	26/18	30/20	30/20	14/11	18/9	16/8
CENTRAL VENOUS PRESSURE (CVP)			20	20	8	8	5
mV O$_2$ SAT	67	73 50	64 40	63	63	72	74

FIGURE 8–18. *A,* Portable chest film that shows a small left pneumothorax (*white arrows*). There is no mediastinal shift. *B,* Hemodynamic manifestations of this patient's early postoperative course as documented in the intensive care unit flow sheet. (PAD = pulmonary artery diastolic pressure [mm Hg]; PAW = pulmonary artery wedge pressure [mm Hg]; MV$_{O_2}$ sat = mixed venous oxygen saturation [%]; X = heart rate.) Cardiotonic infusions are charted according to definitions in the left of the panel. From 4:30 to 6:30 P.M. the patient has adequate cardiac output, although the filling pressures are high and the blood pressure is slightly unstable. At 6:30 P.M. further increases in filling pressure accompanied by decreased cardiac output are noted. Central venous pressure (CVP) was then measured and was found to be equal to the PAW. There was minimal bleeding at this time. Nitroprusside was discontinued, and two inotropic agents were added. At 7:30 P.M. the patient's blood pressure fell to 60 mm Hg, and multiple small boluses of epinephrine were required. The film shown in the *upper panel* was then obtained and showed a pneumothorax. The peak inspiratory pressure was only 45 cm H$_2$O. A left tube thoracostomy was then performed (*black arrow*), which resulted in total resolution of hemodynamic instability and normalization of cardiac function.

sion or defibrillation are directly related to the applied discharge energy, which should be kept at a minimum to achieve the appropriate response. This varies with the type of arrhythmia being treated (Lown and De-Silva, 1982; Resnekov, 1974; Resnekov and McDonald, 1967). Energy requirements may be reduced by 50% using proper electrode position. A posterior electrode placed at the angle of the left scapula with the anterior electrode placed to the right of the sternum is particularly effective. Prolonged asystole, a possible result of cardioversion or defibrillation, is easily treated in the patient who has undergone cardiac surgery by temporary pacing.

Atrial fibrillation is converted in 94% of patients with 200 joules or less (Lown et al., 1964). *Atrial flutter* can be converted successfully in virtually all patients by applying a mean energy of 25 joules (Lown, 1967). Hemodynamically significant narrow QRS complex supraventricular tachyarrhythmias should be treated initially with 75 to 100 joules (Montgomery, 1986).

Ventricular tachycardia can be converted in over 90% of cases with 10 joules or less (Lown et al., 1973) and may be converted successfully with a precordial thump (Caldwell et al., 1985). The recommended treatment for hemodynamically stable ventricular tachycardia is initial cardioversion with 50 joules. Pulseless ventricular tachycardia should be managed with 200-joule cardioversion (Montgomery, 1986), although defibrillation may also be applied.

Ventricular flutter is a wide, complex, bizarre rhythm that should be treated with defibrillation rather than synchronized cardioversion, because synchronization may occur with the T wave or repolarization phase of this arrhythmia and induce ventricular fibrillation (Lown et al., 1973).

Ventricular fibrillation can be converted using maximal device output, although 95% of cases can be treated successfully with discharges of 300 joules or less (Pantridge et al., 1975). Initial defibrillation should be done at 200 joules, with a second at 200 to 300 joules and a third not exceeding 360 joules (Montgomery, 1986).

External Cardiac Massage. Although the American Heart Association's recommended impulse rate for external compression has been raised to 80 to 100 beats per minute (Montgomery, 1986), there is support for use of higher compression rates of about 120 compressions per minute (Feneley et al., 1988; Maier et al., 1984; Newton et al., 1988) (Fig. 8–19). This position is controversial, however (Ornato et al., 1988).

Drug Therapy During Resuscitation. Various antiarrhythmic, inotropic, and metabolically active drugs are usually administered during resuscitation, and they should be delivered centrally to be effective in the low-flow state of artificial circulatory support (Barsan et al., 1981; Hedges et al., 1984; Kuhn et al., 1981). Endotracheal administration of many drugs, including epinephrine and atropine, is possible when intravenous access is not available (Montgomery, 1986). Significant metabolic acidosis rarely occurs in

cardiac arrests involving surgical patients thanks to intensive monitoring and the early institution of support. The need for sodium bicarbonate infusion has increasingly been questioned (Gazmuri et al., 1988). Concerns about worsening of tissue acidosis by excessive administration of sodium bicarbonate have been described (Bircher, 1992). The initial dose of sodium bicarbonate should be 1 mg/kg, followed by no more than half this dose every 10 minutes, although there are few data to suggest that normalization of arterial pH improves outcome (Bircher, 1992; Montgomery, 1986).

The algorithm for ventricular fibrillation drug therapy includes epinephrine followed by lidocaine followed by bretylium (5 mg/kg), followed by bretylium (10 mg/kg) with defibrillations interspersed (Montgomery, 1986). Epinephrine may help alter the character of ventricular fibrillation and lower the defibrillatory threshold (Livesay et al., 1978).

Open Chest Resuscitation. Open cardiac resuscitation should be applied when adequate circulation cannot be established by external massage or when massive hemorrhage and/or sudden tamponade are likely etiologies (Montgomery, 1986). Several retrospective studies have demonstrated that a significant salvage rate is possible, particularly when hemodynamic collapse is sudden and unexpected (Koshal et al., 1986; McKowen et al., 1985). In one large series, the mortality rate was 86% for Class IV cardiogenic shock patients before open resuscitation (McKowen et al., 1985). Superior salvage can be expected in patients with either tamponade or sudden massive bleeding as opposed to primary arrhythmias (Fairman and Edmunds, 1981). The infection rate following survival from open cardiopulmonary resuscitation in the ICU has been reported at 5% regardless of whether sternal rewiring is accomplished in the operating room or in the ICU (Koshal et al., 1986; McKowen et al., 1985).

The criteria of brain death cannot be satisfied during emergency resuscitation, nor can a persistent vegetative state after cardiopulmonary resuscitation be

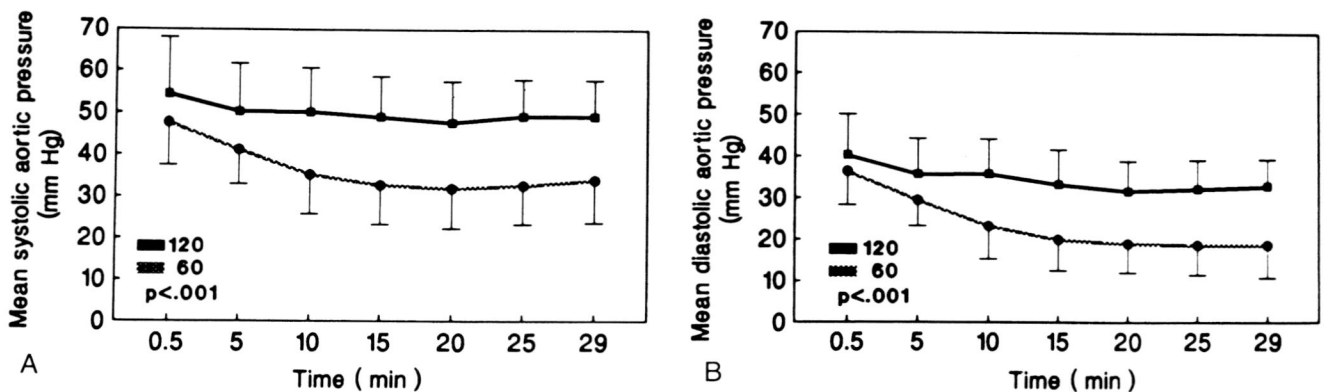

FIGURE 8–19. Hemodynamic data (mean ± SD) obtained in two groups of 13 dogs during manual cardiopulmonary resuscitation. Thirty minutes of compression at rates of 60/min or 120/min was used, which resulted in augmentation of both systolic aortic pressure (*A*) and diastolic aortic pressure (*B*) with higher compression rate. (*A* and *B*, From Feneley, M. P., Maier, G. W., Kern, K. B., et al: Influence of compression rate on initial success of resuscitation and 24 hour survival after prolonged manual cardiopulmonary resuscitation in dogs. *Circulation, 77:*240, 1988. By permission of the American Heart Association, Inc.)

reliably predicted within the first 1 to 2 weeks of unresponsiveness (Safar, 1984). However, prognostic information can be obtained within the first 48 to 72 hours following successful resuscitation (Bertini et al., 1989). Although most patients in the ICU will have experienced cardiac arrest, the time in which cardio-pulmonary function can be restored is predictive in that patients whose flow has been absent for more than 20 minutes are unlikely to recover successfully (Safar, 1988).

Postoperative Bleeding

Postoperative bleeding is always present to some degree following cardiac surgery. Bleeding is related to a combination of *mechanical factors* that are surgically correctable and *coagulopathy*. A surgically correctable cause predominates in less than 3% of cases and is indicated by brisk hemorrhage (>200 ml/hr), normal or near-normal coagulation study results, and the appearance of blood clots in the mediastinal drainage tubes.

Coagulopathy is a common feature of patients placed on the extracorporeal circuit for performance of cardiac procedures. These effects are exacerbated by the preoperative use of antiplatelet agents, thrombolytic agents, and heparin. The predominant cause of abnormal bleeding following CPB is a fall in platelet number and, more important, impaired platelet function (Boldt et al., 1993; Harker, 1986; Wenger et al., 1989). This platelet dysfunction is related to passage through the extracorporeal circuit, resulting in decreased platelet membrane receptors for fibrinogen as well as GpIB and GpIIB/IIIA complex. A second mechanism results from a progressive fibrinolytic state of variable intensity related to the length of CPB. Coagulopathy may be associated with variable or no bleeding and is recognized by the presence of abnormal clotting parameters (prothrombin time [PT], partial thromboplastin time [PTT], fibrinogen level, platelet count) and the absence of solid clot formation in the mediastinal drainage tubes.

The management of patients with excessive mediastinal hemorrhage is complex and may be hazardous. Bleeding predominantly due to coagulopathy is treated by both specific and nonspecific means.

Treatment of Coagulopathy

Specific treatment consists of blood component therapy based on accurate diagnosis and an understanding of changes that occur during CPB. Available resources include fresh frozen plasma (which supplies all coagulation factors except platelets), cryoprecipitate (Factor VIII and fibrinogen), platelet concentrates, and packed red blood cells (Milam, 1983). Guidelines for transfusion support as well as for management of postoperative patients with significant hemorrhage have been suggested (Goodnough et al., 1990) (Fig. 8–20).

Blood Component Resources

Packed Red Blood Cells. Packed red blood cells are the treatment of choice to increase blood oxygen-carrying capacity with minimal increase in circulating blood volume. Each packed red blood cell unit has a hematocrit of approximately 0.66. The following calculation can be used to predict requirements:

$$\frac{(\text{Blood volume} \times \text{Hct}) + (\text{no. of units transfused} \times 200 \text{ ml}) \times 100}{\text{Blood volume} + (\text{no. of units transfused} \times 300 \text{ ml})} = \text{new Hct}$$

$$\text{Women} = \text{body surface area (m}^2) \times 1210,$$
$$\text{men} = \text{body surface area (m}^2) \times 2650$$
or
$$\text{Women} = \text{body weight (kg)} \times 67,$$
$$\text{men} = \text{body weight (kg)} \times 77$$

where Hct = hematocrit; this equation assumes that red blood cells are 300 ml total volume with 200 ml red blood cell mass (Borucki, 1981, p. 33)

Packed red blood cells vary in composition, primarily according to storage technique and length of storage (Table 8–6).

FIGURE 8–20. Management of postoperative bleeding in cardiac surgery patients: an algorithm approach. (DDAVP = deamino-D-arginine vasopressin; PTT = partial thromboplastin time.) (From Goodnough, L. T., et al: Guidelines for transfusion support in patients undergoing coronary artery bypass grafting. Ann. Thorac. Surg., 50:675, 1990. Reprinted with permission from the Society of Thoracic Surgeons [The Annals of Thoracic Surgery].)

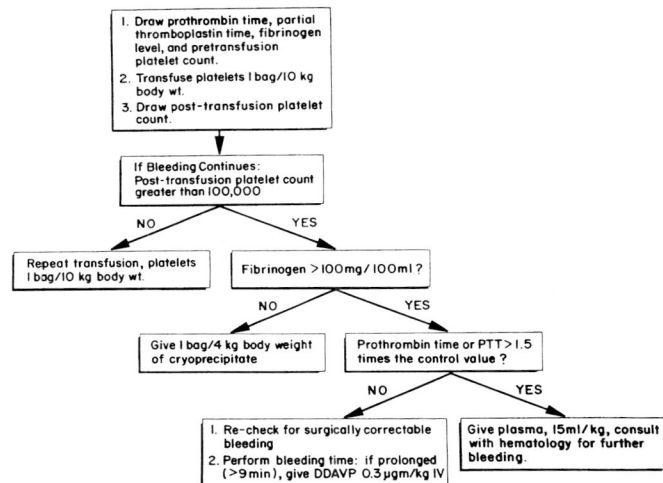

■ **Table 8-6.** EFFECTS OF STORAGE METHOD AND AGE ON PACKED RED BLOOD CELLS

	Storage Medium				
	Citrate-Phosphate-Dextrose			ADSOL (AS-1)	
Days of storage	0	14	28	35	49
Viable cells (%)	100	85	75	87	76
Plasma pH (measured at 37° C)	7.2	6.89	6.78	6.7	6.6
2,3-diphosphoglycerate mutase (% of initial value)	100	50	5		
P_{50} (PO_2 at Hb = HbO_2)	23.5	20	17		
Plasma K (mEq/l)	3.9	17.2	25	49	52
Plasma hemoglobin (mg/dl)	1.7	12.5	28.9	11.9	24.4
Whole blood NH_3 (μg/dl)	282	447	705		

Modified from Miller, W. V. (ed): Technical Manual. 7th ed. Washington, D. C., American Association of Blood Banks, 1977, p. 55.; and Heaton, A., Miripol, J., Aster, R., et al.: 49 to 56 day storage of high hematocrit red cell concentrates using ADSOL preservation solution. Transfusion, 22:4321, 1982.

Platelet Concentrates. Platelet concentrates are prepared from random units of anticoagulated whole blood and contain an average of 5.5×10^{10} platelets. One unit of platelet concentrate can raise the platelet count 9 to 11,000/μl/m² using the following formula:

$$pi = (pc2 - pc1) \times BSA/c$$

where pi = platelet count increment, pc1 = platelet count before transfusion, pc2 = platelet count post transfusion, BSA = body surface area (m²), and c = number of platelet concentrates transfused.

It should be noted that up to one-third of donors may have been on aspirin prior to platelet donation. Thus, platelet counts before and after transfusion do not necessarily reflect functional platelet activity.

Fresh Frozen Plasma. Fresh frozen plasma (FFP) contains all clotting factors, including the labile Factors V and VIII, as well as 250 to 400 mg of fibrinogen (Borucki, 1981). FFP contains naturally occurring antierythrocyte antibodies and is given as a type-specific product. FFP is usually available after a thawing period of 45 minutes, and its supply directly depends on the use of packed red blood cells rather than whole blood. Once thawed, FFP has a shelf life of 24 hours (Reisner et al., 1990). Management consists of administration of 12 ml/kg or 25% of the plasma volume being replaced initially (British Committee for Standardization in Haematology Blood Transfusion Task Force, 1988).

Cryoprecipitate. Cryoprecipitate is the cold insoluble protein fraction of plasma and is rich in Factor VIII (more than 100 units), fibrinogen (more than 150 units), and von Willebrand factor. The volume of one bag is approximately 15 ml. The standard adult dose is a pool of 10 bags and contains approximately 1000 mg of fibrinogen. Cryoprecipitate is also used to produce cryoglue, an adjunct for topical hemostasis used in the operating room.

Diagnosis

Postoperative coagulopathy must be specifically diagnosed by laboratory and clinical evaluation of the coagulation system. Any or all of the following derangements may be present.

Heparin Effect. This effect is demonstrated by a prolonged PTT and/or a prolonged activated clotting time (ACT). The ACT should be measured on admission to the ICU, because the heparin effect is usually seen early in the postoperative course (the half-life of heparin is approximately 1 hour [Estes, 1970; Hattersley, 1984]). Other laboratory parameters are normal. Abnormal laboratory parameters occurring more than 5 hours after the last heparin administration are unlikely to be due to circulating heparin or "heparin rebound" (Ellison et al., 1974). At this time, if heparin effect is suspected, the heparin level should be measured for confirmation. The specific treatment is administration of protamine sulfate, the dosage of which is determined by the dose-response curve established for each patient (Bull et al., 1975) (Fig. 8-21).

Thrombocytopenia. Thrombocytopenia is due to destruction of platelets during CPB or to consumption (Bachmann et al., 1975; Milam, 1983). In the absence of other abnormalities, treatment consists of platelet transfusion (Goodnough et al., 1990). Because many patients are maintained preoperatively on heparin,

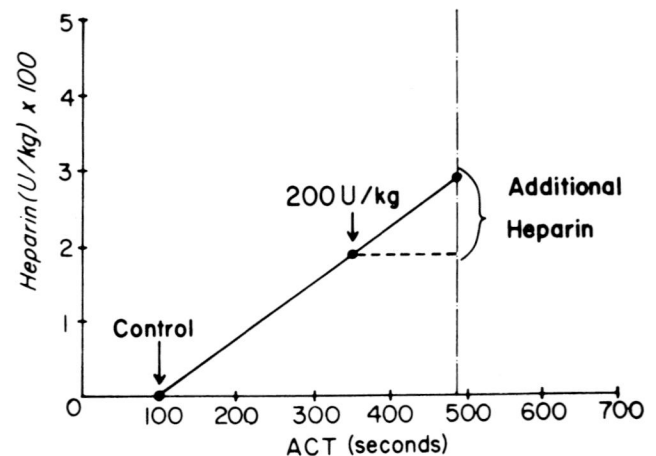

FIGURE 8-21. Relationship between heparin dose and activated clotting time (ACT). A control ACT is determined and a second ACT determined after heparin at 200 units/kg is administered. This yields by extrapolation an additional heparin dose required to elevate the ACT to 480 seconds and can also be used to calculate protamine dose for neutralization. In this instance, 1.3 mg protamine/100 units of heparin is given for neutralization. (From Doty, D. B., Knott, H. W., Hoyt, J. L., and Koepke, J. A.: Heparin dose for accurate anticoagulation in cardiac surgery. J. Cardiovasc. Surg., 20:597, 1979.)

thrombocytopenia may be induced by the presence of heparin-dependent antibodies. In this setting, resulting thromboembolic events as well as significant bleeding have been observed (Hattersley, 1984; Walls et al., 1992). Heparin-induced thrombocytopenia can be diagnosed with heparin-platelet aggregation testing to confirm the presence of antibodies in vitro. All heparin should be discontinued promptly in affected patients.

Thrombasthenia. In this instance, the platelet count is normal, but clot formation is inadequate. This remains a significant problem following cardiac surgery (Harker, 1986). It can be documented by measuring bleeding time using the Ivy method (Koepke, 1984) or more accurately defined using the thromboelastogram (Kang et al., 1985; Spiess et al., 1987). Qualitative defects in platelet function result from CPB (Bagge et al., 1986; British Committee for Standardization in Haematology Blood Transfusion Task Force, 1988; Harker, 1986) or from platelet therapy (Ferraris et al., 1988; Goldman et al., 1988). Aspirin can irreversibly affect platelet function, the life span of which is 6 to 7 days. Therefore, a single dose administered within the 7 days preceding an operation diminishes platelet function (Koepke, 1984). Bleeding complication and transfusion requirements have increased significantly (Sethi et al., 1990; Taggart et al., 1990).

Specific Factor Deficiencies. Specific factor deficiencies are usually manifested by elevation of the PT or the PTT. Abnormalities may be due to a specific genetic disorder, liver disease, prior coumadin therapy, hemodilution, or disseminated intravascular coagulation (DIC). These disorders are generally treated by either specific factor therapy, FFP, or cryoprecipitate.

Defibrination. Defibrination is manifested by abnormalities in the PT, PTT, and fibrinogen level with associated thrombocytopenia. Fibrin split products are moderately elevated. Defibrination is rarely due to inadequate heparinization during CPB and subsequent consumption of coagulation factors (Stoney et al., 1980; Young et al., 1978). Severe defibrination is usually due to the iatrogenic induction of a thrombolytic state with tissue plasminogen activator, urokinase, and particularly streptokinase. Treatment consists of transfusion of platelets, FFP, and cryoprecipitate, which is generally effective if there is no remaining circulating plasminogen activator (Lee et al., 1988).

Disseminated Intravascular Coagulation. The laboratory features of DIC are the same as in defibrination and usually are associated with more than 40 μg/ml of fibrin degradation products (Schmaier, 1984). In DIC, the process may be self-perpetuating and associated with intravascular thrombosis. As in other settings, the underlying cause (an incompatible blood transfusion or, occasionally, prolonged CPB) must be corrected. Specific component therapy, heparinization, and antifibrinolytic therapy (aminocaproic acid) may all be required. DIC is only rarely seen in the early postoperative course and is usually seen after the appearance of other complications (Boyd et al., 1972).

Fibrino(geno)lysis. This process results from activation of the fibrinolytic system, either intrinsically from CPB (Bick, 1976; Bick et al., 1976; Stibbe et al., 1984) or therapeutically. The thrombolytic therapy used preoperatively in patients suffering acute myocardial infarction is the usual circumstance. Streptokinase causes the most severe thrombolytic state when compared with other agents (Marder and Sherry, 1988; Rao et al., 1988). This thrombolytic state is associated with abnormalities of the PT, PTT, whole blood clotting time, and platelet count, as well as with severely low fibrinogen levels. Fibrin split products are mildly elevated. Therapy is the same as for defibrination, and success depends on complete elimination of plasminogen activator. Antifibrinolytic therapy may be helpful in this setting (Lambert et al., 1979; Vander Salm et al., 1988) but is rarely necessary (Wisch et al., 1973).

Protamine Overdosage. Protamine is commonly infused in slight excess, and although an anticoagulant effect can be demonstrated in vitro, this effect is not usually clinically apparent. More commonly, protamine induces an allergic reaction that causes hypotension and occasional cardiovascular collapse with associated pulmonary hypertension. These responses are immunologically mediated through immunoglobulin E (IgE), IgG, and complement activation in high-risk individuals (diabetes patients treated with NPH insulin, patients who have undergone vasectomy, and patients with fish allergy) (Levy et al., 1989).

Complications of Specific Treatment

Transfusion reactions are usually related to immunologic destruction of transfused cells mediated through complement activation with the participation of IgM or IgG antibodies. The estimated risk of hemolytic transfusion reactions is 1 in 6000 units transfused (Goodnough et al., 1990). Hemolysis usually occurs, producing free hemoglobinemia. Hemoglobin is initially bound to haptoglobin, which when depleted is a sensitive indicator of hemolysis. Hemoglobin is eventually removed by the reticuloendothelial system and by renal filtration. Plasma hemoglobin is detectable in the serum when its concentration approaches 20 mg/dl (Simpson, 1984).

Acute hemolytic transfusion reaction is usually due to human error and occurs with a fatality rate that approaches 1 in 100,000 units transfused (Goodnough et al., 1990). Patients undergoing open-heart procedures are among the principal fatalities (Myhre, 1980). In anesthetized patients, classic symptoms may not be apparent with usual signs, including significant hypotension, renal failure, and the sudden occurrence of a diffuse bleeding diathesis. Management includes hemodynamic support, forced alkaline diuresis (which may be stimulated by osmotic diuretic [mannitol]), and administration of sodium bicarbonate.

Other adverse reactions include delayed hemolysis,

passive hemolysis, and reactions causing fever, chills, and urticaria (occurring in approximately 1 in 100 transfusions) (Goodnough et al., 1990). Urticarial reactions are treated supportively and with antihistamines. Anaphylactic reactions are related to transfused IgA and class-specific anti-IgG antibodies in the patient's plasma. This can occur in IgA-deficient patients (1 in 150 to 1 in 700 patients) with infusion of virtually all blood products as well as albumin, plasma protein fraction, and immunoglobulin preparations (Simpson, 1984).

Infectious complications remain a significant concern in blood transfusion. Hepatitis may occur in 8 to 10% of patients given transfusions with a subsequent mortality rate of 0.1% (Grady and Bennett, 1972; Proskey et al., 1970). Fifteen per cent of hepatitis cases may be due to cytomegalovirus (CMV), which may occur in 40% of patients receiving five or more transfusions (Caul et al., 1971; Ho, 1984). CMV is the etiologic agent for "postperfusion syndrome," which occurs in 3 to 8% of patients. The syndrome is manifested by fever, atypical lymphocytosis, and splenomegaly (Kirsh et al., 1970). The incubation period for non-A and non-B hepatitis (the most commonly seen infection after surgery) ranges from 2 to 25 weeks and has an incidence as high as 1 in 100 transfusions (Goodnough et al., 1990). Epstein-Barr virus infection can also occur, causing an infectious mononucleosis-like syndrome 1 to 2 months following exposure (Simpson, 1984). Although great public concern is related to possible transmission of human immunodeficiency virus (HIV) and subsequent seroconversion related to transfusion of blood or blood products, actual cases probably occur in only 1 in 40,000 to 1 in 100,000 exposures (Goodnough et al., 1990).

Metabolic complications include altered hemoglobin-oxygen affinity, hyperkalemia, acid-base imbalance, and fall in calcium ion level due to excess citrate (unusual except in massive transfusion). Thromboembolic complications can occur because of macroaggregate infusion.

Nonspecific Treatment

The major side effects of postoperative bleeding are volume loss and retention of clotted blood within the mediastinum. Nonspecific therapy consists of continuous, adequate volume replacement, maintenance of free drainage, and prevention of hypothermia. Hypothermia has a generalized anticoagulant effect (Goto et al., 1985) that increases PT and PTT in direct accordance with the degree of temperature change (Rohrer and Natale, 1992). Specific anticoagulant effects may be corrected by warming.

Volume replacement can be accomplished by continuous autotransfusion, but this also requires infusion of nonspecific agents. Crystalloid solutions may be provided as normal saline or lactated Ringer's solution. Colloid solutions include serum albumin as a 25% solution, plasma protein fraction (Plasmanate) as a 5% protein solution containing both albumin and alpha- and beta-globulins (Borucki, 1981; Simpson,

1984), or hydroxyethyl starch (Hetastarch). Serum albumin in its 25% solution must recruit extravascular fluid to result in effective volume replacement. Plasmanate may cause a paradoxical hypotension attributed to the use of acetate, present as a buffer (Olinger et al., 1979), or it may lead to the presence of Hageman-factor fragments (Alving et al., 1978). Hydroxyethyl starch provides plasma volume expansion for longer than 24 hours and may be safely used to a total volume of 1.5 liters. Because it has a chemical composition similar to that of dextran, associated urticarial and anaphylactoid reactions may occur (Borucki, 1981; Simpson, 1984). However, unlike the case with dextran, coagulation abnormalities with hydroxyethyl starch generally have been related to hemodilution rather than to a specific anticoagulant effect (Strauss, 1988).

Mechanical means should be used to maintain mediastinal chest tube patency. These means include stripping and the milking of chest tubes, the application of suction, and, occasionally, Fogarty catheter thrombectomy of the mediastinal tubes. Catheter thrombectomy usually precedes reoperation and may prevent significant tamponade. Mechanical stripping of chest tubes can create negative pressures as high as 1500 mm Hg and can damage entrapped tissues.

Other nonspecific measures include strict control of BP and the induction of mild controlled hypotension, which can markedly diminish bleeding rate. However, afterload reduction can be particularly dangerous in the hypovolemic patient with ongoing blood loss and early cardiac tamponade. Levels of PEEP in the range of 10 to 12 cm H_2O have been suggested to reduce postoperative bleeding (Hoffman et al., 1982; Ilabaca et al., 1980; Mills, 1982). The efficacy of PEEP in slowing postoperative bleeding remains controversial (Zurick et al., 1982), and acute reduction in preload with this level of PEEP is potentially dangerous (Smith et al., 1982).

Reoperation

Reoperation is indicated for excessive bleeding (10 ml/kg in the first hour, > 5 ml/kg in each of the next 3 hours) or for the development of cardiac tamponade (Edmunds, 1983). Elective reoperation may be indicated to remove large amounts of retained clot in the mediastinum or pleural cavities (Stevenson et al., 1984, Wareing et al., 1993). Planned reoperation in a stable patient is preferable to resternotomy in the ICU to alleviate hemodynamically significant tamponade. Aggressive normalization of clotting parameters should be attempted while assessing patients with ongoing mediastinal hemorrhage. Presence of clot may increase the incidence of pericarditis. A small margin is often present between normal cardiac function and delayed tamponade, which may be seen as pulmonary dysfunction or ongoing small amounts of bleeding. An additional broad-spectrum perioperative antibiotic is usually prescribed before re-exploration.

Blood Conservation

Continued attempts at blood conservation are an important aspect of the perioperative care of patients undergoing cardiac surgical procedures. Approximately 74% of patients undergoing CABG receive blood or blood product transfusion (Goodnough et al., 1988). Simple, cost-effective blood-conserving efforts have reduced the transfusion requirements in adult patients undergoing open heart procedures (Dietrich et al., 1989; Scott et al., 1990; Tyson et al., 1989). Methods to conserve blood should be considered in the perioperative course of cardiac surgical patients.

Preoperative Considerations

Autologous blood donation before an elective cardiac procedure has been shown to be safe and effective. A national multicenter study of autologous blood donation before elective cardiac and noncardiac procedures determined that only 5% of eligible patients actually predeposited blood (Toy et al., 1987). High-risk patients, excluding those with unstable angina, have safely predonated autologous blood before surgical intervention (Mann et al., 1983). Preoperative discontinuance of aspirin and conversion of warfarin anticoagulation to heparin anticoagulation are also important considerations. In the elective patient who presents for surgical assessment with associated anemia, preoperative erythropoietin may improve blood hemoglobin levels sufficiently to obviate the need for postoperative homologous blood transfusion (Konishi et al., 1993).

Intraoperative Considerations

Intraoperative methods to allow blood conservation include withdrawal of autologous blood before CPB; crystalloid oxygenation priming of the CPB circuit with resultant hemodilution (hematocrit 0.20 to 0.30); blood salvage with retransfusion of ultrafiltered or centrifugated blood remaining in the extracorporeal circuit following separation from CPB; postoperative anemia (hematocrit 0.25); and complete mechanical hemostasis, including application of a topical agent to anastomotic sites, aortotomy sites, and sternal marrow (Schwartz and Moore, 1990; Schwartz and Robertson, 1988; Scott et al., 1990).

Postoperative Considerations

Tolerance of a reduced hematocrit in the postoperative period is important to the avoidance of blood transfusion. Although classic teaching states that the optimal hematocrit is between 0.30 and 0.40 (Asmundsson and Kilburn, 1969; Bryan-Brown, 1988; Czer and Shoemaker, 1978; Wilson and Walt, 1975; Wolfe et al., 1985), this value has not been clearly defined for patients following corrective cardiac surgery. In such patients, no significant difference in mortality rate, morbidity rate, and length of hospital stay has been demonstrated by allowing hematocrits to drop to 0.23 to 0.25 as opposed to maintaining hematocrit at 0.32 or greater (Johnson et al., 1992). Oral iron therapy, and occasionally the prescription of folic acid, restores normal hematocrit 6 weeks following surgery.

An important consideration in postoperative blood conservation is autotransfusion. Since its initial description, autotransfusion has undergone continued refinements that permit safe and effective application to patients who have undergone cardiac surgery. (Cosgrove et al., 1985; Shaff et al., 1978). Autotransfusion can conserve the supply of blood and blood products as well as reduce the complications of transfusion, including adverse reactions to blood components and their infectious complications (Milam, 1983). There are two methods for autotransfusion of shed mediastinal blood in the postoperative period.

Intermittent autotransfusion can be performed by draining shed blood into a separate reservoir; it is then anticoagulated with citrate and, if necessary, reinfused through a micropore filter (pore size of 40 μm) (Sutton et al., 1993; Thurer et al., 1979). This system allows collection of shed mediastinal blood, leaving the option of autotransfusion to clinical discretion. The reinfusion components need be used only if autotransfusion is performed. The main disadvantages of this system include the need for an open system that requires reconfiguration with each "unit" of shed blood and the intermittent nature of autotransfusion in volumes ranging from 200 to 800 ml.

The second method is *continuous autotransfusion*, in which the cardiotomy reservoir is converted into the postoperative drainage container (Hartz et al., 1988; Parker and West, 1978). In this technique, autotransfusion is performed with a closed system using continuous pump/controller infusion from the dependent drainage site of the reservoir. This maintains the patient's blood volume more smoothly than does intermittent autotransfusion. This method requires less additional equipment and allows autotransfusion to be a standard part of each patient's postoperative care. For the processing and reuse of shed mediastinal blood, however, both methods are effective (Sutton et al., 1993). The method used depends to some extent on institutional practice.

Several studies have demonstrated the utility of autotransfusion in both adult and pediatric patients (Bregman et al., 1974; Cosgrove et al., 1985; Hartz et al., 1988; Johnson et al., 1983; Milam, 1983; Schaff et al., 1978, 1979; Scott et al., 1990; Thurer et al., 1979). Potential complications of either method include sepsis, microembolism, air embolism, hemolysis, dilutional anemia, thrombocytopenia, and coagulopathy. Most of these complications have proved to be more theoretical than real, which accounts for the current popularity of autotransfusion (Griffith et al., 1989; Hartz et al., 1988; Thompson and Chant, 1989). Various reports (Hartz et al., 1988; Schaff et al., 1978; Thurer et al., 1979) have shown that the shed blood contains many valuable blood components and is essentially defibrinated (Table 8–7).

■ **Table 8–7.** HEMATOLOGIC ANALYSIS OF SHED MEDIASTINAL BLOOD

Component	Mean Value
Hematocrit	0.2–0.25 ml/dl
Hemoglobin	6.85 g/100 ml
White blood cell count	$5.3 \times 10^3/mm^3$
Red blood cell count	$2.18 \times 10^6/mm^3$
Platelet count	$68 \times 10^3/mm^3$
Plasma hemoglobin	315 mg/100 ml
Factor VIII	11–95%
Fibrinogen	10–19 mg/dl

Data from Schaff, H. V., Hauer, J. M., Bell, W. R., et al.: Autotransfusion of shed mediastinal blood after cardiac surgery. J. Thorac. Cardiovasc. Surg., 75:632, 1978; Thurer, R. L., Lytle, B. W., Cosgrove, D. M., and Loop, F. D.: Autotransfusion following cardiac operations: A randomized, prospective study. Ann. Thorac. Surg., 27:500, 1979; and Hartz, R. S., Smith, J. A., and Green, D.: Autotransfusion after cardiac operation. J. Thorac. Cardiovasc. Surg., 96:178, 1988.

Most patients would benefit from autotransfusion. A risk-and-benefit analysis therefore supports the notion that autotransfusion become standard practice.

Contraindications to autotransfusion include more than 12 to 18 hours administration postoperatively, patients with active mediastinal infection at the time of surgery, and patients in whom potentially dangerous agents could be collected in the shed blood (e.g., kanamycin, fibrin glue). In cardiac operations, a cephalosporin antibiotic applied topically (if an antibiotic is used) at the end of the procedure permits the safe performance of autotransfusion.

Pharmacologic Considerations

As previously noted, abnormalities in platelet function are a significant cause of postoperative mediastinal hemorrhage. Aspirin should be discontinued 1 week before elective surgery in all patients.

Desmopressin (1-deamino-8-D-arginine-vasopressin, or DDAVP), a synthetic analogue of L-arginine vasopressin, has improved platelet function and reduced hemorrhage in a variety of clinical disorders. DDAVP appears to act by increasing the concentration of von Willebrand factor, an important mediator of platelet adhesion. There is no clear consensus on the prophylactic use of DDAVP (Ansell et al., 1992; Lazenby et al., 1990). However, patients with ongoing hemorrhage should be considered for administration of 3 μg/kg given over 15 minutes (Goodnough et al., 1990).

Future considerations for pharmacologic therapy to decrease mediastinal hemorrhage include the use of *epsilon-aminocaproic acid* (Amicar), an antifibrinolytic agent, which has been effective in reducing the amount of postoperative hemorrhage when administered prophylactically. Administration consists of a loading dose of 5 gm (given before incision) and a continuous infusion of 1 gm per hour for 6 hours following separation from CPB (DelRossi et al., 1989; Fremes et al., 1994; Kondo et al., 1994; Vander Salm et al., 1988). *Aprotinin,* a nonspecific serine protease inhibitor extracted from bovine lung, has been sug-

gested as a method of reducing postoperative mediastinal bleeding, and it was approved for this use in December 1993. Pre-CPB administration of aprotinin can preserve platelet function otherwise lost during CPB (de Smet et al., 1990; van Oeveren et al., 1990). It may be administered prior to CPB in low doses (2×10^6 kallikrein-inhibiting units [KIU]) followed by a continuing infusion during bypass in higher doses (5×10^5 KIU). An additional 2×10^6 KIU are also added to the priming fluid of the cardiopulmonary bypass circuit. Numerous reports have demonstrated a reduction in blood loss and transfusion requirements in patients given aprotinin (Bidstrup et al., 1989, 1993; Dietrich et al., 1990; Fremes et al., 1994; Roysten et al., 1987). Although initial success seemed promising, some reports have questioned its safety. Increases in the incidence of perioperative myocardial infarction (with thrombosis of grafts) and significant renal dysfunction have been described (Cosgrove et al., 1992; Westaby, 1993). Aprotinin prolongs the celite ACT owing to its indirect effect on factor XII, thereby making monitored ACT levels during CPB unreliable (Dietrich et al., 1990). Although the contact-mediated activation is slowed, resulting from a diminished factor XIIa production, an effect in clinical hemostasis may not be present. Empiric bolus heparin (based on half-life) or the use of kaolin ACT to monitor heparinization during CPB is recommended if aprotinin is used (Kondo et al., 1994). Overall, aprotinin use should be limited to reoperations and to patients undergoing extensive thoracic aortic procedures until further follow-up verifies its safety.

Blood conservation methods continue to be improved in an attempt to lower the postoperative risk to patients undergoing cardiac operations of transfusion of homologous blood and blood products.

GENERAL POSTOPERATIVE MANAGEMENT

Management of Fluids, Electrolytes, and Acid-Base Balance

Homeostasis requires the maintenance of adequate intravascular volume, normal serum electrolyte concentrations, and normal pH. This must be accomplished in a setting of rapidly changing physiology marked by dramatic changes in cardiac function, respiratory function, and the hormonal environment.

Fluid Administration

The majority of patients following cardiac surgery have a reduced circulating blood volume and an accompanying increase in extracellular fluid (Cleland et al., 1966). The increase in extracellular water is approximately 7%, with an accompanying 12.5% increase in interstitial water. In the postoperative period, sodium and water intake are minimized commensurately with the maintenance of adequate cardiac preload (Pacifico et al., 1970). The daily water allotment is usually limited to 1500 ml/day for several days and is managed through observation of the serum sodium concentration and daily body weight. Insensible water losses vary from 600 to 800 ml/day and may be increased by as much as 300 ml/day for each centigrade degree of elevation in body temperature (Shoemaker, 1984b). During CPB, sodium and water excretion increase (Schaff et al., 1989). The natriuresis that follows separation from CPB appears to be associated with the increase in atrial natriuretic factor (ANF) that has been demonstrated within 30 minutes of CPB (Schaff et al., 1989). Further spontaneous diuresis associated with resolution of surgical stress usually occurs 48 to 72 hours following operation. This may be sufficient to permit normalization of body fluid amount and distribution (Gann and Wright, 1966). However, diuretics commonly are administered to hasten this process. Monitoring of electrolyte and acid-base status is important to prevent complications.

Electrolyte Management

Potassium. Aggressive potassium supplementation is the rule following cardiac operations. A marked kaliuresis is usually present in the postoperative period; if present preoperatively, kaliuresis may exacerbate the depletion of total body potassium (Cox, 1981). Aggressive intravenous administration of potassium (as much as 20 mEq/hr) in the initial postoperative period may be necessary, and oral supplementation may be required until the time of hospital discharge. Frequently used diuretic agents exacerbate kaliuresis, deplete total body potassium, and cause metabolic alkalosis (Cogan et al., 1983). Persistent alkalosis, either respiratory or metabolic, causes an intracellular shift of potassium with a subsequent fall in the measured serum potassium level. Respiratory mechanisms, however, have less effect on potassium balance than do metabolic disturbances (Cox, 1981).

Hyperkalemia, which is most often iatrogenic, must be managed aggressively. The cardiac effects of hyperkalemia depend on the absolute serum potassium concentration and the rate at which this concentration is reached (Fisch et al., 1966). Hyperkalemia may be manifested by peak T wave and alterations of conduction. In extreme cases, intravenous calcium can directly reverse potassium-induced depression of conduction (Fisch, 1973). Induction of alkalosis with sodium bicarbonate ($NaHCO_3$) will shift potassium into cells, causing an acute fall in serum potassium. The administration of insulin and glucose also drives potassium into the cells, lowering the serum concentration. Total body potassium content is effectively reduced by the administration of sodium-potassium exchange resins via the alimentary tract.

Magnesium. Hypomagnesemia (concentration < 1.5 mg/dl) may be present in as many as 58% of ICU patients (Chernow et al., 1988). Its association with cardiac arrhythmias and nonspecific electrocardiographic changes similar to those of hypokalemia are becoming increasingly recognized (Boriss and Papa, 1988). The incidence of postoperative arrhythmias has

been reduced when magnesium concentration is maintained in the normal range (Scheinman et al., 1971). Magnesium levels must be maintained in the normal range for both calcium and potassium repletion to be effective (Boriss and Papa, 1988).

Phosphate. Hypophosphatemia, a common metabolic disorder, can cause leukocyte dysfunction, platelet dysfunction, and depressed ventricular function (Chernow, 1984). Muscle weakness and neurologic dysfunction can also be seen. Intravenous replacement should be initiated if the serum PO_4 level is less than 1 mg/dl. Replacement is contraindicated in hypercalcemia. Both hypokalemia and hypomagnesemia should be corrected before repletion of phosphate.

Acid-Base Management

Arterial pH often ranges widely following cardiac surgery (normal arterial pH is 7.41). Deviations in pH from normal in either direction, regardless of etiology, adversely affect myocardial function (Cook et al., 1965; Darby et al., 1960). Inotropic agents as well as vasopressors less effectively combat significant changes in arterial pH. Acid-base balance is ordinarily determined by the ingestion of fixed acid and disposal of carbon dioxide generated by metabolism. Body buffer systems mitigate the effects of acute and chronic changes, with the kidneys and lungs determining ultimate disposal. Metabolic acidosis ($\geq$ 2 mEq) following cardiac surgery is usually due to hypoperfusion. Low CO, often the underlying cause, must be treated. Mild hyperventilation (P_{CO_2} 30 to 35 mm Hg) may be used to maintain normal pH. Exogenous sodium bicarbonate should be administered when arterial pH is significantly lower. However, administration of sodium bicarbonate, although it is temporarily corrective, produces a significant sodium load.

Respiratory acidosis is usually due to respiratory dysfunction or to ventilator mismanagement. It is rare for metabolic production of carbon dioxide to exceed pulmonary excretion capacity (Laski, 1983). The treatment of respiratory acidosis is pulmonary support and increased ventilation. It is unusual for significant respiratory acidosis to reflect appropriate compensation for metabolic alkalosis.

Metabolic alkalosis is the most common acid-base abnormality seen in cardiac surgical patients, resulting from extracellular volume and potassium depletion (contraction alkalosis). It is often induced by diuretics in the setting of increased mineralocorticoid activity (Cogan et al., 1983). The mainstay of therapy for metabolic alkalosis is the administration of potassium chloride and the repletion of intravascular volume. A carbonic anhydrase inhibitor (acetazolamide) may be used to increase urinary bicarbonate excretion, although aggravation of extracellular volume depletion and metabolic side effects limit the usefulness of such an inhibitor (Brimioulle et al., 1989). Metabolic alkalosis due to excessive gastric loss may be ameliorated by administering a histamine-2 (H_2)-blocker.

Severe metabolic alkalosis may be corrected by continuous infusion of hydrochloric acid, which allows selective correction of the metabolic alkalosis (Brimioulle et al., 1989). Hydrochloric acid (HCl) is administered as a 0.1 normal solution (100 mEq/l) according to the following formula (Wagner et al., 1980):

$$\text{mEq HCl} = \text{weight (kg)} \times 0.3 \times \text{base excess (mEq/l)}$$

This correction should be monitored closely with frequent blood gas determination and central venous administration of the hydrochloric acid.

Respiration

All patients undergoing cardiac surgery require mechanical ventilation, and its management is an important component of early postoperative care. Complications related to mechanical ventilation can be a significant source of morbidity and mortality but may be avoided with proper attention to potential risks. Initial ventilatory parameters can be approximated as follows (Foster et al., 1984):

- Tidal volume of 10 to 12 ml/kg
- Synchronized intermittent mandatory ventilation (SIMV) of 10 to 12 breaths per minute
- Inspired oxygen fraction of 0.6
- PEEP at 5 cm H_2O

The vast majority of patients are suitable for extubation if they meet the following criteria (Foster et al., 1984):

- Appearance: no apprehension or diaphoresis
- Consciousness: alert and responsive to verbal commands
- Mean arterial pressure greater than 80 mm Hg
- Mean left atrial pressure (wedge pressure) less than 18 mm Hg
- Minimal bleeding
- Normal body temperature
- F_{IO_2} less than 0.5 with a P_{O_2} greater than 80 mm Hg
- PEEP at 5 cm H_2O or less
- No untreated arrhythmia
- Spontaneous tidal volume greater than 5 ml/kg
- Spontaneous vital capacity greater than 10 ml/kg
- Spontaneous respiratory rate less than 30 breaths per minute
- Negative inspiratory force greater than 25 cm H_2O

Various studies have shown that 45% of cardiac surgical patients meet extubation requirements within 90 minutes of admission to the ICU (Lichtenthal et al., 1983). Early extubation can lower costs and improve patient comfort (Foster et al., 1984). The mean time to extubation can be decreased by as much as 41% by maintaining the following parameters (Foster et al., 1984):

- PA_{O_2} maintained at greater than 80 mm Hg
- F_{IO_2} set to give a P_{O_2} of 150 mm Hg in the first 2 hours
- F_{IO_2} set to give a P_{O_2} of 110 mm Hg thereafter
- P_{CO_2} maintained at less than 45 mm Hg
- pH maintained between 7.35 and 7.50

This protocol also reduces the arterial blood gas sampling rates.

Early extubation must be planned with appropriate anesthetic management. This may include the use of inhalational anesthetics and reversal of muscle relaxants (Quasha et al., 1980). Chest wall rigidity following early extubation can be a complication of fentanyl redistribution (Caspi et al., 1988; Christian et al., 1983). This phenomenon has been reported with an incidence of 7.5% following fentanyl anesthesia and can be life-threatening even with mechanical ventilation (Caspi et al., 1988). It is specifically treated with naloxone or, in the intubated patient, by administration of a muscle relaxant (Caspi et al., 1988).

Prolonged mechanical ventilation can lead to increased lung water and has adverse effects on cardiac function (Gall et al., 1988; Sladen et al., 1968). Although barotrauma (pneumothorax or subcutaneous emphysema) may occur, especially with preexisting chronic obstructive pulmonary disease, it has not been convincingly correlated with either the magnitude of airway pressure required or the duration of mechanical ventilation (Kumar et al., 1973). Although uncommon, these complications must be avoided.

When patients require mechanical ventilation beyond 24 hours of surgery, particular care must be provided to prevent infectious complications due to violation of the lungs' natural defense mechanisms. Mechanical ventilation predisposes to the development of nosocomial pneumonia, which occurs in approximately 4% of patients undergoing CABG procedures (Gaynes et al., 1991). Gram-negative bacilli are the predominant etiologic agents of postoperative pneumonia, with case fatality rates ranging from 26.6% to as high as 60% (Gaynes et al., 1991; Tuteur, 1991). Supplemental oxygen can adversely affect measured mucus flow at any level deviating from ambient oxygen tension (Laurenzi et al., 1968).

Following extubation, patients undergoing cardiac surgery universally demonstrated hypoxia on breathing room air (Corning et al., 1966). However, when severe hypoxia is present, right-to-left shunting through a patent foramen ovale should be excluded (Streitz and Maggs, 1988). Supplemental oxygen therapy usually is required for several days following surgery because of the development of atelectasis (especially involving the left lower lobe), pleural effusions (seen in as many as 40% of patients), and diaphragmatic dysfunction (Benjamin et al., 1982; Fedullo et al., 1992; MacNaughton et al., 1992; Markand et al., 1985; Shapira et al., 1990; Vargas et al., 1992). The work of breathing normally accounts for 3.7% of resting oxygen consumption, but this may be as high as 7.7% in patients recovering from ventilatory failure and as high as 24.7% in those who cannot be weaned from mechanical ventilation (Lewis et al., 1988).

A severe, reversible, restrictive change in pulmonary function occurs in the early postoperative period following cardiac surgery (Wahl et al., 1993). Lung mechanics are significantly diminished following median sternotomy for open heart procedures. Forced vital capacity, FEV_1, $FEF_{25-75\%}$, and DL_{CO} (a measurement of diffusion capacity) fall compared with preoperative measures. Lung volumes are reduced by as much as 30% when measured at the time of hospital discharge (Shapira et al., 1990). However, these changes are relatively short-lived; pulmonary mechanics and flow rates return to normal when measured 3 postoperative months later (Shapira et al., 1990). Pulmonary compliance also falls significantly (60% decrease) in the preoperative period (Hilberman et al., 1969). Patients with persistent atelectasis or left lower lobe collapse may have more significant impairment of pulmonary function (Vargas et al., 1993). Patients with preexisting chronic obstructive pulmonary disease more frequently experience respiratory complications, including length of stay in the ICU, duration of mechanical ventilation, and development of pulmonary complications (pleural effusions, atelectasis, respiratory infections) (Bevelaqua et al., 1990). The immediate perioperative mortality rate is similar to that of patients without significant chronic obstructive pulmonary disease. However, long-term outlook is less favorable (1-year survival rate of 53% [Burk and George, 1973], 2-year survival rate of 30%, and 5-year survival rate of 16% [Asmundsson and Kilburn, 1974]).

Several noninvasive methods to estimate arterial P_{O_2} and P_{CO_2} have been introduced for use in the ICU. Capnography and the analysis of end-expiratory carbon dioxide may be used to monitor arterial P_{CO_2} during ventilatory weaning (Carlon et al., 1988). Although hypercarbia is found to closely correlate with the arterial P_{CO_2} (Sladen et al., 1985), others have found a 28% sensitivity rate for hypercarbia ($P_{CO_2} > 45$ mm Hg), which makes its use for frequent arterial blood gas determinations problematic (Niehoff et al., 1988).

Pulse oximetry is 100% sensitive in detecting an arterial oxygen saturation of less than 95% (Niehoff et al., 1988) and can be useful in the postoperative period for determining the safe discontinuance of oxygen therapy and obviating the need for frequent arterial blood gas determinations. Pulse oximetry is also useful as a monitor of exercise tolerance in a hospital ward setting (Schnapp and Cohen, 1990).

In intensive care, pulse oximetry is made less accurate by peripheral vasoconstriction (Brunel and Cohen, 1988), where it becomes a measure of peripheral perfusion rather than of oxygen saturation. Reflection pulse oximetry is more accurate in this setting, but the technique is not as yet commonly employed (Palve, 1992). Transcutaneous determinations of P_{O_2} and P_{CO_2} are possible but appear to be effective only in thin-skinned patients with normal peripheral perfusion. However, these methods have been applied successfully in neonatal patients (Shoemaker and Tremper, 1984).

Nutrition

The vast majority of patients undergoing cardiac surgery rapidly progress to oral alimentation in the first 2 to 3 days following cardiac operation. Signifi-

cant preoperative nutritional abnormalities are likely in patients with chronic congestive heart failure (cardiac cachexia) or who have been hospitalized for cardiac complications for more than 2 to 3 days before operation. Thirty-five to 50% of surgical patients present with preoperative abnormalities suggesting malnutrition, including abnormalities of body weight, serum albumin level, transferrin level, and delayed hypersensitivity, all of which are accurate prognostic indicators of increased postoperative morbidity (Albina et al., 1986; Mullen et al., 1979). Postoperative complications were significantly increased in patients undergoing cardiac surgery who presented with weight loss or a body weight less than 15% below ideal (Abel et al., 1976b). In patients with significant preoperative chronic illness or who suffer major complications, supplemental nutritional support is usually necessary. Preoperative nutritional support may not be possible, because the obligate volume and metabolic stress may exceed cardiopulmonary reserve (Heymsfield et al., 1987). In patients with severe malnutrition, preoperative total parenteral nutrition (TPN) for 7 to 10 days can improve patient outcome (Veterans Affairs Study Group, 1991).

A glucose load of approximately 5 mg/kg/min (and a nonprotein calorie load of 30 to 35 kcal/kg/day) with a total calorie load of 40 to 45 kcal/kg/day is necessary. Protein is begun at 0.9 to 2 g/kg/day with at least 100 nonprotein calories provided for each gram of nitrogen. Thirty to 40% of nonprotein calories may be given as an intravenous fat emulsion (Cerra, 1987), although this may adversely affect pulmonary function (Venus et al., 1988).

The preferred route of alimentation is enteral, which can be accomplished safely with placement of a duodenal feeding tube even when there is gastric atony and a moderate ileus (Cerra, 1987). Enteral feedings protect the gastric mucosa from stress ulceration and enhance the integrity of enteral mucosa (Ephgrave et al., 1990; Pingleton and Hadzima, 1983). A nasoenteral tube can be positioned in the ICU without fluoroscopy, but its position should be confirmed by abdominal films. This technique has been shown to be effective, safe, and well tolerated by patients (Harris and Huseby, 1989). Parenteral nutrition (Rombeau and Caldwell, 1986) may be necessary when enteral feeding is not possible, especially in patients suffering central nervous system complications (Abel, 1986).

Most patients advance to a regular diet before hospital discharge. Although adequate caloric intake is important, patients should be started on a low-fat, low-cholesterol diet with moderate sodium restriction while in the hospital. This reinforces postdischarge dietary behavior and provides an opportunity to educate patients about the importance of dietary management (Murphy, 1988).

INFECTIONS AND INFLAMMATORY SYNDROMES

Postoperative recovery from cardiac surgery is often marked by a systemic inflammatory response manifested by fever and leukocytosis. The differentiation of infection from inflammatory response is important and may be difficult in many patients. With normal convalescence, patients may be febrile for 3 to 5 days following operation (Wedley et al., 1975). Fever in the early postoperative course can be destabilizing and should be aggressively managed. Acetaminophen, a cooling blanket, and occasionally, corticosteroids may be required.

Inflammation

CPB nonspecifically activates the inflammatory system (Westaby, 1987). *Biocompatibility* is a term often used to describe the body's inflammatory reaction to different forms of extracorporeal circulation. The type of oxygenator and the extracorporeal circuit itself partly determine the biocompatibility of CPB. Generalized complement activation is seen, with elevations in C3a and C5a anaphylatoxins following discontinuation of CPB (Chenoweth et al., 1981; Kirklin et al., 1983; Moore et al., 1988; Videm et al., 1992). This activation can lead to pulmonary sequestration of leukocytes (Chenoweth et al., 1981; Craddock et al., 1977; Moore et al., 1988) and the production of superoxides and other products of lipoxygenation. This causes further leukocyte activation and the generation of leukotactic circulating factors that increase the local inflammatory response (Dinarello, 1984; McCord et al., 1980). Elevations in tumor necrosis factor, interleukin-1, and prostaglandin E_2 have been described (Butler et al., 1993; Jansen et al., 1992; Markewitz et al., 1993). Additionally, vasoactive substances may be liberated from platelets in response to CPB or protamine infusion, which can cause pulmonary hypertension and systemic hypotension (Jastrzebski et al., 1974). Adverse reaction to protamine may also be complement-mediated and related to prior exposure (Lakin et al., 1978).

The generalized inflammatory reaction that follows CPB may change vascular permeability in the pulmonary bed and cause pulmonary hypertension and bronchial hyperreactivity (Klausner et al., 1989). This inflammatory response may directly reset the hypothalamic thermoregulatory center as the cause of fever following cardiac surgery (Dinarello, 1984). This inflammatory reaction can predict postoperative pulmonary dysfunction and renal dysfunction that is independent of CPB time (Kirklin et al., 1983; Klausner et al., 1989). Amelioration of the inflammatory response by prostaglandin E_1 (Bolanowski et al., 1977) and steroids (MacGregor et al., 1974; Miranda et al., 1982) also suggests that nonspecific inflammation is related to complement activation as well as to elevated interleukin-1 levels.

A specific manifestation of the inflammatory response in cardiothoracic surgery is the *postpericardiotomy syndrome*, which, in 1958, was differentiated from the postcommissurotomy syndrome (Ito et al., 1958). The syndrome, occurring in 10 to 30% of patients, is a self-limited disease beginning in the second or third postoperative week and is associated with fever and pleuritic, precordial, or substernal chest pain (Engle and Ito, 1961). This syndrome has been associated with specific reactive antibodies and may occur following any operation that violates the pericardium (Engle et al., 1974, 1975). It is treated with bed rest and nonsteroidal anti-inflammatory agents, although corticosteroids (nonspecific depression of inflammatory response) may be necessary in severe cases (Horneffer et al., 1990; Kirsh et al., 1970).

Infection

Following cardiac surgery, as many as 73% of patients will develop a temperature of 37° C (rectal) after postoperative day 6. The incidence of fever decreases exponentially throughout the postoperative course (Fig. 8–22). Fevers related to infectious causes are most commonly low-grade (38.9° C, rectal), and most resolve before the fifteenth postoperative day. Fever greater than 38.9° C at any time in the postoperative course is more likely related to a specific infection. The presence or absence of leukocytosis has not been helpful in this differentiation (Livelli et al., 1978). Twenty-five per cent of fevers on postoperative days 4 through 9 may be related to serious infection (Pien et al., 1982).

When infection is suspected, aggressive evaluation is indicated. *Aerobic* and *anaerobic* cultures of blood, urine, sputum, and abnormal fluid collections are mandatory and should precede broad-spectrum antibiotic coverage (Graham, 1984). Indwelling catheters should be considered potential infectious sites; appropriate infection control helps to limit and prevent serious infections from these devices (Norwood et al., 1988, 1991; Wormser et al., 1990). When antibiotics have already been administered, cultures should be

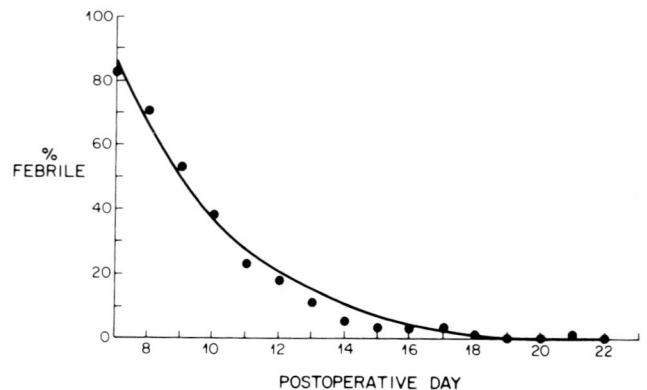

FIGURE 8–22. Prevalence of fever in 118 retrospectively identified patients after cardiac surgery. Patients were considered febrile if any temperature determination on a particular postoperative day was greater than or equal to 37.8° C. The initial prevalence is 83% on the seventh postoperative day, because fever initially developed after the seventh postoperative day in 17% of febrile patients. (From Livelli, F. D., Jr., Johnson, R. A., McEnany, M. T., et al: Unexplained in-hospital fever following cardiac surgery. Circulation, 57:968, 1978. By permission of the American Heart Association, Inc.)

obtained using specific antimicrobe-absorbing resins (Jacobs, 1984).

Soft-tissue infection is most commonly due to *Staphylococcus aureus,* although *S. epidermidis* is emerging as an important pathogen (Williams, 1988). *Pseudomonas* and other gram-negative infections become more common when intensive care exceeds 7 days and in patients receiving broad-spectrum antibiotic therapy (Freeman and McPeake, 1982). Prolonged intensive care and antibiotic use can also cause systemic fungal infections and loss of the gastric mucosal barrier (Ford et al., 1991; Marshall et al., 1988; Stoutenbeek et al., 1984). These infections are particularly difficult to diagnose because of their protean manifestations (Ho, 1984).

Mediastinitis is of particular concern in all cardiac surgical patients. The incidence has been reported to range from 0.8 to 1.86% (Breyer et al., 1984; Culliford et al., 1967; Iberti et al., 1990; Loop et al., 1990; Ottino et al., 1987). Sternal and mediastinal infections must be differentiated from simple subcutaneous fat necrosis, sterile sternal dehiscence, and the postpericardiotomy syndrome. Deep sternal infections and mediastinitis are commonly associated with systemic symptoms (fever, leukocytosis), localized tenderness, severe persistent chest pain, and sternal instability with evidence of perimedian sternotomy (Loop et al., 1990; Sanfelippo and Danielson, 1972; Sarr et al., 1984; Serry et al., 1980; Shafir et al., 1988; Stoney et al., 1978; Ulicny and Hiratzka, 1991). Chest films, computed tomography (which may help to demonstrate a substernal abscess and sternal separation), and indium-111 leukocyte scanning may be used to confirm the clinical diagnosis. Initial treatment consists of operative wound exploration, débridement, and drainage (Serry et al., 1980). Although some infected patients can be treated with reclosure and irrigation (Thurer et al., 1974), diminished morbidity is noted with bilateral pectoral flap closure (Jurkiewicz et al., 1980). Flap closure may be performed as a primary procedure with accompanying sternal débridement (Jeevanadam et al., 1990) or as a staged procedure with sternal débridement followed by muscle flap closure in 3 to 4 days (Johnson et al., 1989; Jurkiewicz et al., 1980).

Soft tissue infections involving saphenous vein harvest, though usually minor, are a significant source of morbidity following coronary revascularization. This complication has been reported to occur in 1% of patients (DeLaria et al., 1981) and is more common in the thigh harvest site. Etiologically, these infections are due to either *S. aureus* or to mixed gram-negative flora. These complications are best prevented by careful selection of harvest sites and meticulous surgical technique. Most of these infections may be treated effectively by simple drainage, dressing changes, and prescription of antibiotics. However, in severe cases, wide débridement and skin grafting may be necessary.

Prevention of Infection

Prophylactic antibiotics are an important component of cardiac surgery; regimens using antistaphylococcal penicillins or cephalosporins significantly reduce the prevalence of postoperative wound infection when compared with placebo (Kreter and Woods, 1992). Wound infection rates (sternal and saphenous vein harvest sites) are reduced from approximately 25% in patients receiving placebo to 5% in antibiotic-treated groups (Kreter and Woods, 1992). Cefamandole is superior to cefazolin with or without an aminoglycoside in cardiac surgical prophylaxis (Kaiser, 1988), although other studies support the use of either cefazolin or cefuroxime (Conklin et al., 1988; Gentry et al., 1988). Preoperative antibiotics must be administered intravenously in the induction room (Petracek, 1988), although the optimal duration of prophylaxis is controversial. In meta-analysis, no difference was shown between short (2 days) and long (3 days or greater) prophylactic regimens (Kreter and Woods, 1992). Although a 2-day course has been shown to be as effective as a 5- to 6-day course (Burnakis, 1984), many surgeons believe that the risk of infection extends until all lines are removed (Moore, 1988; Platt, 1984) and therefore continue antibiotic coverage beyond the second postoperative day (LoCicero, 1990).

The most common nosocomial infection is urinary tract infection from indwelling drainage catheters (40%). Bacteriuria occurs in 80% of patients after 10 days of urinary drainage (DeJongh et al., 1984).

Vascular catheters are an important source of hospital-acquired infections (Maki, 1982). One-third of all hospital-acquired bacteremia cases (Bentley and Lepper, 1968; Harris et al., 1980; Norwood et al., 1991) and most candidemia cases (Rose, 1978) are associated with vascular catheters. One and one-half per cent of cultures of vascular catheters yield positive results, and pulmonary artery catheters have a rate of colonization as high as 2.1% (Damen et al., 1985). Catheter-related sepsis is most commonly due to *S. aureus* and cannot be treated successfully without removing the catheter (Norwood et al., 1991). Following removal, a 7- to 10-day course of appropriate systemic therapy is usually sufficient, although 4 to 6 weeks of therapy may be necessary for central venous septic thrombosis. When central catheter infection has occurred, a latent focus of deep infection resulting from the bacteremia must be carefully sought. Local antimicrobial ointment (combination of polymixin, neomycin, and bacitracin) is superior to iodophor ointments in suppression of line sepsis (Maki and Band, 1981). Infection from invasive lines is most easily prevented by aseptic insertion and dressing technique as well as by changing peripheral lines every 48 hours and central lines every 3 to 7 days, regardless of whether colonization or frank infection is present (DeJongh et al., 1984; Norwood et al., 1991). For central venous access, guidewire exchange appears to be safe if there is no clinical evidence of systemic sepsis (Norwood et al., 1991).

RENAL DYSFUNCTION

Postoperative renal dysfunction has been common following cardiac operation; in some form it has been

■ **Table 8–8.** POSTOPERATIVE RENAL DYSFUNCTION

Study	Postoperative Incidence (%)			Mortality of Severe Renal Failure (%)		
	Moderate	*Severe*	*Total*	*Oliguric*	*Nonoliguric*	*Unspecified*
Yeboah et al., 1972	26.3	4.7	31			70
Abel, 1976a	24.2	7	31.2			88
Bhat et al., 1976	26	4.3	30.3			43
McLeish et al., 1977		1.6		41		
Hilberman et al., 1979	2.5	2.5	5	65	17	

reported at rates of 8 to 44%, with frank acute renal failure occurring in 2 to 13.5% of cases during the 1960s and 1970s (Abel et al., 1974b; McMillan and Maghissi, 1972; Utley, 1982; Yeboah et al., 1972). Improvements in CPB technique and postoperative hemodynamic support have lowered the incidence of renal dysfunction significantly (Weinstein et al., 1989). Renal dysfunction can range from mild to severe and can be oliguric or nonoliguric (Table 8–8). It would appear that any diminution in postoperative renal function is associated with increased mortality (16%, as opposed to 0.9% in patients who show no rise in serum creatinine [Bhat et al., 1976]) and varies with severity of ensuing renal dysfunction (90% with severe acute renal failure, 10 to 20% with mild to moderate renal failure) (Corwin et al., 1989). Acute renal failure is also associated with increased morbidity, increased length of stay, and increased length of ICU stay (Corwin et al., 1989). The mortality rates associated with contrast-induced renal insufficiency (6%) and aminoglycoside-induced renal insufficiency (11%) are much lower than rates associated with other causes (Hou et al., 1983).

Diagnosis

Renal dysfunction is usually heralded by oliguria (urine output < 0.5 ml/kg/hr or < 500 ml/day) and is associated with elevations of blood urea nitrogen and serum creatinine. Hypovolemia and low CO may cause appropriate oliguria ("prerenal") and are usually associated with sodium retention. The stress of operation and associated activation of the renin-angiotensin system, the elevation of serum aldosterone, and the presence of antidiuretic hormone all can contribute to postoperative oliguria, which will respond to fluid resuscitation. Reversible prerenal azotemia is likely when the following are true:

- Urine osmolality is greater than 500 mOsm/l
- Urine sodium (U_{na}) concentration is less than 10 mEq/l
- Urine-plasma urea nitrogen ratio is greater than 100
- Urine-plasma creatinine ratio is greater than 60
- Fractional excretion of sodium (FENa) is less than 1 as calculated by the following formula:

$$FENa = (U_{na}/P_{na})\Pi(U_{cr}/P_{cr}) \times 100$$

where P_{na} = plasma sodium, U_{cr} = urinary creatinine, and P_{cr} = plasma creatinine.

- Urinary specific gravity greater than 1.020

Acute tubular necrosis is manifested by the following:

- Low urine osmolality (less than 350 mOsm/l)
- Urine sodium concentration greater than 25 mEq/l
- Urine-plasma urea nitrogen ratio less than 3
- Urine-plasma creatinine ratio less than 10 (Table 8–9)

Etiology

Postoperative renal failure is associated with preoperative renal insufficiency, age, prolonged CPB and prolonged aortic cross-clamping, combined CABG and valve replacement procedures, and perioperative left ventricular dysfunction (Abel et al., 1976a; Corwin et al., 1989; Hilberman et al., 1979). Perioperative contrast media exposure and the use of aminoglycosides are also causal (Hou et al., 1983). In this study, iatrogenic factors accounted for 55% of all episodes of renal failure. Nonsteroidal anti-inflammatory agents, particularly ibuprofen, can additionally reduce renal function, particularly in salt-depleted patients and patients with renal vascular disease. A similar revers-

■ **Table 8–9.** LABORATORY DIAGNOSIS OF OLIGURIA

Measurement	Physiologic Oliguria	Prerenal Failure	Acute Tubular Necrosis
Urinary sodium	<10 mEq/l	<25 mEq/l	>25 mEq/l
Urinary specific gravity	>1.024	>1.015	>1.01–1.015
Urinary/plasma osmolality	>2.5:1	>1.8:1	1.1:1 or less
Urinary/plasma urea	>100:1	>20:1	3:1, rarely >10:1
Urinary/plasma creatinine	>60:1	>30:1, rarely <10:1	<10:1

From Mazze, R. I.: Critical care of the patient with acute renal failure. Anesthesiology, 47:138, 1977.

ible effect has been specifically related to the ACE inhibitors (Davies, 1985). Diminished renal perfusion and hypotension are commonly implicated causes, although significant hypotension was documented in only 12 of 23 cases in one series (Hou et al., 1983).

Treatment

The most effective treatment is avoidance of renal failure, which is best accomplished by recognition of perioperative risk factors. Exposure to large doses of preoperative iodinated contrast agents and the use of perioperative aminoglycosides (which, if necessary, should be prescribed according to documented serum levels) should be minimized. Postoperative hypotension should be prevented or corrected expediently, particularly in patients with known or suspected fixed renal artery lesions. Hemodilution (Mielke et al., 1966), mannitol (Schuster et al., 1964), and furosemide (Weinstein et al., 1989) have been shown to benefit patients with renal function. Continuous furosemide infusion may be more effective than intermittent bolus administration for patients with significant renal dysfunction (Magovern and Magovern, 1990). Low-dose dopamine (1 to 3 μg/kg/min) improves renal blood flow (Goldberg, 1972; Iaina et al., 1977) and may have prophylactic value.

Once impending renal failure has been recognized, it is imperative to attempt conversion to nonoliguric renal failure (Kron et al., 1985). Optimization of preload, assurance of adequate systemic BP, and the use of diuretics (Magovern and Magovern, 1990) and dopamine may be effective. Once oliguric renal failure is established, dialysis may be indicated for the following conditions:

- Metabolic acidosis
- Hyperkalemia
- Pulmonary edema
- "Uremia" with associated coma or seizure (Raymond, 1990)

Dialysis should be performed to remove toxic metabolites, correct metabolic acidosis, remove endogenous and exogenous nephrotoxins, and maintain normokalemia and fluid balance (Hakim and Lazarus, 1983). Several studies have shown that early and aggressive dialysis to maintain the blood urea nitrogen at a time-average of 70 (Lowrie et al., 1981) improves survival rate (Conger, 1975; Kron et al., 1985). Dialysis should probably be instituted prophylactically at creatinine levels of 8 to 10 with associated blood urea nitrogen of greater than 100 if no other indications become evident (Blachley and Henrich, 1981).

Hemodialysis, peritoneal dialysis, and continuous arteriovenous hemofiltration are current options. Peritoneal dialysis is useful in children, patients with vascular access problems, and patients with hemodynamic instability. It may not be possible after abdominal procedures or in patients with impaired pulmonary function or severe azotemia (Kron et al., 1985).

Hemodialysis may be poorly tolerated in patients with hemodynamic instability following cardiac oper-

ation. Systemic or regional heparinization is necessary but can usually be accomplished without adverse effects (Hakim and Lazarus, 1983).

Continuous arteriovenous ultrafiltration, or hemofiltration, is another option (Darup et al., 1979; Kramer et al., 1977). With low-dose heparin (10 units/kg/hr), it is possible to remove 200 to 600 ml/hr (Kramer et al., 1977). This may significantly benefit patients with pulmonary edema (Susini et al., 1990). This volume may be replaced by the infusion of balanced salt solutions or discarded, depending on fluid status. The technique can be practiced with regional heparinization (Paganini and Nakamoto, 1980) and has the distinct advantage of being well tolerated hemodynamically following cardiac surgery (Kron et al., 1985).

Multisystem support is necessary to achieve optimal results. Particular attention must be paid to depletion of water-soluble vitamins and the effect of dialysis on various drug clearance rates (Hakim and Lazarus, 1983). Nutritional supplementation with the use of TPN has been beneficial (Abel et al., 1973, 1974a, 1974b; Dudrick et al., 1970). In these patients, nearly half the mortality is related to renal failure (Bhat et al., 1976). Residual cardiac dysfunction may also be a significant component of mortality in these patients (Hilberman et al., 1980). Oliguria that persists for more than 3 weeks tends to imply irreversible renal damage (Blachley and Henrich, 1981).

NEUROLOGIC DYSFUNCTION

Neurologic complications can be among the most devastating that follow cardiac operation. These can range in magnitude from mood swings, transient psychosis, and minor self-limited peripheral neuropathies to major, permanent cerebrovascular accidents. The differential diagnosis of delirium in postoperative cardiac patients includes withdrawal from alcohol, hypertensive encephalopathy, hypoglycemia, hypoperfusion, hypoxemia, and drug-induced causes. Intracranial bleeding and meningitis remain remote possibilities. Metabolic causes should also be considered, especially hyponatremia. Endocrinopathies related to adrenal, pancreatic, and parathyroid function must also be excluded. Despite improvements in overall mortality and reduced morbidity in patients undergoing cardiac operations, the prevalence of major neurologic injury or of lesser neuropsychologic disturbances in the early postoperative period does not appear to have declined (Breuer et al., 1983; Shaw et al., 1985).

Postoperative Psychosis

This syndrome was originally reported to occur in 41 to 70% of patients who had undergone cardiac surgery (Blachy and Starr, 1964; Egerton and Kay, 1964; Kornfeld et al., 1965). It is characterized by a lucid postoperative interval followed by a development of frank disorientation, hallucination, and, frequently, paranoia. The patient's age and preoperative psychiatric history and the severity of preoperative and postoperative illness have been identified as relevant factors (Egerton and Kay, 1964; Heller et al., 1970; Sveinsson, 1975). The duration of CPB has not been proven to be a prognostic factor separable from the severity of illness in such cases (Dubin et al., 1979; Sveinsson, 1975). Sleep deprivation and the ICU environment have also been found to be important factors (Blachy and Starr, 1964; Nadelson, 1976; Sveinsson, 1975; Taub and Berger, 1974).

A preoperative interview reduces the incidence of postoperative psychosis by 50% (Dubin et al., 1979; Layne and Yudofsky, 1971). It should be treated by a combination of chemotherapy (alpha-butyrophenone, benzodiazepine, or phenothiazine [Shapiro et al., 1986]) and supportive psychotherapy (Dubin et al., 1979).

In the absence of focal deficit (Javid et al., 1969), neuropsychological testing often reveals impairment immediately following an operation. As many as 28% of patients may have cognitive impairment at 9 postoperative days; persistence beyond 6 months is rare (Savageau et al., 1982; Townes et al., 1989). At long-term follow-up, any cognitive dysfunction has completely resolved in most patients (Hammeke and Hastings, 1988; Townes et al., 1989). The only predictor of negative outcome with respect to cognitive function appears to be advanced age.

Almost all narcotic agents have been shown to cause hallucination and other central nervous system disturbances, particularly in the elderly. Similar effects have been noted with cimetidine, which may be due to central nervous system H_2-receptor blockade (Freston, 1982).

Delirium tremens due to alcohol withdrawal has been reported to carry a 15% mortality rate, although this rate may be less than 6% today. Treatment with midazolam by continuous infusion has the significant advantage of limited respiratory depression and easy titration of effect (Lineaweaver et al., 1988). Adequate pain control is an important aspect of postoperative care. Narcotics and benzodiazepines judiciously administered in bolus injection or by continuous infusion are the mainstays of treatment (Wheeler, 1993).

Focal Central Neurologic Deficit

The incidence of focal neurologic damage varies significantly and appears to depend on the intensity of investigation and changing patterns of patient selection. Stroke rates as low as 0.57% (Gardner et al., 1985) have been reported for CABG procedures. The general incidence of perioperative stroke in patients undergoing CABG is probably 2 to 3% (Hart and Hindman, 1982), although the prevalence gradually rises with increasing age to about 5% in patients over the age of 65 and to as high as 8% in patients over 75 (Cosgrove et al., 1984; Gardner et al., 1985). The presence of carotid disease and significant atherosclerosis

of the ascending aorta also implies an increased risk of perioperative stroke (Wareing et al., 1993). Open heart procedures, especially valve procedures, may produce an incidence of focal neurologic change as high as 43% if such change is specifically sought (Tufo et al., 1970). Delayed presentation of neurologic injury is associated with improved outcome, whereas as many as 70% of patients who are unresponsive immediately after surgery fail to survive (Bojar et al., 1983). Fifteen to 17% of survivors have residual evidence of permanent damage (Kolkka and Hilberman, 1980; Tufo et al., 1970).

Mortality rates following stroke can be as high as 23%, with half of the deaths predominantly due to neurologic dysfunction (Gardner et al., 1985). All deaths were seen in patients who underwent severe changes immediately after operation (Gardner et al. 1985). An increasing percentage of deaths following cardiac surgery are due to neurologic dysfunction rather than cardiac causes (Kouchoukos et al., 1980; Miller et al., 1983). An evaluation of patients with nontraumatic coma demonstrated that good recovery resulted in 10% of cases induced by hypoxia-ischemia; most of the progress occurred in the first month of recovery. Metabolic or diffuse disorders carried the best prognosis. The absence of pupillary light reflex, corneal reflex, caloric reflex, or doll's eyes response is associated with a 5% chance of recovering. After 24 hours, absence of corneal reflex or pupillary light reaction precludes significant recovery (Levy et al., 1981).

The etiology of stroke following cardiac operation is uncertain. Embolic injury (most likely occurring during the redistribution of blood from the heart-lung machine to the patient when the heart is beginning to inject actively), alterations in cerebral blood flow related to the conduct of operation, associated atherosclerosis of the aorta, and pre-existing cerebrovascular disease are all contributing factors (Edmunds, 1983; van der Linden and Casimir-Ahn, 1991; Wareing et al., 1993). Approximately 8% of CABG patients harbor asymptomatic cervical bruits (Balderman et al., 1983). The role of investigation and operative management of asymptomatic extracranial cerebrovascular disease is uncertain at this time (Barnes et al., 1981). The exclusion or inclusion of patients undergoing surgery for symptomatic or asymptomatic carotid disease has made interpretation of many large series difficult. Significant reductions in internal carotid diameter (75%), although considered hemodynamically significant, do not imply a risk for cerebral hyperperfusion during CPB (Johnsson et al., 1991). Aggressive treatment strategies that include carotid endarterectomy and replacement of the ascending aorta in some groups of patients have decreased the incidence of stroke, although this approach is not widely practiced (Wareing et al., 1993).

Treatment of the patient with focal neurologic deficit includes nonspecific measures such as preventing hypoxia and maintaining hypocarbia. Intracranial pressure may be elevated and can be treated with mannitol and diuretics. Of particular concern is the decision to begin anticoagulation in such patients. Approximately 13% of patients who undergo embolic stroke experience a second stroke within 2 weeks if they are not given anticoagulation therapy; an additional 15 to 18% suffer emboli to other organs (Fisher, 1979; Szekely, 1964). Anticoagulation reduces the natural rate of recurrence during this high-risk period (Hart et al., 1983a). Aggregate data suggest that immediate anticoagulation of nonseptic, embolic brain infarction is relatively safe, although approximately 2% of patients experience major secondary brain hemorrhage in the area of prior infarction within 2 weeks (Hart et al., 1983a, 1983b). Neurologic consultation and further investigation with computerized tomography should be done early to assist in this aspect of management.

Injury of the Peripheral Nervous System

Neurologic complications involving the peripheral nervous system that persist beyond the time of discharge occur in approximately 5% of CABG patients (Hart et al., 1983b). Brachial plexus symptoms can occur in 15 to 19% of patients (Vander Salm, 1984). Most patients (92%) are asymptomatic at 3 postoperative months (Morin et al., 1982). The mechanism of injury appears to be related to excessive sternal retraction during operation (Vander Salm, 1984). Unilateral vocal cord paralysis (usually left-sided) may also be due to excessive sternal retraction (Horn and Abouav, 1979; Kirsh et al., 1971) or to prolonged intubation. Although these conditions are usually self-limited, associated abnormalities in swallowing may cause aspiration.

Phrenic nerve damage is also common (1.7 to 11%) and may be due either to direct surgical injury (diathermy or division) or to cold injury caused by the use of topical hypothermia (Benjamin et al., 1982; Markand et al., 1985; Mickell et al., 1978). Many patients sustain peripheral neuropathies as a complication of vascular access in preparation for cardiac procedures. Exposure of the femoral vessels and harvest of saphenous vein may cause nerve injury. A further mechanism is improper patient positioning. Most of these neuropraxic neuropathies will resolve, and their effect can be lessened by appropriate physical therapy and counseling.

ENDOCRINOPATHIES

The postsurgical endocrine environment is complex and multifactorial. Generally, the renin-angiotensin system is activated, and high levels of serum catecholamines are present as a general response to stress. Glucagon is elevated and stimulates the release of endogenous catecholamines (Hall-Boyer et al., 1984). ANF, present in high concentrations in atrial tissue, leads to natriuresis and diuresis despite elevated levels of aldosterone and vasopressin. ANF also acts as a feedback inhibitor of aldosterone secretion and

suppresses vasopressin release (Needleman and Greenwald, 1986). ANF is normally regulated by atrial filling pressure, but this correlation is lost and ANF levels remain high for the initial 24 hours following cardiac surgery (Dewar et al., 1988).

The neurohormonal environment alters cardiac and peripheral vascular function and renal function, and it has complex effects on the blood glucose and serum electrolyte concentrations. An awareness of these normal responses to surgical stress helps the physician to recognize an isolated endocrinopathy that may hinder the physiologic response to stress.

Diabetes Mellitus

The most common endocrine abnormality requiring perioperative management is pre-existing diabetes mellitus. Insulin requirements increase in the perioperative period because of the increases in serum epinephrine (10-fold), serum norepinephrine (4-fold), and serum cortisol levels (3-fold) (Crock et al., 1988). Elevations in serum cortisol may persist for 2 to 3 days after surgery, with a loss of normal circadian rhythm (McIntosh et al., 1981). Insulin secretion is also impaired by hypothermia and sluggishly rises in the postoperative period in diabetic patients (Crock et al., 1988). The exclusion of glucose from the pump priming solution can minimize perioperative hyperglycemia in both insulin-dependent and non–insulin-dependent diabetics. These patients should be given a continuous insulin infusion, which should be started preoperatively. Insulin requirements during hypothermia are low (Kuntschen et al., 1986) but increase during rewarming to as much as 20 to 30 units/hr before stabilizing at between 0.5 units/hr and 10 units/hr (Watson et al., 1986).

Type II (non–insulin-dependent) diabetics can usually be managed perioperatively with diet alone. Oral hypoglycemic agents should be withdrawn and can be reinstituted when the patient tolerates a full diet. For insulin-dependent patients, the euglycemia should be maintained during the perioperative period. Intravenous infusion of insulin with close monitoring of blood sugar is most applicable to the ICU setting. Alternatives, as well as a method for conversion back to subcutaneous insulin requirements, should also be considered (Tables 8–10 and 8–11). Insulin requirements usually decrease by the third postoperative day. Intensive management of serum glucose is often necessary as the patient resumes an oral diet. Non–insulin-dependent diabetics may require subcutaneous insulin administration at the time of discharge, either because of residual changes from surgery or because of the more intensive evaluation of the diabetic disorder prompted by cardiac intervention. Sufficient planning, organization, and education is important to permit timely and safe discharge of such patients.

Hypothyroidism

Thyroid dysfunction can occur in seriously ill patients who were euthyroid preoperatively (Chernow,

■ **Table 8–10.** INSULIN PREPARATIONS* AND REGIMENS

	Peak (Hours)	Duration (Hours)
Rapid-acting—regular†	0.5–4	5–7
Semilente	4–6	12–16
Intermediate—NPH, Lente	4–12	18–24
Long-acting—PZI, Ultralente	18–24	>36

Regimens

1. Intermediate + regular (⅔ + ⅓) in A.M., 0.5 unit/kg ideal body weight. Check blood glucose at 4–5 P.M. to regulate next day's dose.
2. Intermediate ⅔ in A.M. and ⅓ in P.M. plus supplemental regular for late A.M. or bedtime hyperglycemia. *Regular is never given at bedtime.*
3. Single small dose of intermediate in A.M. and 5–10 units subcutaneously before each meal.
4. CSII‡ with an open loop pump set at a basal infusion of 1 unit/hr with 5- to 10-unit bolus 15 minutes before each meal.

From Jonasson, O.: Surgical aspects of diabetes mellitus. *In* Sabiston, D. C., Jr. (ed): Textbook of Surgery. 14th ed., Chap. 8. Philadelphia, W. B. Saunders, 1991.
*Available as pork or beef extracts, semisynthetic, or human recombinant.
†Only regular insulin can be administered intravenously.
‡Continuous subcutaneous insulin infusion.

1984). The euthyroid state is probably important for patients with generalized cellular dysfunction, and a high correlation between low T4 levels and mortality has been found in critical care patients (Slag et al., 1981). The perioperative determination of thyroid function is difficult because of abnormalities of T4 binding (Woeber and Maddux, 1981), and the response of TSH to decreased levels of T3 and T4 is abnormal in critically ill patients (Chernow, 1984; Maturlo et al., 1980). Critical evaluation of thyroid function, with appropriate consultation, is probably indicated in all patients with unexplained hemodynamic dysfunction and in patients who experience a prolonged complicated postoperative course.

■ **Table 8–11.** PERIOPERATIVE MANAGEMENT OF DIABETIC PATIENTS

Discontinue oral hypoglycemic agents 24 hours before operation. Give no intermediate- or long-acting insulin on the day of operation.
Give nothing by mouth after midnight.
Start intravenous infusion of D₅W or D₅NS with 20 mEq KCl/l at 6 A.M. Administer at 100–200 ml/hr.
Start second intravenous infusion of insulin, 25 units/250 ml NS. Run 75 ml through the intravenous tubing (to occupy protein binding sites on tubing), then discard. Administer at 1–2 units/hr via infusion pump.
Monitor blood glucose at 30-minute intervals until stable at 150–200 mg/dl, then monitor hourly until patient is awake, every 4 hours until diet is resumed.
Convert to maintenance regimen when diet has resumed by giving 80% of previous day's total insulin, ⅔ as intermediate and ⅓ as regular. Adjust daily, using blood glucose values (see Table 8–10).

From Jonasson, O.: Surgical aspects of diabetes mellitus. *In* Sabiston, D. C., Jr. (ed): Textbook of Surgery. 14th ed., Chap. 8. Philadelphia, W. B. Saunders, 1991.

Adrenal Insufficiency

Acute adrenal insufficiency has been described in 0.1% of patients undergoing cardiac surgery (Alford et al., 1979). Patients present with symptoms of flank and abdominal pain, delirium, fever, and eventually shock (Alford et al., 1979). The most common cause of hypoadrenalism is preoperative adrenal suppression, although it can arise spontaneously in patients who suffer a long preoperative illness or bilateral adrenal hemorrhage (Dorin and Kearns, 1988; Siu et al., 1990).

Hypoadrenalism causes primary ventricular dysfunction and a failure to maintain peripheral vascular constrictor tone even when catecholamine is administered (Lefer, 1975). The diagnosis can be made by cortisol radioimmunoassay, which would normally show elevated cortisol levels in the immediate postoperative period (Chernow, 1984). One must be looking for hypoadrenalism to diagnose it; it should be considered in any patient with unexplained hypotension, hypothermia, or hyponatremia.

The therapy of documented hypoadrenalism should consist of intravenous glucocorticoid administration. In the absence of documentation, dexamethasone should be used as long as it does not interfere with later cortisol assays. The administration of glucocorticoids can increase systemic vascular resistance by 35% while CO remains stable. A process of synthesis appears to be required, such that response is delayed 30 to 45 minutes (Fig. 8–23). Although a positive inotropic effect of corticosteroids cannot be demonstrated in vitro, such benefit is usually seen in the treated clinical syndrome (Lefer, 1975).

Hypopituitarism

Pituitary apoplexy is a rare complication of cardiac surgery and usually is caused by bleeding into a primary pituitary tumor (Cooper et al., 1986; Peck et al., 1980). Primary pituitary infarction has also been reported (Kovacs and Yao, 1975). Generalized endocrinopathy results from dysfunction of many hormonal systems under pituitary control. Massive diuresis from diabetes insipidus may be the earliest manifestation. When cases result from bleeding into primary pituitary tumors, a mass effect may produce a unilaterally dilated, unresponsive pupil as an early feature. Surgical decompression and endocrine replacement therapy are indicated.

GASTROINTESTINAL COMPLICATIONS

Gastrointestinal complications (Table 8–12) may cause significant postoperative cardiac mortality (10%) (Pinson and Alberty, 1983). Fifty per cent of patients with gastrointestinal complications have a history of previous gastrointestinal disease (Welling et al., 1986). One must look for postoperative gastrointestinal complications to diagnose them, and delayed diagnosis causes excessive mortality. In one series, a

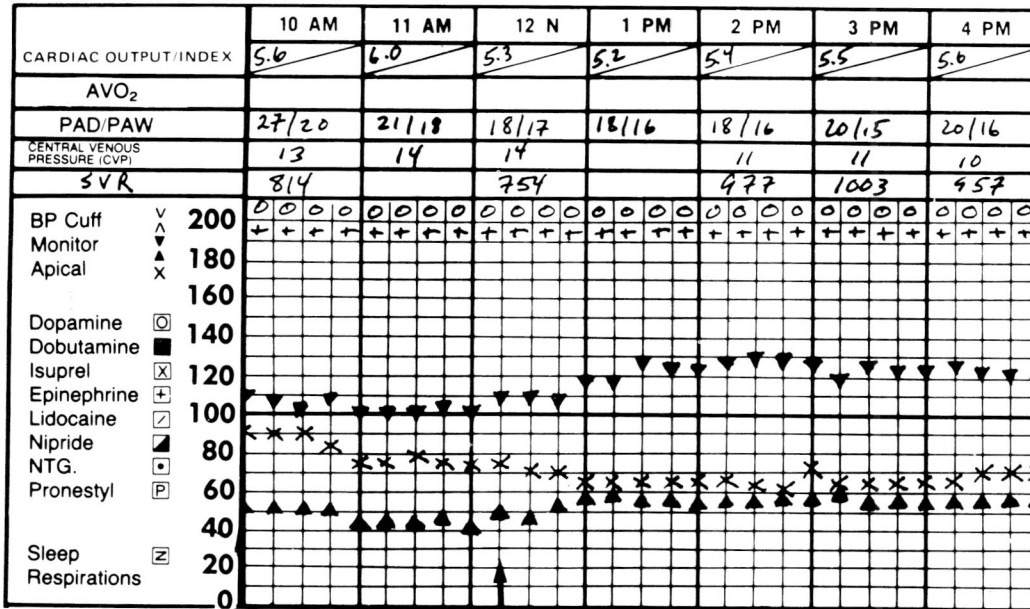

FIGURE 8–23. Hemodynamic data for an 82-year-old patient who had reoperative aortic and mitral valve replacement for prosthetic endocarditis. Manifestations of endocarditis had been present for 2 months preoperatively and were associated with a 40-lb weight loss. His postoperative course was marked by adequately supported cardiac output with high filling pressures and low systemic vascular resistance (SVR). Mean blood pressures in the range of 60 to 70 mm Hg were providing inadequate renal perfusion. A serum cortisol level was drawn, and 250 mg of methylprednisolone was administered (*black arrow*). After approximately 1 hour, an increase in SVR and blood pressure was noted with maintenance of adequate cardiac output and a diminution in filling pressure. These changes occurred without any alterations of cardiotonic agents. The serum cortisol level was below normal, and the patient was placed on maintenance steroids, which resulted in an uneventful recovery.

delay in treatment of 24 hours produced a 75% overall mortality rate (Rosemurgy et al., 1988).

Gastrointestinal complications that mark an otherwise uneventful postoperative recovery are associated with an extremely low mortality rate, whereas those associated with a complex postoperative course and marked by low CO are associated with a high mortality rate (33%) (Rosemurgy et al., 1988). Risk factors for gastrointestinal complications include age, emergency operation, valve operation, long CPB time, significant arrhythmias, the need for inotropic support, or the use of an intra-aortic balloon pump (Leitman et al., 1987; Ohri et al., 1991).

Depressed gastrointestinal motility may be related to low CO and is exacerbated by the associated redistribution of blood flow away from the splanchnic bed (Reilly and Bulkley, 1993). The ileus is mediated by

the renin-angiotensin axis and can be experimentally ameliorated with ACE blockade (Bailey et al., 1982; Bulkley et al., 1983; McNeill et al., 1970; Oshima and Bulkley, 1984; Reilly and Bulkley, 1993). In a hemorrhagic shock model, vasomotor control of splanchnic blood flow was improved with an intra-aortic balloon pump (Landreneau, 1991). Depressed gastrointestinal motility is often manifested by nonspecific alterations in small intestinal motility and by colonic pseudo-obstruction (Wanebo et al., 1971).

Cecal distention may be noted on the plain abdominal film and can lead to cecal necrosis (Hargrove et al., 1978). Cecal diameter normally ranges from 3.5 to 8.5 cm (Lowman and Davis, 1956); aggressive management is indicated when the diameter approaches 12 cm (Lowman and Davis, 1956; Melzig and Terz, 1978; Wanebo et al., 1971; Wojtalik et al., 1973). Colon-

■ **Table 8–12.** POSTOPERATIVE GASTROINTESTINAL COMPLICATIONS

Study	N*	PUD†	Biliary	Intestinal	Total (%)	Mortality Rate (%)
Lawhorne, 1978	2500	4	1	3	11 (0.44)	46
Hanks, 1982	5080	15	6	3	43 (0.85)	63
Pinson and Alberty, 1983	5682	13	50	25	82 (1.4)	22
Welling et al., 1986	1596	4	4	7	18 (1.1)	11
Rosemurgy, 1987	7140	6	2	13	21 (0.29)	24
Leitman et al., 1987	6452	22	11	19	60 (0.94)	59
Ohri, 1991	4629	11	5	4	20 (0.43)	15

*N = total number of patients in each series evaluated for gastrointestinal complications, and the columnar results reflect the number of patients who have each disorder. The incidence of total gastrointestinal complications is expressed as the actual number and as a percentage in parentheses.
†PUD = peptic ulcer disease; intestinal complications include obstruction, perforation, and ischemia of either the small or the large bowel.

oscopic decompression may permit nonoperative management (Bachulis and Smith, 1978; Kukora and Dent, 1977), but operative decompression or resection may be necessary, particularly if focal embolic ischemia or infarction has occurred.

Postoperative cholecystitis (particularly the acalculous type) and cholangitis are difficult to diagnose because of the common presence of mild hyperbilirubinemia and upper abdominal pain and tenderness related to the surgical incision and placement of drainage tubes. Diagnostic evaluation, including the use of computerized tomography and abdominal ultrasonography, can be helpful with specific findings that suggest acute cholecystitis, including a thickened gallbladder (wall thickness greater than 4 mm), pericholecystic fluid or subserosal edema without ascites, intramural gas, or sloughed mucosal membrane (Cornwell et al., 1989). Nuclear scans using iminodiacetic acid derivatives (HIDA), although extremely helpful in the diagnosis of acute calculous cholecystitis, have been shown to have a very low specificity for postoperative cholecystitis (Cornwell et al., 1989). Clinical evaluation and serial abdominal examinations that confirm the diagnosis usually result in operation, which may include a cholecystectomy or cholecystostomy. Percutaneous drainage with image guidance is also possible in hemodynamically unstable patients.

Autopsy series have shown the incidence of pancreatitis to range from 11 to 16% (Rose et al., 1984). Significant elevations in serum amylase with peak levels on the second postoperative day (averaging 446 IU/l), that progressively fall over the ensuing 48 to 72 hours have been described. Hyperamylasemia occurs in over 30% of patients (Rattner et al., 1989; Svensson et al., 1985); approximately 10% of patients manifest subclinical pancreatitis (elevations in amylase and lipase), and 1 to 3% of patients manifest clinically significant pancreatitis (Rattner et al., 1989; Svensson et al., 1985). The renal excretion of amylase appears to be altered in the postoperative period, perhaps accounting for the common finding of hyperamylasemia (Hennings and Jacobson, 1974; Smith and Schwartz, 1983).

The maintenance of gastric pH above 3.5 to 4 is particularly important in the prevention of upper gastrointestinal bleeding or other manifestations of peptic ulcer disease (Baue and Chaudry, 1980). Although H_2-blockers have been used toward such maintenance, antacids generally are required as well (Morris et al., 1988; Priebe et al., 1980). Sucralfate, a complex salt of sucralsulfate and aluminum hydroxide that coats the gastric mucosa and allows ulcerations or erosions to heal, has been effective as a prophylactic agent (Cannon et al., 1987). Mesoprostyl, a prostaglandin E_1 analogue, has been shown to have cytoprotective properties and diminished gastric acid secretion, and it effectively prevents stress ulcerations (Zinner et al., 1989). The institution of enteral feedings in the critical care population has also decreased the incidence of significant gastrointestinal bleeding (Pingleton and Hadzima, 1983).

MULTISYSTEM FAILURE

Although morbidity and mortality can result from single organ system failure, it is becoming increasingly apparent that significant mortality and morbidity are attached to multiple organ system failure (Baue, 1975). Deaths following cardiac surgery that are due to this syndrome increased from 7% in 1974 to 1978 to 21% in 1982 to 1983 (Gardner et al., 1985). Patients with low CO syndrome who develop multisystem organ failure (defined as two or more organ systems that require support for more than 3 days) have poor results, with incrementally increasing mortality rates of 14.7%, 27.7%, 48.8%, 53.7%, 69.7%, and 95.7%, respectively, for each additional organ system failure (Kumon et al., 1986). Multicenter data also clearly demonstrate that both the *number* and the *duration* of organ system failures are important predictors of mortality (Fig. 8–24).

Malnutrition, infection, and hypermetabolism are common features of this disorder, which may have a microcirculatory basis (Fry, 1988) manifested by a failure of peripheral oxygen extraction (Baue, 1993; Cerra, 1987). Tissue injury and inflammation activate vasoactive mediators that can be overwhelming (Baue, 1993) (Fig. 8–25). The primary physiologic change appears to be an increase in oxygen demand with an associated increase in CO and fall in SVR—the "sepsis syndrome." Generalized splanchnic vasoconstriction can occur (Fiddian-Green and Baker, 1987) and cause renal and hepatic dysfunction (Mundth et al., 1967; Notterman et al., 1988; Weber, 1984). Multisystem failure is associated with upper gastrointestinal bleeding (Fiddian-Green and Baker, 1987; Hasting et al., 1978), which occurs in 20% of patients with this syndrome and may be an early sign of its presence (Bumaschny et al., 1988).

Sepsis, a prominent feature of multisystem failure, may be due to a gram-positive organism (*S. epidermidis*), gram-negative organisms (*Enterobacteriaceae*, *Pseudomonas aeruginosa*), or *Candida albicans* (Baue, 1993; Marshall et al., 1988). The gastrointestinal tract is increasingly being recognized as a significant source of infection secondary to bacterial translocation (Baue, 1993). Similar organisms are found in the gastrointestinal tract of patients manifesting clinical sepsis in the ICU and in those who later develop multiple organ failure (Marshall et al., 1993). However, despite the increasing recognition of the gastrointestinal tract as a source of ongoing contamination, a cause-effect relationship with multiple organ failure has been difficult to prove (Carrico, 1993). Immunologic parameters, including complement levels, antibody-producing activity, total peripheral blood lymphocyte count, and T-cell function, are depressed in patients who ultimately succumb to multisystem failure (Nishijima et al., 1986).

A preventive approach is necessary to avoid this syndrome, which has been associated with extensive operation and associated hypotension, multiple blood transfusions, prolonged ventilation, and cardiovascular instability. The support of adequate circulation,

Number of OSF		Day of Failure						
		1st	2nd	3rd	4th	5th	6th	7th
1	Percent Mortality*	22%	31%	34%	35%	40%	42%	41%
	No. Deaths	450	261	204	159	142	118	80
	No. Patients	2070	847	607	455	356	279	195
2	Percent Mortality*	52%	67%	66%	62%	56%	64%	68%
	No. Deaths	239	147	103	118	96	78	56
	No. Patients	458	219	156	191	171	122	82
≥ 3	Percent Mortality*	80%	95%	93%	96%	100%†	100%†	100%†
	No. Deaths	152	70	50	50	38	33	32
	No. Patients	191	74	54	52	38	33	32

FIGURE 8–24. Hospital mortality according to the number and duration of organ system failures (OSF). These data reflect mortality rates for 2719 patients who were admitted to 13 hospitals (and include medical, surgical, and cardiac surgical patients). Five organ systems were assessed for failure: cardiovascular, respiratory, renal, hematologic, and neurologic. Both the duration and the number of organ system failures contribute to increased mortality, and survival becomes extremely unlikely after three or more organ system failures of more than 4 days' duration. Maximal statistical probability of survival is 10% (95% confidence), even though no survivors were found in this series. (From Knaus, W. A., Draper, E. A., Wagner, D. P., and Zimmerman, J. E.: Prognosis in acute organ-system failure. Ann. Surg., 202:685, 1985.)

nutrition, and host defenses, as well as the early management of septic sources, is important.

ADVERSE PHARMACOLOGIC REACTIONS

Intensive care management often becomes a complex, multidrug therapeutic environment, which can involve adverse drug effects and drug interactions (Table 8–13) that cause iatrogenic complications. On a medical service, Steel and co-workers noted 497 episodes that could be considered iatrogenic in 815 patients. Iatrogenic illness was considered major in 9% of patients admitted, contributing to death in 2% (Steel et al., 1981).

Injury/Operation

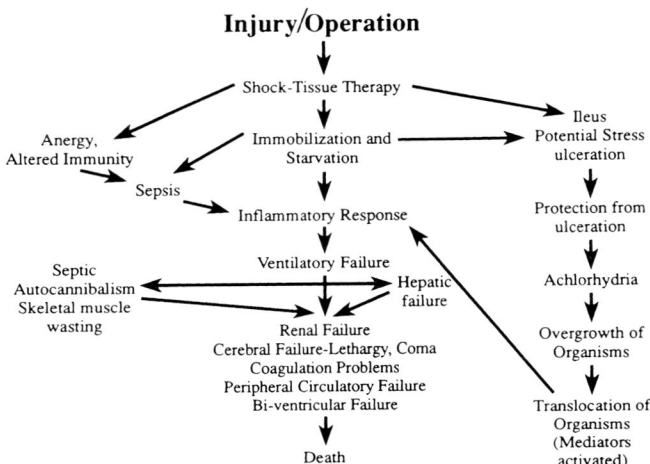

FIGURE 8–25. The sequence of events and relationships that may occur after injury or operation. Death from multiple organ failure may result from this progression of events. (From Baue, A. E.: The role of the gut in the development of multiple organ dysfunction in cardiothoracic patients. Reprinted with permission from the Society of Thoracic Surgeons [The Annals of Thoracic Surgery, 1993, Vol. 55, p. 822].)

Forty-two per cent of iatrogenic occurrences were related to drug therapy (19% of which were considered a major factor in the hospital course), which shows how the adverse effects of drug therapy can significantly contribute to the development of postoperative complications. Drugs most commonly associated with complications include nitrates, digoxin, aminophylline, antiarrhythmic drugs, anticoagulants, penicillins, antihypertensives, propranolol, and benzodiazepines. Digoxin, anticoagulants, antihypertensives, and propranolol were more likely to lead to major complications (Steel et al., 1981).

A heightened awareness of adverse drug effects should simplify drug management, whenever possible, and restrict therapy to definitive indications. Various specific adverse drug effects have been discussed in appropriate sections of this chapter, but two drug-related syndromes merit individual description.

Peripheral Vasodilatation

A number of drugs used in postoperative cardiac care can cause vasodilatation and hypotension. This is a desirable effect with a number of afterload-reducing agents but can be excessive following the administration of prazosin, captopril, and nifedipine. Each of these agents should be instituted initially at low doses, and adequate time for absorption and response should be allowed before therapeutic dosing levels are reached.

Morphine causes significant venodilatation and systemic vascular dilatation through reflex reduction in sympathetic tone (Zelis et al., 1974). It does not appear to have direct cardiac effects (Lowenstein et al., 1969), although it should be used cautiously in patients with borderline hemodynamic stability. Meperidine diminishes vascular resistance only in high doses (Priano and Vatner, 1981). Diazepam may lower BP with intravenous use, although earlier reports as-

■ **Table 8–13.** INTERACTIONS OF DRUGS COMMONLY USED IN POSTOPERATIVE CARDIAC CARE

Interacting Drugs	Possible Effect
Oral Anticoagulants	
Alcohol	Increased anticoagulant effect
Allopurinol	Increased anticoagulant effect
Cimetidine	Increased anticoagulant effect
Steroids	Increased anticoagulant effect
Indomethacin	Increased anticoagulant effect
Quinidine	Increased anticoagulant effect
Salicylates	Increased anticoagulant effect
Metronidazole	Increased anticoagulant effect
Sulfonamide	Increased anticoagulant effect
Hypnotics	Reduced anticoagulant effect
Oral Hypoglycemic Agents	
Beta-blockers	Increased hypoglycemic effect
Anticoagulants	Increased hypoglycemic effect
Propranolol	Increased hypoglycemic effect
Salicylates	Increased hypoglycemic effect
Insulin	
Beta-blockers	Increased hypoglycemic effect
Chlorpromazine	Reduced hypoglycemic effect
Cimetidine	
Diazepam	Inhibition of diazepam metabolism
Phenytoin	Inhibition of phenytoin metabolism
Propranolol	Inhibition of propranolol metabolism
Quinidine	Inhibition of quinidine metabolism
Theophylline	Inhibition of theophylline metabolism
Digitalis	
Sympathomimetics	Cardiac arrhythmias
Erythromycin	Increased risk of toxicity
Quinidine	Increased serum concentration of digoxin
Verapamil	Increased serum concentration of digoxin
Ethacrynic Acid	
Aminoglycosides	Increased nephrotoxicity and ototoxicity
Furosemide	
Aminoglycosides	Increased nephrotoxicity and ototoxicity
Cephalosporins	Increased nephrotoxicity
Sympathomimetics	
Monoamine oxidase inhibitors	Hypertensive crisis
Tricyclic antidepressants	Hypertensive crisis

Data adapted and modified from Davies, D. M. (ed): Textbook of Adverse Drug Reactions. 3rd ed., Appendix 1. New York, Oxford University, 1985, pp. 714–725.

sociated hypotension with diazepam's vehicle of administration rather than the drug itself (Bianco et al., 1971). Chlordiazepoxide can also cause a transient decrease in peripheral vascular resistance (Hitch and Nolan, 1971). Cimetidine has been shown to be a direct vasodilator (Iberti et al., 1986), although ranitidine has been free from this complication (Goelzer et al., 1988).

The vasodilator properties of narcotic and tranquilizing agents are frequently compensated for by generalized elevation of sympathetic tone. When sympathetic tone suddenly is withdrawn (as with reintubation in the combative patient with impending respiratory failure), precipitous hypotension can result from the cumulative effects of these agents.

Anaphylactic Reactions

Anaphylactic reactions are characterized by sudden and dramatic changes in vascular permeability and bronchial hyperreactivity that result from the interaction between an antigen or allergen and IgE antibodies. Anaphylactoid reactions present identically, although they are not mediated through IgE antibodies. Histamine, prostaglandins, and other mediators are released into the extracellular fluid by specific effector cells (mast cells and basophils). The most common symptoms are tachycardia, hypotension, and bronchoconstriction; urticaria and angioedema may also occur. Anaphylaxis is usually associated with antibiotic therapy, particularly with penicillin (15 to 40 per 100,000 patients) and cephalosporins, although it may also occur following the infusion of blood products and many other pharmacologic agents. Anaphylactoid reactions occur in 0.003% of plasma-protein fraction (Plasmanate) infusions, 0.006% of hydroxyethyl starch infusions, and 0.008% of dextran infusions (Ring and Messmer, 1977).

Primary therapy consists of the administration of epinephrine, which reverses bronchoconstriction and hypotension and increases myocardial contractility. Antihistamines can be administered to block the peripheral effects of histamine release. Corticosteroids are available as secondary therapy to increase tissue responsiveness to beta-agonists and to inhibit the synthesis of histamine (Haupt and Carlson, 1984).

BIBLIOGRAPHY

Abel, R. M.: Nutritional support and the cardiac patient. *In* Rombeau, J. L., and Caldwell, M. D. (eds): Clinical Nutrition: Parenteral Nutrition. Chap. 33. Philadelphia, W. B. Saunders, 1986.

Abel, R. M., Beck, C. H., Jr., Abbott, W. M., et al.: Improved survival from acute renal failure after treatment with intravenous essential L-amino acids and glucose. N. Engl. J. Med., *288*:695, 1973.

Abel, R. M., Fischer, J. E., Buckley, M. J., and Austen, W. G.: Hyperalimentation in cardiac surgery. J. Thorac. Cardiovasc. Surg., *67*:294, 1974a.

Abel, R. M., Wick, J., Beck, C. H., Jr., et al.: Renal dysfunction following open-heart operations. Arch. Surg., *108*:175, 1974b.

Abel, R. M., Buckley, M. J., Austen, W. G., et al.: Acute postoperative renal failure in cardiac surgical patients. J. Surg. Res., *20*:341, 1976a.

Abel, R. M., Fischer, J. E., Buckley, M. J., et al.: Malnutrition in cardiac surgical patients. Arch. Surg., *111*:45, 1976b.

ACC/AHA Task Force Report. Guidelines for clinical intracardiac electrophysiologic studies. A report of the American College of Cardiology/American Heart Association Task Force on Assessment of Diagnostic and Therapeutic Cardiovascular Procedures (Subcommittee to Assess Clinical Intracardiac Electrophysiologic Studies). J. Am. Coll. Cardiol., *14*:1827, 1989.

Albina, J. E., Koruda, M. J., and Rombeau, J. L.: Perioperative total parenteral nutrition. *In* Rombeau, J. L., and Caldwell, M. D. (eds): Clinical Nutrition: Parenteral Nutrition. Chap. 20. Philadelphia, W. B. Saunders, 1986.

Alderman, E. L., Matlof, H. J., Shumway, N. E., and Harrison, D. C.: Evaluation of enzyme testing for the detection of myocardial infarction following direct coronary surgery. Circulation, *48*:135, 1973.

Alford, W. C., Jr., Meador, C. K., Mihalevich, J., et al.: Acute adrenal insufficiency following cardiac surgical procedures. J. Thorac. Cardiovasc. Surg., 78:489, 1979.

Alousi, A. A., and Johnson, D. C.: Pharmacology of the bipyridines: Amrinone and milrinone. Circulation, 73:III–10, 1986.

Alving, B. M., Hojima, Y., Pisano, J. J., et al.: Hypotension associated with prekallikrein activator (Hageman-factor fragments) in plasma protein fraction. N. Engl. J. Med., 299:66, 1978.

Angelini, G. D., Fraser, A. G., Koning, M. M., et al.: Adverse hemodynamic effects and echocardiographic consequences of pericardial closure soon after sternotomy and pericardiotomy. Circulation, 82(Suppl.):IV–397, 1990.

Angelini, G. D., Penny, W. J., El-Chamary, F., et al.: The incidence and significance of early pericardial effusion after open heart surgery. Eur. J. Cardiothorac. Surg., 1:165, 1987.

Ansell, J., Klassen, V., Lew, R., et al.: Does desmopressin acetate prophylaxis reduce blood loss after valvular heart operations? A randomized, double-blind study. J. Thorac. Cardiovasc. Surg., 104:117, 1992.

Anstadt, M. P., Anstadt, G., and Lowe, J. E.: Direct mechanical ventricular actuation: A review. Resuscitation, 21:7, 1991.

Antman, E. M., Wenger, T. L., Butler, V. P. Jr., et al.: Treatment of 150 cases of life-threatening digitalis intoxication with digoxin-specific Fab antibody fragments. Final report of a multicenter study. Circulation, 81:1744, 1990.

Appelbaum, A., Blackstone E. H., Kouchoukos, N. T., and Kirklin, J. W.: Effect of afterload reduction on cardiac output in infants after intracardiac surgery. Circulation, 51(Suppl.):II–151, 1975.

Appelbaum, A., Kouchoukos, N. T., Blackstone, E. H., and Kirklin, J. W.: Early risks of open heart surgery for mitral valve disease. Am. J. Cardiol., 37:201, 1976.

Asmundsson, T., and Kilburn, K. H.: Survival after acute respiratory failure. Ann. Intern. Med., 80:54, 1974.

Asmundsson, T., and Kilburn, K. H.: Survival of acute respiratory failure. Ann. Intern. Med., 70:471, 1969.

Assad-Morrell, J. L., Fry, R. L., Connolly, D. L., et al.: Relation of intraoperative or early post-operative transmural myocardial infarction to patency of aortocoronary bypass grafts and to diseased ungrafted coronary arteries. Am. J. Cardiol., 35:767, 1975.

Astiz, M. E., Rackow, E. C., Kaufman, B., et al.: Relationship of oxygen delivery and mixed venous oxygenation to lactic acidosis in patients with sepsis and acute myocardial infarction. Crit. Care Med., 16:655, 1988.

Bachmann, F., McKenna, R., Cole, E. R., and Najafi, H.: The hemostatic mechanism after open-heart surgery. I. Studies on plasma coagulation factors and fibrinolysis in 512 patients after extracorporeal circulation. J. Thorac. Cardiovasc. Surg., 70:76, 1975.

Bachulis, B. L., and Smith, P. E.: Pseudoobstruction of the colon. Am. J. Surg., 136:66, 1978.

Bagge, L., Lilienberg, G., Nystrom, S., and Tyden, H.: Coagulation, fibrinolysis and bleeding after open-heart surgery. Scand. J. Thorac. Cardiovasc. Surg., 20:151, 1986.

Bailey, R. W., Bulkley, G. B., Levy, K. I., et al.: Pathogenesis of nonocclusive mesenteric ischemia: Studies in a porcine model induced by pericardial tamponade. Surg. Forum, 33:194, 1982.

Balderman, S. C., Gutierrez, I. Z., Makula, P., et al.: Noninvasive screening for asymptomatic carotid artery disease prior to cardiac operation. J. Thorac. Cardiovasc. Surg., 85:427, 1983.

Barnes, R. W., Liebman, P. R., Marszalek, P. B., et al.: The natural history of asymptomatic carotid disease in patients undergoing cardiovascular surgery. Surgery, 90:1075, 1981.

Barsan, W. G., Levy, R. C., and Weir, H.: Lidocaine levels during CPR: Differences after peripheral venous, central venous, and intracardiac injections. Ann. Emerg. Med., 10:73, 1981.

Baue, A. E.: Multiple, progressive, or sequential systems failure. A syndrome of the 1970s. Arch. Surg., 110:779, 1975.

Baue, A. E.: The role of the gut in the development of multiple organ dysfunction in cardiothoracic patients. Ann. Thor. Surg., 55:822, 1993.

Baue, A. E., and Chaudry, I. H.: Prevention of multiple systems failure. Surg. Clin. North Am., 60:1167, 1980.

Beller, B. M., Frater, R. W. M., and Wulfsohn, N.: Cardiac pacemaking in the management of postoperative arrhythmias. Ann. Thorac. Surg., 6:68, 1968.

Benjamin, J. J., Cascade, P. N., Rubenfire, M., et al.: Left lower lobe atelectasis and consolidation following cardiac surgery: The effect of topical cooling on the phrenic nerve. Radiology, 142:11, 1982.

Bentley, D. W., and Lepper, M. H.: Septicemia related to indwelling venous catheter. J. A. M. A., 206:1749, 1968.

Bertini, G., Margheri, M., Giglioli, C., et al.: Prognostic significance of early clinical manifestations in postanoxic coma: A retrospective study of 58 patients resuscitated after prehospital cardiac arrest. Crit. Care Med., 17:627, 1989.

Beta-Blocker Heart Attack Trial Research Group: A randomized trial of propranolol in patients with acute myocardial infarction. J. A. M. A., 247:1707, 1982.

Bevelaqua, F., Garritan, S., Haas, F., et al.: Complications after cardiac operations in patients with severe pulmonary impairment. Ann. Thorac. Surg., 50:602, 1990.

Bhat, J. G., Gluck, M. C., Lowenstein, J., and Baldwin, D. S.: Renal failure after open heart surgery. Ann. Intern. Med., 84:677, 1976.

Bhatia, S. J. S., and Smith, T. W.: Digitalis toxicity: Mechanisms, diagnosis, and management. J. Cardiac Surg., 2:453, 1987.

Bianco, J. A., Shanahan, A., Ostheimer, G. W., et al.: Cardiovascular effects of diazepam. J. Thorac. Cardiovasc. Surg., 62:125, 1971.

Bick, R. L.: Alterations of hemostasis associated with cardiopulmonary bypass: Pathophysiology, prevention, diagnosis, and management. Semin. Thromb. Hemost., 3:59, 1976.

Bick, R. L., Schmalhorst, W. R., and Arbegast, N. R.: Alterations of hemostasis associated with cardiopulmonary bypass. Thromb. Res., 8:285, 1976.

Bidstrup, B. P., Harrison, J., Royston, D., et al.: Aprotinin therapy in cardiac operations: A report on use in 41 cardiac centers in the United Kingdom. Ann. Thorac. Surg., 55:971, 1993.

Bidstrup, B. P., Royston, D., Sapsford, R. N., et al.: Reduction in blood loss and blood use after cardiopulmonary bypass with high dose aprotinin (Trasylol). J. Thorac. Cardiovasc. Surg., 97:364, 1989.

Bigger, J. T., and Sahar, D. I.: Clinical types of proarrhythmic response to antiarrhythmic drugs. Am. J. Cardiol., 59:2E, 1987.

Bircher, N. G.: Acidosis of cardiopulmonary resuscitation: Carbon dioxide transport and anaerobiosis. Crit. Care Med., 20:1203, 1992.

Bixler, T. J., Gardner, T. J., Donahoo, J. S., et al.: Improved myocardial performance in postoperative cardiac surgical patients with sodium nitroprusside. Ann. Thorac. Surg., 25:444, 1978.

Blachley, J. D., and Henrich, W. L.: The diagnosis and management of acute renal failure. Semin. Nephrol., 1:11, 1981.

Blachy, P. H., and Starr, A.: Post-cardiotomy delirium. Am. J. Psychiatry, 121:371, 1964.

Bojar, R. M., Najafi, H., DeLaria, G. A., et al.: Neurological complications of coronary revascularization. Ann. Thorac. Surg., 36:427, 1983.

Bolanowski, P. J., Bauer, J., Machiedo, G., and Neville, W. E.: Prostaglandin influence on pulmonary intravascular leukocytic aggregation during cardiopulmonary bypass. J. Thorac. Cardiovasc. Surg., 73:221, 1977.

Boldt, J., Knothe, C., Zickmann, B., et al.: Platelet function in cardiac surgery: Influence of temperature and aprotinin. Ann. Thorac. Surg., 55:652, 1993.

Bolen, J. L., and Alderman, E. L.: Hemodynamic consequences of afterload reduction in patients with chronic aortic regurgitation. Circulation, 53:879, 1976.

Bolooki, H.: Special topic: Instrumentation in cardiology. Med. Instrum., 20:266, 1986.

Boriss, M. N., and Papa, L.: Magnesium: A discussion of its role in the treatment of ventricular dysrhythmia. Crit. Care Med., 16:292, 1988.

Borkon, A. M., Schaff, H. V., Gardner, T. J., et al.: Diagnosis and management of postoperative pericardial effusions and late cardiac tamponade following open-heart surgery. Ann. Thorac. Surg., 31:512, 1981.

Bortolotti, U., Livi, U., Frugoni, C., et al.: Delayed cardiac tamponade following open heart surgery. Analysis of 12 patients. Thorac. Cardiovasc. Surg., 29:233, 1981.

Borucki, D. T. (ed): Blood Component Therapy: A Physician's Handbook. 3rd ed. Washington, D. C., American Association of Blood Banks, 1981.

Boudoulas, H., Lewis, R. P., Vasko, J. S., et al.: Left ventricular function and adrenergic hyperactivity before and after saphenous vein bypass. Circulation, *53*:802, 1976.

Boudoulas, H., Snyder, G. L., Lewis, R. P., et al.: Safety and rationale for continuation of propranolol therapy during coronary bypass operation. Ann. Thorac. Surg., *26*:222, 1978.

Boyd, A. D., Engelman, R. M., Beaudet, R. L., and Lackner, H.: Disseminated intravascular coagulation following extracorporeal circulation. J. Thorac. Cardiovasc. Surg., *64*:685, 1972.

Boyd, A. D., Tremblay, R. E., Spencer, F. C., and Bahnson, H. T.: Estimation of cardiac output soon after intracardiac surgery with cardiopulmonary bypass. Ann. Surg., *150*:613, 1959.

Bregman, D., Parodi, E. N., Hutchinson, J. E., III, et al.: Intraoperative autotransfusion during emergency thoracic and elective open-heart surgery. Ann. Thorac. Surg., *18*:590, 1974.

Bremner, W. F., Taylor, K. M., Baird, S., et al.: Hypothalamo-pituitary-thyroid axis function during cardiopulmonary bypass. J. Thorac. Cardiovasc. Surg., *75*:392, 1979.

Breuer, A. C., Furlan, A. J., Hansom, M. R., et al.: Central nervous system complications of coronary artery bypass graft surgery: Prospective analysis of 421 patients. Stroke, *14*:682, 1983.

Breyer, R. H., Mills, S. A., Hudspeth, A. S., et al.: A prospective study of sternal wound complications. Ann. Thorac. Surg., *37*:412, 1984.

Brimioulle, S., Berre, J., Dufaye, P., et al.: Hydrochloric acid infusion for treatment of metabolic alkalosis associated with respiratory acidosis. Crit. Care Med., *17*:232, 1989.

Bristow, M. R., Ginsburg, R., Minobe, W., et al.: Decreased catecholamine sensitivity and beta-adrenergic-receptor density in failing human hearts. N. Engl. J. Med., *307*:205, 1982.

British Committee for Standardization in Haematology Blood Transfusion Task Force: Guidelines for transfusion for massive blood loss. Clin. Lab. Haematol., *10*:265, 1988.

Broder, G., and Weil, M. H.: Excess lactate: An index of reversibility of shock in human patients. Science, *143*:1457, 1964.

Brown, T. C. K.: The evolution of continuing education in anaesthesia. Anaesth. Intensive Care, *12*:99, 1984.

Brunel, W., and Cohen, N. H.: Evaluation of the accuracy of pulse oximetry in critically ill patients [Abstract]. Crit. Care Med., *16*:432, 1988.

Bryan-Brown, C.: Blood flow to organs: Parameters for function and survival in critical illness. Crit. Care Med., *16*:170, 1988.

Buckberg, G. D., Archie, J. P., Fixler, D. E., and Hoffman, J. I. E.: Experimental subendocardial ischemia during left ventricular hypertension. Surg. Forum, *22*:124, 1971.

Bulkley, G. B., Kvietys, P. R., Perry, M. A., and Granger, D. N.: Effects of cardiac tamponade on colonic hemodynamics and oxygen uptake. Am. J. Physiol., *244*:G604, 1983.

Bull, B. S., Huse, W. M., Brauer, F. S., and Korpman, R. A.: Heparin therapy during extracorporeal circulation. J. Thorac. Cardiovasc. Surg., *69*:674 (Pt. I) and 685 (Pt. II), 1975.

Bumaschny, E., Doglio, G., Pusajo, J., et al.: Postoperative acute gastrointestinal tract hemorrhage and multiple-organ failure. Arch. Surg., *123*:722, 1988.

Burk, R. H., and George, R. B.: Acute respiratory failure in chronic obstructive pulmonary disease. Arch. Intern. Med., *132*:865, 1973.

Burnakis, T. G.: Surgical antimicrobial prophylaxis: Principles and guidelines. Pharmacotherapy, *4*:248, 1984.

Butler, J., Pillai, R., Rocker, G. M., et al.: Effect of cardiopulmonary bypass on systemic release of neutrophil elastase and tumor necrosis factor. J. Thorac. Cardiovasc. Surg., *105*:25, 1993.

Buxton, A. E., Goldberg, S., Harken, A., et al.: Coronary-artery spasm immediately after myocardial revascularization. Recognition and management. N. Engl. J. Med., *304*:1249, 1981.

Buxton, A. E., Hirshfeld, J. W., Jr., Untereker, W. J., et al.: Perioperative coronary arterial spasm: Long-term follow up. Am. J. Cardiol., *50*:444, 1982.

Caldwell, G., Millar, G., Quinn, E., et al.: Simple mechanical methods for cardioversion: Defense of the precordial thump and cough version. Br. Med. J., *291*:627, 1985.

Cannon, L. A., Heiselman, D., Gardner, W., and Jones, J.: Prophylaxis of upper gastrointestinal tract bleeding in mechanically ventilated patients. Arch. Intern. Med., *147*:2101, 1987.

Carlon, G. C., Ray, C., Jr., Miodownik, S., et al.: Capnography in mechanically ventilated patients. Crit. Care Med., *16*:550, 1988.

Carrico, C. J.: The elusive pathophysiology of the multiple organ failure syndrome. Ann. Surg., *218*:109, 1993.

Caspi, J., Klausner, J. M., Safadi, T., et al.: Delayed respiratory depression following fentanyl anesthesia for cardiac surgery. Crit. Care Med., *16*:238, 1988.

Caspi, Y., Safadi, T., Ammar, R., et al.: The significance of bundle branch block in the immediate postoperative electrocardiograms of patients undergoing coronary artery bypass. J. Thorac. Cardiovasc. Surg., *93*:442, 1987.

CASS Principle Investigators and their associates: Coronary artery surgery study (CASS): A randomized trial of coronary artery bypass surgery: Survival data. Circulation, *68*:939, 1983.

CAST Investigators: Preliminary report: Effect of encainide and flecainide on mortality in a randomized trial of arrhythmia suppression after myocardial infarction. The Cardiac Arrhythmia Suppression Trial (CAST) Investigators. N. Engl. J. Med., *321*:406, 1989.

Caul, E. O., Mott, M. G., Clarke, S. K. R., et al.: Cytomegalovirus infections after open heart surgery. Lancet, *1*(703):777, 1971.

Cerra, F. B.: The hypermetabolism organ failure complex. World J. Surg., *11*:173, 1987.

Chatterjee, K., and Parmley, W. W.: The role of vasodilator therapy in heart failure. Prog. Cardiovasc. Dis., *19*:301, 1977.

Chatterjee, K., Parmley, W. W., Swan, H. J. C., et al.: Beneficial effects of vasodilator agents in severe mitral regurgitation due to dysfunction of subvalvular apparatus. Circulation, *48*:684, 1973.

Chenoweth, D. E., Cooper, S. W., Hugli, T. E., et al.: Complement activation during cardiopulmonary bypass: Evidence for generation of C3a and C5a anaphylatoxins. N. Engl. J. Med., *304*:497, 1981.

Chernow, B.: Hormonal and metabolic considerations in critical care medicine. *In* Shoemaker, W. C., Thompson, W. L., and Holbrook, P. R. (eds): Textbook of Critical Care. Chap. 84. Philadelphia, W. B. Saunders, 1984.

Chernow, B., Babberger, S., Stoiko, M., et al.: Hypomagnesemia in postoperative intensive care patients [Abstract]. Crit. Care Med., *16*:441, 1988.

Chesebro, J. H., Clements, I. P., Fuster, V., et al.: A platelet inhibitor drug trial in coronary artery bypass operations: Benefit of perioperative dipyridamole and aspirin therapy on early postoperative vein graft patency. N. Engl. J. Med., *307*:73, 1982.

Chiara, O., Giomarelli, P. P., Biagioli, B., et al.: Hypermetabolic response after hypothermic cardiopulmonary bypass. Crit. Care Med., *15*:995, 1987.

Chiariello, M., Gold, H. K., Leinbach, R. C., et al.: Comparison between the effects of nitroprusside and nitroglycerin on ischemic injury during acute myocardial infarction [Abstract]. Circulation, *54*:766, 1976.

Christian, C. M., II, Waller, J. L., and Moldenhauer, C.: Postoperative rigidity following fentanyl anesthesia. Anesthesiology, *58*:275, 1983.

Chuttani, K., Pandian, N. G., Mohanty, P. K., et al.: Left ventricular diastolic collapse. An echocardiographic sign of regional cardiac tamponade. Circulation, *83*:1999, 1991.

Cleland, J., Pluth, J. R., Tauxe, W. N., and Kirklin, J. W.: Blood volume and body fluid compartment changes soon after closed and open intracardiac surgery. J. Thorac. Cardiovasc. Surg., *52*:698, 1966.

Codd, J. E., Wiens, R. D., Kaiser, G. C., et al.: Late sequelae of perioperative myocardial infarction. Ann. Thorac. Surg., *26*:208, 1978.

Cogan, M. G., Liu, F., Berger, B. E., et al.: Metabolic alkalosis. (Symposium on Acid-Base Disorders). Med. Clin. North Am., *67*:903, 1983.

Cohen, R. D., and Woods, H. F.: Clinical and Biochemical Aspects of Lactic Acidosis. Boston, Blackwell Scientific, 1976.

Cohn, J. N.: Efficacy of vasodilators in the treatment of heart failure. J. Am. Coll. Cardiol., *22*(Suppl. A):135, 1993.

Cohn, J. N., Archibald, D. G., Ziesche, S., et al.: Effect of vasodilator therapy on mortality in chronic congestive heart failure. N. Engl. J. Med., *314*:1547, 1986.

Cohn, J. N., Johnson, G., Ziesche, S., et al.: A comparison of enalapril with hydralamine-isosorbide dinitrate in the treatment of chronic congestive heart failure. N. Engl. J. Med., *325*:303, 1991.

Conger, J. D.: A controlled evaluation of prophylactic dialysis in post-traumatic acute renal failure. J. Trauma, 15:1056, 1975.

Conklin, C. M., Gray, R. J., Neilson, D., et al.: Determinants of wound infection incidence after isolated coronary artery bypass surgery in patients randomized to receive prophylactic cefuroxime or cefazolin. Ann. Thorac. Surg., 46:172, 1988.

Cook, W. A., Webb, W. R., and Unal, M. O.: Myocardial function capacity in response to compensated and uncompensated respiratory alkalosis. Surg. Forum, 16:186, 1965.

Cooper, D. M., Bazaral, M. G., Furlan, A. J., et al.: Pituitary apoplexy: A complication of cardiac surgery. Ann. Thorac. Surg., 41:547, 1986.

Corning, H., Hedley-Whyte, J., and Austen, W. G.: Correlation of blood gas abnormalities and hemodynamic events following cardiac surgery. Ann. Thorac. Surg., 2:783, 1966.

Cornwell, E. E., III, Rodriguez, A., Mirvis, S. E., and Shorr, R. M.: Acute acalculous cholecystitis in critically injured patients. Preoperative diagnostic imaging. Ann. Surg., 210:52, 1989.

Corwin, H. L., Sprague, S. M., DeLaria, G. A., and Norusis, M. J.: Acute renal failure associated with cardiac operations. A case-control study. J. Thorac. Cardiovasc. Surg., 98:1107, 1989.

Cosgrove, D. M.: Evaluation of perioperative risk factors. J. Cardiac Surg., 5:227, 1990.

Cosgrove, D. M., Amiot, D. M., and Meserko, J. J.: An improved technique for autotransfusion of shed mediastinal blood. Ann. Thorac. Surg., 40:519, 1985.

Cosgrove, D. M., III, Heric, B., Lytle, B. W., et al.: Aprotinin therapy for reoperative myocardial revascularization: A placebo-controlled study. Ann. Thorac. Surg., 54:1031, 1992.

Cosgrove, D. M., Loop, F. D., Lytle, B. W., et al.: Primary myocardial revascularization. J. Thorac. Cardiovasc. Surg., 88:673, 1984.

Cox, J. L.: A perspective of postoperative atrial fibrillation in cardiac operations. Ann. Thorac. Surg., 56:405, 1993.

Cox, M.: Potassium homeostasis. Med. Clin. North Am., 65:363, 1981.

Craddock, D. R., Logan, A., and Fadali, A.: Reoperation for hemorrhage following cardiopulmonary bypass. Br. J. Surg., 55:17, 1968.

Craddock, P. R., Fehr, J., Dalmasso, A. P., et al.: Hemodialysis leukopenia. Pulmonary vascular leukostasis resulting from complement activation by dialyzer cellophane membranes. J. Clin. Invest., 59:879, 1977.

Creswell, L. L., Schuessler, R. B., Rosenbloom, M., and Cox, J. L.: Hazards of postoperative atrial arrhythmias. Ann. Thorac. Surg., 56:539, 1993.

Crexells, C., Chatterjee, K., Forrester, J. S., et al.: Optimal level of filling pressure in the left side of the heart in acute myocardial infarction. N. Engl. J. Med., 289:1263, 1973.

Crock, P. A., Ley, C. J., Martin, I. K., et al.: Hormonal and metabolic changes during hypothermic coronary artery bypass surgery in diabetic and nondiabetic subjects. Diabetic Med., 5:47, 1988.

Culliford, A. T., Cunningham, J. N., Jr., Zeff, R. H., et al.: Sternal and costochondral infections following open heart surgery: A review of 2594 cases. J. Thorac. Cardiovasc. Surg., 54:586, 1967.

Culliford, A. T., Girdwood, R. W., Isom, O. W., et al.: Angina following myocardial revascularization. J. Thorac. Cardiovasc. Surg., 77:889, 1979.

Czer, L. S. C., and Shoemaker, W. C.: Optimal hematocrit value in critically ill postoperative patients. Surg. Gynecol. Obstet., 147:363, 1978.

DaLuz, P. L., Forrester, J. S., Wyatt, H. L., et al.: Hemodynamic and metabolic effects of sodium nitroprusside on the performance and metabolism of regional ischemic myocardium. Circulation, 52:400, 1975.

Damen, J., Verhoef, J., Bolton, D. T., et al.: Microbiologic risk of invasive hemodynamic monitoring in patients undergoing open-heart operations. Crit. Care Med., 13:548, 1985.

Darby, T. D., Aldinger, E. E., Gadsden, R. H., and Thrower, W. B.: Effects of metabolic acidosis on ventricular isometric systolic tension and the response to epinephrine and levarterenol. Circ. Res., 8:1242, 1960.

Darup, J., Bleese, N., Kalmar, P., et al.: Hemofiltration during extracorporeal circulation (ECC). Thorac. Cardiovasc. Surg., 27:227, 1979.

Davies, D. M.: Textbook of Adverse Drug Reactions. 3rd ed. New York, Oxford University, 1985.

Davies, D. W., Kadar, D., Steward, D. J., and Munro, I. R.: A sudden death associated with the use of sodium nitroprusside for induction of hypotension during anaesthesia. Canad. Anaesth. Soc. J., 22:547, 1975.

Davis, R. F., Lappas, D. G., Kirklin, J. K., et al.: Acute oliguria after cardiopulmonary bypass: Renal functional improvement with low-dose dopamine infusion. Crit. Care Med., 10:852, 1982.

Davis, R. F., Ribner, H. S., Keung, E., et al.: Treatment of chronic congestive heart failure with captopril, an oral inhibitor of angiotensin-converting enzyme. N. Engl. J. Med., 301:117, 1979.

deJongh, C. A., Caplan, E. S., and Schimpff, S. C.: Infections in the critical care patient. In Shoemaker, W. C., Thompson, W. L., and Holbrook, P. R. (eds): Textbook of Critical Care. Chap. 69. Philadelphia, W. B. Saunders, 1984.

DeLaria, G. A., Hunter, J. A., Goldin, M. D., et al.: Leg wound complications associated with coronary revascularization. J. Thorac. Cardiovasc. Surg., 81:403, 1981.

DelRossi, A. J., Cernaianu, A. C., Botros, S., et al.: Prophylactic treatment of postperfusion bleeding using EACA. Chest, 98:516, 1990.

DeSilva, R. A., Graboys, T. B., Podrid, P. J., and Lown, B.: Cardioversion and defibrillation. Am. Heart J., 100:881, 1980.

de Smet, A. A., Joen, M. C., van Oeveren, W., et al.: Increased anticoagulation during cardiopulmonary bypass by aprotinin. J. Thorac. Cardiovasc. Surg., 100:520, 1990.

Dewar, M. L., Walsh, G., Chiu, R. C.-J., et al.: Atrial natriuretic factor: Response to cardiac operation. J. Thorac. Cardiovasc. Surg., 96:266, 1988.

Dhein, S., Muller, A., Gerwin, R., and Klaus, W.: Comparative study on the proarrhythmic effects of some antiarrhythmic agents. Circulation, 87:617, 1993.

Dietrich, W., Barankay, A., Dilthey, G., et al.: Reduction of blood utilization during myocardial revascularization. J. Thorac. Cardiovasc. Surg., 97:213, 1989.

Dietrich, W., Spannagl, M., Jochum, M., et al.: Influence of high-dose aprotinin treatment on blood loss and coagulation patterns in patients undergoing myocardial revascularization: Anaesthesiology, 73:1119, 1990.

DiLello, F., Mullen, D. C., Flemmon, R. J., et al.: Results of intra-aortic balloon pumping after cardiac surgery: Experience with the Percor balloon catheter. Ann. Thorac. Surg., 46:422, 1988.

Dinarello, C. A.: Interleukin-1 and the pathogenesis of the acute-phase response. N. Engl. J. Med., 311:1413, 1984.

DiSesa, V. J.: The rational selection of inotropic drugs in cardiac surgery. J. Cardiac Surg., 2:385, 1987.

Dixon, S. H., Jr., Limbird, L. E., Roe, C. R., et al.: Recognition of postoperative acute myocardial infarction. Application of isoenzyme techniques. Circulation, 48(Suppl.):III-137, 1973.

Dorin, R. I., and Kearns, P. J.: High output circulatory failure in acute adrenal insufficiency. Crit. Care Med., 16:296, 1988.

Dowing, T. P., Miller, D. C., Stofer, R., et al.: Use of the intra-aortic balloon pump after valve replacement. J. Thorac. Cardiovasc. Surg., 92:210, 1986.

Drop, L. J.: Ionized calcium, the heart, and hemodynamic function. Anesth. Analg., 64:432, 1985.

Drop, L. J., and Scheidegger, D.: Plasma ionized calcium concentration. J. Thorac. Cardiovasc. Surg., 79:425, 1980.

Dubin, W. R., Field, H. L., and Gastfriend, D. R.: Postcardiotomy delirium: A critical review. J. Thorac. Cardiovasc. Surg., 77:586, 1979.

Dudrick, S. J., Steiger, E., and Long, J. M.: Renal failure in surgical patients. Treatment with intravenous essential amino acids and hypertonic glucose. Surgery, 68:180, 1970.

Dupuis, J., Bondy, R., Cattran, C., et al.: Amrinone and dobutamine as primary treatment of low cardiac output syndrome following coronary artery surgery: A comparison of their effects on hemodynamics and outcome. J. Cardiothorac. Vasc. Anesth., 6:542, 1992.

Dyckner, T., and Wester, P. O.: Relation between potassium, magnesium and cardiac arrhythmias. Acta Med. Scand., 647 (Suppl.):163, 1981.

Dyke, C. M., Ding, M., Abd-Elfattah, A. S., et al.: Effects of triiodothyronine supplementation after myocardial ischemia. Ann. Thorac. Surg., 56:215, 1993.

Edmunds, L. H., Jr.: Cardiac surgery. In Dudrick, S. J., Baue, A. E.,

Eiseman, B., et al. (eds): Manual of Preoperative and Postoperative Care. 3rd ed., Chap. 20. Philadelphia, W. B. Saunders, 1983.

Egerton, N., and Kay, J. H.: Psychological disturbances associated with open heart surgery. Br. J. Psychiatry, 110:433, 1964.

Ellis, R. J., Mavroudis, C., Gardner, C., et al.: Relationship between atrioventricular arrhythmias and the concentration of K^+ ion in cardioplegic solution. J. Thorac. Cardiovasc. Surg., 80:517, 1980.

Ellison, L. H., and Kirsh, M. M.: Delayed mediastinal tamponade after open heart surgery. Chest, 65:64, 1974.

Ellison, N., Beatty, C. P., Blake, D. R., et al.: Heparin rebound. J. Thorac. Cardiovasc. Surg., 67:723, 1974.

Emery, R. W., and Joyce, L. D.: Directions in cardiac assistance. J. Cardiac Surg., 6:400, 1991.

Endoh, M., Yanagisawa, T., Tairi, N., et al.: Effects of new inotropic agents on cyclic nucleotide metabolism and calcium transients in canine ventricular muscle. Circulation, 73(Suppl.):III-117, 1986.

Engelman, R. M., Spencer, F. C., Reed, G. E., and Tice, D. A.: Cardiac tamponade following open-heart surgery. Circulation, 41(Suppl.):II-165, 1970.

Engle, M. A., and Ito, T.: The postpericardiotomy syndrome. Am. J. Cardiol., 7:73, 1961.

Engle, M. A., McCabe, J. C., Ebert, P. A., and Zabriskie, J.: The postpericardiotomy syndrome and antiheart antibodies. Circulation, 49:401, 1974.

Engle, M. A., Zabriskie, J. B., Senterfit, L. B., et al.: Immunologic and virologic studies in the postpericardiotomy syndrome. J. Pediatr., 87:1103, 1975.

Ephgrave, K. S., Kleiman-Wexler, R. L., and Adair, C. G.: Enteral nutrients prevent stress ulceration and increase intragastric volume. Crit. Care Med., 18:621, 1990.

Erdmann, E.: The effectiveness of inotropic agents in isolated cardiac preparations from the human heart. Klin. Wochenschr., 66:1, 1988.

Estafanous, F. G., and Tarazi, R. C.: Systemic arterial hypertension associated with cardiac surgery. Am. J. Cardiol., 46:685, 1980.

Estafanous, F. G., Tarazi, R. C., Buckley, S., and Taylor, P. C.: Arterial hypertension in immediate postoperative period after valve replacement. Br. Heart J., 40:718, 1978.

Estes, J. W.: Kinetics of the anticoagulant effect of heparin. J. A. M. A., 212:1492, 1970.

Fairman, R. M., and Edmunds, L. H., Jr.: Emergency thoracotomy in the surgical intensive care unit after open cardiac operation. Ann. Thorac. Surg., 32:386, 1981.

Fedullo, A. J., Lerner, R. M., Gibson, J., and Shayne, D. S.: Sonographic measurement of diaphragmatic motion after coronary artery bypass surgery. Chest, 102:1683, 1992.

Feigl, E. O.: The paradox of adrenergic coronary vasoconstriction. Circulation, 76:737, 1987.

Feldman, R. L.: A review of medical therapy for coronary artery spasm. Circulation, 75(Suppl.):V-96, 1987.

Feneley, M. P., Maier, G. W., Kern, K. B., et al.: Influence of compression rate on initial success of resuscitation and 24 hour survival after prolonged manual cardiopulmonary resuscitation in dogs. Circulation, 77:240, 1988.

Ferraris, V. A., Ferraris, S. P., Lough, F. C., and Berry, W. R.: Preoperative aspirin ingestion increases operative blood loss after coronary artery bypass grafting. Ann. Thorac. Surg., 45:71, 1988.

Fiddian-Green, R. G., and Baker, S.: Predictive value of the stomach wall pH for complications after cardiac operations: Comparison with other monitoring. Crit. Care Med., 15:153, 1987.

Fisch, C.: Relation of electrolyte disturbances to cardiac arrhythmias. Circulation, 67:408, 1973.

Fisch, C., Knoebel, S. B., Feigenbaum, H., and Greenspan, K.: Potassium and the monophasic action potential, electrocardiogram, conduction and arrhythmias. Prog. Cardiovasc. Dis., 8:387, 1966.

Fisher, C. M.: Reducing risks of cerebral embolism. Geriatrics, 34:59, 1979.

Flaherty, J. T., Magee, P. A., Gardner, T. L., et al.: Comparison of intravenous nitroglycerin and sodium nitroprusside for treatment of acute hypertension developing after coronary artery bypass surgery. Circulation, 65:1072, 1982.

Force, T., Hibberd, P., Weeks, G., et al.: Perioperative myocardial infarction after coronary artery bypass surgery. Clinical significance and approach to risk stratification. Circulation, 82:903, 1990.

Ford, E. G., Baisden, C. E., Matteson, M. L., and Picone, A. L.: Sepsis after coronary bypass grafting: Evidence for loss of the gut mucosal barrier. Ann. Thorac. Surg., 52:514, 1991.

Foster, G. H., Conway, W. A., Pamulkov, N., et al.: Early extubation after coronary artery bypass: Brief report. Crit. Care Med., 12:994, 1984.

Fouad, F. M., Estafanous, F. G., Bravo, E. L., et al.: Possible role of cardioaortic reflexes in postcoronary bypass hypertension. Am. J. Cardiol., 44:866, 1979.

Fowler, M. B., Laser, J. A., Hopkins, G. L., et al.: Assessment of the beta-adrenergic receptor pathway in the intact failing human heart: Progressive receptor down-regulation and subsensitivity to agonist response. Circulation, 74:1290, 1986.

Fowler, N. O., Gabel, M., and Buncher, C. R.: Cardiac tamponade: A comparison of right versus left heart compression. J. Am. Coll. Cardiol., 12:187, 1988.

Franciosa, J. A., Limas, C. J., Guiha, N. H., et al.: Improved left ventricular function during nitroprusside infusion in acute myocardial infarction. Lancet, 1:650, 1972.

Freeman, R., and McPeake, P. K.: Acquisition, spread, and control of pseudomonas aeruginosa in a cardiothoracic intensive care unit. Thorax, 37:732, 1982.

Fremes, S. E, Wong, B. I., Lee, E., et al.: Metaanalysis of prophylactic drug treatment in the prevention of postoperative bleeding. Ann. Thorac. Surg., 58:1580, 1994.

Freston, J. W.: Cimetidine. II. Adverse reactions and patterns of use. Ann. Intern. Med., 97:728, 1982.

Fry, D. E.: Multiple system organ failure. Surg. Clin. North Am., 68:107, 1988.

Fuller, J. A., Adams, G. G., and Buxton, B.: Atrial fibrillation after coronary artery bypass grafting. Is it a disorder of the elderly? J. Thorac. Cardiovasc. Surg., 97:821, 1989.

Furnary, A. P., Magovern, J. A., Simpson, K. A., and Magovern, G. J.: Prolonged open sternotomy and delayed sternal closure after cardiac operations. Ann. Thorac. Surg., 54:233, 1992.

Fyke, F. E., Tancredi, R. G., Shub, C., et al.: Detection of intrapericardial hematoma after open heart surgery: The roles of echocardiography and computed tomography. J. Am. Coll. Cardiol., 5:1250, 1985.

Gaffney, F. A., Bastian, B. C., Thal, E. R., et al.: Passive leg raising does not produce a significant or sustained autotransfusion effect. J. Trauma, 22:190, 1982.

Gall, S. A., Jr., Olsen, C. O., Reves, J. G., et al.: Beneficial effects of endotracheal extubation on ventricular performance. J. Thorac. Cardiovasc. Surg., 95:819, 1988.

Gall, W. E., Clark, W. R., and Doty, D. B.: Vasomotor dynamics associated with cardiac operations. I. Venous tone and the effects of vasodilators. J. Thorac. Cardiovasc. Surg., 83:724, 1982.

Gann, D. S., and Wright, H. K.: Increased renal sodium reabsorption after depletion of the extracellular or intravascular fluid volumes. J. Surg. Res., 6:196, 1966.

Gardner, T. J., Horneffer, P. J., Manolio, T. A., et al.: Stroke following coronary artery bypass grafting: A ten year study. Ann. Thorac. Surg., 40:574, 1985.

Gaynes, R., Bizek, B., Mowry-Hanley, J., and Kirsh, M.: Risk factors for nosocomial pneumonia after coronary artery bypass graft operations. Ann. Thorac. Surg., 51:215, 1991.

Gazmuri, R. J., vonPlanta, M., Weil, M. H., and Rackow, E. C.: Absence of acidemia in arterial blood after 12 minutes of cardiac arrest [Abstract]. Crit. Care Med., 16:385, 1988.

Gentry, L. O., Zeluff, B. J., and Cooley, D. A.: Antibiotic prophylaxis in open-heart surgery: A comparison of cefamandole, cefuroxime, and cefazolin. Ann. Thorac. Surg., 46:167, 1988.

Glaubiger, G., and Lefkowitz, R. J.: Elevated beta-adrenergic receptor number after chronic propranolol treatment. Biochem. Biophys. Res. Commun., 78:720, 1977.

Glower, D. D., Spratt, J. A., Snow, N. D., et al.: Linearity of the Frank-Starling relationship in the intact heart: The concept of preload recruitable stroke work. Circulation, 71:994, 1985.

Goelzer, S. L., Farin-Rush, C., and Coursin, D. B.: Ranitidine produces minimal hemodynamic depression in stable intensive care unit patients: A double-blind, prospective study. Crit. Care Med., 16:8, 1988.

Goldberg, L. I.: Cardiovascular and renal actions of dopamine: Potential clinical applications. Pharmacol. Rev., 24:1, 1972.

Goldberg, L. I., and Rajfer, S. I.: Dopamine receptors: Applications in clinical cardiology. Circulation, 72:245, 1985.

Goldberg, M. J., Rubenfire, M., Kantrowitz, A., et al.: Intraaortic balloon pump insertion: A randomized study comparing percutaneous and surgical techniques. J. Am. Coll. Cardiol., 9:515, 1987.

Goldenberg, I. F.: Nonpharmacologic management of cardiac arrest and cardiogenic shock. Chest, 102(Suppl.):596S, 1992.

Golding, L. A. R., Loop, F. D., Peter, M., et al.: Late survival following use of intra-aortic balloon pump in revascularization operations. Ann. Thorac. Surg., 30:48, 1980.

Goldman, S., Copeland, J., Moritz, T., et al.: Improvement in early saphenous vein graft patency after coronary artery bypass surgery with antiplatelet therapy: Results of a Veterans Administration Cooperative Study. Circulation, 77:1324, 1988.

Goldman, S., Probst, P., Selzer, A., and Cohn, K.: Inefficiency of therapeutic serum levels of digoxin in controlling the ventricular rate in atrial fibrillation. Am. J. Cardiol., 35:651, 1975.

Goldstein, R. A.: Clinical effects of intravenous amrinone in patients with congestive heart failure. Circulation, 73(Suppl.):III-191, 1986.

Goldstein, R. E., Stinson, E. B., Scherer, J. L., et al.: Intraoperative coronary collateral function in patients with coronary occlusive disease. Circulation, 49:298, 1974.

Goodnough, L. T., Johnston, M. F., Ramsey, G., et al.: Guidelines for transfusion support in patients undergoing coronary artery bypass grafting. Transfusion Practices Committee of the American Association of Blood Banks. Ann. Thorac. Surg., 50:675, 1990.

Goodnough, L. T., Kruskall, M., Stehling, L., et al.: A multicenter audit of transfusion practice in coronary artery bypass graft (CABG) surgery. Blood, 72:277A, 1988.

Goto, H., Nonami, R., Hamasaki, Y., et al.: Effect of hypothermia on coagulation. Anesthesiology 63(3A):A107, 1985.

Grady, G. F., and Bennett, A. J. E.: Risk of posttransfusion hepatitis in the United States. J. A. M. A., 220:692, 1972.

Graham, R., Jr.: The treatment of serious bacterial infections in the intensive care unit. In Shoemaker, W. C., Thompson, W. L., and Holbrook, P. R. (eds): Textbook of Critical Care. Chap. 70. Philadelphia, W. B. Saunders, 1984.

Gray, R. J., Matloff, J. M., Conklin, C. M., et al.: Perioperative myocardial infarction: Late clinical course after coronary artery bypass surgery. Circulation, 66:1185, 1982.

Grayzel, J.: Clinical evaluation of the Percor percutaneous intra-aortic balloon: Cooperative study of 722 cases. Circulation, 66(Suppl.):I-223, 1982.

Griffith, L. D., Billman, G. F., Daily, P. O., and Lane, T. A.: Apparent coagulopathy caused by infusion of shed mediastinal blood and its prevention by washing of the infusate. Ann. Thorac. Surg., 47:400, 1989.

Grover, F. L., Hammermeister, K. E., and Burchfiel, C.: Initial report of the Veterans Administration Preoperative Risk Assessment Study for Cardiac Surgery. Ann. Thorac. Surg., 50:12, 1990.

Guyton, R. A., Andrews, M. J., Hickey, P. R., et al.: The contribution of atrial contraction to right heart function before and after right ventriculotomy. J. Thorac. Cardiovasc. Surg., 71:1, 1976.

Haber, E.: Antibodies and digitalis: The modern revolution in the use of an ancient drug. J. Am. Coll. Cardiol., 5:111A, 1985.

Hakim, R. M., and Lazarus, J. M.: Hemodialysis in acute renal failure. In Brenner, B. M., and Lazarus, J. M. (eds): Acute Renal Failure. Chap. 25. Philadelphia, W. B. Saunders, 1983.

Hall-Boyer, K., Zaloga, G. P., and Chernow, B.: Glucagon: Hormone or therapeutic agent? Crit. Care Med., 12:584, 1984.

Hammeke, T. A., and Hastings, J. E.: Neuropsychologic alterations after cardiac operation. J. Thorac. Cardiovasc. Surg., 96:326, 1988.

Hammermeister, K. E., Burchfiel, C., Johnson, R., and Grover, F. L.: Identification of patients at greatest risk for developing major complications at cardiac surgery. Circulation, 82(Suppl.):IV-380, 1990.

Hanson, E. L., Kane, P. B., Askanazi, J., et al.: Comparison of patients with coronary artery disease: Intraoperative differences in blood volume and observations of vasomotor response. Ann. Thorac. Surg., 22:343, 1976.

Hardesty, R. L., Thompson, M., Lerberg, D. B., et al.: Delayed postoperative cardiac tamponade: Diagnosis and management. Ann. Thorac. Surg., 26:155, 1978.

Hargrove, W. C., III, Rosato, E. F., Hicks, R. E., and Mullen, J. L.: Cecal necrosis after open-heart operation. Ann. Thorac. Surg., 25:71, 1978.

Harker, L. H.: Bleeding after cardiopulmonary bypass. N. Engl. J. Med., 314:1446, 1986.

Harris, L. F., Alford, R. H., Dan, B. B., et al.: Bacteremia related to IV cannulation: Variability of underlying venous infection. South. Med. J., 73:719, 1980.

Harris, M. R., and Huseby, J. S.: Pulmonary complications from nasoenteral feeding tube insertion in an intensive care unit: Incidence and prevention. Crit. Care Med., 17:917, 1989.

Harris, P. D., Malm, J. R., Bowman, F. O., Jr., et al.: Epicardial pacing to control arrhythmias following cardiac surgery. Circulation, 37(Suppl.):II-178, 1968.

Harris, R. E., Reimer, K. A., Crain, B. J., et al.: Spinal cord infarction following intra-aortic balloon support. Ann. Thorac. Surg., 42:206, 1986.

Hart, R. G., Coull, B. M., and Hart, D.: Early recurrent embolism associated with nonvalvular atrial fibrillation: A retrospective study. Stroke, 14:688, 1983a.

Hart, R. G., and Hindman, B.: Mechanisms of perioperative cerebral infarction. Stroke, 13:766, 1982.

Hart, R. G., Sherman, D. G., Miller, V. T., and Easton, J. D.: Diagnosis and management of ischemic stroke. II. Selected controversies. Curr. Prob. Cardiol., 8:1, 1983b.

Hartz, R. S., Smith, J. A., and Green, D.: Autotransfusion after cardiac operation. Assessment of hemostatic factors. J. Thorac. Cardiovasc. Surg., 96:178, 1988.

Hartzler, G. O., Maloney, J. D., Curtis, J. J., and Barnhorst, D. A.: Hemodynamic benefits of atrioventricular sequential pacing after cardiac surgery. Am. J. Cardiol., 40:232, 1977.

Hashimoto, K., Ilstrup, D. M., and Schaff, H. V.: Influence of clinical and hemodynamic variables on risk of supraventricular tachycardia after coronary artery bypass. J. Thorac. Cardiovasc. Surg., 101:56, 1991.

Hasting, P. R., Skillman, J. J., Bushnell, L. S., and Silen, W.: Antacid titration in the prevention of acute gastrointestinal bleeding. N. Engl. J. Med., 298:1041, 1978.

Hattersley, P. G.: Heparin anticoagulation. In Koepke, J. A. (ed): Laboratory Hematology. Vol. 2., Chap. 31. New York, Churchill Livingstone, 1984.

Haupt, M. T., and Carlson, R. W.: Anaphylactic and anaphylactoid reactions. In Shoemaker, W. C., Thompson, W. L., and Holbrook, P. R. (eds): Textbook of Critical Care. Chap. 12. Philadelphia, W. B. Saunders, 1984.

Hayes, M. A., Yau, E. H., Timmins, A. C., et al.: Response of critically ill patients to treatment aimed at achieving supranormal oxygen delivery and consumption. Relationship to outcome [see comments]. Chest, 103:886, 1993.

Hedges, J. R., Barsan, W. B., Doan, L. A., et al.: Central versus peripheral intravenous routes in cardiopulmonary resuscitation. Am. J. Emerg. Med., 2:385, 1984.

Heller, S. S., Frank, K. A., Malm, J. R., et al.: Psychiatric complications of open-heart surgery. N. Engl. J. Med., 283:1015, 1970.

Heng, M. K., Singh, B. N., Roche, A. H., et al.: Effects of intravenous verapamil on cardiac arrhythmias and on the electrocardiogram. Am. Heart J., 90:487, 1975.

Hennings, B., and Jacobson, G.: Postoperative amylase excretion. Ann. Clin. Res., 6:215, 1974.

Heymsfield, S. B., Casper, K., and Funfar, J.: Physiologic response and clinical implications of nutrition support. Am. J. Cardiol., 60:75G, 1987.

Higgins, C. B., Batner, S. F., and Franklin, D.: Extent of regulation of the heart's contractile state in conscious dog by alteration in the frequency of contraction. J. Clin. Invest., 52:1187, 1973.

Hilberman, M., Derby, G. C., Spencer, R. J., and Stinson, E. B.: Sequential pathophysiological changes characterizing the progression from renal dysfunction to acute renal failure following cardiac operation. J. Thorac. Cardiovasc. Surg., 79:838, 1980.

Hilberman, M., Myers, B. D., Carrie, B. J., et al.: Acute renal failure following cardiac surgery. J. Thorac. Cardiovasc. Surg., 77:880, 1979.

Hilberman, M., Schill, J. P., and Peters, R. M.: On-line digital analysis of respiratory mechanics and the automation of respirator control. J. Thorac. Cardiovasc. Surg., 58:821, 1969.

Hitch, D. C., and Nolan, S. P.: Changes in myocardial performance and total peripheral resistance produced by the administration of chlordiazepoxide. J. Thorac. Cardiovasc. Surg., 61:352, 1971.

Ho, M.: Nonbacterial infections in the ICU. In Shoemaker, W. C., Thompson, W. L., and Holbrook, P. R. (eds): Textbook of Critical Care. Chap. 71. Philadelphia, W. B. Saunders, 1984.

Hodam, R. P., and Starr, A.: Temporary postoperative epicardial pacing electrodes. Ann. Thorac. Surg., 8:506, 1969.

Hoffman, W. S., Tomasello, D. N., and MacVaugh, H.: Control of postcardiotomy bleeding with PEEP. Ann. Thorac. Surg., 34:71, 1982.

Holland, F. W., Brown, P. S., Weintraub, B. D., and Clark, R. E.: Cardiopulmonary bypass and thyroid function: A "euthyroid sick syndrome." Ann. Thorac. Surg., 52:46, 1991.

Hood, W. B., Jr.: Role of converting enzyme inhibitors in the treatment of heart failure. J. Am. Coll. Cardiol., 22(Suppl. A):154A, 1993.

Horn, K. L., and Abouav, J.: Right vocal cord paralysis after open heart operation. Ann. Thorac. Surg., 27:344, 1979.

Horneffer, P. J., Miller, R. H., Pearson, T. A., et al.: The effective treatment of postpericardiotomy syndrome after cardiac operations. A randomized placebo-controlled trial. J. Thorac. Cardiovasc. Surg., 100:292, 1990.

Hou, S. H., Bushinsky, D. A., Wish, J. B., et al.: Hospital-acquired renal insufficiency: A prospective study. Am. J. Med., 74:243, 1983.

Iaina, A., Solomon, S., Gavendo, S., and Eliahou, H. E.: Reduction in severity of acute renal failure (ARF) in rats by dopamine. Biomedicine, 27:137, 1977.

Iberti, T. J., Leibowitz, A. B., Papadakos, P. J., and Fischer, E. P.: Low sensitivity of the anion gap as a screen to detect hyperlactatemia in critically ill patients. Crit. Care Med., 18:275, 1990.

Iberti, T. J., Paluch, T. A., Helmer, L., et al.: The hemodynamic effects of intravenous cimetidine in intensive care unit patients: A double-blind, prospective study. Anesthesiology, 64:87, 1986.

Ilabaca, P. A., Ochsner, J. L., and Mills, N. L.: Positive end-expiratory pressure in the management of the patient with a postoperative bleeding heart. Ann. Thorac. Surg., 30:281, 1980.

Imai, T., Saitoh, K., Kani, H., et al.: Combined dose ratios of dopamine and dobutamine and right ventricular performance after cardiac surgery. Chest, 101:1197, 1992.

Iseri, L. T., Chung, P., and Tobis, J.: Magnesium therapy for intractable ventricular tachyarrhythmias in normomagnesemic patients. West. J. Med., 138:823, 1983.

Ito, T., Engle, M. A., and Goldberg, H. P.: Postpericardiotomy syndrome following surgery for nonrheumatic heart disease. Circulation, 17:549, 1958.

Jacobs, M. R.: Diagnosis of infections. In Shoemaker, W. C., Thompson, W. L., and Holbrook, P. R. (eds): Textbook of Critical Care. Chap. 72. Philadelphia, W. B. Saunders, 1984.

Jansen, N. J., van Oeveren, W., Gu, Y. J., et al.: Endotoxin release and tumor necrosis factor formation during cardiopulmonary bypass. Ann. Thorac. Surg., 54:744, 1992.

Jardin, F., Farcot, J. C., and Boisante, L.: Influence of positive end-expiratory pressure on left ventricular performance. N. Engl. J. Med., 304:387, 1981.

Jastrzebski, J., Sykes, M. K., and Woods, D. G.: Cardiorespiratory effects of protamine after cardiopulmonary bypass in man. Thorax, 29:534, 1974.

Javid, H., Tufo, H. M., Najafi, H., et al.: Neurological abnormalities following open-heart surgery. J. Thorac. Cardiovasc. Surg., 58:502, 1969.

Jeevanadam, V., Smith, C. R., Rose, E. A., et al.: Single-stage management of sternal wound infections. J. Thorac. Cardiovasc. Surg., 90:256, 1990.

Johnson, J. A., Gall, W. E., Gunderson, A. E., and Cogbill, T. H.: Delayed primary closure after sternal wound infection. Ann. Thorac. Surg., 47:270, 1989.

Johnson, R. G., Rosenkrantz, K. R., Preston, R. A., et al.: The efficacy of postoperative autotransfusion in patients undergoing cardiac operations. Ann. Thorac. Surg., 36:173, 1983.

Johnson, R. G., Thurer, R. L., Kruskall, M. S., et al.: Comparison of two transfusion strategies after elective operations for myocardial revascularization. J. Thorac. Cardiovasc. Surg., 104:307, 1992.

Johnsson, P., Algotsson, L., Ryding, E., et al.: Cardiopulmonary perfusion and cerebral blood flow in bilateral carotid artery disease. Ann. Thorac. Surg., 51:579, 1991.

Josephson, M. E.: Treatment of ventricular arrhythmias after myocardial infarction. Circulation, 74:162, 1986.

Jurkiewicz, M. J., Bostwick, J., III, Hester, T. R., et al.: Infected median sternotomy wound. Ann. Surg., 191:738, 1980.

Kaiser, A. B.: Clinical implications of beta-lactamases in surgical prophylaxis. Contemp. Surg., 32(3-A):30, 1988.

Kang, Y. G., Martin, D. J., Marquez, J., et al.: Intraoperative changes in blood coagulation and thromboelastographic monitoring in liver transplantation. Anesth. Analg., 64:888, 1985.

Kaplan, J. A.: Detection and management of perioperative low cardiac output: PDE-III inhibition, inotropy and vasodilation. J. Drug Develop., 4(2):67, October 1991.

Kaplan, J. A.: Amrinone: Contemporary management of the low cardiac output syndrome. J. Cardiothorac. Anesth., 3(Suppl. 2):1, 1989.

Kaplan, J. A., and Levy, J. H. (eds): The management of low cardiac output syndrome. A focus on amrinone. Educational Program (extrapolated from symposia held prior to annual Society of Cardiovascular Anesthesiologists in 1989 and 1990). Califon, Gardiner-Caldwell Synermed, 1990.

Kass, D. A., and Maughan, W. L.: From "E$_{max}$" to pressure-volume relations: A broader view. Circulation, 77:1203, 1988.

Katz, N. M., Ahmed, S. W., Clark, B. K., and Wallace, R. B.: Predictors of length of hospitalization after cardiac surgery. Ann. Thorac. Surg., 45:656, 1988.

Kirklin, J. K., Westaby, S., Blackstone, E. H., et al.: Complement and the damaging effects of cardiopulmonary bypass. J. Thorac. Cardiovasc. Surg., 86:845, 1983.

Kirklin, J. W., and Archie, J. P., Jr.: The cardiovascular system in surgical patients. Surg. Gynecol. Obstet., 139:17, 1974.

Kirsh, M. M., Magee, K. R., Gago, O., et al.: Brachial plexus injury following median sternotomy incision. Ann. Thorac. Surg., 11:315, 1971.

Kirsh, M. M., McIntosh, K., Kahn, D. R., and Sloan, H.: Postpericardiotomy syndrome. Ann. Thorac. Surg., 9:158, 1970.

Klausner, J. M., Morel, N., Paterson, I. S., et al.: The rapid induction by interleukin-2 of pulmonary microvascular permeability. Ann. Surg., 209:119, 1989.

Koepke, J. A. (ed): Laboratory Hematology. Vol. 2, Chap. 42. New York, Churchill Livingstone, 1984.

Kolkka, R., and Hilberman, M.: Neurologic dysfunction following cardiac operation with low-flow, low-pressure cardiopulmonary bypass. J. Thorac. Cardiovasc. Surg., 79:432, 1980.

Kondo, N. I., Madd, R., Ewenstein, B. M. et al.: Anticoagulation and hemostasis in cardiac surgical patients. J. Card. Surg., 9:443, 1994.

Konishi, T., Ohbayashi, T., Kaneko, T., et al.: Preoperative use of erythropoietin for cardiovascular operations in anemia. Ann. Thorac. Surg., 56:101, 1993.

Konstam, M. A., Kronenberg, M. W., Udelson, J. E., et al.: Effect of acute angiotensin converting enzyme inhibition on left ventricular filling in patients with congestive heart failure. Relation to right ventricular volumes. Circulation, 81(Suppl.):III-115, 1990.

Kornfeld, D. S., Zimberg, S., and Malm, J. R.: Psychiatric complications of open-heart surgery. N. Engl. J. Med., 273:287, 1965.

Koshal, A., Murphy, J., and Keon, W. J.: Pros and cons of urgent exploratory sternotomy after open cardiac surgery. Can. J. Surg., 29:186, 1986.

Kosugi, I., and Tajimi, K.: Effects of dopamine and dobutamine on hemodynamics and plasma catecholamine levels during severe lactic acid acidosis. Circ. Shock, 17:95, 1985.

Kouchoukos, N. T., and Karp, R. B.: Management of the postoperative cardiovascular surgical patient. Am. Heart J., 92:513, 1976.

Kouchoukos, N. T., Oberman, A., Kirklin, J. W., et al.: Coronary bypass surgery: Analysis of factors affecting hospital mortality. Circulation, 62(Suppl.):I-84, 1980.

Kovacs, K., and Yao, J.: Pituitary necrosis following major heart surgery. Z. Kardiol., 64:52, 1975.

Kramer, P., Wigger, W., Rieger, J., et al.: Arteriovenous haemofiltration: A new and simple method for treatment of over-hydrated patients resistant to diuretics. Klin. Wochenschr., 55:1121, 1977.

Krauss, X. H., Verdouw, P. D., Hughenholtz, P. G., and Nauta, J.: On-line monitoring of mixed venous oxygen saturation after cardiothoracic surgery. Thorax, 30:636, 1975.

Kreter, B., and Woods, M.: Antibiotic prophylaxis for cardiothoracic operations. Meta-analysis of thirty years of clinical trials. J. Thorac. Cardiovasc. Surg., 104:590, 1992.

Kron, I. L., Joob, A. W., and Van Meter, C.: Acute renal failure in the cardiovascular surgical patient. Ann. Thorac. Surg., 39:590, 1985.

Kron, I. L., Kaiser, D. L., Nolan, S. P., et al.: Who manages the postoperative cardiac patient? J. Thorac. Cardiovasc. Surg., 87:629, 1984.

Kronzon, I., Cohen, M. L., Winer, H. E.: Diastolic atrial compression: A sensitive sign of cardiac tamponade. J. Am. Coll. Cardiol., 2:770, 1983.

Kuhn, G. J., White, B. C., Swetnam, R. E., et al.: Peripheral vs central circulation times during CPR: A pilot study. Ann. Emerg. Med., 10:417, 1981.

Kukora, J. S., and Dent, T. L.: Colonoscopic decompression of massive nonobstructive cecal dilation. Arch. Surg., 112:512, 1977.

Kumar, A., Pontoppidan, H., Falke, K. J., et al.: Pulmonary barotrauma during mechanical ventilation. Crit. Care Med., 1:181, 1973.

Kumon, K., Tanaka, K., Hirata, T., et al.: Organ failures due to low cardiac output syndrome following open heart surgery. Jpn. Circ. J., 50:329, 1986.

Kuntschen, F. R., Galletti, P. M., and Hahn, C.: Glucose-insulin interactions during cardiopulmonary bypass—Hypothermia versus normothermia. J. Thorac. Cardiovasc. Surg., 91:451, 1986.

Kyosola, K., Mattila, T., Harjula, A., et al.: Life-threatening complications of cardiac operations and occurrence of myocardial catecholamine bombs. J. Thorac. Cardiovasc. Surg., 95:334, 1988.

Lahey, S. J., Borlase, B. C., Lavin, P. T., and Levitsky, S.: Preoperative risk factors that predict hospital length of stay in coronary artery bypass patients >60 years old. Circulation, 86(Suppl.):II-181, 1992.

Lakin, J. D., Blocker, T. J., and Strong, D. M.: Anaphylaxis to protamine sulfate mediated by a complement-dependent IgG antibody. J. Allergy Clin. Immunol., 61:103, 1978.

Lambert, C. J., Marengo-Rowe, A. J., Leveson, J. E., et al.: The treatment of postperfusion bleeding using epsilon-aminocaproic acid, cryoprecipitate, fresh-frozen plasma, and protamine sulfate. Ann. Thorac. Surg., 28:442, 1979.

Landow, L.: Splanchnic lactate production in cardiac surgery patients. Crit. Care Med., 21(Suppl.):84, 1993.

Landreneau, R. J.: Splanchnic blood flow response to intra-aortic balloon pump assist of hemorrhagic shock. J. Surg. Res., 51:281, 1991.

Lappas, D. G., Powell, W. M. J., Jr., and Daggett, W. M.: Cardiac dysfunction in the perioperative period: Pathophysiology, diagnosis, and treatment. Anesthesiology, 47:117, 1977.

Laski, M. E.: Normal regulation of acid-base balance. (Symposium on Acid-Base Disorders.) Med. Clin. North Am., 67:771, 1983.

Lassen, N. A.: Brain. In Johnson, P. C. (ed): Peripheral Circulation. New York, John Wiley & Sons, 1978.

Laub, G. W., Janeira, L., Muralidharan, S., et al.: Prophylactic procainamide for prevention of atrial fibrillation after coronary artery bypass grafting: A prospective, double-blind, randomized, placebo-controlled pilot study. Crit. Care Med., 21:1474, 1993.

Lauer, M. S., Eagle, K. A., Buckley, M. J., and DeSanctis, R. W.: Atrial fibrillation following coronary artery bypass surgery. Prog. Cardiovasc. Dis., 31:367, 1989.

Laurenzi, G. A., Yin, S., and Guarneri, J. J.: Adverse effect of oxygen on tracheal mucus flow. N. Engl. J. Med., 279:333, 1968.

Layne, O. L., Jr., and Yudofsky, S. C.: Postoperative psychosis in cardiotomy patients. The role of organic and psychiatric factors. N. Engl. J. Med., 284:518, 1971.

Lazenby, W. D., Russo, I., Zadeh, B. J., et al.: Treatment with desmopressin acetate in routine coronary artery bypass surgery to improve postoperative hemostasis. Circulation, 82(Suppl.):IV-413, 1990.

Lee, K. F., Mandell, J., Rankin, J. S., et al.: Immediate versus delayed coronary grafting after streptokinase treatment. J. Thorac. Cardiovasc. Surg., 95:216, 1988.

Lee, T. H., Salomon, D. R., Rayment, C. M., and Antman, E. M.: Hypotension and sinus arrest with exercise-induced hyperkalemia and combined verapamil/propranolol therapy. Am. J. Med., 80:1203, 1986.

Lefer, A. M.: Corticosteroids and circulatory function. In Greip, R. O., and Astwood, E. B. (eds): Handbook of Physiology, Sect. 7: Endocrinology. Vol. 6. Washington, D. C., American Physiological Society, 1975; pp. 191–206.

Lefkowitz, R. J.: Direct binding studies of adrenergic receptors: Biochemical, physiologic, and clinical implications. Ann. Intern. Med., 91:450, 1979.

Leitman, I. M., Paull, D. E., Barie, P. S., et al.: Intra-abdominal complications of cardiopulmonary bypass operations. Surg. Gynecol. Obstet., 165:251, 1987.

LeJemtel, T. H., and Sonnenblick, E. H.: Heart failure: Adaptive and maladaptive processes. Circulation, 87(Suppl):VII-1, 1993.

Lekven, J., Brunsting, L. A., Jessen, M. E., et al.: Myocardial oxygen use during epinephrine administration to ischemically injured canine hearts. Circulation, 78(Suppl.):III-125, 1988.

Lemmer, J. H., Jr., and Kirsch, M. M.: Coronary artery spasm following coronary artery surgery. Ann. Thorac. Surg., 46:108, 1988.

Levy, D. E., Bates, D., Caronna, J. J., et al.: Prognosis in nontraumatic coma. Ann. Intern. Med., 94:293, 1981.

Levy, J. H., Schwieger, I. M., Zaidan, J. R., et al.: Evaluation of patients at risk for protamine reactions. J. Thorac. Cardiovasc. Surg., 98:200, 1989.

Lewis, W. D., Chwals, W., Benotti, P. N., et al.: Bedside assessment of the work of breathing. Crit. Care Med., 16:117, 1988.

Lichtenthal, P. R., Wade, L. D., Niemyski, P. R., and Shapiro, B. A.: Respiratory management after cardiac surgery with inhalation anesthesia. Crit. Care Med., 11:603, 1983.

Linden, C. H., and Aghababian, R. V.: Further uses of glucagon. Crit. Care Med., 13:248, 1985.

Lineaweaver, W. C., Anderson, K., and Hing, D. N.: Massive doses of midazolam infusion for delirium tremens without respiratory depression. Crit. Care Med., 16:294, 1988.

Lister, J. W., Cohen, L. S., Bernstein, W. H., and Samet, P.: Treatment of supraventricular tachycardias by rapid atrial stimulation. Circulation, 38:1044, 1968.

Little, W. C., Cheng, C.-P., Peterson, T., and Vinten-Johansen, J.: Response of the left ventricular end-systolic pressure-volume relation in conscious dogs to a wide range of contractile states. Circulation, 78:736, 1988.

Livelli, F. D., Jr., Johnson, R. A., McEnany, M. T., et al.: Unexplained in-hospital fever following cardiac surgery. Circulation, 57:968, 1978.

Livesay, J. J., Follette, D. M., Fey, K. H., et al.: Optimizing myocardial supply/demand balance with alpha-adrenergic drugs during cardiopulmonary resuscitation. J. Thorac. Cardiovasc. Surg., 76:244, 1978.

LoCicero, J., III: Prophylactic antibiotic usage in cardiothoracic surgery. Chest, 98:719, 1990.

Lollgen, H., and Drexler, H.: Use of inotropes in the critical care setting. Crit. Care Med., 18(1 Pt 2):S56, 1990.

Loop, F. D., Lytle, B. W., Cosgrove, D. M., et al.: Maxwell Chamberlain memorial paper. Sternal wound complications after isolated coronary artery bypass grafting: Early and late mortality, morbidity, and cost of care. Ann. Thorac. Surg., 49:179, 1990.

Lorenz, R. L., Weber, M., Kotzur, J., et al.: Improved aortocoronary bypass patency by low-dose aspirin: Effects on platelet aggregation and thromboxane formation. Lancet, 1:1261, 1984.

Lotvin, A., and Gorlin, R.: Converting enzyme inhibitors: Current use. ACC Current J. Rev., May/June 1993.

Lowe, J. E., Anstadt, M. P., Van Trigt, P., et al.: First successful bridge to transplantation using direct mechanical ventricular actuation. Ann. Thorac. Surg., 52:1237, 1991a.

Lowe, J. E., Hendry, P. J., Hendrickson, S. C., and Wells, R.: Intraoperative identification of cardiac patients at risk to develop postoperative atrial fibrillation. Ann. Surg., 213:388, 1991b.

Lowenstein, E., Hallowell, P., Levine, F. H., et al.: Cardiovascular response to large doses of intravenous morphine in man. N. Engl. J. Med., 281:1389, 1969.

Lowman, R. M., and Davis, L.: An evaluation of cecal size in impending perforation of the cecum. Surg. Gynecol. Obstet., 103:711, 1956.

Lown, B.: Electrical reversion of cardiac arrhythmias. Br. Heart J., 29:469, 1967.

Lown, B., and DeSilva, R. A.: The technique of cardioversion. In Hurst, J. W. (ed): The Heart. 5th ed., Vol. 2. New York, McGraw-Hill, 1982.

Lown, B., Kleiger, R., and Wolff, G.: The technique of cardioversion. Am. Heart J., 67:282, 1964.

Lown, B., Temte, J. V., and Arter, W. J.: Ventricular tachyarrhythmias. Clinical aspects. Circulation, 47:1364, 1973.

Lowrie, E. G., Laird, N. M., Parter, T. F., and Sargent, J. A.: Effect of the hemodialysis prescription on patient morbidity. N. Engl. J. Med., 305:1176, 1981.

Lytle, B. W., Loop, F. D., Cosgrove, D. M., et al.: Fifteen hundred coronary reoperations; Results and determinants of early and late survival. J. Thorac. Cardiovasc. Dis., 93:847, 1987.

MacCannell, K. L., Giraud, G. D., Hamilton, P. L., and Groves, G.: Haemodynamic responses to dopamine and dobutamine infusions as a function of duration of infusion. Pharmacology, 26:29, 1983.

MacGregor, R. R., Spagnuolo, P. J., and Lentnek, A. L.: Inhibition of granulocyte adherence by ethanol, prednisone, and aspirin, measured with an assay system. N. Engl. J. Med., 291:642, 1974.

Macnaughton, P. D., Braude, S., Hunter, D. N., et al.: Changes in lung function and pulmonary capillary permeability after cardiopulmonary bypass. Crit. Care Med., 20:1289, 1992.

Magovern, J. A., and Magovern, G. J., Jr.: Diuresis in hemodynamically compromised patients: Continuous furosemide infusion. Ann. Thorac. Surg., 50:482, 1990.

Maier, G. W., Tyson, G. S., Jr., Olsen, C. O., et al.: The physiology of external cardiac massage: High-impulse cardiopulmonary resuscitation. Circulation, 70:86, 1984.

Maki, D. G., and Band, J. D.: A comparative study of polyantibiotic and iodophor ointments in prevention of vascular catheter-related infection. Am. J. Med., 70:739, 1981.

Mann, M., Sacks, H. J., Goldfinger, D.: Safety of autologous blood donation prior to elective surgery for a variety of potentially "high-risk" patients. Transfusion, 23:229, 1983.

Manolis, A. S., and Estes, A. M., III: Supraventricular tachycardia. Mechanisms and therapy. Arch. Intern. Med., 147:1706, 1987.

Marcus, M. L., Harrison, D. G., Chilian, W. M., et al.: Alterations in the coronary circulation in hypertrophied ventricles. Circulation, 75(Suppl.):I-19, 1987.

Marder, V. J., and Sherry, S.: Thrombolytic therapy: Current status. N. Engl. J. Med., 318:1512, 1988.

Marini, J.: Respiratory Medicine and Intensive Care for the House Officer. Baltimore, Williams & Wilkins, 1981, pp. 58, 161.

Markand, O. N., Moorthy, S. S., Mahomed, Y., et al.: Postoperative phrenic nerve palsy in patients with open-heart surgery. Ann. Thorac. Surg., 39:68, 1985.

Markewitz, A., Faist, E., Lang, S., et al.: Successful restoration of cell-mediated immune response after cardiopulmonary bypass by immunomodulation. J. Thorac. Cardiovasc. Surg., 105:15, 1993.

Marshall, J. C., Christou, N. V., Horn, S., and Meakins, J. L.: The microbiology of multiple organ failure. Arch. Surg., 123:309, 1988.

Marshall, J. C., Christou, N. V., and Meakins, J. L.: The gastrointestinal tract. The "undrained abscess" of multiple organ failure. Ann. Surg., 218:111, 1993.

Massie, B. M., and Conway, M.: Survival of patients with congestive heart failure: Past, present and future prospects. Circulation, 75(Suppl.):IV-11, 1987.

Massie, B. M., Ports, T., Chatterjee, K., et al.: Long-term vasodilator therapy for heart failure: Clinical response and its relationship to hemodynamic measurements. Circulation, 63:269, 1981.

Matloff, J. M., Wolfson, S., Gorlin, R., and Harken, D. E.: Control

of postcardiac surgical tachycardias with propranolol. Circulation, 37(Suppl.):II-133, 1968.

Maturlo, S. J., Rosenbaum, R. L., Pan, C., and Surks, M. I.: Variable thyrotropin response to thyrotropin-releasing hormone after small decreases in plasma free thyroid hormone concentrations in patients with nonthyroidal diseases. J. Clin. Invest., 66:451, 1980.

McCord, J. M., Wong, K., Stokes, S. H., et al.: Superoxide and inflammation: A mechanism for the anti-inflammatory activity of superoxide dismutase. Acta Physiol. Scand., 492(Suppl.):25, 1980.

McGee, M. G., Zellgitt, S. L., Treno, R., et al.: Retrospective analysis of the need for mechanical circulatory support (intra-aortic balloon pump/abdominal left ventricular assist device or partial artificial heart) after cardiopulmonary bypass: A 44 month study of 14,168 patients. Am. J. Cardiol., 46:135, 1980.

McGeehin, W., Sheikh, F., Donahoo, J. S., et al.: Transthoracic intra-aortic balloon pump support: Experience in 39 patients. Ann. Thorac. Surg., 44:26, 1987.

McGhie, A. I., and Golstein, R. A.: Pathogenesis and management of acute heart failure and cardiogenic shock: Role of inotropic therapy. Chest, 102(Suppl.):626S, 1992.

McIntosh, T. K., Lothrop, D. A., Lee, A., et al.: Circadian rhythm of cortisol is altered in postsurgical patients. J. Clin. Endocrinol. Metab., 53:117, 1981.

McKowen, R. L., Magovern, G. J., Liebler, G. A., et al.: Infectious complications and cost-effectiveness of open resuscitation in the surgical intensive care unit after cardiac surgery. Ann. Thorac. Surg., 40:388, 1985.

McLeish, K. R., Luft, F. C., Kleit, S. A.: Factors affecting prognosis in acute renal failure following cardiac operations Surg. Gynecol. Obstet., 145:28, 1977.

McNeill, J. R., Stark, R. D., and Greenway, C. V.: Intestinal vasoconstriction after hemorrhage: Roles of vasopressin and angiotensin. Am. J. Physiol., 219:1342, 1970.

Mellander, S., and Johansson, B.: Control of resistance, exchange, and capacitance functions in the peripheral circulation. Pharmacol. Rev., 20:117, 1968.

Melzig, E. P., and Terz, J. J.: Pseudo-obstruction of the colon. Arch. Surg., 113:1186, 1978.

Michelson, E. L., Morganroth, J., and MacVaugh, H., III: Postoperative arrhythmias after coronary artery and cardiac valvular surgery detected by long-term electrographic monitoring. Am. Heart J., 97:442, 1979.

Michenfelder, J. D., and Tinker, J. H.: Cyanide toxicity and thiosulfate protection during chronic administration of sodium nitroprusside in the dog: Correlation with a human case. Anesthesiology, 47:441, 1977.

Mickell, J. J., Oh, K. S., Siewers, R. D., et al.: Clinical implications of postoperative unilateral phrenic nerve paralysis. J. Thorac. Cardiovasc. Surg., 76:297, 1978.

Mielke, J. E., Hunt, J. C., Maher, F. T., and Kirklin, J. W.: Renal performance during clinical cardiopulmonary bypass with and without hemodilution. J. Thorac. Cardiovasc. Surg., 51:229, 1966.

Milam, J. D.: Blood transfusion in heart surgery. Surg. Clin. North Am., 63:1127, 1983.

Miller, C. A., Pae, W. E., Jr., and Pierce, W. S.: Combined registry for the use of mechanical ventricular assist devices: Post cardiotomy cardiogenic shock. Trans. Am. Soc. Artif. Intern. Organs, 36:43, 1990.

Miller, D. C., Stinson, E. B., Oyer, P. E., et al.: Discriminant analysis of the changing risks of coronary artery operations: 1971–79. J. Thorac. Cardiovasc. Surg., 85:197, 1983.

Miller, D. C., Stinson, E. B., Oyer, P. E., et al.: Postoperative enhancement of left ventricular performance by combined inotropic-vasodilator therapy with preload control. Surgery, 88:108, 1980.

Miller, L. W.: Mechanical assist devices in intensive cardiac care. Am. Heart. J., 121:1887, 1991.

Mills, N. L.: Postoperative hemorrhage after cardiopulmonary bypass [Editorial]. Ann. Thorac. Surg., 34:607, 1982.

Mills, N. L., and Ochsner, J. L.: Experience with atrial pacemaker wires implanted during cardiac operations. J. Thorac. Cardiovasc. Surg., 66:878, 1973.

Mills, S. A., Poole, G. V., Jr., Breyer, R. H., et al.: Digoxin and propranolol in the prophylaxis of dysrhythmias after coronary artery bypass grafting. Circulation, 68(Suppl.):222, 1983.

Miranda, D. R., Stoutenbeek, C., Karliczek, G., and Rating, W.: Effects of dexamethasone on the early postoperative course after coronary artery bypass surgery. Thorac. Cardiovasc. Surg., 30:21, 1982.

Mizock, B. A., and Falk, J. L.: Lactic acidosis in critical illness. Crit. Care Med., 20:80, 1992.

Moghissi, K., and McMillan, I. K. R.: Acute renal failure in open heart surgery. Br. Med. J., 2:228, 1972.

Montgomery, W. H.: Standards and guidelines for cardiopulmonary resuscitation (CPR) and Emergency Cardiac Care (ECC). Part III: Adult advanced cardiac life support. J. A. M. A., 255:2933, 1986.

Mooney, M. R., Mooney, J. F., Van Tassel, R. A., et al.: The Nimbus hemopump: A new left ventricular assist device that combines myocardial protection with circulatory support. J. Invest. Cardiol., 2:169, 1990.

Moore, C. H., Gordon, F. T., Allums, J. A., et al.: Diagnosis of perioperative myocardial infarction after coronary artery bypass. Ann. Thorac. Surg., 24:323, 1977.

Moore, F. D. Jr., Warner, K. G., Assousa, S., et al.: The effects of complement activation during cardiopulmonary bypass. Ann. Surg., 208:95, 1988.

Moore, W. S.: Antibiotic prophylaxis in clinical practice. Contemp. Surg., 32(3-A):39, 1988.

Morady, F., Nelson, S. D., Kou, W. H., et al.: Electrophysiologic effects of epinephrine in humans. J. Am. Coll. Cardiol., 11:1235, 1988.

Moran, J. M.: Postoperative ventricular arryhthmia. Ann. Thorac. Surg., 38:312, 1984.

Moran, J. M., Opravil, M., Gorman, A. J., et al.: Pulmonary artery balloon counterpulsation for right ventricular failure. II: Clinical experience. Ann. Thorac. Surg., 38:254, 1984.

Morganroth, J., Frishman, W. H., Horowitz, L. N., et al. (eds): Cardiovascular Drug Therapy. Chicago, Year Book Medical, 1986.

Morin, J. E., Long, R., Elleker, M. G., et al.: Upper extremity neuropathies following median sternotomy. Ann. Thorac. Surg., 34:181, 1982.

Morris, D. L., Markham, S. J., Beechey, A., et al.: Ranitidine—Bolus or infusion prophylaxis for stress ulcer. Crit. Care Med., 16:229, 1988.

Mullen, J. C., Miller, D. R., Weisel, R. D., et al.: Postoperative hypertension: A comparison of diltiazem, nifedipine, and nitroprusside. J. Thorac. Cardiovasc. Surg., 96:122, 1988.

Mullen, J. L., Gertner, M. H., Buzby, G. P., et al.: Implications of malnutrition in the surgical patient. Arch. Surg., 114:121, 1979.

Mundth, E. D., Keller, A. R., and Austen, W. G.: Progressive hepatic and renal failure associated with low cardiac output following open-heart surgery. J. Thorac. Cardiovasc. Surg., 53:275, 1967.

Murphy, G. (ed): The latest word on diet and heart disease. Duke University Medical Center, Clin. Nutr. Newslett., 2(1):1, 1988.

Myhre, B. A.: Fatalities from blood transfusion. J. A. M. A., 244:1333, 1980.

Nadelson, T.: The psychiatrist in the surgical intensive care unit. I. Postoperative delirium. II. A consideration of staff roles. Arch. Surg., 111:113. 1976.

Namay, D. L., Hammermeister, K. E., Zia, M. S., et al.: Effect of perioperative myocardial infarction on late survival in patients undergoing coronary artery bypass surgery. Circulation, 65:1066, 1982.

Naunheim, K. S., Fiore, A. C., Wadley, J. J., et al.: The changing profile of the patient undergoing coronary artery bypass surgery. J. Am. Coll. Cardiol., 11:494, 1988.

Nayler, W. G., and Szeto, J.: Effect of verapamil on contractility, oxygen utilization, and calcium exchangeability in mammalian heart muscle. Cardiovasc. Res., 6:120, 1972.

Needleman, P., and Greenwald, J. E.: Atriopeptin: A cardiac hormone intimately involved in fluid, electrolyte and blood-pressure homeostasis. N. Engl. J. Med., 314:828, 1986.

Nelson, R. M., Jenson, C. B., and Smoot, W. M.: Pericardial tamponade following open heart surgery. J. Thorac. Cardiovasc. Surg., 58:510, 1969.

Newton, J. R., Jr., Glower, D. D., Wolfe, J. A., et al.: A physiologic

comparison of external cardiac massage techniques. J. Thorac. Cardiovasc. Surg., 95:892, 1988.

Niehoff, J., DelGuercio, C., LaMorte, W., et al.: Efficacy of pulse oximetry and capnometry in postoperative ventilatory weaning. Crit. Care Med., 16:701, 1988.

Nishijima, M. K., Takezawa, J., Hosotsubo, K. K., et al.: Serial changes in cellular immunity of septic patients with multiple organ-system failure. Crit. Care Med., 14:86, 1986.

Norwegian Multicenter Study Group: Timolol-induced reduction in mortality and reinfarction in patients surviving acute myocardial infarction. N. Engl. J. Med., 304:801, 1981.

Norwood, S. H., Cormier, B., McMahon, N. G., et al.: Prospective study of catheter-related infection during prolonged arterial catheterization. Crit. Care Med., 16:836, 1988.

Norwood, S. H., Ruby A., Civetta, J., and Cortes, V.: Catheter-related infections and associated septicemia. Chest, 99:968, 1991.

Notterman, D., Metakis, L., Dimaio-Hunter, A., et al.: Dopamine elimination in critically ill patients: effect of liver dysfunction [Abstract]. Crit. Care Med., 16:442, 1988.

Novitzky, D., Cooper, D. K. C., Barton, C. I., et al.: Triiodothyronine as an inotropic agent after open heart surgery. J. Thorac. Cardiovasc. Surg., 98:972, 1989.

Novitzky, D., Matthews, N., Shawley, D., et al.: Triiodothyronine in the recovery of stunned myocardium in dogs [see comments]. Ann. Thorac. Surg., 51:10, 1991.

Ohri, S. K., Desai, J. B., Gaer, J. A., et al.: Intraabdominal complications after cardiopulmonary bypass. Ann. Thorac. Surg., 52:826, 1991.

Olinger, G. N., Werner, P. H., Bonchek, L. I., and Boerboom, L. E.: Vasodilator effects of the sodium acetate in pooled protein fraction. Ann. Surg., 190:305, 1979.

Orchard, C. H., Chakrabarti, M. K., and Sykes, M. K.: Cardiorespiratory responses to an i.v. infusion of dobutamine in the intact anaesthetized dog. Br. J. Anaesth., 54:673, 1982.

O'Quinn, R., and Marini, J.: Pulmonary artery occlusion pressure: Clinical physiology, measurement and interpretation. Am. Rev. Respir. Dis., 128:319, 1983.

Ornato, J. P., Gonzalez, E. R., Garnett, A. R., et al.: Effect of cardiopulmonary resuscitation compression rate on end-tidal carbon dioxide concentration and arterial pressure in man. Crit. Care Med., 16:241, 1988.

Oshima, A., and Bulkley, G. B.: Selective reduction of upper gastrointestinal blood flow in cardiogenic shock: Mediation via the renin-angiotensin axis. Surg. Forum, 35:169, 1984.

Ottino, G., De Paulis, R., Pansini, S., et al.: Major sternal wound infection after open-heart surgery: A multivariate analysis of risk factors in 2,579 consecutive operative procedures. Ann. Thorac. Surg., 44:173, 1987.

Pacifico, A. D., Digerness, S., and Kirklin, J. W.: Acute alterations of body composition after open intracardiac operations. Circulation, 41:331, 1970.

Packer, M.: Neurohormonal interactions and adaptations in congestive heart failure. Circulation, 77:721, 1988.

Packer, M.: Part III: New approaches to the treatment of heart failure. J. Am. Coll. Cardiol., 22(Suppl. A):107, 1993.

Packer, M., Kessler, P. D., and Lee, W. H.: Calcium-channel blockade in the management of severe chronic congestive heart failure: A bridge too far. Circulation, 75(Suppl.):V-56, 1987.

Paganini, E. P., and Nakamoto, S.: Continuous slow ultrafiltration in oliguric acute renal failure. Trans. Am. Soc. Artif. Intern. Organs, 26:201, 1980.

Page, P. L., Plumb, V. J., Okumura, K., and Waldo, A. L.: A new animal model of atrial flutter. J. Am. Coll. Cardiol., 8:872, 1986.

Palve, H.: Comparison of reflection and transmission pulse oximetry after open-heart surgery. Crit. Care Med., 20:48, 1992.

Pantridge, J. F., Adgey, A. A., Webb, S. W., et al.: Electrical requirements for ventricular defibrillation. Br. J. Med., 2(5966):313, 1975.

Parker, F. B., Jr., and West, H.: Autotransfusion following open-heart surgery. Ann. Thorac. Surg., 26:559, 1978.

Peck, V., Lieberman, A., Pinto, R., and Culliford, A.: Pituitary apoplexy following open-heart surgery. N. Y. State J. Med., 80:641, 1980.

Pennington, D. G. (moderator), Joyce, L. D., Pae, W. E., Jr., and

Bulkholder, J. A. (panelists). Patient Selection. Ann. Thorac. Surg., 47:77, 1989.

Pennington, D. G., McBride, L. R., Kanter, K. R., et al.: Effect of perioperative myocardial infarction on survival of postcardiotomy patients supported with ventricular-assist devices. Circulation, 78(5 Pt. 2):III-110, 1988.

Pennington, D. G., Swartz, M., Codd, J. E., et al.: Intraaortic balloon pumping in cardiac surgical patients: A nine-year experience. Ann. Thorac. Surg., 36:125, 1983.

Pennock, G. D., Raya, T. E., Bahl, J. J., et al.: Combination treatment with captopril and the thyroid hormone analogue 3,5-diiodothyropropionic acid. A new approach to improving left ventricular performance in heart failure. Circulation, 88:1289, 1993.

Perkins, C. M.: Serious verapamil poisoning: Treatment with intravenous calcium gluconate. Br. Med. J., 2:1127, 1978.

Petracek, M. R.: Surgeons' approach to prevention of wound infections. Contemp. Surg., 32(3-A):24, 1988.

Pichard, A. D., Ambrose, J., Mindich, B., et al.: Coronary artery spasm and perioperative cardiac arrest. J. Thorac. Cardiovasc. Surg., 80:249, 1980.

Pien, F. D., Ho, P. W. L., and Fergusson, D. J. G.: Fever and infection after cardiac operation. Ann. Thorac. Surg., 33:382, 1982.

Pingleton, S. K., and Hadzima, S. K.: Enteral alimentation and gastrointestinal bleeding in mechanically ventilated patients. Crit. Care Med., 11:13, 1983.

Pinson, C. W., and Alberty, R. E.: General surgical complications after cardiopulmonary bypass surgery. Am. J. Surg., 146:133, 1983.

Pitt, B.: Use of converting enzyme inhibitors in patients with asymptomatic left ventricular dysfunction. J. Am. Coll. Cardiol., 22(Suppl. A):158, 1993.

Platt, R.: Antibiotic prophylaxis in surgery. Rev. Infect. Dis., 6(Suppl.):880, 1984.

Plumb, V. J., Karp, R. B., Kouchoukos, N. T., et al.: Verapamil therapy of atrial fibrillation and atrial flutter following cardiac operation. J. Thorac. Cardiovasc. Surg., 83:590, 1982.

Podrid, P. J.: Antiarrhythmic Management: Therapeutic Considerations. A Monograph. Boston, Health Care Communications, 1992.

Priano, L. L., and Vatner, S. F.: Morphine effects on cardiac output and regional blood flow distribution in conscious dogs. Anesthesiology, 55:236, 1981.

Priebe, H. J., Skillman, J. J., Bushnell, L. S., et al.: Antacid versus cimetidine in preventing acute gastrointestinal bleeding. N. Engl. J. Med., 302:426, 1980.

Proskey, V. J., Morrison, G. R., McQuillan, B. P., and Parker, B. M.: Anicteric and icteric hepatitis after open-heart surgery. Gastroenterology, 58:203, 1970.

Prystowsky, E. N.: Antiarrhythmic therapy for asymptomatic ventricular arrhythmias. Am. J. Cardiol., 61:102A, 1988.

Quasha, A. L., Loeber, N., Feeley, T. W., et al.: Postoperative respiratory care: A controlled trial of early and late extubation following coronary artery bypass grafting. Anesthesiology, 52:135, 1980.

Ram, C. V. S., and Kaplan, N. M.: Hypertensive emergencies. In Shoemaker, W. C., Thompson, W. L., and Holbrook, P. R. (eds): Textbook of Critical Care. Ch. 53. Philadelphia, W. B. Saunders, 1984.

Rao, A. K., Pratt, C., Berke, A., et al.: Thrombolysis in myocardial infarction (TIMI) trial—Phase I: Hemorrhagic manifestations and changes in plasma fibrinogen and the fibrinolytic system in patients treated with recombinant tissue plasminogen activator and streptokinase. J. Am. Coll. Cardiol., 11:1, 1988.

Rashkin, M., Boskin, C., and Baughman, R.: Oxygen delivery in critically ill patients. Relationship to blood lactate and survival. Chest, 87:580, 1985.

Rattner, D. W., Gu, Z. Y., Vlahakes, G. J., and Warshaw, A. L.: Hyperamylasemia after cardiac surgery. Incidence, significance, and management. Ann. Surg., 209:279, 1989.

Rawles, J. M.: What is meant by a "controlled" ventricular rate in atrial fibrillation? Br. Heart J., 63:157, 1990.

Raymond, J. R.: Acute renal failure (acute azotemia) (guidelines). Durham, NC, Division of Nephrology, Duke University Medical Center, 1990.

Redwood, D. R., Smith, E. R., and Epstein, S. E.: Coronary artery occlusion in the conscious dog. Circulation, 46:323, 1972.

Reeves, J. T., Grover, R. F., Filley, G. F., and Blount, S. G.: Cardiac output in normal resting man. J. Appl. Physiol., 16:276, 1961.

Reilly, P. M., and Bulkley, G. B.: Vasoactive mediators and splanchnic perfusion. Crit. Care Med., 21(Suppl.):55, 1993.

Reisner, E. G., Telen, M. J., Issitt, L., and Issitt, P. D.: Transfusion Service Manual. Durham, NC, Duke University Medical Center, 1990.

Resnekov, L.: Drug therapy before and after the electroconversion of cardiac dysrhythmias. Prog. Cardiovasc. Dis., 16:531, 1974.

Resnekov, L., and McDonald, L.: Complications in 220 patients with cardiac dysrhythmias treated by phased direct current shock, and indications for electroconversion. Br. Heart J., 29:926, 1967.

Rifkin, R. D., Pandiah, N. E., Funai, J. T., et al.: Sensitivity of right atrial collapse and right ventricular diastolic collapse in the diagnosis of graded cardiac tamponade. Am. J. Noninvasive Cardiol., 1:73, 1987.

Ring, J., and Messmer, K.: Incidence and severity of anaphylactoid reactions to colloid volume substitutes. Lancet, 1:466, 1977.

Roberts, A. J., Woodhall, D. D., Conti, C. R., et al.: Mortality, morbidity, and cost-accounting related to coronary artery bypass graft surgery in the elderly. Ann. Thorac. Surg., 39:426, 1985.

Rodriguez, J. L., Weissman, C., Damask, M. C., et al.: Physiologic requirements during rewarming: Suppression of the shivering response. Crit. Care Med., 11:490, 1983.

Rohrer, M. J., and Natale, A. M.: Effect of hypothermia on the coagulation cascade. Crit. Care Med., 20:1402, 1992.

Rombeau, J. L., and Caldwell, M. D. (eds): Parenteral Nutrition: Clinical Nutrition. Vol. 2. Philadelphia, W. B. Saunders, 1986.

Rose, D. M., Ranson, J. H. C., Cunningham, J. N., Jr., and Spencer, F. C.: Patterns of severe pancreatic injury following cardiopulmonary bypass. Ann. Surg., 199:168, 1984.

Rose, H. D.: Venous catheter-associated candidemia. Am. J. Med. Sci., 275:265, 1978.

Rosemurgy, A. S., McAllister, E., and Karl, R. C.: The acute surgical abdomen after cardiac surgery involving extracorporeal circulation. Ann. Surg., 207:323, 1988.

Rotello, L. C., Warren, J., Jastremski, M. S., and Milewski, A.: A nurse-directed protocol using pulse oximetry to wean mechanically ventilated patients from toxic oxygen concentrations. Chest, 102:1833, 1992.

Royston, D., Bidstrup, B. P., and Taylor, K. M.: Effect of aprotinin on need for blood transfusion after repeat open-heart surgery. Lancet, 2:1289, 1987.

Rubin, D. A., Nieminski, K. E., Reed, G. E., and Herman, M. V.: Predictors, prevention, and long-term prognosis of atrial fibrillation after coronary artery bypass graft operations. J. Thorac. Cardiovasc. Surg., 94:331, 1987.

Ruskin, J. N.: The cardiac arrhythmia suppression trial (CAST). N. Engl. J. Med., 321:386, 1989.

Russo, A. M., O'Connor, W. H., and Waxman, H. L.: Atypical presentation and echocardiographic findings in patients with cardiac tamponade occurring early and late after cardiac surgery. Chest, 104:71, 1993.

Safar, P.: Cardiopulmonary cerebral resuscitation. In Shoemaker, W. C., Thompson, W. L., and Holbrook, P. R. (eds): Textbook of Critical Care. Chap. 2. Philadelphia, W. B. Saunders, 1984.

Safar, P.: Resuscitation from clinical death: pathophysiologic limits and therapeutic potentials. Crit. Care Med., 16:923, 1988.

Sagawa, K., Suga, H., Shoukas, A. A., and Bakalar, K. M.: Endsystolic pressure-volume ratio: A new index of contractility. Am. J. Cardiol., 40:748, 1979.

Sagawa, K., Sunagawa, K., and Maughan, W. L.: Ventricular endsystolic pressure-volume relations. In Levine, H. J., and Gaasch, W. H. (eds): The Ventricle. Boston, Martinus Nijhoff, 1985.

Sanfelippo, P. M., and Danielson, G. K.: Complications associated with median sternotomy. J. Thorac. Cardiovasc. Surg., 63:419, 1972.

Sarnoff, S. J., and Berglund, E.: Starling's law of the heart studied by means of simultaneous right and left ventricular function curves in the dog. Circulation, 9:706, 1954.

Sarr, M. G., Gott, V. L., and Townsend, T. R.: Mediastinal infection after cardiac surgery. Ann. Thorac. Surg., 38:415, 1984.

Savageau, J. A., Stanton, B-A., Jenkins, C. D., and Frater, R. W. M.: Neuropsychological dysfunction following elective cardiac operation. J. Thorac. Cardiovasc. Surg., 84:595, 1982.

Schaff, H. V., Hauer, J. M., Bell, W. R., et al.: Autotransfusion of shed mediastinal blood after cardiac surgery. J. Thorac. Cardiovasc. Surg., 75:632, 1978.

Schaff, H. V., Hauer, J. M., Gardner, T. J., et al.: Routine use of autotransfusion following cardiac surgery: Experience in 700 patients. Ann. Thorac. Surg., 27:493, 1979.

Schaff, H. V., Mashburn, J. P., McCarthy, P. M., et al.: Natriuresis during and early after cardiopulmonary bypass: Relationship to atrial natriuretic factor, aldosterone, and antidiuretic hormone. J. Thorac. Cardiovasc. Surg., 98:979, 1989.

Scheinman, M. M., Sullivan, R. W., Hutchinson, J. C., and Hyatt, K. H.: Clinical significance of changes in serum magnesium in patients undergoing cardiopulmonary bypass. J. Thorac. Cardiovasc. Surg., 61:135, 1971.

Schmaier, A. H.: Diagnosis and therapy of disseminated intravascular coagulation and activated coagulation. In Koepke, J. A. (ed): Laboratory Hematology. Vol. 2, Ch. 25. New York, Churchill Livingstone, 1984.

Schnapp, L. M., and Cohen, N. H.: Pulse oximetry. Uses and abuses. Chest, 98:1244, 1990.

Schuster, S. R., Kakvan, M., Vawter, G. F., and Narter, N.: An experimental study of the effect of mannitol during cardiopulmonary bypass. Circulation 29(Suppl.):I-72, 1964.

Schwartz, S. I., and Moore, E. E.: Techniques in hemostasis: Local hemostasis. Number 6 in a series of 7. Johnson & Johnson Medical, Inc. West Berlin, Innovative Publishing, 1990.

Schwartz, S. I., and Robertson, J. M.: Techniques in hemostasis. Evaluation of patient as hemostatic risk. Number 5 in a series of 7. Johnson & Johnson Patient Care, Inc. Marlton, Innovative Publishing, 1988.

Scott, W. J., Kessler, R., and Wernly, J. A.: Blood conservation in cardiac surgery. Ann. Thorac. Surg., 50:843, 1990.

Selzer, A., and Walter, R. M.: Adequacy of preoperative digitalis therapy in controlling ventricular rate in postoperative atrial fibrillation. Circulation, 34:119, 1966.

Serry, C., Bleck, P. C., Javid, H., et al.: Sternal wound complications. Management and results. J. Thorac. Cardiovasc. Surg., 80:861, 1980.

Sethi, G. K., Copeland, J. G., Goldman, S., et al.: Implications of preoperative administration of aspirin in patients undergoing coronary artery bypass grafting. Department of Veterans Affairs Cooperative Study on Antiplatelet Therapy. J. Am. Coll. Cardiol., 15:15, 1990.

Shabetai, R.: Changing concepts of cardiac tamponade. J. Am. Coll. Cardiol., 12:194, 1988a.

Shabetai, R.: Pericardial and cardiac pressure. Circulation, 77:1, 1988b.

Shafir, R., Weiss, J., Herman, O., et al.: Faulty sternotomy and complications after median sternotomy. J. Thorac. Cardiovasc. Surg., 96:310, 1988.

Shapira, N., Zabatino, S. M., Ahmed, S., et al.: Determinants of pulmonary function in patients undergoing coronary bypass operations. Ann. Thorac. Surg., 50:268, 1990.

Shapiro, J. M., Westphal, L. M., White, P. F., et al.: Midazolam infusion for sedation in the intensive care unit: Effect on adrenal function. Anesthesiology, 64:394, 1986.

Shapiro, W.: Correlative studies of serum digitalis levels and the arrhythmias of digitalis intoxication. Am. J. Cardiol., 41:852, 1978.

Shaw, P. I., Bates, D., Cartilage, N. E. F., et al.: Early neurologic complications of coronary artery bypass surgery. Br. Med. J., 291:1384, 1985.

Shibutani, K., Komatsu, T., Kubul, K., et al.: Critical level of oxygen delivery in anesthetized man. Crit. Care Med., 11:640, 1983.

Shoemaker, W. C.: Fluids and electrolytes in the acutely ill adult. In Shoemaker, W. C., Thompson, W. L., and Holbrook, P. R. (eds): Textbook of Critical Care. Ch. 82. Philadelphia, W. B. Saunders, 1984.

Shoemaker, W. C., Appel, P. L., and Kram, H. B.: Hemodynamic and oxygen transport responses in survivors and nonsurvivors of high-risk surgery. Crit. Care Med., 21:977, 1993.

Shoemaker, W. C., Montgomery, E. S., Kaplan, E., and Elwyn, D. H.: Physiologic patterns in surviving and nonsurviving shock patients. Arch. Surg., 106:630, 1973.

Shoemaker, W. C., Thompson, W. L., and Holbrook, P. R. (eds): Textbook of Critical Care. Philadelphia, W. B. Saunders, 1984, p. 119.

Shoemaker, W. C., and Tremper, K. K.: Transcutaneous Po_2 and Pco_2 monitoring in the adult. In Shoemaker, W. C., Thompson, W. L., and Holbrook, P. R. (eds): Textbook of Critical Care. Chap. 27. Philadelphia, W. B. Saunders, 1984.

Silverman, N. A., DuBrow, I., Kohler, J., and Levitsky, S.: Etiology of atrioventricular-conduction abnormalities following cardiac surgery. J. Surg. Res., 36:198, 1984.

Silverman, N. A., Wright, R., and Levitsky, S.: Efficacy of low-dose propranolol in preventing postoperative supraventricular tachyarrhythmias: A prospective, randomized study. Ann. Surg., 196:194, 1982.

Simpson, M. B., Jr.: Adverse reactions to transfusion therapy: Clinical and laboratory aspects. In Koepke, J. A. (ed): Laboratory Hematology. Vol. 2, Ch. 44. New York, Churchill Livingstone, 1984.

Singh, B. N., Collett, J. T., and Chew, C. Y. C.: New perspectives in the pharmacologic therapy of cardiac arrhythmias. Prog. Cardiovasc. Dis., 22:243, 1980.

Singh, B. N., and Nademanee, K.: Use of calcium antagonists for cardiac arrhythmias. Am. J. Cardiol., 59:153B, 1987.

Singh, B. N., and Williams, E. M. V.: A fourth class of anti-dysrhythmic action? Effect of verapamil on ouabain toxicity, on atrial and ventricular intracellular potentials, and on other features of cardiac function. Cardiovasc. Res., 6:109, 1972.

Singh, S., Wann, L. S., Schuchard, G. H., et al.: Right ventricular and right atrial collapse in patients with pericardial tamponade: A combined echocardiographic and hemodynamic study. Circulation, 70:966, 1984.

Siu, S. C., Kitzman, D. W., Sheedy, P. F., II, and Northcutt, R. C.: Adrenal insufficiency from bilateral adrenal hemorrhage. Mayo Clin. Proc., 65:664, 1990.

Skillington, P. D., Couper, G. S., Peigh, P. S., et al.: Pulmonary artery balloon counterpulsion for intraoperative acute right ventricular failure. Ann. Thorac. Surg., 51:658, 1991.

Skinner, N. S., Jr., Mitchell, J. H., Wallace, A. G., and Sarnoff, S. J.: Hemodynamic effects of altering the timing of atrial systole. Am. J. Physiol., 205:499, 1963.

Sladen, A., Laver, M. B., and Pontoppidan, H.: Pulmonary complications and water retention in prolonged mechanical ventilation. N. Engl. J. Med., 279:448, 1968.

Sladen, R. N., Renaghan, D., Ashton, J. P., and Wyner, J.: Reliability of end-tidal CO_2 monitoring after cardiac surgery [ASA Abstract]. Anesthesiology, 63:A142, 1985.

Sladen, R. N., and Rosenthal, M. H.: Specific afterload reduction with parenteral hydralazine following cardiac surgery. J. Thorac. Cardiovasc. Surg., 78:195, 1979.

Slag, M. F., Morley, J. E., Elson, M. K., et al.: Hypothyroxinemia in critically ill patients as a predictor of high mortality. J. A. M. A., 245:43, 1981.

Smith, C. R., and Schwartz, S. I.: Amylase: Creatinine clearance ratios, serum amylase, and lipase after operations with cardiopulmonary bypass. Surgery, 94:458, 1983.

Smith, P. K., Buhrman, W. C., Ferguson, T. B., Jr., et al.: Conduction block following cardioplegic arrest: Prevention by augmented atrial hypothermia. Circulation, 68(Suppl.):II-41, 1983a.

Smith, P. K., Buhrman, W. C., Ferguson, T. B., Jr., et al.: Relationship of atrial hypothermia and cardioplegic solution potassium concentration to postoperative conduction defects. Surg. Forum, 34:304, 1983b.

Smith, P. K., Buhrman, W. C., Levett, J. M., et al.: Supraventricular conduction abnormalities following cardiac operations: A complication of inadequate atrial preservation. J. Thorac. Cardiovasc. Surg., 85:105, 1983c.

Smith, P. K., Tyson, G. S., Hammon, J. W., Jr., et al.: Cardiovascular effects of ventilation with positive end expiratory pressure. Ann. Surg., 195:121, 1982.

SOLVD (Studies of Left Ventricular Dysfunction). Rationale, design and methods: Two trials that evaluate the effect of enalapril in patients with reduced ejection fraction. Am. J. Cardiol., 66:315, 1990.

Sonnenblick, E. H., Frishman, W. H., and LeJemtel, T. H.: Dobuta-mine: A new synthetic cardioactive sympathetic amine. N. Engl. J. Med., 300:17, 1979.

Sonnenblick, E. H., and Skelton, C. L.: Oxygen consumption of the heart: Physiologic principles and clinical implications. Mod. Conc. Cardiovasc. Dis., 40:9, 1971.

Spencer, F. C., and Skinner, D. B.: The role of the surgeon in the intensive care unit. J. Thorac. Cardiovasc. Surg., 88:483, 1984.

Spiess, B. D., Tuman, K. J., McCarthy, R. J., et al.: Thromboelastogra-phy as an indicator of post-cardiopulmonary bypass coagu-lopathies. J. Clin. Monit., 3:25, 1987.

Spodick, D. H.: The normal and diseased pericardium: Current concepts of pericardial physiology, diagnosis and treatment. J. Am. Coll. Cardiol., 1:240, 1983.

St. John Sutton, M., Pfeffer, M. A., Plappert, T., et al.: Quantitative two-dimensional echocardiographic measurements are major predictors of adverse cardiovascular events after acute myocar-dial infarction. The protective effects of captopril. Circulation, 89:68, 1994.

Stanton, M. S., Prystowsky, E. N., Fineberg, N. S., et al.: Arrhythmo-genic effects of antiarrhythmic drugs: A study of 506 patients treated for ventricular tachycardia or fibrillation. J. Am. Coll. Cardiol., 14:209, 1989.

Steel, K., Gertman, P. M., Crescenzi, C., and Anderson, J.: Iatrogenic illness on a general medical service at a university hospital. N. Engl. J. Med., 304:638, 1981.

Stephenson, L. W., Blackstone, E. H., and Kouchoukos, N. T.: Dopa-mine vs epinephrine in patients following cardiac surgery: Randomized study. Surg. Forum, 27:272, 1976.

Stephenson, L. W., MacVaugh, H., Tomasello, D. N., and Josephson, M. E.: Propanolol for prevention of postoperative cardiac ar-rhythmias: A randomized study. Ann. Thorac. Surg., 29:113, 1980.

Stevenson, L. W., Child, J. S., Laks, H., and Kern, L.: Incidence and significance of early pericardial effusions after cardiac surgery. Am. J. Cardiol., 54:848, 1984.

Stibbe, J., Kluft, C., Brommer, E. J. P., Gomes, M., et al.: Enhanced fibrinolytic activity during cardiopulmonary bypass in open-heart surgery in man is caused by extrinsic (tissue-type) plas-minogen activator. Eur. J. Clin. Invest., 14:375, 1984.

Stinson, E. B., Holloway, E. L., Derby, G. C., et al.: Comparative hemodynamic responses to chlorpromazine, nitroprusside, ni-troglycerin, and trimethaphan immediately after open-heart operations. Circulation, 52(Suppl.)I:26, 1975.

Stinson, E. B., Holloway, E. L., Derby, G. C., et al.: Control of myocardial performance early after open-heart operations by vasodilator treatment. J. Thorac. Cardiovasc. Surg., 73:523, 1977.

Stoney, W. S., Alford, W. C., Jr., Burrus, G. R., et al.: Air embolism and other accidents using pump oxygenators. Ann. Thorac. Surg., 29:336, 1980.

Stoney, W. S., Alford, W. C., Jr., Burrus, G. R., et al.: Median sternotomy dehiscence. Ann. Thorac. Surg., 26:421, 1978.

Stoutenbeek, C. P., van Saene, H. K. F., Miranda, D. R., and Zandstra, D. F.: The effect of selective decontamination of the diges-tive tract on colonisation and infection rate in multiple trauma patients. Intensive Care Med., 10:185, 1984.

Strauss, R. E.: Volume replacement and coagulation: A comparative review. J. Cardiovasc. Anaesth., 2(Suppl.): 24, 1988.

Streitz, J. M., Jr., and Maggs, P. R.: Fatal hypoxemia following mitral valve replacment. Ann. Thorac. Surg., 46:104, 1988.

Strobeck, J. E., and Sonnenblick, E. H.: Myocardial contractile prop-erties and ventricular performance. In Fozzard, H. A., et al. (eds): The Heart and Cardiovascular System. New York, Raven Press, 1986.

Surawicz, B.: Prognosis of ventricular arrhythmias in relation to sudden cardiac death: Therapeutic implications. J. Am. Coll. Cardiol., 10:435, 1987.

Susini, G., Zucchetti, M., Bortone, F., et al.: Isolated ultrafiltration in cardiogenic pulmonary edema. Crit. Care Med., 18:14, 1990.

Sutton, R. G., Kratz, J. M., Spinale, F. G., and Crawford, F. A.: Comparison of three blood-processing techniques during and after cardiopulmonary bypass. Ann. Thorac. Surg., 56:938, 1993.

Sveinsson, I. S.: Postoperative psychosis after heart surgery. J. Thorac. Cardiovasc. Surg., 70:717, 1975.

Svensson, L. G., Decker, G., and Kinsley, R. B.: A prospective study of hyperamylasemia and pancreatitis after cardiopulmonary bypass. Ann. Thorac. Surg., 39:409, 1985.

Swan, H. J. C., Forrester, J. S., and Diamond, G.: Hemodynamic spectrum of MI and cardiogenic shock. Circulation, 45:1097, 1972.

Szekely, P.: Systemic embolism and anticoagulant prophylaxis in rheumatic heart disease. Br. Med. J., 1:209, 1964.

Taggart, D. P., Siddiqui, A., and Wheatley, D. J.: Low-dose preoper-ative aspirin therapy, postoperative blood loss, and transfusion requirements. Ann. Thorac. Surg., 50:424, 1990.

Tajimi, K., Kosugi, I., Hamamoto, F., and Kobayashi, K.: Plasma catecholamine levels and hemodynamic responses of severely acidotic dogs to dopamine infusion. Crit. Care Med., 11:817, 1983.

Task Force on Guidelines, Society of Critical Care Medicine. Recom-mendations for critical care unit design. Crit. Care Med., 16:796, 1988.

Taub, J. M., and Berger, R. J.: Acute shifts in the sleep-wakefulness cycle: Effects on performance and mood. Psychosom. Med., 36:164, 1974.

Taylor, K. M., Brannan, J. J., Bain, W. H., et al.: Role of angiotensin II in the development of peripheral vasoconstriction during cardiopulmonary bypass. Cardiovasc. Res., 13:269, 1979.

Taylor, K. M., Morton, I. J., Brown, J. J., et al.: Hypertension and the renin-angiotensin system following open-heart surgery. J. Thorac. Cardiovasc. Surg., 74:840, 1977.

Thompson, J. F., and Chant, A. D.: Autotransfusion of shed medias-tinal blood. Ann. Thorac. Surg., 48:887, 1989.

Thurer, R. J., Bognolo, D., Vargas, A., et al.: The management of mediastinal infection following cardiac surgery: An experience using continuous irrigation with povidone-iodine. J. Thorac. Cardiovasc. Surg., 68:962, 1974.

Thurer, R. L., Lytle, B. W., Cosgrove, D. M., and Loop, F. D.: Autotransfusion following cardiac operations: A randomized, prospective study. Ann. Thorac. Surg., 27:500, 1979.

Townes, B. D., Bashein, G., Hornbein, T. F., et al.: Neurobehavioral outcomes in cardiac operations. A prospective controlled study. J. Thorac. Cardiovasc. Surg., 98:774, 1989.

Toy, P. T. L. Y., Strauss, R. E., Stehling, L. C., et al.: Predeposited autologous blood for elective surgery. N. Engl. J. Med., 316:517, 1987.

Tufo, H. M., Ostfeld, A. M., and Shekelle, R.: Central nervous system dysfunction following open-heart surgery. J. A. M. A., 212:1333, 1970.

Tuteur, P. G.: Pneumonia after coronary artery bypass grafting: A case for continued evaluation. Ann. Thorac. Surg., 51:177, 1991.

Tyberg, J. V., Taichman, G. C., Smith, E. R., et al.: The relationship between pericardial pressure and right atrial pressure: an intra-operative study. Circulation, 73:428, 1986.

Tyras, D. H., and Willman, V. L.: Paraplegia following intra-aortic balloon assistance. Ann. Thorac. Surg., 25:164, 1978.

Tyson, G. S., Sladen, R. N., Spainhour, V., et al.: Blood conservation in cardiac surgery. Preliminary results with an institutional commitment. Ann. Surg., 209:736, 1989.

Ulicny, K. S., Jr., and Hiratzka, L. F.: The risk factors of median sternotomy infection: A current review. J Cardiac Surg., 6:338, 1991.

Uppal, R., Craig, D., Glower, D., et al.: Right ventricular systolic performance in a porcine model [Abstract]. J. Am. Coll. Cardiol., 21:412A, 1993.

Utley, J. R.: Renal effects of cardiopulmonary bypass. In Utley, J. R. (ed): Pathophysiology and Techniques of Cardiopulmonary Bypass. Vol. I. Baltimore, Williams & Wilkins, 1982, pp. 40–54.

van der Linden, J., and Casimir-Ahn, H.: When do cerebral emboli appear during open heart operations? A transcranial Doppler study. Ann. Thorac. Surg., 51:237, 1991.

Vander Salm, T. J.: Brachial plexus injury after open-heart surgery [Letter]. Ann. Thorac. Surg., 38:660, 1984.

Vander Salm, T. J., Ansell, J. E., Okike, O. N., et al.: The role of epsilon-aminocaproic acid in reducing bleeding after cardiac operation: A double blind randomized study. J. Thorac. Cardiovasc. Surg., 95:538, 1988.

van Oeveren, W., Harder, M. P., Roozendaal, K. J., et al.: Aprotinin protects platelets against the initial effect of cardiopulmonary bypass. J. Thorac. Cardiovasc. Surg., 99:788, 1990.

Van Trigt, P., Spray, T. L., Pasque, M. K., et al.: The influence of time on the response to dopamine after coronary artery bypass grafting: Assessment of left ventricular performance and contractility using pressure/dimension analyses. Ann. Thorac. Surg., 35:3, 1983.

Vargas, F. S., Cukier, A., Terra-Filho, M., et al.: Influence of atelectasis on pulmonary function after coronary artery bypass grafting. Chest, 104:434, 1993.

Vargas, F. S., Cukier, A., Terra-Filho, M., et al.: Relationship between pleural changes after myocardial revascularization and pulmonary mechanics. Chest, 102:1333, 1992.

Vaughn, S., and Puri, V. K.: Cardiac output changes and continuous mixed venous oxygen saturation measurement in the critically ill. Crit. Care Med., 16:495, 1988.

Venus, B., Prager, R., Patel, C. B., et al.: Cardiopulmonary effects of intralipid infusion in critically ill patients. Crit. Care Med., 16:587, 1988.

Vernon, D. D., Garrett, J. S., Banner, W., Jr., and Dean, J. M.: Hemodynamic effects of dobutamine in an intact animal model. Crit. Care Med., 20:1322, 1992.

Veterans Affairs Total Parenteral Nutrition Cooperation Study Group. Perioperative total parenteral nutrition in surgical patients. N. Engl. J. Med., 325:525, 1991.

Videm, V., Fosse, E., Mollnes, T. E., et al.: Time for new concepts about measurement of complement activation by cardiopulmonary bypass? Ann. Thorac. Surg., 54:725, 1992.

Vlay, S. C.: How the university cardiologist treats ventricular premature beats: A nationwide survey of 65 university medical centers. Am. Heart J., 110:904, 1985.

Wade, O. L., and Bishop, J. M.: Cardiac Output in Regional Blood Flow. Oxford, Blackwell Scientific Publications, 1962.

Wagner, C. W., Nesbit, R. R., and Mansberger, A. R., Jr.: The use of intravenous hydrochloric acid in the treatment of thirty-four patients with metabolic alkalosis. Am. Surg., 46:140, 1980.

Wahl, G. W., Swinburne, A. J., Fedullo, A. J., et al.: Effect of age and preoperative airway obstruction on lung function after coronary artery bypass grafting. Ann. Thorac. Surg., 56:104, 1993.

Waldo, A. L., MacLean, W. A. H., Karp, R. B., et al.: Entrainment and interruption of atrial flutter with atrial pacing. Circulation, 56:737, 1977.

Walls, J. T., Curtis, J. J., Silver, D., et al.: Heparin-induced thrombocytopenia in open heart surgical patients: Sequelae of late recognition. Ann. Thorac. Surg., 53:787, 1992.

Wanebo, H., Mathewson, C., and Conolly, B.: Pseudo-obstruction of the colon. Surg. Gynecol. Obstet., 133:44, 1971.

Wareing, T. H., Davila-Roman, V. G., Daily, B. B., et al.: Strategy for the reduction of stroke incidence in cardiac surgical patients. Ann. Thorac. Surg., 55:1400, 1993.

Warltier, D. C., Zyvoloski, M., Gross, G. J., et al.: Redistribution of myocardial blood flow distal to a dynamic coronary arterial stenosis by sympathomimetic amines: Comparison of dopamine, dobutamine and isoproterenol. Am. J. Cardiol., 48:269, 1981.

Watanabe, T., Covell, J. W., Maroko, P. R., et al.: Effects of increased arterial pressure and positive inotropic agents on the severity of myocardial ischemia in the acutely depressed heart. Am. J. Cardiol., 30:371, 1972.

Watson, B. G., Elliott, M. J., Pay, D. A., and Williamson, M.: Diabetes mellitus and open-heart surgery. Anaesthesia, 41:250, 1986.

Weber, F. L., Jr.: Liver dysfunction in critical care medicine. In Shoemaker, W. C., Thompson, W. L., and Holbrook, P. R. (eds): Textbook of Critical Care. Ch. 78. Philadelphia, W. B. Saunders, 1984.

Wedley, J. R., Lunn, H. F., and Vale, R. J.: Studies of temperature balance after open heart surgery. Crit. Care Med., 3:134, 1975.

Weeks, K. R., Chatterjee, K., Block, S., et al.: Bedside hemodynamic monitoring. J. Thorac. Cardiovasc. Surg., 71:250, 1976.

Weigelt, J. A.: A future for surgical critical care? Ann. Surg., 206:809, 1987.

Weil, M. H., and Afifi, A. A.: Experimental and clinical studies on lactate and pyruvate as indicators of the severity of acute circulatory failure. Circulation, 41:989, 1970.

Weiner, B., Rheinlander, H. F., Decker, E. L., and Cleveland, R. J.: Digoxin prophylaxis following coronary artery bypass surgery. Clin. Pharmacol., 5:55, 1986.

Weinstein, G. S., Rao, P. S., Vretakis, G., and Tyras, D. H.: Serial changes in renal function in cardiac surgical patients. Ann. Thorac. Surg., 48:72, 1989.

Weinstein, G. S., Zabetakis, P. M., Clavel, A., et al.: The renin-angiotensin system is not responsible for hypertension following coronary artery bypass grafting. Ann. Thorac. Surg., 43:74, 1987.

Weitzman, L. B., Tinker, P., Kronzon, I., et al.: The incidence and natural history of pericardial effusion after cardiac surgery—an echocardiographic study. Circulation, 69:506, 1984.

Wellens, H. J.: Atrial flutter: Progress, but no final answer [Editorial]. J. Am. Coll. Cardiol., 17:1235, 1991.

Wellens, H. J. J.: A practical approach to proarrhythmic effects of antiarrhythmic drugs. ACC Current Journal Review, April/May 1993.

Welling, R. E., Rath, R., Albers, J. E., and Glaser, R. S.: Gastrointestinal complications after cardiac surgery. Arch. Surg., 121:1178, 1986.

Wenger, R. K., Lukasiewicz, H., Mikuta, B. S., et al.: Loss of platelet fibrinogen receptors during clinical cardiopulmonary bypass. J. Thorac. Cardiovasc. Surg., 97:235, 1989.

Westaby, S.: Aprotinin in perspective. Ann. Thorac. Surg., 55:1033, 1993.

Westaby, S.: Organ dysfunction after cardiopulmonary bypass. A systemic inflammatory reaction initiated by the extracorporeal circuit. Intern. Care Med., 13:89, 1987.

Wheeler, A. P.: Sedation, analgesia, and paralysis in the intensive care unit. Chest, 104:566, 1993.

Whelton, P. K., Flaherty, J. T., MacAllister, N. P., et al.: Hypertension following coronary artery bypass surgery. Role of preoperative propranolol therapy. Hypertension, 2:291, 1980.

Williams, T. W., Jr.: The staphylococcus: A reemerging problem in prosthetic surgery. Contemp. Surg., 32(3-A):15, 1988.

Wilson, R. F., and Walt, A. F.: Blood replacement. In Walt, A. F., and Wilson, R. F. (eds): Management of Trauma: Practices and Pitfalls. Philadelphia, Lea & Febiger, 1975.

Wisch, N., Litwak, R. S., Luckban, S. B., and Glass, J. L.: Hematologic complications of open heart surgery. Am. J. Cardiol., 31:282, 1973.

Woeber, K. A., and Maddux, B. A.: Thyroid hormone binding in nonthyroid illness. Metabolism, 30:412, 1981.

Wojtalik, R. S., Lindenauer, S. M., and Kahn, S. S.: Perforation of the colon associated with adynamic ileus. Am. J. Surg., 125:601, 1973.

Wolfe, J. H. N., Waller, D. G., Chapman, M. B., et al.: The effect of hemodilution upon patients with intermittent claudication. Surg. Gynecol. Obstet., 160:347, 1985.

Woosley, R. L.: Indications for antiarrhythmic therapy: A wealth of controversy, a dearth of data. Ann. Intern. Med., 108:450, 1988.

Wormser, G. P., Onorato, I. M., Preminger, T. J., et al.: Sensitivity and specificity of blood cultures obtained through intravascular catheters. Crit. Care Med., 18:152, 1990.

Yeboah, E. D., Petrie, A., and Pead, J. L.: Acute renal failure and open heart surgery. Br. Med. J., 1:415, 1972.

Young, J. A., Kisker, C. T., and Doty, D. B.: Adequate anticoagulation during cardiopulmonary bypass determined by activated clotting time and the appearance of fibrin monomer. Ann. Thorac. Surg., 26:231, 1978.

Yu, M., Levy, M. M., Smith, P., Takiguchi, S. A., et al.: Effect of maximizing oxygen delivery on morbidity and mortality rates in critically ill patients: A prospective, randomized, controlled study. Crit. Care Med., 21:830, 1993.

Yusuf, S.: Interventions that potentially limit myocardial infarct size: Overview of clinical trials. Am. J. Cardiol., 60:11A, 1987.

Zaloga, G. P., Strickland, R. A., Butterworth, J. F., IV, et al.: Calcium attenuates epinephrine's beta-adrenergic effects in postoperative heart surgery patients. Circulation, 81:196, 1990.

Zeff, R. H., Iannone, L. A., Kongtahworn, C., et al.: Coronary artery spasm following coronary artery revascularization. Ann. Thorac. Surg., 34:196, 1982.

Zelis, R., Mansour, E. J., Capone, R. J., and Mason, D. T.: The cardiovascular effects of morphine. J. Clin. Invest., 54:1247, 1974.

Zinner, M. J., Rypins, E. B., Martin, L. R., et al.: Misoprostol versus antacid titration for preventing stress ulcers in postoperative surgical ICU patients. Ann. Surg., *210*:590, 1989.

Zipes, D. P.: Proarrhythmic events. Am. J. Cardiol., *61*:70A, 1988.

Zoll, P. M.: Resuscitation of the heart in ventricular standstill by external electric stimulation. N. Engl. J. Med., *247*:768, 1952.

Zurick, A. M., Urzua, J., Ghattas, M., et al.: Failure of positive end-expiratory pressure to decrease postoperative bleeding after cardiac surgery. Ann. Thorac. Surg., *34*:608, 1982.

Zwischenberger, J. B., Kirsh, M. M., Dechert, R. E., et al.: Suppression of shivering decreases oxygen consumption and improves hemodynamic stability during postoperative rewarming. Ann. Thorac. Surg., *43*:428, 1987.

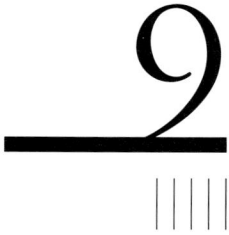

9 Tracheal Intubation and Assisted Ventilation

■ I Tracheal Intubation and Assisted Ventilation: The Anesthesiologist's Viewpoint

Robert N. Sladen, Bret Stolp, and Neil R. MacIntyre

HISTORICAL BACKGROUND

Laryngoscopy and Tracheal Intubation

The first use of elective oral intubation is credited to a Scottish surgeon, William Macewan, who placed flexible metal tubes in patients with airway obstruction to facilitate chloroform anesthesia in 1878 (Macewan, 1880). A few years later, an American surgeon, Joseph O'Dwyer, designed a series of metal tubes first used to relieve vocal cord obstruction during diphtheria, and subsequently modified to provide artificial ventilation during thoracic surgery (Calverly, 1989). O'Dwyer's method was adapted around 1905 for anesthetic use by a German, Franz Kuhn (Fig. 9–1). Kuhn's tubes, made of flexible coiled tubing, were passed blindly into the larynx over an introducer guided by the left hand. Laryngeal gauze packing protected the airway. In describing his experiences with Kuhn's tube in a prisoner-of-war hospital during World War I, Stanley Sykes (Sykes, 1960) commented that it had "one great and solid advantage over modern methods. It does not depend on dry batteries. Kuhn's tube was simple, reliable, durable, immutable, imperishable, insusceptible to damage and absolutely indestructible. There was nothing to go wrong, nothing to damage." Would that we could say the same about modern equipment! Major advances in airway management after World War I were made by the British anesthetists Sir Ivan Magill (1888–1986) and Stanley Rowbotham, who introduced the "sniff" position, blind nasotracheal intubation (first used to deal with military facial injuries), the Magill angulated forceps, red rubber endotracheal tubes, and topical anesthesia with cocaine (Calverley, 1989). In the American Midwest in the 1930s, Arthur Guedel and Ralph Waters pioneered the cuffed endotracheal tube and endobronchial tube. In 1941, Robert Miller in San Antonio, Texas, introduced the straight laryngoscope blade, and in 1943, Robert MacIntosh at Oxford University introduced the curved laryngoscope blade (Calverley, 1989; Miller, 1941). Today, these blades are still used by every anesthesiologist in the world.

Mechanical Ventilation

The brilliant Paduan anatomist, Andreas Vesalius, described a technique of resuscitation of animals via tracheostomy and bellows in 1555 in his great work, *De Humani Corporis Fabrica*. A hundred years later, the experiment was repeated by Robert Hooke in London. However, modern resuscitation stems from the Dutch, who in 1767 formed The Society for the Rescue of Drowned Persons, using mouth-to-mouth breathing to revive citizens of Amsterdam who had had the misfortune to fall into a canal (Mörch, 1985). Initial attempts at long-term mechanical ventilation were based on the application of subambient or negative pressure to the thorax. This led to the development of the first workable tank respirator, or "iron lung," which completely encased the patient's body, by Woillez in Paris in 1876 (Mörch, 1985). Over the next 50 years, refinements were made by Drinker at Harvard, Krogh in Denmark, and J. H. Emerson in Boston that culminated in the iron lungs and cuirass ventilators used for the victims of poliomyelitis from the 1930s to the 1950s.

Positive-pressure ventilation (PPV) remained largely confined to small hand-held resuscitators, culminating in the *air-mask-bag unit* (AMBU) developed in 1955 by Rubin. However, in 1940 in German-occupied Denmark, Ernst Trier Mörch invented the first piston-driven volume ventilator, which was used during thoracic surgery for the next 10 years. An important stimulus to the development of modern positive-pressure ventilators was provided by the severe poliomyelitis epidemic in Denmark in 1952. Under the leadership of Bjørn Ibsen, teams of nurse-anesthetists, interns, and medical students provided round-the-clock manual ventilation to hundreds of intubated patients stricken with respiratory paralysis. The basic principles of suctioning, airway care, and chest physical therapy were established during this time. In the United States, *intermittent positive-pressure breathing* (IPPB) treatments were popularized by the development of the compact and simple Bird pressure-cycled ventilator in Palm Springs and were soon applied to long-term ventilation. Volume ventilators developed

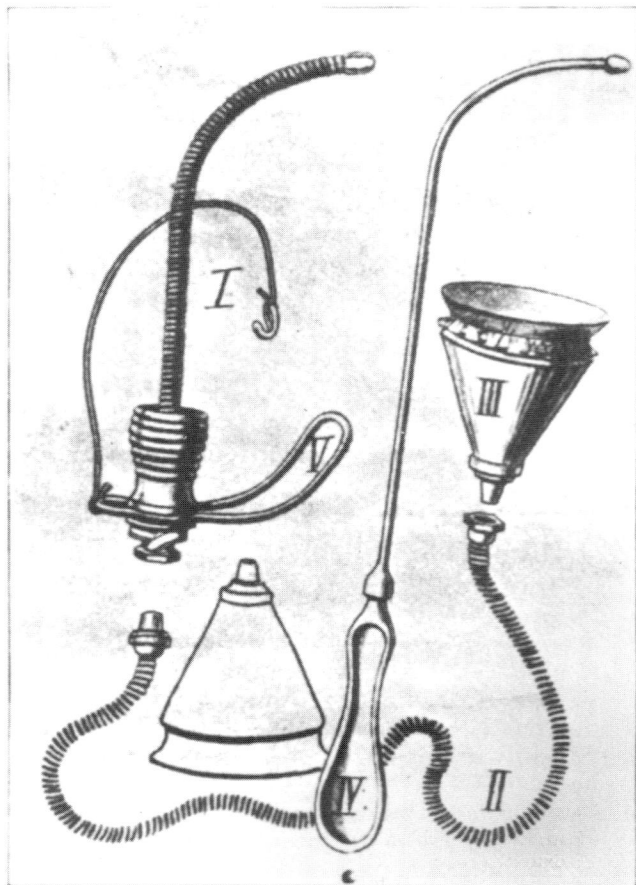

FIGURE 9–1. Franz Kuhn's metal intubating apparatus (1905). *I*, Flexible intratracheal tube with wire loop, string, and hook for fixation (although in practice the tube was kept in place by gauze packed into the pharynx to protect the larynx). The tube was threaded over an introducer *(IV)*, which was guided into the larynx by the index finger of the left hand ("tactile intubation"). *II*, Tube to connect the intratracheal tube to the cone and gauze *(III)* onto which ether or chloroform was poured. (From Sykes, W. S., and Ellis, R. H.: Essays on the First Hundred Years of Anaesthesia. Vol III. Edinburgh, Churchill Livingstone, 1982, p. 109. Used with permission.)

by Bennett in the United States and Engström in Sweden provided fierce competition. Subsequent milestones have included: the introduction of *positive end-expiratory pressure* (PEEP) in anesthesia in 1959 by Frumin and co-workers and its application for the treatment of *adult respiratory distress syndrome* (ARDS) by Ashbaugh and colleagues in 1969; the invention of *intermittent mandatory ventilation* (IMV) in 1971 by Kirby and associates; and the introduction of high-frequency ventilation by Sjöstrand (1977) in Sweden in 1967. Since the mid-1980s, there has been an exponential increase in the pace of development in mechanical ventilation.

TRACHEAL INTUBATION

Airway management is an essential skill for all those caring for critically ill patients. Although anes-

thesiologists and respiratory therapists are frequently close at hand for emergency airway management, all personnel should understand the fundamentals of airway support because initial management may determine the ultimate outcome in critical situations. The most important first step is to secure the airway and provide adequate oxygenation and ventilation prior to tracheal intubation. This may entail simple maintenance of a patent airway in a spontaneously ventilating patient or assisted or controlled ventilation by mask. Premature, futile, or prolonged attempts at tracheal intubation may cause unnecessary hypoxemia, airway irritation, and bleeding and may jeopardize successful resuscitation. In this section, therefore, methods to control the airway without tracheal intubation are described first.

Ventilation Without Tracheal Intubation

Obtaining Access to the Airway

THE "SNIFF" POSITION

The most important consideration in preparation for mask ventilation or tracheal intubation is to align three anatomic axes: oral, pharyngeal, and laryngeal (Fig. 9–2). When the head is in the neutral position, the axes represented by straight lines parallel to the oral, pharyngeal, and laryngeal cavities are about 70 degrees to each other (Fig. 9–2A). The first essential step is to place a pad—pillow, folded towel, or other soft object—under the patient's occiput to flex the neck on the chest. This aligns the pharyngeal and laryngeal axes (Fig. 9–2B). Next, the head should be extended on the neck at the level of the atlanto-occipital joint (head tilt), which aligns the oral axis with the other two axes (Fig. 9–2C). Thus, a straight, open passage is created from the oral aperture to the glottis (the mentum-geniohyoid-hyoid-thyroid line), which provides optimal conditions for both mask ventilation and direct laryngoscopy. Flexion of the neck on the chest coupled with extension of the head on the neck mimics the position assumed "standing before the open bedroom window sniffing the morning air" first described by Sir Ivan Magill (Calverley, 1989); the name *"sniff" position* serves as a useful reminder of the angulation required. A common positioning error made by inexperienced personnel is to extend the head on the neck without flexing the neck on the chest—sometimes to the extent of allowing the patient's head to hang over the end of the bed. As illustrated in Figure 9–2D, the oral axis now forms a right angle with the pharyngeal and laryngeal axes. This may compromise mask ventilation and render visualization of the glottis by laryngoscopy almost impossible without excessive leverage on the upper teeth, gums, and lip (Benumof, 1992).

RELIEF OF UPPER AIRWAY OBSTRUCTION

Loss of consciousness, anesthesia, or the use of muscle relaxants allows the tongue and epiglottis to

Head Position and the Axes of the Upper Airway

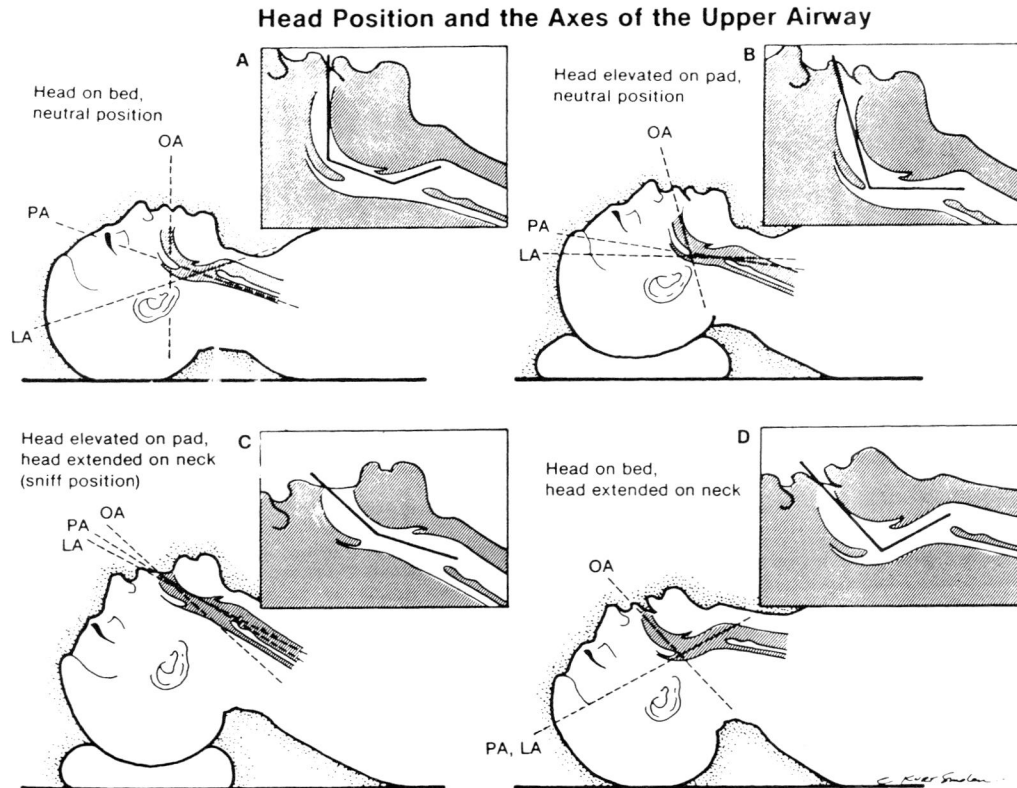

FIGURE 9–2. Alignment of oral, pharyngeal, and laryngeal axes. *A,* Head in neutral position. Note marked angulation of the oral (OA), pharyngeal (PA), and laryngeal (LA) axes. *B,* Back of head elevated on large pad, flexing neck on chest. This aligns the LA with the PA. This is the most important first step in positioning the head. *C,* Second step: Extend head on neck. This brings the OA into alignment with the LA and PA—the "sniff" position. This provides the most patent airway and direct access to the larynx, whether mask ventilation or direct laryngoscopy and tracheal intubation are planned. *D,* A common error: The head is extended on the neck without elevation of the occiput (i.e., without neck flexion). This results in nonalignment of the OA with the PA and LA. (*A–D,* From Benumof, J. L.: Conventional [laryngoscopic] orotracheal and nasotracheal intubation [single-lumen type]. *In* Benumof, J. L. [ed]: Clinical Procedures in Anesthesia and Intensive Care. Philadelphia, J. B. Lippincott, 1992, p. 123.)

fall back and obstruct the pharynx and the glottis, respectively. Partial airway obstruction at the level of the hypopharynx is indicated by snoring, and obstruction at the level of the glottis or larynx is indicated by stridor. Complete airway obstruction obliterates breath sounds or palpable air movement and induces marked subdiaphragmatic, intercostal and suprasternal retraction ("tracheal tug"). Progressive agitation and hypoxemia follow and require urgent relief.

The mouth and pharynx should be swept by a finger or suctioned to clear the airway of foreign objects such as teeth, vomited food particles, or other secretions. The most useful position to open the airway in an emergency situation in an unconscious patient is the triple maneuver (Fig. 9–3), which consists of head tilt, jaw thrust, and mouth opening (McGee and Vender, 1992). The head tilt, described earlier, should be accomplished by pressure on the forehead accompanied by a forward chin lift, which pulls the tongue away from the posterior pharyngeal wall. The jaw thrust is performed by hooking the fingers behind the angles of the mandible, depressing the mentum, and pulling directly anteriorly, thus subluxating the jaw at the temporomandibular joint.

This heightens the movement of the tongue away from the posterior pharyngeal wall. The mouth is opened slightly to facilitate exhalation.

Mask Ventilation

Once the airway has been rendered patent, the adequacy of ventilation should be assessed. If chest and diaphragmatic excursion are poor or discoordinate, and if a satisfactory level of arterial oxygen saturation (90% or greater) cannot be sustained with supplemental oxygen, PPV by face mask must be applied. This may relieve the situation until the patient recovers or may provide a safe level of oxygenation before tracheal intubation.

TECHNIQUE OF MASK VENTILATION

Numerous types of face masks are available, but the following properties are most desirable: First, the mask should be made of clear plastic, so that any regurgitation or vomitus may be immediately visualized. Second, it should have a firm body so that sufficient downward pressure may be applied to the face to obtain a good mask fit, particularly in patients

Triple Airway Maneuver

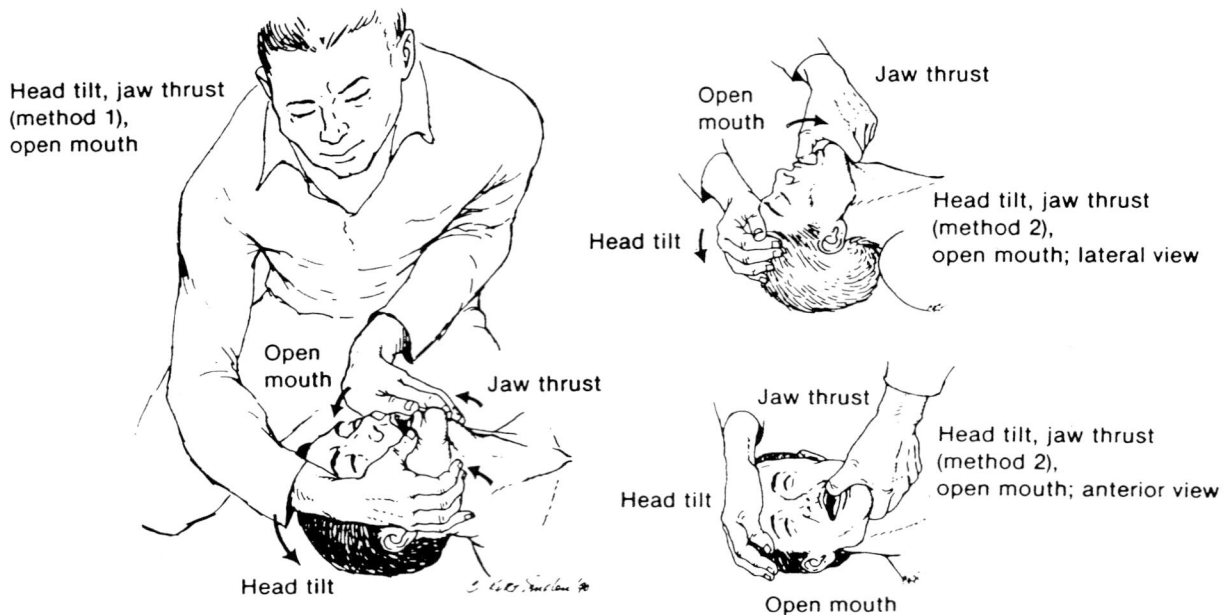

FIGURE 9–3. The triple maneuver. The triple maneuver consists of head tilt, jaw thrust, and mouth opening. In method 1 *(left)*, the hands are positioned in parallel alongside the patient's head. The fourth and fifth fingers curl behind the angles of the jaw, while the thumbs open the mouth and allow the mandible to slide in front of the incisors. Head tilt is provided by pressure from the palms and wrists. In method 2 *(right)*, the right hand presses down on the forehead, while the left hand clasps the mentum and pulls it forward, opening the mouth and providing jaw thrust. (From McGee, J. P., II, and Vender, J. S.: Nonintubation management of the airway. *In* Benumof, J. L. [ed]: Clinical Procedures in Anesthesia and Intensive Care. Philadelphia, J. B. Lippincott, 1992, p. 96.)

with flat facial features or large heads. Third, there should be a high-volume, low-pressure seal or cushion around the rim of its base that can be adjusted to conform to the patient's facial features. The collar of the mask is attached to a self-inflatable bag (AMBU) via a right-angled connector (elbow). The self-inflatable bag should have a reservoir (either a bag or wide-bore tubing) to ensure the delivery of a high-inspired oxygen fraction (FI_{O_2}). Some bags have the capability to provide up to 15 cm H_2O PEEP, which may be extremely helpful in patients with poor lung compliance.

The mask should be held in the left hand and applied to the patient's face with the narrowest part (the bridge) placed at the bridge of the nose. The operator's thumb and forefinger should be placed on either side of the connector and should compress the surface of the mask on the nasal and mental aspects, respectively. The fourth and fifth fingers should be curled around the ramus of the mandible, preferably hooked behind the angle of the jaw to provide forward thrust. Air seal is obtained by attempting to oppose the thumb and forefinger with the fourth and fifth fingers. The right hand holds and squeezes the inflatable bag to provide ventilation.

It is important to obtain a mask of a size appropriate to the patient. Care should be taken to avoid pressure on the eyes at the mask bridge and to avoid compressing the soft tissue under the jaw with the tips of the fourth and fifth fingers (in children, this

may completely obstruct the airway). The chin section of the mask should compress the alveolar ridge of the mandible; if the mask is too large, insertion of an oral airway (see later in this chapter) effectively lengthens the face by 1 to 2 cm (McGee and Vender, 1992).

To assist ventilation in a patient who is still breathing spontaneously, the operator should attempt to synchronize mask ventilation with the patient's own efforts. This is best achieved by closely watching the patient's chest. As soon as it starts to expand, the bag should be gently squeezed and then released to allow exhalation before the next effort. This ensures the maximal augmentation of ventilation, relieves distress in patients who are semiconscious or agitated, and if done appropriately, may allow the operator to gradually increase the size of the tidal volume and slow rapid rates of breathing. If mask ventilation is not timed properly and competes with the patient's own efforts, assistance may not only be quite ineffective but also hyperinflate the stomach, predisposing to regurgitation.

If the patient is apneic, the operator must control ventilation completely. Effectiveness of ventilation should be determined by the adequacy of chest excursion and auscultation of breath sounds by an assistant. If it is difficult to obtain a good seal, first ensure that the patient's head is in the proper "sniff" position, and then attempt to apply increased pressure between the thumb and the fifth finger holding the mask. Oxygen flow should be turned high; excess flow can be decompressed by slight elevation of the lower mask edge once successful ventilation is achieved. In difficult cases, more effective air movement is usually achieved by providing shallow, rapid breaths rather than by attempting large, slower inspirations. If the airway remains partially obstructed, the airway assist devices described later should be used. If it is still impossible to obtain a good seal, the operator should place both hands on the mask, the right hand taking a position the mirror image of the left, while an assistant inflates the bag. In extreme cases, the operator can apply even more pressure on the mask by pressing down on it with his chin.

Care should be taken to avoid progressive gastric distention, which is particularly likely when the airway remains partially obstructed and high oxygen flows are used. If the stomach becomes visibly distended and tympanic, a nasogastric tube may be placed to decompress it. However, the technique is not without hazard, because this in itself may induce regurgitation or vomiting and serve as a "wick" that overcomes the protection of the cardiac sphincter. For this reason, some authors advocate removal of the nasogastric tube after decompression, before inducing anesthesia.

Airway Assist Devices

ORAL AND NASOPHARYNGEAL AIRWAYS

An oral airway functions similarly to the jaw thrust. Its anatomically correct curvature lifts the tongue off the posterior pharynx sufficiently to provide a patent airway. It also serves as a bite block. It is especially helpful in edentulous patients. However, the airway will not be tolerated by a conscious or semiconscious patient without local anesthesia of the oral cavity and tongue. Premature attempts at placement may cause reflex gagging and vomiting or laryngospasm. The correct size must be chosen—in adults, this is usually size 3 or 4. Care must be taken during insertion to avoid trauma to the teeth and oropharynx and not to compress the tongue against the pharynx, which will cause complete airway obstruction. For these reasons, the authors' group prefers to use a tongue blade to flatten the base of the tongue, and then to pass the airway over this along its curvature. Once tracheal intubation has been performed and if prolonged mechanical ventilation is planned, it is preferable to remove the oral airway because it can cause ulceration or pressure necrosis of the lips, gums, or tongue.

The nasopharyngeal airway is a soft red-rubber tube available in French sizes 26 to 32. It has the advantage of being quite well tolerated by semiconscious patients, with no likelihood of disturbing loose teeth. It may be used instead of or in addition to an oral airway; however, used alone, it does not relieve obstruction as reliably. The most important hazards are epistaxis or turbinate avulsion. If there is time before insertion, the nasal mucous membranes may be shrunk with cotton-tipped applicators (Q-Tips) saturated with a 10% solution of phenylephrine or a 4% solution of cocaine (which also provides local anesthesia—but should not be used in patients prone to arrhythmias). The use of nasopharyngeal airways is contraindicated in patients with coagulopathy, cerebrospinal fluid rhinorrhea, or nasal fracture.

ESOPHAGEAL OBTURATOR AND ESOPHAGEAL TRACHEAL DOUBLE–LUMEN AIRWAY

Esophageal tubes have been developed for rapid airway establishment in cardiopulmonary resuscitation by emergency medical technicians in the field. They are contraindicated in patients with known esophageal disease or caustic ingestion.

The *esophageal obturator airway* (EOA) consists of a large endotracheal tube that has had its distal end sealed with a cone, a large 50-ml volume cuff, and a series of lateral eyes that perforate the tube proximal to the cuff. The proximal end clips into a face mask through which oxygen can be delivered by PPV. The design takes into account that, if the tongue and jaw are clasped together and pulled forward with the left hand, it is easier to blindly insert a tube into the esophagus than the trachea. Inflation of the cuff in the esophagus protects against regurgitation while gas delivered by a self-inflatable bag attached to the tube connector is driven into the trachea because of the seal provided by the face mask. Distention of the cuff to pressures greater than 25 mm Hg can damage the esophagus, and it may not be possible to effectively ventilate a patient with poor lung compliance. Withdrawal of the EOA before placing an endotracheal tube predisposes to aspiration. Inadvertent placement of the obturator airway into the trachea will insufflate the stomach and may precipitate regurgitation.

The esophageal tracheal double-lumen airway (Combitube, Sheridan Catheter Corp., Argyle, NY) attempts to improve on the deficiencies of the EOA by providing sufficient ventilation whether the airway is placed in the esophagus or the trachea (Fig. 9–4). The tube consists of a short, clear (No. 2) tube with a distal orifice, conjoined with and embedded in a long, blue (No. 1) tube with lateral fenestrations between a small distal cuff (15 ml) and a large proximal pharyngeal cuff (100 ml). In most cases, blind insertion will place the distal conjoined portion of the tube into the esophagus, which is sealed by the small distal cuff. Inflation of the large proximal cuff occludes the pharynx and allows PPV to be delivered into the trachea via the lateral fenestrations in the blue (No. 1) tube. However, if the conjoined tube is inadvertently inserted into the trachea, inflation is delivered directly via the distal port of the clear (No. 2) tube. This tube has shown promise in trials and has been released for general use in the United States, although in its present form it is suitable for adults only.

LARYNGEAL MASK AIRWAY

The laryngeal mask airway (LMA) is a nondisposable device that was developed and released commer-

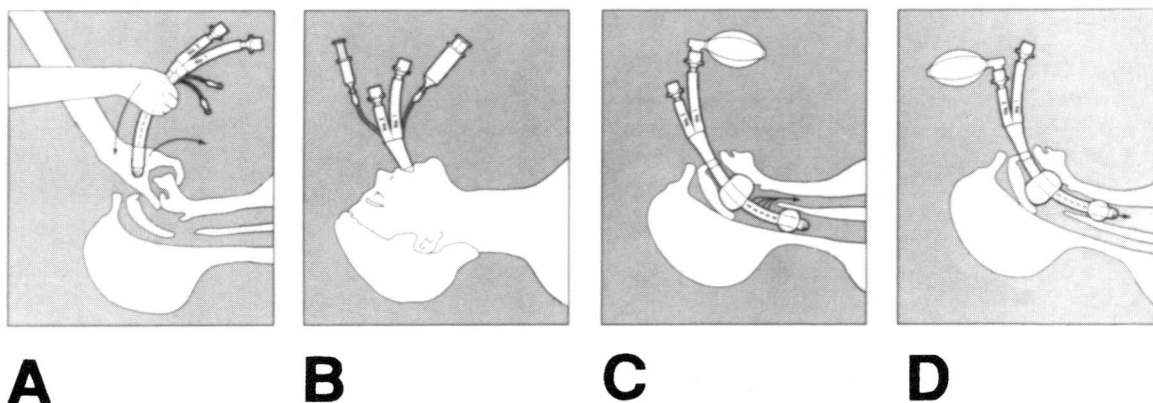

FIGURE 9–4. The esophageal tracheal double-lumen airway (Combitube). *A*, With the left hand, the tongue and lower jaw are lifted upward together. The right hand grips and inserts the Combitube into the natural curve of the pharynx, taking care not to snag the cuffs on the teeth. The tube should be carefully advanced until the printed double ring aligns with the teeth or alveolar ridge. *B*, The blue pilot tube (No. 1) is inflated with 100 ml air, using the supplied 140-ml syringe. This inflates the large proximal cuff and occludes the pharynx; the tube may move slightly outward. The clear pilot tube (No. 2) is inflated with 15 ml air, which inflates the small distal cuff. *C*, Ventilation is commenced by AMBU via the longer, blue connecting tube (No. 1). If breath sounds are auscultated in the chest and no gastric gurgle is heard, the Combitube has been placed in the esophagus and the lungs are being ventilated via the lateral fenestrations. Ventilation is continued in this fashion. The shorter, clear connecting tube (No. 2) may be used to suction gastric contents. *D*, If breath sounds cannot be auscultated in the chest and there is a gastric gurgle, the Combitube has been placed in the trachea. The AMBU should immediately be switched to the shorter, clear connecting tube (No. 2), and insufflation should confirm breath sounds in the chest with no gastric gurgle. In this case, the lungs are being ventilated via the distal port of the Combitube. (*A–D*, © Sheridan Catheter Corp., Argyle, NY. Used with permission.)

cially in the United Kingdom in 1988; it has recently become available in the United States (Pennant and White, 1993). It provides a level of airway support intermediate between mask ventilation and tracheal intubation. The device consists of a silicone rubber tube fused at its distal end to a small, elliptical, spoon-shaped mask rimmed with an inflatable cushion. The mask is constructed at a 30-degree angle to the tube so that, when correctly placed, it pushes the epiglottis up and covers the glottic lumen, allowing gas delivery via fenestrated openings at the distal end of the tube (Fig. 9–5). It also prevents inadvertent esophageal intubation. At present, five mask sizes are available; sizes 3 and 4 are intended for adult use, with tubes having an internal diameter of 10 and 12 mm, respectively. Placement of the LMA is appropriate in patients obtunded or topically anesthetized to a level sufficient to tolerate an oral airway. However, if inserted prematurely, it is far more likely to provoke airway reflexes with gagging, coughing, and laryngospasm.

The LMA has been used predominantly by anesthesiologists to provide general anesthesia or heavy sedation in the operating room. Outside the operating room, the LMA has an important role in the management of the difficult airway (see later in this chapter). Blind insertion, even by less-experienced operators, may effectively secure airway patency and facilitate effective ventilation where mask ventilation or laryngoscopy have been unsuccessful. Once the LMA is in place, access to the trachea can be obtained by a small-caliber fiberoptic bronchoscope, and a size 6 or 6.5 endotracheal tube can be inserted through the adult LMA tube, which is left in situ (McNamee et al., 1991). Alternatively, a bougie or nasogastric tube

can be placed blindly into the trachea and used to guide the passage of a larger-size endotracheal tube once the LMA has been removed.

The LMA does not prevent acute aspiration of stomach contents into the trachea, and its placement in a patient with a full stomach is not generally recommended. The incidence of occult regurgitation is thought to be low, but the risk is increased when the upper esophageal sphincter is included in the mask opening. The application of cricoid pressure during insertion may make initial placement more difficult, and impede subsequent insertion of an endotracheal tube via the LMA (see later in this chapter). The LMA should be removed only when the patient has fully recovered protective airway reflexes. Air leakage around the mask cushion begins to occur when airway pressures exceed 20 cm H_2O, which limits the effective tidal volume in patients with poor lung or chest wall compliance.

Tracheal Intubation

Indications for Tracheal Intubation

Tracheal intubation secures airway patency, protects the airway from gastric reflux, provides a direct route for airway suctioning and pulmonary toilet, and facilitates PPV during anesthesia, cardiopulmonary resuscitation, and acute respiratory failure.

Indications for tracheal intubation during anesthesia are defined largely by the nature and complexity of operation because of necessary access to the head and neck, airway protection during emergency surgery with full stomach, or the requirement for con-

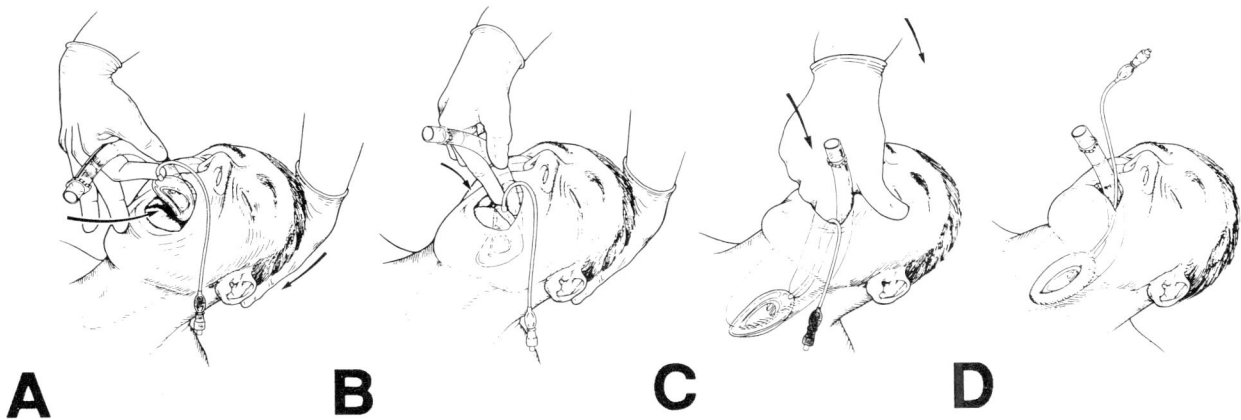

FIGURE 9–5. Placement of the laryngeal mask airway (LMA). *A,* Oral insertion. The left hand elevates the back of the head to achieve a "sniff" position. After the deflated mask cushion is lubricated, the posterior surface of the LMA is pressed firmly against the hard palate to ensure that the tip remains flattened and avoids the tongue. *B,* Pharyngeal advancement. The right index finger guides the LMA down the pharynx, ensuring that it continues to press firmly against the pharyngeal wall. *C,* Insertion into the hypopharynx. The right index finger pushes the mask cushion until the resistance of the upper esophageal sphincter is met. The tube is then grasped firmly by the left hand to retain position while the right index finger is withdrawn. *D,* Inflation of the mask cushion. A volume appropriate for the LMA size is injected via the pilot tube (15 to 30 ml in adult sizes 3 and 4) without the LMA being held. The tube will move outward slightly as it settles into its final position. The black line on the posterior axis of the tube should approximate the midpoint of the upper lip. (*A–D,* From Brain, A. I. J.: The Intavent Laryngeal Mask Instruction Manual. © Brain Medical Limited, Tidmarsh, Berkshire, UK, 1992. Used with permission.)

trolled ventilation and muscle relaxation during major cardiac, thoracic, and abdominal procedures. Tracheal intubation is performed as soon as possible during cardiopulmonary resuscitation because of the necessity to secure and protect the airway in a situation where provision of adequate ventilation and oxygenation is absolutely vital.

In patients with acute respiratory failure, the indications for tracheal intubation may be by no means as clear-cut and depend on careful, serial clinical assessment over a variable period of time. There are two forms of acute respiratory failure. Hypoxemic respiratory failure (e.g., ARDS, pneumonia) implies a primary deficit in oxygenation, and tracheal intubation is needed to facilitate airway pressure therapy (see later in this chapter). Ventilatory respiratory failure (e.g., status asthmaticus, respiratory muscle discoordination, fatigue, or atrophy) implies a primary deficit in the bellows mechanism, and tracheal intubation is needed to decrease or completely remove the work of breathing. Not infrequently, both forms coexist in the same disease process.

Criteria used for tracheal intubation and mechanical ventilation in acute respiratory failure include hypoxemia (Pa_{O_2} less than 55 mm Hg on room air, less than 70 mm Hg on 100% oxygen), hypercarbia (Pa_{CO_2} greater than 60 mm Hg), tachypnea (more than 40 breaths/min), or bradypnea (less than 6 breaths/min). However, these must be interpreted in conjunction with associated clinical signs of acute respiratory distress. These include anxiety, restlessness, agitation, confusion, sympathetic overactivity (sweating, clammy hands, tachycardia, hypertension, tachyarrhythmias), or use of accessory muscles (sternomastoids, pectoralis, flaring alae nasi). Inability to complete sentences because of dyspnea is an important harbinger of collapse. Blood gases may re-

main within relatively normal limits while the patient's work of breathing progressively increases, until just before complete decompensation. The decision to perform tracheal intubation should be based on observation of relentless clinical and laboratory deterioration, rather than on the achievement of set numerical criteria.

Anesthetized Versus Awake Tracheal Intubation

Tracheal intubation is conventionally performed after the induction of general anesthesia with a hypnotic agent (e.g., thiopental, etomidate) and facilitated by complete muscle relaxation with the short-acting depolarizing agent succinylcholine. However, various conditions sensitize the sarcolemma to the potassium-releasing property of succinylcholine, creating the potential for intractable ventricular arrhythmias. These include major trauma to muscle and soft tissue, burns, spinal cord transection, cerebrovascular accidents, and tetanus. Succinylcholine is safe to use within 24 hours of injury, but thereafter a nondepolarizing agent such as pancuronium, vecuronium, or atracurium should be substituted.

Supplemental analgesia with opioids (e.g., fentanyl, sufentanil), amnesia with benzodiazepines (e.g., midazolam), and obtundation of airway reflexes with intravenous lidocaine are frequently provided to enhance circulatory stability and decrease reflex airway hyperreactivity. Rapid-sequence induction with cricoid pressure, which completely avoids the use of mask ventilation, is provided in situations of full stomach and high risk of aspiration.

The use of general anesthesia for tracheal intubation obtunds potentially harmful circulatory responses (tachycardia, hypertension) and airway responses (laryngospasm, bronchospasm), and muscle relaxation facilitates laryngoscopy and passage of the endotracheal tube through the vocal cords. However, it also collapses the tongue and soft tissues of the oropharynx, requiring skilled management to maintain airway patency, and removes the protective reflexes that prevent regurgitation and aspiration of stomach contents. In patients with difficult airways, adequate mask ventilation may be impossible to achieve after the induction of anesthesia. In patients with acute respiratory failure who are hypoxemic and frequently hypovolemic (from diuretic therapy) and have a very high minute ventilation requirement, rapid desaturation and hypotension may occur immediately on anesthetic obtundation of their own ventilatory efforts. Inability to provide equivalent amounts of mask ventilation or rapidly secure tracheal intubation can cause arrythmias or cardiac arrest. Patients with hemodynamic compromise tolerate poorly the combined insult of general anesthesia and PPV (which impedes venous return to the heart) and may be precipitated into circulatory shock. Intravenous access for the rapid administration of fluids and pressor agents must be available.

Consideration should be given to awake tracheal intubation in situations in which difficult intubation is anticipated, or severe acute respiratory failure or hemodynamic instability exist. This requires careful and measured topical anesthesia of the airway (see later in this chapter). Preservation of airway reflexes and spontaneous ventilation maintain airway patency, oxygenation, and hemodynamic stability.

Oral Versus Transnasal Tracheal Intubation

Transnasal tracheal intubation guides the endotracheal tube close to the glottis and greatly facilitates the technique of blind intubation (see later in this chapter). This is particularly useful in patients with acute respiratory failure because it may be performed awake with minimal topical anesthesia and little patient cooperation and mouth opening and without instrumentation of the oral cavity. Once in place, a nasotracheal tube is easily fixated, cannot be occluded by biting, may be better tolerated by the patient, and is less likely to become dislodged or extruded. Mouth care is facilitated.

Nonetheless, some distinct disadvantages to nasotracheal intubation greatly limit its applicability to prolonged airway access. There is a distinct risk of turbinate damage, epistaxis, and pressure necrosis of the intranasal tissues. Placement is contraindicated in patients with abnormal coagulation, maxillofacial trauma, or basilar skull fracture. The nasal passages tolerate a smaller endotracheal tube size than the oral cavity, and the longer, tightly curved tube is more difficult to suction and is predisposed to becoming blocked with inspissated secretions. Most importantly, the nasotracheal tube may block the drainage of the frontal and maxillary sinuses and the eustachian tube (Fig. 9–6) and predispose to bacterial sinusitis or otitis media (Arens, 1974; Gregory, 1980). In critically

ill patients, this may provide a reservoir for nosocomial, especially gram-negative, sepsis.

Tracheal intubation via the oral route is generally accomplished more easily, the largest size tube tolerated can be placed, suctioning is facilitated, and infection is avoided. Patient tolerance is improved and the risk of biting or lip damage is diminished by securing the endotracheal tube against the soft tissue of the angle of the mouth, away from the teeth.

Anatomic Considerations

Tracheal intubation requires the placement of an endotracheal tube through the vocal cords, which lie within the larynx opposite cervical spines 4, 5, and 6. The cords are part of the glottic apparatus, a series of cartilages, ligaments, and muscles arranged as a valve-like conduit between the mouth and the trachea. In the adult, the glottic opening (i.e., the space between the vocal cords) is the narrowest part of the airway, whereas in children, the cricoid ring beyond the glottis has the smallest diameter. The anterior two-thirds of the vocal cords is soft and membranous, but the tougher cartilaginous posterior portion may impede passage of the endotracheal tube. Forced placement of a large endotracheal tube can hook the posterior cords and dislocate the arytenoid cartilages, causing aphonia.

The vocal cords are attached to the arytenoid cartilages on the posterior aspect of the cricoid cartilage and can be tensed, relaxed, or moved from side to side by rotation of the arytenoids. The corniculate (medial) and cuneiform (more lateral) parts of the arytenoids are visualized during laryngoscopy as bulges in the inferior aspects in the glottis.

The epiglottis is a cartilaginous flap attached to the base of the tongue at the vallecula, which protects the glottic opening from aspiration during swallowing, coughing, or vomiting. In childhood, the epiglottis is small and stubby; in the elderly, especially in men, it may become very long and floppy. Tracheal intubation always requires elevation of the epiglottis to expose the glottic opening, either by pulling it anteriorly from the vallecula or by direct lift.

Assessment of the Airway

Careful assessment of the airway is crucial to determine the level of potential difficulty of mask ventilation and tracheal intubation. A catastrophe is much more likely to result when a difficult airway has not been recognized and the operator is left with a paralyzed patient who is unable to be ventilated or intubated. During emergencies, there may be little time to perform a complete and thorough airway assessment. Even so, it is vital to determine potential airway difficulty so that the intubation technique can be appropriately modified and skilled help summoned.

Medical History

It is important to ascertain whether the patient has previously undergone tracheal intubation and, if so,

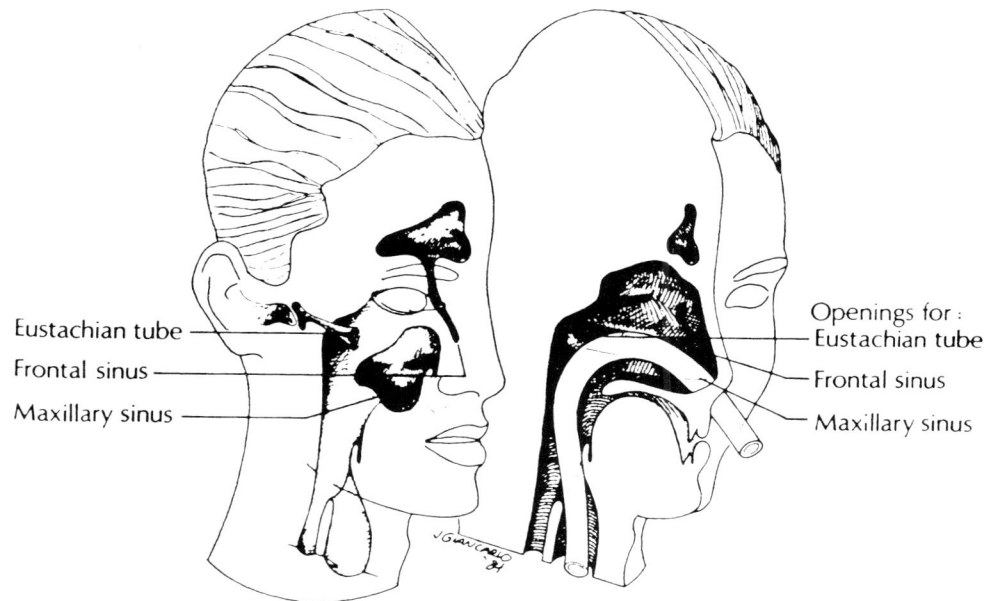

FIGURE 9–6. Hazards of nasotracheal intubation. Schematic diagram illustrating the mechanism of obstruction of frontal and maxillary sinus drainage and of the eustachian tube by a nasotracheal tube. This predisposes to bacterial sinusitis and otitis media, and may serve as a reservoir for nosocomial sepsis. (From Shapiro, B. A., Kacmarek, R. M., Cane, R. D., et al.: Clinical Application of Respiratory Care. 4th ed. St. Louis, Mosby–Year Book, 1991, p. 171. Used with permission.)

the level of ease or difficulty involved. This information can usually be obtained from the patient or from anesthetic records, if available. Medical conditions that predispose to airway difficulty should be recognized and evaluated. In particular, these include rheumatoid arthritis, ankylosing spondylitis, head and neck injury, soft tissue deformity or tumors of the head and neck, and retrosternal thyroid goiter. Symptoms of partial airway obstruction that suggest potential airway difficulty include dyspnea relieved by positional change of the head, hoarseness, dysphonia, stridor, or dysphagia.

Physical Examination

Certain physical characteristics immediately suggest potential difficulty in mask ventilation or laryngoscopy. These include a large head with a short, thick neck, a receding mandible with prominent teeth and overbite, or a small mouth. Inability to open the mouth because of temporomandibular disease (rheumatoid arthritis), trauma, or soft tissue deformity is also an obvious sign. Examination of the exterior landmarks of the larynx indicates whether the tracheal structures are deviated by tumor, trauma, scar tissue, or hematoma. Mobility of the larynx can be assessed by gentle external manipulation. Suspicion of tumor recurrence on the vocal cords or glottis should be assessed by indirect mirror laryngoscopy. The size and patency of the nares should be evaluated by occluding one side and asking the patient to breathe through the other, if transnasal intubation is contemplated. The mouth should be examined for loose or severely carious teeth that could be easily dislodged by laryngoscopy.

It is particularly important to elicit subtle predictors of airway difficulty that may be missed on a cursory examination. Three simple tests are extremely helpful

in this regard: tongue versus pharyngeal size, atlanto-occipital extension, and size of the mandibular space (Benumof, 1991). Prediction of the difficulty of airway management is greatly enhanced if two or more of these tests are used together (Bellhouse and Dore, 1987; Frerk, 1991).

TONGUE VERSUS PHARYNGEAL SIZE (MALLAMPATI'S CLASSIFICATION)

Sitting upright and with the head in the neutral position, the patient is asked to open her mouth as widely as possible and to protrude the tongue maximally. The patient must not phonate (say "ah") or arch the tongue. There is an excellent correlation between the ability to visualize pharyngeal structures and the ease of laryngoscopy (Mallampati et al., 1985) (Fig. 9–7). Visualization of the complete uvula and tonsillar pillars (Class I) virtually ensures straightforward laryngoscopy with a good view of the entire glottic apparatus. Inability to view the uvula at all (Class IV) virtually ensures difficult laryngoscopy with a view of the tip of the epiglottis or the soft palate alone. However, loss of visualization of the tonsillar pillars (Class II) or visualization of the base of the uvula only (Class III) is associated with a wide range of difficulty of laryngoscopy. Thus, used alone, the Mallampati classification does not exclude false-positive or false-negative prediction of airway difficulty.

ATLANTO–OCCIPTAL EXTENSION

This simply tests the ability of the patient to assume the "sniff" position described earlier. This is contraindicated in acute injury to the cervical spine or severe arthritis (e.g., odontoid erosion or cervical spine subluxation in rheumatoid arthritis) and may be impossi-

Class I   Class II   Class III   Class IV

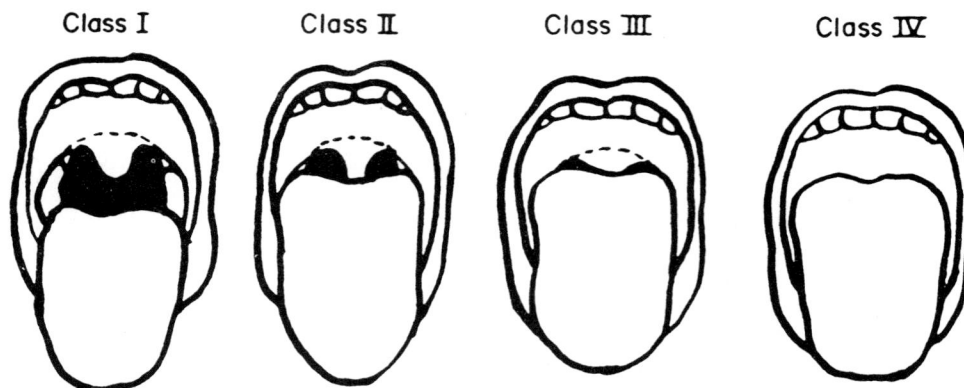

FIGURE 9–7. Tongue vs. pharyngeal size (Mallampati's classification). Class I: The soft palate, fauces, uvula, and anterior and posterior tonsillar pillars are easily visualized. The entire glottic aperture can be seen by laryngoscopy 99 to 100% of the time. Class II: The tonsillar pillars are hidden by the tongue. Class III: Only the base of the uvula can be seen. Class IV: The uvula cannot be visualized at all. During laryngoscopy, only the tip of the epiglottis or the soft palate alone can be seen 100% of the time. (From Benumof, J. L.: Management of the difficult adult airway: With special emphasis on the awake tracheal intubation. Anesthesiology 75:1087–1110, 1991. Used with permission.)

ble when the cervical spine is fused (rheumatoid or osteoarthritis, spondylitis, operative fusion). Range of motion of the neck decreases with age. Inability to extend the atlanto-occipital joint predicts difficulty in aligning the oral, pharyngeal, and laryngeal axes and viewing the glottic opening with laryngoscopy.

SIZE OF THE MANDIBULAR SPACE

In the average-size adult, at least two finger-breadths should be able to be placed in the space anterior to the larynx, between the inside of the mandible and the hyoid bone (Fig. 9–8). A short mandibu-

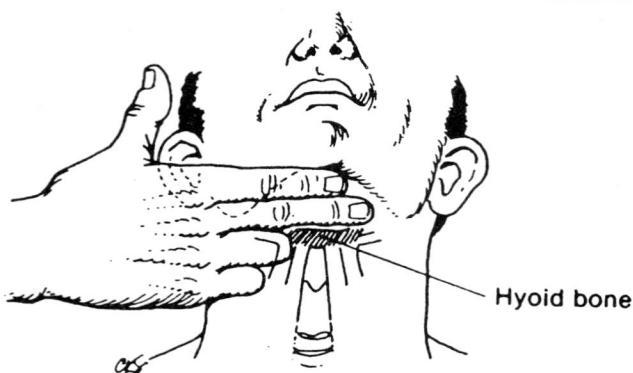

FIGURE 9–8. The mandibular space. The ability to place at least two fingerbreadths between the inside of the mandible and the hyoid bone in an adult patient predicts relatively easy laryngoscopy. This correlates to a distance between the thyroid cartilage and the mentum of greater than 6 cm. A large mandibular space suggests that the laryngeal and the pharyngeal axes will fall in line during the "sniff" position and that the tongue will easily be compressed forward during laryngoscopy, resulting in easy visualization of the glottis. A small space suggests the opposite. (From Benumof, J. L.: Management of the difficult airway: The ASA algorithm. In 1993 Review Course Lectures. Cleveland, International Anesthesia Research Society, 1993, pp. 83–91. Used with permission.)

lar space predicts that the laryngeal axis will not approach the pharyngeal axis during atlanto-occipital extension ("sniff" position), that the tongue must be compressed forward into a small space during laryngoscopy, and that visualization of the glottis will be difficult because it appears to be anteriorly situated. This situation is more likely in a patient with a short, muscular neck or receding chin. A large mandibular space suggests the opposite.

Complicating Factors

Certain preexisting conditions increase the risk of laryngoscopy and tracheal intubation, even if the airway itself does not present any difficulty. Planned techniques should be modified accordingly. The coexistence of a potentially difficult airway represents a major problem, and requires careful planning and skilled assistance.

FULL STOMACH

Acute fulminating pulmonary edema secondary to pulmonary aspiration of regurgitated acid gastric contents has been a complication feared by anesthesiologists since its first description in parturients by Mendelson in 1946. There is general consensus that the precipitating event is aspiration of a large volume (greater than 0.4 ml/kg) of acidic (less than pH 2.5) gastric fluid; particulate matter contributes to airway obstruction and development of pneumonia (Coté, 1990). However, these conclusions are based on animal rather than human studies. The overall incidence of acid aspiration syndrome in healthy patients (American Society of Anesthesiologists [ASA] 1 or 2) is very low, estimated at 1 in 50,000 cases. Risk is considerably greater in patients with a full stomach; with conditions associated with delayed gastric emptying (e.g., pregnancy, diabetes, renal or hepatic failure, obesity, severe sepsis, and trauma); with diseases of the mouth, throat, and esophagus; and with loss of ability to protect the airway (e.g., anesthesia, sedation, intoxication, obtundation and coma, stroke). Mendelson's original series of women undergoing labor and delivery showed an incidence of 0.15% (66 out of 44,016 patients).

The physiologic basis for a 6-hour fast before induction of anesthesia is found in the work of Beaumont in 1833, who observed that, in a man with a gastric fistula secondary to a healed gunshot wound, it took 5 hours for solid food to be converted to chyme and pass through the pylorus. However, Beaumont also noted that clear liquids were emptied "soon after they were received" (Beaumont, 1833; Goresky and Maltby, 1990). There is still general acceptance of the need for a 6-hour fast after solid or fatty foods, but recent studies in children have demonstrated no decrease in pH or increase in volume of gastric juice within 2 to 3 hours of ingestion of clear liquids (Schreiner et al., 1990). Some institutions have changed their preoperative guidelines accordingly.

Premedication administered at least 30 minutes before anesthetic induction may decrease the risk of acid aspiration. These include a nonparticulate antacid such as sodium citrate (15 ml given orally), histamine-2 receptor antagonists to decrease gastric pH and volume (e.g., cimetidine 50 mg, ranitidine 25 mg, or famotidine 10 mg intravenously), or metoclopramide to hasten gastric emptying (5 mg intravenously). If a nasogastric tube is in situ, the stomach should be decompressed. Some physicians advocate placing a nasogastric tube transiently to empty the stomach, and then removing it before induction because it may impair the integrity of the cardiac sphincter. The high-risk patient should be managed with rapid-sequence induction (i.e., no mask ventilation) and cricoid pressure. Control is sacrificed for speed, and there is greater potential for unwanted circulatory responses (e.g., hypotension, hypertension, or tachycardia) and airway responses (e.g., laryngospasm or bronchospasm). Cricoid pressure must be released if retching occurs, because of the possibility of inducing esophageal perforation. Rapid-sequence induction is contraindicated when a difficult intubation is anticipated; awake intubation should be planned (see later in this chapter).

CERVICAL SPINE INJURY

If acute or chronic cervical spine injury is suspected or proved, manipulation of the head into the "sniff" position is contraindicated. The approach to tracheal intubation should follow that for suspected difficult intubation (see later in this chapter). Awake fiberoptic intubation is recommended, but in emergency situations, rapid-sequence induction can be performed if head fixation and traction are provided by the neurosurgeon.

CARDIOVASCULAR DISEASE

In a number of cardiovascular diseases, hypertension and tachycardia in response to tracheal intubation may be extremely deleterious, even life-threatening. These diseases include severe coronary artery disease, particularly when myocardial ischemia is acute, aortic stenosis, idiopathic hypertrophic subaortic stenosis, mitral stenosis, aortic dissection, and aortic aneurysm. Sufficient anesthesia must be provided to obtund circulatory responses without causing excessive myocardial depression. A "cardiac"-type induction with high-dose fentanyl (10 to 20 μg/kg), midazolam (20 to 50 μg/kg), and a nondepolarizing muscle relaxant devoid of vagolytic effects such as vecuronium (0.1 mg/kg) provides ideal conditions. In the case of a full stomach or difficult airway, awake intubation with meticulous local anesthesia is preferred. Rapid-sequence induction should generally be avoided. In all situations, the use of the short-acting beta-blocker esmolol in intravenous bolus doses of 30 to 50 mg can be particularly helpful in controlling tachycardia and hypertension in response to airway manipulation. Myocardial depression and bronchospasm can be precipitated (even though the agent is beta$_1$-receptor-selective), but the drug has a half-life of 9 minutes and its effects dissipate rapidly.

BRONCHOSPASTIC DISEASE

Patients with bronchospastic disease have a significant risk of developing acute bronchospasm with airway manipulation. They provide the anesthesiologist with a considerable challenge, because in some patients, induced bronchospasm may be fulminant and life-threatening. There may be a known history of childhood-onset (atopic, extrinsic) asthma, adult-onset (intrinsic) asthma, or chronic obstructive lung disease with bronchospasm. However, many patients without a history of bronchospasm may have so-called hyperreactive airways and respond poorly to airway instrumentation. Current smoking or a recent upper respiratory tract infection (within the prior 3 weeks) predisposes to this condition.

Skilled assistance should be summoned before attempting tracheal intubation. Premedication with the patient's own bronchodilator aerosols may be very helpful, such as the selective beta$_2$-agonist albuterol and the anticholinergic agent ipratropium. However, cromolyn or steroid inhalers do not provide immediate protection. One of the most useful modes of induction—inhalation of the volatile anesthetic agent halothane, which has potent bronchodilating properties—is obviously not available outside the operating room. Choice of induction agents is less important than the ensurance of adequate depth of anesthesia before airway instrumentation. Intravenous injection of lidocaine (1.5 mg/kg over 2 minutes, prior to induction) protects against airway hyperreactivity. Patients require heavy sedation after tracheal intubation to secure endotracheal tube tolerance without bronchospasm. Rapid-sequence induction is relatively contraindicated; awake intubation carries a high risk of inducing bronchospasm even with the most meticulous local anesthesia.

ELEVATED INTRACRANIAL PRESSURE

The patient presenting with known or suspected elevation in *intracranial pressure* (ICP) due to closed head injury or intracranial hemorrhage is at particular risk for circulatory and respiratory responses to anesthetic induction and tracheal intubation. Respiratory depression caused by opioids or other sedatives increases cerebral blood flow and ICP. Hypertension and tachycardia dramatically increase ICP and may cause cerebral herniation or aneurysmal rupture. The preferred approach is to use an intravenous induction agent (thiopental or etomidate) that rapidly decreases cerebral metabolism and blood flow, together with succinylcholine. A precurarization dose of 1 mg of pancuronium or vecuronium is administered 3 minutes beforehand to suppress succinylcholine-induced fasciculations, which may themselves elevate ICP. Care must be taken to avoid acute hypotension, which will decrease cerebral perfusion pressure, and provision must be made for heavy sedation after tracheal intubation. If awake intubation is required for a difficult airway, meticulous local anesthesia must be provided.

COAGULOPATHIES

Coagulation disorders, known or suspected, provide an absolute contraindication to transnasal tracheal intubation. Uncontrollable epistaxis may occur and can cause fatal asphyxiation. This caveat applies to patients on anticoagulants (e.g., heparin, coumadin), with hematopoietic disease or in renal or hepatic failure. Nerve blocks used to supplement topical anesthesia during awake intubation should be avoided or administered with caution.

Performance of Tracheal Intubation

PREPARATION

The appropriate equipment must be assembled before tracheal intubation, whether elective or emergent. Table 9–1 lists minimal essential equipment required. Of primary importance is the presence of oxygen, suction, pulse oximeter, a variety of sizes of masks, laryngoscopy blades and endotracheal tube, tongue depressors, oral and nasal airways, stethoscope, tape, pillows, and an end-tidal CO_2 monitor or detector. Direct uncluttered access to the head of the bed is essential. Unless contraindicated, the patient should be placed in the "sniff" position.

PREOXYGENATION

The patient should be preoxygenated with 100% oxygen for at least 3 minutes, or until the pulse oximeter gives a consistent reading (SpO_2) as close to 98% as possible. This may simply involve application of a face mask during spontaneous ventilation in an awake patient with adequate minute ventilation or may require forceful mask ventilation in an unconscious, decompensated patient. The goal is to wash

■ **Table 9–1.** MINIMAL ESSENTIAL EQUIPMENT FOR TRACHEAL INTUBATION

I. Preoxygenation and ventilation
  1. Oxygen source on, attached to self-inflating ventilation bag
  2. Small, medium, large anesthesia mask
  3. Small, medium, large oral and nasopharyngeal airways
  4. Tongue depressor
  5. Pulse oximeter attached to patient, functioning
II. Preparation of endotracheal tube
  1. Small, medium, large endotracheal tubes (cut to size if orotracheal intubation planned)
  2. Malleable, lubricated stylet
  3. Three-way stopcock attached to 10-ml syringe
  4. Cuff inflated, checked for leak, then deflated completely
  5. 4% lidocaine jelly and ointment
III. Anesthesia
  1. Intravenous access and fluids (crystalloid or colloid)
  2. Intravenous anesthetics and muscle relaxants, syringes, and needles
  3. Pressor agents (10 ml phenylephrine @ 50 μg/ml)
  4. Atomizer with local anesthetic (e.g., benzocaine [Cetacaine]), 4% lidocaine jelly
IV. Laryngoscopy
  1. Suction apparatus on, Yankauer's catheter attached
  2. Magill's forceps
  3. Functioning light source for laryngoscope blades
  4. MacIntosh's blades sizes 3 and 4, Miller's blades sizes 2 and 3
V. Fixation of endotracheal tube
  1. Tincture of benzoin
  2. Adhesive, umbilical tape
VI. Determination of location of endotracheal tube
  1. Stethoscope
  2. End-tidal CO_2 monitor
  3. Pulse oximeter

Modified from Benumof, J. L.: Conventional (laryngoscopic) orotracheal and nasotracheal intubation (single-lumen type). *In* Benumof, J. L. (ed): Clinical Procedures in Anesthesia and Intensive Care. Philadelphia, J. B. Lippincott, 1992, p. 122.

out lung nitrogen, which delays the onset of hypoxemia during the apneic time period of laryngoscopy and tracheal intubation. Patients dependent on high minute ventilation or in a hypermetabolic state owing to trauma or sepsis tend to desaturate with alarming rapidity with the onset of apnea. If the patient is unable to be ventilated easily by mask, or if regurgitation and possible aspiration have occurred, clinical judgment may dictate that it is more expeditious to immediately attempt tracheal intubation to secure the airway.

LARYNGOSCOPY AND OROTRACHEAL INTUBATION

The operator should wear gloves and eye shields because of the distinct possibility of direct contact with patient secretions. If a malleable stylet is used, it should be thinly lubricated and inserted into the endotracheal tube to a position about 3 cm from the tip. The proximal end should be hooked over the endotracheal tube connector to prevent the stylet from advancing inadvertently. The endotracheal tube should be curved fairly sharply at its distal end to form a "hockey stick" and placed within reach, with suction immediately available. The laryngoscope blade is attached to the handle and the contact and light again checked. The handle is gripped in the left hand, in front of the blade.

The patient's mouth may be opened by tilting the head back with the seat of the right hand, while the fifth finger of the left hand pushes the jaw forward. Alternatively, and usually more successfully, the mouth may be opened widely by using a scissors grip with the right hand. The right thumb is placed on the lower incisor, the second finger on the upper incisor, and pressure is applied. Care should be taken to avoid compressing the lips on the teeth. Once the laryngoscope blade is in good position, the right hand is removed.

Use of Curved Blade (MacIntosh). The curved blade is passed into the mouth to the right of the tongue, and sweeps the tongue aside to the left (Fig. 9–9). The wrist is rotated slightly to bring the blade toward the midline of the base of the tongue, so that the tip can be inserted into the vallecula anterior to the epiglottis. The blade is then lifted up to expose the glottis by pushing the left arm up at a 45-degree angle away from the operator's chest. If this maneuver is performed successfully, the patient's head should be practically elevated off the pillow as the oral, pharyngeal, and laryngeal axes align and the glottis comes into view. It is very important not to use the patient's upper incisors as a fulcrum! If this is done, the handle of the blade will be lowered and the operator will be forced to crouch lower and lower to visualize the glottis—an important sign of incorrect technique.

Use of Straight Blade (Miller). The straight blade provides a major advantage in exposure when the oral cavity is small or it is not possible to open the mouth widely. The blade is flat, without a lateral flange, so that there is a greater tendency for the tongue to flop over the edges and obscure vision. The tip of the blade is inserted under the posterior surface of the epiglottis, which is then lifted up directly (Fig. 9–10). This is helpful when the larynx is anterior (small mandibular space), the epiglottis is large and floppy, or the epiglottis is small, as in children. How-

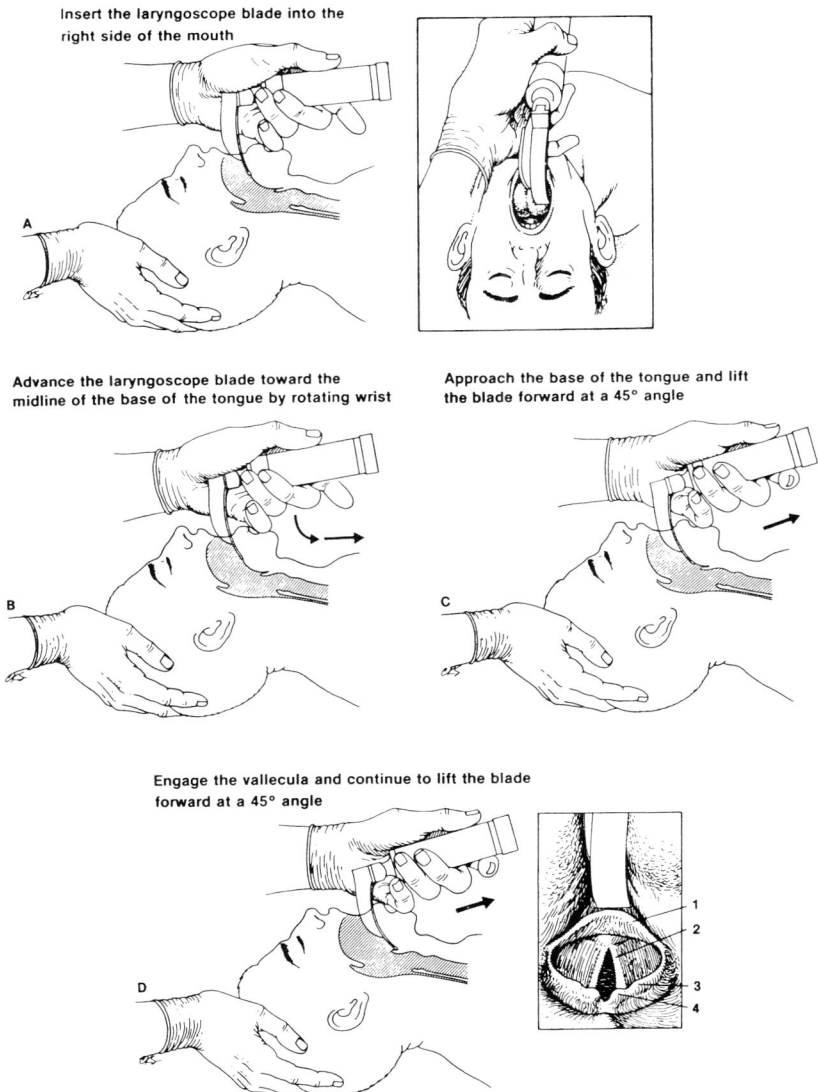

Insert the laryngoscope blade into the right side of the mouth

Advance the laryngoscope blade toward the midline of the base of the tongue by rotating wrist

Approach the base of the tongue and lift the blade forward at a 45° angle

Engage the vallecula and continue to lift the blade forward at a 45° angle

FIGURE 9–9. Laryngoscopy and orotracheal intubation with curved blade. *A,* The curved blade is inserted into the mouth to the right of the tongue, which is swept aside to the left. *B,* The blade is advanced and slightly rotated toward the midline of the base of the tongue. *C,* The blade engages the base of the tongue and the left arm is lifted up and forward at a 45-degree angle. *D,* The blade is seated in the vallecula and the epiglottis is lifted up to expose the view of the glottis. (1 = epiglottis; 2 = vocal cords; 3, 4 = arytenoid cartilage [cuneiform, corniculate parts].) (*A–D,* From Benumof, J. L.: Conventional [laryngoscopic] orotracheal and nasotracheal intubation [single-lumen type]. *In* Benumof, J. L. [ed]: Clinical Procedures in Anesthesia and Intensive Care. Philadelphia, J. B. Lippincott, 1992, pp. 124–127. Used with permission.)

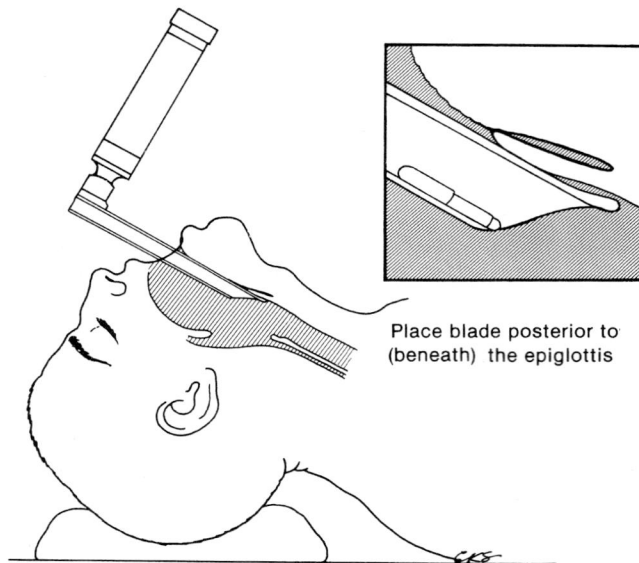

Place blade posterior to
(beneath) the epiglottis

FIGURE 9–10. Laryngoscopy and orotracheal intubation with straight blade. The straight blade is passed down the base of the tongue in the midline, and then lifts the epiglottis directly by its posterior surface to expose the glottic aperture. In all other respects, the procedure is the same as with the curved blade. (From Benumof, J. L.: Conventional [laryngoscopic] orotracheal and nasotracheal intubation [single-lumen type]. In Benumof, J. L. [ed]: Clinical Procedures in Anesthesia and Intensive Care. Philadelphia, J. B. Lippincott, 1992, p. 128. Used with permission.)

ever, stimulation of the posterior surface of the epiglottis (innervated by the superior laryngeal nerve) predisposes to reflex laryngospasm more than does stimulation of the anterior surface (innervated by the glossopharyngeal nerve). Also, it is a little more difficult to pass the endotracheal tube through the oral space provided by the straight blade.

Insertion of the Endotracheal Tube. Once the glottis is exposed by either blade technique, the vocal cords should be kept under direct vision while the endotracheal tube is grasped with the right hand and advanced between them. The malleable stylet, if used, should then be removed to prevent any possibility of injury to the tracheal wall. It is helpful to have an assistant gently palpate the cricoid membrane at this stage. Not only can this confirm that the endotracheal tube is passing through the larynx but mild pressure on the cricoid membrane may also bring an anterior glottis into better view. If resistance is encountered at the level of the vocal cords, a slight clockwise rotation may suffice to pass the endotracheal tube through. However, excessive force must not be used—either the vocal cords are not fully relaxed or a smaller-size endotracheal tube should be chosen. Care should be taken to advance the endotracheal tube only until the cuff is seen just to disappear beyond the cords and no further—this will reduce the risk of inadvertent endobronchial intubation. In most adults, this corresponds to alignment of the 22-cm mark of the endotracheal tube with the patient's lips.

The endotracheal tube cuff is inflated with 8 to 10 ml of air, connected via an elbow to the self-inflating ventilator bag, and hand ventilation provided while the position is confirmed. During this time, the endotracheal tube should be firmly supported with the first finger and thumb of the left hand, while the remaining fingers rest on the patient's face so that they track any sudden movement. Subsequently, the volume of air in the cuff should be adjusted so that "minimal leak" is obtained, and the cuff pressure when checked is less than 25 mm Hg.

Confirmation of Endotracheal Tube Position. These signs help confirm correct placement of the endotracheal tube in the trachea with the first few breaths: no excessive resistance to ventilating bag compression; symmetric and substantial excursion of the chest; bilaterally equal and clear breath sounds; faint transmission of these sounds over the gastric area; condensation in the endotracheal tube with exhalation; palpation of pulsation in the cuff above the sternal notch when the pilot balloon is squeezed; and sustained high (98% or greater) SpO_2 on pulse oximeter. However, the single unequivocal indication of correct endotracheal tube placement is a positive capnogram on an end-tidal CO_2 monitor or evidence of greater than 2% exhaled carbon dioxide on an approved CO_2-sensing device.

Endobronchial intubation invariably involves the right mainstem bronchus because of the relatively obtuse angle it makes with the trachea. Suggestive signs include unilateral chest movement and breath sounds (although these can be misleading), a unilateral wheeze, and high peak airway pressures (greater than 40 cm H_2O) on subsequent mechanical ventilation. The endotracheal tube should be pulled back 1 to 2 cm after cuff deflation, and the signs should be rechecked after repositioning. If doubt remains, endotracheal tube position can be confirmed by fiberoptic bronchoscopy or chest radiograph (see later in this chapter).

Esophageal intubation usually occurs in two situations. The vocal cords may have been well visualized initially, but if the laryngoscope blade is lowered just at the moment of insertion of the endotracheal tube, it slides posteriorly to the larynx. Alternatively, if the larynx is anterior and exposure of the vocal cords is difficult so that only the lower aperture or arytenoid cartilage is seen, the endotracheal tube may glance off the larynx and into the esophagus. Auscultation over the stomach reveals loud, tympanic gurgling sounds with the first breath, associated with gastric distention, poor chest movement and breath sounds, and difficulty in ventilation. All these signs can be misleading, and absence of a capnogram remains the most reliable indicator of esophageal intubation. Occasionally, a capnogram may be created by the exhalation of carbon dioxide if the stomach was inadvertently filled with mixed expired gas during mask ventilation before tracheal intubation. However, endtidal CO_2 levels are low, quickly diminish, and disappear entirely after several breaths. If esophageal intubation is confirmed in a patient with full stomach or delayed gastric emptying, the tube should be left in place to avoid drawing out gastric contents on removal. Once a second endotracheal tube has been correctly placed in the trachea and the cuff inflated, the esophageal tube may be safely withdrawn.

When the correct position of the endotracheal tube has been confirmed, it should be secured by tape to the maxilla, which is anchored, and not the mandible, which may move around. The endotracheal tube is best positioned in the angle of the mouth, away from the teeth and lips, with care taken not to withdraw or advance it. After final taping, breath sounds should be rechecked to assure that they are equal and bilateral. Endotracheal tube position can be confirmed subsequently by fiberoptic bronchoscopy, looking for tracheal rings and the carina 1 to 2 cm below the distal tip, and by chest radiograph, where the tip should be seen at the midtracheal level.

COMMON ERRORS IN LARYNGOSCOPY AND TRACHEAL INTUBATION

The most common cause of poor glottic visualization during laryngoscopy is failure to achieve an adequate "sniff" position. If it is anticipated that the larynx may be anterior, extra padding should be placed under the occiput to accentuate neck flexion. In difficult situations, it may be helpful for an assistant to actually lift up the head while gently pressing the larynx posteriorly by pressure on the cricoid membrane. Second, if the tongue is not swept to the left by the laryngoscope blade, it may flop over the blade and obscure the view (Fig. 9–11). In this situation, it is best to remove the laryngoscope and start again. A third error is to insert the laryngoscope blade so deeply that it lifts up the entire larynx, exposing the esophagus (Fig. 9–12). Finally, if the MacIntosh blade is inserted correctly into the vallecula but advanced too far, the epiglottis may be pushed down over the vocal cords and obscure their exposure.

Difficult Tracheal Intubation

Benumof has constructed a helpful chart of the degree of difficulty in mask ventilation or laryngoscopy, which ranges from zero (extremely easy) to infinite (impossible) (Fig. 9–13).

The most important first step is to recognize a potentially difficult airway (as discussed previously) so that appropriate preparation for awake tracheal intubation may be made. The major advantage of this approach is that it avoids "burning bridges": Spontaneous ventilation, oxygenation, muscle tone, and airway patency are all preserved. However, repeated instrumentation of the airway by any means may cause progressive laryngeal edema, bleeding, and airway obstruction. The most common cause of airway fatality in the operating room is loss of ability to provide effective mask ventilation between persist-

The Tongue Should Be to the Left of the Laryngoscope Blade

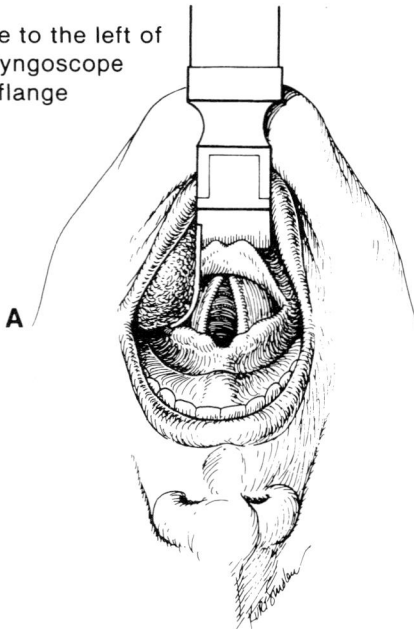

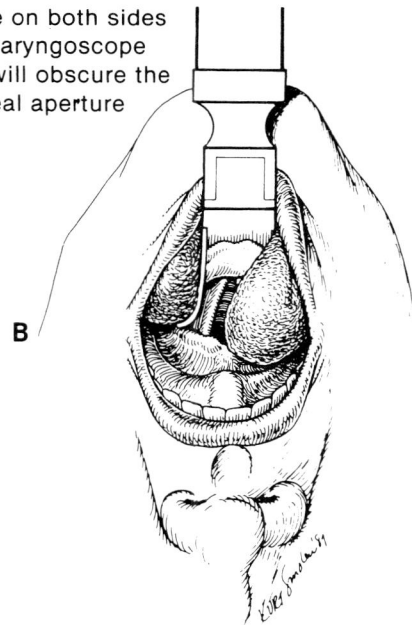

FIGURE 9–11. Malposition of laryngoscope blade—1. A, The lateral flange of the MacIntosh blade should sweep the tongue to the left to provide an unobstructed view of the glottis. B, If the blade slips to the midline too soon, the tongue flops over the right side and obscures the view of the glottis. At this stage, the best course is to withdraw the laryngoscope and start again. (A and B, From Benumof, J. L.: Conventional [laryngoscopic] orotracheal and nasotracheal intubation [single-lumen type]. In Benumof, J. L. [ed]: Clinical Procedures in Anesthesia and Intensive Care. Philadelphia, J. B. Lippincott, 1992, p. 130. Used with permission.)

Insertion of the Laryngoscope Blade Too Deeply into the Pharynx Elevates the Larynx and Exposes the Esophagus

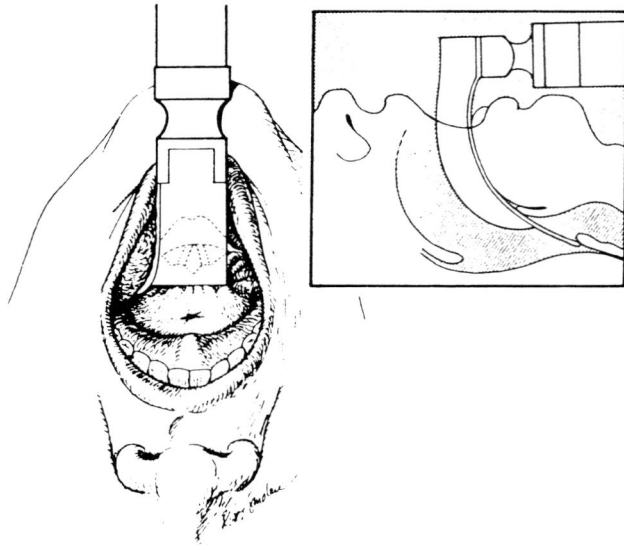

FIGURE 9–12. Malposition of laryngoscope blade—2. If the laryngoscope blade is placed too deeply, it will lift the entire larynx and expose the esophagus, which is a round, puckered structure slightly to the right of the midline. The laryngoscope blade should be slightly withdrawn and moved upward until the epiglottis flops down, then repositioned in the vallecula (curved blade) or under the epiglottis (straight blade). (From Benumof, J. L.: Conventional [laryngoscopic] orotracheal and nasotracheal intubation [single-lumen type]. *In* Benumof, J. L. [ed]: Clinical Procedures in Anesthesia and Intensive Care. Philadelphia, J. B. Lippincott, 1992, p. 129. Used with permission.)

ent, prolonged, and failed attempts at laryngoscopy and tracheal intubation (Caplan et al., 1990).

AWAKE INTUBATION

The initial step is to prepare the patient psychologically by carefully explaining the situation and the planned procedure, while providing reassurance and support. Sedative agents such as fentanyl (50 µg/ml) and midazolam (1 mg/ml) should be prepared, but the sicker the patient, the more important it is to withhold central sedation until the airway has been secured. In a patient in severe acute respiratory failure, as little as 1 mg intravenous midazolam may induce complete apnea. Administration of an anticholinergic agent (atropine 0.4 mg or glycopyrrolate 0.1 mg) will dry secretions, and thereby enhance topical anesthesia and subsequent visualization and decrease airway hyperreactivity.

Topical anesthesia is provided by spraying the tongue with benzocaine (Cetacaine), working progressively toward the base with the aid of a tongue depressor or laryngoscope blade. Anesthesia of the fauces is obtained by soaking gauze in 4% lidocaine and then holding in place with the aid of a spatula, or a bilateral block of the lingual branch of the glosso-

pharyngeal nerve may be provided by direct injection into the fauces with a long needle (Benumof, 1991). Alternatively, the patient can be asked to breathe aerosolized 1% lidocaine via a nebulizer powered by a low flow of oxygen (4 l/min). This is effective, but takes 15 to 20 minutes, and does risk lidocaine overdose. Additional anesthesia of the vocal cords may be obtained by bilateral superior laryngeal nerve block or transtracheal block (2 ml of 2% lidocaine injected via the cricoid membrane after aspiration of air). However, preservation of the cough is desirable in patients with a full stomach.

If transnasal intubation is planned, mucosal vasoconstriction with phenylephrine or 4% cocaine should be provided, as described previously.

BLIND NASOTRACHEAL INTUBATION

This is a reasonable choice in a patient with acute respiratory distress and air hunger, because it usually does not require patient cooperation, opening of the mouth, or laryngoscopic stimulation. However, it is contraindicated in the presence of coagulation disorder or nasal trauma, and may require subsequent change to an orotracheal tube if long-term ventilation is contemplated.

The patient's head must be placed in the "sniff" position. After mucosal anesthesia and constriction, an uncut endotracheal tube (size 8.0 for most adult males, 7.0 for most adult females) should be softened by holding it under a hot-water tap, and then gently inserted into the nares. If there is any difficulty, the opposite nares should be tried. Gentle but firm continuous pressure—not force—should be used to slide the endotracheal tube into the posterior pharynx. If there is persistent difficulty, this route should be abandoned. Proximity to the glottis is revealed by condensation of the endotracheal tube with exhalation and by audible breath sounds. With an ear close to the proximal tube and an eye on the chest, the operator attempts to quickly advance the endotracheal tube into the trachea during a patient inhalation. Firm, "rubbery" resistance or phonation means that the endotracheal tube is impinging on the epiglottis; it should be pulled back until breath sounds via the tube are maximal, and a further attempt should be made. Occasionally, it may be necessary to advance the endotracheal tube with a Magill forceps via the mouth, but great care should be taken not to grasp and puncture the cuff. Successful tracheal intubation is revealed by palpation of air exiting the proximal end of the endotracheal tube; subsequently, its position is confirmed by the standard criteria.

DIRECT LARYNGOSCOPY

This option is possible only if the patient is able to cooperate and open the mouth widely. After topical anesthesia is applied, tracheal intubation is performed in the usual way. A gum elastic bougie or similar device placed through the endotracheal tube may help obtain access to the trachea, after which the

DEFINITION OF DIFFERENT DEGREES OF A DIFFICULT AIRWAY

MASK VENTILATION

0 ——————————————————————————————————————

NATURAL AIRWAY

EASY, CHIN LIFT ONLY

ONE PERSON JAW THRUST/ MASK SEAL

ONE PERSON JAW THRUST/ MASK SEAL
+
OROPHARYNGEAL OR NASOPHARYNGEAL AIRWAY OR BOTH AIRWAYS

TWO PERSON JAW THRUST/ MASK SEAL
+
OROPHARYNGEAL OR NASOPHARYNGEAL AIRWAY OR BOTH AIRWAYS

IMPOSSIBLE, GAS EXCHANGE UNSATISFACTORY OR NONEXISTENT

BRAIN DAMAGE, DEATH

DIRECT VISION LARYNGOSCOPY AND INTUBATION

0 ← GRADE I or II LARYNGOSCOPIC VIEW → * ← GRADE III or IV LARYNGOSCOPIC VIEW →

ONE ATTEMPT, INCREASING LIFTING FORCE

ONE ATTEMPT, INCREASING LIFTING FORCE, USE BETTER SNIFF POSITION

MULTIPLE ATTEMPTS, EXTERNAL LARYNGEAL PRESSURE, MULTIPLE BLADES

MULTIPLE ATTEMPTS, EXTERNAL LARYNGEAL PRESSURE, MULTIPLE BLADES, MULTIPLE LARYNGOSCOPISTS

IMPOSSIBLE, UNSUCCESSFUL

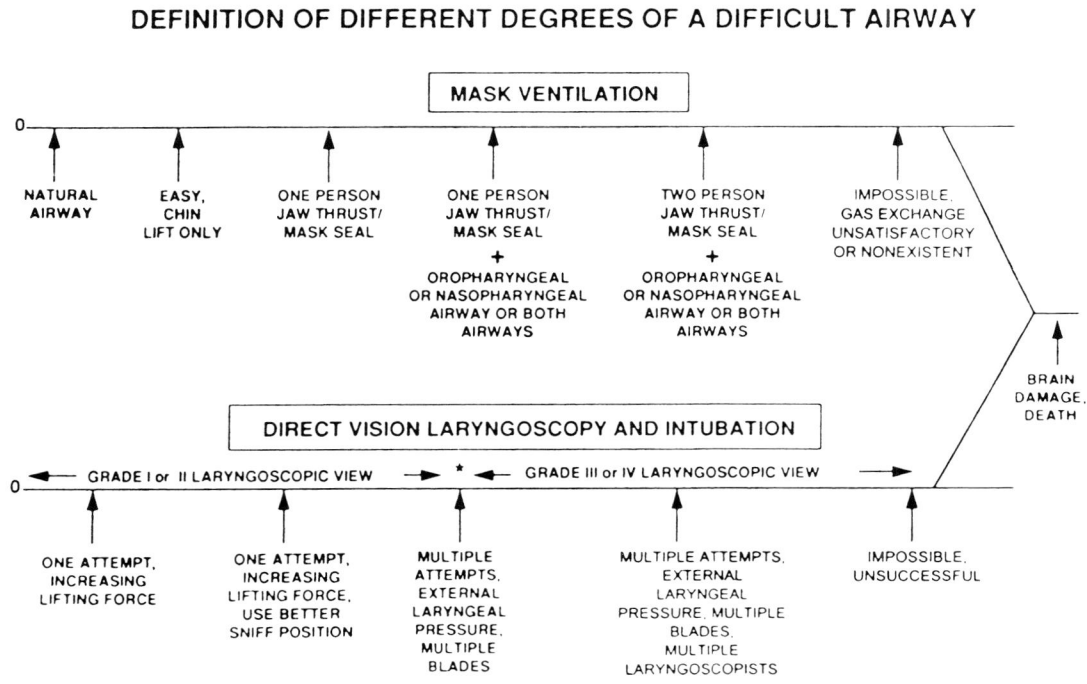

FIGURE 9–13. Definition of difficult airway. Degree of difficulty in mask ventilation or laryngoscopy may vary from zero (extremely easy) to infinite (impossible). The laryngoscopic view is graded as follows—Grade I: entire laryngeal aperture visualized; Grade II: posterior portion of aperture visualized; Grade III: only epiglottis visualized; Grade IV: only soft palate visualized. (From Benumof, J. L.: Management of the difficult adult airway: With special emphasis on the awake tracheal intubation. Anesthesiology 75:1087–1110, 1991. Used with permission.)

endotracheal tube may be guided forward. Repeated failed attempts must be curtailed to avoid edema and bleeding, and an alternative approach selected.

FIBEROPTIC BRONCHOSCOPY

Fiberoptic bronchoscopy is an extremely effective means of securing awake tracheal intubation, via either the nasal or the oral route. The advantages and disadvantages of each route have already been discussed. Use of an antisialogogue and careful topical anesthesia of the nasal or oral passage are important. The connector is removed from a size 8.0 endotracheal tube, which is slid up the fiberoptic scope. In small patients, a size 7.0 endotracheal tube fits over a pediatric bronchoscope, but this is more difficult to maneuver and the arc of vision is more restricted. Once the vocal cords have been entered with the fiberoptic scope and the tracheal rings have been visualized, the endotracheal tube is advanced under direct vision. The fiberoptic scope is then withdrawn, the endotracheal tube connector reattached, and ventilation and confirmation of endotracheal tube position performed in the usual way.

Attachment of an oxygen source at 4 to 6 l/min to the suction port of the fiberoptic scope accomplishes several benefits: The FI_{O_2} to the patient is effectively maintained during manipulation; the fiberoptic tip is kept unfogged; and secretions are blown aside. The fiberoptic scope should be kept at full stretch throughout its advancement, which assures that directional

movement of the tip is faithful to the controls. Orotracheal fiberoptic intubation is greatly facilitated by the use of the Ovassapian oral airway. When the fiberoptic scope is passed through the oral airway, it emerges close to the glottis. The airway is vertically split and easily peels off the endotracheal tube once it has been positioned in the trachea.

LARYNGEAL MASK AIRWAY

The LMA may be extremely helpful in securing a patent airway in an unconscious or semiconscious patient in whom mask ventilation is failing. Tracheal intubation can be accomplished via the LMA by the methods previously described.

RETROGRADE CANNULATION

This technique requires considerable skill and is confined to the patient who is able to maintain adequate oxygenation by spontaneous ventilation. A needle is used to puncture the cricoid membrane, through which a stiff but flexible guidewire is passed retrograde into the pharynx and retrieved from the mouth. The needle is removed, and an endotracheal tube passed anterograde over the wire, which is kept taut. However, the endotracheal tube will not pass completely into the trachea until the wire is withdrawn from the cricoid membrane; at this point, it may become dislodged from the trachea. Greater security is provided by passing the wire retrograde up the suction port of a fiberoptic bronchoscope, so that the endotracheal tube can be placed in the trachea under direct vision.

CRICOTHYROIDOTOMY AND TRACHEOSTOMY

The technical aspects of cricothyroidotomy and tracheostomy are described in the next section of this chapter. The most important consideration is not to delay these interventions so that the patient suffers unnecessary hypoxemia. In certain situations, they may need to be considered at a very early stage. If a high-pressure (50 psi) oxygen source is available, very rapid airway access can be achieved in a desperate situation by transtracheal jet ventilation. A 14-gauge intravenous catheter is inserted through the cricoid membrane, air is aspirated, the needle is withdrawn, and the catheter advanced. A 3-ml syringe is attached to the catheter; the connector from a size 6.0 endotracheal tube fits snugly into the syringe and provides access to high-pressure oxygen, which must be used because of the high resistance of the small-bore airway access.

MECHANICAL VENTILATION

The terms *mechanical ventilation* and *airway pressure therapy* refer to the gamut of artificial means used to support ventilation and oxygenation. They encompass all forms of PPV and those modes used to increase airway pressure above atmospheric during spontaneous ventilation. In this section, we define and characterize the modes of mechanical ventilation and airway pressure therapy used most often in surgical intensive care, discuss their indications and disadvantages, and explore two clinical situations in which they are essential or helpful: postoperative ventilation and the management of hypoxemia.

Classification of Mechanical Ventilation

Determinants of the Ventilator Breath Pattern

The vast majority of mechanical ventilation delivered in the operating room and intensive care unit is provided by PPV. Positive-pressure ventilator modes are defined by inspiratory events. Expiration is treated as an independent entity. The primary expiratory adjustment made, *positive end-expiratory pressure* (PEEP), is one form of airway pressure therapy that can be applied to any of the ventilator modes and is discussed separately. As illustrated in Table 9–2, ventilator breaths may be classified on the basis of three functions (or phase variables) that determine events during inspiration: initiation, limit, and cycle off (Shapiro et al., 1992). Examples of the application of these functions are given in Figure 9–14.

INITIATION

The initiation function defines how inspiration is triggered. For a controlled breath, inspiration is triggered at a predetermined time set by the ventilator rate or frequency (f), regardless of the patient's effort and respiratory cycle. For an assisted or supported breath, inspiration is triggered when the patient initiates a breath that develops a negative airway pressure below a preset threshold, termed the *sensitivity*. If no controlled breaths are provided, the ventilator rate depends on the patient's own respiratory frequency. However, not every patient breath may trigger the ventilator if the sensitivity is turned down too low for the patient's effort (it is usually set at about –2 cm H_2O).

LIMIT

The primary ventilator mode is often described by the preset limit, which defines the goal or target of positive-pressure actuation. In the *volume*-targeted mode, the tidal volume is preset. The ventilator delivers a set flow for a set time until the preset tidal volume limit is achieved. The peak airway pressure that results is variable, depending on airway and tubing flow rate and resistance and lung and chest wall compliance (described later in this chapter). In the *pressure*-targeted mode, the airway pressure is preset. The ventilator delivers a variable (often decelerating) flow to maintain a preset airway pressure limit. The tidal volume that results is variable, depending on airway and tubing flow rate and resis-

■ **Table 9–2.** APPLICATION OF BREATH FUNCTIONS (PHASE VARIABLES)

Function	Mode	Primary Parameter	Secondary Parameters
Initiation	Control	Predetermined time interval	None
	Assist	Patient-triggered, by generation of threshold negative airway pressure	Sensitivity (threshold)
Limit	Volume	Delivery of preset tidal volume	Airway pressure
	Pressure	Attainment of preset airway pressure	Tidal volume
Cycle off	Volume	Preset volume achieved	
	Time	Predetermined time interval passed	Inspiratory pause (zero flow)
	Flow	Decline to preset minimal flow rate	Patient inspiratory flow pattern

The primary parameter is that set by the operator. It determines how each of the three functions (initiation, limit, cycle off) is expressed by the mode used. Secondary parameters are variables that depend on the primary parameters set (e.g., airway pressure in volume-limited mode) or that can be added to the primary parameters (e.g., inspiratory pause).

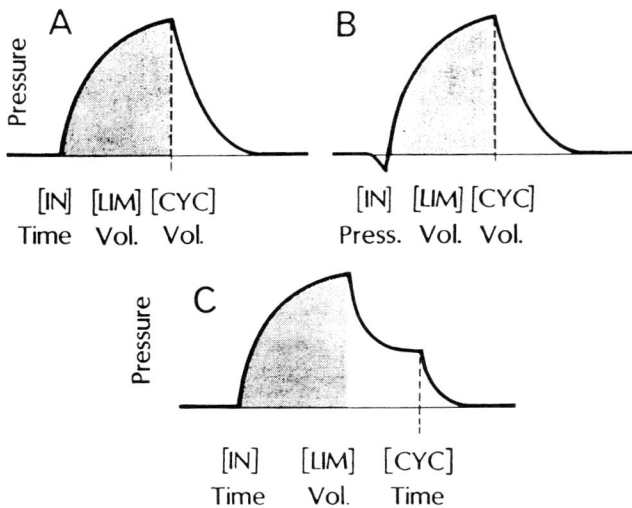

FIGURE 9–14. Characteristics of a ventilator breath. Airway pressure curves illustrating the three basic functions that determine events during inspiration in positive-pressure ventilation. (IN = initiation of the inspiratory cycle; LIM = the preset limit that defines the end-point of delivery of the positive pressure breath; CYC = cycle off—the parameter that determines when the ventilator cycles off into expiration.) *A*, Controlled mechanical ventilation. The breath is initiated at a preset time (time-initiated). The limit is a preset tidal volume; when this is achieved, positive-pressure flow ceases (volume-limited). The ventilator cycles from inspiration to expiration when the preset tidal volume has been delivered (volume-cycled). *B*, Assisted mechanical ventilation. The patient starts to breathe and develops a subatmospheric airway pressure below the baseline. As soon as a preset threshold negative airway pressure is achieved, inspiration is initiated (pressure-initiated, or patient-triggered). The limit is a preset tidal volume; when this is achieved, positive-pressure flow ceases (volume-limited). The ventilator cycles from inspiration to expiration when the preset tidal volume has been delivered (volume-cycled). *C*, Controlled mechanical ventilation with an inspiratory pause. The initiation and limit functions of the ventilator breath are identical to those in *A*: time-initiated, volume-limited. However, after the preset volume has been achieved, there is an inspiratory pause (zero flow) that extends inspiration for a preset time, until the ventilator cycles off into expiration (time-cycled). (*A–C*, From Shapiro, B. A., Kacmarek, R. M., Cane, R. D., et al.: Clinical Application of Respiratory Care. 4th ed. St. Louis, Mosby–Year Book, 1991, p. 277. Used with permission.)

tance, lung and chest wall compliance, and patient effort.

CYCLE OFF

The cycle off function defines the parameter used by the ventilator to cycle from inspiration to expiration. The parameter that is used could be tidal volume, elapsed time, inspiratory flow rate, or airway pressure. Conventional volume-targeted ventilation cycles off to expiration when the preset tidal volume has been delivered to the patient. The inspiratory time can be prolonged by the addition of a phase of zero flow, called an *inspiratory pause*. The ventilator then cycles off when a predetermined time has elapsed. The parameter of time is also used in pressure control ventilation (PCV) and airway pressure release ventilation. During pressure support ventila-

tion (PSV), the ventilator cycles off to expiration when the patient's inspiratory flow rate declines to a predetermined minimal flow rate, usually 25% of the peak flow rate.

Ventilator Modes

In Table 9–3, breath types are defined according to machine or patient control over the phase variables, and in Table 9–4, the various modes of PPV are classified based on the types of breath that are used. Commonly used terms for volume-targeted modes include controlled mechanical ventilation (CMV), assisted mechanical ventilation (AMV), assist-control ventilation (ACV), intermittent mandatory ventilation (IMV), and synchronous intermittent mandatory ventilation (SIMV) (Fig. 9–15). The pressure-targeted modes include pressure support ventilation (PSV), pressure control ventilation (PCV), and pressure assist-control ventilation (PACV) (Fig. 9–16). There is a paucity of controlled, randomized, multicenter studies comparing the different ventilatory modes, so although there are clear differences in their design principles and subjective patient acceptance, no data unequivocally demonstrate that any one of these modes provides a significant benefit over the others in success of treatment, duration of ventilator support, complications, or outcome.

VOLUME–TARGETED MODES

Controlled Mechanical Ventilation. In CMV, all breaths are initiated at a predetermined time (time-initiated) and delivered with a preset flow pattern (flow-limited). The ventilator cycles off to expiration once the tidal volume has been delivered (volume-cycled), unless an inspiratory pause is added for a predetermined time (time-cycled). The tidal volume is delivered regardless of the airway pressure achieved, unless a pressure limit is set as part of the alarm functions. If the pressure limit is exceeded (which

■ **Table 9–3.** BREATH TYPES DEFINED BY MACHINE VERSUS PATIENT CONTROL

Breath Type*	Phase Variable		
	Initiation (Trigger)	Limit	Cycle Off
Mandatory	Machine	Machine	Machine
Assisted	Patient	Machine	Machine
Supported	Patient	Machine	Patient
Spontaneous	Patient	Patient	Patient

Modified from the American Association for Respiratory Care: Consensus Statement on the Essentials of Mechanical Ventilators, 1992. Respir. Care, 37:1000, 1992.

*A *mandatory breath* is triggered, limited, and cycled off by the machine, which does all the ventilatory work. An *assisted breath* is triggered by the patient, and limited and cycled off by the machine. The patient does the work of initiating the breath only, and the ventilator does the rest. A *supported breath* is triggered by the patient, limited by the ventilator, and cycled off by the patient. The patient does the work of initiating the breath, and then interacts with the ventilator to perform a variable amount of the remaining work. A *spontaneous breath* is triggered, limited, and cycled off by the patient, who does all the ventilatory work.

■ **Table 9–4.** MODES OF MECHANICAL VENTILATION

Type of Ventilation	Initiation	Cycle Off
Volume-Targeted		
Controlled mechanical ventilation (CMV)	Control	Volume, time
Assisted mechanical ventilation (AMV)	Assist	Volume, time
Assist-control ventilation (ACV)	Assist/control	Volume, time
Intermittent mandatory ventilation (IMV)	Control (CF)	Volume, time
Synchronized IMV (SIMV)	Assist/control (DF)	Volume, time
Pressure-Targeted		
Pressure support ventilation (PSV)	Assist	Flow
Pressure control ventilation (PCV)	Control	Time
Pressure assist control ventilation (PACV)	Assist/control	Time

CF = continuous flow; DF = demand flow.

could occur with coughing, bucking, bronchospasm, or stiff lungs), an alarm sounds and the ventilator cycles to expiration without delivering the entire pre-set tidal volume. CMV is therefore limited to use in patients who are anesthetized, heavily sedated, or paralyzed or who have severe neuromuscular disorders. Minute ventilation (the product of tidal volume and respiratory rate) is determined solely by the ventilator. The primary advantage of CMV is that it completely eliminates the patient's work of breathing.

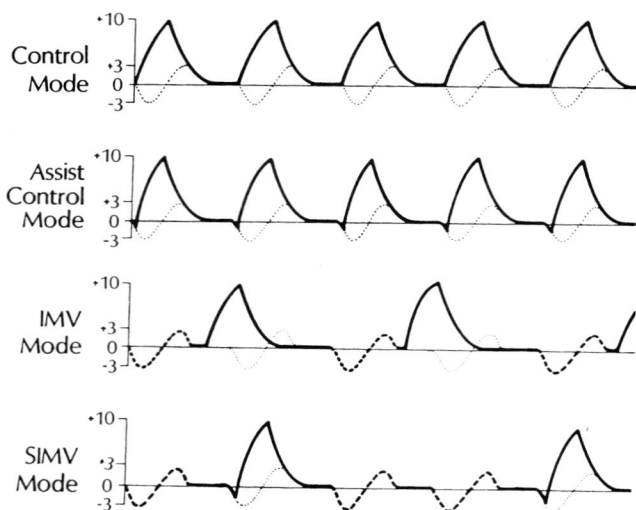

FIGURE 9–15. Volume-targeted modes. Airway pressure tracings of the four commonly used volume-targeted modes. The *thick, solid lines* represent ventilator breaths and the *thick, dotted lines* spontaneous breaths. The *thin, dotted lines* refer to the spontaneous pattern if there were no ventilator breaths. In the control mode, the machine dictates breath initiation (i.e., ventilator rate), limit (i.e., tidal volume), and cycle off (i.e., when the volume has been delivered). Assist-control mode is identical, except that the breath is initiated by negative pressure generated by the patient (i.e., patient can determine ventilator rate). In intermittent mandatory ventilation (IMV), the ventilator inserts mandatory breaths at a set frequency (the IMV rate) over the patient's spontaneous breathing pattern. In synchronous IMV (SIMV), the ventilator allows the patient to trigger the IMV breaths so that they synchronize with the patient's breathing pattern. (From Shapiro, B. A., Kacmarek, R. M., Cane, R. D., et al.: Clinical Application of Respiratory Care. 4th ed. St. Louis, Mosby–Year Book, 1991, p. 304. Used with permission.)

This is important when lung stiffness induces work of breathing that exceeds the patient's cardiopulmonary reserve.

Assisted Mechanical Ventilation. In AMV, all breaths are triggered when the patient's inspiratory effort exceeds the sensitivity threshold of negative pressure (pressure-initiated). In all other respects, AMV is similar to CMV. Inspiratory flow continues until the preset tidal volume is achieved (flow-limited, volume-cycled) regardless of airway pressure, unless a pressure alarm limit is set. An inspiratory pause can be added (time-cycled). The primary advantage of AMV over CMV is that it is well tolerated in the presence of light sedation. Indeed, heavy sedation or muscle relaxation contraindicates the use of AMV. The patient's work of breathing is greater than that on CMV, but breathing is still provided largely by the ventilator. Despite the preset tidal volume, minute ventilation is determined to a large extent by the patient, who sets the respiratory rate. This provides a major limitation for AMV. Patients with central hyperventilation syndromes and tachypnea generate an extremely high minute ventilation, with the potential for dangerous levels of respiratory alkalosis, hypokalemia, and arrhythmias. In contrast, patients who are oversedated with opioids and have an impaired ventilatory response to hypercarbia, or who are too weak to trigger the patient-assisted initiation function, may receive slow ventilator rates and inadequate minute ventilation.

Assist-control Ventilation. The latter problem has been addressed by the development of ACV, which has superseded AMV. In essence, ACV is a combination of AMV and CMV. The ventilator rate that is set by the operator on ACV ensures that the patient receives a *minimal* number of breaths per minute by CMV, while still allowing the patient to receive AMV if the spontaneous respiratory rate exceeds the control rate. It should be noted that ACV does not protect against hyperventilation, only hypoventilation. Also, the patient cannot be weaned from the ventilator by weaning the ACV rate. For example, suppose a patient has a spontaneous rate of 16 breaths per minute, and the ACV rate is set at 12 breaths per minute, with a preset tidal volume of 1 l. The actual minute

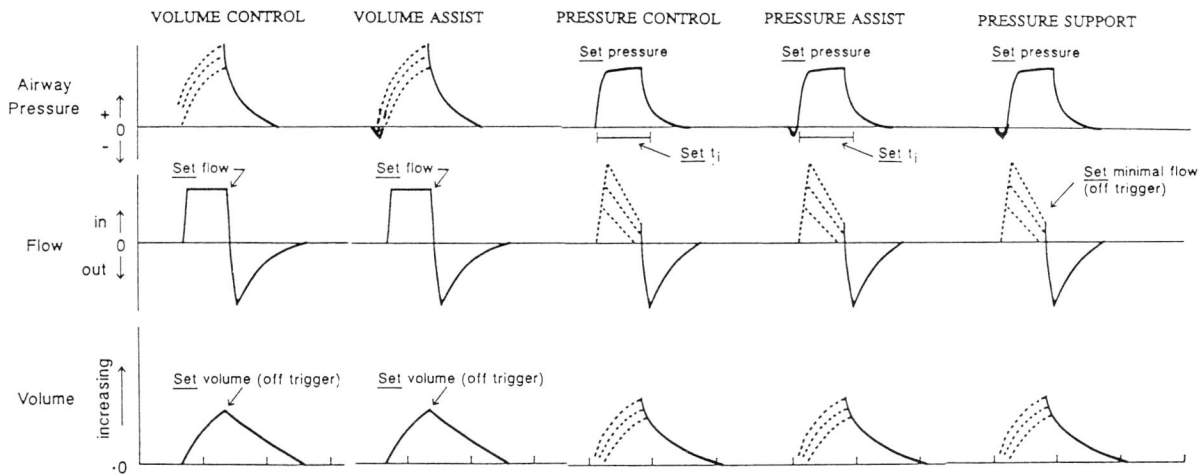

FIGURE 9–16. Comparison of volume and pressure modes. The *top line* represents airway pressure (+ and − indicate above and below atmospheric pressure), the *middle line* represents gas flow (*in* and *out* indicate flow toward and away from the patient), and the *lower line* represents tidal volume. In volume-control mode, or controlled mechanical ventilation (CMV), the tidal volume and inspiratory flow rate are preset. The breath cycles to expiration when the preset tidal volume is reached (off trigger). Airway pressure is variable, depending on lung and chest wall compliance. In volume-assist mode, or assist-control ventilation (ACV), the situation is similar to CMV, except that the patient triggers the breath by generating negative pressure at the start of inspiration. In pressure-control mode, or pressure-control ventilation (PCV), the maximal airway pressure and inspiratory time (t_i) are preset. Gas flow rate can be varied and tidal volume depends on lung and chest wall compliance. In pressure-assist mode, or pressure assist-control ventilation (PACV), the situation is identical except that the patient triggers the breath by generating negative pressure at the start of inspiration. In pressure support mode, or pressure support ventilation (PSV), the situation is similar to PACV, except that the patient is able to increase the delivered tidal volume by continued spontaneous inspiration after the maximal airway pressure has been achieved. The ventilator cycles into expiration (off trigger) when the patient's gas flow declines to about 25% of the peak flow rate.

ventilation the patient will generate is 16 l, whereas the *guaranteed* minute ventilation is 12 l. If the ACV rate is decreased to 8 breaths per minute without any change in the patient's spontaneous ventilatory rate, the patient will still generate a minute ventilation of 16 l. The change in ACV rate will be of consequence only if the patient stops breathing spontaneously, in which case the minute ventilation would decline to the new guaranteed minimum of 8 l.

Intermittent Mandatory Ventilation. IMV is essentially a combination of CMV and spontaneous ventilation. A modified circuit provides a continuous gas flow that allows the patient to breathe spontaneously with minimal work of breathing. At a predetermined frequency (the IMV rate), the ventilator provides a positive-pressure breath to the patient identical to a CMV breath (time-initiated, flow-limited, and volume-cycled, unless an inspiratory pause is added for a predetermined time). The tidal volume is delivered regardless of the airway pressure achieved, unless a pressure limit is set as part of the alarm functions.

Synchronous IMV. In conventional IMV, the IMV breath is delivered regardless of the stage of the patient's spontaneous cycle—for example, it could occur at the end of a spontaneous inspiratory effort (and cause an excessive tidal volume) or during exhalation (and conflict with the patient's effort). SIMV was developed to overcome this problem by allowing the patient to trigger the IMV breath in the assist mode (pressure-initiated). The breath that is delivered is analogous to an AMV breath. However, if the patient does not trigger an SIMV breath within an allotted time, the ventilator delivers a conventional IMV breath (time-initiated)—for example, if the SIMV rate is set to 10 breaths per minute, the ventilator allows the patient a 6-second "window" to trigger an SIMV breath. If there is no spontaneous breath that exceeds the trigger threshold within 6 seconds, the ventilator provides a conventional IMV breath.

Advantages of IMV/SIMV. The primary advantage of IMV is that it allows variation in the relative work of breathing provided by the ventilator versus that provided by the patient, that is, in the ratio of ventilator to spontaneous breaths. In adults at high IMV rates (e.g., 10 to 12 breaths per minute), the patient's work of breathing is usually negligible. Indeed, if the patient does not breathe spontaneously at all, CMV is provided. At low IMV rates (e.g., 4 to 6 breaths per minute), the patient usually contributes a substantial proportion of the work of breathing, and also determines a large component of the minute ventilation. Unlike ACV, IMV does not exacerbate central hyperventilation syndromes because the IMV rate is fixed, and the patient's tachypnea is not augmented by large, machine-delivered tidal volumes.

IMV was initially developed in the early 1970s by Kirby and his associates (1971) at the University of Florida in Gainesville. They observed that neonates with respiratory distress syndrome with respiratory rates of close to 100 breaths per minute required heavy sedation, muscle relaxation, or hyperventilation to induce hypocarbia and abolish the ventilatory drive so that they could tolerate conventional ventilation (CMV or ACV). By designing a circuit that allowed spontaneous ventilation, these authors were able to provide relatively low IMV rates (30 to 40 breaths per minute) and avoid the side effects of sedation, paralysis, or hyperventilation. Similar benefits may be achieved in adults with hypoxemic respiratory failure, albeit at lower IMV rates.

During the spontaneous ventilatory component of IMV, there is improved matching of ventilation and perfusion and enhanced hemodynamic and renal function (these are discussed later). However, these benefits are directly related to the relative preponderance of spontaneous versus IMV ventilation. The physiologic impact of high IMV rates is very similar to that of CMV or AMV.

In patients with chronic obstructive lung disease and carbon dioxide retention, IMV allows the adjustment of minute ventilation to preserve hypercarbia and facilitate ventilatory weaning. For example, a patient with chronic obstructive lung disease has an arterial carbon dioxide tension (Pa_{CO_2}) of 56 mm Hg, and has developed a compensatory metabolic alkalosis with a bicarbonate (HCO_3) of 32 mEq/l so that her pH is 7.38. If, after intubation, she was placed on CMV with ventilator settings that produced a normal Pa_{CO_2} of 40 mm Hg, her pH would increase to 7.51 because the pH increases about 0.08 for an acute decrease in Pa_{CO_2} of 10 mm Hg. (On ACV, this situation may be exacerbated because many patients hyperventilate slightly to a Pa_{CO_2} of around 34 to 36 mm Hg). If mechanical ventilation were continued for several days, the kidneys would attempt to normalize the pH to 7.40 by excreting HCO_3 until its level declined to 24 mEq/l. If this patient was then extubated, her Pa_{CO_2} would once again climb to 56 mm Hg, and her pH would abruptly fall to 7.27 and possibly contribute to acute respiratory failure. In contrast, by appropriate adjustment of the IMV rate in such a patient, it is possible to maintain the Pa_{CO_2} close to 56 mm Hg and preserve the HCO_3, so that there would be no change in pH after tracheal extubation.

Ventilatory Weaning with IMV. Because of the ability to adjust the relative contribution from the patient to the total work of breathing, IMV has become a popular mode for ventilatory weaning, especially in the postoperative period. In most postoperative patients who have relatively normal lung function, IMV serves as a device to allow slower, graded ventilatory weaning with careful patient assessment. Once the patient is fully rewarmed, stable, and emerging from anesthesia, the IMV rate is usually weaned in decrements of 2 breaths per minute (e.g., from 10 to 8 to 6 to 4 breaths per minute). During this phase, two parameters are closely observed. First, the patient should have recovered from the residual effects of opioid anesthesia or sedation. This is evidenced by appropriate "overbreathing" (i.e., the patient's respiratory frequency exceeds that of the IMV rate) and by the absence of respiratory acidosis (pH > 7.35; Pa_{CO_2} < 50 mm Hg) on an arterial blood gas. Second, the patient should be able to sustain a constant level of oxygenation. If the Pa_{O_2} declines as the IMV rate is lowered toward 4 breaths per minute, it suggests that the patient's spontaneous ventilations are shallow and inadequate, and that the functional residual ca-

pacity (FRC) is declining as positive pressure support is being withdrawn. If one or both of these criteria are not met, tracheal extubation should be delayed until the patient has recovered more fully from anesthesia or sedation. Lung mechanics are usually tested at an IMV rate of 4 breaths per minute. It is important to note that excellent muscle strength does not exclude residual narcosis, so the patient must be observed for a period of time (usually 20 to 40 minutes) and an arterial blood gas obtained prior to tracheal extubation.

The original IMV systems provided fresh gas in a continuous-flow mode, which minimized the work that the patient required to open the exhalation valve (usually less than 2 to 3 cm H_2O below baseline pressure). SIMV uses a demand-flow system to actuate the pressure-initiated IMV breath in the form of a patient-triggered assisted breath. This imposes increased work on the patient. Significant work is also performed in overcoming the resistance of the ventilator circuit during spontaneous breathing. This may occur when the IMV rate is weaned down to zero, and the patient breathes spontaneously on PEEP (known as *continuous positive airway pressure* [CPAP] mode). For these reasons, the IMV rate is seldom weaned below 4 breaths per minute. If the patient meets extubation criteria at this setting, tracheal extubation is performed. It has, in fact, become customary to add 5 to 10 cm H_2O pressure support to IMV to minimize the work of breathing used to open the demand valve (decreasing it to the same level as in continuous-flow mode) and overcome the resistance of the endotracheal tube and the ventilator circuit (see later in this chapter). This may also allow increased baseline pressure to be tolerated with negligible increases in work of breathing.

The utility of IMV weaning in patients with severe lung disease or poor lung compliance is less clear. Support of the work of each breath with IMV is an "all or none" phenomenon. Either the ventilator provides nearly 100% of the work (during the IMV breath) or 0% of the work (during spontaneous ventilation). Patients with poor lung compliance commonly develop tachypnea, signs of respiratory fatigue, hemodynamic instability, and increasing anxiety and agitation as IMV rates are decreased below 6 to 8 breaths per minute. In extreme cases, ventilatory weaning with IMV becomes protracted or impossible. This has led to the rapidly increasing popularity of PSV as a weaning mode in patients with intact ventilatory drive but deranged respiratory mechanics (see later in this chapter).

PRESSURE–TARGETED MODES

Pressure Support Ventilation. PSV is a unique pressure-preset, volume-variable mode that allows close tracking of the patient's ventilatory effort and precise decremental withdrawal of ventilatory support of the work of breathing. The PSV breath is triggered by the patient's negative inspiratory effort, as in AMV or ACV, so PSV is applicable only to spontaneously breathing patients. It cannot be used in heavily sedated or paralyzed patients who are not breathing on their own. Once initiated, there is a rapid flow of fresh gas until the predefined airway pressure limit above baseline is achieved. For example, if the patient is on 5 cm H_2O PEEP, and a PSV level of 20 cm H_2O is selected, the ventilator will deliver rapid gas flow until an airway pressure of 25 cm H_2O (5 + 20) is achieved. Thereafter, the ventilator adjusts the inspiratory flow using microprocessor circuitry to keep the airway pressure constant as long as the patient continues to actively inhale. In this manner, the patient is able to increase the delivered tidal volume above that provided by the ventilator alone. The total tidal volume and work of breathing is the sum of that provided by the ventilator and that performed by the patient. The actual tidal volume delivered for a given level of PSV depends on patient effort, airway resistance, and chest wall and lung compliance, and must be measured with each breath. Toward the end of inspiration, when the patient's inspiratory flow rate declines to approximately 25% of the peak flow rate, the ventilator cycles off into expiration (Fig. 9–17). In summary, PSV is pressure-initiated, pressure-limited, and flow-cycled.

The major advantage of PSV over SIMV is that it provides support with *every* breath that the patient takes. An apt analogy is to imagine an anesthesiologist assisting a spontaneously breathing patient's ventilation by manual compression of the reservoir bag. The anesthesiologist is providing a form of PSV, the level of which is proportional to the force with which he compresses the bag once the patient has initiated a breath. Initially, at a high level of PSV, the ventilator provides close to 100% of the work of breathing and the patient's effort is minimal. As the level of PSV is reduced, usually in decrements of 1 to 2 cm H_2O, the relative contributions to the work of the breath by the ventilator and by the patient change inversely to each other. Because part of the tidal volume is generated by the patient's spontaneous effort, peak airway pressure is generally lower with PSV than IMV. However, since maximal inspiratory airway pressure is reached early in the breath, mean airway pressure tends to be higher, which may help oxygenation. Many patients appear to feel more comfortable on PSV than IMV, presumably because of the variable flow pattern and the reduction in their work of breathing with each breath.

Ventilatory Weaning with PSV. PSV is initiated by determining the approximate tidal volume desired. For example, it has been found that the level of PSV that generates a tidal volume of approximately 10 to 12 ml/kg provides about 95% of the work of breathing. Depending on resistance and compliance effects, this level is generally between 20 and 30 cm H_2O. Successful application of PSV to a tachypneic patient with a high work of breathing results in an almost immediate decrease in the patient's spontaneous ventilatory rate, optimally to less than 20 breaths per minute. Ventilatory weaning is performed by gradual reduction in the level of PSV by decrements of 1 to 2 cm H_2O every 8 to 12 hours. The rate of weaning must be individualized to the patient. Weaning of PSV is accompanied by a decrease in the tidal volume generated and an increase in the patient's respiratory frequency. The key to success is to increase the patient's work of breathing at a tolerable rate and allow adequate recruitment of atrophied and discoordinate respiratory musculature.

Most ventilators allow IMV and PSV to be used simultaneously. Some authorities suggest always supplying a low IMV rate of between 2 and 0.5 breaths per minute. The rationale for this is to insert an intermittent fixed, large-volume breath (i.e., a "sigh") to help maintain the FRC. No data suggest that patients do better with or without this maneuver. On the other hand, the IMV mode can be left out altogether, especially in patients who do not tolerate fixed-flow, volume-cycled breaths or large IMV breath volumes. Patients with lung disease may require a PSV of up to 10 cm H_2O to overcome the resistance of the endotracheal tube. Once weaning has reached this level, they should be assessed for endotracheal extubation. Work of breathing at PSV less than 10 cm H_2O may be greater than that incurred after actual tracheal extubation.

Limitations of PSV. PSV depends on the presence of spontaneous ventilation. It cannot be prescribed in association with CMV, AMV, or ACV and will not come into effect if the patient is not spontaneously overbreathing on IMV. It may be inappropriate to use PSV when lung compliance is extremely poor and

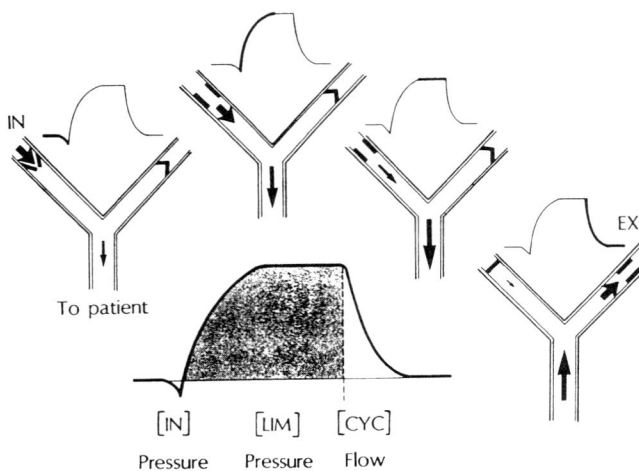

FIGURE 9–17. Pressure support ventilation (PSV). At inspiration (IN), the patient starts to take a spontaneous breath, opens the inflow valve, and gas flows in until the threshold negative airway pressure is achieved, after which the ventilator breath is triggered. The ventilator then delivers gas flow under positive pressure to the patient until the preset maximal airway pressure is reached (determined by the level of pressure support set) (LIM). Thereafter, the ventilator maintains a plateau pressure while allowing the patient to continue to draw in fresh gas spontaneously and increase the total tidal volume. When the patient's inspiratory flow rate declines to less than 25% of the peak flow rate, the ventilator cycles off (CYC) into expiration. EX = expiration. (From Shapiro, B. A., Kacmarek, R. M., Cane, R. D., et al.: Clinical Application of Respiratory Care. 4th ed. St. Louis, Mosby–Year Book, 1991. Used with permission.)

patient efforts are feeble, because high levels of PSV will prematurely terminate and generate small tidal volumes only. Patients with central hyperventilation syndromes tend to develop excessively high minute ventilation and acute respiratory alkalosis on PSV, just as with AMV and ACV. This can be immediately identified by noting the absence of a decrease in spontaneous respiratory frequency when PSV is initiated, together with a large increase in minute ventilation. Occasionally, a low level of PSV (e.g., 10 to 12 cm H_2O) may be titrated that provides meaningful reduction in work of breathing without unacceptable hypocapnia.

Pressure Control Ventilation and Pressure Assist-control Ventilation. PCV is a time-initiated, pressure-limited, and time-cycled mode intended for patients requiring total mechanical ventilatory support. Most ventilators also allow patient triggering of these breaths, producing pressure "assisted" breaths and the capability for PACV. Pressure-limited, time-cycled breaths accomplish two goals that may be very helpful in patients with poor lung compliance and oxygenation. First, the upper limit of peak airway pressure is fixed. This may reduce the risk of barotrauma, although this has not been proved. Moreover, since *alveolar* pressures (i.e., plateau pressures) are comparable for a similar tidal volume with that on a volume-cycled ventilator, there may be no reduction in barotrauma risk. Second, and more important, time cycling with more rapid alveolar filling may increase mean inflation pressure. Alveolar ventilation and oxygenation are thereby improved, allowing reduction of the inspired oxygen fraction (FI_{O_2}). However, the increased mean inflation pressure and very rapid initial flows may themselves induce barotrauma or impair cardiac filling.

Immediately after initiation of any pressure-limited breath, fresh gas flow rapidly achieves the preset pressure limit above baseline. For example, if a pressure control of 25 cm H_2O is prescribed in a patient already on 10 cm H_2O PEEP, the peak airway pressure will be 35 cm H_2O (i.e., 10 + 25). Thereafter flow decelerates and may completely cease with an inspiratory pause. This sustains the airway pressure at the preset limit until the defined time to cycle off into expiration is reached. Time-initiation and time-cycling allows precise definition of inspiratory and expiratory ratios during PCV, but for optimal effect, the ventilatory pattern must be very stable from breath to breath. As with PSV, the delivered tidal volume must be measured continuously. PCV does not allow any patient interaction with the ventilator and is not well tolerated in awake patients. Heavy sedation, often with muscle relaxation, is required, as it is in volume-cycled CMV. On the other hand, an advantage of PACV in the patient with intact ventilatory drive may be improved patient comfort because of the variable flow pattern.

PCV or PACV is initiated by selecting a pressure limit that keeps the peak airway pressure about 40 cm H_2O or less, in the hope that this will limit barotrauma. The actual pressure limit is guided by the level of mean airway pressure that provides the best ratio between the Pa_{O_2} and the FI_{O_2} (P:F ratio). The primary goal is to achieve a safe Pa_{O_2}, that is, above 60 mm Hg (90% hemoglobin saturation), at an FI_{O_2} very unlikely to induce oxygen toxicity, that is, 0.4 or less. If the Pa_{O_2} were 60 mm Hg at an FI_{O_2} of 1.0, the P:F is 60/1.0 = 60. If the FI_{O_2} is 0.3, the P:F is 60/0.3 = 200. A secondary goal is to achieve a P:F greater than 200. The tidal volume, a variable parameter, must be monitored from breath to breath. Any decline in lung or chest wall compliance—such as that caused by inadequate muscle relaxation—decreases tidal volume. Air trapping that results in "auto-PEEP" (intrinsic PEEP) also lowers tidal volume in pressure-limited ventilation (see later in this chapter).

An inadequate level of inspiratory pressure may produce small tidal volumes, decreased P:F, and hypercapnia. On the other hand, excessive levels of inspiratory pressure may so increase alveolar ventilation that acute hypocapnia results despite slow ventilator rates.

Inverse Ratio Ventilation. Inverse ratio ventilation (IRV) is a form of airway pressure therapy, in that mean airway pressure is directly elevated by prolongation of the inspiratory time. It is usually used only with PCV because of its precisely timed inspiratory-to-expiratory (I:E) ratio and control of peak airway pressure. Inspiratory time is increased at the expense of expiratory time by prolongation of the inspiratory pause, which can invert the normal I:E ratio. IRV is increased by small, fixed increments that require precise and interactive manipulations of inspiratory flow and time—for example, I:E may be progressively increased through 1:2, 1.5:2, 1:1, 1.5:1, 2:1, 3:1, to 4:1 or until the desired goal of a Pa_{O_2} greater than 60 mm Hg at an FI_{O_2} of 0.4 or less is achieved.

Inspiratory time prolongation can improve ventilation-perfusion matching by two mechanisms: prolonged inspiratory mixing and development of air trapping ("auto-PEEP" or intrinsic PEEP) (Pepe and Marini, 1982). Air trapping is more likely to develop with the use of high I:E ratios at rapid ventilator rates (Fig. 9–18). As the inspiratory time is prolonged, there may be insufficient time for complete expiration. The next breath is delivered before airway pressure returns to baseline. The new baseline pressure that develops is the intrinsic PEEP. Development of intrinsic PEEP may improve oxygenation by increasing mean airway pressure; indeed, some believe this may be one of the most important benefits of IRV. However, it is usually suggested that the level of PEEP set at the ventilator (extrinsic PEEP) be reduced by the amount of intrinsic PEEP so that the total PEEP remains unchanged. Because the maximal airway pressure is limited, air trapping and intrinsic PEEP reduce the delivered tidal volume and may cause progressive hypercarbia. Paradoxically, a *decrease* in ventilator rate at this stage may actually correct the hypercarbia by allowing a longer expiratory time, reduced air trapping and intrinsic PEEP, and increased delivered tidal volume.

FIGURE 9–18. Air trapping during inverse ratio ventilation (IRV). In this example taken from a pediatric patient receiving PCV with IRV, the *upper graph* indicates delivered tidal volume, the *middle graph* indicates gas flow rate (by convention, above the zero line flow is toward the patient, i.e., inspiration, and below the zero line flow is away from the patient, i.e., expiration), and the *lower graph* indicates airway pressure. Initial ventilator settings include a ventilator rate (f) of 60 breaths/min, inspiratory time (T_I) of 0.6 sec, inspiratory : expiratory ratio (I : E) of 1 : 0.7, tidal volume (V_T) of 95 ml, and minute ventilation ($\dot{V}_E$) of 5.5 l/min. Pressure limit or relief (Press. Relief) is set at 25 cm H_2O, peak airway pressure (P_{AW}) is 25 cm H_2O and mean P_{AW} is 12.1 cm H_2O. Baseline P_{AW} (i.e., the airway pressure at end-expiration) is 0 cm H_2O. An increase in IRV with an increase in I : E to 1 : 0.3 induces air trapping, illustrated to the right of the broken line. Inspiration commences before the previous expiration is complete, so that airway pressure never declines to zero during expiration, and a new baseline (+ 2 cm H_2O) is set. This is instrinsic positive end-expiratory pressure ($PEEP_i$). Because the pressure limit is fixed at 25 cm H_2O, inflation pressure (peak − baseline) is reduced. There is a decrease in delivered V_T and V_E to 85 ml and 5.2 l/min, respectively. Progressive air trapping results in hypercarbia. Mean P_{AW} is increased to 15.4 cm H_2O by $PEEP_i$, which may improve oxygenation but impede cardiac function. (From MacIntyre, N. R., and Hagus, C. K.: Graphical analysis of flow, pressure and volume during mechanical ventilation. © Bear Medical Systems, Inc., Riverside, CA, 1989, p. 80. Used with permission.)

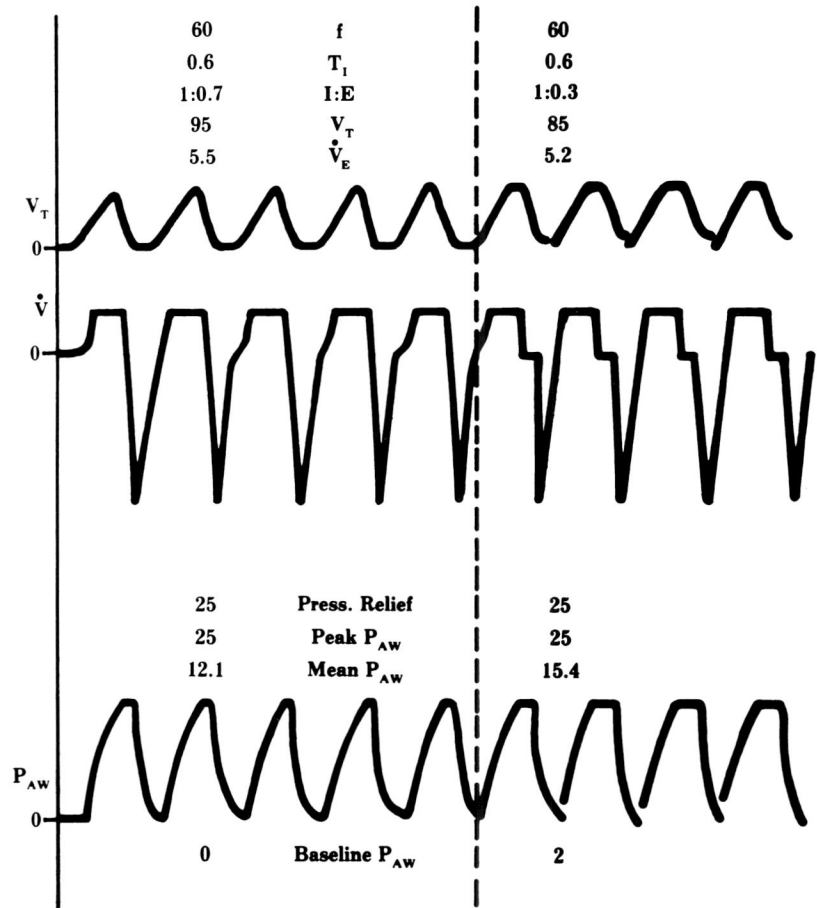

60	f		60
0.6	T_I		0.6
1:0.7	I:E		1:0.3
95	V_T		85
5.5	$\dot{V}_E$		5.2

25	Press. Relief		25
25	Peak P_{AW}		25
12.1	Mean P_{AW}		15.4
0	Baseline P_{AW}		2

Limitations of PCV and IRV. A major limitation of PCV-IRV is that it requires heavy sedation, usually with the addition of skeletal muscle relaxants, to ensure complete ventilatory control and timing. Conscious patients do not tolerate the prolonged inspiratory phase of IRV. Emergence from sedation may be associated with rapid decline in delivered tidal volume and desaturation. Effects on venous return, cardiac output, and renal function may be substantial at high levels of IRV and be poorly tolerated in patients with cardiac dysfunction. The development of air trapping and intrinsic PEEP may be subtle and is technically difficult to monitor. Transport of patients out of the intensive care unit requires the use of an AMBU fitted with a PEEP valve to maintain mean airway pressure close to its original setting and the placement of a suitable ventilator in the operating room or the radiology suite. Sudden release of mean airway pressure through the use of standard AMBUs or anesthesia ventilators may have disastrous consequences.

POSITIVE END–EXPIRATORY PRESSURE

PEEP is the most established means of providing airway pressure therapy. It is applied during expiration and can be added to every type of mechanical ventilation, from spontaneous ventilation (where it is referred to as CPAP) to PCV-IRV. The primary goals of the use of PEEP are to increase FRC (Shapiro et al., 1984), distend patent alveoli (at levels less than 10 cm H_2O), and recruit previously collapsed alveoli (at levels greater than 10 cm H_2O). In pulmonary edema, PEEP may redistribute extravascular lung water, and thereby improve FRC, lung compliance, and oxygen diffusion (Paré et al., 1983). However, PEEP does not decrease total extravascular lung water; in fact, it may increase it (Demling et al., 1975). PEEP appears to move extravascular lung water from the alveolar-capillary interstitium to the peribronchial and perihilar interstitium, and thus renders the alveoli more compliant.

A low level of PEEP (5 cm H_2O) is routinely used to maintain FRC during postoperative mechanical ventilation as a substitute for the "physiologic PEEP" provided by glottic closure in the nonintubated patient. It seldom, if ever, causes any adverse effects. Moderate levels of PEEP (6 to 10 cm H_2O) are used to reverse atelectasis during postoperative mechanical ventilation (see later in this chapter). Higher levels of PEEP (>10 cm H_2O) are used to treat acute respiratory failure, as discussed in the section on the use of airway pressure therapy. Under these circumstances, PEEP is generally titrated to achieve the best compliance or best P:F ratio (see later in this chapter).

Adverse Effects and Limitations of PEEP. Because PEEP directly increases all airway pressures (peak, mean, and baseline), it exacerbates the circulatory and barotrauma effects of mechanical ventilation, discussed later. Adverse effects are related to the magnitude of increased airway and alveolar pressures. By causing alveolar distention, PEEP can increase intrapulmonary dead space. Ultimately, this causes air trapping, carbon dioxide retention, and hypercapnia. This is especially liable to occur in patients with emphysema or acute bronchospasm (Pepe and Marini, 1982).

PEEP is distributed uniformly throughout the lungs. Normal, compliant alveoli are more likely to be distended by PEEP than collapsed, stiff alveoli. For this reason, PEEP may not be very effective in patients with localized lung disease, because it overdistends normal lung zones rather than diseased areas (Horton and Cheney, 1975). Airway pressure increases, but oxygenation does not improve, and hypercarbia results.

Finally, the application of PEEP in spontaneously breathing patients may provide an unacceptable increase in the work of breathing if a demand valve is utilized, as in SIMV.

Adverse Effects of Mechanical Ventilation and Airway Pressure Therapy

Ventilation-Perfusion Mismatch

Gravity augments perfusion to the dependent zones of the lung, but gas delivered by PPV follows the path of least resistance, so that ventilation is greatest in the nondependent zones. During normal spontaneous breathing, the diaphragm actively ventilates dependent lung zones. When the diaphragm is paralyzed, it is passively pushed cephalad by the abdominal viscera into the dependent lung zone, further impeding ventilation to that area (Froese and Bryan, 1974). Therefore, PPV invariably results in mismatched ventilation and perfusion, especially when used with skeletal muscle relaxants (Fig. 9–19). This mismatch in ventilation and perfusion induces an increased alveolar-arterial oxygen gradient, requiring a higher inspired oxygen fraction (FI_{O_2}).

Circulatory Impairment

EFFECTS ON CARDIAC OUTPUT

During the inspiratory phase of normal spontaneous ventilation, venous return to the heart is augmented by the generation of negative intrapleural pressure. All modes of PPV increase intrathoracic pressure, decreasing venous return of blood to the heart and decreasing cardiac output (Pinsky et al., 1985). Intravascular measures of cardiac preload (central venous pressure, pulmonary artery wedge pressure [PAWP]) increase during PPV. However, the true distending ventricular pressure (the transmural pressure) declines, because it equals the intravascular pressure minus the intrapleural pressure (Jardin et al., 1981).

Circulatory effects are directly proportional to the degree of elevation of mean airway pressure and intrathoracic pressure and are exacerbated by hypovolemia (Qvist et al., 1975). For example, during IMV, the adverse effect on the circulation is greater the higher the IMV rate and the smaller the contribution of spontaneous ventilation. The effect of PSV on intrathoracic pressure depends on the relative ventilator and patient contributions to inspiration. Controlled modes (CMV, PCV), which allow no spontaneous patient effort, have the greatest effect on venous return and cardiac output. The addition of IRV to PCV further limits the expiratory time during which venous return occurs. Finally, PEEP, which may be used with any ventilatory mode, increases mean airway pressure proportional to the level applied. Paradoxically, in the presence of severe disease and stiff, noncompliant lungs, the transmission of intra-alveolar pressure to the intravascular space is less, and the adverse circulatory effects of PPV are attenuated.

Other lung-heart interactions contribute to circulatory effects. The use of PEEP at levels greater than 10 cm H_2O may compress the pulmonary capillary bed, increase right ventricular afterload and pressure, and cause the intraventricular septum to shift and impede left ventricular filling (Jardin et al., 1981). Decreased left ventricular filling also occurs as a consequence of the direct transmission of elevated intrathoracic pressure to the heart.

EFFECTS ON RENAL FUNCTION

Mechanical ventilation and airway pressure therapy suppress renal function by a complex series of mechanisms (Doherty and Sladen, 1989). About 25% of the total cardiac output is directed to the kidneys, and renal blood flow declines pari passu with a decline in cardiac output. In addition, the baroreceptor response to hypotension induced by PPV triggers the release of catecholamines, activation of the renin-angiotensin-aldosterone system, and antidiuretic hormone (Annat et al., 1983; Sellden et al., 1986). The net effect of these responses is to cause renal vasoconstriction; decrease renal blood flow, glomerular filtration rate, and urine flow; and promote salt and water retention. The decrease in atrial transmural pressure induced by airway pressure therapy appears to inhibit the release of atrial natriuretic factor, which also impedes glomerular filtration rate and urine flow rate (Andrivet et al., 1988; Kharasch et al., 1988). If intrathoracic pressure is increased sufficiently to increase renal vein pressure, renal blood flow and glomerular filtration rate are further impaired (Mullins et al., 1984).

EFFECTS ON BRAIN AND LIVER

The use of airway pressure therapy during mechanical ventilation impairs venous return from the head and may thereby increase ICP and worsen neurologic

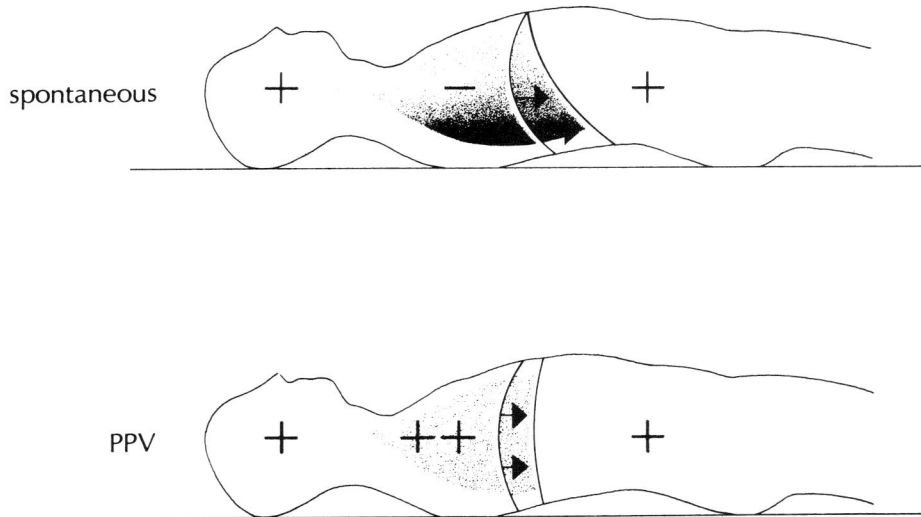

FIGURE 9–19. Ventilation-perfusion matching. During spontaneous ventilation (*top diagram*), active contraction of the diaphragm overcomes the pressure of the abdominal contents and creates subatmospheric pressure in the pleural space. This draws air into the lungs. Ventilation is greater in the dependent portion of the lung because the net change in alveolar size is greater than in nondependent regions. This provides optimal ventilation-perfusion matching because gravity dictates that perfusion is greatest in the dependent region as well. In addition, venous return to the heart is augmented by the relatively negative intrathoracic pressure. During positive-pressure ventilation (PPV), especially if the diaphragm is paralyzed, the weight of the abdominal contents compresses the dependent region and gas distribution is greater to the nondependent lung zones, resulting in ventilation-perfusion mismatch and increased alveolar-arterial O_2 gradient. Venous return to the heart is hindered by the relatively positive intrathoracic pressure and cardiac output declines. (From Shapiro, B. A., Kacmarek, R. M., Cane, R. D., et al.: Clinical Application of Respiratory Care. 4th ed. St. Louis, Mosby–Year Book, 1991, p. 282. Used with permission.)

injury (Doblar et al., 1981). However, elevation of the head of the bed usually attenuates the effect of PEEP on ICP and improves lung function. Impairment of hepatic vein outflow by airway pressure therapy may cause passive congestion of the liver (Bonnet et al., 1982).

THERAPEUTIC STRATEGIES

Two therapeutic strategies address the impairment of cardiac and renal function induced by PPV. The first is to choose a mode of ventilation that provides the lowest mean airway pressure while still sustaining adequate levels of oxygenation. Thus, patients on a high IMV rate who are hypovolemic may benefit from a reduction of the IMV rate to the lowest rate tolerated. The second is to enhance cardiac and renal function by the use of preload augmentation, inotropic agents, or vasodilator therapy. Careful fluid administration reverses the effects of airway pressure therapy (Venus et al., 1985) and renal function is restored when cardiac output reaches only 70% of control values (Priebe et al., 1981). Both the cardiac and the renal effects of PEEP can be reversed by modest doses (5 μg · kg^{-1} · min^{-1}) of dopamine (Hemmer and Suter, 1979).

Barotrauma

PATHOGENESIS

The term *barotrauma* refers to physical damage done to the lungs by pressure applied in the airways and alveoli. Studies on animals revealed that this includes epithelial desquamation and necrosis, increased microvascular permeability, and inflammatory changes indistinguishable from ARDS. However, the earliest and most common consequence of barotrauma is rupture of the fragile alveolar epithelium, so that air enters the interstitium (Cullen and Caldera, 1979). Pulmonary interstitial emphysema is identified on chest film as dark, linear shadows emanating along the perivascular spaces, on the periphery of the lung fields, and surrounding the cardiac contour (Fig. 9–20). The most sensitive means of identifying all forms of pulmonary barotrauma is computed tomography scanning. Air tracks back to the mediastinum (pneumomediastinum), then cephalad to the thoracic inlet. From there, it follows tissue planes between the strap muscles of the neck, the pectoralis muscle, and subcutaneous tissue. Subcutaneous emphysema may be detected clinically by finding crepitus in the skin and soft tissues of the neck, face, and upper body, which on occasion may become grotesquely deformed. In severe cases, it may spread to the trunk, abdomen, and legs as far as the knees. Pneumomediastinum may also track caudad and manifest as subdiaphragmatic air on x-ray, where it may be confused with that due to visceral rupture (Hillman, 1982). It is important to identify widespread barotrauma in this context to avoid unnecessary laparotomy. Pneumoperitoneum may ultimately outline most abdominal viscera. Pneumopericardium, which implies penetration of the pericardium, is not caused by barotrauma—the air that is seen around the heart is extrapericardial. Interstitial and subcutaneous emphysema is not in itself harmful, but it is a harbinger of the most dreaded complication of barotrauma, pneumo-

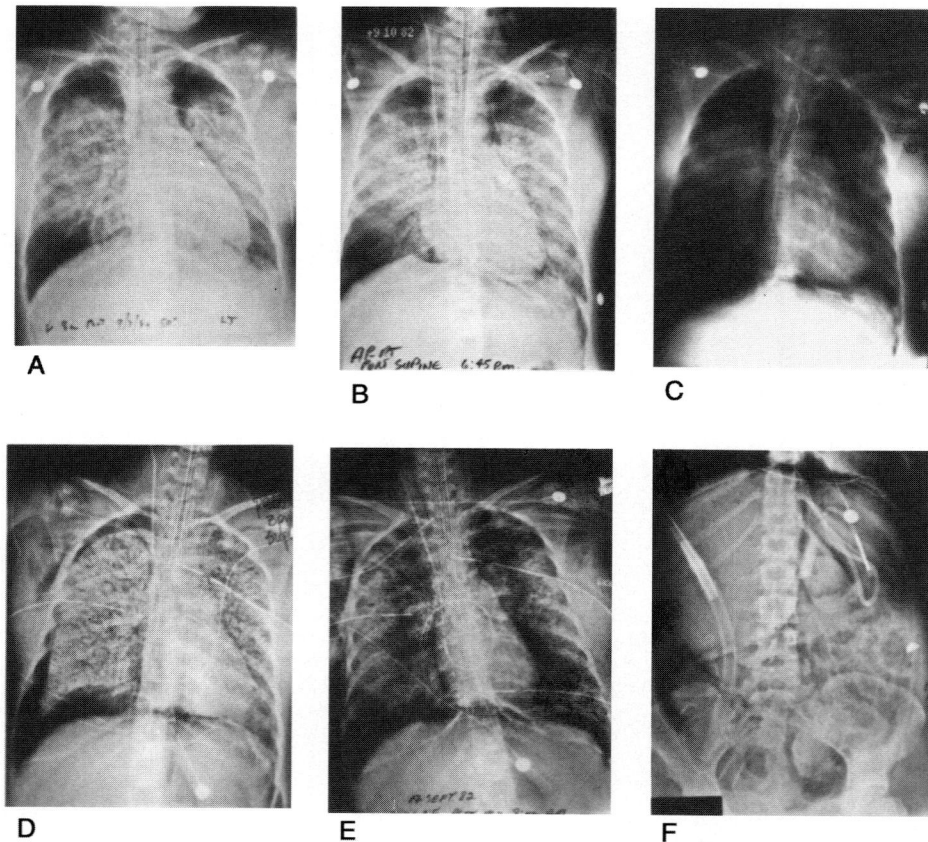

FIGURE 9–20. Pulmonary barotrauma. This series of radiographs illustrates the progression of pulmonary barotrauma in a patient with severe adult respiratory distress syndrome (ARDS), who required high levels of airway pressure therapy to maintain minimal safe levels of Pa_{O_2}. Volume-controlled ventilation with PEEP was used, as PCV had not yet been developed. Peak airway pressures consistently reached 80 cm H_2O. The changes occurred over a period of about 1 week. After a protracted course, the patient ultimately recovered and left the hospital. *A,* Dense, bilateral pulmonary infiltrates with early signs of pulmonary interstitial emphysema and pneumomediastinum (pencil-thin shadows around the cardiac border). *B,* Pneumomediastinum has extended superiorly. Subcutaneous air can be seen outlining the strap muscles of the neck and the pectoralis muscles. *C,* Pneumothorax. A large, right pneumothorax has developed, with slight mediastinal shift to the left. Note the increase in subcutaneous air around the neck and pectoralis muscles. *D,* Pneumothorax persists despite placement of a right chest tube, although tension has been relieved. A left chest tube has been placed prophylactically. *E,* Worsening barotrauma. Bilateral pneumothoraces persist despite the presence of two chest tubes on each side. Subdiaphragmatic air represents air that has tracked down the mediastinum, and does not in this circumstance indicate a visceral perforation. *F,* Pneumoperitoneum. The liver, spleen, kidneys, and other viscera are outlined by a large amount of peritoneal air that has tracked down from the thorax via the mediastinum.

thorax, which results when the tougher visceral pleura finally tears. In patients on high levels of mean airway pressure, the risk of immediate tension pneumothorax is extremely high. When airway pressure is moderate, the pneumothorax may be stable or even become completely loculated.

Barotrauma appears to be directly related to the severity of lung disease and the magnitude of the pressure applied to the airway and alveoli. Most clinical studies suggest that, at a peak airway pressure of greater than 40 cm H_2O, the incidence of barotrauma markedly increases. However, when airway pressure is measured at the proximal end of the endotracheal tube, it may be considerably higher than the actual pressure in the large airways because of the small caliber and high resistance of the endotracheal tube. The mean airway pressure may be a more important parameter to follow. Factors that increase airway pressure include excessive tidal volume with alveolar overdistention, elevated pleural pressures, increased impedance to flow in the endotracheal tube or ventilator, increased airway resistance (bronchospasm, mucus plugging), and high levels of PEEP (extrinsic or intrinsic, or both). High inspiratory flow rate elevates the peak airway pressure, but this is not necessarily transmitted to the small airways and alveoli. Coughing and bucking generate instantaneous high airway pressures that may cause sudden pneumothorax. The most frequent cause of severe barotrauma is inadvertent endobronchial intubation, because a large tidal volume is forced into a single lung.

The effect of a given pressure on the airway appears to depend most on the nature and severity of the lung disease process. Airway pressure therapy that improves FRC and lung compliance may actually decrease the risk of barotrauma (Suter et al., 1975). Disease entities most commonly associated with barotrauma on mechanical ventilation include ARDS, chronic obstructive lung disease (especially with emphysematous blebs and bullae), necrotizing pneumonia, neoplasm, and chemotherapy and radiation pneumonitis.

PREVENTION AND MANAGEMENT

Unfortunately, there are no prospective controlled studies that indisputably show that any one method of ventilation is superior to any other with respect to the incidence of barotrauma. On volume preset ventilators, peak airway pressure can be lowered by minimizing the inspiratory flow rate to 25 to 30 l/min. Ventilator modes that incorporate spontaneous ventilation, such as SIMV, may decrease the risk of barotrauma by reducing mean airway pressure despite higher peak airway pressures and PEEP than CMV (Mathru et al., 1983). One of the goals of PCV is to limit the peak airway pressure in patients with noncompliant lungs. However, mean airway pressure is usually increased above that provided by volume preset modes, and there are as yet no data that demonstrate that the incidence of barotrauma is reduced.

A promising development in the control of barotrauma in patients with extremely stiff lungs or status asthmaticus has been the use of permissive hypercapnia (Darioli and Perret, 1984; Hickling et al., 1990). Tidal volume is fixed at less than 10 ml/kg to keep peak airway pressures lower than 40 cm H_2O. If the Pa_{CO_2} is allowed to slowly rise over 3 to 5 days and the pH is kept greater than 7.25, there are no adverse effects and renal compensation causes gradual retention of bicarbonate. Patients tolerate a Pa_{CO_2} of 60 to 110 mm Hg with slight increases in pulmonary artery pressure and vascular resistance but little other hemodynamic change (Toth et al., 1992). Although it has been claimed that barotrauma and mortality are lower than expected with permissive hypercapnia (Darioli and Perret, 1984; Hickling et al., 1990), this has not been proved with controlled studies.

Pulmonary interstitial emphysema, pneumomediastinum, subcutaneous emphysema, and pneumoperitoneum are not in themselves dangerous and do not require any specific therapy. However, they are all harbingers of potentially life-threatening pneumothorax. In the light of present knowledge, attempts should be made to control peak and mean airway pressure by limiting inspiratory flow rate and the size of tidal volume. Heavy sedation and muscle relaxation, PCV, and permissive hypercapnia provide control of airway pressures even if there is no guarantee that further barotrauma will be halted. In the presence of severe barotrauma, it may be reasonable to accept an increased (but unknown) risk of oxygen toxicity by limiting increases in airway pressure and accepting a higher FI_{O_2}, up to 0.7.

Debate exists on whether it is justifiable to place prophylactic thoracostomy tubes in the hope of preventing catastrophic tension pneumothorax. This maneuver is not without risk of causing direct lung injury producing hemorrhage, further pneumothorax, and marked exacerbation of subcutaneous emphysema along the tube track. In extreme cases, a bronchopleural fistula may be created. It is the authors' practice to have a thoracostomy set and drainage system ready at the bedside and to commence pleural drainage only when clinically or radiologically indicated.

Applications of Mechanical Ventilation

Postoperative Mechanical Ventilation

RATIONALE

Prolonged postoperative tracheal intubation with mechanical ventilation is potentially hazardous. Patients require sedation and analgesia to tolerate the endotracheal tube; otherwise coughing, bronchorrhea, and bronchospasm occur, especially with hyperreactive airways. The most assiduous endotracheal suctioning is less effective in clearing airway secretions than an adequate spontaneous cough. The circulatory and barotrauma effects of PPV discussed previously remain an ever-present danger. Several studies on patients undergoing cardiac or vascular surgery indicated that there is no detectable benefit in providing prolonged prophylactic postoperative ventilation if patients are hemodynamically stable and have recovered fully from the effects of anesthesia (Prakash et al., 1977; Quasha et al., 1981; Shackford et al., 1981).

The important point, then, is to decide when the benefits of postoperative mechanical ventilation outweigh the adverse effects. There are several reasons to consider postoperative mechanical ventilation, even if only for a period as short as 1 to 4 hours. It provides time for careful assessment of the patient's readiness for tracheal extubation, a judgment that must be made rapidly and often under duress in the operating room. In patients with limited pulmonary reserve, it provides an opportunity to reverse the adverse effects on lung function induced by anesthesia and surgery. It allows aggressive pain control without concern for respiratory depression, which is particularly important in patients with myocardial ischemia. In patients who are hemodynamically unstable, it ensures effective and appropriate ventilation and reduces the number of variables in management.

Assessment of Readiness for Extubation. In the operating room, readiness for tracheal extubation is assessed by the adequacy of reversal of the anesthetic (volatile agents, opioids, or muscle relaxants). This is based on the response to verbal commands and the depth and frequency of ventilation, and by arterial oxygen saturation and end-tidal capnometry. In most patients, this assessment is quite adequate and the patient's trachea is extubated in the operating room without incident. However, patients with preexisting lung disease may require a period of stabilization and observation to ensure that they will have adequate spontaneous ventilation, cough, and deep breathing. Delayed emergence from anesthesia may be caused by advanced age, hypothermia, debilitation, severe systemic disease, renal or hepatic dysfunction, alcoholism and drug abuse, or simply a large dose of anesthetic agents. Postoperative mechanical ventilation should be continued in the postanesthetic care unit or intensive care unit until the patient has fully emerged from anesthesia.

In cases of delayed emergence from anesthesia, the patient whose trachea is intubated should not be placed on a T tube apparatus. This provides a high F_{IO_2} and secure airway, but does nothing to guarantee the adequacy of ventilation. Reversal of opioid-induced narcosis with naloxone is effective. However, too large a dose will abruptly reverse analgesia and may cause acute pain, hypertension, and even myocardial ischemia and pulmonary edema. Respiratory depression may return when the effect of a single dose of naloxone wears off in 30 minutes or so. A similar caveat applies to the use of flumazenil to antagonize benzodiazepines. The best way to manage this situation is to provide a short period of postoperative mechanical ventilation. This guarantees the adequacy of tidal volume and minute ventilation and prevents hypoxemia and hypercarbia while the patient is recovering from the effects of anesthesia. It facilitates careful assessment of the patient's level of consciousness and observation for relapse of opioid or relaxant effects and allows a graded withdrawal of ventilatory support through IMV or PSV.

Restoration of FRC. The most constant and predictable alteration in pulmonary function caused by anesthesia and surgery is a significant decrease in *functional residual capacity* (FRC). As discussed previously, PPV invariably causes ventilation-perfusion mismatch, with preferential ventilation of the nondependent lung zones. In the underventilated dependent lung zones, progressive microatelectasis occurs, and is not simply reversed by restoration of spontaneous ventilation. Unless, after tracheal extubation, the patient can generate large tidal volumes and cough adequately, microatelectasis tends to spread, causing decreased lung compliance, increased work of breathing, and further alveolar collapse and retention of secretions. Left uncorrected, these events predispose the patient to postoperative pneumonia and acute respiratory failure.

During normal spontaneous breathing in an awake, unsedated patient, FRC is maintained by periodic sighs, which open up areas of microatelectasis. The residual effect of volatile or opioid anesthesia abolishes the normal sigh mechanism and results in a monotonous pattern of ventilation that leads to progressive microatelectasis and decline in the FRC.

Many other factors predispose to postoperative reduction in FRC through collapse of small airways and alveoli. Cigarette smoking impairs cilial clearance of secretions, causes mucus retention, and inhibits surfactant production. In chronic bronchitis, goblet-cell hyperplasia produces sheets of tacky mucus. Adequate clearance of secretions is further compromised by tracheal intubation, blind suctioning (with selective right lung clearance), and inadequate warming and humidification of inspired anesthetic gases. Obese patients suffer from alveolar hypoventilation;

lung expansion is impeded by the weight of the abdomen, markedly reducing expiratory reserve volume and FRC. Direct manipulation and compression of the lungs by surgical retraction, weight of viscera, pleural effusion and hematoma, or induced collapse may all cause an injury akin to pulmonary contusion, with persistent atelectasis and localized edema.

It has been demonstrated that, following tracheal extubation after major surgery, FRC declines up to 60 to 70% from preoperative values. Postoperative complications are likely when the FRC is reduced more than 40% from preoperative values (Meyers et al., 1975). After cardiac surgery, FRC reaches a nadir about 12 to 18 hours postoperatively and does not return to preoperative levels for a week (Turnbull et al., 1974).

When alveoli collapse, surfactant quickly dissipates. It takes a great deal more effort to reexpand a collapsed alveolus than to expand an alveolus that is already open. Low lung volumes cause increased lung stiffness, that is, a decreased lung volume change for a given change in transpulmonary pressure. Not only is it harder for a patient to expand the lungs when there is diffuse atelectasis, but the patient's ability to cough and deep breathe—the most helpful means of improving FRC—is hampered by all the factors mentioned previously, as well as by the residual effects of anesthesia.

A period of postoperative mechanical ventilation provides an opportunity to reexpand the lungs by the use of large tidal volumes and PEEP. Because FRC invariably declines after tracheal extubation, it seems rational to extubate patients from the best possible FRC.

Provision of Pain Relief. Pain after thoracic or upper abdominal surgery characteristically causes a restrictive defect, with splinting of the chest and diaphragm caused by wound pain. The patient breathes rapidly and shallowly, which predisposes to basal atelectasis. Deep breathing and coughing are difficult, and respiratory therapy may need to be quite aggressive. This in turn may provoke hypoxemia, arrhythmias, and myocardial ischemia. Postoperative pain is effectively treated with epidural or intrathecal analgesia, which facilitates early tracheal extubation and rapid recovery of lung mechanics. However, if epidural or intrathecal analgesia is not available or not possible, postoperative mechanical ventilation allows adequate sedation and analgesia to be provided without concern for respiratory depression.

PLANNED POSTOPERATIVE MECHANICAL VENTILATION

Postoperative mechanical ventilation may be planned or unplanned. It should be planned based on the nature of the surgical procedure, the presence of existing lung dysfunction, or airway compromise. Unplanned mechanical ventilation may be required for unexpected hypothermia, cardiopulmonary or surgical complications, or delayed emergence from anesthesia.

Based on the Nature of the Surgical Procedure

Cardiac Surgery. Many factors cause deterioration in the FRC during cardiac surgery (Sladen, 1982). Effective surgical exposure during cardiopulmonary bypass (CPB) requires complete lung collapse. The routine use of 100% oxygen during cardiac surgery further decreases FRC by absorption atelectasis. Extravascular lung water, which predisposes toward atelectasis, is increased by preexisting pulmonary edema, CPB-induced capillary leak, or hypersensitivity reactions. It is further increased when a high cardiac preload is required after CPB. Surfactant production is inhibited during CPB by lung collapse and pulmonary hypoperfusion. Passive compression of the left lung by the heart during CPB, and by pleural fluid and chest tubes, may further cause localized atelectasis, especially of the left lower lobe. After cardiac surgery, the routine provision of a period of postoperative mechanical ventilation with modest amounts of PEEP (5 to 10 cm H_2O) restores the FRC to that prior to tracheal extubation.

It also facilitates the use of a high-dose opioid anesthetic technique that suppresses sympathetic responses that predispose to myocardial ischemia, avoids the hazards of reversal agents, and safeguards the transition from the operating room to the intensive care unit. Postoperative rewarming and shivering after hypothermic CPB can markedly increase the work of breathing, oxygen consumption, and carbon dioxide production. With appropriate sedation, mechanical ventilation allows the use of muscle relaxants to suppress shivering and adjustment of minute ventilation to ensure adequate oxygen supply and avoid acute respiratory acidosis.

In the early postoperative period, control of ventilation reduces the number of physiologic variables, allowing aggressive volume resuscitation to stabilize cardiac and renal function with less concern for its effect on pulmonary function. This is particularly important for patients who have had complicated procedures with prolonged CPB or residual myocardial ischemia, with requirement for potent inotropic support, intra-aortic balloon counterpulsation, and ongoing arrhythmias. The presence of excessive postoperative bleeding is a contraindication to ventilatory weaning and extubation, because of hemodynamic instability and requirement for rapid transfusion of blood and blood products. The risk of ARDS is high. Maintenance of mechanical ventilation allows a smooth and safe transition back to the operating room if surgical reexploration is required for bleeding.

Nonetheless, once the patient is fully rewarmed and hemodynamically and hemostatically stable, there is no reason not to proceed to ventilatory weaning and tracheal extubation. In most uncomplicated cases, mechanical ventilation can be discontinued within 6 to 9 hours after operation, and there is no advantage to continuing it beyond this time.

Major Vascular Surgery. Patients with peripheral vascular disease requiring operation frequently have associated risk factors for coronary artery disease (diabetes, smoking, obesity, hypertension), a high inci-

dence of underlying myocardial ischemia (Raby et al., 1989), and other manifestations of diffuse atherosclerosis, including cerebrovascular and renovascular disease. They are at risk of many complications postoperatively, including acute myocardial infarction, atelectasis, stroke, acute renal failure, and peripheral thrombosis. In any patient in whom major blood loss or hemodynamic instability is anticipated, a period of postoperative mechanical ventilation should be planned for many of the reasons that have already been elucidated.

Ruptured or leaking aortic aneurysm provides a particular indication for postoperative mechanical ventilation. Even if repair is timely and successful, there is a period of splanchnic ischemia that causes capillary leak. If shock has occurred, there is a high incidence of multisystem organ damage, including acute lung injury. The abdomen may be tense and distended and, together with a large, painful abdominal incision, can markedly impair adequate ventilation, deep breathing, and cough.

In recent years, the use of intrathecal or lumbar and thoracic epidural opioids (e.g., morphine, hydromorphone, meperidine, and fentanyl) with or without low-dose local anesthetic agents (e.g., bupivacaine, lidocaine) has become commonplace after major vascular surgery. Potential advantages include excellent pain control, suppression of catecholamine release, improved hemodynamic stability, decreased risk of arterial and venous thrombosis, and decreased catabolic stress response. Concerns remain about the possible risk of epidural hematoma associated with intraoperative anticoagulation, but this complication appears to be extraordinarily rare. Epidural or intrathecal analgesia usually facilitates rapid emergence from anesthesia and early tracheal extubation, although patients who are hypothermic, unstable, or bleeding still benefit from a period of postoperative mechanical ventilation.

Procedures with Major Blood Loss. Postoperative mechanical ventilation should be planned for any procedure in which major blood loss is anticipated, to reduce the physiologic variables, facilitate adequate sedation, ensure oxygenation and ventilation, and allow recovery from hypothermia. Fluid, blood, and blood products may be administered rapidly with less concern for the patient's pulmonary function. Particular attention should be given to major trauma, liver transplantation, tumor exenteration (especially urologic and gynecologic tumor debulking), or major back procedures.

High-risk Surgical Incisions. The site and type of the surgical incision markedly affects the incidence of postoperative pulmonary complications. Pain from the surgical wound causes splinting, shallow respirations, and impaired cough. This decreases the expiratory reserve volume and leads to a progressive decline in FRC. Upper abdominal incisions impair coughing the most and may cause the FRC to decrease by 60%, whereas a lateral thoracotomy causes it to decrease by about 40%. Impairment is much less after sternotomy and lower abdominal incisions and negligible after peripheral and limb procedures (Ali et al., 1974). An abdominothoracic incision is more detrimental to pulmonary function than two separate abdominal and thoracic incisions, and a midline incision is more detrimental than a subcostal one. Incisions that involve diaphragmatic fibers impair the adequacy of cough (Black et al., 1977). After thoracotomy, negative pressure to generate cough is decreased to 30% of preoperative values, and requires up to 3 weeks for resolution (Byrd and Burns, 1975).

Good postoperative analgesia provided by intrathecal, thoracic, or lumbar epidural opioids is the most effective way to deal with a high-risk surgical incision. This is especially so after lateral thoracotomy for lung surgery, when there is a concern to discontinue the effect of PPV on the bronchial stump or lung margin as soon as possible. Nonetheless, postoperative mechanical ventilation may be indicated when patients with limited pulmonary reserve have a large upper abdominal or thoracoabdominal incision.

Patients who undergo complex head and neck, plastic reconstructive, or distant flap procedures may benefit from 24 to 48 hours of postoperative mechanical ventilation because this allows heavy sedation and muscle relaxation and protects the fragile wounds and grafts from inadvertent disruption.

Based on Abnormal Lung Function

Neuromuscular and Mechanical Dysfunction. In patients in whom the mechanical or bellows function of the ventilatory apparatus is compromised, anesthesia and operation may precipitate postoperative acute ventilatory failure. Anesthesia in patients with neurologic disorders (e.g., Guillain-Barré syndrome, polio, tetanus) or myopathies may cause critical loss of ventilatory function for a considerable period of time. In thymectomy for myasthenia gravis, even when excellent analgesia is provided by epidural opioids, a short period of postoperative ventilation is helpful to allow careful assessment of the adequacy of neuromuscular function (Gorback, 1990). Severe kyphoscoliosis causes restrictive lung disease, with or without pulmonary hypertension, that is not immediately reversed by surgical correction. Patients undergoing acoustic neuroma resection, which involves the brain stem ventilatory center, may require postoperative ventilatory support. Marked obesity predisposes to alveolar hypoventilation, decreased FRC, and atelectasis. Malnutrition and cachexia produce diminished forced vital capacity (FVC), cough, and tidal volume.

Parenchymal Lung Disease. In restrictive lung disease, whether caused by diffuse fibrosis, pneumoconioses, or pleural disease, the characteristic pattern of breathing is shallow and rapid, with decreased FVC and impaired cough. Predictive risk factors of postoperative morbidity have been developed that may be helpful in planning elective postoperative ventilation (Tisi, 1979), although these must be combined with clinical evaluation of the patient during and after operation.

Patients with chronic obstructive lung disease fall in a different category because of their potential for airway hyperreactivity, air trapping, and pneumothorax. In chronic bronchitis, the primary pathologic abnormality is mucus cell hyperplasia, which increases tenacious secretions, predisposing to small airway collapse and atelectasis. Such patients generally tolerate tracheal intubation poorly and emphysematous patients in particular have an increased risk of barotrauma because of blebs and bullous disease. Every effort should be made to proceed to ventilatory weaning and tracheal extubation as soon as possible after the procedure.

Acute Lung Injury. Lung injury with poor compliance and oxygenation should be anticipated after procedures such as transthoracic esophagogastrectomy, thoracic aortic aneurysm resection, repair of traumatic thoracic aortic tears, or operation on trauma patients who have pulmonary contusion. In these situations, postoperative mechanical ventilation should be given a high priority.

Multisystem Failure. When neurologic, hepatic, or renal failure exists, there is always uncertainty about the patient's response to anesthesia. There may be untoward effects on neurologic and ventilatory function or delayed emergence. A period of postoperative mechanical ventilation allows appropriate assessment of these responses before tracheal extubation.

Based on Airway Compromise.

When the surgical procedure predictably compromises the airway, postoperative tracheal intubation is mandatory. This includes mandibular surgery with jaw wiring, procedures causing airway edema (e.g., head and neck surgery of the oropharynx, prolonged surgery in the prone position), and burns with smoke inhalation. In these situations, the main priority is to protect the airway. However, until the patient is fully awake, alert, and capable of deep breathing, mechanical ventilatory support should be provided to maintain the FRC and ensure adequate oxygenation and minute ventilation. Patients with a history of sleep apnea, whether central or obstructive, have abnormal responses to hypoxemia and hypercapnia. Uvulopalatopharyngoplasty, or any other procedure performed on the airway, should be followed by a period of controlled ventilation until the patient is absolutely awake. Premature tracheal extubation may engender complete airway obstruction.

UNPLANNED POSTOPERATIVE MECHANICAL VENTILATION

Hypothermia. Inadvertent intraoperative hypothermia (central temperature less than 34° C) depresses the central nervous system, which impairs airway protection and ventilatory responses to hypoxemia and hypercarbia. Elimination of volatile anesthetic agents and nondepolarizing muscle relaxants is delayed. Vasoconstriction induced by hypothermia gives a false sense of security about the patient's intravascular volume status. During subsequent rewarming, rapid vasodilatation can induce acute hypotension, tachycardia, and myocardial ischemia. Oxygen consumption and carbon dioxide production increase by 100% or more if rewarming is associated with shivering. As described in the previous section on management of patients after cardiac surgery, postoperative mechanical ventilation ensures the adequacy of oxygenation and minute ventilation until the patient is fully rewarmed.

Cardiopulmonary Complications

Acute Myocardial Ischemia. Intraoperative myocardial ischemia may be diagnosed by new ST changes on the electrocardiogram, elevated PAWP, ventricular irritability, or regional wall motion abnormalities on transesophageal echocardiography. Any of these findings should warn against the danger of allowing rapid, painful emergence from anesthesia, with its attendant risks of hypertension, tachycardia, hypoxemia, and hypercarbia. The presence of effective intrathecal or epidural opioid analgesia may be sufficiently protective. However, if this is unavailable or incomplete, or if spontaneous ventilation is borderline, mechanical ventilation should be continued postoperatively. Systemic opioids such as fentanyl may then be given to control pain and catecholamine release and prevent tachycardia and hypertension. In the extubated patient, respiratory depression may occur owing to the residual effects of anesthesia or may be induced by attempts at analgesia. Hypoxemia exacerbates acute myocardial ischemia. Once a sufficient load of opioid has been given, it is usually possible later to allow the patient to emerge slowly from sedation without coughing and bucking on the endotracheal tube.

Arrhythmias. Arrhythmias may be provoked by myocardial ischemia, hypoxemia, hypercarbia, or acid-base and electrolyte imbalance. There is good reason to avoid emergence and tracheal extubation until these factors have been evaluated. If there is any possibility that the patient may require cardioversion in the postoperative period, tracheal intubation and mechanical ventilation should be continued until the arrhythmias are resolved.

Pulmonary Edema. Pulmonary edema may be associated with elevated cardiac filling pressures in acute heart failure (cardiogenic) or with normal cardiac filling pressures in acute lung injury (noncardiogenic). Regardless of the primary mechanism, interstitial edema leads to closure of small airways, diffuse alveolar flooding and collapse, lung stiffness, impaired lung defense mechanisms, and acute respiratory failure. Increasing intrapulmonary shunting causes progressive hypoxemia despite increasing F_{IO_2}. The signs of acute pulmonary edema include decreased lung compliance, increased peak airway pressure, frothy pink endotracheal secretions, crackles on lung auscultation, and decreasing Pa_{O_2}. Postoperative mechanical ventilation is mandatory to support oxygenation with airway pressure therapy until the underlying cause of pulmonary edema has resolved (see later in this chapter).

Severe Bronchospasm. Although there is always a concern that new onset of severe bronchospasm may have been provoked by irritation caused by the endotracheal tube, there are a number of indications for postoperative mechanical ventilation. First, reversal should be avoided in any patient given nondepolarizing muscle relaxants. Even with the use of anticholinergic agents, anticholinesterases such as neostigmine or edrophonium can cause an excessive buildup of acetylcholine, which will exacerbate bronchospasm when the effect of the anticholinergic agent has worn off. Indeed, with very severe bronchospasm, the continued use of muscle relaxants may be required to ensure adequate alveolar ventilation. Bronchodilator therapy with phosphodiesterase inhibitors or adrenergic agents is ineffective in the presence of respiratory acidosis and pH less than 7.25. Mechanical ventilation allows appropriate pharmacologic therapy (such as aminophylline infusion, albuterol aerosol treatments) to be given to gain control of bronchospasm while maintaining safe levels of ventilation before tracheal extubation.

Lobar Atelectasis or Lung Collapse. If lobar atelectasis or lung collapse occurs during anesthesia (as indicated by lung stiffness, high peak airway pressures, hypoxemia with large alveolar-arterial oxygen gradient, and chest film), postoperative ventilation is warranted, even after thoracotomy (Gallagher et al., 1990). With major atelectasis or collapse, the work of breathing is markedly increased, and the patient may not be able to generate a sufficient FVC to expel the mucus plug or secretions and to maintain adequate ventilation. Treatment requires positioning with the good lung down (to enhance ventilation-perfusion matching and allow drainage of secretions from the affected lung), frequent suctioning, and fiberoptic bronchoscopy, all of which are facilitated by endotracheal intubation. Mechanical ventilation and PEEP are required to open up the collapsed lobe or lung before extubation.

Surgical Complications

Hemorrhage. If major hemorrhage has occurred or is ongoing, the patient should be kept sedated and mechanically ventilated postoperatively. This removes ventilation as a variable while resuscitation to treat hypotension, tachycardia, oliguria, hypothermia, and metabolic acidosis is continued or completed. Total oxygen consumption is reduced, which decreases the risk of ischemia caused by acute hypovolemic anemia. Mechanical ventilation should be continued until there is no longer a prospect of immediate surgical reexploration for bleeding.

Other Complications. Unanticipated surgical complications may include cardiac contusion during transmediastinal esophagogastrectomy, phrenic nerve injury during thoracic operations, bowel ischemia during manipulation of the gut, or visceral perforation during pelvic operations. If any of these complications are suspected during the case, the patient should be left sedated and mechanically ventilated in the postoperative period so that adequate steps can be taken to evaluate the problem and stabilize the patient. A return to the operating room for surgical reexploration may be required.

Failure of the patient to emerge from anesthesia, or the presence of focal neurologic signs or seizures on emergence, may reveal an intraoperative cerebrovascular accident. Continued endotracheal intubation with mechanical ventilatory support is necessary if neurologic dysfunction impairs airway protection and clearance of secretions.

Intraoperative Catastrophes. Unexpected intraoperative catastrophes that produce major circulatory instability are absolute indications for a period of postoperative mechanical ventilation to allow stabilization, evaluation, and further management of the patient. These include acute acid aspiration syndrome, major anaphylactic reactions (to antibiotics, protamine, methyl methacrylate), mismatched ABO blood transfusion with hemodynamic instability and intravascular hemolysis, malignant hyperthermia, intraoperative cardiac arrest, and venous air embolism causing hemodynamic instability.

Inadequate Reversal of Anesthesia

Inadequate Elimination of Volatile Anesthetic Agents. All volatile anesthetic agents (e.g., halothane, enflurane, isoflurane) depress the ventilatory response to hypoxemia and hypercarbia even at subanesthetic concentrations (Knill et al., 1979). Delayed emergence may occur with hypothermia, advanced age, cachexia, respiratory disease (especially emphysema, where increased dead space slows elimination), anemia, or hypothyroidism. Concomitant sedative drugs such as clonidine and tricyclic antidepressants enhance the depressant effect of all anesthetic agents.

Inadequate Reversal of Opioid Anesthesia. A primary effect of opioid anesthetic agents (such as morphine, meperidine, fentanyl, or sufentanil) is to depress the ventilatory response to hypercarbia (Weil et al., 1975). Respiratory depression outlasts analgesia. Depression may range from complete apnea to obvious bradypnea to subtle hypercarbia revealed only by an arterial blood gas. Characteristically, the patient awakens readily when stimulated but subsides into stupor when left undisturbed. Muscle strength is unaffected, and lung mechanics may be quite normal despite substantial narcosis. Residual narcosis occurs with simple overdose, as an additive effect in combination with volatile anesthetic agents, in the elderly, and in uremia, liver disease, or congestive heart failure. Although opioid-induced respiratory depression is readily reversible by the specific antagonist naloxone, sudden loss of analgesia may precipitate acute hypertension, tachyarrhythmias, myocardial ischemia, and pulmonary edema. The duration of naloxone's effect is short-lived, about 30 minutes, so close surveillance and repeated doses are required. In most cases, it is safer to continue mechanical ventilation and maintain good analgesia until the patient has recovered to a level appropriate for tracheal extubation.

Inadequate Reversal of Muscle Relaxants. Residual muscle relaxation is usually recognized by shallow, rapid, ineffectual respirations. A patient who awakens while still paralyzed may exhibit panic, with hypertension, tachycardia, lacrimation, and sweating. Attempts to move produce ineffectual wriggling or jerking movements, particularly of the hands and feet. Diaphragmatic function returns before upper or lower intercostal movement. A useful sign is the inability to sustain a head lift for more than 5 seconds. A successful head lift requires use of the neck and back muscles and correlates with a FVC of greater than 15 ml/kg.

Prolonged muscle relaxation induced by succinylcholine may be caused by overdose, abnormal pseudocholinesterase (a genetic abnormality), or deficient pseudocholinesterase (severe malnutrition or liver disease). There is no antidote, and sedation and mechanical ventilation are required until recovery, although this seldom takes more than 6 hours. There are many causes of delayed recovery from nondepolarizing agents such as pancuronium or vecuronium. The most important include overdose (synergism exists with enflurane and isoflurane), hypothermia, respiratory acidosis (induced by opioids or the relaxant itself), hypokalemia, hypermagnesemia (important in the treatment of toxemia of pregnancy), renal and liver failure, myopathy, and concomitant aminoglycoside antibiotic administration. If full reversal does not occur despite the maximal dose of neostigmine (about 5.0 mg) or edrophonium (about 80 mg), sedation and mechanical ventilation must be continued until recovery is complete.

MANAGEMENT OF POSTOPERATIVE MECHANICAL VENTILATION

Ventilator Prescription. Patients undergoing postoperative mechanical ventilation for less than 24 hours, most of whom do not have significant lung disease, require simple volume preset ventilators only. CMV is provided for patients who are still anesthetized, paralyzed, or heavily sedated. Frequently, SIMV is set up on admission to the intensive care unit so that, as the patient emerges from anesthesia and sedation, he is able to resume spontaneous ventilation on the ventilator. Patient-triggered modes (AMV, ACV, or PSV) are seldom required.

A primary goal of postoperative mechanical ventilation is to restore the FRC. This is best achieved by the use of a large tidal volume (15 ml/kg) and moderate levels of PEEP (5 to 10 cm H_2O). The tidal volume may need to be reduced in patients with restrictive lung disease or to avoid disruption of an internal mammary artery graft. Slow inspiratory flow rates (25 to 30 l/min) and resulting longer inspiratory times promote peripheral gas distribution and keep peak airway pressure low. The $F_{I_{O_2}}$ should be adjusted to maintain safe levels of arterial hemoglobin oxygen saturation (i.e., >96%), and the ventilator rate adjusted to maintain normal pH (i.e., 7.35 to 7.45). Capnometry is a useful guide to the adequacy of minute ventilation and ventilator rate. In most patients, the alveolar-arterial CO_2 gradient is less than 4 mm Hg. Maintenance of an end-tidal CO_2 of less than 36 mm Hg usually ensures a Pa_{CO_2} of less than 40 mm Hg. End-tidal CO_2 is unreliable when the alveolar-arterial CO_2 gradient is increased because of low flow (shock, hypotension), high dead space, or air-trapping (bronchospasm, emphysema).

Hypoxemia on admission to the intensive care unit

(e.g., Pa_{O_2} less than 100 mm Hg on 60% oxygen) should induce an immediate evaluation for endobronchial intubation, pneumothorax, or pulmonary edema. The most common cause of postoperative hypoxemia is atelectasis, which should be treated by incremental increases in PEEP, although more than 10 cm H_2O is seldom required. PEEP is contraindicated during severe hemodynamic instability, acute bronchospasm, or severe emphysema or when pneumothorax is present or suspected.

Ventilator Weaning and Tracheal Extubation. Weaning from postoperative mechanical ventilation should commence if the patient is hemodynamically stable, normothermic, fully emerged from the effects of anesthesia, and neurologically intact. Once the patient meets weaning criteria, a simple SIMV wean can be performed, usually in decrements of 2 breaths per minute. Criteria for tracheal extubation are based on intact neurologic status, lung mechanics, and recovery from opioid-induced respiratory depression (see later in this chapter). Serial clinical evaluation over a period of time provides more reliable prediction of success of withdrawal from ventilatory support than a quick, one-time assessment of lung mechanics. Failure to tolerate ventilatory weaning may be heralded by deterioration in arterial blood gases (hypoxemia, hypercarbia). However, arterial blood gases may be preserved at the expense of increased work of breathing demonstrated by tachypnea, tachycardia, hypertension, arrhythmias, agitation, diaphoresis, and vasoconstriction. SIMV rate should be increased until the patient is comfortable, underlying causes such as pulmonary edema or bronchospasm reevaluated and treated, and ventilatory weaning recommenced when appropriate. Management of the difficult-to-wean patient is discussed later.

Management of Hypoxemia

AIRWAY PRESSURE THERAPY

Airway pressure therapy refers to interventions that elevate the mean airway pressure to treat the alveolar collapse that induces hypoxemic acute respiratory failure. In the postoperative period, the most important causes include pneumonia, acute lung injury (usually known as the *adult respiratory distress syndrome* [ARDS]), and blunt chest trauma (pulmonary contusion). Causes of hypoxemia not related to alveolar collapse do not respond to airway pressure therapy and, in fact, may be exacerbated by its application. These include endobronchial intubation, pneumothorax, acute bronchospasm, and pulmonary embolism. These entities must always be excluded before instituting airway pressure therapy.

Today there are two interventions available: PEEP and IRV. The primary effect of airway pressure therapy is to enhance alveolar patency, augment the *functional residual capacity* (FRC), and improve matching of ventilation with perfusion (increased $\dot{V}_A/\dot{Q}$ ratio) (Falke et al., 1972). This increases oxygenation and reverses life-threatening hypoxemia. Reduction of the required inspired oxygen fraction (FI_{O_2}) decreases the potential for oxygen toxicity. However, airway pressure therapy must be applied in such a way as to minimize complications related to circulatory compromise and barotrauma.

For more than 2 decades, PEEP has been the only form of airway pressure therapy available. At one time, its application to extraordinarily high levels (30 to 40 cm H_2O) was advocated, but in most institutions, levels of more than 20 cm H_2O are seldom used because of the concern for barotrauma. The major advantage of IRV over PEEP is that peak airway pressures are controlled by PCV, and that weaning of the FI_{O_2} can usually be accomplished at a lower mean airway pressure. However, heavy sedation, often accompanied by muscle relaxation, is required for the proper administration of PCV-IRV. In the authors' practice, institution of IRV is considered when significant hypoxemia persists despite the use of 15 cm H_2O PEEP, or when peak airway pressures consistently exceed 40 cm H_2O.

There is no evidence that airway pressure therapy alters the natural history of ARDS, but it prevents death from primary respiratory failure and sustains the patient until the pathophysiologic process burns out.

Indications for Airway Pressure Therapy. The degree of hypoxemia that warrants a trial of PEEP or IRV is defined by the ratio of the arterial oxygen tension (Pa_{O_2}) to the inspired oxygen fraction (FI_{O_2}), known as the P to F ratio (P:F). A P:F of less than 150 (if the patient is not on PEEP or IRV) or less than 200 (if the patient is already on PEEP or IRV, and the FI_{O_2} is greater than 0.4) implies a need for airway pressure therapy. Examples consistent with these indications would be a patient not on PEEP, with a Pa_{O_2} of 65 mm Hg on an FI_{O_2} of 0.5 (P:F = 130), or a patient on PEEP, with a Pa_{O_2} of 95 mm Hg on an FI_{O_2} of 0.5 (P:F = 180).

Alternatively, the presence of a decreasing Pa_{O_2} in a patient with suspected ARDS would be a compelling indication for airway pressure therapy. This diagnosis should be considered when hypoxemia is associated with clinical and radiographic evidence of noncardiogenic pulmonary edema—that is, diffuse infiltrates in the presence of a PAWP of less than 18 mm Hg.

Limitations of Airway Pressure Therapy. In addition to the limitations mentioned, airway pressure therapy should be used with great caution in patients with head injury, because it may increase ICP, and in patients with uncorrected hypovolemic or cardiogenic shock, because it may further impair venous return to the heart and exacerbate hemodynamic instability. However, this effect is mitigated in patients with poor lung compliance (who would be receiving airway pressure therapy) because less pressure is transmitted from the alveolar to the intravascular space. In the presence of unilateral lung disease or emphysema, the increase in mean airway pressure causes excessive distention of compliant normal or emphysematous lung units. Not only does this not improve hypoxemia, but it increases dead space (causing air trapping and CO_2 retention) and potentiates barotrauma.

TRIAL OF PEEP OR IRV

The principle of the trial approach is to evaluate the effect of incremental increases in airway pressure on oxygenation, ventilation, hemodynamic performance, and overall tissue oxygen delivery (Bolin and Pierson, 1986; Craig et al., 1985). It is predicated on the fact that these changes are usually readily apparent within 20 to 30 minutes after each increment, although continued slow improvement in oxygenation may occur for many hours. Close surveillance of the patient by the respiratory therapy, nursing, and medical staff is essential. Invasive hemodynamic monitoring with an indwelling arterial catheter and pulmonary artery catheter is a prerequisite. Continu-

ous display of the mixed venous oxygen saturation ($S\bar{v}_{O_2}$) provides a very useful real-time guide to the overall effects of airway pressure therapy on oxygenation and oxygen delivery.

Therapeutic Goals. The primary goal of airway pressure therapy is to improve oxygenation so that the FI_{O_2} can be decreased to nontoxic levels, or less than 0.4. This is usually associated with an improvement in P:F to greater than 200.

While this is in progress, monitoring should be directed to ensure that static lung compliance (Fig. 9–21) consistently improves, that dead-space ventilation and progressive air trapping do not occur, and that there are no adverse effects on cardiac output or oxygen delivery.

While all other ventilator settings and hemodynamic therapy are kept constant, PEEP is increased in increments of 2 to 3 cm H_2O. With IRV, the inspira-

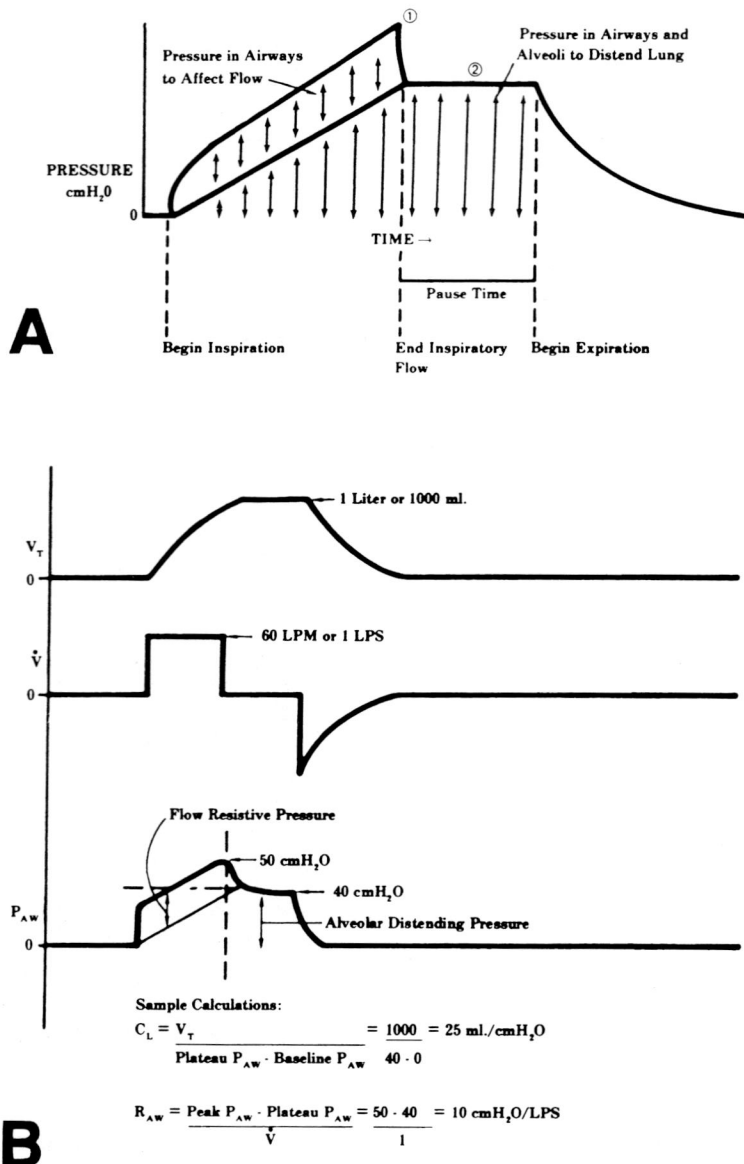

A

B

FIGURE 9–21. Static lung compliance. *A*, Components of inflation pressure during a single ventilator breath. The inflation pressure required to deliver a tidal volume has two components, flow resistive pressure and lung distending pressure. ① = the peak proximal airway pressure (P_{AW}) achieved at end-inspiration. When flow is stopped to provide an inspiratory pause, the proximal airway pressure decreases slightly to a plateau pressure ②. The pressure gradient between the peak P_{AW} and the plateau P_{AW} depends on the proximal airway resistance and peak flow rate. The pressure gradient between the plateau P_{AW} and the end-expiratory pressure depends on the compliance of the alveoli and the chest wall. Compliance may be thought of as the inverse of stiffness, i.e., the more compliant the lung, the greater the tidal volume achieved for a given lung-distending pressure. *B*, Calculation of static lung compliance and proximal airway resistance. In this illustration of a single ventilator breath, the *top line* represents the tidal volume (V_T), in this case 1000 ml, the *middle line* represents airway flow ($\dot{V}$), in this case 60 l/min (LPM) or 1 l/sec (LPS), and the *bottom line* represents proximal airway pressure (P_{AW}). Static lung compliance (C_L) is calculated by dividing the exhaled tidal volume (V_T) by the alveolar-distending pressure, which is the difference between the plateau P_{AW} and the baseline P_{AW}. In this example, the alveolar-distending pressure is 40 cm H_2O (40 − 0 cm H_2O) and $C_L = 1000/40 = 25$ ml/cm H_2O. Normal C_L is 80 − 100 ml/cm H_2O, so this example indicates very poor lung compliance, as encountered in the adult respiratory distress syndrome. (Note: The presence of chest wall rigidity or shivering prevents the accurate calculation of lung compliance.) Proximal airway resistance (R_{AW}) is calculated by dividing the flow resistive pressure, which is the difference between the peak P_{AW} and the plateau P_{AW}, by the peak flow rate ($\dot{V}$). In this example, the flow resistive pressure is 10 cm H_2O (50 − 40 cm H_2O), the peak flow rate is 1 LPS, and $R_{AW} = 10/1 = 10$ cm H_2O/LPS. Normal R_{AW} is 2 − 6 cm H_2O/LPS, so this example indicates elevated proximal airway resistance, as encountered in acute bronchospasm. (*A* and *B*, From MacIntyre, N. R., and Hagus, C. K.: Graphical analysis of flow, pressure and volume during mechanical ventilation. © Bear Medical Systems, Inc., Riverside, CA, 1989, pp. 12, 89. Used with permission.)

tion-expiration (I:E) ratio is increased serially from, for example, 1:2 to 1:1, then to 1.5:1, 2:1, 3:1, and 4:1, or in smaller increments. This is done by increasing total inspiratory time through manipulation of the inspiratory flow rate and end-inspiratory pause time. After approximately 20 to 30 minutes, a set of respiratory and hemodynamic measurements is made. The results are tabulated in a grid that allows rapid assessment of all the parameters followed and the choice of the optimal level of airway pressure (Fig. 9–22). In most cases, airway pressure therapy is not rapidly incremented to the highest levels tolerable (e.g., 20 to 25 cm H_2O PEEP, 4:1 IRV), but instead, is carefully increased to a level at which a definite positive response is seen, after which the $F_{I_{O_2}}$ is progressively weaned as long as arterial saturation (Sa_{O_2}) is greater than 90% and Pa_{O_2} greater than 60 mm Hg.

Adverse Effects of Airway Pressure Therapy. Adverse effects of airway pressure therapy include a paradoxic decrease in oxygenation, worsened lung compliance, decreased cardiac output, and air trapping. Barotrauma and tension pneumothorax are constant risks in these patients and equipment for immediate chest tube placement should be available at the bedside.

A decrease in oxygenation may occur through one of two mechanisms. Inflated alveoli may become overdistended and compress the adjacent capillaries, diverting blood flow to underventilated areas and increasing the intrapulmonary shunt. This may or may not be associated with a decrease in static lung compliance. At the same time, if cardiac output is decreased, $S\bar{v}_{O_2}$ declines and increases the effect of venous admixture on lowering the Pa_{O_2} in the presence of a substantial intrapulmonary shunt. If the blood pressure abruptly decreases within a short time after an increase in airway pressure therapy, PEEP or IRV should be returned to the previous setting.

Oxygenation may be improved by augmenting pulmonary blood flow and cardiac output with judicious fluid challenge if PAWP is less than 12 to 15 cm H_2O, or by the use of inotropic agents such as dopamine or dobutamine. If the Pa_{O_2} does not improve, the level of airway pressure therapy previously associated with the best oxygenation should be chosen.

Air trapping is usually recognized by an increase in Pa_{CO_2}, by identifying an increase in intrinsic PEEP, or by calculating an increase in the dead space–tidal volume ratio (V_D/V_T). If intrinsic PEEP is increased, the amount of extrinsic PEEP applied should be decreased to restore the total PEEP to its former level. The use of fluid or inotropic support will also improve V_D/V_T by increasing pulmonary blood flow. Alternatively, a certain degree of air trapping and hypercarbia may be tolerable if they are associated with an airway pressure that enhances oxygenation (permissive hypercapnia).

WEANING AIRWAY PRESSURE THERAPY

Once the patient's clinical status has been stable or improving for at least 12 hours, consideration can be

SICU Hypoxia Protocol
PEEP/Reverse I:E Trial Flowsheet

FIGURE 9–22. Trial of airway pressure therapy. Example of a flow sheet used for a trial of PEEP or IRV. (I : E ratio = inspiration : expiration ratio; Pa_{O_2} = arterial oxygen tension.) Oxygen delivery (D_{O_2}) in ml/min is calculated by multiplying cardiac output (l/min) by arterial oxygen content (ml O_2/l blood). Oxygen consumption (V_{O_2}) in ml/min is calculated via the Fick equation, and equals cardiac output (l/min) times the difference between arterial and venous oxygen content (ml O_2/l blood). Carbon dioxide tension (Pa_{CO_2}) may be added to the table to document hypercarbia caused by air trapping (auto-PEEP). The "best" PEEP or I : E ratio is that which achieves maximal Pa_{O_2}, without excessive increase in peak inflation pressure or air trapping, and without excessive decrease in static compliance, cardiac output, and oxygen delivery. Fluid administration or inotropic support may be added to restore impaired cardiac output and oxygen delivery. (Courtesy of R. Lawrence Reed III, M.D.)

Patient name: _____
History number: _____ ____ ____
Date: _____

F_IO_2: _____

(*Note:* Do not change F_IO_2 during PEEP trial unless a severe deterioration in P_aO_2 occurs.)

Time*	PEEP	I:E Ratio	Cardiac Output	Static Compliance	Peak Inflation Pressure	P_aO_2	Oxygen Delivery (D_{O_2})	Oxygen Consumption (V_{O_2})

* Only 3-5 minutes allowed from time of PEEP or I:E ratio change to measurement of Cardiac Output, Compliance, and Peak Inflation Pressure following the change. At least 20 minutes must elapse before P_aO_2 sample obtained on new PEEP or I:E ratio setting.

given to weaning airway pressure therapy. Active processes such as septic shock, aspiration, excessive secretions and circulatory instability should be under control. The P:F ratio should be constantly greater than 200 or increasing, with an Fi_{O_2} of less than 0.4 and Pa_{O_2} greater than 80 mm Hg. The lower the Fi_{O_2} prior to weaning of airway pressure therapy, the greater the chance of success, because a greater proportion of nitrogen fills unstable alveoli, acting as a "strut" to prevent atelectasis after the adsorption of oxygen.

Premature withdrawal of airway pressure therapy may rapidly worsen oxygenation through acute airway collapse, making it necessary to again increase Fi_{O_2}. It may also require levels of airway pressure *higher* than the previous settings to be applied for more than 24 hours to restore the FRC and oxygenation to their former levels (Luterman et al., 1978). This unnecessarily exposes the patient to oxygen toxicity and barotrauma. A "window" on the instability of alveoli may be obtained by decreasing the level of PEEP or IRV for no longer than 3 minutes before returning it to its former level. Any derecruitment of alveoli that occurs in this short period of time is reversed within 5 minutes (DeCampo and Civetta, 1979). An arterial blood gas is obtained immediately before the pressure decrement and at the end of 3 minutes. If the Pa_{O_2} declines by less than 20% of baseline, the new lower level of airway pressure is adopted once the result is known. On the other hand, if the Pa_{O_2} declines by more than 20% of baseline, the level of airway pressure is kept at its previous setting. For example, a patient has a Pa_{O_2} of 72 mm Hg on an Fi_{O_2} of 0.3 and 16 cm H_2O PEEP. The PEEP is decreased to 14 cm H_2O for 3 minutes, and then returned to 16 cm H_2O. If the Pa_{O_2} at the end of 3 minutes was 68 mm Hg (a 5% decrease), the PEEP is reset at its new level, 14 cm H_2O. However, if the Pa_{O_2} was 56 mm Hg (a 22% decrease), the PEEP is left at 16 cm H_2O. Whether or not the attempt at decreasing the level of airway pressure is successful, further attempts are not repeated any more frequently than every 6 to 8 hours, and then only if the P:F ratio has been stable or has continued to improve.

In practice, the authors usually wean IRV first, until the I:E ratio returns to 1:1 or 1:2, and then proceed with weaning PEEP by 1 to 2 cm H_2O decrements to 6 cm H_2O. At this stage, if the mean airway pressure is less than 16 to 18 cm H_2O, the authors attempt to convert the patient to PSV and then proceed with a pressure support wean.

Difficult Ventilatory Weaning

Rationale

Weaning is the gradual process of removing mechanical ventilatory support. By definition, weaning uses *partial* ventilatory support so that the patient and ventilator share the work of breathing. As weaning progresses, the share of the workload provided by the patient gradually increases and that provided by the ventilator gradually decreases. When the patient is finally able to perform all the work of breathing independently, weaning is complete and mechanical ventilation can be removed.

After routine, uncomplicated postoperative mechanical ventilation, weaning is rapid, and once extubation criteria are met, the patient can undergo tracheal extubation from a low level of ventilatory support—for example, an IMV rate of 4 breaths per minute and 5 cm H_2O PEEP. This provides a work of breathing similar to that required after tracheal extubation. Gradual reduction in ventilatory support is indicated in those patients who are slowly recovering from a respiratory system injury. Such patients might have slowly resolving infections, slowly resolving ARDS (Marini, 1986a), phrenic nerve injuries, slowly resolving heart failure, or similar conditions. Weaning can usually progress only as fast as these underlying disease processes resolve. Pushing patients to do unacceptable or intolerable work in an attempt to "get the patient off the ventilator as fast as possible" may often precipitate muscle fatigue and unnecessarily delay the weaning process. Weaning thus should be gauged according to patient tolerance and not according to some arbitrary time schedule (see later) (Marini, 1986b).

INDICATIONS FOR GRADUAL VENTILATOR WEANING

The argument is sometimes made that weaning is an unnecessary process. This argument states that total support should be given to patients until they can breathe entirely on their own. At this point, ventilatory support is discontinued. This approach is certainly appropriate for rapidly resolving processes such as emergence after anesthesia. However, it is probably inappropriate in patients with much slower recovery processes, for two reasons. First, partial mechanical ventilatory support induces less intrathoracic pressure increase than total support and decreases the risk of hemodynamic compromise or barotrauma. Second, partial support demands some patient activity, which helps prevent muscle atrophy and may contribute to muscle conditioning. Total ventilatory support causes progressive atrophy of the respiratory musculature and increases the likelihood of muscle fatigue and discoordination when spontaneous ventilation is resumed.

Techniques for Partial Support and Weaning

At least three established methods provide partial support during the weaning process (MacIntyre, 1988). The oldest technique is to alternate periods of total mechanical ventilatory support with *intermittent spontaneous breathing* on a T piece system. The patient assumes the total work of breathing, but the T piece ensures a consistent Fi_{O_2} and provides a very low resistance to breathing. Weaning progresses by having the patient take longer and longer periods of spontaneous breathing. In between these periods, the ventilator takes over all the work of breathing and allows the patient to rest. This is an all-or-none situation: Either the ventilator provides 100% of the work of breathing or it provides none at all. A second technique is IMV. During IMV, patients breathe spontaneously and mandatory ventilator breaths are intermittently interspersed. Weaning progresses by decreasing the frequency of ventilator breaths (i.e., the IMV rate) so that an increasing proportion of the minute ventilation and work of breathing is provided by the patient. A variation on this approach is SIMV, which uses volume-assisted breaths along with backup volume control breaths. With regard to patient work, IMV is also an all-or-none situation, although the periods during which the patient performs 100% of the work of breathing are much shorter than during T piece breathing. The third technique is stand-alone PSV. With this technique, partial support is provided with every breath by using a pressure-limited, patient-triggered breath. Weaning progresses from a high level of pressure support, enough to provide virtually all the work of each breath (usually associated with tidal volumes of 8 to 10 ml/kg) to lower levels of pressure support in which the patient contributes substantial work to each breath. However, the patient never provides 100% of the work of breathing until pressure support is completely withdrawn.

The use of T piece breathing trials or IMV offers the advantage that a certain mandatory minute ventilation is ensured by the ventilator, which is not the case with PSV. However, PSV does offer the theoretical advantage of being a more comfortable and physiologic way to have the muscles work, since a pressure "boost" is provided with each ventilatory effort (Brochard et al., 1989; MacIntyre, 1986). In addition, it is a logical method to use in weaning patients with muscle atrophy who have been sedated and paralyzed for PCV and IRV, because PSV can initially provide close to 100% of the work of breathing, and then gradually and smoothly allow the patient's contribution to increase. However, clinical studies comparing the outcome of these different approaches to ventilatory weaning are not available. The choice of mode is usually based on the clinician's experience and assessment of the patient's physiologic needs regarding a minimal minute ventilation and comfort. In fact, these modes are frequently combined or used sequentially. For example, in the SIMV mode, 5 to 10 cm H_2O pressure support is commonly added to the spontaneous breaths taken by the patient to reduce or eliminate the work of breathing imposed by narrow endotracheal tubes. Patients who have undergone tracheostomy may be weaned to a low IMV rate (e.g., 4 breaths per minute) or level of pressure support (e.g., 10 cm H_2O), and then started on sequential intermittent spontaneous breathing trials on a T piece system.

MONITORING THE WEANING PROCESS

Regardless of the technique used, appropriate monitoring of the weaning process is crucial to facilitate an adequate rate of progress. Since the goal is to return ventilatory work to the patient as quickly as possible, indicators of patient load tolerance should be the best parameters to monitor during weaning (Yang and Tobin, 1986). The respiratory rate is a particularly useful sign of how well the patient is tolerating the loads placed on the ventilatory muscles during partial ventilatory support and weaning. Tachypnea is one of the earliest signs of respiratory muscle overload and fatigue and is an excellent guide to the adjustment of the appropriate level of partial support. Although it is usually helpful to monitor arterial blood gases during the weaning process, it should be noted the changes in Pa_{CO_2} and Pa_{O_2} may not occur until long after respiratory muscle fatigue has begun to develop, and they should not be the exclusive guide to weaning. Indirect indications of a patient tolerance of the weaning process include stable hemodynamics, subjective comfort, and a regular breathing pattern. Sympathetic overactivity—tachycardia, hypertension, diaphoresis, and ultimately, tachyarrhythmias—is an invaluable sign of excessive work of breathing and may considerably precede any alteration in arterial blood gases.

Newer monitors allow actual measurements of patient work of breathing and pressure-time product during partial ventilatory support (Brochard et al., 1989; Collett et al., 1985). These measurements can be used to make subtle adjustments to the level of partial support by the consistent provision of a normal ventilatory workload or by maintaining the pressure-time product less than 15% of the maximal diaphragmatic pressure, which minimizes fatigue. However, these approaches require expensive equipment and the information provided has not been shown to help the decision-making process any more than the simple observation of respiratory rate and patient comfort.

ASSESSING THE LIKELIHOOD OF EXTUBATION SUCCESS

When the weaning process has progressed to a fairly low level of partial support (spontaneous breathing trials lasting 30 to 60 minutes, IMV rates less than 4 breaths per minute, pressure support levels less than 10 cm H_2O), the patient's ability to protect the airway, tolerate spontaneous breathing, and generate an adequate cough needs to be assessed. So-called lung mechanics are performed during spontaneous ventilation on room air, so the patient must be able to safely tolerate this situation, at least for a limited time, when these are ordered.

The *negative inspiratory force maximum* (NIFM) measures the negative airway pressure generated when the patient attempts to inspire against an occluded airway. The normal level is -80 to -100 cm H_2O, and a NIFM of greater than -25 cm H_2O is the criterion of adequacy generally used. The NIFM depends on reflex, rather than voluntary activity, and can be performed on obtunded patients. The *forced vital capacity* (FVC) measures the exhaled volume when a maximal expiration follows a maximal inspiration. The normal FVC is 50 to 70 ml/kg, and an FVC of greater than 15 ml/kg is the criterion of adequacy usually used. Performance of the FVC depends on patient alertness and cooperation and also predicts the ability of the patient to cooperate with respiratory therapy after tracheal extubation. The NIFM and FVC are important indicators of the patient's ability to reflexively clear airway secretions and voluntarily cough and deep breathe. However, they measure effort during a single breath and do not predict endurance or fatigability with repetitive breathing.

The spontaneous minute ventilation, which is the product of the tidal volume and the respiratory rate, can be more helpful in predicting ongoing work of breathing and the potential for fatigue. Normal minute ventilation is 120 ml/kg, or about 10 l/min in an 80-kg patient (minute ventilation changes about 10% for each degree centigrade change in temperature). A minute ventilation of greater than 15 l/min, whether due to hyperventilation (i.e., associated with hypocarbia) or hyperpnea (i.e., associated with a normal Pa_{CO_2}) implies a high ventilatory demand on the patient, which will usually cause fatigue and decompensation after several hours.

The spontaneous ventilatory pattern may be the best single predictor of outcome. A patient with a rapid respiratory rate and shallow tidal volume is likely to develop progressive atelectasis, increasing lung stiffness and work of breathing, and ultimately, acute respiratory failure. A ventilatory frequency–tidal volume (f/V_T) ratio of greater than 100 appears to be a reliable predictor of failure (Yang and Tobin, 1986). For example, a patient breathing at 30 breaths per minute with a tidal volume of 0.2 l would have a f/V_T of 150, predictive of failure, whereas a patient breathing at 20 breaths per minute with a tidal volume of 0.5 l would have a f/V_T of 40, predictive of success. However, the f/V_T does not provide information on the patient's ability to cough and clear secretions.

Some have tried to combine several criteria into a nomogram, such as the CROP index (compliance, respiratory rate, oxygenation, [negative inspiratory] pressure), which is actually less predictive than the f/V_T ratio (Yang and Tobin, 1986). Rather, the combination of tests of the ability to cough and clear secretions (NIFM, FVC) together with the spontaneous minute ventilation and ventilatory pattern (f/V_T) provide the most realistic assessment of the likelihood of success in withdrawal of ventilatory support and tracheal extubation. Observation of the patient for cooperation, cyanosis, fatigue, or sympathetic overactivity during the tests makes the interpretation of the numbers much more meaningful. In borderline cases, the serial performance of lung mechanics every 12 or 24 hours can demonstrate gradual improvement or lack thereof and further discriminate between success or failure.

General Management Issues in the Difficult-to-Wean Patient

In addition to treating the underlying disease and setting the proper level of partial ventilatory support, a number of other aspects of care must be considered for total management of the patient requiring prolonged support. The ventilator mode should be a comfortable one for the patient. Specifically, required triggering efforts should be small and ventilator flows should be provided in accordance with patient demand. Airway toilet must be meticulous, with proper suctioning techniques, aspiration precautions, humidification, and circuit hygiene. The patient should obtain adequate rest between periods of exercise. Forward progress in ventilatory weaning is helped by active withdrawal of support during the day, followed by an increase in support at night to a level that decreases the patient's work of breathing and facilitates sleep. As the patient grows stronger, the nocturnal rest period is gradually shortened and finally omitted.

Cardiovascular and fluid management should be designed to achieve an appropriate cardiac output while reducing the accumulation of extravascular lung water. During the weaning, the ventilatory muscles are being asked to take over an increasing workload, and the adequacy of oxygen delivery is critical. Use of an inotropic agent such as dobutamine and a renal vasodilator such as low-dose dopamine ($3 \mu g \cdot kg^{-1} \cdot min^{-1}$) may help to minimize the preload required for an adequate cardiac output, while maintaining high urine flow rate.

Nutritional support is essential, particularly in a patient whose lean body mass is depleted by the catabolic stress of major trauma, operation, or sepsis. Starvation or inadequate feeding perpetuates somatic protein deficit (ventilatory muscle weakness) and visceral protein deficit (surfactant depletion and atelectasis, impaired immune response, and pneumonia). On the other hand, excessive carbohydrate intake induces hepatic lipogenesis, markedly increases CO_2 production, and may actually induce acute respiratory failure (Amene et al., 1987). In difficult cases, a decrease in carbohydrate intake for 3 or 4 days may sufficiently decrease CO_2 production to facilitate ventilatory weaning.

At some point in the difficult weaning process—either after a failed trial of tracheal extubation or if weaning progress is very slow—tracheostomy should be considered because it improves secretion clearance and decreases dead space. However, it is not necessary to proceed with tracheostomy simply based on the duration of tracheal intubation. Soft-cuffed endotracheal tubes are well tolerated for many days—as long as the patient is heavily sedated or paralyzed. Indeed, it is risky to undertake tracheostomy in the early stages of acute respiratory failure, when lung compliance and oxygenation are poor, because removal from high levels of $F_{I_{O_2}}$ and airway pressure therapy is not tolerated for even short periods of time. Later, especially when the patient is again breathing spontaneously and the $F_{I_{O_2}}$ is relatively low, tracheostomy greatly improves patient comfort, mobility, and psychological status. It takes away the angst associated with extubation of the trachea, facilitates movement out of bed, and promotes rapid progression to T piece weaning.

Finally, patience is needed on the part of the clinician. Ventilatory weaning can progress no faster than healing of the respiratory system itself. On occasion, it may be beneficial to set aside ventilatory weaning for a few days and concentrate on building up the patient's overall muscle strength through physical therapy, weight bearing, and mobilization. Thereafter, weaning often proceeds more quickly because diaphragmatic strength has improved pari passu with the rest of the body. The goal of ventilatory management is not to "cure" the lung, but rather to provide an adequate level of support while recovery proceeds and to not hinder the process with iatrogenic complications.

SELECTED BIBLIOGRAPHY

Benumof, J.: Conventional (laryngoscopic) orotracheal and nasotracheal intubation (single-lumen type). *In* Benumof, J. (ed): Clinical Procedures in Anesthesia and Intensive Care. Philadelphia, J. B. Lippincott, 1992, p. 115.

This is an excellent review of standard approaches to uncomplicated airway management and tracheal intubation. The author emphasizes the importance of positioning and airway aids in ensuring adequate oxygenation and ventilation before attempts at tracheal intubation and explains and corrects common errors committed during laryngoscopy and intubation.

Benumof, J.: Management of the difficult adult airway: With special emphasis on the awake tracheal intubation. Anesthesiology, 75:1087, 1991.

The author provides a succinct approach to the clinical assessment of the patient with a potentially difficult airway and a systematic approach to managing this situation, with emphasis on techniques of awake tracheal intubation. The algorithm for management of the difficult airway developed by the American Society of Anesthesiologists is presented.

MacIntyre, N. R.: Respiratory function during pressure support ventilation. Chest, 89:677, 1986.

The author presents the effects of pressure support ventilation (PSV) on 15 patients, comparing and contrasting it with synchronous intermittent mandatory ventilation. In patients with spontaneous ventilatory drive, PSV improved patient comfort, decreased work of breathing, and provided a more balanced pressure and volume change form of muscle work to the patient. The article provides a clear explanation of the mechanisms and potential benefits of PSV.

Shapiro, B. A., Cane, R. D., and Harrison, R. A.: Positive end-expiratory pressure therapy in adults with special reference to acute lung injury: A review of the literature and suggested clinical correlations. Crit. Care Med., 12:127, 1984.

This is a classic review of the mechanisms of action of positive end-expiratory pressure (PEEP), which explains its mechanisms of action, particularly in adult respiratory distress syndrome, and its potentially detrimental effects on the cardiovascular system and alveoli. Therapeutic issues such as prophylactic use of PEEP, "physiologic PEEP," and spontaneous breathing with PEEP are also addressed (168 references).

Shapiro, B. A., Vender, J. S., and Peruzzi, W. T.: Airway pressure therapy for cardiac surgical patients: State of the art and clinical controversies. J. Cardiothorac. Vasc. Anesth., 6:735, 1992.

The authors provide a clear exposition of the major functions of a ventilator breath (initiation, limit, and cycle off) and use it to provide a logical and helpful classification of ventilator modes. This classification is then applied to the use of mechanical ventilation in the postoperative period after cardiac surgery, emphasizing interactions between positive-pressure ventilation and the cardiovascular system.

BIBLIOGRAPHY

Ali, J., Weisel, R. D., Layug, A. B., et al.: Consequences of postoperative alterations in respiratory mechanics. Am. J. Surg., 128:376, 1974.

Amene, P. C., Sladen, R. N., Feeley, T. W., et al.: Hypercapnia during total parenteral nutrition with hypertonic dextrose. Crit. Care Med., 15:171, 1987.

Andrivet, P., Adnot, S., Brun-Buisson, C., et al.: Involvement of ANF in the acute antidiuresis during PEEP ventilation. J. Appl. Physiol., 65:1967, 1988.

Annat, G., Viale, J. P., Xuan, B. B., et al.: Effect of PEEP ventilation on renal function, plasma renin, aldosterone, neurophysins and urinary ADH, and prostaglandins. Anesthesiology, 58:136, 1983.

Arens, J. F.: Maxillary sinusitis: A complication of tracheal intubation. Anesthesiology, 40:415, 1974.

Ashbaugh, D. G., Petty, T. L., Bigelow, D. B., et al.: Continuous positive pressure breathing (CPPB) in adult respiratory distress syndrome. J. Thorac. Cardiovasc. Surg., 57:31, 1969.

Beaumont, W.: Gastric Juice and the Physiology of Digestion. Plattsburgh, NY, Allen, 1833, p. 159.

Bellhouse, C. P., and Dore, C.: Criteria for estimating likelihood of difficulty of endotracheal intubation with MacIntosh laryngoscope. Anaesth. Intensive Care, 42:329, 1987.

Benumof, J.: Conventional (laryngoscopic) orotracheal and nasotracheal intubation (single-lumen type). *In* Benumof, J. (ed): Clinical Procedures in Anesthesia and Intensive Care. Philadelphia, J. B. Lippincott, 1992, p. 115.

Benumof, J.: Management of the difficult adult airway: With special emphasis on the awake tracheal intubation. Anesthesiology, 75:1087, 1991.

Black, J., Kalloor, G. J., and Collis, J. L.: The effect of the surgical approach on respiratory function after esophageal resection. Br. J. Surg., 64:624, 1977.

Bolin, R. W., and Pierson, D. J.: Ventilatory management in acute lung injury. Crit. Care Clin., 2:585, 1986.

Bonnet, F., Richard, C., Glaser, P., et al.: Changes in hepatic flow induced by continuous positive pressure ventilation in critically ill patients. Crit. Care Med., 10:703, 1982.

Brochard, L., Harf, A., Lorino, H., et al.: Pressure support prevents diaphragmatic failure during weaning from mechanical ventilation (MV). Am. Rev. Respir. Dis., 139:513, 1989.

Byrd, R. B., and Burns, J. R.: Cough dynamics in the post-thoracotomy state. Chest, 67:654, 1975.

Calverley, R. K.: Anesthesia as a specialty: Past, present and future. *In* Barash, P. G., Cullen, B. F., and Stoelting, R. K. (eds): Clinical Anesthesia. Philadelphia, J. B. Lippincott, 1989, p. 3.

Caplan, R. A., Posner, K. L., Ward, R. J., et al.: Adverse respiratory events in anesthesia: A closed claims analysis. Anesthesiology, 72:828, 1990.

Collett, P. W., Perry, C., and Engel, L. A.: Pressure-time product, flow, and oxygen cost of resistive breathing in humans. J. Appl. Physiol., 58:1263, 1985.

Coté, C. J.: NPO after midnight for children—A reappraisal [Editorial]. Anesthesiology, 72:589, 1990.

Craig, K. C., Pierson, D. J., and Carrico, C. J.: The clinical application of positive end-expiratory pressure (PEEP) in the adult respiratory distress syndrome (ARDS). Respir. Care, 30:184, 1985.

Cullen, D. J., and Caldera, D. L.: The incidence of ventilator-induced pulmonary barotrauma in critically ill patients. Anesthesiology, 50:185, 1979.

Darioli, R., and Perret, C.: Mechanical controlled ventilation in status asthmaticus. Am. Rev. Respir. Dis., 129:385, 1984.

DeCampo, T., and Civetta, J. M.: The effect of short-term discontinuation of high-level PEEP in patients with acute respiratory failure. Crit. Care Med., 7:49, 1979.

Demling, R. H., Staub, N. C., and Edmunds, L. H. J.: Effect of end-expiratory pressure on accumulation of extravascular lung water. J. Appl. Physiol., 38:907, 1975.

Doblar, D. D., Santiago, T. V., Kahm, A. U., et al.: Effect of positive end-expiratory pressure ventilation (PEEP) on cerebral blood flow and cerebrospinal fluid pressure in goats. Anesthesiology, 55:244, 1981.

Doherty, D., and Sladen, R. N.: Effects of positive airway pressure on renal function. Probl. Respir. Care, 2:369, 1989.

Falke, K. J., Pontoppidan, H., Kumar, A., et al.: Ventilation with end-expiratory pressure in acute lung disease. J. Clin. Invest., 51:2315, 1972.

Frerk, C. M.: Predicting difficult intubation. Anaesthesia, 46:1005, 1991.

Froese, A. B., and Bryan, A. C.: Effects of anesthesia and paralysis on diaphragmatic mechanism in man. Anesthesiology, 44:247, 1974.

Frumin, M. J., Lee, A. S. J., and Papper, E. M.: New valve for nonrebreathing systems. Anesthesiology, 20:383, 1959.

Gallagher, C., Sladen, R. N., and Lubarsky, D.: Thoracotomy: Postoperative complications. Probl. Anesthesiology, 4:393, 1990.

Gorback, M. S.: Analgesic management after thymectomy. Anesth. Rep., 2:262, 1990.

Goresky, G. V., and Maltby, J. R.: Fasting guidelines for elective surgical patients. Can. J. Anaesth., 37:493, 1990.

Gregory, G. A.: Respiratory care of the child. Crit. Care Med., 8:582, 1980.

Hemmer, M., and Suter, P. M.: Treatment of cardiac and renal effects of PEEP with dopamine in patients with acute respiratory failure. Anesthesiology, 50:399, 1979.

Hickling, K. G., Henderson, S. J., and Jackson, R.: Low mortality associated with low-volume pressure-limited ventilation with permissive hypercapnia in severe adult respiratory distress syndrome. Intensive Care Med., 16:372, 1990.

Hillman, K. M.: Pneumoperitoneum: A review. Crit. Care Med., 10:476, 1982.

Horton, W. G., and Cheney, F. W.: Variability of effect of positive end-expiratory pressure. Arch. Surg., 110:395, 1975.

Jardin, F., Forest, J. C., Boisante, L., et al.: Influence of positive end-expiratory pressure on left ventricular performance. N. Engl. J. Med., 304:387, 1981.

Kharasch, E. D., Yeo, K., Kenny, M. A., et al.: Atrial natriuretic factor may mediate the renal effects of PEEP ventilation. Anesthesiology, 69:862, 1988.

Kirby, R. R., Robison, E. J., Schulz, J., et al.: A new pediatric volume ventilator. Anesth. Analg., 50:533, 1971.

Knill, R. L., Manninen, P. H., and Clement, J. L.: Ventilation and chemoreflexes during enflurane sedation and anaesthesia in man. Can. Anaesth. Soc. J., 26:353, 1979.

Luterman, A., Horovitz, J. H., Carrico, C. J., et al.: Withdrawal from positive end-expiratory pressure. Surgery, 83:328, 1978.

Macewan, W.: Clinical observations on the introduction of tracheal tubes by mouth instead of performing tracheotomy or laryngotomy. Br. Med. J., 2:122, 1880.

MacIntyre, N. R.: Respiratory function during pressure support ventilation. Chest, 89:677, 1986.

MacIntyre, N. R.: Weaning from mechanical ventilatory support: Volume-assisting intermittent breaths versus pressure-assisting every breath. Respir. Care, 33:121, 1988.

Mallampati, S. R., Gatt, S. P., Gugino, L. D., et al.: A clinical sign to predict difficult tracheal intubation: A prospective study. Can. J. Anaesth., 32:429, 1985.

Marini, J. J.: Exertion during ventilator support: How much and how important? Respir. Care, 31:385, 1986a.

Marini, J. J.: The physiologic determinants of ventilator dependence. Respir. Care, 31:271, 1986b.

Mathru, M., Roat, K., and Venus, B.: Ventilator-induced barotrauma in controlled mechanical ventilation versus intermittent mechanical ventilation. Crit. Care Med., 11:359, 1983.

McGee, J. P. I., and Vender, J. S.: Nonintubation management of the airway. In Benumof, J. L. (ed): Clinical Procedures in Anesthesia and Intensive Care. Philadelphia, J. B. Lippincott, 1992, p. 89.

McNamee, C. J., Meyns, B., and Pagliero, K. M.: Flexible bronchoscopy via the laryngeal mask: A new technique. Thorax, 46:141, 1991.

Mendelson, C. L.: The aspiration of stomach contents into the lungs during obstetric anesthesia. Am. J. Obstet. Gynecol., 52:191, 1946.

Meyers, J. R., Lembeck, L., O'Kane, H., et al.: Changes in functional residual capacity of the lung after operation. Arch. Surg., 110:576, 1975.

Miller, R. A.: A new laryngoscope. Anesthesiology, 2:317, 1941.

Mörch, E. T.: History of mechanical ventilation. In Kirby, R. R., Smith, R. A., and Desautels, D. A. (eds): Mechanical Ventilation. New York, Churchill Livingstone, 1985, p. 1.

Mullins, R. J., Dawe, E. J., Lucas, C. E., et al.: Mechanisms of impaired renal function with PEEP. J. Surg. Res., 37:189, 1984.

Paré, P. D., Warriner, B., Baile, M., et al.: Redistribution of pulmonary extravascular water with positive end-expiratory pressure in canine pulmonary edema. Am. Rev. Respir. Dis., 127:590, 1983.

Pennant, J. H., and White, P. F.: The laryngeal mask airway: Its uses in anesthesiology. Anesthesiology, 79:144, 1993.

Pepe, P. E., and Marini, J. J.: Occult positive end-expiratory pressure in mechanically ventilated patients with airflow obstruction: The auto-PEEP effect. Am. Rev. Respir. Dis., 126:166, 1982.

Pinsky, M. R., Matuschak, G. M., and Klain, M.: Determinants of cardiac augmentation by elevations in intrathoracic pressure. J. Appl. Physiol., 58:1189, 1985.

Prakash, O., Jonson, B., Meij, E., et al.: Criteria for early extubation after intracardiac surgery in adults. Anesth. Analg., 56:703, 1977.

Priebe, H., Heimann, J. C., and Hedley-Whyte, J.: Mechanisms of renal dysfunction during PEEP ventilation. J. Appl. Physiol., 50:643, 1981.

Quasha, A. L., Loeber, N., Feeley, T. W., et al.: Postoperative recovery care: A controlled trial of early and late extubation following coronary artery bypass grafting. Anesthesiology, 51:499, 1981.

Qvist, J. H., Pontoppidan, H., Wilson, R. S., et al.: Hemodynamic response to mechanical ventilation with PEEP. Anesthesiology, 42:45, 1975.

Raby, K. E., Goldman, L., Creager, M. A., et al.: Correlation between preoperative ischemia and major cardiac events after peripheral vascular surgery. N. Engl. J. Med., 321:1296, 1989.

Rubin, H.: A new nonrebreathing valve. Anesthesiology, 16:643, 1955.

Schreiner, M. S., Triebwasser, A., and Keon, T. P.: Oral fluids compared to preoperative fasting in pediatric outpatients. Anesthesiology, 72:593, 1990.

Sellden, H., Sjovall, H., and Ricksten, S.: Sympathetic nerve activity and central hemodynamics during mechanical ventilation in rats. Acta Physiol. Scand., 127:51, 1986.

Shackford, S. R., Virgilio, R. W., Peters, R. M., et al.: Early extubation vs. prophylactic ventilation for the high-risk patient: A comparison of postoperative management in the prevention of respiratory complications. Anesth. Analg., 29:463, 1981.

Shapiro, B. A., Cane, R. D., and Harrison, R. A.: Positive end-expiratory pressure therapy in adults with special reference to acute lung injury: A review of the literature and suggested clinical correlations. Crit. Care Med., 12:127, 1984.

Shapiro, B. A., Vender, J. S., and Peruzzi, W. T.: Airway pressure therapy for cardiac surgical patients: State of the art and clinical controversies. J. Cardiothorac. Vasc. Anesth., 6:735, 1992.

Sjöstrand, U.: Review of the physiological rationale for and development of high-frequency positive pressure ventilation (HFPPV). Acta Anaesthesiol. Scand. Suppl., 64:165, 1977.

Sladen, R. N.: Management of the adult cardiac patient in the intensive care unit. In Ream, A. K., and Fogdall, R. P. (eds): Acute Cardiovascular Management: Anesthesia and Intensive Care. Philadelphia, J. B. Lippincott, 1982, pp. 528–548.

Suter, P. M., Fairley, H. B., and Isenberg, M. D.: Optimum end-expiratory pressure in patients with acute pulmonary failure. N. Engl. J. Med., 292:284, 1975.

Sykes, W. S.: Essays on the First Hundred Years of Anaesthesia. Vol. 2. London, Churchill Livingstone, 1960.

Tisi, G. M.: Preoperative evaluation of pulmonary function: Validity, indications and benefits. Am. Rev. Respir. Dis., 119:293, 1979.

Toth, J. L., Capellier, G., Walker, P., et al.: Lung emphysematous changes in ARDS. Am. Rev. Respir. Dis., 145(Suppl.):A184, 1992.

Turnbull, K. W., Miyagishima, R. T., Gerein, A. N., et al.: Pulmonary complications and cardiopulmonary bypass: A clinical study in adults. Can. Anaesth. Soc. J., 21:181, 1974.

Venus, B., Mathru, M., Smith, R. A., et al.: Renal function during application of positive end-expiratory pressure in swine: Effects of hydration. Anesthesiology, 62:765, 1985.

Weil, J. V., McCollough, R. E., Kline, J. S., et al.: Diminished ventilatory response to hypoxia and hypercapnia after morphine in normal man. N. Engl. J. Med., 292:1103, 1975.

Yang, K. L., and Tobin, M. J.: A prospective study of indexes predicting the outcome of trials of weaning from mechanical ventilation. N. Engl. J. Med., 324:1445, 1986.

■ II Tracheal Intubation and Mechanical Ventilation: The Surgeon's Viewpoint

Arthur D. Boyd, Greg H. Ribakove, and Robert J. Sparaco

The practice of thoracic surgery has progressed alongside advances in equipment and techniques for mechanical ventilation and intubation of the respiratory tract. Although these technologic advances are critical to refinements in thoracic surgery, some surgeons have difficulty in staying abreast of changes in methodology and instrumentation. Such difficulty occurs when respiratory care department personnel and physicians who have specialized in this area of medicine assume responsibility for in-hospital delivery of respiratory care, clinical research, and product and technique development.

Regular communication between physicians specializing in respiratory care and respiratory care department personnel can provide surgeons with an excellent source of current information and with major assistance in the management of patients who have airway or respiratory problems. Recovery rooms and *intensive care units* (ICUs) now offer specialized care for patients who require intubation and mechanical ventilation. As originally recognized by Gold and Shin in 1974, respiratory care teams directed by physicians (e.g., ICU and recovery room nurses, respiratory therapists, and physiotherapists) provide patients with the most current techniques for treating respiratory failure. Changes in surgical management have led to a remarkable increase in the need for ventilatory support in patients following surgery. As a result, many patients undergoing thoracic surgery remain intubated and receive ventilatory support for several postoperative days. This treatment requires continuous respiratory care services to monitor *intracuff pressures* (ICPs) and to manage patients and equipment.

The primary purpose of tracheal intubation, whether from above, through the larynx, or by direct incision through the cricothyroid membrane or cervical trachea, is to gain access to and ensure patency of the airway. The most common indications for tracheal intubation are to establish a route for mechanical ventilatory support, to allow removal of tracheobronchial secretions (mucus, blood, or pus) or aspirated material that the patient is unable to clear spontaneously, to prevent aspiration of regurgitated gastric contents, to relieve upper airway obstruction, and to reduce anatomic dead space. Some of the major indications for tracheal intubation are listed in Table 9–5.

In the past, tracheostomy was the standard procedure for tracheal intubation. More recently, routine translaryngeal intubation has been recommended for the 24 to 48 hours that precede tracheostomy, which has made tracheostomy an elective, controlled procedure with fewer complications (Mulder and Marelli, 1992). Intubation of the trachea from above, by either the oral or the nasal route, for as long as several weeks before considering tracheostomy has become a widely accepted practice. This approach frequently permits extubation before a tracheostomy is required and has greatly reduced the number of tracheostomies. When the primary indication for intubation is

■ **Table 9–5.** INDICATIONS FOR TRACHEAL INTUBATION

Upper airway obstruction
  Congenital malformations
  Head and neck trauma, laryngeal injuries, respiratory tract burns
  Infections: acute epiglottitis, tetanus
  Neoplasms: oropharyngeal carcinoma, respiratory tract tumors
Control of secretions
  Neurologic disease or injury: stroke, poliomyelitis, after neurosurgery
  Acute or chronic pulmonary disease: obstructive airway disease (secretions, suppuration)
Ventilatory support
  Respiratory failure: massive pulmonary infection, post-traumatic pulmonary insufficiency
  Neurologic disease or injury: Guillain-Barré syndrome, cervical cord trauma
  Postoperative hypoventilation, after cardiothoracic or major abdominal surgery
Prevention of aspiration
  Loss of protective oropharyngeal reflexes
  Coma

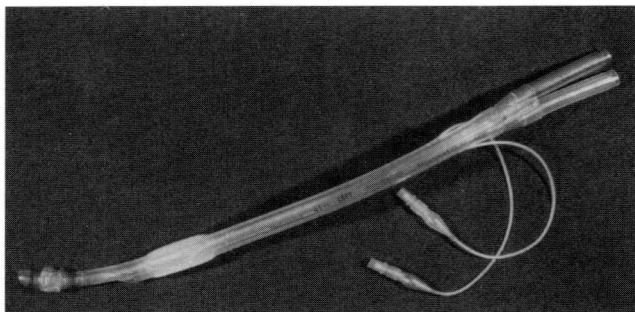

FIGURE 9–23. A Broncho-Cath Left (endobronchial tube) (Mallinckrodt Anesthesia Products, St. Louis, MO). (Courtesy of Will Stewart, VITAID.)

the need for ventilatory support, tracheostomy should be avoided if possible. Nasal or oral tracheal tubes function well as airways for several weeks. However, when it appears likely that prolonged control of the airway will be required, tracheostomy should be done promptly to minimize tube-related laryngeal trauma.

If potential or actual airway obstruction is the indication for tracheal intubation, the decision to intubate from above rather than to perform a cricothyroidotomy or tracheostomy depends on several factors, including the etiology and degree of the obstruction, the level of the obstruction in the respiratory tract, the facilities available, and the experience of the surgeons and nurses. In most cases, translaryngeal tracheal intubation is safer and more expeditious and appropriate. Patients who have suffered major head or facial trauma with facial fractures, cervical spine injuries, or tracheal division present a special challenge, and safe translaryngeal intubation may not be possible.

If the tracheobronchial tree is being flooded with fluid (blood, pus, or pleural fluid) from a tumor, pulmonary infection, or bronchopleural fistula, the site of entrance of the fluid into the airway must be separated from the normal tracheobronchial tree. This allows ventilation to be maintained and prevents aspiration and possible asphyxiation. A double-lumen endobronchial tube (Fig. 9–23), a Univent tube (Fig. 9–24), or a balloon catheter (see Chapter 3) can be used for this purpose. One or more of these instruments should be available in every emergency room, recovery room, and ICU.

If a patient with partial obstruction is cooperative, a skilled surgeon may be able to accomplish intubation from above without difficulty using sedation and local anesthesia. If intubation from above is not possible and the airway obstruction is life-threatening, it must be managed by immediate cricothyroid puncture and jet ventilation, cricothyroidotomy, or tracheostomy. These techniques are discussed later in this chapter.

The safe duration of translaryngeal tracheal intubation depends on the type of tracheal tube used, the proper control of ICP, adequate humidification, careful tracheobronchial suctioning, and correct nursing and airway care. Currently, tracheal tubes are left in

position for 3 to 4 weeks in numerous hospitals (Lewis et al., 1978; Orringer, 1980). One series described six patients who were intubated translaryngeally for 50 to 155 days without serious complications (Via-Reque and Rattenborg, 1981). A prospective study that compared tracheostomy and translaryngeal intubation for up to 3 weeks showed fewer complications after translaryngeal intubation than after tracheostomy (Stauffer et al., 1981). A more recent study, however, compares patients who underwent tracheostomy within 7 days of translaryngeal intubation with patients who were left intubated for longer periods; the morbidity and mortality rates were similar, but the time on a respirator and in the ICU was shorter for the patients who underwent early tracheostomy (Rodriguez et al., 1990). The timing of an elective tracheostomy in a patient with an endotracheal tube in place thus remains controversial since no data are available that clearly demonstrate the maximal safe duration of translaryngeal intubation (Applebaum et al., 1989; Heffner, 1991).

If low-durometry (soft), thermolabile, biocompatible, polyvinylchloride (PVC) tracheal tubes fitted with large-diameter, thin-walled, low-pressure compliant cuffs are used, translaryngeal intubation may be continued safely for a least 2 weeks. However, if it is anticipated from the outset that tracheal intubation will be needed for more than 2 weeks, it is wise to proceed with tracheostomy promptly, because mucosal alterations in the larynx and trachea can develop within 12 to 48 hours of intubation (Donnelly, 1969).

TECHNIQUE OF INTUBATION

Intubation of the trachea by the oral or nasal route is the most rapid and most common method of establishing a secure airway. An appropriate size of tracheal tube, a straight (Miller) blade, a curved (McIntosh) blade, McGill grasping forceps for tube direction, and a functioning laryngoscope must be available. The application of topical vasoconstrictors in the nose may facilitate nasotracheal intubation and may reduce bleeding. If tube insertion is not required immediately, intravenous sedation and topical anes-

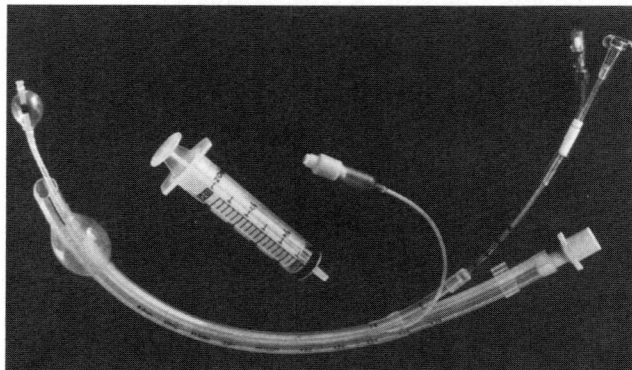

FIGURE 9–24. A Univent Tube (Fuji Systems Corporation, Tokyo). (Courtesy of Will Stewart, VITAID.)

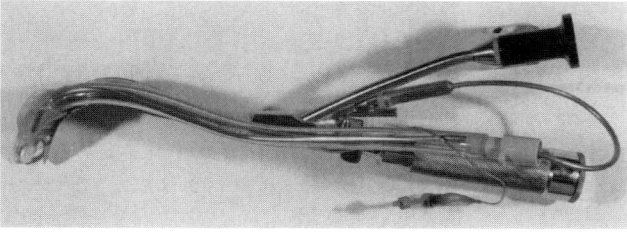

FIGURE 9–25. A Bullard laryngoscope (Circon ACMI, Stamford, CT). (Courtesy of Will Stewart, VITAID.)

thesia, which is applied to the nasal passages, mouth, pharynx, and vocal cords, will enhance patient comfort. Cocaine, tetracaine (Pontocaine), and lidocaine (Xylocaine) have all been recommended as topical anesthetics. We prefer lidocaine because it is a safe, effective, and rapidly acting local anesthetic. Two per cent lidocaine is used to spray the nasal passages, mouth, and pharynx. Cotton pledgets soaked in anesthetic may be applied to the piriform sinuses, and 2% or 4% lidocaine solution is sprayed onto the vocal cords and into the trachea. These maneuvers abolish the gag and cough reflex and allow exposure of the vocal cords for tube insertion. Local nerve block anesthesia of the glossopharyngeal and superior laryngeal nerves has also been advocated for intubing the trachea (DeMeester et al., 1977), but our clear preference is topical anesthesia.

If the patient is uncooperative and exposure of the cords is impossible, a rapidly acting muscle relaxant (e.g., succinylcholine) may be required. Use of this drug is hazardous, however, because once it is given, spontaneous ventilation stops and a patent airway must be secured immediately. Muscle relaxants should not be used unless the surgeon is adept at exposing the vocal cords and inserting an endotracheal tube. Intubation through the mouth is usually accomplished more easily than nasal intubation. For long-term use, however, the nasal route is preferred because the tube can be placed in position more securely and because it causes less laryngeal trauma (Dubick and Wright, 1978). Although patients tolerate these tubes better, associated sinus infections may complicate nasotracheal intubation.

For oral intubation, the laryngoscope blade is gently used to expose the cords, and a cuffed tracheal tube of appropriate size is inserted. Care is taken to place the top of the cuff at least 2 cm below the vocal cords. Laryngeal trauma may result from movement of the tube and cuff with flexion and extension of the neck. Nasotracheal intubation can often be done "blindly." If blind intubation is unsuccessful, the cords should be exposed with a laryngoscope blade, and McGill grasping forceps should be used to guide the tip of the tube into the trachea.

Tracheal intubation may be difficult because of the anatomic configuration of the mouth and pharynx or because of facial bone injuries or cervical spine trauma that contraindicates motion of the neck. In such situations, special techniques and instruments must be used for tracheal intubation (Benumof, 1991), or a cricothyroidotomy or tracheostomy must be performed.

A blade in which a fiberoptic channel (Fig. 9–25) is incorporated (Saunders and Geisecke, 1989) or a blade with a built-in prism (Bellhouse, 1988) (Fig. 9–26) allows the cords to be visualized when they cannot be seen with a Miller or McIntosh blade. These specialized blades frequently are not readily available, however. Another technique is to pass the endotracheal tube over a guidewire that has been passed from the cricothyroid membrane retrograde through the mouth or nostril. The most useful technique, however, once it is mastered, is to pass a tracheal tube over a flexible fiberoptic bronchoscope, the tip of which has been inserted into the trachea.

Once the trachea has been intubated, uniform bilateral pulmonary ventilation must be observed by chest auscultation and by absence of "gastric breath sounds." Radiographic confirmation of the position of the tip of the tube is necessary, but it is not urgent if the cuff has visually been placed 2 cm below the vocal cords and if the tube has been taped securely in place.

TECHNIQUE OF TRACHEOSTOMY

Tracheostomy should be done as a planned surgical procedure, preferably in an operating room, with the patient intubated from above and with the assistance of anesthesia personnel. If necessary, the procedure can be done in an ICU or emergency room. Every effort should be made, however, to duplicate conditions of an operating room: Operating-room personnel should participate, auxiliary lighting should be used, and oxygen should be administered during the operation. Regardless of where the tracheostomy is done, continuous electrocardiographic monitoring and oximetry are essential, preferably with an oscilloscope and pulse oximeter that are visible to both the surgeon and the anesthesiologist. Continuous monitoring of the patient's airway, ventilation, blood pressure, heart rate, cardiac rhythm, and oxygen saturation maximizes the patient's safety.

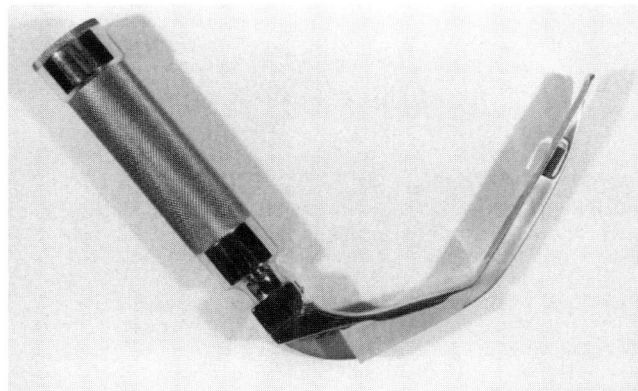

FIGURE 9–26. A Belscope laryngoscope (International Medical Inc., Burnsville, MN). (Courtesy of Will Stewart, VITAID.)

With the patient in the supine position, the neck is moderately hyperextended by placing a folded sheet beneath the shoulders and by adjusting the headpiece of the operating-room table. Total hyperextension should be avoided because it may lead the inexperienced surgeon to position the tracheal stoma such that it falls behind the manubrium when the head and neck return to a neutral or flexed position. With a low stoma, replacement of the tracheostomy tube is difficult, and risk of erosion into the innominate artery is greatly increased.

Before preparing the operative field, it is useful to palpate anatomic landmarks, particularly the cricoid cartilage and thyroid isthmus. The goal is to place the tracheostomy tube through an opening that is centered over the third tracheal ring (Fig. 9–27). If a transverse incision is made over the third ring or thyroid isthmus, it should be located no less than one finger's breadth above the clavicular heads. A low incision may allow the tube flange to impinge on the clavicles or on the sternum. An alternative guide is

to place the incision 1.5 to 2 cm below the cricoid cartilage. The scar from a vertical incision may be no less cosmetically acceptable than the scar that follows a transverse incision (Trimble and Yao, 1966).

After the neck is cleansed and draped, the operative area should be infiltrated with 1% lidocaine if a general anesthetic has not been given. A transverse incision, which is 4 to 5 cm in length, should be extended through the platysmal layer. The strap muscles are separated vertically from the inferior edge of the cricoid cartilage to the lower border of the thyroid isthmus. Division of pretracheal fascia facilitates an accurate count of tracheal rings and identification of the thyroid isthmus. If the thyroid isthmus cannot be reflected superiorly or inferiorly, it should be doubly clamped and divided, and its ends should be oversewn.

At this point, the anesthesiologist should deflate the cuff and retract the tracheal tube so that the tip lies at the level of the second or third cartilaginous ring. Before the trachea is opened, the surgeon should be prepared by having a large catheter for tracheal and bronchial suctioning, an appropriate tracheostomy tube, and a length of flexible tubing with a suitable swivel connector to attach the seated tracheostomy tube to a ventilating device. The third tracheal ring is identified and is divided in the midline. The second and fourth rings may be divided if necessary. The first tracheal ring should be preserved, however, in an effort to prevent injury to the cricoid cartilage. An alternative technique is to place a sharp tracheal hook around the third tracheal ring and to excise a 5-mm segment of this cartilage. The stoma can be quickly enlarged by gently spreading the blades of a hemostat against the margins of the tracheal opening. A lubricated, thermolabile, PVC tracheostomy tube fitted with a large-diameter, low-pressure, thin-walled compliant cuff is inserted through this opening. The tracheostomy cuff should be collapsed completely around the tube before it is inserted through the stoma. Transtracheal injection of 2% or 4% lidocaine before the stoma is made reduces coughing, which often accompanies tube placement. A sample of tracheal secretions is collected for bacteriologic examination. The tracheostomy tube should be fitted with spacers or with an adjustable neck plate so that the distal end of the tube is at least 2 cm above the carina. One should particularly note whether the inflated cuff remains within the trachea when the patient's head is extended after the shoulder pad is removed. If the tracheostomy has been performed to augment ventilation or to protect the respiratory tract from aspiration, the cuff should be filled to the minimal occluding volume (usually an ICP of 20 to 25 torr) at peak inspiratory pressure during positive-pressure ventilation. This should be done with the stoma in direct view under a thin layer of saline while the patient is quiet. ICP should be measured and recorded carefully in the patient's record.

Generally, it is unnecessary to close the incision. A simple dry gauze dressing is usually adequate.

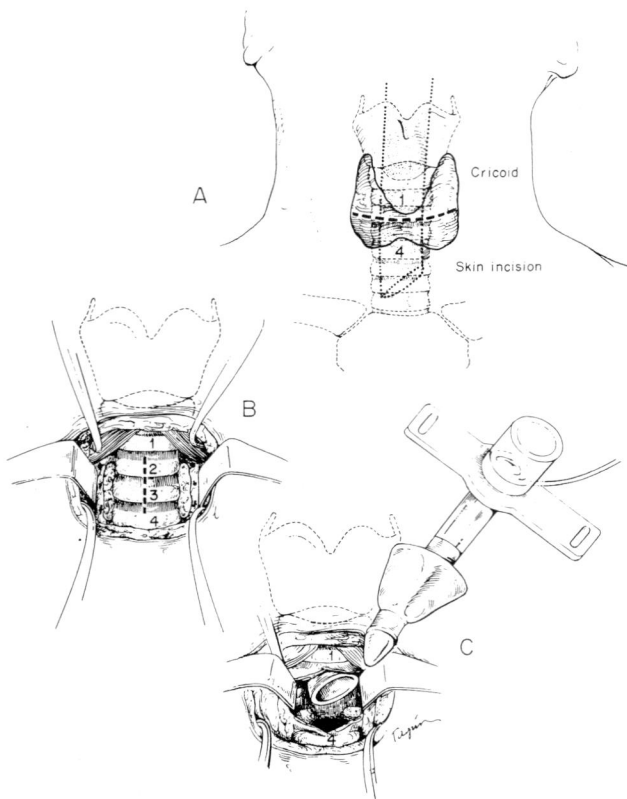

FIGURE 9–27. *A*, With an endotracheal tube in position, the neck is hyperextended, and a transverse incision is made over the third tracheal ring. *B*, After separation of the strap muscles in the midline, the thyroid isthmus is divided or retracted inferiorly or superiorly, exposing the trachea. *C*, The third tracheal ring is identified and divided. The second and fourth rings are divided, if necessary. The first tracheal ring, however, should be preserved in an effort to prevent injury to the cricoid cartilage above. A high-volume, low-pressure cuffed tracheostomy tube is inserted. (*A–C*, From Grillo, H. C.: Tracheostomy and its complications. *In* Sabiston, D. C., Jr. [ed]: Davis-Christopher Textbook of Surgery. 12th ed. Philadelphia, W. B. Saunders, 1981.)

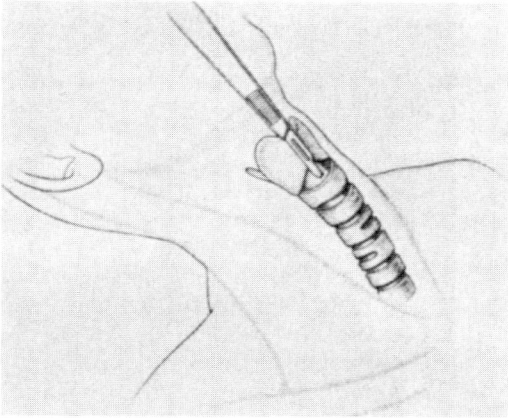

FIGURE 9–28. Cricothyroid membrane is divided. (From Boyd, A. D., Romita, M. C., Conlan, A. A., et al.: A clinical evaluation of cricothyroidotomy. Surg. Gynecol. Obstet., *149:365, 1979.*)

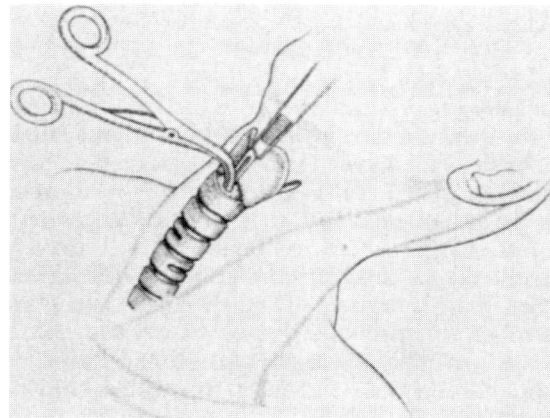

FIGURE 9–29. A dilator is inserted and is opened longitudinally. (From Boyd, A. D., Romita, M. C., Conlan, A. A., et al.: A clinical evaluation of cricothyroidotomy. Surg. Gynecol. Obstet., *149:365, 1979.*)

With uncooperative patients, one should not rely solely on cotton tapes but should secure the tube in position with sutures through the flange of the neck plate.

TECHNIQUE OF CRICOTHYROIDOTOMY

Brantigan and Grow (1976) reported excellent results with 566 cricothyroidotomies. Their results were the first large series that advocated the use of cricothyroidotomy since Jackson condemned its use in 1921. We have studied 198 patients who underwent cricothyroidotomy at New York University Medical Center (Boyd et al., 1979), and the results were similar to those reported by Brantigan and Grow. Cricothyroidotomy should be done over a translaryngeal tracheal tube. After the patient's neck is extended moderately, the operative area is cleansed, draped, and infiltrated with 1% lidocaine. With the finger of the surgeon's left hand stabilizing the larynx, the cricothyroid space is identified. A transverse incision is made through the skin and subcutaneous tissues that lie over the cricothyroid space (Fig. 9–28). Any venous bleeding points are clamped and tied with absorbable suture material. After the endotracheal tube cuff is deflated and the tube is retracted, a transverse stab wound is made through the cricothyroid membrane. A Trousseau dilator or fine clamp is inserted into the trachea and is spread vertically to separate the thyroid and cricoid cartilages (Fig. 9–29). Scissors are inserted through this opening and are spread transversely (Fig. 9–30), which opens the cricothyroid membrane sufficiently to allow insertion of a lubricated tracheostomy tube. The technique of tying off subcutaneous veins has reduced the incidence of troublesome postoperative bleeding.

The precise role of cricothyroidotomy is still evolving. Many surgeons are reluctant to use it because they fear that subglottic stenosis may develop, whereas other surgeons use it enthusiastically (Branti-

gan and Grow, 1980). O'Connor and associates (1985) endorsed cricothyroidotomy and reported its use in 49 patients after an average of 7 days of endotracheal intubation. The average period of intubation was 38 days in 30 survivors, none of whom developed subglottic stenosis. However, Esses and Jafek (1987) from Denver are more restrictive in the use of cricothyroidotomy. They reported on 78 patients who underwent cricothyroidotomy. Of these patients, 42 (59%) survived, 22 (28%) developed complications, and 2 (2.6%) developed subglottic stenosis. Cricothyroidotomy should be used in emergency situations and in patients with fresh median sternotomy incisions. The cricothyroidotomy wound can be separated from the median sternotomy incision, thus reducing the incidence of mediastinal infection. In other situations, we tend to perform standard tracheostomies. Cricothyroidotomy is contraindicated if a translaryngeal tube has been in position for more than 7 days or if there is evidence of laryngeal inflammation or injury (Boyd et al., 1979). In our experience, subglottic stenosis occurred three times in this setting.

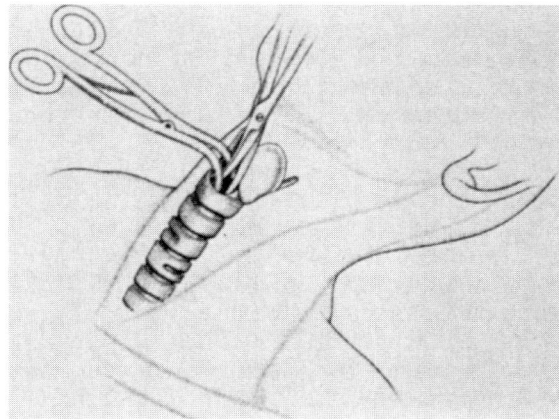

FIGURE 9–30. Cricothyroid membrane is opened transversely with heavy scissors. (From Boyd, A. D., Romita, M. C., Conlan, A. A., et al.: A clinical evaluation of cricothyroidotomy. Surg. Gynecol. Obstet., *149:365, 1979.*)

EMERGENCY CRICOTHYROIDOTOMY AND TRACHEOSTOMY

In emergency situations in which the trachea cannot be intubated from above, cricothyroidotomy is preferred to slash tracheostomy. Emergency cricothyroidotomy (Boyd and Conlan, 1979) is performed exactly as described under standard cricothyroidotomy, excep that a stab wound is made over the cricothyroid space through the skin, subcutaneous tissue, and cricothyroid membrane without taking time to tie off bleeders. A clamp is used to separate the cricoid and thyroid cartilages. Scissors are spread transversely, the membrane is opened, and the tracheostomy tube is inserted immediately. It has not been necessary to convert emergency cricothyroidotomies to standard tracheostomies unless a patient has undergone prolonged translaryngeal intubation or shows evidence of laryngeal inflammation.

For urgent cervical tracheostomy, a vertical incision is made, and the cricoid cartilage and thyroid isthmus are taken as guide points. The surgeon's left hand is used to stabilize the larynx while the incision is made from the level of the cricoid cartilage to the suprasternal notch. Every effort is made to maintain the incision in the midline as it is deepened to the level of the strap muscles. An electrocautery unit is used for hemostasis, but the urgency of the procedure dictates the need for control of the small blood vessels. Advantage is taken of the superficial position of the cricoid cartilage to begin separation of the strap muscles and division of the pretracheal fascia at that level. The incision is then developed inferiorly to expose the thyroid isthmus for a third-ring tracheostomy, but the first tracheal ring must not be divided. A short segment of the second ring may be excised, or the second and third rings may be divided vertically in the midline to allow intubation. We believe strongly that emergency or slash tracheostomy should not be used and that emergency cricothyroidotomy is the preferred procedure unless the trachea has been severed completely or is obstructed below the level of the cricothyroid membrane.

In an extreme emergency, jet ventilation with oxygen through a No. 14 gauge Teflon intravenous catheter, which is inserted through the cricothyroid membrane or trachea, may stabilize a patient temporarily until tracheal intubation, cricothyroidotomy, or tracheostomy can be performed.

TRACHEAL INTUBATION IN CHILDREN

Refined intensive pediatric nursing care, increased experience in managing intubated children, and concern over the complications of tracheostomy have made tracheostomy in pediatric patients a relatively infrequent procedure. This is particularly true for infants and children who require airway control for augmented ventilation after a neurologic or cardiothoracic operation. Nasotracheal intubation combined with a meticulous suctioning technique, humidification of inspired gases, and prevention of tube displacement may delay the need for a tracheostomy for 2 to 3 weeks. The safety of prolonged intubation depends on the skill and competence of the people who care for the child. Neonatologists are particularly reluctant to subject their patients to tracheostomy and prefer many weeks of tracheal intubation before resorting to tracheostomy (Allen and Stevens, 1972). Laryngeal trauma, vocal cord ulceration, and glottic or subglottic stenosis are potential hazards of tracheal intubation, even when an infant or child is managed under ideal circumstances. Unfortunately, overemphasis of the problems of decannulation sometimes delays the decision to perform tracheostomy.

The major indications for tracheostomy in children are the same as those in adults. Fewer tracheostomies are performed for inflammatory conditions, whereas more tracheostomies are performed for congenital anomalies and respiratory insufficiency (Dempster et al., 1986). Patients with acute laryngotracheobronchitis (croup) rarely require tracheostomy. Racemic epinephrine usually controls soft tissue swelling and thus prevents respiratory obstruction. If this method is unsuccessful, tracheal intubation from above is preferred to tracheostomy. Nasotracheal intubation under emergency circumstances requires considerable skill, and in a critical situation, orotracheal intubation is probably the preferred method to establish an airway. Cricothyroidotomy may be indicated in some situations. In small children, we convert the cricothyroidotomy to a formal tracheostomy within 24 hours, whereas in older children, cricothyroidotomy can be continued.

There are minor differences in the operative technique of tracheostomy used in children from that used in adults. The cricoid cartilage lies at the level of the third cervical vertebra and descends with growth to the level of the fifth or sixth vertebra at puberty. Because the thyroid isthmus maintains its relation to upper tracheal rings, the tracheal stoma is generally made below or at the same level as the thyroid isthmus. Use of a transverse incision is not as important in young children as it is in adults; the surgeon should choose the type of incision she or he feels will give the best exposure. General anesthesia is most often necessary and has the advantage of providing a quiet patient and facilitating dissection in tissue planes that have not been distorted by infiltration of local anesthetic solutions. After separation of strap muscles in the midline, the position of the thyroid isthmus should be evaluated in relation to the suprasternal notch. Tracheal rings should be identified carefully so that the first and second rings are not disturbed. In infants, the isthmus generally can be retracted cephalad without division. After accurate identification, the third and fourth tracheal rings are incised vertically, and the stoma is opened gently. Tracheal cartilage should not be excised in any child. The child's neck should be returned to a neutral position before tapes are tied carefully to secure the tracheostomy tube in position.

■ **Table 9–6.** ESTIMATED TRACHEAL TUBE SIZES

Population	Bore (OD)
Premature infants	2.5–3 mm
Infants	3–4 mm
Children	$\dfrac{\text{Age in years} + 16}{4}$ = usual size
Adults	
Men	8–9 mm
Women	7–8 mm

TUBE SELECTION

Tracheal Tubes

A tracheal tube that slides loosely through the cricoid cartilage should be chosen. The tube should be no larger than 8 mm in women or 9 mm in men (Berlauk, 1986) because a tube that is too tight may abrade mucosa and may cause subglottic stenosis (Table 9–6). A large tube also has a more traumatic effect on the nose, pharynx, and larynx.

In 1990, The American Society for Testing Materials published "Standard Specifications for Cuffed and Uncuffed Tracheal Tubes" (cited in Colice, 1991), which addressed five aspects of tube construction: materials used, cuff characteristics, tube dimensions, tube markings, and packaging and labeling. Producers of tracheal tubes have voluntarily complied with the specifications in this publication, which has more or less standardized tracheal tubes internationally.

The ideal tube should be soft, thermolabile, kink-resistant, and collapse-resistant, and it should be fitted with a large-diameter, thin-walled, soft, compliant cuff (Fig. 9–31). Studies by Bernhard and associates have shown that to prevent aspiration and to achieve "just-seal" at a low ICP, a PVC cuff must be thin, compliant, strong enough to resist perforation, and greater in diameter than the trachea. The PVC cuff of an adult's tube should have a diameter larger than 28 mm; it should be less than 0.06 mm thick and it should have a compliance of more than 0.15 ml/cm H_2O. Although several currently available cuffed

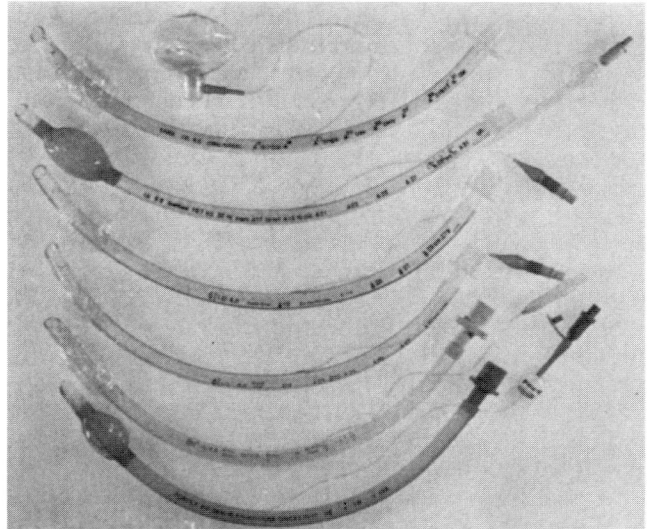

FIGURE 9–31. Various tracheal tubes in current use.

tracheal tubes are satisfactory, no cuffed tube is completely atraumatic (Bernhard et al., 1982, 1985).

Tracheostomy Tubes

A tracheostomy tube should also be thermolabile and soft (Table 9–7). This tube should have a soft tip and should be fitted with a large-diameter, thin-walled, compliant cuff (Fig. 9–32). Cuffless tubes with inner cannulas should be reserved for healthy, alert patients with protective oropharyngeal reflexes who undergo permanent tracheostomy. A removable inner cannula facilitates regular cleaning and is important to prevent tube obstruction in patients who must take care of themselves and who are not breathing humidified air. The tubes that are currently available have a removable inner cannula and usually have relatively hard bodies and tips. These "hard tubes" may erode the tracheal wall. Fenestrated tracheostomy tubes, which allow phonation when the inner cannula is removed and the tube is closed, should be reserved for special circumstances.

■ **Table 9–7.** SPECIFICATIONS FOR SEVERAL COMMONLY USED CUFFED TRACHEOSTOMY TUBES

Tube	Size Designation	Outside Diameter (mm)	Inside Diameter (mm)	Length (mm)
Shiley's pediatric	00	4.5	3.1	39
	0	5.0	3.4	40
	1	5.5	3.7	41
	2	6.0	4.1	42
	3	7.0	4.8	44
Shiley	6	10.0	7.0	68
	8	12.0	8.5	71
Portex	10	10.0	7.5	72
	11	12.0	9.0	82
Mallinckrodt	7	9.6	7.0	78
	9	12.3	9.0	88

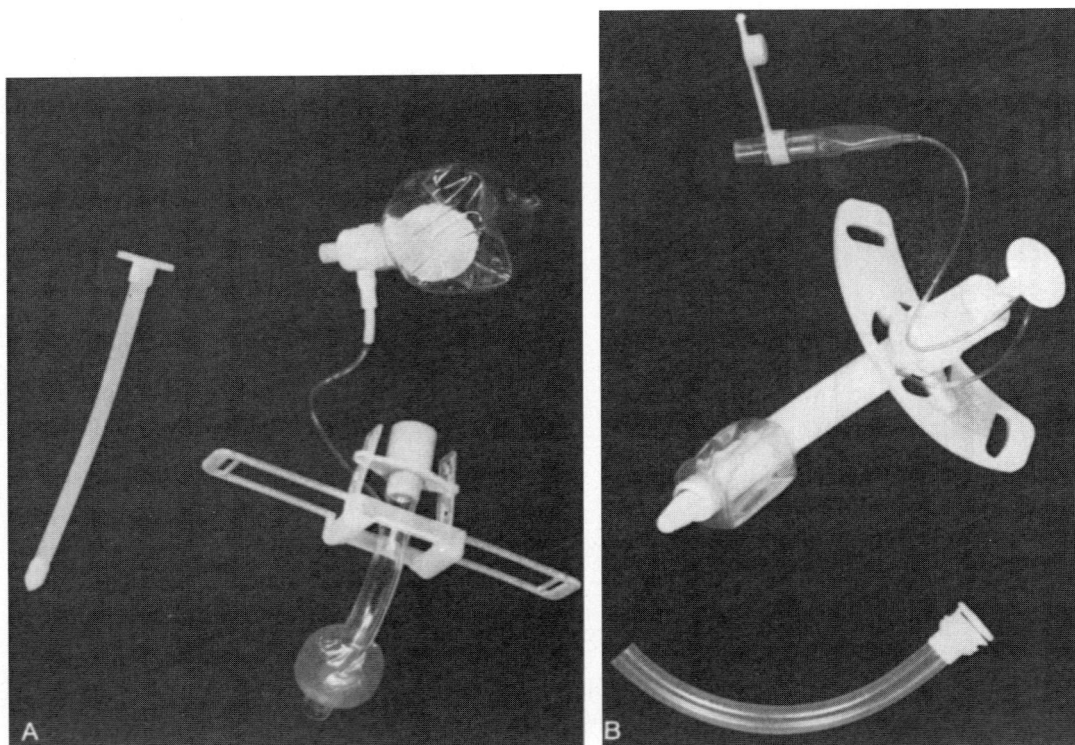

FIGURE 9–32. *A,* Mallinckrodt tracheostomy tube. *B,* Portex tracheostomy tube.

In the ICU, tracheostomy tubes that are fitted with low-pressure, large-diameter, thin-walled, compliant cuffs should be used, and inhaled gases should be humidified. When ventilation is spontaneous, a tracheostomy collar provides a reservoir of humidified gas and allows head and body motion without traction on the tracheostomy tube. Tracheal and innominate artery perforations can be associated with tube-tip trauma that is secondary to traction from ventilator hoses and connectors. When patients must be connected to ventilator circuits, a swivel adapter and a small piece of flexible tubing should be used between the tracheostomy tube and the Y connector. Cameron and associates (1973) reported aspiration in most patients in the ICU who had undergone tracheostomy but noted that high-volume, low-pressure, large-diameter cuffs minimized this complication significantly (Bone et al., 1974). A cuffed tube that allows positive-pressure ventilation and prevents significant aspiration should be used in patients who undergo tracheostomy in the ICU.

Concentrated efforts to reduce the frequency of serious tracheal damage at the cuff site have led to the development of several disposable tubes with large-diameter, thin-walled, high-volume, low-pressure, compliant cuffs. The previous generation of cuffs had small diameters and resting volumes, so they contained little air at atmospheric pressure and often inflated asymmetrically, with pressures well in excess of capillary pressure. To produce a seal in the normal, irregularly shaped trachea, high-pressure cuffs often stretched and distorted the trachea at the cuff site

(Fig. 9–33). Any gas that was added to or diffused into the cuff beyond the just-seal intracuff volume produced high ICP and cuff-to-tracheal wall pressure (Cooper and Grillo, 1969). This was shown to be the principal mechanism of pressure necrosis and subsequent tracheoesophageal fistula, tracheal stenosis, and tracheal malacia during the 1960s and the early 1970s (Grillo et al., 1971; Pearson and Andrews, 1971).

Dramatic differences in ICP at just-seal intracuff volume resulted from changes in cuff design and pressure-regulating valves (Ching et al., 1974). The relationship among cuff volume, ICP, and cuff-to-tracheal wall pressure was reviewed in detail by Carroll and associates in 1974. They noted that large-diameter, large-residual-volume cuffs automatically adjusted ICP during positive-pressure mechanical ventilation. Thus, a large-diameter, large-residual-volume cuff can cycle automatically from an ICP of 18.4 torr (25 cm H_2O), which is adequate to prevent aspiration (Bernhard et al., 1979), up to the minimal pressure adequate for just-seal intracuff volume during positive-pressure ventilation. In patients with stiff lungs, low ICPs may not prevent gas leaks during mechanical ventilation. The cuff should be filled to the point of minimal leak at peak inspiratory pressure. The cuff must have a diameter greater than that of the trachea to function at low ICPs. ICP approximates cuff-to-tracheal wall pressure in large-diameter, large-residual-volume cuffs.

Kamen and Wilkinson introduced a departure from the traditional concept of air-filled cuffs in 1971. They developed a foam-filled cuff that expands by elastic

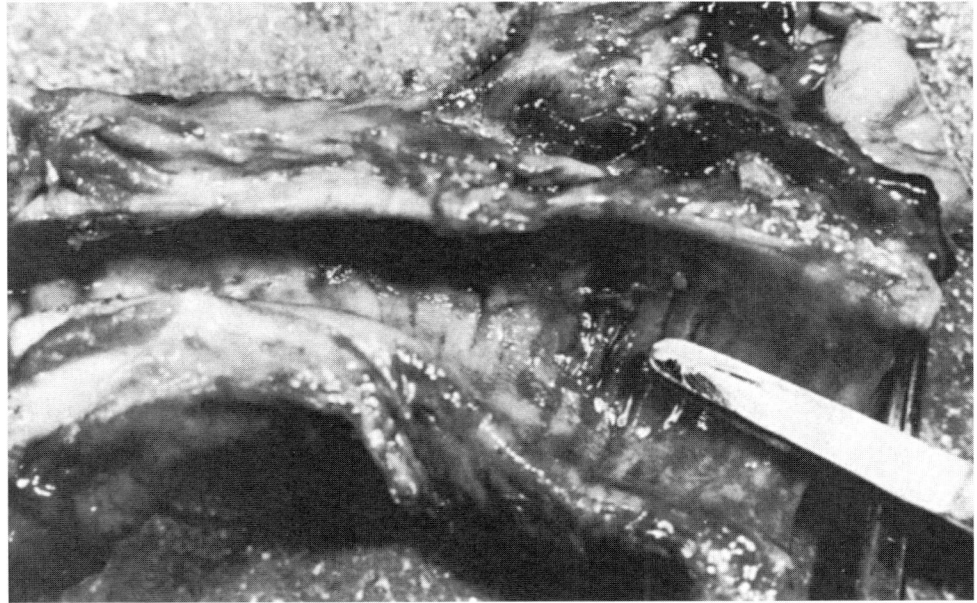

FIGURE 9–33. Mucosal ulceration and tracheal dilatation at the site of a high-pressure cuff.

recoil of the foam against the cuff and tracheal wall. Lateral tracheal wall pressure varies because lateral pressure depends on the distance that the foam has to expand to push the cuff against the tracheal mucosa (Fig. 9–34).

The frequency of stomal stenosis has led to the tendency to use tracheostomy tubes of a diameter smaller than that of tracheal tubes. No clear relationship between tube size and stenosis at the stoma has been established, however, and one should not hesitate to use large tracheostomy tubes in adults with thick secretions. Insertion depth should be regu-

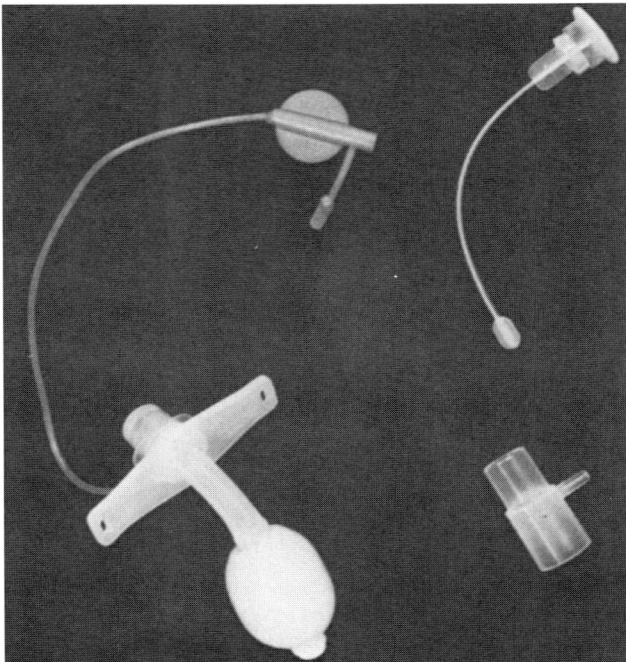

FIGURE 9–34. Bivona foam-cuff tracheostomy tube.

lated with an adjustable neck plate or a spacer that is placed between the skin and the tracheostomy tube collar. Stomal size and complications may be reduced by minimizing tube motion with appropriate fixation.

Opinions differ about the value of an inner cannula. With good nursing care and humidification of inhaled gases, an inner cannula is unnecessary. Because the inner cannula reduces internal tube diameters, it may not be possible to use a small tracheostomy tube. Disposable tubes are rapidly replacing metal tracheostomy tubes in most institutions.

For infants and young children, tube selection is less difficult. Only an exceptional patient under 5 years of age requires a cuffed tracheostomy tube for positive-pressure ventilation, unless excessively high inspiratory pressures are required. Shiley's silastic pediatric tubes are preferred by some surgeons (Fig. 9–35). A tube with an outer diameter of 5 mm, size 0, is generally satisfactory for newborn infants (Table 9–7). For premature infants who weigh less than 2.5 kg, a 4.5-mm, size 00 tube should fit.

TUBE CARE

Care for patients with tracheal or tracheostomy tubes should include (1) humidification of inspired gases, (2) cuff inflation, (3) flexible connection to ventilator hoses, (4) aspiration of bronchopulmonary secretions, (5) bacteriologic cultures, (6) wound cleansing and tube replacement, (7) proper management of patients, and (8) termination of intubation (decannulation).

Humidification of Inspired Gases

During the first week or more following tracheostomy, it is important to humidify inspired gases. Hu-

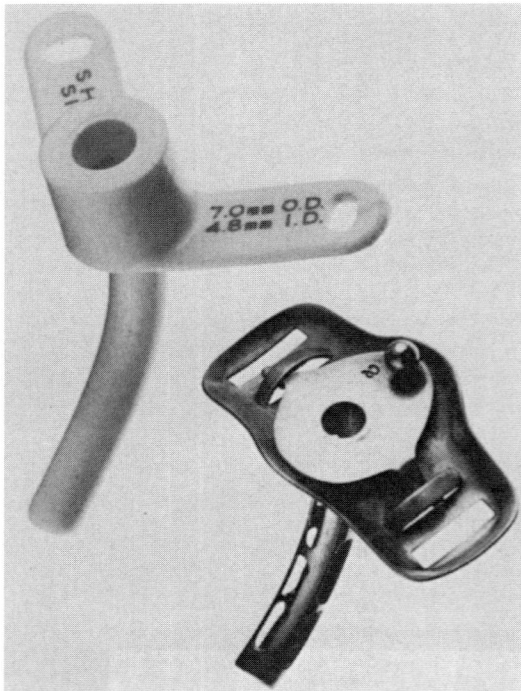

FIGURE 9–35. Shiley pediatric tracheostomy tube *(left)* is satisfactory for infants and young children. The cannula of the metal tube has been fenestrated to facilitate the process of decannulation *(right).*

midification refers to both molecular (water vapor) and particulate (aerosol) water. If inspired gases are not saturated with water vapor at or near body temperature, the respiratory tract gives up water to the inspired gas, drying the secretions. Such drying impairs mucosal defense mechanisms and produces tenacious secretions that may be difficult to cough up or aspirate. If the patient is breathing spontaneously, inhaled gases should be humidified (nebulizer or cascade-type humidifier) and delivered to the patient through a tracheostomy collar. Water vapor is provided by both nebulizers and humidifiers, but only nebulizers produce fine particles of water. An aerosol preserves the natural source of vapor for humidification and provides water particles for liquefaction of bronchial secretions. Particles that measure 3 μm or smaller reach the small distal airways. Because a considerable volume of water may be delivered to the respiratory tract by ultrasonic nebulizers, overhydration must be considered when such nebulizers are used in small children and infants.

Cuff Inflation

Cuff inflation is intended to provide tracheal seal while exerting minimal pressure against the mucosa. After a cuff has been filled to 20 to 25 torr or to just-seal intracuff volume, the addition of more gas to the cuff by diffusion (Bernhard et al., 1978) or filling risks injury to the trachea if the resultant cuff-to-tracheal

wall pressure exceeds capillary perfusion pressure. Routine care of any cuffed tracheal airway should include periodic measurement and adjustment of ICP, unless a pressure-regulating valve that maintains ICP between 20 and 25 torr is incorporated into the system. A blood pressure monitor connected at the side of the bed with a three-way stopcock can be used for pressure regulation, but it is more convenient and accurate to use a small aneroid unit such as a Portex pressure manometer for ICP measurement.

Because of the possibilities of accidental overinflation, diffusion of oxygen and nitrous oxide into the cuff (Bernhard et al., 1978), and possible accumulation of secretions in the cul-de-sac above the cuff, it is useful to deflate the tracheostomy cuff two or three times daily while positive pressure is being delivered to the trachea. After tracheal and oropharyngeal suctioning, the cuff should be reinflated with a just-seal intracuff volume, usually with an ICP of 20 to 25 torr (Bernhard et al., 1979). The technique of hourly cuff deflation and reinflation for the purpose of reducing tracheal injury should not be used.

Ventilator Connection

It is generally agreed that tube and cuff movement traumatizes the tracheal wall at points of contact. With tracheostomies and cricothyroidotomies, this motion may also contribute to stomal enlargement and possibly to tracheal stenosis at the stomal level. Therefore, a swivel adapter and a flexible tube should be used to connect a tracheostomy tube to the ventilatory Y to minimize transmission of motion or force from ventilator hoses and connections to the tracheostomy tube (Fig. 9–36).

Aspiration

Removal of bronchopulmonary secretions by suctioning is simpler in patients who are not receiving mechanical ventilation. Swivel adapters (Portex) are available, and they provide a suction port with or without a suction catheter seal. They produce less interference with positive-pressure ventilation during suctioning and less risk of trauma when the adapter is disconnected from the tracheal tube. Hazards that are associated with suctioning include hypoxia, arrhythmia, and even cardiac arrest from prolonged suctioning or use of excessive negative pressure

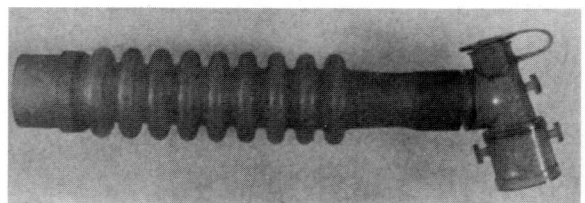

FIGURE 9–36. Swivel trach adapter and flexible tubing for connecting the respirator to the tube.

(> 150 torr); repeated mucosal trauma from suction catheter manipulation; and introduction of pathogenic bacteria into the airway.

Only a sterile catheter approximately one-half the diameter of the tube should be passed into the airway. To accomplish this, a fresh catheter must be used for each aspiration, and the nurse or therapist must hold the catheter with either a sterile glove or a clamp. Less than 150 torr of negative pressure should be applied only when the catheter is being withdrawn. Suctioning should last less than 10 seconds. T connectors or catheters with a thumbhole allow proper selective control of suctioning.

Improved humidification with current humidifiers has reduced the need for frequent tracheal instillation of saline to help loosen bronchopulmonary secretions. However, judicious use of tracheal lavage with 3 to 5 ml of saline may be needed to remove secretions. The difficulty with aspiration of secretions from the left bronchial tree is well known. With an angled-tip (coudé) suction catheter, it is possible to cannulate the left main bronchus in approximately 90% of attempts. If an attempt is unsuccessful, a flexible fiberoptic bronchoscope can be inserted through an adult tracheal or tracheostomy tube for suctioning the left bronchial tree.

Although numerous attempts have been made to design an atraumatic suction catheter (Fig. 9–37), none has been completely successful. Tracheobronchial trauma results each time that a suction catheter is inserted, even if secretions are copious. Muto has developed a double-lumen lavage catheter (Fig. 9–38) that may be less traumatic and more efficient than other catheters (Mann et al., 1987). The TRACH-CARE suction system (Figs. 9–39 and 9–40), a self-contained suction system that can be used repeatedly

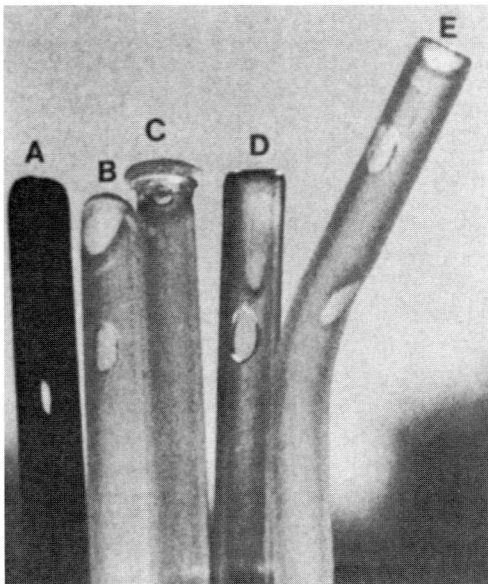

FIGURE 9–37. Various catheter tips are shown. A, Open-ended. B, Whistle-tip. C, Argyle Airflow. D, Modified whistle-tip. E, Coudé. (A–E, From Burton, G. G., and Hodgkins, J. E.: Respiratory Care. 2nd ed. Philadelphia, J. B. Lippincott, 1984.)

for up to 24 hours, is now widely used. It is thought to limit tracheal contamination with repeated suctioning (Caldwell and Sullivan, 1984).

Bacteriologic Cultures

Considerable effort is required to minimize contamination of the respiratory tract in patients with tracheal or tracheostomy tubes in position. Airway infection is more common with tracheostomy than with translaryngeal tracheal tubes. Poor suctioning technique, contaminated nebulizers and ventilator hose assemblies, and inadequate handwashing by personnel are probably the main sources of infecting bacteria. The bronchopulmonary secretions of intubated patients should be collected in a sterile trap on alternate days for culture and sensitivity testing. In many patients, potential pathogens colonize within a few days, but this must not be equated with significant respiratory infection (Bryant et al., 1972). On the contrary, administration of topical or systemic antibiotics for simple colonization or for uncomplicated tracheobronchitis may cause serious superinfection with resistant organisms.

Despite adequate suctioning and humidification, encrusted secretions may accumulate on the inner and outer surfaces of tubes and cuffs. This material provides a culture medium for bacteria and may reach proportions that are significant enough to obstruct the tube. A fiberoptic bronchoscope may be used to observe obstructing secretions and tube-related trauma.

Tube Replacement and Wound Cleansing

A tube should be changed only if complications or problems develop. The frequency of translaryngeal tracheal tube replacement depends on tube function and on the nature and amount of bronchopulmonary secretions. If tube and pulmonary care is optimal, it is not unusual for a tracheal tube to remain in position for several weeks. Because tracheostomy wounds become contaminated within a few days, wound cultures should be compared with cultures of the bronchopulmonary secretions. Povidone-iodine solution or ointment applied two or more times daily on gauze sponges is especially effective for controlling suppuration of these wounds. For many patients, daily cleansing of the wound with saline and hydrogen peroxide allows satisfactory healing.

Management of Patients

Cameron and associates (1973) reported that some degree of aspiration occurs frequently in patients who have undergone tracheostomy. The ability of patients with tracheostomies to swallow without significant aspiration can be evaluated by oral administration of small amounts of dilute methylene blue solution.

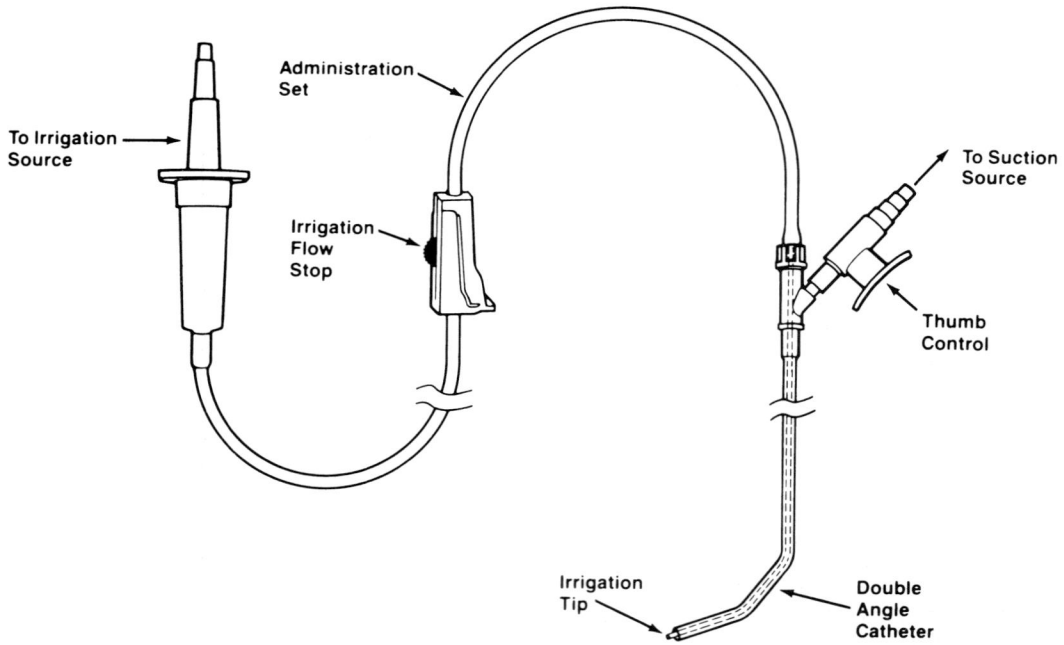

FIGURE 9–38. A disposable suction-irrigation catheter for continuous tracheobronchial irrigation and suctioning for lavage or sampling of secretions. (Courtesy of Portex, Inc.)

Obvious aspiration or recovery of significant amounts of dye in the tracheal aspirate necessitates exclusion of a tracheoesophageal fistula and consideration of temporary nasogastric tube feedings. Soft, pureed foods should also be considered, because they are often swallowed more efficiently than liquids. A patient may occasionally be unable to swallow normally until the tracheostomy tube is removed.

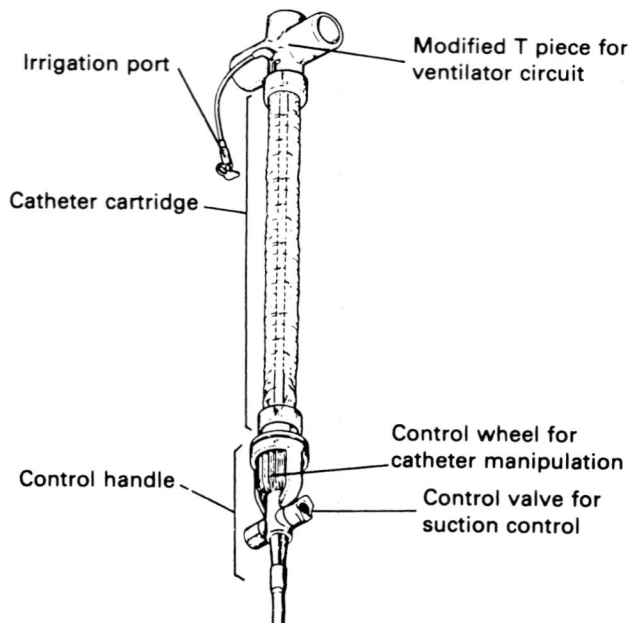

FIGURE 9–39. Schema of the TRACH-CARE closed trachea suction system (Ballard Medical Products). (From Burton, G. G., and Hodgkins, J. E.: Respiratory Care. 2nd ed. Philadelphia, J. B. Lippincott, 1984.)

Decannulation

The decision to decannulate implies that the patient is gaining strength, no longer needs augmentation of ventilation, has protective oropharyngeal reflexes, and has diminished tracheobronchial secretions or has recovered from the respiratory problem that required intubation. Although no precise measurements predict successful decannulation, a measured vital capacity that is three times the predicted tidal volume suggests that the patient will be able to cough, breathe deeply, and effectively clear airway secretions. Evidence of coordinated swallowing must also be present. With most adults, the tracheostomy tube can be

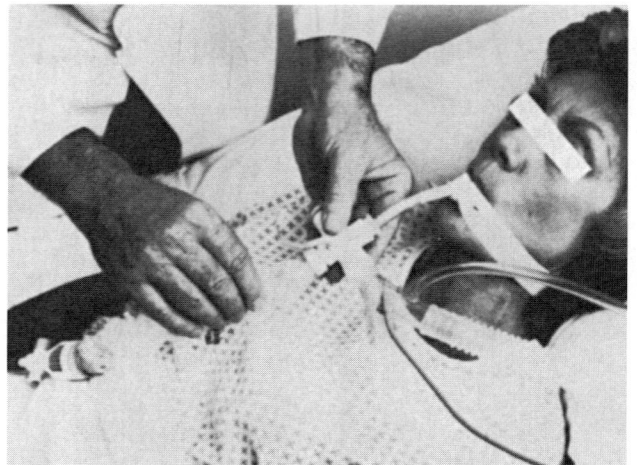

FIGURE 9–40. The TRACH-CARE continuous suction system in use (Ballard Medical Products). (From Burton, G. G., and Hodgkins, J. E.: Respiratory Care. 2nd ed. Philadelphia, J. B. Lippincott, 1984.)

removed when conditions for decannulation are met. It may be necessary to trim away excessive granulation tissue. In addition, when a tracheostomy tube has been in position for more than 3 weeks, a bronchoscopy should be done through the larynx at the time of decannulation to observe the stoma and the extent of trauma to the trachea.

Occasionally, patients continue to produce excessive bronchopulmonary secretions, and it is unclear whether the initial attempt to decannulate them will succeed. In these circumstances, the tube tract and tracheal stoma can be kept open with a tracheal stomal button (Fig. 9–41) or a fenestrated tracheostomy tube. The tracheal button is adjusted so that its flange lies just inside the tracheal stoma with minimal obstruction to airflow. A one-way valve in the button allows inspiration through the tube and permits the patient to talk and to cough. Both metal and plastic fenestrated tubes are available. Use of fenestrated tubes with the tube capped is hazardous, however, because secretions may block the fenestration and obstruct the airway. Portex and Shiley fenestrated tracheostomy tubes are supplied with an accessory cannula for occlusion of the fenestration.

For both children and adults, failure to achieve decannulation mandates bronchoscopy to determine whether an obstructing lesion is present. When a tracheostomy tube is removed, the wound must be closed tightly so that coughing is effective. This requires the application of benzoin to the skin that surrounds the tracheostomy wound. Waterproof tape should be used to approximate wound edges snugly, and the wound should be inspected frequently for air leaks. Decannulation difficulties in infants and children have been overemphasized, and most children are weaned successfully from the tube at the first properly planned attempt. In children 4 years of age and older, there is rarely any problem if the factors that led to tracheostomy have subsided. In a

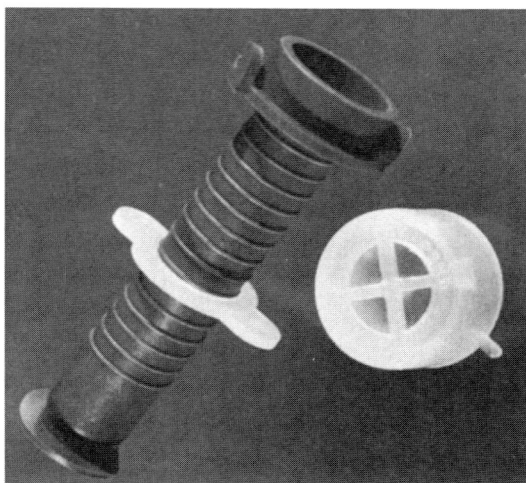

FIGURE 9–41. Kistner tracheostomy tube serves to maintain the tube tract and stoma in patients who may not tolerate sudden decannulation. Phonation and coughing are facilitated when the one-way valve is in position.

review of 274 tracheostomies in children of all ages, Oliver and associates (1962) noted a 9.5% rate of decannulation problems. An excellent review by Wind in 1971 considers the interplay of anatomic and physiologic factors that may cause decannulation failure in young children and infants. In young children and infants, we perform bronchoscopy at least several days before decannulation to ensure that no granulation tissue or other obstructive lesion is present in the area of the tracheal stoma. A tube one or two sizes smaller than the tube that is being used is then inserted 24 hours before decannulation to allow air to pass through the vocal cords and to rule out laryngeal dysfunction. Decannulation is performed, and the patient is observed carefully for several days to ensure that no respiratory difficulty arises. Reinsertion of a nasotracheal tube for 24 to 48 hours in addition to administration of steroids to reduce laryngeal and subglottic edema has also been used for decannulation in some infants.

All of the maneuvers directed to decannulation in the young child may fail, and it may be necessary to leave the tracheostomy tube in position for weeks or months. In that event, it is generally necessary to teach tracheostomy care to the parents so that the child can be managed as an outpatient. Depending on circumstances, the interval between discharge and the next attempt at decannulation may vary from a few weeks to several months.

COMPLICATIONS OF TRANSLARYNGEAL INTUBATION

Immediate complications of translaryngeal intubation are caused primarily by direct trauma to the nose, larynx, trachea, or esophagus. If a flexible stylet has been used for tube insertion, intubation complications are more likely to occur. Fortunately, serious complications from tube insertion are uncommon. Delayed complications are more frequent (Table 9–8). The prolonged presence of an oral or nasotracheal tube through the larynx often ulcerates the medial side of the arytenoid cartilages, the interarytenoid region, the posterior portion of the true vocal cords, and the posterior aspect of the cricoid cartilage (Lindholm, 1970). Most of these ulcers heal without serious sequelae. Granulation may form if the ulcer extends to the basement membrane of the mucosa. The granulation tissue is self-limited in most cases, and excision of the granulations is necessary in only a small percentage of patients.

Glottic stenosis is a rare complication of translaryngeal intubation (Podoshin et al., 1978). When seen, it almost invariably occurs when prolonged translaryngeal intubation is followed immediately by cricothyroidotomy or tracheostomy. The cuffed tracheostomy tube may cause ulcerated cords to heal together in the midline, owing to the absence of airflow passing between the cords, which would normally keep them separated. To prevent glottic stenosis, one should allow air to flow through the cords in patients who have undergone tracheostomy or cricothyroidotomy

■ **Table 9–8.** SELECTED COMPLICATIONS OF ENDOTRACHEAL INTUBATION

Complications During Tube Placement

Patient discomfort
Dental accidents
Facial trauma
Nasal/oral soft tissue injuries (hemorrhage, laceration, edema)
Pharyngeal soft tissue injuries (hematoma, perforation, laceration)
Retropharyngeal/hypopharyngeal perforation
Esophageal intubation
Laryngeal trauma

Laryngospasm
Intubation of the right mainstem bronchus
Bronchospasm
Pulmonary aspiration
Barotrauma
Cardiac/respiratory arrest
Cardiac arrhythmias
Hypoxemia
Cervical spine and cord injuries

Complications While Tube Is in Place

Patient discomfort (pain, retching, salivation, difficulty in
  communicating)
Malnutrition
Nasal/oral soft tissue injury (mucosal ulceration, infection, edema,
  hemorrhage)
Lip ulceration
Sinusitis
Otitis media
Laryngeal injury (ulceration, edema, inflammation, submucosal
  hemorrhage)
Laryngeal muscle dysfunction
Subglottic edema
Pneumonia
Pulmonary aspiration
Mechanical problems with the tube (kinking, obstruction,
  disconnection from ventilator, biting the tube, difficulty in
  suctioning secretions)

Mechanical problems with the cuff (cuff laceration, cuff leak,
  herniation over tube tip, compression of the shaft of the tube,
  excessive pressure)
Tracheal injury (ulceration, inflammation, submucosal hemorrhage,
  tracheomalacia, cartilage and mucosal necrosis)
Laryngeal/tracheal web formation
Laryngeal/tracheal granuloma
Tracheal dilatation
Irritation of the carina
Tracheoesophageal fistula
Spontaneous dislocation of the tube (into right mainstem
  bronchus, too high in trachea, self-extubation)
Atelectasis
Reduction in mucociliary transport
Squamous metaplasia of respiratory epithelium
Ineffective cough

Complications During Extubation

Patient discomfort (hoarseness, sore throat, dysphagia)
Upper-airway obstruction (laryngospasm, laryngeal edema)
Bronchospasm

Aspiration
Glottic injury
Cardiac arrest

Complications After Extubation

Nasal stricture
Dysphagia
Laryngeal/tracheal granuloma
Laryngeal stenosis (glottic, subglottic)
Laryngeal motor dysfunction (vocal cord paralysis)
Cricoarytenoid ankylosis

Laryngeal/tracheal web
Laryngeal chondritis, perichondritis
Tracheal stenosis
Tracheomalacia
Tracheal dilatation

From Stauffer, J. L., and Silvestri, R. C: Complications of endotracheal intubation, tracheostomy, and artificial airways. Respir. Care, 27:417, 1982.

and who previously had been intubated from above. Separation of the cords can be accomplished by delivering positive pressure to the trachea after suctioning and deflating the cuff, allowing air to flow up through the larynx.

Subglottic stenosis also occurs rarely after translaryngeal intubation for as short a time as 24 hours (Hawkins, 1977). Although tracheal stenosis, tracheoinnominate artery fistula, and tracheoesophageal fistula can occur, these complications are related more to cuff pressure than to the route of intubation, and they are discussed later.

COMPLICATIONS OF CRICOTHYROIDOTOMY

Esses and Jafek evaluated 78 patients who had undergone cricothyroidotomy. Of these patients, 22 (28%) developed complications. Three patients (2.6%)

developed subglottic stenosis (Esses and Jafek, 1987). However, subglottic stenosis was not encountered in 30 patients who were reported by O'Connor and associates (1985). The complication rate with 298 cricothyroidotomies performed at the New York University Medical Center was 6.9% (Boyd et al., 1979). Stomal bleeding and postdecannulation hoarseness were the most commonly encountered complications. In two patients, inexperienced surgeons placed the cricothyroidotomy tube above the thyroid cartilage rather than through the cricothyroid membrane. Glottic stenosis and subglottic stenosis were encountered in three patients, all of whom had laryngeal inflammation from previous translaryngeal intubation. Because of this experience, we believe that cricothyroidotomy is contraindicated in patients who have laryngeal injury or inflammation or a tracheal tube in place for more than 7 days. In these circumstances, we prefer standard tracheostomy.

Complications occurred in 2 of 19 patients who

underwent emergency cricothyroidotomy (Boyd and Conlan, 1979). One patient had stomal bleeding, and in another patient, the tube had to be replaced after it was initially inserted above the thyroid cartilage. A complication rate of approximately 10% is superior to the rate associated with slash tracheostomy.

COMPLICATIONS OF TRACHEOSTOMY

An apparent reduction in the frequency of tracheostomy complications has been credited to two factors (Table 9–9). First is widespread acceptance of the concept that tracheostomy should be preceded by orotracheal or nasotracheal intubation; second is the development of improved tracheostomy tubes and cuffs.

■ **Table 9–9.** SELECTED COMPLICATIONS OF TRACHEOSTOMY

Complications During the Operation

Hemorrhage	Pneumothorax
Thyroid injury	Placement of the tube in
Tracheostomy too low or too	pretracheal space
high	Tracheoesophageal fistula
Injury to recurrent laryngeal	Cuff laceration during tube
nerve	placement
Subcutaneous emphysema	Cardiac arrest
Mediastinal emphysema	

Complications While Tracheostomy Tube Is in Place

Patient discomfort	Pseudomembrane formation
Infection of wound	Irritation of the carina
Infection of trachea	Tracheoesophageal fistula
Hemorrhage (mild: skin	Mediastinitis
vessel; major:	Sepsis
tracheoarterial fistula)	Atelectasis
Tracheal injury (inflammation,	Pneumonia
submucosal hemorrhage,	Pulmonary aspiration
ulceration, cartilage and	Subcutaneous emphysema
mucosal necrosis)	Mediastinal emphysema
Tracheal dilatation	Pneumothorax
Tracheal granuloma	Self-decannulation
Tracheal web formation	Reduction in mucociliary
Tracheal perforation	transport
Mechanical problems with the	Squamous metaplasia of
tube (obstruction,	respiratory epithelium
disconnection from	Ineffective cough
ventilator, difficulty in	
suctioning secretions)	
Mechanical problems with the	
cuff (same as for	
endotracheal intubation)	

Complications During Decannulation

Difficult decannulation	Patient discomfort
(tight stoma)	

Complications After Decannulation

Scar	Tracheomalacia
Keloid	Tracheal granuloma
Persistent open stoma	Tracheal web formation
Dysphagia	Tracheal dilatation
Tracheal stenosis	

From Stauffer, J. L., and Silvestri, R. C.: Complications of endotracheal intubation, tracheostomy, and artificial airways. Respir Care, 27:417, 1982.

By converting the procedure to a planned operation under proper conditions, the incidence of injury to the recurrent laryngeal nerve, esophagus, and large neck veins has been decreased. Serious cardiac arrhythmias or cardiac arrest may occur during the operation, even though the airway is controlled. Although introduction of the tracheostomy tube into the trachea might occasionally precipitate reflexes that affect cardiac rhythm, it is more likely that hypoxia secondary to improper suctioning (too high a suctioning pressure—greater than 150 cm H_2O—for too long a period—greater than 10 seconds) precipitates arrhythmias.

Misplacement of the tracheal incision may cause serious complications. An incision into the first tracheal ring involves a high risk of subsequent inflammation or pressure injury to the cricoid cartilage. A subglottic stricture or tracheal stenosis at the level of the first ring is more difficult to repair than stenosis at a lower level, and there is greater risk of injury to the recurrent laryngeal nerve. An incision made below the fourth tracheal ring may cause the stoma to lie posterior to the sternum when the patient's neck is flexed. The result may be difficult or impossible recannulation if the tracheostomy tube is inadvertently displaced, and the possibility of tracheo-innominate artery fistula is increased.

Mediastinal emphysema and pneumothorax are more common complications in children than in adults (Chew and Cantrell, 1972). The principal mechanism of pneumothorax in children is air drawn in through the tracheostomy incision and dissected into the mediastinum, with rupture into the pleural cavity (Oliver et al., 1962). Operative injury to a high-lying pleural space is considered a less frequent cause.

Inadvertent extubation before a tube tract is well formed is hazardous in small children and infants. Blind attempts to reinsert a displaced tube may create a false passage with asphyxia in adults as well. The use of a suction catheter, or guide, inserted into the trachea to aid in tube replacement has been advocated, but occasionally it is necessary to reintubate through the larynx to secure an airway. With a low-lying stoma, unrecognized tube displacement may be confused with sudden tube obstruction due to thick, encrusted secretions. In such cases, however, there has generally been an indication of difficulty with suctioning or suction catheter insertion. Proper humidification should reduce the likelihood of complete tube obstruction with dried mucus.

An alert patient who has undergone tracheostomy can be carefully introduced to a diet of soft food 2 to 5 days after the procedure. Some patients have a swallowing dysfunction that either is transient or increases in severity so that saliva and ingested foods spill over into the larynx. Bonanno (1971) concluded from a perspective evaluation of swallowing before and after tracheostomy that the dysfunction was the result of a check-rein effect of the tracheostomy tube on the hypomandibular muscle complex. The resultant limitation of laryngeal motion allowed spillage into the larynx and trachea during swallowing. Cameron and associates (1973) and Bone and associates (1974) confirmed a high incidence of aspiration in patients with tracheostomy. The incidence and the extent of aspiration have been greatly reduced, but not entirely eliminated, by newer large-diameter, large-volume, low-pressure, thin-walled cuffs (Bone et al., 1974). Because atelectasis and respiratory infection occur frequently in patients who require tracheostomy, they may be related to the frequency and severity of aspiration. For patients with preexisting pulmonary disease, it may be safer to use the methylene blue dye test to check for aspiration before allowing oral intake of food.

Tracheal obstruction at the cuff site or tracheostomy stoma and tracheoesophageal fistula are the complications that have received the most attention in recent years. These injuries occurred frequently with use of small-diameter, high-pressure cuffs available before 1971 and led directly to the development of the high-volume, low-pressure cuffs that are now used. The newer cuffs have reduced the incidence of fistula formation.

In 1969, Cooper and Grillo showed the evolution of the pathologic changes at the cuff site, proceeding from mucosal erosion and ulceration to exposure and fragmentation of the cartilages (Fig. 9–42). As little as 3 or 4 days of cuff inflation produced sufficient ischemic necrosis to bare the cartilage rings and ulcerate the posterior tracheal wall. With continuing pressure posteriorly, a fistula between the trachea and the esophagus can develop. An indwelling nasogastric tube increases this likelihood. Fortunately, the incidence of tracheoesophageal fistula has been lower than the incidence of tracheal stenosis; the incidence of the former should decrease greatly with the general

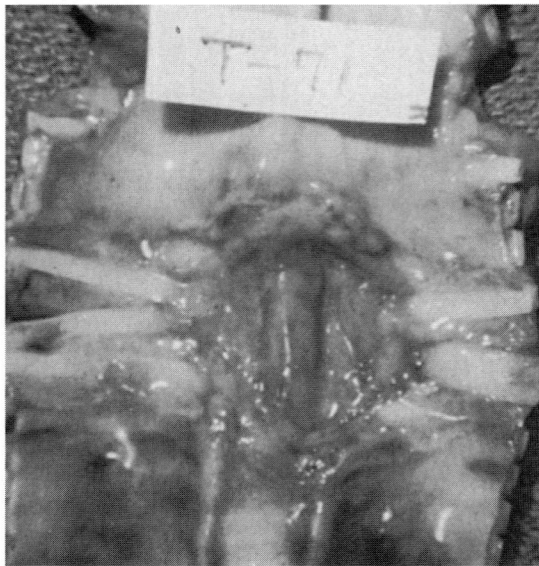

FIGURE 9–42. A laboratory example of tracheal injury from an overinflated cuff of the high-pressure type. The trachea, from a dog with an indwelling cuffed tracheostomy tube for 3 days, has been opened anteriorly to show the denuded cartilage rings and a circular area of deep erosion in the posterior wall.

availability of large-diameter, high-volume, low-pressure cuffs.

Although it has been accepted that fistula formation is the direct result of pressure, there may be cases in which the communication results from trauma from the tube tip or from suction catheters (Hardy, 1973; Harley, 1972). Development of a fistula rarely occurs until the second or third week after tracheostomy, and fistula recognition may be delayed because their symptoms are similar to those of the swallowing dysfunction described earlier. Depending on the relationship of the cuff to the opening of the fistula, material from the esophagus may enter the trachea above the cuff to appear around the tube, or it may enter below the cuff and be suctioned from the distal tracheobronchial tree. In some cases, the fistula is functional only when the cuff is deflated, and occasionally the presenting symptom is gastrointestinal distention.

Repeated aspiration through the fistula may cause severe progressive pneumonia, or a massive episode may produce rapid death by asphyxiation. If a fistula is suspected, a cine-esophogram may establish the diagnosis, or the patient can be given an oral dose of methylene blue solution. However, these maneuvers cannot distinguish absolutely between a fistula and spillover through the larynx. The definitive diagnostic procedures are esophagoscopy and bronchoscopy, using Hopkins' rod-lens telescopes to identify the fistulous opening. Thomas (1973) recommended prompt closure of these fistulas, using a muscle flap to close the tracheal end. Grillo and associates (1976) recommended resection of the abnormal segment of trachea with end-to-end anastomosis and esophageal repair. More recently, tracheoesophageal fistulas have been closed by bronchoscopic application of fibrin glue to the fistula (Antonelli et al., 1991). This approach is still under evaluation.

Tracheal obstruction after decannulation becomes apparent either immediately or gradually over a period of days or weeks. If the inflated cuff produces deep circumferential necrosis, healing may result in a circumferential fibrous stricture, which is often accompanied by granulation tissue. Obstruction is frequently severe. The stenosis may vary from a membrane-like constriction to a narrowing several centimeters in length. With less severe tracheal injury, reduction in the diameter of the lumen may produce mild obstruction and symptoms of dyspnea only with effort. Tracheomalacia is a type of partial tracheal obstruction that occurs less frequently in which a segment of trachea becomes thin-walled and collapsible. This may occur at the cuff or stomal site and is rarely the entire cause of tracheal obstruction. After extubation, obstruction may develop at the tracheostomy stoma owing to fibrous stricture, granulation tissue, or a combination of the two. This is the most common site of stenosis. Several factors have been implicated in the occurrence of stomal stenosis, and the obvious conclusion is that the greatest obstruction is most likely to follow the largest stoma (Bardin et al., 1974). Surprisingly, no data show conclusively that one type of tracheal incision produces a smaller stoma than any other. Some studies have suggested routine use of a vertical incision through two or three tracheal rings (Bardin et al., 1974; Dobrin et al., 1974), whereas other clinical and laboratory studies oppose that recommendation (Bryant et al., 1978). Enlargement of the initial tracheal opening always occurs as a result of motion of the tracheostomy tube, infection, and perhaps other factors, such as protrusion of the cuff into the stoma. Although the development of large-diameter, high-volume, low-pressure cuffs has significantly reduced the occurrence of stenosis at the cuff site, there is still no way to predict a trend for stomal obstruction (Fig. 9–43).

Granulation formation where the tip of the tracheostomy tube traumatizes the tracheal wall is occasionally significant and may produce symptoms of obstruction before or soon after decannulation. Use of tracheostomy tubes with soft tips should reduce the incidence of this complication. The symptoms of post-tracheostomy obstruction may be apparent in some patients, but in other patients with mild obstruction, such obstruction is discovered only by direct questioning and bronchoscopy. Perhaps all patients who have undergone tracheostomy should have radiologic studies of the trachea during the first 4 to 6 weeks after extubation. Computed tomographic scans or tomograms of the neck and upper chest and oblique views of the chest can be used to confirm the clinical diagnosis and to locate the level of a lesion. Tracheograms that are made with a small amount of contrast material are especially helpful in defining the extent and dynamic behavior of a stenotic segment. Although bronchoscopy is needed to determine the presence and severity of obstruction, care must be taken to avoid precipitation of critical airway obstruction. Unfortunately, some patients are not examined until they have reached the stage at which tracheostomy is urgent—a situation that makes subsequent resection and repair more difficult and more likely to fail (Dobrin et al., 1974; Pearson and Andrews, 1971). Grillo (1973) showed conclusively that resection with end-to-end anastomosis is the ideal method of handling tracheal stenosis. Dilatation is rarely successful in the treatment of tracheal stenosis, but in 1974, Otherson reported the successful management of four children by a combination of intraluminal, systemic, and local steroid administration together with dilatation.

Massive hemorrhage due to a tracheo–innominate artery fistula is an infrequent, but often fatal, complication of tracheostomy. It occurs most often with a tracheostomy below the fourth tracheal ring and results from direct erosion of the inner curve of the tube into the medial wall of the innominate artery. Less frequently, an erosion of a hard tube tip through the tracheal wall or overdistention of a cuff causes a fistula to develop. Unfortunately, improvements in plastic tubes have not completely prevented this type of injury. Hemorrhage may occur within a few days of tracheostomy or many months later in the presence of a continuously indwelling tube. Some patients have one or more brief episodes of bleeding a few hours or even several days before massive hemorrhage fills the respiratory tract and mouth. If bleeding begins during deflation of the cuff, the cuff should be reinflated while adjusting the tube position, if necessary, in the hope of temporarily occluding the fistula. At the same time, preparation should be made to insert an orotracheal tube, because it can provide greater mobility along the length of the trachea in an effort to block the fistula. If bleeding is not controlled completely by these methods, the hemorrhage may be controlled by inserting a finger through the tracheostomy wound and by compressing the innominate artery against the undersurface of the sternum while the patient is transferred to the operating room. A median sternotomy is performed immediately to expose the innominate artery and its branches. The

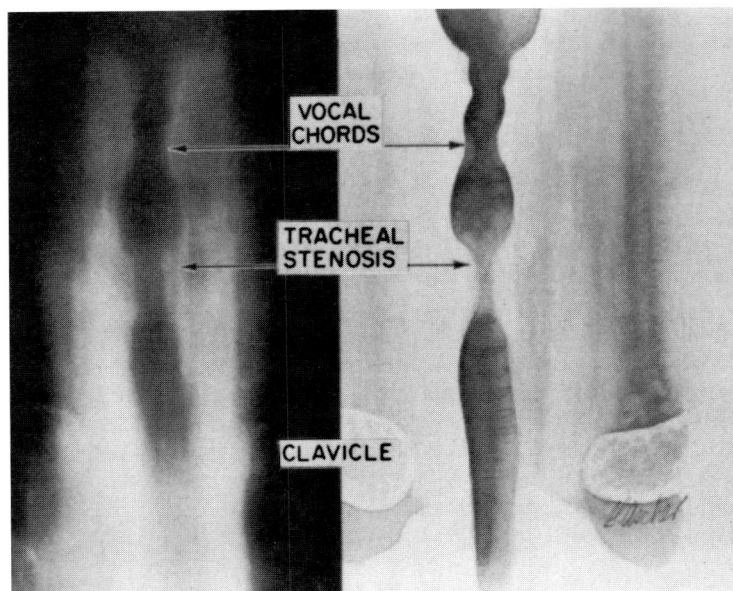

FIGURE 9–43. The tracheal stenosis shown in this laminogram followed 12 days of assisted ventilation through a disposable plastic tracheostomy tube that was inserted with a vertical incision in the second and third tracheal rings.

damaged portion of the artery should be excised, and the ends should be oversewn. Arterial repair or insertion of a graft should not be attempted. The incidence of neurologic damage from this procedure has not been precisely defined, but most survivors have had no neurologic defects (Cooper, 1977).

Complete spontaneous closure of a tracheostomy opening sometimes fails to occur in a patient whose tracheostomy tube has remained in position for many weeks or months. This can usually be managed by limited excision of the skin and soft tissue scar that have fused with the margins of the tracheal opening. The fascia of the strap muscles may be approximated over the tracheal opening, followed by loose closure of the subcutaneous tissues. Subsequent healing usually proceeds rapidly without recurrence of the fistula. For large defects in the tracheal wall and for cosmetic improvement of depressed or unsightly tracheostomy scars, techniques used in plastic surgery are required (Kulber and Passy, 1972).

SELECTED BIBLIOGRAPHY

Bernhard, W. N., Yost, L., Joynes, D., et al.: Intracuff pressure in endotracheal and tracheostomy tubes. Chest, 87:720, 1985.

The ICPs and cuff physical characteristics of various currently used tracheostomy tubes are compared, and the recommended cuff characteristics are reported. The physical characteristics of tracheostomy tubes are also evaluated. The authors recommend the use of endotracheal and tracheostomy tubes fitted with cuffs that seal with low ICPs and tracheostomy tubes that are soft, nonrigid, and thermolabile.

Benumof, J. L.: Management of the difficult adult airway. Anesthesiology, 75:1087, 1991.

Comprehensive review of the difficult adult airway; its causes, classification, and recognition; and the various means of its management.

Brantigan, C. O., and Grow, J. B.: Cricothyroidotomy: Elective use in respiratory problems requiring tracheostomy. J. Thorac. Cardiovasc. Surg., 72:72, 1976.

The authors report 566 patients who undergo cricothyroidotomies with excellent results. This is the first article that advocated the use of cricothyroidotomy since Jackson's classic article (1921) condemned the use of the procedure. None of the patients developed subglottic stenosis; this article renewed interest in the use of cricothyroidotomy.

Cooper, J. D., and Grillo, H. C.: Experimental production and prevention of injury due to cuffed tracheal tubes. Surg. Gynecol. Obstet., 129:1235, 1968.

In this important report, the authors confirmed that pressure necrosis from the inflated balloon cuff was a primary cause of tracheal stenosis, and they demonstrated its prevention via large-volume, low-pressure cuffs.

Grillo, H. C.: Reconstruction of the trachea: Experience in 100 consecutive cases. Thorax, 28:667, 1973.

This publication clearly showed that resection of an abnormal segment of trachea with end-to-end anastomosis is the preferred treatment for tracheal pathology. The concepts and techniques used in tracheal resections are described in this classic article.

Orringer, M. B.: Endotracheal intubation and tracheostomy. Surg. Clin. North Am., 60:1447, 1980.

This concise review clearly outlines the indications, techniques, and complications of intubation of the trachea from above or by means of cricothyroidotomy or tracheostomy.

Rodriguez, J. L., Steinberg, S. M., Luchetti, F. A., et al.: Early tracheostomy for primary airway management in the surgical critical care setting. Surgery, 108:655, 1990.

This study shows that the risk of early (1 to 7 days) tracheostomy is low (mortality rate 0%, morbidity rate 4%). It also suggests that early tracheostomy shortens the number of days on a ventilator, in the ICU, and in the hospital as compared with tracheostomy performed after 7 days.

Stauffer, J. L., Olson, D. E., and Petty, T. L.: Complications and consequences of endotracheal intubation and tracheostomy. Am. J. Med., 70:65, 1981.

A prospective study of the complications and consequences of translaryngeal endotracheal intubation and tracheostomy in 150 critically ill adult patients. Adverse consequences occurred in 62% of all patients undergoing tracheostomy. The complications of tracheostomy were judged to be more severe than the complications of endotracheal intubation. The data contained in this study failed to support the value of tracheostomy over endotracheal intubation for periods as long as 3 weeks.

BIBLIOGRAPHY

Allen, T. H., and Stevens, I. M.: Prolonged nasotracheal intubation in infants and children. Br. J. Anaesth., 44:835, 1972.

Antonelli, M., Cicconetti, F., Vivino, G., and Gasparetto, A.: Closure of a tracheoesophageal fistula by bronchoscopic application of fibrin glue and decontamination of the oral cavity. Chest, 100:578, 1991.

Applebaum, E. L., Astrachan, D., Barker, A., et al.: Symposium: Consensus Conference on Artificial Airways in Patients Receiving Mechanical Ventilation. Chest, 96:178, 1989.

Bardin, J., Boyd, A. D., Hirose, H., and Engelman, R. M.: Tracheal healing following tracheostomy. Surg. Forum, 25:210, 1974.

Bellhouse, C. P.: A new laryngoscope for routine and difficult intubations. Anesthesiology, 69:126, 1988.

Benumof, J. L.: Management of the difficult adult airway. Anesthesiology, 75:1087, 1991.

Berlauk, J. F.: Prolonged endotracheal intubation vs. tracheostomy. Crit. Care Med., 14:742, 1986.

Bernhard, W. N., Cottrell, J. E., Sivakumaran, C., et al.: Adjustment of intracuff pressure to prevent aspiration. Anesthesiology, 50:363, 1979.

Bernhard, W. N., Yost, L., Joynes, D., et al.: Intracuff pressure in endotracheal and tracheostomy tubes. Chest, 87:720, 1985.

Bernhard, W. N., Yost, L. C., Turndorf, H., and Danziger, F.: Cuffed tracheal tube—Physical and behavioral characteristics. Anesth. Analg., 61:36, 1982.

Bernhard, W. N., Yost, L. C., Turndorf, H., et al.: Physical characteristics of and rates of nitrous oxide diffusion into tracheal tube cuffs. Anesthesiology, 48:413, 1978.

Bonanno, P. C.: Swallowing dysfunction after tracheostomy. Ann. Surg., 174:29, 1971.

Bone, D. K., Davis, J. L., Zuidema, G. D., and Cameron, J. L.: Aspiration pneumonia: Prevention of aspiration in patients with tracheostomies. Ann. Thorac. Surg., 18:30, 1974.

Boyd, A. D., and Conlan, A. A.: Emergency cricothyroidotomy: Is its use justified? Surg. Rounds, 2:19, 1979.

Boyd, A. D., Romita, M. D., Conlan, A. A., et al.: A clinical evaluation of cricothyroidotomy. Surg. Gynecol. Obstet., 149:365, 1979.

Brantigan, C. O., and Grow, J. B.: Cricothyroidotomy: Elective use in respiratory problems requiring tracheostomy. J. Thorac. Cardiovasc. Surg., 71:72, 1976.

Brantigan, C. O., and Grow, J. B.: Cricothyroidotomy revisited again. Ear Nose Throat J., 59:26, 1980.

Bryant, L. R., Mugia, D., Greenberg, S., et al.: Evaluation of tracheal incisions for tracheostomy. Am. J. Surg., 135:675, 1978.

Bryant, L. R., Trimble, J. K., Mobin-Uddin, K., and Griffen, W. O.: Interpretation of tracheal cultures in patients with intubation and mechanical ventilation. Am. Surg., 38:537, 1972.

Caldwell, S. L., and Sullivan, K. N.: Artificial airways. In Burton, G. B., and Hodgkin, J. D. (eds): Respiratory Care: A Guide to Clinical Practice. 2nd ed. Philadelphia, J. B. Lippincott, 1984.

Cameron, J. L., Reynolds, J., and Zuidema, G. D.: Aspiration in patients with tracheostomies. Surg. Gynecol. Obstet., 136:68, 1973.

Carroll, R. G., McGinnis, G. E., and Grenvik, A.: Performance characteristics of tracheal cuffs. Int. Anesthesiol. Clin., 12:111, 1974.

Chew, J. Y., and Cantrell, R. W.: Tracheostomy complications and their management. Arch. Otolaryngol., 96:538, 1972.

Ching, N. P., Ayres, S. M., Spina, R. C., and Nealon, T. F., Jr.: Endotracheal damage during continuous ventilatory support. Ann. Surg., 179:123, 1974.

Colice, G. L.: Technical standards for tracheal tubes. Clin. Chest Med., *12*:433, 1991.

Cooper, J. D.: Tracheo–innominate artery fistula: Successful management of 3 consecutive patients. Ann. Thorac. Surg., *24*:439, 1977.

Cooper, J. D., and Grillo, H. C.: Experimental production and prevention of injury due to cuffed tracheal tubes. Surg. Gynecol. Obstet., *129*:1235, 1969.

DeMeester, T. R., Skinner, D. B., Evans, R. H., and Benson, D. W.: Local nerve block anesthesia for peroral endoscopy. Ann. Thor. Surg., *24*:278, 1977.

Dempster, J. H. Dykes, E. H., Brown, W. C., and Raine, P. A. M.: Tracheostomy in childhood. J. R. Coll. Surg. Edinb., *31*:359, 1986.

Dobrin, P. B., Goldberg, E. M., and Lunfield, T. R.: Endotracheal cuff: A comparative study. Anesth. Analg., *53*:456, 1974.

Donnelly, W. H.: Histopathology of endotracheal intubation: An autopsy study of 99 cases. Arch. Pathol., *88*:511, 1969.

Dubick, M. W., and Wright, B. D.: Comparison of laryngeal pathology following long-term oral and nasal endotracheal intubation. Anesth. Analg., *57*:663, 1978.

Esses, B. A., and Jafek, B. W.: Cricothyroidotomy: A decade of experience in Denver. Ann. Otol. Rhinol. Laryngol., *96*:519, 1987.

Gold, M. I., and Shin, B.: Respiratory care in the absence of a respiratory care unit. Chest, *65*:388, 1974.

Grillo, H. C.: Reconstruction of the trachea: Experience in 100 consecutive cases. Thorax, *28*:667, 1973.

Grillo, H. C., Cooper, J. D., Geffin, B., and Pontopiddan, H.: A low pressure cuff for tracheostomy tubes to minimize tracheal injury. J. Thorac. Cardiovasc. Surg., *62*:898, 1971.

Grillo, H. C., Moncure, A. C., and McEnany, M. T.: Repair of inflammatory tracheo-esophageal fistula. Ann. Thorac. Surg., *22*:112, 1976.

Hardy, K. L.: Tracheostomy: Indications, technics and tubes. Am. J. Surg., *126*:300, 1973.

Harley, J. R.: Ulcerative tracheo-esophageal fistula during treatment by tracheostomy and intermittent positive pressure ventilation. Thorax, *27*:338, 1972.

Hawkins, D. B.: Glottic and subglottic stenosis from endotracheal intubation. Laryngoscope, *87*:339, 1977.

Heffner, J. E.: Timing of tracheostomy in ventilator-dependent patients. Clin. Chest Med., *12*:611, 1991.

Jackson, C.: High tracheostomy and other errors, the chief causes of chronic laryngeal stenosis. Surg. Gynecol. Obstet., *32*:392, 1921.

Kamen, J. M., and Wilkinson, C. J.: A new low-pressure cuff for endotracheal tubes. Anesthesiology, *34*:482, 1971.

Kulber, H., and Passy, V.: Tracheostomy closure and scar revisions. Arch. Otolaryngol., *96*:22, 1972.

Lewis, F. R., Schlobohm, R. M., and Thomas, A. N.: Prevention of complications from prolonged tracheal intubation. Am. J. Surg., *135*:452, 1978.

Lindholm, C. E.: Prolonged endotracheal intubation. Acta Anaesthesiol. Scand., *33*(Suppl.):1, 1970.

Mann, J. M., Altus, C. S., Webber, C. A., et al.: Non-bronchoscopic lung lavage for diagnosis of opportunistic infections in AIDS. Chest, *91*:319, 1987.

Mulder, D. S., and Marelli, D.: The 1991 Fraser Gurd Lecture: Evolution of airway control in the management of injured patients. J. Trauma, *33*:856, 1992.

O'Connor, J. V., Reddy, K., Ergin, M. A., and Griepp, R. B.: Cricothyroidotomy for prolonged ventilatory support after cardiac operations. Ann. Thorac. Surg., *39*:353, 1985.

Oliver, P., Richardson, J. R., Clubb, R. W., and Flake, C. G.: Tracheostomy in children. N. Engl. J. Med., *267*:631, 1962.

Orringer, M. B.: Endotracheal intubation and tracheostomy. Surg. Clin. North Am., *60*:1447, 1980.

Otherson, H. B., Jr.: Steroid therapy for tracheal stenosis in children. Ann. Thorac. Surg., *17*:254, 1974.

Pearson, F. G., and Andrews, M. J.: Detection and management of tracheal stenosis following cuffed tube tracheostomy. Ann. Thorac. Surg., *12*:359, 1971.

Podoshin, L., Gertner, R., and Fardis, M.: Postintubation glottic stenosis. Ear Nose Throat J., *57*:46, 1978.

Rodriguez, J. L., Steinberg, S. M., Luchetti, F. A., et al.: Early tracheostomy for primary airway management in the surgical critical care setting. Surgery, *108*:655, 1990.

Saunders, P. A., and Geisecke, A. H.: Clinical assessment of the adult Bullard (TM) Laryngoscope. Can. J. Anaesth., *36*:S118, 1989.

Stauffer, J. L., Olson, D. E., and Petty, T. L.: Complications and consequences of endotracheal intubation and tracheostomy. Am. J. Med., *70*:65, 1981.

Thomas, A. N.: The diagnosis and treatment of tracheoesophageal fistula caused by cuffed tracheal tubes. J. Thorac. Cardiovasc. Surg., *65*:612, 1973.

Trimble, A. S., and Yao, J.: Tracheostomy: Surgical technique and sequelae in 50 cardiovascular patients. J. Thorac. Cardiovasc. Surg., *51*:569, 1966.

Via-Reque, E., and Rattenborg, C. C.: Prolonged oro- or nasotracheal intubation. Crit. Care Med., *9*:637, 1981.

Wind, J.: Reflections on difficult decannulation. Arch. Otolaryngol., *94*:426, 1971.

■ III Respiratory Support in Infants

James M. Steven, Russell C. Raphaely, L. Henry Edmunds, Jr., and John J. Downes

Disease or injury to structures involved in external respiration—the transfer of gas between ambient atmosphere and pulmonary capillary blood—which include the respiratory center and the brainstem, spinal cord, peripheral nerves, muscles, and skeletal structures of the respiratory bellows, gas-conducting passages, and acini, frequently causes respiratory failure in neonates and infants. Disorders of the cardiovascular and gastrointestinal systems may also impair respiratory function, which leads to a need for respiratory support.

In recent years, a great deal has been learned about the anatomy, development, physiology, and biochemistry of the lung. Careful morphometrics and histologic studies of both normal and pathologic fetal and postnatal lungs have provided anatomic details of the development of the lung and its pathologic processes. Such studies have provided new insights into the pathologic physiology of the idiopathic respiratory distress syndrome, oxygen toxicity, response of the lung to injury, *congenital diaphragmatic hernia* (CDH), cardiac lesions that increase or reduce pulmonary blood flow, and acute and chronic pulmonary infections.

Methods have evolved to monitor and support the diseased respiratory system of infants and adults. Pulse oximeters and end-tidal carbon dioxide manometers, which help to make a continuous estimation of arterial blood-gas conditions; reliable electrodes, which measure blood-gas tensions in small blood-sample volumes; long-term indwelling arterial catheters; nontoxic tracheal tubes; reliable ventilators; effective and safe methods to control airway pressure throughout the respiratory cycle; humidifiers; chest physiotherapy; and neuromuscular blockers have provided methods to support failing respiratory function.

The prevalence of respiratory disease in newborns and infants, new knowledge of disease processes, and new techniques of respiratory support have created the need for experts in pediatric respiratory disease. These experts work in intensive care units in which skilled personnel and specialized equipment are concentrated. These individuals must maintain a thorough and current knowledge of the critically ill infant, be experienced in doing physical examinations, have technical skill, be specially trained in cardiopulmonary care, and dedicate themselves to the challenge of achieving optimal outcome for these patients.

This section discusses some of the anatomic and physiologic differences in the respiratory systems of infants and adults, some common respiratory problems of newborns and infants, and the reasons and current methods for providing respiratory support.

ANATOMY

Structure influences function; thus, the structure of the infant's respiratory system must be considered. The newborn's respiratory system is not a miniature model of an adult's respiratory system and differs in many important aspects (Table 9–10).

At birth, gas exchange occurs in clusters of terminal saccules of the respiratory bronchioles. Although all of the conducting airways are formed by the 16th week of gestation, true alveoli develop after birth. The saccules are lined with epithelial cells, and the alveolar-capillary barrier is only 0.5 μm, as in adults. Type II epithelial cells, which produce surfactant, are present. All pulmonary and bronchial arteries and veins are formed. The lung contains approximately 20 million respiratory units (saccules) and 1.5 million respiratory bronchioles and weighs 60 g (Dunhill, 1962; Inselman and Mellins, 1981). Tissue constitutes 24% of the total pulmonary volume of 200 ml (Dun-

hill, 1962). As alveoli are formed, the initial diameter measures only 40 to 120 μm and the total surface area of the blood-gas barrier is only 2.8 m^2. These measurements contrast with those found in infants and adults (see Table 9–10).

During the first 18 months after birth, respiratory units multiply rapidly (Hislop and Reid, 1974). Septa partition terminal saccules into alveolar ducts and alveoli that contain a single rather than a double capillary network. Pulmonary arteries and veins proliferate and form intra-acinar branches. While the lung grows, respiratory bronchioles, alveolar ducts, and alveoli multiply; the length of each acinus increases; the ratio of tissue volume to total pulmonary volume decreases; and the diameter of each alveolus increases (Reid, 1979). Formation of new alveoli is completed by approximately 8 years (Dunhill, 1962).

In late gestation, the walls of the pulmonary arteries are relatively thick and constitute 14 to 20% of the external diameter of the vessel. During the first 3 to 28 days after birth, internal and medial layers of intrapulmonary arteries less than 200 μm in diameter decrease so that wall thickness is only 6% of the external diameter of the vessel (Hislop and Reid, 1974). This process results from the onset of breathing (Reid, 1979), is independent of gestational age, and reduces pulmonary vascular resistance and increases pulmonary blood flow as the foramen ovale and ductus arteriosus close during the first week after birth.

The newborn breathes principally with the diaphragm, and respiration is rapid and shallow. Because the thoracic wall is elastic (Karlberg, 1968) and ribs are aligned horizontally, the thoracic cavity does not expand when ribs are elevated (Engel, 1962). In addition, abdominal organs crowd thoracic space from below. Deep inspirations are more difficult, and vital capacity, adjusted for size, is less than that of an adult. At 6 to 8 months of age, when the ribs begin to stiffen and slope (Engel, 1962), the thoracic wall begins to augment inspiratory volume.

The newborn has a short, wide trachea that is approximately one-third of the diameter of the adult trachea and is consequently disproportionately large for the size of both lung and infant (Dawes, 1968; Engel, 1962). During infancy and childhood, the cross-sectional area of the trachea increases 10 times, whereas pulmonary volume increases almost 30 times (Dunhill, 1962). Major bronchi of newborns are also large in relation to pulmonary volume but are thin and collapsible because elastic tissues and smooth muscle are sparse and poorly developed. Elastic tissue develops rapidly during the first year after birth, but bronchial smooth muscle does not increase until the third or fourth year (Engel, 1962). In infants and young children, peripheral airways beyond the 18th generation are disproportionately narrow (Hogg et al., 1970). Large central airways facilitate rapid respiration; however, narrow peripheral airways are more susceptible to obstruction and closure by disease (Hogg et al., 1970).

Mucous glands are sparse and poorly developed within neonatal bronchi, but they develop rapidly

■ **Table 9–10.** MEASUREMENTS OF ANATOMIC UNITS OF THE RESPIRATORY SYSTEM AT DIFFERENT AGES

Anatomic Unit	Newborn	2 Years	Adult
Body surface area (m²)	0.21	0.52	1.9
Lung weight (g)	60		800
Lung volume (ml)	200	700	5500
Tracheal diameter (mm)	6.0	9.4	16.5
Diameter of terminal bronchioles (mm)	0.1	0.13	0.3
Number of airways	1.5×10^6	7.2×10^6	14×10^6
Alveolar diameter (μm)	40–120	230	300
Number of alveoli	20×10^6	170×10^6	300×10^6
Alveolar surface area (m²)	2.8	15	75
Mucous glands	Few	Many	Many
Bronchial elastic tissue	Poorly developed	Poorly developed	Well developed
Musculature of bronchial walls	Sparse fibers	Sparse fibers	Thick fibers
Basement membrane small bronchi	Poorly developed in bronchi and bronchioles	Developed in most bronchi and bronchioles	Present in all bronchi
Medial thickness of pulmonary arterioles	Thick	Thin	Thin

during the first year after birth. This paucity of mucous glands and airway mucus may interfere with mucus transport and the ability of the neonate to clear inhaled particles and resist infection.

The newborn lacks well-defined alveoli, but alveolar surfactant is present (Gluck and Kulovich, 1973) and gas diffusion is normal because the blood-gas barrier is not increased. As alveoli form, they are initially smaller in diameter than those of older infants and are therefore more likely to collapse in accordance with Laplace's law. Disproportionately smaller peripheral airways, paucity of airway mucus, and smaller alveoli all combine to render the newborn's lung more susceptible to atelectasis than lungs of older infants and children.

PHYSIOLOGY

Birth produces dramatic changes in the circulation and initiates the respiratory function of the lung. Expansion of the lungs with air and increased pulmonary arterial oxygen tension reduce pulmonary vascular resistance (Dawes, 1968). Pulmonary blood flow increases. Separation of the low-resistance placental vasculature and increased systemic arterial oxygen tension (Pa_{O_2}) and pH increase systemic vascular resistance (Heymann and Rudolph, 1972). Raised systemic vascular resistance and reduced pulmonary vascular resistance cause left ventricular end-diastolic and left atrial pressures to exceed those in the right side of the heart. Thus, the foramen ovale functionally closes within a few hours after birth. The overlapping atrial septal tissue flaps that constitute the foramen ovale remain probe patent in as many as 50% of children at age 5 and in 20 to 25% of adults (Hagen et al., 1984; Scammon and Norris, 1918). Although usual physiologic conditions effectively keep the foramen ovale closed, circumstances that cause selective right ventricular or tricuspid valve dysfunction may promote right-to-left interatrial shunting of blood. The withdrawal of placental prostaglandin E_2 and an increase in systemic Pa_{O_2} above 50 torr causes constriction of the ductus arteriosus and functional

closure within 10 to 15 hours after birth (Dawes, 1968; Heymann and Rudolph, 1972). Prostaglandin E_1 dilates the ductus, and infusions at 0.05 to 0.1 μg/kg/min can maintain ductal patency for several weeks if the infusion is started before anatomic closure occurs at 7 to 10 days of age (Freed et al., 1981). Closure of the ductus arteriosus and foramen ovale converts the parallel pulmonary and systemic circulations of the fetus to a separated circulation in series.

Pulmonary arterial pressure decreases if blood oxygen tension increases. Normally, pulmonary arterial pressure in newborns is higher than in adults (Fig. 9–44). As the media of pulmonary vessels thin, pulmonary vascular resistance and pulmonary arterial pressure decrease (Fig. 9–45). By 2 to 3 weeks of age,

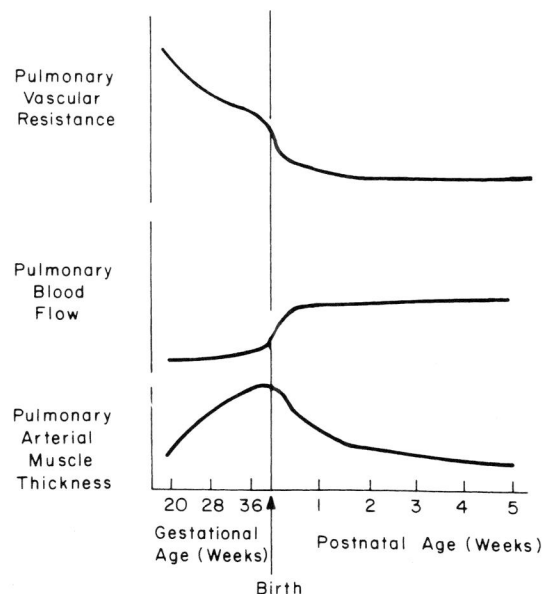

FIGURE 9–44. Relative changes in pulmonary vascular resistance, pulmonary blood flow, and pulmonary arterial wall thickness before and shortly after birth. Normally, pulmonary vascular resistance reaches adult levels within 2 to 3 weeks of birth. (Adapted from Heymann, M. A., and Rudolph, A. M.: Effects of congenital heart disease on fetal and neonatal circulations. Prog. Cardiovasc. Dis., 15:115, 1972.)

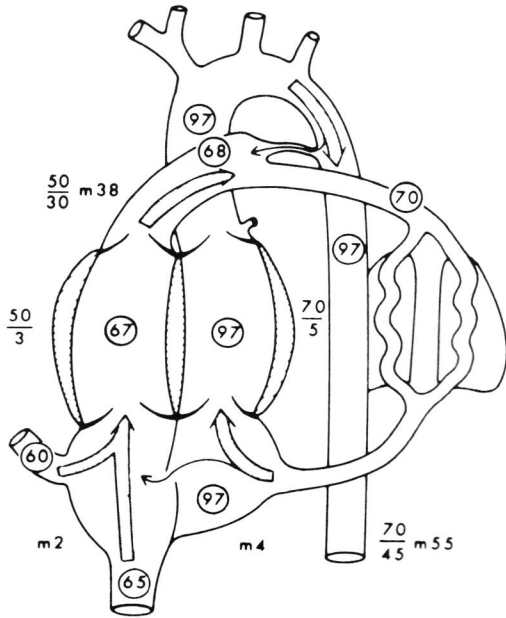

FIGURE 9–45. Cardiac catheterization findings in normal infants during the first few days after birth. Systolic and diastolic pressures are separated by a horizontal line; *m* indicates mean pressure. Percentage of oxygen saturation appears within circles. (Adapted from Heymann, M. A., and Rudolph, A. M.: Effects of congenital heart disease on fetal and neonatal circulations. Prog. Cardiovasc. Dis., *15*:115, 1972.)

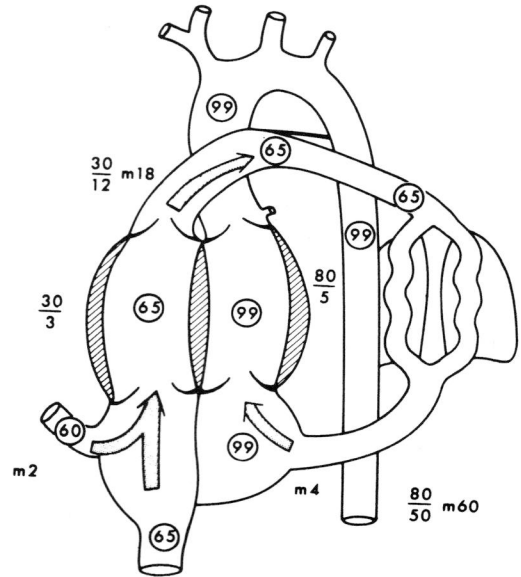

FIGURE 9–46. Cardiac catheterization findings in normal infants approximately 1 month after birth. Symbols as in Figure 9–45. (Modified from Heymann, M. A., and Rudolph, A. M.: Effects of congenital heart disease on fetal and neonatal circulation. Prog. Cardiovasc. Dis., *15*:115, 1972.)

pulmonary arterial pressure has reached normal adult levels and systemic arterial pressure has increased (Fig. 9–46).

During the neonatal period, the pulmonary vasculature is labile and responds to many factors (Dawes, 1968). Acidosis, hypoxia, hypercapnia, atelectasis, epinephrine, norepinephrine, serotonin, angiotensin, and methoxamine increase pulmonary vascular resistance in neonates as well as in adults (Dawes, 1968; Duke and Lee, 1963). Isoproterenol, bradykinin, acetylcholine, and prostaglandins E_1 and E_2 cause pulmonary vasodilatation of previously constricted vessels in newborns (Coceani and Olley, 1973; Heymann and Rudolph, 1972), but bradykinin has little effect on adults (Dawes, 1968). The lung also produces converting enzyme, which inactivates bradykinin and converts angiotensin I to angiotensin II. Activity of this enzyme is proportional to the progressive development of the pulmonary vasculature (Stalcup et al., 1978). The lung also produces superoxide dismutase and glutathione peroxidase, which protect the neonatal lung against oxygen toxicity (Autor et al., 1976).

The normal hematocrit at birth is approximately 53%, and the blood contains fetal hemoglobin, which binds oxygen more avidly than does adult hemoglobin. The oxyhemoglobin dissociation curve is shifted to the left; thus, oxygen is released to the tissues less easily than in adults. Fetal hemoglobin begins to disappear shortly after birth, and the amount is less than 2% of the total hemoglobin within a few months (Comroe, 1965).

The first breath is initiated by somatic stimuli and perhaps by hypoxemia, hypercapnia, and acidosis coincident with parturition. With negative intrapleural pressures up to 70 cm of water (Karlberg, 1968), the newborn inhales 20 to 80 ml and rapidly establishes the residual volume and functional residual capacity necessary for adequate gas exchange. Initially, the infant hyperventilates and metabolic acidosis is present (Table 9–11). Blood P_{CO_2} and pH reach normal adult values by 7 to 10 days after birth. Reflex mechanisms, such as chemoreceptors and Hering-Breuer reflexes, are present in newborns (Dawes, 1968). With increased arterial P_{CO_2} or decreased arterial P_{O_2}, the newborn increases minute volume, alveolar ventilation, and respiratory frequency. However, when placed in a hypoxic environment ($F_{I_{O_2}}$ 0.15), the newborn only transiently responds with hyperventilation. A significant depression of minute ventilation follows, persisting well beyond the restoration of normal

■ **Table 9–11.** NORMAL INFANT pH, BLOOD-GAS TENSIONS, AND HEMATOCRIT (MEAN ± [SD])

	Age		
Measurements	*1 hr**	*24 hr**	*1–24 mo†*
pH	7.33 (0.06)	7.37 (0.03)	7.4 (0.03)
Pa_{CO_2} (torr)	36 (4)	33 (3)	34 (4)
BE‡ (mEq/l)	−6 (1)	−5 (1)	−3 (3)
Pa_{O_2} ($F_{I_{O_2}}$ = 0.21 torr)	63 (11)	73 (10)	
Hematocrit (vol %)	54 (5)	55 (7)	35 (2.5)

*Koch, G., and Wendel, H.: Adjustment of arterial blood gases and acid base balance in the normal newborn infant during the first week of life. Biol. Neonat., 12:136, 1968.
†Albert, M. S., and Winters, R. W.: Acid-base equilibrium of blood in normal infants. Pediatrics, 37:728, 1966.
‡BE = base excess.

ambient oxygen tension (Rigatto, 1982). This paradoxical ventilatory depression occurs even when carbon dioxide is added to the hypoxic environment. Although ventilatory depression in response to hypoxia ceases to occur once the neonate reaches 3 weeks of age, the normal hyperventilatory response does not mature until later in infancy. In newborns, control of respiration is more susceptible to change in body temperature than it is in adults. Respiratory irregularities may occur if body temperature falls below 36° C.

The metabolism, oxygen consumption, and carbon dioxide production per kilogram of body weight in newborns are nearly twice those in adults (Dawes, 1968) (Table 9–12). To provide this higher oxygen consumption, the newborn primarily increases respiratory rate and does not change proportionate tidal volume. Minute ventilation and alveolar ventilation are 2.5 to 3 times those of adults. Proportionate volumes of dead space and functional residual capacity are approximately equal. Thus, the newborn provides a higher rate of metabolism by increasing respiratory frequency rather than by changing proportionate pulmonary volume. During childhood and adolescence, respiratory frequency decreases (Fig. 9–47).

Although it is more cellular, the newborn's lung has a specific compliance that does not differ from that of an adult (Cook et al., 1957). During quiet breathing, transpulmonary pressure changes do not differ. The newborn's airway flow resistance is approximately 15 times that of the adult, but because an adult's actual tidal volume is more than 30 times that of an infant, the work of breathing per breath is similar. Because the newborn's respiratory rate is greater, the minute work of breathing is proportionately greater (see Table 9–12).

INDICATIONS FOR INTENSIVE RESPIRATORY THERAPY

We consider that respiratory failure exists when arterial oxygen tension falls below and carbon dioxide tension rises above the lower and upper limits of normal, respectively, for age and peer group (ACCP-ATS Joint Committee on Pulmonary Nomenclature, 1975). Severity depends on the magnitude of the reduction or increase in Pa_{O_2} and Pa_{CO_2} and influences caretakers in the choice of therapy. Common causes of respiratory failure in the neonate and infant are shown in Table 9–13. Although diagnosis of respiratory failure depends on arterial gas tensions, the physical examination, roentgenographic features, and certain pulmonary volume and airway pressure measurements may precede and provide advanced warning that respiratory failure will occur (Belani et al., 1980; Shimada et al., 1979). Criteria that are used to judge the severity of respiratory failure are shown in Table 9–14. Hypoxemia, hypercapnia, increased work of breathing, and inability to expel tracheobronchial secretions effectively are the principal reasons for undertaking intensive respiratory therapy. Early detection of hypoxemia and hypercapnia prevents clinical

■ **Table 9–12.** RESPIRATORY PHYSIOLOGIC MEASUREMENTS IN NORMAL NEWBORN AND ADULT

	Newborn	Adult (21-yr-old)
Body weight (kg)	3.0	70.0
Surface area (m²)	0.21	1.7
Basal metabolic rate (cal/kg/hr)	2.0	1.0
Oxygen consumption (ml/kg/min)	6.5	3.5
CO_2 production (ml/kg/min)	6.0	3.0
Respiratory frequency (per min)	35.0	12.0
Tidal volume (ml/kg)	6.0	6.0
Minute volume (ml/kg/min)	200.0	85.0
Alveolar ventilation (ml/kg/min)	150.0	60.0
Dead space (ml/kg)	2.2	2.2
Functional residual capacity (ml/kg)	30.0	34.0
Vital capacity (ml/kg)	35.0	70.0
Specific compliance (l/cm H_2O/FRC [l])	0.05	0.06
Transpulmonary pressure change at rest (cm H_2O)	5.0	5.0
Pulmonary work (g/cm/min/kg)	460.0	224.0
Specific conductance $\dfrac{(l/sec/cm\ H_2O)}{FRC[l]}$	0.28	0.24

cyanosis, bradycardia, feeble pulses, gasping respiratory efforts, apnea, and central nervous system depression and progression to cardiopulmonary arrest.

Three types of respiratory failure are now considered to occur (Hall and Wood, 1987). In Type I, hypoxemia is the dominant finding. Processes such as pneumonia, pulmonary hemorrhage, or edema fill the alveoli with fluid, cells, and other substances, which deny gas entry to the alveoli and most often lead to this type of respiratory failure. Hypoventilation, which leads to hypercarbia, is characteristic of Type II respiratory failure. Depression of the respiratory center, neuromusculoskeletal disorders, and airway obstruction classically lead to Type II respiratory failure. An increase in closing volume, the lung volume at which substantial small-airway closure occurs, with the result that it falls within the tidal range of respiration and leads to atelectasis and decreases in ventilation-perfusion ratios, is considered the principal disturbance in Type III respiratory failure. This type of respiratory failure occurs most often after operations.

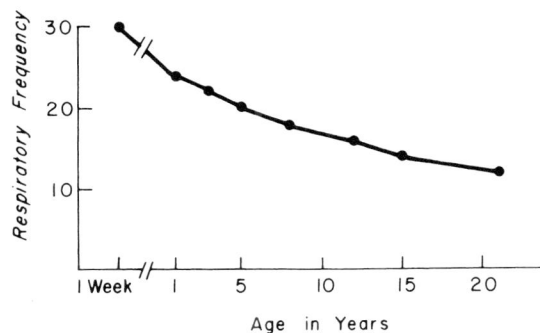

FIGURE 9–47. Respiratory frequency plotted as a function of age. (Data from Cook, C. D., and Montoyama, E. K.: Respiratory physiology in infants and children. *In* Smith, R. M. [ed]: Anesthesia for Infants and Children. 3rd ed. St. Louis, C. V. Mosby, 1968.)

■ **Table 9–13.** COMMON CAUSES OF ACUTE CARDIOPULMONARY FAILURE IN INFANCY

Neonate (0–30 Days)	Infant (1–24 Mo)
Gasway Obstruction	
Extrathoracic	
Choanal atresia	Subglottic swelling
Cord paralysis	Infection
Congenital web, cyst	Trauma
Pierre Robin syndrome	Subglottic stenosis
Laryngomalacia, hypoplasia	Congenital
Tracheomalacia	Postintubation
Arnold-Chiari malformation	Foreign body
Intrathoracic	
Tracheobronchobronchiolitis	Tracheobronchobronchiolitis
Chemical (meconium)	Viral (Bronchiolitis)
Bacterial	Bacterial
Viral	Parasitic
Parasitic	Chemical
Bronchopulmonary dysplasia	Bronchopulmonary dysplasia
Edema	Asthma (age ≥6 mo)
Interstitial emphysema	Edema
Compression	Interstitial emphysema
Vascular	Cystic fibrosis
Cardiac	Compression
	Vascular
	Cardiac
	Neoplastic
Acinar Disorders	
Surfactant deficiency (IRDS)	Pneumonitis
Pneumonitis	Bacterial
Chemical (meconium)	Parasitic
Bacterial	Edema
Viral	Cardiogenic
Parasitic	Permeability
Edema	Hypo-oncotic
Cardiogenic	
Permeability	
Hypo-oncotic	
Extrapulmonary Disorders	
Neuromusculoskeletal Dysfunction	
Prematurity (<36 wk; gestation <2.5 kg)	
Hypoperfusion	Hypoperfusion
Hypoglycemia	Sudden infant death syndrome
Hypothermia	Hypoglycemia
Drugs: depressants, muscle relaxants	Hypothermia
Central nervous system hemorrhage	Drugs: depressants, muscle relaxants
Diaphragmatic defects	Spinal cord injury
	Neuropathies
Miscellaneous Abnormalities	
Pneumothorax	
Pleural effusion	
Abdominal distention	

IRDS = idiopathic respiratory distress syndrome.

RESPIRATORY INSUFFICIENCY ASSOCIATED WITH CARDIAC SURGERY

Many infants show evidence of acute respiratory insufficiency before or after cardiac operations

■ **Table 9–14.** SEVERITY OF RESPIRATORY FAILURE

Degree of Failure	Characteristics
Mild	Failure between 67 and 95% confidence limits for age* Mild intercostal or subcostal retractions Pa_{O_2}/FI_{O_2} 285–150 neonate 330–150 infant Pa_{CO_2} 43–49†
Moderate	Failure outside 95% confidence limits for age Moderate intercostal retractions Nasal flaring Pa_{O_2}/FI_{O_2} 150–120 infant Pa_{CO_2} 50–55‡ Grunting
Severe	Gasping Marked intercostal and subcostal retractions $Pa_{O_2}/FI_{O_2} < 120$ infant $Pa_{CO_2} > 55$‡ pH < 7.35

*Phelan, P. D., and Williams, H. E.: Ventilatory studies in healthy infants. Pediatr. Res., 3:425, 1969.
†Albert, M. S., and Winter, R. W.: Acid-base equilibrium of blood in normal infants. Pediatrics, 37:728, 1966.
‡No metabolic alkalosis.

(Downes et al., 1970; Manners et al., 1980). Cardiac dysfunction often causes pulmonary dysfunction and vice versa. Hypoxia, hypercapnia, and acidosis adversely affect myocardial contractility and cardiac output. Raised left atrial pressure increases pulmonary venous resistance, which causes capillary leakage of fluid and interstitial edema. Interstitial pulmonary water reduces dynamic pulmonary compliance and vital capacity and increases venoarterial shunting by promoting ventilation-perfusion imbalances (Robin et al., 1973). Severe pulmonary edema involves obstruction of terminal airways because of extravasation of fluid around bronchi and pulmonary vessels in the bronchovascular pedicle; eventually, proteinaceous or bloody fluid appears in the alveoli and airways. Acute distention of the left atrium and ventricle during or immediately after cardiopulmonary bypass can cause hemorrhagic pulmonary edema.

Pulmonary blood flow also affects pulmonary function. Excessive pulmonary blood flow increases ventilation-perfusion imbalance and physiologic dead space (Downes et al., 1970; Yates, 1987), increases venoarterial shunting with reduced arterial oxygen saturation (Lees et al., 1967), decreases compliance (Bancalari et al., 1977), and causes profuse, thick bronchial secretions and atelectasis. Diminished pulmonary blood flow causes hypoxia and, in extreme conditions, hypercapnia; produces ventilation-perfusion inequalities within the lungs (Lees et al., 1968); and usually causes an increase in physiologic dead space, minute volume, and alveolar ventilation (Nicodemus and Downes, 1969). When pulmonary blood flow is less than optimal but may vary in relation to pulmonary vascular resistance, systemic oxygen saturation may be favorably influenced by deliberate hyperventilation.

After cardiopulmonary bypass, polymorphonuclear white blood cells accumulate in pulmonary capillaries adjacent to swollen endothelial cells and Type I pneumocytes (Ratliff et al., 1973). Cardiopulmonary bypass activates polymorphonuclear cells, perhaps through activation of complement (C5a) (Hammerschmidt et al., 1981). It is not known whether or not these white blood cells release lysosomal enzymes (Addonizio et al., 1982) and vasoactive substances that could increase capillary permeability. Kirklin and associates (1983) have even suggested that the magnitude of postoperative respiratory dysfunction can be gauged by C3a levels obtained 3 hours after an operation.

In rare instances, the patient who has undergone cardiac surgery manifests the findings of acute lung injury unrelated to elevated pulmonary venous pressure. This disorder strongly resembles the *adult respiratory distress syndrome* (ARDS) initially described in trauma victims (Ashbaugh et al., 1967), which results when altered pulmonary capillary permeability enables fluid to leak into the interstitium of the lung. The ensuing extravasation of formed and nonformed blood elements into the interstitium and alveolus creates a life-threatening impairment of gas exchange. Despite the name, ARDS has been described in children and infants only a few days old (Faix et al., 1989; Katz, 1987; Lyrene and Truog, 1981). Although ARDS occurs as a consequence of a variety of illnesses and injuries, including viral infection, sepsis, near drowning, and trauma, it follows a remarkably reproducible sequence of manifestations. Early clinical manifestations include tachypnea, hypoxemia, and alveolar radiodensities that progress to respiratory failure with markedly diminished pulmonary compliance. The pathologic findings are consistent, with early pulmonary congestion, pneumocyte desquamation, and hyaline membrane formation ultimately giving way to fibrosis by the second week.

Current evidence suggests that this wide spectrum of initiating lung injuries together form a reproducible pathophysiologic sequence by triggering a common cascade of inflammatory mediators. Possibly initiated by complement, activated neutrophils become sequestered in the lung, where they exert toxic effects by three mechanisms: Release of potent proteolytic enzymes and production of free radical oxidants both disrupt tissue integrity, while arachidonic acid metabolites such as leukotriene B_4 act as potent neutrophil chemotactic factors (Sarnaik and Lieh-Lai, 1994). Despite the strong association of neutrophils with ARDS, reports of the syndrome in neutropenic children suggest that neutrophils are not essential (Sivan et al., 1990). However, macrophages probably play a central role in the development of ARDS: In addition to free radical formation and arachidonic acid metabolite liberation, they produce cytokines, such as *tumor necrosis factor* (TNF) and *interleukin-1* (IL-1), that are capable of mediating a fulminant inflammatory response. *Platelet activating factor* (PAF), a mediator known to promote platelet aggregation, systemic and pulmonary vaso-

constriction, and capillary permeability, also arises from the macrophage. The relationship of ARDS to cardiac surgery may involve mediator release in response to cardiopulmonary bypass or massive transfusion of blood products.

After cardiopulmonary bypass, alveolar-arterial oxygen differences are usually greater than before operation. In addition, postoperative pulmonary function tests indicate decreased alveolar ventilation, reduced compliance (Ellison et al., 1967), an increase in airways resistance, and an increase in the work of breathing. These changes are consistent with an increase in extravascular pulmonary water and imbalance between ventilation and perfusion of units of the lung (Parker et al., 1972). DiCarlo and co-workers (1992) demonstrated diminished lung compliance in 26 neonates examined 1 day after open heart surgery. However, the 46% of neonates who did not tolerate withdrawal of mechanical ventilatory support exhibited substantially higher total lung resistance (> 75 cm $H_2O/l/sec$). The mechanism of this abnormality likely resides with interstitial fluid accumulation that may reflect loss of capillary integrity, perhaps related to an inflammatory process. The cohort requiring prolonged mechanical ventilation gained more weight perioperatively, and the lungs of the two infants in this group who died revealed nearly twice-normal weight, denuded epithelium, and alveoli filled with macrophages, proteinaceous material, and hyaline membranes.

Many factors may cause increased pulmonary water after cardiopulmonary bypass. Often, the degree of respiratory dysfunction is proportional to the degree of heart failure and elevation of pulmonary venous pressures. Vincent and associates (1984) demonstrated a threefold increase in extravascular lung water immediately following cardiac surgery in 12 children who had experienced increased pulmonary blood flow and heart failure preoperatively. Increased capillary hydrostatic pressures and reduced plasma colloid osmotic pressure (from hemodilution) (Beattie et al., 1974) increase the net movement of fluid into the pulmonary interstitial spaces even if capillary permeability does not change. Animal studies confirm that interstitial edema impairs lung compliance (Noble et al., 1975), whereas pulmonary venous pressure elevations between 15 and 20 mm Hg cause vascular engorgement that narrows peripheral airways and increases airway resistance (Hogg et al., 1972). Although these changes in airway resistance are reversible if pulmonary venous pressure falls, extreme (30 mm Hg) or protracted venous pressure elevations cause alveolar fluid accumulation and irreversible increases in airway resistance (Ishii et al., 1985).

Respiratory support can aid the failing heart during the early postoperative period. Mechanical ventilation and pharmacologic muscle paralysis reduce oxygen consumption by approximately 20% when pulmonary mechanics are normal and significantly more when pulmonary compliance or airway resistance abnormalities are substantial. Furthermore, hypoxia, hypercarbia, and acidosis increase pulmonary vascular resistance (Cassin et al., 1964; Park et al., 1969; Rudolph and Yuan, 1966), thereby imposing a pressure load on the right ventricle while creating a biochemical milieu that promotes myocardial irritability and impairs contractility. Measures designed to reduce pulmonary vascular resistance relieve the failing right ventricle. Hyperventilation with high concentrations of oxygen remains the mainstay of such therapy (Drummond et al., 1981; Peckham and Fox, 1978). Although pharmacologic agents such as isoproterenol, nitroprusside, nifedipine, prostaglandin E_1, prostacyclin, and tolazoline all have demonstrated some efficacy in selected circumstances, they often promote undesired vasodilation of the systemic vasculature as well (Bush et al., 1988; Prielipp et al., 1991; Rubis et al., 1981; Soifer, 1993). Although it is limited to investigational use at present, inhaled nitric oxide holds great promise as a selective pulmonary vasodilator, at least for infants plagued by elevated pulmonary vascular resistance that is not caused by fixed anatomic reduction of the cross-sectional area of the pulmonary vascular bed (Roberts et al., 1993; Soifer, 1993; Wessel, 1993). Conversely, when the heart is failing because of the excessive volume load imposed by a massive left-to-right shunt, measures should be directed to normalize ventilation and minimize $F_{I_{O_2}}$. In selected circumstances, such as the infant with a single ventricle perfusing both the systemic and the pulmonary circulations in parallel, the addition of carbon dioxide to the inspired gas mixture may ameliorate the physiology (Jobes et al., 1993).

MANAGEMENT OF RESPIRATORY SUPPORT

Personnel, Equipment, and Physical Plant

Neonates and infants who require intensive respiratory therapy are cared for preferably in an intensive care unit that is primarily dedicated to that task. The unit should be staffed on a 24-hour basis by a team of physicians and nurses who are specially trained in infant care and who are free of other responsibilities. They should be thoroughly familiar with the recognition and therapy of respiratory insufficiency and with the resuscitative, supportive, and monitoring equipment used in that unit. Physicians in the unit must work closely with each infant's surgeon or pediatrician, who may not be physically in the unit at all times. The unit should have a full-time medical director who is responsible for its administration, control of the environment, which includes aseptic practices, and other matters vital to the care of critically ill infants. Nurses must also be trained specially in the care of these infants and must be assigned full time to the unit. Ideally, one nurse should be assigned to each infant around the clock. The unit needs to be equipped with extensive cardiovascular and respiratory monitoring equipment; wall outlets for air, vacuum, and oxygen; and resuscitative equipment for both respiratory and cardiac emergencies (Table 9–15).

■ **Table 9–15.** RECOMMENDED CONTENTS FOR A PEDIATRIC RESUSCITATION CART

Airway Equipment
1. Bag of 0.5-, 1-, or 2-liter capacity; masks of neonate, infant, toddler sizes; T piece and gas exhaust valves with 15-mm and 22-mm fittings for universal sequencing to provide circuit for manual ventilation
2. Oropharyngeal airways (Guedel's sizes 00, 0, 1, 2)
3. Tracheal tubes 2.5 mm internal diameter (ID) to 4.5 ID uncuffed sterile at least two of each size with appropriate size straight 15-mm male connectors; two of each size in extra-long lengths for use in pathologically narrowed airways
4. Laryngoscope
   Handle: C batteries
   Handle: AA batteries
   Blades: Miller 0 and Wis-Hipple 1 and 1.5
            Flagg 2
            1 reserve light for each blade
5. Magill's forceps: Pediatric
6. Stylets (Teflon-coated for tubes 2.5–4.5 mm ID)
7. Aspiration equipment
   Yankauer aspirator
   Disposable sterile plastic suction catheters sizes, 6, 8, 10, 14

Drugs

Sodium bicarbonate (1 mEq/ml)	Atropine sulfate (0.4 mg/ml)
Epinephrine (1 mg/ml)	Dopamine (40 mg/ml)
Isoproterenol (0.2 mg/ml)	Dextrose (500 mg/ml)
Calcium gluconate (100 mg/ml)	0.9% Saline (for dilution)

Defibrillator
Direct current with range of 20 to 400 joules
0.9% Saline for soaking 4 × 4 in. gauze pads stored with external paddles
Conducting paste
Infant (3 cm diameter), pediatric (5 cm diameter), and adult (8 cm diameter) external paddles

Miscellaneous
Intracardiac needles: 20 and 22 gauge, 6 to 8 cm length
Plastic intravenous cannulas (16, 18, 20, 22, 24 gauge) and butterfly needles (19, 21, 23, 25, 27 gauge)
Tongue blades, alcohol swabs, sterile hemostat, sterile 4 × 4 in. gauze sponges
Scissors, syringes (plastic disposable), needles
Thoracostomy set
Thoracotomy set

Commonly used supplies should be stocked in or immediately adjacent to the unit. Measurements of blood gases, pH, and hematocrit must be available on a 24-hour basis with a response time of less than 15 minutes.

Initial Evaluation and Therapy

We believe that patients are best served when caretakers follow two types of management: One identifies the cause and selects specific therapy, if available, to reverse the process; the other focuses on managing the altered physiology and achieves arterial gas tensions that permit normal organ function. Historical information, physical examination, and laboratory evaluation, which includes radiographic techniques, are considered in determining the nature of a problem in the respiratory system.

At the same time as the search is being made for a primary cause, correction or compensation for disturbed physiology must receive attention. In mild Types I and III respiratory failure in which hypoxemia is the dominant feature, enrichment of inspired gas with oxygen may be all that is necessary to achieve acceptable arterial oxygen tensions. Most experts consider an $F_{I_{O_2}}$ of less than 0.5 to be well tolerated; oxygen toxicity can be avoided, and absorption atelectasis can be minimized.

When $Pa_{O_2}/F_{I_{O_2}}$ falls below 100 in the absence of hypoventilation, most caretakers use increased transpulmonary distending pressure to improve matching of ventilation with perfusion, which often has a dramatic effect on oxygen transfer efficiency. However, when alveoli filled with material prevent gas entry, minimal improvement in arterial oxygen tension occurs. In Type II, and when respiratory mechanics become severely abnormal in Types I or III respiratory failure, manual or mechanical ventilation augments or substitutes for a patient's respiratory bellows function to correct alveolar hypoventilation.

When acute cardiopulmonary failure is recognized, pulmonary gas exchange must be improved immediately. Severe hypoxemia, bradycardia, or systemic arterial hypotension demands the use of 100% oxygen by bag and mask with assisted ventilation, aspiration of upper airway secretions, establishment of an adequate intravenous route with a plastic cannula, monitoring of precordial heart tones and electrocardiogram, and the use of intravenous sodium bicarbonate to restore arterial pH to 7.25 or higher. Manually assisted or controlled ventilation for a brief period while cardiovascular function is restored provides time to assess the need for more complex respiratory support. Unless ventilation and blood-gas tensions immediately improve, an orotracheal tube should be inserted and ventilation should be controlled.

AIRWAY MANAGEMENT

Establishing the Airway

After at least 1 minute of manually controlled ventilation with 100% oxygen, direct laryngoscopy with a blade appropriate for the patient's age should be done and an orotracheal tube of appropriate diameter for age (Table 9–16) should be inserted. Most of these patients have retained gastric secretions or food that can be regurgitated and readily aspirated. Thus, an individual skilled in laryngoscopy and intubation should do the maneuver while an assistant applies cricoid pressure to occlude the esophagus. The conscious patient usually tolerates and benefits from administration of a small dose of intravenous thiopental or ketamine and neuromuscular blockade.

After orotracheal intubation, full lung expansion and the removal of secretions from the central airways should be attempted. Stomach contents should be aspirated with a nasogastric tube.

■ **Table 9–16.** DIMENSIONS OF TRACHEAL TUBES*

Age	Internal Diameter ID (mm)	Connector ID (mm)	Minimal Length (Oral)† (cm)
Premature	2.5	3	10–11
Full term	3.0	3	10–11
3 Months	3.5	4	11–12
6 Months	4.0	4	13
12 Months	4.0	4	14
18–24 Months	4.5	5	15

*Tubes that conform to ANSI Standard Z-79.1 are recommended.
†For nasal tubes, add 2 to 3 cm to length.
ID = internal diameter.

Selection of Airway

Nasotracheal intubation and tracheostomy are elective procedures that are accomplished after initial orotracheal intubation. If an artificial tracheal airway is needed for more than 12 hours, a nasotracheal tube is preferred to an orotracheal tube. A nasotracheal tube that is placed correctly provides more stable fixation, less danger of inadvertent extubation (Black et al., 1990), and fewer oropharyngeal secretions, and it facilitates care of the mouth and oropharynx. Nasotracheal intubation should be accomplished with the orotracheal tube in position while an assistant ventilates the lungs. When the nasotracheal tube is visualized at the level of the larynx and is advanced anteriorly toward the glottis, the orotracheal tube is removed. Occasionally, small Magill's forceps or another type of forceps is required to grasp the tube in the hypopharynx and bring it anterior for advancement into the glottis.

Cuffed tubes are not necessary in infants whose narrow, tapered, subglottic tracheal diameter ensures an adequate tracheal seal. To reduce the risk of injury resulting from excessive pressure of the tube on the airway mucosa, most pediatric anesthesiologists and intensivists place tubes that permit the audible leak of gas at airway pressures less than 40 cm H_2O (Finholt et al., 1985; Lee et al., 1980). The risks of laryngeal and tracheal injury posed by large tubes must be analyzed individually for patients, because smaller tubes that permit a leak have disadvantages, particularly in the infant with markedly diminished pulmonary compliance or increased airway resistance. The principal hazards of smaller tubes are increased resistance to gas flow, tendency to occlude, and variation in delivered tidal volume due to the leak. Once the tube is secured, its position should be evaluated with a chest film.

Tracheostomy may be necessary in infants and children who have intrinsic laryngeal disease or thick or bloody tracheobronchial secretions. Some anesthesiologists and surgeons also prefer tracheostomy in infants who require an artificial tracheal airway for more than 2 to 4 weeks.

Airway Care

An artificial tracheal airway interferes considerably with normal mucociliary transport (Wanner, 1977).

Not only does the tube itself denude the ciliated, columnar epithelium of the trachea with which it has contact, but also cilia remain paralyzed for a millimeter or more beyond the tip of the tube (Hilding, 1965). Cold, dry inspired air further inhibits ciliary function, disrupts cellular integrity (Chalon et al., 1972), and increases the viscosity of the mucous carpet. Inspired gas should be humidified to provide 35 to 44 mg of water vapor per liter of gas flow at 37° C (80 to 100% relative humidity) in the trachea. Secretions in the smaller bronchi and bronchioles can be mobilized and moved toward the trachea by changes in the patient's position, chest vibration, and percussion every 1 to 2 hours. These maneuvers should be followed by sterile aspiration using a catheter with a proximal thumb-hole and an end hole with a molded tip and multiple distal side holes. To minimize tracheal mucosal damage, the catheter is inserted to the maximal depth but is retracted 2 to 3 mm before applying suction. Vacuum pressure limited to 50 to 100 torr may reduce the extent of mucosal damage by the catheter. Before and after tracheal aspiration, the patient's lungs should be inflated intermittently with oxygen to a volume near vital capacity for 1 to 3 minutes to protect against hypoxemia and to reexpand atelectatic segments. Culture of tracheobronchial secretions, using a Lukens' trap to obtain an adequate sample, enables the physician to detect the tracheobronchial pathogens when infection is suspected.

Inspired Gases

Except for infants with cyanotic congenital heart disease, inspired oxygen-air mixtures that provide a Pa_{O_2} between 60 and 80 torr are usually satisfactory. Because masks are poorly tolerated by most infants less than 18 months old, head hoods for infants less than 6 months of age and oxygen tents for older infants or nasal cannulae for either age group are preferable for inspired oxygen concentrations up to 75%. Higher concentrations of oxygen are generally delivered by means of a tracheal tube or tracheostomy. Oxygen-air mixing valves (blenders) are used to control oxygen concentrations, but for accuracy and estimation of alveolar-arterial oxygen differences, the concentration of inspired oxygen near the mouth or at the tracheal connector must be measured.

Infants, particularly those born at gestational ages less than 36 weeks, are susceptible to the toxic effects of oxygen. Retinopathy of prematurity (ROP) may result from elevated or even normal arterial blood oxygen tension in the preterm newborn (James and Lanman, 1976). However, the most significant risk factor in the development of retinopathy is not the level of hyperoxemia but the degree of immaturity of the retina in any given infant (Flynn, 1987). Increased alveolar oxygen tension causes alveolar injury directly proportional to the concentration and duration of oxygen exposure. Pulmonary oxygen toxicity in adults begins to occur if 100% oxygen is inspired for more than 12 hours or if 80% oxygen is breathed for

more than 24 hours. Oxygen concentrations below 40 to 50% appear to be tolerated indefinitely by both infants and adults (Deneke and Fanburg, 1980).

MECHANICAL RESPIRATORY SUPPORT

Continuous Positive Airway Pressure (CPAP)

In the spontaneously breathing hypoxic infant whose trachea has been intubated and Pa_{CO_2} is less than 50 torr, arterial oxygenation may be improved by providing end-expiratory airway pressures from 2 to 15 cm of water (CPAP) above atmospheric pressure (Gregory et al., 1971). This method can be used in conjunction with, but not as a substitute for, mechanical ventilation. CPAP increases functional residual capacity (FRC) and often increases Pa_{O_2} in hypoxic infants who have poorly ventilated but perfused alveoli (Gregory et al., 1975; Hatch et al., 1973; Stewart et al., 1973). The increase in FRC is proportional to the transpulmonary pressure at end-expiration. At higher transpulmonary pressures, inflated alveoli have large diameters, which tend to stabilize adjacent alveoli and the smaller airways and prevent their collapse. Because alveolar ventilation is minimally affected, Pa_{CO_2} does not change appreciably. If previously collapsed alveoli are reinflated and remain inflated at the higher transpulmonary pressures, pulmonary capillary blood passing through these alveoli becomes oxygenated and the venoarterial shunt decreases. In normovolemic infants, CPAP causes little or no depression of systemic arterial pressure. Infants can be fed by gavage while receiving CPAP, but the feedings should be small and should be preceded by aspiration of residual gastric fluid. These same comments apply to positive end-expiratory pressure (PEEP) in conjunction with mechanical ventilation.

Ventilators

If CPAP alone proves to be insufficient to restore adequate oxygenation, or if Pa_{CO_2} exceeds 50 torr, mechanical ventilation should be instituted. In the presence of adverse changes in pulmonary mechanics, volume-preset ventilators provide more consistent and effective alveolar ventilation than pressure-preset or time-flow-preset types (Table 9–17). A major problem with many commercially available ventilators for infants is their large internal compliance (compression volume). Internal compliance is defined as the volume of gas compressed in the ventilator system per unit of peak airway pressure; this gas does not participate in minute ventilation of the patient. For example, if the internal compliance is 4 ml/cm H_2O pressure and an infant is ventilated with a tidal volume that produces a peak airway pressure of 15 cm H_2O, 60 ml of gas is compressed within the ventilator, tubing, humidifier, water trap, and alarm system. Thus, a volume setting of 60 ml results in almost no inspired gas reaching the patient's lungs. A higher ventilator

■ **Table 9–17.** MECHANICAL VENTILATORS COMMONLY USED IN INFANTS

Volume Preset
Siemens Servo 900C
Siemens Servo 300
Bird VIP
Newport E100i

Pressure Preset
Bear Cub
Sechrist IV 100B
Sechrist IV 200 Savi System
Infrasonic Infant Star 500
Drager Babylog 8000
Premi Care 105
Bird VIP

High-Frequency Jet
Bunell Lifepulse

High-Frequency Oscillator
Sensor Medics 3100A

High-Frequency Flow Interrupter
Infrasonics Infant Star 500

volume setting is required to compensate for the internal compliance.

Apparatus dead space has received considerable attention in the past but, if not excessive, can be overcome by increasing the tidal volume. Usually, visual and auscultatory evidence of ventilation must be relied on during initial adjustments of the ventilator. Tidal volume and respiratory frequency are readjusted according to serial arterial Pa_{CO_2} and Pa_{O_2} determinations. Delivered tidal volumes (excluding compression volume) of 12 to 15 ml/kg and a respiratory frequency approximately two-thirds normal for the patient's age will serve to correct arterial blood-gas tensions toward normal.

Controlled ventilation or *intermittent mandatory ventilation* (IMV) has proved to be effective in ultimately restoring gas exchange in most infants with acute cardiopulmonary failure. IMV exists when unassisted, unrestricted spontaneous breathing is supplemented by mechanical ventilator breaths. Gas flow equal to or greater than the neonate's or infant's peak inspiratory flow rate most effectively provided by a continuous fresh gas flow into the breathing circuit spares the infant work to trigger demand values and prevents rebreathing during spontaneous ventilation (Downs et al., 1973). The ventilator delivers preset tidal volumes at 1 to 40 times per minute, which depend on the patient's ability to maintain adequate ventilation. These ventilator breaths may be synchronized with the initiation of a spontaneous breath (synchronous IMV) or may be delivered at any time in the patient's respiratory cycle. Synchronous IMV is not used in infants because they cannot trigger the machine and because they readily accept the mandatory tidal breath without agitation or difficulty.

Current developments in ventilatory support of infants focus on methods of more homogeneous distribution of gas in order to promote expansion and ventilation of diseased regions without overdistending and injuring normal lung tissue. Reversal of the I/E ratio and, more recently, pressure release ventilation are two methods by which lower peak inflating pressures are held for more extended periods. Unfortunately, no published studies have demonstrated that these methods are more effective or less injurious in infants, whereas sustained intrathoracic pressure often has demonstrable effects on hemodynamics. Pressure support ventilation, in which a preset pressure accompanies all spontaneous inspirations, was designed to reduce the work of spontaneous breathing that arises from resistance to gas flow in the circuit and tracheal tube (Brochard et al., 1989). As with synchronous IMV, the major obstacle to this technique resides in the technical difficulties posed by detecting the onset of the infant's breath and cycling on and off with sufficiently rapid response time so as to avoid lung overdistention and increased work exhaling against the ventilator. Traditional means of determining spontaneous activity by pressure changes within the circuit are woefully inadequate in infants. These methods are finally being challenged by prototypes using such methods as hot-wire anemometers to detect flow, esophageal balloons to detect changes in intrathoracic pressure, and even diaphragmatic electromyography to provide the sensitivity and response time necessary to make these ventilatory techniques useful in infants (Truog and Jackson, 1992). In the ultimate infant ventilator, these exquisite sensors of spontaneous activity will be combined with microprocessor-driven breath-by-breath analysis of flow and pressure delivery characteristics in order to constantly adjust the pattern of delivery to satisfy preset minute ventilation requirements with minimal distending pressure (Hazelzet et al., 1993) in a manner that mimics manual ventilation (DiCarlo and Steven, 1994).

Synchronization of the patient's breaths with the mechanical ventilator is often achieved by providing adequate alveolar ventilation and oxygenation. Diazepam (0.1 mg/kg intravenously) or morphine (0.05 to 0.2 mg/kg intravenously) in repeated doses or by continuous infusion produces adequate sedation and depression of respiratory drive in the restless infant. In hemodynamically fragile infants, even small doses of morphine and benzodiazepines often create unacceptable cardiovascular depression. When warranted by the clinical circumstances, sedation with infusions of synthetic opioids, such as fentanyl and sufentanil, appears to cause fewer hemodynamic changes. No matter what regimen is selected, tolerance develops over a few days, necessitating ever-increasing doses. In infants with severe bronchospasm (e.g., in bronchiolitis) or in whom severe pneumonia has caused a marked reflex tachypnea, neuromuscular blockade by continuous infusion of pancuronium bromide provides minimal chest wall resistance to ventilation and appears to reduce the hazards of pneumothorax or pneumomediastinum. Continuous infusion of sedatives and muscular relaxants in infants with profound cardiovascular failure or intense lower airways obstruction evenly controls activity and reduces the infant's oxygen consumption.

High levels of PEEP (10 to 20 cm H_2O) with IMV are required in infants with an extraordinary loss of pulmonary volume who need high inspired oxygen concentrations (F_{IO_2} over 0.75). Patients who receive high PEEP require frequent assessment of cardiac output and vascular filling pressures (Kirby et al., 1975). Raised systemic venous pressures may be needed to maintain adequate pulmonary and systemic perfusion. Infusion of dopamine or other inotropic drugs often proves necessary to maintain cardiac output. Many of these patients develop interstitial pulmonary emphysema and pneumomediastinum, for which little can be done; more than 25% of them incur a pneumothorax (which may be bilateral), which necessitates thoracic drainage tubes.

An alternative way to reduce the toxicity of positive-pressure ventilation entails acceptance of abnormal arterial gas tensions. The movement toward "permissive" hypercapnia acknowledges the reality that clinicians confront in balancing the risks and benefits that achieving normal gas tensions poses to patients with markedly abnormal respiratory mechanics. Reynolds and associates (1993) described a 3-year-old child who developed ARDS following inhalation injury in whom they arbitrarily defined a maximal inflating pressure of 40 cm H_2O and tolerated mean Pa_{CO_2} values of 89 mm Hg with maximal values of 160 mm Hg. The Pa_{O_2} range during this period was 58 to 121 mm Hg (mean 82 mm Hg). No specific measures were undertaken to neutralize the respiratory acidosis. Unlike the case in many patients with such severe ARDS, in this patient 6-month follow-up revealed normal electrocardiographic and pulmonary function test results, suggesting that the avoidance of extreme positive-pressure ventilation limits pulmonary fibrosis and improves long-term functional outcome. Although such anecdotes are tantalizing, more systematic study should define the safety, efficacy, and limits of this strategy.

High-Frequency Ventilation

Except for a few well-defined indications, the precise role of high-frequency ventilation remains controversial after more than a decade of use in infants (Marchak et al., 1981). Uncertainties persist partly because "high-frequency" ventilation incorporates at least three types of ventilators (jet, oscillator, and flow interrupter), the efficacy of which probably varies with the method. Although a common strategy unites all methods (i.e., to deliver small tidal volumes [V_T] at high frequency in order to lower peak and, in some instances, mean airway pressures, thereby preserving satisfactory lung volume with less toxicity), the methods employed to accomplish this goal vary (Bancalari and Goldberg, 1987; Truog and Jackson, 1992; Wetzel and Gioia, 1987). Jet ventilators typically employ V_T greater than dead space (V_D) at rates near 4 to 10 Hz, whereas flow interrupters and oscillators deliver V_T

less than V_D at rates between 10 and 20 Hz. Jet ventilators deliver the preset V_T via a small coaxial channel to the distal orifice of a specially designed tracheal tube. The flow interrupter employs a fixed inspiratory flow rate, with V_T and rate adjusted by manipulating the expiratory time. High-frequency oscillators use active inspiratory and expiratory phases in order to reduce the risk of gas trapping.

In clinical trials on neonates with respiratory failure, these devices have achieved varying success. Although the high-frequency jet ventilator (HFJV) effectively reduced the morbidity rate in neonates with demonstrated air leaks, no difference in mortality or the incidence of chronic lung disease occurred (Keszler et al., 1991). In a large multicenter trial of the high-frequency oscillator ventilator (HFOV) for respiratory failure in preterm neonates, no demonstrable differences in mortality, incidence of bronchopulmonary dysplasia (BPD), or level of ventilatory support at 28 days were detected (HIFI Study Group, 1989). Nevertheless, advocates of HFOV cite their own experience and subsequent smaller studies demonstrating reduced incidence of BPD (Clark et al., 1990; Frantz, 1993). Laboratory observations in premature baboons, which showed reduced volumes of proteinaceous pulmonary edema and improved gas exchange at 6 hours when HFOV was employed exclusively, support the possibility that lung injury occurred in the 12 hours of conventional ventilation permitted in the HIFI study before randomization (Jackson et al., 1991). Experience with these devices in older infants with respiratory failure remains limited, but they deserve consideration as rescue therapy, particularly when vexing air leaks develop.

By altering the intrathoracic pressure necessary to achieve a given degree of ventilation, high-frequency ventilators may promote pulmonary blood flow. In dogs following right-sided ventriculotomy, HFJV lowered pulmonary vascular resistance and increased cardiac output (Lucking et al., 1986). Similar changes were observed in infants and small children ventilated with HFJV following the Fontan operation (Meliones et al., 1991).

Negative Pressure Ventilation

Negative or, more precisely, subatmospheric pressure ventilation provides mechanical support under more natural physiologic conditions. Although they are more cumbersome logistically than positive-pressure ventilation devices, subatmospheric pressure ventilation devices permit relatively normal V_T, flow patterns, and rates for infants who lack the cardiovascular reserve to satisfy the load placed by their respiratory mechanics (DiCarlo and Steven, 1994). Although this technique affords demonstrable hemodynamic benefits in selected circumstances, such as promoting pulmonary blood flow in children following the Fontan operation (Penny et al., 1991), the principal advantage accrues from reducing the cycle of airway inflammation and injury that occurs with positive pressure ventilation via a tracheal tube (Jardine et al., 1992).

Liquid Ventilation

Ventilation by instilling a liquid, usually perfluorochemical, in which both oxygen and carbon dioxide are highly soluble, is a promising experimental method of achieving pulmonary gas exchange (Greenspan et al., 1990). The advantage to pulmonary mechanics is the elimination of the gas-liquid interface that creates surface tension. The decrease in interfacial surface tension significantly increases pulmonary compliance, lowers necessary distending pressure, and promotes homogeneous gas exchange.

Adjuncts to Ventilatory Support

Surfactant

Surfactant is a mixture of phospholipids and proteins secreted by the Type II alveolar epithelial cell. Although most widely recognized for their ability to modulate the surface tension forces acting on the alveoli in order to stabilize alveolar units of varying sizes, surfactant proteins also diminish the alveolar permeability to the serum proteins that promote lung injury (Lacaze-Masmonteil, 1993). Immaturity of the Type II pneumocyte, with resulting surfactant deficiency, is considered central to the pathogenesis of *idiopathic respiratory distress syndrome* (IRDS) in premature infants. In 1980, Fujiwara and associates reported the initial administration of exogenous surfactant to a premature infant with IRDS. Although many surfactant preparations exist, the two most prevalent are a synthetic combination of phospholipids and spreading substances (Exosurf Neonatal) and a natural extract derived from bovine lung (Survanta). Gortner (1992) summarized the results of 17 controlled trials of natural surfactant administration in IRDS and concluded that differences in survival were small, but survival without BPD increased from 41 to 56%. Reduced incidences of pneumothorax (26 to 12%) and pulmonary interstitial edema (37 to 17%) were the only other benefits of surfactant therapy. The optimal dose of surfactant and the timing of its administration (i.e., prophylaxis or rescue) are still controversial.

Secondary surfactant deficiency follows a number of pulmonary insults. Meconium inhibits surfactant activity, whereas inflammatory mediators such as TNF suppress synthesis of surfactant protein. Despite the logic of administering exogenous surfactants to infants stricken with any of these pathologic processes that cause secondary surfactant depletion, too little experience has accrued outside the realm of IRDS to support such application (Gortner, 1992).

Hemofiltration and Ultrafiltration

The respiratory compromise that accompanies many disease states relates, at least in part, to the pulmonary mechanical abnormalities caused by the accumulation of interstitial fluid. Preliminary reports suggest that extracorporeal methods of fluid removal may indeed benefit pulmonary function. DiCarlo and associates (1990) reported a series of eight children with multiple organ failure and ARDS in whom they used continuous arteriovenous hemofiltration to achieve a mean weight loss of 5 kg. With that weight loss came a significant increase in the Pa_{O_2}/Fi_{O_2} ratio (137 to 208). Naik and associates (1991) conducted a controlled study of 10 minutes of ultrafiltration at the completion of cardiopulmonary bypass in 50 children undergoing open heart surgery. This intervention significantly reduced the magnitude of total body water increase and appreciably reduced 24-hour blood loss. In infants repaired by the use of deep hypothermia and low-flow cardiopulmonary bypass, ultrafiltration significantly reduced the duration of mechanical ventilation (2 days vs. 7 days in control subjects). Myocardial performance improved as well, with a 49% increase in arterial pressure during ultrafiltration. It is unknown whether these methods achieve benefit purely on the basis of extracellular water removal or if the elimination of inflammatory mediators is involved as well.

Extracorporeal Membrane Oxygenation (ECMO)

Extracorporeal circulation using a membrane oxygenator can treat newborns with idiopathic respiratory distress syndrome, meconium aspiration, and persistent fetal circulation (Bartlett et al., 1977). The technique involves cannulation of the internal jugular vein and carotid artery and requires systemic heparinization. ECMO has become an accepted therapy for neonates whose predicted mortality rate exceeds 80% with conventional respiratory therapy, provided they are afflicted by a disease process from which one would anticipate recovery in 10 to 14 days (Bartlett et al., 1985; O'Rourke et al., 1989). Despite early successful ECMO support of older children (Hicks et al., 1977), a multicenter trial of ECMO in adults that demonstrated no improved survival (Zapol et al., 1979) discouraged application outside the neonatal period until recently.

ECMO has been used to treat various types of respiratory insufficiency since the first successful use of prolonged extracorporeal bypass was reported by Hill and associates in 1972 in an adult who had severe respiratory failure associated with multiple traumatic injuries (Hill et al., 1972). Efficacy of ECMO in patients with reversible pulmonary disease was soon successfully shown in neonates. Bartlett and associates (1976) reported successful use of venoarterial ECMO after the *meconium aspiration syndrome* (MAS) in a newborn in 1975. This group continued their interest and by 1982 were able to report 45 moribund newborns treated by ECMO with a survival rate of 55% (Bartlett et al., 1977; 1982). The technique used for ECMO includes cannulation of the right atrium via the right internal jugular vein under local anesthesia. Venous drainage is accomplished by a siphon to a small collapsible bladder, which serves to regulate a roller pump, a membrane lung to exchange oxygen and carbon dioxide, with a small heat exchanger, and return of arterialized blood to the aorta through the right common carotid artery as a venoarterial bypass or to the venous circulation if venovenous bypass is desired (Bartlett et al., 1986). Double-lumen venovenous ECMO cannulas enable withdrawal of 30% of the venous return, principally to achieve carbon dioxide removal in children capable of oxygenation via their own lungs and in whom cardiovascular support is unnecessary.

The entry criteria for ECMO remain somewhat controversial. In reporting data from the Extracorporeal Life Support Organization (ELSO) on 7667 neonatal patients who underwent ECMO between 1973 and 1993, Zwischenberger and associates (1994) found that 28% of neonates met the criteria on the basis of oxygenation index (OI).

$$OI = \frac{F_{I_{O_2}} \times \text{mean airway pressure} \times 100}{Pa_{O_2}}$$

The University of Michigan group reported 80 to 90% mortality when OI was 40 or greater (Ortiz et al., 1987). Another 26% of neonates met ECMO criteria on the basis of failure to respond to maximal therapy, 21% on the basis of acute deterioration, 17% on the basis of excessive alveolar arterial oxygen gradient, and 2% on the basis of barotrauma.

The overall survival rate of neonates in the ELSO study receiving ECMO was 81%. Table 9–18 lists the frequency of diagnoses and their specific survival rates. Neurologic complications occurred most commonly (35%), principally seizures (14%) and infarction (13%). Intracranial hemorrhage complicated the course of 12% of neonates over 35 weeks of gestational age and of 36% of infants who were more premature. The survival rate following venovenous ECMO (91%) exceeded that of the ECMO population

as a whole, and complications occurred less frequently, perhaps because this patient subset required less support. Nearly 18% of patients on venovenous ECMO required conversion to a venoarterial system. Neonates with *congenital diaphragmatic hernia* (CDH) often die even with ECMO. Although some authors advocate ECMO stabilization of neonates with CDH and severe gas exchange abnormalities even before operation, in practice the degree of pulmonary underdevelopment usually means that the infant probably will not survive if maximal conventional ventilation fails to achieve a Pa_{CO_2} of less than 40 mm Hg (Bohn et al., 1987) or when infants are less than 35 weeks of gestational age (Walker, 1993).

Growing acceptance of neonatal ECMO has rekindled an interest in extending this therapy to older infants and children with severe respiratory failure (Fuhrman and Dalton, 1992). In the ELSO experience from 1982 to 1991, O'Rourke and associates (1993) reported 285 children from 14 days to 17 years of age. Viral pneumonia (32%) and ARDS (28%) were the most frequent diagnoses; aspiration pneumonia (11%) and bacterial pneumonia (8%) were less common. Because the value of predictive scores, such as OI and $P(A-a)O_2$, is unknown in the pediatric population, they were far less commonly cited as the entry criteria (12 and 5%, respectively). Far more commonly cited were failure to respond to therapy (49%) and barotrauma (16%). In the absence of controlled studies or standardized entry criteria, one is left to presume that the survival rate of 47% in this population represents an improvement in outcome.

DISCONTINUING MECHANICAL SUPPORT

A program for discontinuing mechanical ventilation can usually be initiated when the following criteria are met: (1) cardiovascular stability has been achieved with minimal or no use of inotropic drugs; (2) Pa_{O_2} exceeds 100 torr at an $F_{I_{O_2}}$ of 0.50; (3) Pa_{CO_2} remains less than 45 torr with peak inspiratory pressure less than 25 to 30 cm H_2O; and (4) the chest radiograph shows consistent improvement. In infants who have uncorrected cyanotic congenital cardiac lesions, a Pa_{O_2} of more than 30 torr at an $F_{I_{O_2}}$ of 0.5 indicates that the infant is eligible for discontinuation of mechanical respiratory support. Because these criteria are not infallible, patients are weaned from ventilatory support by gradually decreasing the frequency of IMV while maintaining PEEP. Progress is monitored by frequent determinations of arterial pH, blood-gas tensions, continuous estimation of arterial hemoglobin saturation by pulse oximetry (SpO_2), end-tidal carbon dioxide, daily chest radiographs, and physical examination. Often tachypnea, tachycardia, pallor, and perspiration precede deterioration of blood-gas values. They indicate excessive work of breathing and the need for increased ventilatory support.

When the neonate or infant can tolerate spontane-

■ **Table 9–18.** SUMMARY OF THE EXTRACORPOREAL LIFE SUPPORT ORGANIZATION EXPERIENCE WITH NEONATAL EXTRACORPOREAL MEMBRANE OXYGENATION (ECMO), 1973–1993 (n = 7667)

	Frequency (%)	Survival (%)	ECMO duration (hrs)
Meconium aspiration	38	94	124 ± 64
PPHN/PFC	12	84	128 ± 87
RDS/HMD	12	83	127 ± 72
Pneumonia/sepsis	15	77	133 ± 85
CDH	19	59	189 ± 118
Mean of all patients		81	141 ± 89

From Zwischenberger, J. B., Nguyen, T. T., Upp, R., et al.: Complications of neonatal extracorporeal membrane oxygenation. Collective experience from the Extracorporeal Life Support Organization. J. Thorac. Cardiovasc. Surg., *107*:838–849, 1994.

PPHN/PFC = persistent pulmonary hypertension/persistent fetal circulation; RDS/HMD = respiratory distress syndrome/hyaline membrane disease; CHD = congenital diaphragmatic hernia.

ous ventilation or infrequent (e.g., 6) ventilator breaths, PEEP is gradually reduced by 1 to 2 cm H_2O decrements. Inspired oxygen concentration is maintained constant, and Pa_{O_2} is observed before each change in PEEP. A Pa_{O_2} of 70 torr or greater (Fi_{O_2} of 0.40 or less) is required before PEEP is reduced further. To maintain optimal functional residual capacity and Pa_{O_2}, PEEP is not reduced below 2 to 3 cm H_2O before extubation (Berman et al., 1976).

Tracheal extubation should be done when secretions are minimal and of thin consistency, the chest radiograph shows continuing improvement, and the patient's cardiovascular condition is satisfactory. After extubation, humidified oxygen or air should be delivered by mask or cannula to ensure adequate moisture in the airway.

SUPPLEMENTARY SUPPORT

Appropriate intravenous fluid and electrolyte therapy, sufficient calories to prevent further catabolism, and antibiotic therapy based on specific clinical and laboratory indications of infection are essential for the recovery of the child with cardiopulmonary failure. Normal body temperature must be maintained by using automated heating and cooling blankets or radiant overhead warming devices; the latter can induce exceptionally large evaporative fluid losses in infants, however. These losses can be detected by precise daily weights and measurements of serum osmolality. Caloric deprivation and catabolism usually accompany an acute critical illness. Because 5% intravenous glucose provides less than one-fourth of the basic caloric requirement of 100 to 120 kcal/kg/day, supplementary gastrointestinal feedings or intravenous alimentation is necessary when cardiopulmonary stability has been achieved. Infection and sepsis are the most common fatal complications that occur as a result of the treatment of acute cardiopulmonary failure; careful attention to handwashing by physicians and nurses and meticulous practice in the handling of airway connections, vascular puncture sites, and surgical wounds will reduce the incidence of bacterial contamination. Frequent changes of position, passive range of motion exercises, and judicious use of orthopedic splints serve to prevent skin pressure lesions and muscle contractures.

MONITORING

Commercially available adult monitoring systems can be adapted for continuous surveillance of infants and children. These systems should have bedside display units and appropriate alarms for heart rate, respiratory rate (impedance pneumograph), direct arterial and central nervous pressures (strain gauges), and body temperature (thermistor probe for esophagus or rectum). Cannulation of a peripheral artery (radial, femoral, dorsalis pedis, or posterior tibial) by percutaneous or cutdown technique permits continuous measurement of arterial pressure and frequent blood sampling for pH and blood-gas tensions as well as other data. Teflon-coated catheters appear to produce the least tissue reaction and least incidence of long-term arterial occlusion. Continuous infusion of a dilute heparin solution (1 ml/hr; 1 unit of heparin/ml) using a calibrated pump maintains patency of the cannula for many days without altering the pressure waveform.

Fluid and electrolyte balance is monitored in infants by measurements of hourly urine volume, accurate daily weights, frequent measurements of serum osmolality, pH, and electrolytes, and careful measurements of fluid intake and output. This is required in infants who need mechanical ventilatory support because application of CPAP and PEEP induces abnormal water retention. This renal dysfunction most probably is related to reduced intravascular volume (Priebe et al., 1981).

Continuous pulse oximetry provides an estimation of arterial hemoglobin saturation and reduces the likelihood of harmful transitory hypoxemic episodes due to disconnections or obstruction of gas lines or airways. Inspired oxygen concentrations are monitored continuously. Adequacy of alveolar ventilation is judged by end-expired carbon dioxide tension monitoring. These measurements can be made with low dead-space sampling devices and either an infrared analyzer or a mass spectrometer.

Quadrilumen, No. 5 French Swan-Ganz catheters may be inserted by percutaneous or cutdown techniques into the internal jugular or femoral veins of infants weighing over 5 kg. For infants who weigh under 5 kg, double-lumen, No. 3.5 French catheters can be used to measure pulmonary arterial and right atrial pressures. The quadrilumen catheter permits continuous measurements of central venous and pulmonary arterial pressures and intermittent measurements of pulmonary capillary wedge pressure, cardiac output by thermodilution, and mixed venous P_{O_2}. These measurements provide reliable data for determining preload of both the right and left ventricles and calculation of pulmonary and systemic vascular resistance. The mixed venous P_{O_2} reflects the adequacy of tissue perfusion; a measurement of less than 30 torr indicates inadequate cardiac output.

Small dedicated microcomputers that can be transported readily to the bedside or operating room are becoming useful adjuncts in the surveillance and assessment of critically ill infants. Various indices of cardiopulmonary performance such as pulmonary and systemic vascular resistance, stroke volume, cardiac work, physiologic shunt and dead space, arteriovenous oxygen difference, airway resistance, and dynamic pulmonary compliance can be calculated quickly according to predetermined programs from monitored and measured data. These data can be compared with normal values and expected treatment responses. Computers can also be used as "smart alarms" to detect ominous combinations of various analogue and digital signals. Eventually, computers may be used to initiate treatments, such as fluid infusions and drugs, in response to deviations in monitored measurements.

COMPLICATIONS

Airway Complications

Accidental tracheal extubation or obstruction of the tracheal airway by mucus or blood can be prevented by proper airway care and adequate humidification of inspired gas. Clinical signs of tracheal tube obstruction include suprasternal and subcostal retractions, lack of expansion of the chest with inspiration, flaring nares, restlessness, bradycardia, cyanosis, and inability to pass a suction catheter easily beyond the end of the tube. An obstructed tube is an emergency that must be treated immediately by aspiration of the oropharynx, removal of the tube, bag and mask ventilation with 100% oxygen, and reintubation.

Prolonged nasotracheal intubation has been associated with postextubation subglottic bands, tracheal granuloma, and fibrotic bands. The incidence varies considerably with different diseases and from one institution to another (Hatch, 1968; Striker et al., 1967). Subglottic obstruction occurs in 3 to 5% of children who are intubated over 24 hours (Hatch, 1968). These subglottic complications cause partial upper airway obstruction and may appear as late as 6 weeks after extubation. However, with the use of implant-tested polyvinylchloride tubes, atraumatic insertion, and an appropriate tracheal fit determined by "leak pressure," this complication may be less common.

Leak pressure provides a reliable method of matching artificial airway size to tracheal cross-sectional area and should be used to link the tightness of fit of tubes to laryngeal or tracheal damage (Finholt et al., 1985; 1986). However, data do not exist that enable identification of harmful conditions. Some studies suggest that tight-fitting tubes result in less postintubation stridor (Lee, 1980). We therefore assign the highest priority to choosing the artificial airway that ensures adequate ventilation.

Severe subglottic stenosis may respond to repeated subglottic dilatations at 1- to 2-month intervals with concomitant growth and development of the infant. When this proves to be ineffective and decannulation of the trachea cannot be accomplished, a tracheoplasty procedure should be considered.

Tracheostomy may lead to granuloma formation distal to the end of the tracheostomy tube and at the cephalad margin of the tracheostomy incision. Difficulties in extubation of small infants after tracheostomy result from instability of the anterior tracheal wall and granulomas. Tracheal stenosis secondary to tracheostomy is rare in infants and children because cuffed tracheostomy tubes are not used and the surgical technique does not involve excision of cartilage (Aberdeen and Downes, 1974). Severe tracheal stenosis may be improved with intermittent dilatations and growth; however, life-threatening stenosis requires resection of the stenotic segment and reanastomosis of the trachea or carina or both. Unfortunately, partial recurrence of stricture at the anastomosis site may occur.

Tracheomalacia with weakened or incomplete cartilaginous rings associated with vascular rings, tracheoesophageal fistula, or mediastinal masses can cause acute respiratory failure, requiring prolonged tracheal intubation or tracheostomy, and precludes early removal of the artificial tracheal airway. Although management of an infant tracheostomy at home is difficult, some patients improve with growth and can be successfully decannulated at age 18 months to 2 years. Others require surgery to provide external support of the flail tracheal segment (Johnston et al., 1980).

Pulmonary Complications

Major intrapulmonary complications are caused by infection, barotrauma, excessive pulmonary extravascular water, and oxygen toxicity.

Sudden deterioration in the circulatory status or blood-gas tensions of a patient who receives CPAP or mechanical ventilation requires immediate examination to exclude tension pneumothorax. The danger of pneumothorax is increased and interstitial emphysema may occur when peak airway pressure exceeds 40 cm H_2O or when CPAP exceeds 15 cm H_2O. Interstitial tears can occlude terminal bronchioles, blood vessels, and lymphatic channels (Srouji et al., 1981). If the patient survives, interstitial tearing may contribute to the development of interstitial peribronchiolar fibrosis that is associated with bronchopulmonary dysplasia.

Some infants who require prolonged mechanical ventilation retain water, which reduces Pa_{O_2}, with or without radiographic evidence of interstitial pulmonary edema. These infants require fluid restriction, diuretics, and sometimes albumin to improve Pa_{O_2} and the findings on the chest radiograph.

Prolonged exposure to high concentrations of oxygen can damage alveolar capillary membranes and produce congested edematous lungs with intra-alveolar hemorrhage and exudate (Deneke and Fanburg, 1980). Although concentrations of oxygen below 50% can probably be tolerated indefinitely by normal lungs, lungs that are immature or damaged by disease may be more sensitive to oxygen. Oxygen toxicity is suggested by increasing alveolar-arterial oxygen difference and the absence of pulmonary fluid accumulation. Use of the lowest concentration of inspired oxygen to prevent arterial hypoxemia is the best method to avoid pulmonary oxygen toxicity.

As a consequence of successful life support in the neonate and young infants over the past 25 years, a new disease entity, bronchopulmonary dysplasia, has developed in some infants who have survived the most severe forms of cardiopulmonary failure (Northway, 1979; Northway et al., 1967). In infants with congenital anomalies amenable to surgical correction (including cardiovascular defects) who require mechanical ventilation for more than 4 weeks, the incidence is approximately 4% (Ziegler et al., 1979). Factors contributing to BPD include the basic lung disorder; pulmonary immaturity; high inspired oxygen concentrations; interstitial emphysema; recurrent pulmonary infection; poor nutritional state; and persistence of these factors for more than 1 month. BPD is characterized by severe impairment of pulmonary mechanics and ventilation-perfusion mismatch (Loeber et al., 1980).

In a series of 193 infants with chronic respiratory failure treated since 1967, Downes and Pilmer (1993) reported a survival rate of 80% in children without congenital heart disease. Only 14% of those with heart disease survived. Once chronic respiratory failure developed, mechanical ventilation continued for an average of 12 months (Schreiner et al., 1987). Testing of patients who reached the age of 2 showed normal development to mild delay in 66%. Roughly the same proportion were successfully weaned from mechanical support and decannulated.

Infection

Infection is a major risk in the treatment of acute cardiopulmonary failure. Trauma to the tracheal mucosa, which is associated with catheter aspiration and inadvertent breaks in aseptic technique, is responsible for the high incidence of bacterial tracheitis and pneumonia. Because of possible emergence of virulent gram-negative pathogens or antibiotic-resistant strains, prophylactic antibiotics are not recommended, except in the immediate postoperative period. However, frequent cultures are obtained. If fever or new pulmonary infiltrates develop, a Gram's stain and culture of an airway aspirate should be obtained and appropriate antibiotics should be administered immediately.

Gram-negative septicemia is the most common fatal complication in infants who require prolonged respiratory support. The artificial airway and multiple intravascular catheters represent the routes of contamination, and the hands of professional personnel are the major vectors. The incidence of infection and sepsis can be reduced by careful handwashing technique using a bactericidal agent; limited examination of the patient by personnel not directly involved; strict aseptic practice in the handling of the patient's vascular catheters; correct care of the patient's skin; daily dressing changes; and daily changes of respiratory tubing and water containers.

An increase in the pH in gastric secretions by antacids or histamine-receptor antagonists may permit intestinal overgrowth with colonic flora and may increase the likelihood of pneumonia with enteric organisms (Cerra, 1988). In addition, intestinal translocation of enteric bacteria when gut hypoperfusion or malnutrition exists may be a factor in septicemia (Baker et al., 1987; Deitch, 1987).

Substituting mucosal barrier or cytoprotection for antacids and histamine-2 (H_2) blockers for modulation of gastric acidity, early and aggressive enteral nutrition and intestinal decontamination procedures may prove to be helpful in reducing the incidence of infections.

Other Complications

Fever and muscular work increase oxygen demand, carbon dioxide excretion, and cardiac output. If cardiac output is limited by cardiac disease, the circulation may not be adequate for the increased tissue metabolism. Fever, regardless of cause, should be controlled and appropriately and vigorously treated. Excessive muscular activity can be controlled by relief of pain, attention to the patient's comfort, sedation, and, occasionally, muscle relaxants.

PEEP increases intrathoracic pressure and reduces systemic venous return and cardiac output. PEEP may cause a shift to the left of the interventricular septum and may thus reduce left ventricular stroke work (Jardin et al., 1981). In infants, the effects of PEEP on cardiac output can be overcome usually by increasing blood volume; however, high central venous pressures can lead to acute hepatomegaly and ascites.

Other circulatory consequences of mechanical ventilation are seldom serious in infants and children. Hypocapnia (Pa_{CO_2} less than 25 torr) and alkalosis (pH over 7.5) may cause decreased cerebral blood flow and cardiac output; however, quantitative data are lacking, and no ill effects have been observed. However, inadequate alveolar ventilation has dire consequences.

Retinopathy of prematurity has been associated with prematurity and oxygen administration and leads to various degrees of visual impairment from mild myopia to blindness. Vascular maturity of the retina is not achieved until 48 weeks after conception. Because vascular immaturity is the dominant, predisposing factor to retrolental fibroplasia (Flynn, 1987) and oxygen is the major inciting factor, infants less than this age should be considered susceptible. Administration of raised inspired oxygen concentrations, however, is not absolutely necessary for the retinal damage to occur, because retrolental fibroplasia has been observed in infants who do not receive supplemental oxygen and in infants with cyanotic congenital heart disease (Kalina et al., 1972). The duration of abnormally high Pa_{O_2} necessary to produce this lesion remains undetermined; elevated Pa_{O_2} for as brief as 2 hours during anesthesia has been associated with retrolental fibroplasia (Betts et al., 1977). Although the disease is clearly multifactorial (Gunn et al., 1980), a consensus exists that a Pa_{O_2} compatible with appropriate cardiopulmonary adaptation and effective tissue oxygenation with a minimal risk of retrolental fibroplasia is between 60 and 80 torr (James and Lanman, 1976).

RESULTS OF RESPIRATORY SUPPORT

From July 1990 to June 1992, 1529 infants and children with respiratory failure were admitted to the pediatric intensive care unit of the Children's Hospital of Philadelphia. The outcome of these patients bore a direct relationship to their principal physiologic disturbance. The survival rate of those presenting with primary respiratory failure was 96.4%; those in whom respiratory failure was secondary to either circulatory or neurologic failure exhibited significantly less satisfactory outcomes (56.2 and 52.7% survival rates, respectively). Among survivors, nearly 1% have developed chronic respiratory failure, which is defined as requiring mechanical ventilatory support for more than 1 month.

SELECTED BIBLIOGRAPHY

Deneke, S. M., and Fanburg, B. L.: Normobaric oxygen toxicity of the lung. N. Engl. J. Med., 303:76, 1980.

A comprehensive review of the clinical, pathologic, biochemical, and pharmacologic aspects of human oxygen toxicity.

DiCarlo, J. V., and Steven, J. M.: Respiratory failure in congenital heart disease. Pediatr. Clin. North. Am., 41:525–542, 1994.

A recent clinical review of the topic with emphasis on the impact of various disease entities and methods of support on pulmonary mechanics.

Fishman, A. P., and Renkin, E. M. (eds): Pulmonary Edema. Bethesda, MD, American Physiological Society, 1979.

A comprehensive, scientific description of the anatomy, physiology, and pathology of pulmonary edema with reference to its clinical consequences. This monograph deserves the attention of any physician who is treating patients with cardiopulmonary failure.

Heymann, M. A., and Rudolph, A. M.: Effects of congenital heart disease on fetal and neonatal circulations. Prog. Cardiovasc. Dis., 15:115, 1972.

A concise description of the fetal and neonatal circulations and of the changes that occur at birth and in early infancy in normal infants and in those with common forms of heart disease.

Hirschl, R. B., and Bartlett, R. H.: Extracorporeal membrane oxygenation support in cardiorespiratory failure. Adv. Surg., 21:189, 1987.

The term *ECMO* is used to describe prolonged extracorporeal circulatory bypass via extrathoracic cannulation in patients who have acute, reversible cardiac or respiratory failure that has proved to be refractory to conventional medical or pharmacologic therapy. In this review, the history, techniques, indications, and results of the use of ECMO are considered in detail.

Inselman, L. S., and Mellins, R. B.: Growth and development of the lung. J. Pediatr., 98:1, 1981.

A comprehensive but concise review of the prenatal and postnatal growth and development of the normal lung. Excellent bibliography.

Polin, R. A., and Fox, W. W. (eds): Fetal and Neonatal Physiology. Philadelphia, W. B. Saunders, 1992.

An authoritative consideration of developmental human physiology of the fetus and neonate with special emphasis on respiratory and cardiovascular physiology.

Scarpelli, E. M. (ed): Pulmonary Physiology of the Fetus, Newborn and Child. Philadelphia, Lea & Febiger, 1975.

A concise, informative review of developmental morphology and physiology of the human cardiopulmonary systems by experts.

Scarpelli, E. M., Auld, P. A. M., and Goldman, A. S. (eds): Pulmonary Disease of the Fetus, Newborn and Child. Philadelphia, Lea & Febiger, 1978.

A logical and thorough approach to the pathophysiology, diagnosis, and management of the disorders that lead to respiratory failure in infants and children.

Weibel, E. R.: The Pathway for Oxygen. Cambridge, MA, Harvard University Press, 1984.

A thorough, logical treatise on the evolutionary, anatomic, and physiologic factors that contribute to the delivery of oxygen from the environment to the cell.

BIBLIOGRAPHY

Aberdeen, E., and Downes, J. J.: Artificial airways in children. Surg. Clin. North Am., 54:1155, 1974.

Addonizio, V. P., Jr., Strauss, J. F., III, Chang, L. G., et al.: Release of lysosomal hydrolases during simulated extracorporeal circulation. J. Thorac. Cardiovasc. Surg., 84:28, 1982.

Albert, M. S., Rahill, W. J., Vega, L., and Winters, R. W.: Acid-base changes in cerebrospinal fluid of infants with metabolic acidosis. N. Engl. J. Med., 274:719, 1966.

American College of Chest Physicians, American Thoracic Society (ACCP-ATS) Joint Committee on Pulmonary Nomenclature: Pulmonary Terms and Symbols. Chest, 67:583, 1975.

Ashbaugh, D. E., Bigelow, D. B., Petty, T. L., et al.: Acute respiratory distress in adults. Lancet, 2:319, 1967.

Autor, A. P., Frank, L., and Roberts, R. J.: Developmental characteristics of pulmonary superoxide dismutase: Relationship to idiopathic respiratory distress syndrome. Pediatr. Res., 10:154, 1976.

Baker, J. W., Deitch, E. A., Berg, R., et al.: Hemorrhagic shock impairs the mucosal barrier, resulting in bacterial translocation from the gut and sepsis. Surg. Forum, 38:73, 1987.

Bancalari, E., and Goldberg, R. N.: High-frequency ventilation in the neonate. Clin. Perinatol., 14:581–597, 1987.

Bancalari, E., Jesse, M. J., Gelband, H., et al.: Lung mechanics in congenital heart disease with increased and decreased pulmonary blood flow. J. Pediatr., 90:192–199, 1977.

Bartlett, R. H., Andrews, A. F., Toomasian, J. M., et al.: Extracorporeal membrane oxygenation (ECMO) for newborn respiratory failure: 45 cases. Surgery, 92:425, 1982.

Bartlett, R. H., Gazzaniga, A. B., Huxtable, R. F., et al.: Extracorporeal circulation (ECMO) in neonatal respiratory failure. J. Thorac. Cardiovasc. Surg., 74:826, 1977.

Bartlett, R. H., Gazzaniga, A. B., Jefferies, R., et al.: Extracorporeal membrane oxygenation (ECMO) cardiopulmonary support in infancy. Trans. Am. Soc. Artific. Intern. Organs, 22:80, 1976.

Bartlett, R. H., Gazzaniga, A. B., Toomasian, J., et al.: Extracorporeal membrane oxygenation (ECMO) in neonatal respiratory failure: 100 cases. Ann. Surg., 204:236, 1986.

Bartlett, R. H., Roloff, D. W., Cornell, R. G., et al.: Extracorporeal circulation in neonatal respiratory failure: A prospective randomized study. Pediatrics, 76:479–487, 1985.

Beattie, H. W., Evans, G., Garnett, E. S., et al.: Albumin and water fluxes during cardiopulmonary bypass. J. Thorac. Cardiovasc. Surg., 67:926, 1974.

Belani, K. G., Gilmour, I. J., and McComb, R. C.: Pre-extubation ventilatory measurements in newborns and infants. Anesth. Analg., 59:47, 1980.

Berman, L. S., Fox, W. W., Raphaely, R. C., and Downes, J. J.: Optimum levels of CPAP for tracheal extubation of newborn infants. J. Pediatr., 89:109, 1976.

Betts, E. K., Downes, J. J., Schaffer, D. B., and Johns, R.: Retrolental fibroplasia and oxygen administration during general anesthesia. Anesthesiology, 6:47, 1977.

Black, A. E., Hatch, D. J., and Nauth-Misir, N.: Complications of nasotracheal intubation in neonates, infants and children: A review of 4 years' experience in a children's hospital. Br. J. Anaesth., 65:461, 1990.

Bohn, D., Tamura, M., Perrin, D., et al.: Ventilatory predictors of pulmonary hypoplasia in congenital diaphragmatic hernia, confirmed by morphometric assessment. J. Pediatr., 111:423–431, 1987.

Brochard, L., Harf, A., Lorino, H., et al.: Inspiratory pressure support prevents diaphragmatic fatigue during weaning from mechanical ventilation. Am. Rev. Resp. Dis., 139:513, 1989.

Bush, A., Busst, C. M., Knight, W. B., and Shinebourne, E. A.: Comparison of the haemodynamic effects of epoprostenol (prostacycline) and tolazoline. Br. Heart. J., 60:141–148, 1988.

Cassin, S., Dawes, G. S., Mott, J. C., et al.: The vascular resistance of the foetal and newly ventilated lung of the lamb. J. Physiol., 171:61–79, 1964.

Cerra, F. B.: The multiple organ failure syndrome. In Gallagher, T. J., and Shoemaker, W. C. (eds): Critical Care. Fullerton, Society of Critical Care Medicine, 1988.

Chalon, J., Loew, D. A. Y., and Malebranche, J.: Effects of dry anesthetic gases on tracheobronchial and ciliated epithelium. Anesthesiology, 37:338, 1972.

Clark, R. H., Gerstmann, D. R., Null, D. M., et al.: High-frequency oscillatory ventilation reduces incidence of severe chronic lung disease in respiratory distress syndrome. Am. Rev. Respir. Dis., 141:A686, 1990.

Coceani, F., and Olley, P. M.: The response of the ductus arteriosus to prostaglandins. Can. J. Physiol. Pharmacol., 51:220, 1973.

Comroe, J. H.: Physiology of Respiration. Chicago, Year Book Medical Publishers, 1965.

Cook, C. D., and Motoyama, E. K.: Respiratory physiology in infants and children. In Smith, R. M. (ed): Anesthesia for Infants and Children, 3rd ed. St. Louis, C. V. Mosby Co., 1968.

Cook, C. D., Sutherland, J. M., Segal, S., et al.: Studies of respiratory physiology in the newborn infant. III: Measurements of mechanics of respiration. J. Clin. Invest., 36:440, 1957.

Dawes, G. S.: Foetal and Neonatal Physiology. Chicago, Year Book Medical Publishers, 1968.

Deitch, E. A., Winterton, J., and Berg, R.: The gut as a portal of entry for bacteremia: Role of protein malnutrition. Ann. Surg., 205:682, 1987.

Deneke, S. M., and Fanburg, B. L.: Normobaric oxygen toxicity of the lung. N. Engl. J. Med., 303:76, 1980.

DiCarlo, J. V., Dudley, T. E., Sherbotie, J. R., et al.: Continuous arteriovenous hemofiltration/dialysis improves pulmonary gas exchange in children with multiple organ system failure. Crit. Care Med., 18:822–826, 1990.

DiCarlo, J. V., Raphaely, R. C., Steven, J. M., et al.: Pulmonary mechanics in infants after cardiac surgery. Crit. Care Med., 20:22–27, 1992.

DiCarlo, J. V., and Steven, J. M.: Respiratory failure in congenital heart disease. Pediatr. Clin. North Am., 41:525–542, 1994.

Downes, J. J., Nicodemus, H. F., Pierce, W. S., and Waldhausen, J. A.: Acute respiratory failure in infants following cardiovascular surgery. J. Thorac. Cardiovasc. Surg., 59:21, 1970.

Downes, J. J., and Pilmer, S. L.: Chronic respiratory failure—Controversies in management. Crit. Care Med., 21(Suppl.): 363–364, 1993.

Downs, J. B., Klein, E. F., Sesautels, D., et al.: Intermittent mandatory ventilation. Chest, 64:331, 1973.

Drummond, W. H., Gregory, G. A., Hyman, M. A., et al.: The independent effects of hyperventilation, tolazoline, and dopamine on infants with persistent pulmonary hypertension. J. Pediatr., 98:603–611, 1981.

Duke, H. N., and Lee, G. de J.: The regulation of blood flow through the lungs. Br. Med. Bull., 19:71, 1963.

Dunhill, M. S.: Postnatal growth of the lung. Thorax, 17:329, 1962.

Ellison, L. T., Duke, J. F., and Ellison, R. G.: Pulmonary compliance following open heart surgery and its relationship to ventilation and gas exchange. Circulation, 35(Suppl. 1):217, 1967.

Engel, S.: Lung Structure. Springfield, IL, Charles C Thomas, 1962.

Epstein, R. A.: Sensitivities and response times of ventilatory assistors. Anesthesiology, 34:321, 1971.

Faix, R. G., Viscardi, R. M., DiPetro, M. A., et al.: Adult respiratory distress syndrome in full-term newborns. Pediatrics, 83:971, 1989.

Finholt, D. A., Audenaert, S. M., Stirt, J. A., et al.: Endotracheal tube leak pressure and tracheal lumen size in swine. Anesth. Analg., 65:667, 1986.

Finholt, D. A., Henry, D. B., and Raphaely, R. C.: The "leak" test—A standard method for assessing tracheal tube fit in pediatric patients. Can. Anaesth. Soc. J., 32:326, 1985.

Flynn, J. T.: Retinopathy of prematurity. Pediatr. Clin. North Am., 34:1487–1516, 1987.

Frantz, I. D.: High-frequency ventilation. Crit. Care Med., 21 (Suppl.):370, 1993.

Freed, M. D., Heymann, M. A., Lewis, A. B., et al.: Prostaglandin E₁ in infants with ductus arteriosus-dependent congenital heart disease. Circulation, 64:899, 1981.

Fuhrman, B. P., and Dalton, H. J.: Progress in pediatric extracorporeal membrane oxygenation. Crit. Care Clin., 8:191–202, 1992.

Fujiwara, T., Chinda, S., Watabe, Y., et al.: Artificial surfactant therapy in hyaline-membrane disease. Lancet, 1:55, 1980.

Gluck, L., and Kulovich, M. V.: Fetal lung development. Pediatr. Clin. North Am., 20:367, 1973.

Gortner, L.: Natural surfactant for neonatal respiratory distress syndrome in very premature infants: A 1992 update. J. Perinatol. Med., 20:409–419, 1992.

Greenspan, J. S., Wolfson, M. R., Rubenstein, S. D., and Shaffer, T. H.: Liquid ventilation of human preterm neonates. J. Pediatr., 117:106–111, 1990.

Gregory, G. A.: Respiratory Failure in the Child. New York, Churchill Livingstone, 1981.

Gregory, G. A., Edmunds, L. H., Jr., Kitterman, J. A., et al.: The effect of continuous positive pressure breathing on pulmonary and circulatory function after cardiac surgery in infants less than three months of age. Anesthesiology, 43:426, 1975.

Gregory, G. A., Herman, K., Phibbs, J. A., et al.: Treatment of the idiopathic respiratory-distress syndrome with continuous positive airway pressure. N. Engl. J. Med., 284:1333, 1971.

Gunn, T. R., Easdown, J., Outerbridge, E. W., and Aranda, J. V.: Risk factors in retrolental fibroplasia. Pediatrics, 65:1096, 1980.

Hagen, P. T., Scholz, D. G., and Edwards, W. D.: Incidence and size of patent foramen ovale during the first 10 decades of life: An autopsy of 965 normal hearts. Mayo Clin. Proc., 59:17–20, 1984.

Hall, J. B., and Wood, L. D. H.: Liberation of the patient from mechanical ventilation, J.A.M.A., 257:1621, 1987.

Hammerschmidt, D. E., Stroncek, D. F., Bowers, T. K., et al.: Complement activation and neutropenia occurring during cardiopulmonary bypass. J. Thorac. Cardiovasc. Surg., 81:370, 1981.

Hatch, D. J.: Prolonged nasotracheal intubation in infants and children. Lancet, 1:1272, 1968.

Hatch, D. J., Taylor, B. W., Glover, W. J., et al.: Continuous positive-airway pressure after open-heart operations in infancy. Lancet, 2:469, 1973.

Hazelzet, J. A., Petru, R., Den Ouden, C., and van der Voort, E.: New modes of mechanical ventilation for severe respiratory failure. Crit. Care Med., 21(Suppl.):366–367, 1993.

Heiss, K., Manning, P., Oldham, K. T., et al.: Reversal of mortality for congenital diaphragmatic hernia with ECMO. Ann. Surg., 209:225, 1989.

Heymann, M. A., and Rudolph, A. M.: Effects of congenital heart disease on fetal and neonatal circulations. Prog. Cardiovasc. Dis., 15:115, 1972.

Hicks, R. E., Kinney, T., Raphaely, R. C., et al.: Successful treatment of varicella pneumonia in a leukemic child with prolonged extracorporeal membrane oxygenation. J. Thorac. Cardiovasc. Surg., 73:297, 1977.

HIFI Study Group: High frequency oscillatory ventilation compared with conventional mechanical ventilation in the treatment of respiratory failure in preterm infants. N. Engl. J. Med., 320:88–93, 1989.

Hilding, A. C.: Regeneration of respiratory epithelium after minimal surface trauma. Ann. Otol. Rhinol. Laryngol., 74:903, 1965.

Hill, D., O'Brien, T. G., Murray, J. J., et al.: Extracorporeal oxygenation for acute post-traumatic respiratory failure (shock-lung syndrome): Use of the Bramson membrane lung. N. Engl. J. Med., 286:629, 1972.

Hirschl, R. B., and Bartlett, R. H.: Extracorporeal membrane oxygenation support in cardiorespiratory failure. Adv. Surg., 21:189, 1987.

Hislop, A., and Reid, L.: Development of the acinus in the human lung. Thorax, 29:90, 1974.

Hogg, J. C., Agarwal, J. B., Gardiner, A. J. S., et al.: Distribution of airway resistance with developing pulmonary edema in dogs. J. Appl. Physiol., 32:20–24, 1972.

Hogg, J. C., Williams, J., Richardson, J. B., et al.: Age as a factor in the distribution of lower-airway conductance and in the pathologic anatomy of obstructive lung disease. N. Engl. J. Med., 282:1283, 1970.

Inselman, L. S., and Mellins, R. B.: Growth and development of the lung. J. Pediatr., 98:1, 1981.

Ishii, M., Matsumoto, N., Fuyuki, T., et al.: Effects of hemodynamic edema formation on peripheral vs. central airway mechanics. J. Appl. Physiol., 59:1578–1584, 1985.

Jackson, J. C., Truog, W. E., Standaert, T. A., et al.: Effect of high-frequency ventilation on the development of alveolar edema in premature monkeys at risk for hyaline membrane disease. Am. Rev. Respir. Dis., 143:865–871, 1991.

James, S., and Lanman, J. T. (eds): History of oxygen therapy and retrolental fibroplasia. Prepared by the American Academy of Pediatrics, Committee on Fetus and Newborn. Pediatrics, 57:591, 1976.

Jardin, F., Farcot, J. C., Boisante, L., et al.: Influence of positive end-expiratory pressure on left ventricular performance. N. Engl. J. Med., 304:387, 1981.

Jardine, D. S., and Costarino, A. T.: Negative pressure ventilation for infants with respiratory failure after cardiac surgery. Paediatr. Anaesth., 2:45–50, 1992.

Jobes, D. R., Nicolson, S. C., Steven, J. M., et al.: Carbon dioxide prevents pulmonary overcirculation in hypoplastic left heart syndrome. Ann. Thorac. Surg., 54:150–151, 1993.

Johnston, M. R., Loeber, N., Hillyer, P., et al.: External stent for correction of secondary tracheomalacia. Ann. Thorac. Surg., 30:291, 1980.

Kalina, R. E., Hodson, W. A., and Morgan, B. C.: Retrolental fibroplasia in a cyanotic infant. Pediatrics, 50:765, 1972.

Karlberg, P.: Developmental anatomy and physiology of the lungs. In Cooke, R. E.(ed): The Biologic Basis of Pediatric Practice. New York, McGraw-Hill, 1968, pp. 283–295.

Katz, R.: Adult respiratory distress syndrome in children. Clin. Chest Med., 8:635, 1987.

Keszler, M., Donn, S. M., Bucciarelli, R. L., et al.: Multi-center controlled trial comparing high frequency jet ventilation and conventional mechanical ventilation in newborn infants with pulmonary interstitial emphysema. J. Pediatr., 119:85, 1991.

Kirby, R. R., Downs, J. B., Civetta, J. M., et al.: High level positive end expiratory pressure (PEEP) in acute respiratory insufficiency. Chest, 67:16, 1975.

Kirklin, J. K., Westaby, D., Blackstone, E. H., et al.: Complement and the damaging effects of cardiopulmonary bypass. J. Thorac. Cardiovasc. Surg., 86:845, 1983.

Lacaze-Masmonteil, T.: Pulmonary surfactant proteins. Crit. Care Med., 21(Suppl):376–379, 1993.

Lee, K. W., Dougal, R. M., Templeton, J. J., and Downes, J. J.: Selection of endotracheal tubes in infants and children. Abstracts of American Academy of Pediatrics Annual Meeting, Section on Pediatric Anesthesia, April, 1980.

Lees, M. H., Burnell, R. H., Morgan, C. L., and Ross, B. B.: Ventilation-perfusion relationships in children with heart disease and diminished pulmonary blood flow. Pediatrics, 42:778, 1968.

Lees, M. H., Way, R. C., and Ross, B. B.: Ventilation and respiratory gas transfer of infants with increased pulmonary blood flow. Pediatrics, 40:259, 1967.

Loeber, N. V., Morray, J. P., Kettrick, R. G., and Downes, J. J.: Pulmonary function in chronic respiratory failure of infancy. Crit. Care Med., 8:596, 1980.

Lucking, S. E., Fields, A. I., Mahfood, S., et al.: High-frequency ventilation versus conventional ventilation in dogs with right ventricular dysfunction. Crit. Care Med., 14:798, 1986.

Lyrene, R. K., and Truog, W. E.: Adult respiratory distress syndrome in a pediatric intensive care unit: Predisposing conditions, clinical course and outcome. Pediatrics, 67:790, 1981.

Manners, J. M., Monro, J. L., Edwards, J. C.: Corrective cardiac surgery in infants. Anaesthesia, 35:1149–1156, 1980.

Marchak, B. E., Thompson, W. K., Duffty, P., et al.: Treatment of RDS by high-frequency oscillatory ventilation: A preliminary report. J. Pediatr., 99:287, 1981.

Markestad, T., and Fitzhardinge, P. M.: Growth and development in children recovering from bronchopulmonary dysplasia. J. Pediatr., 98:597, 1981.

Meliones, J. N., Bove, E. L., Dekeon, M. K., et al.: High-frequency jet ventilation improves cardiac function after the Fontan procedure. Circulation, 84(Suppl. III):364–368, 1991.

Naik, S. K., Knight, A., and Elliott, M.: A prospective randomized study of a modified technique of ultrafiltration during pediatric open-heart surgery. Circulation, 84(Suppl. III):422–431, 1991.

National Heart, Lung and Blood Institute: Extracorporeal Support for Respiratory Insufficiency. Washington, D.C., U.S. Government Printing Office, 1979.

Nicodemus, H. F., and Downes, J. J.: Ventilatory alterations associated with operation for tetralogy of Fallot. Anesthesiology, 31:265, 1969.

Noble, W. H., Kay, J. C., and Obdrazalek, J.: Lung mechanics in hypervolemic pulmonary edema. J. Appl. Physiol., 38:681–687, 1975.

Northway, W. H. (ed): Workshop on bronchopulmonary dysplasia—National Heart, Lung and Blood Institute. J. Pediatr., 85:815, 1979.

Northway, W. H., Rosan, R. C., and Porter, D. Y.: Pulmonary disease following respiratory therapy of hyaline-membrane disease. N. Engl. J. Med., 276:357, 1967.

O'Rourke, P. P., Crone, R. K., Vacanti, J. P., et al.: Extracorporeal membrane oxygenation and conventional medical therapy in neonates with persistent pulmonary hypertension of the newborn: A prospective randomized study. Pediatrics, 84:957–963, 1989.

O'Rourke, P. P., Stolar, C. J. H., Zwischenberger, J. B., et al.: Extracorporeal membrane oxygenation: Support for overwhelming pulmonary failure in the pediatric population. Collective experience from the Extracorporeal Life Support Organization. J. Pediatr. Surg., 28:523–529, 1993.

Ortiz, R. M., Cilley, R. E., and Bartlett, R. H.: Extracorporeal membrane oxygenation in pediatric respiratory failure. Pediatr. Clin. North Am., 34:39–46, 1987.

Park, C. D., Nicodemus, H. F., Downes, J. J., et al.: Changes in pulmonary vascular resistance following closure of ventricular septal defects. Circulation, 39(Suppl. 1):193, 1969.

Parker, D. J., Karp, R. B., Kirklin, J. W., and Bedard, P.: Lung water and alveolar and capillary volumes after intracardiac surgery. Circulation, 45(Suppl. 1):139, 1972.

Peckham, G. J., and Fox, W. W.: Physiologic factors affecting pulmonary artery pressure in infants with persistent pulmonary hypertension. J. Pediatr., 93:1005–1010, 1978.

Penny, D. J., Hayek, Z., and Redington, A. N.: The effects of positive and negative extrathoracic pressure ventilation on pulmonary blood flow after the total cavopulmonary shunt procedure. Int. J. Cardiol., 30:128, 1991.

Phelan, P. D., and Williams, H. E.: Ventilatory studies in healthy infants. Pediatr. Res., 3:425, 1969.

Pollitzer, M. J., Whitehead, M. D., Reynolds, E. O. R., and Delpy, D.: Effect of electrode temperature and in vivo calibration on accuracy of transcutaneous estimation of arterial oxygen tension in infants. Pediatrics, 65:515, 1980.

Priebe, H., Heimann, J. C., and Hedley-Whyte, J.: Mechanisms of renal dysfunction during positive end-expiratory pressure ventilation. J. Appl. Physiol., 50:643, 1981.

Prielipp, R. C., McLean, R., Rosenthal, M. H., and Pearl, R. G.: Hemodynamic profiles of prostaglandin E₁, isoproterenol, prostacyclin, and nifedipine in experimental porcine pulmonary hypertension. Crit. Care Med., 19:60–67, 1991.

Ratliff, N. B., Young, W. E., Jr., Hackel, D. B., et al.: Pulmonary injuries secondary to extracorporeal circulation. J. Thorac. Cardiovasc. Surg., 65:425, 1973.

Reid, L. M.: The pulmonary circulation: Remodeling in growth and disease. Am. Rev. Respir. Dis., 119:531, 1979.

Reynolds, E. M., Ryan, D. P., and Doody, D. P.: Permissive hypercapnia and pressure-controlled ventilation as treatment of severe adult respiratory distress syndrome in a pediatric burn patient. Crit. Care Med., 21:944–947, 1993.

Rigatto, H.: Apnea. Pediatr. Clin. North Am., 29:1105–1116, 1982.

Roberts, J. D., Lang, P., Bigatello, L. M., et al.: Inhaled nitric oxide in congenital heart disease. Circulation, 87:447–453, 1993.

Robin, E., Cross, C. E., and Zelis, R.: Pulmonary edema. N. Engl. J. Med., 288:239, 1973.

Rubis, L. J., Stephenson, L. W., Johnston, M. R., et al.: Comparison of effects of prostaglandin E₁ and nitroprusside on pulmonary vascular resistance in children after open heart surgery. Ann. Thorac. Surg., 32:563, 1981.

Rudolph, A. M., and Yuan, S. Response of the pulmonary vasculature to hypoxia and H⁺ ion concentration changes. J. Clin. Invest., 45:399–411, 1966.

Sarnaik, A. P., and Lieh-Lai, M.: Adult respiratory distress in children. Pediatr. Clin. North Am., 41:337–363, 1994.

Scammon, R. E., and Norris, E. H.: On the time of obiteration of the fetal blood passages (foramen ovale, ductus arteriosus, ductus venosus). Anat. Rec., 15:165–180, 1918.

Scarpelli, E. M., Auld, P. A. M., and Goldman, A. S. (eds): Pulmonary Disease of the Fetus, Newborn and Child. Philadelphia, Lea & Febiger, 1978.

Schreiner, M. S., Downes, J. J., Kettrick, R. G., et al.: Chronic respiratory failure in infants with prolonged ventilator dependency. J. A. M. A., *258*:3398–3404, 1987.

Shimada, Y., Yoshiya, I., Tanaka, K., et al.: Crying vital capacity and maximal inspiratory pressure as clinical indicators of readiness for weaning of infants less than a year of age. Anesthesiology, *51*:456, 1979.

Sivan, Y., Mor, C., Al-Jundi, S., et al.: Adult respiratory distress syndrome in severely neutropenic children. Pediatr. Pulmonol., *8*:104, 1990.

Soifer, S. J.: Pulmonary hypertension: Physiologic or pathologic disease? Crit. Care Med., *21*(Suppl.):370–374, 1993.

Srouji, M. M., Buck, B., and Downes, J. J.: Congenital diaphragmatic hernia: Deleterious effects of pulmonary interstitial emphysema and tension extrapulmonary air. J. Pediatr. Surg., *16*:45, 1981.

Stalcup, J. A., Pong, L. M., Lipset, J. S., et al.: Gestational changes in pulmonary converting enzyme activity in the fetal rabbit. Circ. Res., *43*:705, 1978.

Stewart, S., III, Edmunds, L. H., Kirklin, J. W., and Allarde, R. R.: Spontaneous breathing with continuous positive airway pressure after open intracardiac operation in infants. J. Thorac. Cardiovasc. Surg., *65*:37, 1973.

Striker, T. W., Stool, S. E., and Downes, J. J.: Prolonged nasotracheal intubation in infants and children. Arch. Otolaryngol., *85*:210, 1967.

Truog, W. E., and Jackson, J. C.: Alternative modes of ventilation in the prevention and treatment of bronchopulmonary dysplasia. Clin. Perinatol., *19*:621–647, 1992.

University of Michigan ECMO Manual, Ann Arbor, MI.

Vincent, R. N., Lang, P., Elixson, E. M., et al.: Measurement of extravascular lung water in infants and children after cardiac surgery. Am. J. Cardiol., *54*:161–165, 1984.

Walker, L. K.: Use of extracorporeal membrane oxygenation for preoperative stabilization of congenital diaphragmatic hernia. Crit. Care Med., *21*(Suppl.):379–380, 1993.

Wallgren, G., Ganbrelle, F., and Koch, G.: Studies of the mechanics of breathing in children with congenital heart lesions. Acta Paedriatr. Scand., *49*:415, 1960.

Wanner, A.: Clinical aspects of mucociliary transport. Am. Rev. Respir. Dis., *116*:73, 1977.

Wessel, D. L.: Inhaled nitric oxide for the treatment of pulmonary hypertension before and after cardiopulmonary bypass. Crit. Care Med., *21*(Suppl.):344–345, 1993.

Wetzel, R. C., and Gioia, F. R.: High frequency ventilation. Pediatr. Clin. North Am., *34*:15–38, 1987.

Yates, A. P., Lindahl, S. G. E., and Hatch, D. J.: Pulmonary ventilation and gas exchange before and after correction of congenital cardiac malformations. Br. J. Anaesth., *59*:170, 1987.

Zapol, W. M., Snider, M. T., Hill, J. D., et al.: Extracorporeal membrane oxygenation in severe acute respiratory distress: A randomized prospective study. J. A. M. A., *242*:2193, 1979.

Ziegler, M. M., Shaw, S., Goldberg, A. I., et al.: Sequelae of prolonged ventilatory support for pediatric surgical patients. J. Pediatr. Surg., *14*:768, 1979.

Zwischenberger, J. B., Nguyen, T. T., Upp, R., et al.: Complications of neonatal extracorporeal membrane oxygenation. J. Thorac. Cardiovasc. Surg., *107*:838–849, 1994.

10 Cardiopulmonary Resuscitation

J. Scott Rankin

Cardiopulmonary arrest is an emergency common to all medical practice, and each physician should be knowledgeable about and proficient with resuscitation techniques. Most health care providers should gain experience with resuscitation methods through structured course work and also during supervised clinical emergencies. This chapter reviews current concepts in *cardiopulmonary resuscitation* (CPR) from both basic and clinical viewpoints.

HISTORICAL DEVELOPMENT

CPR has been described in various forms since antiquity. Reference to ancient Hebrew practices exists in the Bible (Rosen and Davidson, 1972), and Galen employed bellows to inflate the lungs of a dead animal (DeBard, 1980). During the 18th century, techniques for performing mouth-to-mouth ventilation were standardized, and in 1786, John Sherwin suggested that "the surgeon should go on inflating the lungs and alternately compressing the sternum" (Julian, 1975). Dr. Franz Koenig, professor of surgery at Göttingen, Germany, is credited as the father of external cardiac compression, reporting, in 1885, six successful resuscitations in humans (Jude et al., 1961). Further application of the closed chest technique was reported by Maas in 1892 (Jude et al., 1964), and Igelsrud successfully employed direct cardiac massage in 1901 (Keen, 1904). Crile (1914) studied adrenaline injections in the treatment of cardiac arrest and later applied this method on the battlefields of World War I. In 1947, Beck and associates reported the first successful internal electrical defibrillation, which was followed by the development of external cardioversion in 1956 (Zoll et al., 1956).

Kouwenhoven and co-workers (1960) initiated the modern era of CPR, by combining the techniques of mechanical ventilation, external cardiac massage, and electrical defibrillation, and this method soon became established clinically. In 1963, the American Heart Association formed the Committee on Cardiopulmonary Resuscitation, which currently publishes and periodically updates guidelines for CPR (American Heart Association, 1992). In recent years, a standardized approach to CPR has been emphasized and the importance of extensive training at the community level has been stressed. Experience indicates that large numbers of cardiac arrest victims can be salvaged by early and effective application of CPR followed by transport and appropriate hospital therapy.

ETIOLOGY

Approximately one million individuals experience acute myocardial infarction annually in the United States, and roughly half of this number die each year of ischemic heart disease. It is estimated that over 300,000 of these deaths occur before hospital admission, most commonly from sudden ventricular fibrillation. Experiences in coronary care units and supervised exercise programs indicate that many sudden death victims could be salvaged by immediate CPR and defibrillation at the scene. Thus, it is essential that a large portion of the public be trained to initiate CPR immediately and that paramedical teams be organized to respond with a defibrillator within 3 minutes. With this type of system, over 40% of out-of-hospital arrest victims with documented ventricular fibrillation can be resuscitated (Cobb et al., 1980; Copley et al., 1977; Eisenberg et al., 1979), and it is estimated that 100,000 lives could be saved annually by providing effective on-site CPR.

The most common cause of sudden cardiac arrest is ventricular fibrillation associated with ischemic heart disease (Cobb et al., 1980). Fibrillation may occur as the end result of cardiac decompensation after myocardial infarction or may be a primary electrical event occurring coincident with coronary thrombosis or transient coronary insufficiency. Early resuscitation in the last category may be associated with little permanent damage, and even in patients with coronary thrombosis, successful resuscitation now can be followed by definitive therapy, such as pharmacologic thrombolysis, coronary balloon angioplasty, or coronary artery bypass grafting (Tenaglia et al., 1991). Thus, the current availability of effective methods for treating acute ischemic heart disease makes successful resuscitation more important than ever. In addition, emphasis should also be placed on identifying ischemic heart disease patients who are at risk for sudden death and on applying appropriate therapy at an earlier stage (Cobb et al., 1980). Other primary cardiac causes of sudden death, such as ventricular tachycardia or fibrillation associated with left ventricular aneurysms or Wolff-Parkinson-White syndrome, can also be treated routinely with a high degree of success.

Another common cause of sudden cardiac arrest is inadequate ventilation or pulmonary gas exchange. The resultant hypoxia, hypercarbia, and systemic acidosis produce acute circulatory decompensation and ventricular fibrillation. Many such conditions are encountered in daily practice, such as suffocation, drowning, drug overdosage, foreign-body aspiration, electrocution, or hypoventilation from primary pulmonary or neurologic disease. Early recognition of acute pulmonary insufficiency is essential so that ventilatory support can be provided before the development of cardiac arrest. With adequate monitoring of (1) ventilatory patterns, (2) work of breathing, (3) mental alertness, (4) arterial blood gases, and (5) capillary pulse oximetry, respiratory support should be initiated before cardiac decompensation occurs.

The final general causes of cardiopulmonary arrest are metabolic disorders. Hyperkalemia leading to ventricular fibrillation or asystole is associated with a very low rate of recovery and is best treated by prevention. Whenever the serum potassium approaches 6.0 mg/dl or the rate of increase in serum potassium is rapid, aggressive therapy with intravenous glucose (25 g) and insulin (20 units) or sodium bicarbonate (44 mEq) is indicated. At that point, the situation can be assessed further, the cause corrected, and ion exchange resin therapy (Kayexalate) or dialysis initiated. Other metabolic disturbances such as hypocalcemia or metabolic acidosis are more rarely associated with cardiac arrest, but these should also be treated at an early stage, before circulatory standstill occurs.

Independent of the causative factor, cardiopulmonary arrest is manifested by ineffective cardiac output and arterial blood pressure. Cessation of oxygenated blood flow to the body is associated with rapid progression of tissue hypoxia and acidosis. Because of high metabolic demands, the central nervous system is most vulnerable and can tolerate no more than 5 to 7 minutes of normothermic ischemia in adults before permanent neurologic injury ensues. After longer arrest periods, successful resuscitation may produce recovery of other organs, but return of central nervous system function is unlikely. Thus, one important goal of initial CPR is to preserve neurologic integrity until cardiac function can be restored.

DIAGNOSIS

The diagnosis of cardiac arrest should be considered whenever a previously alert patient collapses or becomes unconscious. The first step in approaching the problem is direct questioning and documenting total loss of consciousness. In addition, complete arrest is usually accompanied by initial tonic muscular movements and rolling back of the eyes. After transient agonal respiratory motion, spontaneous breathing stops if the sequence progresses untreated. In a mechanically ventilated patient, thoracic motion and breath sounds obviously persist after cardiac arrest, and respiratory movements are of little help. If ventilator malfunction is suspected, the patient should be removed from the ventilator and manually ventilated with 100% oxygen.

The presumptive diagnosis of cardiac arrest is made whenever a previously palpable central arterial pulse is lost. Palpation of either the carotid or the femoral artery is adequate to establish the diagnosis, and in monitored patients, loss of the electrocardiogram or arterial pressure waveform can confirm. Occasionally, patients continue to have a normal-appearing electrocardiogram, even though the pulse is absent and systolic blood pressure is severely diminished. In this event, resuscitation should be initiated anyway, because of ineffective circulatory performance. On more than one occasion, however, resuscitation has been instituted because electrocardiographic leads became disconnected or for other erroneous reasons. Inappropriate resuscitation should be avoided whenever possible by approaching each patient slowly and thoughtfully. A 15-second period of careful diagnostic attention, including the documentation of absent pulses, is prudent. In emergency situations, the tendency is often to proceed with haste; however, a short evaluation does not delay therapy significantly, and the potentially harmful complications of an unnecessary resuscitation can be avoided. This concept is especially important in postoperative cardiac surgical patients, in whom chest compression can produce sternal disruption, suture line hemorrhage, or perforation of the ventricles by artificial valves. Conversely, if arrested circulation is firmly indicated, one should not hesitate to begin resuscitation while further evaluation is pursued. Coincidentally, a call for help is issued, since effective CPR requires the coordinated efforts of multiple individuals.

RESUSCITATION METHODS

As defined by the subcommittee on Emergency Cardiac Care of the American Heart Association, CPR can be divided into two categories: basic life support and advanced life support. During in-hospital resuscitation, basic and advanced techniques are not distinct but proceed simultaneously. For the sake of clarity, however, each is discussed individually as if used sequentially.

Basic Life Support

Ventilation

After cardiac arrest is diagnosed, initial efforts are directed toward maintaining cardiopulmonary function and flow of oxygenated blood to the body. If evidence exists of isolated airway obstruction, such as produced by meat impaction of the larynx, a combination of back blows and abdominal thrusts frequently can dislodge the impaction (American Heart Association, 1992). Otherwise, the patient is placed supine in a hospital bed or on the ground. With a complete cardiopulmonary arrest, the mouth is opened and inspected; foreign objects such as dentures or chewing gum are removed. An airway is established by extending the neck and tilting the victim's head backward. If difficulty is encountered in opening the airway, the jaw can be extended by applying forward pressure behind the mandibular angles. Ventilation is begun with a valved mask system, taking care to maintain an airtight seal around the face. If a mask is unavailable, mouth-to-mouth breathing is employed while the patient's nostrils are occluded with one hand. With either technique, respirations should be delivered at 12 to 15 breaths per minute.

Ventilatory pressure should be great enough to raise the chest and produce satisfactory breath sounds, but not forceful enough to distend the stomach. Gastric dilatation can produce vomiting, aspiration, and long-term pulmonary complications. Mask ventilation is entirely satisfactory in most cases, and intubation should not be attempted until satisfactory mask ventilation has first been established and until trained personnel are available. Unsuccessful attempts at endotracheal intubation can diminish the chances of resuscitation or can directly injure the patient by lacerating the pharynx or vocal cords.

Endotracheal intubation of a semiconscious patient can be performed nasally, and this method may be preferred if ventilatory efforts are still present. In an arrest victim, intubation is accomplished orally with the aid of a laryngoscope. The blade of the laryngoscope is inserted into the mouth and upper pharynx while the instrument is held with delicacy (Fig. 10–1A). With steady forward pressure, the blade is advanced in the midline until the epiglottis comes into

view (Fig. 10–1B). At that point, the laryngoscope is passed further until the tip lies behind the epiglottis, and the entire tongue and mandible are elevated by a gentle upward and forward movement of the laryngoscope (Fig. 10–1C). Excessive force or a prying motion should never be necessary, and with proper technique, the glottis and vocal cords should come clearly into view just beyond the tip of the blade. It is often helpful to have a suction catheter available for clearing secretions. With the balloon cuff deflated, the endotracheal tube is passed precisely through the vocal cords into the upper trachea (Fig. 10–1D). Care is taken to advance the tube only 5 to 6 cm beyond the vocal cords, so that the right mainstem bronchus is not intubated. The cuffed endotracheal balloon is inflated until an airtight seal with the trachea is obtained, and the patient is ventilated manually throughout the resuscitation at 12 breaths per minute, preferably with 100% oxygen. Mechanical ventilatory support with a respirator is begun only after cardiovascular performance is stabilized.

Circulation

Before chest compression is begun in a patient with documented cardiac arrest, a precordial thump is delivered in an effort to restore cardiac rhythm. If the thump is unsuccessful, circulatory support is initiated with external cardiac massage. The patient is placed supine in the horizontal position, and a board or

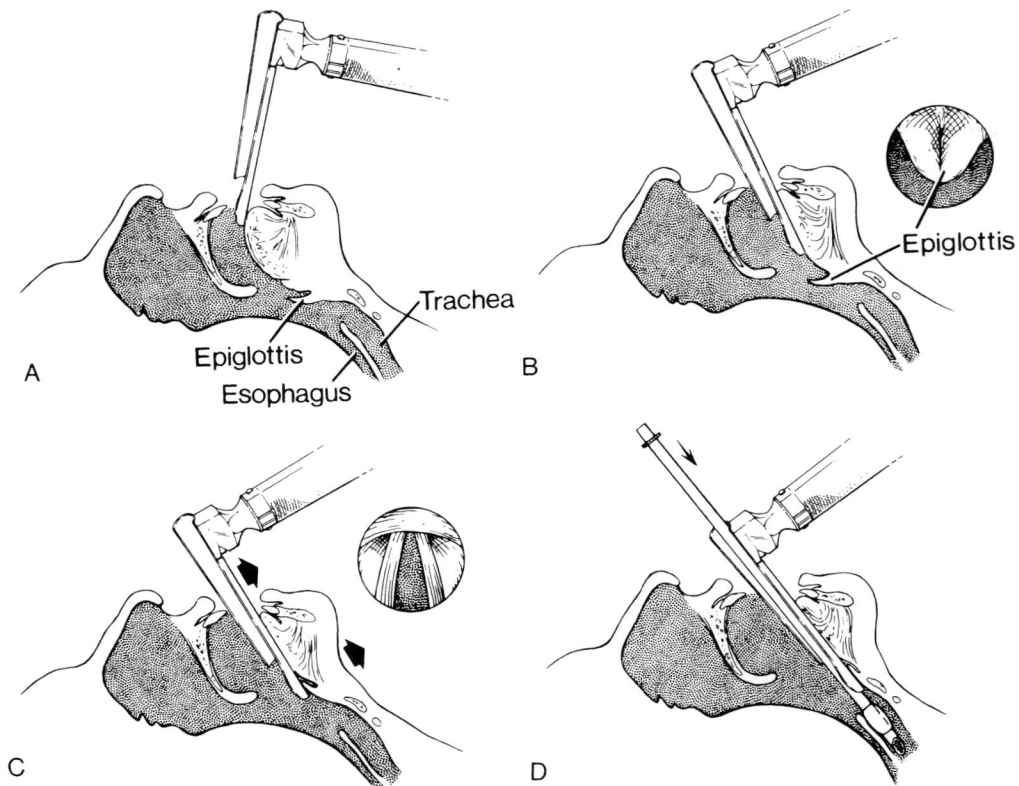

FIGURE 10–1. The standard technique of laryngoscopic endotracheal intubation. *A,* The laryngoscope is inserted into the mouth. *B* and *C,* The blade is advanced to expose the epiglottis and vocal cords. *D,* The trachea is intubated.

other rigid surface is interposed behind the back to provide support. The heel of one hand is placed over the other, and force is applied rhythmically over the lower half of the sternum (Fig. 10–2). The arms are locked to transmit the full momentum of the resuscitator's upper body to the patient's chest.

Although the topic of external chest compression has been somewhat controversial, recent studies have clarified many issues (Feneley and Rankin, 1988; Maier et al., 1984, 1986). First, systemic blood flow during manual external cardiac massage seems to be generated both by *direct* transmission of compression force to the heart through the chest wall (cardiac pump) and by *indirect* transmission of force to the vasculature through an increase in intrathoracic pressure (thoracic pump) (Rudikoff et al., 1980). Although both mechanisms are operative in most situations, manual external chest compression seems to use primarily the *direct* or cardiac component. To illustrate the physiology of external chest compression, measurements of ventricular dimensions, aortic blood flow, and cardiac chamber pressures from an anesthetized dog are shown in Figure 10–3 in the control state *(left panels)* and during CPR with an arrested circulation *(right panels)*. Several important principles are evident. First, a flattening of ventricular shape is observed with external massage, consistent with di-

rect chamber compression. Second, peak aortic flow velocity and stroke volume are reduced significantly during CPR as compared with control. Finally, peak ventricular and aortic pressures approach normal values with external compression, but diastolic and mean aortic perfusion pressures remain low because of reduced cardiac output. Thus, circulatory support provided by external cardiac massage is marginal at best.

Stroke volume during manual CPR seems to be optimized by chest compressions of high velocity, moderate force, and brief duration (high-impulse CPR). When compression rate is increased (Fig. 10–4), ventricular filling is not impaired, and in fact, the heart remains distended because of ineffective chamber emptying. Stroke volume stays constant with increasing manual compression rate, so that cardiac output and diastolic aortic pressure are significantly improved.

Coronary blood flow seems to occur primarily during noncompression or diastolic periods, and falls to zero or even slightly negative values during compression. This finding reflects a vascular waterfall phenomenon, in which pressure generated in the ventricular cavity resists coronary blood flow through the ventricular wall. Because of this finding, chest compression should be not prolonged but brief, to provide

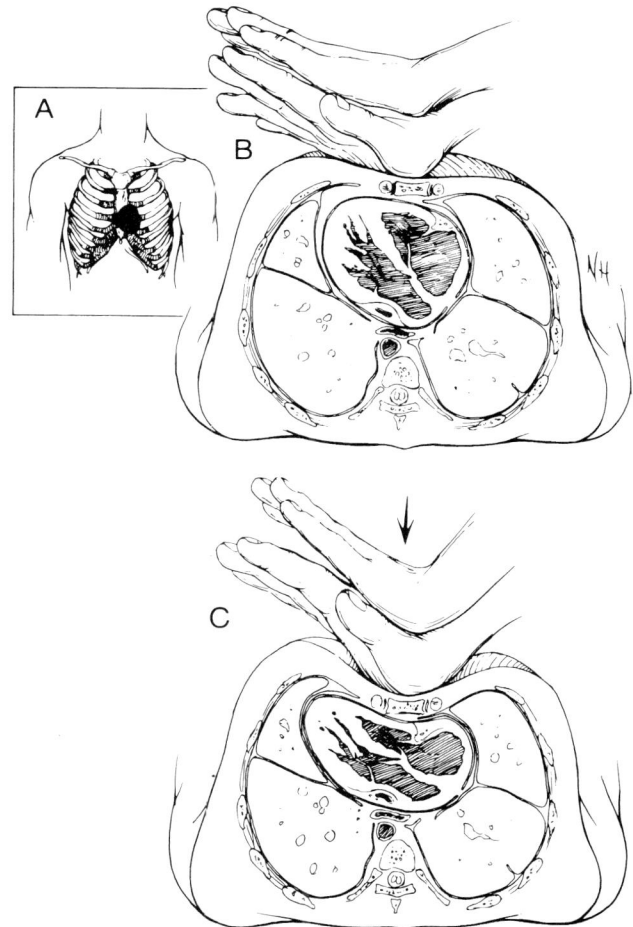

FIGURE 10–2. *A,* Manual compression is performed over the lower sternum. *B,* The position of the hands on the sternum is shown. *C,* External cardiac massage is performed with high-velocity compressions of moderate force and brief duration.

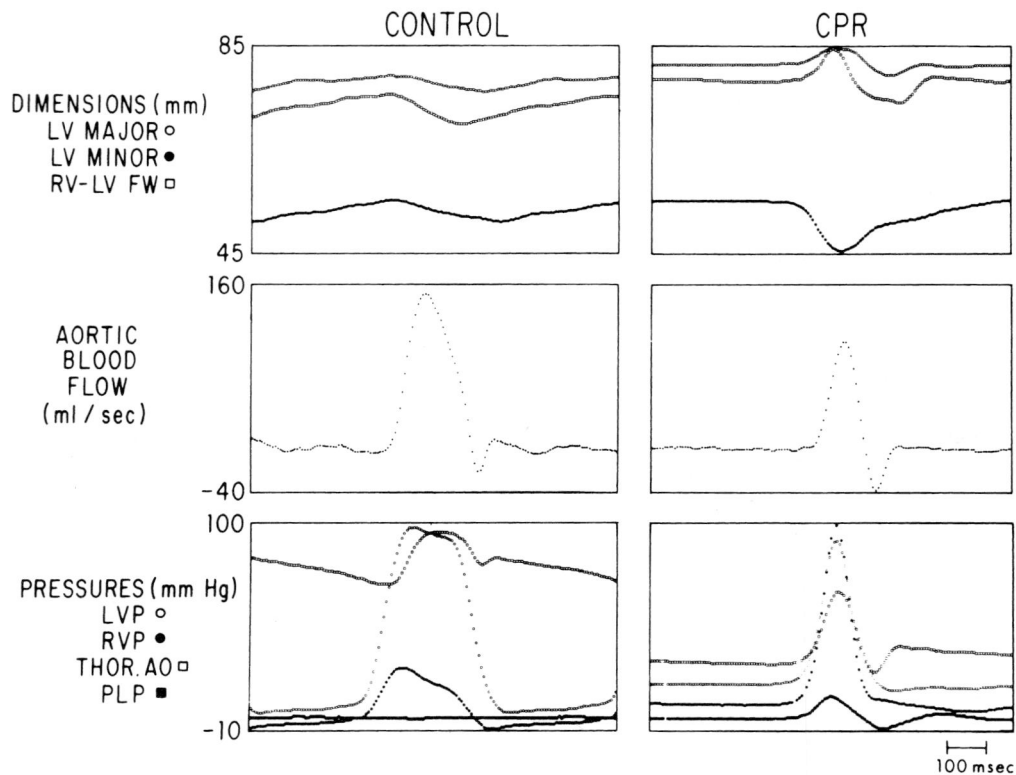

FIGURE 10–3. Digital measurements of left ventricular dimensions, aortic blood flow, and cardiac chamber pressures during control *(left panels)* and during cardiac pulmonary resuscitation (CPR) in the arrested state *(right panels)* in a chronically instrumented dog. LV = left ventricular; major = major axis diameter; minor = minor axis diameter; RV-LV FW = right-to-left ventricular free wall diameter; THOR. AO = thoracic aorta; PL = pleural; P = pressure.

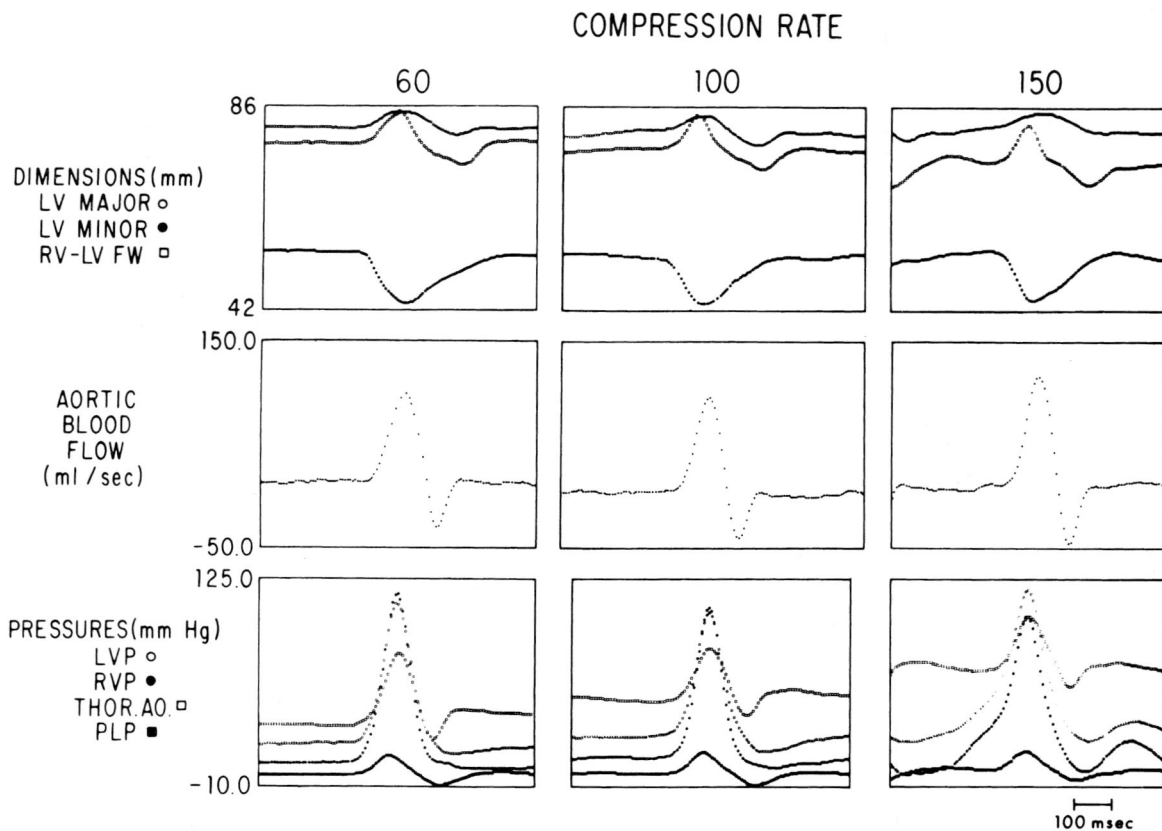

FIGURE 10–4. Representative digital data from a compression rate study in an arrested chronically instrumented dog. Rate of manual compression was varied from 60 to 100 to 150/min while compression force was held constant at moderate levels. Abbreviations are the same as in Figure 10–3. See text for details.

372

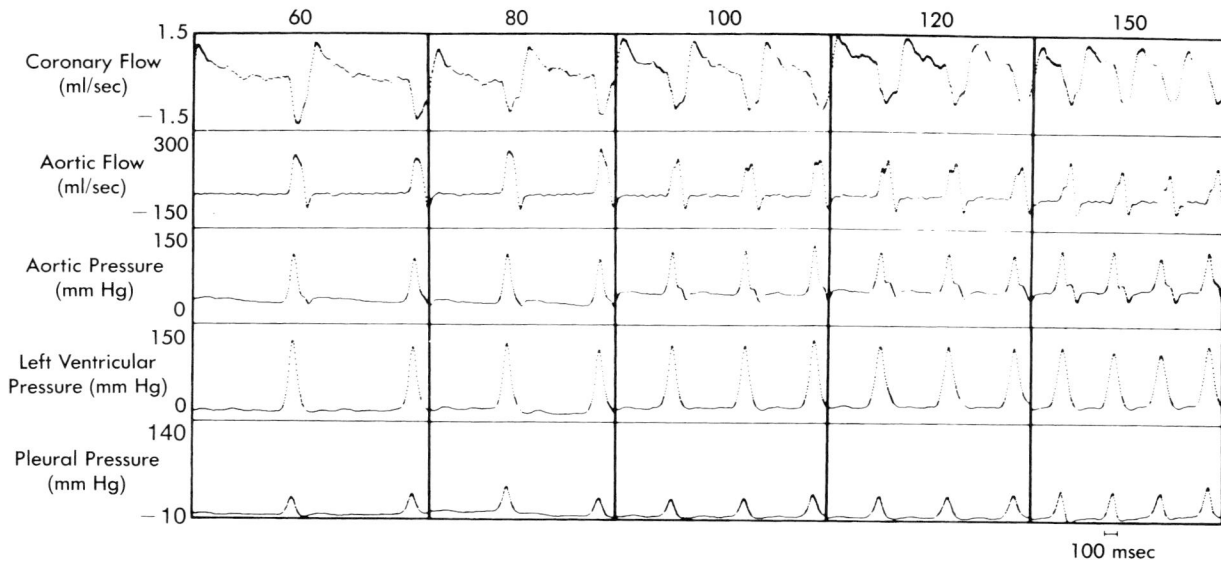

FIGURE 10–5. Coronary and aortic blood flow, and aortic, left ventricular, and pleural pressures measured in an arrested chronically instrumented dog during a high-impulse manual compression rate study. See text for details.

sufficient diastolic time for coronary perfusion (Dean et al., 1991; Wolfe et al., 1988). Increasing the rate of manual chest compression (Fig. 10–5) improves overall cardiac output, aortic perfusion pressure, and coronary blood flow velocity. However, diastolic perfusion time declines linearly with an increasing rate, so that total coronary blood flow is optimized at a manual compression rate of 100 to 120 per minute (Fig. 10–6). The values for coronary blood flow observed with high-impulse CPR at 120 per minute are the highest reported with any resuscitation technique, and improved coronary perfusion may be especially important in providing the best possible conditions for successful early defibrillation.

Mitral valve motion may be a key factor in optimizing hemodynamics during external cardiac massage. With the onset of sternal compression, both left ventricular and left atrial pressures rise as force is transmitted across the chest wall to the heart (Fig. 10–7). Soon into the compression phase, a pressure gradient develops from the left ventricle to the left atrium that is associated echocardiographically with mitral valve closure (Feneley et al., 1987). The aortic valve opens during compression to eject a "stroke volume," as illustrated in Figures 10–3 to 10–5. During the release phase, the aortic valve closes and maintains a coronary arterial perfusion gradient, while the mitral valve opens, allowing left ventricular filling. Thus, cardiac valve function during manual chest compression is essentially physiologic, again supporting the importance of direct cardiac compression during manual CPR. Experimental and clinical studies have confirmed this principle (Hackl et al., 1990; Kuhn et al., 1991; Kuhn and Juchems, 1991). Significantly, mitral valve closure directs the transthoracic energy of compression into forward perfusion pressure and blood flow, maintaining the efficient unidirectionality of the circulation.

When manual external chest compression with the high-impulse technique is compared with other types of CPR (Fig. 10–8), the high-impulse method produces significantly better cardiac output, bracheocephalic blood flow, and coronary perfusion (Newton et al., 1988). As a result, early and late survival in dogs

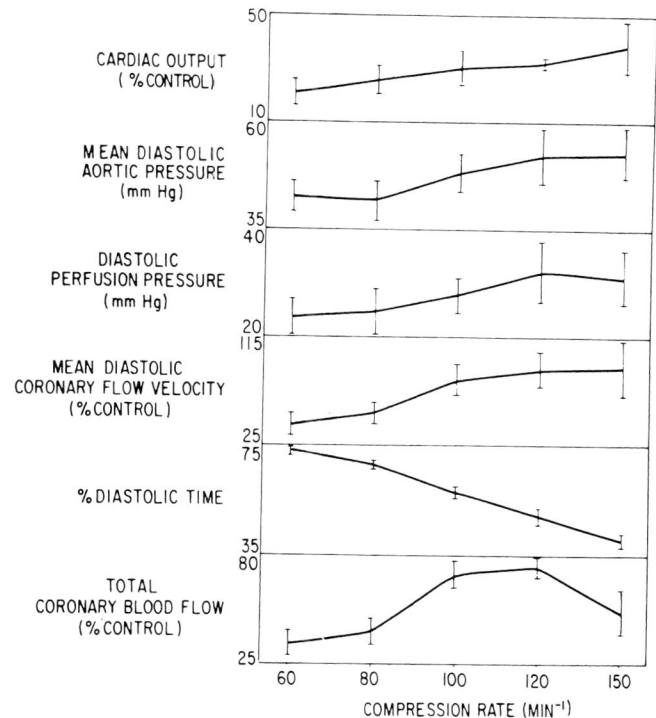

FIGURE 10–6. Cumulative hemodynamic data from a compression rate study (mean ± SEM). Changes in cardiac output, per cent diastolic time, and total coronary blood flow with each increase in compression rate were significant by multivariate analysis ($p < .05$). Changes in other parameters were not significant.

HIGH-IMPULSE COMPRESSION

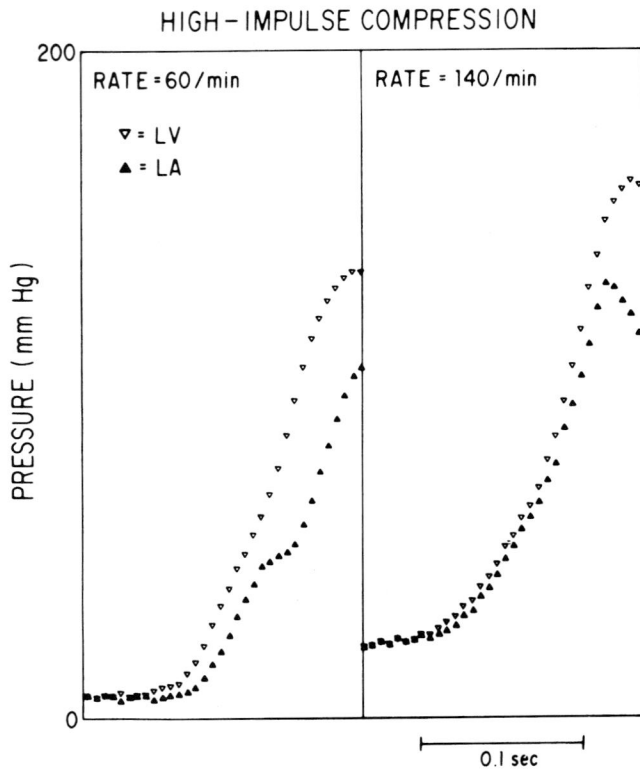

FIGURE 10–7. Segments of the left ventricular (LV) and left atrial (LA) digital pressure data points at 5-msec intervals from the early phase of two high-impulse chest compressions in the arrested dog model. *Both panels* demonstrate the early onset of a left ventriculo-atrial pressure gradient associated with mitral valve closure during compression and illustrate the maximal observed variation in the pattern of the gradient during early compression.

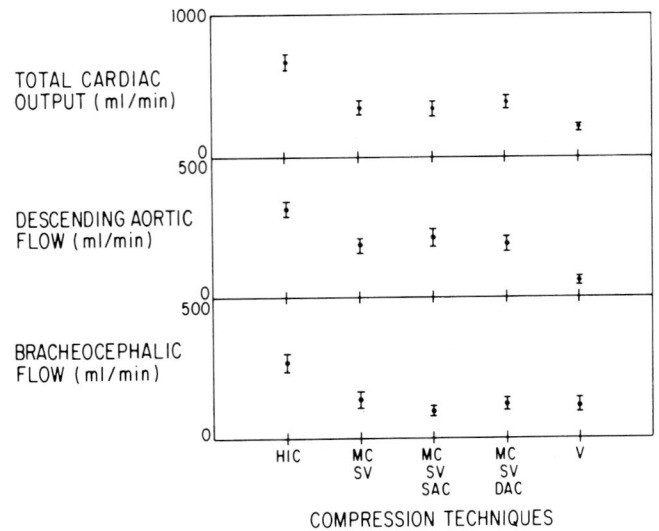

FIGURE 10–8. Mean ± SEM blood flow data from eight studies randomly comparing five chest compression methods during cardiac arrest. Methods other than HIC employed compression rates of 60/min and 50% duty cycles. HIC = high-impulse manual compression at 150/min; MC SV = mechanical compression and simultaneous ventilation; SAC = interposed systolic abdominal compression; DAC = interposed diastolic abdominal compression; V = pneumatic vest compression with simultaneous ventilation and abdominal compression.

arrested for 30 minutes is significantly improved with high-impulse CPR as compared with conventional methods at 60 per minute (Feneley et al., 1988) (Fig. 10–9). Again, the primary factors associated with improved survival seemed to be better cardiac output and mean coronary perfusion pressure (Fig. 10–10). Clinical reports have confirmed the importance of optimizing both of these variables (Paradis et al., 1990; Sanders et al., 1989). Additionally, hemodynamic observations in humans (Fig. 10–11) as well as end-tidal carbon dioxide concentrations during human CPR (Kern et al., 1992) have supported increasing the manual chest compression rate toward 120 per minute. Studies have also supported the clinical efficacy of CPR methods that emphasize direct cardiac compression rather than thoracic pump mechanisms (Krischer et al., 1989). These data led the American Heart Association to recommend brisk manual external chest compression during CPR at a rate of 100 per minute (American Heart Association, 1992).

In summary, available data suggest that sternal compression during manual CPR should be of *high velocity, moderate force,* and *brief duration.* A compression rate of *100 to 120 per minute* and a compression duration of 250 msec (50% duty cycle) have been shown to optimize cardiac output and coronary blood

flow. High-impulse techniques introduce a fatigue factor for the resuscitator, and with in-hospital arrests, frequent changes of personnel are required. In current practice, ventilations are interspersed randomly at 12 to 15 breaths per minute. Newer methods of chest compression, such as active compression-decompression, are currently under investigation, and these may further improve resuscitation rates in the future (Cohen et al., 1992a, 1992b).

In hospitalized arrest victims, effective circulatory dynamics occasionally cannot be achieved with external chest compression. In this case or if a question of pericardial tamponade exists, open chest cardiac

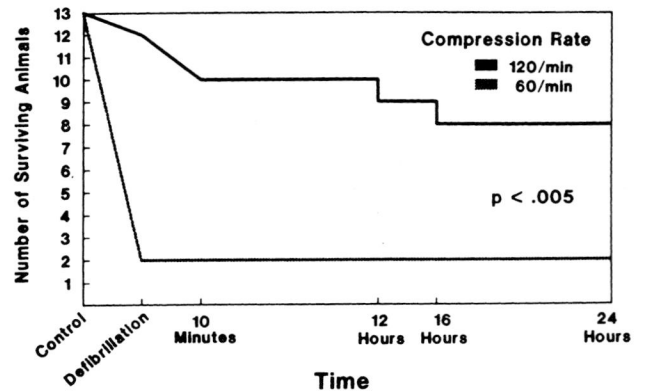

FIGURE 10–9. Comparison of 24-hour survival curves after manual CPR for 30 minutes at a compression rate of 60/min or 120/min in two groups of 13 dogs each. The *p* value refers to the statistical significance of the difference in survival between the two compression rates over the entire 24-hour observation period.

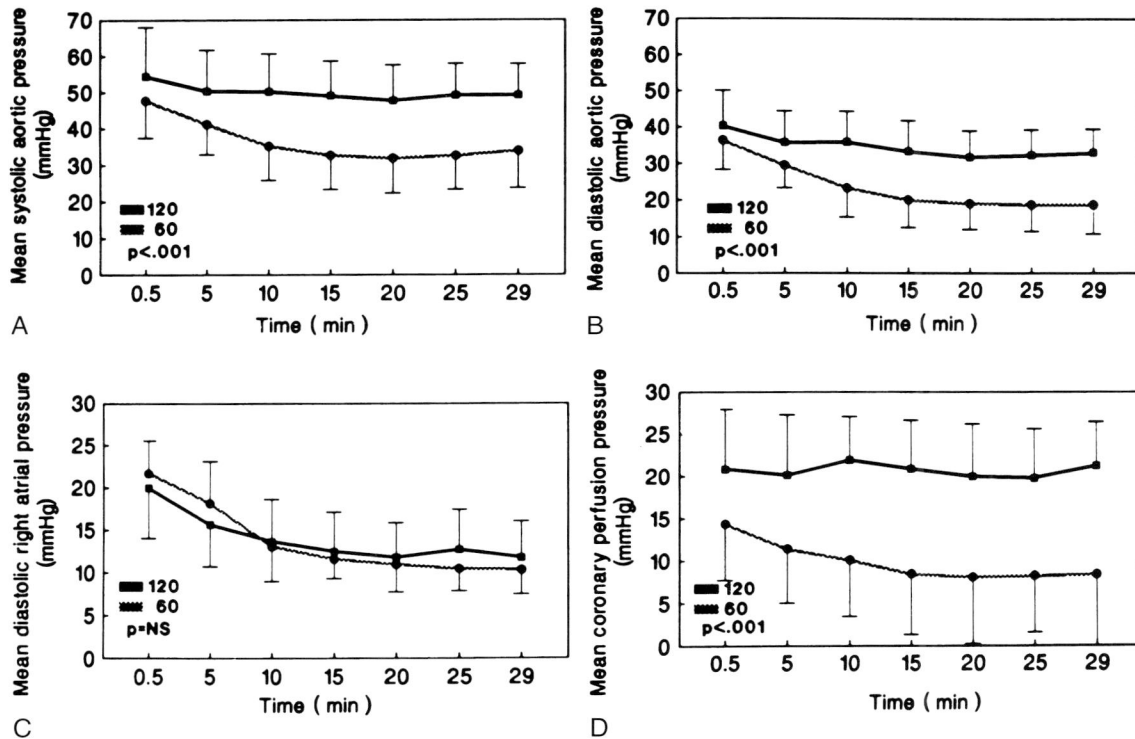

FIGURE 10–10. Mean ± SD hemodynamic data obtained during manual CPR for 30 minutes at a compression rate of 60/min or 120/min in two groups of 13 dogs each. *A,* The mean systolic aortic pressures. *B,* The mean diastolic aortic pressures. *C,* The mean diastolic right atrial pressures. *D,* The mean coronary perfusion pressures, which were maintained at a significantly higher level at a compression rate of 120/min because of the higher mean diastolic aortic pressures in this group; there was no significant difference between the mean diastolic right atrial pressures at 120/min and those at 60/min.

massage should be initiated. It has been clearly demonstrated that cardiac output and diastolic aortic perfusion pressure respond better to open chest techniques, and manual cardiac massage provides the ultimate direct cardiac compression. Open methods are commonly used when arrest occurs after cardiac surgery, where access to the heart is available through the sternotomy incision. In other situations, the left anterior side of the chest is entered surgically after application of antiseptic solution, and a rib retractor

FIGURE 10–11. Analogue femoral arterial pressure data from a patient undergoing manual external chest compression early after cardiac arrest. The *upper panel* represents a rate of 60/min, the *center panel* a rate of 100/min, and the *lower panel* a rate of 150/min. Mean and diastolic arterial pressures improved with increased compression rate.

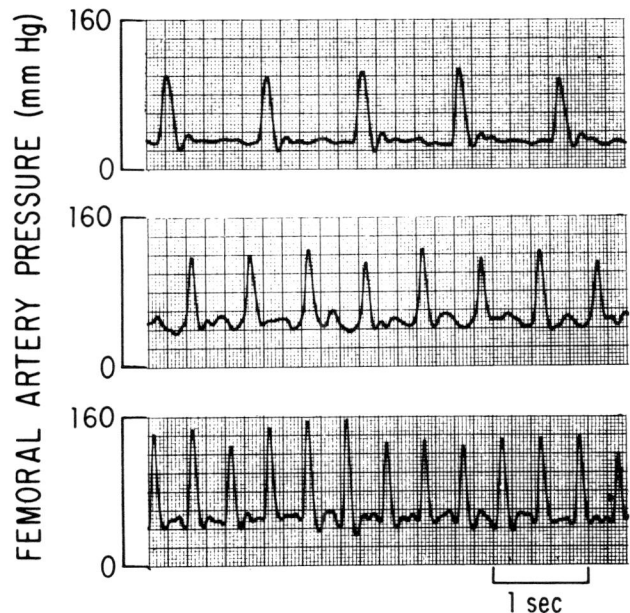

is inserted (Fig. 10–12). The heart is compressed directly by squeezing the ventricles with the hands, and pericardiotomy is not always necessary. Ventricular emptying is more complete with open massage, so that a compression rate of 60 to 80 per minute is used to allow adequate diastolic filling. Defibrillation is accomplished by direct application of cardioversion paddles to the heart; if resuscitation is successful, the patient is taken to the operating room for chest closure. A surprisingly low incidence of thoracic infection exists with this technique, and little is lost by converting to the open chest method. Data suggest that, after 10 to 15 minutes of unsuccessful closed chest CPR, one should convert to open chest resuscitation and that resuscitation success can be improved by this policy (Badylak et al., 1986; Kern et al., 1987a, 1987b; Paradis et al., 1992).

When cardiac arrest occurs in the community with only one witness, single-rescuer CPR can be performed after making a call for help. With the single-rescuer method, it is more difficult to optimize resuscitation conditions, since the same person performs mouth-to-mouth ventilation and external cardiac massage. Sternal compression proceeds at a rate of 80 to 100 per minute, and after each five compressions, two breaths are interposed by the rescuer during a brief pause in compressions. Needless to say, this method is not ideal and should be used only as a last resort. Finally, it should be emphasized that external cardiac massage is relatively ineffective, providing only 25 to 40% of the normal cardiac output, even under the best of conditions, and the primary goal of any resuscitation should be the restoration of a normal heartbeat.

Advanced Life Support

Because the cardiac output attainable with CPR is inadequate, efforts should be made primarily to restore intrinsic cardiac function as soon as possible. The senior physician or most experienced person takes charge of coordinating the care, and as the resuscitation continues, an electrocardiogram is obtained to document the cardiac rhythm. In most cases, the paddles of the defibrillator also serve as electrocardiographic electrodes, and the rhythm can be assessed initially without other equipment. If ventricular tachycardia or fibrillation is present, cardioversion is immediately attempted, using a maximal energy setting of 400 joules. Direct current countershock across the chest simultaneously depolarizes all myocardial cells and interrupts disorganized electrical activity. After repolarization, sinus node pacemaker activity resumes, and a coherent wavefront of depolarization spreads over the heart. Most defibrillators have two handheld paddles that are positioned to the right of the upper sternum and to the left of the nipple in the anterior axillary line. To maximize current transmission to the heart, a low-impedance gel is applied to the paddle-skin interface. Occasionally, placing one defibrillator paddle behind the back improves the efficacy of cardioversion. Chest compression should be discontinued for no more than 5 to 10 seconds during diagnosis or defibrillation. To diminish the chances of inadvertent electrical shock, all personnel should stand well away from the patient during defibrillation. If initial attempts are unsuccessful, CPR is continued, and further interventions to improve the chances of cardioversion are initiated. During complex resuscitations or after defibrillation, a standard electrocardiograph monitor should also be employed.

Venous access is obtained by inserting a large-bore plastic catheter into the subclavian or femoral vein or a large antecubital vein. If central or pulmonary artery lines are present, drugs are administered centrally to diminish the transit time to the coronary circulation. Because of the transit time, 10 to 20 seconds of CPR are provided after drug administration before further cardioversions are attempted. Periodically, CPR is discontinued briefly to assess changes in electrocardiographic rhythm and hemodynamics.

Restoration of coronary blood flow by CPR and correction of myocardial hypoxia and acidosis often improve the coarseness of fibrillation and make successful cardioversion more likely. Sodium bicarbonate is administered intravenously to correct metabolic acidosis. Arterial blood gases are drawn periodically to evaluate the adequacy of bicarbonate therapy as well as arterial gas exchange. Intravenous or intracardiac cardiotonic drugs such as calcium chloride and epinephrine may improve the success of defibrillation. Both drugs produce arterial vasoconstriction, which increases arterial blood pressure at a given cardiac output and thereby improves coronary blood flow. If ventricular tachycardia or fibrillation persists, intravenous antiarrhythmic agents may be helpful. Intravenous lidocaine or procainamide, or both, are employed as first-line drugs; in especially refractory cases, bretylium may be required. Detailed dosages

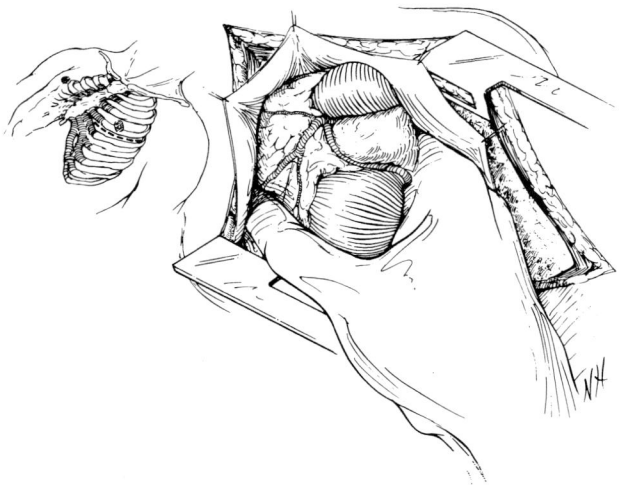

FIGURE 10–12. Open cardiac massage is performed through a short left anterior thoracotomy. The ventricles are compressed directly with the hands at 60 to 80/min.

and protocols for drug therapy are given elsewhere (American Heart Association, 1992).

If cardiac arrest occurs during induction of anesthesia for noncardiac operations, resuscitation is accomplished (using open chest techniques if necessary), and the operation is terminated. The patient is transferred to an intensive care unit where hemodynamics are monitored with a thermodilution Swan-Ganz catheter to measure pulmonary capillary wedge pressure and cardiac output. Once the patient is stabilized, a cardiologist is consulted, and coronary arteriography is considered when evidence of coronary artery disease exists. When cardiac arrest occurs during anesthetic induction for cardiac procedures, the operation is initiated immediately, and the patient is placed rapidly on cardiopulmonary bypass. Similarly, if arrest occurs after the conclusion of a cardiac operation, bypass is reinstituted as quickly as possible. When circulatory dynamics have been stabilized by the bypass circuit, the cause of the problem is investigated, and further therapy is initiated accordingly. In many ways, cardiopulmonary bypass is the ultimate resuscitation technique and should be used primarily whenever it is available. Percutaneous cardiopulmonary bypass support is being investigated for general cardiac arrest victims in several centers. Results have not been good to date (Rees et al., 1992) but may improve with technical refinements.

RESULTS

Two important factors that determine the success of resuscitation are the severity and reversibility of the patient's underlying disease and the time from arrest to defibrillation. With improved intensive care monitoring of high-risk patients with myocardial infarction, and with more rapid response times for defibrillation, the incidence of in-hospital sudden death from primary cardiac electrical events is now extremely low. In the overall hospital population, approximately half of the patients sustaining sudden cardiac arrest can be resuscitated, and half of these survive to discharge. Results obviously depend on the patient population, however, and are not as good in chronic medical patients with end-stage illness (Landry et al., 1992). Improved paramedical response times and better public education in immediate bystander CPR have enhanced resuscitation rates for outpatient arrests. With paramedical response times averaging 2.9 minutes in the Seattle program, 60% of out-of-hospital arrest victims were resuscitated and transported to the hospital for further evaluation. Half of this group survived to discharge (Cobb et al., 1980). Hospital management after admission is designed to diagnose and treat the underlying cause of the cardiac arrest. If ischemic heart disease is suspected, cardiac catheterization is recommended. For patients with coronary obstruction, the options of coronary thrombolysis, balloon angioplasty, and coronary artery bypass grafting offer excellent prospects for long-term survival.

External cardiac massage is associated with a significant incidence of costochondral fractures, and chest injury becomes more problematic with lengthening time of resuscitation. Occasionally, a flail sternal segment is produced that interferes with subsequent ventilatory function. Lacerations of the liver, spleen, lung, or other viscera can also occur. In patients after cardiac surgery, vascular suture line disruption, great vessel injury, or cardiac perforation should be considered. In victims of sudden cardiac arrest, however, these risks must be incurred if the patient is to be saved, and experienced personnel can minimize complications by exercising care with external chest massage. As shown experimentally (Maier et al., 1984), additional stroke volume is not generated by using excessive force, so that compressions performed with brief, high-velocity, high-frequency strokes and only *moderate* compression force are effective and potentially less injurious. Finally, adequate training and proficiency with other techniques, such as central line placement and intubation, minimize the well-known complications of these procedures.

Because CPR is ineffective in maintaining circulation, the chances of resuscitation diminish directly with time after arrest. Therefore, the goal of every resuscitation should be to restore the patient's own cardiac function as quickly as possible. As the time of arrest increases, progressive and generalized ischemic injury occurs throughout the body, causing permanent organ dysfunction and worsening vasodilatation. As systemic arterial resistance deteriorates, the aortic blood pressure attainable with CPR also diminishes, so that coronary and cerebral perfusion decline. Generally, persistent cardiac arrest after 1 hour of full CPR (including open chest techniques when feasible) is unlikely to be reversible, and resuscitation should be discontinued at that point.

CPR has evolved into a highly technical and effective form of therapy for sudden cardiopulmonary arrest. With acquisition of additional knowledge in future years and with better medical and community training, results should improve even further.

SELECTED BIBLIOGRAPHY

American Heart Association, Emergency Cardiac Care Committee and Subcommittees: Guidelines for cardiopulmonary resuscitation and emergency cardiac care. I: Introduction. J. A. M. A., *268*:2172, 1992.

This publication is an important reference on current topics in CPR. Detailed information about CPR techniques is given as well as exact dosage schedules for pharmacologic therapy. Every physician should be familiar with this paper.

Cobb, L. A., Werner, J. A., and Trobaugh, G. B.: Sudden cardiac death. I. Experience with out-of-hospital resuscitation. II. Outcome of resuscitation, management, and future directions. Mod. Concepts Cardiovasc. Dis., *49*:31, 1980.

This paper is a classic description of an extensive clinical experience with CPR by leaders in the field. Detailed information about current results of CPR is given along with recommendations for future development.

Kern, K. B., Sanders, A. B., Raife, J., et al.: A study of chest compression rates during cardiopulmonary resuscitation in humans. The importance of rate-directed chest compressions. Arch. Intern. Med., *152*:145, 1992.

This clinical study confirmed the importance of more rapid chest compression rates to hemodynamic support in humans. An excellent discussion of CPR mechanisms is provided.

Kouwenhoven, W. B., Jude, J. R., and Knickerbocker, G. G.: Closed chest cardiac massage. J. A. M. A., *173*:1064, 1960.

This paper initiated the modern era of CPR. The history of CPR to that date (1960) is given, as well as the original experimental data on modern closed chest cardiac massage. The methods of artificial ventilation, external chest compression, and external defibrillation were combined in five patients and reported for the first time. This landmark paper is highly recommended.

Maier, G. W., Tyson, G. S., Jr., Olsen, C. O., et al.: The physiology of manual external cardiac massage: High-impulse cardiopulmonary resuscitation. Circulation, *70*:86, 1984.

This article examines in detail the physiology of closed chest cardiac massage. Ventricular dynamics, cardiac output, and coronary blood flow were investigated during a variety of different compression techniques. In this study, the method of high-impulse chest compression was developed.

BIBLIOGRAPHY

American Heart Association, Emergency Cardiac Care Committee and Subcommittees: Guidelines for cardiopulmonary resuscitation and emergency cardiac care. I: Introduction. J. A. M. A., *268*:2172, 1992.

Badylak, S. F., Kern, K. B., Tacker, W. A., et al.: The comparative pathology of open chest vs. mechanical closed chest cardiopulmonary resuscitation in dogs. Resuscitation, *13*:249, 1986.

Beck, C. S., Pritchard, W. H., and Feil, H. S.: Ventricular fibrillation abolished by electric shock. J. A. M. A., *135*:985, 1947.

Cobb, L. A., Werner, J. A., and Trobaugh, G. B.: Sudden cardiac death. I. Experience with out-of-hospital resuscitation. II. Outcome of resuscitation, management, and future directions. Mod. Concepts Cardiovasc. Dis., *49*:31, 1980.

Cohen, T. J., Tucker, K. J., Lurie, K. G., et al.: Active compression decompression. A new method of cardiopulmonary resuscitation. Cardiopulmonary Resuscitation Working Group. J. A. M. A., *267*:2916, 1992a.

Cohen, T. J., Tucker, K. J., Redberg, R. F., et al.: Active compression decompression resuscitation: A novel method of cardiopulmonary resuscitation. Am. Heart J., *124*:1145, 1992b.

Copley, D. P., Mantle, J. A., Rogers, W. J., et al.: Improved outcome for prehospital cardiopulmonary collapse with resuscitation by bystanders. Circulation, *56*:901, 1977.

Crile, G.: Anemia and Resuscitation: An Experimental and Clinical Research. New York, Daniel Appleton & Co., 1914.

Dean, J. M., Koehler, R. C., Schlein, C. L., et al.: Improved blood flow during prolonged cardiopulmonary resuscitation with 30% cycle in infant pigs. Circulation, *84*:896, 1991.

DeBard, M. L.: The history of cardiopulmonary resuscitation. Ann. Emerg. Med., *9*:273, 1980.

Eisenberg, M. S., Gergner, L., and Hallstrom, A.: Cardiac resuscitation in the community: Importance of rapid provision and implication for program planning. J. A. M. A., *241*:1905, 1979.

Feneley, M. P., Maier, G. W., Gaynor, J. W., et al.: Sequence of mitral valve motion and transmitral blood flow during manual cardiopulmonary resuscitation in dogs. Circulation, *76*:363, 1987.

Feneley, M. P., Maier, G. W., Kern, K. B., et al.: Influence of compression rate on initial success of resuscitation and 24-hour survival after prolonged manual cardiopulmonary resuscitation in dogs. Circulation, *77*:240, 1988.

Feneley, M. P., and Rankin, J. S.: Mechanisms of blood flow during cardiopulmonary resuscitation: Analysis of recent experimental observations concerning the importance of the chest compression technique. *In* Califf, R. M., and Wagner, G. S. (eds): Acute Coronary Care in the Thrombolytic Era. Boston, Martinus Nijhoff, 1988.

Hackl, W., Simon, P., Mauritz, W., and Steinbereithner, K.: Echocardiographic assessment of mitral valve function during mechanical cardiopulmonary resuscitation in pigs. Anesth. Analg., *70*:350, 1990.

Jude, J. R., Kouwenhoven, W. B., and Knickerbocker, G. S.: Cardiac arrest. J. A. M. A., *128*:1063, 1961.

Jude, J. R., Kouwenhoven, W. B., and Knickerbocker, G. S.: External cardiac resuscitation. Monogr. Surg. Sci., *1*:59, 1964.

Julian, D. G.: Cardiac resuscitation in the eighteenth century. Heart Lung, *4*:46, 1975.

Keen, W. W.: A case of total laryngectomy (unsuccessful) and a case of abdominal hysterectomy (successful) in both of which massage of the heart for chloroform collapse was employed, with notes on 25 other cases of cardiac massage. Therap. Gaz., *28*:217, 1904.

Kern, K. B., Sanders, A. B., Badylak, S. F., et al.: Long-term survival with open chest cardiac massage after ineffective closed chest compression in a canine preparation. Circulation, *75*:498, 1987a.

Kern, K. B., Sanders, A. B., and Ewy, G. A.: Open chest cardiac massage after closed chest compression in a canine model: When to intervene. Resuscitation, *15*:51, 1987b.

Kern, K. B., Sanders, A. B., Raife, J., et al.: A study of chest compression rates during cardiopulmonary resuscitation in humans. The importance of rate-directed chest compressions. Arch. Intern. Med., *152*:145, 1992.

Kouwenhoven, W. B., Jude, J. R., and Knickerbocker, G. G.: Closed chest cardiac massage. J. A. M. A., *173*:1064, 1960.

Krischer, J. P., Fine, E. G., Weisfeldt, M. L., et al.: Comparison of prehospital conventional and simultaneous compression-ventilation cardiopulmonary resuscitation. Crit. Care Med., *17*:1263, 1989.

Kuhn, C., and Juchems, R.: Opening and closing movements of the heart valves in cardiopulmonary resuscitation. Confirmation of the cardiac pump theory. Dtsch. Med. Wochenschr., *116*:734, 1991.

Kuhn, C., Juchems, R., and Frese, W.: Evidence for the "cardiac pump theory" in cardiopulmonary resuscitation in man by transesophageal echocardiography. Resuscitation, *22*:275, 1991.

Landry, F. J., Parker, J. M., and Phillips, Y. Y.: Outcome of cardiopulmonary resuscitation in the intensive care setting. Arch. Intern. Med., *152*:2305, 1992.

Maier, G. W., Newton, J. R., Wolfe, J. A., et al.: The influence of manual chest compression rate on hemodynamic support during cardiac arrest: High-impulse cardiopulmonary resuscitation. Circulation, *74*(Suppl. IV):IV-51, 1986.

Maier, G. W., Tyson, G. S., Jr., Olsen, C. O., et al.: The physiology of manual external cardiac massage: High-impulse cardiopulmonary resuscitation. Circulation, *70*:86, 1984.

Newton, J. R., Glower, D. D., Wolfe, J. A., et al.: A physiologic comparison of external cardiac massage techniques. J. Thorac. Cardiovasc. Surg., *95*:892, 1988.

Paradis, N. A., Martin, G. B., and Rivers, E. P.: Use of open chest cardiopulmonary resuscitation after failure of standard closed chest CPR: Illustrative cases. Resuscitation, *24*:61, 1992.

Paradis, N. A., Martin, G. B., Rivers, E. P., et al.: Coronary perfusion pressure and the return of spontaneous circulation in human cardiopulmonary resuscitation. J. A. M. A., *263*:1106, 1990.

Rees, M. R., Browne, T., Sivananthan, U. M., et al.: Cardiac resuscitation with percutaneous cardiopulmonary support. Lancet, *340*:513, 1992.

Rosen, Z., and Davidson, J. T.: Respiratory resuscitation in ancient Hebrew sources. Anesth. Analg., *51*:502, 1972.

Rudikoff, M. T., Maughan, W. L., Effron, M., et al.: Mechanisms of blood flow during cardiopulmonary resuscitation. Circulation, *61*:345, 1980.

Sanders, A. B., Kern, K. B., Otto, C. W., et al.: End-tidal carbon dioxide monitoring during cardiopulmonary resuscitation. A prognostic indicator for survival. J. A. M. A., *262*:1347, 1989.

Tenaglia, A. N., Califf, R. M., Candela, R. J., et al.: Thrombolytic therapy in patients requiring cardiopulmonary resuscitation. Am. J. Cardiol., *68*:1015, 1991.

Wolfe, J. A., Maier, G. W., Newton, J. R., et al.: Physiologic determinants of coronary blood flow during external cardiac massage. J. Thorac. Cardiovasc. Surg., *95*:523, 1988.

Zoll, P. M., Paul, M. H., Linenthal, A. J., et al.: The effects of external electric currents on the heart. Control of cardiac rhythm and induction and termination of cardiac arrhythmias. Circulation, *14*:745, 1956.

11

Computer Applications in Cardiothoracic Surgery

Peter K. Smith

The development of the electronic computer was a complicated process in which the evolution of ideas (in logic and mathematics) generally preceded the development of suitable technology. Now, particularly in cardiothoracic surgery, technology is advancing more rapidly than the application of ideas.

The first application of an electronic computer, as we know it, was made in 1944. At that time, 200 individuals were used to calculate weapon trajectories for the Army Ordnance Department in order to solve a practical problem of war (Augarten, 1984). The Electronic Numerator, Integrator, Analyzer, and Computer (ENIAC), which was funded by the Army, eventually reduced the time required for this calculation to 20 seconds.

A useful analogy can be made to present-day problems of obtaining and manipulating data related to the practice of cardiac surgery. In his Presidential Address at the Twelfth Annual Meeting of The Western Thoracic Surgical Association, Peters (1987) summarized these problems:

Unfortunately, the ICU [intensive care unit] sheet is an exception to our usual totally disorganized methods of collecting and recording data. Our present clinical clerk and house staff training takes a select group of people with the most expensive education in the world and wastes their time in the pursuit of more trivia, scheduling procedures and collecting results. . . . House officers must have strong legs, know whom to telephone, be expert sleuths, and be good at diplomatic negotiations. These data are then stored in a record devised a century ago. . . . The academic curse of wasting the talents of these skilled trainees with our obsolete systems leads to the present myth of deans and hospital administrators that house staff are an expensive luxury. Exploiting and wasting the time and talents of house staff is expensive because it fosters abysmally inefficient hospitals and clinics.

Unfortunately, these thoughts remain true today despite tremendous progress in informatic hardware and ever-increasing demands for information. This chapter reviews accomplishments in computer applications related to the care of patients and emphasizes problems associated with cardiothoracic surgery. It also projects developments that are likely to be essential for continued progress in overall management of patients.

CURRENTLY FUNCTIONAL COMPUTER APPLICATIONS

Although the computer is widely accepted as a useful tool in almost all academic and professional environments and is conspicuous in most hospitals, there are surprisingly few generally accepted applications of computers in the care of patients. Even in academic medical centers, computer applications designed for the daily care of patients are limited.

Hospital Information Systems

Hospital information systems (HISs) have been implemented successfully in virtually all institutions. Their success has depended primarily on their ability to operate as accounting and inventory maintenance systems (Kwon et al., 1983). Installation has been widespread primarily because of the direct relationship between the funding of these computer applications and the limited goals on which they are based.

HIS operations generally involve a mainframe computer and many "dumb" terminals. The data are entered predominantly by nonmedical personnel with secretarial or accounting backgrounds who are reliable in a structured environment. System architecture and software development have been oriented toward maintaining database integrity and the hospital's balance sheet. Attempts to expand into the daily practice of medicine have had mixed results.

The underlying problems in this approach are exemplified in the processing of laboratory information by the *Duke Hospital Information System* (DHIS). The DHIS was established in 1975 and is a prototype for more than 60 systems marketed by International Business Machines (IBM) as *Patient Care Systems* (PCSs). It is now based on an IBM 3090-200 mainframe computer and has 550 terminals and 175 printers. It maintains information for almost 1000 inpatients daily and is the focal point for almost all service activities for patients (Kirby et al., 1987) (Fig. 11–1).

The following data steps occur in tracking a laboratory test from entry of the order to reporting of the result:

1. A handwritten order is entered by the physician.
2. The order is transcribed by a data terminal operator.

379

Duke Hospital Information System—Interactions

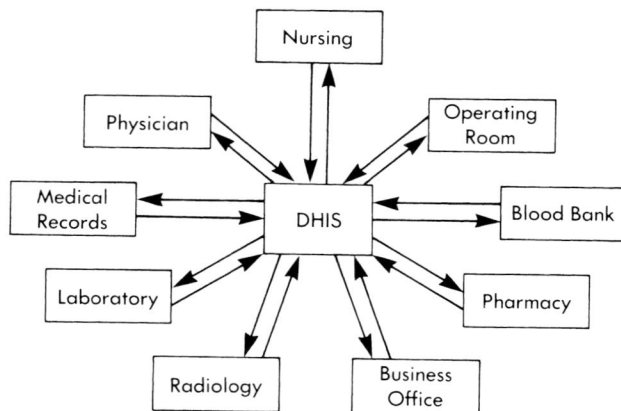

FIGURE 11–1. Diagrammatic representation of information flow in the Duke Hospital Information System (DHIS). Two-way communication for data transfer and query among departments is supported.

3. The order is transmitted to the laboratory. A routing sheet is printed locally for attachment to the sample, or the blood collection service is notified to collect and deliver the blood sample. A standard multiple chemistry test may be done in any one of many different locations (sublaboratories), depending on the time of day and the urgency of the test.

4. The test is done by an automated machine, and the results are assessed against internal laboratory standards. The data are then entered into a clinical laboratory information system.

5. The results are transferred to the HIS via a specialized interface.

6. The results are printed at the terminal that originated the order, and the printout is placed in the chart or in a local report bin.

From the hospital's point of view, the transaction is complete and satisfies all perceived needs. The hospital can show that the test was ordered and the blood was drawn. An audit trail can be followed if the result is erroneous or unavailable because of problems with the laboratory, the blood collection service, or the physician. Billing is ensured, and differential billing for the same test can be done because the sublaboratory that performed the test has been identified (e.g., a test in the "stat" laboratory may cost more than the same test in the routine laboratory). A hard copy of the results has been delivered to the originating nursing station, which absolves the "system" of responsibility for notification. Promptness of service can be checked by observation of the times of order entry, the sample receipt in the laboratory, and the report of results.

The inadequacies of this system begin with a question of time. From the physician's point of view, the actual time at which the blood sample was drawn and the delay in reporting the results are important. Because there is no standard method of notification, the physician must inspect the report bin (or the HIS itself through a terminal) periodically to obtain results. This system leads to an automatic and indeterminate delay, which is repeated for each different laboratory test ordered, regardless of whether the report contains normal or abnormal results. Physicians commonly delay daily report gathering until all results ordered are likely to be available.

The physician is then presented with the problem of analysis. The reports are not time-oriented or organized and are "noisy" (i.e., they contain irrelevant information). The physician is not concerned with such details as the machine that produced a particular set of results, which are of interest only to the accountant or the laboratory professional, and is not interested in which sublaboratory did the test, although the report of the results may differ greatly from sublaboratory to sublaboratory even when a test is done on the same machine. This extraneous information and lack of organization leave the physician with the task of organizing the data logically in terms of the diagnostic thought process and temporally for trend detection.

The HIS does not perform these processes for two fundamental reasons. First, it has not been considered important to organize the data (there is no monetary gain). Second, it is difficult to organize the data because the database was designed to optimize other goals. Generally, a system designed for a hospital's billing (wherein time is measured in days to weeks) would not respond in a time frame appropriate for the care of patients (wherein time is measured in minutes). Because the original goals of the HIS were not directly related to the care of patients and the need for such development was not considered, it is generally futile to expect such development to occur at the mainframe level. It is probably also erroneous to expect the original funding agency (the hospital) to agree to fund such efforts or to accept the diminution in accounting or inventory power that would accompany such a shift in emphasis.

An interesting irony of this example is that the laboratory information system (a departmental system) has built-in result-reporting capabilities that resolve many of the problems outlined above. Unfortunately, these features are not available to clinicians because they are lost in the data transfer to the HIS.

Clinical Databases

A clinical database can be described as a well-defined, discrete, and continuous series of data elements regarding patients (Pryor et al., 1985). These data elements are combined with descriptors of outcome and are well organized. Databases designed to aid in management have descriptors of the management process and emphasize care assistance for patients, data collection, report generation, and clinical research. Research databases collect descriptors that are useful for examining hypotheses, which are defined at the outset if possible.

Information is collected, entered, and stored as data

elements and is subsequently recalled for either individuals or groups. The four common features of a database (collection, entry, storage, and recall of data) have separate and conflicting attributes. In the process of data collection, it is necessary to decide which variables will be collected, the length of collection, and the methods of collection.

Data entry should use a coding system for time efficiency and clarification of data. Some flexibility in data entry is needed, but "free-text" data entry should be minimized. Data recall must be on-line, efficient, and rapid, and it must use common terminology.

In implementing clinical databases, clinicians or others trained in the clinical arena should be involved to ensure collection of appropriate data and to define long-term goals. Biostatisticians and computer scientists are needed to maintain the data structure and quality as well as the hardware and software. The paucity of common ground between information scientists and clinicians can lead to insurmountable communication problems and is a major impediment to implementation (Pryor et al., 1985).

Clinical databases have been implemented successfully when the emphasis has been on a well-defined medical problem and the impetus for establishing the database originates from the physician. With clearly defined objectives, the database can then be limited to data of medical importance. By limiting the patients involved, further simplification is possible.

TMR (The Medical Record)

At Duke University Medical Center, TMR was developed in 1975 to support both inpatient and outpatient services and the Cardiovascular Disease Databank (Hammond et al., 1980, 1983; Jelovsek, 1983; Stead et al., 1983a).

TMR has a modular design and contains demographic, financial, and appointment data, problem lists, procedures, subjective and physical findings, study results, and therapies. Data can be retrieved in problem-oriented, time-oriented, or encounter-oriented formats. The following six major groups use TMR:

Administration
Business office
Laboratory
Pharmacy
Nurses
Physicians

Despite their different needs, these groups demand access to all information, which supports the concept that a consolidated system is needed for computerization of the medical record (Stead and Hammond, 1983).

The system has interactive questionnaires and permits free-text entry, exclusive response from a list, or multiple responses from a list. Programming that is independent of data and applications is possible with the use of data definition tables or dictionaries. More than 90% of the data is coded. A nonprogrammer can

define the characteristics of a report using structured English (Hammond et al., 1984). TMR is currently linked to the DHIS through IBM personal computers with an immunoradiometric assay (IRMA) connection (Hammond and Stead, 1986).

A TMR workstation with a link to the DHIS can serve as the focal point in the development of a physician workstation (Kirby et al., 1987). Important aspects include time-oriented flow sheets, problem-oriented displays, and multiple formatting for the same data elements (Stead and Hammond, 1987).

TMR provides the means by which the Cardiovascular Disease Databank has been maintained at Duke University Medical Center. TMR is maintained on a VAX 6210 computer with 100 terminals. Information about all patients evaluated by the Division of Cardiology or the Division of Cardiothoracic Surgery is contained in 45,000 records. The operation of TMR, as compared with that of an HIS, emphasizes the medical meaning of data rather than administrative functions (Stead and Hammond, 1983).

TMR is being replaced by a networked microcomputer application for the Cardiovascular Disease Databank. The fundamental reason for this is that TMR has not withstood advancement at the same pace as commercial hardware and software and is deficient in the areas of database structure, user interface, and connectivity.

This replacement seems to be a natural outcome for many applications and occurs for both commercial products and those developed locally. Because resources for continued development cannot be allocated, many applications probably will be unable to survive transitions imposed by newly introduced technology.

Other Clinical Databases

The *Computer-Stored Ambulatory Record* (COSTAR) (Barnett et al., 1978) is designed to replace the traditional medical chart and to make information in the medical record more accessible to physicians. This system has administrative and research functions. Alternatives are the Regenstrief Medical Record System, which was developed in 1973 (McDonald, 1976), and the HELP system (Waki et al., 1982), which was developed at Latter-Day Saints Hospital with the assistance of the faculty of the University of Utah. HELP is a comprehensive computer system designed to provide clinical information, assist medical decision making, and perform administrative and research functions (Clayton et al., 1987).

Microcomputer Clinical Databases

The rapid evolution of microcomputer network applications is best exemplified by the Duke experience in developing an *Operating Room Information System* (ORIS).

Originally developed in 1983, as a microcomputer database, ORIS basically functioned as a repository for case information (demographic, procedural, and operative timing). Data input was centrally provided from data entry forms, and various reports (such as the operating room [OR] schedule) were generated. Data analysis was performed retrospectively, yielding statistics for volume and use. Procedural data were derived from centrally maintained data dictionaries.

In 1988, surgical scheduling was decentralized at the surgical division level, moving the responsibility for data dictionary maintenance to the various divisions. This produced better information content in the schedule at the expense of a cumbersome integration of divisional schedules into a master schedule.

In 1992, an intensive in-house development created a fully networked ORIS with features that yield the benefits of both distributed and centralized elements. As currently implemented, ORIS is composed of 70 microcomputer workstations located in all operating rooms, in all divisional offices, and in several administrative locations. The database is Sybase SQL Server, a client server database operating in an OS2 environment over the Medical Center's fiberoptic Common Services Network. An object-oriented programming language (SmallTalk Applications) was used to create the user front-end to the database.

All data are entered through a graphical user interface, and the vast majority of entries are codified from look-up tables using a pointing device (track ball or mouse) (Figs. 11–2, 11–3, and 11–4). The system is robust and permits real-time interaction of all users with the "live" database. Demographic information is provided through an interface with a dedicated server on the Common Services Network, which synchronizes the data for many patient care applications.

The "instantaneously correct" OR schedule is available at all ORIS workstations, which permits the scheduling process to be highly distributed. Divisions now are able to identify and use OR resources that were previously centrally controlled to prevent double-posting. Additionally, the OR schedule is continuously uploaded to the HIS to permit viewing and printing access for all Medical Center employees.

The National Library of Medicine

If practitioners attempted to keep up with the literature by reading two articles per day, by the end of one year, they would be 55 centuries behind.

Bernier and Yerkey, 1979

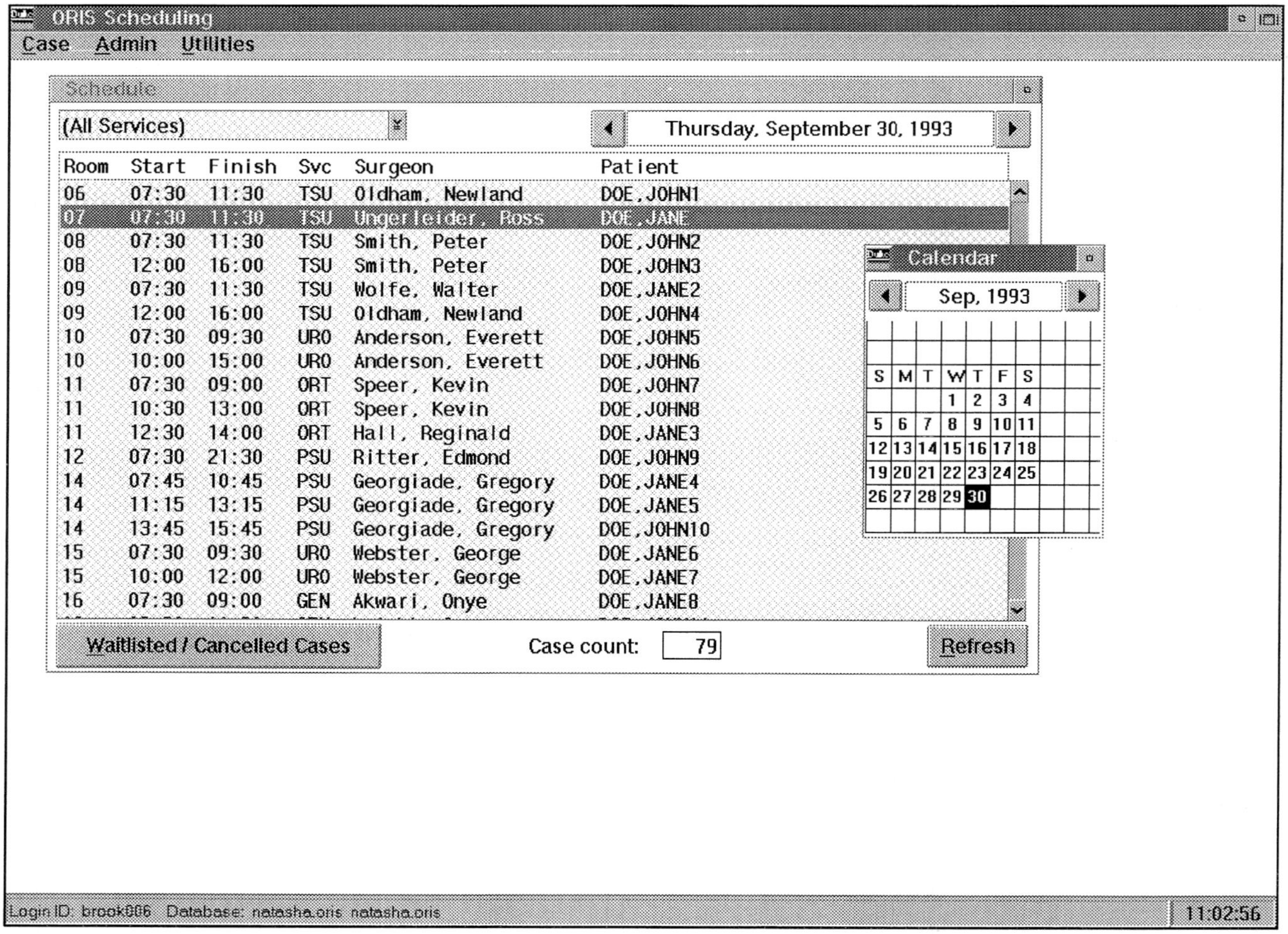

FIGURE 11–2. The basic "surgical list" screen within operating room information system (ORIS) scheduling. A pop-up calendar is used to select the date for display, which shows the operating schedule ordered by operating room and start time. A case is highlighted to show selection, which leads to the screen presented in Figure 11–3.

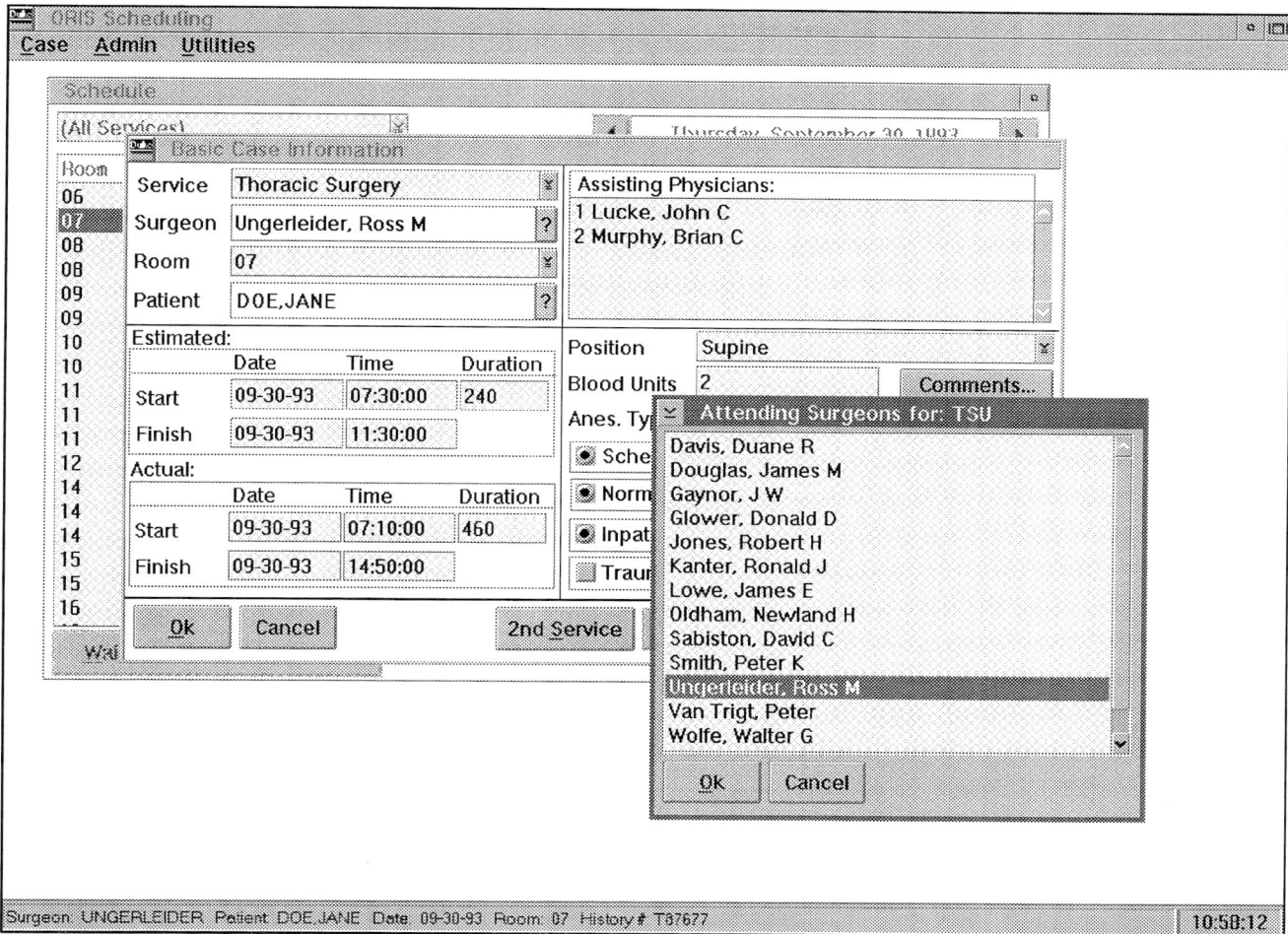

FIGURE 11–3. The basic case information, including assisting physicians and related time estimates. The attending surgeon is highlighted on a pop-up window, which leads to a window depicted in Figure 11–4 to select procedural and diagnostic information.

The medical literature contains a large and expanding database on the management of heart disease (Figs. 11–5 and 11–6). This information must be correlated with the information gathered for an individual patient, a process that involves the application of each physician's knowledge and thought to these data when acquired. This process cannot be accomplished by an unaided individual physician.

Gathering information for individual patients often requires reference to published material. Ideally, such reference and the material itself would be put in the medical record to document and justify diagnosis and therapy. In practice, it is impractical to locate appropriate information and impossible to place it in the record without assistance.

The databases (e.g., Medical Literature Analysis and Retrieval System [MEDLARS]) of the National Library of Medicine (NLM) can be accessed through a microcomputer, a telephone modem, and communication software. MEDlars onLINE (MEDLINE) can be accessed by using NLM's GRATEFUL MED software package, which helps the user to formulate a search with the almost 16,000 medical subject headings (MeSH) terms and submits the user's query as a batch directly to NLM computers. Other searching aids have been developed (Adams and Gray, 1987); with MicroMeSH, which was developed at the MGH Laboratory of Computer Science (Lowe and Barnett, 1987), the information (e.g., title, author, abstract) can be returned for local viewing and disk storage. Other resources include Paperchase (Bleich et al., 1985; Underhill and Bleich, 1986), Dialogue, BRS/Information Technologies, and miniMEDLINE (Broering, 1985).

Duke University Medical Center maintains a self-service network of electronic health sciences databases based on CD Plus Technologies hardware and software. A Unix server supports local storage of large volumes of data that are available through the Common Services Network or by telephone dial-in 24 hours per day. There are currently 5000 password holders performing an average of 314 sessions (105 session hours) each day.

Intensive Care Unit Computerization

Computer applications to the ICU have been divided into five broad areas (Martin and Jeffreys, 1987); computers are used

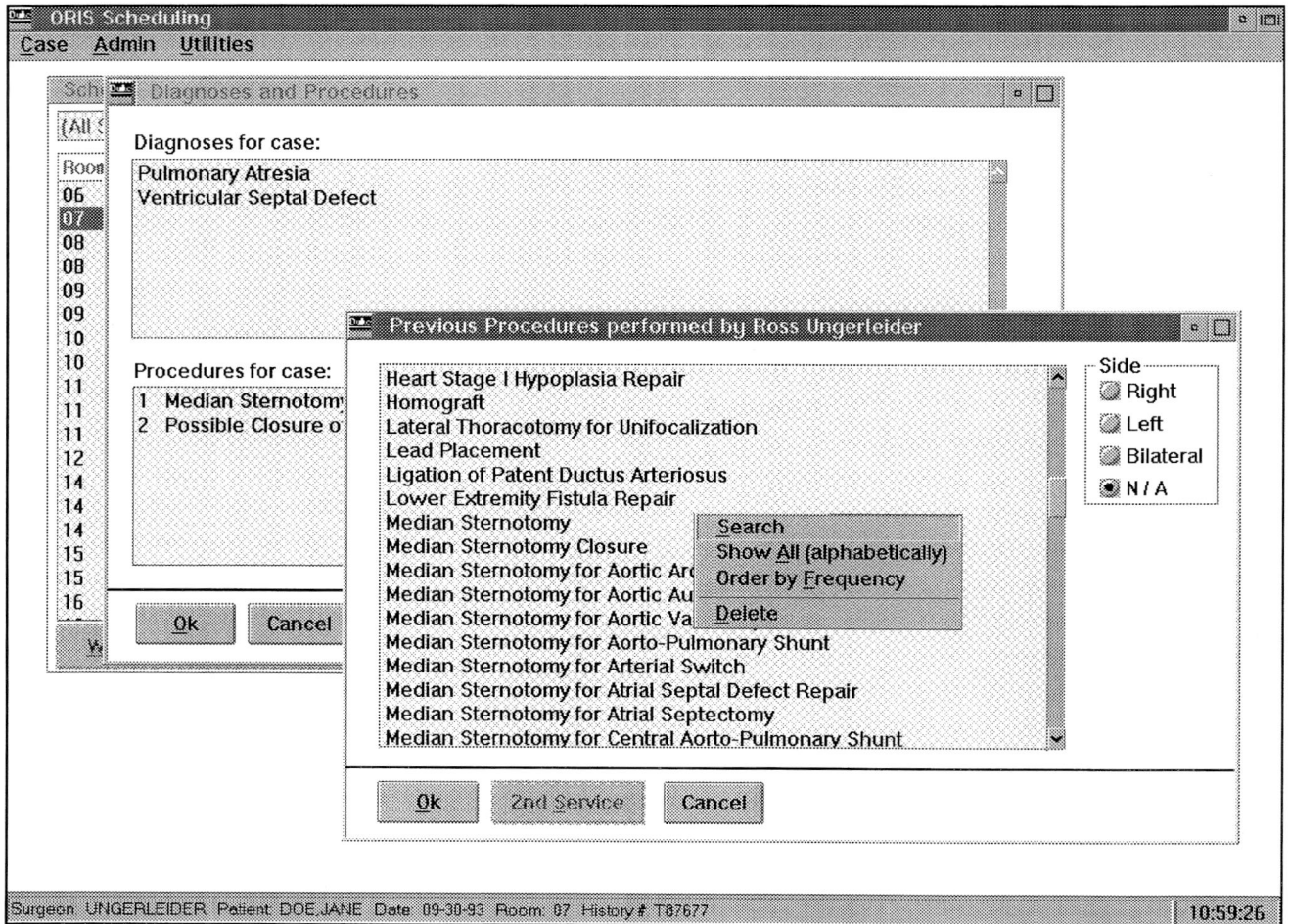

FIGURE 11–4. A pop-up window displays a historical list of procedures performed by the surgeon selected, which exist in a data dictionary. Behind this window, several diagnoses and procedures have been selected to be applied to the proposed operation.

1. For online monitoring of physiologic data
2. For controlling equipment
3. For communications with a hospital laboratory computer system
4. As terminals for commercial databases
5. As stand-alone machines to use with individual programs (e.g., pharmacologic interaction, blood-gas interpretation, hemodynamic calculation, tutorials, and intravenous dosage calculation)

Cardiac surgical ICUs were among the first to use computers to simplify the care of patients and decrease the need for specialized nursing support. Sheppard and Kirklin, at the University of Alabama at Birmingham, developed a centralized minicomputer system that has streamlined postoperative care. They first used the system for 124 patients from July 1, 1967, to March 15, 1968 (Sheppard et al., 1968). At the University of Alabama, the norm for postoperative nursing care is one nurse for every two patients. This is made possible in part by the timesaving online computer system. Although nurse staffing has not always been decreased by ICU computer installation, nursing efficiency almost always improves (Crew et al., 1987; Leyerle et al., 1985; Miller et al., 1978).

Many other institutions have installed computers in their ICUs (Glaeser et al., 1975; Goldwyn et al., 1971; Halford et al., 1987; Mortensen and Anderson, 1968; Osborn et al., 1968, 1969; Robicsek et al., 1977; Shubin et al., 1971; Shubin and Weil, 1966; Warner et al., 1968). Acceptance and implementation of computers in the future are expected for various reasons:

1. Continued application of cardiac surgical procedures is now being associated with the need to reduce the cost of care. The maintenance of a high level of critical care will require labor-saving and time-saving measures.
2. Computer systems improve the quality of intensive care and decrease the average length of stay in the ICU (Sheppard and Kouchoukos, 1977). Computer monitoring can detect critical low-probability events (Maloney, 1968) and has been associated with improved survival (Jurado et al., 1977).
3. The organization and storage of ICU information improve the education of physicians and nurses (Burridge and Skakun, 1983) and the ICU work environment (Hammond et al., 1991; Johnson et al., 1987).
4. The relationship between ICU resource use and

HEART 1976-1992
(total 387,007)

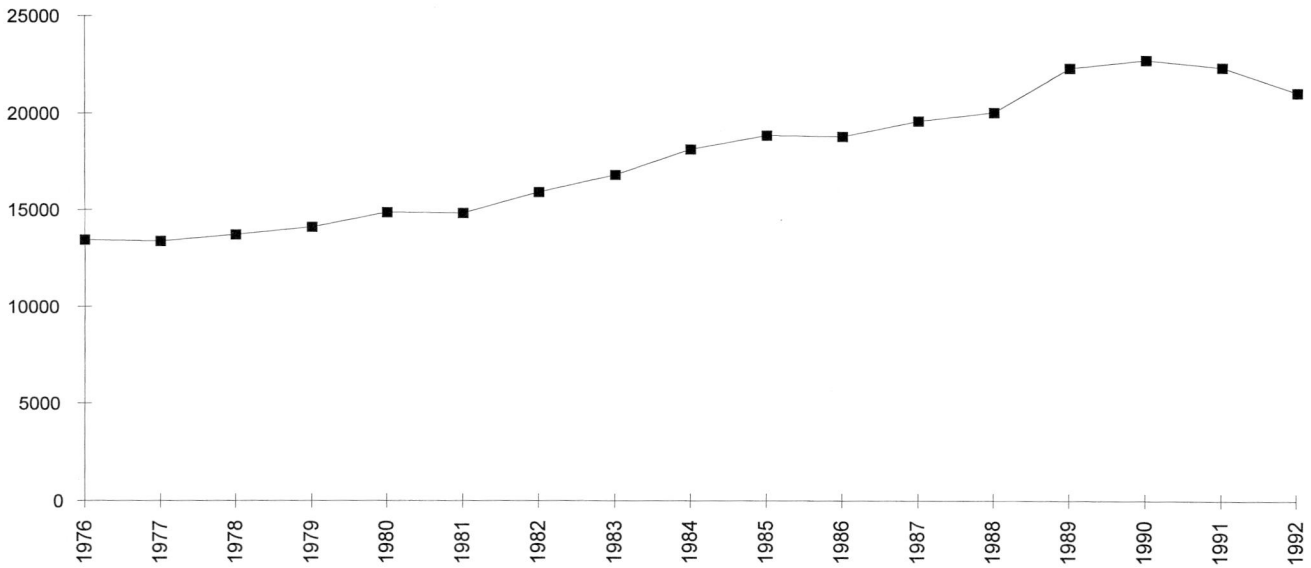

FIGURE 11–5. Number of articles on the heart published from 1976 to 1992 found by searching MEDLINE for articles in which the major key word was "heart." A personal computer and BRS/Information Technologies were used. The number of articles published per year ranged from 13,441 in 1976 to 22,420 in 1991, with a slight decline in 1992 to 21,121.

CORONARY-ARTERY-BYPASS.MJ or
AORTO CORONARY BYPASS or
CORONARY DISEASE (SU).MJ.
1976-1992
(total 9,775)

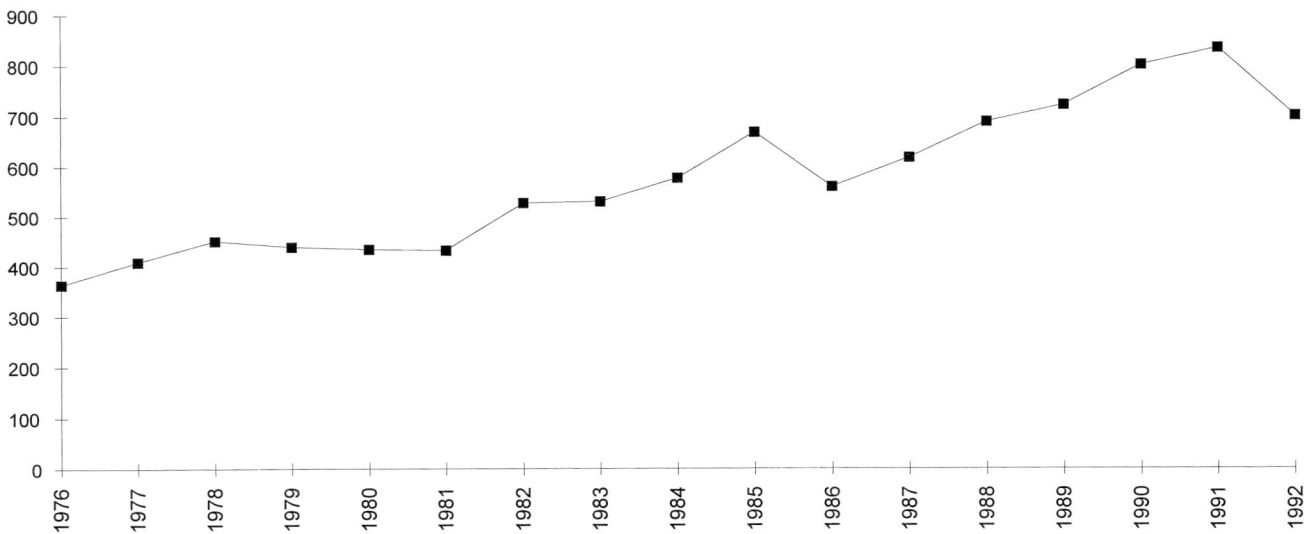

FIGURE 11–6. Number of articles published in which "coronary-artery-bypass" or "aortocoronary bypass" or "coronary disease: surgery" was used as a major index term by the National Library of Medicine. The number of articles published in this area increased in the early and late 1980s, with a downward trend in 1992.

clinical outcome must be defined explicitly in reference to individual patient risk factors to respond appropriately to local and national economic objectives.

The manufacturers of most monitoring systems have introduced microprocessors to provide digital output of the information from the monitors. Companies have developed computer systems that can interpret the output of numerous monitors in the ICU. These hardware and software packages are based on either a minicomputer with multiple terminals at the bedside or a distributed system with microcomputers at the bedside linked to a microcomputer server that is a central point for the database and data transmission (Martin and Jeffreys, 1987).

The computer enables one to do many complex calculations that reduce and simplify data, and the resultant data can show adverse hemodynamic conditions that may not be apparent from raw physiologic data (Caceres et al., 1962; Civetta, 1977; Kouchoukos et al., 1969; Lewis et al., 1966; Siegel et al., 1968; Stoodley et al., 1987). Data from the monitors alone, along with laboratory information and automatically acquired intake and output values, generate the critical care flow sheet. These data can be used to automate therapy, which has been accomplished for postoperative blood volume therapy (Kouchoukos et al., 1971; Sheppard, 1980b, 1986), the control of postoperative hypertension (Kouchoukos et al., 1971; Sheppard, 1980a; Sheppard et al., 1974; Sheppard and Sayers, 1977), and infusion of insulin for management of diabetes (Watson et al., 1986).

DEVELOPING COMPUTER APPLICATIONS

Various computer applications have been developed by motivated individuals for specialized and often entrepreneurial purposes. These applications are often based on microcomputers and are nearing acceptance.

Each application requires formal mechanisms for information gathering and processing for physician-oriented display and analysis. Information processing is done automatically by computer to compress massive amounts of data, to assess the data for accuracy, and possibly to emphasize particularly important information. This level of processing is controlled by arbitrary rules that are generally accepted. Changes in the care of patients on the basis of these data would require approval by the physician.

In caring for the individual patient, a large amount of material is gathered and must be organized and processed by the physician. The data include the medical history, results of the physical examination, laboratory determinations, physician's orders, and imaging results, which are all quantifiable to some extent. Variable amounts of basic physiologic data are also recorded. The rest of the material consists of the impressions and thoughts of care providers during the patient's stay in the hospital.

These data are stored in a document (the medical record) that is poorly organized, incomplete, and "noisy" (i.e., contains much material that is required for nonmedical, often legal, reasons) (Anderson, 1988). The record does not include or refer to resource documents such as medical literature, medical research databases, codification aids, information about prescribing pharmaceuticals, or warnings about drug interactions. It does not enumerate the thought processes guiding the patient's care. There is no mechanism for detecting errors in the data entered or for checking the completeness of the document or the appropriateness of a particular entry.

These deficiencies must be corrected, which will involve acceptance of computer assistance at all levels in this process. Physicians, nurses, and hospitals must participate in the development of the required software (which is the present limiting factor) and in the purchase and installation of the hardware (which, it appears, will be accomplished last).

Cardiothoracic surgery is likely to be a leader in this field. The pertinent anatomy and physiology of the cardiac patient are well defined. The number of potential principal diagnoses and outcomes is limited. The procedures done are highly stylized and thus relatively easy to encode. The complications of surgery are limited in number and easily defined. These features tend to make practical the acquisition of a computerized database on patients.

Cardiothoracic surgery is labor- and information-intensive. A large amount of quantitative information is accumulated for each patient, and attention to each item is critical. Detection of low-probability events (abnormalities of individual data items or trends) in such a situation is a task that the computer performs well. Computer assistance is likely to be well received and has practical value.

Finally, cardiothoracic surgeons have been leaders in the field of "applied medical informatics." The surgical environment has tended to foster the development of computer applications (Watson, 1974). This environment, more than any other factor, is necessary for progress in this area.

The next section reviews computer applications that concern management of the individual patient and considers the methods used for information gathering, processing, and reporting.

History and Physical Examination Databases

This evaluation of any patient must be codified (or encoded) to create a meaningful database. For the average patient, many signs and symptoms are possible. Those pertinent to cardiac disease have been categorized so that databases can be created.

The Duke Databank for Cardiovascular Disease is the oldest and largest functioning cardiovascular database collecting historical, procedural, and longitudinal follow-up information on more than 85,000 patients undergoing over 300,000 cardiovascular procedures (coronary and peripheral artery angioplasty, coronary artery bypass surgery, exercise or stress tests, and a number of new evolving technologies) since 1969. The information in the database has been the subject of over 600 scientific papers. The database housing this information was traditionally hierarchical in architecture but was recently restructured in a normalized relational database format. The relational database is SQL Server from Sybase Corporation.

The cardiology division of the databank has evolved from a 50-user Novell 3.11 local area network (LAN) in 1990 to a 400-user distributed network with six Windows NT Advanced Servers (three file and printer servers [Compaq Proliant 2000—dual 486/50 with 64-MB DRAM and 8-GB hard drives] and three applications [SQL Servers—Compaq Proliant 4000 dual 66-MHZ Pentiums and 8-GB mirrored hard drives]). The activities of this group support a wide variety of research interests ranging from statistical analysis to image analysis of cardiovascular disease. The cardiology division databank end-users number approximately 400 and are using Windows 3.1 IBM-compatible personal computers.

A user interface based on the programming language Visual C++ has been developed (Fig. 11–7). Concern over long-term maintenance of the interface prompted a search of available technology. A search is under way for multiplatform (X-windows, Windows, and Macintosh) development tools that have a shallow learning curve. The promise of portability

among different platforms would permit greater flexibility in the implementation of any future revisions to the database.

When the demographic information, physical findings, and historical information for the patient have been coded, the patient can be categorized on the basis of the constellation of features defined. The outcome for the patient is tracked during long-term follow-up. Records for individual patients in the Cardiovascular Disease Databank can be compared with those for cohorts of patients with similar profiles (based on demographic data and results of cardiac catheterization). The results of medical or surgical therapy can thus be projected within confidence limits.

Procedural Databases

Nothing (except possibly the history and physical examination) more clearly defines the status of a surgical patient than the procedures that are done and the results of those procedures. This is particularly true in cardiothoracic surgery, wherein most of the potential outcomes of an operation (such as complications) can be forecast accurately.

The operative note for a cardiac operation generally consists of discrete factual data (e.g., aortic cross-

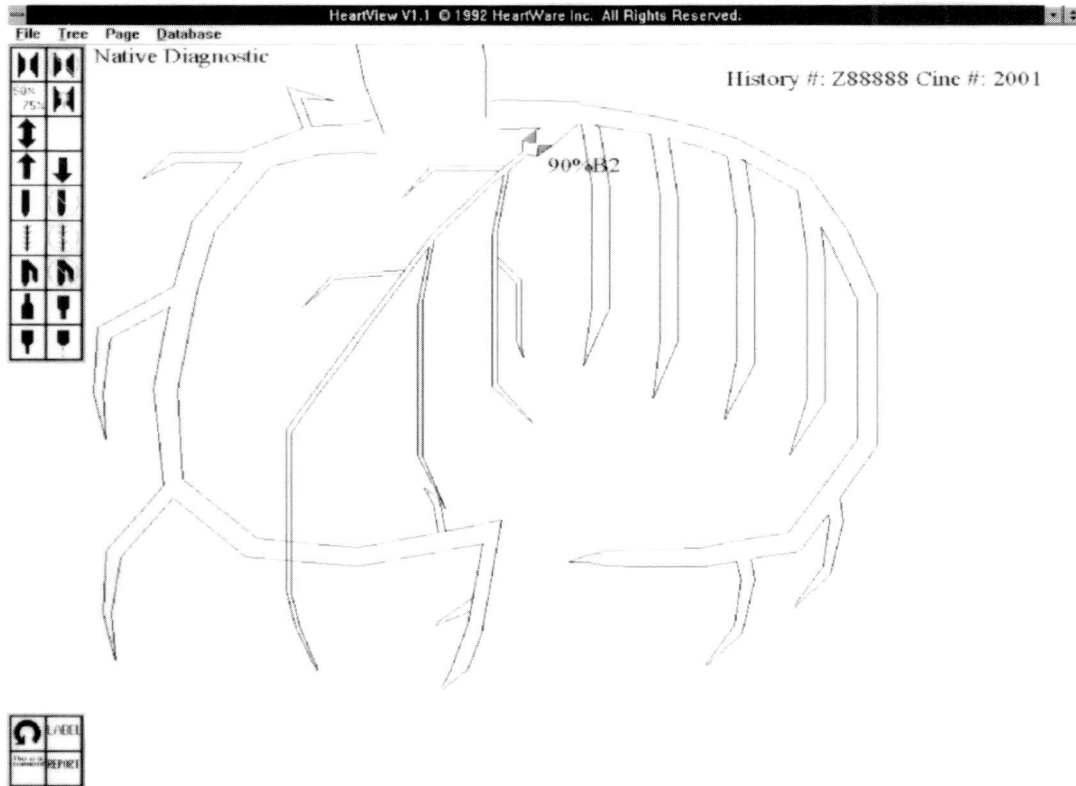

FIGURE 11–7. Coronary tree diagram: A sophisticated interface has been developed for entering the large number of details regarding coronary anatomy. This page represents what would be seen for a diagnostic cardiac catheterization. Similar pages exist with a context-sensitive tool box for adding information on bypass grafts as well as on interventional procedures. This information is stored in an underlying relational database for subsequent analysis. (Courtesy of Heartware, Inc.)

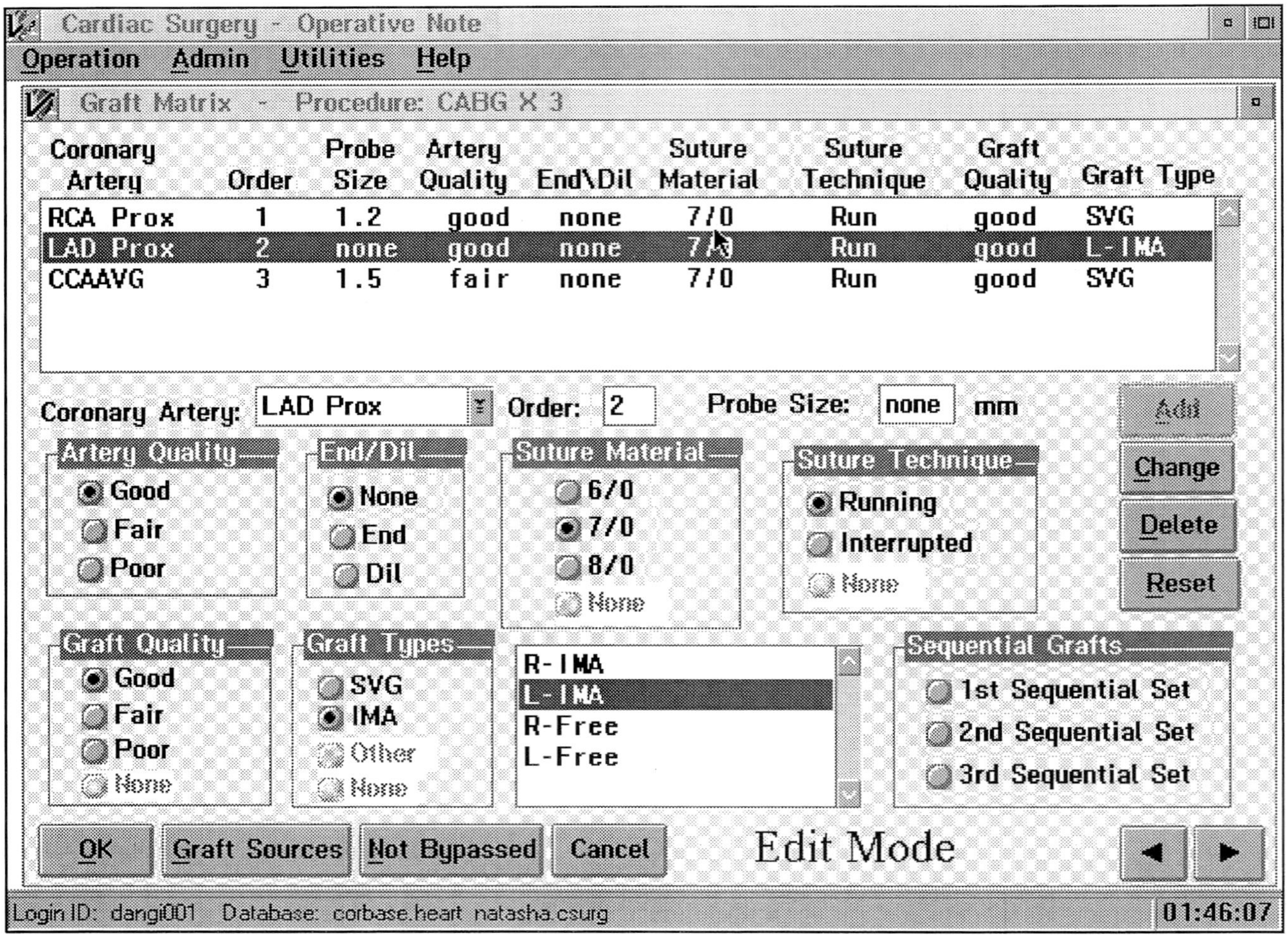

FIGURE 11–8. Details of a coronary artery bypass grafting procedure are recorded in this pop-up window, which feeds information from multiple data dictionaries into the Cardiovascular Disease Database. Similar screens exist for valvular and other cardiac procedures. Other similar screens are used to document preoperative patient characteristics and other information that characterizes the conduct of the procedure.

clamp time, cardiopulmonary bypass time, vessels grafted), which are presented in a narrative format. To maintain consistency in reporting and to generate a database regarding the procedure performed, these data elements have been stored at Duke University Medical Center for the last 20 years. In the past, a form that contains a series of questions was completed as the operation proceeded. The data were collected by the perfusionists, who recorded demographic and anesthesia information at the beginning of the procedure, information on extracorporeal circulation during the procedure, and information from the surgeon about the operative procedure itself at the end of the procedure.

Duke University has developed a new application to capture cardiac operative information in the OR using ORIS workstations. These workstations, located in each operating room, are used by surgeons and perfusionists to enter relevant information directly into a Sybase database (Fig. 11–8). Patient demographic information and posted procedural information "preload" the data entry screens to narrow the

choice of responses through the graphical user interface. Error-checking algorithms ensure that entered data are internally consistent and conform to established standards.

A tabular operative note is then printed for signature in the operating room (Fig. 11–9). The note is then uploaded to the HIS and is available for general viewing throughout the hospital.

Critical Pathways

Critical pathways are gaining popularity as cardiac surgeons seek methods to improve use management in cardiac services. A critical pathway outlines certain expectations for resource use and treatment for a defined disease process. By making explicit the expectations for the average patient, it is possible to predict resource use and analyze departures from the pathway to promote continuous quality improvement.

Computerization will be an integral step in deployment of such pathways. Duke University Medical

THORACIC SURGERY SERVICE
DUKE UNIVERSITY MEDICAL CENTER

DOB: 05-12-28

WOLFE
SURGERY (DUKE UNIVERSITY HOSPITAL)

Print Date: 12-30-93

OPERATIVE NOTE - CARDIAC SURGERY

NAME:

HX#:

DIAGNOSIS: Coronary Artery Disease, Mitral Regurgitation

PROCEDURES: CABG X 3 Redo
                        Mitral Valve Replacement

DATE OF SURGERY: 11-12-93

SSN:

SURGEON: Walter G. Wolfe, M.D.

ANESTHESIOLOGIST: Thomas E. Stanley, M.D.

ASSISTANT: Scott J. Kabas, M.D.

     PA: Lewis Newman, PA-C

CLINICAL HISTORY

Patient Age: 65 years old.

Gender: Male

Disease History: Coronary Artery Disease, Mitral Regurgitation

Coronary Artery Status: 2 vessel, left main.

Indications for Surgery: Unstable Angina
                                          Acute Evolving MI
                                          Failed Angioplasty

Valve Disease Origin: Degenerative
                                        Ischemic
                                        Calcific

CCS Class for Angina: III

NYHA Class for Congestive Heart Failure: II

Ventricular ejection fraction: 61%

The patient was taken to surgery directly from the ACU.

The operation was performed as a coronary artery redo procedure.

FIGURE 11–9. Tabular representation of the initial portion of a computer-generated operative note, which is used for all patients undergoing cardiac surgery.

Center has developed a pilot program in this area, which uses a point-of-care clinical workstation based on a standard Intel 486 personal computer running the NEXTSTEP Mach Unix operating system. The software design is object-oriented and interacts with a Sybase database server. This platform is intended to house numerous applications, including access to laboratory results, MEDLINE, and, by emulation, the HIS.

The application employs a graphical user interface and is a central source of patient information to facilitate communication among the health care staff (Fig. 11–10). It provides methods to customize and update a care map template for a given encounter and generates lists of nursing tasks for a period covered by the care map (Fig. 11–11). It also produces standard order sets generated from the care map template and allows the recording and tracking of variance from that template.

Laboratory Databases

Laboratory reports include data that are needed for the evaluation of a patient. When the data have been categorized and checked for error, they are analyzed by computer algorithms to detect values out of physiologic range that would require medical intervention. National or local laboratory standards may be applied before reporting the results (Lincoln and

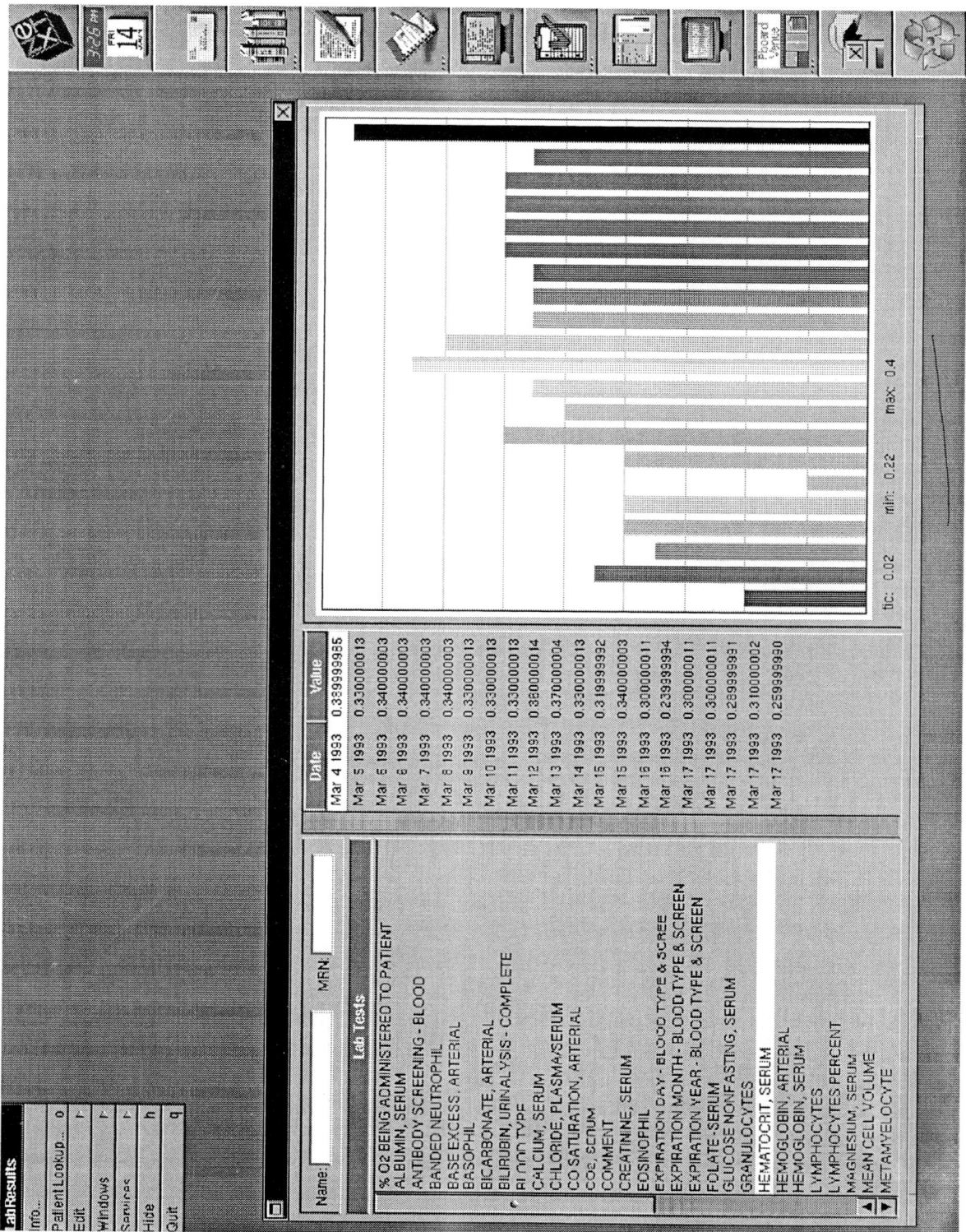

FIGURE 11–10. A pop-up window from the care map application permits the user to graphically trend laboratory information for an individual patient.

390

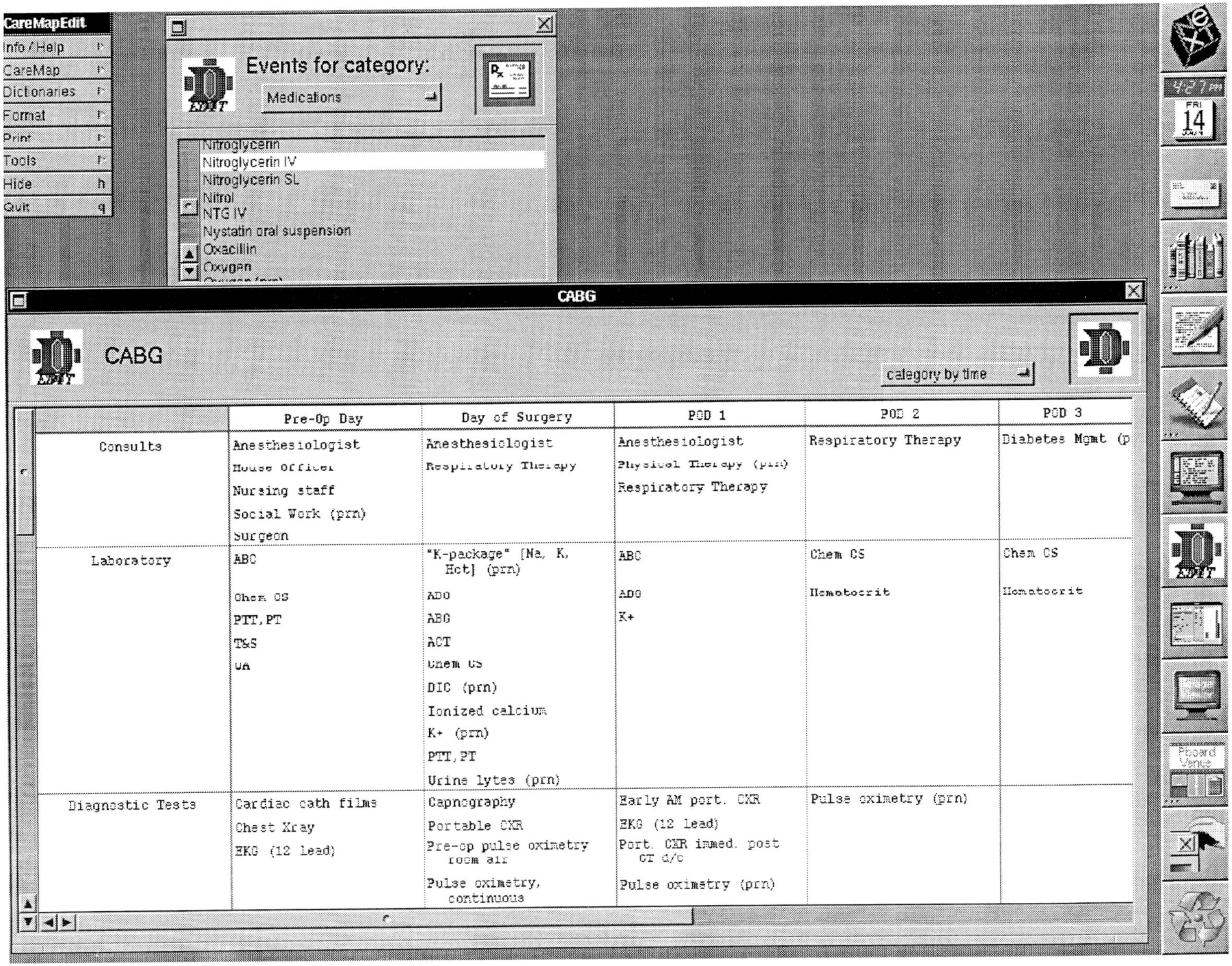

FIGURE 11-11. A portion of the care map for coronary artery bypass grafting is seen in a pop-up window. Elements within the spreadsheet are linked to data dictionaries and can be "selected" for action individually or along columns to generate standard order sheets.

CareMapEdit
Info / Help
CareMap
Dictionaries
Format
Print
Tools
Hide
Quit

Events for category:
Medications

Nitroglycerin
Nitroglycerin IV
Nitroglycerin SL
Nitrol
NTG IV
Nystatin oral suspension
Oxacillin
Oxygen

CABG

category by time

	Pre-Op Day	Day of Surgery	POD 1	POD 2	POD 3
Consults	Anesthesiologist	Anesthesiologist	Anesthesiologist	Respiratory Therapy	Diabetes Mgmt (p
	House Officer	Respiratory Therapy	Physical Therapy (prn)		
	Nursing staff		Respiratory Therapy		
	Social Work (prn)				
	Surgeon				
Laboratory	ABG	"K-package" [Na, K, Hct] (prn)	ABG	Chem 0S	Chem 0S
	Chem 0S	ABG	ABG	Hematocrit	Hematocrit
	PTT, PT	ABG	K+		
	T&S	ACT			
	UA	Chem 0S			
		DIC (prn)			
		Ionized calcium			
		K+ (prn)			
		PTT, PT			
		Urine lytes (prn)			
Diagnostic Tests	Cardiac cath films	Capnography	Early AM port. CXR	Pulse oximetry (prn)	
	Chest Xray	Portable CXR	EKG (12 lead)		
	EKG (12 lead)	Pre-op pulse oximetry room air	Port. CXR immed. post OT d/c		
		Pulse oximetry, continuous	Pulse oximetry (prn)		

CABG

Blume, 1986). These data are recodified to reflect the physician's analytic patterns rather than the more common organizational schemes (e.g., results from the same machine reported together or results of the same test from different sublaboratories reported separately).

Local organizational patterns can be recognized. The cardiac surgeon may wish to see the results for blood urea nitrogen, creatinine, potassium, hematocrit, and bilirubin at one time, even though the results are reported from three different locations. Time-oriented displays of serial results are essential (a fact that is considered only in accounting terms in most systems). Finally, the reported results should be presented to the physician in real time through computer-based surveillance of outstanding requests and receipt notification. Many hospitals have purchased departmental laboratory computer systems that satisfy most of these requirements. Unfortunately, most laboratory systems are interfaced to a HIS mainframe to distribute the information to health care providers. This inevitably decreases apparent functionality, which cannot be duplicated at the mainframe level.

Image Databases

Imaging material can be collected in a computer for application to bedside care only after codification and interpretation of the data at the imaging site. Thus, electronic transmission of the imaging "report" is possible in near real time. The encoding of these reports involves almost as many possibilities as there are in generally accepted diagnostic code lists. In the encoding, simplification (stress on the principal diagnosis) is likely to be more effective than all-inclusiveness.

Various imaging methods, from the conventional x-ray film to *magnetic resonance imaging* (MRI), are used in cardiothoracic surgery. The actual images obtained in echocardiography, computed tomography, MRI, and many other modalities can be stored electronically. Conventional x-ray films can also be digitally scanned and stored (Dayhoff, 1987; Huang, 1986). Optical disks are expected to replace hard-copy film (Thoma et al., 1987).

Image display is improved by using digital images. Interpretation of image sequences is facilitated by depiction of motion with display in a cine-loop manner. Color or pseudocolor can be used to show subtle variations in images. In the future, depiction of three-dimensional images in a two-dimensional format will be essential (Collins and Skorton, 1987), and the images will be transmitted over fiberoptic links to distributed viewing stations (Hauser and Crocker, 1987).

Pharmaceutical Databases

Pharmacologic information (e.g., drug type, dose, and dose interval) is kept in the medical record in the form of drug orders in the patient's chart. This information is usually also kept in the HIS for purposes of inventory, supply, and billing. Results such as drug levels and values that indicate adverse drug effects are located in the laboratory reports. Pharmaceutical information (appropriate dosing schemes, pharmacokinetic information, adverse reactions, and incompatibilities) is found in manuals or obtained from the pharmacy department. All this information is encoded and could be incorporated in an individual database by entering the physician's orders directly (Klee and Harris, 1985).

Information on drug pharmacokinetics is obtained from studies of the volume of distribution and its clearance mechanism of individual agents. A preferable method for displaying information would be a time-oriented projection of the effect of the drug on serum levels. The National Biomedical Simulation Resource has developed a program generator (SCoP) that can solve this problem. For various drugs, the dosage, dose frequency, volume of distribution, renal function, and function of other organs responsible for drug clearance can be defined as parameters. Published data on the kinetics of individual drugs are used. The SCoP interface establishes the pharmacokinetic formula that applies, and a graphical display of anticipated serum levels over time can be generated (Kootsey et al., 1986). The physician can use this information to choose the initial dose of a drug, anticipate the peak and trough serum levels that will be achieved, and time the determinations of serum levels to monitor therapy (Nicholson and Jelliffe, 1983; Seifert, 1985).

Numerous software packages are available for the evaluation of various pharmacologic agents in relation to characteristics of patients. This software can be obtained for Coumadin (private development), theophylline (private development), and a number of aminoglycosides (drug manufacturers). Private developers have produced software that can evaluate several drugs used in ICUs and eliminate the need for repeated entry of the patient's weight, height, creatinine level, and so forth to predict separate drug regimens for the same patient. Because a universal program that can be used to prescribe all common drugs is unavailable at this time, it is necessary to maintain a large library of software to achieve this goal. Similar software is available for automatic writing of prescriptions (Allen et al., 1985).

Automated Discharge Summary

The development of an automated discharge summary would do much to improve the care of patients. A timely, accurate document helps the care provider, both locally and in referral situations. The discharge summary is a list of the patient's problems and subjective and objective information provided by the physician and the hospital. This basic document for quality assurance describes the discovery of these problems and the methods used to resolve them. The coding of such documents is becoming a source of remuneration for both hospitals and physicians.

Attempts to provide automated discharge summaries have had various degrees of success. Johns Hopkins Hospital developed the AUTRES Report (Lenhard et al., 1985). In a pilot system, discharge reports are produced from records entered in a database. Attempts were made to integrate work done by ancillary services for automatic entry of data into the system.

Lexical problems are impediments to the development of computerized report generators that can produce automated discharge summaries (McGray et al., 1987). Natural language text processing is discussed by Gabrieli and Speth (1987), who note that the inpatient chart is "an undisciplined diary without standards." Gabrieli and Speth developed 362 formalized data fields and a word lexicon containing 126,000 different words—and they noted that William Shakespeare, in all his plays, used only 29,000 words.

An automated discharge summary will probably also generate progress notes to ensure daily input of information and decrease the work of physicians entering data. This approach has been used at the Ontario Cancer Treatment and Research Foundation (Matte and Murphy, 1985).

Computerized medical records are beneficial, particularly if codification of diagnoses and treatments is done by the professional care provider and it is not necessary to train coding clerks. When the care provider interacts with a microcomputer, accuracy improves, and the computer's memory and sorting ability are available to the individual most qualified to use them. The presentation of choices based on diagnosis and observation of discrepancies between data entered and data previously acquired from cohorts of patients should make the data more complete and accurate. Elimination of repetitive transcription and report collation will reduce clerical work. Fewer charges will be missed, and cash flow will improve (Jelovsek and Stead, 1986). The limiting factors are problems in codification of diagnoses and lack of acceptance by physicians.

Decision Making/Artificial Intelligence

The underlying assumption that there is a well-defined, monolithic diagnostic process is almost certainly simplistic and fundamentally misleading.

Barnett, 1982

Decision making regarding the care of an individual patient is the area in which computer applications are most controversial. Diamond and associates (1987) noted the following ways in which such applications can be useful:

1. Failure to apply a broader perspective to personal experience because of ignorance of a larger repository of clinically relevant information can be corrected by computers.

2. Hidden assumptions in decision making can be made explicit by computers.

3. Decisions that do not appear consistent with these hidden assumptions can be pointed out.

When presented with a patient who has a poorly characterized illness with a large differential diagnosis, the human mind is superior to a computer in weighing the possibilities and eliminating the unlikely ones. When the clinical possibilities have been limited to a small subset, computerized decision making supported by accurate data is more efficient (Blois, 1980; Diamond et al., 1987). A study of diagnostic errors showed that 57% are due to factors other than knowledge deficiencies (Bordage and Allen, 1982).

For example, Cadenza is a microcomputer program based on Bayes' theorem. It was developed to help physicians interpret clinical data to diagnose and evaluate coronary artery disease. Estimates of sensitivity and specificity are made from published medical experience with more than 60,000 patients (Diamond et al., 1983). An evaluation of Cadenza showed that the higher the probability of disease, the greater the severity of angiographic disease. Cadenza was as effective as a cardiologist in the differential diagnosis of anginal pain (Hlatky et al., 1982; Wong et al., 1982).

Physicians are both intrigued by and reluctant to accept computer assistance in decision making (Diamond et al., 1987; Langlotz, 1987; Long et al., 1987; Siegel and Strom, 1974; Singer et al., 1983; Weaver, 1987). Physicians will use expert systems to assist in the diagnosis and management of disease only if the reasoning process used by the computer is in full view of the physician at all times. The method by which the computer makes the decision must be obvious and subject to "physician override" (Greenes et al., 1969; Moskowitz and Pauker, 1985; Weed et al., 1985). Only when there is clear-cut and universal agreement (e.g., in computation of a mean blood pressure from digital data describing an analog waveform) should the computer be allowed to manipulate data and present information without explanation or override capacity.

A computer application must not attempt to alter the way in which physicians assess problems. Presenting the computer as a "consultant" will ensure acceptance (Bleich, 1971). However, physicians using expert systems must recognize that computers are never 100% accurate (Kerr, 1983). The final necessary quality of a decision-making program is that it saves the physician time and effort (Weaver, 1987).

HOSPITAL APPLICATIONS

Use of computers throughout the hospital can have a large impact on the level of care for all patients. Computer applications in hospitals are now diverse, based on various computer methodologies, and not structured so that data flow and sharing are universal. Because large proportions of a hospital's bed capacity and income are related to cardiovascular disease, this area is an attractive one in which to restructure computer applications.

Use of Scarce Resources

The cardiovascular patient uses various resources that are scarce within the hospital. Not necessarily in the order of importance, these include the following:

Physician time
Nursing time
Bed space
Catheterization laboratory space
Operating room space
Laboratory resources
Blood bank resources

These resources are all expensive and must be used efficiently. In most hospitals, management of cardiovascular patients is dictated by a system in which availability is on a first come, first served basis. Advanced planning and scheduling are not standard, and communication is inefficient and often obstructive.

The only attractive solution is to maintain patient information in a centralized data repository from the time of hospital entry to the time of discharge. Access to information about the patient at each step by all individuals concerned will permit the development of scheduling algorithms that operate in near real time to anticipate local needs. The central repository would be updated automatically so that all team members can adjust schedules to accommodate changing needs. When two-way communication with the database is possible, requests by physician and nurses and the needs of the patient can be communicated and addressed. When a time-oriented record of requests and response to services is available, use of resources can be assessed in real time as well as in retrospect. Only by continuous tracking of these data can alterations in the inventory of scarce resources be assessed and appropriately managed.

Communication

A centralized repository that contains all relevant information on patients is essential to efficient communication. An essential component of this information is a unique patient identifier to link multiple independent clinical databases. By providing universal access to information electronically, interpersonal communication can be limited to the essential decision-making process. Decisions can be made more efficiently if the involved individuals have equal and timely access to information; remote communication with the database would provide 24-hour access.

Efficient communication is especially important in the transition from hospital care to home care. In cardiac surgery, this transition is often associated with transfer of responsibility for care of the patient to another physician (the referring physician). At discharge, information is transferred in the form of the hospital discharge summary. This document has many serious limitations. Generating the discharge summary from a computerized database would ensure the quality, completeness, and timeliness of the summary. The ultimate goal would be to supersede the discharge summary by providing direct access to the database to obtain information about all aspects of the patient's care and compare the patient's characteristics and outcome with those of a similar group of patients.

Quality Assurance—Analyzed Results

Prospective assignment of risk is an effective method of quality assurance. SYN·OP·SYS is a computerized information system that is used for quality assurance and risk management. Data regarding occurrences and associated clinical data are collected and used for accreditation by the Joint Commission for the Accreditation of Hospital Organizations (JCAHO), peer review organization (PRO) assessments, and liability concerns. The data can also be used for institutional purposes such as credentialing and cost containment. SYN·OP·SYS was developed on a mainframe computer by the Medical Mutual Liability Insurance Society of Maryland. This system can organize occurrence data according to medical specialty and thus reduce the set of possibilities (Thomas et al., 1985). The creation of large automated files of standards of compliance that can be used hospital-wide presents many technical problems (Downey et al., 1983).

Microcomputers are used in infection control to provide surveillance of positive cultures. All information flows through a single point, the microbiology laboratory, which permits accurate and complete case control (Wise, 1987). Statistical reports can be enumerated easily, and the hospital flora can be evaluated continuously for the emergence of resistant strains and unusual occurrences.

Quality control requires an extensive database to normalize morbidity and mortality rates and identify events that fall outside established norms (Shabot et al., 1987). In the surgical ICU, an outcome score can be devised and converted to an outcome index to compare actual mortality with predicted mortality as a method of monitoring patient care (Gilbert et al., 1987). The fundamental problems in quality control seem to be an inability to identify variables that can predict outcome and an incomplete ability to record the data in an ongoing manner to establish a database of normal outcomes. Such norms will be established only through consistent and universal application of computer data collection (Shoemaker et al., 1992).

In the interim, published statistics from large institutional studies are the only available standard. In these studies, a limited number of parameters are recorded to define the control group. Comparisons with these statistics are always subject to criticism because of differences between the control population and the patients under study, differences in methodology of enrollment, and differences in the baseline characteristics of patients. These data are also biased by the tendency to encode for maximal reimbursement, rather than to classify patients properly by disease and severity.

Quality assurance in cardiac surgery is mainly an analysis of complications related to patient selection and outcomes. A centralized database that contains salient features of a patient's diagnosis, evaluation, and treatment would permit individual outcomes to be analyzed and compared with outcomes for similar groups of patients. Potential outcomes are limited in number and can be predicted from information about diagnoses and operative procedures. The acquisition of a large demographic and medical database for each patient would make it possible to quantify the incidence and prevalence of complications associated with a particular procedure.

Administration

Computerization of the operative schedule and information about operations performed is useful for many administrative functions in the academic institution. The information allows the divisional director to keep an up-to-date record of the operative experience of residents to ensure adequate training. The categorization of departmental or divisional procedures provides information regarding the allocation of operating room facilities among various groups of surgeons.

The final administrative requirement is the development of cost-containment and marketing strategies related to preoperative diagnoses and related diagnostic groups. When this development is combined with data on outcomes and length of stay, it can be used to improve the financial status of the institution (Blum, 1986).

INTEGRATION OF CURRENT TECHNOLOGY

Open Architecture

The transformation of the HIS from a centralized to an open architecture is the critical next step for hospital information processing.

Duke University Medical Center has chosen to pursue parallel development of an open-architecture system composed of the following key elements (Fig. 11–12):

1. *Common services network* (CSN): A broad-based fiberoptic backbone network distributed to all areas of the medical center connects multiple systems, servers, and workstations. There are currently approximately 4000 workstations in 100 LANs, as well as several departmental systems, served by the CSN.

2. *Message router:* Information originating from many disparate systems must be acquired, converted, and appropriately distributed. The message router performs these functions to relieve users and donor systems from the continued need to perform these tasks and modify task performance as technology advances. An HL7 standard is in place for new purchases, whereas older systems already in place are given centrally maintained translation protocols. Rules for information distribution also are centrally maintained.

3. *Common data repository:* The repository is designed to accept data from widely distributed applications and then to reformat and organize the data for defined access by all users. The central repository database will support the transactional nature of the clinical process and the analytic function required for administration and management. It will be insulated from departmental systems to ease technologic transition, which has become an operational reality for information systems managers.

This model allows for the building or purchasing of departmental systems (e.g., ORIS, a pharmacy system, or laboratory system) and maintenance of universal access to selected information. This permits the end-user to realize the advantages inherent in a system optimized for local use without compromising the ability to distribute locally acquired information.

Clinical and administrative workstations are being developed and will perhaps co-exist at points-of-care and in administrative areas. Varying views of the CDR, either for individual patients or for groups of patients with common characteristics, will permit effective data presentation for clinical decision support.

INHIBITORY FACTORS

Legal Considerations

Various medicolegal issues have arisen from the application of computers to patient care problems. Confidentiality is not clearly defined even for medical records as they exist today (Brannigan, 1983). Computer databases can be encrypted, and security measures can prevent access to the entire system or to selected subsets of the system. Despite these capabilities, computer systems are generally considered incapable of preventing determined access by unauthorized users. Progress in this area can be anticipated.

Software designed to analyze patients' data, to assist in medical diagnosis, and to advise in medical therapy will be less than 100% accurate (Victoroff, 1985). This opens the question of assignment of legal responsibility for an incorrect diagnosis or an unacceptable therapeutic result (Peterson, 1988). The tort system is likely to inhibit the growth of computer applications, particularly software design. In the numerous legal decisions that have been made, software authors generally have been found liable, but the question of responsibility has not been answered completely (Adams and Gray, 1987; Brannigan, 1986).

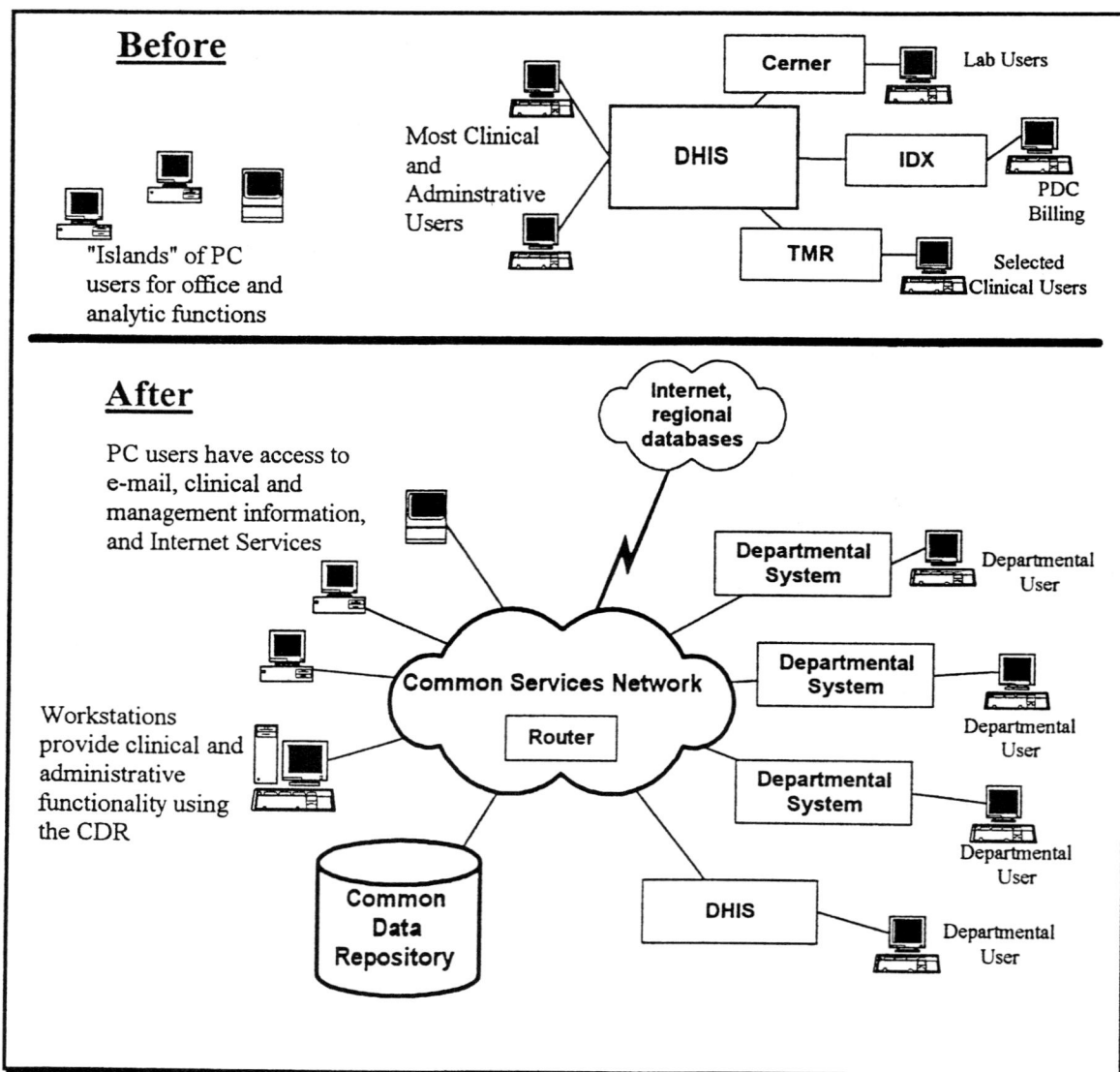

FIGURE 11–12. "Before" and "after" versions of Duke University Medical Center administrative system. CDR = common data repository; DHIS = Duke Hospital information system; IDX = scheduling/billing system; TMR = the medical record. (Courtesy of Wes Rischel, Wes Rischel Consulting.)

Language of Medicine

The language of medicine must undergo changes for computer implementation. The NLM is developing a *unified medical language system* (UMLS) that will be suitable for codification of the medical literature and reports of our daily care of patients (National Library of Medicine, 1987; Shute et al., 1991). Since the initial attempt by Billings, in 1879, to codify the medical literature, this process has developed into two trends (Lindberg and Schoolman, 1986). The NLM and practitioners of medical informatics have attempted to structure the language of medicine to facilitate translation of medical terms into common denominators suitable for categorization (Gabrielli, 1989). Simultaneously, physicians and others have expanded the vocabulary of medicine, making it more

descriptive but at the same time more inaccessible. As a result of these trends, an entire work force has been developed for the purpose of codifying medical information.

Various elements of this work force often are involved in redundant efforts. For instance, coding is done at the NLM, in medical record departments for research and for the assignment of diagnosis-related groups, in organizations that review medical resources, and in professional offices to assign fees for services. In addition to the overlap, the encoded information is not mutually compatible.

One significant problem in codification is the physician's distance from the process. Codification procedures themselves are just becoming computerized, and as an aid for trained encoders, not for physicians. Software to make encoding by physicians practical is not being developed (Stead et al., 1983b). Participation by physicians would simplify the process, make it self-correcting, and ensure accuracy and timely availability of medical information. This applies at the levels of care of individual patients and of indexing of the medical literature.

Lack of Academic Credit

Although the field of medical informatics has been defined since the early 1970s (Collen, 1986), academic credit for software development by academic physicians is not yet a reality (Greenes and Shortliffe, 1990). This has inhibited participation by physicians in software development.

For over a decade, annual Symposia on Computer Applications in Medical Care (SCAMC) have been a major forum for this field. An analysis of the submissions to the symposium in 1986 (Stead, 1987) showed interest in artificial intelligence, systems and organizations, and database methods (Fig. 11–13). Support for clinical decisions and development of computer-based medical records was predominant in the applications (Fig. 11–14). Overall, 70% of the submissions were related to care of patients or to facilities for care of patients (Stead, 1987).

Perceptions and Attitudes

Attitudes of physicians and nurses have both supported and inhibited the development of computer applications. These attitudes should become more positive as health care experts are exposed to computer applications through training (Jelovsek, 1986). Negative attitudes have resulted from premature implementation of computer applications that created more work without perceptible advantage, whereas current applications should have obvious and immediate advantages to users.

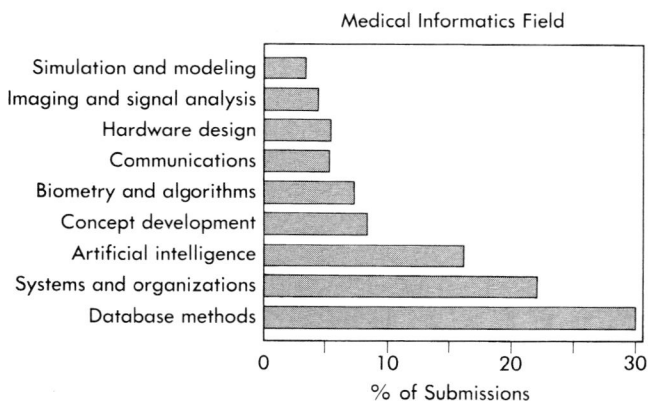

FIGURE 11–14. Articles submitted to the 11th SCAMC meeting expressed as percentage of submissions and categorized according to type of application area addressed by each article. (From Stead, W. W.: A window on medical informatics. Proc. Symp. Comput. Appl. Med. Care, 1987. Washington, DC, IEEE Computer Society Press, 1987, p. 5.)

Reviews of computer applications in the care of patients have shown limited acceptance, particularly by practicing physicians (Teach and Shortliffe, 1981). Physicians were more concerned than were residents about the potential effects of computers on their style of practice (Anderson et al., 1986). At the same time, physicians complained about the increasing "data density" in processing paper records (Anderson, 1988).

Physicians who are knowledgeable about computers are more likely to accept computer assistance (Anderson et al., 1985). A physician who enters practice today is more likely to have had formal education in computer programming and use, to own a personal computer, and to use a computer in practice.

Computer applications must enhance rather than interfere with the physician's role as "chief architect" in the care of patients. The physician's judgment and autonomy should be augmented, not interfered with (Kerr, 1983; Singer et al., 1983). Issues of dehumanization and disruption of the doctor-patient relationship must be addressed (Kaplan, 1985).

Funding Considerations

A final inhibitory factor is cost-accountability. The financial benefits of the institution are distributed across traditional funding lines. The beneficiaries are not only the patients but also physicians, nurses, other hospital employees, hospital administrators, insurance companies, granting agencies, and, eventually, taxpayers. These entities tend to consider com-

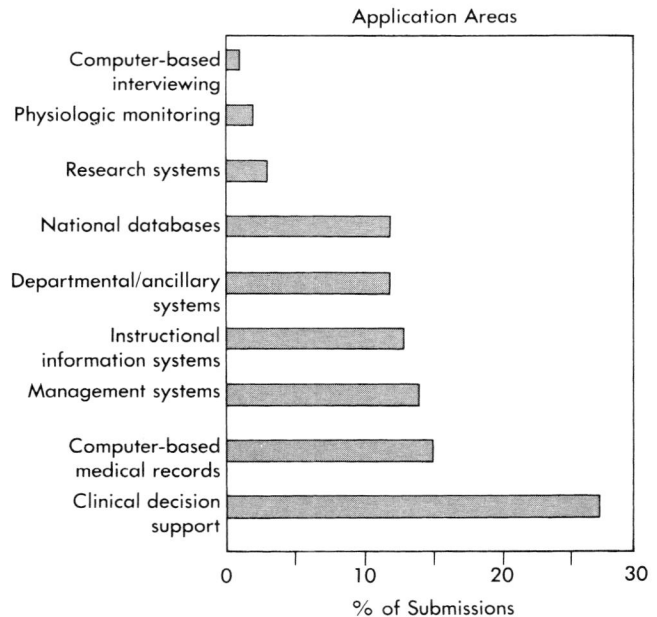

FIGURE 11–13. Separate submissions to the 11th SCAMC meeting expressed as a percentage of total submissions and categorized by major topics in the field of medical informatics. (From Stead, W. W.: A window on medical informatics. Proc. Symp. Comput. Appl. Med. Care, 1987. Washington, DC, IEEE Computer Society Press, 1987, p. 4.)

puter applications and partial funding in terms of their area of interest. It will be difficult to cultivate an attitude of shared fiscal responsibility before actual implementation is begun. In the past, when computer costs were exorbitant and anticipated benefits were subject to rigid cost-accounting procedures, this problem was insurmountable. The exponential increases in computer power and sharp decreases in hardware costs should make shared fiscal responsibility more acceptable. The major costs of computer applications are in software development, which should be fostered as both an academic and a proprietary pursuit.

ANNOTATED BIBLIOGRAPHY

Greenes, R. A., and Shortliffe, E. H.: Medical Informatics. An emerging academic discipline and institutional priority. J. A. M. A., *263*:1114, 1990.

The authors thoughtfully summarize the issues relevant to the development of medical informatics as a valid institutional role for physicians.

Maloney, J. V. Jr.: The trouble with patient monitoring. Ann. Surg., *168*:605, 1968.

This is an early assessment of the impact of monitoring and computers on intensive care. Presented before the American Surgical Association in 1968, the discussion that follows this paper provides interesting insights into the thoughts of the time. Most of the comments are equally applicable to today's intensive care unit.

Pryor, D. B., Califf, R. M., Harrell, F. E. Jr., et al.: Clinical data bases. Med. Care, *23*:623, 1985.

This excellent review article describes clinical databases and their characteristics. The article contains a description of the Duke Data Bank for Cardiovascular Disease and comprehensive reviews of other available systems.

Sheppard, L. C., and Kouchoukos, N. T.: Automation of measurements and interventions in the systematic care of postoperative cardiac surgical patients. Med. Instrum., *11*:296, 1977.

This article provides a more recent description of the Alabama system and an initial report of the use of a computer-controlled infusion of vasodilating agents.

Sheppard, L. C., Kouchoukos, N. T., Kurtis, M. A., and Kirklin, J. W.: Automated treatment of critically ill patients following operation. Ann. Surg., *168*:596, 1968.

The initial report of the continuous use of an automated intensive care unit monitoring system at the University of Alabama describes the utility of this system in the management of 124 patients.

BIBLIOGRAPHY

Adams, E. S., and Gray, M. W.: Strict liability for the malfunction of a medical expert system. Proc. Symp. Comp. Appl. Med. Care, 1987, p. 93.

Allen, S. I., Johannes, R. S., Brown, C. S., et al.: Prescription-writing with a PC. Proc. IEEE, 1985, p. 54.

Anderson, B. Jr.: The "noisesome" hospital chart. N. C. Med. J., *49*:105, 1988.

Anderson, J. G., Jay, S. J., Schweer, M. M., and Anderson, M. M.: Perceptions of the impact of computer on medical practice and physician use of a hospital information system. Proc. IEEE, 1985, p. 565.

Anderson, J. G., Jay, S. J., Schweer, H. M., and Anderson, M. M.: Why doctors don't use computers: Some empirical findings. J. R. Soc. Med., *79*:142, 1986.

Augarten, S.: Bit by Bit. New York, Ticknor and Fields, 1984, p. 109.

Barnett, G. O.: The computer and clinical judgement. N. Engl. J. Med., *307*:493, 1982.

Barnett, G. O., Winickoff, R., Dorser, J. L., et al.: Communication: Quality assurance through automated monitoring and concurrent feedback using a computer-based medical information system. Med. Care, *16*:962, 1978.

Bernier, C. L., and Yerkey, A. N.: Cogent Communication: Overcoming Information Overload. Westport, CT, Greenwood Press, 1979, p. 39.

Bleich, H. L.: The computer as a consultant. N. Engl. J. Med., *284*:141, 1971.

Bleich, H. L., Jackson, J. D., and Rosenberg, H. A.: Paperchase: A program to search the medical literature. Proc. IEEE, 1985, p. 595.

Blois, M. S.: Clinical judgment and computers. N. Engl. J. Med., *303*:192, 1980.

Blum, B. I.: Clinical information systems—A review. In Medical Informatics [Special Issue]. West. J. Med., *145*:791, 1986.

Bordage, G., and Allen, T.: The etiology of diagnostic errors: Process or content? An exploratory study. Twenty-first Proceedings of Conference on Research in Medical Education. Washington, DC, Association of American Medical Colleges, 1982.

Brannigan, V. M.: Patient privacy: A consumer protection approach. Proc. IEEE, 1983, p. 648.

Brannigan, V.: The regulation of medical computer software as a "device" under the Food, Drug, and Cosmetic Act. Proc. IEEE, 1986, p. 347.

Broering, N. C.: The miniMEDLINE System (TM) and the Library Information System. Proc. IEEE, 1985, p. 601.

Burridge, P. W., and Skakun, E. N.: A computerized bedside clinical information system for an intensive care unit teaching service. Proc. IEEE, 1983, p. 171.

Caceres, C. A., Steinberg, C. A., Abraham, S., et al.: Computer extraction of electrocardiographic parameters. Circulation, *25*:356, 1962.

Civetta, J. M.: Cardiopulmonary calculations: A rapid, simple and inexpensive technique. Int. Care Med., *3*:208, 1977.

Clayton, P. D., Delaplaine, K. H., Jensen, R. D., et al.: Integration of surgery management and clinical information systems. Proc. Symp. Comp. Appl. Med. Care, 1987, p. 393.

Collen, M. F.: Origins of medical informatics. In Medical Informatics [Special Issue]. West. J. Med., *145*:778, 1986.

Collins, S. M., and Skorton, D. J.: Computers in cardiac imaging. J. Am. Coll. Cardiol., *9*:669, 1987.

Crew, A. D., Stoodley, K. D. C., Old, S., et al.: A sampling study of bedside nursing activity in a cardiac surgical intensive care unit. Int. Care Med., *13*:119, 1987.

Dayhoff, R. E.: A medical image database system utilizing a write once optical disk. Proc. Symp. Comp. Appl. Med. Care, 1987, p. 549.

Diamond, G. A., Pollock, B. H., and Work, J. W.: Seminar on computer applications for the cardiologist—VI. Clinician decisions and computers. J. Am. Coll. Cardiol., *9*:1385, 1987.

Diamond, G. A., Staniloff, H. M., Forrester, J. S., et al.: Computer assisted diagnosis in the noninvasive evaluation of patients with suspected coronary artery disease. J. Am. Coll. Cardiol., *1*:444, 1983.

Downey, J. E., Walczak, R. M., and Hohri, W. M.: Evaluating hospital compliance with the JCAH quality assurance standards. Proc. IEEE, 1983, p. 94.

Gabrieli, E. R.: A new biomedical nomenclature. Proceedings of the American Association for Medical Systems and Informatics, 1989, pp. 336–346.

Gabrieli, E. R., and Speth, D. J.: Computer processing of discharge summaries. Proc. Symp. Comp. Appl. Med. Care, 1987, p. 137.

Gilbert, J., Schoolfield, J., and Gaydou, D.: Improved medical quality assurance in special care areas through computer management data collection. Proc. Symp. Comp. Appl. Med. Care, 1987, p. 662.

Glaeser, D. H., Trost, R. F., Brown, D. B., et al.: A hierarchical minicomputer system for continuous postsurgical monitoring. Comput. Biomed. Res., *8*:336, 1975.

Goldwyn, R. M., Friedman, H. P., and Siegel, J. H.: Iteration and interaction in computer data bank analysis: A case study in the physiologic classification and assessment of the critically ill. Comput. Biomed. Res., *4*:607, 1971.

Greenes, R. A., Pappalardo, A. N., Marble, C. W., et al.: Design and implementation of a clinical data management system. Comput. Biomed. Res., *2*:469, 1969.

Greenes, R. A., and Shortliffe, E. H.: Medical Informatics. An emerging academic discipline and institutional priority. J. A. M. A., *263*:1114, 1990.

Halford, G., Pryor, T. A., and Burkes, M.: Measuring the impact of bedside terminals. Proc. Symp. Comp. Appl. Med. Care, 1987, p. 359.

Hammond, J., Johnson, H. M., Varas, R., and Ward, C. G.: A qualitative comparison of paper flowsheets vs a computer-based clinical information system. Chest, 99:155, 1991.

Hammond, W. E., and Stead, W. W.: TLS—The Laboratory System: A networked patient care system and laboratory system. Proc. Symp. Comp. Appl. Care, 1987, p. 778.

Hammond, W. E., Stead, W. W., Straube, J. M., et al.: A clinical database management system. Policy Inform., 4:79, 1980.

Hammond, W. E., Stead, W. W., Straube, M. J., Lutz, M.: TMR—Meeting the demand for the variety of report modalities. Proc. Symp. Comp. Appl. Med. Care (IEEE), 1984, p. 421.

Hauser, S. E., and Crocker, M. A.: A performance study of an ethernet-based image transmission protocol. Proceedings of the Twelfth Conference on Local Computer Networks (IEEE), October, 1987, p. 86.

Hlatky, M., Botvinick, E., Brundage, B.: Diagnostic accuracy of cardiologists compared with probability calculations using Bayes' rule. Am. J. Cardiol., 49:1927, 1982.

Huang, H. K.: Ten years' progress in image processing technology related biomedical application. Proc. IEEE, 1986, p. 203.

Jelovsek, F. R.: The Medical Record—Session overview. Proc. IEEE, 1983, p. 99.

Jelovsek, F. R.: Learning resources for medical computing. In Medical Informatics [Special Issue]. West. J. Med., 145:869, 1986.

Jelovsek, F. R., and Stead, W. W.: Computerized medical records. In Javitt, J. (ed): Computers in Medicine: Applications and Possibilities. Philadelphia, W. B. Saunders, 1986, p. 234.

Johnson, D. S., Burkes, J., Sittig, D., et al.: Evaluation of the effects of computerized nurse charting. Proc. Symp. Comp. Appl. Med. Care, 1987, p. 363.

Jurado, R. A., Fitzkee, H. L., De Asla, R. A., et al.: Reduction of unexpected, life-threatening events in postoperative cardiac surgical patients: The role of computerized surveillance. Circulation, 56(Suppl. 2):44, 1977.

Kaplan, B.: Barriers to medical computing: History, diagnosis, and therapy for the medical computing "lag." Proc. IEEE, 1985, p. 400.

Kerr, C. P.: Computers in medicine. A Practitioner's comment. J. A. M. A., 249:2027, 1983.

Kirby, J. D., Pickett, M. P., Boyarsky, M. W., and Stead, W. W.: Distributed processing with a mainframe-based hospital information system: A generalized solution. Proc. Symp. Comp. Appl. Med. Care, 1987, p. 764.

Klee, B. M., and Harris, R. B.: A microcomputer based pharmacy information system. Proc. IEEE, 1985, p. 341.

Kootsey, J. M., Kohn, M. C., Feezar, M. D., et al.: SCoP: An interactive simulation control program for micro- and mini-computers. Bull. Mathematical Biol., 48:427, 1986.

Kouchoukos, N. T., Sheppard, L. C., and Kirklin, J. W.: Automated patient care following cardiac surgery. Cardiovasc. Clin., 3:109, 1971.

Kouchoukos, N. T., Sheppard, L. C., McDonald, D. A., and Kirklin, J. W.: Estimation of stroke volume from the central arterial pressure contour in postoperative patients. Surg. Forum, 20:180, 1969.

Kwon, I. W., Vogler, T. K., and Kim, J. H.: Computer utilization in health care. Proceedings of the American Association for Medical Systems and Informatics Congress, 83(AAMSI: Bethesda, MD):538, 1983.

Langlotz, C. P.: Advice generation in an axiomatically-based expert system. Proc. Symp. Comp. Appl. Med. Care, 1987, p. 49.

Lenhard, R. Jr., Patilla, J., Horbiak, P., et al.: AUTRES: The Johns Hopkins Hospital automated clinical resume. Proc. IEEE, 1985, p. 427.

Lewis, F. J., Shimizu, T., Scofield, A. L., and Rosi, P. S.: Analysis of respiration by an on-line digital computer system: Clinical data following thoracoabdominal surgery. Ann. Surg., 164:547, 1966.

Leyerle, B. J., Nolan-Avila, L. S., and Shabot, M. M.: Implementation of a comprehensive computerized ICU data management system. Proc. IEEE, 1985, p. 386.

Lincoln, T. L., and Blume, P.: Laboratory medicine in the age of information. In Medical Informatics [Special Issue]. West. J. Med., 145:840, 1986.

Lindberg, D. A. B., and Schoolman, H. M.: The National Library of Medicine and medical informatics. In Medical Informatics [Special Issue]. West. J. Med., 145:786, 1986.

Long, W. J., Naimi, S., Criscitiello, M. G., and Jayes, R.: The development and use of a causal model for reasoning about heart failure. Proc. Symp. Comp. Appl. Med. Care, 1987, p. 30.

Lowe, H. J., and Barnett, G. O.: MicroMeSH: A microcomputer system for searching and exploring the National Library of Medicine's medical subject headings (MeSH) vocabulary. Proc. Symp. Comp. Appl. Med. Care, 1987, p. 717.

Maloney, J. V. Jr.: The trouble with patient monitoring. Ann. Surg., 168:605, 1968.

Martin, L., and Jeffreys, B.: Microcomputers in intensive care. In Geisow, M. J., and Barrett, A. N. (eds): Microcomputers in Medicine. New York, Elsevier, 1987, p. 263.

Matte, W. B., and Murphy, B. A.: An automated progress note application. Proc. IEEE, 1985, p. 431.

McDonald, C. J.: Protocol-based computer reminders, the quality of care and the nonperfectability of man. N. Engl. J. Med., 295:1351, 1976.

McGray, A. T., Sponsler, J. L., Brylawski, B., and Browne, A. C.: The Role of Lexical Knowledge in Biomedical Text Understanding. Bethesda, MD, Lister Hill National Center for Biomedical Communications, 1987.

Miller, J., Preston, T. D., Dann, P. E., et al.: Charting vs. computers in a postoperative cardiothoracic ITU. Nursing Times, August 24, 1978, p. 1423.

Mortensen, J. D., and Anderson, L. H.: Clinical experiences with computerized monitoring of cardiovascular variables in the postoperative thoracic patient. J. Thorac. Cardiovasc. Surg., 56:510, 1968.

Moskowitz, A. J., and Pauker, S. G.: The decision to repair an abdominal aortic aneurysm in a patient with severe coronary artery disease. Proc. IEEE, 1985, p. 212.

National Library of Medicine Executive Summary, Long Range Plan, January, 1987.

Nicholson, W. F., and Jelliffe, R. W.: "Smart" infusion apparatus for computation and automated delivery of loading, tapering, and maintenance infusion regimens of lidocaine, procainamide, and theophylline. Proc. IEEE, 1983, p. 212.

Osborn, J. J., Beaumont, J. O., Raison, J. C. A., and Abbott, R. P.: Computation for quantitative on-line measurements in an intensive care ward. In Stacy, R. W., and Waxman, B. D. (eds): Computers in Biomedical Research. Vol. 3. New York, Academic Press, 1969, p. 207.

Osborn, J. J., Beaumont, J. O., Raison, J. C. A., et al.: Measurement and monitoring of acutely ill patients by digital computer. Surgery, 64:1057, 1968.

Peters, R. M.: Trivial pursuit or education? J. Thorac. Cardiovasc. Surg., 93:487, 1987.

Peterson, I.: A digital matter of life and death. Science News, 133:170, 1988.

Pryor, D. B., Califf, R. M., Harrell, F. E. Jr., et al.: Clinical data bases. Med. Care, 23:623, 1985.

Robicsek, F., Masters, T. N., Reichertz, P. L., et al.: Three years' experience with computer-based intensive care of patients following open heart and major vascular surgery. In Collected Works on Cardio-Pulmonary Disease. Vol. 21. Charlotte, The Heinemann Medical Research Center, 1977, p. 48.

Seifert, S. A.: Computer-aided prescribing of aminoglycosides: Bedside determination of volume of distribution and elimination rate constant. Proc. IEEE, 1985, p. 103.

Shabot, M. M., LoBue, M., and Leyerle, B. J.: Use of automatic computerized intensity-intervention scores to measure the appropriateness of ICU utilization. Proc. Symp. Comp. Appl. Med. Care, 1987, p. 671.

Sheppard, L. C.: Computer control of the infusion of vasoactive drugs. Ann. Biomed. Eng., 8:431, 1980a.

Sheppard, L. C.: Computer control of blood and drug infusions in patients following cardiac surgery. J. Biomed. Eng., 2:83, 1980b.

Sheppard, L. C.: Computer based clinical systems: Automation and integration. Thirty-ninth Annual Conference in Engineering and Medicine in Biology, September 1986, p. 73.

Sheppard, L. C., Kirklin, J. W., and Kouchoukos, N. T.: Computer-controlled interventions for the acutely ill patient. In Stacey,

R. W., and Waxman, B. D. (eds): Computers in Biomedical Research. Vol. 4. New York, Academic Press, 1974, p. 135.

Sheppard, L. C., and Kouchoukos, N. T.: Automation of measurements and interventions in the systematic care of postoperative cardiac surgical patients. Med. Instrum., 11:296, 1977.

Sheppard, L. C., Kouchoukos, N. T., Kurtis, M. A., and Kirklin, J. W.: Automated treatment of critically ill patients following operation. Ann. Surg., 168:596, 1968.

Sheppard, L. C., and Sayers, B. McA.: Dynamic analysis of the blood pressure response to hypotensive agents, studied in postoperative cardiac surgical patients. Comput. Biomed. Res., 10:237, 1977.

Shoemaker, W. C., Patil, R., Appel, P. L., and Kram, H. B.: Hemodynamic and oxygen transport patterns for outcome prediction, therapeutic goals, and clinical algorithms to improve outcome. Feasibility of artificial intelligence to customize algorithms. Chest, 102(Suppl 2): 617–625, 1992.

Shubin, H., and Weil, M. H.: Efficient monitoring with a digital computer of cardiovascular function in seriously ill patients. Ann. Intern. Med., 65:453, 1966.

Shubin, H., Weil, M. H., Palley, N., and Afifi, A. A.: Monitoring the critically ill patient with the aid of a digital computer. Comput. Biomed. Res., 4:460, 1971.

Shute, C. G., Yang, P. H., and Evans, D. A.: Latent semantic indexing of medical diagnoses using UMLS semantic structures. Fifteenth Annual Symposium on Computer Applications in Medical Care, 1991, pp. 185–189.

Siegel, J. H., Greenspan, M., Coh, J. D., and Del Guercio, L. R. M.: A bedside computer and physiologic nomograms. Arch. Surg., 97:480, 1968.

Siegel, J. H., and Strom, B. L.: An automated consultation system to aid the physician in the care of the desperately sick patient. In Stacy, R. W., and Waxman, B. D. (eds): Computers in Biomedical Research. Vol. 4. New York, Academic Press, 1974, p. 115.

Singer, J., Sacks, H. S., Lucente, F., and Chalmers, T. C.: Physician attitudes toward applications of computer data base systems. J. A. M. A., 249:1610, 1983.

Stead, W. W.: A window on medical informatics. Proc. Symp. Comp. Appl. Med. Care, 1987, p. 3.

Stead, W. W., and Hammond, W. E.: Demand-oriented medical records: Toward a physician work station. Proc. Symp. Comp. Appl. Med. Care, 1987, p. 275.

Stead, W. W., and Hammond, W. E.: Functions required to allow TMR to support the information requirements of a hospital. Proceedings of the Seventh Annual Symposium on Computer Applications in Medical Care (IEEE), 1983, p. 106.

Stead, W. W., Garrett, L. E. Jr., and Hammond, W. E.: Practicing nephrology with a computerized medical record. Kidney Int., 24:446, 1983a.

Stead, W. W., Hammond, W. E., and Straube, M. J.: A chartless record—Is it adequate? J. Med. Sys., 7:103, 1983b.

Stoodley, K. D. C., Crew, A. D., Lu, R., and Naghdy, F.: A microcomputer implementation of status and alarm algorithms in a cardiac surgical intensive care unit. Int. J. Clin. Mon. Comput., 4:115, 1987.

Teach, R. L., and Shortliffe, E. H.: An analysis of physician attitudes regarding computer-based clinical consultation systems. Comput. Biomed. Res., 14:542, 1981.

Thoma, G. R., Harris, T. R., Hauser, S. E., and Walker, F. L.: Design considerations affecting throughput in an optical disk-based document storage system. Proc. ASIS, 24:225, 1987.

Thomas, D. J., Weiner, J., Lippincott, R. C.: SYN-OP-SYS: A computerized management information system for quality assurance and risk management. Proc. IEEE, 1985, p. 864.

Underhill, L. H., and Bleich, H. L.: Bringing the medical literature to physicians. In Medical Informatics [Special Issue]. West. J. Med., 145:853, 1986.

Victoroff, M. S.: Ethical expert systems. Proc. IEEE, 1985, p. 644.

Waki, R., Clayton, P. D., Jensen, R. L., et al.: HELP-based decision analysis applied to coronary artery disease. Comput. Biomed. Res., 15:188, 1982.

Warner, H. R., Gardner, R. M., and Toronto, A. F.: Computer-based monitoring of cardiovascular functions in postoperative patients. Circulation, 37:(Suppl. 2):68, 1968.

Watson, B. G., Elliot, M. J., Pay, D. A., and Williamson, M.: Diabetes mellitus and open heart surgery. Anaesthesia, 41:250, 1986.

Watson, R. J. Medical staff response to a medical information system with direct physician-computer interface. In Anderson, J., and Forsythe, J. M. (eds): Medinfo. 74. Oxford, North-Holland Publications, 1974, p. 299.

Weaver, R. R.: Editorial Comments, 1974–1986: The case for and against the use of computer-assisted decision making. Proc. Symp. Comp. Appl. Med. Care, 1987, p. 143.

Weed, L. L., Hertzberg, R. Y., and Weed, C.: Construction and use of knowledge couplers and networks and a POMR on a personal computer. Proc. IEEE, 1985, p. 600.

Wise, W. S.: Microcomputers in infection control. In Geisow, M. J., and Barrett, A. N. (eds): Microcomputers in Medicine. New York, Elsevier, 1987, p. 115.

Wong, D. F., Tibbits, P., O'Donnell, J., et al.: Computer-assisted Bayesian analysis in the diagnosis of coronary artery disease [Abstract]. J. Nucl. Med., 23:P83, 1982.

12
Congenital Lesions, Neoplasms, Inflammation, Infections, Injuries, and Other Lesions of the Trachea

Hermes C. Grillo

EVOLUTION OF TRACHEAL SURGERY

Tracheostomy is one of the oldest procedures in surgery, but controversy continues about technique for the procedure. Reconstruction of the trachea as predictably effective methodology has evolved largely since the mid-1960s. Faced with an obstructive lesion of the trachea, the surgeon previously had little alternative but to insert a tracheostomy below a high lesion, or through it, if it was low. Primary tumors sometimes were treated by bronchoscopic morcellation for palliation. Although circumferential resection was accepted as theoretically ideal treatment, authorities believed that only 2 cm at most could be removed and the trachea still be reconstructed end-to-end dependably (Belsey, 1950). Longer lesions were managed by lateral resection, leaving as wide a bridge of tracheal tissue as possible to maintain rigidity and patency of the airway. Because the defects were usually too large to be closed by suture, various materials were used as patches. Dermal grafts supported with wires, fascia lata similarly supported, pericardium, and various types of plastic sheets and meshes, such as Marlex, were all used (Grillo, 1970). Some of these methods established an airway for various periods. In many cases, early leakage with fatal mediastinitis or obstruction due to scar and granulation tissue occurred. The tumor usually recurred because the surgeon, concerned about salvaging enough tracheal wall to keep the airway open, accepted insufficient margins.

Search for a solution to these problems led early to prosthetic replacement of the tubular airway. Grillo (1970) reviewed the enormous variety of materials that have been used, including solid and meshwork tubes of many materials, such as metal, glass, plastic, and, more recently, polytetrafluoroethylene (PTFE). Tissue composites, with and without supporting materials, were also used. Although most materials were tried in experimental animals, usually dogs, some were used clinically. Some early successes and fewer long-term successes were reported. Borrie and co-workers (1973) reported promising results with a cuffed prosthesis in sheep. Neville and colleagues (1990) described surprisingly favorable results in humans, using a similar device. The failure of prostheses results from basic problems in tissue biology. Success-

ful surgical prostheses, such as cardiac, vascular, and orthopedic devices, are buried in potentially sterile mesenchymal tissue. However, placement of prostheses to join epithelium-lined tracts, whether intestinal, respiratory, or urologic, has failed. The bed of mesenchymal tissue in which the foreign body lies becomes, in effect, a chronic ulcer, which responds characteristically because it is adjacent to a bacterially contaminated epithelial surface. The situation is basically unstable. Granulation tissue that proliferates in an attempt to heal the area may produce obstruction or stricture. Inflammatory erosion and migration of inlying tubular prostheses have often produced fatal hemorrhage from great vessels.

Complex reconstructions that use the patient's own tissues generally have been successful only in the neck, where delayed healing can be accepted and multistaged procedures are possible. Reconstruction in the mediastinum requires that a fully fashioned rigid tube with an epithelial lining be present at conclusion of the initial operation.

Multiple experiments have been performed to replace the trachea with homografts (Grillo, 1970). No matter how the transplanted tissue is treated, ultimately scar tissue has replaced the graft. Even autografts of the trachea do not regularly take on a blood supply rapidly enough to maintain a complex structure. In many cases, the tissue slowly necroses and is gradually replaced by scar tissue, with inevitable stenosis. Even if success is attained using omental or other vascular pedicles, the patient is condemned to an immunosuppressive regimen.

Belsey's (1950) placement of the limitation of tracheal resection with primary repair in humans at four rings (2 cm) was supported by Rob and Bateman (1949) in dissections of cadavers. Numerous studies of the limits of tracheal reconstruction in experimental animals have little applicability to the different gross anatomy of the human trachea.

However, indications based on anatomic dissections, radiologic observations, and scattered clinical cases showed that more trachea might be removed in humans. After canine experiments and observations of elasticity in 10 human tracheas, Ferguson and associates (1950) suggested that one-third of the trachea might be removed and anastomosis effected. Radiologic studies (Harris, 1959) showed a 2.6-cm difference in length of the supraclavicular trachea at the extremes of flexion and extension. Barclay and co-workers (1957) successfully reconstructed the tracheas in two patients after excision of 5 cm of trachea, accomplished by extensive dissection of the trachea and reimplantation of the left main bronchus into the bronchus intermedius. In extensive and detailed experiments, Michelson and colleagues (1961) found that 4 to 6 cm of trachea could be removed in cadavers and that the ends could be approximated by mobilizing the cervical and intrathoracic trachea. An additional 2.5 to 5 cm was added by dividing the inferior pulmonary ligament and left main bronchus. One pound of tension was used for approximation. The authors noted half as much mobility in patients over 50 years of age compared with those from 30 to 50 years of age.

Grillo and associates (1964) and Mulliken and Grillo (1968) systematically explored the amount of trachea that could be removed from the cadaver with thoracic and cervicomediastinal approaches and approximation done without excessive tension or destruction of vital blood supply. Approximately one-half of the adult human trachea could be removed and approximation effected. The length varied with individual anatomy, age, posture, and other factors. With such observations, techniques of surgical resection with primary reconstruction moved rapidly forward and proved their worth in significant series of cases (Grillo, 1973, 1978, 1979b; Mathey et al., 1966; Naef, 1973; Pearson and Andrews, 1971; Perelman and Koroleva, 1980). Grillo (1989) reviewed these developments. Although the problem of reconstruction of the subtotally resected trachea where the larynx yet remains potentially functional has not been solved ideally, few patients require such extensive reconstruction if their initial operation is performed appropriately. Few benign lesions involve more than half of the trachea when first seen, and there are few primary tumors of the trachea larger than this that have not already metastasized widely or have extended laterally into the mediastinum too far to permit resection. Nonetheless, a replacement technique is needed, particularly for infiltrating adenoid cystic carcinoma.

ANATOMY

The adult trachea averages 11 cm in length from the inferior border of the cricoid cartilage to the carinal spur. It ranges from 10 to 13 cm, depending on the size of the individual. There are 18 to 22 cartilaginous rings in the human trachea, with approximately 2 rings per centimeter (Grillo et al., 1964). The internal diameter also varies: In the adult male, it measures about 2.3 cm laterally and 1.8 cm anteroposteriorly (Grillo et al., 1964); it is smaller in adult females. The airway is roughly elliptical in the adult. In the infant, the anteroposterior diameter is the greater. The reverse configuration gradually emerges as the child grows (Engel, 1959). Histologic evidence suggests that

growth occurs at the lateral margins of the cartilages (Maeda and Grillo, 1972). In some adults with severe chronic obstructive lung disease and emphysema, the trachea gradually assumes a cross-sectional shape in which the anteroposterior diameter is the greater of the two and is called a "saber-sheath" trachea (Greene and Lechner, 1975).

The only complete cartilaginous ring in the normal airway is the cricoid cartilage of the larynx, which has a broad posterior plate and resembles a reversed signet ring. The first ring of the trachea is partly recessed or set into the broader ring of the cricoid. The endoscopist does not always appreciate that the vocal cords are in approximately midlaryngeal position, so that the trachea does not begin just below the cords but is really 1.5 to 2 cm distal to the cords in the adult. The initial portion of the subglottic airway is actually intralaryngeal. The posterior wall of the trachea, the membranous wall, is applied to the esophagus throughout its extent with a plane of loose connective tissue between the structures. The trachea has considerable flexibility but normally will remain open even in extremes of coughing and forced respiration. A degree of lateral approximation is observed fluoroscopically and bronchoscopically. Tracheomalacia shows dynamic collapse of a greater degree in comparison with normal. The trachea is not very extensible even in youth, and it becomes more rigid with age. Calcification of the cricoid is not unusual, and there may be calcification of other cartilaginous rings with age. Calcification also occurs in response to such local trauma as tracheostomy and intubation injuries.

The blood supply and connective tissue attachments of the trachea are such that vertical movement is easily possible in relation to other anatomic structures. The most fixed point below the cricoid lies where the aortic arch forms a sling over the left main bronchus, although the trachea can be drawn up slightly from that position. A surgeon usually thinks of the trachea as it lies when the patient is in position for thyroid procedures, with the neck hyperextended. For a young person in this position, more than half of the trachea may be above the suprasternal notch. If the neck is severely flexed forward, almost the entire trachea becomes intramediastinal and the cricoid devolves down to the level of the sternal notch. In the aged, the trachea is less mobile, and the position of the larynx does not vary greatly with extension and flexion. Indeed, palpation of the neck in an aged patient in the extended position may show that the larynx is already down at the suprasternal position.

The trachea is only 11 cm long, but in that short distance, it courses from an immediately subcutaneous position in the neck to a position against the esophagus and prevertebral fascia at the carinal level. In lateral projection, the trachea lies obliquely. In an aged patient who is kyphotic and has an increased anteroposterior thoracic diameter, the trachea may approach the horizontal position in lateral projection. The distance between the anterior surface of the neck and the anterior surface of the vertebral bodies in the thorax is greatly increased, and the trachea has to traverse this distance. This change in position accounts mainly for the lack of tracheal mobility in such patients. These points are important when determining the extent of resection possible in individual patients and the procedures that may be needed.

The relationships of the trachea to adjacent structures are obvious. Anteriorly, the thyroid isthmus crosses the trachea at approximately the level of the second or third tracheal ring. The thyroid is fixed to the trachea laterally by connective tissue and vessels. Shortly below this, the innominate artery courses obliquely across the anterior wall of the trachea. The innominate veins are anterior to this. The anterolateral surface of the trachea below lies behind the aortic arch, which passes over the left main bronchus. Posteriorly, the esophagus lies close to the membranous wall of the trachea throughout. The azygos vein arches over the right main bronchus and is adjacent to the tracheobronchial angle on that side. Laterally, the pleura is applied on the right with fibrofatty node-containing tissue intervening. The greatest masses of lymph nodes are in the right paratracheal plane, particularly above the azygos vein, pretracheally on the right, with a smaller collection of nodes on the left, close to the tracheobronchial angle. Inferiorly, there are anterior and posterior subcarinal lymph nodes. Although extensive studies of the lymphatic drainage

of various regions of the trachea have not been performed, it would appear that the drainage goes fairly directly to the paratracheal and subcarinal lymph nodes. The left recurrent nerve is juxtaposed to the trachea along almost its entire length in the tracheo-esophageal groove. On the right, the nerve approaches the trachea superiorly but ends in essentially the same position. The nerves enter the larynx medial to the inferior cornua of the thyroid cartilage.

The blood supply of the trachea is shared with the esophagus laterally and with the main bronchi below. Above, the supply comes from the inferior thyroid artery, which has branches coursing down to supply both esophagus and trachea (Fig. 12–1). Usually, there are three principal fine branches on either side of the upper trachea (Miura and Grillo, 1966). Salassa and co-workers (1977) fully described the contributions of the subclavian, supreme intercostal, internal thoracic, innominate, and superior and middle bronchial arteries. Fine lateral longitudinal anastomoses exist, and from these, transverse vessels travel between the cartilages and feed the submucosa and the cartilages.

Because the blood supply of the trachea comes mainly from end vessels and segments, it becomes important in surgical procedures not to devascularize the trachea over any extent by total circumferential dissection. Only 1 or 2 cm of trachea that is to remain in the patient is circumferentially dissected to avoid

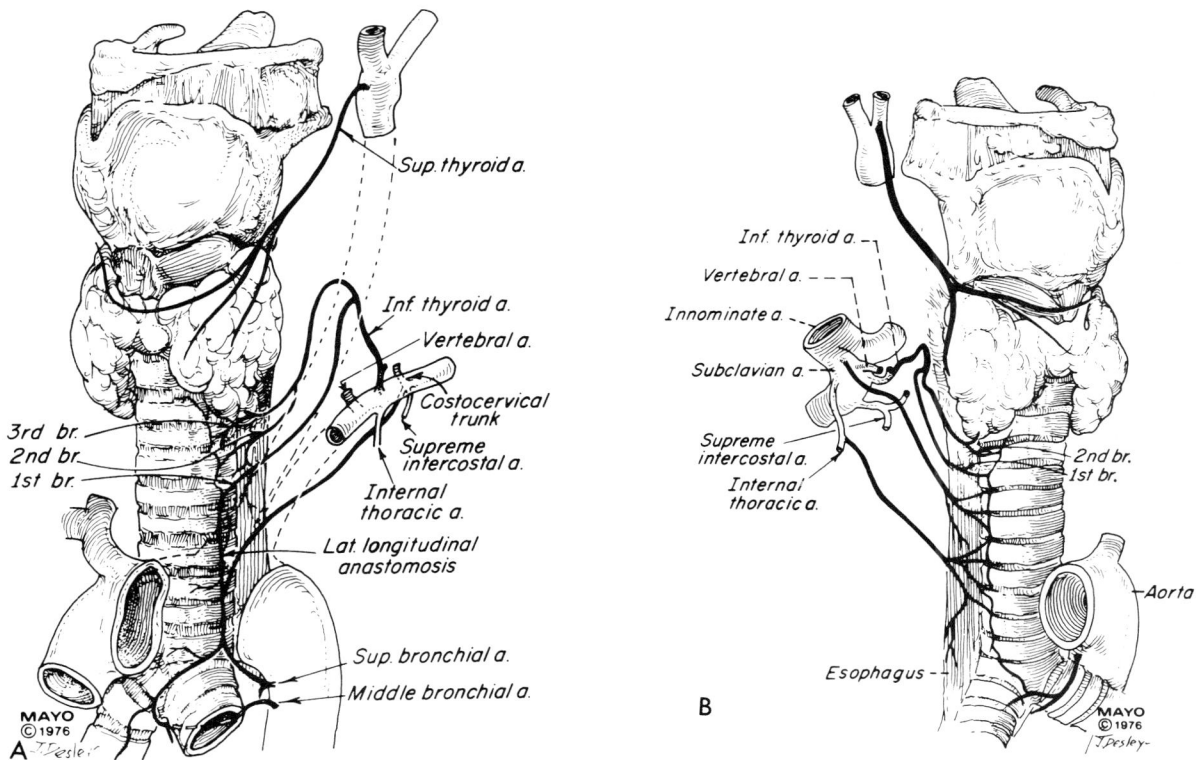

FIGURE 12–1. A, Left anterior view of arteries supplying the trachea. In this specimen, the lateral longitudinal anastomosis links branches of the inferior thyroid, costocervical trunk, and bronchial arteries. B, Right anterior view of vessels supplying the trachea. In this specimen, the lateral longitudinal anastomosis links branches from the inferior thyroid, the subclavian, the internal thoracic, and the superior bronchial arteries. (A and B, From Salassa, J. R., Pearson, B. W., and Payne, W. S.: Gross and microscopic blood supply of the trachea. Reprinted with permission from the Society of Thoracic Surgeons [The Annals of Thoracic Surgery, 1977, Vol. 24, p. 100].)

later ischemic necrosis. Because the blood supply enters laterally, it is possible to dissect the entire pretracheal plane safely. The membranous wall of the trachea may also be separated from the esophagus posteriorly without encountering significant vessels. These maneuvers are important in permitting the trachea to slide more easily for reconstruction.

The tracheal mucosa is columnar and ciliated. It is closely applied to the tracheal cartilages and to the interannular tissues between them. Mucous glands are liberally present. In patients with chronic bronchitis, particularly in heavy smokers, squamous metaplasia may be found to a variable extent and sometimes with absence of ciliated cells.

Several surgical implications of tracheal anatomy have been identified in this section. In addition, the unpaired nature of the organ and its relatively short course and nonextensibility present problems to the surgeon. The trachea's close relationship to major vessels and its relative inaccessibility throughout its entire course by any single incision demand great care in planning surgical approaches.

CONGENITAL LESIONS

Congenital lesions of the trachea are rare. Tracheal *agenesis* or *atresia* is most often fatal at birth. In these patients, the larynx and the lungs may be normally formed (Gray and Skandalakis, 1972), with or without bronchial communication to the esophagus. Fonkalsrud and colleagues (1963) described a case of atresia with bronchoesophageal fistula, in which short-term survival was obtained by using the esophagus as an airway. In the more common anomaly of tracheoesophageal fistula (see Chapter 25), the tracheal problem usually is managed easily by suture closure, and the reconstructive challenge is esophageal. Rarely is there an accompanying tracheal stenosis.

Congenital stenosis of the trachea presents in several principal patterns with many variants (Holinger et al., 1950). Web-like diaphragms are seen in the neonatal and juvenile trachea, most often at the subcricoid level. Intralaryngeal webs also occur. These webs do not involve any length of trachea. Apart from webs, three main types of stenosis have been described (Cantrell and Guild, 1964): generalized hypoplasia, funnel-like narrowing, and segmental stenosis (Fig. 12–2). In the first type, the airway has a normal diameter to the level of the bottom of the cricoid and then severely narrows to 1 to 3 mm (in the newborn) to a point just above the carina. The main bronchi are most often normal in diameter. In the second, the trachea begins with a normal diameter but funnels to a stenosis of varied length above the carina. The bronchi may or may not be normal in size. Segmental stenoses of various length (third type) occur at any level in the trachea. Funnel-type stenoses may also be segmental in involvement. Not infrequently, there may be bronchial anomalies that include such malformations as a right upper lobe bronchus that arises from the trachea above the stenosis. Most often, the

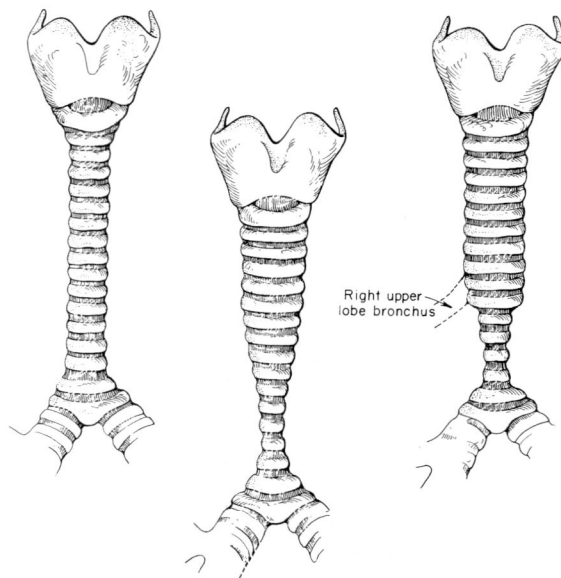

FIGURE 12–2. Congenital tracheal stenosis. *Left,* Type I: Generalized hypoplasia of the trachea. The airway has a normal caliber at the level of the cricoid cartilage and also in the main bronchi. *Center,* Type II: Funnel-like narrowing. The trachea has a normal caliber immediately below the cricoid cartilage but funnels to its narrowest point most frequently just above the carina. *Right,* Type III: Segmental stenosis may be accompanied by bronchial anomalies. The segmental stenosis may vary in length and may be at various levels. (Redrawn from Cantrell, J. R., and Guild, H. C.: Congenital stenosis of the trachea. Am. J. Surg., *108*:297, 1964, with permission.)

cartilaginous rings in the stenotic segment form complete circles, rather than the normal C-shape. Various degrees of cartilaginous disorganization occur, which include longitudinal ridges posteriorly. The main bronchi may also be characterized by complete cartilaginous rings. Congenital tracheal stenosis may be isolated or may accompany a wide range of other anomalies throughout the body. Lower tracheal stenosis is seen in association with an aberrant left pulmonary artery (Clarkson et al., 1967). In these cases of "pulmonary artery sling," the left pulmonary artery originates from the proximal portion of the right artery and passes behind the trachea to the left lung. Completely circular tracheal rings are common in this anomaly (Jacobson et al., 1960) (Fig. 12–3). Release of the artery and its reimplantation anteriorly will not correct the airway obstruction under these latter circumstances. About half of the cases of pulmonary sling are accompanied by this tracheal anomaly (Sade et al., 1975).

When respiratory difficulty in the newborn is due to *vascular ring* malformations compressing the trachea and esophagus, without an associated primary tracheal anomaly, release of the encirclement provides relief. Tracheal compromise of this type occurs with double aortic arch, right aortic arch with patent ductus arteriosus or ligamentum arteriosum, aberrant subclavian artery, and abnormal innominate artery (Gross, 1953; Lincoln et al., 1969).

Congenital chondromalacia of the trachea without compressive vascular origin occurs, but some re-

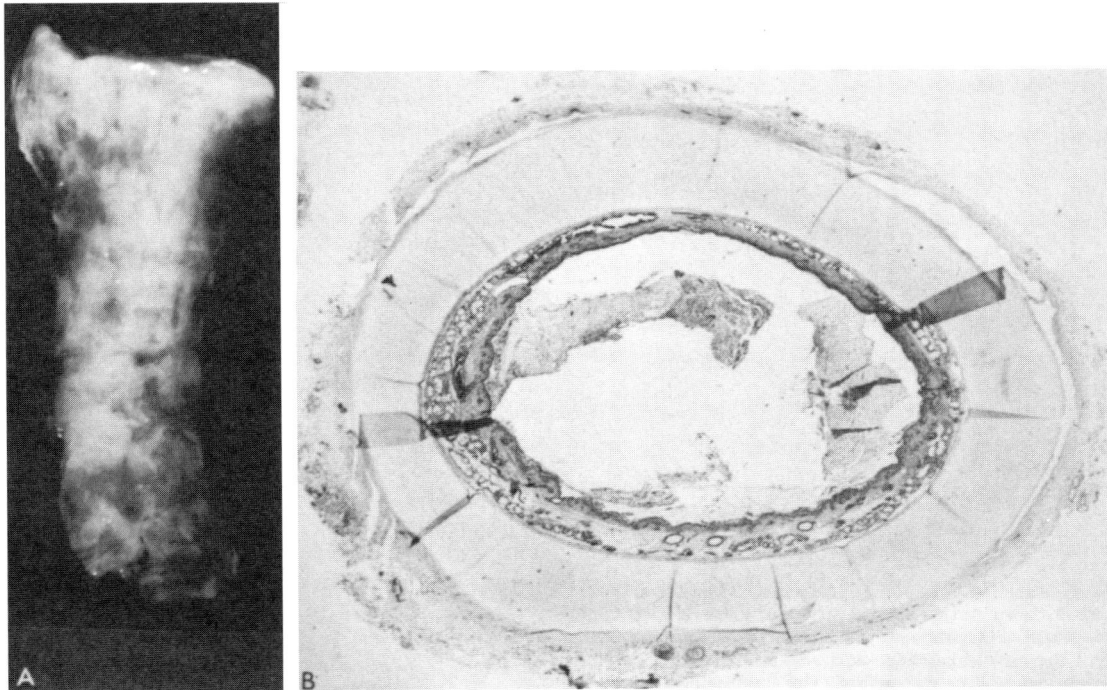

FIGURE 12–3. Segmental congenital stenosis of the lower trachea in association with an aberrant left pulmonary artery. A, Resected specimen of the stenotic segment, a rigid tube. B, Photomicrograph of a cross-section that shows a completely circular cartilaginous ring.

ported cases suggest stenosis rather than true malacia (Cox and Shaw, 1965). In true malacia, the potential diameter of the trachea is normal, but the wall is collapsible. It may be segmental or not. *Tracheobronchomegaly,* Mounier-Kuhn disease, presents with a hugely dilated trachea and main bronchi characterized also by severe cartilaginous deformation and resultant obstruction. It usually becomes clinically manifest in adult life.

The diagnosis of congenital stenosis of the trachea and other obstructive anomalies is based on a high degree of suspicion in infants with respiratory distress. Inspiratory and expiratory stridor may be present and may be accompanied by wheezing and retraction. Dyspnea may be paroxysmal rather than continuous. The patients often have feeding difficulties and, consequently, may fail to develop normally. Frequent and obstinate respiratory infections may lead to death.

Air tracheograms and fluoroscopy provide precise information on the presence and type of an anomaly (Evans, 1949). Contrast media may prove to be dangerous when used in patients with tiny stenotic airways. Bronchoscopy performed with great delicacy and use of magnifying pediatric bronchoscopes helps greatly, but undue trauma and the secretions incited by the procedure can obstruct the trachea.

Differential diagnosis requires that intrinsic tracheal lesions be distinguished from extrinsic lesions such as vascular rings or mediastinal compressive masses, and that concurrent and related anomalies such as "pulmonary sling" be identified. *Computed tomography* (CT) and *magnetic resonance imaging* (MRI) delineate vascular components clearly.

Surgical procedures on the infant trachea carry high risks. Although anastomoses of systemic vessels may be performed successfully in infancy, because the column of blood then splints the anastomosis, and although gut anastomosis may be done with reasonable expectation of function, great hazards attend the attempt to anastomose tiny airways where a few millimeters of postoperative edema can easily cause total obstruction. Intubation and ventilation of a patient who has just had tracheal anastomosis may lead to separation of the anastomosis or to stenosis. Moreover, the juvenile trachea tolerates anastomotic tension less well than the adult trachea (Maeda and Grillo, 1973).

For these reasons, a conservative approach seems judicious in management of congenital lesions of the trachea. Tracheal "webs" are divulsed or removed bronchoscopically with biopsy forceps and, occasionally, with the help of fine insulated cauterizing electrodes (Kim and Hendren, 1976) or lasering. If this fails, tracheostomy done below a web is a temporary solution that allows the patient to grow until an age when definitive resection may be performed. Tracheostomy may be used in patients with strictures of the upper trachea. If the lesion is segmental, it is preferable to put the tracheostomy through the narrowest part of the stenosis, because in a future reconstruction, this part of the trachea will be removed. The normal trachea should not be injured, if possible. Tracheostomies have also been used for temporization in patients with distal tracheal stricture who have respiratory difficulty in infancy. In such patients, if the stenosis extends to the immediately supracarinal region, a tube cannot be placed all the way through the stenosis, because it will then impinge on the carina. T-Y tubes may be used but are difficult to manage in the infant or small child.

Dilatation of congenital stenoses other than webs is unlikely to help and may split the trachea, which then incites granulations. Intramural steroid injection in the management of such lesions is unlikely to help. Empirically, it appears to be useful in patients in whom a diaphragm has been resected transbronchoscopically. The purpose in this case is to minimize the immediate inflammatory response owing to surgical trauma.

For some patients, cautious and concerned observation is the best course, while waiting for the infant to grow. The stenotic area appears to grow but only in proportion to the general growth of the trachea, and it remains a point of relative narrowing. Tracheal anastomosis in infancy is followed by adequate growth at the anastomotic site. Maeda and Grillo (1972, 1973) showed that, in puppies, the average growth rate at the anastomotic site was 82% of normal sagittally and 75% coronally, which produced a 20% narrowing of the lumen in the adult. Tension on the suture line caused greater degrees of resultant narrowing in puppies than in adult dogs. Although the gross anatomy of the human trachea is different, these studies of healing are probably valid for humans. Resections of more than one-third of the tracheal length may lead to stenosis in the small child—a lesser tolerance for anastomotic tension than in the adult.

Congenital stenosis and other tracheal lesions in infants and children have been increasingly recognized and treated surgically by resection and reconstruction (Carcassonne et al., 1973; Grillo and Zannini, 1984; Nakayama et al., 1982). Patch techniques using pericardium or cartilage have been applied successfully where the length of stenosis contraindicates resection and anastomosis (Heimansohn et al., 1991; Idriss et al., 1984), but with significant complications (Dunham et al., 1994) related to the use of a mesenchymal patch. Apparently, satisfactory growth occurs. Repetitive bronchoscopy may be required to remove the granulation tissue that often forms on the mesenchymal bed of pericardium or other connective tissue "gussets." The author has also used the technique of "slide tracheoplasty" described by Tsang and associates (1989) with success to treat long congenital stenosis. The circumference is doubled, creating a nearly fourfold increase in cross-sectional area (Grillo, 1994). The rare anomaly of laryngotracheoesophageal cleft, with failure of formation of the septum between aerodigestive components near the carina, may be repaired by painstaking technique (Donahoe and Gee, 1984).

NEOPLASTIC LESIONS

Primary Neoplasms

Primary neoplasms of the trachea are rare. Between 1962 and 1989, 198 patients with primary tumors of the trachea (excluding laryngeal tumors and tumors of the main bronchi) were seen at Massachusetts General Hospital (Grillo and Mathisen, 1990b). Eschapasse (1974) collected 152 patients with primary tumors from 12 French and 2 Soviet groups. Perelman and Koroleva's (1987) experience consisted of 90 malignant and 45 benign tumors. Pearson and co-workers (1984) surgically treated 44 primary tumors over 20 years. Adenoid cystic carcinoma and squamous cell carcinoma were the two most common and comprised about three-quarters of all primary tumors of the trachea. Various other rarer tumors occur, including carcinoid, carcinosarcoma, pseudosarcoma, mucoepidermoid carcinoma, basal cell adenoma, squamous papilloma, fibroma, hemangioma, chondroma, chondrosarcoma, granular cell tumor, leiomyoma, neurofibroma, and paraganglioma. This by no means exhausts the list of possibilities. Chondromas occur more commonly in the larynx at cricoid level (Weber et al., 1978b).

Adenoid cystic carcinoma was formerly called "cylindroma," which gives a false impression of benignity (Fig. 12–4A). The neoplasm was seen between ages 13 and 79 years and quite evenly in males and females. In the era preceding radical excision of adenoid cystic carcinoma, the lesion was almost invariably fatal, although it sometimes had a prolonged course (Grillo, 1978). The lesion grows so slowly in many patients that it appears to be benign in behavior, even after metastases have occurred to the lungs. Initially in its spread it tends to displace mediastinal structures rather than invade them directly. However, adenoid cystic carcinoma infiltrates the airway submucosally for longer distances than are grossly evident. Perineural spread is also common. Some lesions are highly malignant and spread to pleura and lungs before they are discovered. Remote metastasis is most often to lung and bone. Almost all patients with this diagnosis who have had previous attempts at local excision or repeated intrabronchial excisions have shown metastases when considered later for possible cure. The best opportunity for complete removal of the tumor is at the initial therapeutic effort, as is borne out by encouraging statistics after primary resection and reconstruction (Eschapasse, 1974; Grillo and Mathisen, 1990b; Pearson et al., 1984; Perelman and Koroleva, 1987).

Squamous cell carcinoma of the trachea may present as a well-localized lesion of exophytic type or as an ulcerating lesion (Fig. 12–5). Multiple lesions with interspersed normal trachea also occur, as well as superficial infiltrating carcinoma, which may extend over the whole length of the trachea. About one-third of the patients examined by the author had mediastinal or pulmonary metastases at the time of initial diagnosis. It appears that squamous cell carcinoma of the trachea spread first to the regional lymph nodes adjacent to the trachea and then by direct extension to mediastinal structures. Squamous cell carcinoma of the trachea is distributed comparably to squamous bronchogenic carcinoma with respect to age (principally 50 to 70 years) and sex (52 male, 17 female). All of our patients have been cigarette smok-

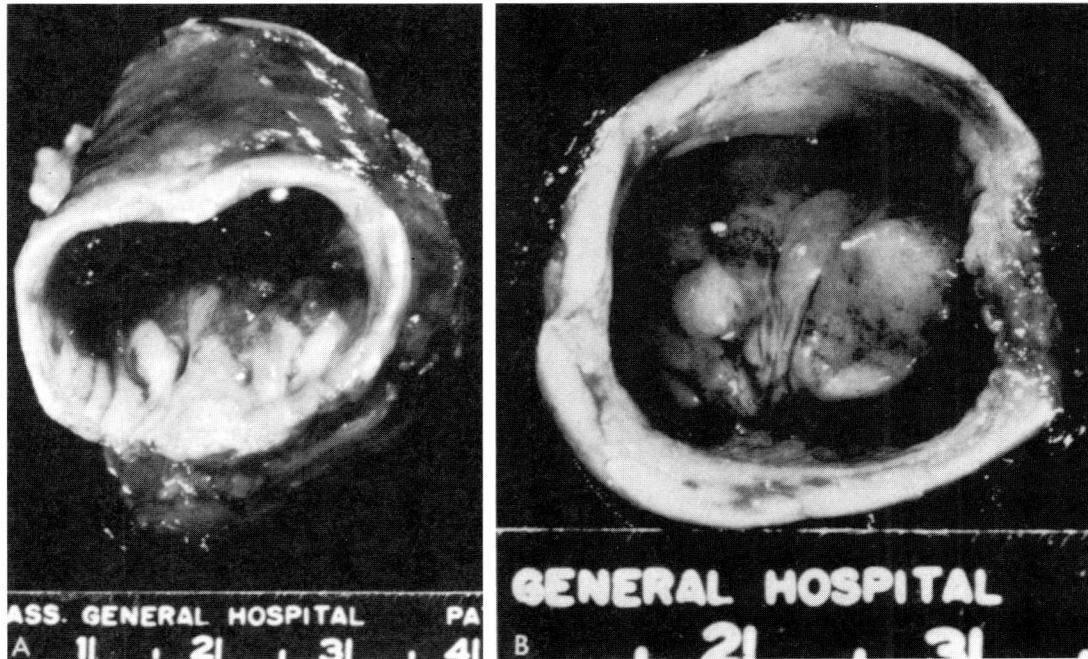

FIGURE 12–4. *A,* Adenoid cystic carcinoma of the trachea. In this case, the lesion presented largely intraluminally. There may often be a large mediastinal component. This is the most common primary tumor of the trachea. *B,* Carcinoid tumor of the trachea. This tumor is rare in the trachea. In its typical form, it has a low-grade malignant potential in comparison with the rather aggressive adenoid cystic carcinoma. This patient presented with recurrent bilateral pneumonia caused by obstruction. (*B,* From Grillo, H. C.: Surgery of the trachea. Curr. Probl. Surg., July 1970, p. 28.)

ers. Forty per cent had prior, concurrent, or later carcinoma of oropharynx, larynx, or lung (Grillo and Mathisen, 1990b).

There is not sufficient experience with any numbers of other primary tracheal tumors to make firm generalizations about their natural history. Benign tumors are, of course, cured by resection. Carcinoid tumors of the trachea (Fig. 12–4*B*) can usually be cured, un-less they are of aggressive atypical variety (Briselli et al., 1978; Grillo and Mathisen, 1990b; Wilkins et al., 1984). Carcinosarcoma and chondrosarcoma (Fig. 12–6) probably can be cured by resection, or long-term palliation can be provided. In the past, these patients died from strangulation obstruction due to local growth or recurrence. Other sarcomas have a poor prognosis.

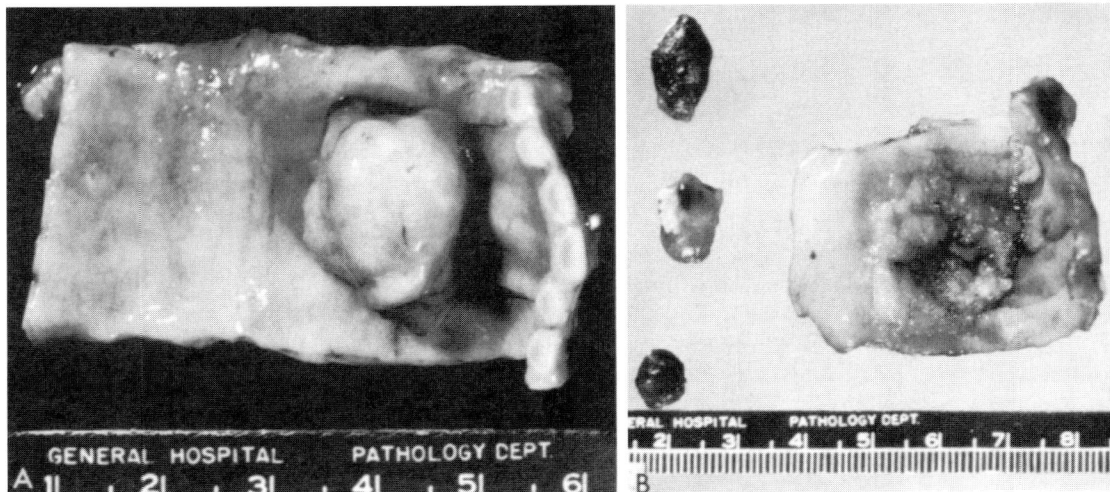

FIGURE 12–5. Squamous cell carcinoma of the trachea. *A,* A surgical specimen showing exophytic lesion. The lesion was removed in 1964, and the patient had no recurrence. *B,* An ulcerative lesion is shown in this seven-ring specimen. Cancer recurred extratracheally 2½ years later on the side where node removal had not been performed. Irradiation gave an additional year of palliation. (*A,* From Grillo, H. C.: Circumferential resection and reconstruction of mediastinal and cervical trachea. Ann. Surg., *162*:347, 1965; *B,* From Grillo, H. C.: Surgery of the trachea. Curr. Probl. Surg., July 1970, p. 28.)

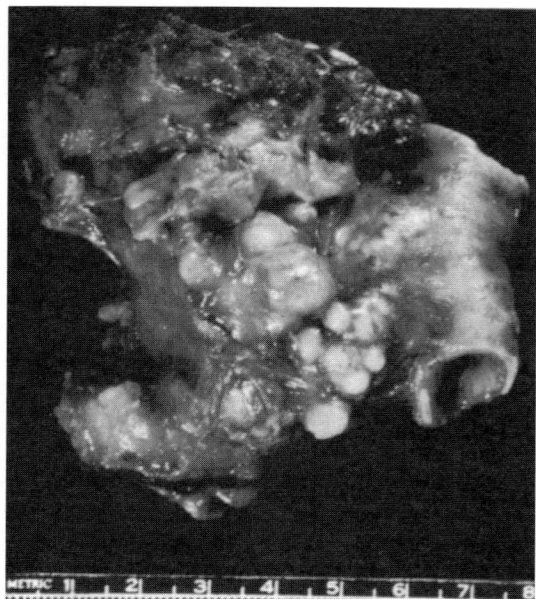

FIGURE 12–6. Chondrosarcoma of the trachea. Chondrosarcoma is rare in the trachea and is usually of low-grade malignancy. This huge tumor could be palpated in the supraclavicular space and involved a large extent of trachea, which displaced the great vessels and partially occluded the innominate veins. One recurrent nerve was destroyed by tumor. Primary anastomosis along with carotid endarterectomy for high-grade stenosis was performed in this 71-year-old man. The result was good, but the tumor recurred in his lungs years later.

The *clinical presentation* of primary tumors of the trachea may occur in several ways (Weber and Grillo, 1978b). The patient's first symptom may be shortness of breath on activity, which gradually worsens, usually at a relatively slow pace. One patient was unable to breathe except when sitting upright and could not even finish a sentence. Delay in diagnosis had occurred because the pulmonary fields remained normal on a film. Wheezing and stridor are often seen. The patient may have repeated attacks of respiratory obstruction owing to secretions. At this point, the patient's airway is usually greatly narrowed. If the patient has hemoptysis, it is more likely that a diagnosis will be made, because bronchoscopy will be performed even in the presence of a "normal" chest film. Another presentation is with repeated episodes of either unilateral or bilateral pneumonitis or pneumonia that respond to antibiotics and physiotherapy. If the lesion is at the tracheobronchial angle on one side, unilateral pneumonia may be seen, even though the degree of organic obstruction is small. If the lesion is centrally located, bilateral pneumonitis has been seen but with higher degrees of obstruction. A persistent and troublesome cough may also be a manifestation of primary tracheal tumors. In the absence of hemoptysis, too often a diagnosis of "adult-onset asthma" is made, and treatment is long delayed.

Secondary Neoplasms

Carcinoma of the larynx may involve the upper trachea by direct extension. Recurrence of invasive laryngeal carcinoma is not uncommon in the end tracheostomy site. Attempts at radical removal of such recurrences, with concurrent mediastinal tracheostomy, rarely lead to cure (Krespi et al., 1985). The recurrences are probably due to lymphatic permeation so that there is tumor at any level of transection, no matter how distal.

Bronchogenic carcinoma may involve the trachea or the origin of the main bronchus, especially on the right. Carinal resection may be considered if there is no mediastinal lymph node involvement (Dartevelle et al., 1988; Deslauriers, 1985; Jensik et al., 1982; Mathisen and Grillo, 1991). Pneumonectomy is usually required, but reimplantation of the lower lobe is occasionally possible. Mortality from carinal pneumonectomy is higher than that from standard pneumonectomy, principally owing to acute and unexplained adult respiratory distress syndrome (ARDS). The long-term survival ranged between 19 and 23%.

Carcinoma of the esophagus notoriously invades the tracheal wall. Tracheoesophageal fistula, caused either by direct erosion and necrosis of carcinoma of the esophagus or by necrosis induced by irradiation treatment of a carcinoma that involves the common wall, is too frequently seen. Surgical excision or bypass is usually not justified. Rarely, carcinoma of the esophagus requires a concurrent tracheal resection as part of combined adjuvant therapy and surgical attempt at extirpation. About the only circumstances under which such extension appears justified are if the lesion is otherwise totally resectable and the last point of involvement or adherence is the adjacent trachea. Although this may control local disease, distant recurrence remains common.

In several patients, inadequately resected carcinoid of the main bronchus has required later carinal resection, with good results.

The greatest field for tracheal operations in secondary neoplasia is for thyroid malignancy (Grillo et al., 1992c; Grillo and Zannini, 1986; Ishihara et al., 1991). Differentiated papillary or follicular carcinoma may be locally invasive, especially in older patients. If the lesion is producing tracheal obstruction or is found anatomically to be invading trachea at the time of resection of the thyroid, the optimal treatment is removal of the segment of involved airway at the time of initial resection (Fig. 12–7A and B) or soon thereafter. The author has also operated on numerous patients with late recurrences of carcinoma at points where tumor had been "shaved off" the trachea at a previous operation. In these patients, resection provided excellent and prolonged palliation, often for many years (Fig. 12–7C), but rarely a cure. Resection when, or soon after, airway involvement is first discovered, however, can cure. Less commonly partial laryngectomy is required, with laryngotracheoplastic reconstruction. Massive recurrent differentiated carcinoma or, rarely, localized undifferentiated lesions are indications for cervicomediastinal exenteration.

Various other tumors can involve the trachea, including metastases from other forms of head and neck carcinoma or carcinoma of the breast, which

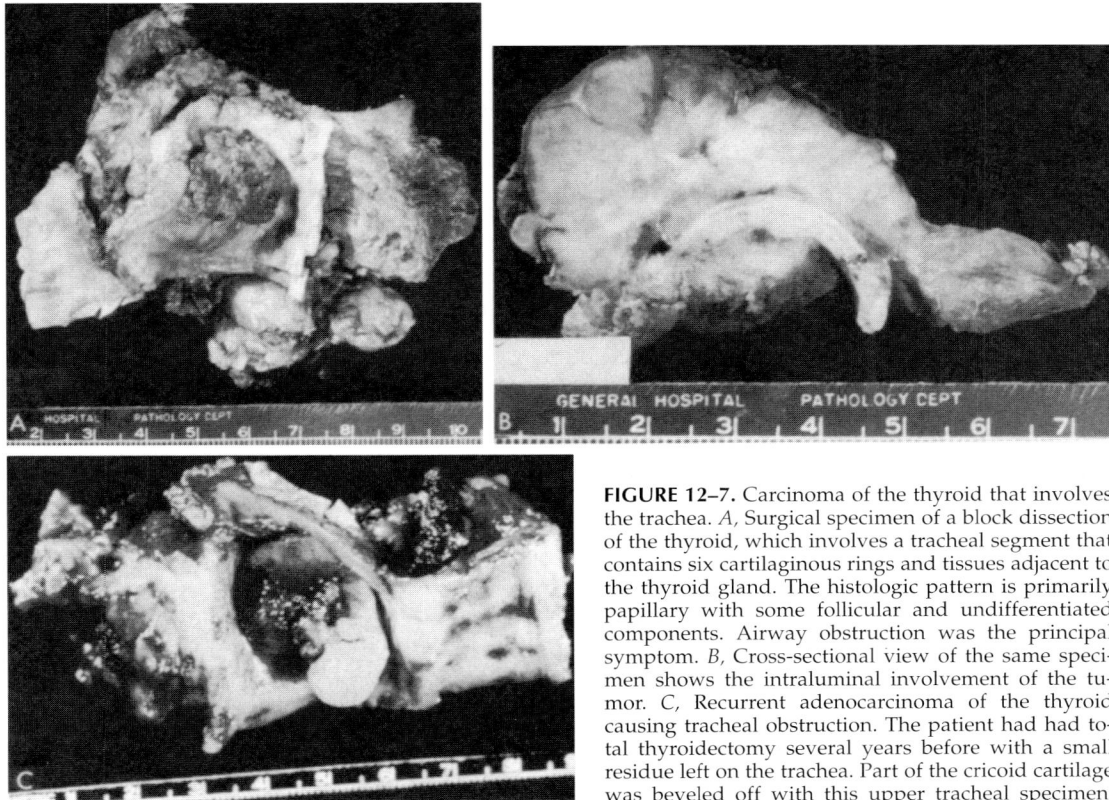

FIGURE 12–7. Carcinoma of the thyroid that involves the trachea. *A*, Surgical specimen of a block dissection of the thyroid, which involves a tracheal segment that contains six cartilaginous rings and tissues adjacent to the thyroid gland. The histologic pattern is primarily papillary with some follicular and undifferentiated components. Airway obstruction was the principal symptom. *B*, Cross-sectional view of the same specimen shows the intraluminal involvement of the tumor. *C*, Recurrent adenocarcinoma of the thyroid causing tracheal obstruction. The patient had had total thyroidectomy several years before with a small residue left on the trachea. Part of the cricoid cartilage was beveled off with this upper tracheal specimen, and a primary anastomosis was performed with a good resultant airway and preservation of voice. Later recurrences were distant, occurring in bone. (*B*, From Grillo, H. C.: Circumferential resection and reconstruction of mediastinal and cervical trachea. Ann. Surg., *162*:374, 1965.)

invades the mediastinum, and lymphoma. In none of these is primary tracheal resection usually indicated.

INFECTION, INFLAMMATION, AND TRAUMA

Infection

Tuberculosis of the upper airway principally involves the lower trachea or main bronchi. As acute ulcerative tuberculous tracheitis, treated medically, heals, stenosis may result. Submucosal, circumferential fibrosis markedly narrows or occludes the airway. The tracheal cartilages appear to be intact, but peritracheal fibrosis is found. Active tuberculosis must be arrested before surgical resection and reconstruction are performed. Long lesions may be irresectible. In patients with mature stenosis, carinal resection and reconstruction have been done, sometimes with excision of the right upper lobe as well and reimplantation of the bronchus intermedius. Complete stenosis of the left main bronchus has been managed by its total excision and reimplantation of the bifurcation of the left upper and lower lobes into the carina (Newton et al., 1991).

Histoplasmosis may produce massive mediastinal fibrosis with involvement of distal trachea, carina, and main bronchi, or it may involve principally the right bronchial tree in relation to lymph nodes in the right paratracheal and pretracheal area or in the middle lobe sump. The fibrosis may involve the right pulmonary artery within pericardium. The airway lesions may result from compression and intrinsic fibrosis. Subcarinal histoplasmoma may also compress the airway. Fibrotic and calcified subcarinal and precarinal lymph nodes may invade and erode through the walls of the trachea, carina, or bronchi, producing broncholithiasis. Infection and hemorrhage may follow (Mathisen and Grillo, 1992). The organism *Histoplasma capsulatum* is identified by special stains of pathologic material removed at surgery more often than from cultures. Organisms have been identified in fewer than 50% of patients who are presumed to have pathology owing to histoplasmosis. The continuing fibrotic process is believed to be a reaction to products of infection rather than to viable organisms. Diagnosis must often remain presumptive, based on pathologic and radiologic findings as well as on history of exposure and clinical evolution of the disease.

Diphtheria in childhood may be followed years later with tracheal stenosis or laryngotracheal stenosis. Since most of these patients had tracheostomies in infancy or early childhood for treatment of the acute disease, it is difficult to know whether late stenosis is due to the disease or to the treatment. *Scleroma*, found in Mexico and Central America, is a rare disease that may involve the airways as well as the nasopharynx

(Acuña, 1973). Necrosing *mucormycosis* involving the trachea or carina as well as the lungs may occur in diabetics or in patients who are immunosuppressed or undergoing chemotherapy, particularly for lymphoma. Prompt and radical surgical excision under protection of vigorous and prolonged treatment with amphotericin may save some of these patients (Tedder et al., 1994).

Trauma

Direct injury to the trachea can result from penetrating or blunt injuries (Besson and Saegesser, 1983; Mathisen and Grillo, 1987). Penetrating injuries to the trachea, as expected, are often cervical. One of the earliest descriptions of a tracheal injury was that of a sword wound treated by Ambroise Paré (1960). Relatively clean and fresh knife wounds may be sutured primarily. If the wound is extensive, the function of the vocal cords should be noted. The central location of the intrathoracic trachea makes its injury by gunshot wound or by other penetrating injury infrequent in a surviving patient.

Various blunt injuries may damage the trachea: for example, the force of an external blow to the neck may be sufficient to lacerate the trachea or to sever it. The patient initially may have a satisfactory airway, but then develop difficulty after arrival at hospital. Intubation may be impossible, and bronchoscopy may show a confusing and bloody situation in which the airway cannot be found. At emergency tracheostomy, the trachea may be totally severed and the distal end may have slipped down into the mediastinum after separation. If an injury is fresh and the damage is not too extensive, débridement and primary suture are performed. Nonfunction of the recurrent nerves may be temporary or permanent. Repair of the trachea under such circumstances should usually be accompanied by a distal tracheostomy for security. However, it may be better not to attempt the repair of complex, shattering tracheal lesions if the surgeon has no experience in tracheal and laryngeal reconstruction. The necessary accompanying tracheostomy and the extensive operation performed initially may compromise what otherwise would be an excellent possibility for later repair after the inflammation has regressed and any laryngeal problem has been solved or clarified. In such a circumstance, it is preferable to insert a tracheostomy tube into the severed end of the trachea rather than to make another opening distally through otherwise undamaged trachea (Mathisen and Grillo, 1987).

In injuries of the type described, the larynx may also be fractured. Concurrent injuries in the larynx with or without detachment of the trachea require expert otolaryngologic care. The placement of laryngeal molds and keels to restore the form of the larynx and allow it to heal in a functional state is best accomplished immediately after the acute injury (Montgomery, 1968; Ogura and Powers, 1964).

The intrathoracic trachea may be lacerated in closed chest trauma. Bronchi and trachea may both be ruptured by such trauma. Also seen is a vertical split through the carina, which extends up the membranous wall of the trachea. Such injury is usually manifested by unilateral or bilateral pneumothorax that fails to respond completely to tube thoracostomy and suction. If injury is suspected despite an initial good response to chest suction, bronchoscopy should be performed promptly. Early repair should be performed. Anesthesia may be critical, and guidance of a tube into the left main bronchus may be necessary for low lesions repaired via right thoracotomy. Generally, thoracic tracheal, right main bronchial, or bilateral main bronchial injuries—when fresh—are best approached through right thoracotomy. Left main bronchial avulsion is approached from the left. Median sternotomy with cervical extension may be useful, especially when the great vessels branching from the aortic arch are also injured (Symbas et al., 1992). Later repair should always be attempted if the lung has not become infected or fibrotic. Pulmonary function returns in approximately inverse proportion to the length of time without functioning (Deslauriers et al., 1982).

Severe closed injury may also lacerate the esophagus and trachea in their common wall, with the establishment of a traumatic tracheoesophageal fistula. Identification of such a fistula should be followed by prompt repair. If the fistula is not identified initially, secondary inflammatory changes may make repair difficult and may even require temporary defunctioning of the esophagus before reconstruction is possible. If the leak is not diagnosed, fatal mediastinitis may follow.

Late stenosis of the trachea due to blunt trauma and separation in the neck may present as a stenosis with or without previous attempts at repair (Couraud et al., 1989; Mathisen and Grillo, 1987). It is vital under these circumstances to establish the functional status of the larynx and to wait a sufficient length of time to determine whether this malfunction is permanent or temporary. Once it is clear that the patient will not regain laryngeal function, assuming bilateral cord palsies, it may be necessary to do arytenoidectomy, arytenoidesis, or lateralization of a vocal cord to establish a functional airway in the larynx. Laryngotracheal or tracheotracheal anastomosis may then be performed. Even a paralyzed larynx can produce a better voice than an esophageally motivated pharyngeal voice. A traumatic separation of the trachea that appears extensive on film may really represent little loss of substance but simply distraction of the ends of the severed trachea. Repair under these circumstances has usually not been difficult from the standpoint of length. More difficult is the blunt injury in which pharyngoesophageal disruption has occurred as well as laryngotracheal separation. Vertebral and spinal injury may also be present in such cases. Repair—early or late—is most demanding. Pharyngoesophageal or esophageal rupture must always be repaired primarily.

Inhalation Burns

Severe inhalation burns of larynx, trachea, and bronchi are particularly difficult to manage. The agent may be chemical or thermal, or a combination. These patients often show little damage to the pharynx or supraglottic larynx once the initial reaction to injury has subsided. Persistent damage commences in the subglottis just below the vocal cords and extends down the airway in gradually diminishing intensity. The depth of injury as well as the length of airway injured probably relates to the dose received as well as to the actual injury potential of the agent. In 18 patients treated for tracheal stenosis due to inhalation injury, 14 had subglottic strictures as well and 2 had main bronchial stenosis. Although it is sometimes difficult to differentiate burn damage from later injuries owing to the intubation with which the patients were treated acutely, 3 patients had laryngotracheal strictures without any history of intubation (Gaissert et al., 1993).

In most cases, the tracheal rings were not destroyed and the injuries were confined to various depths of mucosal and submucosal damage. Attempts to resect injuries, especially in their early phase, should not be made. First, involvement often commences immediately below the cords and involves the entire subglottic larynx, making repair almost impossible. Second, the burned airway responds poorly to early surgery, even where the lesion appears to be limited, much in the way that burned skin elsewhere in the body does—by the re-formation of massive scarring. With appropriately placed splinting silicone T tubes and a great deal of patience, a stable and open airway may usually be obtained in most of these patients in time.

Postoperative Stenosis

Stenosis of the trachea following tracheal reconstruction is due in most cases to excessive tension on the anastomosis, and this is related to overzealous resection of too great a length of trachea. Dangerous tensions in tracheal resection may be reached generally at a resection level of 50% of tracheal length in an adult and at a level of 30 to 40% in a child. These figures vary greatly with age, body habitus, pathology, and prior intervention. Carinal resections are particularly at risk because of their complex nature. Patients chronically on high doses of prednisone are endangered if extensive tracheal resection is performed. Unnecessary disturbance of the blood supply to the trachea by extensive circumferential dissection will also lead to stenosis or separation. Profuse, hypertrophic granulations at the anastomosis, which were seen when nonabsorbable sutures were used for tracheal repair, have vanished since the introduction of absorbable Vicryl sutures.

Stenoses may also result from *radiation therapy* and *laser injury*. Stenosis due to irradiation may appear years following therapy. *Brachytherapy* has also contributed a number of main bronchial stenoses. The contribution of lasering to tracheal damage is difficult to assess because the lasering is often used to treat preexisting stenosis and, in conjunction with distal tracheostomy, performed to "safeguard" the airway. Whereas laser injury may be treated by subsequent resectional surgery if the lesion is not too extensive, irradiation injury may be either surgically incorrectable when first seen or correctable only with considerable risk depending on radiation dosage and the interval following irradiation. Omental advancement is advisable to support healing, which otherwise may fail completely (Muehrcke et al., 1995).

Postintubation Injuries

Oral or nasal endotracheal tubes or tracheostomy tubes are most commonly used to deliver mechanical ventilatory support in respiratory failure. Assistance supplied through cuffed tubes has thus far proved to be the only practicable method of management for adults with poor pulmonary or chest wall compliance. High-flow respirators with uncuffed tubes, electrophrenic respirators, and negative-pressure tank respirators have not been satisfactory to manage these severe problems. High-frequency ventilation for long-term use remains developmental. A spectrum of tracheal lesions resulting from such treatment was discerned (Andrews and Pearson, 1971; Grillo, 1969) (Fig. 12–8). Despite improvements in equipment and technique, these lesions continue to provide the principal indication for tracheal reconstruction. Because a single patient may have more than one lesion and because the treatment of these lesions differs, precise definition of the pathologic state is essential in planning treatment.

Lindholm (1970) showed that endotracheal tubes may cause obstruction at the *laryngeal level* even after only 48 hours of endotracheal intubation: glottic edema, vocal cord granulomas, erosions particularly over the arytenoids, formation of granulation tissue, polypoid obstructions, and stenosis, anterior or posterior commissural and particularly at the subglottic intralaryngeal level. Whited (1984) confirmed the sequelae of long-term endotracheal intubation in a prospective study. Subglottic injury, although most commonly the result of endotracheal tube damage, is also produced by cricothyroidostomy and by cricoid erosion due to high tracheostomy in the presence of kyphosis. Subglottic stenosis may be difficult to correct, and is sometimes impossible. The multiplicity of complex procedures proposed to correct subglottic stenosis attests to the difficulty of the problem (Grillo, 1982b). The importance of defining the state of the larynx before embarking on corrective tracheal procedures cannot be emphasized enough. The larynx should be examined carefully, the function of the cords should be noted, and observations should be confirmed by fluoroscopic and radiologic examination as well. Such examinations must also define as precisely as possible the level at which pathology presents. An upper tracheal lesion just below cricoid level

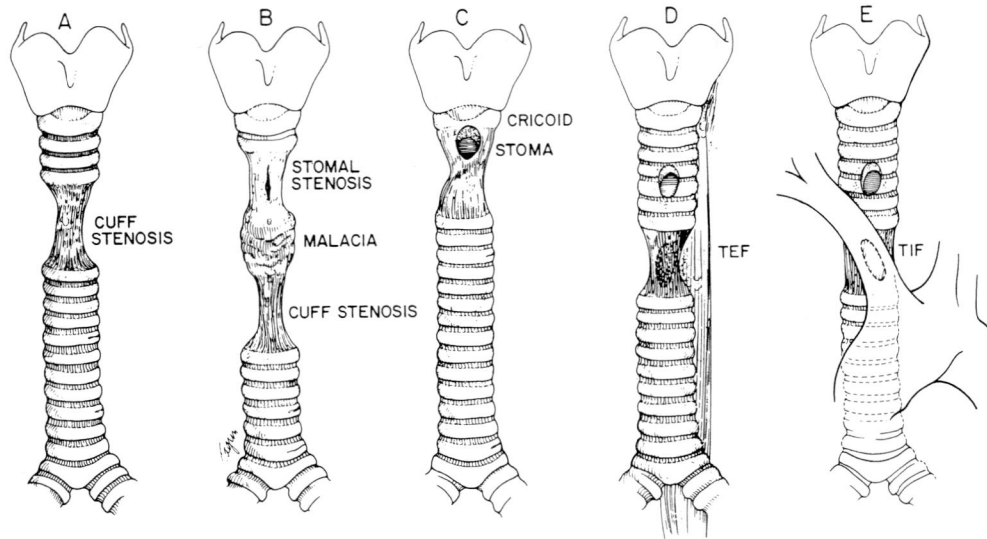

FIGURE 12–8. Principal postintubation tracheal lesions. *A,* Lesion at the cuff site in a patient who has been treated with an endotracheal tube alone. The lesion is high in the trachea and is circumferential. Sometimes the external tracheal surfaces look almost normal. *B,* Lesions that occur with tracheostomy tubes. At the stomal level, anterolateral stenosis is seen. At the cuff level, which is lower than with an endotracheal tube, circumferential cuff stenosis occurs. The segment between is often inflamed and malacic. Malacia may also occur at cuff level. *C,* Damage to the subglottic larynx. A high tracheostomy or one that erodes back by virtue of the patient's anatomy may damage the inferior cricoid and produce a low subglottic stenosis as well as an upper tracheal injury. *D,* Tracheoesophageal fistula (TEF). The level of fistulization is usually where the cuff has eroded posteriorly. There is also usually severe circumferential damage at this level by the cuff. Occasionally, angulation of the tube may produce erosion from the tip. *E,* Tracheo–innominate artery fistula (TIF). A high-pressure cuff frequently rests on the trachea directly behind the innominate artery. Erosion may occur, although rarely. The more common innominate artery injury is from a low tracheostomy in which the inner portion of the curve of the tube rests in proximity to the artery and causes direct erosion. Laryngeal injuries due to endotracheal tubes or cricothyroidostomy are not shown. (*A–E,* From Grillo, H. C.: Surgical treatment of postintubation tracheal injuries. J. Thorac. Cardiovasc. Surg., *78:*860, 1979.)

may be separated with difficulty from a subglottic intralaryngeal lesion. The surgical management differs and may be difficult in the latter case.

At the *tracheostomy site,* granulomas that obstruct the airway may form during healing. If the tracheostomy stoma has been made too large by turning a large flap or excising a large window during tracheostomy, or most commonly, if erosion is caused by sepsis and heavy prying equipment, cicatricial healing of this defect may produce an anterior A-shaped stenosis that can severely compromise the airway (Fig. 12–9). The posterior wall of the trachea is usually relatively intact in these patients. Another lesion that occurs at stomal level, especially in children, is posterior depression of a flap of trachea by the tracheostomy tube.

At the level of the inflatable *cuff,* whether it is placed on a tracheostomy tube or an endotracheal tube, circumferential erosion of the tracheal wall may occur. If this erosion is deep enough, all the anatomic layers of the trachea may be destroyed, so that cicatricial repair creates a tight circumferential stenosis (Fig. 12–10). Malacia may result instead, much less commonly. Below this level, at the point where the tip of the tube may pry against the tracheal wall, additional erosion may occur with formation of a granuloma, especially in children, in whom uncuffed tubes are used. In the segment between the stoma and the cuff level, varying degrees of chondromalacia with resulting tracheomalacia may occur. Here the carti-

lages are not totally destroyed but only thinned. Bacterial infection in this segment of the trachea during the period of ventilatory support probably contributes to this process.

The *cause* of cuff stenosis has been attributed variously to pressure necrosis by the cuff, to the irritative quality of materials in rubber and plastic cuffs and tubes, to irritant products from gas sterilization, to hypotension, and to bacterial infection. Autopsy studies of patients who had been on ventilators with inflated cuffs (Cooper and Grillo, 1969a; Florange et al., 1965) (Fig. 12–11), prospective studies (Andrews and Pearson, 1971), analysis of surgically removed lesions caused by cuffs (Grillo, 1969), and experimental reproduction of these lesions under controlled conditions (Cooper and Grillo, 1969b) point to pressure necrosis as the principal causative agent. When high-pressure Rusch cuffs were inflated to provide just a seal at ventilatory pressures of 25 cm H_2O, intracuff pressures rose to 180 to 250 mm Hg (Grillo et al., 1971). Although these pressures are not exactly those exerted on the tracheal mucous membrane, high pressures are indeed exerted (Carroll et al., 1969). The trachea has an elliptical form, so it becomes deformed at the point where a seal is obtained. If perfusion pressures in the patient are lower than normal, necrosis can occur even more easily. The mucosa overlying the cartilage is initially destroyed. The bared cartilages become necrotic and ultimately slough. Attempts at repair following full-thickness damage to

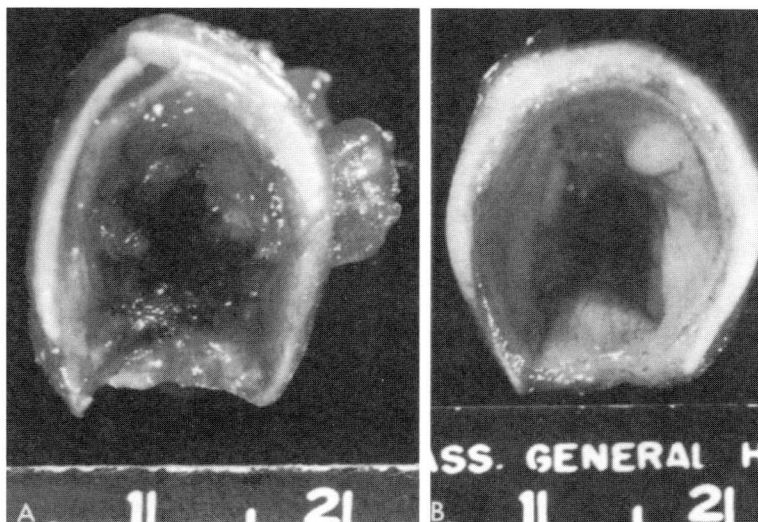

FIGURE 12–9. Stenosis at the stomal site. Surgical specimens. *A,* The roughly triangular shape of the stenosis is evident with the apex anteriorly. The principal cicatricial and granulomatous changes are anterolateral. In this case of a relatively fresh stricture, there are some granulations posteriorly as well. *B,* A more "mature" stomal stricture shows the same triangular narrowing with firm cicatricial changes in the anterolateral wall. The membranous wall is relatively intact, although it is squeezed together by the lateral processes.

the tracheal wall lead only to scar formation. Because the erosion is circumferential, so are the resultant strictures (Fig. 12–12). Even further erosive damage can lead to tracheoesophageal fistula posteriorly or to perforation of the innominate artery anteriorly.

Clinical Manifestations

Most of these lesions manifest themselves as obstruction of the trachea (Weber and Grillo, 1978a). The patient presents with dyspnea on effort, wheezing that progresses to stridor, and later, episodes of obstruction with even minimal amounts of mucus. All too often, when such patients have normal lung fields radiographically, a diagnosis of "asthma" is made. Treatment may extend to high doses of steroids for alleged asthma before the true diagnosis is made. A few present with unilateral or bilateral pneumonia.

Any patient who develops symptoms of airway obstruction who has been intubated and ventilated in the recent past must be considered to have an organic lesion until it is proved otherwise.

Another danger to these patients is that many remain sedentary from the original disease that caused respiratory failure. Because the patients do not exert themselves, very severe stenoses may evolve before dyspnea is recognized. Clinically and experimentally, it has been noted that the peak expiratory flow rate dropped to approximately 80% of normal at airway diameters below 10 mm (Al-Bazzaz et al., 1975). However, the flow drops to about 30% of normal at diameters of 5 to 6 mm. Below this, the drop in flow is rapid.

Diagnosis is accomplished by relatively simple radiologic studies. Bronchoscopic confirmation is usually deferred to the time of proposed corrective ther-

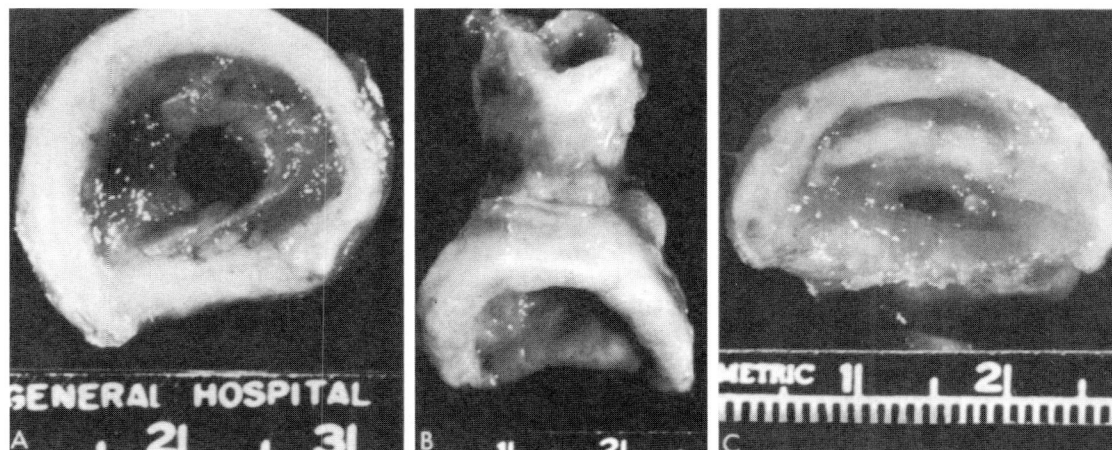

FIGURE 12–10. Tracheal stenosis at cuff level. Surgical specimens. *A,* Typical circumferential stenosis with an effective airway of 5 mm. These are not soft granulations but are rather firm fibrous strictures. Seen end-on, the full extent of destruction of the tracheal wall at the level of the stricture is not clearly visible. *B,* Stenotic segment. In many cases, the external appearance of the stricture is not as "wasp-waisted" as this one because most of the thickening is inside, although rings are absent for the length of the stricture. In this case, additional trachea was taken above to reach a normal size of lumen. *C,* The tiny size of the remaining airway in this patient precipitated acute obstruction, although the patient was still sedentary and hospitalized. The results of resection in all of these patients were good.

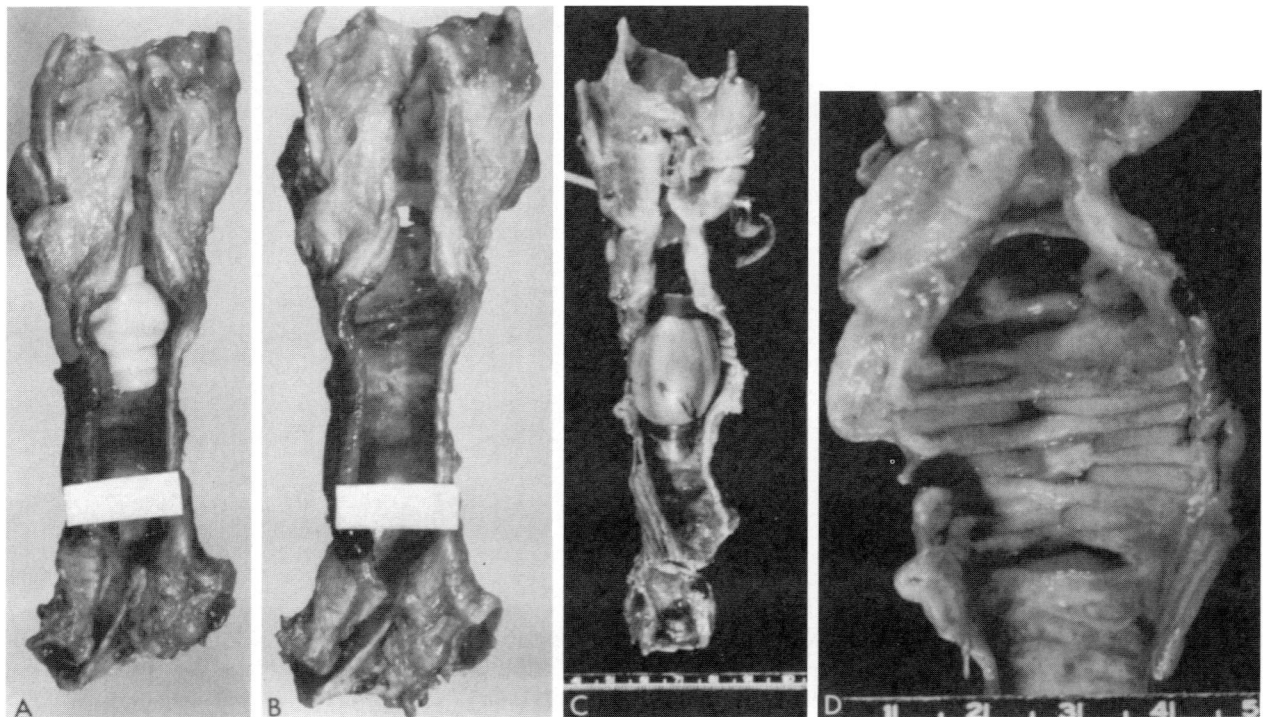

FIGURE 12–11. Injury due to cuffed tracheostomy tubes of prior design that produced high intracuff pressures. *A*, Autopsy specimen of a patient who had received ventilatory treatment with a Portex tube in place. The wall is thinned at the site of the cuff. There is tracheitis below it. *B*, Beneath the cuff there has been mucosal erosion baring the tracheal cartilages. *C*, Another trachea with an inlying metal tracheostomy tube and standard rubber cuff. *D*, Detail shows not only baring of cartilage but also evidence of missing fragments. (*A–D*, From Cooper, J. D., and Grillo, H. C.: The evolution of tracheal injury due to ventilatory assistance through cuffed tubes: A pathologic study. Ann Surg., *196:*334, 1969.)

apy unless airway obstruction is severe or operation should be deferred. Flow-volume curves are interesting but provide little practical help in management.

Tracheoesophageal fistula due to cuff erosion is usually manifested by increasing difficulty in ventilating the patient, gastric dilatation, or more often, the sudden appearance of large amounts of secretions in the tracheobronchial tree (Hedden et al., 1969). Tracheoesophageal fistula occurs most commonly in patients who have a ventilating cuff in the trachea for a long time, along with a feeding tube in the esophagus. The two foreign bodies pincer the "party wall" between trachea and esophagus, producing first inflammation, which seals one wall against the other, and then perforation, which may enlarge to include the entire membranous wall of the trachea. There is usually concomitant circumferential injury to the trachea as well, since this is basically a cuff lesion. The patient may develop pneumonitis, pneumonia, or abscess. Feedings appear promptly in the tracheobronchial tree, and methylene blue appears promptly in the trachea.

Anterior erosion of the trachea may lead to *innominate artery fistula*. A small number of anterior erosions were seen in the past due to angulation of a tube tip or a high-pressure cuff itself eroding directly into the artery. More common, although fortunately still rare, are erosions of the artery that occur at the inferior margin of a low-placed tracheostomy stoma that is

immediately contiguous with the artery. The inner curve of the tube erodes its way through the arterial wall. It is seen most often in children and young adults in whom tracheostomy is placed too low because, on hyperextension, more than half the trachea rises up into the neck, and the artery with it. If the stoma is placed with respect to the sternal notch rather than to the cricoid cartilage, the tracheostomy will then reside just above the elevated innominate artery (Deslauriers et al., 1975). Tracheoinnominate fistula is manifested by sudden exsanguinating hemorrhage into the tracheobronchial tree (Deslauriers et al., 1975; Grillo, 1979a). Occasionally, there are smaller premonitory hemorrhages. Such hemorrhages must be differentiated from bleeding resulting from severe tracheitis. If the lesion is caused by cuff erosion, emergency control can be attained by prompt insertion of an endotracheal tube with inflation of a high-pressure cuff to tamponade the opening. If the erosion occurred because the tube itself rests on the artery, packing plus digital pressure anterior to the stoma is needed for emergency control. Repair must be done immediately.

Treatment

The preferred treatment of postintubation stenosis of the trachea is resection and reconstruction when the patient can tolerate it. With careful evaluation,

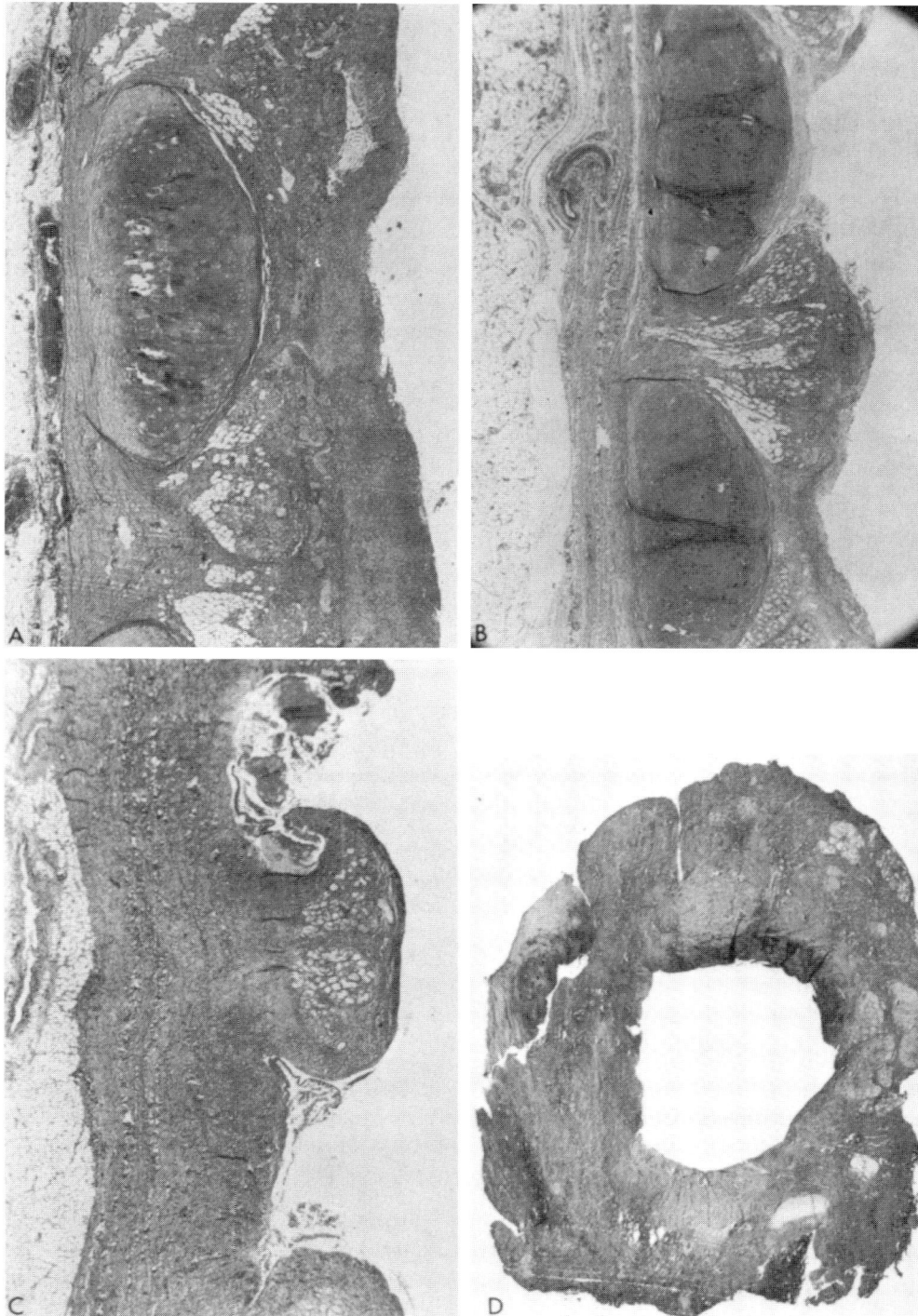

FIGURE 12–12. Development of stenosis at the cuff site. Photomicrographs of stages. *A,* The surface epithelium has become ulcerated, especially overlying the individual cartilages where the tissue is squeezed between the high-pressure cuff and the firm surface of cartilage. *B,* The superficial ulceration has progressed to destruction of the epithelium and underlying soft tissues so that the cartilages are bared. *C,* The cartilage has become necrotic and fragmented above and the area below it has been destroyed. Inflammatory response has penetrated deeply into the wall of the trachea. The next stage would be a loss of the tissue between the cartilages so that the tracheal wall loses all identifying anatomy and becomes an ulcer bed. *D,* Cross-sectional view of a stenotic lesion. Almost all of the normal tracheal microscopic anatomy has been destroyed, and all that is left is the cicatricial response of the new connective tissue formed in the ulcerated area in an attempt at healing. (*A–C,* From Cooper, J. D., and Grillo, H. C.: The evolution of tracheal injury due to ventilatory assistance through cuffed tubes. Ann. Surg. *169*:334, 1969; *D,* From Grillo, H. C.: The management of tracheal stenosis following assisted respiration. J. Thorac. Cardiovasc. Surg., *57*:52, 1969.)

planning, and execution, most patients can be treated successfully by operation when they have recovered from the primary disease that led to the stenosis. A properly conducted anesthesia and operative repair from the anterior approach does not have great physiologic impact. Nonoperative methods of temporizing are, however, available. Since the disease is not malignant, risks must not be taken. Very rarely, the patient's medical condition may not permit even the relatively benign procedure required. If the patient has serious neurologic or psychiatric deficits that will prevent cooperation postoperatively, reconstruction is best deferred. The patient and her anesthesia must be selected to avoid the need for ventilatory support postoperatively. If ventilatory support is needed postoperatively in a shortened trachea, the cuff may rest against the anastomosis and this could lead to dehiscence.

The temporizing methods available are repetitive bronchoscopic dilatation of a stenosis or reinstitution of a tracheostomy, dilatation of the stricture, and passage of a tracheostomy tube or a Silastic T tube through the lesion to splint the airway. Lesions in the immediate supracarinal position are not easily managed in this way. A tube long enough to remain seated may cause obstruction when it rests on the carina, and a T-Y tube may lead to bronchial granulations. Generally, however, it is wiser to use a T tube for a permanent airway than to undertake a hazardous reconstruction which has a high risk for failure (Cooper et al., 1989; Gaissert et al., 1994).

Repeated dilatation and stenting have been proposed as definitive methods for treating tracheal stenosis. In most severe lesions in which the whole thickness of the tracheal wall has been converted to scar tissue, even prolonged stenting for many years will not lead to permanent recovery. Numerous patients have been treated this way. Despite repeated trials, it has been impossible, with only rare exceptions in less severe strictures, to permanently remove the splinting tube. Laser treatment can lead only to cure of granuloma—also easily removed by bronchoscopy—and thin, web-like stenosis (Dumon, 1985; Toty et al., 1987). Such stenoses are very rare. In the usual postintubation stenosis, definitive opening by laser would lead to tracheal perforation. The principal effect of use of the laser for these lesions has been to delay definitive treatment and, sometimes, to worsen the lesion. Particularly to be deplored is reestablishment of tracheostomy in order to permit laser treatment.

Few, if any, patients with postintubation tracheal stenosis cannot be repaired successfully when first identified. It is only successive failure of inappropriate therapies (e.g., successive tracheostomies, failed reconstruction, cartilage grafts, laser treatment) that make such patients nonreconstructible.

Prevention of Postintubation Tracheal Stenosis

The incidence of stenosis at the *stomal level* can be reduced by careful placement of the stoma, avoidance of large apertures, meticulous care of the tracheostomy, and most importantly, elimination of heavy and prying ventilatory connecting equipment.

Many proposals have been made to reduce the formerly inevitable occurrence of some *stenoses at the cuff level*. These methods included use of double-cuff tubes, changes in materials and sterilization techniques, attempts to avoid cuffs altogether, use of disk and sponge seals instead of cuffs, use of spacers to relocate the cuff level periodically, prestretching of plastic cuffs, and intermittent inflation of cuffs cycled to the respirator. The development of large-volume, low-pressure cuffs that conform to the shape of the trachea, rather than deforming it, provides a means of avoiding cuff stenosis (Cooper and Grillo, 1969b; Grillo et al., 1971) (Fig. 12–13). The cuff provides a seal at intracuff pressures of 33 mm Hg, compared with 270 mm Hg in a comparative Rusch (formerly) standard cuff. In a series of 45 patients in whom such a cuff was compared, on a randomized basis, with standard cuffs, 25 patients with the soft cuff showed half as much damage—scaled on the basis of endoscopic observations at the time of deflation of the cuff—as 20 patients with standard cuffs. All severe damage was in the standard group. Incidence of cuff stenosis has dropped markedly as equipment has improved. Since the identification of this cause over 25 years ago, not a single cuff stenosis has been produced in the Massachusetts General Hospital. However, since all available (large-volume) cuffs are uniformly made from plastic, which is relatively inextensible after resting maximal volume is attained, additional volume causes steeply rising intracuff pressures. Such incorrect use continues to produce circumferential cuff tracheal stenosis.

Cricothyroidostomy should be avoided. Although laryngeal injury is rare, it may not be correctable when it occurs. In contrast, tracheal injuries—also rare—almost always are reparable when they first occur. Inappropriate treatment makes some incorrectable.

EXTRINSIC LESIONS

Goiter

Large goiters, either cervical or mediastinal, may gradually compress the airway sufficiently to cause symptoms. The slow growth of the goiter may deform cartilaginous rings without destroying them. When the goiter is removed, the trachea may remain distorted in shape and narrowed, but clinically significant airway obstruction rarely persists. Removal of the goiter usually leads to immediate relief of respiratory symptoms. Rarely, if sufficient softening of the cartilages has occurred owing to prolonged compression, removing the supporting mass of thyroid tissue allows the trachea to collapse with respiratory effort. This is determined by intraoperative bronchoscopy, local examination and palpation in the operative field, and finally, by observation of the patient in the op-

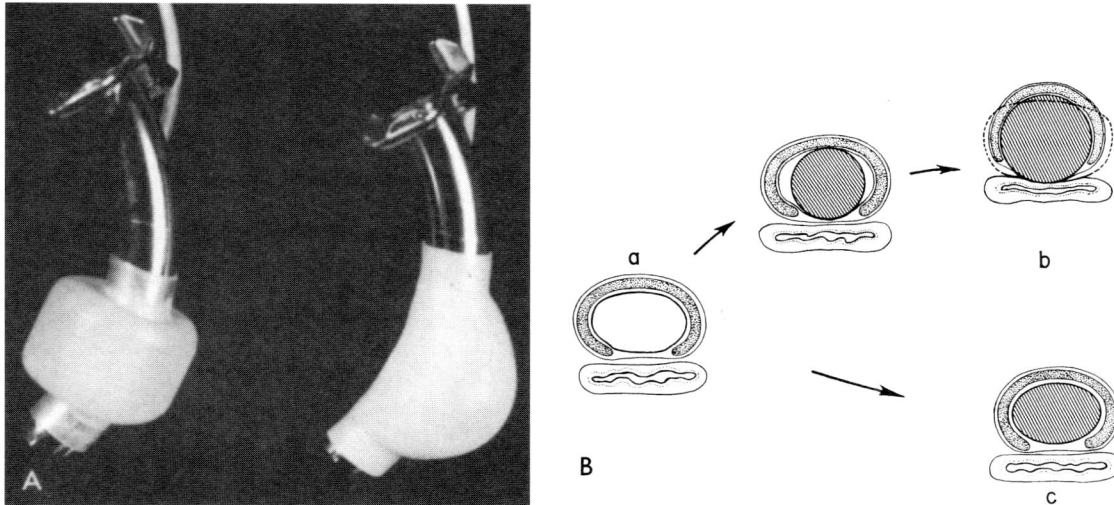

FIGURE 12–13. Tracheostomy tube cuffs. *A,* On the left is a large-volume, high-compliance latex cuff applied to a metal tube. The cuff contains the same volume of air as the high-pressure cuff at the right, but this is also the resting volume of the cuff before exerting any stretch on the material of which it is made. On the right, the cuff has been distended from its normally collapsed position of close application to the tube. It is tense, has a high intracuff presssure, and exerts high pressure on the tracheal wall. Furthermore, it distends eccentrically. *B,* Diagram showing the mechanism effecting tracheal seal with standard high-pressure cuff and with high-compliance, low-pressure cuff. The eccentrically shaped trachea *(a)* is not sealed when the high-pressure cuff first distends enough to reach the anterior and posterior walls. It must continue to be distended and gives a seal when the airway is occluded *(b).* At this point, there is high intracuff pressure that is transmitted to the tracheal wall. In *c,* a large-volume cuff with high compliance has simply flowed into the shape of the trachea and provides occlusion without exerting significant pressure. *(A,* From Grillo, H. C., Cooper, J. D., Geffin, B., and Pontoppidan, H.: A low-pressure cuff for tracheostomy tubes to minimize tracheal injury: A comparative clinical trial. J. Thorac. Cardiovasc. Surg., *62:*898, 1971; *B,* From Cooper, J. D., and Grillo, H. C.: Experimental production and prevention of injury due to cuffed tracheal tubes. Surg. Gynecol. Obstet., *129:*1235, 1969.)

erating room following extubation. Several methods of managing this problem have evolved, including intubation with an uncuffed tube followed by tracheostomy, preferably with insertion of a silicone T tube several days later when the wound planes are sealed or immediate buttressing of the trachea with specially made polypropylene plastic rings or by utilizing traction sutures from the tracheal wall tied over either internal or external buttons. An anterior substernal goiter usually does not exert pressure on the trachea because of its position in front of the great vessels. The trachea is more likely to be compressed by posterior descending goiters that enter the thoracic strait lateral to the esophagus and trachea (Katlic et al., 1985).

Vascular Compression

Symptoms of tracheal compression may be produced by congenital vascular rings (see Chapter 33, part II) or aneurysms of the innominate artery or of an anomalous subclavian artery that passes behind the trachea and esophagus. In children, the trachea may be compressed by the innominate artery.

Mediastinal Masses

Most mediastinal masses that compress the trachea are malignant neoplasms. However, bronchogenic cysts located at the carina may cause cough and, rarely, compress the airway (Suen et al., 1993).

Postpneumonectomy Syndrome

Following right pneumonectomy, the mediastinum may move completely over to the right axilla and posteriorly. In so doing, the aortic arch becomes rotated horizontally. This may lead to angulation and compression of the remaining tracheobronchial tree, with obstruction either at the carina or in the proximal left main bronchus. Less commonly, lobar bronchi are affected. The bronchus is actually compressed between the pulmonary artery, which is stretched in front of it, and either the aorta or the vertebral bodies posteriorly (Fig. 12–14). It is difficult to predict which patients will suffer this distortion following pneumonectomy. It was formerly believed that this was principally seen in children, but the problem has appeared following pneumonectomy in adult life (Grillo et al., 1992b). The reverse situation may be seen after left pneumonectomy in the presence of a right aortic arch, with flattening of the right bronchial tree. The patient's symptoms may be rapidly progressive and lead to a total disability. Malacia of the compressed airway may result secondarily over an undetermined span of time.

MISCELLANEOUS LESIONS

Relapsing polychondritis is a disease of unknown origin and unpredictable course. Nasal and ear cartilages

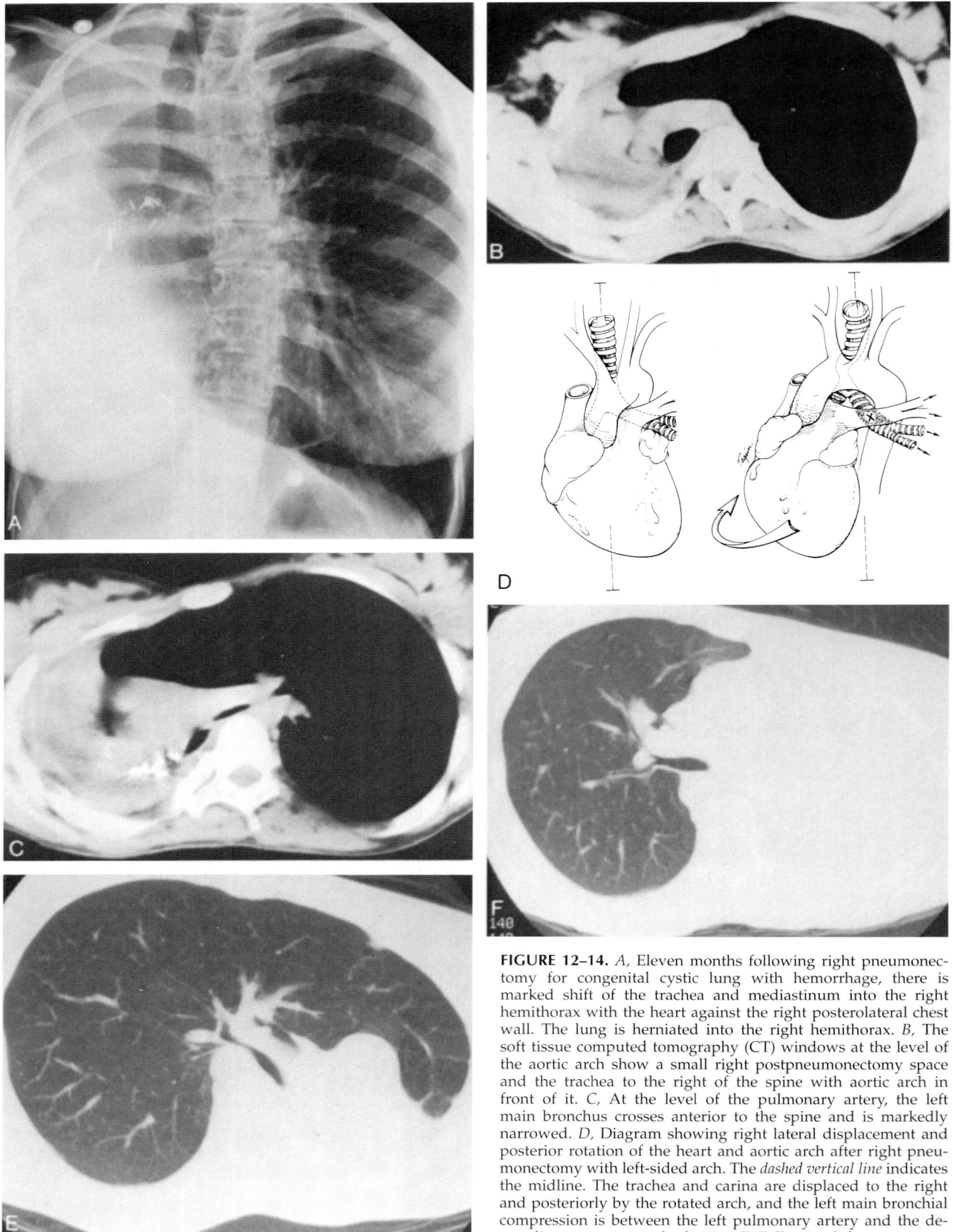

FIGURE 12–14. *A,* Eleven months following right pneumonectomy for congenital cystic lung with hemorrhage, there is marked shift of the trachea and mediastinum into the right hemithorax with the heart against the right posterolateral chest wall. The lung is herniated into the right hemithorax. *B,* The soft tissue computed tomography (CT) windows at the level of the aortic arch show a small right postpneumonectomy space and the trachea to the right of the spine with aortic arch in front of it. *C,* At the level of the pulmonary artery, the left main bronchus crosses anterior to the spine and is markedly narrowed. *D,* Diagram showing right lateral displacement and posterior rotation of the heart and aortic arch after right pneumonectomy with left-sided arch. The *dashed vertical line* indicates the midline. The trachea and carina are displaced to the right and posteriorly by the rotated arch, and the left main bronchial compression is between the left pulmonary artery and the descending aorta or vertebral spine. *E,* Following left pneumonectomy in a patient with a right aortic arch, mirror image distortion occurs. There is no postpneumonectomy space. The right main bronchus is compressed between the right pulmonary artery and the aorta and spine. *F,* After mediastinal repositioning, CT in the same patient shows the bronchial tree returned to normal position and the compression relieved. (*A–F,* From Grillo, H. C., Shepard, J. O., Mathisen, D. J., and Kanarek, D. J.: Postpneumonectomy syndrome: Diagnosis, management, and results. Reprinted with permission from the Society of Thoracic Surgeons [The Annals of Thoracic Surgery, 1992, Vol. 54, p. 638].)

and those of the tracheobronchial tree are most commonly affected. The airway changes may precede by years the more characteristic changes in the nose and ears. When the lower trachea and bronchi are affected first, the disease manifests itself by progressive malacic airway obstruction, difficulty in clearing secretions, and pulmonary infection. The process may extend into segmental bronchi. Relapsing polychondritis may also affect the larynx and uppermost trachea, where the cartilages become inflamed and thickened. Constrictive narrowing of the subglottic and subcricoid airways results. The disease may then progress distally, but without predictability. Surgical therapy is not usually applicable. Sometimes it is necessary to provide an airway with a tracheostomy tube, and sometimes stenting with a T tube or T-Y tube may provide temporary palliation. The disease is unrelenting.

Wegener's granulomatosis may affect the larynx and trachea with inflammatory lesions that lead to airway obstruction. The rate and extent of involvement are highly unpredictable. With response to medical treatment, an apparently stable stenosis may result and, on rare occasions, be suited to surgical treatment.

Sarcoid may produce airway obstruction by massive enlargement of mediastinal lymph nodes compressing and distorting the airway and also by intrinsic fibrotic changes in the wall of the trachea and bronchi. A circumferential stenosis results that usually involves a long segment of trachea and main bronchi. It may also involve more distal bronchi. These lesions are not amenable to surgical treatment because of diffuseness and extent, but periodic dilatation will tide the patient over for some time.

Amyloid disease on rare occasions involves the trachea and main bronchi in a very extensive process leading to narrowing throughout the tracheobronchial tree. The lesions are usually too extensive to permit surgical resection and reconstruction.

Tracheopathia osteoplastica manifests itself pathologically by the formation of calcified nodules beneath the mucosa, adjacent to but not actually originating from the cartilages (Young et al., 1980). Involvement may commence in the subglottic larynx and extend throughout the trachea and bronchi. It appears in adults, progressing insidiously. As the disease progresses, patients have difficulty in raising tenacious secretions. Ultimately, severe obstructive symptoms may ensue. In many patients, however, the disease remains a curiosity and does not seriously impair them. It may be discovered only incidentally at autopsy. Surgical relief is obtained by reshaping the airway over a Silastic T-Y tube (Mark et al., 1992).

Tracheobronchiomegaly (Mounier-Kuhn syndrome) is probably of congenital origin, although it usually becomes clinically manifest in adult life. The symptoms are progressive dyspnea on exertion and difficulty in raising secretions. The trachea may be hugely widened on x-ray. The cartilages are elongated and markedly deformed, and the membranous wall is redundant and thickened. The cartilages gradually tend to assume a reverse curve that brings the redundant

membranous wall up against the cartilages, causing obstruction. The main bronchi are also involved. A T tube can provide relief.

Saber-sheath tracheal deformity is usually an incidental finding in patients with varying degrees of chronic obstructive pulmonary disease later in their lives (50s and 60s). The lower two-thirds of the trachea—the intrathoracic trachea—gradually assumes a configuration in which the side-to-side diameter diminishes progressively and the anteroposterior diameter increases (Greene and Lechner, 1975). The cartilages are not malacic. In early stages, the change in airway configuration causes no difficulty, but as it becomes more and more marked, the posterior part of the cartilages approximate with attempts to cough and breathe deeply. The patient finds that he cannot clear the thickened secretions. The proximal cervical portion of the trachea usually remains quite normal. Internal or external tracheal splinting permits the patient to raise secretions with cough.

Idiopathic tracheal stenosis presents over a wide spectrum of age, principally in women, with progressive dyspnea on exertion and wheezing. These patients are usually found to have a short stenosis (about 2 to 3 cm) involving the uppermost trachea and, in many cases, the subglottic larynx as well. Distally, the trachea is quite normal in appearance (Fig. 12–15). The patients have no history of trauma, infection, inhalation injury, intubation for ventilation, or any other tracheal or airway disease. In a series of 49 patients, only 3 had any systemic symptoms (Grillo et al., 1993). Two had mild arthralgias and 1 had poorly defined arteritis. Most who had been followed for as long as 15 years had never developed any systemic symptoms or evolved into other defined diseases. The stricture itself is roughly circumferential and pathologically shows only chronic inflammation with marked submucosal fibrosis. The cartilages are uninvolved. The pathology is distinct from polychondritis, Wegener's granulomatosis, or any of the conditions described previously. The patients do not have mediastinal fibrosis or pathologic processes involving mediastinal lymph nodes. Only 1 patient showed progression of stenosis following surgical resection.

A small number of patients will also be seen with stenosis involving a large part of the trachea and others in whom the carina or main bronchi are involved in an undefined inflammatory fibrotic process. The causes remain unidentified.

Tracheal and tracheobronchial malacia remains poorly defined for the most part. A segmental area of malacia may result from postintubation injury either at the level of a cuff lesion or in the segment between the stoma and the cuff lesion. With chronic obstructive pulmonary disease, including emphysema and chronic bronchitis, malacia may develop in the lower trachea, main bronchi, and sometimes the more distal bronchi. In this situation, the tracheal rings take on the shape of an archer's bow with elongation of the membranous wall. When the patient attempts to expire forcefully or to cough, the membranous wall approximates to the anterior softened and flattened

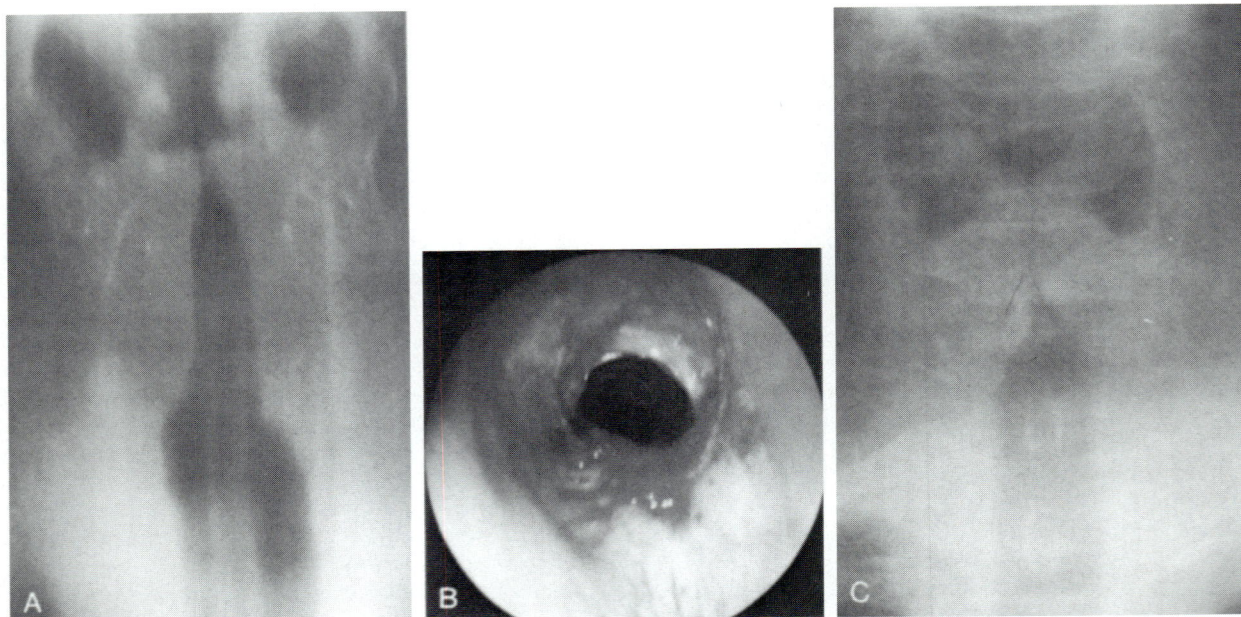

FIGURE 12–15. Idiopathic laryngotracheal stenosis. *A,* Roentgenogram showing severe stenosis involving subglottic larynx and proximal trachea. *B,* Bronchoscopic view of typical subglottic concentric stenosis. Normal tracheal rings are seen distally. *C,* Postoperative view of *A.* The subglottic conus is much improved. (*A–C,* From Grillo, H. C., Mark, E. J., Mathisen, D. J., and Wain, J. C.: Idiopathic laryngotracheal stenosis: The entity and its management. Reprinted with permission from the Society of Thoracic Surgeons [The Annals of Thoracic Surgery, 1993, Vol. 56, p. 80].)

cartilage, causing nearly total obstruction (Herzog et al., 1987). It will respond to posterior membranous wall splinting of the lower two-thirds of trachea and main bronchi. This is entirely different from the characteristics of saber-sheath trachea. A smaller number of patients have been seen who have malacia involving a large portion of or even the entire trachea, wherein the rings are thinned to such an extent that they no longer support the airway. The airway takes on almost the appearance of the esophagus. In these patients, the malacia is in total contrast with the picture just described of anteroposterior collapse.

DIAGNOSTIC STUDIES

Tracheal lesions too often are recognized late despite prolonged symptoms. Radiologically clear lung fields divert the physician. A diagnosis of adult-onset asthma should be made only after excluding the possibility of tracheal obstruction. Appropriate but simple radiographic examinations will reveal almost all tracheal lesions.

Radiographic Examination of the Trachea

Radiographic studies of the trachea are used not only to rule in or out the presence of a tracheal lesion but also to define the location, extent, and sometimes the character of the lesion (Momose and Macmillan, 1978) (Figs. 12–16 and 12–17). Further, these studies demonstrate the involvement of paratracheal structures by neoplastic lesions.

Lateral films of the neck with the chin raised demonstrate most lesions of the upper trachea. Careful technique shows the cartilaginous structures of the larynx as well as the trachea and the relationship of the trachea to the vertebral column posteriorly. Anteroposterior views of the airway from larynx to carina, using a copper filter, provide useful overall assessment. Oblique views throw the tracheal air column into relief. Fluoroscopy demonstrates malacia and clarifies vocal cord function.

If the studies discussed previously do not provide sufficient information, tracheal laminograms help measure precisely the extent of lesions and their relative distances from landmarks such as the vocal cords and the carina. Radiograms are magnified, but at the same time, the trachea is foreshortened in the anteroposterior view because of its oblique passage through the chest. It should be noted in viewing all radiograms, as well as during bronchoscopy, that the vocal cords do not mark the border between larynx and trachea. There are approximately 1.5 to 2 cm of larynx between the vocal cords and the inferior border of the cricoid cartilage. Dye-contrast studies of the trachea add little information except with tracheo-esophageal fistula, which is better shown by barium esophagogram.

CT is valuable only in showing the cervical or mediastinal extent of a tumor. It is of little use in assessing benign stenosis except in special cases such as goiter, vascular lesions, or histoplasmosis. Inspiratory and expiratory CT scans help to clarify dynamic

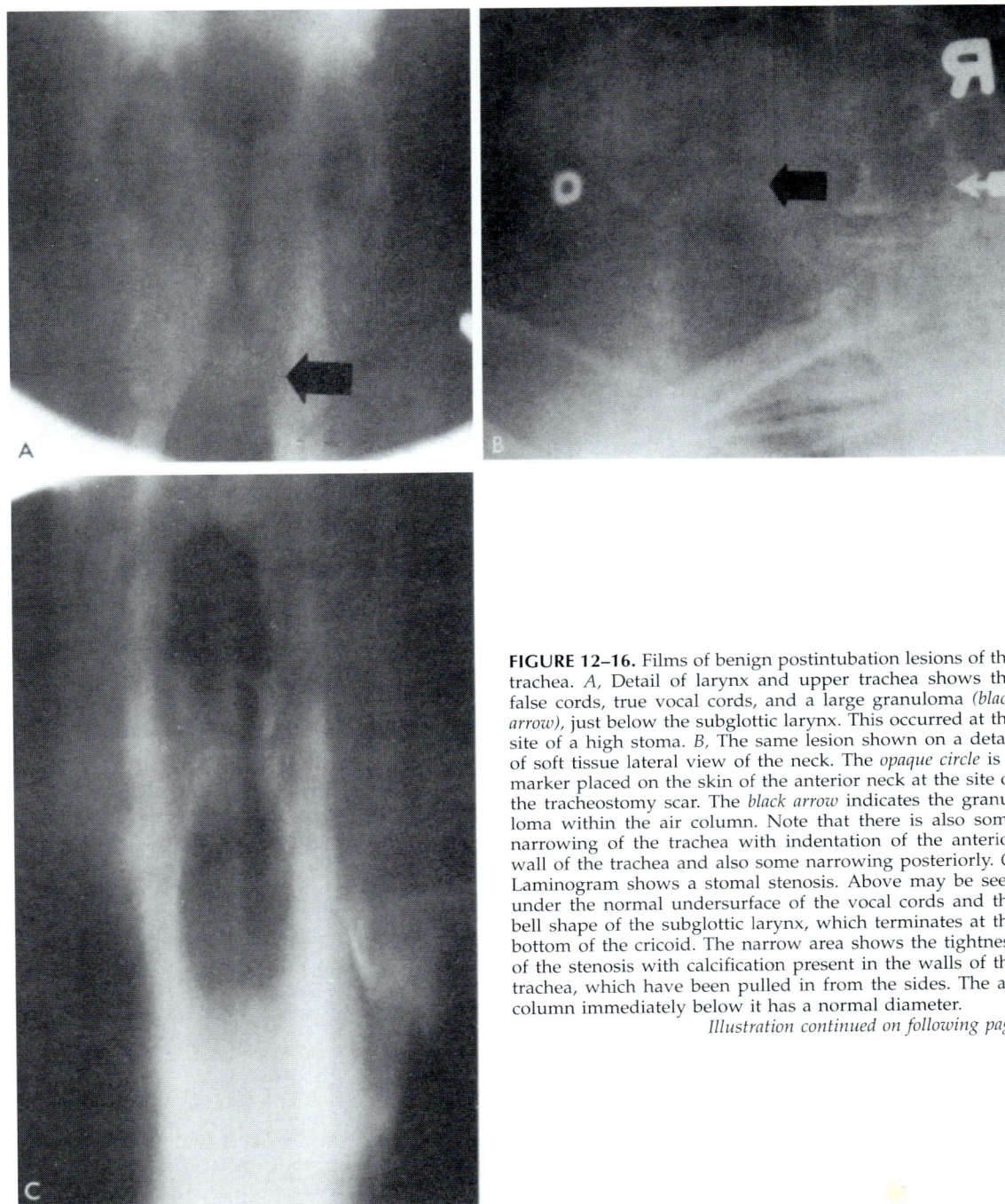

FIGURE 12–16. Films of benign postintubation lesions of the trachea. *A*, Detail of larynx and upper trachea shows the false cords, true vocal cords, and a large granuloma *(black arrow)*, just below the subglottic larynx. This occurred at the site of a high stoma. *B*, The same lesion shown on a detail of soft tissue lateral view of the neck. The *opaque circle* is a marker placed on the skin of the anterior neck at the site of the tracheostomy scar. The *black arrow* indicates the granuloma within the air column. Note that there is also some narrowing of the trachea with indentation of the anterior wall of the trachea and also some narrowing posteriorly. *C*, Laminogram shows a stomal stenosis. Above may be seen under the normal undersurface of the vocal cords and the bell shape of the subglottic larynx, which terminates at the bottom of the cricoid. The narrow area shows the tightness of the stenosis with calcification present in the walls of the trachea, which have been pulled in from the sides. The air column immediately below it has a normal diameter.

Illustration continued on following page

states such as tracheobronchomalacia and postpneumonectomy syndrome (Shepard et al., 1986; Stern et al., 1993). MRI has not shown special value in the study of tracheal problems.

If a patient with tracheal stenosis still has a tracheostomy tube in place, it must be removed during radiographic examination in order to obtain useful information, regardless of the composition of the tube. Even if a tube has been in place for many months, it should be removed cautiously, with provision made for immediate reinsertion. Emergency equipment, including suctioning devices and a range of replacement tubes, should be available. The physician must be competent to perform such intubation under difficulty. The airway may become nearly totally obstructed within 20 to 30 minutes following removal of such a tube. Occasionally, considerable force is required to reinsert an airway.

Angiographic studies occasionally may be useful for patients who have had previous operations, who previously had correction that involved major vessels in the mediastinum, who have large tumors that may displace or involve major vessels, or who have angiomatous malformation that involves the trachea.

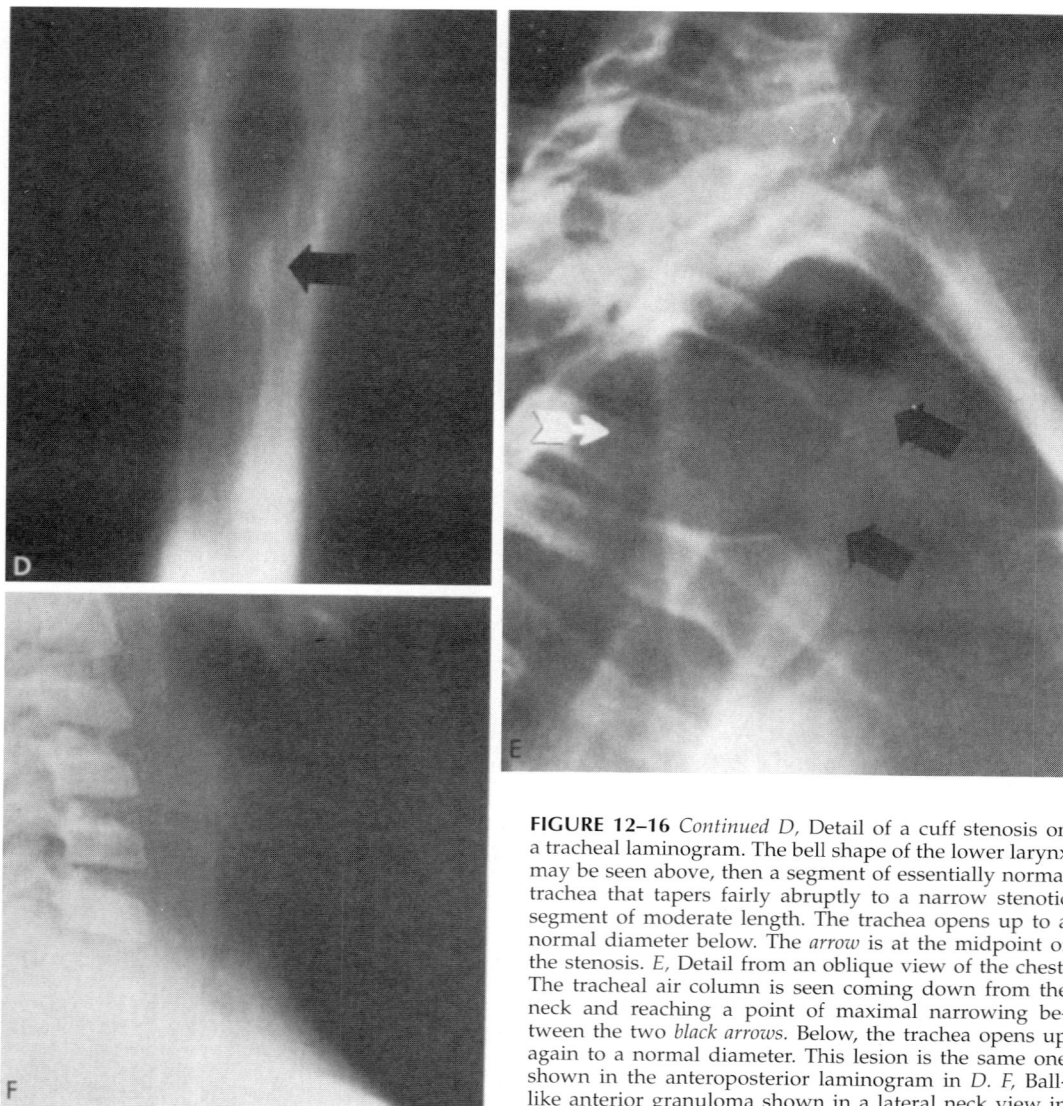

FIGURE 12–16 *Continued D,* Detail of a cuff stenosis on a tracheal laminogram. The bell shape of the lower larynx may be seen above, then a segment of essentially normal trachea that tapers fairly abruptly to a narrow stenotic segment of moderate length. The trachea opens up to a normal diameter below. The *arrow* is at the midpoint of the stenosis. *E,* Detail from an oblique view of the chest. The tracheal air column is seen coming down from the neck and reaching a point of maximal narrowing between the two *black arrows.* Below, the trachea opens up again to a normal diameter. This lesion is the same one shown in the anteroposterior laminogram in *D. F,* Ball-like anterior granuloma shown in a lateral neck view in the lower part of the rather long cervical trachea of a child who was ventilated through a tracheostomy tube without a cuff. This granuloma formed at the site of an anterior erosion where the tip of the tube had pried against the tracheal wall. (*A–F,* From Grillo, H. C.: Surgery of the trachea. Curr. Probl. Surg., July 1970, pp. 3–59.)

Bronchoscopy

Bronchoscopic examination is required, sooner or later, for all patients. When a lesion is known to be present, whether it is neoplastic or inflammatory, and when all else points to its surgical correctability, bronchoscopy is deferred until treatment is decided. The trauma of bronchoscopy in a patient who is subtotally obstructed may precipitate complete obstruction. Frozen sections may be obtained for histologic diagnosis. In the presence of most obstructive lesions, the requirements for resection are clear at the outset. In patients with highly complicated conditions who may have had unsuccessful tracheal surgery before referral, bronchoscopic examination as an occasional independent procedure is performed, because so many factors may be involved and because such a patient

may well be unreconstructable. Biopsy of lesions such as carcinoid tumors may rarely be hazardous owing to vascularity. It is preferred, therefore, to defer biopsy to the time of operation, when everything is prepared to move ahead if difficulty arises. If resection is indicated in any case, biopsy may be omitted if it seems hazardous. The bronchoscopy is performed with the patient under general anesthesia, permitting unhurried, atraumatic examination and manipulation. Rigid bronchoscopy is preferred, for diagnostic precision and airway control.

Other Diagnostic Studies

Pulmonary function studies in patients with obstructing lesions of the trachea confirm a high degree

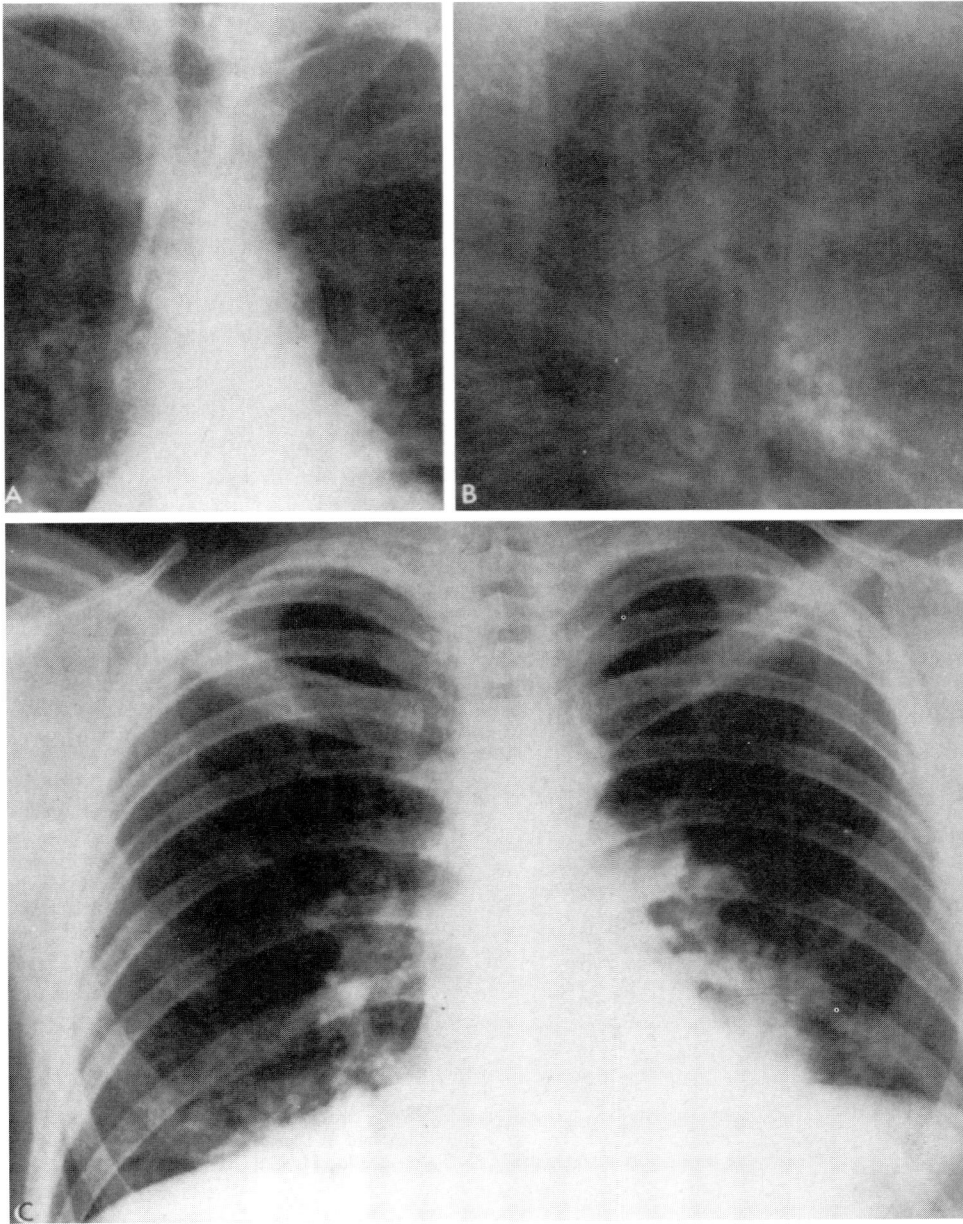

FIGURE 12–17. Films of neoplasms in the trachea. *A* and *B*, Details of posteroanterior and lateral chest films of a patient with a squamous cell carcinoma of the lower trachea. This lesion, which produced relatively high-grade obstruction, might be overlooked on a cursory examination of the chest film because the lung fields are clear. *C*, Chest film shows bilateral pneumonitis that has recurred several times in a young patient.

Illustration continued on following page

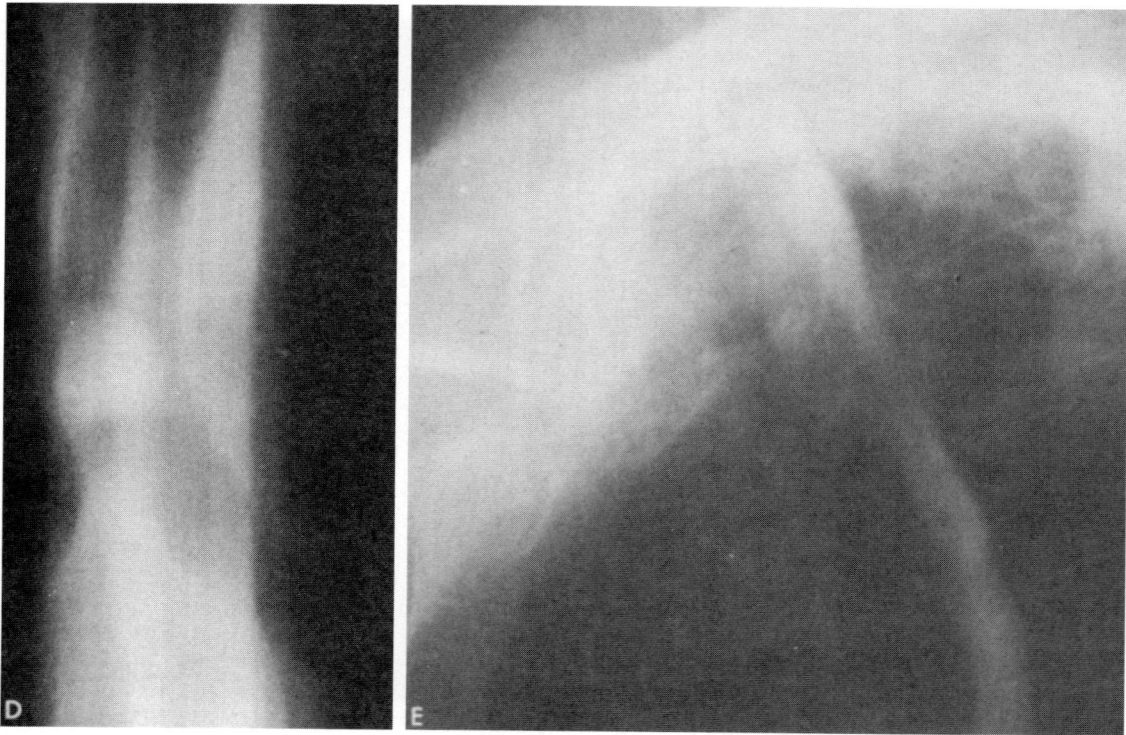

FIGURE 12–17 *Continued D,* The lesion is shown. Carcinoid tumor of the lower trachea is clearly revealed in this detail of a laminogram of the lower trachea and carina. *E,* Squamous cell carcinoma of the lower trachea. This detail of a spot film taken during fluoroscopy with a swallow of barium outlines the lesion, which narrows the tracheal lumen and slightly indents the esophagus by extrinsic pressure. (*A* and *B,* From Grillo, H. C.: Circumferential resection and reconstruction of mediastinal and cervical trachea. Ann. Surg., *162:*374, 1965.)

of airway obstruction. Measurements are sometimes useful in clarifying the presence of parenchymal disease and could alter the extent of the operative approach. Obstructing lesions generally require surgical relief in any case. Function studies, especially 1-second forced expiratory volume (FEV_1), peak expiratory flow rate (PEFR), and flow-volume loops, provide a useful basis for measurement of results.

Bacteriologic cultures are made of tracheal secretions and of tracheostomy wounds. Antibiotic sensitivities guide the prophylactic program for perioperative protection.

MANAGEMENT OF ACUTE OBSTRUCTION

Trauma

Intubation may be attempted, preferably over a flexible bronchoscope, because the separated trachea may be offset. An attempt at intubation, however, may obstruct the tenuous airway that courses across the discontinuous portion of the trachea. Therefore, the surgeon should be prepared to do an emergency tracheostomy immediately. The severed trachea is sometimes considered to be one of the few remaining indications for emergency tracheostomy as the primary method for establishing an airway. The distal trachea has usually retracted into the mediastinum. The surgeon uses her finger to find the lumen, the

edge of the trachea is grasped with a clamp, and a tube is placed directly into the distal end of trachea.

Postintubation Injuries

Although it is possible, if the lesion is low enough in the trachea, to intubate above a lesion, to suction out the airway, and to provide hand ventilation on an emergency basis, it is usually preferable to dilate the severely obstructed airway in the operating room with the patient under general anesthesia. Inhalation anesthesia is used without paralyzing agents to provide a margin of safety. The surgeon must be immediately available with appropriate equipment, which includes rigid pediatric bronchoscopes of different sizes and bougies, which may be passed through the adult rigid bronchoscope. Dilatation should not be attempted with the patient under local anesthesia. The lesion is visualized with the adult bronchoscope, and a dilatation may be commenced with Jackson-type dilators through the bronchoscope. Dilatation is continued by using rigid pediatric bronchoscopes with rounded tips, such as the classic Jackson bronchoscopes. These bronchoscopes are passed serially by using a "corkscrewing" motion, and great care is taken not to use excessive force. A normal membranous wall yields before a firm fibrous stricture does, and perforation may result (Grillo, 1987).

Dilatation provides various periods of respite before a definitive procedure is required. Tracheostomy is instituted if a prolonged period is needed before correction of a stenosis. If the lesion is accessible in the neck, the tracheostomy should be made through the damaged trachea at the level of the stenosis, not above or below it. If the lesion is distal to the sternal notch, the tracheostomy should be performed at the conventional level and a sufficiently long tube should be passed, which extends through the stricture and does not simply lie above it.

There is no advantage to lasering for the emergency establishment of an airway. It has no benefits over the technique described.

Neoplasms

It is always possible to intubate between the neoplasm and the uninvolved tracheal wall, even where it is cartilaginous. In the rare circumferential tumor, the bronchoscope may be passed in a manner similar to that described for benign stricture, and intubation is accomplished through the dilated lumen.

If the tracheal lumen is severely obstructed and needs to be opened either to permit safe anesthesia for resection or to temporize in order to assess or treat the patient otherwise, this is accomplished most easily and safely with the patient under general anesthesia by using the rigid bronchoscope as a coring device (Mathisen and Grillo, 1989). Successive amounts of tumor are removed with the tip of the bronchoscope, strong suction, and biopsy forceps. In 56 consecutive patients "cored out" for airway obstruction in trachea and bronchi, improvement in the airway was accomplished in 90%, by a single bronchoscopy in 96%, with no deaths, and with bleeding that was easily controlled in 3 patients. In the other patients, the lesion was too peripheral to permit much relief.

Contrary to widespread belief, this procedure does not cause hemorrhage that endangers life. Most bleeding that occurs is easily controlled in a brief time by normal coagulation, by suctioning, and sometimes by pressure with the bronchoscope. The use of laser techniques has no more to offer in safety, speed, or cost over this dependable method.

TRACHEAL RECONSTRUCTION

Before resection, the tracheal lesion is precisely evaluated. The nature, location, and extent, as well as the amount of apparently normal trachea that remains for reconstruction, are determined from radiologic studies. If carinal reconstruction or concomitant pulmonary resection is necessary, pulmonary function studies may be useful, including ventilation-perfusion quantitation. Sputum or tracheostomy cultures are obtained and sensitivities determined. Appropriate antibiotics are selected on the basis of these studies and are started in the morning before operation. A good tissue level of antibiotic should be present be-

fore the incision because many patients have pathogens present at the site of inflammatory lesions or stomas. Antibiotic coverage is continued for 4 days after operation.

If there is a high degree of obstruction, *anesthesia* is induced slowly and gently by using inhalation technique. The patient should breathe without assistance at the conclusion of the operation to avoid the hazard of intubation injury to the suture line. Therefore, the patient is maintained as much as possible on spontaneous respiration (Wilson, 1987). Induction may take a long time if there is a high degree of obstruction. The surgeon should be present at the bronchoscopic table in the event that airway obstruction increases during induction. Topical anesthetic is applied to the larynx and is sprayed through the vocal cords. The lesion is then further appraised by bronchoscopy. If the lesion is a stricture, it is dilated if the airway measures less than 5 mm in diameter. The risk of dilatation is balanced against the greater risk of carbon dioxide retention during operation before full dissection of the trachea is possible at a point below the obstruction. Dilators passed through large bronchoscopes with care may be used to initiate dilatation. Dilatation is done serially with pediatric ventilating bronchoscopes under direct vision. If the airway measures more than 5 mm in diameter, the endotracheal tube is passed only to a point above the stricture. It is not pressed against the stricture because this in turn may lead to obstruction. Patients may be ventilated easily with such a system. Tumors present fewer problems because few are circumferential and a small tube can usually be passed beside the tumor, if necessary. High-grade obstruction may be relieved easily by coring-out tumor with the rigid bronchoscope, aided with biopsy forceps (Mathisen and Grillo, 1989). High-frequency jet ventilation is useful in tracheal procedures (El-Baz et al., 1982), especially in the case of complex carinal reconstructions.

The only *incision* that will expose the entire trachea is one that begins in the neck, passes down along the midline of the sternum, and then angles out through the fourth interspace on the right to the posterior axillary line. This allows access both to the anterior trachea in the neck and larynx, if necessary, and to the carina posteriorly. Initially, this incision was used for transthoracic approach to the trachea (Grillo et al., 1963). It does not, however, offer as good an exposure of the trachea posteriorly and inferiorly as does a high posterolateral thoracotomy through the fourth interspace. The author now uses two basic incisions to approach the trachea. An anterior collar incision with or without a vertical partial sternal division is used for most lesions of the upper half of the trachea, whether benign or malignant, and for almost all stenoses, including those at supracarinal levels. Exploration is performed initially through the collar incision. Partial sternal division, only through the angle of Louis, is added later, if necessary. Full sternal division adds nothing to upper tracheal exposure. The trachea passes posteriorly in the mediastinum; the reason for the partial sternal division is to provide working space for hands and instruments at the thoracic inlet.

Lesions of the lower half of the trachea are approached through a posterolateral thoracotomy incision in the fourth interspace or the bed of the fifth rib. In complex lesions, where it is thought that further mobilization might be required, the neck is also prepared, and the arm is draped and prepared so that it can be moved into the field for easier access to the neck. A collar incision can then be added to free the trachea if there has been previous tracheostomy or, rarely, to perform laryngeal release.

Full median sternotomy is occasionally selected for midtracheal tumors. Laryngeal release is performed more easily in this position, if it is required. Although laryngeal release does not aid carinal resection, it does give length to the upper trachea or midtrachea after resection. If the pericardium is opened anteriorly and posteriorly between the vena cava and the aorta, the carina may be visualized in a deep space, which is also bordered by the innominate artery and pulmonary artery. Although intraluminal lesions may be approached by this route, it is difficult to do adequate dissection of larger lesions that may, for example, involve the esophagus or to do complex carinal reconstructions well in such a constricted field. Even with pleural opening, left-sided hilar release is not feasible through this approach, since the heart prevents access. Bilateral anterolateral thoracotomy in the fourth interspace and across the sternum is useful for special problems of carinal, tracheal, and left main bronchial involvement. Initially, one side may be opened, including horizontal sternal transection, to determine operability and also because it may prove to be sufficient for resection.

In special cases of extensive or unusual lesions or where there has been extensive previous surgery, preparations are also made so that the incision can be continued in one or another direction. A vertical anterior incision can be extended into the right fourth interspace and can be carried laterally or a posterolateral incision and a cervical incision can be joined across the sternum. On rare occasions, sternal division is done beneath a broad bipedicled bridge of anterior chest wall skin in case there is a possibility of needing a skin tube interposition between the larynx and the trachea or a mediastinal tracheostomy. These possibilities must be considered in advance in any given case, and steps should be taken sequentially without destroying possible routes of further access or approach. Cardiac and oxygen saturation monitoring are essential during all of these procedures, and frequent blood-gas determinations are made.

The patient who is undergoing tracheal surgical procedures should be under full control at all times. No hurried maneuvers should be required. Several authors have proposed that cardiopulmonary bypass be used for tracheal reconstruction. Subsequent descriptions of operative procedures show that no simplification of the operation is obtained under cardiopulmonary bypass. Indeed, the complexities that are introduced by that technique are unjustified even in relatively complex cases of tracheal reconstruction. In the most complex and unusual cases, in which many hours of operation and much manipulation of the lungs are required, cardiopulmonary bypass introduced enormous dangers owing to anticoagulants. In one patient in whom such an attempt was made, death ensued from hemorrhage into the pulmonary parenchyma on the right, when insufficient residual pulmonary tissue remained on the opposite side. Even in patients with only one lung, it is preferable to do a tracheal reconstruction with ventilatory control rather than cardiopulmonary bypass.

Reconstruction of the Upper Trachea

The patient is usually in the supine position with an inflatable bag beneath the shoulders to provide controlled cervical extension. If it is thought necessary to extend the incision into the right side of the chest, the patient is placed obliquely in a 45-degree position, with the bag still in position for extension of the neck and with the table tilted laterally so that the patient is in a horizontal position in the initial phase of the operation. A low, short, collar incision is made, so that if a T is necessary, it will not extend vertically far across the neck (Fig. 12–18A). Occasionally, the incision is placed a little higher to circumscribe an existing tracheostomy. If the tracheostomy is too high, it is removed independently, and the result is a small horizonal incision that is closed separately. If a cuff stenosis lies at some distance below a tracheostomy, the skin may not need to be detached from the stoma. In that case, the stoma serves as an access point for postoperative suctioning and is allowed to close spontaneously. If, however, extensive resection has to be done, it will be necessary to detach the skin from the stoma to allow the trachea to slide. In that case, the stoma is reexteriorized and allowed to close spontaneously. If the stoma is pulled behind the sternum and if cutaneous inversion is not feasible, a flap of a strap muscle is used to seal it in its new position.

Anterior dissection of the trachea is usually carried from the cricoid cartilage to the carina (Fig. 12–18B). The dissection may be difficult if the inflammatory process is recent. The innominate artery is often densely adherent to the anterior trachea, but in almost every case, unless it has been previously injured surgically, it can be dissected free without incident. Dissection is kept close to the trachea to avoid arterial trauma. Dissection around the back of the trachea is done at a point inferior to an inflammatory lesion, because it may be difficult to separate the lesion from the esophagus. If the patient has not been intubated through the stricture, dissection must be done with delicacy to avoid obstructing the airway. In inflammatory lesions, dissection is kept close to the trachea to avoid injuring the recurrent laryngeal nerves. The author has avoided identifying the nerves in dissection for inflammatory strictures and believes that this would be more likely to cause injury. Great care is required when the tracheal lesion is just below the

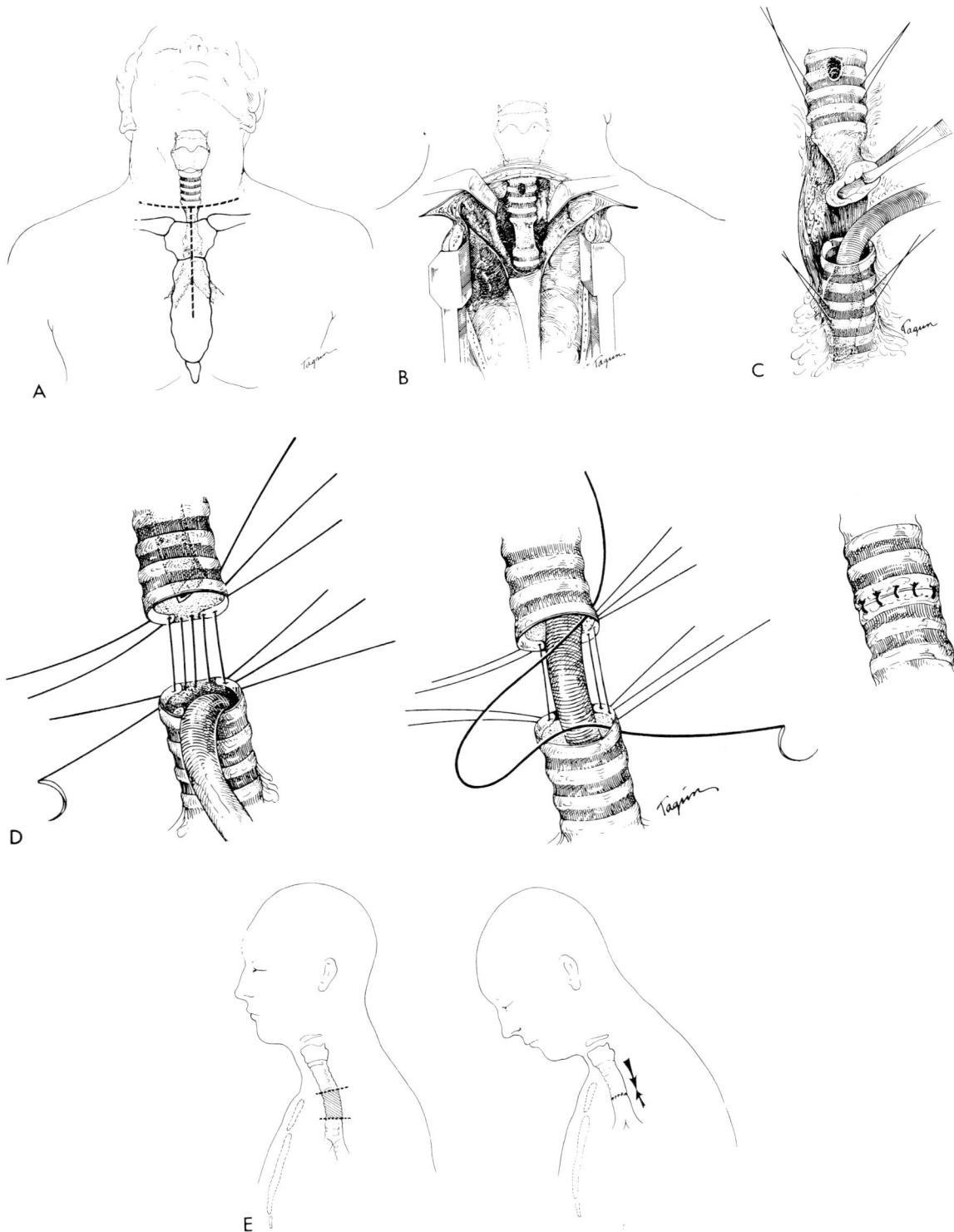

FIGURE 12–18. Reconstruction of the upper trachea. *A,* Collar incision and extension for upper sternotomy. Essentially all benign strictures as well as upper tracheal neoplasms may be most easily resected through this approach. The vertical incision need be carried only 1 cm below the sternal angle. *B,* Dissection is carried anteriorly to the level of the carina. Nothing is gained by dividing the innominate vein. The innominate artery may be gently retracted downward with all of its investments intact. The pleura is intact. *C,* Circumferential dissection has been accomplished only immediately beneath the lowermost level of the pathology. Traction sutures are in place, and the patient has been intubated distal to the lesion. The lesion is now being retracted upward to facilitate dissection from the underlying esophagus. *D,* Details of anastomotic technique. The sutures are placed beginning posteriorly and working anteriorly. Now all of the sutures are placed before advancing the tube from above into the distal trachea. All the knots are on the outside. This diagrammatic representation must be recognized as not indicating complete circumferential dissection of the lengths of trachea shown. *E,* This diagram indicates that in the anterior approach the greater amount of approximation is obtained by cervical flexion rather than by upward traction on the carina. (*A–D,* From Grillo, H. C.: Surgery of the trachea. Curr. Probl. Surg., July 1970, pp. 36–37.)

larynx. Obviously, a different approach is taken for neoplasms. Dissection is begun more laterally and includes adjacent paratracheal tissue. The nerves must be identified. If a vocal cord is already palsied, that nerve will probably be sacrificed when the tumor is removed.

Once a tape has been placed around the trachea below the lesion, lateral traction sutures of 2-0 Vicryl are placed through the full thickness of the tracheal wall in the midline on either side at a point no more than 2 cm below the expected point of division of the trachea. Similar sutures are placed now or later above the lesion in the midlateral position. If the lesion is a high one, these sutures will be in laryngeal tissue, namely cricoid. The sutures do *not* pass into the subglottic lumen. The trachea is transected below the lesion, and care is taken not to remove excessive trachea, but at the same time to divide the trachea where the tissue is essentially normal. Division through an area of severe inflammatory change invites restenosis. If the lesion is supracarinal, transection is performed initially above the lesion for convenience. The distal trachea is intubated across the operative field by using a flexible, armored Tovell tube. The necessary connecting equipment and additional corrugated tubing have been previously prepared and are available on the field. The endotracheal tube must not be inserted too far so that its tip rests in the right main bronchus. The lesion is grasped and is lifted upward to facilitate dissection from the esophagus (Fig. 12–18C). Dissection is carried a short distance proximally between normal esophagus and trachea. The lesion is removed. The distal trachea is freed from the esophagus posteriorly for a short distance. Great care is taken not to disturb the lateral tissue that contains the blood supply of the trachea, either proximally or distally. Only 1.5 cm of trachea proximal or distal to the line of transection is circumferentially dissected. This amount is necessary to allow room for anastomosis.

The surgeon and assistant now draw the traction sutures together from above and below, each on her own side after the anesthesiologist flexes the cervical spine. If tracheal approximation is possible without excessive tension, no further mobilization needs to be done. If the ends will not reach without tension, more mobilization is required. Mulliken and Grillo (1968) found in cadavers that 4.5 cm of trachea could be removed by this anterior route and that reanastomosis could be effected with 35 degrees of flexion and 1000 g of pull. This amount of tension on the anastomosis should be within a safe level, which was shown by Cantrell and Folse (1961). The figure varies considerably depending on the age and build of the patient. Further blunt dissection over the anterior surface of the left main bronchus beneath the aortic arch may provide further release. Bands of scar tissue that hold the distal trachea down can be divided, but care must be taken not to destroy the lateral blood supply.

If the ends will not approximate now despite marked flexion, two alternatives are possible. One is extension of the incision into the right fourth in-

terspace with mobilization of the right lung and carina. This, however, is a drastic procedure and is contraindicated in the case of patients with poor pulmonary function. Under these circumstances, a laryngeal devolvement procedure may be useful (Ogura and Powers, 1964). Dedo and Fishman (1969) released the larynx by dividing the thyrohyoid muscles, the thyrohyoid membrane, and the superior cornua of the thyroid cartilage to allow the thyrohyoid ligaments to retract. Great care must be taken not to injure the superior laryngeal nerves, or else the patient's swallowing function will be destroyed. In any case, many patients will have great difficulty in swallowing postoperatively but will eventually recover. Montgomery (1974) has described a suprahyoid procedure that reduces these swallowing difficulties. In 521 tracheal reconstructions for postintubation stenosis, laryngeal release was required in 49 patients. The amount of trachea that can be removed without these additional maneuvers is extremely variable. The author has removed up to 60% of the trachea with an anterior approach without even sternal division in young patients with relatively long necks. Difficulty has been encountered with even a 4-cm resection in an older patient without much tissue resiliency and with severe kyphosis.

Once it has been shown that the ends will approximate, the neck is allowed to fall back into extension, and the anastomotic sutures are placed (Fig. 12–18D). The first suture is placed in the midline posteriorly by using fine, absorbable suture material (4-0 Vicryl). The suture is placed from outside to inside through the full thickness of the tracheal wall approximately 3 mm from the cut edge. The knot is tied on the outside of the tracheal lumen. Successive sutures are placed individually at approximately 3-mm intervals, each starting from the posterior one. When the cartilaginous ring is reached, sutures pass through the cartilage. As much as possible, the line of division of the trachea is in the tissue between the cartilaginous rings, but this is not essential. The sutures are carefully held by hemostats, which in turn are clamped by other hemostats in a radial manner around the field, placing them so that the most posterior sutures on either side are at the head of the field and so that the successive ones radiate distally. When all sutures have been placed, the distal Tovell tube is removed, and the endotracheal tube is advanced from above into the distal trachea. The endotracheal tube must not be pushed down too far, because when the trachea is approximated, it will be pushed into the right main bronchus. Suctioning is performed frequently during the procedure to minimize leakage of blood past the occluding cuff. Excessive blood in the lungs causes shunting postoperatively and increases the dangers of needing respiratory support after reconstruction. After all sutures have been placed and the tube is readjusted, the inflatable bag is deflated, the patient's neck is flexed, and the head is supported firmly in this position (Fig. 12–18E). The lateral traction sutures are drawn together simultaneously by the surgeon and the assistant and then tied in position so that the ends of the trachea are approximated but are not intussuscepted. The anastomotic sutures are tied, beginning anteriorly. As each suture is tied, the ends are cut. The posterior sutures cannot be seen and are tied entirely by touch. The lateral traction sutures, which can be absorbed, are left in position to minimize tension on the anastomosis. The anastomosis is tested under saline for leakage. Suction drainage catheters are placed in the wound. Occasionally, the thyroid isthmus, which has been divided in the original dissection, is reapproximated, or other tissue is brought over the suture line anteriorly. The strap muscles are lightly approximated over the reconstructed trachea. Special protection has not been necessary for the innominate artery, although several surgeons have reported postoperative hemorrhages from this source. This probably results from dissecting the artery out of its protective surrounding connective tissues. If there is a special problem, a strap muscle or a lobe of thymus is pedicled and interposed between the artery and the trachea. Coverage is required if it has been necessary to dissect out the brachiocephalic artery, which occurs in a secondary tracheal repair, or when the artery adhered to the stenosis.

An especially difficult problem is offered by resection of a high stomal stricture that impinges on the lower cricoid. In this case, it is necessary to bevel off the lower part of the cricoid, especially anteriorly. In such cases, the trachea is sutured to the larynx, but essentially the same technique is used. Sutures are placed so that mucosal approximation will result as nearly as possible. Some sutures are not passed through the full thickness of the cricoid but are angled up into the midpoint of the cut inferior surface and out into the lumen through the mucosa of the lower larynx and then back out again through the wall of the trachea that is to be approximated. Some patients also have a degree of submucosal fibrosis in the larynx, which may narrow the lumen so that a perfect approximation of the airway cannot be obtained.

When the stenosis involves the subglottic larynx more extensively, repair is more difficult. Results with various complex, multistaged procedures have not been consistently good. Gerwat and Bryce (1974), Pearson and colleagues (1975), Couraud and associates (1979), and Grillo (1982b) described one-stage operations for correction of these stenoses. The lower anterior larynx is resected with the stricture, and the trachea is anastomosed to the thyroid cartilage anteriorly. The posterior lamina of the cricoid is retained to protect the recurrent laryngeal nerves. If the stenosis extends posteriorly, a further plastic variation is necessary (Fig. 12–19). Grillo and co-workers (1992a) reported 69 good and 8 satisfactory results in 79 of these difficult cases.

When tumors of the proximal trachea invade the subglottic larynx unilaterally, it is often possible to conserve laryngeal function by an individually tailored resection, which is applicable particularly with locally invasive differentiated carcinoma of the thyroid (Grillo and Zannini, 1986) (Fig. 12–20). Unlike inflammatory disease, the larynx proximal to transection is normal and healing is fraught with fewer difficulties.

After completion of the operation, the patient should be breathing spontaneously and should be under light anesthesia. The drapes are removed, and a heavy suture is placed from just beneath the chin to the anterior sternal skin and is tied with the neck in flexion. This suture serves to guard the patient in the postoperative phase against sudden movements that might put stress on the unhealed incision. The suture is left in position 7 days, at which point early healing has begun and the patient has already become accustomed to maintaining flexion. After another week, full movement is begun. This program is empirically based and appears to be effective.

At the conclusion of the operation, the patient is extubated, preferably in the operating room, so that the quality of breathing may be noted. Early in this work, the author met occasional difficulties, which had not been noticed preoperatively, that arose in the larynx, at the site of another tracheal lesion, or occasionally, with the anastomosis itself. If there is any question, flexible bronchoscopy is performed. The time for recognition and correction of problems is at this point rather than later. In a few cases with laryngeal edema, it has been necessary to leave a tube in position and, in even fewer cases, to give some measure of ventilatory support. If this has to be done, it is important that the endotracheal tube be placed so that the cuff, even though it is a low-pressure cuff, does not rest on the anastomosis. In patients who have had laryngotracheal repair, a small distal tracheostomy is occasionally needed. In most patients, it is both unnecessary and potentially harmful to "splint" the anastomosis, if the anastomosis is adequate.

Reconstruction of the Lower Trachea

The basic incision for approach to the lower trachea has been discussed. The patient is placed in a lateral position but with the adjustments described, so that further extension is possible, if necessary. Dissection of the trachea is performed around the lesion before opening the trachea. Insofar as possible, the degree of mobilization that is thought necessary is better done before dividing the trachea (Fig. 12–21).

In initial studies, Grillo and associates (1964) showed that about half of the trachea could be resected and the ends could be brought together by intrathoracic mobilization. In those dissections, without the use of cervical flexion, it was found that 3 cm of lower trachea could be removed and approximation could be effected by dissecting out the hilus of the lung and by loosening the attachments around the carina. A further length of almost 1 cm could be obtained by taking the major vessels out of the pericardium so that the inferior vein no longer held the lung downward. Division of the left main bronchus and its reimplantation in the bronchus interme-

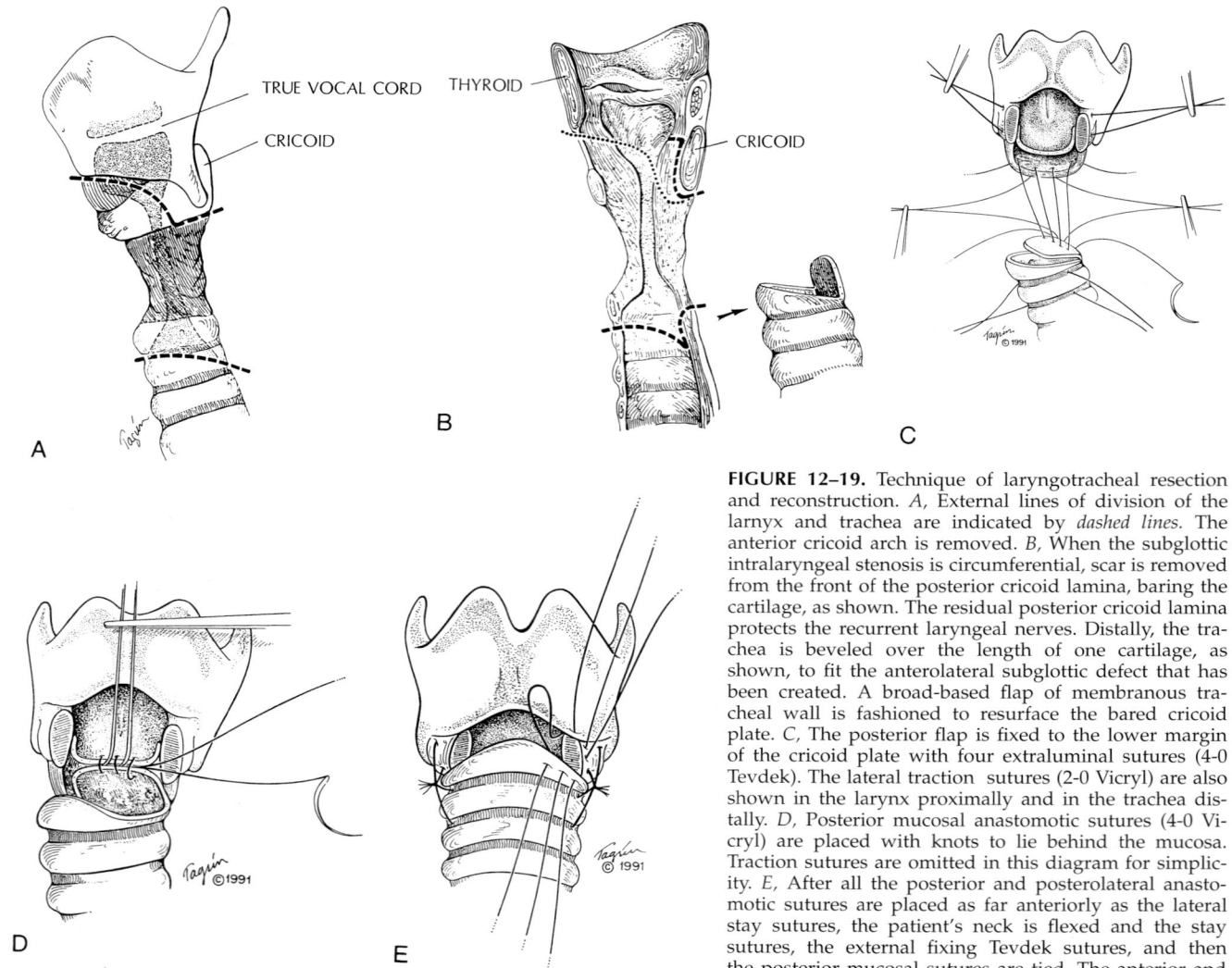

FIGURE 12–19. Technique of laryngotracheal resection and reconstruction. *A,* External lines of division of the larnyx and trachea are indicated by *dashed lines.* The anterior cricoid arch is removed. *B,* When the subglottic intralaryngeal stenosis is circumferential, scar is removed from the front of the posterior cricoid lamina, baring the cartilage, as shown. The residual posterior cricoid lamina protects the recurrent laryngeal nerves. Distally, the trachea is beveled over the length of one cartilage, as shown, to fit the anterolateral subglottic defect that has been created. A broad-based flap of membranous tracheal wall is fashioned to resurface the bared cricoid plate. *C,* The posterior flap is fixed to the lower margin of the cricoid plate with four extraluminal sutures (4-0 Tevdek). The lateral traction sutures (2-0 Vicryl) are also shown in the larynx proximally and in the trachea distally. *D,* Posterior mucosal anastomotic sutures (4-0 Vicryl) are placed with knots to lie behind the mucosa. Traction sutures are omitted in this diagram for simplicity. *E,* After all the posterior and posterolateral anastomotic sutures are placed as far anteriorly as the lateral stay sutures, the patient's neck is flexed and the stay sutures, the external fixing Tevdek sutures, and then the posterior mucosal sutures are tied. The anterior and anterolateral anastomotic sutures are then placed and finally tied serially. (*A* and *B,* Reproduced with permission from Grillo, H. C.: Primary reconstruction of airway after resection of subglottic laryngeal and upper tracheal stenosis. Reprinted with permission from the Society of Thoracic Surgeons [The Annals of Thoracic Surgery, 1982, Vol. 33, pp. 3–18]; *C–E,* From Grillo, H. C., Mathisen, D. J., and Wain, J. C.: Laryngotracheal resection and reconstruction for subglottic stenosis. Reprinted with permission from the Society of Thoracic Surgeons [The Annals of Thoracic Surgery, 1992, Vol. 53, p. 54].)

dius were also done in these early experiments to gain maximal length. Later, the information obtained from upper tracheal studies was applied to intrathoracic resection. The addition of cervical flexion, even though the patient is in the lateral thoracotomy position, makes 4.5 to 5 cm of trachea removable without extreme maneuvers, such as bronchial reimplantation, being needed. Every effort is made to preserve bronchial blood supply. The cervical trachea is thus pushed down into the mediastinum and helps to close the gap to the carina. The trachea may be dissected along its anterior surface well up into the neck with the finger from the transthoracic approach unless previous tracheostomy has been performed. In that case, a cervical incision is needed in addition to the thoracotomy. Laryngeal release translates nothing to the carina.

Once the trachea is divided, it is intubated distally.

The flexible armored tube that is passed via the operative field is preferentially sited in the left main bronchus in order to collapse the right lung. In the presence of chronic lung disease, it may be necessary, if PO_2 determinations indicate, to eliminate the arterial shunt through the unventilated right lung. An atraumatic clamp is placed on the right pulmonary artery, and the shunt is removed from the circuit. If for some reason, such as unrecognized previous obstruction of the left pulmonary artery, oxygenation is not maintained, it is possible to ventilate the right lung as well by using a second anesthesia machine that operates intermittently until reconstruction is effected. High-frequency jet ventilation is useful here since the right lung will not be so fully expanded. Sutures are placed much as they are in the neck, and a pedicled pleural flap or pericardial fat flap is wrapped around the anastomosis (see Fig. 12–21).

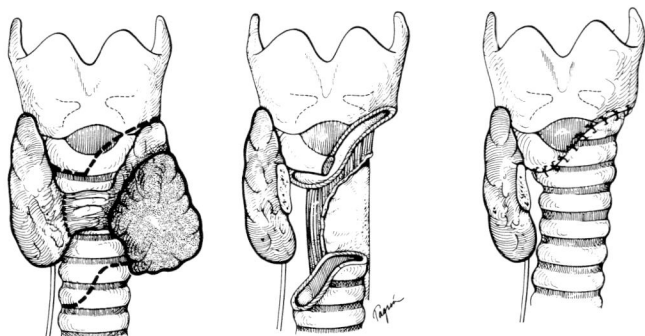

FIGURE 12–20. Complex resection was used for primary treatment of a patient with mixed papillary and follicular carcinoma that invaded the junction of cricoid and trachea. The left recurrent laryngeal nerve was paralyzed by tumor invasion. A portion of muscular esophageal wall was removed and repaired. The reconstruction provided an excellent airway and a functional larynx. (Reproduced with permission from Grillo, H. C., and Zannini, P.: Resectional management of airway invasion by thyroid carcinoma. Reprinted with permission from the Society of Thoracic Surgeons [The Annals of Thoracic Surgery, 1986, Vol. 42, p. 287].)

Carinal Reconstruction

Carinal resection and reconstruction present special difficulties not only in anesthetic maintenance during the procedure but also in the selection and accomplishment of the anatomic reconstructive techniques. Furthermore, there are many more difficulties postoperatively in the clearing of secretions and in the maintenance of well-expanded lungs (Grillo, 1982a).

Over 75 carinal resections and reconstructions have been done by the author and his colleagues for primary neoplasms, over 50 for bronchogenic carcinoma involving main bronchi or carina, and numerous additional resections for various inflammatory diseases. When both lungs were salvaged after resection of the carina, the most common reconstruction was anastomosis of the trachea to the left main bronchus with elevation of the mobilized right lung and implantation of the right main bronchus into the side of the trachea (Fig. 12–22B). Where a greater length of trachea must be resected, leaving a gap between trachea and left main bronchus greater than 4 cm, it is usually not possible to approximate the trachea and left main bronchus, and therefore the right main bronchus must be raised by intrapericardial release and anastomosed to the trachea. The left main bronchus is then brought across the mediastinum to be implanted in the bronchus intermedius (Barclay et al., 1957) (Fig. 12–22C). Rarely is the resection so limited that the carina may be reconstituted with suturing of the left and right main bronchi together and devolvement of the trachea to this newly constructed carina (Fig. 12–22A). When a long length of both the trachea and the left main bronchus are involved by tumor—usually adenoid cystic—the left lung must be sacrificed and the right advanced to the trachea. This is accomplished best through bilateral thoracotomy. The most difficult problems that involve the carina are the lengthy ade-

noid cystic tumors and also inflammatory processes such as fibrosing mediastinitis (Eschapasse, 1974; Grillo, 1982a; Pearson et al., 1984; Perelman and Koroleva, 1980).

Complex Reconstructions

In complicated situations in which there is excessive destruction of trachea and loss due to either extensive tumor or previous operation, it is necessary, in order to reconstitute the mediastinal trachea, to drop a segment of cervical trachea with intact blood supply into the mediastinum by dividing it below the first cartilaginous ring. This extreme maneuver is to be used only under the most urgent circumstances, where even laryngeal release is insufficient. In these cases, a first-stage skin tube is interposed between the still-functional larynx and the devolved trachea, which then emerges as a tracheostomy just behind the sternal notch. A skin tube with buried plastic rings may be used later to join the two ends of the airway in the neck (Grillo, 1965). Mortality or technical failure in such procedures has been high (Grillo, 1978). It should rarely, if ever, be used and is considered to be a trial procedure only (Grillo, 1982a).

The problem of subtotal trachiectomy remains unsolved. When the larynx also has to be sacrificed because of disease involvement, mediastinal tracheostomy suffices. However, in rare cases, the larynx may be saved functionally yet most of the trachea is involved by the disease process, with little more than 2 or 3 cm of relatively normal trachea remaining. The airway consists of a tracheostomy tube lying in a channel of scar tissue. Some adenoid cystic or squamous cancers present similar problems. For these patients, no dependable reconstructive solution has yet evolved.

For benign stenosis, surgical recanalization and placement of a long, tailored T tube (Hood Laboratories, Pembroke, MA) seem best at present (Gaissert et al., 1994). In the few neoplastic cases, the use of a prosthesis would be desirable.

The hazards of prosthesis with respect to granulation tissue obstruction and erosive hemorrhage from great vessels appear to negate the use of any yet developed (Grillo, 1970; Neville et al., 1990). Combinations and sequence of radiotherapy, brachytherapy, laser, core-out and T tubes at present offer prolonged palliation.

Laryngotrachiectomy

Destructive resection of the trachea is required when disease, usually neoplastic, involves the larynx as well as a large part of the upper trachea. Attempts to establish a mediastinal tracheostomy are fraught with numerous difficulties. The lower trachea lies behind the innominate artery in the posterior mediastinum. An attempt to pull it to the surface puts too much tension on a suture line. Creation of tubed skin

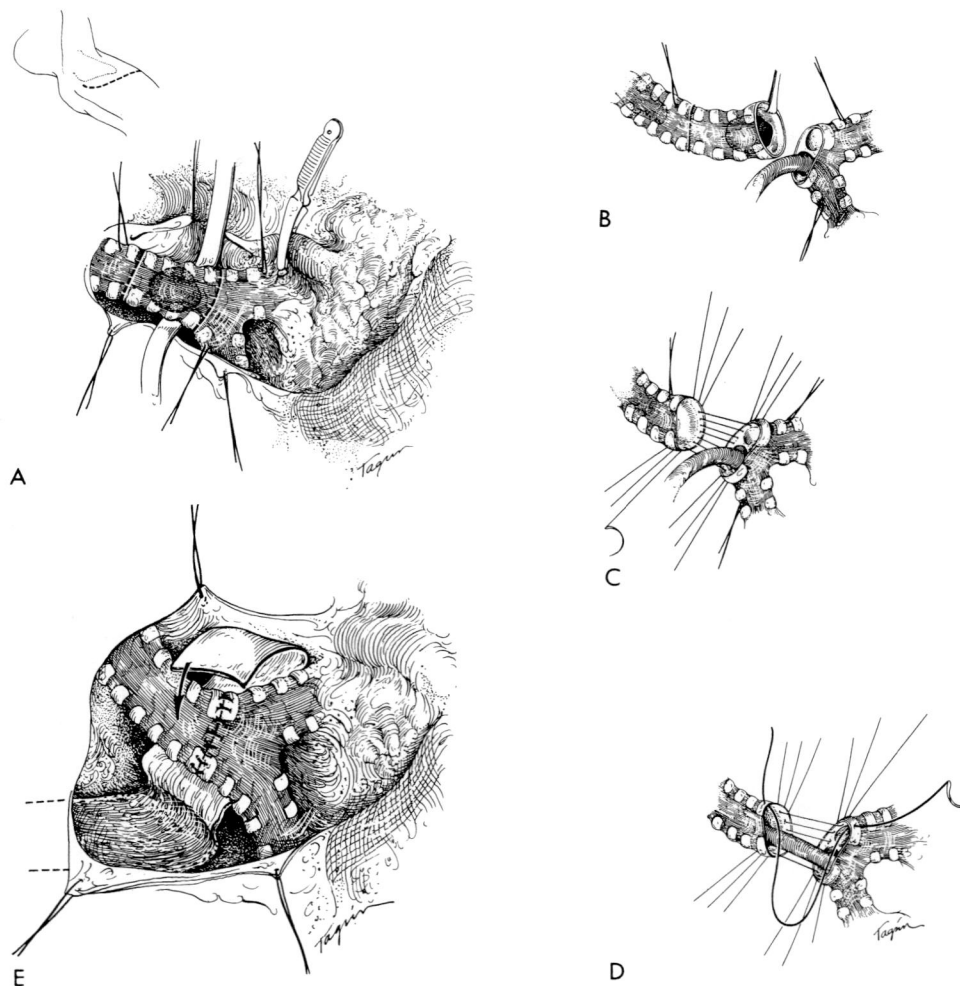

FIGURE 12–21. Transthoracic approach for resection of the lower trachea. *A,* As much mobilization as is thought to be necessary is performed before the division of the trachea. The drawing shows the placement of a clamp on the pulmonary artery, but this is not done routinely. Proximal and distal traction sutures are placed as in the cervical procedure. The lateral blood supply of the trachea is preserved. *B,* The trachea has been divided just above the carina, and the left main bronchus is intubated. *C,* Details of anastomotic suture placement. *D,* At a certain point, the tube from above is advanced distally and the rest of the sutures placed or all sutures may be placed before the endotracheal tube is advanced. *E,* Once the anastomosis has been demonstrated to be airtight, a pedicled flap is placed over the anastomosis for security. The author's group most often uses the pericardial fat pad. (*A–E,* From Grillo, H. C.: Surgery of the trachea. Curr. Probl. Surg., July 1970, p. 41.)

with long flaps produces complex suture lines that are more likely to have healing difficulties (Waddell and Cannon, 1959). Any failure of healing in the mediastinum is likely to produce sepsis, and the subsequent possibility of erosion and bleeding from the innominate artery or arch of the aorta is often fatal. Sisson and colleagues' (1962) solution to this problem was to bring muscle flaps into the mediastinum to protect the vessels.

In an attempt to meet this problem, the author developed an approach of removing a plaque of sternum to the second interspace level, the heads of the clavicles, and the cartilages of the first and second ribs (Grillo, 1966). The anterior skin surface was dropped down to the trachea without pull on the stoma. This was performed through a large horizontal bipedicled skin flap with excellent blood supply. An opening in

the midflap served for anastomosis to the trachea, the simplest possible suture line (Fig. 12–23).

On the whole, this approach has worked well. When the anastomosis lies behind the innominate artery, however, the possibility of anastomotic separation exists, and in a few cases, hemorrhage occurred. For this reason, the innominate artery is divided electively with *electroencephalographic* monitoring in such patients. The omentum is advanced substernally to cover the great vessels (Grillo and Mathisen, 1990a; Mathisen et al., 1988). This obviates the need for more complex myocutaneous flaps unless the lesion requires extensive cutaneous resection. Transposition of a short stump of trachea to the right of the innominate artery has also been recommended (Orringer, 1992; Waddell and Cannon, 1959), but the author's group has not found it useful.

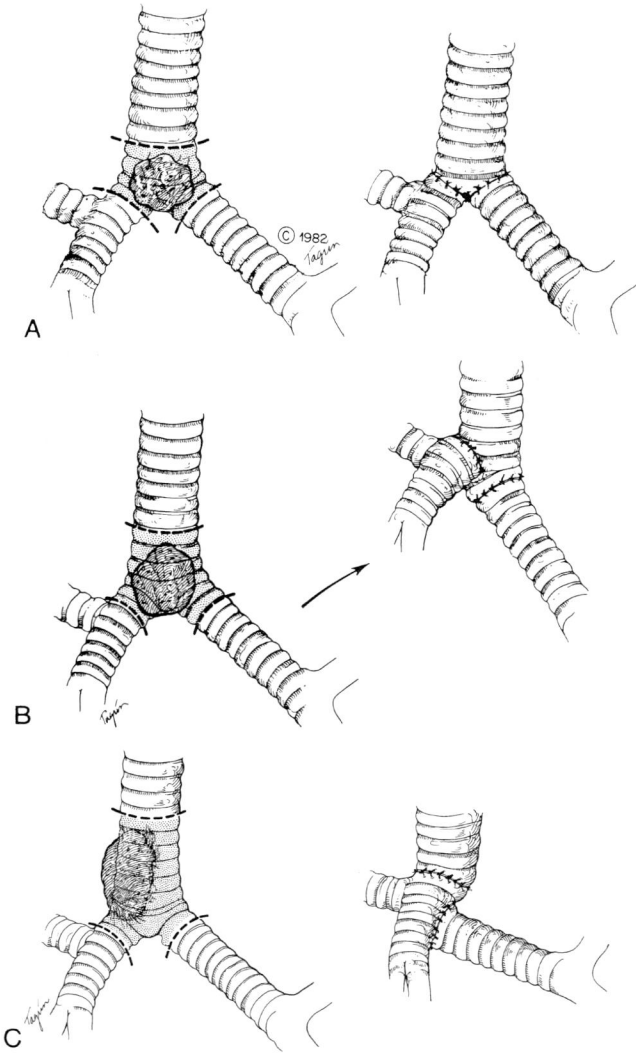

FIGURE 12–22. *A,* Resection with restitution of carina. This technique is applicable only for small, centrally placed tumors. *B,* For greater extent of tracheal resection, but not exceeding 4 cm of trachea, the left main bronchus is anastomosed end-to-end to the trachea. After hilar mobilization, the right main bronchus is implanted in the side of the trachea above the end-to-end anastomosis. *C,* With more extensive tracheal resection, the mobilized right main bronchus is elevated for end-to-end anastomosis to the stump of the trachea. The left main bronchus, which is tethered by the presence of the aortic arch, is anastomosed to the bronchus intermedius across the mediastinum. (*A,* From Grillo, H. C.: Carinal reconstruction. Reprinted with permission from the Society of Thoracic Surgeons [The Annals of Thoracic Surgery, Vol. 34, 1982, p. 356]; *B* and *C,* From Grillo, H. C.: Tracheal tumors: Surgical management. Reprinted with permission from the Society of Thoracic Surgeons [The Annals of Thoracic Surgery, 1978, Vol. 26, p. 112].)

Tracheostomy

Although tracheostomy is an ancient operation, it has never become standardized. The principal indication for tracheostomy remains that of upper airway obstruction, although intubation is now done in the acute phase in most patients. The second indication is the management of secretions, particularly in patients with neurologic deficits. This indication is managed by endotracheal tubes for prolonged periods. When a patient is going to receive respiratory support for a prolonged period, tracheostomy is usually resorted to after a week or more of trial with an endotracheal tube. A tracheostomy is rarely used for emergency airway. With the development of flexible fiberoptic intubating laryngoscopes, even the rare patient with cervical arthritis whose cords cannot be visualized may now be intubated perorally. Tracheostomy, therefore, has become an urgent rather than an emergent procedure. A large number of what were described in the past as the immediate and early complications of tracheostomy have been eliminated. These complications include hypoxia with cardiac arrest during the procedure; injury to adjacent structures, which include recurrent nerves, esophagus, and great vessels; pneumothoraces; and hemorrhage either during the procedure or shortly after (Mulder and Rubush, 1969).

With an endotracheal tube in position, the procedure is performed through a short horizontal cutaneous incision placed at the level of the second ring (Fig. 12–24). Strap muscles are separated in the midline, and the thyroid isthmus is deliberately divided and sutured. Specific identification is made of the exact ring that is to be opened by counting down from the easily palpable cricoid cartilage. The second and third rings are divided vertically in the midline, and sometimes the fourth ring if more space is needed. The tracheostomy tube should be placed so that it will not erode the first ring and then press against the cricoid cartilage. The opening must not be placed too low in case the tip of the tube and its cuff are seated close to the carina. Low placement of the tracheostomy tube is also hazardous, particularly in the child or the young adult, because the innominate artery is high. A window of trachea does not have to be removed and flaps do not have to be turned because this can cause even greater loss of tracheal wall and predispose to stenosis. The sides of the tracheal opening are held back with thyroid pole retractors to avoid tearing the cuff on the tube with the sharp edges of cartilage. The endotracheal tube is then drawn back but not out of the airway to a point above the new stoma. The tracheostomy tube is inserted, preferably using a relatively small tube—No. 6 or 7 in an average adult—because larger tubes may increase tracheal damage (Andrews and Pearson, 1971). A low-pressure cuff is used to prevent damage to the trachea. After the tube is well seated and the airway is shown to be adequate, suctioning is performed and the endotracheal tube is removed. The wound is closed loosely. The flanges of the tracheostomy tube are sutured to the skin for security in addition to the usual tracheostomy tape.

A late complication of tracheostomy is *persistence of a stoma* 3 to 6 months after the removal of the tracheostomy tube. This occurs when the tube has been left in position for a very long time, the patient has been malnourished or has been given high doses of steroids for a long time, or there has been infection around the stoma. In these patients, it is found that

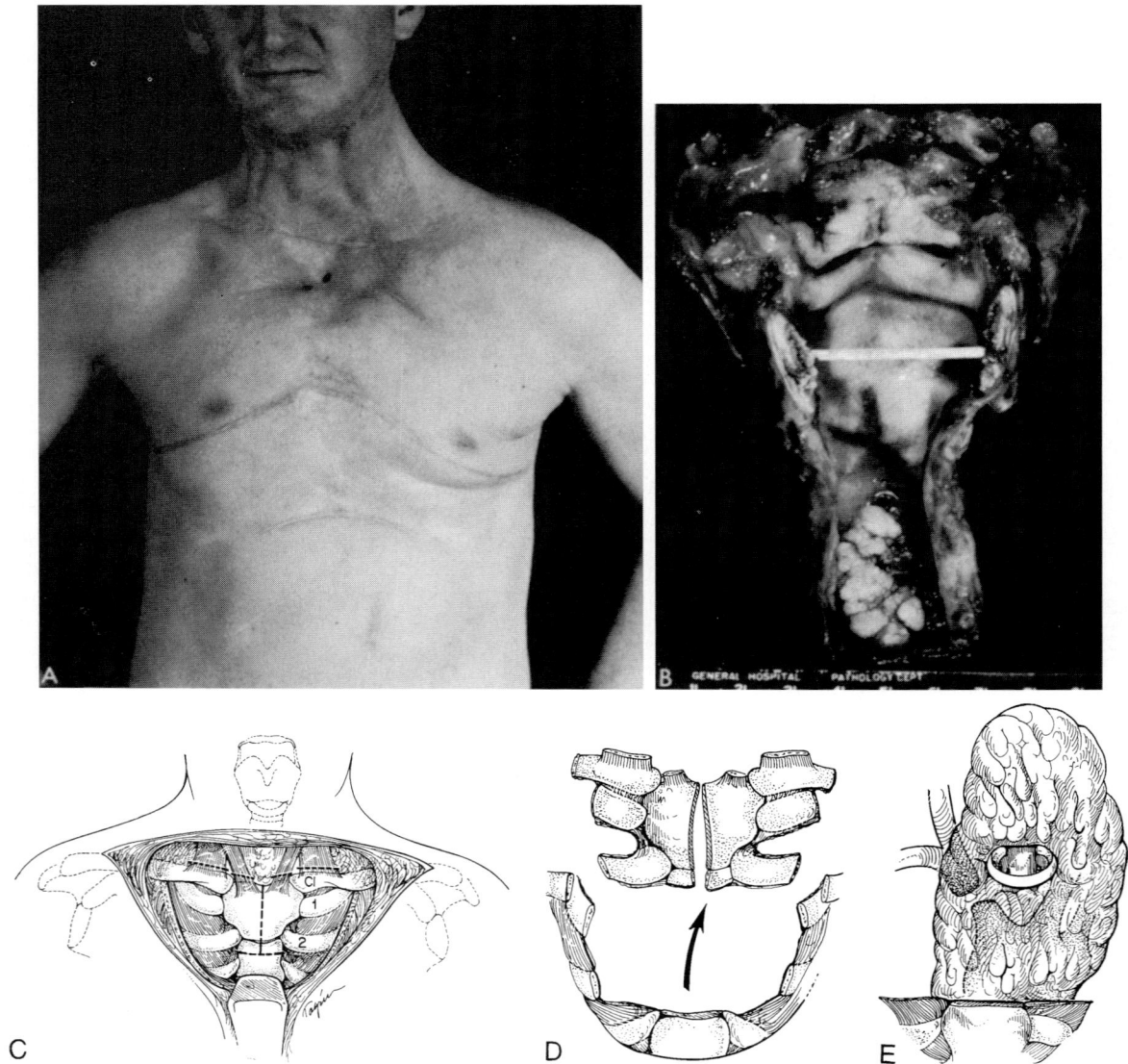

FIGURE 12–23. Laryngotracheal resection with low mediastinal tracheostomy. *A,* The upper sternum, heads of clavicles, and cartilages of ribs one and two have been resected. One long incision is at the clavicular level, and the other incision is below the nipples. The skip flap has been dropped to the stump of the trachea. The lowermost incision was a relaxing incision done at the time of the original procedure. *B,* The specimen has been removed and shows epidermoid carcinomas of the larynx and trachea that are present simultaneously.

　Details of operation: C, Elevation of the superior horizontal incision along the level of the clavicles (Cl) permits dissection of the neck by elevation of the superior flap and exposes the sternum and anterior chest wall by elevation of the lower flap, as shown here. The line of sternal division in an inverted T permits exploration of the upper mediastinum for resectability. *D,* Once the need for mediastinal tracheostomy is known and the resectability of the lesion ascertained, a plate of sternum, the heads of clavicles, and the first and second costal cartilages are removed. This is facilitated by the prior midline division of the sternum. Removal of the bony plate permits the skin to be depressed to the trachea. *E,* The omentum, which has been brought up substernally, surrounds the trachea, separates the trachea from the innominate artery, and buttresses the esophageal closure or anastomosis. In this case, the innominate has been divided and the omentum covers these arterial closures. (*A,* From Grillo, H. C.: Tracheal anatomy and surgical approaches. *In* Shields, T. W. [ed]: Textbook of General Thoracic Surgery, Philadelphia, Lea & Febiger, 1972; *B,* From Grillo, H. C.: Surgery of the trachea. Curr. Probl. Surg., July 1970, p. 45; *C–E,* From Grillo, H. C., and Mathisen, D. J.: Cervical exenteration. Reprinted with permission from the Society of Thoracic Surgeons [The Annals of Thoracic Surgery, 1990, Vol. 49, p. 401].)

the skin epithelium has healed to the tracheal epithelium around the margins of the stoma. After an adequate period of observation, it is advisable to close these stomas surgically. They are closed easily enough using the well-healed stomal margins as the base of a first-stage skin flap (Lawson and Grillo, 1970) (Fig. 12–25). A circular incision is made around the stoma, raising the margins of the flap but not sufficiently to destroy its blood supply. This ring is then inverted and the stoma is closed with a subcuticular suture. The epidermal surface of this circular flap now presents a smooth lining inside the trachea. With short lateral extensions of the incision, the strap muscles are freed and approximated in the midline to fill any defect. The platysma is approximated and the skin is closed horizontally using subcuticular sutures. An

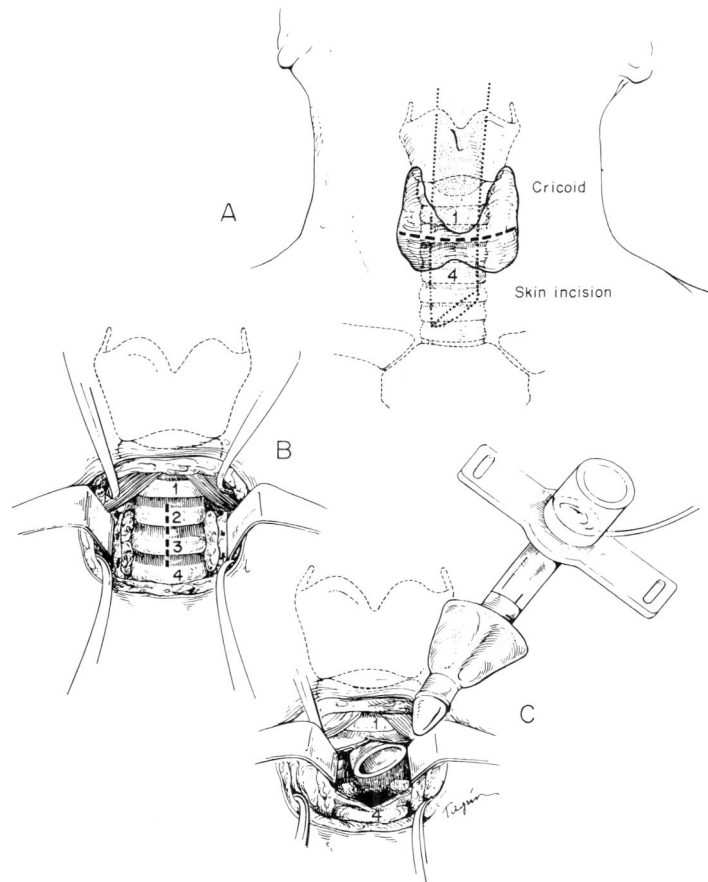

FIGURE 12–24. Technique of tracheostomy. *A*, Because an airway is already in place, the preferred horizonal incision may be made. This is placed between 1 and 2 cm below the cricoid cartilage. The cricoid, not the sternal notch, is the point of reference. *B*, The platysma has been divided horizontally, the strap muscles spread in the midline, and the thyroid isthmus is divided. Precise identification is made of the tracheal cartilages, and an incision is made in the second and third cartilages; if more space is necessary, an incision is made in the fourth cartilage. The first cartilage must be protected against injury. *C*, With small thyroid pole retractors holding back the cut edges of cartilage to avoid injury to the cuff, a tracheostomy tube is gently inserted. The endotracheal tube is withdrawn to a point above the tracheostomy opening but is not actually removed until the tracheostomy is functional. (*A–C*, From Grillo, H. C.: Tracheostomy and its complications. *In* Sabiston, D. C., Jr. [ed]: Textbook of Surgery. 13th ed. Philadelphia, W. B. Saunders, 1986.)

excellent cosmetic closure is thus obtained with a completely sealed epithelium on the inside of the trachea at the onset. Although simple approximation of the strap muscles may work equally well in many cases, occasionally the presentation of a mesenchymal surface to the inside of the trachea may cause formation of a granuloma, which requires further attention.

Tracheoinnominate Fistula

Acute tracheoinnominate artery fistula is frequently a lethal lesion (Silen and Spieker, 1965). When it occurs owing to the erosion of a cuff through the tracheal wall into the innominate artery, emergency management is by tamponade with a high-pressure cuff on an endotracheal tube (Fig. 12–26). If the tube has eroded the artery inferior to the stoma, packing and digital pressure are needed. The patient must be operated on promptly (Deslauriers et al., 1975; Grillo, 1979a). Because there is inflammatory change, it is usually safest to resect the segment of involved innominate artery and to oversew both proximal and distal ends with fine, nonabsorbable arterial sutures. Thymus, fat, or muscle is placed over these suture lines for protection. In cuff lesions, there is usually sufficient damage to the trachea at this point so that the segment is best resected and end-to-end anasto-

mosis is performed. Tracheal resection is not necessary for stomal erosion, but it is necessary to establish a proper proximal stoma and muscle flap closure of the original low stoma. Although reconstruction of the artery would be attractive, the placement of a foreign body or an autograft in this infected field is probably unwise. Occasionally, a patient will have neurologic sequelae, but in the author's experience with patients who for various reasons required innominate artery interruption, no neurologic deficits have been seen.

Tracheoesophageal Fistula

Acute tracheoesophageal fistula may be repaired if the patient is no longer on a ventilator. Techniques have been described that use muscle flaps to plug the hole in the trachea with a primary suture of the esophageal opening. Patients who have sustained enough damage from a cuff to produce a tracheoesophageal fistula usually have circumferential damage of the trachea that will likely progress to a stenosis, which was the case in several patients described (Thomas, 1972).

If repair is attempted in a patient who is still using a ventilator, it is likely to fail. Such patients are managed by extraction of any inlying nasogastric tubes,

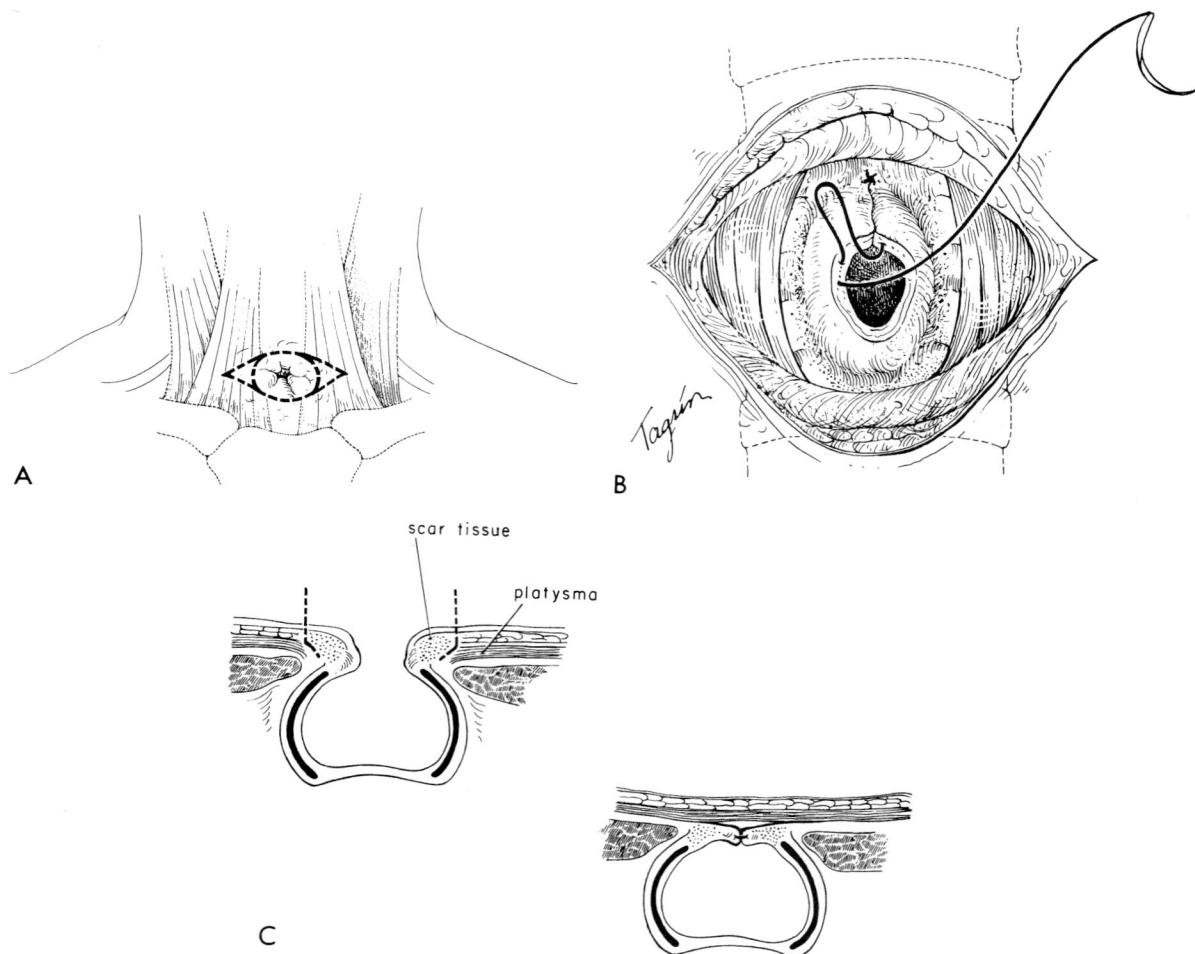

FIGURE 12–25. Closure of a persistent tracheal stoma. *A,* The existing stoma is carefully circumcised, and this doughnut-shaped skin flap is raised carefully so that the blood supply entering from the margin of the tracheostomy opening is not harmed. Additional skin segments are excised laterally to provide a short horizontal incision through which plastic closure is accomplished. *B,* The preexisting skin flap is tailored and inverted and is closed in the midline with a running subcuticular absorbable suture. The strap muscles are next approximated vertically over this closure, and the skin and platysma are then closed horizontally as a final layer. *C,* Diagram of the technique of closure that presents an immediately epithelialized surface to the trachea at the conclusion of the procedure. The diagram fails to show approximation of the strap muscles, which helps to fill the soft tissue defect before platysmal and skin closure. (*A–C,* From Lawson, D. W., and Grillo, H. C.: Closure of a persistent tracheal stoma. Surg. Gynecol. Obstet., *130:*995, 1970.)

insertion of a low-pressure cuffed tube into the trachea, and placement of a draining gastrostomy to prevent reflux and a feeding jejunostomy for nutrition. After weaning, a single-stage repair of trachea and esophagus is accomplished (Grillo et al., 1976). The esophageal side of the fistula is closed in layers, a pedicled strap muscle is interposed, and the trachea is reanastomosed after resection of the damaged segment (Fig. 12–27). Results have been excellent. Resection is not necessary in patients who do not have circumferential tracheal damage, such as those resulting from foreign bodies. The esophageal and tracheal walls are separately closed, borrowing tissue from the esophageal side, if necessary, to accomplish tension-free closure of the membranous tracheal wall. An important point is the interposition of healthy tissue between tracheal and esophageal closure (Hilgenberg and Grillo, 1983; Mathisen et al., 1991).

In special cases, individual treatment must be planned. In one patient with double fistulas that involved two-thirds of the trachea, probably due to external trauma, it was necessary to divide the esophagus in the neck and to bring out the proximal end as a temporary stoma by inverting the distal end to allow regression of the marked inflammatory changes and to protect the lungs. Later, when the tissues had repaired sufficiently, it was possible to excise the fistulas, close the trachea by longitudinal suture, and reanastomose the esophagus.

RESULTS OF TREATMENT

Primary Neoplasms

In a 26-year period, 198 patients with primary tracheal tumors were examined. Approximately one-quarter had disease that was too extensive for resec-

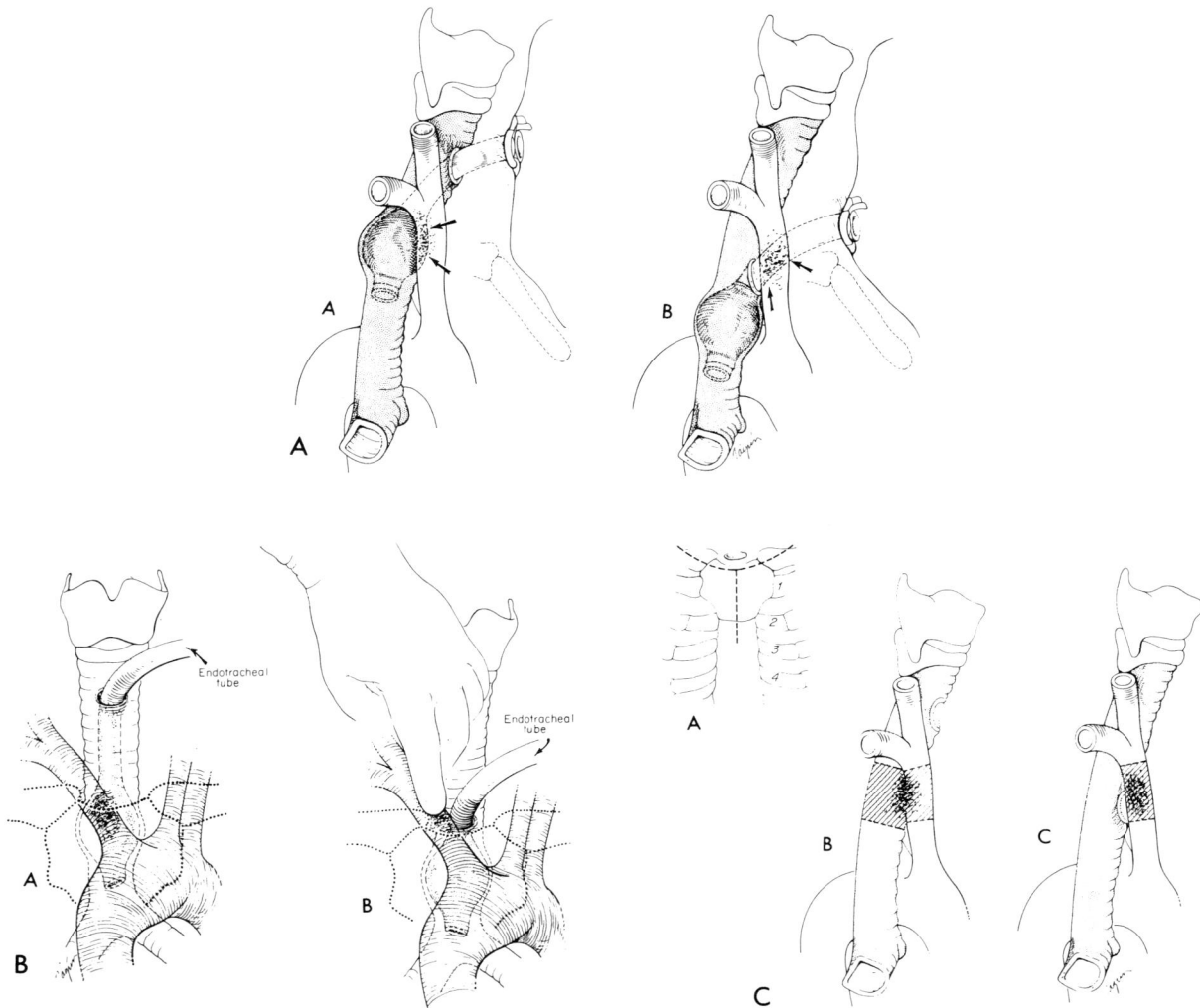

FIGURE 12–26. *A,* Etiology of the two principal types of tracheo–innominate artery fistulas due to tracheostomy tubes. Less commonly, especially now, the tip of the tube or a high-pressure cuff will erode directly through the tracheal wall into the overlying innominate artery. On the right is the more common type of fistula, in which erosion of the artery occurs at the stomal level where the stoma has been placed too low in the trachea. Direct pressure by the tube causes the erosion. This is more common in children and young adults in whom the trachea rises up into the neck as does the innominate artery. *B,* Emergency treatment of hemorrhage. In the first type, the fistula is too distal to be reached for emergency tamponade except by inserting an endotracheal tube and blowing up a balloon tightly against the fistula. In the type that occurs at the stoma, control is obtained by downward and outward pressure on the fistula itself. An endotracheal tube provides further tamponade and seals the airway. *C,* Definitive management in the type of fistula that has occurred by erosion of the tracheal wall; especially where a cuff has caused this erosion, there is circumferential tracheal damage. The eroded artery is excised. A cuff of trachea is resected, and an anastomosis is performed. Muscle tissue is interposed. In the more common type, the artery is excised. Because the erosion at the stomal site does not necessarily severely damage the trachea, tracheal resection is unnecessary. A tracheostomy tube may often be placed higher up with a long enough tube that will bypass the area of the offending stoma. The tracheal defect is sealed with adjacent tissue, as described.

tion to be considered when first seen. These patients were either irradiated or given tracheostomies for airway, or given no treatment at all, if terminal. Sixteen had complex staged resections and reconstructions or laryngotrachiectomies. One hundred thirty-two patients were treated by resection with single-stage reconstruction. Eighty-two had cylindrical resections and 50 had carinal reconstructions (Grillo and Mathisen, 1990b).

In the group who had primary reconstruction, 41 patients had squamous cell cancer, 50 had adenoid cystic carcinoma, and 41 had other types of primary tumors. Seven deaths occurred in the hospital following resection and reconstruction (5%), 6 related to complex carinal reconstruction. An additional 5 patients died after staged reconstruction, which was abandoned, and 3 following exploration only.

The number of patients with a single histology remains small and the natural history of adenoid cystic carcinoma is so long that oncologic results are at present indicative at best (Grillo and Mathisen, 1990b). Of 135 patients surviving resection (including both primary and staged reconstruction), 70% were alive without tumor—49% of those with squamous

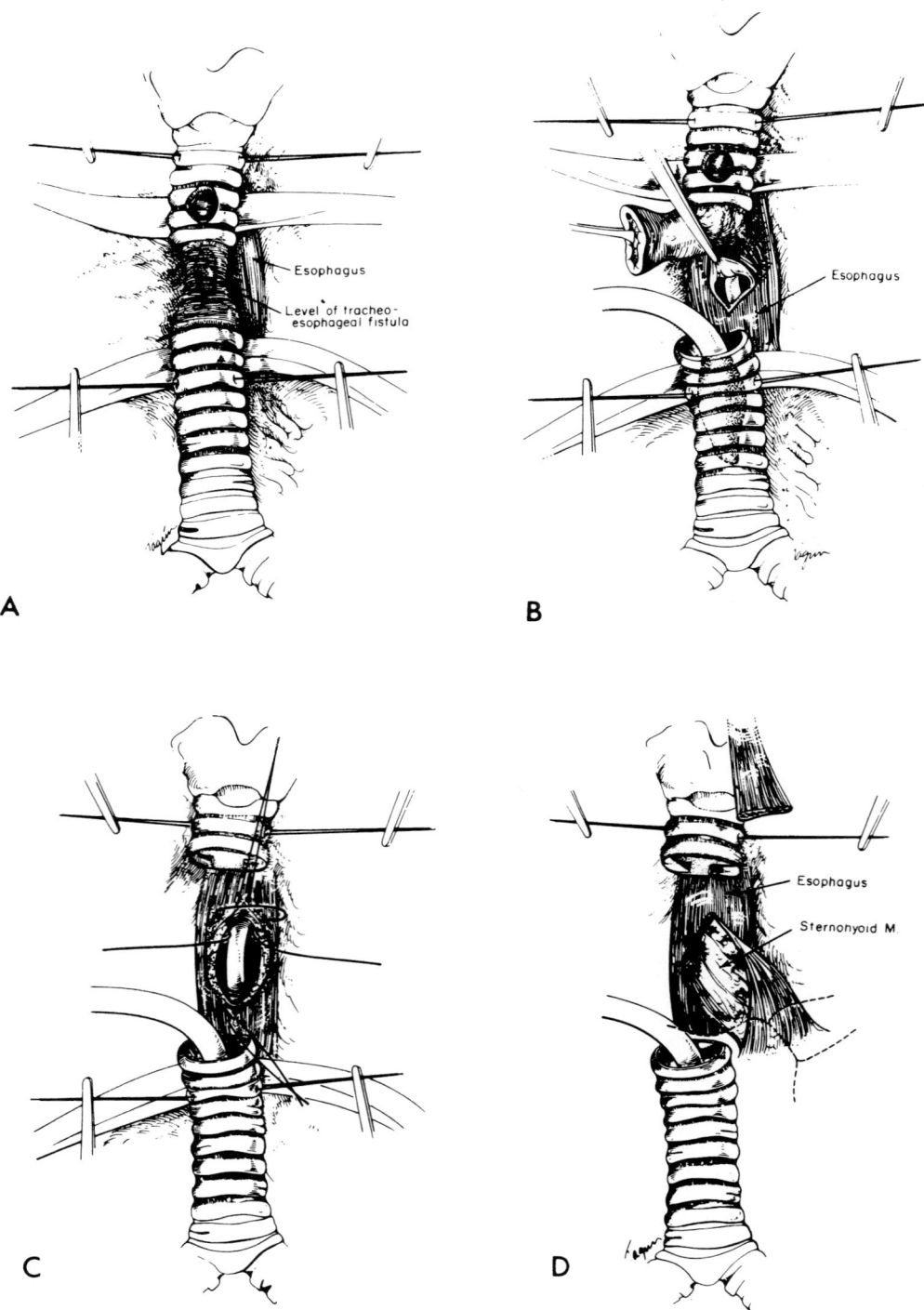

FIGURE 12–27. Postintubation tracheoesophageal fistula. *A,* Dissection has been extended to expose the trachea in the midline. This dissection remains close to the trachea and esophagus to avoid injury to the recurrent laryngeal nerves; these nerves are not exposed. Stay sutures are placed above and below the lines of planned resection. Although it is not always necessary to resect the segment of trachea that contains the stoma, this is often so close to the area of injury that the trachea below is of too poor quality to be used successfully for anastomosis. Tapes have been passed around the trachea above and below the fistula, but care is taken not to dissect excessive lengths of tracheal circumferentially. *B,* The trachea is transected, and the patient is intubated across the operative field. With the proximal end of the divided trachea elevated, the area of the fistula can be identified. The esophagus is entered at the lowermost border of the fistula. The edges of the fistula are then excised elliptically by continuing upward on both sides *(dotted lines). C,* The trachea has been excised above the level of the stoma. The fistula in the esophagus is closed using fine interrupted sutures that invert the musosa and a second layer is made with Lembert's sutures. *D,* The sternohyoid muscle is detached superiorly, and a pedicle is inserted across the esophageal closure. This is carefully sutured into place with 4-0 silk to cover the closure completely. End-to-end tracheal repair is performed by the author's group's usual technique. *(A–D,* From Grillo, H. C., Moncure, A. C., and McEnany, M. T.: Repair of inflammatory transesophageal fistula. Reprinted with permission from the Society of Thoracic Surgeons [The Annals of Thoracic Surgery, 1976, Vol. 22, p. 112].)

and 75% of those with adenoid cystic carcinoma. As might be expected, those patients with miscellaneous tumors, largely benign, showed 83% disease-free survival. Recurrence of squamous carcinoma was seen principally in the first 3 postoperative years and a few between 3 and 5 years, with none thereafter—much like squamous carcinoma of the lung. Adenoid cystic carcinoma continues to show recurrence many years later (up to 17).

Almost all patients with malignant tumors received 4500 to 6500 cGy postoperatively. Many patients with squamous cell cancer who had either positive regional lymph nodes or invasive microscopic tumor at resection margins suffered recurrence. In contrast, those with similar findings with adenoid cystic carcinoma had few recurrences. However, those patients with adenoid cystic carcinoma who were treated with irradiation only because of linear extent of gross tumor uniformly had recurrence despite an initially excellent response to irradiation. In both tumors, resection plus irradiation produced threefold prolongation of life over irradiation alone in those who died of recurrence (squamous, 31 versus 11 months; adenoid cystic: 107 versus 39 months).

Secondary Neoplasms

Fifty-two patients were encountered who had thyroid cancer invading the airway (Grillo et al., 1992c). Thirty-four were resectable—27 with reconstruction (1 wedge excision, 10 sleeve tracheal resections, 6 tracheal resections with a portion of cricoid, and 10 complex laryngotracheal resections) and 7 by cervicomediastinal exenteration and mediastinal tracheostomy. Nineteen were papillary, 6 follicular, 4 mixed papillary and follicular, and 5 various undifferentiated lesions. Thirteen of 31 operative survivors died from cancer ¼ to 10¼ years later and 4 died from other diseases. Only 2 developed airway recurrence. It is important that 9 of 13 survivors (over 1 year) underwent airway resection either at the time of initial thyroidectomy for cancer or soon after discovery of airway invasion at thyroidectomy. Some may truly represent cures. Those who underwent airway resection for late recurrence of previously noted airway invasion (tumor "shaved off" the trachea) often obtained prolonged palliation, but usually presented later with metastatic disease. Although such surgery is performed widely in Japan, this is unfortunately not yet the case in North America.

Carinal pneumonectomy or, less commonly, carinal resection with lobectomy and reimplantation of the bronchus intermedius or right lower lobe bronchus for *bronchogenic carcinoma* seems logical, but remains in an exploratory state. Five-year survival ranges from 15 to 23%, but unfortunately, operative mortality ranged from 11 to 29% (Dartevelle et al., 1988; Deslauriers, 1985; Jensik et al., 1982; Mathisen and Grillo, 1991). Deaths from respiratory failure have accounted for much of the excess mortality—a particularly unresponsive form of noncardiogenic pulmonary edema appearing 36 to 48 hours after uneventful surgery. Hypotheses about perioperative fluid overload, lymphatic interruption, and barotrauma have not thus far been substantiated.

Comparison of these limited results with results obtained before the more aggressive surgical approach to tracheal neoplasms seems to justify the following conclusions: (1) Resection of benign primary tumors of the trachea and low-grade malignant tumors of the trachea appears to offer excellent palliation and a high probability of cure. (2) Resection and reconstruction, when possible in a single-stage procedure, appear to offer the best palliation and a significant chance for cure in squamous cell carcinoma and adenoid cystic carcinoma of the trachea. Adjunctive irradiation is indicated. The results reported by Eschapasse in a collected series (1974), by Pearson and co-workers (1984), and by Perelman and Koroleva (1987) support these conclusions. (3) Tracheal resection and reconstruction for certain secondary tumors that involve the trachea may provide good palliation and opportunity for cure in carefully selected patients.

Postintubation Lesions

The results of treatment of benign strictures have been satisfactory. From 1965 to 1992, 503 patients had tracheal resection and reconstruction for postintubation injuries (Grillo et al., 1995). Fifty-three had had previous attempts at surgical reconstruction. Many patients had laryngeal injuries. Five hundred twenty-one reconstructions were done, 13 for restenosis after initial resection. The cervical or cervical mediastinal approach was used in 495 patients. The length of resection extended to 7.5 cm. There were 12 deaths in the series (2.4%). Twenty failures (3.9%) occurred. Ninety-four per cent (471) of patients showed good (440) or satisfactory (31) results. Granulations at the suture line, necessitating bronchoscopy, were the most common complication, now eliminated by the use of absorbable polymeric sutures. Five patients in this series had postoperative innominate arterial hemorrhage. Twenty-nine suffered dehiscence or restenosis. Seven died. Eight needed permanent tracheostomy, T tube, or dilatations. Fourteen attained good results.

Grillo and co-workers (1992a) described the results of single-stage laryngotracheal resection and repair of *postintubation subglottic stenosis* involving larynx and upper trachea in 50 patients. An additional 30 patients had stenoses in the same location from other causes: trauma, 7; idiopathic, 19; miscellaneous, 4. Long-term results were excellent in 18 patients, good in 51, satisfactory in 8, and failed in 2. One patient died from acute myocardial infarction. Maddaus (1992) and Couraud (1979) and their colleagues have produced similar encouraging results.

Excellent results followed repair of 27 *postintubation tracheoesophageal fistulas*, but 1 death followed anastomotic separation consequent to extensive tracheal resection. Three deaths also occurred after transthoracic repair of very distal post-traumatic fistulas in the presence of established mediastinal sepsis. All 3 required postoperative ventilation. Prompt recognition and repair following the initial injury would likely have been successful (Mathisen et al., 1991).

Trauma

Mathisen and Grillo (1987) found that 16 of 17 patients treated for *laryngotracheal stenosis resulting from trauma*, acute and chronic, attained good airways and voices, despite the initial presence of vocal cord paralysis in 14. Four also had esophageal injury requiring repair. Eight needed intralaryngeal procedures prior to laryngotracheal repair.

Complex *laryngotracheal strictures due to burns* responded well in many cases to prolonged stenting (mean, 28 months), with recovery of a functional airway and voice in most patients (Gaissert et al., 1993). In a few, resection of subglottic stenosis was necessary. Early tracheal resection was best avoided. Of 16 patients treated, 9 require no airway support, 4 have permanent tracheal tubes, 2 died—1 from respiratory failure and 1 from unrelated cause—and 1 was lost to follow-up.

Miscellaneous

Histoplasmosis can present nearly insuperable problems in airway management. Nine patients underwent tracheobronchoplastic procedures: right carinal pneumonectomy, 4; carinal reconstruction, 1; sleeve lobectomy, 3; main bronchial sleeve resection, 1. Three died postoperatively, 1 from anastomotic separation after extended resection, and 2 from postpneumonectomy adult respiratory distress syndrome (Mathisen and Grillo, 1992).

Severe *postpneumonectomy syndrome* was treated in 11 adults (Grillo et al., 1992b). Ten underwent mediastinal repositioning. Five who had not also developed tracheobronchomalacia did well. Another died from presumed pulmonary embolism. Four suffered malacic obstruction unrelieved by repositioning. Aortic division with bypass to relieve compression and resection of malacic airway in these desperately ill patients produced only 1 success. Clearly, correction must be done early, before malacia develops.

Extrinsic compression due to *substernal or intrathoracic goiter* was generally relieved by total thyroidectomy, without need for tracheal procedure (Katlic et al., 1985) in a series of 80 patients. Dyspnea was present preoperatively in 28% and stridor in 16%. Seventy-nine per cent had tracheal deviation. Flow-volume loops showed tracheal obstruction. There were no deaths. The procedure is well tolerated even by frail and aged patients. Only a few patients in the past required tracheal splinting. There is no effective medical treatment.

The clinical and pathologic characteristics of *idiopathic laryngotracheal stenosis* were defined, and results

of surgical treatment in 35 patients reported (Grillo et al., 1993). Twenty-nine patients underwent single-stage laryngotracheal resection and reconstruction and 6 patients had cricotracheal segmental resection and reconstruction. Thirty-two achieved good or excellent results in voice and airway, 2 needed annual dilatations, and 1 has a permanent tracheostomy. This disease entity had not been fully described previously.

SELECTED BIBILIOGRAPHY

Grillo, H. C.: Notes on the windpipe. Ann. Thorac. Surg., *47*:9, 1989.

This is a personal account of 25 years of development of tracheal surgery that enumerates problems and solutions in the field. The bibliography directs the reader to important contributions.

Grillo, H. C., Donahue, D. M., Mathisen, D. J., et al.: Postintubation tracheal stenosis: Treatment and results. J. Thorac. Cardiovasc. Surg., *109*:486, 1995.

Experience in the management of 503 patients who had tracheal resection and reconstruction for postintubation stenosis is described. The lesions included those from endotracheal tubes alone due to cuff pressure and from stomal and cuff injuries from tracheostomy tubes as well as laryngeal injuries from endotracheal tubes and cricothyroidotomy. Operative approach was predominantly cervical or cervicomediastinal. Factors studied include prior treatment, anastomotic levels, presence of tracheoesophageal fistula, tracheomalacia, and need for postoperative tracheostomy or intubation. Complications included granulations, dehiscence, restenosis, laryngeal dysfunction, hemorrhage, and infection.

Grillo, H. C., and Mathisen, D. J.: Primary tracheal tumors: Treatment and results. Ann. Thorac. Surg., *49*:69, 1990.

Experience in management of 198 primary tumors of trachea is detailed, with analysis of surgical and oncologic results, and comparison is made between squamous cell carcinoma and adenoid cystic carcinoma.

Grillo, H. C., Zannini, P., and Michelassi, F.: Complications of tracheal reconstruction. J. Thorac. Cardiovasc. Surg., *91*:322, 1986.

The complications that occurred in 365 patients who had resection and primary reconstruction for either neoplasm or postintubation lesions are analyzed. Failures of diagnosis included 2 patients in whom due to cuff incompetence was not recognized preoperatively and 3 in whom residual malacia was left unresected. The technical complications included granulations, separation, air leak, restenosis, hemorrhage, tracheoesophageal fistula, and vocal cord dysfunction. Miscellaneous complications included wound infection, laryngeal edema, respiratory failure, and pneumonia.

The results of resection of postintubation lesions were: mortality, 1.8%; good results, 83.2%; satisfactory results, 9.6%; and failure, 4%. With resections done for primary and secondary tumors, there were: deaths, 9%; good results, 90%; and failure, 1%. The treatment of complications is discussed and particular attention is given to the prevention of complications. Thus, in the second half of the series, there were fewer complications than in the first half.

BIBLIOGRAPHY

Acuña, R. T.: Endoscopy of the air passages with special reference to scleroma. Ann. Otol. Rhinol. Laryngol., *82*:765, 1973.

Al-Bazzaz, F., Grillo, H. C., and Kazemi, H.: Response to exercise in upper airway obstruction. Am. Rev. Resp. Dis., *111*:631, 1975.

Andrews, M. J., and Pearson, F. G.: The incidence and pathogenesis of tracheal injury following cuffed tube tracheostomy with assisted ventilation: An analysis of a two-year prospective study. Ann. Surg., *173*:249, 1971.

Barclay, R. S., McSwan, N., and Welsh, T. M.: Tracheal reconstruction without the use of grafts. Thorax, *12*:177, 1957.

Belsey, R.: Resection and reconstruction of the intrathoracic trachea. Br. J. Surg., *38*:200, 1950.

Besson, A., and Saegesser, F.: Trauma of the trachea and major bronchi. *In* Besson, A., and Saegesser, F. (eds): Color Atlas of Chest Trauma and Associated Injuries. Vol. 2. Oradell, NJ, Medical Economics, 1983.

Borrie, J., Redshaw, N. R., and Dobbinson, T. L.: Silastic tracheal bifurcation prosthesis with subterminal Dacron-suture cuffs. J. Thorac. Cardiovasc. Surg., *65*:956, 1973.

Briselli, M., Mark, E. J., and Grillo, H. C.: Tracheal carcinoids. Cancer, 42:2870, 1978.

Cantrell, J. R., and Folse, J. R.: The repair of circumferential defects of the trachea by direct anastomosis: Experimental evaluation. J. Thorac. Cardiovasc. Surg., 42:589, 1961.

Cantrell, J. R., and Guild, H. G.: Congenital stenosis of the trachea. Am. J. Surg., 108:297, 1964.

Carcassonne, M., Dor, V., Aubert, J., and Kreitman, P.: Tracheal resection with primary anastomosis in children. J. Pediatr. Surg., 17:854, 1973.

Carroll, R., Hedden, M., and Safar, P.: Intratracheal cuffs: Performance characteristics. Anesthesia, 31:275, 1969.

Clarkson, P. M., Ritter, D. G., Rahimtoola, S. H., et al.: Aberrant left pulmonary artery. Am. J. Dis. Child., 113:373, 1967.

Cooper, J. D., and Grillo, H. C.: The evolution of tracheal injury due to ventilatory assistance through cuffed tubes: A pathologic study. Ann. Surg., 169:334, 1969a.

Cooper, J. D., and Grillo, H. C.: Experimental production and prevention of injury due to cuffed tracheal tubes. Surg. Gynecol. Obstet., 129:1235, 1969b.

Cooper, J. D., Pearson, F. G., Patterson, G. A., et al.: Use of silicone stents in the management of airway problems. Ann. Thorac. Surg., 47:371, 1989.

Couraud, L., Martigne, C., Houdelette, P., et al.: Intérêt de la résection cricoïdienne dans le traitement des sténoses cricotrachéales après intubation. Ann. Chir. Thorac. Cardiovasc., 33:242, 1979.

Couraud, L., Velly, J. F., Martigne, C., and N'Diaye, M.: Posttraumatic disruption of the laryngotracheal junction. Eur. J. Cardiothorac. Surg., 3:441, 1989.

Cox, W. L., and Shaw, R. R.: Congenital chondromalacia of the trachea. J. Thorac. Cardiovasc. Surg., 49:1033, 1965.

Dartevelle, P. G., Khalife, J., Chapelier, A., et al.: Tracheal sleeve pneumonectomy for bronchogenic carcinoma: Report of 55 cases. Ann. Thorac. Surg., 46:68, 1988.

Dedo, H. H., and Fishman, N. H.: Laryngeal release and sleeve resection for tracheal stenosis. Ann. Otol. Rhinol. Laryngol., 78:285, 1969.

Deslauriers, J.: Involvement of the main carina. In Delarue, N., and Eschapasse, H. (eds): International Trends in General Thoracic Surgery. Vol. 1. Philadelphia, W. B. Saunders, 1985.

Deslauriers, J., Beaulieu, M., Archambault, G., et al.: Diagnosis and long-term follow-up of major bronchial disruptions due to nonpenetrating trauma. Ann. Thorac. Surg., 33:32, 1982.

Deslauriers, J., Ginsberg, R. J., Nelems, J. M., et al.: Innominate artery rupture: A major complication of tracheal surgery. Ann. Thorac. Surg., 20:671, 1975.

Donahoe, P. K., and Gee, P. E.: Complete laryngotracheoesophageal cleft: Management and repair. J. Pediatr. Surg., 19:143, 1984.

Dumon, V. F.: YAG Laser Bronchoscopy. New York, Praeger, 1985.

Dunham, M. E., Holinger, L. D., Backer, C. L., and Mavroudis, C.: Management of severe congenital tracheal stenosis. Ann. Otol. Rhinol. Laryngol., 103:351, 1994.

El-Baz, N., Kensik, R., Faber, L. P., et al.: One-lung high-frequency ventilation for tracheoplasty and bronchoplasty. Ann. Thorac. Surg., 34:564, 1982.

Engel, S.: The Child's Lung. Ann Arbor, MI, University Microfilms, 1959.

Eschapasse, H.: Les tumeurs trachéales primitives: Traitement chirurgical. Rev. Fr. Malad. Resp., 2:425, 1974.

Evans, W. A., Jr.: Congenital obstructions of the respiratory tract. I: Tracheal malformations. Am. J. Roentgenol., 62:167, 1949.

Ferguson, D. J., Wild, J. J., and Wangensteen, O. H.: Experimental resection of the trachea. Surgery, 28:597, 1950.

Florange, W., Muller, J., and Forster, E.: Morphologie de la nécrose trachéale après trachéotomie et l'utilisation d'une prothèse respiratoire. Anesth. Analg., 22:693, 1965.

Fonkalsrud, E. W., Martelle, R. R., and Maloney, J. V., Jr.: Surgical treatment of tracheal agenesis. J. Thorac. Cardiovasc. Surg., 45:520, 1963.

Gaissert, H. A., Grillo, H. C., Mathisen, D. J., and Wain, J. C.: Temporary and permanent restoration of airway continuity with the tracheal T tube. J. Thorac. Cardiovasc. Surg., 107:600, 1994.

Gaissert H. A., Lofgren, R. H., and Grillo, H. C.: Upper airway compromise after inhalation injury: Complex strictures of larynx and trachea and their management. Ann. Surg., 218:672, 1993.

Gerwat, J., and Bryce, D. P.: The management of subglottic laryngeal stenosis by resection and direct anastomosis. Laryngoscope, 84:940, 1974.

Gray, S. W., and Skandalakis, J. E.: Embryology for Surgeons. Philadelphia, W. B. Saunders, 1972.

Greene, R. E., and Lechner, G. L.: "Saber-sheath" trachea: A clinical and functional study of marked coronal narrowing of the intrathoracic trachea. Radiology, 115:265, 1975.

Grillo, H. C.: Carinal reconstruction. Ann. Thorac. Surg., 34:356, 1982a.

Grillo, H. C.: Circumferential resection and reconstruction of mediastinal and cervical trachea. Ann. Surg., 162:374, 1965.

Grillo, H. C.: Complications of tracheal operations. In Cordell, A. R., and Ellison, R. G. (eds): Complications of Intrathoracic Surgery. Boston, Little, Brown, 1979a.

Grillo, H. C.: The management of tracheal stenosis following assisted respiration. J. Thorac. Cardiovasc. Surg., 57:52, 1969.

Grillo, H. C.: Notes on the windpipe. Ann. Thorac. Surg., 47:9, 1989.

Grillo, H. C.: Primary reconstruction of airway after resection of subglottic laryngeal and upper tracheal stenosis. Ann. Thorac. Surg., 33:3, 1982b.

Grillo, H. C.: Reconstruction of the trachea: Experience in 100 consecutive cases. Thorax, 28:661, 1973.

Grillo, H. C.: Slide tracheoplasty for long segment congenital tracheal stenosis. Ann. Thorac. Surg., 58:613, 1994.

Grillo, H. C.: Surgical treatment of postintubation tracheal injuries. J. Thorac. Cardiovasc. Surg., 78:860, 1979b.

Grillo, H. C.: Surgery of the trachea. Curr. Probl. Surg., July 1970, p. 3.

Grillo, H. C.: Terminal or mural tracheostomy in the anterior mediastinum. J. Thorac. Cardiovasc. Surg., 51:422, 1966.

Grillo, H. C.: Tracheal tumors: Surgical management. Ann. Thorac. Surg., 26:112, 1978.

Grillo, H. C.: The urgent treatment of tracheal obstruction. In Grillo, H. C., and Eschapasse, H. (eds): International Trends in General Thoracic Surgery. Vol. 2. Philadelphia, W. B. Saunders, 1987.

Grillo, H. C., Bendixen, H. H., and Gephart, T.: Resection of the carina and lower trachea. Ann. Surg., 158:889, 1963.

Grillo, H. C., Cooper, J. D., Geffin, B., and Pontoppidan, H.: A low-pressure cuff for tracheostomy tubes to minimize tracheal injury: A comparative clinical trial. J. Thorac. Cardiovasc. Surg., 62:898, 1971.

Grillo, H. C., Dignan, E. F., and Miura, T.: Extensive resection and reconstruction of mediastinal trachea without prosthesis or graft: An anatomical study in man. J. Thorac. Cardiovasc. Surg., 48:741, 1964.

Grillo, H. C., Donahue, D. M., Mathisen, D. J., et al.: Postintubation tracheal stenosis: Treatment and results. J. Thorac. Cardiovasc. Surg., 109:486, 1995.

Grillo, H. C., Mark, E. J., Mathisen, D. J., and Wain, J. C.: Idiopathic laryngotracheal stenosis and its management. Ann. Thorac. Surg., 56:80, 1993.

Grillo, H. C., and Mathisen, D. J.: Cervical exenteration. Ann. Thorac. Surg., 49:401, 1990a.

Grillo, H. C., and Mathisen, D. J.: Primary tracheal tumors: Treatment and results. Ann. Thorac. Surg., 49:69, 1990b.

Grillo, H. C., Mathisen, D. J., and Wain, J. C.: Laryngotracheal resection and reconstruction for subglottic stenosis. Ann. Thorac. Surg., 53:54, 1992a.

Grillo, H. C., Moncure, A. C., and McEnany, M. T.: Repair of inflammatory tracheoesophageal fistula. Ann. Thorac. Surg., 22:112, 1976.

Grillo, H. C., Shepard, J. O., Mathisen, D. J., and Kanarek, D. J.: Postpneumonectomy syndrome: Diagnosis, management, and results. Ann. Thorac. Surg., 54:638, 1992b.

Grillo, H. C., Suen, H. C., Mathisen, D. J., and Wain, J. C.: Resectional management of thyroid carcinoma invading the airway. Ann. Thorac. Surg., 54:3, 1992c.

Grillo, H. C., and Zannini, P.: Management of obstructive tracheal disease in children. J. Pediatr. Surg., 19:414, 1984.

Grillo, H. C., and Zannini, P.: Resectional management of airway invasion by thyroid carcinoma. Ann. Thorac. Surg., 42:287, 1986.

Grillo, H. C., Zannini, P., and Michelassi, F.: Complications of tracheal reconstruction. J. Thorac. Cardiovasc. Surg., 91:322, 1986.

Gross, R. E.: The Surgery of Infancy and Childhood. Philadelphia, W. B. Saunders, 1953.

Harris, R. S.: The effect of extension of the head and neck upon the infrahyoid respiratory passage and the supraclavicular portion of the human trachea. Thorax, 14:176, 1959.

Hedden, M., Ersoz, C. J., and Safar, P.: Tracheoesophageal fistulas following prolonged artificial ventilation via cuffed tracheostomy tubes. Anesthesiology, 31:281, 1969.

Heimansohn, D. A., Kesler, K. A., Turrentine, M. W., et al.: Anterior pericardial tracheoplasty for congenital tracheal stenosis. J. Thorac. Cardiovasc. Surg., 102:710, 1991.

Herzog, H., Heitz, M., Keller, R., and Graedel, E.: Surgical therapy for expiratory collapse of the trachea and large bronchi. In Grillo, H. C., and Eschapasse, H. (eds): International Trends in General Thoracic Surgery. Vol. 2. Philadelphia, W. B. Saunders, 1987.

Hilgenberg, A. D., and Grillo, H. C.: Acquired nonmalignant tracheoesophageal fistula. J. Thorac. Cardiovasc. Surg., 85:492, 1983.

Holinger, P. H., Johnston, K. C., and Basinger, C. E.: Benign stenosis of the trachea. Ann. Otol. Rhinol. Laryngol., 59:837, 1950.

Idriss, F. S., DeLeon, S. Y., Ilbani, M. N., et al.: Tracheoplasty with pericardial patch for extensive tracheal stenosis in infants and children. J. Thorac. Cardiovasc. Surg., 88:527, 1984.

Ishihara, T., Lybayaski, K., Kikuchi, K., et al.: Surgical treatment of advanced thyroid carcinoma invading the trachea. J. Thorac. Cardiovasc. Surg., 102:171, 1991.

Jacobson, J. H., II, Morgan, B. C., Anderson, D. H., and Humphreys, C. H., II: Aberrant left pulmonary artery. J. Thorac. Cardiovasc. Surg., 39:602, 1960.

Jensik, R. J., Faber, L. P., Kittle, C. F., et al.: Survival in patients undergoing sleeve pneumonectomy for bronchogenic carcinoma. J. Thorac. Cardiovasc. Surg., 84:482, 1982.

Katlic, M. R., Grillo, H. C., and Wang, C. A.: Substernal goiter: Analysis of 80 Massachusetts General Hospital cases. Am. J. Surg., 149:283, 1985.

Kim, S. H., and Hendren, W. H.: Endoscopic resection of obstructing airway lesions of children. J. Pediatr. Surg., 11:431, 1976.

Krespi, Y. P., Wurster, C. F., and Sisson, G. A.: Immediate reconstruction after total laryngopharyngoesophagectomy and mediastinal dissection. Laryngoscope, 95:156, 1985.

Lawson, D. W., and Grillo, H. C.: Closure of a persistent tracheal stoma. Surg. Gynecol. Obstet., 130:995, 1970.

Lincoln, J. C. R., Deverall, P. B., Stark, J., et al.: Vascular anomalies compressing the oesophagus and trachea. Thorax, 24:295, 1969.

Lindholm, C. E.: Prolonged endotracheal intubation. Acta Anaesth. Scand. 33(Suppl.):1, 1970.

Maddaus, M. A., Toth, J. L. R., Gullane, P. J., and Pearson, F. G.: Subglottic tracheal resection and synchronous laryngeal reconstruction. J. Thorac. Cardiovasc. Surg., 104:1443, 1992.

Maeda, M., and Grillo, H. C.: Tracheal growth following anastomosis in puppies. J. Thorac. Cardiovasc. Surg., 64:304, 1972.

Maeda, M., and Grillo, H. C.: Effect of tension on tracheal growth after resection and anastomosis in puppies. J. Thorac. Cardiovasc. Surg., 65:658, 1973.

Mark, E. J., Patterson, G. A., and Grillo, H. C.: Case records of the Massachusetts General Hospital. N. Engl. J. Med., 327:1512, 1992.

Mathey, J., Binet, J. P., Galey, J. J., et al.: Tracheal and tracheobronchial resections. J. Thorac. Cardiovasc. Surg., 51:1, 1966.

Mathisen, D. J., and Grillo, H. C.: Carinal resection for bronchogenic carcinoma. J. Thorac. Cardiovasc. Surg., 102:16, 1991.

Mathisen, D. J., and Grillo, H. C.: Clinical manifestations of mediastinal fibrosis and histoplasmosis. Ann. Thorac. Surg., 54:1053, 1992.

Mathisen, D. J., and Grillo, H. C.: Endoscopic relief of malignant airway obstruction. Ann. Thorac. Surg., 48:469, 1989.

Mathisen, D. J., and Grillo, H. C.: Laryngotracheal trauma. Ann. Thorac. Surg., 43:254, 1987.

Mathisen, D. J., Grillo, H. C., Wain, J. C., and Hilgenberg, A. D.: Management of acquired nonmalignant tracheoesophageal fistula. Ann. Thorac. Surg., 52:759, 1991.

Mathisen, D. J., Grillo, H. C., Vlahakes, G., and Daggett, W. M.: The omentum in the management of complicated cardiothoracic problems. J. Thorac. Cardiovasc. Surg., 95:677, 1988.

Michelson, E., Solomon, R., Maun, L., and Ramirez, J.: Experiments in tracheal reconstruction. J. Thorac. Cardiovasc. Surg., 41:748, 1961.

Miura, T., and Grillo, H. C.: The contribution of the inferior thyroid artery to the blood supply of the human trachea. Surg. Gynecol. Obstet., 123:99, 1966.

Momose, K. J., and Macmillan, A. S., Jr.: Roentgenologic investigations of the larynx and trachea. Radiol. Clin. North. Am., 16:321, 1978.

Montgomery, W. W.: The surgical management of supraglottic and subglottic stenosis. Ann. Otol., 77:534, 1968.

Montgomery, W. W.: Suprahyoid release for tracheal stenosis. Arch. Otolaryngol., 99:255, 1974.

Muehrcke, D. D., Grillo, H. C., and Mathisen, D. J.: Reconstructive airway surgery after irradiation. Ann. Thorac. Surg., 59:14, 1995.

Mulder, D. S., and Rubush, J. L.: Complications of tracheostomy: Relationship to long-term ventilatory assistance. J. Trauma, 9:389, 1969.

Mulliken, J., and Grillo, H. C.: The limits of tracheal resection with primary anastomosis: Further anatomical studies in man. J. Thorac. Cardiovasc. Surg., 55:418, 1968.

Naef, A. P.: Tracheobronchial reconstruction. Ann. Thorac. Surg., 15:301, 1973.

Nakayama, D. K., Harrison, M. R., de Lorimier, A. A., et al.: Reconstruction surgery for obstructing lesions of the intrathoracic trachea in infants and small children. J. Pediatr. Surg., 17:854, 1982.

Neville, W. E., Bulanowski, P. J. P., and Kotia, G. G.: Clinical experience with the silicone tracheal prosthesis. J. Thorac. Cardiovasc. Surg., 99:604, 1990.

Newton, J. R., Grillo, H. C., and Mathisen, D. J.: Main bronchial sleeve resection with pulmonary conservation. Ann. Thorac. Surg., 52:1272, 1991.

Ogura, J. H., and Powers, W. E.: Functional restitution of traumatic stenosis of the larynx and pharynx. Laryngoscope, 74:1081, 1964.

Orringer, M. B.: Anterior mediastinal tracheostomy with and without cervical exenteration. Ann. Thorac. Surg., 54:628, 1992.

Paré, A.: The Case Reports and Autopsy Records of Ambroise Paré (ed. by W. B. Hamby). Springfield, IL, Charles C. Thomas, 1960.

Pearson, F. G., and Andrews M. J.: Detection and management of tracheal stenosis following cuffed tube tracheostomy. Ann. Thorac. Surg., 12:359, 1971.

Pearson, F. G., Cooper, J. D., Nelems, J. M., and Van Nostrand, A. W. P.: Primary tracheal anastomosis after resection of the cricoid cartilage with preservation of recurrent laryngeal nerves. J. Thorac. Cardiovasc. Surg., 70:806, 1975.

Pearson, F. G., Todd, T. R. J., and Cooper, J. D.: Experience with primary neoplasms of the trachea and carina. J. Thorac. Cardiovasc. Surg., 88:511, 1984.

Perelman, M. I., and Koroleva, N. S.: Surgery of the trachea. World J. Surg., 4:583, 1980.

Perelman, M. I., and Koroleva, N. S.: Primary tumors of the trachea. In Grillo, H. C., and Eschapasse, H. (eds): International Trends in General Thoracic Surgery. Vol. 2. Philadelphia, W. B. Saunders, 1987.

Rob, C. G., and Bateman, G. H.: Reconstruction of the trachea and cervical esophagus. Br. J. Surg., 37:202, 1949.

Sade, R. M., Rosenthal, A., Fellows, K., and Castanada, A. R.: Pulmonary artery sling. J. Thorac. Cardiovasc. Surg., 69:333. 1975.

Salassa, J. R., Pearson, B. W., and Payne, W. S.: Gross and microscopic blood supply of the trachea. Ann. Thorac. Surg., 24:100, 1977.

Shepard, J. O., Grillo, H. C., McLoud, T. C., et al.: Right pneumonectomy syndrome: Radiologic findings and CT correlation. Radiology, 161:661, 1986.

Silen, W., and Spieker, D.: Fatal hemorrhage from the innominate artery tracheostomy. Ann. Surg., 162:1005, 1965.

Sisson, G. A., Straehley, C. J., Jr., and Johnson, N. E.: Mediastinal dissection for recurrent cancer after laryngectomy. Laryngoscope, 72:1064, 1962.

Stern, E. J., Graham, C. M., Webb, W. R., and Gamsu, G.: Normal trachea during forced expiration: Dynamic CT measurements. Radiology, 187:27, 1993.

Suen, H. C., Mathisen, D. J., Grillo, H. C., et al.: Surgical management and radiological characteristics of bronchogenic cysts. Ann. Thorac. Surg., 55:476, 1993.

Symbas, P. N., Justicz, A. G., and Ricketts, R. R.: Rupture of the airways from blunt trauma: Treatment of complex injuries. Ann. Thorac. Surg., 54:199, 1992.

Tedder, M., Spratt, J. A., Anstadt, M. P., et al.: Pulmonary mucormycosis: Results of medical and surgical therapy. Ann. Thorac. Surg., 57:1044, 1994.

Thomas, A. N.: Management of tracheoesophageal fistula caused by cuffed tracheal tubes. Am. J. Surg., 124:181, 1972.

Toty, L., Personne, C., Colchen, A., et al.: Laser treatment of postintubation lesions. In Grillo, H. C., and Eschapasse, H. (eds): International Trends in General Thoracic Surgery. Vol. 2. Philadelphia, W. B. Saunders, 1987.

Tsang, V., Murday, A., Gillbe, C., and Goldstraw, P.: Slide tracheoplasty for congenital funnel-shaped tracheal stenosis. Ann. Thorac. Surg., 48:632, 1989.

Waddell, W. R., and Cannon, B.: Technic for surgical excision of the trachea and establishment of sternal tracheostomy. Ann. Surg., 149:1, 1959.

Weber, A. L., and Grillo, H. C.: Tracheal stenosis: An analysis of 151 cases. Radiol. Clin. North Am., 16:291, 1978a.

Weber, A. L., and Grillo, H. C.: Tracheal tumors: A radiological, clinical, and pathological evaluation of 84 cases. Radiol. Clin. North Am., 16:277, 1978b.

Whited, R. E.: A prospective study of laryngotracheal sequelae in long-term intubation. Laryngoscope, 94:367, 1984.

Wilkins, E. W., Scannell, J. G., Grillo, H. C., and Moncure, A. C.: Changing times in surgical management of bronchopulmonary carcinoid tumor. Ann. Thorac. Surg., 38:339, 1984.

Wilson, R. S.: Anesthetic management for tracheal reconstruction. In Grillo, H. C., and Eschapasse, H. (eds): International Trends in General Thoracic Surgery. Vol. 2. Philadelphia, W. B. Saunders, 1987.

Young, R. H., Sandstrom, R. E., and Mark, E. J.: Tracheopathia osteoplastica: Clinical, radiologic, pathologic, and histogenetic features. J. Thorac. Cardiovasc. Surg., 79:537, 1980.

13

Management of Infants and Children Undergoing Thoracic Surgery

Bradley M. Rodgers

HISTORICAL DEVELOPMENTS

The early attempts at thoracic surgery in children paralleled closely the advances made in chest surgery in general. Historically, pediatric patients played an important role in the development of techniques of pulmonary resection and cardiac surgery. In 1931, Nissen reported the first successful staged pneumonectomy, performed with mass ligature of the hilar structures in a 12-year-old girl with bronchiectasis (Nissen, 1931). Two years later, Rienhoff initiated the modern era of pulmonary resection when he performed the first successful pneumonectomy with individual ligation of the hilar structures on a 3-year-old girl with a benign tumor of the left bronchus (Rienhoff, 1933). The decades between 1935 and 1955 witnessed the birth of cardiac surgery, and children were important participants. In 1939, Gross and Hubbard described the first successful ligation of a patent ductus arteriosus in a 7-year-old child (Gross and Hubbard, 1939). Six years later, in 1945, Gross reported the successful division of a constricting vascular ring in a 4-month-old infant (Gross, 1945b), and Gross and Crawford independently corrected coarctation of the aorta in children (Crawford and Nylin, 1945; Gross, 1945a). Also in 1945, Blalock and Taussig reported the first successful systemic-to-pulmonary artery shunt for relief of cyanosis in a 15-month-old infant with tetralogy of Fallot (Blalock and Taussig, 1945). The modern era of intracardiac correction was initiated in 1954 with the report by Gibbon of the first successful open heart procedure using complete cardiopulmonary bypass in an 18-year-old girl with an atrial septal defect (Gibbon, 1954). Extracorporeal membrane oxygenation (ECMO), an outgrowth of this technology and that of the membrane oxygenator, was initially described and perfected in pediatric patients, although it has been applied more recently to adult patients in respiratory distress (Anderson et al., 1992; White et al., 1971).

The decades of the 1980s and 1990s have seen refinement of surgical and anesthetic management of children: Few cardiothoracic anomalies cannot be corrected completely. Indeed, many of these anomalies are now diagnosed before birth with prenatal ultrasound (Reece et al., 1987), which increases flexibility in planning for surgery in the perinatal period. Phar-macologic manipulations of the cardiovascular and pulmonary systems with drugs, such as indomethacin, prostaglandins, and artificial surfactant, present thoracic surgeons with smaller, but more stable infants to treat.

The interval between birth and adolescence is clearly one of remarkable growth and development. The "pediatric patient" spans a range of body weight from less than 500 g to more than 70 kg. This chapter concentrates on some of the important anatomic and physiologic changes occurring in the pediatric patient within this interval and discusses their contributions to successful surgical management.

RESPIRATORY SYSTEM

The lungs undergo the most dramatic changes in function of any organ system in the perinatal period. Within minutes, they must make the transition from organs with essentially no function in utero to providing for the entire oxygen needs of the newborn infant. The ability of the newborn to expand the collapsed parenchyma and maintain alveolar ventilation depends on production of sufficient quantities of surfactant, produced by the Type II alveolar cells. These cells are first noted at 21 weeks of gestation, and they increase in numbers to the time of delivery. Without sufficient surfactant, the volume of the infant's lung at the end of expiration is smaller than the closing volume, causing atelectasis and *respiratory distress syndrome* (RDS). The classic studies by Gregory and co-workers demonstrated the benefit of continuous positive airway pressure in these patients, but the mortality rate, particularly in premature infants, remained high (Gregory et al., 1971). In 1980, Fujiwara and associates reported the first use of bovine surfactant as replacement therapy in human neonates (Fujiwara et al., 1980). They noted a decrease in the F_{IO_2} requirements of these infants and a higher alveolar-arterial oxygen gradient for a given mean alveolar pressure. Since the introduction of bovine and synthetic surfactant, several clinical studies have demonstrated a significant increase in *functional residual capacity* (FRC) and an increase in static compliance in infants given surfactant replacement (Jobe, 1993; Kelly et al., 1993; Vidyasagar et al., 1987). The reduced peak ventilator pressures as well as inspired oxygen concentrations in most of these infants have significantly improved the survival of infants with respiratory distress syndrome and other respiratory disorders.

Pulmonary function studies consistently have demonstrated a high closing volume in infants, often overlapping the FRC (Fig. 13–1). The FRC acts as a gas reservoir, preventing wide fluctuations in Pa_{O_2} and Pa_{CO_2} during respiration. The FRC also maintains a partially expanded air space that requires less effort to re-expand than one that has totally collapsed. Maintenance of FRC with surfactant and positive airway pressures therefore reduces the work of breathing. The total pulmonary resistance of the term infant is approximately 6 times greater than that of the adult, and, unlike in the adult, the majority of the resistance is in the small terminal airways (Hogg et al., 1970). Anatomic studies have demonstrated that the pores of Kohn, which connect the peripheral alveolar units, and the canals of Lambert, which extend from respiratory bronchioles to alveolar ducts, are absent or poorly developed in infants and young children. These structures are thought to represent significant avenues of collateral ventilation of the peripheral alveoli; their absence, in conjunction with obstruction of the small terminal airways with edema or mucus, makes these small patients particularly prone to develop refractory atelectasis (Griscom et al., 1978; Machkem, 1971). Judicious use of airway suctioning and chest physiotherapy is especially important for children undergoing thoracic surgical procedures to maintain the patency of these peripheral airways. When secretions are suctioned from the endotracheal tube of infants, the catheter should be passed only 1 to 2 cm beyond the end of the endotracheal tube to avoid perforation of the airway (Anderson and Chandra, 1976). Wide fluctuations in Pa_{O_2} have been noted in preterm and term infants during suctioning and chest physiotherapy, and these patients should be treated aggressively and monitored carefully during these interventions.

The normal neonate spends 20 hours of the day in sleep, compared to 8 hours for an adult. More important, however, 80% of the sleep of a neonate is *rapid eye movement* (REM) sleep, as opposed to 20% for the adult (Muller and Bryan, 1979). During REM sleep, the eyes are closed but move rapidly, and there are frequent movements of the extremities and sucking activity. In REM sleep, the muscles of proprioception, such as the intercostal muscles, lose tone. In the infant, the intercostal muscles stabilize the chest wall during contraction of the diaphragm; therefore, loss of this function makes the action of the diaphragm less efficient. This causes a significant fall in tidal volume and alveolar ventilation during sleep, requiring a compensatory increase in the respiratory rate and oxygen consumption. Clinical studies have demonstrated that during REM sleep in the neonate, there is a 30% reduction in FRC, increasing the work of breathing and reducing Pa_{O_2} (Bolton and Herman, 1974; Hathorn, 1974). The sleep state, usually considered to be a state of rest and recovery in the adult, may therefore be costly to the infant in terms of respiratory efficiency and oxygen consumption. Vigorous support, including administration of humidified oxygen and chest physiotherapy, must be continued during this interval to combat the natural changes that occur during REM sleep.

The pulmonary vasculature of the neonate maintains the thickened muscular wall noted in the fetus. Perhaps because of this, the neonatal pulmonary circulation appears particularly sensitive to hypoxia, acidosis, hypercarbia, and hypothermia for the first several weeks of life. The pulmonary vasoconstriction stimulated by these conditions elevates pulmonary vascular resistance and pulmonary artery pressure, creating right-to-left shunting at the level of the foramen ovale and ductus arteriosus, with resultant systemic hypoxia. Attention should be directed in the perioperative period to preventing these conditions wherever possible. Occasionally, alkalization of the patient with sodium bicarbonate infusion will provide some relief from pulmonary vasoconstriction. The increased capillary permeability and low interstitial oncotic pressure in the lung predispose the infant to accumulation of pulmonary interstitial fluid, with an increase in the diffusion gradient. Slight excesses in fluid replacement may produce hypoxia in these patients and precipitate pulmonary vasoconstriction. Following most thoracic surgical procedures, the initial fluid intake should be maintained at two-thirds to three-quarters of the calculated maintenance volumes, with further adjustments being made on the basis of urine output and cardiorespiratory function. In cases

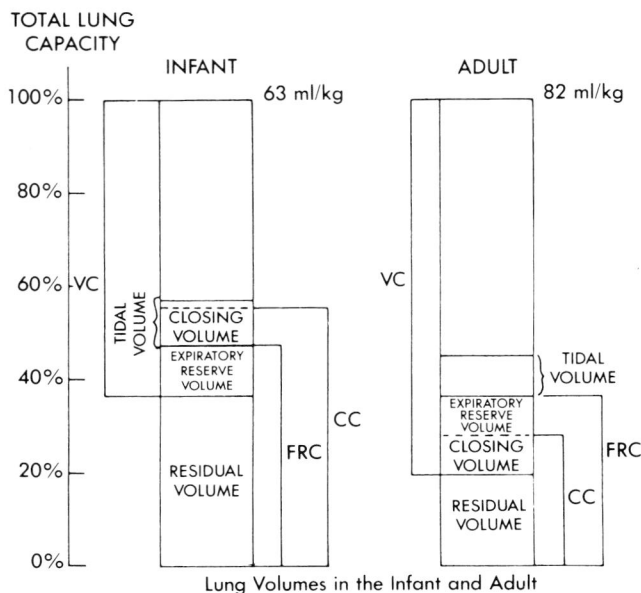

FIGURE 13–1. Pulmonary volumes in the infant and adult. The infant has a high closing volume that overlaps the tidal volume. Accordingly, even during quiet tidal breathing, some of the infant's dependent airways are collapsed. (FRC = functional residual capacity; CC = closing capacity; VC = vital capacity.) (From Smith, C. A., and Nelson, N. M.: The Physiology of the Newborn Infant. 4th ed. Springfield, IL, Charles C Thomas, 1976, p. 207.)

of "persistent fetal circulation," as seen in infants with congenital diaphragmatic hernia, ECMO may improve survival (Short et al., 1987).

Several anatomic peculiarities of the airway of the neonate are important to thoracic surgeons. The larynx of the infant is high in the neck, at the level of the fourth cervical vertebra, and the plane of the vocal cords is angled to make direct visualization of the entire glottic opening difficult during intubation. The use of a rigid stylet in the endotracheal tube facilitates successful orotracheal intubation of these patients. The narrowest portion of the airway in the adult is at the level of the vocal cords, whereas in the child it is at the cricoid cartilage. Endotracheal tubes that pass through the cords in a child may be too tight in the subglottic area. One must be familiar with the appropriate endotracheal tube size before intubating a child (Table 13–1). A leak of air should be audible, with a peak inspiratory pressure of 20 to 25 mm Hg with a properly sized endotracheal tube (Koka et al., 1977). The loose areolar tissue of the larynx makes it especially susceptible to forming edema through endotracheal tube trauma or excessive hydration, and postintubation "croup" is common. Inspiratory stridor in this setting may respond to dexamethasone (1 mg/kg administered intravenously) and racemic epinephrine aerosol treatment. The trachea of the neonate is short, and the angles of origin of the right and left mainstem bronchi are equivalent, making right or left mainstem bronchial intubation equally likely. Finally, the mediastinum is mobile in children, and a seemingly insignificant pneumothorax may rapidly progress to a tension pneumothorax with resultant respiratory distress.

Apnea of the newborn is a potentially lethal event. The premature newborn is particularly susceptible to central apnea: cessation of breathing activity for longer than 20 seconds is associated with hypoxia and bradycardia. The carbon dioxide response curve for central ventilation has been shown to be flatter than that of older and more mature infants (Rigatto, 1982). Usually this apnea responds to simple physical stimulation of the infant, although occasionally atropine (0.02 mg/kg) and ventilatory support are neces-

sary. Studies of children undergoing general anesthesia have indicated that infants younger than 40 to 50 weeks of gestational age have an increased risk of central apnea on awakening from general anesthesia (Kurth et al., 1987). These patients must be carefully monitored for 12 to 24 hours in the hospital until they have fully recovered from surgery, even though the operation usually is performed on an outpatient basis. This tendency to unmask central apnea following surgery does not seem to hold for infants undergoing procedures under spinal anesthesia, but it is probably prudent to monitor these infants as well until further data are acquired (Welborn et al., 1990).

CARDIOVASCULAR SYSTEM

Successful transition from fetal to extrauterine life involves several familiar changes in cardiovascular function. With the first several breaths of the newborn, circulation through the pulmonary vascular bed must increase markedly as pulmonary vascular resistance falls. The ductus arteriosus becomes functionally occluded within minutes of the initiation of respiratory activity to establish normal circulatory dynamics. Experimental studies with fetal and newborn myocardial tissue have demonstrated significant differences from such tissue in the adult. Friedman found that fetal myocardium contains a higher proportion of noncontractile mass, such as nuclei and surface membranes (Friedman, 1972). Seventy per cent of adult myocardium is composed of myofibrils, which constitute only 40% of fetal myocardium. As a result, at all muscle lengths along the length-tension curve, there is a significant decrease in the active tension generated by fetal papillary muscle compared with that of the adult. The fetal myocardium was also noted to be less compliant than that of the adult. Wallgren and associates studied the effects of graded hemorrhage on human infants (Wallgren et al., 1967). They concluded that the newborn was less able than the adult to adapt to loss of intravascular volume. The increase in pulse rate and decline in blood pressure noted after losses of 7.5 and 15% of the total

■ **Table 13–1.** PEDIATRIC ENDOTRACHEAL TUBES

Age	Body Weight (kg)	Internal Diameter (mm)	Minimal Length (cm) Oral	Minimal Length (cm) Nasal	Suction Catheter (French)
Premature	2.5	2.5–3.0	11	13	3
Term newborn	3.5	3.0–3.5	12	13.5	5
3 Mo	6.0	3.5–4.0	12.5	14	5
1 Yr	10.0	4.0	13	15	5
2 Yr	12.5	4.5	14	16	6
4 Yr	17.0	5.0	15	17	6
6 Yr	20.0	5.5	17	19	6
8 Yr	25.0	6.0	19	21	6
10 Yr	32.0	6.5*	20	22	8
12 Yr	40.0	7.5*	22	23	8
14 Yr	50.0	8.0*	23	24	10

*When using cuffed tubes, select the size with a 0.5 cm smaller inner diameter.

blood volume were significantly greater in the neonate than in the adult. The diminished compliance of the ventricle of the newborn and increased capacity of the venous system creates a situation wherein augmentation of cardiac output is achieved principally by increase in heart rate. More rapid heart rates are associated with a shorter diastolic interval, however, and coronary perfusion is impaired, reducing myocardial oxygen delivery.

Maintenance of adequate cardiac output is obviously of prime importance in the postoperative interval. Cardiovascular shock in infants and children most often is due to reduced preload secondary to volume loss. Restoration of intravascular volume, monitored by urine output and central venous pressure, should be the immediate aim of therapy. Intravenous fluid may be administered in repetitive boluses of 10 to 20 ml/kg until blood pressure and central venous pressure increase and heart rate falls. If urine output is less than 1 ml/kg/hr or hypotension persists with a central venous pressure of greater than 10 mm Hg, then positive inotropic support should be provided. Shock in the child frequently is associated with glycogen depletion and hypoglycemia. Despite the tendency to avoid glucose administration for adults in shock, severe hypoglycemia may develop in infants and young children, and these patients should be given 1 to 2 ml/kg of 25% dextrose solution early in resuscitation.

The response of the neonatal myocardium to inotropic agents varies, and there are wide differences in the metabolism, volume of distribution, and biotransformation of drugs in the pediatric patient. It is well known that infants and children require larger doses of digoxin (0.01 mg/kg/day), but appropriate doses of beta- and alpha-adrenergic drugs are harder to ascertain. Experimental studies have suggested that the neonatal myocardium is relatively less sensitive to the positive inotropic effects of isuprel than to those of dopamine and relatively more sensitive to the negative inotropic effects of propranolol (Driscoll, 1987). The appropriate doses of all of the drugs used in cardiac resuscitation should be determined at the time of admission of these patients and displayed in a prominent place at the bedside. The drugs should be titrated within the recommended dose range to achieve the expected cardiovascular effect (Table 13–2).

MUSCULOSKELETAL SYSTEM

The thoracic cage of the newborn and young child differs in several important aspects from that of the adult. The rib cage must be pliable and relatively easily compressible in order to allow the infant to safely traverse the birth canal. This flexibility, however, becomes a liability to the newborn because it compromises the ability to produce a large tidal volume. The increased compliance of the chest wall, in association with decreased pulmonary compliance of the infant, produces greater distortion of the chest wall with respiratory fluctuations and reduces the efficiency of ventilation. The ribs of the infant are oriented in a horizontal plane and have a circular configuration, unlike those of the adult, which are at a more oblique angle, allowing them to contribute to thoracic expansion by a "bucket handle" effect. The diaphragm of the infant inserts horizontally onto the chest wall and resides at a higher level in the thorax. This flat configuration of the diaphragm creates a shorter fiber length and diminishes the force that can be generated (Davis and Bureau, 1987).

In addition to the anatomic inefficiencies of the diaphragm, there appear to be physiologic deficits as well. Keens and co-workers noted a smaller proportion of Type I muscle fibers in the diaphragm of the infant (Keens et al., 1978). Type I muscle fibers, identified by characteristic straining properties, are high-oxidative, slow-twitch fibers with considerable resistance to fatigue. The proportion of these fibers in the diaphragm of preterm infants is only 10%; in term infants, 25%. The proportion of Type I fibers increases progressively to reach adult values (55%) by 8 months of life. Developmental changes in the contractile protein myosin have also been demonstrated in the diaphragm muscle (Albis et al., 1989). During postnatal development, adult-type myosins with the same light chain as neonatal myosins, but with a different heavy chain, gradually replace neonatal myosins. The transition from neonatal to adult myosin heavy chain forms appears to be nearly complete within several weeks

■ **Table 13–2.** PEDIATRIC EMERGENCY DRUGS

Drug	Dose (IV)	Stock Concentration
Atropine	0.02 mg/kg	0.1 mg/ml
Calcium chloride	20 mg/kg	100 mg/ml (10%)
Calcium gluconate	100 mg/kg	100 mg/ml (10%)
Dopamine	2–20 μg/kg/min	40 mg/ml
Dobutamine	5–20 μg/kg/min	250 mg/ml
Epinephrine (1:10,000)	0.1 ml/kg	0.1 mg/ml
Isoproterenol	0.1–1.5 μg/kg/min	0.2 mg/ml
Lidocaine	1 mg/kg	10 mg/ml (1%)
Sodium bicarbonate	1 mEq/kg	1 mEq/ml
Succinylcholine	1 mg/kg	20 mg/ml

IV = intravenous.

of birth. In vitro studies of baboon diaphragm muscles have shown a longer time to peak tension and longer relaxation time in premature muscle, as compared with the adult diaphragm (Maxwell et al., 1983). The efficiency of the diaphragm in the neonate diminishes progressively with increasing respiratory rate, and rates above 85 breaths per minute do not allow complete relaxation of the diaphragm and are not tolerated for prolonged periods. In addition, the percentage of maximum isometric contraction that any skeletal muscle can exert without fatigue is inversely proportional to the rate of contraction of that muscle (Muller and Bryan, 1979). The relatively rapid respiratory rate of the young patient predisposes the diaphragm to early fatigue. Extrathoracic derangements interfering with the movement of the diaphragm, such as gastric distention following thoracic surgery, may cause respiratory insufficiency. Respiratory insufficiency may progress rapidly in these patients as the muscles of ventilation fatigue. Awareness of these facts should prompt early intubation and mechanical ventilatory support.

RENAL SYSTEM

The term infant is born with a full complement of renal glomeruli, but they are small and functionally immature. The *glomerular filtration rate* (GFR) of the term infant is 2.24 ml/min, as opposed to that of the adult, 120 ml/min (Arant, 1978). The diminished GFR is caused by an increased resistance of the afferent arteriole of the glomerulus and the lower systemic blood pressure of the neonate. This contributes to the decreased ability of the term infant to excrete a sodium load. In contrast to the term newborn, the very premature infant (less than 35 weeks' gestational age), who may require thoracic surgery, tends to be a sodium waster. Careful attention must be paid to the sodium administered to these patients in the perioperative period, and frequent electrolyte determinations should be made. Krummel and co-workers noted the occurrence of significant hypernatremia in the first 12 hours following operation in preterm and term infants, presumably complicated by large sodium loads administered during the operation (Krummel et al., 1985). The renal tubules at birth also are functionally immature and have a limited capacity for concentrating urine. The newborn is unable to concentrate the urine beyond 600 mOsm/kg, whereas the normal adult may reach levels of 1200 mOsm/kg. Normally, this is of minimal clinical importance, because the infant's diet contains a large percentage of free water. When a normal diet is not being consumed, however—such as postoperatively—this concentrating defect renders the infant more susceptible to dehydration. Paradoxically, although the term infant is able to produce urine as dilute as that of the adult (30 mOsm/kg), the restricted GFR limits the ability to excrete large water loads. The fluid balance of the infant must be evaluated especially closely in the postoperative period to avoid overhydration or

dehydration. Fluid status may be monitored by hourly measurement of total fluid intake and urine output, daily measurement of body weight, and frequent determination of serum electrolytes. The hourly urine volume should be maintained at 2 ml/kg. Because of the changing concentrating ability of the nephron in the newborn and altered permeability of the glomerulus, measurement of urinary specific gravity and osmolality are less useful when one is monitoring fluid status in these patients. Glomerular and tubular function mature progressively following birth, such that by the age of 1 or 2 months, the immaturity of the kidney is no longer a limiting factor in water and sodium metabolism, although adult levels of renal function may not be reached until considerably later in life.

The total body water of the infant is proportionally high, measuring between 75 and 85% of body weight at birth and gradually declining to reach adult levels (65%) by 1 year of age (Bell and Oh, 1987). This change in total body water is attributable largely to the growing child's accumulation of hydrophobic fat stores. In addition, when compared with an adult, an infant of less than 6 months of age has a proportionately higher extracellular fluid volume. The ratio between extracellular and intracellular volume declines progressively with growth and reaches adult values by the end of the first year of life. Because the extracellular fluid space is most vulnerable to rapid depletion through abnormal fluid losses, the young child is more susceptible than the adult to dehydration from these mechanisms. The smaller intracellular volume of the infant makes rapid correction of this dehydration less effective. The infant can sustain a loss of approximately 7% of body weight before clinical signs of dehydration occur, but further losses produce tachycardia, oliguria, and diminished skin turgor. In trying to balance the infant's inability to excrete large water loads and the propensity for dehydration, the surgeon does best by slightly *under*estimating the infant's total fluid needs. Bell and associates have shown that providing newborns with a total fluid intake of more than 140 mg/kg/day increases both the incidence of patent ductus arteriosus and the frequency of necrotizing enterocolitis (Bell et al., 1980).

The newborn has a marked tendency to develop hypocalcemia. Serum levels of parathormone are insufficient for the first several days following delivery, whereas calcitonin levels are elevated for a more prolonged period (Root and Harrison, 1976). Mild hypocalcemia may be asymptomatic in the neonatal period; frequent measurements of total and ionized calcium are necessary to detect it. More severe hypocalcemia may present with twitching of the facial muscles and extremities, laryngospasm, and diminished cardiac output (Perkin and Levin, 1980). Serum levels of ionized calcium below 3.0 mg/dl should be treated with intravenously administered calcium (2 ml/kg 10% calcium gluconate). Calcium should be administered intravenously through a central venous catheter, if available, because extravasation into the tissues with an infiltrated peripheral intravenous line may cause tissue slough.

HEMATOLOGIC SYSTEM

The red blood cell of the newborn infant contains both fetal and adult hemoglobin. At term, 65% of the hemoglobin is in the fetal form, and 35% is in the adult form (Bard and Prosmanne, 1982). By 12 months of age, the percentage of fetal hemoglobin has fallen to 2%. The level of *2,3-diphosphoglycerate* (2,3-DPG) in the red blood cell of the newborn appears to be the same as in the adult, but fetal hemoglobin interacts poorly with 2,3-DPG. The 2,3-DPG is responsible for the release of oxygen from hemoglobin, and fetal hemoglobin has a stronger oxygen affinity than adult hemoglobin does. The affinity of hemoglobin for oxygen is expressed as the P_{50}, the partial pressure of oxygen at 50% saturation. The oxygen dissociation curve for fetal hemoglobin is shifted to the left of that for adult hemoglobin and its P_{50} is 20 mm Hg, compared with 27 mm Hg for the adult (Fig. 13–2). Nonetheless, under normal circumstances, the infant, with an elevated hemoglobin concentration and a high cardiac output, is well adapted to oxygen transport. However, when hemoglobin levels are reduced or oxygen demands increase—such as might be seen following thoracic surgical procedures—oxygen availability may not meet oxygen demands, and metabolic acidosis may result. Replacement of operative blood loss should be more liberal in infants in whom significantly increased metabolic needs are anticipated. Transfusion with red blood cells containing adult hemoglobin will immediately facilitate oxygen release in these patients by shifting the hemoglobin dissociation curve back toward the right.

SPECIAL CONSIDERATIONS

Thermal Regulation

The lability of the child's body temperature is appreciated by most surgeons. Erroneously considered poikilothermic, infants have all of the essential responses necessary to achieve homeothermia but are able to do so only over a very limited temperature range. The absolute lower limit of thermal regulation in a term infant is approximately 22° C; in the adult, this limit reaches nearly 0° C (Heiser and Downes, 1984). Homeothermia implies that the patient's metabolic rate may be varied to maintain normal body temperature under various environmental conditions, and that, under basal conditions, there must be a balance between heat production and heat loss. Heat loss may occur through conduction, convection, radiation, or evaporation. Conduction, the loss of heat to adjacent structures, accounts for less than 5% of heat loss in the human infant. Convection, loss of heat to the surrounding environment, accounts for approximately 35% of the heat loss from an infant. Loss by convection is proportional to the surrounding air temperature and velocity. Radiation is loss of heat to a nearby surface, such as the walls of an incubator. Radiation accounts for almost 45% of heat loss in an infant and is proportional to the temperature of the presenting surface. Under basal conditions, evaporation accounts for about 15% of heat loss and is proportional to the air speed about the patient and the relative humidity (Hey and Scopes, 1987). The newborn, especially if premature, is particularly susceptible to increases in evaporative losses because of the increased permeability of the immature epidermis. Evaporative heat losses are especially costly to the patient, because the latent heat of vaporization of water is 0.58 kcal/ml. The metabolic cost of evaporative heat loss in the premature infant may reach 4 kcal/hr. In general, heat loss by all methods is greater in the infant and child than in the adult for several reasons: the larger ratio of surface area to body mass, the lack of thermal insulation in the form of subcutaneous fat, the thinner epidermis, and the smaller radius of curvature of the exchange surfaces of the infant.

Heat production in the newborn proceeds principally by *nonshivering thermogenesis* (NST). Although shivering has been observed in term infants, it does not occur until NST has been induced to its full extent and the body temperature has fallen considerably (Hey and Scopes, 1987). NST occurs in specialized fat, known as brown fat. These cells contain many small vacuoles surrounded by mitochondria. They are rich in blood supply and nerve endings and have a considerably higher metabolic activity than the more prevalent white fat. Brown fat accounts for 2 to 6% of the term infant's body weight and is located principally

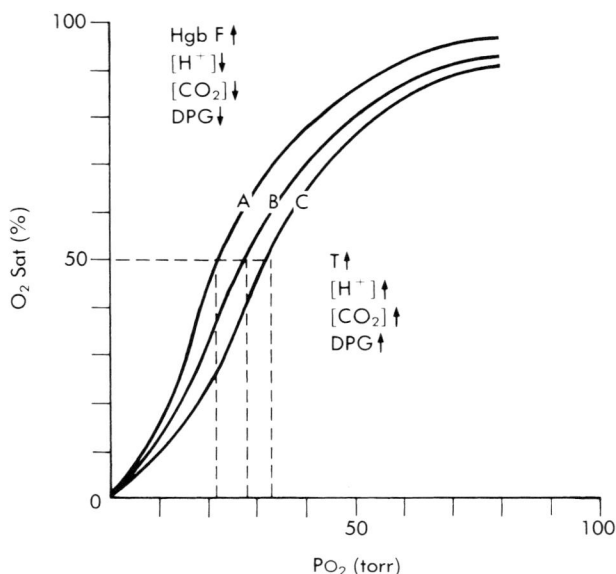

FIGURE 13–2. Hemoglobin dissociation curves. An increase in the proportion of fetal hemoglobin (Hgb F) shifts the curve to the left and decreases the P_{50}. Fever and acidosis shift the curve to the right and increase the P_{50}. (From Talner, N. S., and Lister, G.: The pathophysiology of disorders of oxygen transport in the infant. Curr. Probl. Pediatr., *11*:1, 1981.)

in the interscapular region and the posterior triangle of the neck and axilla. It is thought that this location of the brown fat facilitates transfer of heat to the blood returning to the thoracic cavity. Release of norepinephrine, induced by cold stress, initiates NST. The norepinephrine activates beta-adrenergic receptors in the brown fat, releasing tissue lipase, which begins a cycle of hydrolysis and resynthesis of triglycerides (Heiser and Downes, 1984). This highly exothermic reaction uses fatty acids, glucose, and oxygen to produce heat. The increased oxygen consumption of NST correlates best with the temperature gradient between the infant's skin and the environment (Fig. 13–3). The metabolic cost of NST for the infant is exceptionally high: Even if it succeeds in defending against hypothermia, metabolic acidosis may result. The process of NST is rendered inactive in many situations encountered frequently in thoracic surgical patients. Most anesthetic agents, certain drugs, systemic acidosis, and malnutrition often block NST, forcing the infant to rely on less efficient shivering mechanisms for heat production to avoid hypothermia (Stein et al., 1987).

Knowledge of the mechanisms and maturation of heat conservation and production in the infant is essential for the perioperative management of these patients. Because considerable heat may be lost by the patient while in the operating room, measures should be initiated to minimize such loss before and during the operation. Transport of the infant to the operating room in a heated isolette or foil swaddling suit minimizes heat loss. Warming the operating room to 30 to 32° C before the patient arrives allows the walls and equipment to warm and reduces radiant heat loss. Use of overhead radiant warmers during the induction phase of anesthesia and warmed skin preparation solutions reduces loss by convection. A warming blanket maintained at 40° C and covered with two layers of cotton blankets placed under the patient effectively reduces heat loss by conduction in patients weighing less than 10 kg but is less effective for larger patients. Warming of all intravenous fluids and anesthetic gases further reduces heat loss. Postoperatively, most infants are nursed in open, radiant-heated bassinets to allow more ready access to the patient. Marks demonstrated significant increases in *insensible water loss* (IWL) in infants maintained in these warmers (Marks et al., 1980). The IWL of term infants nursed in an enclosed incubator was 0.97 to 0.78 ml/kg/hr, whereas that in an open radiant warmer was 1.98 to 0.75 ml/kg/hr. The addition of phototherapy to the infant in a radiant warmer increased IWL even further (Bell et al., 1979). There was no significant increase in oxygen consumption noted in these infants, however, because the heat lost through evaporation was balanced by heat gained from the radiant warmer. Nevertheless, the surgeon must be aware of these changes in IWL and make appropriate corrections in postoperative fluid administration. The metabolic expense of homeothermia requires frequent or continuous recording of body temperature in these patients and careful control of the environment to maintain a basal state. The appropriate neutral thermal environment is determined by the age and weight of the patient (Fig. 13–4B). For the naked term infant, this neutral thermal environment is 34° C with 50% humidity (Sauer et al., 1984).

Nutrition

The infant's glucose balance is precarious. Severe hyperinsulinemia and hypoglycemia are often seen in infants of diabetic mothers and in infants who are large for gestational age. The normal term neonate is also susceptible to hypoglycemia, however. Stores of hepatic glycogen begin to accumulate only late in gestation. Ninety per cent of the glycogen stored in the newborn's liver is released in the first 2 to 3 hours after birth, with cessation of the nutrition derived from placental circulation. The remaining glycogen is depleted within the next 48 hours, and significant accumulation of glycogen occurs only in the second postnatal week (Thaler, 1981). During this interval, exogenous glucose must be supplied in order to avoid profound hypoglycemia and its neurologic consequences. Following surgery, all of these children must be maintained on 5% dextrose solutions, and many may require 10% solutions to compensate for the stress of surgery. Dextrostix monitoring of blood glucose should be performed at least every 4 hours in the immediate postoperative period.

The importance of providing adequate caloric intake for the pediatric patient undergoing an operation cannot be overstated. Short-term starvation in the adult surgical patient is well tolerated because of the

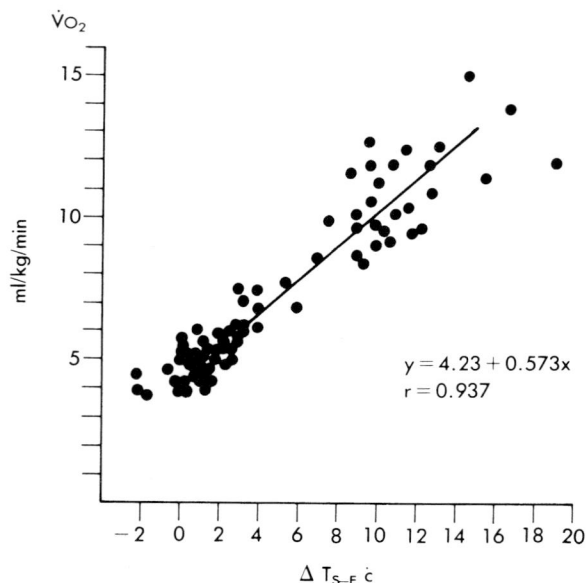

$$y = 4.23 + 0.573x$$
$$r = 0.937$$

FIGURE 13–3. Relationship between the oxygen consumption of newborn human infants (ml/kg/min) and the gradient between body surface (skin) and environmental temperature (ΔT_{S-E}). (From Adamsons, K., Jr., Gandy, G. M., and James, L. S.: The influence of thermal factors upon oxygen consumption of the newborn human infant. J. Pediatr., 66:495, 1965.)

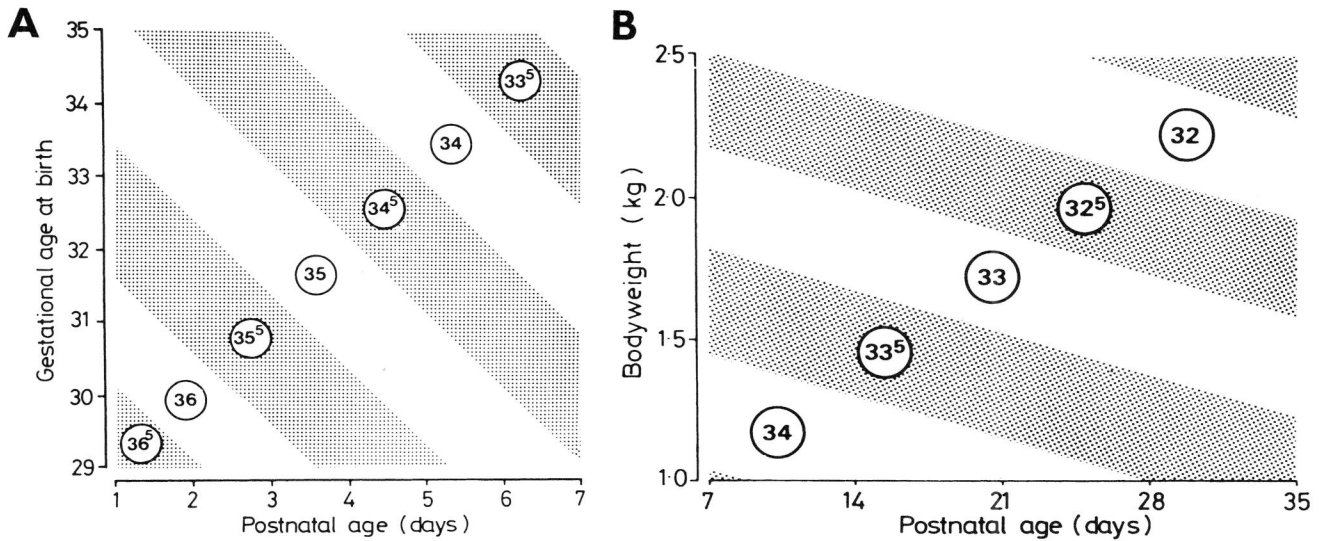

FIGURE 13–4. *A*, Neutral thermal environment for the human infant during the first week of life. *B*, Neutral thermal environment from day 7 to day 35 of life. (Dew point of the air 18° C, airflow 10 ml/min). (From Sauer, P. J. J., Dane, H. J., and Visser, H. K. A.: New standards for neutral thermal environment of healthy very low birthweight infants in week one of life. Arch. Dis. Child., *59*:18, 1984.)

abundant fat and protein stores available for metabolism. The infant has limited carbohydrate and protein stores and virtually no fat stores on which to rely for metabolic needs. It is estimated that there are only 460 calories available to the newborn for metabolic expenditure without additional replacement (Swyer and Heim, 1987). This would be sufficient for only 4 days of survival. By 1 year of life, there are sufficient body stores of fat and protein to allow 40 to 50 days of survival, and the adult can survive for an estimated 2 to 3 months without external nutritional support. In the first 4 months of life, fully one-third of the infant's total caloric intake is used for growth, including the brain and other vital organs. By the end of the second year of life, this expenditure has been reduced to 1% or 2% of the total caloric intake. Although nutritional balance is reasonable for most children undergoing thoracic surgery, some may be depleted by the metabolic cost of chronic illnesses such as bronchiectasis or cardiac disease. A study of a large number of children with congenital heart disease indicated that 55% were below the 16th percentile for weight and that 52% were below this level for height (Mehrizi and Drash, 1962). Children with cyanotic congenital heart disease appeared to have the greatest growth failure. Lees and associates evaluated oxygen consumption in undernourished children with congenital heart disease and found it to be nearly 50% higher than in infants with congenital cardiac disease who were better nourished (Lees et al., 1965). Significantly, the increase in oxygen consumption noted in these patients did not decrease immediately following surgical repair.

Infants and children expected to require intravenous therapy for more than 48 hours should be considered candidates for intravenous alimentation. Calculation of the metabolic expenditure in these patients under basal conditions estimates total caloric needs

in these circumstances. The most convenient estimate is based on body weight (Table 13–3). These estimates may need modification in patients with increased metabolic needs caused by fever, sepsis, trauma, or surgery. These caloric needs may be met with parenterally administered hypertonic glucose-amino acid solutions and intravenously administered lipids. A solution of 20% dextrose and 5% amino acids provides 1 kcal/ml. In the neonate, the amino acid concentration is reduced to 2.5% to minimize the complication of hepatic cholestasis. These solutions must be administered through a central venous catheter to avoid sclerosis and thrombosis of peripheral veins. The intravenous addition of 10% lipid solution provides an additional 1.1 kcal/ml. Many excellent reviews describe the details of intravenous nutrition in infants and children (Swyer and Heim, 1987; Zlotkin et al., 1985). Special precautions should be taken in

■ **Table 13–3.** PEDIATRIC MAINTENANCE REQUIREMENTS

Weight	Calories	Fluids
For each kg ≤ 10 kg	100 kcal/kg/24 hr	D₅¼ NS 100 ml/kg/24 hr
For each kg = 11–20 kg	Add 50 kcal/kg/24 hr	Add 50 ml/kg/24 hr
For each kg < 20 kg	Add 20 ml/kg/24 hr	Add 20 ml/kg/24 hr

Electrolytes	
Sodium	3–4 mEq/kg/24 hr
Potassium	2–3 mEq/kg/24 hr
Chloride	2–4 mEq/kg/24 hr
Calcium	50–100 mg/kg/24 hr
Magnesium	0.4–0.9 mEq/kg/24 hr
Glucose	100–200 mg/kg/hr

Adapted from Perkin, R. M., and Levin, D. L.: Common fluid and electrolyte problems in the pediatric intensive care unit. Pediatr. Clin. North Am., *27*:567, 1980.

administering concentrated carbohydrate alimentation to patients who have significant respiratory insufficiency following thoracic surgery. An increase in the provision of intravenous glucose from resting use of 7.2 g/kg/day to 24 g/kg/day with hyperalimentation increases carbon dioxide production 2-fold, increasing alveolar ventilation and work of breathing (Swyer and Heim, 1987). The net change is an increase in oxygen consumption by 33%; patients unable to increase alveolar ventilation may become hypercarbic and acidotic. Under these circumstances, replacement of some of the glucose calories with intravenously administered lipid entails less carbon dioxide production and energy expenditure.

Monitoring

One of the most striking clinical differences between children and adults is the unpredictable lability of the child. Physiologic changes occur rapidly, so these patients require careful monitoring to detect these changes before disastrous consequences occur. The smaller the patient, the greater the lability and the greater the need for close monitoring. There are, however, more technical difficulties in achieving this goal in small infants. New technologic developments have enhanced the ability to monitor the pediatric patient through all phases of surgical care. As an absolute minimum, all children undergoing thoracic surgical procedures should be monitored for blood pressure, pulse, respiratory rate, oxygen saturation, body temperature, and urine output. More severely ill children may require more extensive monitoring with measurement of central venous pressure, pulmonary capillary wedge pressure, cardiac output, and blood gases.

Monitoring blood pressure in small children traditionally has been performed by palpating the arterial pulse distal to a pneumatic cuff. This technique accurately reflects arterial pressure but is difficult to perform serially and is cumbersome in the operating room. In 1979, Ramsey developed an instrument that determined the blood pressure from the oscillations of cuff pressure with each heartbeat (Ramsey, 1979). This device, the Dinamap, measures systolic and diastolic blood pressure as well as mean arterial pressure. The correlation with direct intra-arterial pressure measurements is excellent if a cuff of the appropriate size is used. The width of the pneumatic cuff should be one-half of the circumference or 1.2 times the diameter of the extremity. Wider cuffs tend to underestimate the pressure (Darnall, 1985). The Dinamap has the advantage of allowing serial measurements of blood pressure without operator intervention and without disturbing the patient, and the frequency of measurement can be varied over a wide range. This device is especially useful for intraoperative monitoring, because it noninvasively measures mean arterial pressure.

Monitoring of arterial blood gases may be essential following many thoracic and cardiac procedures.

Percutaneous radial arterial catheters—22- or 24-gauge—may be placed in most infants and children. Frequent sampling of arterial blood gases is time-consuming, however, and often causes significant blood loss for small infants. In addition, instantaneous events are often missed because of the delay in obtaining readings. Transcutaneous measurements of oxygen tension or oxygen saturation offer the advantage of continuous monitoring of these parameters without blood sampling. Huch and associates described the first practical apparatus for transcutaneous measurement of oxygen tension in 1972 (Huch et al., 1972). This method takes advantage of the fact that the oxygen tension on the skin surface (TcP_{O_2}) approaches arterial oxygen tension (PA_{O_2}) as local hyperemia is produced. The oxygen electrode is attached to a small thermistor, which is used to heat the skin under the probe. In healthy infants without hypotension, there is a very close correlation between TcP_{O_2} and measured PA_{O_2} (Peabody and Emery, 1985). Factors interfering with local blood flow, such as anemia, acidosis, and hypotension, impair the passage of oxygen across the skin and cause the transcutaneous measurement to underestimate true arterial oxygen tension. For this reason, it is important to calibrate the transcutaneous sensor intermittently with arterial samples. The presence of a right-to-left shunt through a patent ductus arteriosus can be identified and followed using two transcutaneous oxygen electrodes. One electrode is placed on the right shoulder to sense preductal oxygen tension, while the second is placed on the abdomen or lower extremity to reflect postductal oxygen. Differences of greater than 10 mm Hg confirm the presence of a right-to-left shunt. The electrode also may be used to monitor oxygen tension in older children. In these patients, the electrode should be placed in areas of thin skin, along the volar aspect of the forearm or the inner thigh. The temperature of the heating element should be increased to 43 to 43.5° C in these patients to achieve better local warming. The correlation between TcP_{O_2} and PA_{O_2} is 95% in the neonate and 80% in older patients (Cassady, 1983).

Similar transcutaneous electrodes are available to measure arterial carbon dioxide tension (PA_{CO_2}). The transcutaneous carbon dioxide (TcP_{CO_2}) measurement is always greater than the PA_{CO_2} because of production of carbon dioxide within the skin itself (Cassady, 1983). Shock states, which produce local hypoxia, will increase the TcP_{CO_2} measurement even further. Because of these variabilities, more frequent calibration of the transcutaneous carbon dioxide electrode with directly measured PA_{CO_2} is necessary.

Undoubtedly, the most significant advance in patient monitoring since the 1980s has been the development of pulse oximetry as a method of noninvasive measurement of oxygen saturation. Hemoglobin saturation may be measured continuously by application of a simple, nonheated, cutaneous probe. The pulse oximetry probe detects the absorption of two wavelengths of light through a pulsating arterial bed. This equipment can be used with equal facility on patients of all ages. Several studies have shown a close correlation between oxygen saturation measured transcutaneously and that measured from arterial blood samples (Duran and Ramanathan, 1986; Friedman, 1972). An elevated fetal hemoglobin level does not appear to interfere with the accuracy of these readings. The continuous nature of pulse oximetry monitoring allows instantaneous detection of events causing hypoxia. Because it depends on detection of transmitted light, the pulse oximetry probe may be interfered with by high-intensity lighting in the environment. This may be a particular problem in the operating room, so the probe should be shielded from the light by covering it with a drape or foil. Similarly, alterations of skin color with pigment or jaundice may interfere with the pulse oximeter. As with transcutaneous oxygen monitoring, hypofusion may render the pulse oximeter inaccurate, but this is usually detected by the absence of correlation of the oximeter pulse with the electrocardiogram (ECG). Because of the shape of the hemoglobin dissociation curve, measurements of oxygen saturation are sensitive indicators of PA_{O_2} in states of hypoxia. The flattening of the curve at higher oxygen tensions makes measurement of oxygen saturation somewhat less useful in detecting hyperoxia. Nonetheless, it has been shown that when oxygen saturation levels are kept at or below 95%, PA_{O_2} is not likely to exceed 100 mm Hg (Solimano et al., 1986). Thus, pulse oximetry can be used to monitor sick neonatal patients while avoiding dangerous hyperoxia.

Measurement of end-tidal PCO_2 (PET_{CO_2}) continuously and noninvasively estimates arterial PCO_2. This apparatus may be especially helpful in monitoring patients on a respirator to access adequacy of ventilation. A small amount of gas is continuously withdrawn from the endotracheal tube, and PET_{CO_2} is measured with an infrared sensor. Uniform sampling difficulties in small infants with rapid respiratory rates and small tidal volumes may make measurement of PET_{CO_2} somewhat less accurate in this patient population (McEvedy et al., 1990). Currently, the PET_{CO_2} device is somewhat bulky, but technical advances in this area will make this a very useful technique for patient monitoring in thoracic surgery.

Pain

The proper management of the postoperative pain of infants and children has received increasing attention in the last several years. Pain is a particular problem following a thoracotomy because it may significantly limit ventilatory function and clearance of airway secretions. Several widely held, but invalid, assumptions have prevented the administration of appropriate postoperative analgesia in children. It was once thought that the delay in myelinization of the nervous system in the newborn blunted the infant's perception of pain. Current evidence indicates that myelinization of the sensory nerve tracts of the spine is complete at birth and that cutaneous sensory organs are fully intact. It has been thought that children require less analgesia than adults because they don't feel pain as intensely as older individuals do; supposedly they lack a negative perception of pain because they lack past experiences. It is difficult to quantify pain in young children who may not communicate well, but clinical studies have indicated that these patients may perceive postoperative pain as severe pain. Changes in physiologic parameters, such as pulse and respiratory rate, would confirm these observations. There is a widely held belief, particularly among nurses, that children have a greater potential for addiction to narcotic analgesics. True addiction following the use of narcotic analgesics for postoperative pain is extraordinarily rare, and there is no evidence for an increased frequency in children.

Beyer and co-workers evaluated the postoperative use of analgesia in 50 children with a mean age of 5.2 years following cardiac surgery (Beyer et al., 1983). These patients were compared with 50 adults also undergoing cardiac surgery. No orders for postoperative analgesia were written for six of the children (12%). Orders for narcotic analgesics were written for 58% of the children; similar orders were written for 73% of the adults. Nonetheless, the children received only 30% of the analgesia ordered by the physicians, whereas the adults received 70% of the analgesia ordered. Mather and Mackie studied 170 children with a mean age of 8 years who had just undergone surgery (Mather and Mackie, 1983). Sixteen per cent of these patients were given no orders for analgesia. When the nurses were allowed discretion in using narcotic or non-narcotic analgesia, the non-narcotic medication was chosen in almost every instance, despite the fact that only 25% of these children indicated that they were pain-free and 40% indicated that they felt moderate to severe pain.

Several additional methods of postoperative analgesia administration have been described. The *patient-controlled analgesia* (PCA) system uses an apparatus that allows the patient to initiate doses of analgesia in amounts and at intervals prescribed by the physician. PCA has been used successfully for the relief of postoperative pain in children older than 10 years (Rodgers et al., 1988). These patients use more morphine than control patients treated in a more standard manner for the first postoperative day but receive less medication over the entire postoperative period than do the control patients. Preliminary studies indicate that intrapleural bupivacaine, administered through an indwelling catheter, may be useful for relief of post-thoracotomy pain. This method appears safe and has been shown to provide excellent analgesia (Seltzer et al., 1987). Thoracic epidurally administered analgesia has been successfully used in some older children following thoracic procedures (Badner et al., 1990).

The ability of the current generation of thoracic surgeons to treat a wide variety of thoracic abnormalities in children is far superior to that of our predecessors. Advances in the understanding of cardiopulmonary physiology in infants and children have improved the perioperative management of these patients. The prognosis for infants and children with most thoracic anomalies is now excellent. Yet there are still areas in which our therapies are not adequate, particularly in the management of pulmonary insufficiency and the syndrome of "persistent fetal circulation" in the neonate. Pharmacologic manipulation of the cardiovascular system and the pulmonary vasculature offers considerable hope for improving our surgical results for these disorders.

SELECTED BIBLIOGRAPHY

Rogers, M. C. (ed): Textbook of Pediatric Intensive Care. 2nd ed. Baltimore, Williams & Wilkins, 1992.

This two-volume edition covers a broad range of topics in pediatric critical care. Each chapter provides an extensive physiologic background of the topic and concludes with considerable practical information to facilitate the diagnosis and management of these patients. The authors have considerable experience in this field and have compiled the state-of-the-art knowledge in pediatric intensive care in this volume. Each chapter is very well illustrated, and the bibliographies are extensive and current. This is an excellent reference source for the physician managing critically ill infants and children.

Talner, N. S., and Lister, G.: The pathophysiology of disorders of oxygen transport in the infant. Curr. Probl. Pediatr., 11:1, 1981.

This monograph thoroughly discusses the physiology of oxygen transport. The authors describe the developmental physiology of the respiratory and cardiovascular systems, which includes the central control of their function. A general discussion of the physiology of oxygen transport in the infant is followed by discussion of derangements in each of the component systems. A uniform schematic diagram illustrates the consequences of these disorders, and each section concludes with strategies for the management of patients. This is an excellent review of pulmonary and cardiovascular physiology and contains information that is important to thoracic surgeons.

BIBLIOGRAPHY

Adamsons, K., Jr., Gandy, G. M., and James, L. S.: The influence of thermal factors upon oxygen consumption of the newborn human infant. J. Pediatr., 66:495, 1965.

Albis, A., Couteaux, R., Janmot, C., et al.: Specific programs of myosin expression in the postnatal development of rat muscles. Eur. J. Biochem., 183:583, 1989.

Anderson, H. L. III, Delius, R. E., Sinard, J. M., et al.: Early experience with adult extracorporeal membrane oxygenation in the modern era. Ann. Thorac. Surg., 53:553, 1992.

Anderson, K. D., and Chandra, R.: Pneumothorax secondary to perforation of segmental bronchi by suction catheters. J. Pediatr. Surg., 11:687, 1976.

Arant, B. S., Jr.: Developmental patterns of renal functional maturation compared in the human neonate. J. Pediatr., 92:705, 1978.

Badner, N. H., Sandler, A. N., Koren, G., et al.: Lumbar epidural fentanyl infusions for post-thoracotomy patients: Analgesia, respiratory, and pharmacokinetic effects. J. Cardiothorac. Anesth., 4:543, 1990.

Bard, H., and Prosmanne, J.: Postnatal fetal and adult hemoglobin synthesis in preterm infants whose birth weight was less than 1000 grams. J. Clin. Invest., 70:50, 1982.

Bell, E. F., Neidich, G. A., Cashore, W. J., and Oh, W. M.: Combined effect of radiant warmer and phototherapy on insensible water loss in low-birth-weight infants. J. Pediatr., 94:810, 1979.

Bell, E. F., and Oh, W.: Fluid and electrolyte management. In Avery, G. B. (ed): Neonatology: Pathophysiology and Management of the Newborn. 3rd ed. Philadelphia, J. B. Lippincott, 1987, Chapter 34.

Bell, E. F., Warburton, B., Stonestreet, B. S., and Oh, W.: Effect of fluid administration on the development of symptomatic patent ductus arteriosus and congestive heart failure in premature infants. N. Engl. J. Med., 302:598, 1980.

Beyer, J. E., DeGood, D. E., Ashley, L. C., et al.: Patterns of postoperative analgesic use with adults and children following cardiac surgery. Pain, 17:71, 1983.

Blalock, A., and Taussig, H. B.: Surgical treatment of malformations

of the heart in which there is pulmonary stenosis or pulmonary atresia. J. A. M. A., 128:189, 1945.

Bolton, D. P. G., and Herman, S.: Ventilation and sleep state in the newborn. J. Physiol., 240:67, 1974.

Cassady, G.: Transcutaneous monitoring in the newborn infant. J. Pediatr., 103:837, 1983.

Crawford, C., and Nylin, G.: Congenital coarctation of the aorta and its surgical treatment. J. Thorac. Surg., 14:347, 1945.

Darnall, R. A. J. R.: Noninvasive blood pressure measurement in the neonate. Clin. Perinatol., 12:31, 1985.

Davis, G. M., and Bureau, M. A.: Pulmonary and chest wall mechanics in the control of respiration in the newborn. Clin. Perinatol., 14:551, 1987.

Driscoll, D. J.: Use of inotropic and chronotropic agents in neonates. Clin. Perinatol., 14:931, 1987.

Duran, M., and Ramanathan, R.: Pulse oximetry for continuous oxygen monitoring in sick newborn infants. J. Pediatr., 109:1051, 1986.

Friedman, W. F.: The intrinsic physiologic properties of the developing heart. Prog. Cardiovasc. Dis., 15:87, 1972.

Fujiwara, T., Chida, S., Watabe, Y., et al.: Artificial surfactant therapy in hyaline-membrane disease. Lancet, 1:55, 1980.

Gibbon, J. H., Jr.: Application of a mechanical heart and lung apparatus to cardiac surgery. Minn. Med., 37:171, 1954.

Gregory, G. A., Kitterman, J. A., Phibbs, R. H., et al.: Treatment of the idiopathic respiratory distress syndrome with continuous positive airway pressure. N. Engl. J. Med., 284:1333, 1971.

Griscom, N. T., Wohl, M. E. B., Kirkpatrick, J. A., Jr.: Lower respiratory infections: How infants differ from adults. Radiol. Clin. North Am., 16:367, 1978.

Gross, R. E., and Hubbard, J. P.: Surgical ligation of a patent ductus arteriosus. Report of first successful case. J. A. M. A., 112:729, 1939.

Gross, R. E.: Surgical correction for coarctation of the aorta. Surgery, 18:673, 1945a.

Gross, R. E.: Surgical relief for tracheal obstruction from a vascular ring. N. Engl. J. Med., 233:586, 1945b.

Hathorn, M. K. S.: The rate and depth of breathing in newborn infants in different sleep states. J. Physiol., 243:101, 1974.

Heiser, M. S., and Downes, J. J.: Temperature regulation in the pediatric patient. Semin. Anesth., 3:37, 1984.

Hey, E., and Scopes, J. W.: Thermoregulation in the newborn. In Avery, G. B. (ed): Neonatology: Pathophysiology and Management of the Newborn. 3rd ed. Philadelphia, J. B. Lippincott, 1987, Chapter 12.

Hogg, J. C., Williams, J., Richardson, B., et al.: Age as a factor in the distribution of lower-airway conductance and in the pathologic anatomy of destructive lung disease. N. Engl. J. Med., 282:1283, 1970.

Huch, R., Lubbers, D. W., and Huch, A.: Quantitative continuous measurement of partial oxygen pressure on the skin of adults and newborn babies. Pflugers Arch., 337:185, 1972.

Jobe, A. H.: Pulmonary surfactant therapy. N. Engl. J. Med., 328:861, 1993.

Keens, T. G., Bryan, A. C., Levison, H., and Ianuzzo, C. D.: Developmental pattern of muscle fiber types in human ventilatory muscles. J. Appl. Physiol., 44:909, 1978.

Kelly, E., Bryan, H., Possmayer, F., et al.: Compliance of the respiratory system in newborn infants pre- and postsurfactant replacement therapy. Pediatr. Pulmonol., 15:225, 1993.

Koka, B. V., Jeon, I. S., Andre, J. M., et al.: Postintubation croup in children. Anesth. Analg., 56:501, 1977.

Krummel, T. M., Lloyd, D. A., and Rowe, M. I.: The postoperative response of the term and preterm newborn infant to sodium administration. J. Pediatr., 20:803, 1985.

Kurth, C. B., Spitzer, A. R., Broennie, A. M., et al.: Postoperative apnea in preterm infants. Anesthesiology, 66:483, 1987.

Lees, M. H., Bristow, J. F., Griswold, H. E., and Olmsted, R. W.: Relative hypermetabolism in infants with congenital heart disease and undernutrition. Pediatrics, 36:183, 1965.

Machkem, P. T.: Airway obstruction and collateral ventilation. Physiol. Rev., 51:368, 1971.

Marks, K. H., Gunther, R. C., Rossi, J. A., et al.: Oxygen consumption and insensible water loss in premature infants under radiant heaters. Pediatrics, 66:228, 1980.

Mather, L., and Mackie, J.: The incidence of postoperative pain in children. Pain, 15:271, 1983.

Maxwell, L. C., McCarter, R. J. M., Kuehl, T. J., et al.: Development of histochemical and functional properties of baboon respiratory muscles. Am. Physiol. Soc., 54:551, 1983.

McEvedy, B. A. B., McLeod, M. E., Kirpalani, H., et al.: End-tidal carbon dioxide measurements in critically ill neonates: A comparison of side-stream and mainstream capnometers. Can. J. Anaesth., 37:322, 1990.

Mehrizi, A., and Drash, A. L.: Growth disturbance in congenital heart disease. J. Pediatr., 61:418, 1962.

Muller, N. L., and Bryan, A. C.: Chest wall mechanics and respiratory muscles in infants. Pediatr. Clin. North Am., 26:503, 1979.

Nissen, R.: Extirpation eines gansen Lungenflugels. Zbl. Chir., 47:3003, 1931.

Peabody, J. L., and Emery, J. R.: Noninvasive monitoring of blood gases in the newborn. Clin. Perinatol., 12:147, 1985.

Perkin, R. M., and Levin, D. L.: Common fluid and electrolyte problems in the pediatric intensive care unit. Pediatr. Clin. North Am., 27:567, 1980.

Ramsey, M. III: Noninvasive automatic determination of mean arterial pressure. Med. Biol. Eng. Comput., 17:11, 1979.

Reece, E. A., Lockwood, C. J., Rizzo, N., et al.: Intrinsic intrathoracic malformations of the fetus: Sonographic detection and clinical presentation. Obstet. Gynecol., 70:627, 1987.

Rienhoff, W. F., Jr.: Pneumonectomy: A preliminary report of the operative technique in two successful cases. Bull. Johns Hopkins Hosp., 53:390, 1933.

Rigatto, H.: Apnea. Pediatr. Clin. North Am., 29:1105, 1982.

Rodgers, B. M., Webb, C. J., Sergios, D., and Newman, B. M.: Patient-controlled analgesia in pediatric surgery. J. Pediatr. Surg., 23:259, 1988.

Root, A. W., and Harrison, H. E.: Recent advances in calcium metabolism, I. Mechanisms of calcium homeostasis. J. Pediatr., 88:1, 1976.

Sauer, P. J. J., Dane, H. J., and Visser, H. K. A.: New standards for neutral thermal environment of healthy very low birthweight infants in week one of life. Arch. Dis. Child., 59:18, 1984.

Seltzer, J. L., Larijani, G. E., Goldberg, M. E., Marr, A. T.: Intrapleural bupivacaine—A kinetic and dynamic evaluation. Anesthesiology, 67:798, 1987.

Short, B. L., Miller, M. K., and Anderson, K. D.: Extracorporeal membrane oxygenation in the management of respiratory failure in the newborn. Clin. Perinatol., 14:737, 1987.

Smith, C. A., and Nelson, N. M.: The Physiology of the Newborn Infant. 4th ed. Springfield, IL, Charles C Thomas, 1976, p. 207.

Solimano, A. J., Smyth, J. A., Mann, T. K., et al.: Pulse oximetry advantages in infants with bronchopulmonary dysplasia. Pediatrics, 78:844, 1986.

Stein, J., Chèu, H., Lee, M., et al.: Effects of muscle relaxants, sedatives, narcotics and anesthetics on neonates' thermogenesis. Surg. Forum, 38:76, 1987.

Swyer, P. R., and Heim, T.: Nutrition, body fluids, and acid-base homeostasis. In Fanaroff, A. A., and Martin, R. J. (eds): Neonatal-Perinatal Medicine: Diseases of the Fetus and Infant. 4th ed. St. Louis, C. V. Mosby, 1987, Chapter 25, Part I.

Thaler, M.: Liver function and maturation in the perinatal period. In Lebenthal, E. (ed): Textbook of Gastroenterology and Nutrition in Infancy. New York, Raven Press, 1981, Chapter 16.

Vidyasagar, D., Raju, T. N. K., Shimada, S., and Maeta, H.: Surfactant replacement therapy: Clinical and experimental studies. Clin. Perinatol., 14:713, 1987.

Wallgren, G., Hanson, J. S., and Lind, J.: Quantitative studies of the human neonatal circulation. Acta Paediatr. Scand. Suppl., 179:44, 1967.

Welborn, L. G., Rice, L. J., Hannaliah, R. S., et al.: Postoperative apnea in former preterm infants: Prospective comparison of spinal and general anesthesia. Anesthesiology, 72:838, 1990.

White, J. J., Andrews, H. G., Risenberg, H., et al.: Prolonged respiratory support in newborn infants with membrane oxygenator surgery, 70:288, 1971.

Zlotkin, S. H., Stallings, V. A., and Pencharz, P. B.: Total parenteral nutrition in children. Pediatr. Clin. North Am., 32:381, 1985.

14 Trauma to the Chest

David H. Wisner

A useful division of trauma is into *blunt* and *penetrating* mechanisms of injury. Motor vehicle accidents are the most common blunt mechanism. Others include motorcycle accidents, pedestrians hit by cars, bicycle accidents, and assaults with blunt objects such as fists or baseball bats. Increasing traffic speed has increased the frequency of severe thoracic injury suffered from motor vehicle accidents; chest injuries occur in approximately 25% of motor vehicle accident victims (LoCicero and Mattox, 1989). It is difficult to estimate the contribution of thoracic injury to morbidity and mortality in blunt trauma victims, but it is clearly an important factor. Development of air bags in motor vehicles and the institution of mandatory seat belt laws in many states are recent examples in which the epidemiology of injury has been applied to product development and public policy.

Gunshot and stab wounds are the most common penetrating mechanisms of injury to the chest. Widespread availability of high-velocity and large-caliber guns has increased the frequency of high-energy missile wounds of the chest, but most injuries are still caused by relatively low-caliber handguns (Mattox et al., 1989; Symbas et al., 1976).

Regardless of the mechanism of injury, chest trauma is common and takes many different forms. Some injuries, such as rib fractures in the elderly, blunt diaphragmatic rupture, and penetrating esophageal injuries, can be subtle in their initial presentation and are diagnostic dilemmas. Other thoracic injuries, such as penetrating cardiac wounds and tension pneumothorax, are among the most immediately serious and life-threatening of all traumatic injuries.

HISTORICAL ASPECTS

References to thoracic wounds are found in the oldest medical writings. The Smith papyrus (3000 B.C.) contains notations about chest injuries treated by the Egyptian physician Imotep (Breasted, 1930), which underscores the fact that many thoracic injuries can be treated with relatively simple techniques.

In the fourth century B.C., Hippocrates, aware that rib fractures can be associated with hemoptysis, prescribed rest and bloodletting for patients with broken ribs (Hippocrates, 1959). He also advocated stabilization of the chest wall with binding, a technique that may have been appropriate in an age in which adequate pain control was impossible. The Greeks and Romans considered penetrating injuries of the chest almost uniformly fatal. Aristotle, writing in the third century B.C., felt that "The heart alone of all the viscera cannot withstand injury" (Aristotle, 1937). Galen, in the second century A.D., wrote of packing open chest wounds suffered by gladiators in ancient Rome (Pickard, 1991).

In the 16th century, Ambroise Paré described subcutaneous emphysema associated with chest wall injury and advocated débriding segments of broken ribs. In the 17th century, Riolanus successfully treated cardiac injuries in animals (Riolanus, 1649), and Scultetus described empyema as a complication of penetrating thoracic injury (Scultetus, 1674).

Scultetus also advocated drainage tubes and irrigation for established intrapleural infections. Drainage tubes generally functioned as passive conduits. The importance of suction was recognized, however, especially in the treatment of infection. In the absence of an efficient mechanical means of aspiration, oral aspiration of wounds by professional "wound suckers" arose as a means of treating chest infections. Anel, a military surgeon who wrote a treatise entitled *The Art of Sucking Wounds* in 1707, noted that the professional wound suckers suffered (not surprisingly) from frequent oral infections (Anel, 1707) (Fig. 14–1).

The use of water seal to drain the pleural cavity was first practiced in rudimentary form in the nineteenth century (Playfair, 1872). Thoracentesis was associated with a high mortality rate, probably because of a lack of antibiotics and anesthesia. One of the leading surgeons of the day, Dupuytren of Paris, reportedly performed thoracentesis on 50 patients with only two long-term survivors. Dupuytren himself, when he subsequently developed an empyema, refused thoracentesis, saying that he would rather die by the hand of God than by that of surgeons (Guthrie, 1848).

There was debate about the treatment of injuries to the heart. No less a figure than Theodore Billroth stated in 1885 that "the surgeon who should attempt to suture a wound of the heart would lose the respect of his colleagues" (Billroth, 1913). Despite such sentiments, the first repair of a penetrating cardiac wound in a human being was performed in 1896 (Rehn, 1897).

Much of the 20th-century history of the treatment of thoracic trauma centers on developments in anesthesia, antibiotics, and radiology. Positive pressure ventilation permitted more aggressive surgical management of thoracic wounds. Refinements in equipment and technique allowed for radiography of the

456

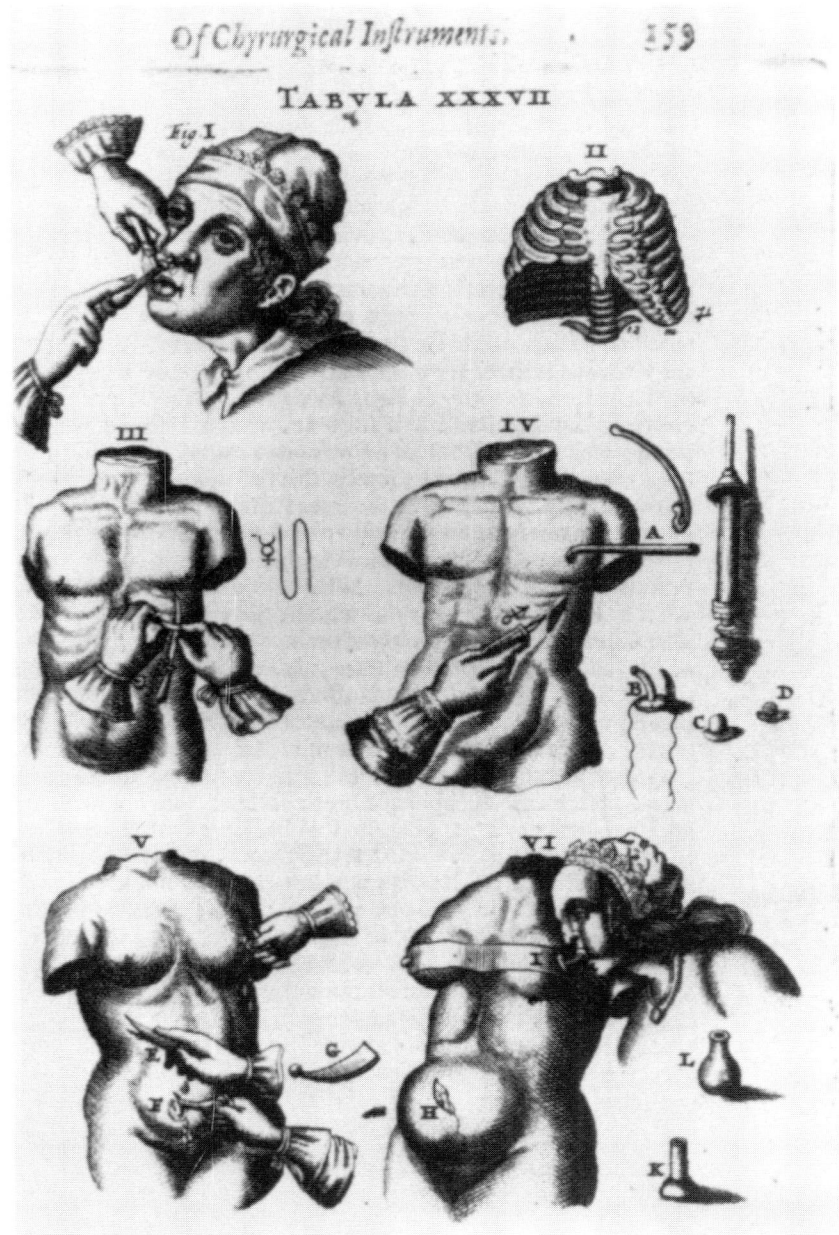

FIGURE 14–1. A 17th-century illustration taken from *The Surgeon's Storehouse* by Scultetus (1674). Wound sucking is seen in the lower right corner. Also included are figures of irrigation devices and the location for incisions for the drainage of empyema.

chest, which rapidly became widely available (Graham, 1957). Graham and Bell, as an outgrowth of experience with casualties during World War I, advocated routine drainage of the chest for empyema (Graham and Bell, 1918). The development of antibiotics and widespread acceptance of the importance of drainage of the pleural cavity for hemothorax or pneumothorax markedly improved the prognosis for both penetrating and blunt injuries.

During the last several decades, the availability of cardiopulmonary bypass has allowed treatment of intracardiac defects, and further improvements in anesthesia (selective lung ventilation) and radiology (computed tomography [CT] of the chest) have been introduced. In critical care, prolonged survival of patients with injuries that previously had been fatal led to the formal description of the adult respiratory distress syndrome. Increasing organization of trauma care delivery and efforts at injury prevention have also reduced morbidity and mortality (West, 1988).

INITIAL RESUSCITATION

The initial resuscitation of patients with thoracic injuries follows the same principles as for the resuscitation of any trauma patient: these have been dubbed the "ABCs" as an acronym for *a*irway, *b*reathing, and *c*irculation (American College of Surgeons, 1989; Wood and Lawler, 1992). Some elements of the ABCs have particular significance for thoracic injury.

The first priority is to ensure an adequate airway

(Barone et al., 1986; Grande et al., 1990; Rhee et al., 1990). In some patients, this requires endotracheal intubation, the one therapeutic maneuver of proven benefit when done in the prehospital arena. Nasotracheal or orotracheal intubation usually can be accomplished with relative ease. In some patients, however, intubation is complicated by the presence of an injury to the larynx or trachea. Emergent cricothyrotomy should be performed in such cases to ensure a reliable airway (Fig. 14–2). If the tracheal injury is large, the simplest and most expedient means of management is to place an endotracheal tube through the defect.

The second priority of initial resuscitation is to assure adequate ventilation. Although some intubated trauma patients are able to spontaneously ventilate, most require mechanical ventilation. Also, some patients with patent airways require intubation and mechanical ventilation because of a loss of respiratory drive or because the severity of injury is such that optimizing oxygenation and ventilation is paramount.

Several aspects of mechanical ventilation are particularly important to the patient with thoracic injury. If the lung has been injured, positive pressure ventilation increases the risk of a tension pneumothorax. The important pathophysiology in tension pneumothorax is compromise of venous return and a corresponding decrease in cardiac output. Treatment is rapid decompression of the chest with a needle followed by tube thoracostomy. Even if a pneumothorax is not present, positive pressure ventilation decreases venous return, and increased infusion of intravenous fluid may be required to maintain cardiac preload.

The third priority in trauma management is circulation. Intravenous catheters should be placed, and several liters of fluid should be infused rapidly. Catheters should be placed at peripheral sites. The saphenous vein at the ankle will admit a very large intravenous line; we use intravenous tubing in the form of an extension tube. Central venous lines should not be inserted during emergent resuscitation. Other procedures in the area of the head and neck, such as intubation and neurologic assessment, are of higher priority, and many central venous catheters are small in caliber. In addition, hypovolemic patients have collapsed central veins due to volume loss, so chances of a complication are increased.

Intrapleural hemorrhage usually can be suspected on physical examination and confirmed with a chest film. Most patients with blunt trauma from assaults or motor vehicle accidents and any patients with penetrating trauma to the chest should undergo chest radiography early in initial management if at all possible. When the film is interpreted, the position of the patient should be considered. Large pneumothoraces usually are easy to diagnose, but blood in the chest will not necessarily layer out in the pleural sulcus if the patient is supine.

Blood should be drawn while the ABCs of resuscitation are performed. Essential initial tests are arterial blood gases, a hematocrit, and a sample for typing and cross-matching. Urinary catheter placement is valuable in many patients, and the urine should be checked for gross hematuria. After initial resuscitation, a primary and secondary survey are done. Further diagnostic and therapeutic maneuvers are individually based on the findings of these examinations, the laboratory and radiographic data, and the status of the patient.

EMERGENCY DEPARTMENT THORACOTOMY

Improvements in prehospital care have increased the number of trauma patients with markedly de-

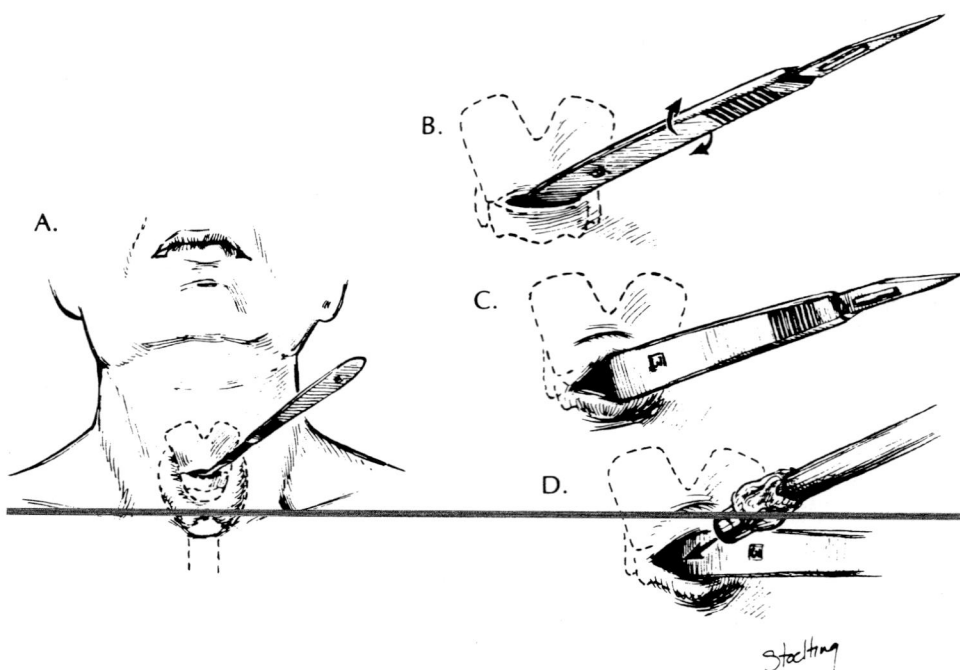

FIGURE 14–2. Cricothyrotomy is the procedure of choice for placement of an emergent surgical airway. The cricothyroid membrane is located between the lower margin of the thyroid cartilage and the upper margin of the cricoid cartilage. A short transverse skin incision should be made, and the knife blade should be inserted directly through the membrane into the airway (A). The knife handle should then be inserted through the hole and twisted 90 degrees to widen the aperture (B and C). An indwelling tube is then inserted (D). (A–D, From Blaisdell, F. W., and Trunkey, D. D.: Trauma Management. Vol. III. Cervicothoracic Trauma. New York, Thieme, 1986.)

ranged physiology. The most severely injured of these patients have no blood pressure, pulse, or spontaneous respiration. The prognosis for such patients is poor, but some can be successfully resuscitated. Because closed-chest cardiopulmonary resuscitation is ineffective in hypovolemic patients, it makes sense to perform emergency thoracotomy if resuscitation is to be attempted. Emergency thoracotomy is also diagnostic in that entry into one or both pleural cavities may disclose a life-threatening injury amenable to temporizing treatment in the emergency setting (Bodai et al., 1983).

Prognosis for trauma patients without vital signs relates to two factors: mechanism of injury and length of time without vital signs (Attar et al., 1991; Baker et al., 1980; Bodai et al., 1982; Boyd et al., 1992; Esposito et al., 1991; Ivatury et al., 1991a). Blunt trauma victims have a negligible survival rate, and emergency department thoracotomy is rarely indicated. Patients with penetrating trauma to the abdomen fare only slightly better, with a survival rate of approximately 5%. The best prognosis is for patients with penetrating chest injuries, who survive approximately 25% of the time. Because it is difficult in the initial emergency department evaluation to determine exactly which parts of the body have been violated by a penetrating injury, no distinction should be made between penetrating injuries to the chest and penetrating injuries to the abdomen.

The other important factor in determining outcome from emergency thoracotomy is the length of time without vital signs (Durham et al., 1992; Ivatury et al., 1991a; Lorenz et al., 1992). Patients who do not have vital signs when emergency field personnel arrive have a poor prognosis; those who lose their vital signs while under observation by medical personnel do better. Arbitrary lengths of time without vital signs have been proposed as cutoffs beyond which no further interventions should be undertaken. Prehospital information is sometimes unreliable, however, and should not be used in making decisions about emergency department thoracotomy.

In blunt trauma victims, the patient should be placed immediately on a cardiac monitor. If there is minimal cardiac activity, nothing further should be done. Patients with penetrating thoracic injury should undergo thoracotomy. If, when the chest is opened, there is no apparent thoracic visceral injury and no response to open cardiac massage, clamping of the aorta, and control of external bleeding, resuscitation should be stopped. If the patient responds to these measures, resuscitation should be continued, and the patient should be taken to the operating room for definitive control of bleeding. Some injuries, such as large-caliber gunshot wounds with multiple cardiac holes or multiple chamber involvement, are obviously hopeless, and resuscitation efforts should be brief.

Emergency thoracotomy incisions should be anterolateral, with the patient in a supine position. This maintains access to the abdomen and does not require repositioning of the patient. The incision should be in the fourth or fifth intercostal space and should be large, from the sternum to the surface of the gurney (Fig. 14–3). There should be minimal concern about incisional bleeding, even from named arteries such as the internal mammary; bleeding from the incision is minimal in patients without a blood pressure, and the top priority is rapid access to the chest. The thoracotomy should be done on the side of penetrating injury to optimize access to any easily controllable injuries that might be found. If the patient does not immediately respond to emergency department thoracotomy, the contralateral pleural space should be decompressed, either with a chest tube or by pushing a finger through the contralateral pleura via the thoracotomy incision.

The pericardium should always be opened. Grasping the pericardium in a patient with tamponade is difficult; in such circumstances, the most expedient way to relieve the tamponade is to make an initial hole in the pericardium with scissors or the tip of a knife blade. After the tamponade has been partially relieved, it is possible to enlarge the opening with scissors. Cross-clamping of the aorta in the chest first requires incision of the overlying pleura. For immediate control before this is done, the aorta can be compressed against the underlying vertebral column and ribs.

BLUNT TRAUMA

Chest Wall Injury

Blunt chest wall injury is the most common form of thoracic trauma (Beeson and Spegesser, 1983; Newman and Jones, 1984). The chest wall, consisting of the ribs, sternum, clavicles, and scapulae, is designed to protect the underlying viscera, but in some patients serious intrathoracic injuries are present even in the absence of obvious chest wall injury. This is particularly likely in children and young adults, because they have very pliable and compressible chest walls that can deform significantly without inducing breaks in any of the bony elements.

Rib fractures are the most common form of chest wall injury (Beeson and Spegesser, 1983; LoCicero and Mattox, 1989; Newman and Jones, 1984). Rib fracture is a clinical rather than a radiographic diagnosis, and the important diagnostic findings are pain with respiration and tenderness on palpation. The pain and tenderness are usually well localized to the area of injury, and a rib fracture should be assumed in the presence of such findings even if there is no fracture visible on the film. Many of the fractures are linear and are easily missed by standard chest films. Such fractures are seen on specialized views of individual ribs, but obtaining such views serves little diagnostic or therapeutic purpose. Fractures that *are* visible on the chest film, however, are relatively severe and may be associated with chest wall instability, longer healing times, and more profound and lasting chest wall pain. Rib fractures can also be diagnosed by the presence of crepitus or deformity at the fracture site.

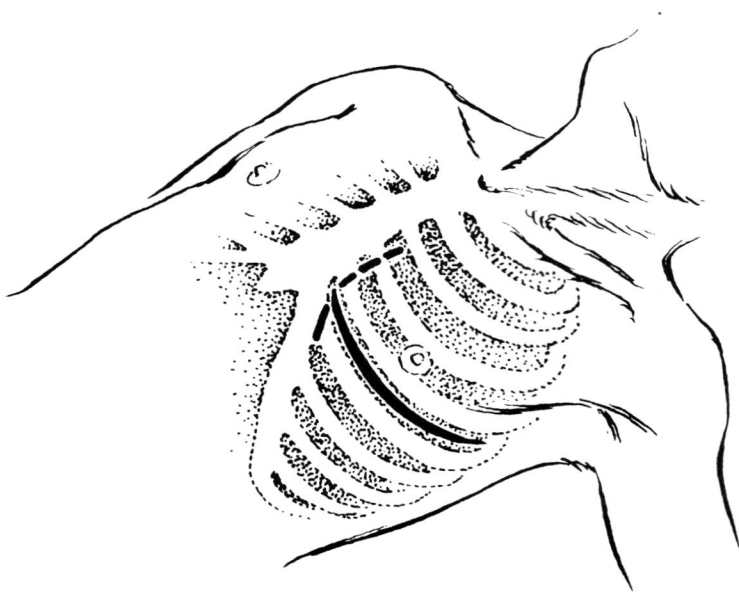

FIGURE 14–3. Emergency thoracotomies should be done in the fourth or fifth intercostal space with the patient supine. The costal cartilages superior to the medial portion of the incision can be cut to improve exposure. The incision can also be extended to the other side of the chest if necessary. (From Blaisdell, F. W., and Trunkey, D. D.: Trauma Management. Vol. III. Cervicothoracic Trauma. New York, Thieme, 1986.)

Along with a chest film, this may be the only means of making the diagnosis in patients with altered mental status.

Blood loss also occurs from rib fractures. The amount varies, but bleeding from the fracture site and adjacent intercostal vessels can be as much as 100 to 150 ml per rib. The blood sometimes leaks through injured parietal pleura into the pleural space as a hemothorax or can remain in the subpleural space between the parietal pleura and the chest wall if the pleura remains intact.

Sternal fractures are most common in drivers of motor vehicles in whom the anterior chest hits the steering wheel during sudden deceleration. As with rib fractures, the diagnosis is best made clinically. There is often ecchymosis overlying the sternum, and the degree of injury runs the spectrum from mildly painful sternal contusion to a severely displaced fracture. As with rib fractures, the emphasis of treatment is pain control. Anterior mediastinal bleeding is associated with fractures of the sternum and can look like a wide mediastinum on an anteroposterior chest film, suggesting the possibility of a torn thoracic aorta.

Fractures of the clavicle are relatively common and are usually treated with temporary immobilization of the arm and observation. Most of these injuries heal well with time, although on occasion there is a cosmetic deformity at the site of the fracture. Rarely, dislocation of the sternoclavicular joint compresses the underlying vasculature in the superior mediastinum. These cases are best treated with relocation or resection of the medial portion of the clavicle. Scapular fractures usually are treated conservatively unless the articular surface with the humerus is involved. Such fractures, however, are a marker for significant force applied to the chest wall.

The primary focus of treatment for all forms of chest wall trauma is relief of pain and clearance of pulmonary secretions. Persistent pain leads to atelectasis and hypoventilation, predisposing the patient to

pneumonia. If it is extreme, untreated chest wall pain causes hypoxemia, hypoventilation, carbon dioxide narcosis, and even respiratory arrest. This is particularly likely to occur in elderly patients with multiple rib fractures (Shorr et al., 1989; Wisner, 1990).

There are a variety of approaches to controlling pain in patients with chest wall trauma. Patients with trivial injuries may not require any pain medication at all, or a nonsteroidal anti-inflammatory agent may suffice. Orally administered narcotics may be adequate in young patients with relatively minor injuries; such patients sometimes may be treated as outpatients. There should be low threshold for admission in older patients, however, and they should generally be treated with parenterally administered analgesia. Parenterally administered medications, besides relieving pain, also cause respiratory depression. Their use requires careful titration of enough medication to control pain without undue inhibition of respiratory drive. *Patient-controlled analgesia* (PCA) devices that allow the patient, within limits, to administer his own analgesia are valuable. When properly managed, PCAs allow adequate pain relief with minimal respiratory depression and prevent intermittent periods of inadequate pain relief.

Intercostal nerve blocks are another approach to analgesia for chest wall injury (Engberg, 1978). An advantage of intercostal blocks is that they are locally administered and provide pain relief without associated respiratory depression. There are many disadvantages, however (Pederson et al., 1983; Wisner, 1990). The degree to which the blocks relieve pain depends on the experience of the person who administers them. There are associated complications, such as intravascular injection of the anesthetic agent or creation of a pneumothorax. Probably the most important disadvantage of intercostal procedures is that the injections must be repeated frequently. If this is difficult, the patient experiences pain while waiting. Avoiding episodic loss of adequate analgesia is critically important in providing effective pain relief and improving outcome from injury (Mackersie et al., 1987; Wisner, 1990).

Epidural analgesia is another alternative in managing chest wall pain (Johnston and McCaughey, 1980; Wisner, 1990; Worthley, 1985). In skilled hands, epidural catheters can be placed safely, are effective in controlling pain without causing associated respiratory depression, and can reduce morbidity and mortality. Delayed respiratory depression due to slow cephalad migration of the analgesic into a central location, where it affects the respiratory drive, is a concern with epidural analgesia. This complication can be minimized by placement of epidural catheters in a lumbar rather than a thoracic location. In most instances, particularly in patients with chest wall trauma to the mid or lower chest, a lumbar approach is effective. Another means of minimizing delayed respiratory depression is the use of analgesics such as fentanyl, which have a short half-life and therefore cannot migrate cephalad (Mackersie et al., 1987).

Epidural catheters are not without complications. Although rare, epidural hematomas and infections occur. Some patients develop pruritus or ileus. Urinary retention, especially in elderly males with prostatic disease, is also a possibility, so a urinary catheter should be left in place until the epidurally administered analgesic has been discontinued.

Severe chest wall injury can create chest wall instability, or "flail chest." In flail chest, a free-floating segment of the chest wall moves paradoxically with spontaneous respiration (Fig. 14–4). When the patient inspires and the intrapleural pressure decreases, the paradoxical segment retracts instead of expanding with the rest of the chest wall. When the patient exhales, the paradoxical segment "balloons" out in the opposite direction from the rest of the chest wall. Flail segments can occur either laterally or anteriorly. The posterior chest wall is relatively protected from this type of injury by the presence of the vertebral column and strong surrounding musculature. Production of a lateral flail segment requires multiple breaks in multiple ribs in order to create a free-floating segment. Anteriorly, a sternal flail segment can be produced by bilateral disruption of multiple costochondral junctions.

Disruption of the mechanics of chest wall function is a minor contributor to the morbidity of a flail chest. A more likely explanation for the significant morbidity associated with flail chest is contusion of

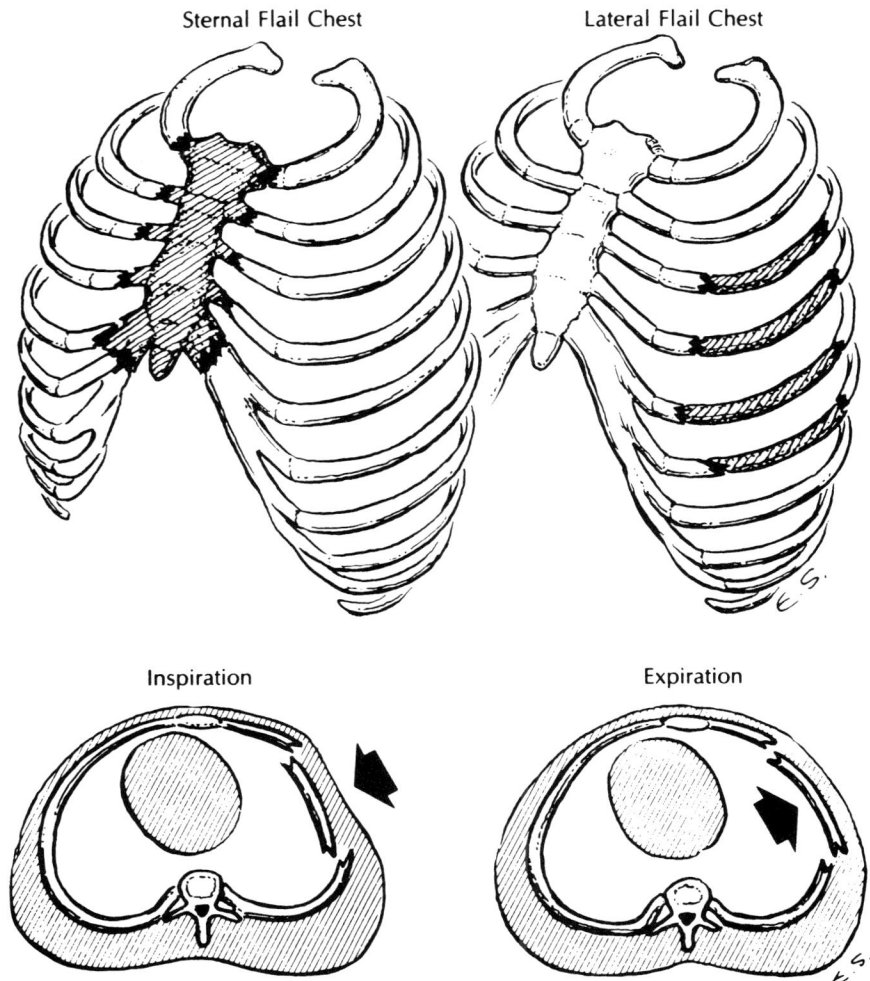

FIGURE 14–4. Flail chest can occur either anteriorly or laterally. Anteriorly, there is disruption of multiple costal cartilages, and the sternum is the free-floating segment. Laterally, there are multiple breaks of multiple ribs. Paradoxical motion of the free-floating segment of the chest wall is seen with spontaneous respiration. (From Blaisdell, F. W., and Trunkey, D. D.: Trauma Management. Vol. III. Cervicothoracic Trauma. New York, Thieme, 1986.)

Sternal Flail Chest

Lateral Flail Chest

Inspiration

Expiration

the underlying lung parenchyma, which produces arteriovenous shunting and hypoxemia (Duff et al., 1968; Maloney et al., 1961; Roscher and Bittner, 1974). Another contributing factor is the pain associated with chest wall trauma, likely to be severe in patients with enough chest wall trauma to produce a flail segment. Severe chest wall pain results in hypoventilation and carbon dioxide retention. The combination of pulmonary contusion and chest wall pain therefore leads to derangements in both oxygenation and ventilation (Parham et al., 1978; Sankaran et al., 1970).

Adequate pain control for patients with flail chest is critical. Epidural catheters are ideal for this purpose because there is minimal associated respiratory depression. Avoiding atelectasis with incentive spirometry and mobilization is also important. In some patients with flail chest, these measures successfully forestall the need for mechanical ventilation. In others, intubation and positive pressure ventilation are necessary to treat hypoxemia, hypoventilation, or both. The approach to initial ventilation of such patients is to rest them on the ventilator by providing complete ventilatory support. After the patient has been ventilated for 4 to 5 days, other modes of ventilation more conducive to weaning can be used.

Pneumothorax

Pneumothorax, like chest wall injury, is a common sequela of blunt thoracic injury. Because the intrapleural pressure is normally negative during inspiration, any communication with atmospheric pressure causes accumulation of air in the pleural space. Communications can occur through either the chest wall or the lung.

Communication with air at atmospheric pressure through a hole in the chest wall is less common than communication by way of a hole in the lung. When a patient has a persistent hole in the chest wall, air is drawn in through the "sucking" chest wound when the patient inspires (Fig. 14–5). Such wounds are rare. When they do occur, they are most commonly associated with blast injuries, severe avulsion injuries, or close-range shotgun wounds (Bender and Lucas, 1990). Sucking chest wounds can be emergently treated by covering them with an occlusive dressing, which prevents further ingress of air from the outside. Because the presence of an underlying lung injury is likely and pneumothorax or hemopneumothorax may develop, a tube thoracostomy should also be done. Definitive treatment is usually relatively simple and involves either surgical closure or continued application of an occlusive dressing until the wound heals. In severe cases, complex closures may ultimately be required, but initial closure can usually be obtained by mobilizing surrounding skin and subcutaneous tissue (Bender and Lucas, 1990). Patients with extremely large defects of the chest wall that might be difficult to close usually do not survive to reach the hospital.

Pneumothoraces in which air enters the pleural

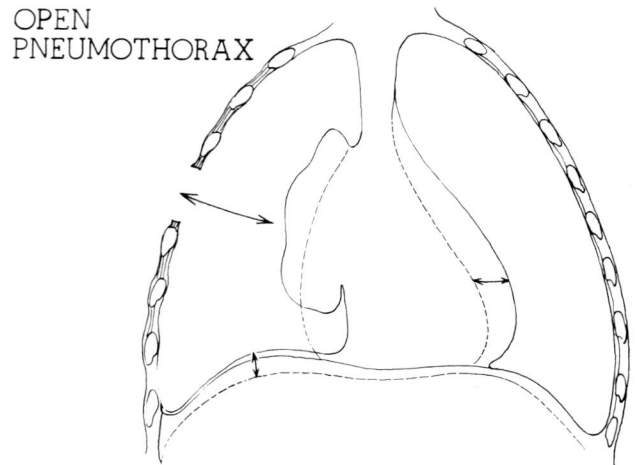

FIGURE 14–5. Pathophysiology of open pneumothorax. The lung on the ipsilateral side collapses, and respiration is ineffectual until the defect is covered or repaired.

cavity via a hole in the lungs are common. The lungs are often injured on their surface by fragments of broken ribs. Compression of the chest, especially against a closed glottis, can lead to a "blowout" of the lung. In either of these circumstances, a communication is formed between the airways and the pleural space, and air pulled into the pleural space forms a pneumothorax. Increased pressure in the pleural space collapses the lung. As the lung collapses, the hole on its surface decreases in size and ultimately closes. When the patient inspires, the hole in the lung surface reopens as the lung expands, but with expiration the hole again closes. As pressure in the pleural space increases, the hole in the pulmonary surface is less and less likely to open with inspiratory effort. In most cases, the lung collapses to the point at which intrapleural air no longer accumulates with inspiration, and the pneumothorax is stable.

Sometimes, however, air continues to accumulate in the pleural space with each inspiratory effort. The fact that the hole opens with inspiration and closes with expiration produces a valve-like mechanism that causes the pneumothorax to increase in size with each respiratory cycle and produces a tension pneumothorax. Although tension pneumothorax is possible during spontaneous ventilation, it is more common when a patient is on positive pressure ventilation, because a constant tidal volume is delivered despite increasing intrapleural pressures. Accordingly, when a patient deteriorates hemodynamically with the institution of positive pressure ventilation, the possibility of a tension pneumothorax should be considered.

If the pressure in the pleural space with tension pneumothorax becomes high enough, both respiration and hemodynamics are impaired. High intrapleural pressures on the side of injury minimize effective expansion of the lungs. As the pressure in the ipsilateral pleural cavity increases, the heart is pushed toward the other side of the chest, venous return is compromised, and cardiac output decreases (Fig. 14–6). This pathophysiology is easily and quickly reversed with decompression of the pneumothorax.

Some of the physical findings associated with tension pneumothorax are the same as those seen with any pneumothorax, but may be more pronounced. There are no breath sounds on the injured side, and subcutaneous air may develop. The trachea may be deviated away from the side of the injury. Shock may also be present and, because there is interference with venous return to the right atrium, neck veins may be distended. Distention of the neck veins is not a particularly sensitive sign, however, because it is not necessarily present in patients who are also hypovolemic.

Almost all pneumothoraces from blunt mechanisms of injury should be treated with a chest tube, particularly sucking chest wounds and pneumothoraces in patients who are also being treated with positive pressure ventilation. There are occasional small pneumothoraces that can be followed with serial chest films and do not necessarily require an emergent chest tube if minimal dead space appears in the pleural cavity. Chest films are two-dimensional studies, however, and there is a tendency to underestimate the size of what appear to be "rim" pneumothoraces (Fig. 14–7). The presence of dead space and fluid in the chest are a potent combination for the development of empyema. In addition, some element of lung function may be permanently lost if the lung is not re-expanded. For these reasons, a low threshold for tube thoracostomy should be maintained.

In many patients, CT of the abdomen after blunt trauma has discovered pneumothoraces visible on

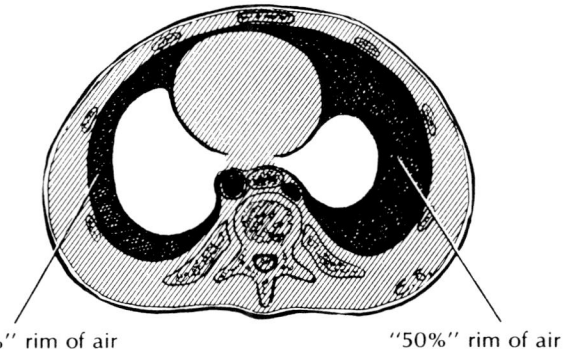

"10%" rim of air "50%" rim of air

FIGURE 14–7. A cross-section of the chest depicts the large amount of lung volume lost even with pneumothoraces that appear small on a two-dimensional radiographic view of the chest. Small rim pneumothoraces on the chest film that measure only 10% in two dimensions actually result in a loss of approximately 50% of lung volume. A "50%" pneumothorax on chest film corresponds to a 90% loss of lung volume. (From Blaisdell, F. W., and Trunkey, D. D.: Trauma Management. Vol. III. Cervicothoracic Trauma. New York, Thieme, 1986.)

the upper cuts of the abdominal CT scan that were not visible on chest film (Nelson et al., 1992; Wing et al., 1985). Most of these patients do well without placement of a chest tube. The presence of a pneumothorax on CT scanning, however, should prompt serial repeat films of the chest to ensure that the pneumothorax does not increase in size (Garramone et al., 1991).

Tube thoracostomy for traumatic pneumothorax should generally be placed in the fourth or fifth intercostal space in the midaxillary line (Fig. 14–8). Tubes should be large enough (at least No. 32 French) to adequately drain any associated hemothorax. An open technique should be used, and trocars should be avoided. This is particularly important in the injured patient, because the hemidiaphragm is sometimes quite high in the lower chest, or it may be ruptured with abdominal viscera in the pleural cavity. The tube should be placed only after a finger has been inserted into the chest. In truly emergent settings, a generous skin incision should be made and, to save time, the tube should not be tunneled.

Data conflict about whether patients with chest tubes placed for trauma should routinely receive antibiotics. The argument for antibiotic coverage of common skin pathogens is that it prevents empyema. The argument against routine antibiotic coverage is that it produces resistant organisms and does not prevent empyema. Although there is no consensus on this issue, there is some evidence that prophylactic antibiotics are of benefit (Fallon and Wears, 1992; LoCicero and Mattox, 1989; LoCurto et al., 1986).

Hemothorax

Like pneumothorax, hemothorax is a common finding after blunt chest trauma; not surprisingly, the two are often found together. Physical findings are

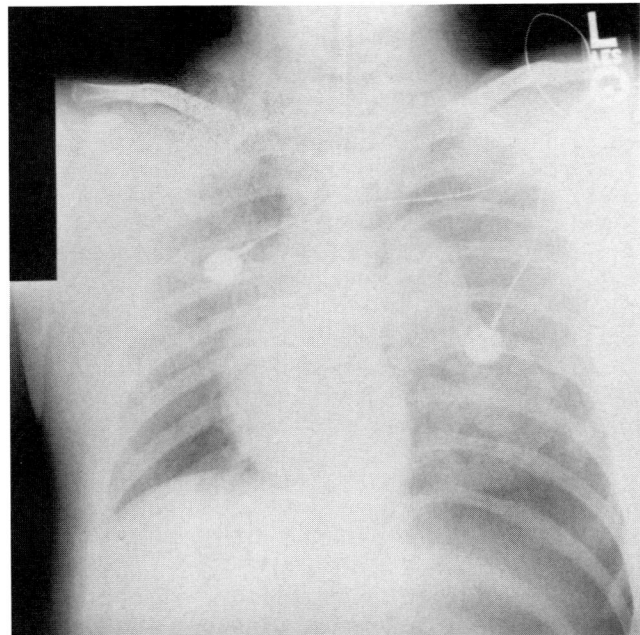

FIGURE 14–6. An example of tension pneumothorax. The left lung is collapsed, and the heart is shifted to the contralateral side of the chest. Venous return is compromised.

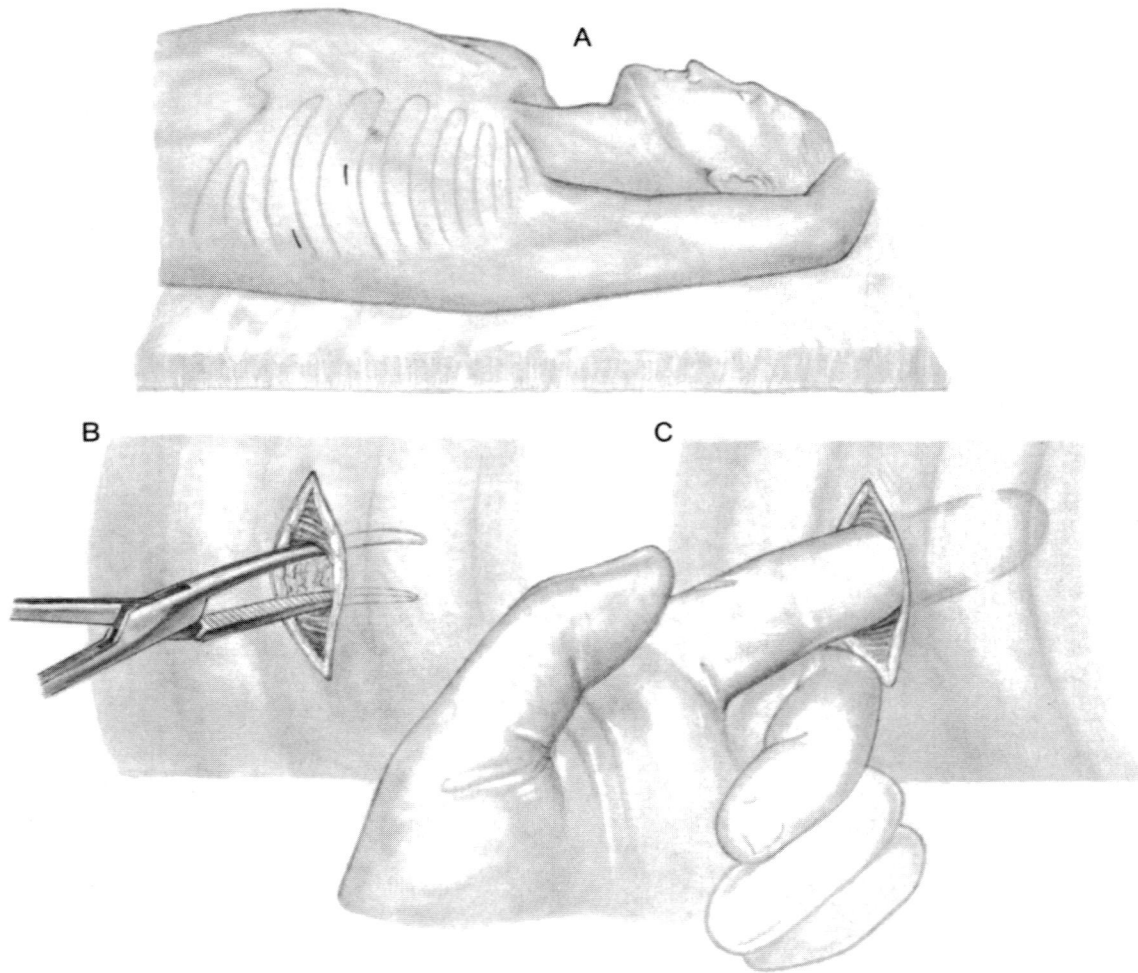

FIGURE 14–8. Chest tube insertion. *A,* Two sites for chest tube insertion. The upper site is in the anterior axillary line in the fourth interspace and is the site preferred for pneumothorax. The lower site is in the fifth or sixth interspace in the posterior axillary line. This site can be used for drainage of a hemothorax. *B,* After a skin incision has been made, a clamp should be used to enlarge the wound, separate the musculature, and penetrate the pleural space. *C,* A finger should always be placed through the hole into the pleural space prior to placement of the chest tube. (*A–C,* From Hood, R. M.: Techniques in General Thoracic Surgery. Philadelphia, W. B. Saunders, 1985.)

not very sensitive for the presence of hemothorax except in cases of massive intrapleural blood; the diagnosis is usually radiographic. Hemothoraces of 500 to 1000 ml can be missed on the admission chest film, particularly if the film is taken with the patient in the supine position. Blood in the chest does not layer out at the base of the pleural cavity, as it would on an upright film, and a fluid level is not necessarily seen. In some cases, even those with massive hemothorax, findings on the admission chest film may be subtle. If the hemothorax is partially clotted, as is often the case, it may look flocculent.

As with pneumothorax, small traumatic hemothoraces are sometimes missed on a chest film and are seen later on the upper cuts of a computerized tomographic study of the abdomen (Nelson et al., 1992; Wing et al., 1985) (Fig. 14–9). Some of these patients can be treated without chest drainage. A very low threshold should be maintained for placement of a chest tube in such circumstances, however, because persistent blood in the chest increases the risk of

empyema and loss of lung function. Delay in placement of a chest tube allows the blood to clot and consolidate so that later attempts at drainage are more difficult.

Initial treatment of hemothorax should be with tube thoracostomy. In emergent circumstances, the tube should be placed via the fourth or fifth intercostal space. In more elective circumstances, the tube can be placed via the sixth intercostal space in the posterior axillary line for better access to the sulcus. A right-angle chest tube directed toward the sulcus is ideal, but, because blood accumulates posteriorly rather than interiorly if the patient is supine, a straight tube directed toward the apex, as for pneumothorax, may suffice. Regardless of whether a straight or a right-angle tube is used, it should be large caliber (No. 32 to No. 36 French) to ensure optimal drainage of partially clotted blood and liquefying clot.

Early placement of a tube thoracostomy can help greatly in the drainage of blood from the pleural cavity, but the natural tendency is for the blood to

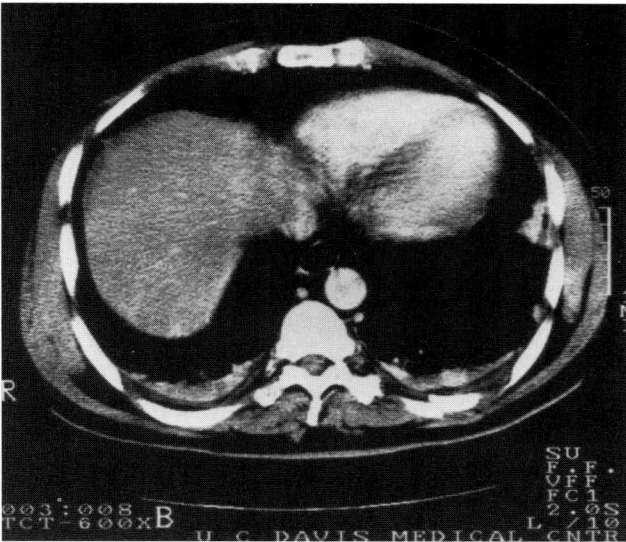

FIGURE 14–9. An example of small bilateral hemothoraces seen on the upper cuts of an abdominal computed tomography scan of a blunt trauma patient. Neither hemothorax was visible on chest film. Some of these hemothoraces can be treated expectantly.

clot. Small amounts of residual hemothorax on a chest film taken shortly after placement of a chest tube is therefore fairly common. In most instances, this blood liquifies over the next several days and drains via the tube. Sometimes, however, the clot persists and organizes in the chest. One course of action in such circumstances is to accept the residual organizing clot, remove the chest tube, and follow the patient. This is an acceptable management plan in patients with small residual hemothoraces (Condon, 1968; Coselli et al., 1984). In cases of larger residual hemothoraces, however, expectant management greatly increases the risk of empyema (Arom et al., 1977).

When drainage from the tube is minimal and the radiographic findings demonstrate persistent hemothorax, continued attempts at drainage are rarely successful because of the semisolid nature of the organizing clot. Definitive treatment of significant hemothorax that persists beyond several days involves a limited thoracotomy, evacuation of the clot, removal of whatever organized peel has developed on the pleural surfaces, and placement of new thoracostomy tubes. The thoracotomy should not be delayed unduly, because as the hemothorax continues to organize it becomes increasingly difficult to remove. Thoracotomy as early as 2 to 3 days after trauma is advisable in cases of large persistent hemothoraces in which further attempts at thoracostomy drainage are obviously futile.

Thoracoscopy is a new alternative to thoracotomy for residual hemothorax. Experience with this approach is limited but shows promise. The scope is placed in the chest and blood is removed by a combination of suction, irrigation, and instillation of lytic agents. Timing of thoracoscopy for residual hemothorax is probably important. When done immediately after the trauma, it is unlikely to succeed because of

difficulties with ongoing bleeding. Delaying thoracoscopy beyond several days may also decrease the chances of success. Because it is more difficult to remove peel and organized clot from the chest thoracoscopically than with an open technique, it is important to do the procedure before the hemothorax becomes too organized. The low morbidity rate of thoracoscopy as opposed to thoracotomy permits a low threshold for the procedure and makes a strong argument for early intervention before a prolonged trial of tube thoracostomy drainage has run its course. Further experience with thoracoscopy for the treatment of residual hemothorax is necessary to better define timing and technique, but its role may grow in the treatment of this problem.

Pulmonary Contusion

Some of the damage in a contused lung is the result of disruption of the vasculature and hemorrhage into the pulmonary parenchyma. In other areas, injury is more subtle, with damage to the pulmonary microvasculature but no extravasation of red blood cells. This range of injury is analogous to contusion in other areas of the body. Part of the fluid accumulation associated with contusion is related to hemorrhage, but much of it is due to extravasation of fluid from the intravascular to the extravascular space as a consequence of increased pulmonary microvascular permeability seen with an inflammatory response. Increased permeability promotes diapedesis of inflammatory cells and diffusion of inflammatory mediators necessary to combat infection and begin repair.

In the lungs as well as in other areas of the body, accumulation of edema fluid is a natural consequence of increased permeability. Although edema formation may help with resisting infection and initiating repair, edema can harm organ function. In areas such as skeletal muscle and soft tissue, these functional side effects are of minimal importance. In the lungs, however, interstitial and alveolar edema causes arteriovenous shunting and hypoxemia.

The diagnosis of pulmonary contusion on the basis of radiographic and blood gas findings can be difficult. On chest film, pulmonary contusion appears as patchy areas of pulmonary infiltrate and is usually localized to areas of the lung that underlie obvious chest wall injury. Other entities, such as hemothorax, aspiration, and the presence of subpleural blood associated with rib fractures, can be easily confused with pulmonary contusion. Blood gas analyses, in the presence of an established contusion, are manifested by hypoxemia. The diagnosis is best made by the combination of suspicious radiographic findings and difficulties with oxygenation. Although other entities (e.g., aspiration) can still be confused with contusion when this sort of definition is used, the distinction between the two is largely moot in the emergent setting, because the initial treatment of each is the same.

Because loss of pulmonary capillary membrane integrity is part of the pathogenesis of pulmonary contusion, the amount of pulmonary edema and physiologic derangement may evolve over time, and the degree of abnormality seen on chest film may also increase over the first 24 to 48 hours after injury. It can be difficult to distinguish contusion from adult respiratory distress syndrome or pneumonia. Repeated films and blood gas analyses are important in patients in whom pulmonary contusion is suspected.

Whether patients with pulmonary contusion should receive prophylactic antibiotics is controversial. The evidence that antibiotics help prevent pneumonia is not particularly convincing, and antibiotics should not be given routinely unless aspiration pneumonia is likely. Another contentious issue in the treatment of pulmonary contusion is fluid management (Trinkle et al., 1975; Wisner and Sturm, 1986). It seems logical to administer primarily colloid-containing fluids to maintain intravascular colloid osmotic pressure and discourage movement of fluid from the intravascular to the extravascular space. Colloid administration is sometimes augmented by diuretic agents in an attempt to "dry out" the contused, edematous lung. Unfortunately, damaged pulmonary microvasculature cannot maintain a colloid osmotic gradient, and contusion is not effectively treated by this approach (Fig.

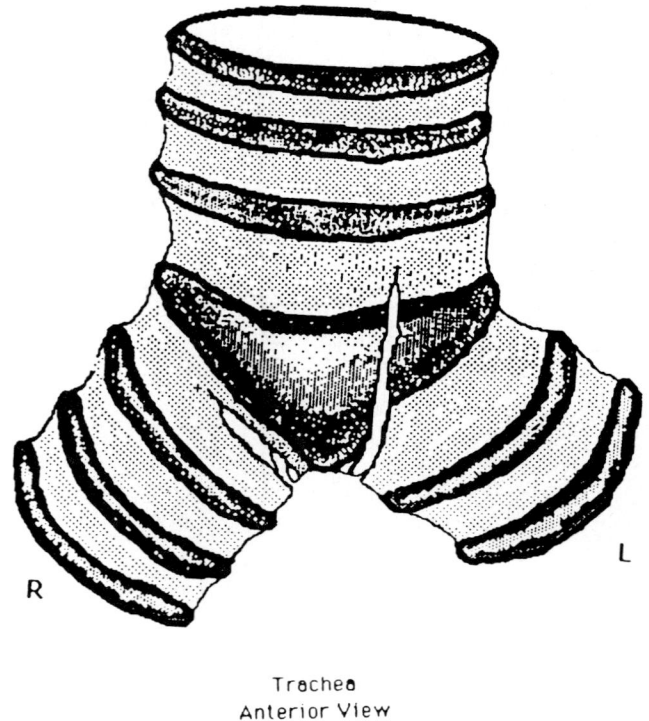

Trachea
Anterior View

FIGURE 14–11. An example of a complex tear of the trachea and mainstem bronchi in a victim of blunt trauma. Most such injuries are located within 2.5 cm of the carina. (From Millham, F. H., Rajii-Khorasani, A., Birkett, D. F., et al.: Carinal injury: Diagnosis and treatment—Case report. J. Trauma, 31:1420, 1991.)

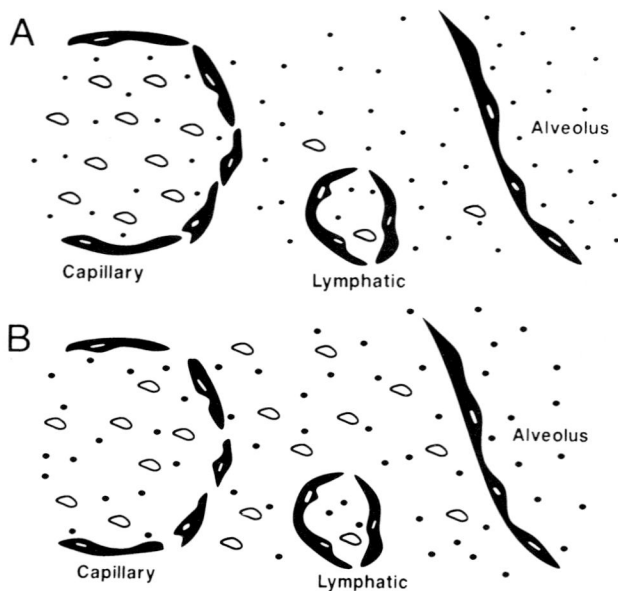

FIGURE 14–10. Comparison of "high-pressure" (A) and "low-pressure" (B) pulmonary edema. In high-pressure pulmonary edema, the capillary endothelial junctions are intact and relatively tight. When intravascular pressure is elevated, water (small dots) crosses from the intravascular space into the interstitium, but albumin and other protein molecules (large circles) leak into the extravascular space to a minimal degree. In low-pressure pulmonary edema, such as that seen in pulmonary contusion, the primary defect is to the vascular endothelium, and both water and colloid leak out into the extravascular space. Administration of colloid solutions is of minimal benefit in the setting of low-pressure pulmonary edema. (A and B, From Wisner, D. H., and Holcroft, J. W.: Surgical critical care. Curr. Probl. Surg., 27:467, 1990.)

14–10). Furthermore, the use of diuretics and overly stringent restriction of fluids in the acutely traumatized patient can compromise intravascular volume and perfusion.

In patients with pulmonary contusion, there should be a low threshold for placement of a pulmonary artery catheter, with close monitoring of filling pressures, cardiac output, and oxygen extraction so that a balance can be maintained between administration of adequate fluid for perfusion and prevention of pulmonary edema from inappropriate volume loading. The type of fluid administered is less important than ensuring adequate perfusion.

Injuries to the Trachea and Major Bronchi

Blunt injuries of the trachea and major bronchi are rare (Flynn et al., 1989; Grover et al., 1979; Symbas et al., 1992). The trachea can be injured anywhere along its course, but the most common locations are the neck and near the carina. Injuries to the major bronchi are usually within 2.5 cm of the carina, and right-sided injuries may be more common than those on the left (Millham et al., 1991) (Fig. 14–11).

In the neck, the pathophysiology of blunt injury to the trachea is a "clothesline" mechanism in which there is sudden and violent tracheal compression. Sometimes there is associated injury to the larynx or esophagus. There are several theories about the mechanism of injury in the chest. One is that the chest is crushed in its anteroposterior dimension, and the lungs, in contact with the parietal pleura of the chest wall, are stretched transversely with disruption at the carina secondary to the stretching mechanism. Another theory is that chest compression against a closed glottis disrupts the airway from increased intraluminal pressure. Because wall tension is directly proportional to the diameter of the airway, it is greatest in the larger airways, in keeping with the empiric observation that most blunt injuries of the thoracic trachea or bronchi occur near the carina. A final theory about the pathogenesis of tears of the thoracic trachea and bronchi is similar to the theory for pathogenesis of tears of the thoracic aorta. According to this theory, the trachea is fixed relative to the lungs. With sudden deceleration, shear forces are generated near the carina that can disrupt the airway.

The diagnosis of blunt injury to the trachea or bronchi is sometimes missed initially because many of the associated findings are nonspecific (Jones et al., 1984). Patients who can communicate often describe dyspnea. If laryngeal injury is present, speech may be altered or impossible. Most patients have subcutaneous emphysema, sometimes quite extensive, but this finding is not invariably present or may not become manifest until after the institution of positive pressure ventilation. On chest film, the presence of pneumomediastinum is a clue to the presence of major airway injury. Pneumomediastinum is common but, like subcutaneous emphysema, is not invariably present. A large pneumothorax is another finding that can aid diagnosis. This is particularly suspicious if the pneumothorax is not relieved by a tube thoracostomy or if there is a massive air leak after chest tube placement. The presence of a round, undeformed endotracheal cuff balloon in an intubated patient is a subtle radiographic finding related to the passage of the endotracheal tube out through the airway defect.

Although the above clinical and radiographic findings suggest a major airway injury, definitive diagnosis should be made with bronchoscopy, if time permits. In some cases, there is no time for bronchoscopy, and emergent thoracotomy is required because of massive air leak and the inability to ventilate the patient. If a major airway injury is suspected at the time of emergent thoracotomy, a right-sided incision should be made to optimize access to the distal trachea and right mainstem bronchus. If, as is often the case, the nature of the life-threatening injuries is initially unclear and a left thoracotomy is first performed, it is necessary to extend the thoracotomy to the right side unless the injury is limited to the left mainstem bronchus. Fortunately, most patients who survive to reach the hospital are stable enough to permit bronchoscopy. Both rigid and fiberoptic bronchoscopy can be used, but the injuries can be missed if the bronchoscopist is not experienced (Baumgartner et al., 1990; Jones et al., 1984).

The first aim of therapy is to stabilize the airway (Symbas et al., 1992). A trial of nonoperative management may be attempted for small injuries that encompass less than one-third of the airway circumference. Short longitudinal tears of a single airway are particularly likely to be managed successfully in this way. Nonoperative management should not be attempted, even if the injury is less than one-third the circumference of the airway, if the air leak is massive and ventilation is difficult. If nonoperative treatment is attempted, ventilator management should be designed to minimize airway pressures. Results with high-frequency ventilation have been mixed (Carlson et al., 1980; MacIntyre, 1988).

Injuries to the cervical trachea should be approached via a transverse neck incision. Tears to the thoracic trachea and major bronchi can be transverse or longitudinal, simple or complex. If the injury is to the distal trachea or right mainstem bronchus, it should be approached via a right thoracotomy. If the injury is limited to the left mainstem bronchus, a left posterolateral thoracotomy should be used. Intubation should be cautious and should take into account the location of the injuries seen on bronchoscopy. If there is injury to only one mainstem bronchus, the endotracheal tube should be positioned in the contralateral mainstem bronchus to allow for ventilation of the patient while the injured side is repaired. Sometimes it is necessary to manipulate placement of the distal end of the endotracheal tube under direct vision after the chest has been opened and the airway has been visualized. Relatively simple repair techniques suffice in most patients, but some patients with complex injuries involving the carina or both mainstem bronchi can only be safely controlled and repaired with cardiopulmonary bypass (Symbas et al., 1992).

Major airway injuries generally should be closed with interrupted sutures, but a running suture can be used for longitudinal tears. Although the choice of suture is variable, there is some evidence that absorbable suture reduces the development of granulation tissue and subsequent stricture (Gibbons et al., 1981; Urschel and Razzuk, 1973). After closure of the airway defect, the endotracheal tube should be positioned so that the cuff of the tube does not press against the repair. Whenever possible, a tissue flap of pleura, pericardium, or muscle should be placed over the suture line. Postoperative ventilator management should minimize airway pressures.

Great Vessels

Blunt trauma can injure the aorta or the branches of the aortic arch. Approximately 95% of patients with blunt tears of the thoracic aorta die before reaching the hospital (Feczko et al., 1992). In the small percentage who survive the initial postinjury period, bleeding is tamponaded in the periaortic and other mediastinal tissues (Parmley et al., 1958; Pickard et al., 1977).

Pseudoaneurysms of the innominate, common carotid, and subclavian arteries are rare and probably are related to a stretch mechanism of injury. One of the more common of these injuries is disruption of a vessel at its origin from the aorta (Fig. 14–12). The

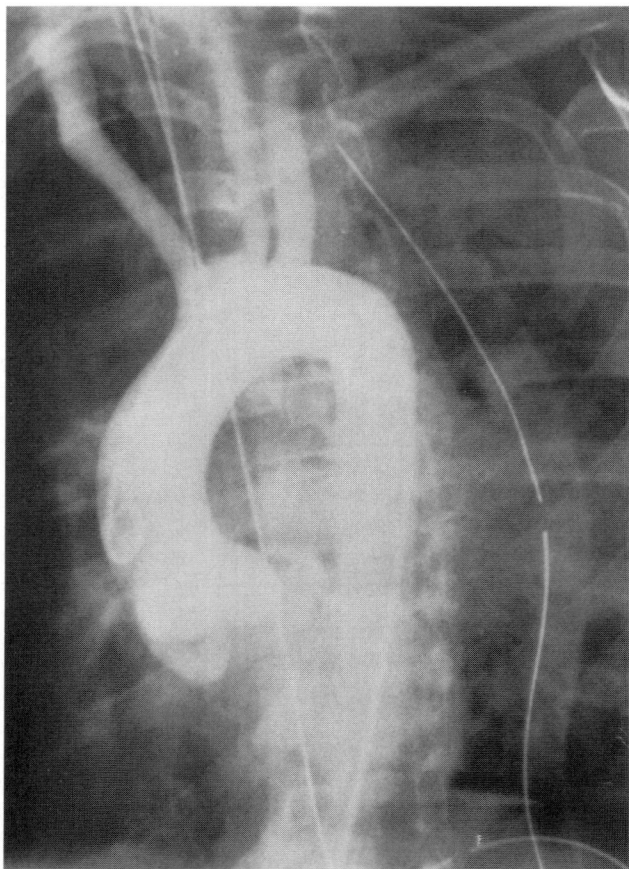

FIGURE 14–12. Angiogram demonstrating a pseudoaneurysm secondary to blunt trauma involving the origin of the innominate and left common carotid arteries. The patient also had a pseudoaneurysm of the origin of the left subclavian artery not seen on preoperative angiography and discovered at surgery. There were also pseudoaneurysms of the left internal mammary artery and of the origin of the left vertebral artery and left thyrocervical trunk (not shown). (From Gubler, K. D., Wisner, D. H., and Blaisdell, F. W.: Multiple vessel injury to branches of the aortic arch: Case report. J. Trauma, 31:1566, 1991.)

pression and spasm of that artery. The result on physical examination is a diminished blood pressure in the left arm as compared with the right. Similar pathophysiology of the descending aorta can lead to differential pulses and blood pressures in the lower as compared with the upper extremities. Both of these blood pressure findings are uncommon and occasionally occur in the absence of a thoracic aortic tear.

Findings on a chest film are somewhat more helpful than the physical examination in patients with a torn thoracic aorta. Some findings are related to the fact that a tear of the thoracic aorta usually causes extravasation of blood into the mediastinum (Gundry et al., 1983; Richardson et al., 1990). There may be a widened superior mediastinum. The definition of "widened" varies, but a superior mediastinal width of more than 8 cm on an anteroposterior view of the chest in an adult is suspicious.

Although a widened superior mediastinum is the most sensitive radiographic finding associated with a torn thoracic aorta, there are some patients in whom there has been minimal extravasation of blood into the mediastinum and in whom the superior mediastinum is not appreciably widened on chest film. A widened superior mediastinum can also be absent in patients with tears of the thoracic aorta at the diaphragm. The finding of a wide mediastinum is also not very specific; only 10 to 20% of patients with this finding have a torn thoracic aorta. Several factors contribute to this low specificity. Mediastinal hematomas can occur in patients in association with sternal trauma or venous bleeding. A poor inspiratory effort can make the superior mediastinum appear artifactually wide. Anteroposterior views and supine positioning also make the superior mediastinum seem wider than normal.

Other possible findings on the admission chest film are less sensitive but more specific than the finding of a widened superior mediastinum (Fig. 14–13). A

thoracic aorta can tear at a variety of locations, including in its ascending portion and at the diaphragm. In patients who survive to reach the hospital, the most common site of disruption is just distal to the origin of the left subclavian artery at the ligamentum arteriosum. This site is the juncture of the mobile aortic arch and immobile descending thoracic aorta, tethered by the intercostal arteries. The aorta is further tethered by the ligamentum arteriosum. In a sudden deceleration, the descending aorta stops with the rest of the body while the heart and aortic arch continue moving forward. Shear force develops at the juncture of these two segments of the aorta, creating a tear (Feczko et al., 1992). Tears range from partial to complete disruption. When partial, the tear usually includes the posteromedial aorta in the vicinity of the ligamentum arteriosum.

In most patients with tears of the thoracic aorta, there are no specific physical findings. Occasionally, blood from the aortic tear dissects distally along the course of the left subclavian artery and causes com-

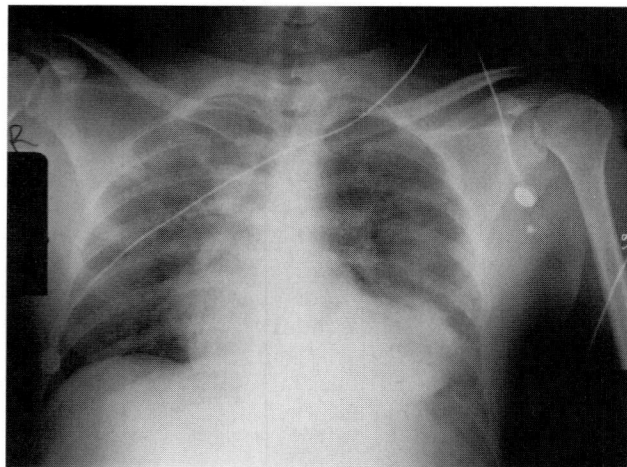

FIGURE 14–13. In addition to a wide superior mediastinum, this patient had some of the secondary findings associated with a torn thoracic aorta. There is a left hemothorax, the trachea is deviated to the right, and the left mainstem bronchus is depressed compared with normal.

mediastinal hematoma in the area of the ligamentum arteriosum can depress the left mainstem bronchus or the trachea to the right, or it can blur the aortic knob. The esophagus is not normally visible on a chest film, but if a nasogastric tube is in place it, too, can be deviated to the right by the hematoma. Mediastinal blood that dissects distally along the course of the left subclavian artery in the subpleural space can create a left apical cap (Fig. 14–14). A left hemothorax is often associated with a torn thoracic aorta but is a very nonspecific finding. Several findings on chest film merely indicate that the degree of force exerted on the chest was extreme enough to have torn the aorta. Not surprisingly, these findings are neither very sensitive nor specific. They include the presence of a first or second rib fracture and the presence of a scapular fracture.

It is sometimes difficult to decide on the basis of an admission chest film which patients require further work-up (Gundry et al., 1983). A reasonable approach is to look first for the presence of a widened superior mediastinum. If this condition is present, the possibility of a torn aorta should be further investigated. If this finding is absent or questionable, further work-up should still be done if there are specific secondary findings such as a depressed mainstem bronchus, deviated trachea, or left apical cap.

If further investigation is warranted, a decision must be made about what imaging procedure should be used. Rapid diagnosis is important, because if the diagnosis is not made and the aorta is not repaired, the tamponaded pseudoaneurysm can rupture and the patient can exsanguinate (Parmley et al., 1958;

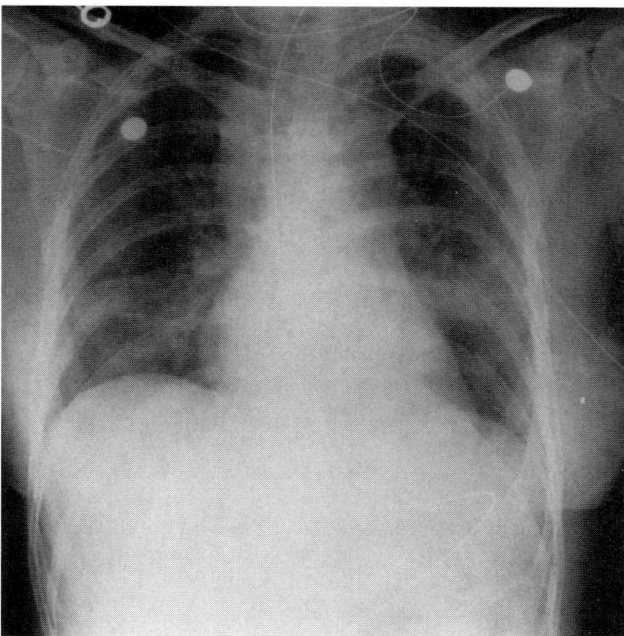

FIGURE 14–14. The superior mediastinum is wide in this chest film of a patient with torn thoracic aorta. In addition, the aortic knob is indistinct, and there is a left apical "cap" secondary to blood in the subpleural space along the course of the left subclavian artery.

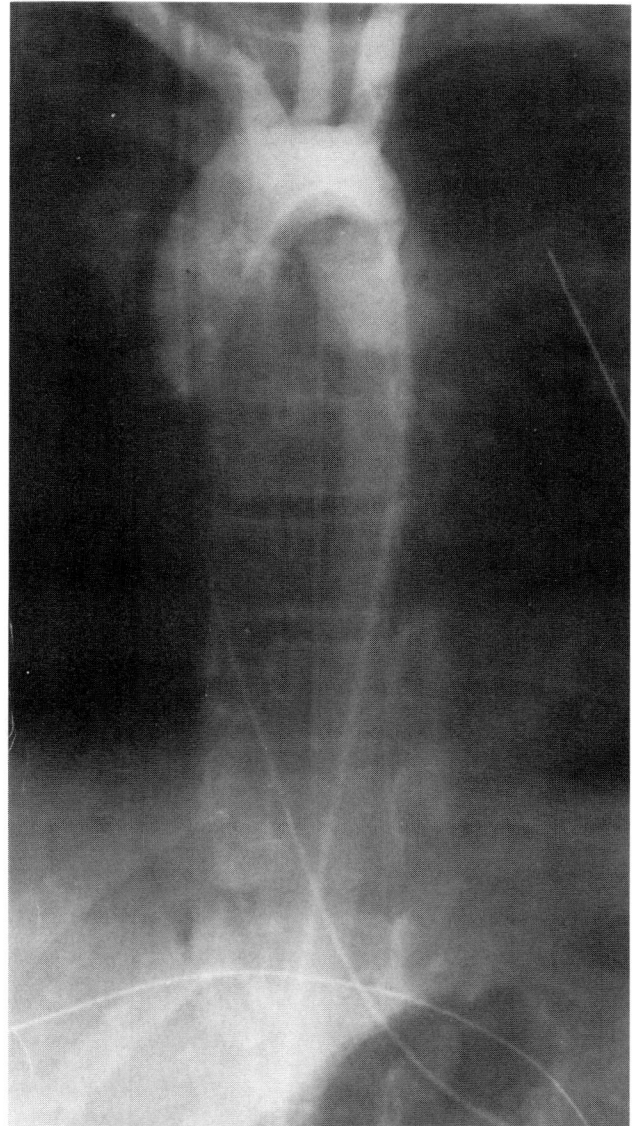

FIGURE 14–15. An angiographic example of torn thoracic aorta. The tear is at the usual location just distal to the origin of the left subclavian artery and is seen as a pseudoaneurysmal widening of the caliber of the aorta.

Pickard et al., 1977). Patients with a suspected torn thoracic aorta should therefore be kept under close observation during diagnostic imaging studies to quickly detect a deterioration in vital signs or increase in chest tube output that might signify rupture into the pleural cavity. If this should occur, further attempts at imaging should be abandoned, and the patient should undergo immediate thoracotomy for both diagnosis and treatment.

Angiography is the commonly accepted approach to the definitive diagnosis of a torn thoracic aorta (Fig. 14–15). The false-positive and false-negative rates for angiography are low. In some patients, however, the aortic injury is quite subtle and will only be detected as a very small intimal tear (Fig. 14–16). In other cases, there is a mild kinking or stenosis of the aorta

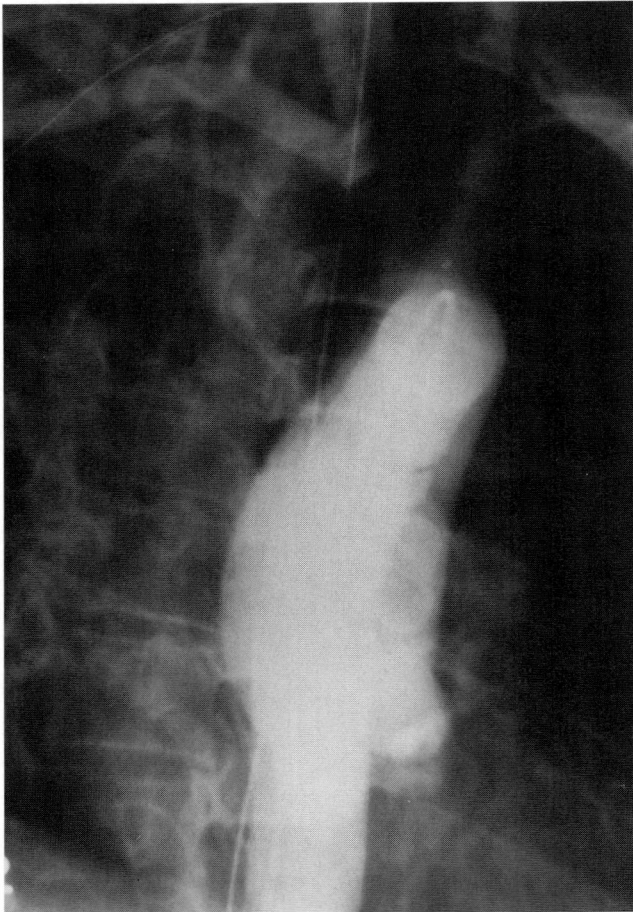

FIGURE 14–16. Some tears of the thoracic aorta are subtle, even on angiography. In this case, the angiogram showed only the intimal tear and flap seen on this single view. At surgery, there was a partial tear of the aorta at the ligamentum arteriosum.

at the site of the ligamentum arteriosum with a resultant poststenotic dilatation that can be mistaken for a pseudoaneurysm (Fig. 14–17).

Aortography is expensive, labor-intensive, and somewhat invasive. When it is done for the indication of a wide mediastinum, the percentage of positive results is low. For these reasons, a less costly, less invasive, and simpler diagnostic imaging study is desirable. CT is one possibility. The advantages of CT as an alternative to angiography are obvious (Agee et al., 1992; Heiberg et al., 1983; Ishikawa et al., 1989). It can be performed more quickly and is less invasive. It is also more likely to be available in many hospitals and is less labor-intensive. There are also potential disadvantages: If the computed tomographic study is not definitive and the patient requires angiography anyway, more contrast agent is necessary and there is a delay in diagnosis. There are also questions about the accuracy of CT; some series have a disturbingly high percentage of false-negative results (Agee et al., 1992; McLean et al., 1991; Miller et al., 1989a). Better results are seen with dynamic contrast-enhanced scans than with other techniques, but there is still inconclusive evidence that computed tomographic

work-up is as sensitive for the diagnosis of thoracic pseudoaneurysms as angiography is.

Although CT should not be used routinely as a screening test in patients with a wide mediastinum, it may have a role for some patients. If the index of suspicion is low and there is a good possibility that a wide mediastinum seen on a chest film is related to radiographic technique, poor inspiratory effort, or patient positioning, CT is appropriate. If a mediastinal hematoma is not seen on the scan, no further work-up is necessary. If a mediastinal hematoma is seen, the patient should undergo angiography (Brooks et al., 1988; Ishikawa et al., 1989).

Because of their propensity for rupture, traumatic pseudoaneurysms of the thoracic aorta should be treated surgically. A major complication of such repairs is the development of paraplegia as a result of spinal cord ischemia during aortic cross-clamping. None of the measures developed to prevent this complication are proven but they make intuitive sense and should be employed if they are available and if time permits (McCroskey et al., 1991; Merrill et al., 1988; Van Norman et al., 1991).

Distal perfusion can be maintained by several methods (Young et al., 1989). One is the placement of a heparin-bonded Gott shunt from the ascending aorta to the femoral artery or the aorta distal to the cross-clamp. Although this technique is relatively simple, it can be cumbersome to work around the shunt during the aortic repair, the shunt can clot, and flow rate through the shunt cannot be adjusted.

Another alternative is the use of femoro-femoral bypass. This is relatively easy to institute and the cannulas do not interfere with the operative field. The bypass cannulas can be placed before dissection around the aorta is begun so that if rapid aortic cross-clamping is necessary, bypass can be instituted immediately. The flow rates through the bypass can be regulated, and minimal heparin is necessary to keep the bypass circuit open. A disadvantage is that the venous cannula may be too small or poorly positioned so that venous outflow is low and distal perfusion is compromised. Another disadvantage is that an oxygenator is required.

Yet another alternative is to use left-sided heart bypass with a centrifugal pump (Grosso et al., 1991; Oliver et al., 1984) (Fig. 14–18). Blood can be drawn from the left atrium, left ventricle, or aortic root. After being sent through the pump, the blood can be reinfused via a femoral artery or the distal thoracic aorta. Advantages of this approach are the assurance of adequate volumes for the inflow cannula, absence of an oxygenator, and the ability to control flow through the bypass circuit. Disadvantages are the need to cannulate the aortic root or left side of the heart and the fact that the tubing is sometimes in the way during the aortic repair.

It is fairly obvious that ischemia may occur with aortic cross-clamping because of lack of arterial inflow. An additional factor can compromise blood supply to the spinal cord. When the aortic cross-clamp is applied, proximal hypertension develops, which leads

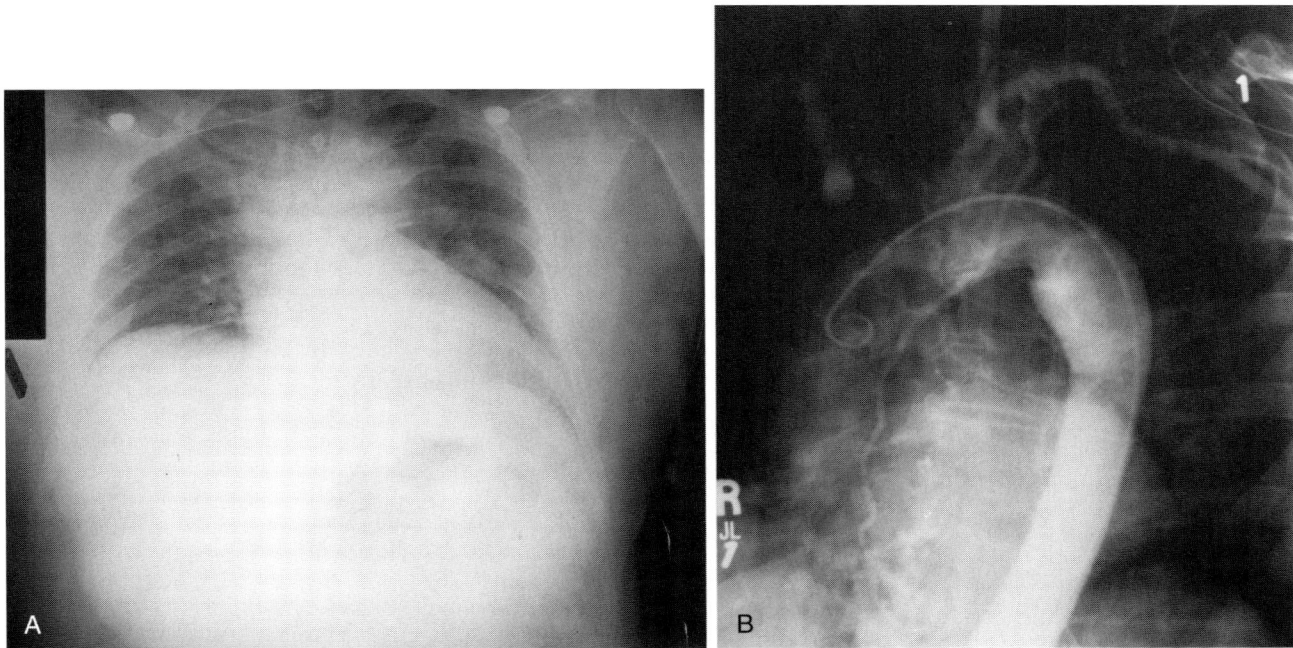

FIGURE 14–17. An example of a false-positive angiogram for torn thoracic aorta. The chest film (*A*) demonstrated a wide mediastinum, and on this basis, an angiogram (*B*) was obtained. The chest film is a good example of the difficulties of interpreting a wide mediastinum in a supine patient with poor inspiratory effort. At surgery, there was no tear of the aorta, and the abnormality seen on angiography was attributed to a mild coarctation of the aorta with poststenotic dilatation.

to increased cerebrospinal fluid pressure. This increased pressure, when transmitted to the spinal cord, may decrease cord perfusion. Use of bypass techniques to shunt blood helps minimize this problem by controlling proximal hypertension. High cerebrospinal fluid pressure can also be treated by placement of a lumbar subarachnoid catheter, which can be used to monitor cerebrospinal fluid pressure and to withdraw fluid as necessary for pressure control.

Thoracic aortic pseudoaneurysms should generally be approached via a left-sided posterolateral thoracotomy, but in emergent cases an anterolateral thoracotomy may already have been done. If the pseudoaneurysm is not actively bleeding and some form of bypass is planned, the thoracotomy incision should be in place so that if aortic cross-clamping is subsequently necessary, bypass can be instituted rapidly. After bypass cannulas are in place, the aorta distal to the pseudoaneurysm should be dissected and encircled with a vessel loop. Proximal control is then obtained, first with dissection and encirclement of the proximal left subclavian artery and then with encirclement of the aorta between the left common carotid and left subclavian arteries. This technique of proximal control is preferred because it gives the best chance of obtaining control without entering the pseudoaneurysm and because there is often a very short cuff between the origin of the left subclavian artery and the tear. Obtaining proximal control is the most difficult part of the operation. The left recurrent laryngeal nerve is in the area of dissection and should be protected.

After proximal and distal control have been ob-

tained, the bypass circuit should be started, the pseudoaneurysm entered, and the free edges of the aorta defined. Most patients require placement of a graft, but in occasional cases of partial tears, a primary repair can be done. If a graft is used, woven Dacron is the graft material of choice.

Perioperative antibiotics covering skin flora are appropriate. If there is a severe associated pulmonary injury with an air leak, the antibiotic course should be longer and broader in spectrum. If hypertension is a problem postoperatively, it should be controlled with beta-blockade rather than peripheral vasodilators. Peripheral dilation has the theoretical disadvantage of increasing the pressure gradient across the anastomosis and thereby increasing rather than decreasing the shear forces across the anastomosis.

Sometimes, patients with a remote history of trauma present with an abnormal routine chest film or with symptoms of compression of the airway, left recurrent laryngeal artery, or left subclavian artery. On work-up, they are found to have a chronic aortic pseudoaneurysm. Surgical repair is indicated as outlined above, even in asymptomatic patients. Repair is more difficult secondary to chronic scarring and inflammation.

Heart

Blunt injuries of the myocardium range from mild asymptomatic contusion to cardiac rupture (Brathwaite et al., 1990; Fulda et al., 1991; Nirgiotis et al.,

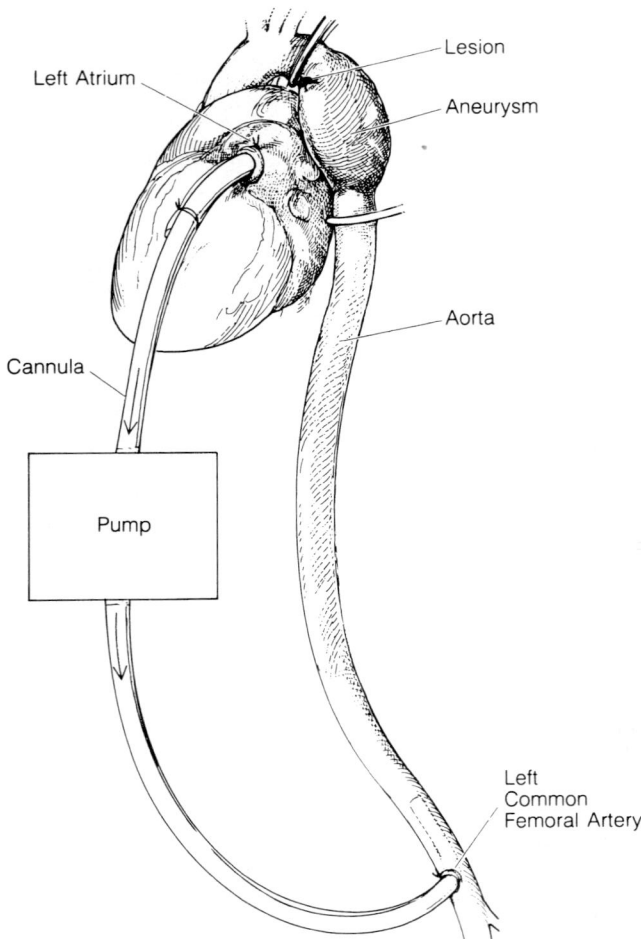

FIGURE 14–18. Left-sided heart bypass used during the repair of a torn thoracic aorta. Cannulas are placed in the left atrium and the left common femoral artery. A centrifugal pump is used to circulate the blood from the heart to the systemic circulation below the aortic cross-clamps necessary for the repair. No oxygenator and minimal heparin are needed. (From Holcroft, J. W., and Blaisdell, F. W.: Trauma to the torso. Scientific American Surgery, Wilmore, D. W., Cheung, L. Y., Harken, A. H., et al. (eds). Section IV, Subsection 1. © 1995 Scientific American, Inc. All rights reserved.)

1990). Nonmyocardial cardiac injuries are also possible. Rupture of the pericardium can occur with or without associated cardiac injury. Laceration or thrombosis of the coronary arteries from blunt trauma is rare but also possible. Diagnosis is best made by electrocardiogram and, if time permits, coronary angiography. Treatment is selective; repair is indicated if ischemia and myocardial dysfunction are severe and there is salvageable myocardium.

Blunt rupture of the heart is not that uncommon, but most patients with such a condition do not survive to reach medical attention. Occasionally, however, bleeding is tamponaded in the pericardial sac, or temporary hemostasis occurs at the site of rupture after hemorrhage has decreased cardiac filling. Most patients present in shock from a combination of hemorrhage and cardiac tamponade (Pevec et al., 1989), but in some patients the admission blood pressure is normal. When an admission chest film is possible, it sometimes reveals a wide cardiac shadow.

The mechanism of injury is probably sudden, severe compression of the chest at the end of diastole. Blunt rupture occurs with equal frequency to all of the cardiac chambers, but injuries to the right atrium are associated with the most favorable prognosis because it is a low-pressure chamber and is relatively easy to access. The prognosis of left atrial and right ventricular injuries is intermediate; survivors of left ventricular injuries are rare.

Blunt cardiac ruptures should be treated surgically. Either sternotomy or thoracotomy can be used, with left-sided thoracotomy the best approach for left-sided lesions, particularly of the left atrium, and sternotomy the best approach for right atrial and right ventricular lesions. Most injuries can be repaired without cardiopulmonary bypass. Ruptures of the atria, particularly at the atrial appendage, can initially be controlled with a vascular clamp (Fig. 14–19). Ruptures of the ventricles sometimes can be temporized by balloon tamponade with a urinary catheter placed through the defect.

Nonabsorbable sutures should be used for repair. The type of suture is less important than the size and type of needle. An atraumatic needle should be used, and it should be big enough to take moderately large bites of the myocardium for approximation but not so large that there are large needle holes after the repair is done. Pledget material should be used to reinforce the repair and to keep the sutures from pulling through the myocardium. The pledget mate-

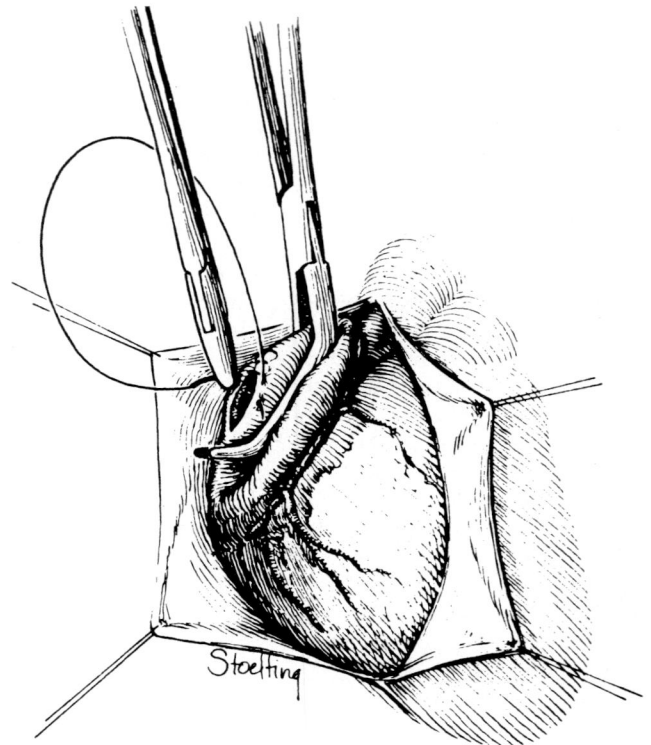

FIGURE 14–19. Control of an atrial tear with a vascular clamp. The tear can then be repaired in a bloodless field. (From Blaisdell, F. W., and Trunkey, D. D.: Trauma Management. Vol. III. Cervicothoracic Trauma. New York, Thieme, 1986.)

rial can be used as individual pledgets for each suture or as a rectangle long enough to extend the length of the repair.

Blunt trauma can also bruise the myocardium—myocardial contusion. In experimental animals, this can lead to serious arrhythmias and cardiac pump failure. In most animals, these effects occur within seconds to minutes of the blunt injury, but the possibility of delayed manifestation of myocardial contusion is a concern (Tenzer, 1985).

There is no reliable "gold standard" diagnostic test for myocardial contusion (Fabian et al., 1988; Mattox et al., 1992; McLean et al., 1992; Miller et al., 1989b; Shapiro et al., 1991; Sturaitis et al., 1986). There is no doubt that blunt trauma can cause a contusion of the heart; autopsy series readily document these injuries. The clinical dilemma is how to predict which patients are at risk for deleterious sequelae (Flancbaum et al., 1986). A number of different diagnostic tests have been proposed (Dubrow et al., 1989; Nirgiotis et al., 1990; Tenzer, 1985). For many of these tests, however, positive results do not correlate with any untoward consequences attributable to a contused myocardium in the vast majority of patients. Conversely, patients with negative results still develop complications possibly related to myocardial contusion. Creatine phosphocreatine levels and echocardiography are examples of such low-sensitivity, low-specificity tests and are not helpful in diagnosis or treatment planning.

Sequelae of myocardial contusion are uncommon in patients who demonstrate hemodynamic and cardiac stability on admission (Fabian et al., 1988; Wisner et al., 1990). Obviously unstable patients declare the severity of their illness early in the emergency department course and are triaged to an intensive care setting, where they receive treatment for possible myocardial contusion with monitoring and cardiac support as needed. In hemodynamically stable patients, the admission rhythm strip electrocardiogram is a simple and reliable way to make triage decisions in the emergency department (Fig. 14–20). If there is a marked rhythm strip disturbance (heart block, premature ventricular contractions, paroxysmal atrial tachycardia), the patient should be placed in a monitored bed for 48 hours. This approach detects not only patients with possible myocardial contusion but also some patients with preexisting cardiac disease. If no further arrhythmias are apparent for 48 hours, the patient can be transferred to an unmonitored bed or discharged. Patients without a rhythm disturbance on admission can be admitted to an unmonitored bed (Wisner et al., 1990).

Diaphragm

Blunt injuries of the diaphragm are becoming more common with higher automotive speeds and increased use of seat belt restraints (Beal and McKennan, 1988; Ilgenfritz and Stewart, 1992; Kearney et al.,

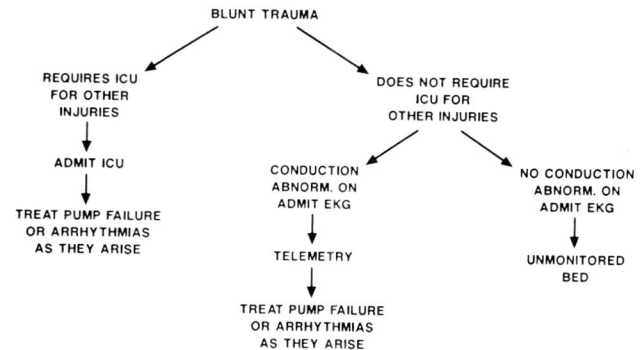

FIGURE 14–20. An algorithm for the management of blunt trauma patients with the possibility of myocardial contusion. If the patient requires admission to an intensive care unit (ICU) bed for other reasons, there is no triage dilemma, and the management is expectant. If the patient does not require ICU disposition for other injuries, the admission rhythm strip should be used for a decision as to whether a monitored bed is needed. (ABNORM. = abnormal; EKG = electrocardiogram.) (From Wisner, D. H., Reed, W. H., and Riddick, R. S.: Suspected myocardial contusion: Triage and indications for monitoring. Ann. Surg., 212:82, 1990.)

1989). When a seat belt is in place, sudden deceleration can lead to marked increases in intra-abdominal pressure, which is secondarily transmitted to the diaphragm.

Blunt rupture of the diaphragm occurs more commonly on the left than on the right (Beal and McKennan, 1988). The liver protects the right hemidiaphragm and distributes pressure evenly across its surface. It is also easier to make the diagnosis on the left side because radiographic findings are more obvious; right-sided ruptures are therefore more likely to be missed because the liver prevents abdominal visceral herniation, and small tears on the right side are of minimal consequence. Rarely, both hemidiaphrams are ruptured. The diaphragm can rupture in any location, but ruptures of the central tendon and the lateral attachments to the torso wall are most common. The size varies, but most of the tears that are diagnosed are at least several centimeters long. On the left side, abdominal viscera can herniate through the diaphragmatic defect, but this does not universally occur, and herniation of abdominal viscera is less likely in patients on controlled positive-pressure ventilation.

The diagnosis of diaphragmatic rupture is usually made either by radiographic findings or incidental discovery at surgery. Herniation of abdominal viscera has already been mentioned, and when hollow viscera such as the stomach, small bowel, and colon herniate, abnormal air densities can sometimes be seen in the pleural cavity (Fig. 14–21). When solid viscera such as the liver or spleen herniate, the hemidiaphragm may appear elevated. Bleeding from associated intra-abdominal injuries is common, and when this blood is sucked into the pleural cavity, it may be apparent as a hemothorax. Subtle blunting of the costophrenic angle and a "fuzzy" quality to the hemidiaphragm are common radiographic findings (Fig. 14–22). Persistence of the blunting after chest tube

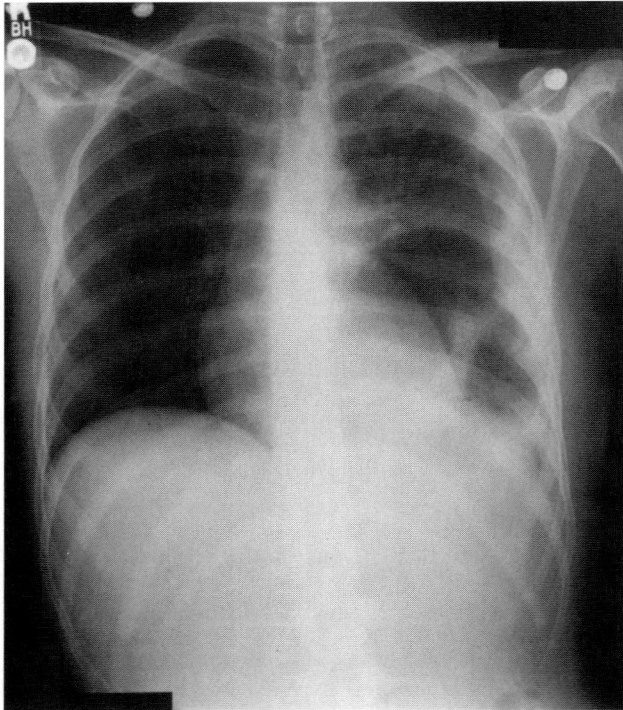

FIGURE 14–21. Admission chest film of a patient who was involved in a motor vehicle accident. There is obvious herniation of the stomach into the left chest. The diagnosis of blunt diaphragmatic rupture was confirmed at laparotomy.

placement and drainage of the ipsilateral pleural cavity is a clue to differentiating diaphragmatic rupture from simple hemothorax. If a chest tube has been placed in a suspicious case, chest tube output should be monitored for lavage fluid if there is subsequent diagnostic peritoneal lavage.

In some patients, bleeding from associated intraabdominal injuries is severe and manifests itself as a large hemothorax or high chest tube output. In the absence of a definitive diagnosis of blunt diaphragmatic rupture, the decision about whether to perform thoracotomy or laparotomy is difficult. Although thoracotomy may be appropriate on rare occasions when an intrathoracic source of hemorrhage is most likely, it is prudent to position the patient so that a laparotomy can also be done if the chest is opened and bleeding is seen to be coming through a ruptured hemidiaphragm.

It is important to inspect the diaphragm closely during exploratory laparotomy, whether or not the diagnosis of diaphragmatic rupture has been made preoperatively. Some of the tears are subtle and hidden by folds of the diaphragm, which can balloon and collapse with the cycle of positive pressure ventilation. When the tear is located, any herniated viscera should be pulled back into the abdomen and inspected for bleeding or ischemia. The rent should then be repaired. There is no commonly agreed-on method for repair, but we have had good results using a large running absorbable suture. If not already present, a chest tube should be placed on the

affected side; there is often considerable drainage over the first several postoperative days until the diaphragmatic repair has healed and become watertight.

Occasionally, the diagnosis of blunt rupture of the diaphragm is initially missed. If a hemidiaphragm is elevated in the early postinjury period and the diagnosis is suspected, CT of the lower chest and upper abdomen sometimes aids diagnosis. Detection of visceral herniation can be delayed, even years after the traumatic event. Herniation may be asymptomatic and only appear on a chest film obtained for other reasons, or the herniated viscera may become strangulated and cause symptoms. If the diagnosis is delayed and the patient is asymptomatic, repair can be effected by either an abdominal or a thoracic approach. If the patient is symptomatic and there is the possibility of visceral ischemia or perforation, the approach should be abdominal.

Esophagus

Blunt injuries to the esophagus are rare (Beal et al., 1988; Stothert et al., 1980). When they do occur, they are almost always either in the cervical esophagus or at the gastroesophageal junction. Blunt injuries to the cervical esophagus are often associated with tracheolaryngeal injuries. They can be difficult to diagnose but may be detected on work-up of the associated

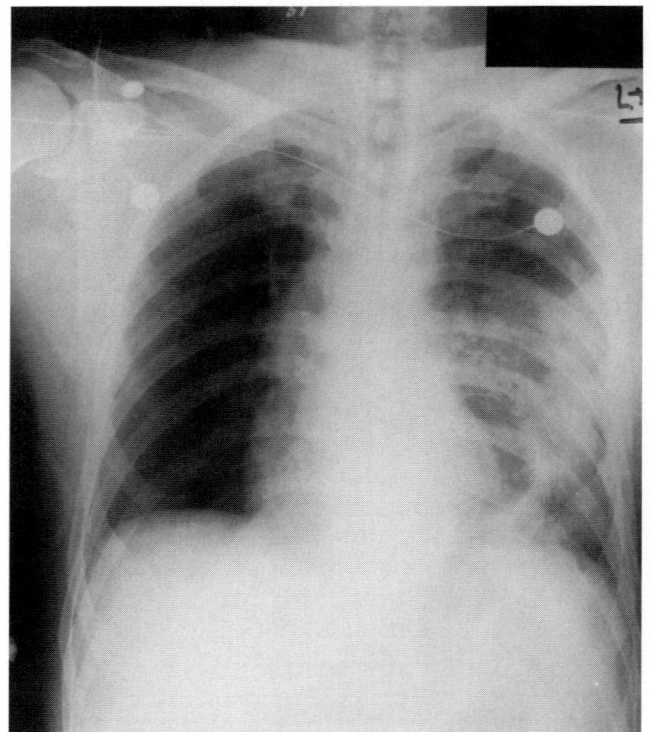

FIGURE 14–22. In this patient with blunt rupture of the left hemidiaphragm, the diagnosis is not clearly apparent on an admission chest film. Abdominal findings and hypotension prompted exploratory laparotomy, which revealed the diaphragmatic injury and a ruptured spleen.

Bullet Path

Entrance
Wound

Trajectory

Exit
Wound

FIGURE 14–23. An example of how a gunshot wound can be confusing when the patient is examined in the emergency department while in the anatomic position. In the example shown, wounds will be seen in the left elbow and medial aspect of the left knee. (From Holcroft, J. W., and Blaisdell, F. W.: Trauma to the torso. Scientific American Surgery, Wilmore, D. W., Cheung, L. Y., Harken, A. H., et al. (eds). Section IV, Subsection 1. © 1995 Scientific American, Inc. All rights reserved.)

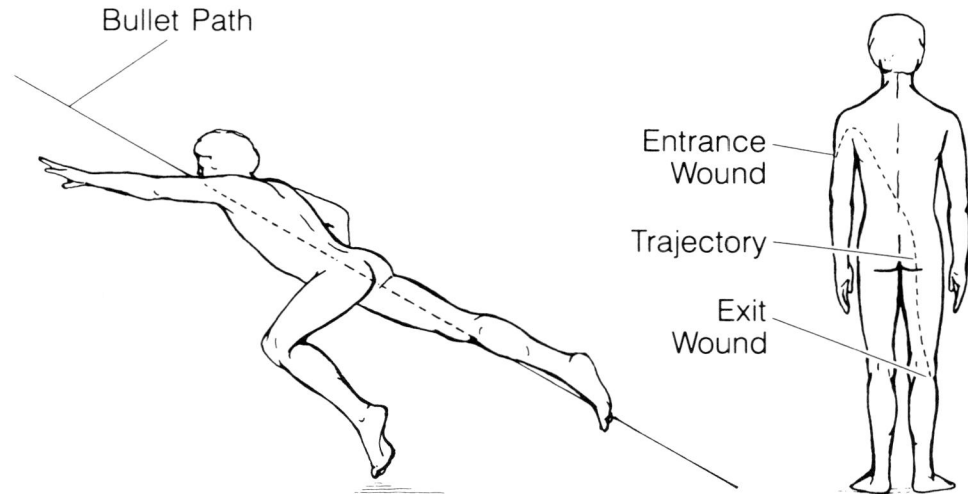

tracheolaryngeal injury. When diagnosis is delayed, the only clue to the presence of the lesion may be unexplained neck pain, crepitance, or mediastinitis. When injuries are located at the gastroesophageal junction, diagnostic clues are abdominal or lower chest pain and subdiaphragmatic air on chest film. Contrast studies or esophagoscopy confirms the diagnosis.

Cervical esophageal injuries should be approached from the left side via an incision along the anterior border of the sternocleidomastoid muscle. The distal pharynx and proximal esophagus are exposed. Visualization of small holes can be difficult. Sometimes the only clue to the presence of an injury is a "greasy" feel on the surgical gloves due to salivary amylase in the wound. Cervical esophageal injuries should be closed in one layer and drained.

PENETRATING CHEST TRAUMA

Victims of penetrating trauma are not always injured while in the anatomic position; no assumptions can be made about the direction of the knife or bullet; also, it cannot be assumed that only the structures immediately underlying the skin wound have been wounded (Fig. 14–23). It is easy to miss small puncture or gunshot wounds if the skin is not closely inspected.

An early chest film should be obtained in patients with gunshot wounds of the chest in order to try to estimate the path of the bullet. It is helpful to mark all skin wounds with a radiopaque marker before obtaining a chest film to relate wounds to one another or to retained bullets (Fig. 14–24). The chest film should also be used for an inspection of the type and state of any retained bullets. Bullet fragmentation should be noted; this tells the surgeon that the bullet either hit a hard structure such as a rib or had soft elements that fragmented on impact. Sometimes the caliber of the bullet is apparent and the degree of wounding can be inferred.

Ballistic theory dictates that the kinetic energy of a missile is proportional to the mass and the square of the missile velocity. High-velocity missiles from rifles and military weapons therefore have a much higher energy than do lower-velocity missiles such as those from most hand guns. High-speed photographs of high-velocity missiles hitting gelatin analogues of human tissue demonstrate a marked cavitation effect. From this, it has been inferred that high-energy and low-energy missile wounds should be treated differently, with much more aggressive débridement for high-energy missile tracts. Newer ballistic research argues against such an approach and suggests that treatment for all wounds should be based on their

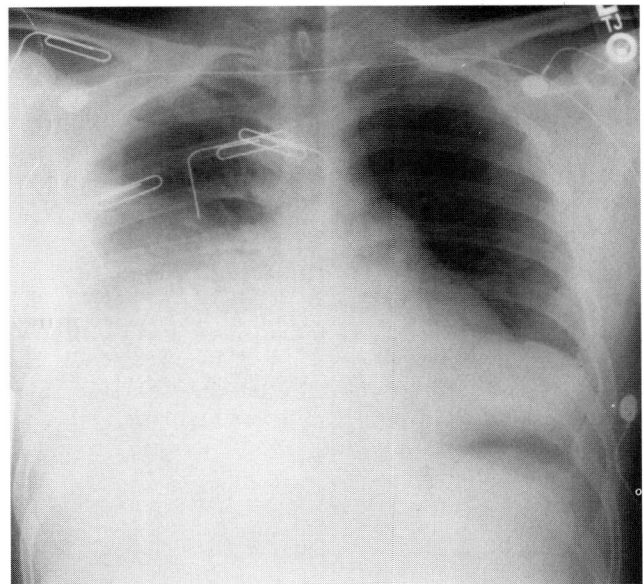

FIGURE 14–24. This patient suffered multiple stab wounds to the right chest and right upper extremity. Before a chest film was obtained, all of the wounds were marked with radiopaque markers. The markers are nothing more sophisticated than paper clips taped to the skin and bent so that the free end of the metal is at the site of the wound.

appearance at surgery. Débridement should be done as with any other wound, and wide débridement of tissue that is not obviously devitalized should not be done just because the wound was caused by a high-velocity projectile.

CHEST WALL INJURY

Most penetrating chest wall injuries are relatively innocuous; morbidity usually relates to underlying visceral injury. Shotgun injuries to the chest wall, however, especially when delivered at close range, can be highly destructive, and chest wall integrity can be disrupted (Bender and Lucas, 1990). Both gunshot and stab wounds to the chest wall can injure an intercostal or internal mammary artery. When this occurs, bleeding into the pleural cavity is more common than external bleeding because the intercostal and mammary vessels are immediately adjacent to the parietal pleura. Massive intrapleural bleeding after penetrating trauma is more commonly derived from the chest wall than from the lungs because the intercostal and mammary arteries are systemic vessels with relatively high systemic arterial pressure, whereas the pulmonary vasculature is a low-pressure system.

One of the important early decisions necessary in patients who have suffered penetrating chest injuries is which patients require early thoracotomy. Objective guidelines to help in this decision-making process have been advocated (Table 14–1). These numerical guidelines are useful but should always be combined with the clinical status of the patient and the appearance of repeated chest films; they should not be followed blindly (Mansour et al., 1992). For example, if a chest tube is placed for hemothorax and 800 ml is drained, the patient should still undergo thoracotomy if there is a large undrained hemothorax on follow-up chest film or if the patient remains hemodynamically unstable and other sources of bleeding are unlikely.

Pneumothorax and Hemothorax

Most of the principles of diagnosis and treatment described for pneumothorax and hemothorax after blunt trauma also pertain to pneumothoraces and hemothoraces from penetrating trauma. Air embolus and bullet embolus are unique to penetrating trauma, however.

Air embolus occurs when air moves from the airway into the pulmonary venous system through a

■ **Table 14–1.** INDICATIONS FOR URGENT THORACOTOMY FOR HEMOTHORAX

1000–1500 ml with initial tube thoracostomy
> 100 ml/hr for 4 hours after tube thoracostomy placement

---

traumatic fistula (Meier et al., 1979; Thomas and Roe, 1973). Although this is uncommon, the consequences can be devastating. Air emboli delivered to the systemic circulation can cause mortality or major morbidity if delivered to critical arteries such as those in the cerebral or coronary circulation. Because the pathophysiology of air embolism is the movement of air from the airway to the pulmonary venous system, increases in the pressure difference across the traumatic communication worsen the problem. Hypovolemia decreases pressure in the pulmonary venous system and increases the gradient. Similarly, increased airway pressure with institution of positive-pressure ventilation increases the likelihood of air embolus. In a patient with penetrating chest trauma, air embolus should be suspected if there is evidence of a stroke or cardiac failure shortly after initiation of positive-pressure ventilation. If the pressures used for positive-pressure ventilation are kept low, air embolus is less likely to occur (Graham et al., 1977).

Treatment of air embolus begins with control of the bronchopulmonary venous fistula. This is done via thoracotomy and placement of a hilar cross-clamp. The heart should then be exposed, and the left atrium, left ventricle, and root of the aorta should be vented with needles. To deal with air already in the coronary circulation, the aortic root should be compressed via the transverse sinus and the heart should be massaged to push the emboli through the coronary circulation. After the air has been vented, the bronchopulmonary venous fistula should be repaired or the affected area of lung should be resected to prevent further embolization.

Bullet embolus is also unique to penetrating trauma. Rarely, a bullet or bullet fragments enter the venous system via an iliac vein, inferior vena cava, or another large vein. Once in the venous system, they can pass through the right side of the heart and into the pulmonary vasculature. Bullet embolus should be expected if there are an unequal number of wounds in the skin and if a bullet or fragments are not in an expected location. A chest film reveals the bullet or fragments in the chest. If there is no other potential route for the bullet to have directly entered the chest and the patient has no history of prior gunshot wounds, the diagnosis is made. If embolization of an intact bullet occurs, the bullet should be removed because of the danger of erosion of the pulmonary vasculature and potential pulmonary infarct. Occasionally, the bullet is removed radiographically, but usually the approach is surgical, with isolation of the affected portion of pulmonary artery, arteriotomy, and removal of the bullet. Bullet fragments sometimes can be left in place (Fig. 14–25).

Pulmonary Injuries

Gunshot wounds and stab wounds to the pulmonary parenchyma can usually be treated with observation and a chest tube for associated hemopneumo-

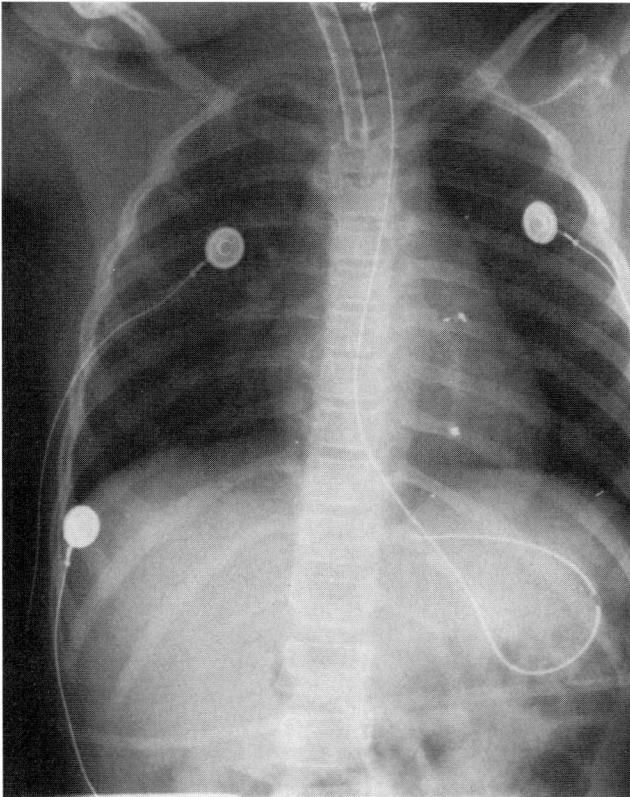

FIGURE 14–25. Multiple bullet fragment emboli in a patient with a gunshot wound of the left iliac vein. Because they were small, the fragments in this case were not removed.

thorax (Graham et al., 1979). An occasional wound, particularly from a bullet, requires pulmonary repair or resection. Exposure of the peripheral tract of a bullet or knife can be facilitated by opening the tract with a stapling device, which exposes the length of the tract and allows for suture ligation of bleeding points and parenchymal repair as necessary. A running locked absorbable suture should be used for parenchymal repairs. Small tears can be successfully repaired in this fashion, but more severe injuries require resection.

Severe peripheral injuries with a great deal of bleeding or air leak are appropriately treated with a wedge resection. This is best done with stapling devices and is particularly appropriate if there are a number of associated injuries. Lobectomy or even pneumonectomy are occasionally needed if the injury is hilar and there has been major destruction to the airway or the vasculature.

Pulmonary vascular injuries in the hilum are often fatal, and most patients exsanguinate before arrival in the emergency department (Mattox et al., 1989). In patients who survive to reach medical attention, diagnosis is suggested by hemodynamic instability and a large hemothorax. The most important aspect of surgical management is rapid vascular control. For both pulmonary arterial and venous injuries, pressure may be the best means of immediately staunching hemorrhage. Alternatively, a hilar cross-clamp pro-

vides initial hemorrhage control. Pressure or cross-clamping cannot be used for definitive control, however, because both interfere with exposure. Therefore, it is sometimes helpful to open the pericardium for proximal control in the pericardial space.

Repair can be made once there is adequate exposure and vascular control. If the injury is relatively straightforward and the patient has minimal associated injuries, repair should be done using standard techniques and nonabsorbable vascular suture. It is important to adequately mobilize the lung before repair by dividing the inferior pulmonary ligament. In patients with complex or severe injuries, the affected portion of lung should be resected.

Injuries to the Trachea and Major Bronchi

Penetrating injuries to the trachea and major bronchi are more common than blunt injuries (Grover et al., 1979; Symbas et al., 1976). Most of the principles of diagnosis and management are the same. Injuries to the cervical trachea are more common than injuries to the thoracic trachea in patients who survive to reach the emergency department. The most common symptoms are shortness of breath and hoarseness or a voice change if the larynx is involved. The most common associated findings on physical examination are neck crepitus and "bubbling" of air from the wound with respiration. Sometimes the skin wound immediately overlies the trachea. On a film of the neck, there may be evidence of subcutaneous air.

In some patients with penetrating injuries to the cervical trachea, the airway is compromised by blood or loss of structural integrity, and immediate intervention is necessary. If the situation is emergent and the tracheal injury is obvious, the injury itself should be intubated and converted to a tracheostomy. Otherwise, orotracheal intubation should be done to protect the airway and allow unhurried neck exploration. Once an airway has been assured, the neck should be explored and the trachea should be repaired, but any vascular injuries have priority over the tracheal injury. The trachea should be repaired with a series of interrupted absorbable mattress sutures. The trachea can usually be repaired simply, but when there are relatively large defects and loss of tissue, more complex procedures may be necessary.

Patients with injuries to the thoracic trachea or major bronchi usually present with a large pneumothorax; there may also be subcutaneous crepitus. Although many of these patients are in extremis on presentation, sometimes the diagnosis is more subtle, and there should be a low threshold for diagnostic bronchoscopy in stable patients. A single bronchoscopy is not completely reliable and may need to be repeated. When the patient is in extremis, the need for surgical intervention is obvious. When the chest is entered, the presence of a large air leak is a clue to the presence of major airway injury. Associated vascular injuries are common and should be treated as necessary. If the patient has multiple penetrating injuries or severe associated injuries to the vasculature, it is sometimes best to treat bronchial injuries with resection, even if this requires pneumonectomy. The possibility of bronchopulmonary venous fistula and the risk of air embolus should be kept in mind.

Great Vessels

Most blunt injuries to the great vessel involve the descending thoracic aorta. In contrast, penetrating injuries to the great vessels can occur in any location. The entrance sites of many wounds to intrathoracic great vessels actually are in the base of the neck. This is particularly true for stab wounds, which can injure the innominate, subclavian, or axillary arteries as well as the carotid arteries in the neck. Wounds to the base of the neck can also injure the subclavian or innominate veins. These wounds are not as serious as those to the adjacent arteries because of the low pressure of the venous system and its tendency to tamponade.

Many patients with penetrating injuries to the chest or base of the neck that involve a major arterial vessel are bleeding massively on presentation and require emergency thoracotomy. Others are initially more stable hemodynamically but have massive hemothorax or ongoing bleeding and are candidates for urgent thoracotomy. Although the location of arterial injury may be guessed prior to thoracotomy or sternotomy, the definitive diagnosis is made at surgery.

Patients with occult traumatic pseudoaneurysms of a major intrathoracic arterial vessel are usually stable on arrival. In a stable patient with a wound or missile track involving the base of the neck, immediate angiography is mandatory to rule out a vascular injury (Fig. 14–26). A missed injury can decompress into the pleural cavity, with disastrous consequences.

Injuries to the descending aorta should be approached through a left-sided thoracotomy. If there is time and if it is certain that there are no associated injuries to the right side of the neck or the abdomen, a left-sided posterolateral thoracotomy is the incision of choice. If time is limited or injuries to other areas are possible, an anterolateral thoracotomy should be done with the patient "bumped up" on the left side. Injuries to the proximal aortic arch, the innominate artery, and the proximal left common carotid artery should be approached via a median sternotomy. It is sometimes necessary to divide and suture ligate the left innominate vein for exposure. Cardiopulmonary bypass is helpful on occasion, but the timing of such injuries usually does not permit its use, and the need for heparin is problematic in the face of associated injuries.

Sternotomy provides good exposure to the innominate artery, the origin of the right common carotid artery, and the proximal right subclavian artery (Fig. 14–27). Supraclavicular or anterior sternocleidomastoid extensions may be necessary for distal carotid or subclavian injuries. Distal subclavian and axillary artery injuries can be approached via infraclavicular

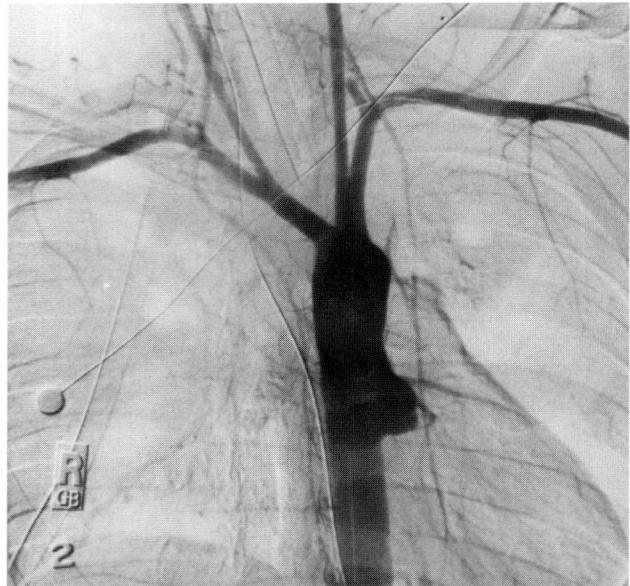

FIGURE 14–26. This patient had a gunshot wound to the base of the left side of the neck. The bullet was located in the right lower chest. A bullet fragment can be seen in the right side of the chest on this angiogram. The patient was asymptomatic and hemodynamically stable. There was a small amount of blood in the right side of the chest. Angiography revealed an injury to the proximal left vertebral artery. The vertebral artery was ligated at surgery.

incisions; if necessary, proximal control can be obtained via a separate supraclavicular incision. To adequately expose portions of the axillary artery, it is often necessary to divide portions of the insertions of the pectoralis major and pectoralis minor muscles (Fig. 14–28). During exposure of the subclavian and axillary arteries, the phrenic nerve and the brachial plexus should be protected.

Although exposure and operative repair of the innominate artery and the proximal portions of the right subclavian, right common carotid, and left common carotid arteries can be obtained via a median sternotomy, exposure of the proximal left subclavian artery requires an approach through a left-sided posterolateral thoracotomy (Fig. 14–29). If the injury is to the subclavian artery in the chest, such an approach is adequate for both control and repair. However, if the injury is to the subclavian artery at the thoracic outlet, thoracotomy provides proximal control only, and a neck incision is also necessary (Fig. 14–30). For this reason, the patient should be positioned so that there is ready access to both the left neck and the left chest.

The left subclavian artery can be exposed by several other methods (Graham et al., 1980). With "trap door" incision, a thoracotomy and a supraclavicular incision are connected by a partial sternotomy so that the upper portion of the chest wall can be elevated and the underlying vasculature can be exposed (Fig. 14–31). An alternative is to resect the medial third of the clavicle, which provides good exposure of the subclavian artery and its major branches, can be done

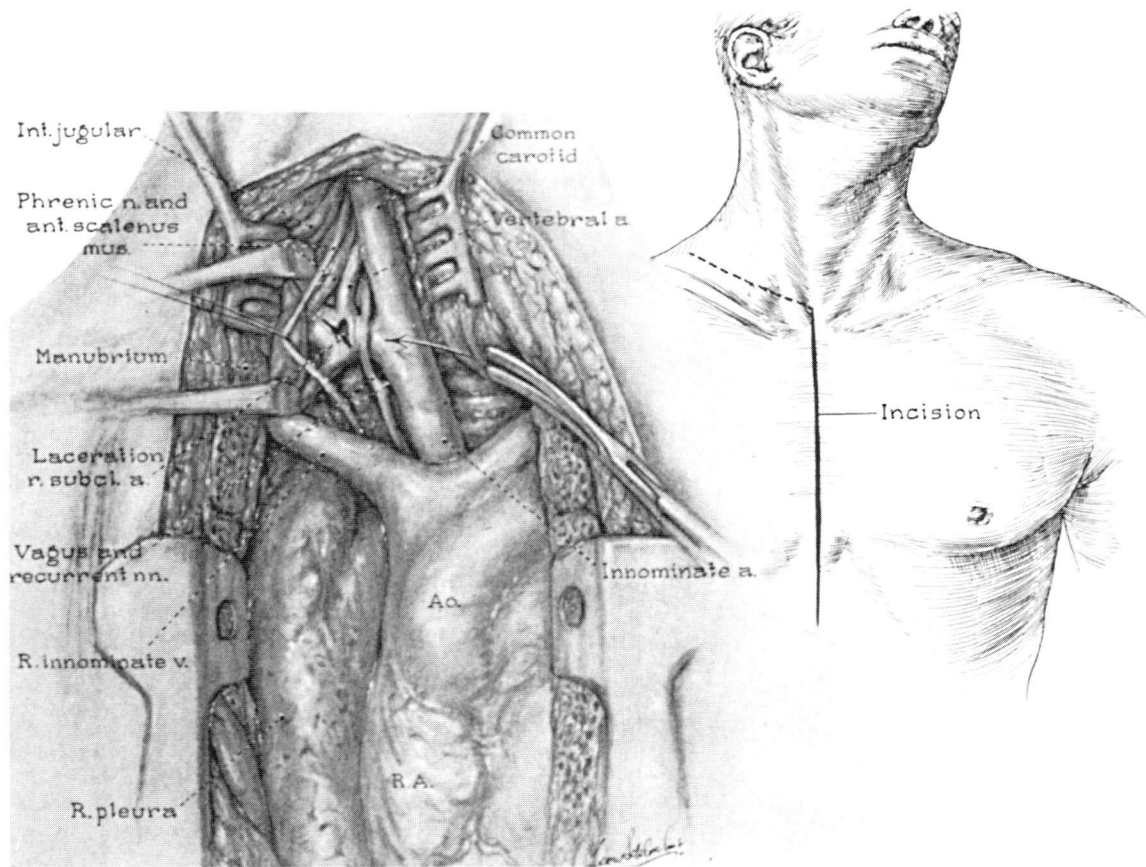

A

Int. jugular
Phrenic n. and ant. scalenus mus.
Common carotid
Vertebral a.
Manubrium
Laceration r. subcl. a.
Vagus and recurrent nn.
Ao.
Innominate a.
R. innominate v.
R. A.
R. pleura
Incision

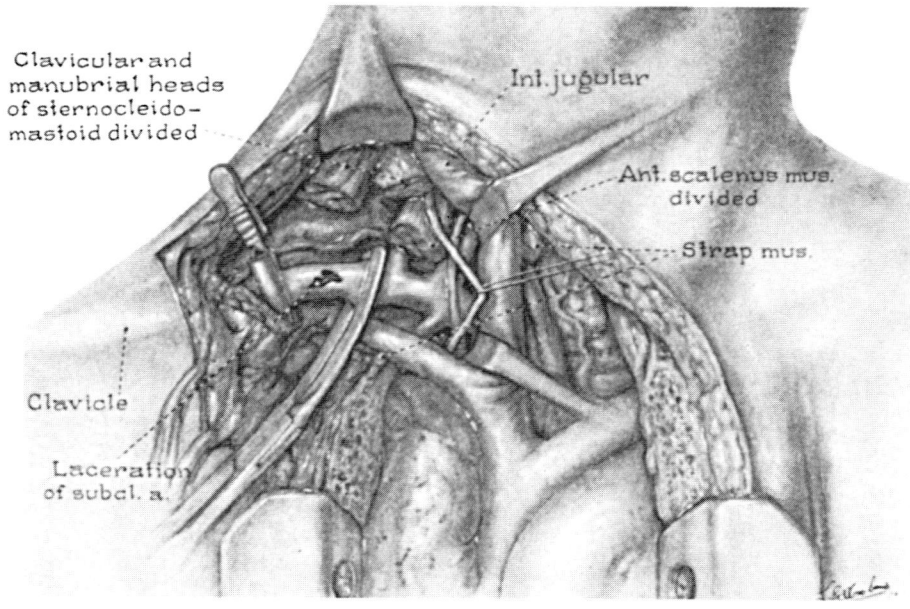

B

Clavicular and manubrial heads of sternocleido-mastoid divided
Int. jugular
Ant. scalenus mus. divided
Strap mus.
Clavicle
Laceration of subcl. a.

FIGURE 14–27. Exposure of a proximal right subclavian arterial injury obtained via a median sternotomy extended into the right side of the neck (*A*). This incision also provides access to the innominate artery and the proximal right common carotid artery and vertebral arteries. The more distal portion of the right subclavian artery is exposed by dividing the sternocleidomastoid, anterior scalene, and strap muscles (*B*). (*A* and *B*, From Brawley, R. K., Murray, G. F., Crisler, C., et al.: Management of wounds of the innominate, subclavian, and axillary blood vessels. Surg. Gynecol. Obstet., *131*:1130, 1970.)

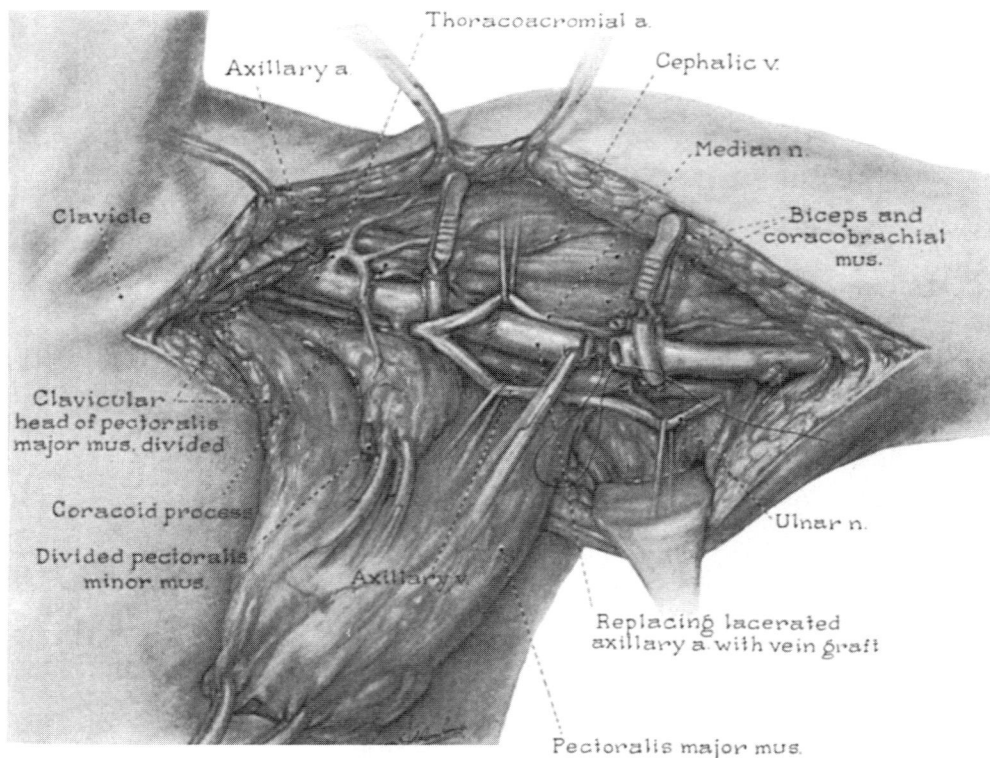

FIGURE 14–28. With division and inferior retraction of the pectoralis major and minor muscles, wide access to injuries of the axillary artery is obtained. (From Brawley, R. K., Murray, G. F., Crisler, C., et al.: Management of wounds of the innominate, subclavian, and axillary blood vessels. Surg. Gynecol. Obstet., *131*:1130, 1970.)

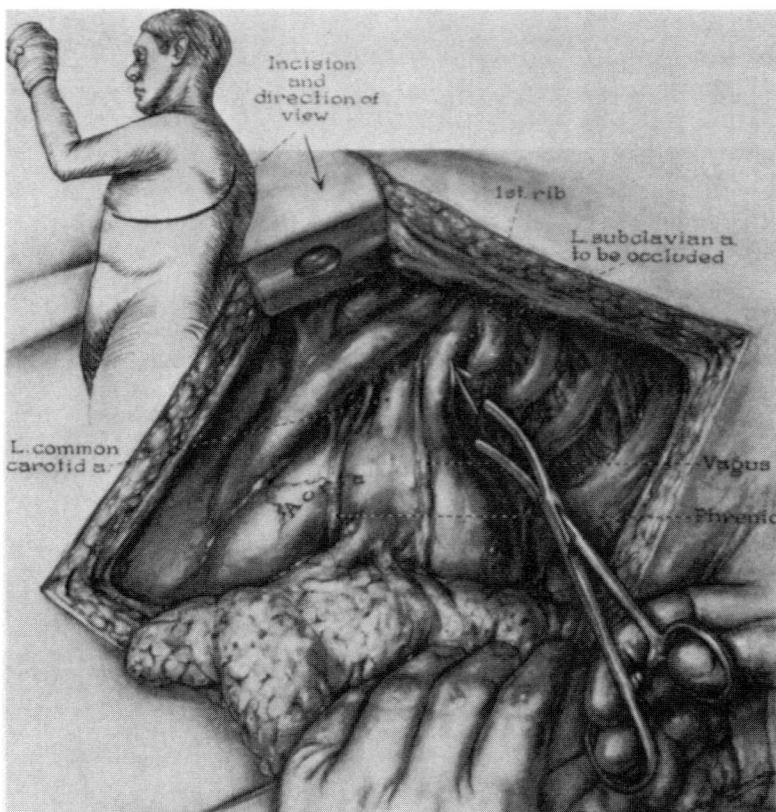

FIGURE 14–29. The proximal left subclavian is best approached via a left posterolateral thoracotomy. The incision can be used for both exposure and repair of proximal injuries and for vascular control if the injury is more distal. (From Schaff, H. V., and Brawley, R. K.: Operative management of penetrating vascular injuries of the thoracic outlet. Surgery, *82*:182, 1977.)

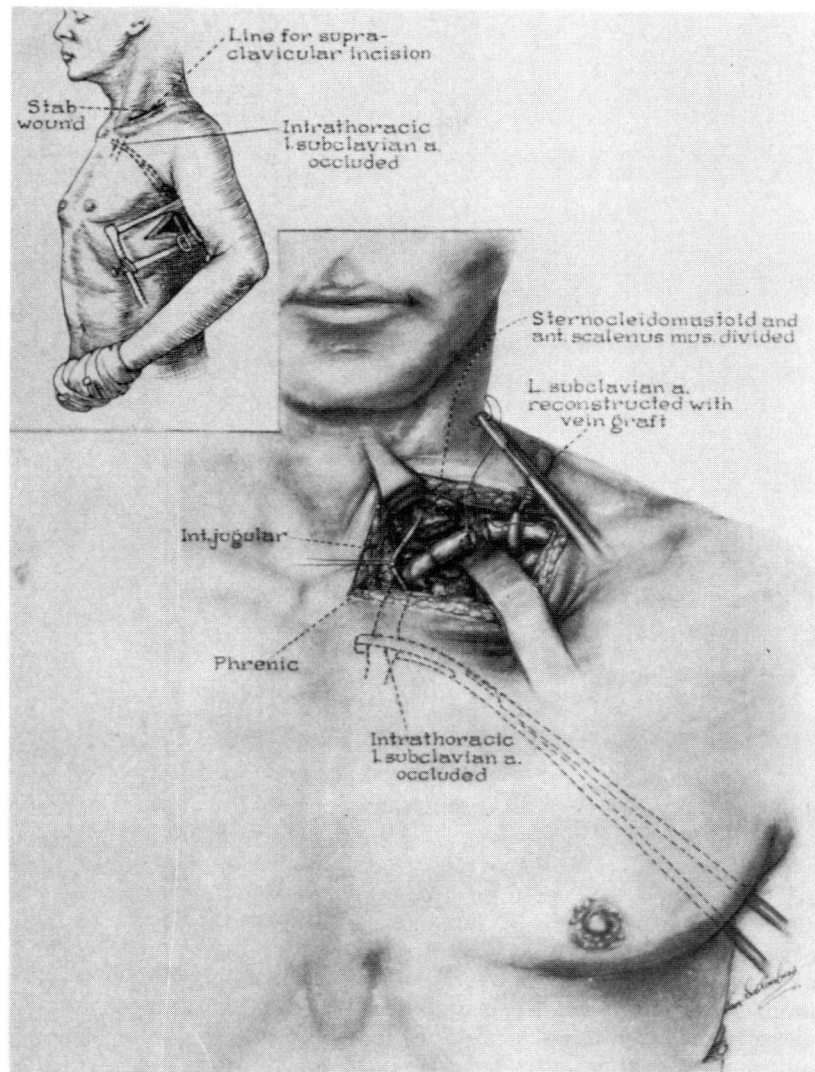

FIGURE 14–30. Proximal control of the left subclavian artery has been obtained through a left posterolateral thoracotomy before approaching a more distal subclavian artery injury via a supraclavicular incision.

relatively quickly, and is associated with minimal long-term morbidity.

Regardless of the incision or incisions used, the approach to left-sided subclavian injuries should be the same as the approach to any other arterial injury. Accordingly, initial attention should be directed to proximal and distal control. If it is readily apparent that the only effective means of obtaining proximal control is via left-sided thoracotomy, this should be done early. After control has been obtained, repair should be made using standard vascular surgical technique.

Heart

The heart, like any other intrathoracic structure, may be injured by a penetrating knife or missile (Attar et al., 1991; Knott-Craig et al., 1992; Marshall et al., 1984; Naughton et al., 1989; Symbas et al., 1973; Trinkle et al., 1975). When the wounding agent is a knife, the skin wound is usually anterior, although the entry site of deep wounds is sometimes lateral in the chest. Posterior stab wounds that injure the heart are uncommon. Bullet wounds that injure the heart are associated with skin wounds almost anywhere in the body.

If the heart is perforated by a knife, bullet, or other penetrating object, one of two pathophysiologic events may occur. Blood may leak from the heart into the adjacent pleural cavity and present as a hemothorax. This diagnosis is suspected when there is hemodynamic instability from hemorrhagic shock or persistent bleeding from a chest tube. The other possibility is that blood will accumulate in the pericardial space. For this to occur, the hole in the pericardial space must tamponade. The pericardial membrane is thick and elastic, and the hole created in it often becomes occluded, which prevents the patient from exsanguinating. Unfortunately, continued pericardial blood accumulation also leads to pericardial tamponade. Characterizing the response of cardiac wounds as either bleeding or tamponade is something of an oversimplification, because most wounds actually do both.

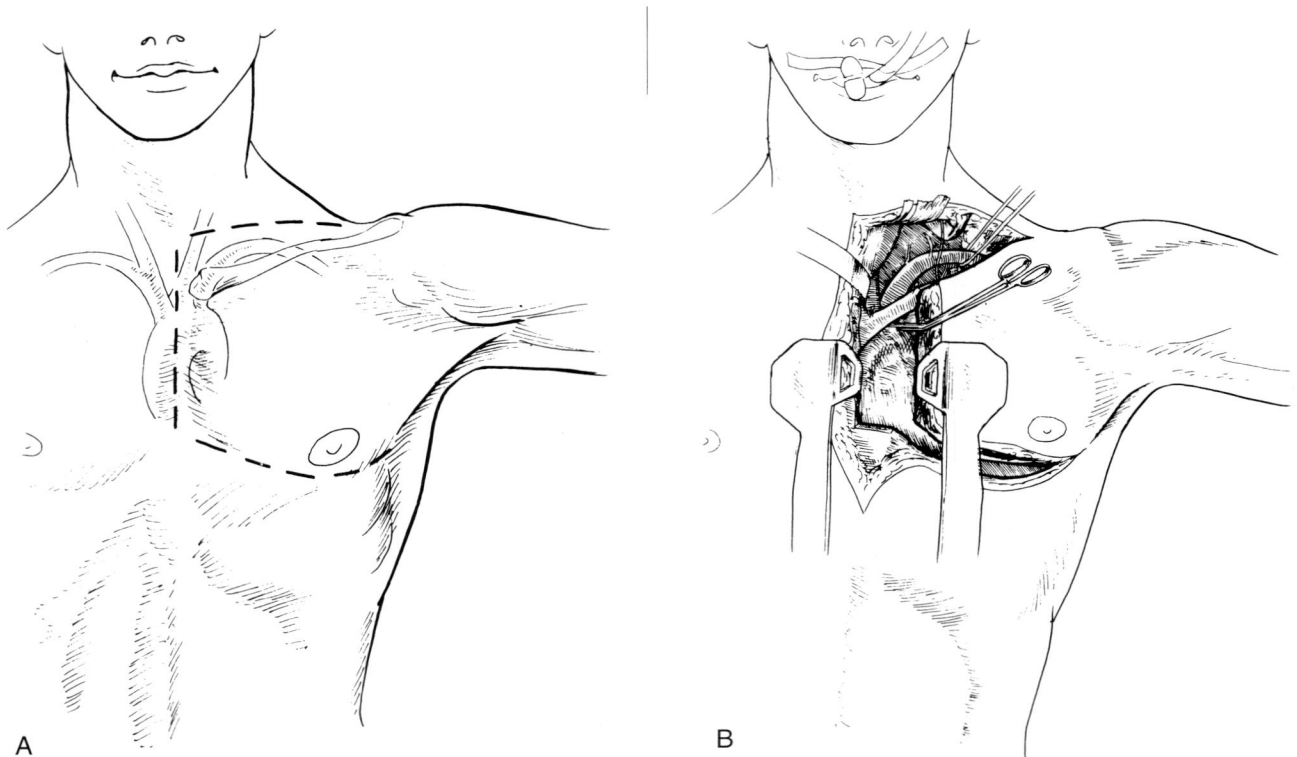

FIGURE 14–31. The "trap door" incision for repair of injuries to the left subclavian artery. The incision includes a left anterolateral thoracotomy, a supraclavicular incision, and a partial sternotomy connecting the two (*A*). Once the incision has been accomplished and the sternum has been partially divided, a portion of the chest wall can be elevated to provide exposure to the subclavian artery (*B*). (*A* and *B*, From Wind, G. G., and Valentine R. J.: Anatomic Exposures in Vascular Surgery. Baltimore, Williams & Wilkins, 1991.)

Penetrating injuries to the heart can occur to any of the four chambers, but are most common in the right ventricle. The right ventricle is anteriorly located and therefore more vulnerable. Because right-sided pressures are lower than left-sided pressures, the bleeding of injuries to the right side of the heart is more likely to tamponade and allow patients to survive to reach medical attention. Although most injuries involve only one chamber of the heart, injuries to multiple chambers are possible.

Many patients with penetrating injuries to the heart present with obvious hemodynamic compromise from hemorrhagic shock, pericardial tamponade, or a combination of the two (Sugg et al., 1968). When the compromise is severe enough, there are no vital signs and the patients are candidates for emergent thoracotomy. Regardless of whether or not tamponade is present, the pericardium should be opened and the heart should be visualized. This maneuver relieves tamponade, if present, and allows digital control of the cardiac wound. Attempts at suture of the heart in an emergency setting should be avoided; if sutures are not carefully placed and pledgeted, they can tear through the myocardium, enlarge the traumatic defect, and convert a salvageable wound into one that cannot be repaired.

An alternative to suturing cardiac wounds in the emergency department is to employ stapling devices (Shamoun et al., 1989). Special wide staples can be placed quickly in the emergency department to control bleeding until the patient has been transported to the operating room for definitive repair. Experience with this technique is limited, but published results of its use are impressive.

Assuming that stapling is not attempted, the wound should be controlled digitally while the patient is transported to the operating room. Occasionally, a urinary catheter can be inserted through the defect for control. If this is done, the balloon should be filled with only enough fluid to control most of the bleeding. If the balloon is overfilled, chamber volume and cardiac output may be compromised. Our experience with this technique has been mixed. In general, if the defect is small enough to respond well to this technique, it will also respond well to digital control.

Although many patients with penetrating cardiac injuries present in extremis, some are stable hemodynamically on presentation. In most patients, bleeding in the pericardial space has tamponaded, and venous return to the right heart is compromised. Intravenous administration of fluid counteracts this effect, although in most cases it only improves the situation temporarily. Administration of intravenous fluid increases intracavitary pressures in the heart, which increases cardiac output but at the same time increases bleeding through the cardiac defect (Gyhra et al., 1992). A cycle is created in which administration of fluid temporarily improves hemodynamics but needs to be vigorously continued because of further deterioration. If this sequence of events occurs, the possibility of pericardial tamponade should be considered.

Similar pathophysiology may cause acute deterioration upon initiation of positive pressure mechanical ventilation because of increased intrapleural pressure and decreased venous return. The effect of positive pressure ventilation, when added to pericardial tamponade, can lead to critical hemodynamic compromise. If tamponade is suspected and the patient is to be intubated in the operating room, the chest should be prepared and draped before intubation so that tamponade can be relieved rapidly if the patient deteriorates with the institution of positive-pressure ventilation.

Few reliable physical findings point to the diagnosis of pericardial tamponade. The elements of Beck's triad (hypotension, venous distention, and quiet heart sounds) are sometimes present individually but are rarely seen in combination. If neck veins are distended, a diagnosis of tamponade should be presumed until proven otherwise. If the patient is hypovolemic in addition to having tamponade, however, neck vein distention may not be present. Auscultation is difficult in the emergency department, and distant heart sounds or pulsus paradoxus are unreliable signs. Diffusely decreased amplitude on an admission electrocardiogram is a subtle finding that is easily missed. On chest film, the finding of a globular cardiac silhouette sometimes aids the diagnosis in a stable patient with tamponade (Fig. 14–32).

Because simple, noninvasive diagnostic tests are neither sensitive nor specific for the diagnosis of cardiac injury, other more elaborate or invasive means of diagnosis are employed. Echocardiography is a logical approach in the stable patient with a penetrat-

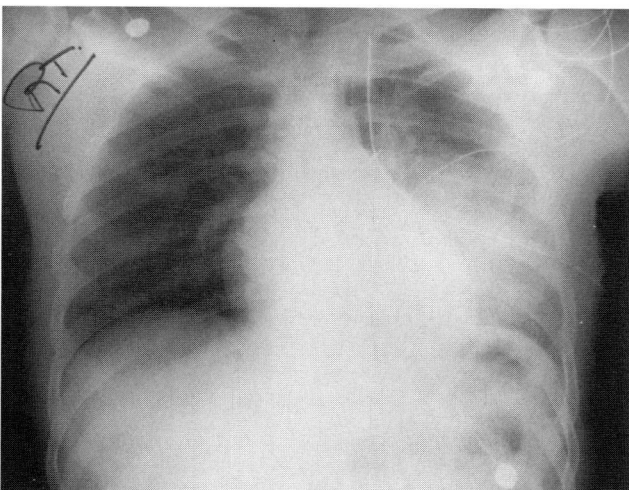

FIGURE 14–32. This patient sustained a stab wound to the left side of the chest (note the paper clip marking the entrance wound). He was hypotensive, and there was a suggestion of neck vein distention. The chest film reveals a globular cardiac silhouette. At surgery, the patient underwent cardiac laceration and pericardial tamponade.

ing injury that might involve the heart. Experience with this technique has been limited, but it holds promise (Freshman et al., 1991; Jimenez et al., 1990). One center has trained residents and emergency department physicians to perform echocardiograms for the diagnosis of pericardial fluid and tamponade. This approach addresses one of the major problems with the use of echocardiography: lack of availability at nights and on weekends.

Pericardiocentesis is a more invasive approach to the diagnosis of cardiac injury and the presence of pericardial blood (Fig. 14–33A). A needle is placed in the subxiphoid position and directed toward the left shoulder at a 30- to 40-degree angle from the skin surface. While the needle is advanced, constant aspiration is maintained. An electrocardiogram lead can be attached to the hub of the advancing needle to detect myocardial contact with the needle tip. If blood is aspirated, the result is positive. The importance of checking the aspirated blood for clot has been emphasized, because if the needle is advanced too far into a cardiac chamber the blood will clot, whereas if the aspirated blood is from the pericardial sac it is defibrinated and will not clot.

Pericardiocentesis is somewhat controversial (Trinkle et al., 1975). If the result is positive, there is nothing definitive that can be done if an expert surgeon is not immediately present (Demetriades, 1984; Ivatury et al., 1987; Marshall et al., 1984). Removal of only a small amount of blood from the pericardial sac, however, can temporarily improve the hemodynamic status, and repeated aspirations may be of some use. In the hands of an expert surgeon, pericardiocentesis is appropriate if the surgeon is comfortable with the procedure to rule out the presence of pericardial blood in a stable patient. Pericardiocentesis is also reasonable when performed by emergency department or other physicians if an expert surgeon is not immediately available.

Creation of a subxiphoid pericardial window is another approach to the stable patient with a wound that may have injured the heart (Fig. 14–33B) (Jimenez et al., 1990; Mayor-Davies and Britz, 1990; Trinkle et al., 1975). A small subxiphoid incision is made through which the diaphragmatic portion of the pericardial surface is grasped and incised. If a small amount of normal serous pericardial fluid is seen, the test result is negative and the wound is closed. Return of blood is a positive test result, and the patient should undergo sternotomy or thoracotomy for repair of the cardiac injury. Subxiphoid pericardial windows are both sensitive and highly specific.

Many of the wounds that raise the possibility of cardiac injury also suggest underlying abdominal injury. The abdominal viscera, depending on the patient's positioning and phase of respiration at the time of injury, can rise as high as the fourth or fifth intercostal space (Fig. 14–34); in many cases of penetrating precordial trauma, abdominal exploration is necessary. If a laparotomy is performed and there is concern about the possibility of a penetrating injury to the heart, it is simple to make a small hole in

CARDIAC TAMPONADE

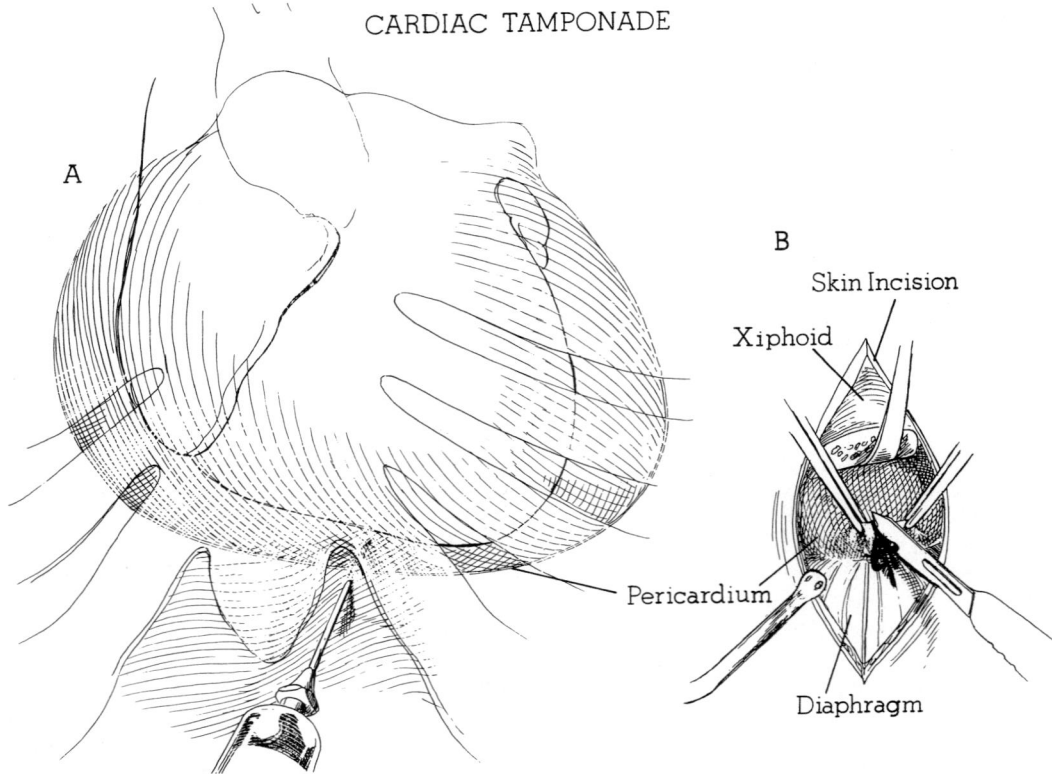

FIGURE 14–33. *A*, Demonstration of the subxiphoid approach to pericardiocentesis. *B*, Limited pericardial exploration via a subxiphoid window for diagnosis and temporary relief of hemopericardium with tamponade.

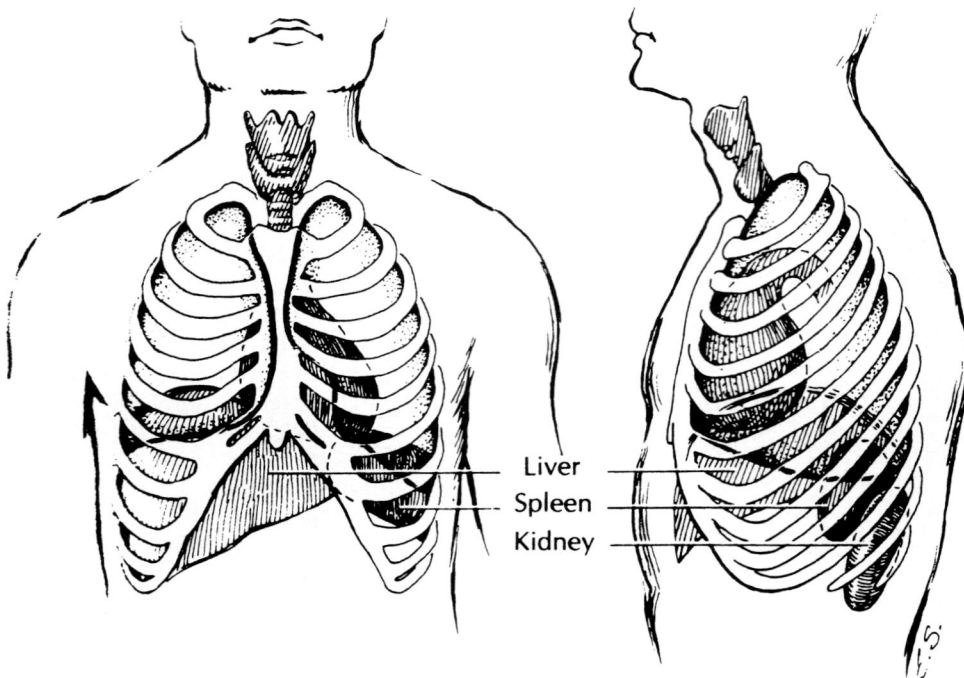

FIGURE 14–34. The lower six ribs overlie the abdominal viscera, which are subject to penetrating injury of the lower chest. Such wounds should therefore be thought of as abdominal injuries as well as chest injuries. (From Blaisdell, F. W., and Trunkey, D. D.: Trauma Management. Vol. III. Cervicothoracic Trauma. New York, Thieme, 1986.)

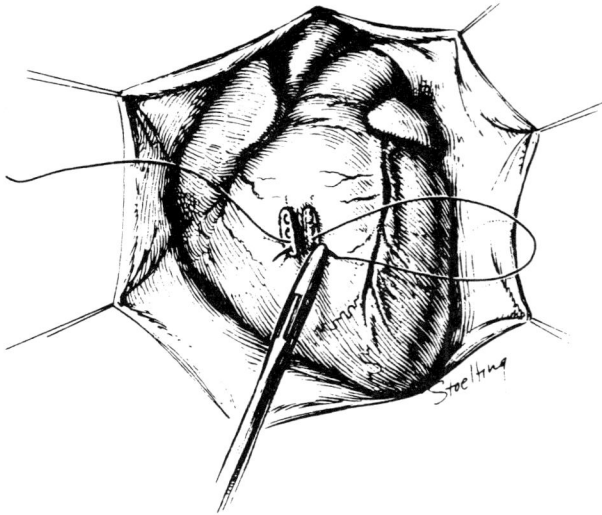

FIGURE 14–35. Suture repair of cardiac lacerations should usually be done with interrupted, pledgeted horizontal mattress sutures. Individual pledgets or a strip of pledget material can be used. (From Blaisdell, F. W., and Trunkey, D. D.: Trauma Management. Vol. III. Cervicothoracic Trauma. New York, Thieme, 1986.)

the diaphragmatic surface of the pericardium via the laparotomy incision. Blood from the pericardiotomy should prompt a sternotomy for repair of a presumed cardiac injury. Bleeding from the edges of the pericardiotomy secondary to small diaphragmatic vessels should be controlled with electrocautery. Such bleeding can be confused with intrapericardial blood but is much smaller in amount and does not persist after electrocautery has been applied.

Either thoracotomy or sternotomy can be used to repair cardiac injuries. In patients who arrive without vital signs or deteriorate in the emergency department, an emergency thoracotomy should be done on the side of injury. If exposure of the cardiac injury is inadequate, the thoracotomy should be extended across the sternum to the other side of the chest. The pericardium should be opened widely so that access to the heart is adequate.

For wounds of the left side of the heart, particularly wounds of the left atrium, a left-sided posterolateral thoracotomy is preferred because minimal manipulation of the heart is necessary for exposure. Unfortunately, there is rarely enough time preoperatively to determine the location of the wound and to place the patient in the lateral decubitus position. In addition, lateral decubitus positioning and entry into the chest through a thoracotomy incision limits the possibilities for operative exposure of the right side of the heart, the right chest, and the abdomen. For these reasons, the usual incision of choice for relatively stable patients with penetrating cardiac injuries is a sternotomy.

Sternotomy provides ready access to the right-sided chambers of the heart. For injuries to the left-sided chambers, particularly the left atrium (rare) or the posterior aspect of the left ventricle, exposure requires more cardiac manipulation. Because the heart is fixed

at its attachments to the superior and inferior venae cavae, elevating it out of the pericardial sac in a left-to-right direction results in axial twisting and occlusion of venous return. Loss of venous return and resultant cardiac dysfunction usually resolve with return of the heart to its normal position (Hunt et al., 1992). Decreases in cardiac activity and venous return can, in fact, help in the repair, because they create a quieter, relatively blood-free field.

Repair of most cardiac injuries is straightforward. In some wounds of the atria, a side-biting vascular clamp can be used for control during repair. Alternatively, the area of injury can be compressed with a finger while it is being sutured. Nonabsorbable suture should be used and should be pledgeted. Precise location of each initial suture is difficult in a bleeding, beating heart and is not as important as gaining some degree of control of the bleeding so that refinements of the repair can be performed in a relatively bloodless field (Fig. 14–35).

When the wound is immediately adjacent to a major coronary artery, the defect should be repaired without damaging or occluding the coronary circulation. Horizontal mattress sutures should be placed under the coronary artery and the knots tied at a distance from the artery (Fig. 14–36).

When a major coronary artery has been damaged and there is cardiac dysfunction, cardiopulmonary bypass should be initiated and the artery repaired (Reissman et al., 1992). Other potential situations in which cardiopulmonary bypass is necessary are in patients in whom initial attempts at repair of the cardiac injury are unsuccessful and patients who have evidence of large intracardiac defects requiring immediate repair. Intraoperative transesophageal echocardiography, if available, is a helpful diagnostic adjunct after the external cardiac injury has been repaired,

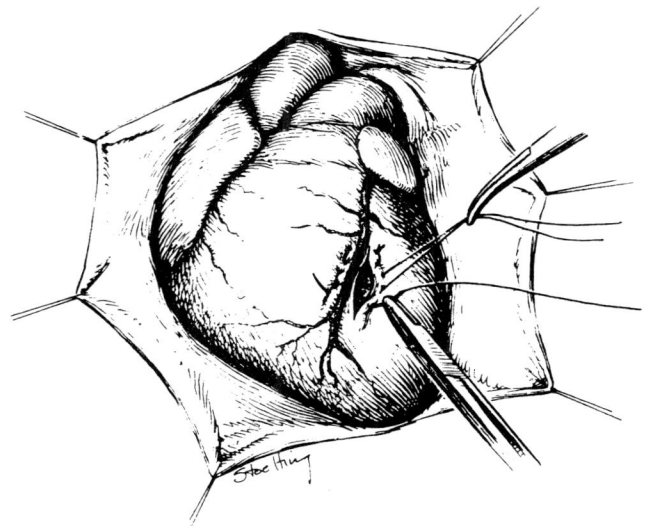

FIGURE 14–36. Technique for repair of a cardiac laceration adjacent to a coronary artery. (From Blaisdell, F. W., and Trunkey, D. D.: Trauma Management. Vol. III. Cervicothoracic Trauma. New York, Thieme, 1986.)

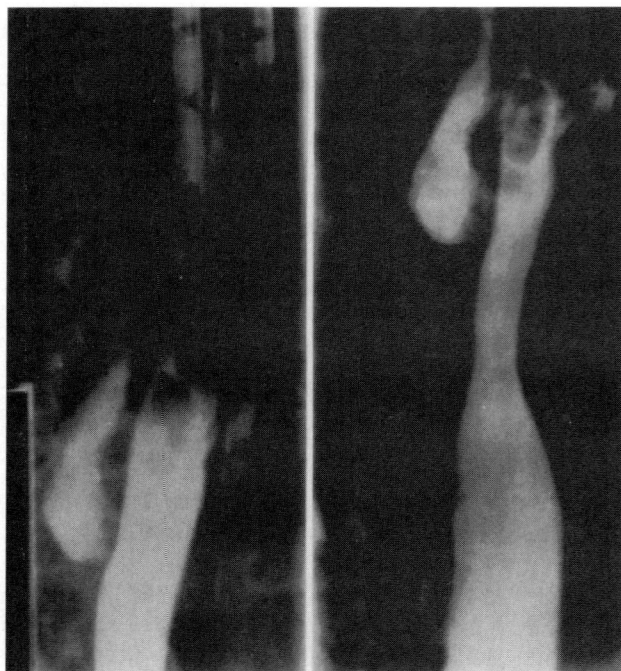

FIGURE 14–37. This patient with suspected esophageal injury underwent a water-soluble contrast study, which revealed extravasation of contrast at the T1–T2 level.

especially if the patient remains compromised or shows signs of an intracardiac shunt.

There is a surprisingly low incidence of postoperative infection, even after emergent operations. All patients who have not undergone intraoperative echocardiography should have it performed in the postoperative period. Small intracardiac defects not seen in the immediate postoperative period may become more significant and visible with time. If the patient's status and the size and character of the defect mandate it, repair of intracardiac defects should be performed on a delayed basis (Rayner et al., 1977; Symbas, 1991). As with any other procedure in which the pericardium has been violated, postpericardiotomy syndrome can occur (Symbas, 1991).

Diaphragm

The primary emergent concern with penetrating diaphragmatic injuries is the possibility of associated injuries to abdominal viscera (Mariadason et al., 1988). In addition, blood or visceral contents from the abdomen can enter the chest because of the difference in pressure between the abdomen (positive pressure during inspiration) and the chest (negative pressure during inspiration). This is a particular concern in patients with combined injuries to the stomach and diaphragm (Durham et al., 1991). When the stomach is injured and there is an immediately adjacent hole in the diaphragm, the stomach contents are drawn into the pleural cavity. Because of the particulate nature of the stomach contents, empyema is common if the chest is not thoroughly cleaned. The gastric injury should be closed as quickly as possible, and the pleu-

ral cavity should be irrigated. Sometimes, adequate irrigation of the chest requires enlarging the hole in the diaphragm. It may even prove necessary to do a small left-sided anterolateral thoracotomy to adequately wash out the pleural cavity after the diaphragm has been repaired and the abdominal operation has been completed.

Laparoscopy and thoracoscopy show some promise in the diagnosis of diaphragmatic injuries (Ivatury et al., 1991b; Livingston et al., 1992; Smith et al., 1993). Because insufflation of gas into the abdominal cavity is necessary as part of the laparoscopic approach, a chest tube should be placed early in the course of the work-up.

If diaphragmatic injuries are not diagnosed and treated, intra-abdominal viscera can gradually herniate through the defect. Incarceration and strangulation occur in some cases, sometimes not becoming manifest until years after the trauma. Surgery is the treatment of choice for chronic diaphragmatic hernias. Unlike the acute treatment of these lesions, which should be approached via an abdominal incision, chronic lesions can be approached via the chest.

Esophagus

The esophagus can be injured by penetrating trauma at any location throughout its course (Cohn et al., 1989; Jones and Samson, 1975; Nesbitt and Sawyers, 1987) (Fig. 14–37). Injuries to the pharynx and cervical esophagus are more commonly seen than are injuries to the thoracic or abdominal esophagus. The cervical esophagus is more exposed, and the thoracic esophagus is closely associated with the aorta and pulmonary vasculature, so patients with injuries

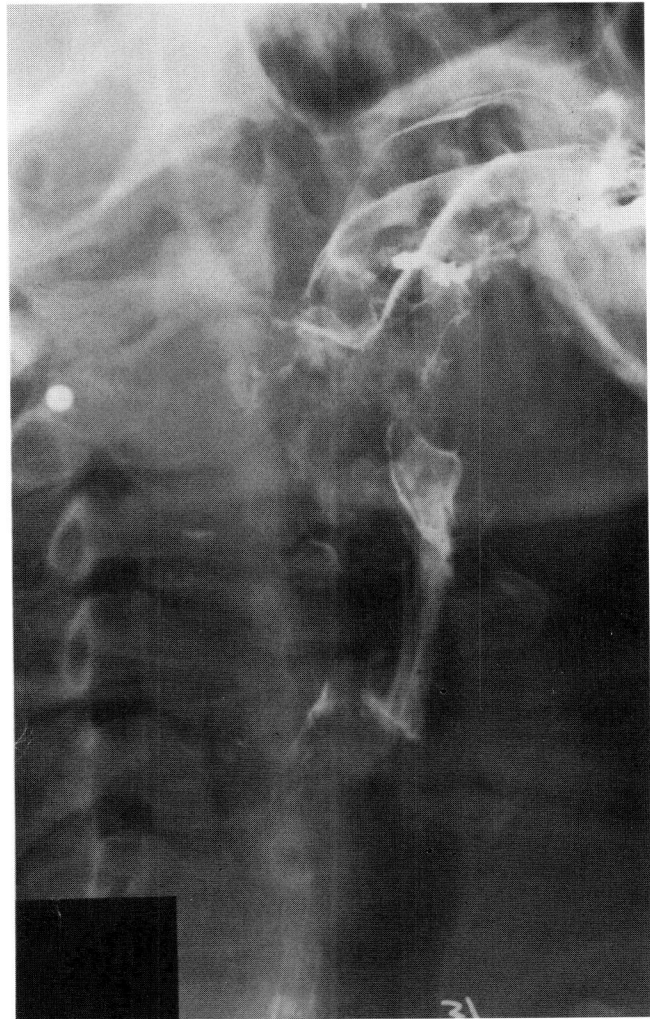

FIGURE 14–38. A contrast study demonstrating extravasation of contrast in a patient with a cervical esophageal injury.

to the esophagus in the chest are more likely to exsanguinate before receiving medical attention (Symbas, 1991; Winter and Weigelt, 1990).

Injuries to the pharynx are more common than are injuries to the cervical esophagus. Clues to the diagnosis are hematemesis and hemoptysis; many of these injuries can be seen by looking into the oropharynx and hypopharynx for a source of bleeding. If the patient is stable and there is no need for urgent neck exploration, the pharynx should be examined, and an esophageal contrast study should be performed (Fig. 14–38). If an esophageal injury is highly suspected and the contrast study results are negative, esophagoscopy should also be done, because contrast studies have an approximately 10% false-negative rate (Symbas, 1991). Esophagoscopy also has a 10% false-negative rate; if a patient has mediastinitis or clinical findings that suggest an esophageal injury, a missed esophageal injury should be considered even if the initial work-up results were negative (Merion et al., 1981).

Cervical esophageal injuries should be approached via an incision along the anterior border of the sterno-cleidomastoid on the side of the injury (Fig. 14–39). A large bougie should be placed in the esophagus to help localize the injury, and repair should be made in one or two layers with absorbable suture used on the inner layer. If the injury is large or the diagnosis is delayed, primary repair may not be feasible, and the area should be widely drained.

Upper thoracic esophageal injuries should be approached via a right-sided thoracotomy. Lower thoracic esophageal injuries should be approached through the left chest unless preoperative imaging studies clearly demonstrate the esophageal leak to be right-sided. A pleural or intercostal patch should be placed over the repair whenever possible (Fig. 14–40), and the chest should be drained with chest tubes. As with cervical injuries, large defects or lesions in which the diagnosis was delayed are sometimes repairable at the time of operation, and it may be necessary to defunctionalize the esophagus to allow the area to heal (Urschel and Razzuk, 1973) (Fig. 14–41). Reestablishment of gastrointestinal continuity is delayed if the wound heals. If the esophageal injury does not heal, esophageal replacement is necessary.

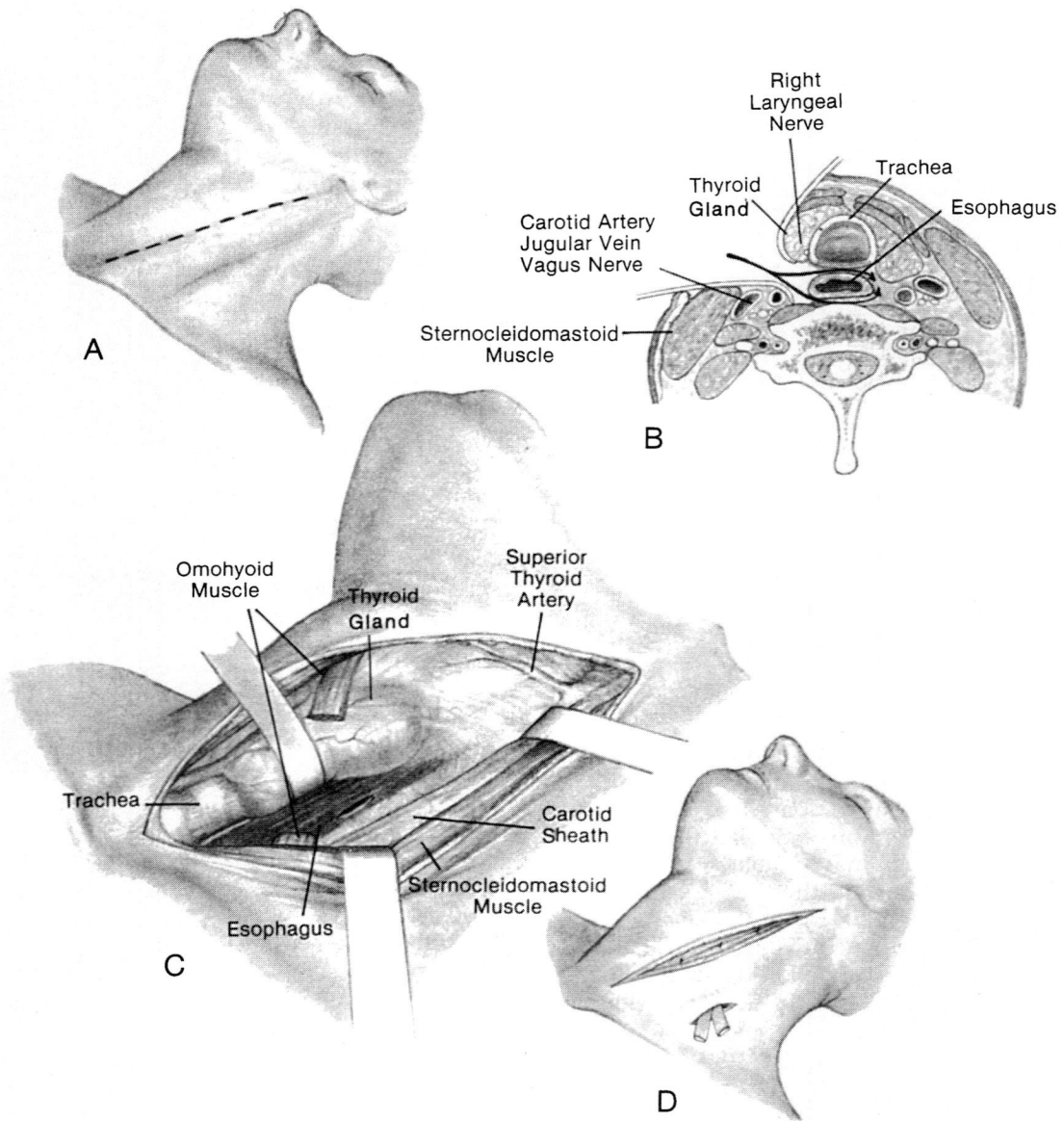

FIGURE 14–39. Surgical drainage after injury to the cervical esophagus. *A,* The incision should be along the anterior border of the sternocleidomastoid muscle. *B,* The plane of drainage is posterior to the thyroid gland and anterior to the carotid sheath and the sternocleidomastoid muscle. *C,* An exposed injury. *D,* Drainage should be done with a Penrose or closed drainage system. The wound can be left at least partially open. (*A–D,* From Hood, R. M.: Techniques in General Thoracic Surgery. Philadelphia, W. B. Saunders, 1985.)

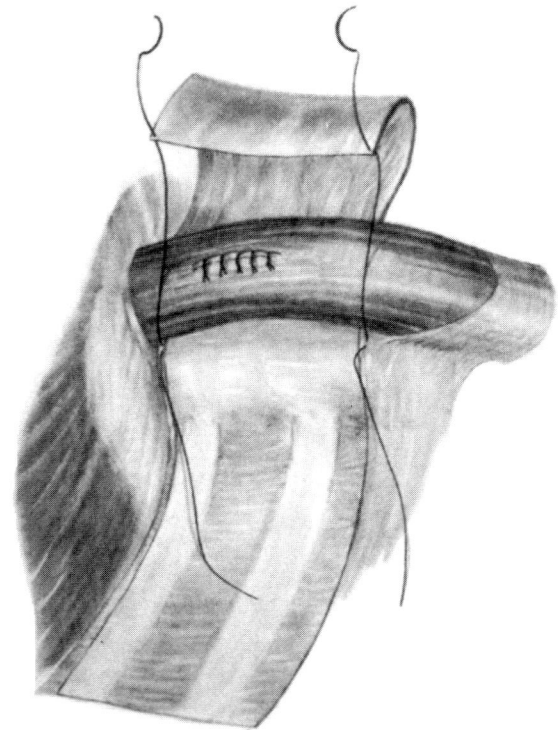

FIGURE 14–40. When possible, a pedicled flap of parietal pleura should be wrapped around the area of repair to serve as a buttress. (From Hood, R. M., Boyd, A. D., and Culliford, A. T.: Thoracic Trauma. Philadelphia, W. B. Saunders, 1989.)

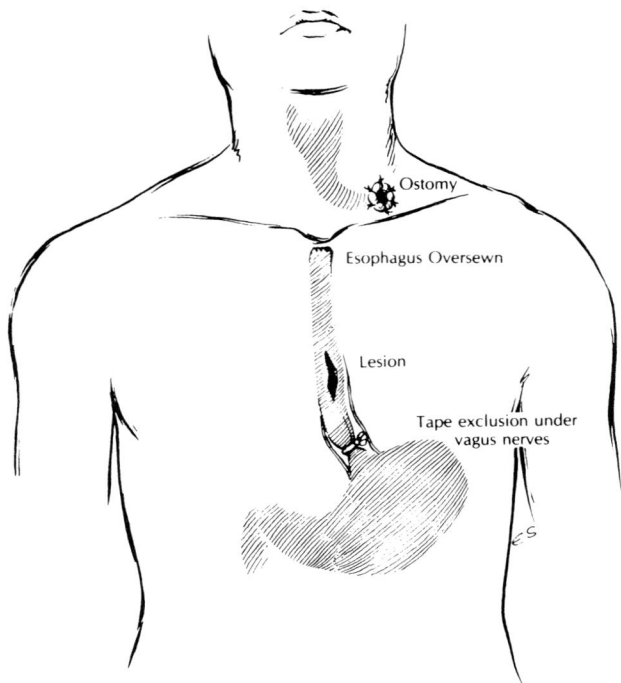

FIGURE 14–41. Esophageal exclusion for large esophageal defects or injuries in which there has been a delay in diagnosis. A cervical esophagostomy is combined with transabdominal ligation of the distal esophagus. A feeding gastrostomy should also be done. (From Blaisdell, F. W., and Trunkey, D. D.: Trauma Management. Vol. III. Cervico-thoracic Trauma. New York, Thieme, 1986.)

SELECTED BIBLIOGRAPHY

Beal, S. L., and McKennan, M.: Blunt diaphragm rupture: A morbid injury. Arch. Surg., *123*:828, 1988.

A large series of blunt diaphragmatic ruptures is reviewed. Epidemiologic characteristics of this relatively uncommon injury are discussed, and some of the pitfalls of diagnosis are highlighted. There are also several good radiographic examples of subtle findings associated with the diagnosis.

Bodai, B. I., Smith, J. P., Ward, R. E., et al.: Emergency thoracotomy in the management of trauma, a review. J. A. M. A., *249*:1891, 1983.

This is a relatively old review of the state of the art with respect to management of trauma patients who arrive in the emergency department in extremis, but the management principles outlined have not changed appreciably since the review was published. There is a good compilation of existing studies examining this topic, and a sound statistical basis is established for the principles outlined.

Cohn, H. E., Hubbard, A., and Patton, G.: Management of esophageal injuries. Ann. Thorac. Surg., *48*:309, 1989.

Only some of the patients in this series of 39 esophageal injuries had trauma as their mechanism of injury, but the principles of management for esophageal injury from other mechanisms are applicable to traumatic injuries. Management of cervical, thoracic, and abdominal esophageal injuries is discussed.

Fallon, W. F., and Wears, R. L.: Prophylactic antibiotics for the prevention of infectious complications including empyema following tube thoracostomy for trauma: Results of meta-analysis. J. Trauma, *33*:110, 1992.

The statistical technique of meta-analysis is applied to six clinical trials of antibiotic prophylaxis in patients requiring chest tubes for trauma. When results of the individual trials are considered separately, the results are conflicting. When analyzed in combination, the prophylactic effect of antibiotic coverage is significant.

Garramone, R. R., Jacobs, L. M., and Sahdev, P.: An objective method to measure and manage occult pneumothorax. Surg. Gynecol. Obstet., *173*:257, 1991.

This paper discusses the management of small pneumothoraces seen on abdominal computerized tomography and provides quantitative guidelines as to which of these occult lesions can be treated expectantly.

Ishikawa, T., Nakajima, Y., and Kaji, T.: The role of CT in traumatic rupture of the thoracic aorta and its proximal branches. Semin. Roentgenol., *24*:38, 1989.

This paper presents an algorithm for the use of computed tomography in the work-up of patients whose chest film suggests torn thoracic aorta. The number of cases is relatively small and there is a heavy reliance on CT in selected subgroups of patients, but the algorithm is logical.

Ivatury, R. R., Simon, R. J., Weksler, B., et al.: Laparoscopy in the evaluation of the intrathoracic abdomen after penetrating injury. J. Trauma, *33*:101, 1992.

The authors report laparoscopic experience in the work-up of patients with penetrating injury. There was a relatively high frequency of diaphragmatic injuries in this series, and laparoscopy proved reliable in making this diagnosis.

Lorenz, H. P., Steinmetz, B., Lieberman, J., et al.: Emergency thoracotomy: Survival correlates with physiologic status. J. Trauma, *32*:780, 1992.

In this series of emergency thoracotomies done for trauma, the physiologic status of patients is emphasized. The authors conclude that emergency thoracotomy is not indicated if there have been no signs of life in the field and that there should be a low threshold for performance of emergency thoracotomy in patients with penetrating mechanisms of injury.

Mattox, K. L. (ed): Thoracic trauma. Surg. Clin. North Am., 69(1), 1989.

This entire issue of *Surgical Clinics of North America* is devoted to thoracic injury. There are excellent articles on the history of thoracic trauma and the epidemiology of thoracic injury. The editor is quite knowledgeable on the subject, and the review is quite good.

Mattox, K. L., Flint, L. M., Carrico, C. J., et al.: Blunt cardiac injury. J. Trauma, *33*:649, 1992.

In this editorial on the subject of myocardial contusion, the authors summarize the current state of knowledge and make specific recommendations about the management of patients suspected of such injury. They also discuss the relevant terminology and injury severity scoring of this entity.

Pevec, W. C., Udekwu, A. O., and Peitzman, A. B.: Blunt rupture of the myocardium. Ann. Thorac. Surg., *48*:139, 1989.

This is an excellent and comprehensive review of these relatively uncommon injuries that includes discussion of their diagnosis and management. The mechanisms of injury and pitfalls in making the diagnosis in subtle cases are particularly interesting. The bibliography is thorough.

Symbas, P. N.: Cardiothoracic trauma. Curr. Prob. Surg., *28*:742, 1991.

This is a comprehensive review of the subject by a knowledgeable author with a great deal of personal experience. The sections on penetrating trauma are especially good and excellently describe the epidemiology and treatment of these injuries.

Symbas, P. N., Justicz, A. G., and Ricketts, R. R.: Rupture of the airways from blunt trauma: Treatment of complex injuries. Ann. Thorac. Surg., *54*:177, 1992.

These injuries are uncommon, but the authors nicely review their own experience and the available literature on this topic. Specific principles of diagnosis and operative management are discussed.

Wisner, D. H., Reed, W. H., and Riddick, R. S.: Suspected myocardial contusion: Triage and indications for monitoring. Ann. Surg., *212*:82, 1990.

Review of a large blunt trauma experience done to determine reliable guidelines for the diagnosis and work-up of myocardial contusion in patients with blunt chest trauma. A sensible algorithm is presented.

BIBLIOGRAPHY

Agee, C. K., Metzler, M. H., Churchill, R. J., and Mitchell, F. L.: Computed tomographic evaluation to exclude traumatic aortic disruption. J. Trauma, *33*:876, 1992.

American College of Surgeons: Advanced Trauma Life Support Course. Chicago, American College of Surgeons, 1989.

Anel, D.: L'Art de Sucer les Plaies. Amsterdam, 1707.

Aristotle: De Partibus Animalum. Peck, A. (trans). Cambridge, MA, Harvard University Press, 1937.

Arom, K. V., Grover, F. L., Richardson, J. D., and Trinkle, J. K.: Posttraumatic empyema. Ann. Thorac. Surg., *23*:254, 1977.

Attar, S., Suter, C. M., Hankins, J. R., et al.: Penetrating cardiac injuries. Ann. Thorac. Surg., *51*:711, 1991.

Baker, C. C., Thomas, A. N., and Trunkey, D. D.: The role of emergency room thoracotomy in trauma. J. Trauma, *20*:848, 1980.

Barone, J. E., Pizzi, W. F., Nealon, T. F., Jr., and Richman, H.: Indications for intubation in blunt chest trauma. J. Trauma, *26*:334, 1986.

Bassett, J. S., Gibson, R. D., and Wilson, R. F.: Blunt injuries to the chest. J. Trauma, *8*:418, 1968.

Baumgartner, F., Sheppard, B., de Virgilio, C., et al.: Tracheal and main bronchial disruptions after blunt chest trauma: Presentation and management. Ann. Thorac. Surg., *50*:569, 1990.

Beal, S. L., and McKennan, M.: Blunt diaphragm rupture. A morbid injury. Arch. Surg., *123*:828, 1988.

Beal, S. L., Pottmeyer, E. W., and Spisso, J. M.: Esophageal perforation following external blunt trauma. J. Trauma, *28*:1425, 1988.

Beeson, A., and Spegesser, F.: Color Atlas of Chest Trauma and Associated Injuries. Oradell, NJ, Medical Economics Books, 1983.

Bender, J. S., and Lucas, C. E.: Management of close-range shotgun injuries to the chest by diaphragmatic transposition: Case reports. J. Trauma, *30*:1581, 1990.

Billroth, T. (Quoted by Jeger, E.): Die Chirurgie der Blutgefass und des Herzens. Berlin, Hirschwal, 1913, p. 295.

Bodai, B. I., Smith, J. P., and Blaisdell, F. W.: The role of emergency thoracotomy in blunt trauma. J. Trauma, *22*:487, 1982.

Bodai, B. I., Smith, J. P., Ward, R. E., et al.: Emergency thoracotomy in the management of trauma. J. A. M. A., *249*:1891, 1983.

Boyd, M., Vanek, V. W., and Bourguet, C. C.: Emergency room resuscitative thoracotomy: When is it indicated? J. Trauma, *33*:714, 1992.

Brathwaite, C. E. M., Rodriguez, A., Turney, S. Z., et al.: Blunt traumatic cardiac rupture. Ann. Surg., *212*:701, 1990.

Breasted, J. H.: The Edwin Smith Papyrus. Vol. 1. Chicago, University of Chicago Press, 1930.

Brooks, A. P., Olson, L. K., and Shackford, S. R.: Computed tomography in the diagnosis of traumatic rupture of the thoracic aorta. Clin. Radiol., 40:133, 1988.

Carlson, G. C., Ray, C., and Klain, M.: High frequency positive pressure ventilation in management of patients with bronchopleural fistula. Anesthesiology, 52:160, 1980.

Cohn, H. E., Hubbard, A., and Patton, G.: Management of esophageal injuries. Ann. Thorac. Surg., 48:309, 1989.

Condon, R. E.: Spontaneous resolution of experimental clotted hemothorax. Surg. Gynecol. Obstet., 126:505, 1968.

Coselli, J. S., Mattox, K. L., and Beall, A. C., Jr.: Reevaluation of early evacuation of clotted hemothorax. Am. J. Surg., 148:786, 1984.

Demetriades, D.: Cardiac penetrating injuries: Personal experience of 45 cases. Br. J. Surg., 71:95, 1984.

Dubrow, T. J., Mihalka, J., Eisenhauer, D. M., et al.: Myocardial contusion in the stable patient: What level of care is appropriate? Surgery, 106:267, 1989.

Duff, J. H., Goldstein, M., McLean, A. P. H., et al.: Flail chest: A clinical review and physiological study. J. Trauma, 8:63, 1968.

Durham, L. A. III, Richardson, R. J., Wall, M. J., et al.: Emergency center thoracotomy: Impact of prehospital resuscitation. J. Trauma, 32:775, 1992.

Durham, R. M., Olson, S., and Weigelt, J. A.: Penetrating injuries to the stomach. Surg. Gynecol. Obstet., 172:298, 1991.

Engberg, G.: Relief of postoperative pain with intercostal blockage compared with the use of narcotic drug. Acta Anaesth. Scand. 70(Suppl.):36, 1978.

Esposito, T. J., Jurkovich, G. J., Rice, C. L., et al.: Reappraisal of emergency room thoracotomy in a changing environment. J. Trauma, 31:881, 1991.

Fabian, T. C., Mangiante, E. C., Patterson, C. R., et al.: Myocardial contusion in blunt trauma: Clinical characteristics, means of diagnosis, and implications for patient management. J. Trauma, 28:50, 1988.

Fallon, W. F., Jr., and Wears, R. L.: Prophylactic antibiotics for the prevention of infectious complications including empyema following tube thoracostomy for trauma: Results of meta analysis. J. Trauma, 33:110, 1992.

Feczko, J. D., Lynch, L., Pless, J. E., et al.: An autopsy case review of 142 nonpenetrating (blunt) injuries of the aorta. J. Trauma, 33:846, 1992.

Flancbaum, L., Wright, J., and Siegel, J. H.: Emergency surgery in patients with post-traumatic myocardial contusion. J. Trauma, 26:795, 1986.

Flynn, A. E., Thomas, A. N., and Schecter, W. P.: Acute tracheobronchial injury. J. Trauma, 29:1326, 1989.

Freshman, S. P., Wisner, D. H., and Weber, C. J.: 2-D echocardiography: Emergent use in the evaluation of penetrating precordial trauma. J. Trauma, 31:902, 1991.

Fulda, G., Brathwaite, C. E. M., Rodriguez, A., et al.: Blunt traumatic rupture of the heart and pericardium: A ten-year experience (1979–1989). J. Trauma, 31:167, 1991.

Garramone, R. R., Jr., Jacobs, L. M., and Sahdev, P.: An objective method to measure and manage occult pneumothorax. Surgery, 173:257, 1991.

Gibbons, J. A., Peniston, R. L., Diamond, S. S., and Aaron, B. L.: A comparison of synthetic absorbable suture with synthetic nonabsorbable suture for construction of tracheal anastomoses. Chest, 79:340, 1981.

Graham, E. A.: A brief account of the development of thoracic surgery and some of its consequences. Surg. Gynecol. Obstet., 104:241, 1957.

Graham, E. A., and Bell, R. D.: Open pneumothorax: Its reaction to the treatment of empyema. Am. J. Med. Sci., 156:839, 1918.

Graham, J. M., Beall, A. C., Jr., Mattox, K. L., and Waughan, G. D.: Systemic air embolism following penetrating trauma to the lung. Chest, 72:449, 1977.

Graham, J. M., Feliciano, D. V., Mattox, I. L., et al.: Management of subclavian vascular injuries. J. Trauma, 20:537, 1980.

Graham, J. M., Mattox, K. L., and Beall, A. C., Jr.: Penetrating trauma of the lung. J. Trauma, 19:665, 1979.

Grande, C. M., Stene, J. K., and Bernhard, W. N.: Airway management: Considerations in the trauma patient. Crit. Care Clin., 6:37, 1990.

Grosso, M. A., Brown, J. M., Moore, E. E., and Moore, F. A.: Repair of the torn descending thoracic aorta using the centrifugal pump with partial left heart bypass: Technical note. J. Trauma, 31:395, 1991.

Grover, F. L., Ellestad, C., Arom, K. V., et al.: Diagnosis and management of major tracheobronchial injuries. Ann. Thorac. Surg., 28:384, 1979.

Gundry, S. R., Burney, R. E., MacKenzie, J. R., et al.: Assessment of mediastinal widening associated with traumatic rupture of the aorta. J. Trauma, 23:293, 1983.

Guthrie, G. J.: On Wounds and Injuries of the Chest. London, Renshaw and Churchill, 1848.

Gyhra, A., Pierart, J., Torres, P., and Prieto, L.: Experimental cardiac tamponade with a myocardial wound: The effect of rapid intravenous infusion of saline. J. Trauma, 33:25, 1992.

Heiberg, E., Wolverson, M. K., Sundaram, M., and Shields, J. B.: CT in aortic trauma. A. J. R., 140:1119, 1983.

Hippocrates: Works. Vol. III. Withington, E. T. (trans). Cambridge, MA, Harvard University Press, 1959, p. 307.

Hunt, G. B., Malik, R., Bellenger, C. R., and Pearson, M. R. B.: Total venous inflow occlusion in the normothermic dog: A study of hemodynamic, metabolic and neurological consequences: Res. Vet. Sci., 52:371, 1992.

Ilgenfritz, F. M., and Stewart, D. E.: Blunt trauma of the diaphragm: A 15-county, private hospital experience. Am. Surg., 6:334, 1992.

Ishikawa, T., Nakajima, Y., and Kaji, T.: The role of CT in traumatic rupture of the thoracic aorta and its proximal branches. Semin. Roentgenol., 24:38, 1989.

Ivatury, R. R., Kazigo, J., Rohman, M., et al.: "Directed" emergency room thoracotomy: A prognostic prerequisite for survival. J. Trauma, 31:1076, 1991a.

Ivatury, R. R., Rohman, M., Steichen, F. M., et al.: Penetrating cardiac injuries: Twenty-year experience. Am. Surg., 53:310, 1987.

Ivatury, R. R., Simon, R. J., Weksler, B., et al.: Laparoscopy in the evaluation of the intrathoracic abdomen after penetrating injury. J. Trauma, 33:101, 1991b.

Jimenez, E., Martin, M., Krukenkamp, I., and Barrett, J.: Subxiphoid pericardiotomy versus echocardiography: A prospective evaluation of the diagnosis of occult penetrating cardiac injury. Surgery, 108:676, 1990.

Johnston, J. R., and McCaughey, W.: Epidural morphine. A method of management of multiple fractured ribs. Anaesthesia, 35:155, 1980.

Jones, W. S., Mavroudis, C., Richardson, J. D., et al.: Management of tracheobronchial disruption resulting from blunt trauma. Surgery, 95:319, 1984.

Jones, R. J., and Samson, P. C.: Esophageal injury. Ann. Thorac. Surg., 19:216, 1975.

Kearney, P. A., Rouhana, S. W., and Burney, R. E.: Blunt rupture of the diaphragm: Mechanism, diagnosis, and treatment. Ann. Emerg. Med., 18:1326, 1989.

Knott-Craig, C. J., Dalton, R. P., Rossouw, G. J., and Barnard, P. M.: Penetrating cardiac trauma: Management strategy based on 129 surgical emergencies over 2 years. Ann. Thorac. Surg., 53:1006, 1992.

Livingston, D. H., Tortella, B. J., Blackwood, J., et al.: The role of laparoscopy in abdominal trauma. J. Trauma, 33:471, 1992.

LoCicero, J., and Mattox, K. L.: Epidemiology of chest trauma. Surg. Clin. North Am., 69(1):15, 1989.

LoCurto, J. H., Jr., Tischler, C. D., Swan, K. G., et al.: Tube thoracostomy and trauma—Antibiotics or not? J. Trauma, 26:1067, 1986.

Lorenz, H. P., Steinmetz, B., Liberman, J., et al.: Emergency thoracotomy: Survival correlates with physiologic status. J. Trauma, 32:780, 1992.

MacIntyre, N. R.: New forms of mechanical ventilation in the adult. Clin. Chest Med., 9:47, 1988.

Mackersie, R. C., Shackford, S. R., Hoyt, D. B., and Karagianes, T. G.: Continuous epidural fentanyl analgesia: Ventilatory function improvement with routine use in treatment of blunt chest injury. J. Trauma, 27:1207, 1987.

Maloney, J. V., Jr., Schnutzer, K. L., and Raschke, F.: Paradoxical respiration and "pendelluft." J. Thorac. Cardiovasc. Surg., 41:291, 1961.

Mansour, M. A., Moore, E. E., Moore, F. A., and Read, R. R.: Exigent postinjury thoracotomy analysis of blunt versus penetrating trauma. Surg. Gynecol. Obstet., 175:97, 1992.

Mariadason, J. G., Parsa, M. H., Ayuyao, A., and Freeman, H. P.: Management of stab wounds to the thoracoabdominal region. A clinical approach. Ann. Surg., 207:335, 1988.

Marshall, W. G., Jr., Bell, J. L., and Kouchoukos, N. T.: Penetrating cardiac trauma. J. Trauma, 24:147, 1984.

Mattox, K. L., Feliciano, D. V., Beall, A. C., et al.: Five thousand seven hundred sixty cardiovascular injuries in 4459 patients. Ann. Surg., 209:698, 1989.

Mattox, K. L., Flint, L. M., Carrico, C. J., et al.: Blunt cardiac injury [Editorial]. J. Trauma, 33:649, 1992.

Mayor-Davies, J. A., and Britz, R. S.: Subxiphoid pericardial windows—Helpful in selected cases. J. Trauma, 30:1399, 1990.

McCroskey, B. L., Moore, E. E., Moore, F. A., and Abernathy, C. M.: A unified approach to the torn thoracic aorta. Am. J. Surg., 162:473, 1991.

McLean, R. F., Devitt, J. H., McLellan, B. A., et al.: Significance of myocardial contusion following blunt chest trauma. J. Trauma, 33:240, 1992.

McLean, T. R., Olinger, G. N., and Thorsen, M. K.: Computed tomography in the evaluation of the aorta in patients sustaining blunt chest trauma. J. Trauma, 31:254, 1991.

Meier, G. H., Symbas, P. N., Wood, W. J.: Systemic air embolization for penetrating lung injury. Ann. Thorac. Surg., 27:161, 1979.

Merion, R. M., Harness, J. K., Ramsburgh, S. R., and Thompson, N. W.: Selective management of penetrating neck trauma. Cost implications. Arch. Surg., 116:691, 1981.

Merrill, W. H., Lee, R. B., Hammon, J. W., Jr., et al.: Surgical treatment of acute traumatic tear of the thoracic aorta. Ann. Surg., 207:699, 1988.

Miller, F. B., Richardson, J. D., and Thomas, H. A.: Role of CT in the diagnosis of major arterial injury after blunt thoracic trauma. Surgery, 106:596, 1989a.

Miller, F. B., Shumate, C. R., and Richardson, J. D.: Myocardial contusion. Arch. Surg., 124:805, 1989b.

Millham, F. H., Rajii-Khorasani, A., Birkett, D. F., and Hirsch, E. F.: Carinal injury: Diagnosis and treatment. J. Trauma, 31:1420, 1991.

Naughton, M. J., Brissie, R. M., Bessey, P. Q., et al.: Demography of penetrating cardiac trauma. Ann. Surg., 209:675, 1989.

Nelson, J. B., Bresticker, M. A., and Nahrwold, D. L.: Computed tomography in the initial evaluation of patients with blunt trauma. J. Trauma, 33:722, 1992.

Nesbitt, J. C., and Sawyers, J. L.: Surgical management of esophageal perforation. Am. Surg., 53:183, 1987.

Newman, R. J., and Jones, I. S.: A prospective study of 413 consecutive car occupants with chest injuries. J. Trauma, 24:129, 1984.

Nirgiotis, J. G., Colon, R., and Sweeney, M. S.: Blunt trauma to the heart: The pathophysiology of injury. J. Emerg. Med., 8:617, 1990.

Oliver, H. E., Jr., Maher, T. D., Liebler, G. A., et al.: Use of the biomedicus centrifugal pump in traumatic tears of the thoracic aorta. Ann. Thorac. Surg., 38:586, 1984.

Paré, A.: Collected Works (A.D. 1582). Johnson, I. (trans). London, 1634, p. 571.

Parham, A. M. L., Yarbrogh, D. R. III, and Redding, J. S.: Flail chest syndrome and pulmonary contusion. Arch. Surg., 113:900, 1978.

Parmley, L. F., Mattingly, T. W., and Manlow, W. C.: Non-penetrating traumatic injury to the aorta. Circulation, 17:1096, 1958.

Pederson, V. M., Schulze, S., Hoier-Madsen, K., et al.: Air-flow meter assessment of the effect of interstitial nerve blockage on respiratory function in rib fractures. ACTF Chir. Scand., 149:119, 1983.

Pevec, W. C., Udekwu, A. O., and Peitzman, A. B.: Blunt rupture of the myocardium. Ann. Thorac. Surg., 48:139, 1989.

Pickard, L. R., and Mattox, K. L.: Thoracic Trauma General Considerations and Indications for Thoracotomy in Trauma. 2nd ed. Norwalk, CT, Appleton & Lange, 1991, p. 319.

Pickard, L. R., Mattox, K. L., Espada, R., et al.: Transection of the descending thoracic aorta secondary to blunt trauma. J. Trauma, 17:749, 1977.

Playfair, W. S.: On the treatment of empyema in children. Obstet. Soc. London Trans., 14:4, 1872.

Rayner, A. V. S., Fulton, R. L., Hess, P. J., and Daicoff, G. R.: Post-traumatic intracardiac shunts. Report of two cases and review of the literature. J. Thorac. Cardiovasc. Surg., 73:728, 1977.

Rehn, L.: Veber penetrierende Herzwunder und Herznaht. Arch. Klin. Chir., 55:315, 1897.

Reissman, P., Rivkind, A., Jurim, O., and Simon, D.: Case report: The management of penetrating cardiac trauma with major coronary artery injury—Is cardiopulmonary bypass essential? J. Trauma, 33:773, 1992.

Rhee, K. J., Green, W., Holcroft, J. W., and Mangili, J. A.: Oral intubation in the multiply injured patient: The risk of exacerbating spinal cord injury. Ann. Emerg. Med., 19:511, 1990.

Richardson, J. D., Wilson, M. E., and Miller, F. B.: The widened mediastinum. Diagnostic and therapeutic priorities. Ann. Surg., 211:731, 1990.

Riolanus, J.: En cheiridium anatomicum et pathologicum, in quo ex naturali constitutione partium, recessus, a naturale statu demonstratur; Ad usum theatri anatomici adornatum. Lugd Bat, A Wynegaerden, 1649.

Roscher, R., and Bittner, R.: Pulmonary contusion: Clinical experience. Arch. Surg., 109:500, 1974.

Sankaran, S., and Wilson, R. F.: Factors affecting prognosis in patient with flail chest. J. Thorac. Cardiovasc. Surg., 60:402, 1970.

Scultetus, J.: The Surgeon's Storehouse. London, Starkey, 1674, p. 159.

Shamoun, J. M., Barraza, K. R., Jurkovich, G. J., and Salley, R. K.: In extremis use of staples for cardiorrhaphy in penetrating cardiac trauma: Case report. J. Trauma, 29:1589, 1989.

Shapiro, M. J., Yanofsky, S. D., Trapp, J., et al.: Cardiovascular evaluation in blunt thoracic trauma using transesophageal echocardiography (TEE). J. Trauma, 31:835, 1991.

Shorr, R. M., Rodriguez, A., Indeck, M. C., et al.: Blunt chest trauma in the elderly. J. Trauma, 29:234, 1989.

Smith, R. S., Tsoi, E. K. M., Fry, W. R., et al.: Laparoscopic evaluation of abdominal trauma: A preliminary report. Contemp. Surg., 42:13, 1993.

Stothert, J. C., Jr., Buttorff, J., and Kaminski, D. L.: Thoracic esophageal and tracheal injury following blunt trauma. J. Trauma, 20:992, 1980.

Sturaitis, M., McCallum, D., Sutherland, G., et al.: Lack of significant long-term sequelae following traumatic myocardial contusion. Arch. Intern. Med., 146:1765, 1986.

Sugg, W. L., Rea, W. J., Ecker, R. R., et al.: Penetrating wounds of the heart: Analysis of 459 cases. J. Thorac. Cardiovasc. Surg., 56:531, 1968.

Symbas, P. N.: Cardiothoracic trauma. Curr. Prob. Surg., 28:747, 1991.

Symbas, P. N., Diorio, D. A., Tyras, D. H., et al.: Penetrating cardiac wounds: Significant residual and delayed sequelae. J. Thorac. Cardiovasc. Surg., 66:526, 1973.

Symbas, P. N., Harlaftis, N., and Waldo, W. J.: Penetrating cardiac wounds: A comparison of different therapeutic methods. Ann. Surg., 183:377, 1976.

Symbas, P. N., Justicz, A. G., and Ricketts, R. R.: Rupture of the airways from blunt trauma: Treatment of complex injuries. Ann. Thorac. Surg., 54:177, 1992.

Tenzer, M. L.: The spectrum of myocardial contusion: A review. J. Trauma, 25:620, 1985.

Thomas, A. H., and Roe, B. B.: Air embolism following penetrating injuries. J. Thorac. Cardiovasc. Surg., 66:533, 1973.

Trinkle, J. K., Richardson, J. D., and Franz, J. L., et al.: Management of flail chest without mechanical ventilation. Ann. Thorac. Surg., 19:355, 1975.

Urschel, H. C., and Razzuk, M. A.: Management of acute traumatic injuries of tracheobronchial tree. Surg. Gynecol. Obstet., 136:113, 1973.

Van Norman, G. A., Pavlin, E. G., Eddy, A. C., and Pavlin, D. J.: Hemodynamic and metabolic effects of aortic unclamping following emergency surgery for traumatic thoracic aortic tear in shunted and unshunted patients. J. Trauma, 31:1007, 1991.

West, J. G., Williams, M. J., Trunkey, D. D., and Wolferth, C. C., Jr.: Trauma systems. Current status—Future challenges. J. A. M. A., 259:3597, 1988.

Wing, V. W., Federle, M. P., Morris, J. A., Jr., et al.: The clinical impact of CT for blunt abdominal trauma. A. J. R., *145:*1191, 1985.

Winter, R. P., and Weigelt, J. A.: Cervical esophageal trauma. Arch. Surg., *125:*849, 1990.

Wisner, D. H.: A stepwise logistic regression analysis of factors affecting morbidity and mortality after thoracic trauma: Effect of epidural analgesia. J. Trauma, *30:*799, 1990.

Wisner, D. H., Reed, W. H., and Riddick, R. S.: Suspected myocardial contusion. Triage and indications for monitoring. Ann. Surg., *212:*82, 1990.

Wisner, D. H., and Sturm, J. A.: Symposium paper. Controversies in the fluid management of post traumatic lung disease. Injury, *17:*295, 1986.

Wood, P. R., and Lawler, P. G. P.: Managing the airway in cervical spine injury. A review of the Advanced Trauma Life Support protocol. Anaesthesia, *47:*792, 1992.

Worthley, L. I. G.: Thoracic epidural in the management of chest trauma. Intens. Care Med., *11:*312, 1985.

Young, J. N., Stallone, R. J., Iverson, L. I. G., et al.: Surgical management of traumatic disruption of the descending aorta. West. J. Med., *150:*662, 1989.

15

Disorders of the Sternum and the Thoracic Wall

■ I Congenital Deformities of the Chest Wall

Kevin P. Landolfo and David C. Sabiston, Jr.

The growing appreciation that congenital chest wall deformities are often associated with clinically significant, surgically correctable, physiologic derangements has heightened awareness of these problems in both the medical and the surgical communities. The psychological impact on patients with these conditions often overshadows physical limitations, and surgical correction can be expected to yield positive results. Much of the management strategy and surgical technique for correction of chest wall deformities has been pioneered by Ravitch, whose extensive publications in this field are well known (Ravitch, 1949, 1951, 1952, 1960, 1961, 1962, 1965, 1966, 1972a, 1972b, 1977a, 1977b, 1979, 1980, 1981, 1986, 1988; Ravitch and Matzen, 1968).

PECTUS EXCAVATUM

Pectus excavatum is the most common congenital deformity of the sternum, occurring in as many as 1 in 300 to 1 in 400 live births (Ravitch, 1977b). This condition is seen as a continuum, from a very mild deformity to one that is severe (Fig. 15–1), and although a number of grading systems have been proposed, none has been universally accepted (Haller et al., 1987; Hummer and Willital, 1984; Welch, 1980).

Theories regarding the etiology of this defect have included functional abnormalities of the anterior diaphragm (Brodkin, 1953) and a short central tendon (Brown, 1939), as well as failure of osteogenesis and chondrogenesis (Mullard, 1967). However, the currently accepted cause of pectus excavatum is an excessive, misdirected growth of the lower costal cartilages, which form congenitally in a concave manner because of rapid growth and create a depressed sternum (Garcia et al., 1989; Ochsner and DeBakey, 1939). The first and second ribs, as well as the corresponding costal cartilages, are often uninvolved, with the most severe depression just above the xiphoid process and continuing cephalad to the sternomanubrial junction. In extreme cases, the sternum may be depressed laterally to the vertebral gutter. As the prevertebral space is reduced, the heart is usually depressed to the left, as shown on the chest film (Fig. 15–2), and the extent of the cardiac depression that may occur is seen on the

computed tomography (CT) scan (Fig. 15–3). Although this deformity is usually present at birth, sporadic cases have occurred as late as adolescence (Shamberger et al., 1988). In most patients, the severity of the defect increases with time. To date there have been no reliable indicators, other than clinical reevaluation, as to which defects progress and which defects remain static. Although a familial incidence of pectus excavatum has been described (Leung and Hoo, 1987; Welch, 1980), many cases are sporadic.

Clinical Manifestations

Symptomatic improvement following surgical correction of a pectus deformity was documented as early as 1913 in an 18-year-old man presenting with dyspnea and palpitations. After the operation, his exercise tolerance improved such that he could return to heavy manual labor (Sauerbruch, 1920). However, most infants and young children with pectus excavatum are asymptomatic. When questioned carefully, older children and teenagers may become aware that they do not have the same respiratory reserve as their peers. This finding is most noticeable when heavy and continuous exercise is performed. After a corrective surgical procedure, it is common for these patients to notice increased stamina, now that they are fully aware of their preoperative exercise limitation. In some patients, serious cardiorespiratory problems improve after surgical correction (Ravitch, 1951). Frequent and recurrent lower respiratory tract infections and asthma may be seen in as many as 32% of patients with this deformity (Fonkalsrud et al., 1994).

Scoliosis may be found in association with anterior chest wall deformities (Iseman et al., 1991; Waters et al., 1989). One review (Waters et al., 1989) cited a 21.5% incidence of scoliosis in patients with pectus excavatum. Paraspinal muscle imbalance and asymmetric pneumatic thoracic pressures may be the etiologic factors in these children. The abnormality usually involves a single thoracic curve originating between T4 and T9, inclusive. Although only a small number of these patients require specific therapy (18%), the relative frequency of this association suggests that children with pectus excavatum should be screened for scoliosis.

494

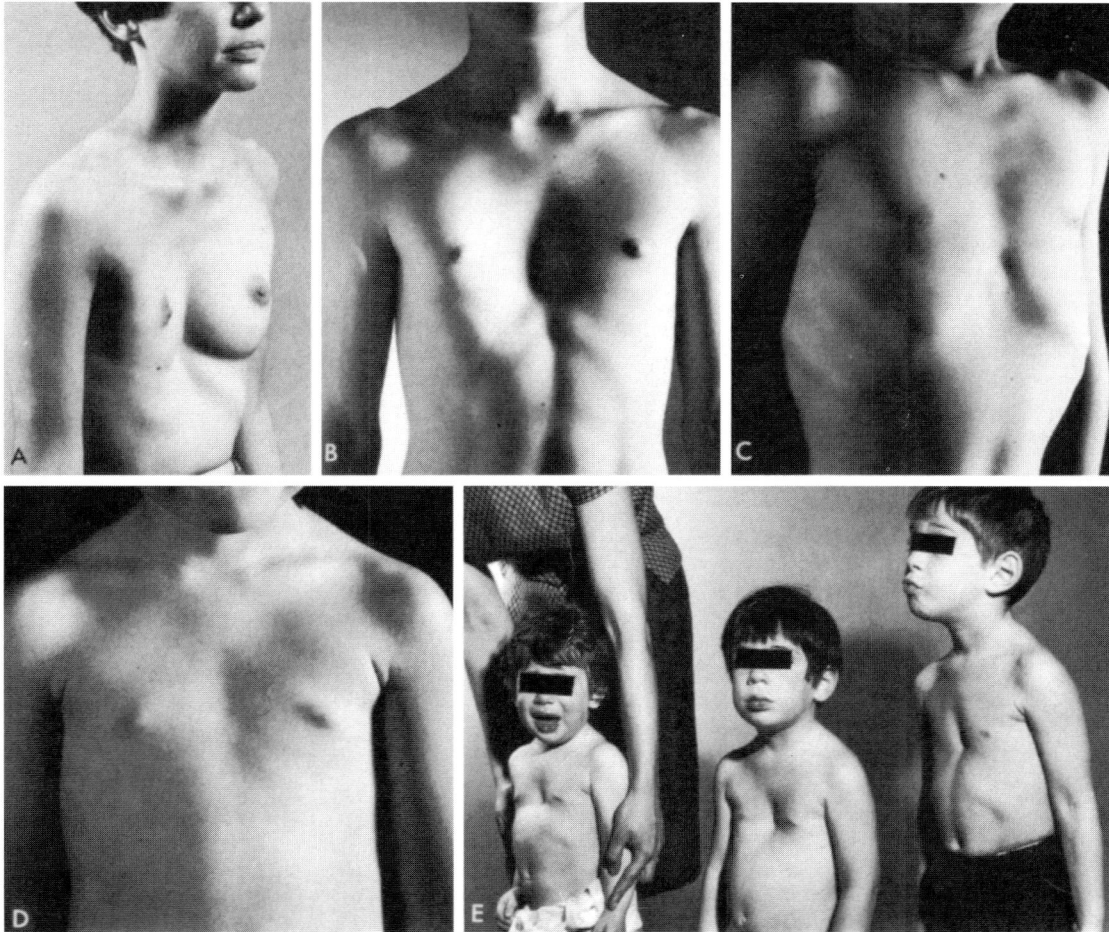

FIGURE 15–1. Pectus excavatum has a variety of appearances in two families. Although most of the patients have been sporadic, the authors have frequently operated on pairs of siblings. There is often a familial history and the authors have operated on one parent-and-child combination. The varieties of expression of pectus deformities in two families are seen here. *A*, The oldest sister has a deep asymmetric deformity (note that the right nipple points obliquely to the left). She was modestly symptomatic. As is not uncommon, the right breast is smaller and less well developed than the left breast, and the rotation of the sternum is to the right. *B*, Her teenage brother has a progressive deformity and no obvious symptoms. *C* and *D*, Younger children in the same family. The two older children underwent operations with satisfactory restoration of thoracic contour. The younger children's deformities were not severe enough to require an operation. The boy with a broad, shallow deformity (*C*) may well show a progression that will require an operation in the future. We believe that his young sister (*D*) will not require an operation. *E*, Three brothers showing the characteristic posture, rounded shoulders, and potbelly (in the two younger brothers).

Mitral valve prolapse has also been observed, either clinically or echocardiographically, in 40 to 65% of patients whose pectus deformities were subsequently corrected (Bon Tempo et al., 1975; Roman et al., 1989; Saint-Mézard et al., 1986; Salomon et al., 1975; Shamberger et al., 1987). The cause of the mitral valve prolapse has not been completely defined, but because postoperative resolution has been demonstrated in many cases, there may be a mechanical etiology (Shamberger et al., 1987, 1988).

The physiologic effect of pectus excavatum has been the topic of much debate; there is no consensus on the degree of cardiopulmonary impairment produced. Although it was previously believed that few, if any, patients had respiratory or cardiac insufficiency (Haller et al., 1970), several studies have provided evidence that both cardiac and respiratory functions are slightly below normal, and that these abnormali-

ties are exacerbated by exercise and position (Shamberger et al., 1988).

In a study of Air Force recruits with pectus excavatum who complained of exercise intolerance, significant decreases were found both in the force of the expiratory flow and in maximal voluntary ventilation when compared with unselected recruits (Weg et al., 1967). Additional reports suggest a restrictive pulmonary abnormality attributable to an extrapulmonary cause. This was manifested by a decrease in transpulmonary and transdiaphragmatic pressures, which did not improve following surgical correction of the chest wall abnormality (Derveaux et al., 1988, 1989; Kaguraoka et al., 1992).

Lung volumes were measured both preoperatively and postoperatively in another series of patients. Children with pectus excavatum demonstrated low normal vital capacities that were unchanged by opera-

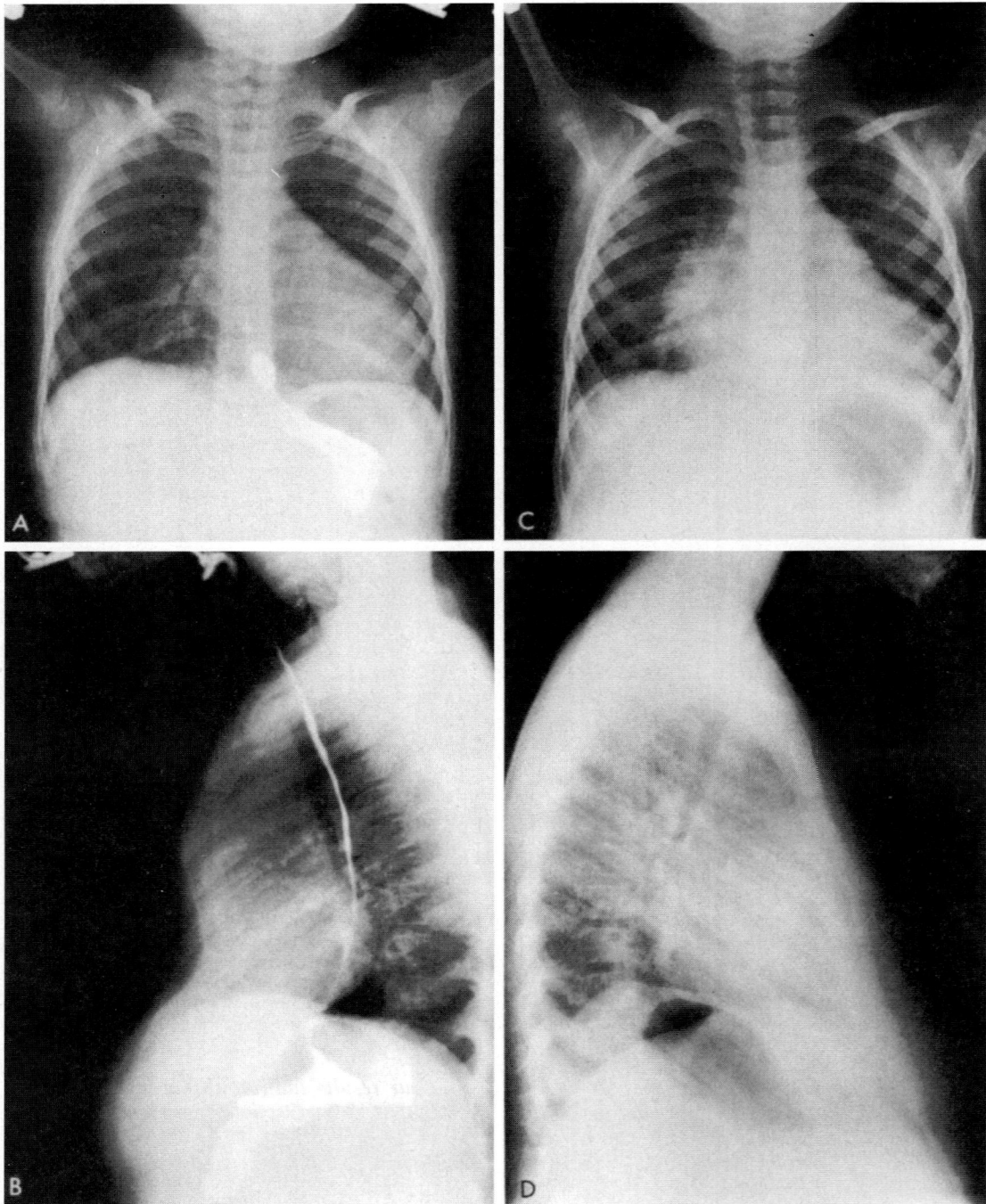

FIGURE 15–2. Posteroanterior (PA) and lateral views before and after operation in a 6-year-old girl with pectus excavatum. In the preoperative films (*A* and *B*), note the substantial displacement of the heart to the left in the PA view and the concavity of the sternum, the position of the posterior border of the sternum behind the anterior border of the heart, and the overlapping of the anterior borders of the vertebrae and the posterior borders of the heart in the lateral view. In the postoperative films of this young child (*C* and *D*), the heart has shifted back in the PA view, although this usually requires time for complete correction; in the lateral view, the correction of the sternum and the substantial forward movement of the heart are obvious.

tion; however, total lung capacity and maximal voluntary ventilation significantly improved with corresponding increases in exercise capacity and maximal oxygen consumption (Cahill et al., 1984). Abnormal preoperative pulmonary function assessed by xenon perfusion and ventilation scintigraphy has also significantly improved with surgical correction of the chest wall deformity in some series (Blickman, 1985).

The working capacity of patients with pectus excavatum was normal in the supine position but significantly reduced when sitting. The stroke volume was 40% lower in the sitting position than in the supine

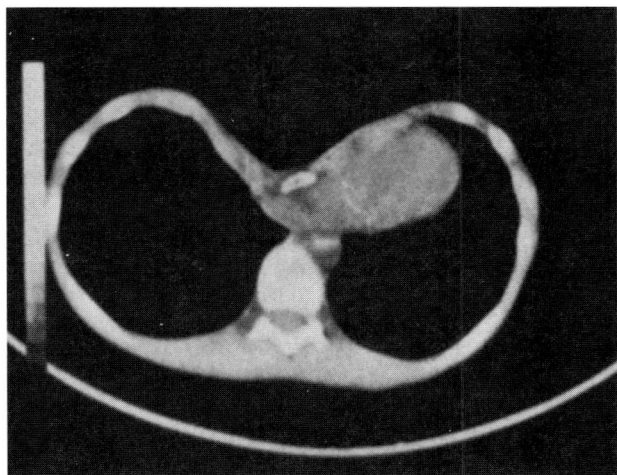

FIGURE 15–3. Computed tomographic image of the chest of a symptomatic 15-year-old boy with severe pectus excavatum. The heart is considerably displaced to the left, and the right ventricle is deformed by compression between the depressed chest wall and the vertebral column. (From Ravitch, M. M.: Disorders of the chest wall. *In* Sabiston, D.C. [ed]: Textbook of Surgery. 14th ed. Philadelphia, W. B. Saunders, 1991.)

position. Moreover, stroke volume increase with exercise was blunted in patients with pectus deformity when measured in the sitting position and was believed to be due to impaired ventricular filling (Bevegard, 1985). In another study, patients with mild restrictive ventilatory defects underwent cardiac catheterization at rest in the supine position. Normal right atrial, right ventricular, pulmonary arterial, and pulmonary wedge pressures were observed, and cardiac index was normal. However, in some patients, cardiac output during upright exercise was below the normal range, primarily because of a subnormal increase in the stroke volume. From these studies, Beiser and associates (1972) at the National Heart, Lung, and Blood Institute concluded:

Our results indicate that a mild to moderate pectus-excavatum deformity interferes importantly with cardiac function, primarily when exercise is performed in the upright position. These results appear to explain the disparity between operative reports describing marked clinical improvement in patients after correction of pectus excavatum deformities and hemodynamic reports indicating little or no cardiac abnormality in such patients.

Changes in cardiac function have been demonstrated during rest and exercise after the pectus deformity was corrected using single-pass radionuclide angiocardiography. Exercise studies done on patients in the upright position on a bicycle at 6 months or more after correction showed that the operation did not change left ventricular ejection fraction or cardiac index at rest or during exercise. However, the left ventricular end-diastolic volume index and stroke volume index increased at rest after surgical correction. The estimated right ventricular end-diastolic volume also increased greatly after operation and was associated with a reduction in ventricular ejection fraction.

The increase in right and left ventricular volumes after operation suggests that, if present, cardiac compression may be improved by operative correction (Peterson et al., 1985).

On balance, sufficient evidence indicates a cardiopulmonary impairment in patients with pectus excavatum. However, many issues remain unresolved, including an accurate correlation between the severity of the deformity and extent of the cardiopulmonary dysfunction, as well as comparison of various repair techniques and corresponding improvement in postoperative cardiopulmonary function.

Indications for Operation

Increasing numbers of patients with the pectus excavatum deformity are being considered for surgical correction. In most patients, the primary indication for referral is the desire for cosmetic improvement. Patients with this disorder may develop a negative self-image when they begin school. The inquisitive attitude of other children may lead to embarrassment and recognition that the pectus deformity makes them different. These children almost always wear shirts and are seldom comfortable when their chests must be uncovered—for example, during swimming. Unless the condition is surgically corrected before daily attendance at school begins, many of these patients become withdrawn and shy, and they have a significantly different social life from that of their peers. Therefore, the presence of a pectus excavatum in all but very mild cases is an indication for correction. Patients with evidence of respiratory insufficiency, exercise limitation, and recurrent respiratory infections also require operation.

As many as two-thirds of patients with Marfan's syndrome may have associated pectus excavatum deformities (Arn et al., 1989; Scherer et al., 1988; Seliem et al., 1992). Marfan's syndrome was once thought to be a contraindication to operation; however, although patients with this syndrome have a higher recurrence rate, surgical correction of their pectus deformity has been safe and effective (Arn et al., 1989; Scherer et al., 1988).

The timing of the surgical intervention depends partly on the patient's age at the time of consultation. If a significant deformity is present at 1 or 2 years of age, operation can be performed at that time. However, the best results are obtained when the operation is performed on a child 2 to 5 years old. At this age, the deformity usually is limited to the costal cartilages, with minimal rib involvement. Additionally, thoracogenic stress that may lead to secondary scoliosis has not yet occurred (Waters et al., 1989).

Whenever possible, correction should be made before a child reaches school age (approximately 5 years old) to minimize the psychological impact of the deformity. Although surgical correction is possible in patients of any age, the operation is technically easier and may have the best results when performed in younger patients.

Operative Technique

We prefer the technique described by Ravitch (1949, 1977b). The results of this approach have been excellent, and few complications have been encountered. Schlossberg's drawings of the operation as done by Ravitch are classic and are presented here with a description of each technical step. A midline incision is generally made in males (Fig. 15–4A). However, in girls or if the patient prefers a more cosmetic incision, a transverse inframammary incision can be used. This incision requires more dissection and makes adequate exposure more difficult. The skin incision should be made with a scalpel, but the remainder of the dissection should be done with fine needle-tip electrocautery. Through a midline approach, the incision is extended down to the periosteum of the sternum. The pectoralis major muscle on each side is then reflected laterally to expose all costal cartilages (Fig. 15–4B). The lower costal cartilages are often covered by the rectus muscles, which must be split for adequate exposure. The costal cartilages are bilaterally resected subperichondrially for the full length of the deformed segments. The perichondrium is left to form new costal cartilages (Fig. 15–4C). The resected cartilages regenerate rapidly, generally within several months, and a firm anterior wall develops adjacent to the sternum. The stepwise technique and instruments used for resection of the costal cartilages are shown in Figure 15–4C.

After removal of the costal cartilages, the xiphisternal joint is transected (Fig. 15–4D), and a finger can then be passed beneath the sternum into the mediastinum to separate the parietal pleura bilaterally (Fig. 15–4E). The intercostal muscles are then divided. The sternum has now been entirely freed of all attachments except for the sternomanubrial joint. The second, and sometimes the third, costal cartilages may be divided obliquely if they are not deformed, allowing the entire sternum to be lifted anteriorly. A transverse osteotomy is made on the posterior surface of the sternum through the sternomanubrial joint, allowing overcorrection of the sternum. To fix the sternum correctly in this position, a wedge of bone or costal cartilage can be placed in the osteotomy and secured (by two trans-sternal sutures of synthetic monofilament) (Fig. 15–4F). The pectoralis fascia is then approximated with interrupted sutures, and the subcutaneous tissue is closed. Absorbable subcuticular sutures are preferred to skin sutures in children.

In older patients as well as in those with Marfan's syndrome, a Kirschner's wire is usually placed beneath the sternum and underneath the pectoral muscles. The wire should protrude laterally into the subcutaneous tissue on each side to allow palpation, so that the wire can be easily identified later for removal under local anesthesia (Fig. 15–4G). A closed suction drain with multiple perforations is left in the mediastinum. Some surgeons prefer to use multiple needle aspirations of the mediastinum, particularly in infants and young children.

Postoperatively, serous drainage may occur for several days, generally in small amounts. Blood transfusion is rarely necessary. A mild fever may occur during the first 24 hours (38° or 39° C), most frequently because of pulmonary atelectasis. Fortunately, wound infections are rare. The patients are allowed to walk soon after operation. At the time of discharge, these patients are advised to avoid body-contact sports for several months or until the pin has been removed (if one is in place).

Alternatives to Ravitch's technique have been described. A "sternal turnover" was initially proposed by Judet (1954) and Jung (1956). The procedure was modified and popularized in Japan by Wada and coworkers (1970). In this technique, the entire deformed portion of the sternum together with the associated costal cartilages or ribs was excised en bloc with the intercostal muscles. This free graft was then turned over and sutured in place. Wada and associates demonstrated in 271 patients that this large free graft remains viable, an observation supported by other surgeons (Davis and Shah, 1974).

An alternative technique provides a vascular pedicle to supply the sternum after it has been immobilized and inverted. The vascular supply to the sternal graft is based on the internal mammary pedicle (Hawkins et al., 1984). These operative techniques are illustrated and described in Figure 15–5. The authors of this approach have described 26 patients, in 21 of whom (81%) results were good. Results were fair in 4 patients (15%), and two patients with Marfan's syndrome experienced a partial recurrence. In addition, one patient had skin necrosis, and another developed a hypertrophic scar. The last patient had a poor early result due to wound infection and distal sternal necrosis, which required reoperation. Other authors have described the use of vascularized rib struts for correction of pectus (Hayashi and Maruyama, 1992; Nakanishi et al., 1992). A purely cosmetic correction by the subcutaneous application of silastic molds has also been suggested (Allen and Douglas, 1979; Rudolph, 1986; Sorenson, 1988). However, implant migration and failure to correct the structural abnormality limit the usefulness of this technique. Nonoperative techniques using orthotic support during childhood have also produced satisfactory results in small groups of patients (Haje and Bowen, 1992).

Our approach has been consistently to use the technique described by Ravitch. Although alternative methods exist, most surgeons favor this technique or a modification thereof to correct pectus excavatum deformities (Crump, 1992; Fonkalsrud et al., 1994; Golladay and Wagner, 1991; Haller, 1988; Haller et al., 1989; Mansour et al., 1993; Morshuis et al., 1992; Robicsek et al., 1974; Shamberger et al., 1988).

STERNAL FISSURE

In embryo, the sternum originates from the same lateral plate mesoderm that gives rise to the pectoral muscles. At 6 weeks, the migrating cells form two bands on either side of the anterior chest wall, and

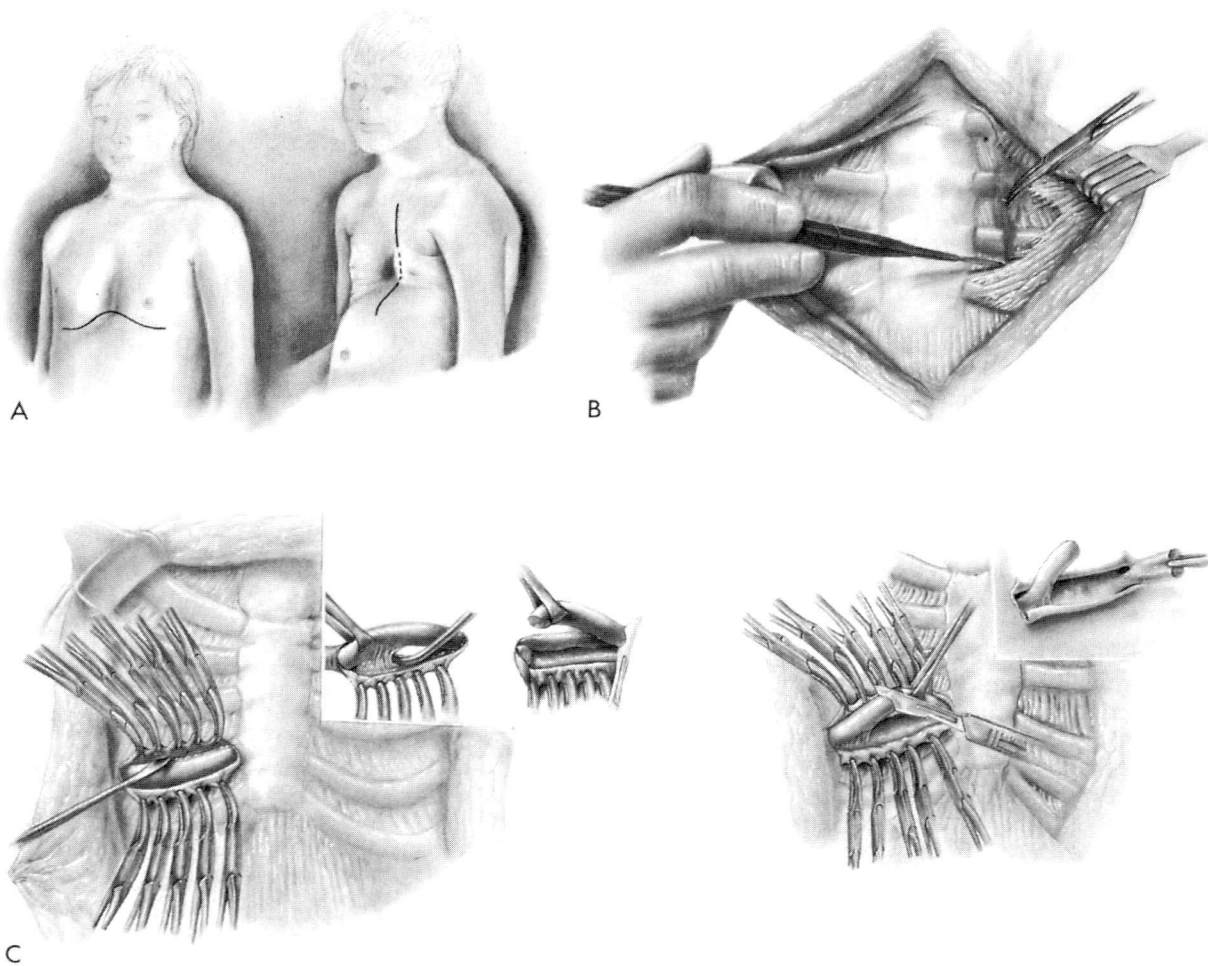

FIGURE 15–4. Operative technique for the correction of pectus excavatum. *A, The incision.* The incision in males and in all adults is midline from well up on the sternum to well down on the epigastrium. In girls, the authors use a transverse submammary incision that arches upward in the midline. This incision yields a superior cosmetic result but involves more dissection. There is some risk to the vascular supply of the edge of the upper flap and additional loss of time and blood. *B, Exposure of costal cartilages (vertical incision).* Traction on the skin and fat is transmitted to the pectoralis major, the muscular slips of which are divided from the sternum and costal cartilages, preferably with the electrocautery. (The artist has used license in the amount of smoke and has shown a knife-tip electrode rather than the fine-needle tip that the authors use.) The perforating branches of the internal mammary vessels are clamped and coagulated before division, and there should be little blood loss. Inferiorly, the cartilages that underlie the rectus abdominis are exposed by cutting the sheath and by splitting the muscle fibers. All the involved cartilages are exposed for the full extent of their deformity, which, particularly in older children, may be beyond the costochondral junctions. Superiorly, the lowest apparently normal cartilage is laid bare, and the sternum is exposed in the interspace above this. *C, Resection of deformed cartilages.* Rectangular flaps of perichondrium are reflected after a longitudinal incision is made with a scalpel or cautery on the entire length of the cartilage to be resected, and transverse incisions are made at either end. The application of multiple, fine, curved clamps to the edge of the incised perichondrium will serve to peel the anterior surface of the cartilage. A Freer elevator is shown (*left*) dissecting the cartilage. The *insets* show the cartilage raised and a blunt elevator placed beneath it to complete the stripping of the cartilage, which is then divided laterally with a scalpel and medially with a small Doyen elevator (not shown). When it is difficult to free the perichondrium posteriorly, as it often is in older children and adults, an alternative method (*right*) is employed. The cartilage is grasped with a Kocher or Allis forceps and is raised while being gingerly cut through until the cut end pulls away from the intact posterior perichondrium. The two halves of the cartilage are then removed separately.

Illustration continued on following page

D

E

F

G

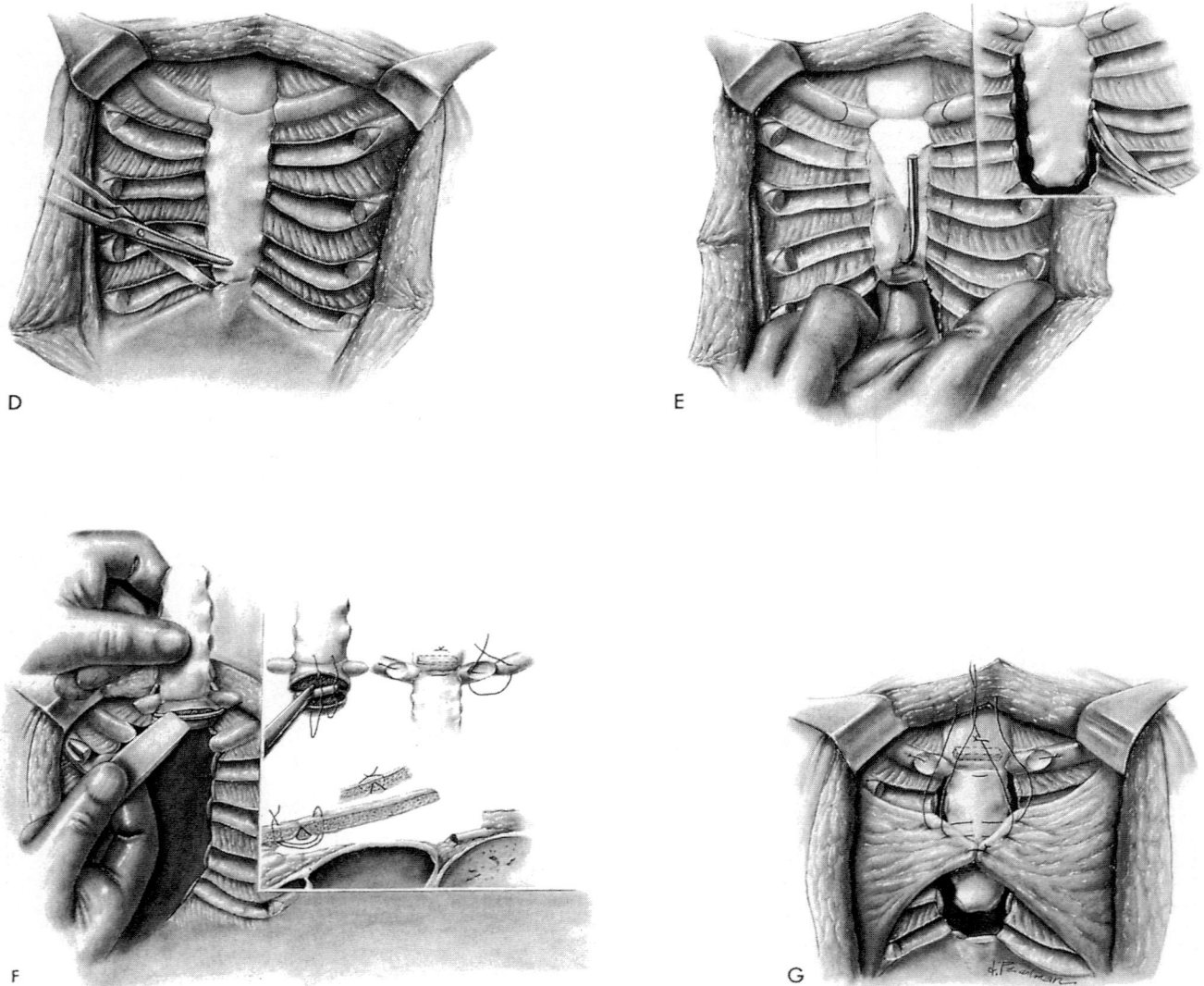

FIGURE 15–4 *Continued D, Division of the xiphoid.* Five deformed cartilages have been removed subperichondrially for the full extent of their deformity, and the xiphoid is divided from the sternum with heavy scissors. Sometimes it is necessary to divide the lowest intercostal bundle from the sternum to gain access to the xiphisternal junction. The xiphoid occasionally comes off the posterior surface of the sternum in this deformity. There is usually an arterial vessel on each side of the xiphoid, which may bleed vigorously if not controlled. *E, Freeing the sternum.* The sternum is raised with a bone hook by an assistant, and the operator's index finger is inserted into the mediastinum and swept from one side to the other, reflecting the pleural envelopes to either side. The intercostal bundles are then completely divided from the sternum with scissors or cautery, and an attempt is made (not always successfully) to cut medial to the internal mammary vessels. The lowest normal cartilage encountered is incised obliquely from in front and medially to behind and laterally, usually only after the intercostal bundles have been divided. *F, Sternal osteotomy and repair.* While the sternum is held forward, a wire is passed around it to serve as a guide to an accurate transverse osteotomy. The posterior cortical lamella is scored with the corner of a sharp osteotome until the sternum fractures forward. A bone graft has been cut from the bony ends of one of the ribs. The *inset* shows this bone graft being inserted into the osteotomy as a chock block held by circumferential sutures. Alternatively, a technique is shown for passing the suture through the wedge of bone before it is inserted. The authors now generally fix the wedge of bone securely in place by passing a suture through it and through the anterior sternal periosteum. The medial stump of the obliquely divided cartilage on either side overlies the lateral end and is fixed to it with a silk suture, which further supports the overcorrection. In some cases, the sternum is so scaphoid that the distal end projects too far anteriorly, and a second transverse osteotomy is required in the anterior sternum at the level of the beginning of this curvature, so that the distal end may be depressed. A wedge of bone may be fixed in this anterior osteotomy. *G, The closure.* The pectoral muscles are tacked back to each other and to the sternal midline with suture, completely covering the sternum, except possibly the distal portion of the gladiolus. The intercostal bundles are not tacked back to the sternum, because this tends to tether the sternum and re-create the defect. At least two layers of subcutaneous sutures are placed to effect a good closure before the skin is closed with either subcuticular sutures or continuous nylon. The authors do not use any rigid internal fixation in children. In an adult, the authors pass a Kirschner wire through the sternal marrow from one side to the other and bend the ends in a small circle, which allows the wire to lie comfortably under the pectoral muscles and on the ribs laterally. The wire is usually not removed. The authors do not generally use drains or suction catheters, but rather either incise the right pleura to allow the mediastinal blood to be absorbed in the pleural cavity or aspirate the substernal space when required with a syringe and needle. (*A–G,* From Ravitch, M. M.: *In* Rob, C., and Smith, R. [eds]: Operative Surgery. 3rd ed. London, Butterworth, 1977.)

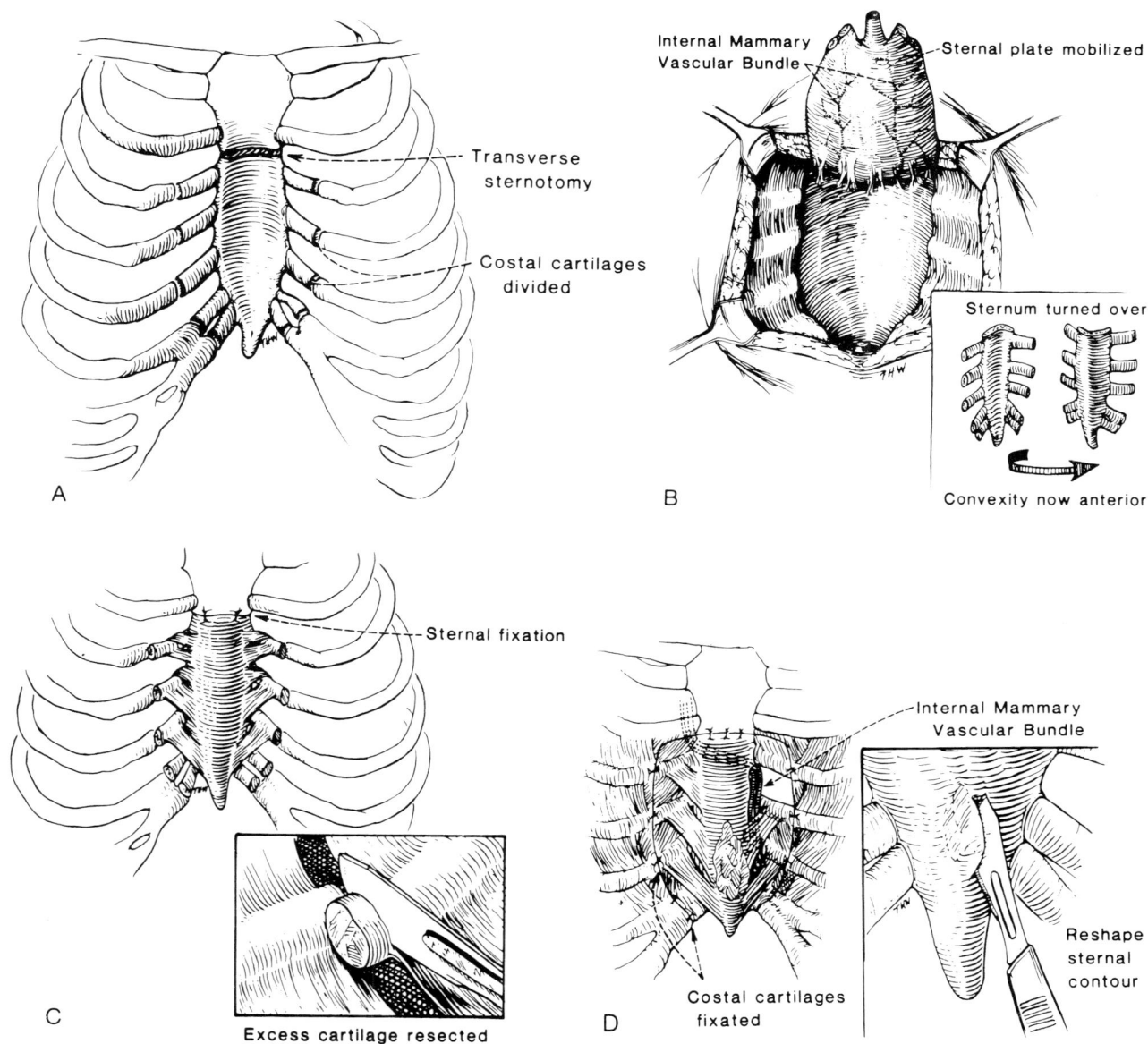

FIGURE 15–5. *A,* Sternal eversion technique for repair of pectus excavatum. The sternum is divided transversely in the second intercostal space, just above the beginning of the sternal deformity. The costal cartilages and intercostal muscles (not shown) are divided vertically, just lateral to the beginning of the cartilage deformity. *B,* Elevation of the sternal graft in sternal eversion repair of pectus excavatum. The internal mammary vessels are preserved as the sternum and attached costal cartilages are separated from mediastinal tissues. The sternal graft is based on one internal mammary pedicle and is rotated 180 degrees axially so that the convexity is anterior. *C,* Reapproximation of the sternal graft in sternal eversion repair of pectus excavatum. After the sternum has been repaired with wire, the costal cartilages are trimmed. This procedure allows precise reapproximation of the costal cartilages to the ribs laterally and helps to correct asymmetric deformities. *D,* Final shaping of the sternal graft in sternal eversion repair of pectus excavatum. The costal cartilages have been sutured to the lateral ribs by using wire. The internal mammary vessels can now be seen coursing on the anterior surface of the turned-over sternum through the interspace channel to their origin from the subclavian vessels. A scalpel is used to shave thin layers of cartilage and bone to achieve a symmetric contour of the anterior chest wall. (*A–D,* From Hawkins, J. A., Ehrenhaft, J. L., and Doty, D. B.: Repair of pectus excavatum by sternal eversion. Reprinted with permission from The Society of Thoracic Surgeons [The Annals of Thoracic Surgery, 1984, Vol. 38, p. 368].)

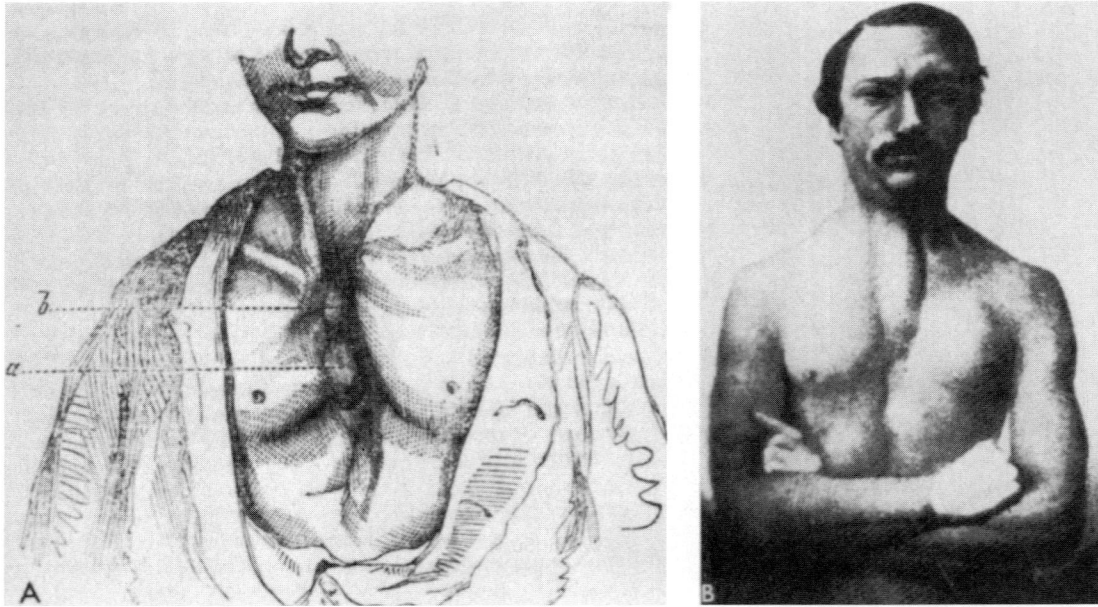

FIGURE 15–6. Groux, who came from Hamburg, put himself on display in universities and hospitals and for individual physicians. His visible and palpable cardiac pulsations were studied physiologically by physicians who used the current methods of the day. *A,* Contemporary woodcut reproduction of a photograph. Pavy, lecturing at Guy's Hospital, pointed out that the swelling (*a*) was pulsatile and that there was at *b* "another pulsatile swelling, which can scarcely be seen, but may be felt. It is doubtless formed by the arch of the aorta." *B,* When Groux placed his arms thusly and executed Valsalva's maneuver, the pulsating swelling bulged forward. (*A,* From Pavy, F. W.: Congenital fissure of the sternum. Medical Times & Gazette, Nov. 21, 1957, pp. 522, 523; *B,* From deGroot, J. W. C., and Huizenga, J. C.: Fissure sterni congenita. Maandschr. Kindergeneesk., 22:203, 1954.)

these bands become fused by the tenth week. Subsequently, the manubrium is formed by primordia between the ventral ends of the developing clavicles. In rare cases, the sternal bars do not become joined or become joined only in the lower portion and leave a defect superiorly.

The most widely known patient with sternal fissure was Groux. He visited many centers and allowed himself to be examined for an appropriate fee in major clinics, at medical societies, and at other gatherings in the nineteenth century (Fig. 15–6). He exhib-

ited his condition in Germany, France, Spain, Russia, and Great Britain.

There are three principal types of sternal fissure. In the *superior sternal cleft,* the heart is orthotopic, although it may appear to be in the cervical region. Skin covers the midline defect, and the pericardium, pleural envelopes, and diaphragm are intact. The superior cleft is usually broad and has the appearance of a U (Fig. 15–7). It commonly extends to the fourth costal cartilage and is occasionally V-shaped (Fig. 15–8). The defect can be closed in the midline by reap-

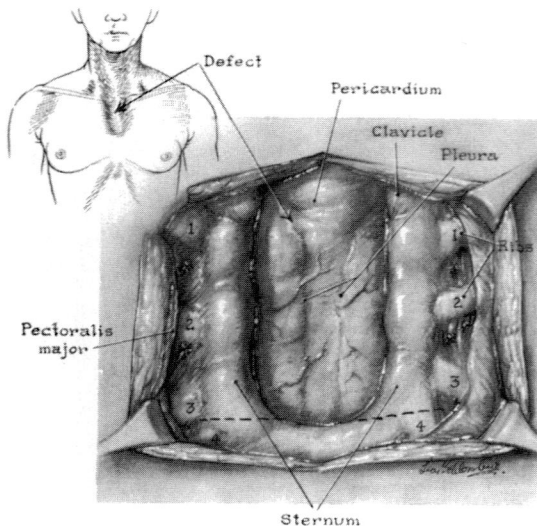

FIGURE 15–7. Cleft of upper sternum. An 11-year-old girl with a striking pulsation that appeared to be in her neck. The exploration showed a U-shaped deformity of the sternum. Transection of the limbs of the U, which is indicated by the *dotted lines,* did not allow the sternal halves to come together. Oblique chondrotomies of the three involved cartilages did allow the sternum to be pulled together, but the heart was compressed by the decreased circumference of the chest wall, which then caused hypotension and bradycardia. The sternal halves were replaced and covered satisfactorily with stainless-steel wire mesh that was folded over twice to produce a four-ply covering that widely overlapped the sternal border so that the risk of fragment erosion into the great vessels was reduced. The result has been excellent.

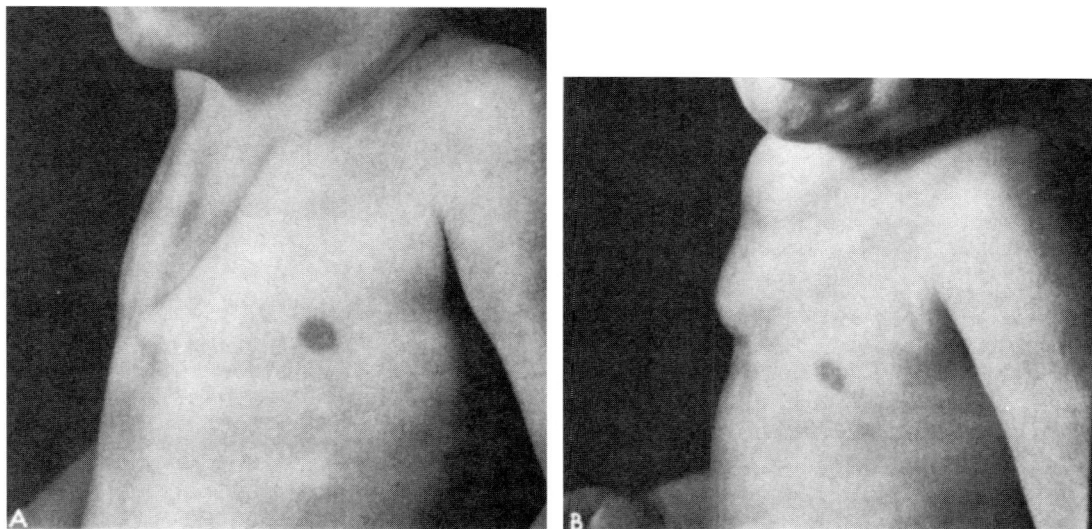

FIGURE 15–8. Cleft sternum. *A,* At rest. *B,* During forced expiration. Superior clefts of the sternum are variously V- or U-shaped. The appearance of the child as he cries explains the term *ectopia cordis,* although the heart is actually not displaced. In the newborn, defects of this kind can be corrected by direct apposition of the sternal halves. In this child, closure of the defect was made possible by sliding chondrotomies on either side. (*A* and *B,* From Sabiston, D. C., Jr.: The surgical management of congenital bifid sternum with a partial ectopia cordis. J. Thorac. Surg., *35*:118, 1958.)

proximating the two sternal bands with encircling sutures after oblique chondrotomies have been performed (Figs. 15–9 through 15–11). In the more severe defects of this type, oblique chondrotomies may not be sufficient because closure may excessively compress the heart, producing hypotension and bradycardia. Under these circumstances, a prothesis of Marlex or Gore-Tex is required to close the defect (Fig. 15–12).

Repair during the perinatal period may allow direct approximation in some patients (Firmin et al., 1980; Samarrai et al., 1985). In one such technique, a superior sternal cleft can be corrected in the newborn by a V excision of the inferiorly joined bars with direct

closure of the bars using an encircling suture (Salley and Stewart, 1985).

Complete clefts of the sternum are more complex defects, and they require an extensive procedure for closure because there is usually no bone between the hyoid and the pubis. An associated crescentic anterior defect in the diaphragm and a wide diastasis recti are also present. This allows free communication between the pericardial and peritoneal cavities. The surgical correction described by Ravitch is shown in Figure 15–13.

Cantrell's pentalogy is the third type of sternal deformity in this category (Cantrell et al., 1958). This pen-

FIGURE 15–9. The defect after dissection of the skin flaps. The sternal bands are shown, and the periosteum is being freed from the anterior surface. Incisions have been made into the perichondrium of the first, second, third, and fourth costal cartilages. The *inset* shows the incisions in the costal cartilage. (From Sabiston, D. C., Jr.: The surgical management of congenital bifid sternum with a partial ectopia cordis. J. Thorac. Surg., *35*:118, 1958.)

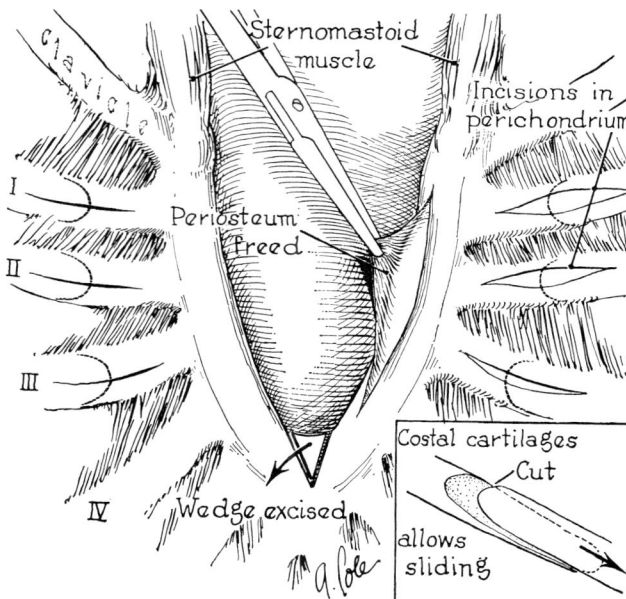

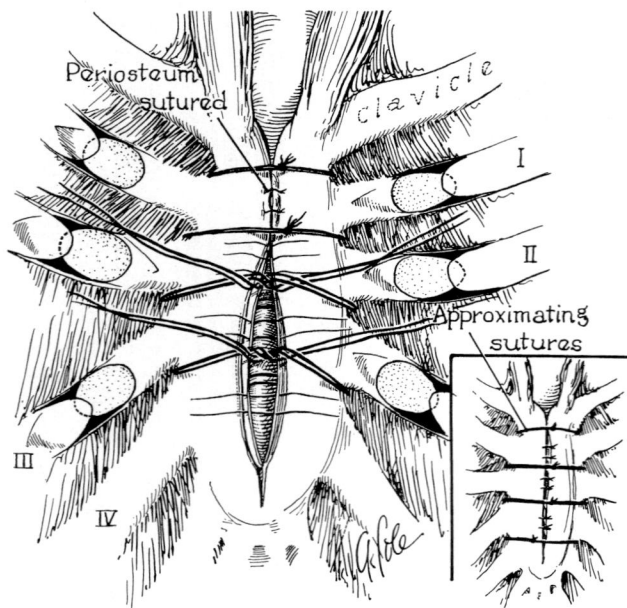

FIGURE 15–10. Approximation of sternal bands with encircling sutures after the oblique incisions in the costal cartilages. Multiple fine silk sutures are shown in the periosteal flaps. The *inset* shows the final appearance. (From Sabiston, D. C., Jr.: The surgical management of congenital bifid sternum with a partial ectopia cordis. J. Thorac. Surg., *35*:118, 1958.)

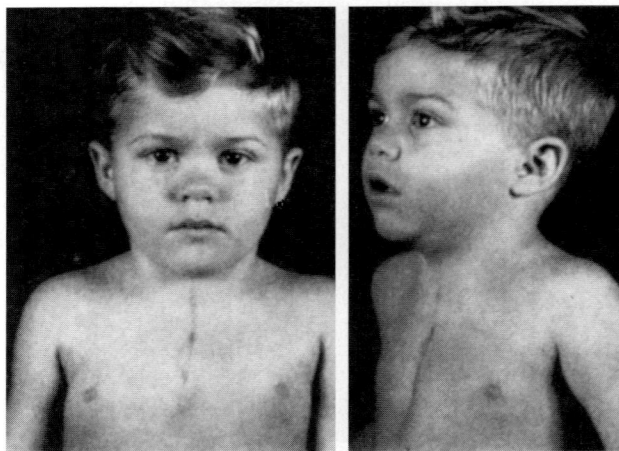

FIGURE 15–11. Correction of the sternal cleft. *Left*, Postoperative photograph. *Right*, Postoperative photograph (*oblique*). (From Sabiston, D. C., Jr.: The surgical management of congenital bifid sternum with a partial ectopia cordis. J. Thorac. Surg., *35*:118, 1958.)

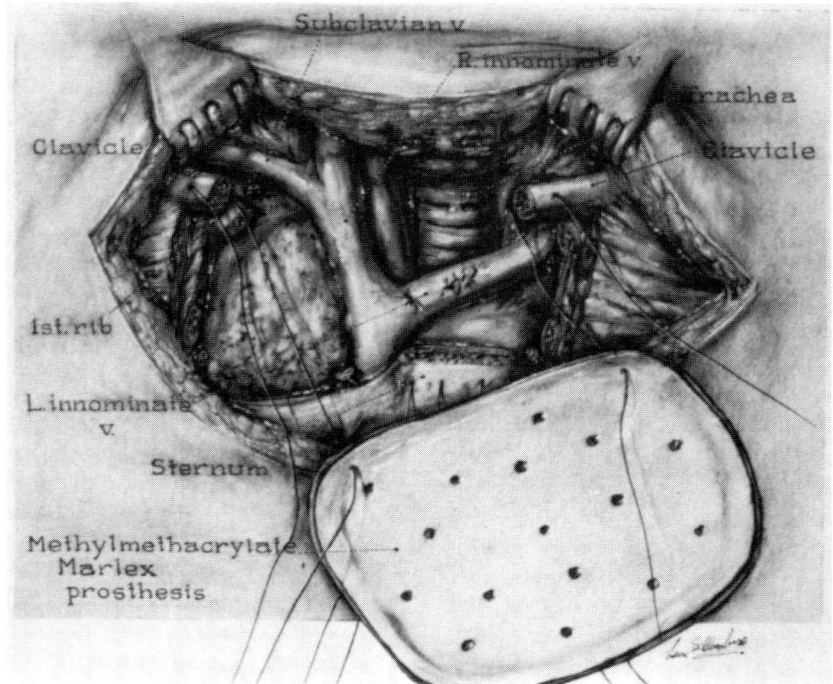

FIGURE 15–12. The methyl methacrylate sandwich, between two layers of Marlex, has several drill holes to prevent accumulation of fluid and to permit ingrowth of granulation tissue. A free margin of Marlex beyond the acrylic facilitates suture fixation to the chest wall. (From Sabiston, D. C., Jr.: Disorders of the chest wall. *In* Sabiston, D. C., Jr. [ed]: Essentials of Surgery. Philadelphia, W. B. Saunders, 1987.)

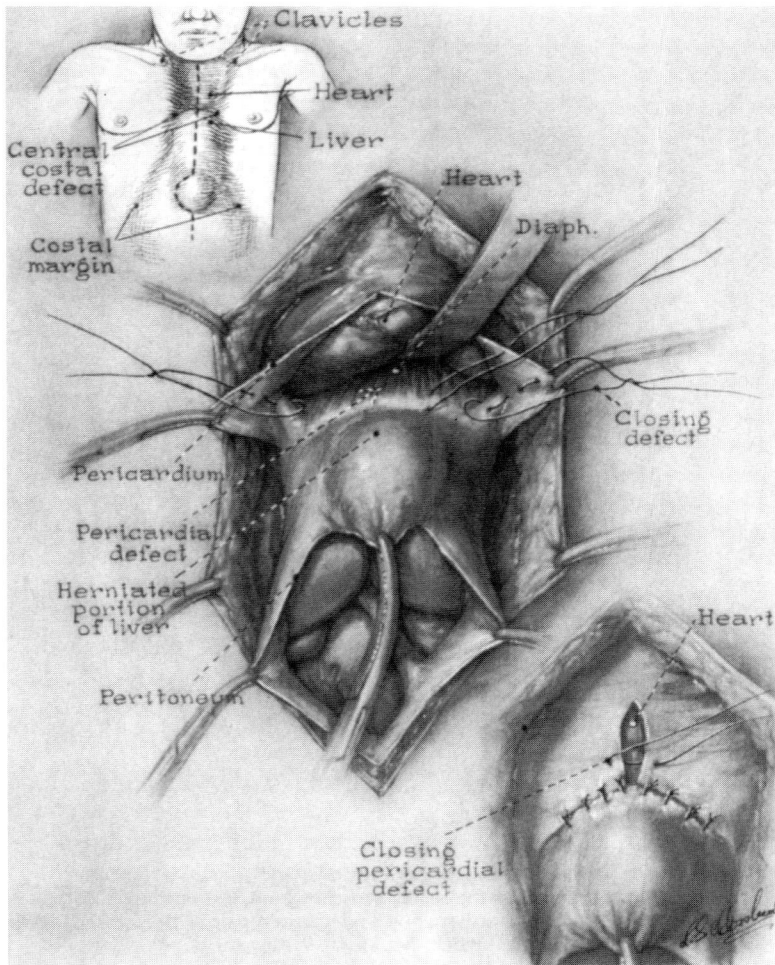

FIGURE 15–13. Complete cleft of the sternum in an infant with no bone between the hyoid and the pubis and a large midline ventral abdominal defect. Even at operation, the authors were not sure that the sternum was present. Films in subsequent years clearly showed a sternum. Shown are the heart, uncovered by any sternum; the globular liver, which had lain in the ventral hernia; the diaphragm, which comes no further anteriorly than the posterior pericardium; and the free communication between the pericardial and the peritoneal cavities. Herniation of bowel into the pericardium has been reported in these cases. The pericardium was readily closed. The sheaths of the recti were swung medially for the abdominal closure, and the sternal gap was covered with Teflon felt. One year later, it was seen that the Teflon felt had not gone high enough cephalad. An additional sheet of Teflon felt was inserted, with two autogenous rib grafts beneath it, between the bony borders at the upper end of the defect.

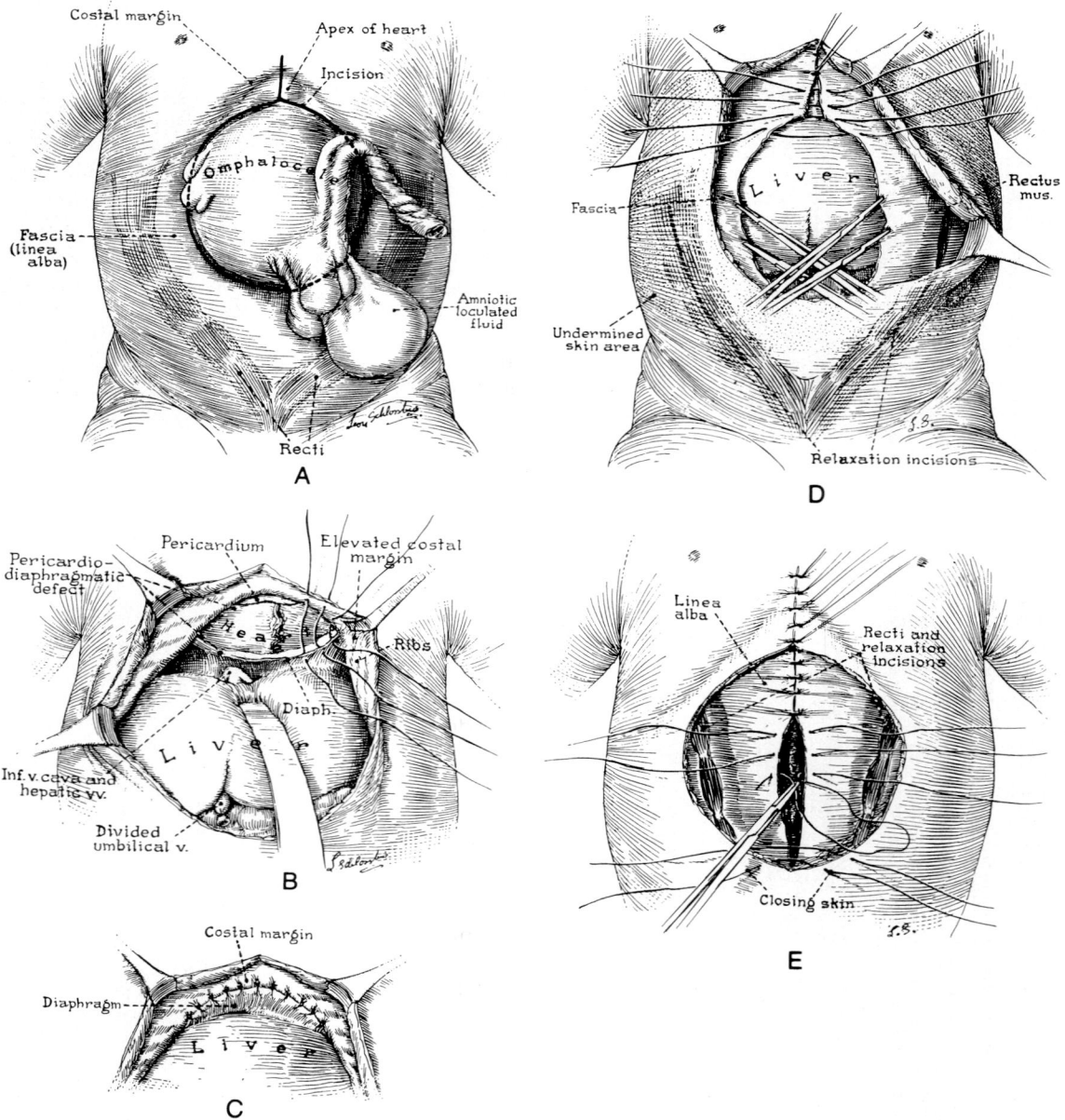

FIGURE 15–14. *A,* Note the wide separation of the rectus muscles, the abnormalities of the sternum and rib cage, and the exposed position of the heart. *B* and *C,* Note the defects of the diaphragm, pericardium, and thorax, and the repair of the diaphragmatic defect. *D,* Closure of the midline defect by using fascia medial to the rectus muscle. Note the relaxing incisions in the anterior rectus sheath and lateral undermining of the skin. *E,* Completed closure that shows adequate repair of the defect despite the lateral position of the rectus muscles. (*A–E,* From Cantrell, J. R., Haller, J. A., and Ravitch, M. M.: A syndrome of congenital defects involving the abdominal wall, sternum, diaphragm, pericardium, and heart. Surg. Gynecol. Obstet., *107:*602, 1958.)

talogy is characterized by a cleft in the distal sternum, an omphalocele, a crescentic deficiency of the anterior diaphragm, a deficiency of the diaphragmatic portion of the pericardium with free communication between the pericardial and peritoneal cavities, and a congenital heart defect. The cardiac anomaly most often involves a ventricular septal defect, tetralogy of Fallot, an atrial septal defect, or a left ventricular diverticulum (Toyama, 1972). A one-stage repair is technically feasible in this rare syndrome (Bogers et al., 1993). The correction of this defect is shown in stepwise illustrations (Figs. 15–14 through 15–17).

POLAND'S SYNDROME

This condition was first described in 1841 by Alfred Poland, a medical student at Guy's Hospital, after anatomic dissection of a convicted murderer. His initial description noted the absence of the sternum, absence of the costal portions of the pectoralis major and minor muscles, and absence of the serratus anterior muscles, as well as ipsilateral abnormality of the hand, including brachysyndactyly. Poland did not describe abnormalities of the ribs or costal cartilages, and his illustration showed that both the ribs and cartilages were present.

The incidence of Poland's syndrome is estimated to be between 1 in 30,000 and 1 in 50,000 live births (Der Kaloustian et al., 1991; McGillivary and Lowry, 1977). The syndrome is 3 times more common in males and involves the right side in 75% of cases (Smith, 1982). Most cases are sporadic, but familial cases have been reported (David, 1982; Darian et al., 1989; Der Kaloustian et al., 1991; Fraser et al., 1989).

The etiology of this condition remains unknown, although an in utero vascular pathogenetic mechanism is favored. A disruption in the subclavian or vertebral blood flow during the sixth to seventh weeks of gestation has been suggested as the cause of Poland's syndrome (Baunick and Weaver, 1986). Support for this theory includes the syndrome's association with the Adams-Oliver syndrome, a single gene mutation that predisposes to in utero vascular disruption with highly variable phenotypic results (Fraser et al., 1989; Hoyme, 1992). Vascular abnormalities are more common on the right side, in both syndromes (Darian et al., 1989). Real-time ultrasonography (Doppler Duplex scans) demonstrates significant differences in the subclavian diameter (reduced by 50%) and blood flow velocity when comparing the normal with the affected side in patients with Poland's syndrome (Merlob et al., 1989).

Clinical Features

This syndrome includes congenital absence of the pectoralis major muscle, with or without loss of the pectoralis minor, and associated absence of nerve supply to this musculature. Also involved are the pectoral girdle and abdominal muscles, including the rectus abdominus, the serratus anterior, and the latissimus dorsi. Absence or hypoplasia of ipsilateral ribs and costal cartilages, loss of subcutaneous tissue, and hypomastia or amastia, particularly in females, may also be present. Abnormalities of the upper extremity frequently occur, including hypoplasia or agenesis as well as brachydactyly and syndactyly (Darian et al., 1989; Garcia et al., 1989; Haller, 1988; Marks et al., 1991; Ohijimi et al., 1989; Seyfer et al., 1988; Shamberger et al., 1989; Wright et al., 1992). Rare associations with dextrocardia and certain forms of leukemia also have been described (Darian et al., 1989; Lodha et al., 1992; Hicsonmez and Ozsoylu, 1982).

Because the degree of this malformation may vary—from simple absence of the costosternal portion of the pectoralis major muscle to the fully developed syndrome involving the chest wall—the extent of the abnormality should be defined before surgical correction. Evaluation using CT and *magnetic resonance imaging* (MRI) has been suggested (Bainbridge et al., 1991; Merlob et al., 1989). Advantages of MRI include multiplanar imaging, avoidance of ionizing radiation, and coronal scanning to assess the latissimus dorsi muscle used for reconstruction in some patients with Poland's syndrome (Wright et al., 1992).

Operative Technique

There is little physical disability associated with Poland's syndrome, although the cosmetic defect may be severe. As children with this syndrome grow older, the defect usually becomes more pronounced. Several operative procedures have been described, but the procedure advocated by Ravitch is the preferred approach and is shown in Figure 15–18. In one series of 24 patients, 11 were men and 10 had right-sided lesions. Four patients had syndactyly, 5 patients had brachydactyly, and 3 patients had absence of the phalanges or digits (Ravitch, 1983).

This deformity has also been corrected by reconstruction of the chest wall and simultaneous augmentation mammoplasty, with transfer of a myocutaneous flap of latissimus dorsi muscle as an island pedicle (Marks et al., 1991; Urschel et al., 1984). In one patient with a co-existent pectus carinatum, the repair was accomplished by resection of the costal cartilages and osteotomy of the sternum with a breast implant and myocutaneous flap of latissimus dorsi muscle.

One report describes 33 patients with Poland's syndrome who underwent anatomic correction with a latissimus dorsi flap transferred to the anterior chest wall with preservation of the neurovascular pedicle. In women, the procedure was accompanied by insertion of a mammary prosthesis (Seyfer et al., 1988).

The largest reported series describes 75 patients treated over 33 years. Repair in patients with muscle and chest wall abnormalities included correction of the abnormal position and rotation of the sternum as well as replacement of the aplastic ribs. One concern was potential functional loss of shoulder strength when latissimus dorsi muscle flaps were used. This

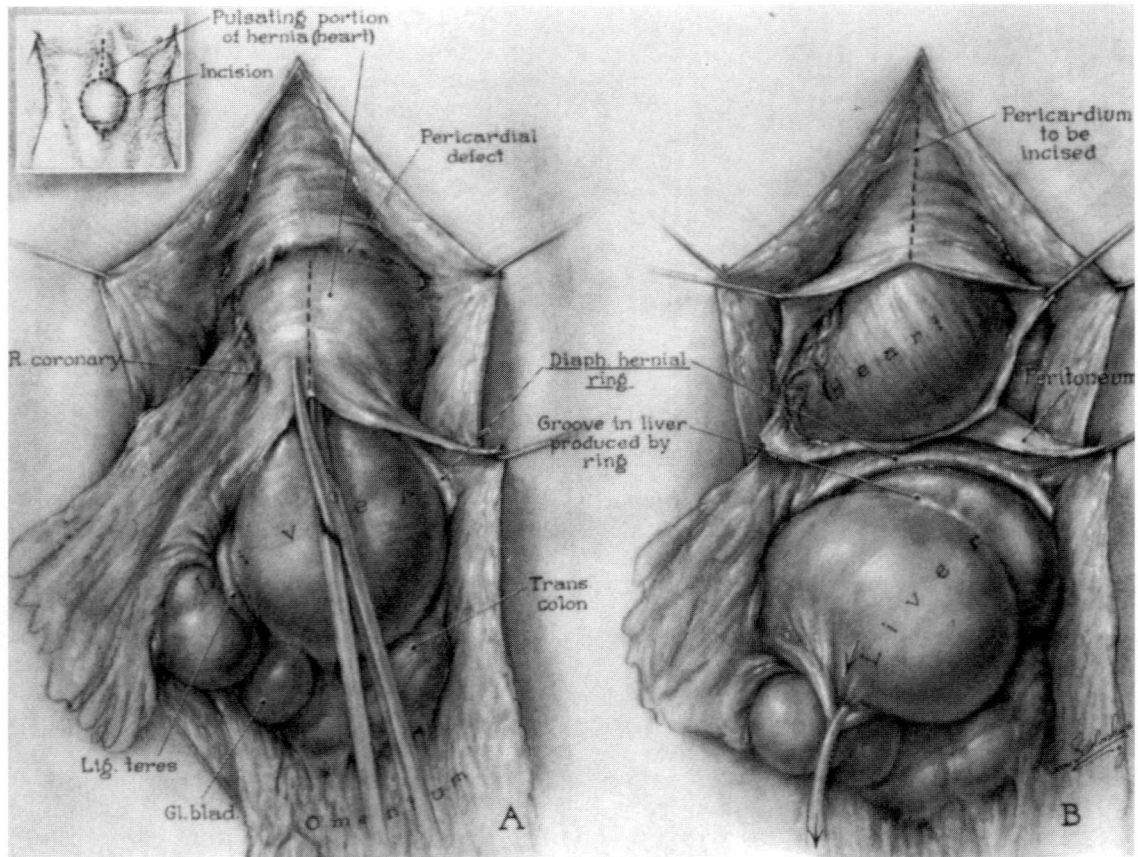

FIGURE 15–15. Note the exposed position of the heart produced by the sternal and abdominal wall defects and the diaphragmatic and pericardial defects. (From Cantrell, J. A., and Ravitch, M. M.: A syndrome of congenital defects involving the abdominal wall, sternum, diaphragm, pericardium, and heart. Surg. Gynecol. Obstet., *107*:602, 1958.)

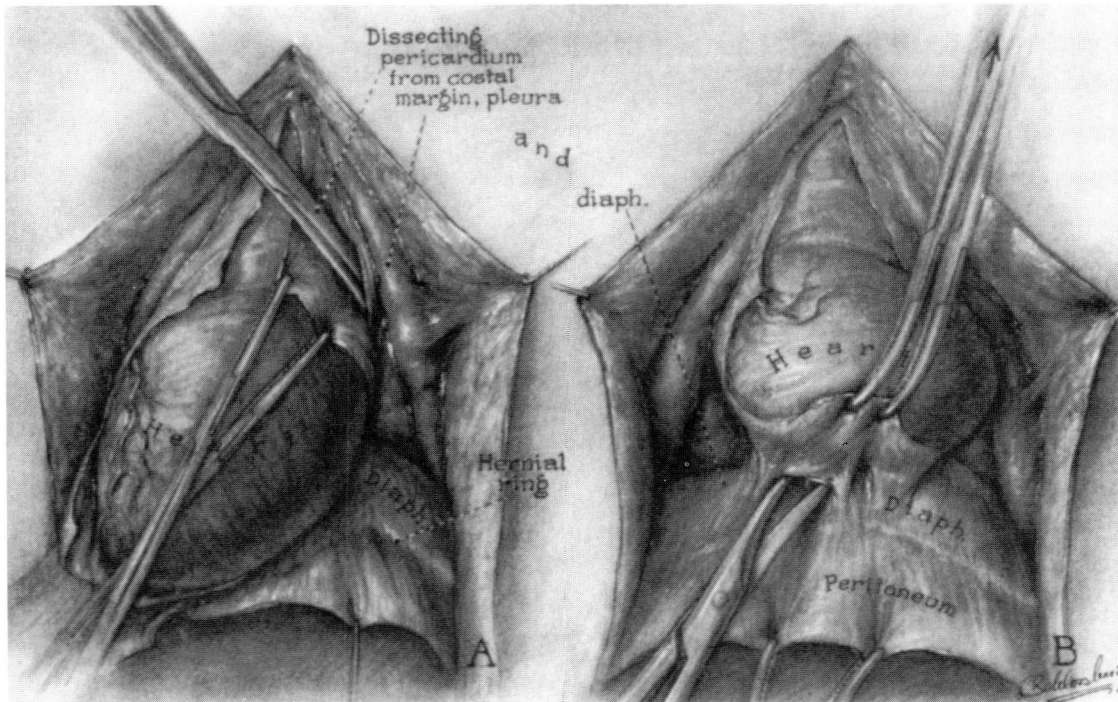

FIGURE 15–16. Dissection of heart and pericardium from surrounding structures allows the heart to retract slightly within the thoracic cavity. (From Cantrell, J. R., Haller, J. A., and Ravitch, M. M.: A syndrome of congenital defects involving the abdominal wall, sternum, diaphragm, pericardium, and heart. Surg. Gynecol. Obstet., *107*:602, 1958.)

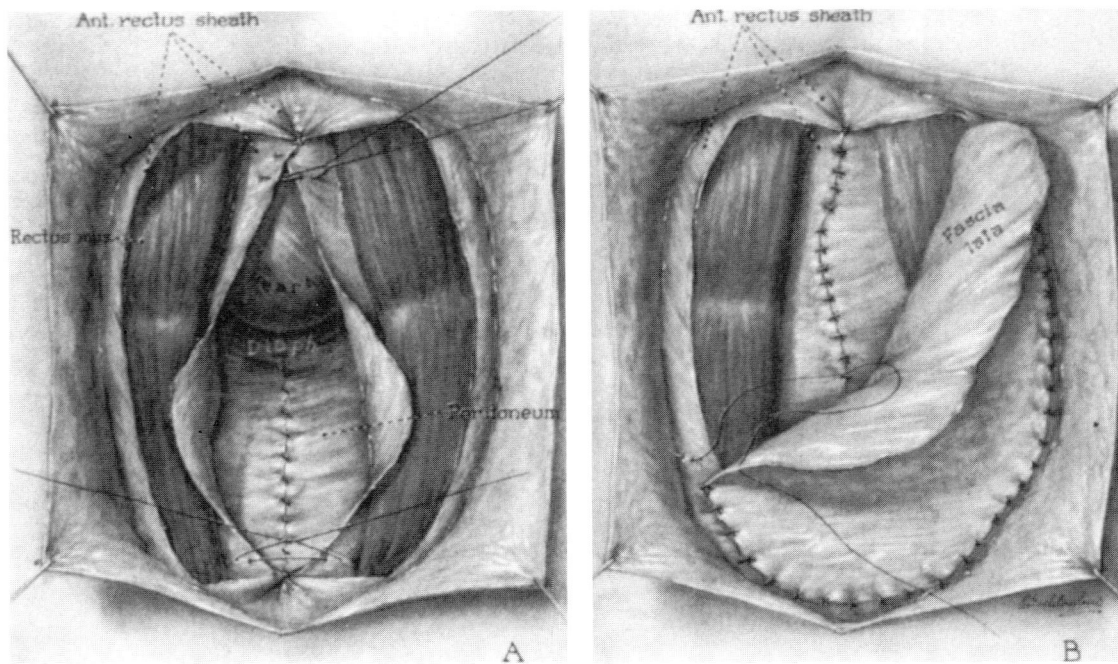

FIGURE 15–17. *A,* Fascial closure is effected by reflecting flaps of the anterior rectus sheath to the midline. *B,* Closure is reinforced by autogenous fascia lata. (*A* and *B,* From Cantrell, J. R., Haller, J. A., and Ravitch, M. M.: A syndrome of congenital defects involving the abdominal wall, sternum, diaphragm, pericardium, and heart. Surg. Gynecol. Obstet., *107*:602, 1958.)

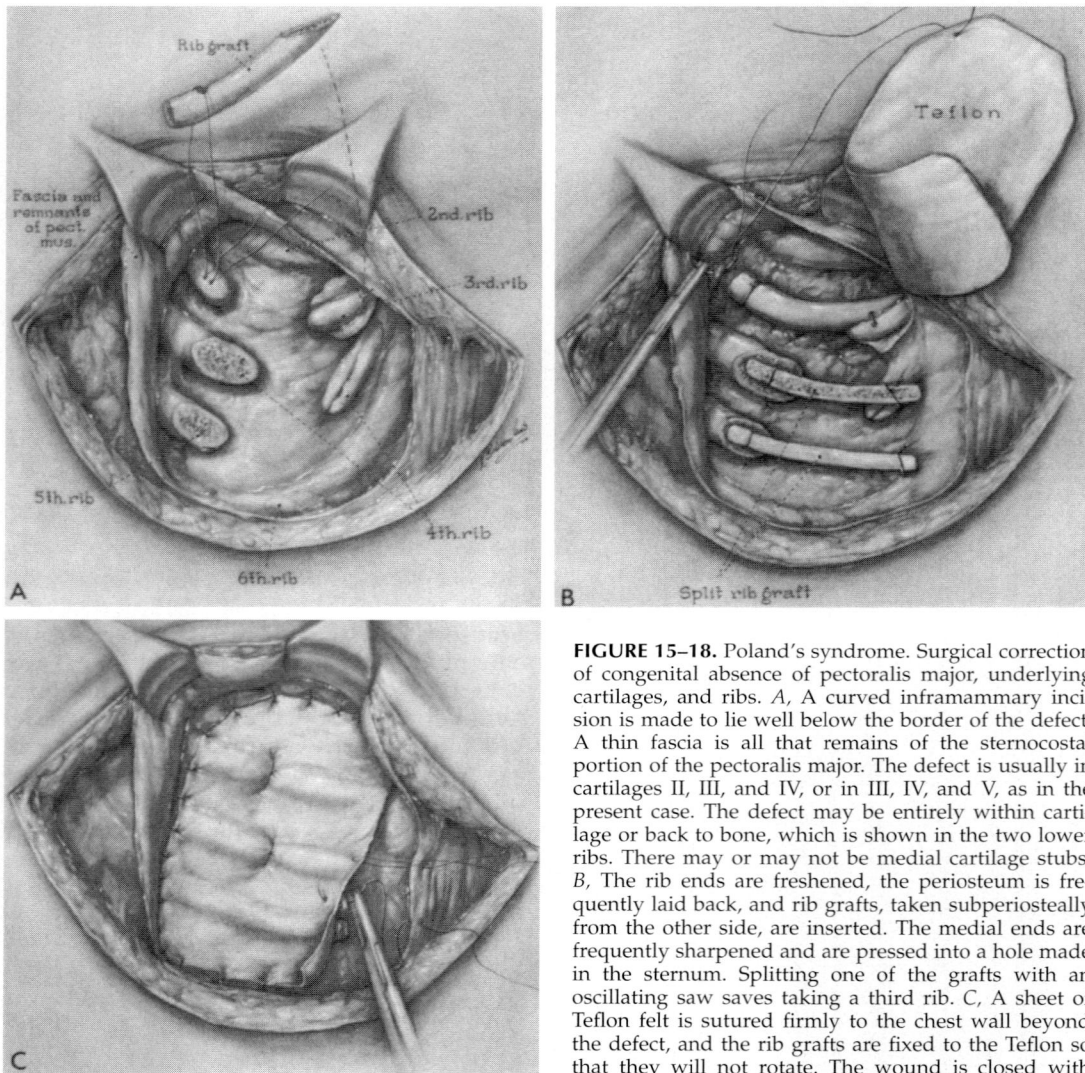

FIGURE 15–18. Poland's syndrome. Surgical correction of congenital absence of pectoralis major, underlying cartilages, and ribs. *A,* A curved inframammary incision is made to lie well below the border of the defect. A thin fascia is all that remains of the sternocostal portion of the pectoralis major. The defect is usually in cartilages II, III, and IV, or in III, IV, and V, as in the present case. The defect may be entirely within cartilage or back to bone, which is shown in the two lower ribs. There may or may not be medial cartilage stubs. *B,* The rib ends are freshened, the periosteum is frequently laid back, and rib grafts, taken subperiosteally from the other side, are inserted. The medial ends are frequently sharpened and are pressed into a hole made in the sternum. Splitting one of the grafts with an oscillating saw saves taking a third rib. *C,* A sheet of Teflon felt is sutured firmly to the chest wall beyond the defect, and the rib grafts are fixed to the Teflon so that they will not rotate. The wound is closed with suction drainage. (*A–C,* From Ravitch, M. M.: Atypical deformities of the chest wall—Absence and deformities of the ribs and costal cartilages. Surgery, *59:*438, 1966.)

method was used only in females with associated hypomastia or amastia to facilitate breast reconstruction (Shamberger et al., 1989).

THORACIC DYSTROPHY

Thoracic dystrophy, also called asphyxiating thoracic infantile thoracic-pelvic-phalangeal dystrophy, or Jeune's disease, is a rare and often fatal condition. This inherited autosomal recessive deformity is characterized by a constricted thorax, short extremities, and associated changes such as polydactyly. Although some patients die in infancy of severe respiratory insufficiency, others survive with respiratory assistance and may be considered for possible surgical intervention. A median sternotomy that allows the chest to expand by holding the sternal halves apart with autogenous rib has been successful. Fortunately, these patients are rare. The ultimate choice for such patients is between a premature operation, which might be unnecessary in a desperately ill infant, and an operation in an older child who might benefit from operative intervention.

PECTUS CARINATUM

Pectus carinatum ("pigeon breast") comprises protrusion deformities of the chest. The deformity is more common in males, and associated musculoskeletal abnormalities, of which scoliosis is most common, are seen in up to 21.4% of patients (Waters et al., 1989). A family history of the deformity may also be present (Shamberger and Welch, 1987). The condition is characterized by protrusion of the sternum caused by an upward curve in the lower costal cartilages, generally the fourth to the eighth cartilages, so that the sternum is moved forward (Fig. 15–19). Pectus carinatum is not a single entity but a spectrum of abnormal thoracic development, which may be classified into three types of deformities. The most common type (90%) consists of anterior displacement of the body of the sternum with symmetric concavity of the costal cartilages. Less frequent (9%) are asymmetric deformities consisting of unilateral displacement of costal cartilages. The least common type (1%) is the chondromanubrial deformity. This deformity involves synostosis of the sternum (Currarino Silverman syndrome), which causes protrusion of the manubrium and depression of the body of the sternum.

Symptoms are sometimes present and include exertional dyspnea and cardiac arrhythmias. Associated congenital heart defects have been observed in patients with chondromanubrial deformity (Chidambaram and Mehta, 1992; Shamberger and Welch, 1987). The reduced flexibility of the chest wall limits chest expansion during inspiration by the anteriorly displaced sternum and abnormal cartilages. However, in a study of preoperative and postoperative pulmonary function tests in patients with pectus carinatum together with progressive work exercise perfor-

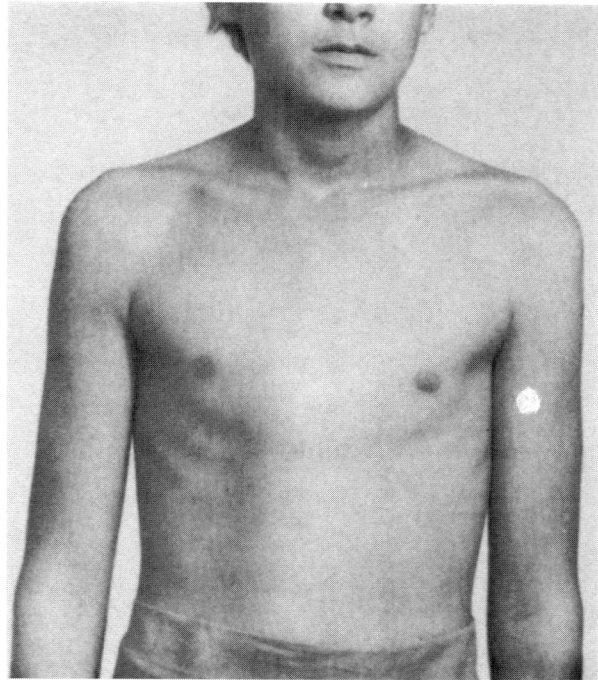

FIGURE 15–19. Pectus carinatum. (From Sabiston, D. C., Jr.: Disorders of the chest wall. *In* Sabiston, D. C., Jr. [ed]: Essentials of Surgery. Philadelphia, W. B. Saunders, 1987.)

mances, no significant changes were found (Cahill et al., 1984).

Operative Techniques

The operation may be performed through either a midline or a submammary transverse incision (Fig. 15–20A). The skin flaps are dissected, and the muscles along the entire length of the deformity are exposed. The pectoral muscles are then stripped laterally as described earlier to correct a pectus excavatum, except that the rectus muscles are separated from the lower cartilages and the xiphoid (Fig. 15–20B). As in the procedure for pectus excavatum, each deformed cartilage is removed subperichondrially, and multiple reefing sutures are placed to remove the redundancy in the perichondrial beds (Fig. 15–20D).

The operative results are generally excellent, with few, if any, complications. In one series of 150 patients with pectus carinatum deformities, good or satisfactory results were achieved in 138 (Robicsek et al., 1974).

Shamberger and Welch (1987) described 152 patients with pectus carinatum with a low morbidity rate of 3.9% that included pneumothorax, atelectasis, and local tissue necrosis. Only three patients required reoperation, and all patients ultimately achieved a satisfactory result.

ASYMMETRIC CONGENITAL DEFORMITY OF THE RIBS (COLLAPSE OF THE RIGHT SIDE OF THE CHEST)

The chest wall in normal individuals is symmetric, although some congenital abnormalities produce

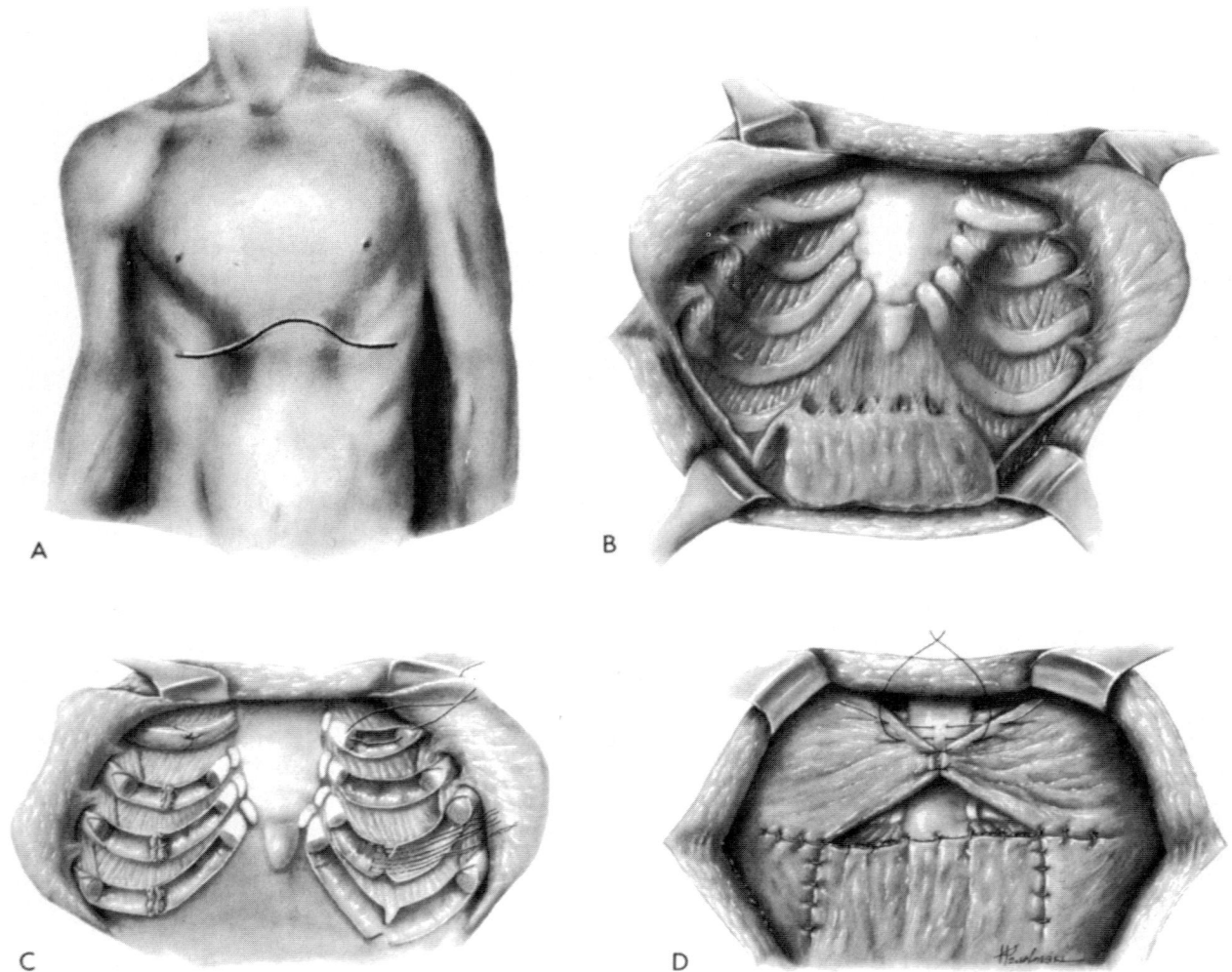

FIGURE 15–20. Operative technique for correction of pectus carinatum. *A, Incision.* The authors use a long transverse incision with some upward bowing in the center for cosmetic reasons, to reduce the length of the midportion of the upper flap, and to provide maximal exposure. Skin and fat are dissected widely to expose the deformed costal cartilages and ribs to the full extent of their deformity, which is highly variable. *B, Reflection of muscles.* The pectoral muscles are detached, precisely as in the operation for pectus excavatum, and the upper deformed cartilages are exposed completely. The recti are dissected free and are reflected inferiorly. *C, Reefing the perichondral beds.* The deformed portions of the cartilages and ribs have been removed subperichondrially and subperiosteally. The lower three cartilages on each side were abnormally prominent at their sternal junctions. Anomalous articulations were found when the prominences were cut away. The perichondral beds, lifted forward by the heart and lung as each cartilage is removed, are now redundant and shortened by reefing sutures placed as shown, which puts the entire perichondral bed more or less on a plane from one end of the resected rib-cartilage element to the other. Rarely, as shown in the highest cartilage, a segment that is so small is resected so that the gap can be closed. *D, Reattachment of muscles.* The pectoral muscles are reattached to the sternum and to each other in the midline. The rectus is drawn up and sutured to the sternum, perhaps a little higher than its point of origin, and is sutured to the lower borders of the pectoral muscles. No drains or tubes are necessary, and reaccumulation of fluid has not been a problem. (From Ravitch, M. M.: Pectus excavatum: Pectus carinatum. *In* Rob, C., and Smith, R.: Operative Surgery. 3rd ed. London, Butterworth, 1977.)

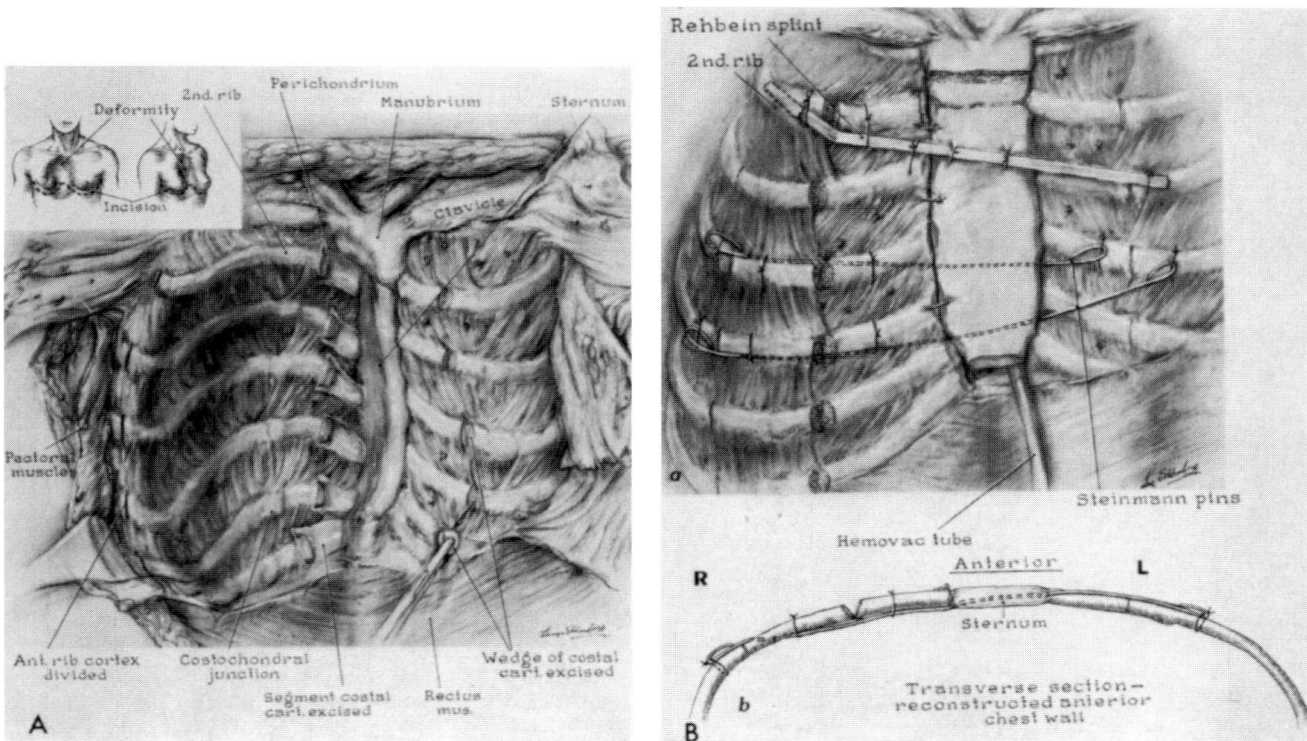

FIGURE 15–21. *A,* Correction of the unilateral costal depression. The minimally involved first rib is not disturbed. There are deep angulations of the second to seventh ribs and, in this patient, a very sharp rotation of the sternum to the right. There is no depression of the sternum. The apex of the deformity is in the ribs lateral to the costochondral junction, whereas in pectus excavatum it is in the sternum, or, if the sternum is rotated, at the chondrosternal junction. Through a bilateral, submammary incision, the pectoral muscles have been reflected laterally. On the right, short segments of the costal cartilages are removed subperichondrially adjacent to the sternum, and anterior osteotomies are done with a bone cutter at the depth of the depression and in the rib lateral to the depression. The posterior cortex is retained to permit a greenstick fracture when the rib segments are lifted forward. The cartilages on the left are not deformed, except when they turn to meet the rotated sternum. Small wedge chondrotomies are done on the left to permit derotation of the sternum. *B,* The chest wall has been reconstructed. Two Steinmann's pins through the sternal marrow lie on the chest wall and extend beyond the transections of the costal elements. The wires pass under the chest wall on the right and emerge medial to the lateral osteotomy in the rib. The ends are looped to prevent migration. The costochondral elements on the right are secured to the Steinmann pins with heavy synthetic sutures. Superiorly is a Rehbein splint, the end of which enters the marrow of the second rib on the right. The arched spring steel, which is sutured to the sternum and ribs, tends to lift it all forward. Superiorly, one can see the sternal osteotomy, which is across the sternum anteriorly but involves only the posterior cortex on the right side, thus permitting derotation. A suction drainage catheter has been placed in the mediastinum, although it is equally satisfactory to incise the pleura on the right and to insert an intercostal tube to collect the drainage that results from the multiple osteotomies. (From Ravitch, M. M.: Asymmetric congenital deformity of the ribs. Ann. Surg., *191*:534, 1980.)

asymmetric deformities. This deformity occurs on the right side, and inspection reveals a chest that is deeply sunken with an associated and variable rotation of the sternum to the right. The defect causes significant deformity. The procedure for surgical correction is shown in Figure 15–21. This technique usually yields generally good results.

SELECTED BIBLIOGRAPHY

Haller, J. A., Jr.: Operative management of chest wall deformities in children: Unique contributions of southern thoracic surgeons. Ann. Thorac. Surg., 46:4, 1988.

This paper chronicles the important historical developments that led to our understanding of chest wall deformities. This address recognizes the important contributions of individuals who developed the surgical principles that underlie management of these patients.

Ravitch, M. M.: Congenital Deformities of the Chest Wall and Their Operative Correction. Philadelphia, W. B. Saunders, 1977.

This definitive monograph on all congenital deformities of the chest wall is written by the primary contributor in this field. The monograph consid-

ers each of the deformities in detail. It is superbly illustrated and is highly recommended for supplementary reading on this subject.

Robicsek, F., Daugherty, H. K., Mullen, D. C., et al.: Technical considerations in the surgical management of pectus excavatum and carinatum. Ann. Thorac. Surg., 18:549, 1974.

An extensive experience in a large group of patients reviewed over a 25-year period is reported. The management principles and surgical approach offer a clear strategy for treating these patients.

Shamberger, R. C., and Welch, K. J.: Cardiopulmonary function in pectus excavatum. Surg. Gynecol. Obstet., 166:383, 1988.

The authors review the large body of literature on the physiologic impairment of patients with pectus excavatum.

Shamberger, R. C., and Welch, K. J.: Surgical correction of pectus excavatum. J. Pediatr. Surg., 23:615, 1988.

The authors describe a large, well-analyzed cohort of patients with pectus excavatum. This paper is written by a group with extensive experience in the surgical management of patients affected with this deformity.

Shamberger, R. C., Welch, K. J., and Upton, J.: Surgical treatment of thoracic deformity in Poland's syndrome. J. Pediatr. Surg., 24:760, 1989.

The authors report a large series of patients with a relatively rare congenital deformity. Important clinical observations and results of surgical correction are described.

BIBLIOGRAPHY

Allen, R. G., and Douglas, M.: Cosmetic improvement of thoracic wall defects using a rapid-setting Silastic mold: A special technique. J. Pediatr. Surg., 14:745, 1979.

Arn, P. H., Scherer, L. R., Haller, A., and Pyeritz, R. E.: Outcome of pectus excavatum in patients with Marfan syndrome and in the general population. J. Pediatr., 115:954, 1989.

Bainbridge, L. C., Wright, A. R., and Kanthan, R.: Computed tomography in the preoperative assessment of Poland's syndrome. Br. J. Plast. Surg., 44:604, 1991.

Baunick, J. B., and Weaver, D. D.: Subclavian artery disruption sequence: Hypothesis of vascular etiology for Poland, Klippel-Feil, and Mobius anomalies. Am. J. Med. Genet., 23:903, 1986.

Beiser, G. C., Epstein, S. E., Stamper, M. D., et al.: Impairment of cardiac function with pectus excavatum with improvement after operative correction. N. Engl. J. Med., 287:267, 1972.

Bevegard, S.: Postural circulatory changes at rest and during exercise in patients with funnel chest, with special reference to factors affecting stroke volume. Acta. Med. Scand., 171:695, 1985.

Blickman, J. G., Rosen, P. R., Welch, K. J., et al.: Pectus excavatum in children: Pulmonary scintigraphy before and after corrective surgery. Radiology, 156:781, 1985.

Bogers, A. J., Hazebroek, F. W., and Hess, J.: Left and right ventricular diverticula, ventricular septal defect and ectopia cordis in a patient with Cantrell's syndrome. Eur. J. Cardiothorac. Surg., 7:334, 1993.

Bon Tempo, C. P., Ronan, J. A., deLeon, A. C., et al.: Radiographic appearance of the thorax in systolic click-late systolic murmur syndrome. Am. J. Cardiol., 36:27, 1975.

Brodkin, S. H.: Pectus excavatum: Surgical indications and time of operation. Pediatrics, 11:582, 1953.

Brown, S. L.: Pectus excavatum. J. Thorac. Surg., 9:164, 1939.

Cahill, J. L., Lees, G. M., and Robertson, H. T.: A summary of preoperative and postoperative cardiorespiratory performance in patients undergoing pectus excavatum and carinatum repair. J. Pediatr. Surg., 19:430, 1984.

Cantrell, J. R., Haller, J. A., Jr., and Ravitch, M. M.: A syndrome of congenital defects involving the abdominal wall, sternum, diaphragm, pericardium, and heart. Surg. Gynecol. Obstet., 107:602, 1958.

Chidambaram, B., and Mehta, A. V.: Currarino-Silverman syndrome (pectus carinatum type 2 deformity) and mitral valve disease. Chest, 102:780, 1992.

Crump, H. W.: Pectus excavatum. Am. Fam. Physician, 46:173, 1992.

Darian, V. B., Argenta, L. C., and Pasyk, K. A.: Familial Poland's syndrome. Ann. Plast. Surg., 23:531, 1989.

David, T. J.: Familial Poland anomaly. J. Med. Genet., 19:293, 1982.

Davis, M. V., and Shah, H. H.: Sternal turnover operation for pectus excavatum. Ann. Thorac. Surg., 17:268, 1974.

Der Kaloustian, V. M., Hoyme, H. E., Hogg, H., et al.: Possible common pathogenetic mechanisms for Poland sequence and Adams-Oliver syndrome. Am. J. Med. Genet., 38:69, 1991.

Derveaux, L., Clarysse, I., Ivanoff, I., and Demedts, M.: Preoperative and postoperative abnormalities in chest x-ray indices and in lung function in pectus deformities. Chest, 95:850, 1989.

Derveaux, L., Ivanoff, I., Rochette, F., and Demedts, M.: Mechanism of pulmonary function changes after surgical correction for funnel chest. Eur. Respir. J., 1:823, 1988.

Firmin, R. K., Fragomeni, L. S., and Lennox, S. C.: Complete cleft sternum. Thorax, 35:303, 1980.

Fonkalsrud, E. W., Salman, T., Guo, W., and Gregg, J. P.: Repair of pectus deformities with sternal support. J. Thorac. Cardiovasc. Surg., 107:37, 1994.

Fraser, F. C., Ronen, G. M., and O'Leary, E.: Pectoralis major defect and Poland sequence in second cousins: Extension of the Poland sequence spectrum. Am. J. Med. Genet., 33:468, 1989.

Garcia, V. F., Seyfer, A. E., and Graeber, G. M.: Reconstruction of congenital chest-wall deformities. Surg. Clin. North Am., 69:1103, 1989.

Golladay, E. S., and Wagner, C. W.: Pectus excavatum: A 15-year perspective. South. Med. J., 84:1099, 1991.

Haje, S. A., and Bowen, J. R.: Preliminary results of orthotic treatment of pectus deformities in children and adolescents. J. Pediatr. Orthop., 12:795, 1992.

Haller, J. A., Jr., Kramer, S. S., and Lietman, S. A.: Use of CT scans in selection of patients for pectus excavatum surgery: A preliminary report. J. Pediatr. Surg., 22:904, 1987.

Haller, J. A., Jr., Peters, G. N., Mazur, D., and White, J. J.: Pectus excavatum: A 20-year surgical experience. J. Thorac. Cardiovasc. Surg., 60:375, 1970.

Haller, J. A., Jr., Scherer, L. R., Turner, C. S., and Colombani, P. M.: Evolving management of pectus excavatum based on a single institutional experience of 664 patients. Ann. Surg., 209:578, 1989.

Hawkins, J. A., Ehrenhaft, J. L., and Doty, D. B.: Repair of pectus excavatum by sternal eversion. Ann. Thorac. Surg., 38:368, 1984.

Hayashi, A., and Maruyama, Y.: Vascularized rib strut technique for repair of pectus excavatum. Ann. Thorac. Surg., 53:346, 1992.

Hicsonmez, E., and Ozsoylu, S.: Poland's syndrome and leukemia. Am. J. Dis. Child., 136:1098, 1982.

Hoyme, H. E.: Possible common pathogenetic mechanisms for Poland sequence and Adams-Oliver syndrome. Am. J. Med. Genet., 42:398, 1992.

Hummer, H. P., and Willital, G. H.: Morphologic findings of chest deformities in children corresponding to the Willital-Hummer classification. J. Pediatr. Surg., 19:562, 1984.

Iseman, M. D., Buschman, D. L., and Ackerson, L. M.: Pectus excavatum and scoliosis. Am. Rev. Respir. Dis., 144:914, 1991.

Judet, J., and Judet, R.: Thorax en entonnoir. Un procede operatoire. Rev. Orthop., 40:248, 1954.

Jung, A.: Le traitement du thorax en entonnoir par le "retournement pedicule" de la cuvette sterno-chondrale. Mem. Acad. Chir., 82:242, 1956.

Kaguraoka, H., Ohnuki, T., Itaoka, T., et al.: Degree of severity of pectus excavatum and pulmonary function in preoperative and postoperative periods. J. Thorac. Cardiovasc. Surg., 104:1483, 1992.

Leung, A. K. C., and Hoo, J. J.: Familial congenital funnel chest. Am. J. Med. Genet., 26:887, 1987.

Lodha, A., Mody, P., Singh, S., et al.: Poland syndrome with dextrocardia. Ind. Pediatr., 29:1301, 1992.

Mansour, K. A., Anderson, T. M., and Hester, T. R.: Sternal resection and reconstruction. Ann. Thorac. Surg., 55:838, 1993.

Marks, M. W., Argenta, L. C., Izenberg, P. H., et al.: Management of the chest-wall deformity in male patients with Poland syndrome. Plast. Reconstr. Surg., 87:674, 1991.

McGillivray, B. C., and Lowry, R. B.: Poland syndrome in British Columbia: Incidence and reproductive experience of affected persons. Am. J. Med. Genet., 1:65, 1977.

Merlob, P., Schonfeld, A., Ovadia, Y., et al.: Real-time echo-Doppler duplex scanner in the evaluation of patients with Poland sequence. Eur. J. Obstet. Gynecol. Reprod. Biol., 32:103, 1989.

Morshuis, W. J., Mulder, H., Wapperom, G., et al.: Pectus excavatum. A clinical study with long-term postoperative follow-up. Eur. J. Cardiothorac. Surg., 6:318, 1992.

Mullard, K.: Observation of the etiology of pectus excavatum and other chest deformities and a method of recording them. Br. J. Surg., 54:115, 1967.

Nakanishi, Y., Nakajima, T., Sakakibara, A., and Nishiyama, T.: A vascularised rib strut technique for funnel chest reconstruction. Br. J. Plast. Surg., 45:364, 1992.

Ochsner, A., and DeBakey, M.: Chone-chondrosternon: Report of a case and review of the literature. J. Thorac. Surg., 8:469, 1939.

Ohijimi, Y., Shioya, N., Ohijimi, H., and Kamiishi, H.: Correction of a chest wall deformity utilizing latissimus dorsi with a turnover procedure. Anesth. Plast. Surg., 13:199, 1989.

Peterson, R. J., Young, W. G., Jr., Godwin, J. D., et al.: Noninvasive assessment of exercise cardiac function before and after pectus excavatum repair. J. Thorac. Cardiovasc. Surg., 90:251, 1985.

Ravitch, M. M.: Associated anomalies in infants and children with congenital defects of the thoracic wall. In el Shafie, M., and Klippel, C. H., Jr. (eds): Associated Congenital Anomalies. Baltimore, Williams & Williams, 1981.

Ravitch, M. M.: Asymmetric congenital deformity of the ribs, collapse of the right side of the chest. Ann. Surg., 191:534, 1980.

Ravitch, M. M.: Atlas of General and Thoracic Surgery. Philadelphia, W. B. Saunders, 1988.

Ravitch, M. M.: Atypical deformities of the chest wall—Absence and deformities of the ribs and costal cartilages. Surgery, 59:438, 1966.

Ravitch, M. M.: Congenital Deformities of the Chest Wall and Their Operative Correction. Philadelphia, W. B. Saunders, 1977a.

Ravitch, M. M.: Disorders of the sternum and thoracic wall. In Sabiston, D. C., Jr., and Spencer, F. C. (eds): Gibbon's Surgery of the Chest. 4th ed. Philadelphia, W. B. Saunders, 1983.

Ravitch, M. M.: Disorders of the sternum and the thoracic wall. In Sabiston, D. C., Jr. (ed): Davis-Christopher Textbook of Surgery. 10th ed. Philadelphia, W. B. Saunders, 1972a.

Ravitch, M. M.: Disorders of the sternum and the thoracic wall. In Sabiston, D. C., Jr. (ed): Textbook of Surgery. 13th ed. Philadelphia, W. B. Saunders, 1986.

Ravitch, M. M.: Operative treatment of congenital deformities of the chest. Am. J. Surg., 101:588, 1961.

Ravitch, M. M.: Pectus excavatum and heart failure. Surgery, 30:178, 1951.

Ravitch, M. M.: Pectus excavatum: Pectus carinatum. In Rob, C., and Smith, R. (eds): Operative Surgery. 3rd ed. London, Butterworth, 1977b.

Ravitch, M. M.: Technical problems in the operative correction of pectus excavatum. Ann. Surg., 162:29, 1965.

Ravitch, M. M.: The chest wall. In Benson, C. L., et al. (eds): Pediatric Surgery. Chicago, Year Book Medical, 1962.

Ravitch, M. M.: The chest wall. In Ravitch, M. M., et al. (eds): Pediatric Surgery. 3rd ed. Chicago, Year Book Medical, 1979.

Ravitch, M. M.: The chest wall. In Shields, T. W. (ed): General Thoracic Surgery. Philadelphia, Lea & Febiger, 1972b.

Ravitch, M. M.: The operative correction of pectus carinatum (pigeon breast). Ann. Surg., 151:705, 1960.

Ravitch, M. M.: The operative treatment of pectus excavatum. Ann. Surg., 128:429, 1949.

Ravitch, M. M.: Unusual sternal deformity with cardiac symptoms—Operative correction. J. Thorac. Surg., 23:138, 1952.

Ravitch, M. M., and Matzen, R. N.: Pulmonary insufficiency in pectus excavatum associated with left pulminary agenesis, congenital clubbed feet and ectromelia. Dis. Chest, 54:58, 1968.

Roman, M. J., Devereux, R. B., Kramer-Fox, R., and Spitzer, M. C.: Comparison of cardiovascular and skeletal features of primary mitral valve prolapse and Marfan syndrome. Am. J. Cardiol., 63:317, 1989.

Rudolph, R.: Buried transverse abdominal myocutaneous flap and silicone implants to reconstruct pectus excavatum and bilateral mastectomy deformity. Plast. Reconstr. Surg., 78:817, 1986.

Saint-Mézard, G., Duret, J. C., Chanudet, X., et al.: Prolapsus valvulaire mitral et pectus excavatum: Association fortuite ou groupement syndromique? Presse Med., 15:439, 1986.

Salley, R. K., and Stewart, S.: Superior sternal cleft: Repair in the newborn. Ann. Thorac. Surg., 39:582, 1985.

Salomon, J., Shah, P. M., and Heinle, R. A.: Thoracic skeletal abnor-

malities in idiopathic mitral valve prolapse. Am. J. Cardiol., 36:32, 1975.

Samarrai, A. A., Charmockly, H. A., and Attra, A. A.: Complete cleft sternum: Classification and surgical repair. Int. Surg., 70:71, 1985.

Sauerbruch, F: Die chirurgie der brustorgane. Berlin, Von Julius Springer, 1920, pp. 437–444.

Scherer, L. R., Arn, P. H., Dressel, D. A., et al.: Surgical management of children and young adults with Marfan syndrome and pectus excavatum. J. Pediatr. Surg., 23:1169, 1988.

Seliem, M. A., Duffy, C. E., Gidding, S. S., et al.: Echocardiographic evaluation of the aortic root and mitral valve in children and adolescents with isolated pectus excavatum: Comparison with Marfan patients. Pediatr. Cardiol., 13:20, 1992.

Seyfer, A. E., Icochea, R., and Graeber, G. M.: Poland's anomaly: Natural history and long-term results of chest wall reconstruction in 33 patients. Ann. Surg., 208:776, 1988.

Shamberger, R. C., and Welch, K. J.: Surgical correction of pectus carinatum. J. Pediatr. Surg., 22:48, 1987.

Shamberger, R. C., Welch, K. J., and Sanders, S. P.: Mitral valve prolapse associated with pectus excavatum. J. Pediatr., 111:404, 1987.

Shamberger, R. C., Welch, K. J., Castaneda, A. R., et al.: Anterior chest wall deformities and congenital heart disease. J. Thorac. Cardiovasc. Surg., 96:427, 1988.

Smith, D.: Recognizable Patterns of Human Malformations. Philadelphia, W. B. Saunders, 1982.

Sorenson, J. L.: Subcutaneous silicone implants in pectus excavatum. Scand. J. Plast. Reconstr. Surg. Hand Surg., 22:173, 1988.

Toyama, W. M.: Combined congenital defects of the anterior abdominal wall, sternum, diaphragm, pericardium, and heart: A case report and review of the syndrome. Pediatrics, 50:778, 1972.

Urschel, H. C., Jr., Byrd, S., Sethi, S. M., and Razzuk, M. A.: Poland's syndrome: Improved surgical management. Ann. Thorac. Surg., 37:204, 1984.

Wada, J., Ikeda, K., Ishida, T., and Hasegawa, T.: Results of 271 funnel chest operations. Ann. Thorac. Surg., 10:526, 1970.

Waters, P., Welch, K., Micheli, L. J., Shamberger, R., et al.: Scoliosis in children with pectus excavatum and pectus carinatum. J. Pediatr. Orthop., 9:551, 1989.

Weg, J. G., Krumkolz, R. A., and Harkleroad, L. E.: Pulmonary dysfunction in pectus excavatum. Am. Rev. Respir. Dis., 96:936, 1967.

Welch, K. J.: Chest wall deformities. In Holder, I. M., and Ashcraft, K. W. (eds): Pediatric Surgery. Philadelphia, W. B. Saunders, 1980.

Wright, A. R., Milner, R. H., Bainbridge, L. C., and Wilsdon, J. B.: MR and CT in the assessment of Poland syndrome. J. Comput. Assist. Tomogr., 16:442, 1992.

15

■ II Surgical Management of Neoplasms of the Chest Wall

Peter C. Pairolero

Neoplasms of the chest wall encompass various bone and soft tissue disorders. Primary and metastatic neoplasms of both the bony skeleton and the soft tissues are included, as well as primary neoplasms that invade the thorax from adjacent structures such as the breast, lung, pleura, and mediastinum. Almost all of these neoplasms have been irradiated as the treatment of choice, or have been irradiated in combination with chest-wall resection. It is not uncommon for patients to present with a postradiation necrotic chest-wall neoplasm. The thoracic surgeon is frequently asked to evaluate and diagnose the condition of most of these patients, to treat some patients for cure, and to manage a few patients for necrotic chest-wall malignant ulcers. All of these patients present a diagnostic and therapeutic challenge. For many patients, surgical extirpation is frequently the only remaining method of treatment; such treatment may be compromised by incorrect diagnosis or an inability to reconstruct large chest-wall defects.

From a practical standpoint, however, chest-wall resection most often is used to treat primary chest-wall neoplasms (Pairolero and Arnold, 1985). Because primary neoplasms are uncommon, relatively few series have been reported. Moreover, most previous reports have included only patients with bone tumors (Groff and Adkins, 1967). When bone neoplasms are combined with primary soft tissue tumors, however, the soft tissues become a major source of chest-wall neoplasms and account for almost half of these resected tumors (Eng et al., 1990; Evans et al., 1990; Farley and Seyfer, 1991; Graeber et al., 1982; King et al., 1986; Pairolero and Arnold, 1985).

The incidence of malignancy in primary chest-wall neoplasms varies and has been reported to be in the range of 50 to 80%. The higher malignancy rates are found in the series that include soft tissue tumors. When combined, malignant fibrous histiocytoma (fibrosarcoma), chondrosarcoma, and rhabdomyosarcoma are the most common primary malignant neoplasms that the thoracic surgeon is asked to manage, whereas cartilaginous tumors (osteochondroma and chondroma) and desmoid tumors are the most common primary benign tumors (Table 15–1).

CLINICAL PRESENTATION

Chest-wall neoplasms generally present as slowly enlarging, asymptomatic masses. With continued growth, pain invariably occurs. Initially, the pain is often generalized, and the patient frequently is treated for a neuritis or for a musculoskeletal complaint. Almost all malignant neoplasms eventually become painful, compared with only two-thirds of benign tumors. In some cases of rib tumors, a mass may not be apparent on physical examination but is detected on a chest film.

Evaluation of patients with suspected chest-wall tumors should include a careful history, physical examination, and laboratory examination followed by conventional plain and tomographic chest films. Previous chest films are important to determine the rate of growth. In general, *magnetic resonance imaging* (MRI) is the preferred method of imaging chest-wall tumors. Not only does MRI distinguish the tumor from nerves and blood vessels, but it also allows visualization in different planes, such as caronal or sagittal planes. However, MRI does not accurately assess pulmonary nodules or the extent of calcification within the lung. Thus, if the lung parenchyma needs evaluation for metastatic disease, computed tomography is preferable.

SURGICAL MANAGEMENT

Chest-wall neoplasms that are clinically suspected of being a metastasis from a known primary neoplasm elsewhere can be accurately diagnosed by incisional or needle biopsy. However, if a primary chest-wall neoplasm (either benign or malignant) is suspected, an excisional biopsy rather than an incisional or needle biopsy should be done. Limited

■ **Table 15–1.** PRIMARY CHEST–WALL NEOPLASM

Malignant	Benign
Myeloma	Osteochondroma
Malignant fibrous histiocytoma	Chondroma
Chondrosarcoma	Desmoid
Rhabdomyosarcoma	Lipoma
Ewing's sarcoma	Fibroma
Liposarcoma	Neurilemoma
Neurofibrosarcoma	
Osteogenic sarcoma	
Sarcoma	
Hemangiosarcoma	
Leiomyosarcoma	
Lymphoma	

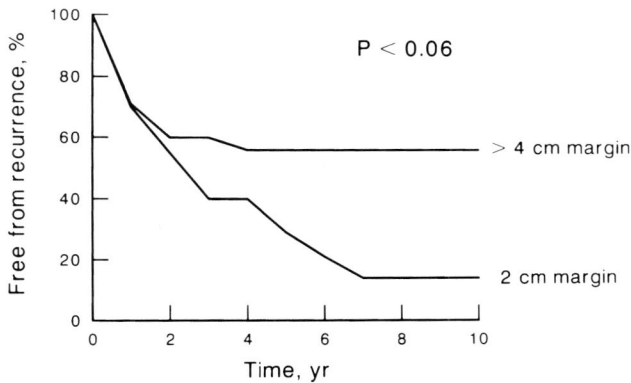

FIGURE 15–22. Percentage of patients with malignant chest-wall tumors free from recurrent tumor by extent of resection margin. Zero time on abscissa represents day of chest-wall resection. (From King, R. M., Pairolero, P. C., Trastek, V. F., et al.: Primary chest wall tumors: Factors affecting survival. Reprinted with permission from the Society of Thoracic Surgeons [The Annals of Thoracic Surgery, 1986, Vol. 41, pp. 597–601].)

biopsies tend to underdiagnose certain low-grade malignancies, such as chondrosarcoma, as benign neoplasms. Consequently, wide resection is invariably not done, and the patient is denied the opportunity for a cure. However, the biopsy should not interfere with subsequent treatment. An improperly placed biopsy site, extensive soft tissue dissection, and wound infection can all complicate subsequent treatment by delaying definitive resection, radiation, or chemotherapy. If frozen tissue diagnosis of a primary chest wall malignancy cannot be established at the time of excisional biopsy, the chest wound should be closed, most often without skeletal reconstruction, because the chest-wall defect is usually small. If the neoplasm is determined subsequently to be benign, no further surgical therapy is required. If, however, a malignancy is diagnosed, wide resection is then required, which must also include en-bloc resection of the entire biopsy site (skin, subcutaneous tissue, and muscle) because of potential contamination by a tumor of the overlying muscle, subcutaneous tissue, and skin.

CHEST–WALL RESECTION

Wide resection of a primary malignant chest-wall neoplasm is now recognized as essential to successful management. However, the extent of resection should not be compromised because of an inability to close large chest-wall defects (Arnold and Pairolero, 1979, 1984; Pairolero and Arnold, 1985, 1986). Opinions differ as to what constitutes wide resection. In a report from the Mayo Clinic (King et al., 1986), which analyzed the effect of the extent of resection on long-term survival in patients with primary malignant chest-wall neoplasm, 56% of patients with a margin of resection 4 cm or greater remained free from cancer at 5 years, compared with only 29% for patients with a 2-cm margin (Fig. 15–22). Many surgeons consider a resection margin of 2 cm adequate. Although this margin may be adequate for chest-wall metastases,

benign tumor, and certain low-grade malignant primary neoplasms such as chondrosarcoma, a 2-cm margin for resection is inadequate for more malignant neoplasms, such as osteogenic sarcoma and malignant fibrous histiocytoma. These neoplasms can spread within the marrow cavity or along tissue planes such as the periosteum or parietal pleura. Consequently, all primary malignant neoplasms that are initially diagnosed by excisional biopsy should be resected further to include at least a 4-cm margin of normal tissue on all sides. The entire involved bone should be resected for high-grade malignancies. For neoplasms of the rib cage, this includes removal of the involved ribs and the corresponding anterior costal arches if the tumor is located anteriorly, as well as several partial ribs above and below the neoplasm. For tumors of the sternum and manubrium, resection of the entire involved bone and corresponding costal arches bilaterally is indicated. Any attached structures, such as lung, thymus, pericardium, or chest-wall muscles, should also be excised.

CHEST–WALL RECONSTRUCTION

The ability to close large chest-wall defects is of prime importance in the surgical treatment of chest-wall neoplasms. The critical questions of whether the reconstructed thorax will support respiration and protect the underlying organs must be answered when considering both the extent of resection and the method of reconstruction. Adequate resection and dependable reconstruction are the mandatory ingredients for successful treatment. These two important items are accomplished most safely by the joint efforts of a thoracic and a plastic surgeon (Arnold and Pairolero, 1984).

Reconstruction of chest-wall defects involves many factors (Table 15–2). The location and size are of utmost importance, but the past medical history and local conditions of the wound may drastically alter a reconstructive choice. Primary closure remains the best option, when possible. If full-thickness recon-

■ **Table 15–2.** FACTORS TO CONSIDER FOR RECONSTRUCTION OF CHEST–WALL DEFECTS

Location
Size
Depth
Partial thickness
Full thickness
Duration
Condition of local tissue
Irradiation
Infection
Residual tumor
Scarring
General condition of patient
Chemotherapy
Corticosteroid
Chronic infection
Life-style and type of work
Prognosis

struction is required, as it is with most primary neo-plasms that have not been previously treated, both structural stability of the thorax and soft tissue cover-age must be considered.

Skeletal Reconstruction. Reconstruction of the bony thorax is controversial. Opinions differ as to who should undergo reconstruction and what type of reconstruction should be used. In general, all full-thickness skeletal defects that could result in pneumo-thorax should be reconstructed. The decision not to reconstruct the skeleton depends on the size and loca-tion of the defect. Defects smaller than 5 cm in great-est diameter anywhere on the thorax usually are not reconstructed. Likewise, high posterior defects smaller than 10 cm do not require reconstruction, because the overlying scapula provides support. However, if the defect is located near the tip of the scapula, the defect should be closed to avoid impinge-ment of the tip of the scapula into the chest with movement of the arm. Alternatively, the lower half of the scapula could be resected. Finally, all larger de-fects located anywhere on the chest should be recon-structed, and either autogenous tissue, such as fascia lata or ribs, or prosthetic material, such as the various meshes, metals, or methyl methacrylate, may be used.

Stabilization of the bony thorax is accomplished best with prosthetic material such as Prolene mesh (Ethicon, Somerville, NJ) or 2-mm-thick Gore-Tex (polytetrafluoroethylene) soft tissue patch (W. L. Gore & Associates, Elkton, MD). Placing either of these materials under tension improves the rigidity of the prosthesis in all directions. Currently, the Gore-Tex soft tissue patch is superior, because this material has the added advantage of preventing movement of fluid and air across the reconstructed chest wall. Mar-lex mesh (Daval, Providence, RI) is used less fre-quently, because when placed under tension, it is rigid in one direction only. Reconstruction with rigid material, such as methyl methacrylate–impregnated meshes, is not necessary.

All large full-thickness skeletal defects resulting from resection of neoplasm in both the sternum and lateral chest wall should be reconstructed if the wound is not contaminated. If the wound is contami-nated from previous radiation necrosis or necrotic neoplasm, reconstruction with prosthetic material is not advised, because the prosthesis may subsequently become infected and require removal. In this situa-tion, reconstruction with a musculocutaneous flap alone is preferred. Similarly, resection of full-thickness bony thorax in a patient who has been previously irradiated may not require skeletal reconstruction, be-cause the lung frequently adheres to the underlying parietal pleura, and pneumothorax may not occur with chest-wall resection.

Soft Tissue Reconstruction. Both muscle and omentum can be used to reconstruct soft tissue chest-wall defects (Table 15–3). Muscle can be transposed as muscle alone or as a musculocutaneous flap; it is the tissue of choice for closure of most full-thickness soft tissue defects. All of the major chest-wall muscles can be mobilized on a single axis of rotation and

■ Table 15–3. AUTOGENOUS TISSUE AVAILABLE FOR CHEST–WALL RECONSTRUCTION

Muscle
Latissimus dorsi
Pectoralis major
Rectus abdominis
Serratus anterior
External oblique
Trapezius
Omentum

transposed to another location on the chest wall (McGraw and Arnold, 1986). The omentum should be reserved for partial-thickness reconstruction or as a backup procedure when muscle is either not available or has failed in a previous full-thickness repair.

Latissimus Dorsi. The latissimus dorsi muscle is the largest flat muscle on the thorax. Its dominant thoracodorsal neurovascular leash has an arc of rota-tion that allows coverage of the lateral and central back as well as the anterolateral and central front of the thorax (Bostwick et al., 1979; Campbell, 1950). Its dependable musculocutaneous vascular connections permit it to be used also as a reliable musculocuta-neous flap. This muscle flap can cover huge chest-wall defects, because virtually one-half of the back can be elevated on the blood supply of a single latissi-mus dorsi muscle in the uninjured, nonirradiated pa-tient. The donor site posteriorly may require skin grafting when large musculocutaneous flaps are ele-vated, but this is a small disadvantage, considering that large, robust flaps can be transposed to either the anterior or the posterior chest for full-thickness reconstruction. If the dominant blood supply has been compromised from previous trauma or surgery, the muscle can still be dependably transposed on the branch of the adjacent serratus anterior muscle (Fisher et al., 1983).

Pectoralis Major. The pectoralis major muscle is the second-largest flat muscle on the chest wall and in many respects is the mirror image of the latissimus dorsi muscle. Its dominant thoracoacromial neurovas-cular leash, which enters posteriorly about mid-clavi-cle, allows both elevation of the muscle as either a muscle or a musculocutaneous flap (Arnold and Pairolero, 1979) and rotation centrally for chest-wall reconstruction. The pectoralis major flap is just as reliable as the latissimus dorsi flap. It is of major benefit in reconstruction of anterior chest-wall defects such as those resulting from sternal tumor excisions (Arnold and Pairolero, 1978; Pairolero and Arnold, 1984, 1986). Generally, only the muscle is transposed, thereby avoiding the distortion created by centraliz-ing the breast. Reconstruction in this manner is more symmetric and more aesthetically acceptable. If cen-tral skin must be excised, symmetry of the breast can still be maintained, because the transposed muscle readily accepts and supports an overlying skin graft. If necessary, the muscle may also be transposed on its secondary blood supply via the perforators from the internal mammary vessels.

Rectus Abdominis. Use of the rectus abdominis muscle for chest-wall reconstruction is based on the internal mammary neurovascular leash. The inferior epigastric vessels must be divided to allow rotation to the chest wall. This muscle can be mobilized and moved either as a muscle or as a musculocutaneous flap with the skin component oriented horizontally, vertically, or both ways. The vertical skin flap, however, is more reliable, because it is oriented along the long axis of the muscle and thus maintains more musculocutaneous perforators. The donor site usually is closed primarily.

The rectus abdominis muscle is most useful in reconstruction of lower sternal wounds. Either muscle can be used, because their arcs of rotation are identical. Care must be taken to choose the muscle that has patent and uninjured internal mammary vessels. Angiographic demonstration of vessel patency may help determine which musculocutaneous unit would be most reliable, particularly in previously irradiated patients or in patients who have undergone coronary artery bypass surgery.

Serratus Anterior. The serratus anterior muscle is a smaller, flat muscle located along the midaxillary chest wall. Its blood supply comes from the serratus branch of the thoracodorsal vessels and from the long thoracic artery and vein. Although this muscle can be used alone, it is more commonly used in chest-wall reconstruction as an adjunctive muscle in tandem with either the pectoralis major or the latissimus dorsi muscle to close larger defects. The muscle also augments the skin-carrying ability of either adjacent muscle (Arnold et al., 1984). This muscle is particularly useful as an intrathoracic muscle flap (Arnold et al., 1984).

External Oblique. The external oblique muscle may also be transposed as either a muscle or a musculocutaneous flap, and it is most useful in closing defects of the upper abdomen and lower thorax. It reaches the inframammary fold without tension but does not readily extend higher (Hodgkinson and Arnold, 1980). The primary blood supply is from the lower thoracic intercostal vessels. The advantage of this muscle is that lower chest-wall defects can be closed without distortion of the breast.

Trapezius. The trapezius muscle has been useful in closing defects at the base of the neck or the thoracic outlet, but it is not a consistently useful muscle for the remainder of chest-wall reconstruction sites. Its primary blood supply is the dorsal scapular vessels.

Omentum. Omental transposition has been very useful in reconstruction of partial-thickness chest-wall defects that may occur with certain soft tissue neoplasms or radiation necrosis (Arnold and Pairolero, 1986; Jurkiewicz and Arnold, 1977). In the latter situation, the skin and soft tissue are debrided down to what remains of the thoracic skeleton, which may be either bone or cartilage but frequently is only irradiated ischemic scar. The transposed omentum, with its excellent blood supply from the gastroepiploic vessels, adheres to the irradiated wound and readily accepts and supports an overlying skin graft. The omentum has no structural stability of its own, and

thus it is not useful in full-thickness defects, because additional support with fascia lata, bone, or prosthetic material would be necessary.

Omental transposition is exceedingly helpful when planned muscle flaps have been used but have failed because of partial necrosis. Generally, this results in only a soft tissue defect, and pleural seal with respiratory stability is not required, thus allowing a most threatening situation to be salvaged.

CLINICAL EXPERIENCE

Since the early 1980s, nearly 500 chest-wall resections for primary neoplasms were performed at the Mayo Clinic by one team of surgeons (unpublished data). Approximately two-thirds of these neoplasms were malignant. Malignant fibrous histiocytoma and chondrosarcoma were the most common malignant neoplasms, and desmoid tumor was the most common benign tumor. Ages ranged from 12 to 81 years, with a median of 44.3 years. An average of 3.8 ribs were resected per patient. Total or partial sternectomies were performed in 21 patients. Skeletal defects were closed with prosthetic material in 63 patients and with autogenous ribs in 5. Eighty-four patients underwent 108 muscle transpositions, including 42 pectoralis major, 33 latissimus dorsi, 10 serratus anterior, 3 external oblique, 2 rectus abdominis, 2 trapezius, and 16 other muscles. The omentum was transposed in 11 patients. Median hospitalization was 9 days. There were no 30-day postoperative deaths. Patients were generally extubated during the evening of the operation or on the following morning. Three patients required tracheostomy. Most other patients showed only minor changes in pulmonary function (Meadows et al., 1985).

Long-term survival of patients with primary chest-wall malignant neoplasm depends on cell type and the extent of chest-wall resection. In the Mayo Clinic,

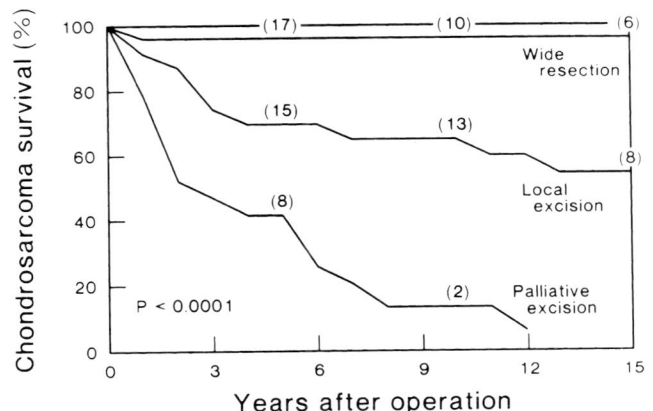

FIGURE 15–23. Survival of patients with chest-wall chondrosarcoma by extent of operation. Zero time on abscissa represents day of chest-wall resection. (From McAfee, M. K., Pairolero, P. C., Bergstralh, E. J., et al.: Chondrosarcoma of the chest wall: Factors affecting survival. Reprinted with permission from the Society of Thoracic Surgeons [The Annals of Thoracic Surgery, 1985, Vol. 40, pp. 535–541].)

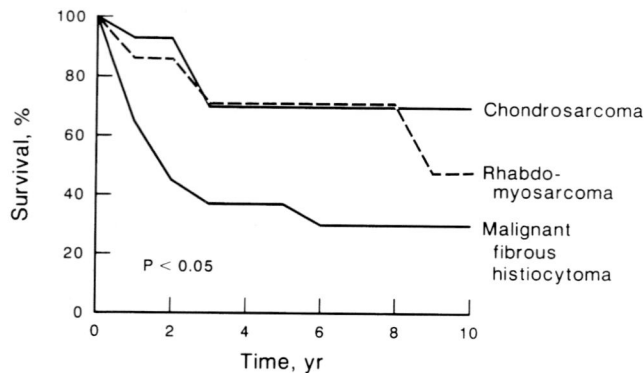

FIGURE 15–24. Survival rate for patients with chondrosarcoma and rhabdomyosarcoma compared with that of patients with malignant fibrous histiocytoma. Zero time on abscissa represents day of chest-wall resection. (From King, R. M., Pairolero, P. C., Trastek, V. F., et al.: Primary chest wall tumors: Factors affecting survival. Reprinted with permission from the Society of Thoracic Surgeons [The Annals of Thoracic Surgery, 1986, Vol. 41, pp. 597–601].)

the series overall 5-year survival rate was 57% (King et al., 1986). Wide resection for chondrosarcoma resulted in a 5-year survival rate of 96% (McAfee et al., 1985), compared with only 70% for patients who underwent local excision (Fig. 15–23). The 5-year overall survival rate for patients with either chondrosarcoma or rhabdomyosarcoma was 70% (King et al., 1986), in contrast with a survival rate of only 38% for patients with malignant fibrous histiocytoma (Fig. 15–24). Recurrent neoplasm, however, was an ominous sign: only 17% of patients whose neoplasms recurred survived 5 years.

SUMMARY

The key to successful treatment of primary chest-wall neoplasms remains early diagnosis and aggressive surgical resection. This procedure generally can be performed in one operation with minimal respiratory insufficiency and with a low operative mortality rate. With current methods of reconstruction, cure is likely for most patients with primary chest-wall neoplasm.

SELECTED BIBLIOGRAPHY

Graeber, G. M., Snyder, R. J., Fleming, A. W., et al.: Initial and long-term results in the management of primary chest wall neoplasms. Ann. Thorac. Surg., 34:664, 1982.

These authors present the Armed Forces Institute of Pathology's experience with 110 patients with primary chest-wall neoplasms. Included are both soft tissue and bone neoplasms. Fifty-four per cent of patients had malignant neoplasms. The most common malignancies were fibrosarcoma, chondrosarcoma, and myeloma. Bone neoplasms were the most common type of benign tumor. No deaths were associated with primary definitive therapy, which included surgical resection, chemotherapy, and radiation therapy. The 5-year survival rate for patients with chondrosarcoma was 89%; with fibrosarcoma, 53%; and with myeloma, 25%. The role of chemotherapy and radiation therapy for each type of malignant neoplasm is discussed.

King, R. M., Pairolero, P. C., Trastek, V. F., et al.: Primary chest wall tumors: Factors affecting survival. Ann. Thorac. Surg., 41:597–601, 1986.

This series represents a 20-year experience of chest-wall tumors treated at the Mayo Clinic from 1955 to 1975, and includes both soft tissue and bony tumors. A painful mass was the most common sign and symptom. Eighty per cent of the tumors were malignant. Malignant fibrous histiocytoma, chondrosarcoma, and rhabdomyosarcoma were the most common malignant tumors. Most malignancies were treated by wide resection. There were no operative deaths. Overall, 1-, 5-, and 10-year survival rates were 89%, 57%, and 49% respectively. Recurrent tumor developed in 52% and clearly depended on the extent of chest-wall resection. The 5-year survival rate after recurrence was only 17%. Cell type also significantly influenced survival. Both chondrosarcoma and rhabdomyosarcoma had a better prognosis than malignant fibrous histiocytoma.

McAfee, M. K., Pairolero, P. C., Bergstralh, E. J., et al.: Chondrosarcoma of the chest wall: Factors affecting survival. Ann. Thorac. Surg., 40:535–541, 1985.

These authors present a single institution's experience (96 patients) with chondrosarcoma of the chest wall. Tumor involved the rib in 78 patients and the sternum in 18. During this study, patients were treated by palliative excision, local excision, and wide resection. There was one operative death. The 10-year chondrosarcoma survival rate for patients treated by wide resection was 96%, by local excision 65%, and by palliative excision 14%. Tumor grade, tumor diameter, tumor location, and date of operation all significantly influenced survival. This series is the largest series of chest-wall chondrosarcoma reported to date, and clearly demonstrates that the natural history of chondrosarcoma is one of slow growth and local recurrence.

McCraw, J. B., and Arnold, P. G.: McCraw and Arnold's Atlas of Muscle and Musculocutaneous Flaps. Norfolk, VA, Hampton Press, 1986.

The anatomy, indications for, and technique of commonly used muscle flaps in all areas of the body are each summarized, illustrated by color photographs of fresh cadaver dissections, and then supplemented by appropriate intraoperative color photographs of clinical cases. All of the major chest-wall muscles are demonstrated, including their use intrathoracically. The axial blood supply and arc of rotation for each muscle are clearly shown. Each muscle flap is compared with other regional flaps according to its strengths and weaknesses. Complications and pitfalls are also discussed. This atlas should be read by every surgeon interested in reconstruction of the chest wall.

Pairolero, P. C., and Arnold, P. G.: Chest wall tumors: Experience with 100 consecutive patients. J. Thorac. Cardiovasc. Surg., 90:367–372, 1985.

This series represents the experience of a single team of surgeons in the management of 100 consecutive patients with chest-wall tumors. Fifty patients had primary malignant neoplasms, 32 had metastases, and 18 had benign tumors. The tumors were located in the ribs in 78 patients and in the sternum in 22. Primary malignancy was treated with wide resection; metastases and benign tumor were treated with local excision. The median number of ribs resected was 3.4. Sternectomy was performed in 22 patients. Reconstruction was with prosthetic material in 57 patients and with autogenous ribs in 11. Soft tissue reconstruction used torso muscle in 81 patients and omentum in 3. Median hospitalization was 9.6 days. Complications occurred in 9 patients. Only 1 patient required tracheostomy. There was one operative death. Ninety-five per cent of patients with primary malignant neoplasms were alive at a median follow-up of 2.5 years. This series of patients demonstrates that aggressive resection for chest-wall tumor with reliable reconstruction can be accomplished safely, and that early wide resection can be curative.

Pairolero, P. C., and Arnold, P. G.: Thoracic wall defects: Surgical management of 205 consecutive patients. Mayo Clin. Proc., 61:557–563, 1986.

This series represents one surgical team's experience with over 200 consecutive chest-wall reconstructions. Reconstruction was for chest-wall tumors in 114 patients, radiation necrosis in 56, infected median sternotomy wounds in 56, and costochondritis in 8. Twenty-nine of these patients had multiple conditions. Total or partial sternectomies were performed in 60 patients. Skeletal defects were closed with prosthetic material in 66 patients and with autogenous rib in 12. One hundred sixty-eight patients underwent 244 muscle flap transpositions, including 149 pectoralis major, 56 latissimus dorsi, 14 rectus abdominis, 13 serratus anterior, 8 external oblique, 2 trapezius, and 2 advancements of the diaphragm. The omentum was transposed in 20 patients. The mean number of operations per patient was 1.9. Mean hospitalization was 16.5 days. One perioperative death occurred at 29 days. Four patients required tracheostomy. During a mean follow-up of nearly 3 years there were 49 late deaths, predominantly due to malignant disease. All patients who were alive 30 days after operation had well-healed wounds at last follow-up examination or at the time of death. This series demonstrates that nearly all chest-wall afflictions can be successfully treated with current methods of chest-wall resection and reconstruction.

BIBLIOGRAPHY

Arnold, P. G., and Pairolero, P. C.: Chest wall reconstruction: Experience with 100 consecutive patients. Ann. Surg., *199*:725–732, 1984.

Arnold, P. G., and Pairolero, P. C.: Chondrosarcoma of the manubrium. Resection and reconstruction with pectoralis major muscle. Mayo Clin. Proc., *53*:54–57, 1978.

Arnold, P. G., and Pairolero, P. C.: Surgical management of the radiated chest wall. Plast. Reconstr. Surg., *77*:605–612, 1986.

Arnold, P. G., and Pairolero, P. C.: Use of pectoralis major muscle flaps to repair defects of anterior chest wall. Plast. Reconstr. Surg., *63*:205–213, 1979.

Arnold, P. G., Pairolero, P. C., and Waldorf, J. C.: The serratus anterior muscle: Intrathoracic and extrathoracic utilization. Plast. Reconstr. Surg., *73*:240–248, 1984.

Bostwick, J. III, Nahai, F., Wallace, J. G., and Vasconez, L. O.: Sixty latissimus dorsi flaps. Plast. Reconstr. Surg., *63*:31–41, 1979.

Campbell, D. A.: Reconstruction of the anterior thoracic wall. J. Thorac. Surg., *19*:456–461, 1950.

Eng, J., Sabanathan, S., Pradhan, G. N., and Meams, A. J.: Primary bony chest wall tumours. J. R. Coll. Surg. Edinb., *5*:44–47, 1990.

Evans, K. G., Miller, R. R., Muller, N. L., and Nelems, B.: Chest wall tumours. Can. J. Surg., *33*:229–232, 1990.

Farley, J. H., and Seyfer, A. E.: Chest wall tumors: Experience with 58 patients. Milit. Med., *156*:413–415, 1991.

Fisher, J., Bostwick, J., and Powell, R. W.: Latissimus dorsi blood supply after thoracodorsal vessel division: The serratus collateral. Plast. Reconstr. Surg., *72*:502–509, 1983.

Graeber, G. M., Snyder, R. J., Fleming, A. W., et al.: Initial and long-term results in the management of primary chest wall neoplasms. Ann. Thorac. Surg., *34*:664, 1982.

Groff, D. B., and Adkins, P. C.: Chest wall tumors. Ann. Thorac. Surg., *4*:260, 1967.

Hodgkinson, D. J., and Arnold, P. G.: Chest-wall reconstruction using the external oblique muscle. Br. J. Plast. Surg., *33*:216–220, 1980.

Jurkiewicz, M. J., and Arnold, P. G.: The omentum: An account of its use in the reconstruction of the chest wall. Ann. Surg., *185*:548–554, 1977.

King, R. M., Pairolero, P. C., Trastek, V. F., et al.: Primary chest wall tumors: Factors affecting survival. Ann. Thorac. Surg., *41*:597–601, 1986.

McAfee, M. K., Pairolero, P. C., Bergstralh, E. J., et al.: Chondrosarcoma of the chest wall: Factors affecting survival. Ann. Thorac. Surg., *40*:535–541, 1985.

McCraw, J. B., and Arnold, P. G.: McCraw and Arnold's Atlas of Muscle and Musculocutaneous Flaps. Norfolk, VA, Hampton Press, 1986.

Meadows, J. A. III, Staats, B. A., Pairolero, P. C., et al.: Effect of resection of the sternum and manubrium in conjunction with muscle transposition on pulmonary function. Mayo Clin. Proc., *60*:604–609, 1985.

Pairolero, P. C., and Arnold, P. G.: Chest wall tumors: Experience with 100 consecutive patients. J. Thorac. Cardiovasc. Surg., *90*:367–372, 1985.

Pairolero, P. C., and Arnold, P. G.: Management of recalcitrant median sternotomy wounds. J. Thorac. Cardiovasc. Surg., *88*:357–364, 1984.

Pairolero, P. C., and Arnold, P. G.: Primary tumors of the anterior chest wall. Surg. Rounds, November 1986, pp. 19–24.

Pairolero, P. C., and Arnold, P. G.: Thoracic wall defects: Surgical management of 205 consecutive patients. Mayo Clin. Proc., *61*:557–563, 1986.

16 The Pleura

Robbin G. Cohen, Tom R. DeMeester, and Edwin Lafontaine

HISTORICAL ASPECTS

Experience with battle injuries over the centuries demonstrated to physicians the rapid lethal effects that ensued when a gaping hole in the chest collapsed the lung. As a consequence, surgeons feared to enter the pleural cavity and devised ways to approach parts of the thorax without violating the pleura. Early in the 20th century, this fear was dispelled by an understanding of how expansion of the lungs could be maintained with an open chest. Since then, advances in anesthesiology have permitted transpleural operations to be performed with great safety and minimal morbidity.

Before the antibiotic era, pleural empyema was a common problem in thoracic surgery and an Empyema Commission was formed during World War I. Publications from this group contributed to present-day understanding and management of pleural space infection (Graham and Bell, 1918). With the availability of antibiotics, the incidence of pleural infections and of empyema decreased. Today, thoracic surgeons rarely see a fully developed pneumococcal empyema, but they encounter pleural fluid infected with organisms that were unheard of a century ago.

The development of pulmonary resection for various pulmonary diseases and the application of surgical therapy to lesions of the esophagus and heart have caused an increase in postoperative pleural complications. These complications are some of the most difficult problems encountered by thoracic surgeons.

The increase in knowledge of pulmonary, cardiac, and esophageal physiology has led to an appreciation of the important role of the pleura and the pleural space environment and to fresh interest in the study of the pleura and pleural space.

ANATOMY OF THE PLEURA

Each lung is invested by and enclosed within the pleura. Consequently, the pleural space has the form of a closed, invaginated, serous sac (Fig. 16–1). During development, the lung buds grow as diverticula of the foregut. As they enlarge bilaterally into the thoracic coelom, they invaginate the pleural sac. The resulting closed, mesothelium-lined pleural space contains the two parts of the pleura: the outer parietal pleura, which retains its original relationship to the thoracic wall, and the visceral pleura, which intimately invests the lung (see Fig. 16–1). The visceral pleura adheres to the lung and covers its entire surface including the fissures and indentations of the lobes. The mesothelial lining of the opposed surfaces of the two pleural layers secretes a small amount of lubricating serous fluid that minimizes friction between them during respiration.

The parietal pleura lines the thoracic cavity and is divided into four areas: the *costal pleura*, which lies against the ribs and intercostal muscles; the *diaphragmatic pleura*, which covers the thoracic surface of the diaphragm; the *mediastinal pleura*, which covers the mediastinum; and the *cervical pleura*, which covers the superior aspect of the pleural space in the plane of the first rib. These terms designate regional parts of the contiguous pleural sac that extends beyond the lung and provides potential space for maximal expansion of the lung during forced ventilation. Beyond the lung margins, parts of the parietal pleura are in contact until they are separated by excursions of the lung with deep inspiration. These potential spaces include the *costodiaphragmatic sinus* (Fig. 16–2), where the diaphragmatic and costal pleurae are in contact at the sides of the diaphragm, and the *costomediastinal sinus* (see Fig. 16–1), where the costal and mediastinal pleurae are in contact behind the sternum. The costomediastinal sinuses may extend medially over the heart such that inadvertent entry of the pleural space may occur with a sternotomy incision.

Anteriorly, the mediastinal pleura follows the curvature of the pericardium to the root of the lung. Posteriorly, it overlies the bodies of the thoracic vertebrae, the thoracic aorta, and the esophagus (see Fig. 16–1). The mediastinal pleura reflects over the root of the lung and onto the lung surface to become the visceral pleura. From the inferior border of the root of the lung to the diaphragmatic surface, the anterior and posterior reflections of the pleura join to form the

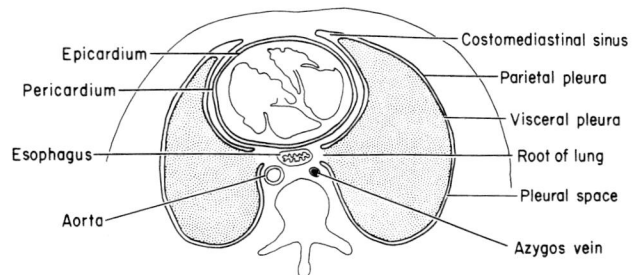

FIGURE 16–1. Schematic cross-section of the thorax. The shape of the pleural space is shown by the invagination of the lung buds, and the pleura is divided into its parietal and visceral parts. Note the location of the costomediastinal sinus anteriorly.

523

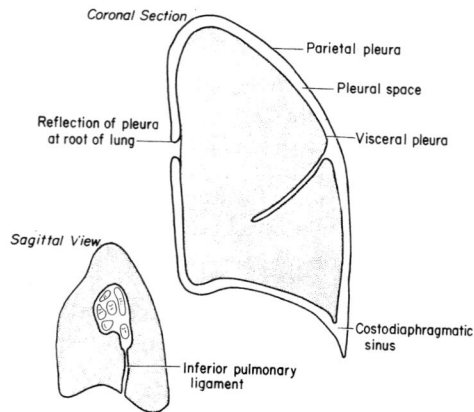

FIGURE 16–2. Schematic coronal section of a hemithorax and sagittal view of the root of the lung showing the pleural coverings. Note the location of the costodiaphragmatic sinus.

inferior pulmonary ligament (see Fig. 16–2, sagittal view).

The arterial blood supply to the parietal pleura is from branches of the posterior intercostal, internal mammary, superior phrenic, and anterior mediastinal arteries. The veins of the parietal pleura correspond to these arteries. The visceral pleura is supplied by radicles of the bronchial and pulmonary arteries, the veins of which are tributaries of the pulmonary veins. No bronchial veins drain the visceral pleura. The costal and peripheral parts of the diaphragmatic pleura are innervated by the intercostal nerves. The central portion of the diaphragmatic pleura and probably the mediastinal pleura are innervated by the phrenic nerves. Vagal and sympathetic twigs also reach the visceral pleura through branches from the pulmonary plexus. Unlike the parietal pleura, which is extremely sensitive to contact and inflammatory changes, the visceral pleura is insensitive because it receives no nerves of general sensation.

The lymphatic vessels of the pleura are located in the connective tissue beneath the mesothelial lining. The lymphatics of the visceral pleura combine with the superficial efferent lymphatics of the lung to form an extensive subpleural lymphatic plexus. Lymphatics from the subpleural plexus and remaining lung drain into the mediastinal lymph nodes. The lymphatics from the parietal pleura drain regionally; those from the costal pleura drain into intercostal and substernal nodes, those from the diaphragmatic pleura drain into phrenic nodes, and those from the mediastinal pleura drain into anterior and posterior mediastinal nodes. A few superolateral lymphatic channels from the cervical to the costal pleurae reach the axillary nodes. Eventually, the lymphatic drainage from the parietal and visceral pleurae is returned to the vascular system by the right lymphatic duct or the left thoracic duct.

The pleura maintains the environment of the pleural space in which the organs of the chest function. The pleural space and pleura are susceptible to disease that affects not only their own function but also that of organs invested by them. Diseases that affect

the pleural space are essentially mechanical in pathophysiology and consist of pneumothorax, hemothorax, chylothorax, pleural effusions, empyema, bronchopleural fistula, fibrothorax, and iatrogenic space problems. Diseases that affect the pleura are essentially cellular and include tuberculosis, pleural plaques, and pleural tumors.

DISEASES OF THE PLEURAL SPACE

Pneumothorax

A pneumothorax is an accumulation of gas in the pleural space and was the first disorder recognized to affect the pleural space (Lindskog and Halasz, 1957). In 1623, Paré described the presence of subcutaneous emphysema secondary to a rib fracture without mention of the presence of an associated pneumothorax. In 1724, in his report of spontaneous rupture of the esophagus, Boerhaave described the presence of a large amount of air in the pleural cavity with collapse of the lungs and was the first person to report the occurrence of a pneumothorax in the absence of external chest trauma. In 1803, Etard first used the term *pneumothorax* to describe a pathologic entity, and in 1826, Laënnec described its clinical features. For many years, the abnormality was thought to be a complication of tuberculosis. In 1932, Kjaergaard was the first to emphasize a nontuberculous etiology in most patients.

Pathophysiology

A pneumothorax may be spontaneous or secondary to a traumatic, diagnostic, or therapeutic event. A spontaneous pneumothorax can be "primary" and occur without known etiology or clinical evidence of an underlying disease or "secondary" to a disease process that predisposes to pneumothorax (Lindskog and Halasz, 1957) (Table 16–1). Regardless of the cause, the physiologic consequences are similar.

During quiet breathing, the intrapleural pressure fluctuates between -8 and -9 mm Hg during inspiration and -3 and -6 mm Hg during expiration. Because of the elastic recoil of the lung, the intrabronchial pressure in the lungs is greater than the intrapleural pressure throughout the respiratory cycle and fluctuates between -1 and -3 mm Hg during inspiration and $+1$ and $+5$ during expiration (Killen and Gobbell, 1968) (Fig. 16–3). The pressure gradient between the intrabronchial and the intrapleural pressures, separated by the alveolar walls and visceral pleura, holds the visceral pleura of the lungs against the parietal pleura of the chest wall.

Pneumothorax occurs when air enters the pleural space as a result of disruption of one of the pleural surfaces. This disruption may cross the visceral pleura secondary to a ruptured pulmonary bleb, the parietal pleura secondary to trauma, or the mediastinal pleura from an injured airway or esophagus. Loss of the negative intrapleural pressure and collapse of the

■ **Table 16–1.** CAUSES OF SECONDARY SPONTANEOUS PNEUMOTHORAX

Airway Disease

Bullous disease
Chronic obstructive pulmonary disease
Asthma
Cyst (congenital)
Pneumatocele
Cystic fibrosis

Interstitial Disease

Idiopathic pulmonary fibrosis
Eosinophilic granuloma
Sarcoidosis
Tuberous sclerosis
Collagen vascular diseases

Infections

Anaerobic pneumonia
Staphylococcal pneumonia
Gram-negative pneumonia
Lung abscess
Actinomycosis
Nocardiosis
Tuberculosis
Atypical mycobacteria
Pneumocystis carinii pneumonia

Neoplasms

Primary
Metastatic

Others

Endometriosis
Ehlers-Danlos syndrome
Pulmonary embolism
Marfan's syndrome

20 cm H_2O can shift the mediastinum, mechanically interfere with venous return to the heart, and decrease cardiac output (Fig. 16–4).

A pneumothorax reduces pulmonary volumes, pulmonary compliance, and diffusing capacity. The pathophysiologic consequences depend on the size of the pneumothorax, the presence of tension, and the condition of the underlying lung. Arterial hypoxemia usually occurs with collapse of 50% or more and is secondary to continued perfusion of the poorly ventilated areas. If the contralateral lung is normal, the hypoxemia is usually transient and disappears as perfusion to the collapsed lung decreases. Patients whose vital capacity is decreased by underlying pulmonary disease are less able to compensate for the loss of functional lung and may die from an untreated pneumothorax. On the other hand, patients with underlying pulmonary disease that has destroyed the elastic recoil of the lung have a smaller alveolar-pleural gradient. Under these conditions, collapse may be slow and less extensive, although even this small reduction in vital capacity can increase the work of breathing and precipitate respiratory failure.

Clinical Presentation and Roentgenographic Diagnosis

The clinical history and physical findings in patients with pneumothorax depend on the underlying cause, extent of lung collapse, and the presence or absence of preexisting pulmonary disease. In some

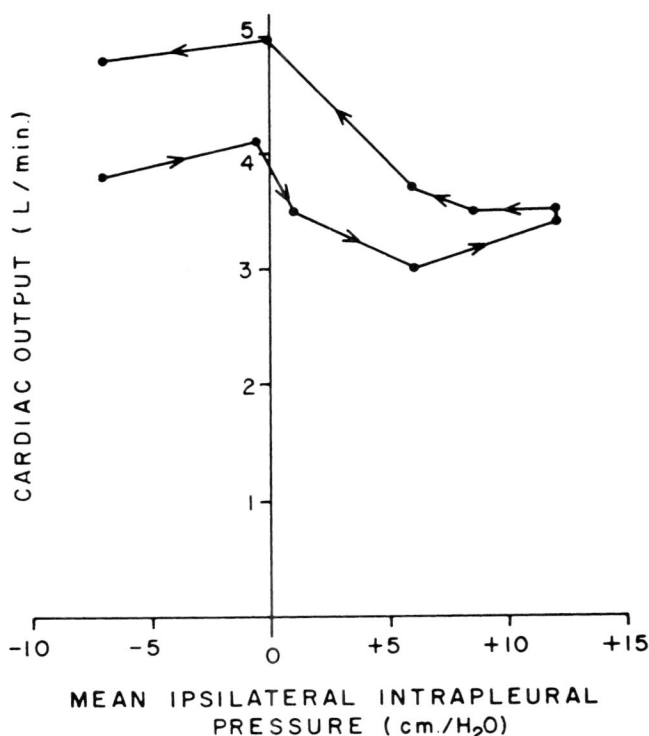

lung ensue until the disruption seals or the pressures between the communicating spaces become equalized. A check-valve effect at the site of the pleural rupture may permit entry but not exit of air. Progressively deeper and more labored inspiration produces a greater negative intrapleural pressure and further accumulation of air within the pleural space, which cannot escape. During expiration, this becomes a positive pressure that results in a tension pneumothorax. A positive intrapleural pressure as small as 15 to

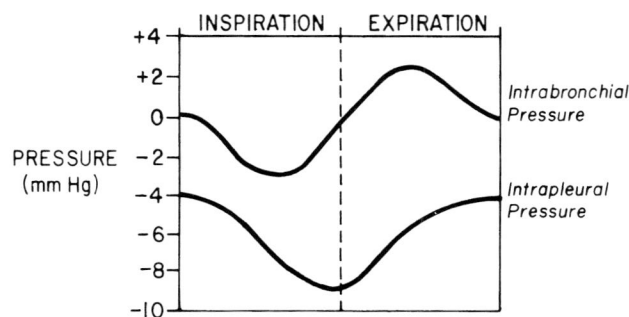

FIGURE 16–3. Pressure tracing of the intrabronchial and intrapleural pressures during inspiration and expiration, showing the constant pressure gradient between the bronchus and the pleural space.

FIGURE 16–4. Reduction in cardiac output caused by increasing intrapleural pressure. A positive pleural pressure interferes with venous return to the heart.

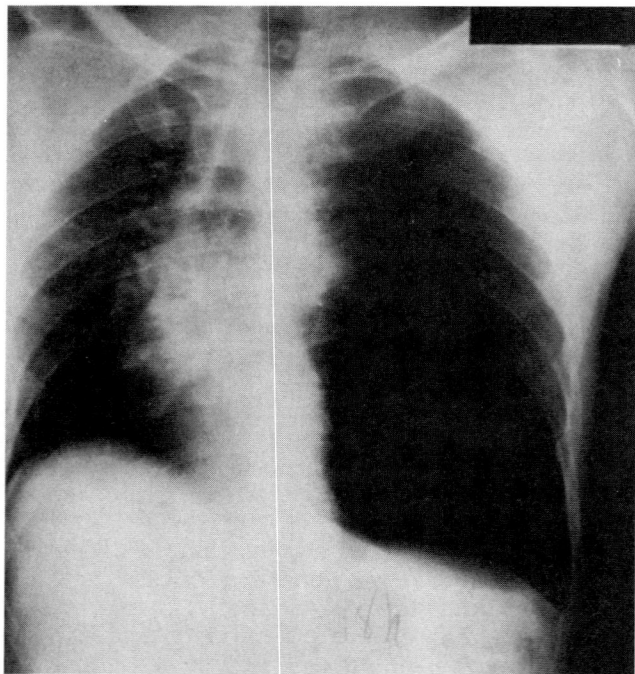

FIGURE 16–5. Chest film of a patient with severe dyspnea from a tension pneumothorax. Note the shift of the trachea and mediastinum to the left, absence of vascular markings in the left hemithorax, and depression of the left diaphragm.

ent, a crunching sound (Hamman's sign) is heard with cardiac auscultation.

Patients with tension pneumothorax may appear cyanotic and in marked respiratory distress. The veins of the neck are distended, and the trachea and cardiac apex are deviated toward the uninvolved side (Fig. 16–5). If the pressure on the involved side is not urgently relieved by needle aspiration or tube thoracostomy, death from cardiovascular collapse ensues.

A pneumothorax can usually be seen on the standard posteroanterior chest film taken with deep inspiration. The radiographic hallmark is displacement of the visceral pleura from the parietal pleura by air in the pleural space. This appears as a hyperlucent area with absent pulmonary markings in the periphery of the hemithorax. The visceral pleura is visualized as a thin white line outlined by air in the outer pleural space on one side and air within pulmonary parenchyma on the other (Fig. 16–6). If the clinical manifestations strongly suggest a pneumothorax and no abnormality is seen on the chest film taken with inspiration, an expiratory study should be performed. With expiration, the size of a pneumothorax appears to increase on a chest film because the lung volume is reduced during maximal forced expiration. Expiration also increases the radiographic density of the lung, increasing the contrast between the lung and the air in the pleural space.

When attempting to estimate the size of a pneumo-

patients, the pneumothorax may be asymptomatic. Serementis (1970) reported that 18% of patients did not seek medical attention for more than 1 week and some may never seek medical attention. A pneumothorax that occurs after central venous line placement or percutaneous needle biopsy of a pulmonary lesion is frequently asymptomatic, and is detected on a routine chest film after the procedure. In 80% of patients with spontaneous pneumothorax, the symptoms occur at rest or during normal activity (Adkins and Smyth, 1960; Brooks, 1973; Clark et al., 1972). Pain is the most frequent complaint and may be the only symptom if the pneumothorax is small. The pain is initially sharp and pleuritic in nature but, with time, may become dull and persistent. Dyspnea is the second most frequent symptom and may be pronounced, depending on the degree of pulmonary collapse and the presence of underlying pulmonary disease. A tension pneumothorax causes severe dyspnea, often followed by cardiovascular collapse. Less frequent symptoms of pneumothorax are orthopnea, hemoptysis, and nonproductive cough (DeVries and Wolfe, 1980; Leach, 1945).

A patient with a small pneumothorax may have no abnormal physical findings. Those with larger pneumothoraces may have diminished to absent motion of the chest wall with respiration, hyperresonance and tympany to percussion, and reduced or absent tactile fremitus, all on the affected side. Breath sounds are reduced or absent on the involved side. Cyanosis may be present, especially with underlying pulmonary disease. When mediastinal emphysema is pres-

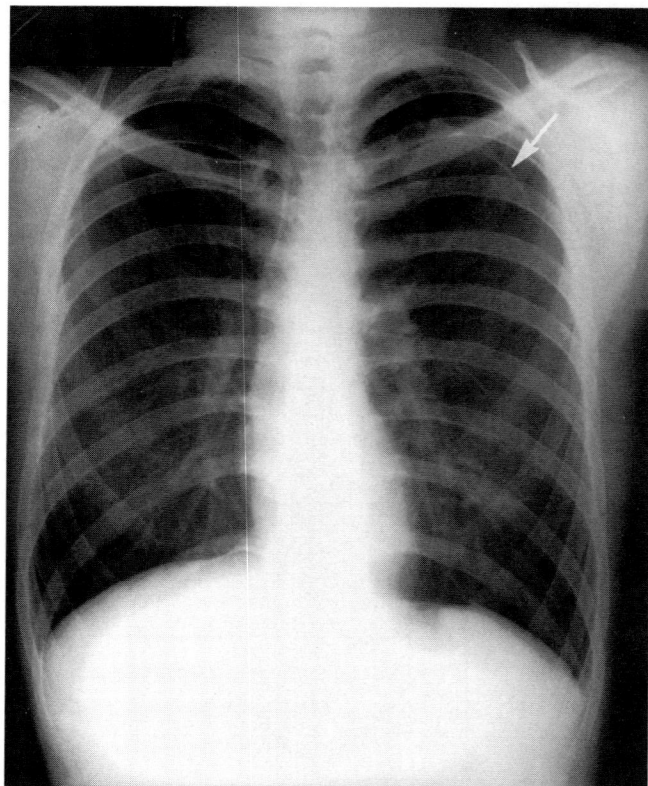

FIGURE 16–6. Chest film of a patient wth moderate left pneumothorax. The *arrow* denotes white line of visceral pleura, with air in the pleural space on one side and pulmonary parenchyma on the other side. (Courtesy of Indiana Reformatory, Pendleton, IN.)

thorax from a two-dimensional chest film, it is important to remember that the air in the pleural space may surround the lung on all sides. Hence, a pneumothorax that is seen only along the periphery of the chest film can occupy 30% of the volume of the pleural cavity. Rhea and associates (1982) reported a method for calculating the size of a pneumothorax by dividing by 3 the sum of three roentgenographic measurements (Fig. 16–7A). This value is plotted on a nomogram, and the size of the pneumothorax is estimated as a percentage of the volume of the hemithorax on the affected side (Fig. 16–7B). The size of a pneumothorax is then classified as small (<20%), moderate (20 to 40%), or large (>40%).

Certain clinical situations may make a pneumothorax difficult to recognize. Portable chest films taken in the critically ill or the trauma patient in the supine or semirecumbent position may obscure a pneumothorax. Rather than being visualized in the apex or areas lateral to the lung, air accumulates in the anteromedial and subpulmonic areas, which are the least dependent pleural spaces in this position (Chiles and Ravin, 1986; Tocino et al., 1985). Pneumothorax is also difficult to visualize in patients with bullous emphysema. Differentiation of a pneumothorax from a large bulla is a common clinical problem (Fig. 16–8).

Mistaking a bulla for a pneumothorax could lead to inappropriate insertion of a chest tube. A *computed tomography* (CT) scan that shows the septa of bullae filling the hyperlucent area excludes the diagnosis of a pneumothorax (Fig. 16–9). CT scanning may also be necessary to identify a loculated pneumothorax in patients with multiple pleural adhesions secondary to pleural disease, trauma, or previous surgery.

An air fluid level seen with a pneumothorax on chest film represents a pleural effusion. Accumulation of large quantities of pleural fluid within hours of the onset of a pneumothorax suggests an associated hemothorax. This is usually secondary to bleeding from a torn parietal pleural adhesion or, more rarely, from the lung surface. When a sizable air fluid level or pneumomediastinum accompanies a pneumothorax, spontaneous rupture of the esophagus must be considered. The diagnosis can be confirmed by obtaining a meglumine diatrizoate (Gastrografin) swallow with the patient in the lateral decubitus position. When a patient is upright, small esophageal injuries may be overlooked.

Roentgenographic findings that may accompany a pneumothorax include pulmonary blebs, interstitial pulmonary disease, pleural adhesions, and pulmonary parenchymal nodules. After reexpansion of the

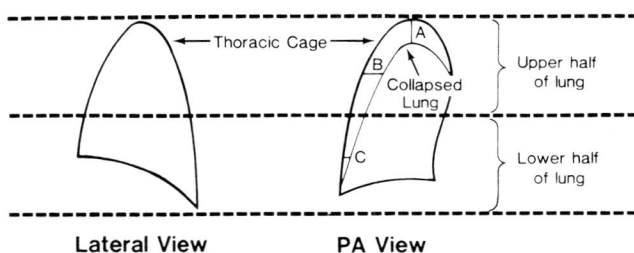

A = Maximum apical interpleural distance

B = Interpleural distance at midpoint of upper half of lung

C = Interpleural distance at midpoint of lower half of lung

A   **Average Interpleural Distance** $= \dfrac{A + B + C}{3}$

AVERAGE INTERPLEURAL DISTANCE (cm) $=$ PNEUMOTHORAX SIZE (%)

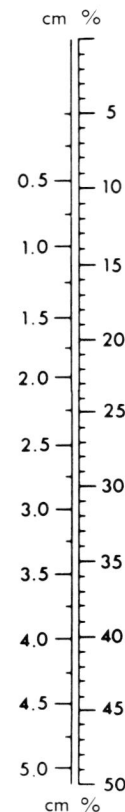

FIGURE 16–7. *A,* Schematic drawing showing how to calculate the average distance between the visceral and the parietal pleurae from a chest film showing a pneumothorax. *B,* Nomogram used to predict the size of a pneumothorax from the average intrapleural distance measured on the chest film. (*A* and *B,* From Rhea, J. T., DeLuca, S. A., and Greene, R. E.: Determining the size of pneumothorax in the upright patient. Radiology *144:*733, 1982.)

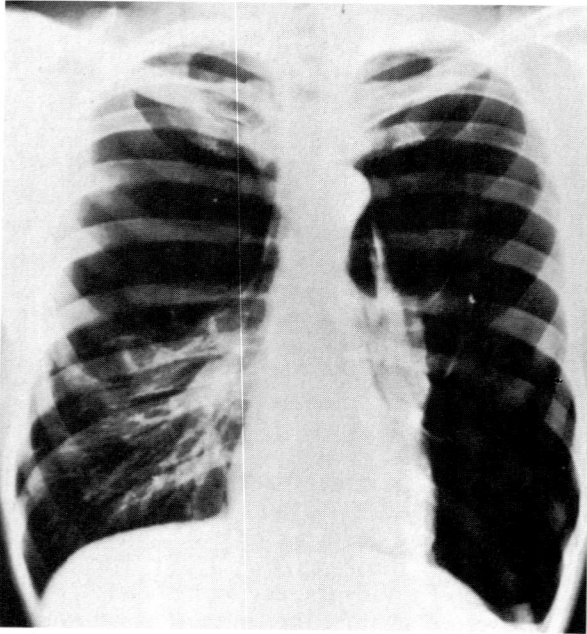

FIGURE 16–8. Chest film of a patient with severe dyspnea secondary to a large left pneumothorax in the presence of giant bullous disease in the right lung.

lung, CT scanning may further define any underlying pulmonary pathology. Bronchoscopy is indicated when the lung fails to reexpand after the insertion of an appropriately placed chest tube (Fig. 16–10).

The clinical syndrome produced by a spontaneous pneumothorax is usually so typical that other conditions can be excluded by the history, physical examination, and radiographic findings. Occasionally, pneumothorax must be differentiated from myocardial ischemia, acute aortic dissection, spontaneous rupture of the esophagus, or a perforated peptic ulcer.

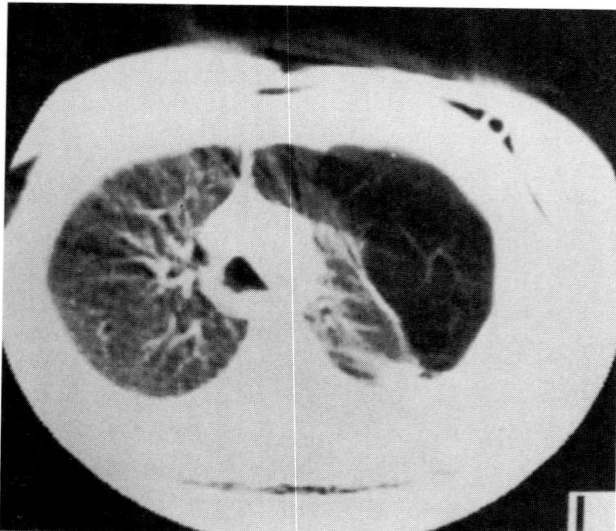

FIGURE 16–9. Computed tomography (CT) scan showing the septa of bullae filling the area of hyperlucent lung. This is helpful in differentiating a pneumothorax from bullous disease.

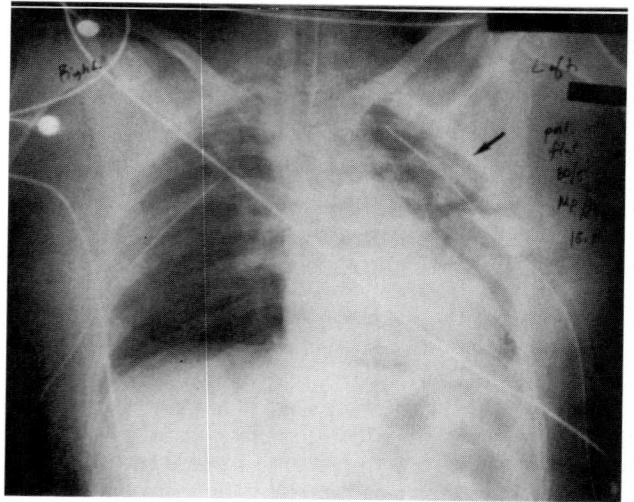

FIGURE 16–10. Portable chest film of patient after blunt trauma to the chest. The persistence of a pneumothorax (arrow) despite good thoracostomy tube position and function suggested a rupture of the left mainstem bronchus. Bronchoscopy confirmed the diagnosis.

Primary Spontaneous Pneumothorax

Primary spontaneous pneumothorax is a disease of young adults. Most patients are between the ages of 20 and 30 years, with 85% under the age of 40 years. The disease has an annual incidence of 9 cases per 100,000 population (Melton et al., 1979), with men outnumbering women by a ratio of 4 to 6 : 1. There is an increased incidence among cigarette smokers. The disease is slightly more common on the right side, and simultaneous bilateral pneumothoraces are seen in 10% of patients. Familial spontaneous pneumothorax has been reported sporadically since it was first described (Faber, 1921), and a positive family history for primary spontaneous pneumothorax has been shown to occur in 11.5% of patients (Abolnik et al., 1993).

Primary spontaneous pneumothorax results from rupture of a pulmonary bleb. The bleb is an air-filled space between the parenchyma of the lung and the visceral pleura, and develops from rupture of an alveolar wall with intrapulmonary dissection of the free air to the pleural surface. The observation that these blebs have no epithelial lining supports their acquired etiology, although their true pathogenesis is unknown. One explanation is that the mechanical stresses caused by the weight of the upright lung are not distributed uniformly throughout the lung, but are stronger in the apices than in the bases. According to the law of Laplace, the tension in the walls of the apical alveoli is increased and the walls are prone to enlarge, causing the alveoli to overexpand and rupture. The alveolar gas then dissects along the lobular septa either centrally to produce a pneumomediastinum or peripherally to collect as blebs beneath the visceral pleura (Fig. 16–11).

The incidence of radiographically demonstrable blebs is approximately 15%. They are most often located in the apices of the upper lobes and occasionally

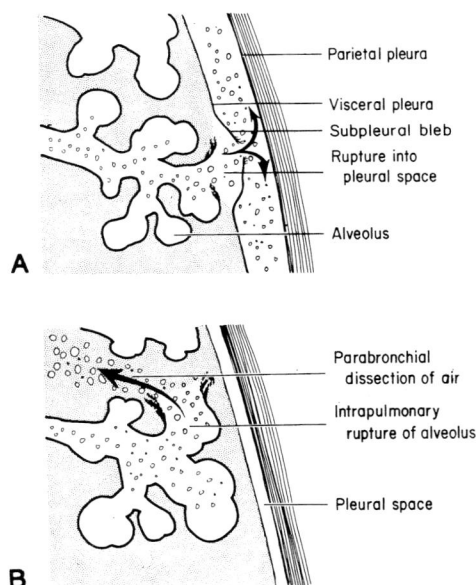

FIGURE 16–11. Schematic drawing of the distended apical alveoli caused by mechanical stress from the weight of the upright lung. Alveolar rupture allows alveolar gas to dissect peripherally and form blebs that eventually rupture into the pleural space and cause a pneumothorax (A) or dissect centrally along lobular septa and produce a pneumomediastinum (B).

along the fissures. In cases requiring surgical therapy, blebs are found approximately 85% of the time (Macklin and Macklin, 1944; West, 1971).

Follow-up studies show a 20 to 50% recurrence rate of primary spontaneous pneumothorax after the initial episode. Ninety per cent of recurrences occur on the same side as the previous episode. After a second episode, the recurrence rate increases to 60 to 80% (Gaensler, 1956; Gobbell et al., 1963). Risk factors for recurrence include more than one previous episode, large cysts seen on roentgenograms, and increased height:weight ratio (Lippert et al., 1991).

Secondary Spontaneous Pneumothorax

In 20% of patients with spontaneous pneumothorax, the event is related to localized or generalized underlying pulmonary disease (Dines et al., 1967; Steier et al., 1974) (see Table 16–1). The pneumothorax may precipitate respiratory failure because the patients are older and usually have compromised pulmonary function. The recurrence rate with secondary pneumothorax is reported to be similar to that of a primary pneumothorax (Dines et al., 1970).

The most common pulmonary pathology associated with secondary spontaneous pneumothorax is chronic obstructive pulmonary disease (COPD). This entity accounts for the second peak in the incidence of spontaneous pneumothorax between the ages of 45 and 65 years (Dines et al., 1970). A pneumothorax that occurs in older individuals as a complication of severe emphysema often goes unnoticed because the signs and symptoms resemble those of the underlying pulmonary disease (George et al., 1975). The bullae in these

patients are formed not by alveolar rupture, as in primary spontaneous pneumothorax, but by progressive destruction of alveolar walls (Fitzgerald et al., 1974). Because the underlying disease process destroys the elastic recoil of the lung, the pneumothorax develops more slowly. Even though these pneumothoraces are slow to develop, they can cause severe respiratory compromise because these patients lose pulmonary reserve. Unlike primary spontaneous pneumothorax, which has a low mortality, spontaneous pneumothorax in patients with underlying severe COPD has a mortality of 16% (Fitzgerald et al., 1974).

Malignant neoplasms, particularly metastatic sarcomas, can cause a secondary spontaneous pneumothorax (Dines et al., 1973). Most commonly, the pneumothorax is secondary to osteogenic sarcoma in children and may be the first evidence of pulmonary metastasis. Two mechanisms by which a malignant lesion can cause a pneumothorax have been proposed: First, malignant lesions associated with a pneumothorax are subpleural, and their rapid growth leads to ischemic necrosis and perforation into the pleural space. Similarly, chemotherapy leading to tumor necrosis can cause a pneumothorax in patients with pulmonary metastasis (Janetos and Ochsner, 1963; Schulman et al., 1979). Second, tumors in the lung can cause expiratory bronchial obstruction and lead to alveolar distention, intrapulmonary rupture, bleb formation, and rupture into the pleural space (Ayres et al., 1980).

Spontaneous pneumothorax can be secondary to tuberculosis in patients with advanced cavitary disease. Such symptoms as cough, expectoration, debility, fever, and weight loss usually precede the onset of pneumothorax by many months. The pneumothorax commonly develops into tuberculous empyema and can be diagnosed from smears and cultures of pleural fluid (Kjaergaard, 1932, 1933). Of patients felt to have primary spontaneous pneumothorax, 2 to 3% subsequently develop active pulmonary tuberculosis and may have had active occult tuberculosis at the time of their pneumothorax.

Neonatal Spontaneous Pneumothorax

In the neonate, pneumothorax has been associated with hyaline membrane disease, renal malformation, Potter's syndrome, and meconium aspiration (Boer and Andrews, 1977; Luck et al., 1977). In children, spontaneous pneumothorax can be secondary to cystic fibrosis.

Catamenial Spontaneous Pneumothorax

A spontaneous pneumothorax that occurs during menstruation was described by Maurer and colleagues (1968) and was named catamenial pneumothorax by Lillington and co-workers (1972). The highest incidence is in the third and fourth decades of life and the pneumothorax occurs on the right side in 90% of patients. Onset is usually within 48 to 72 hours after the beginning of menses. The pneumothorax never occurs during periods of nonovulation, as in pregnancy or while taking oral contraceptives. Four possible causes of this condition have been proposed: rupture of a pulmonary bleb; alveolar rupture due to high levels of prostaglandin F_2 during menstruation; ingress of air into the pleural cavity through the uterus, fallopian tubes, and diaphragmatic fenestrations with loss of the uterine mucous plug during menses; and pleural or pulmonary endometriosis. There is no single explanation for all occurrences of catamenial pneumothorax. Only the temporal relationship between the pneumothorax and menstruation is irrefutable (Schoenfeld et al., 1986).

Complications of Spontaneous Pneumothorax

Pleural fluid in the presence of spontaneous pneumothorax can be seen on the chest film in approximately 20% of patients. This fluid is a true hemothorax in only 3% of patients (Lindskog and Halasz, 1957). Bleeding is usually from the parietal pleura at the site of a torn adhesion or occasionally from a torn subclavian vein. Bleeding from the visceral pleura is rare because of the low pulmonary vascular pressure and the reduction in pulmonary blood flow to the lung when collapse occurs. When the hemorrhage is massive or continuous, exploratory thoracotomy is indicated.

Respiratory failure as a consequence of a pneumothorax is rare in healthy individuals, but is a frequent complication in older patients with COPD. These patients may have minimal pulmonary reserve, and a small pneumothorax can precipitate respiratory failure.

Empyema is rare with a primary spontaneous pneumothorax, but may be associated with a pneumothorax secondary to an abscess in the lung, tuberculosis, or a ruptured esophagus. In some patients the lung is difficult to reexpand after several weeks of therapy and a trapped lung results. This tends to occur in older patients who have associated pulmonary diseases, and it can persist with moderate disability for years. It is usually caused by an epithelialized bronchopleural fistula, a ruptured congenital cyst with a large bronchial communication, or an endobronchial obstruction that prevents aeration of part of the lung. A chronic bronchopleural fistula develops in only 3 to 4% of patients (Serementis, 1970).

A tension pneumothorax occurs in only 2 to 3% of patients and produces profound circulatory disturbances owing to displacement of the mediastinum and interference with the venous return to the heart (Brooks, 1973).

Management of Spontaneous Pneumothorax

Treatment of a spontaneous pneumothorax aims to alleviate symptoms, recognize complications, and prevent recurrences. The choice of therapy is based on the severity and duration of symptoms, presence of underlying pulmonary disease, history of previous episodes, and occupation of the patient. Possible ther-

apeutic approaches include observation, thoracentesis, chest tube insertion with or without suction, chemical pleurodesis via chest tube, thoracotomy with blebectomy plus pleural abrasion or pleurectomy, and more recently, thoracoscopic blebectomy and pleurodesis. The therapy that is most likely to return the patient to a normal life with the least inconvenience and delay and the lowest recurrence rate should be chosen. Observation or tube drainage is sufficient in 80 to 90% of initial episodes (Hamilton and Archer, 1983; Jones, 1985; Mercier et al., 1976).

OBSERVATION

A stable, small pneumothorax (approximately 20% or less) in an asymptomatic patient can be observed. Alhough hospitalization may not be indicated in otherwise healthy, stable patients, close follow-up with a repeat chest film in 24 to 48 hours is indicated to ensure that the pneumothorax does not enlarge. Patients should be instructed to limit their activity, to stay within reasonable range of a medical facility, and to return with persistent or increased symptoms. Approximately 1.25% of the intrapleural air is absorbed daily from the pleural cavity. As a result, it may take weeks for the lung to fully reexpand with observation (Clark et al., 1972). Delayed pulmonary expansion, progressive pneumothorax, and development of symptoms are indications for insertion of a thoracostomy tube.

THORACENTESIS

Needle or small catheter aspiration of a small to moderate pneumothorax occasionally can be accomplished to hasten reexpansion of the lung and relieve symptoms. Advocates of this approach report success rates of 30 to 70% (Hamilton and Archer, 1983; Jones, 1985; Raja and Labor, 1981). Disadvantages of this method are that it is difficult to evacuate the entire pneumothorax in order to completely reexpand the lung, it is not applicable in patients who have an active air leak, and it may delay definitive therapy with a thoracostomy tube. It is occasionally useful in patients who have sustained a small to moderate pneumothorax secondary to central venous line placement or percutaneous needle biopsy of the lung.

THORACOSTOMY

Tube drainage is the most successful therapy for pneumothorax. The thoracostomy tube should be placed in the fourth or fifth intercostal space just behind the anterior axillary fold. An alternative site is the second intercostal space in the midclavicular line. Complete reexpansion of the lung can be achieved, even in the presence of a continuous air leak. Adherence between the visceral and the parietal pleura can then occur, which may be promoted by inflammation secondary to the presence of the tube. Suction can be applied to the thoracostomy drainage system if reexpansion is incomplete, or if air is leaking into the pleural cavity faster than it can be removed by a chest tube connected to underwater seal drainage (So and Yu, 1982). Once the two pleural surfaces are apposed, the air leak usually seals. The chest tube is left in position for at least 24 hours after the air leak stops. If the patient has a history of trauma or instrumentation, a persistent large air leak and failure to completely reexpand the lung despite the use of suction suggest rupture of a mainstem bronchus and the need for operative repair.

Some patients with primary spontaneous pneumothorax who have complete reexpansion of the lung after tube thoracostomy may be treated as outpatients with a Heimlich valve attached to the thoracostomy tube (Bernstein et al., 1973; Heimlich, 1968). Ideal patients for this regimen are otherwise healthy and are able to understand and comply with instructions concerning care of the tube and valve. The tube usually can be removed 3 to 4 days later. Patients with significant underlying pulmonary disease or other medical problems and those with incomplete reexpansion or continuous air leak after placement of a thoracostomy tube should be treated as inpatients (Mercier et al., 1976).

Complications from insertion of a thoracostomy tube are infrequent if careful technique is employed. Pulmonary injury can occur if part of the lung adheres to the chest wall, or if a tube perforates a large bulla that was mistaken for a pneumothorax. Injury to the diaphragm and abdominal viscera is possible if the tube is placed too low on the chest wall. This can occur with a tension pneumothorax where initial decompression relieves the tension and allows the diaphragm to rise, covering the entry site; subsequent tube placement becomes difficult and may cause diaphragmatic injury. Hemorrhage can occur from injury to the intercostal artery or vein that runs along the inferior surface of the rib. Infectious complications, including abscess at the insertion site or empyema, are uncommon. Unilateral pulmonary edema after lung expansion with chest tube placement occurs rarely and is poorly understood (Paulin and Cheney, 1979). Prolonged air leaks are more common in patients with secondary than in those with primary spontaneous pneumothorax. With time and patience, most air leaks stop if the pleural space is adequately decompressed and the lung is fully expanded.

CHEMICAL PLEURODESIS

In 1906, Spengler described chemical pleurodesis by injection of silver nitrate into the pleural cavity. Since then a number of other agents have been used, including tetracycline hydrochloride, quinacrine, talcum powder, nitrogen mustard, iodized oil, and hypertonic glucose (Thorsrud, 1965). Quinacrine is less painful than other agents but causes a high incidence of fever and side effects of the central nervous system (Larrieu et al., 1979). Tetracycline has been very effective when compared with other agents (Austin and Flye, 1979), but is extremely painful on injection into the pleural space, and is no longer commercially available. Doxycycline continues to be available and works similarly to tetracycline.

In contrast to its role in the treatment of recurrent pleural effusions, chemical pleurodesis has a limited role in the treatment of primary pneumothorax (Keagy and Wilcox, 1989). In fact, results obtained with chemical pleurodesis have not necessarily been superior to those obtained with chest tube insertion alone. Some authors feel that chemical pleurodesis is indicated for the treatment of secondary spontaneous pneumothorax because the mortality and recurrence rates in these patients are high (Larrieu et al., 1979; Nandi, 1980; Tanaka et al., 1993). Further information regarding the technique of chemical pleurodesis is found in the discussion of pleural effusions.

Surgery for Spontaneous Pneumothorax

Nine to 20% of patients with spontaneous pneumothorax require surgical therapy (Brooks 1973; Ruckley and McCormack, 1966; Serementis, 1970). The indications for operation are listed in Table 16–2. Surgical treatment includes ablation or resection of blebs when identified, followed by pleurodesis. Pleurectomy has been advocated by some in order to ensure symphysis of the lung and chest wall. However, it is probably no more effective than mechanical pleural abrasion and has a 5 to 35% rate of complication that includes fibrothorax, hemothorax, and Horner's syndrome. It also makes subsequent thoracotomy for unrelated disease more difficult (Gaensler, 1956; Singh, 1979). Transaxillary apical pleurectomy has fewer major complications than other approaches (Weeden and Smith, 1983). Unlike pleurectomy, pleural abrasion has a complication rate of only 3% and a recurrence rate of 3 to 5%. Recurrence of pneumothorax pleurectomy is less than 1% (Brooks, 1973; DesLauriers et al., 1980; Ruckley and McCormack, 1966; Youmans et al., 1970).

Operative incisions that have been successful in treating spontaneous pneumothorax include anterior, lateral thoracotomy, and transaxillary thoracotomy or median sternotomy. The limited transaxillary ap-

■ **Table 16–2.** INDICATIONS FOR THORACOTOMY IN PATIENTS WITH SPONTANEOUS PNEUMOTHORAX

Massive air leak that prevents lung reexpansion
Persistent air leak for more than 5 days
Recurrent pneumothorax (second episode)
Complications of pneumothorax:
  Hemothorax
  Empyema
  Chronic pneumothorax
Specific surgical indications for conditions causing secondary spontaneous pneumothorax
Occupational indications after first episode:
  Airline pilots
  Scuba divers
  Individuals living in remote areas
Previous contralateral pneumothorax
Bilateral simultaneous pneumothorax
Presence of large cysts visible on chest roentgenogram

proach creates a small incision across the lower axilla, which provides access to the chest via the third intercostal space (Murray et al., 1993). Because the incision is made between the pectoralis major and the latissimus dorsi muscles, only a small portion of the serratus anterior muscle is divided. This approach produces little postoperative morbidity and an excellent cosmetic result, but access to the entire pleural space is somewhat limited by this incision. Because the blebs are commonly found near the apex of the lung, resection with adequate pleurodesis can usually be performed. More traditional incisions are often necessary in patients who have had a previous thoracic surgical procedure or who have blebs in locations other than the apex of the lung (Keagy and Wilcox, 1989). Bilateral pneumothoraces can be treated with sequential unilateral procedures or with a single operation via a median sternotomy.

Thoracoscopic Surgery for Spontaneous Pneumothorax

Thoracoscopy for the management of pneumothorax is not new. Sattler (1937) first described the use of the pleuroscope in the management of pneumothorax, and Keller and colleagues (1974) discussed its use before thoracotomy in patients with persistent air leaks. Weissberg and associates (1980) used pleuroscopy to detect subpleural blebs and pleural adhesions that impeded expansion of the lung. If reexpansion was achieved, talc pleurodesis was performed through the pleuroscope. If reexpansion failed, thoracotomy was performed.

Technologic advances in imaging devices and instrumentation have made video-assisted thoracoscopic surgery a widely accepted treatment of spontaneous pneumothorax. Whereas previous thoracoscopic techniques visualized the thorax directly through a narrow straight tube, the operative field is now projected onto a video monitor using a camera connected to a solid fiberoptic operating telescope. As the entire surgical team views the operation on color video monitors, specialized instruments are inserted through 2-cm incisions, enabling the surgeon to identify and resect or obliterate pulmonary blebs and perform pleurodesis using a variety of techniques. Advantages of thoracoscopic surgery over conventional open techniques for spontaneous pneumothorax may include shorter hospital stays, less postoperative pain, and earlier return to work.

Techniques of Thoracoscopic Blebectomy and Pleurodesis

After induction of general anesthesia, endotracheal intubation is performed using a double-lumen tube. The patient is placed in the lateral decubitus position with the ipsilateral arm abducted at right angles to the chest (Fig. 16–12A). The lung on the operative side is allowed to collapse. The thoracoscopy trocar for the 10-mm video telescope is placed through a 2-cm incision in the anterior axillary line at the level of

the fifth intercostal space. Before the trocar and telescope are placed, a finger should be inserted through the incision into the pleural space to confirm that the lung falls away freely and that the trocar can be placed safely. Brief exploration of the chest is then performed with the operating telescope, noting the location and number of blebs. Two other trocar sites are usually necessary, and should be angled anteriorly and posteriorly to the initial site to form a triangle. Trocar sites should be at least 5 cm away from each other to avoid "dueling" instruments. The area of lung containing the blebs is grasped with an endoscopic lung clamp and excised using an endoscopic stapling device (Fig. 16–12B). The stapling device may have to be reloaded and fired more than once to complete the resection.

Blebs are found in as many as 85% of operative procedures for spontaneous pneumothorax (Macklin and Macklin, 1944; West, 1971). Whereas most surgeons prefer to resect them using stapling devices, others have used electrocautery, carbon dioxide laser, or neodymium:yttrium-aluminum-garnet (Nd:YAG) laser ablation (Torre and Belloni, 1989; Wakabayashi, 1989; Wakabayashi et al., 1990) with mixed results.

Endoscopic pleurodesis has been performed most frequently with mechanical abrasion using a Kitner sponge on an endoscopic clamp. Other devices include electrocautery, the Nd:YAG laser, and the argon beam coagulator (Torre and Belloni, 1989), although these are expensive and have not shown significant advantages over mechanical abrasion (Bresticker et al., 1993). Endoscopic parietal pleurectomy has been successfully performed, but it is more time-consuming and probably unnecessary (Nathanson et al., 1991). Talc can be instilled using the thoracoscope with excellent results, but its use is not recommended in young patients who may require a thoracic procedure later in life. These techniques are all applied under direct visualization using the video telescope. Usually, pleurodesis of the apical pleura alone is sufficient.

Thoracoscopic treatment of secondary spontaneous pneumothorax is more difficult. These patients may have diffuse pulmonary disease, which makes it difficult to identify the site of air leak. The lung is more friable, so manipulation can cause tearing and prolonged air leaks. The role of endoscopic surgery in this setting should consist primarily of pleurodesis to control the air leak. Since many of these patients are older, talc pleurodesis may be used more liberally (Daniel and Wyatt, 1993). After management of the pneumothorax, treatment focuses on the underlying disease.

Pneumothorax in Patients with Acquired Immunodeficiency Syndrome

Spontaneous pneumothorax in patients with *acquired immunodeficiency syndrome* (AIDS) usually occurs in the setting of *Pneumocystis carinii* pneumonia (PCP) (Sepkowitz et al., 1991). Approximately 6% of AIDS patients with PCP develop pneumothorax (Ger-

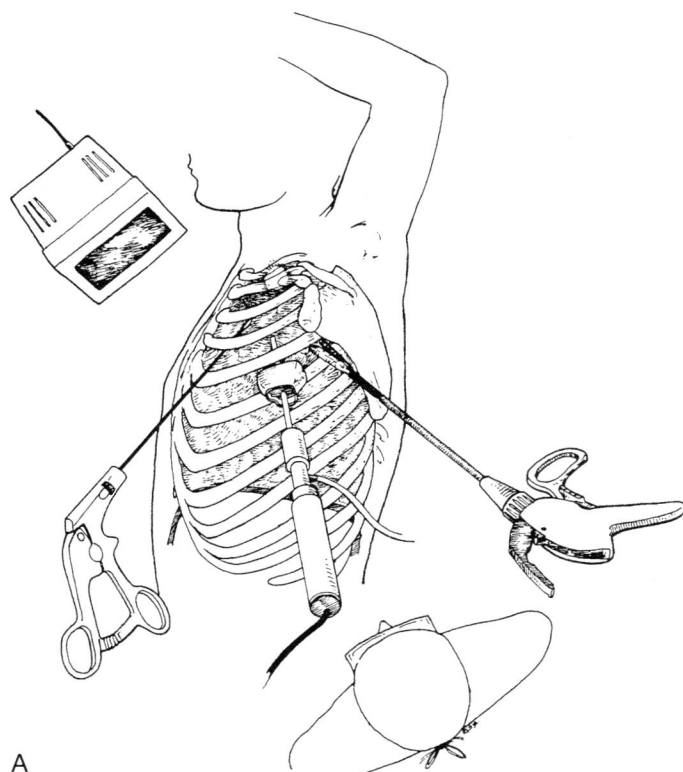

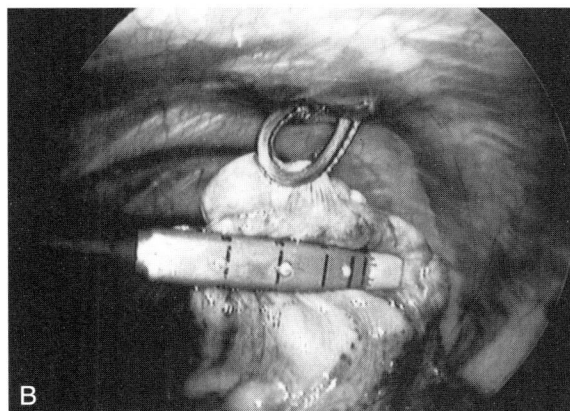

FIGURE 16–12. *A,* Operative positioning of the patient and the equipment for thoracoscopic bleb resection. The instruments, from left to right, are the endograsper, video camera, and endoscopic stapler. The patient is in the lateral decubitus position with the arm abducted. *B,* Thoracoscopic blebectomy using the endoscopic stapler. (*A,* From Daniel, T. M., and Wyatt, D. A.: Pneumothorax and bullous disease. *In* Kaiser, L. R., and Daniel, T. M. [eds]: Thoracoscopic Surgery. Boston, Little, Brown, 1993, p. 88; *B,* From Kaiser, L. R., and Daniel, T. M. [ed]: Thorascopic Surgery. Boston, Little, Brown, Company, 1993. Published by Little, Brown and Company.)

ein et al., 1991). *Pneumocystis carinii* produces a necrotizing pneumonia with diffuse subpleural blebs, causing pneumothoraces that are frequently refractory, recurrent, and bilateral (Crawford et al., 1992). Prolonged air leak is common, and recurrent pneumothorax occurs in as many as 65% of these patients after conservative management (Sepkowitz et al., 1991). Approximately one-third of patients manifest synchronous or asynchronous spontaneous bilateral pneumothorax. The rate of bilaterality is higher in patients who receive positive-pressure ventilation (PPV) (Byrnes et al., 1989; Gerein et al., 1991). PCP in AIDS patients that is complicated by pneumothorax can have a hospital mortality as high as 50%, with mortality approaching 90% in patients requiring ventilatory support (Byrnes et al., 1989; Walker et al., 1993). Patients who respond to medical therapy may survive a year or more after pneumothorax; however, most die of their disease within 5 months after pneumothorax occurs (Gerein et al., 1991).

Observation is appropriate for AIDS patients with small pneumothoraces who are asymptomatic and are not receiving PPV (McClellan et al., 1991). Treatment by tube thoracostomy alone has been successful in over 50% of patients. Those with prolonged air leaks have been managed as outpatients with Heimlich valves (Crawford et al., 1992; Gerein et al., 1991; Walker et al., 1993). Unfortunately, the durability of conservative management is limited by the high recurrence rate.

Chemical pleurodesis has been ineffective in controlling prolonged air leaks or recurrence. Crawford

and Gerein and their associates reported excellent results with parietal pleurectomy in selected patients. Patients were considered candidates for surgical intervention if their PCP was controlled, if they could tolerate a general anesthetic, if they had no ongoing extrapulmonary infections, if they had persistent air leaks for greater than 10 days, or if they had recurrent pneumothorax. Generally, these patients' hospital discharge is prevented only by their ongoing air leak. Before surgical therapy, patients should be evaluated for the presence of bilateral disease. Contralateral disease can be assessed with CT. If disease is present, bilateral pleurectomies can be performed via a median sternotomy (Gerein et al., 1991). Pleurectomy should be accompanied by diaphragmatic abrasion to prevent subpulmonic recurrence. Concurrent pulmonary wedge resection or stapling of blebs or cysts can be done if indicated (Gerein et al., 1991). Video-assisted thoracoscopy may provide a preferable technique in these patients, whose survival is measured in months.

Iatrogenic Pneumothorax

Mechanical ventilation is a recognized cause of iatrogenic pneumothorax. PPV increases the incidence of pneumothorax in patients with asthma, emphysema, pulmonary infarction, multiple trauma, and necrotizing pneumonia. The incidence of pneumothorax in patients on ventilators is approximately 3 to 4%. This increases significantly with the addition of *positive end-expiratory pressure* (PEEP). Many of these patients develop tension pneumothorax and rapidly deteriorate. A thoracoscopy tube must be inserted without delay to prevent death from hemodynamic collapse.

Other causes of iatrogenic pneumothorax include thoracentesis, pleural biopsy, needle aspiration biopsy of pulmonary lesions, and insertion of central venous catheters. A chest film should be taken after these procedures to exclude pneumothorax. If pneumothorax is present, treatment is similar to that for a spontaneous pneumothorax. Unusual causes of iatrogenic pneumothorax are bronchial rupture from a malpositioned nasogastric tube, use of an esophageal obturator airway, acupuncture, stellate ganglion block, esophageal perforation, and transbronchial lung biopsy (Vukich, 1983). After percutaneous biopsy of the lung, 98% of iatrogenic pneumothoraces become evident within 1 hour, and only 2% are seen on delayed radiographs (Perlmutt et al., 1986).

Spontaneous Hemothorax

Blood in the pleural space is called a *hemothorax*. There is no agreement on distinction between a bloody pleural effusion and a hemothorax. The clinical signs of a spontaneous hemothorax depend on its etiology, and causes are shown in Table 16–3. Sponta-

■ **Table 16–3.** ETIOLOGY OF SPONTANEOUS HEMOTHORAX

Pulmonary

Bullous emphysema
Necrotizing infections
Pulmonary embolus with infarction
Tuberculosis
Arteriovenous malformation
Hereditary hemorrhagic telangiectasia

Pleural

Torn pleural adhesions secondary to spontaneous pneumothorax
Neoplasms
Endometriosis

Pulmonary Neoplasms

Primary
Metastases
　Melanoma
　　Trophoblastic tumors (Johnson et al., 1979)

Blood Dyscrasias

Thrombocytopenia (Fromke and Schmidt, 1972)
Hemophilia (Rasaretnam et al., 1976)
Complication of systemic anticoagulation (Rostand et al., 1977)
von Willebrand's disease

Abdominal Pathology

Pancreatic pseudocyst (Cochran, 1978)
Splenic artery aneurysm
Hemoperitoneum (Pratt and Shamblin, 1968)

Thoracic Pathology

Ruptured thoracic aortic aneurysm

neous hemothorax occurs most commonly with a spontaneous pneumothorax or pulmonary arteriovenous malformation, and most patients are young men in the third decade of life (Abyholm and Storen, 1973; Calvert and Smith, 1955; Gula et al., 1981; Spear et al., 1975). A family history or the presence of mucosal and cutaneous lesions suggests hereditary hemorrhagic telangiectasia as the cause (Deaton and Johnston, 1962). Patients with pulmonary arteriovenous malformations may have a history of cyanosis, clubbing, and polycythemia and a continuous extracardiac murmur on auscultation of the lungs. Spontaneous hemothorax in the newborn is associated with the trauma of childbirth (Aaron and Doohen, 1970). The bleeding seems to occur only if there is an underlying pulmonary lesion, such as arteriovenous malformation, hemangioma, or pulmonary sequestration, or a defect in the blood clotting mechanism.

The onset of bleeding may be sudden or insidious and is unrelated to the activity of the patient. Typically, the patient has dyspnea and chest pain that may radiate to the neck, back, or upper abdomen. Syncope may follow, depending on the amount and rate of bleeding. Irritation of the diaphragmatic pleura may produce signs of an acute abdominal emergency.

Pathophysiology

When blood enters the pleural cavity, it coagulates rapidly but eventually becomes defibrinated and leaves fluid that is radiologically indistinguishable from a pleural effusion. The bloody pleural fluid, if free of contaminants and bacteria, is absorbed spontaneously in most patients (Wilson et al., 1960). In a few patients, hemothorax can progress to fibrothorax and a trapped lung that requires decortication for reexpansion. This is more likely to occur after trauma when the pleural space is contaminated with bacteria. Inadequate drainage in this situation causes deposition of fibrin over the pleural surface of the compressed lung, which usually occurs within several days of the hemorrhage. Early on, the thin membrane has little substance, but by the seventh day, angioblastic and fibroblastic proliferation occurs. Within weeks, the outer fibrin film is fully organized and a thick inelastic membrane develops. Unless infection is present, the underlying pleura remains normal, and a dissection plane lies between the pleura and the membranous peel.

Management

Initial treatment of a hemothorax is volume resuscitation to maintain the blood pressure and drainage of the pleural cavity with tube thoracostomy. If brisk hemorrhage continues, a thoracotomy is performed to control the bleeding and evacuate all blood from the pleural cavity (Borrie, 1953; Clyne and Hutter, 1955). If hemorrhage has ceased and evacuation of the chest with reexpansion of the lung has not been complete, surgical therapy should be undertaken by the seventh to 10th day. After this interval, a peel will have formed on the pleural surface and may require decortication to reexpand the lung. In some patients, the hemothorax will resolve over time without surgical therapy (Fig. 16–13).

If a pulmonary arteriovenous malformation has caused the bleeding, the lesion, which is usually just beneath the visceral pleura, can be locally excised with a wedge resection. Metastatic melanoma and trophoblastic tumor are the neoplasms that most commonly cause a spontaneous hemothorax, and the hemorrhage is usually managed by local resection of the lesion (DeFrance et al., 1974; Johnson et al., 1979).

Chylothorax

Chylothorax is the presence of lymph in the pleural space, a condition that has become more common with the increased incidence of chest trauma and surgical procedures performed via the pleural space.

The anatomy of the thoracic duct is constant only in its variability (Davis, 1915). The duct originates from the cisterna chyli, passes through the chest, and ends at or near the left jugulosubclavian junction (Fig. 16–14). The cisterna chyli is a globular structure 3 to 4 cm long and 2 to 3 cm in diameter that usually lies adjacent to the vertebral column between L3 and T10, just to the right of the aorta. In 2% of individuals, the cisterna chyli is absent. Usually, a single thoracic duct enters the chest through the aortic hiatus, at the level of T12 to T10, just to the right of the aorta. Above the diaphragm, the duct lies on the anterior surface of the vertebral column behind the esophagus and between the aorta and the azygos vein. Approximately 25% of individuals have multiple ducts at this level. At the level of T5, the duct courses to the left, ascends behind the aortic arch into the left side of the posterior mediastinum, and passes superiorly adjacent to the left side of the esophagus. In the root of the neck, the thoracic duct passes behind the left carotid sheath and jugular vein, and enters the venous system at the left jugulosubclavian junction. There are several lymphaticovenous anastomoses between the duct and the azygos, intercostal, and lumbar veins, so that the duct can be ligated safely at any point in its thoracic or cervical course. This "normal" anatomic description is observed in slightly more than half of individuals. In the remainder, two or more main ducts are present in some part of its course (Kausel et al., 1957; Van Pernis, 1949).

The rate of flow of lymph is approximately 1.5 ml/kg body weight/hr. The volume varies with meals and the fat content of food (Shafiroff and Kan, 1959). Thoracic duct pressure at maximal flow is 10 to 28 cm H_2O (Shafiroff and Kan, 1959). Ninety-five per cent of thoracic duct lymph comes from the liver and intestinal lymphatics. Spontaneous rhythmic contractions of the thoracic duct, retroperitoneal lymphatics, and cisterna chyli have been seen independent of respiratory movements and are probably the main

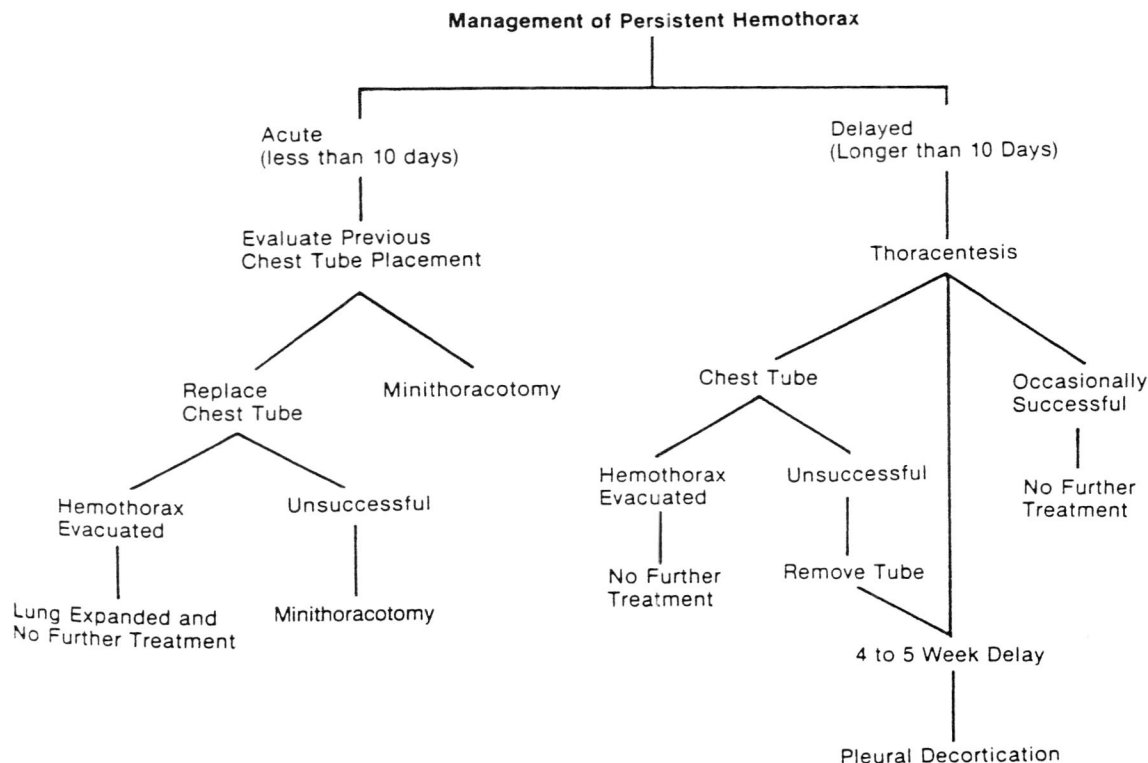

FIGURE 16–13. Algorithm for the management of persistent hemothorax. (From Boyd, A. D.: Pneumothorax and hemothorax. *In* Hood, R. M., [ed]: Surgical Diseases of the Pleura and Chest Wall. Philadelphia, W. B. Saunders, 1986, p. 225.)

THORACIC DUCT

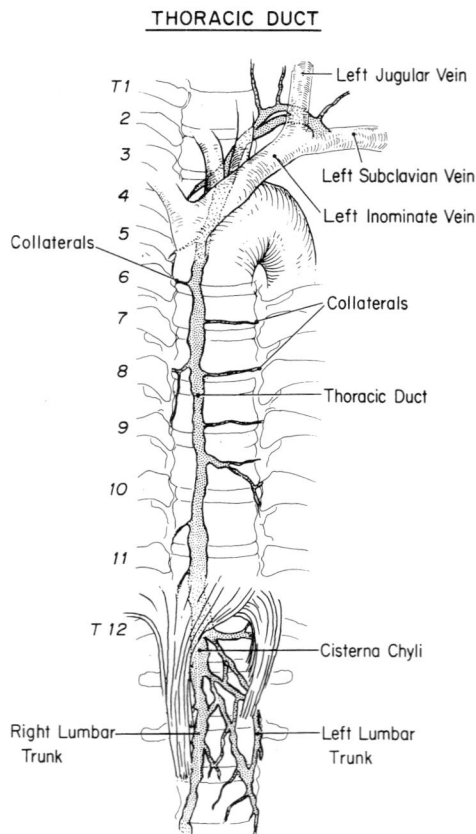

FIGURE 16–14. Schematic drawing of the most usual pattern and course of the thoracic duct. The single duct that enters the chest through the aortic hiatus between T12 and T10 is a relatively consistent finding and the usual site for surgical ligation.

contributor to the forward flow (Ross, 1961) (Fig. 16–15). These contractions empty the duct at intervals of 10 to 15 seconds into the subclavian vein. Forward flow may be aided by respiration, which causes both an increase in intra-abdominal pressure, with subsequent intermittent compression of the cisterna chyli, and an increase in negative intrathoracic pressure, which increases the pressure gradient between the abdomen and the thorax. The thoracic duct has valves, primarily in its upper portion, that permit only unidirectional flow. The most consistent of the valves prevents reflux of blood into the ductal system at the junction of the duct with the veins of the neck.

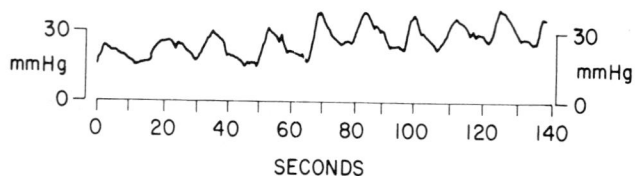

FIGURE 16–15. Pressure tracing from a human thoracic duct showing the frequency of rhythmic pressure waves caused by contraction of the muscular wall of the duct and the progressive buildup in pressure from 20 to 40 mm Hg in 140 seconds after ligation. (Modified from Ross, J. K.: A review of the surgery of the thoracic duct. Thorax, 16:12, 1961.)

Thoracic duct lymph contains 0.4 to 6.0 g of fat/100 ml. Sixty to 70% of ingested fat is absorbed by the intestinal lymphatic system and conveyed to the bloodstream via the thoracic duct. This fat consists of neutral fat, free fatty acids, phospholipid, sphingomyelin, cholesterol, and cholesterol esters. Fatty acids with fewer than 10 carbon atoms in the chain are absorbed directly by the portal venous system. These medium-chain triglycerides can be used as an oral diet in the conservative management of patients with chylothorax. Neutral fat is found in the lymph as minute globules, or chylomicrons, 0.5 mm or less in diameter (Ross, 1961).

The protein content of the thoracic duct is 2.5 to 6 g/ml, roughly half of that in plasma. The thoracic duct is also the main pathway for return of extravascular plasma to the bloodstream (Nix et al., 1957; Ross, 1961; Roy et al., 1967). The thoracic duct fluid contains 300 to 6000 lymphocytes/ml, of which 90% are T cells (Hyde et al., 1974). The role of T cells in cellular immunity is well known, and prolonged drainage of the thoracic duct can impair the immune system. The thoracic duct is also the route for fat-soluble vitamins, and a long-standing fistula can cause vitamin K deficiency and coagulation anomalies.

Etiology and Pathophysiology

Trauma and neoplasms are the most frequent causes of chylothorax (Randolph and Gross, 1957; Roy et al., 1967) (Table 16–4). The thoracic duct can be injured by blunt and penetrating trauma, exaggerated physiologic maneuvers, or iatrogenic injury during surgical procedures (Cevese et al., 1978). The most common mechanism of nonpenetrating injury is sudden hyperextension of the spine owing to blast or blunt trauma with rupture of the duct just above the diaphragm. Vomiting episodes or violent coughing have been known to tear the thoracic duct. Spontaneous rupture of the duct is more likely when it is distended after a fatty meal. There is usually an interval of 2 to 10 days between rupture and the onset of a chylous pleural effusion. This delay is due to accumulation of lymph in the posterior mediastinum until the mediastinal pleura ruptures, usually on the right side at the base of the inferior pulmonary ligament. The fistula seals spontaneously in 50% of patients. The remainder require surgical therapy to prevent serious complications, including death (Ross, 1961).

Penetrating injury to the thoracic duct from a gunshot or stab wound is unusual and is apt to be overshadowed by injury to other structures in the vicinity of more immediate importance. Injury to the duct has occurred in almost every known thoracic operation. The duct is most vulnerable in the upper part of the left side of the chest, particularly during procedures that involve mobilization of the aortic arch, left subclavian artery, or esophagus (Higgins and Mulder, 1971). The course of the duct explains why injury below the level of T5 or T6 usually causes a right-

■ Table 16–4. ETIOLOGY OF CHYLOTHORAX

Congenital

Atresia of the thoracic duct
Thoracic duct—pleural fistula space
Birth trauma

Traumatic

Blunt
Penetrating
Surgery
  Cervical—Excision of lymph nodes; radical neck dissection
  Thoracic
    Patent ductus arteriosus
    Coarctation of the aorta
    Vascular procedure reinvolving the origin of left subclavian
      artery
    Esophagectomy
    Sympathectomy
    Resection of thoracic aneurysm
    Resection of mediastinal tumors
    Left pneumonectomy
  Abdominal—Sympathectomy; radical lymph node dissection
Diagnostic procedures
  Translumbar arteriography
  Subclavian vein catheterization
  Left-sided heart catheterization

Neoplasms

Infections

Tuberculous lymphadenitis
Nonspecific mediastinitis
Ascending lymphangitis
Filariasis

Miscellaneous

Venous thrombosis
  Left subclavian-jugular veins
  Superior vena cava
Pulmonary lymphangiomatosis

---

sided chylothorax, whereas injury above this level results in a left-sided effusion.

Chylothorax can be caused by benign tumors of the lymphatic system that involve the thoracic duct, such as lymphangiomas and mediastinal hygromas. Tumor is responsible for more than 50% of chylothoraces in adults and should be suspected whenever a nontraumatic chylothorax is discovered. The chylous effusion can be unilateral or bilateral. In 75% of patients, an unsuspected mediastinal retroperitoneal lymphoma is found (Roy et al., 1967). Lymphosarcoma and carcinoma of the lung are other causes. Abdominal and thoracic malignancies can cause chylothorax from invasion of the thoracic duct, lymphatic permeation of the duct, or tumor embolus obstructing the main duct. The distended tributaries rupture because of back pressure from the obstruction, or the main duct ruptures secondary to direct tumor erosion. Malignant chylous leaks can fill the pericardial sac with chyle and produce cardiac tamponade.

Thrombosis of the great veins into which the thoracic duct drains can also produce chylous effusion (Ross, 1961). In adults, most cases of idiopathic chylothorax are probably caused by minor trauma, such as

coughing or stretching after ingestion of a fatty meal. Pulmonary lymphangiomyomatosis, a rare condition seen in women of reproductive age, is associated with a 75% incidence of chylothorax. This disease is characterized by proliferation of immature smooth muscles in the peribronchial, perivascular, and perilymphatic regions of the lung, which results in obstructed lymphatics. These women usually die of pulmonary insufficiency within 10 years (Bradley et al., 1980).

Congenital chylothorax is rare, but it is the leading cause of pleural effusion in infancy. Although its cause is unknown, increased venous pressure resulting from trauma at birth has been suggested as one etiology. Another possibility is congenital malformations of the lymphatic system. These include atresia of the thoracic duct and fistulas between the thoracic duct and the pleural space.

The clinical manifestations of accumulation of chyle in the pleural space initially are caused by mechanical compression of the ipsilateral lung and mediastinum, producing dyspnea, fatigue, and discomfort on the affected side. Because of the bacteriostatic nature of chyle, infectious complications are rare. A chronic thoracic duct–pleural fistula can result in serious losses of fats, proteins, fat-soluble vitamins, and antibodies. Protein loss may cause falling plasma protein levels, wasting, and edema (Ross, 1961). Fluid losses can be enormous—up to 2500 ml of chyle in 24 hours—and can produce cardiovascular instability if replacement is not timely (Ross, 1961). When conservative measures fail, severe debilitation and death can occur unless the fistula closes spontaneously or is treated surgically.

Diagnosis

The key to diagnosing a chylothorax is to recognize the pleural fluid as chyle. The characteristics of chyle are listed in Table 16–5. The fluid is milky and non-clotting, and contains fat globules that clear with alkali and ether, and stain with Sudan III. Chylothorax may develop 1 to 2 weeks after a surgical procedure in the region of the aorta, esophagus, or posterior

■ Table 16–5. CHARACTERISTICS OF CHYLE

Milky appearance with creamy layer on standing; clears when fat
  is extracted by alkali and ether
Fat globules stain with Sudan III
Alkaline, odorless
Sterile, bacteriostatic
Specific gravity: 1.012–1.025

Lymphocytes	400–7000/mm^3
Erythrocytes	50–600/mm^3
Total fat	0.4–5.0 gms/dl
Total cholesterol	65–220 mg/dl
Triglycerides	>110 mg/dl
Cholesterol-triglyceride ratio	<1
Total protein	2–6 g/dl
Albumin	1–4 g/dl
Glucose	50–100 g/dl
Electrolytes	Similar to plasma

mediastinum. Once a chest tube is placed, drainage may exceed 1 to 2 1/24 hr. Chylothorax must be differentiated from pseudochylothorax, which also gives a milky, turbid fluid related to high levels of cholesterol or lecithin globulin complexes, and usually occurs in the presence of pleura thickened or calcified by chronic infections. Pseudochylothorax can be seen with tuberculosis, rheumatoid arthritis, diabetes, and malignancy (Bower, 1968). Cholesterol and triglyceride levels of the fluid help differentiate chylous fistula from other causes of pleural effusion. Most chylous effusions have a cholesterol:triglyceride ratio greater than 1. A triglyceride level of more than 110 mg/dl indicates a 99% probability that the fluid is chyle. If the triglyceride level is less than 50 mg/dl, the probability is less than 5% (Staats et al., 1980). Intermediate values require a lipoprotein analysis to verify the presence of chylomicrons in chylous effusions (Seriff et al., 1977). The diagnosis can be further confirmed by having the patient ingest a fatty meal or olive oil and observing the drainage of pleural fluid.

Management

With the introduction of thoracic duct ligation in 1948, the mortality from chylothorax decreased from 50 to 15% (Lampson, 1948). Current mortality rates are less than 10% (Dulchavsky et al., 1988). Today, the crucial decision in managing these patients is when to intervene surgically. Conservative therapy consists of thoracostomy tube drainage of the chylous effusion with expansion of the lung to avoid fibrothorax or loculated fluid collections; correction of fluid losses and prevention of electrolyte imbalance; and nutritional support. Most patients should receive nutrition parenterally, with nothing by mouth. Oral feedings usually increase the output through the fistula, although clear liquids and medium-chain triglycerides can occasionally be given to patients with low-volume fistulas.

There is no consensus regarding the duration of conservative treatment, but a maximum of 14 days seems appropriate (Selle et al., 1973; Williams and Burford, 1964). Other indications for operation include drainage greater than 1500 ml/day for adults or greater than 100 ml/year-age/d for children older than 5 years, as well as metabolic complications (Marts et al., 1992). If the fistula appears to have closed spontaneously, a high-fat meal should be administered before removing the chest tube to confirm that closure is complete. Conservative management may be prolonged when thoracotomy is contraindicated, such as in patients with vertebral fractures or multiple organ injuries. When chylothorax is secondary to lymphoma or other malignancies, radiation or chemotherapy may be considered. Early operation is recommended if the ipsilateral lung is trapped, a malignant etiology is suspected, or multiple loculated fluid collections are present. Approximately 20 to 50% of patients will require surgical therapy.

Operative Management

Surgical therapy is indicated when a chylous effusion does not respond to conservative management, and there are no contraindications to operation. In unilateral chylothorax, the chest should be opened on the side of the effusion. With bilateral effusion, the right side should be explored first, with ligation of the duct low in the chest, and the left side explored later, if necessary. To locate the duct and the leakage point, the patient is given 100 to 200 ml of olive oil through a nasogastric tube 2 to 3 hours before the operation (Ross, 1961). Olive oil that remains in the stomach at the time of anesthetic induction can be removed by the nasogastric tube. The olive oil causes the duct to fill with milky chyle, which can be recognized throughout the operation.

Three techniques are combined to control the leak of chyle: direct closure of the fistula, suture of the leaking mediastinal pleura, and supradiaphragmatic ligation of the duct. Suture closure of the point of leakage should be performed if possible; however, the duct is thin-walled and tears easily. If repair is not possible, ligation above and below the tear is acceptable, combined with ligation at the diaphragmatic hiatus. If the leak cannot be visualized, the duct should be ligated at the diaphragm and the mediastinal pleura oversewn. If the duct cannot be identified at the hiatus, a mass ligature encircling all tissue between the azygos vein and the aorta is performed. This procedure is successful in 80% of patients (Patterson et al., 1981). If the site of leak is not identified, some surgeons add pleurectomy and pleurodesis to ligation of the thoracic duct.

Ligation of the thoracic duct at the diaphragmatic hiatus can be performed without side effects because of the minor lymphatic-venous anastomoses between the thoracic duct system and the azygos, intercostal, and lumbar veins (Patterson et al., 1981; Seriff et al., 1977). Even extirpation of the thoracic duct and removal of the cisterna chyli in humans have not had harmful effects. Distal intraductal pressure can rise as high as 50 mm Hg when the proximal duct is ligated (see Fig. 16–15), although the pressure gradually falls as collateral vessels open (Ross, 1961). Ligation of the thoracic duct is not followed by outward signs of nutritional disturbances, but serum lipid levels fall temporarily. Studies in experimental animals show that after hemorrhage of 25% of the blood volume, animals who had thoracic duct ligation took 8 days for plasma protein levels to return to normal, compared with 2 days for the nonligated group (Ross, 1961).

Pleuroperitoneal shunts have been used in some patients with persistent chylothorax. Most have been children who have had operation for congenital heart disease, or who have had caval thrombosis from central venous catheters. Success rates of 75 to 90% have been reported with this modality (Murphy et al., 1989; Rheuban et al., 1992). Pleuroperitoneal shunting may also be useful for patients with chylothorax and malignancies who are not candidates for thoracic duct ligation.

Pleural Effusions

A pleural effusion is an accumulation of fluid in the pleural space from excessive transudation or exudation of interstitial fluid from the pleural surfaces. A pleural effusion is not a disease entity, but a sequelae of systemic or pleural disease. Symptoms include pleuritic chest pain and dyspnea. Pleuritic chest pain is a sharp, stabbing sensation that may be minimal with quiet respiration but intensified with full inspiration. When the effusion is large, pleuritic chest pain tends to disappear. When the effusion is due to involvement of the parietal pleura by tumor, the pain is usually constant, dull, and independent of respiration.

The abnormal presence of pleural fluid can alter pulmonary function by mechanically inhibiting expansion of the lung, causing dyspnea. When chronic, it may cause atelectasis, intercurrent pulmonary infections, and lung trapping. The effect of unilateral or bilateral pleural effusions on overall pulmonary function depends on the size of the effusion and the functional status of both lungs. Patients with significant underlying pulmonary disease may become symptomatic with only small to moderate pleural effusions, and may improve dramatically with drainage.

Pathophysiology

Passage of protein-free fluid through the pleural membrane depends on the hydrostatic and colloid osmotic pressures across the pleura (Agostini et al., 1957) (Fig. 16–16). The net hydrostatic pressure that moves the fluid from the parietal pleura into the pleural space is the sum of the systemic capillary pressure (30 cm H_2O) and the negative pleural pressure (5 cm H_2O), which equals approximately 35 cm H_2O. Opposing this pressure is the colloid osmotic pressure of the blood (34 cm H_2O) minus that of the

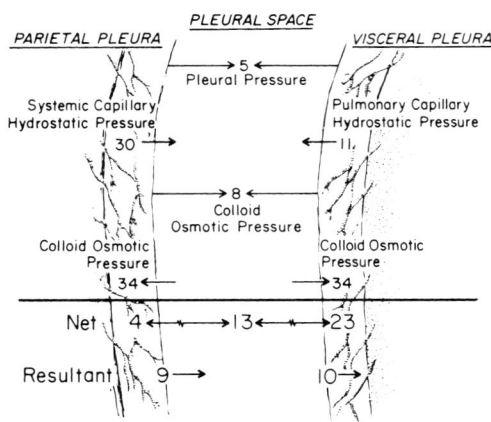

FIGURE 16–16. Diagrammatic representation of the pressures involved in the formation and absorption of pleural fluid. Arrows show the direction of fluid movement exerted by the numerary pressure. The result of all these pressures under physiologic conditions is flow of fluid from the parietal pleura to the visceral pleura.

pleural fluid (8 cm H_2O). The net pressure difference of 9 cm H_2O favors movement of fluid from the parietal pleura into the pleural space.

Unlike the parietal pleura, the capillaries of which respond to systemic pressures, the capillaries of the visceral pleura have the pressure of the pulmonary circulation. Thus, the hydrostatic pressure is lower and the net force across the visceral pleura is 10 cm H_2O, favoring absorption of pleural fluid. Protein-free fluid normally flows from the systemic capillaries in the parietal pleura into the pleural space, and then to the pulmonary capillaries in the visceral pleura. Five to 10 l of fluid normally traverse the pleural space over a 24-hour period.

Normally, only 2 to 3 ml of fluid with a protein content of approximately 1.5 g/100 ml is present in the pleural space (Agostini, 1972). If protein leaks from the pleural capillaries into the pleural space and accumulates there, the colloid osmotic pressure of the pleural fluid increases and the pressure gradients favor fluid movement from both the visceral and the parietal pleura into the pleural space. The pleural fluid accumulates until the protein is diluted or the pleural pressure increases to restore conditions for fluid absorption. Because the protein concentration in serum is greater than that of pleural fluid, protein is never removed from pleural fluid by simple diffusion. This is accomplished by lymphatic drainage from the pleural space. Lymphatic drainage accounts for 150 to 500 ml/24 hr, which is less than 10% of the clearance of protein-free fluid, but is important for clearing the protein that enters the pleural space from parietal and visceral pleural surfaces (Stewart, 1963).

The mechanisms of abnormal accumulation of pleural fluid are (1) increased hydrostatic pressure, such as in congestive heart failure; (2) increased capillary permeability, as in pneumonia or inflammatory pleuritis; (3) decreased plasma colloid oncotic pressure, as in hypoalbuminemia; (4) increased intrapleural negative pressure, as in atelectasis; and (5) impaired lymphatic drainage of the pleural space, usually owing to obstruction of the lymphatics by tumor, radiation, or fungal disease.

Pleural effusions are divided into transudates and exudates. A *transudate* occurs with the alteration of systemic factors that influence the formation or absorption of pleural fluid. Examples are decreased plasma colloid osmotic pressure in hypoalbuminemia or increased hydrostatic pressure in congestive heart failure. The pleural surfaces are not involved in the primary pathologic process. An *exudate* results from disease of the pleural surface or lymphatics. Pleural disease leads to the accumulation of pleural fluid because the capillaries' permeability increases through inflammation caused by bacterial pneumonia, tuberculosis, or tumor. Lymphatic obstruction secondary to lymphoma or metastatic tumor also causes an exudative effusion. Once the diagnosis of pleural effusion has been made, it should be further characterized as a transudate or an exudate. If the effusion is a transudate, no further diagnostic procedures are necessary and the underlying systemic cause is treated. If

■ **Table 16–6.** CAUSES OF TRANSUDATES

Congestive heart failure	Peritoneal dialysis
Cirrhosis	Hypoproteinemia
Nephrotic syndrome	Meigs' syndrome
Myxedema	Sarcoidosis

the effusion is an exudate, further evaluation is needed to elucidate the etiology of the pleural or lymphatic disease.

A pleural effusion has been considered an exudate when the protein level exceeded 3 g/100 ml or the specific gravity was more than 1.016. But these values alone can lead to an error in diagnosis in 10% of cases

because the protein concentration of long-standing transudates increases as fluid is absorbed in excess of protein, hence making them seem like exudates. Simultaneous determination of protein and *lactic acid dehydrogenase* (LDH) levels in pleural fluid and serum correctly differentiates transudative from exudative effusions 99% of the time. A pleural effusion with one or more of the following characteristics is an exudate (Light et al., 1972):

1. Pleural fluid protein/serum protein > 0.5
2. Pleural fluid LDH/serum LDH > 0.6
3. Pleural fluid LDH > two-thirds of the upper limit of normal for serum LDH.

The differentiation of pleural fluid into transudates

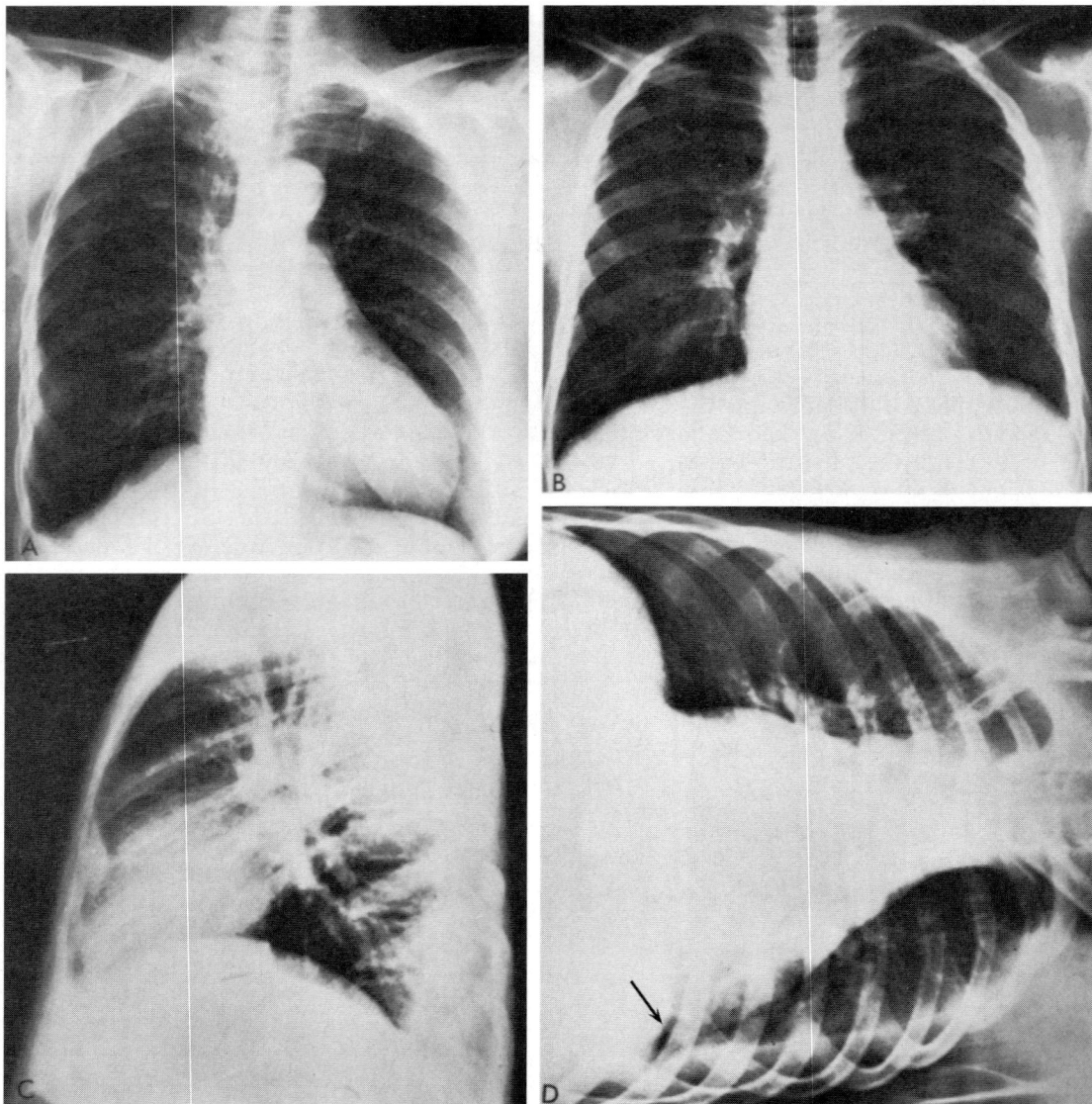

FIGURE 16–17. Patterns of roentgenographic recognition of pleural effusion. *A,* Upright chest film showing a concave meniscus in the right costodiaphragmatic sinus in a patient who previously had a mastectomy for carcinoma of the right breast. *B* and *C,* Upright posteroanterior and lateral chest films suggesting a subpulmonic effusion between the left lung and the left diaphragm by the apparent elevation of the left diaphragm and shallow costodiaphragmatic sinus *(B)* and the large distance between the stomach air shadow and the top of the diaphragm plus the flattening of the contour of the diaphragm anteriorly *(C)*. *D,* Chest film of the patient in *B* and *C,* taken in the lateral decubitus position, confirms the presence of fluid *(arrow)* by its accumulation along the dependent costal surface.

and exudates is less valuable today; nevertheless, approximately 43% of patients with an exudate have malignant disease and 83% of patients with a transudate have congestive heart failure (Light et al., 1972). Other causes of transudates are listed in Table 16–6.

Diagnosis of Pleural Effusion

The presence of abnormal fluid in the pleural space is almost always suggested by the chest film (Vix, 1974) (Fig. 16–17). On the upright chest film, pleural effusion is usually seen as a density on the diaphragm, with a concave meniscus in the costodiaphragmatic sinus (see Fig. 16–17A). Approximately 250 ml of fluid must be present to obliterate the costodiaphragmatic sinus. Unless other films show a recent change, obliteration of the costodiaphragmatic sinus by pleural thickening may be indistinguishable from obliteration by fluid. A film taken with the patient in the lateral decubitus position allows differentiation between these conditions because fluid gravitates to the dependent part of the pleural space (Fig. 16–17D). A homogeneous density with a relatively straight horizontal superior border along the dependent chest wall identifies the free pleural effusion. Large effusions that appear as confusing densities in other positions are apparent with this technique. With the patient in the supine position, a considerable amount of pleural fluid must be present to be detected. In this position, presence of pleural fluid is

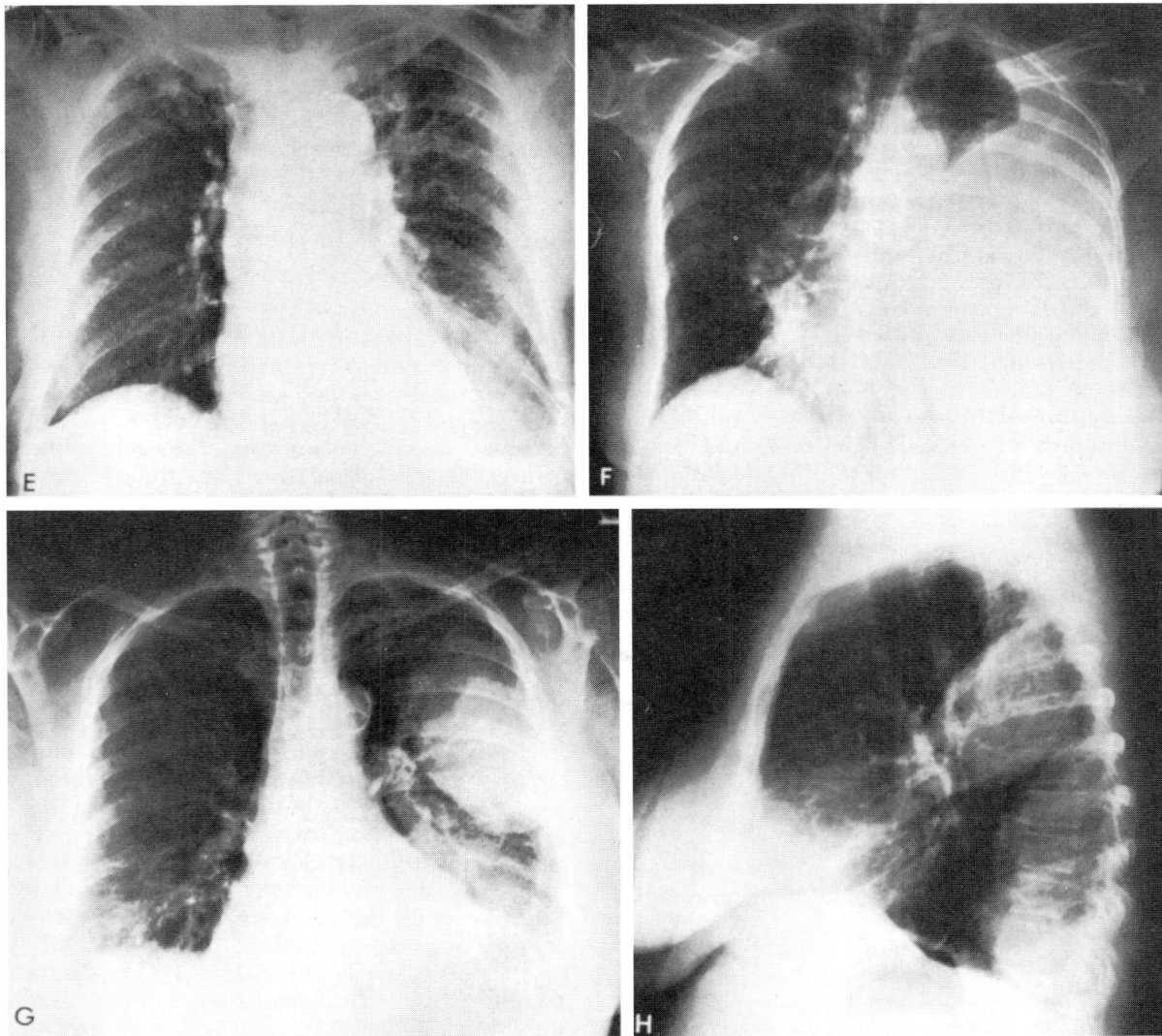

FIGURE 16–17 *Continued E,* Supine chest film suggesting a left pleural effusion by the diffuse increase in density of the left hemithorax. Note that the vascular structures are readily visible through the density. *F,* Upright chest film showing how a massive left pleural effusion can be differentiated from complete atelectasis of the left lung by causing complete opacity of the hemithorax and shifting of the mediastinum away from the involved side. This was shown to be a serous effusion from an ovarian carcinoma. *G* and *H,* Upright posteroanterior and lateral chest films showing loculated pleural fluid in the left costovertebral area and left major fissure. Note the "raindrop on a windowpane" configuration of the loculation along the chest wall and the tapered anterior end of the loculation in the left major fissure on the lateral view *(H).* (*A–H,* Courtesy of Dr. John Courtney, Radiology Department of the University of Chicago Hospitals and Clinics.)

suggested by a diffuse hazy density in one hemithorax in which the vascular structures of the lung are visible and there are no parenchymal infiltrates or air bronchograms (Fig. 16–17E). An intrapulmonic disease that produces a similar density obliterates the vascular structures by the "silhouette effect." Chest-wall edema, hematoma, or a large dressing can produce a similar effect. Lateral decubitus views or a thoracic ultrasound may help establish the diagnosis.

Free pleural fluid may have an atypical distribution. Accumulation of an effusion between the lung and the diaphragm, a subpulmonic effusion, is suggested by an apparent elevation of one hemidiaphragm, a shallow costodiaphragmatic sinus, a large distance between the stomach air shadow and the top of the diaphragm on the lateral view, or a small spur of fluid projecting from the diaphragm into the major fissure (Wilson, 1955). Subpulmonic effusions simulating an elevated hemidiaphragm are frequently overlooked, especially when they are bilateral.

A spur-like projection into a fissure may occur where a fissure meets the diaphragm or chest wall and is an additional sign of pleural fluid. The diaphragm may be inverted by a large pleural effusion so that its normally convex superior border becomes concave. Inversion occurs almost exclusively on the left side and is suspected when the stomach gas shadow is displaced downward and medially (Fig. 16–17B–D).

A large pleural effusion may be confused with atelectasis of an entire lung (Fig. 16–17F). Pleural effusion alone seldom fills the entire hemithorax, but leaves some visible lung superiorly. Although mediastinal shift away from the involved side is common, it may be prevented by mediastinal fixation. Atelectasis, with loss of volume and overexpansion to the contralateral lung, produces an enlarged retrosternal clear space on the lateral view. Unless fixed, the mediastinum shifts toward the affected side on the posteroanterior view.

Pleural effusions can be encapsulated by adhesions between the parietal and the visceral pleurae anywhere within the pleural space (Figs. 16–17G and H). Loculated fluid collections have tapered edges and are best identified in a lateral view. Occasionally, CT scanning is necessary to document the presence and location of a loculated pleural effusion.

Air fluid levels in the pleural space can be detected only with a horizontal x-ray beam. Differential diagnosis of air fluid levels in the chest includes iatrogenic injection of air, pulmonary laceration, spontaneous hemopneumothorax, bronchopleural fistula, and rupture of the esophagus into the pleural space.

Clinical and Laboratory Diagnosis in Pleural Effusions

Numerous physical and chemical characteristics of a pleural effusion help determine its etiology. These have been comprehensively described by Sahn (1987). Fluid can be safely obtained for analysis by thoracentesis. Although a definitive diagnosis based on pleural fluid analysis can be made in only 20% of cases, the fact that infection can often be eliminated as a potential cause of the effusion makes pleural fluid analysis clinically helpful in up to 90% of patients (Collins and Sahn, 1987). Diagnoses that can be established by thoracentesis are listed in Table 16–7. Tests that are cost-effective and should be obtained routinely on pleural fluid after thoracentesis include total protein, LDH, white blood cell count and differential, glucose, and pH. Simultaneous serum total protein, LDH, and glucose should also be measured. If the pH of the pleural fluid is less than 7.30, arterial pH should be obtained to exclude acidemia. Culture, Gram's stain, and acid-fast bacillus smear should be obtained if infection is suspected, such as when specimens are cloudy or foul-smelling. Pleural fluid cytology should be performed when malignancy or an undiagnosed exudate is suspected. Lipid studies will help in the evaluation of possible chylothorax, and immunologic studies are performed for possible rheumatoid or lupus pleuritis. Pleural fluid amylase is useful if pancreatitis, pancreatic pseudocyst, or esophageal rupture is suspected. Malignant mesothelioma may be associated with increased levels of hyaluronic acid in the pleural fluid.

VOLUME, COLOR, AND CELL CONTENT OF PLEURAL FLUID

Clinical assessment of the volume of pleural fluid can have diagnostic value. Massive pleural effusions that occupy an entire hemithorax are infrequent, but 70% are secondary to malignant involvement of the pleura. Less frequent causes of massive pleural effusions are tuberculosis, empyema, chylothorax, or transudates from congestive heart failure or cirrhosis of the liver (Maher and Berger, 1972).

■ **Table 16–7.** DIAGNOSES THAT CAN BE ESTABLISHED BY THORACENTESIS

Diagnosis	Diagnostic Pleural Fluid Tests	Usual Time Course
Empyema	Observation (pus, putrid odor); stain or culture	Immediately to 48 hr
Malignancy	Cytology	24–48 hr
Lupus pleuritis	Lupus erythematosus cells present	Minutes to hours
Tuberculous pleurisy	Stain, culture	Minutes to 3 wk
Esophageal rupture	Amylase, pH	Hours
Fungal pleurisy	Stain, culture	Minutes to days
Chylothorax	Centrifugation, triglycerides, lipoprotein electrophoresis	Minutes to 48 hr
Hemothorax	Centrifugation	Minutes
Urinothorax	Creatinine (pleural fluid and serum)	Hours

From Sahn, S. A.: Pleural fluid analysis: Narrowing the differential diagnosis. Reprinted with permission from Seminars in Respiratory Medicine, 9:23, 1987, Thieme Medical Publishers, Inc.

The fluid of most transudates is straw-colored, clear, and odorless. Most exudates are cloudy because they contain white blood cells. The white blood cell count of most transudates is less than 1000 cells per mm³. When the white blood cell count reaches empyemic levels (>10,000 per mm³), the fluid becomes opaque. Neutrophils predominate in effusions associated with pneumonia, pulmonary infarction, pancreatitis, and early tuberculosis. A predominance of lymphocytes occurs with more advanced tuberculosis, lymphoma, or malignancy. If small lymphocytes make up 50% of cells in an undiagnosed exudate, a pleural biopsy should be done. Pleural fluid eosinophilia (10% of total lymphocytes) occurs with parasitic disease and benign asbestos effusion, but can indicate a benign, self-limited pleural effusion associated with air or blood in the pleural space (Campbell and Webb, 1964). Lupus erythematosus cells in pleural fluid are diagnostic (Andrews et al., 1981; Carel et al., 1977).

Yellow or tan, creamy, viscous fluid indicates a chronic empyema. Milky-white fluid suggests a chylous effusion, particularly if the patient has been eating. Although an empyema can appear similar to a chylothorax, the two can be differentiated by centrifugation, which gives a clear supernatant in empyema fluid. Black pleural fluid is consistent with *Aspergillus* invasion of the pleura, whereas brownish fluid may be observed secondary to rupture of an amebic liver abscess into the pleural space.

Grossly bloody pleural effusions with red blood cell counts of more than 100,000 per mm³ are usually due to trauma, pulmonary infarction, or malignancy. When trauma and pulmonary infarction are excluded, neoplasms cause 90% of the remaining hemorrhagic effusions.

Blood-tinged pleural fluid has limited diagnostic implications (Light et al., 1973a). Only 5000 to 10,000 red blood cells per mm³ impart a red color to a pleural effusion. If an effusion has a total volume of 500 ml and the red blood cell count in the peripheral blood is 5 million per mm³, then only 1 ml of blood in the pleural space at thoracentesis can produce red fluid. If the red discoloration of the pleural fluid removed from the chest is not uniform, the fluid is probably secondary to trauma from the thoracentesis needle.

AMYLASE

If the amylase level in the pleural fluid is several times that of the serum level, acute pancreatitis or rupture of a pancreatic pseudocyst should be suspected (Goldman et al., 1962; Kaye, 1968). Esophageal perforation can elevate amylase in both the pleural fluid and the serum by leakage of swallowed saliva into the pleural space and reabsorption of the amylase. The salivary origin of the amylase can be determined by fractionation (Sherr et al., 1972).

GLUCOSE AND LIPID

A glucose level in the pleural fluid lower than the serum level can occur in tuberculosis, rheumatoid arthritis, empyema, and malignancy. The low glucose level may be due to a large number of free cells that use glucose in an environment of decreased pleural circulation. This condition is further exacerbated by glucose diffusion due to thickened, diseased pleural membranes (Berger and Maher, 1971; Glenert, 1962). Lipid analysis of the pleural fluid to measure the triglyceride-cholesterol concentration and analysis of the lipoprotein for the presence of chylomicrons help identify a chylothorax (Seriff et al., 1977; Staats et al., 1980).

PLEURAL FLUID pH

The pH of pleural fluid may be a prognostic index for patients with acute bacterial pneumonia and a pleural effusion because the pH decreases before organisms are visible with Gram's stain. A low pH (<7.2) suggests that the effusion is contaminated with bacteria and will not resolve without chest tube drainage. Because drainage of the pleural space is more difficult when loculation from bacterial infection develops, early thoracostomy drainage is indicated.

Parapneumonic effusions that are turning to empyema have low glucose, low pH, and higher LDH levels. Usually the pH falls before the glucose and is a more sensitive indicator of empyema. The pH is lowered by phagocytotic activity of the white blood cells and bacterial metabolism. If the pleural fluid glucose is above 40 g/dl, the pH above 7.2, and the LDH below 1000 units/l, the effusion will likely resolve with the treatment of the pneumonia. If the pleural fluid pH is less than 7.2 or the serum glucose is less than 40 mg/dl, a thoracostomy tube should be inserted (Light et al., 1973b; Potts et al., 1976). This applies only with parapneumonic effusions. Usually, the pH of the pleural fluid parallels that of arterial blood. Exceptions occur with rheumatoid arthritis, tuberculosis, or malignant effusions, where the pH is routinely less than 7.20 (Light et al., 1973b) and a thoracoscopy tube is not needed. The pleural fluid pH must be collected with the same care as the arterial pH; the fluid must be withdrawn anaerobically into a heparinized syringe and maintained at 0 °C until the pH is measured.

CYTOLOGY

Malignancy is a common cause of pleural effusions. In patients with malignant pleural effusions, the initial pleural fluid specimen is positive for malignant cells in approximately 60% of patients. This rises to 90% if three separate, sequential specimens are obtained. Obtaining more than one sample on separate occasions increases the diagnostic yield because the repeat samples contain fresher cells, the older degenerated cells having been removed during the earlier thoracentesis (Light et al., 1973a). Malignancies can cause pleural effusions by mechanisms other than direct pleural involvement, such as lymphatic or bronchial obstruction, or hypoproteinemia. As a result, not all pleural effusions associated with malignancies have positive cytopathology. Cytologic examination is unreliable in diagnosing lymphoma. In the presence of inflammation, cytologic studies may be inconclusive because marked variation occurs in mesothelial cells. Monoclonal antibodies against carcinoembryonic antigen and chromosome markers can be determined and flow cytometry can be done on pleural fluid, but their usefulness is not clear (Dewald et al., 1982; Vladutiu et al., 1981).

PLEURAL BIOPSY

Needle biopsy of the pleura helps identify two common causes of pleural effusions: tuberculous pleuritis and tumor involving the pleura. The yield is usually higher in tuberculosis because of generalized pleural involvement. Histologic analysis of the pleural biopsy shows granulomas or mycobacteria in up to 80% of patients. The tuberculous bacillus grows in cultures of the pleural fluid from 20 to 25% of those with the disease, whereas cultures of pleural biopsy specimens are positive in more than 75%. A combination of pleural histology and cultures establishes the diagnosis in 70 to 95% of tuberculous effusions (Levine et al., 1970).

The diagnostic yield of pleural biopsy for malignancy, where pleural involvement is localized, is approximately 46%. A combination of cytology of the effusion and pleural biopsy increases the success rate to 60 to 90% (Prakash and Reiman, 1985; Salyer et al., 1975).

THORACOSCOPY FOR PLEURAL EFFUSIONS OF INDETERMINATE CAUSE

Video-assisted thoracoscopy is extremely useful for increasing the diagnostic yield in patients with pleural effusions that remain undiagnosed after conventional evaluation. Thoracoscopy allows for examination of the entire pleural space with biopsy of suspicious lesions of the pleura, lung, and pericardium. It has been performed successfully with good results with the patients under local and general anesthesia. A diagnosis can be made in 80 to 96% of patients who have pleural effusions that have remained undiagnosed after thoracentesis and needle biopsy of the pleura (Hucker et al., 1991; Menzies and Charbonneau, 1991). In addition, talc pleurodesis can be performed for malignant pleural effusions diagnosed at thoracoscopy. Lymphoma and mesothelioma are the most common diagnoses.

Before the advent of video-assisted thoracoscopy, thoracotomy was occasionally performed in order to obtain a diagnosis in patients with pleural effusions of indeterminate cause. When a definite diagnosis could not be made, 61% of patients had no further problem with their effusion and 39% showed a benign or malignant disease within 6 years (Ryan et al., 1981).

CAUSES OF TRANSUDATIVE EFFUSIONS (See Table 16–6)

Clinical disorders secondary to an increase in systemic or pulmonary capillary pressure, a reduction in plasma colloid osmotic pressure, and a sharp decrease in intrapleural pressure cause accumulation of transudate in the pleural space. Congestive heart failure is the most frequent cause. Increases in systemic and pulmonary venous pressures increase the formation and reduce the absorption of pleural fluid. The patients usually have other clinical manifestations of heart failure and the chest film generally shows cardiomegaly and bilateral effusions. If a unilateral pleural effusion is present, it is usually on the right side. If the heart is of normal size and the effusion is bilateral, causes such as neoplasia, cirrhosis, and pulmonary embolism must be considered. Congestive heart failure is a major cause of bizarre loculated interlobar pleural fluid, sometimes called *phantom tumor*. The pleural effusions generally disappear with treatment of the heart failure.

Five to 6% of patients with cirrhosis and ascites have an accompanying pleural effusion. In 70%, the effusion is right-sided and enters the pleural cavity through diaphragmatic defects, which are more numerous on the right, or through transdiaphragmatic lymphatics. Treatment is directed at management of the ascites.

In 1934, Meigs described a rare syndrome that consisted of a benign solid ovarian tumor, ascites, and pleural effusion (Meigs, 1957). The pleural effusion is usually on the right side and can be a transudate or an exudate. The ovarian tumor can be a fibroma, thecoma, granulosa cell, or Brenner cell type. The ascites and the pleural effusion resolve spontaneously after removal of the tumor. This is important because the clinical findings may suggest that the patient has an inoperable malignant disease. The ascitic fluid is presumably a transudate from the surface of the tumor. The pleural effusion is thought to arise from passage of ascitic fluid through microscopic defects in the diaphragm. The pleural fluid is usually straw-colored and may be tinged with blood.

Causes of Exudative Effusions (Table 16–8)

MALIGNANT EFFUSIONS

Malignancy is the major cause of both exudative pleural effusions and massive pleural effusions. Such malignancies usually have an insidious onset. In the absence of trauma and pulmonary infarction, malignant involvement of the pleura is the most frequent cause of a grossly bloody pleural effusion (Leff et al., 1978).

The most common causes of malignant pleural effusions are carcinoma of the lung in men and carcinoma of the breast in women. Less common causes are lymphomas and carcinoma of the ovary, kidney, and colon. The effusion is usually associated with scattered metastatic tumor implants on the parietal and visceral pleurae, and free tumor cells are frequently recovered from the pleural fluid. In lymphomas, malignant cells are not as common in the pleural fluid because the effusion derives from lymphatic obstruction rather than tumor implants. Lung cancer also can

■ **Table 16–8.** CAUSES OF EXUDATES

Neoplastic Diseases	Gastrointestinal Diseases
Metastatic disease	Pancreatitis
Mesotheliomas	Pancreatic pseudocyst
Lymphomas	Esophageal rupture
Chest wall tumors	Subphrenic abscess
Meigs' syndrome	Hepatic abscess
Infectious Diseases	**Trauma**
Tuberculosis	Hemothorax
Viral (adenovirus, coxsackie	Chylothorax
group B mycoplasma)	**Miscellaneous**
Fungal (coccidioidomycosis)	
Parasitic (amebiasis)	Postradiation therapy
Bacterial pneumonia	Postmyocardial infarction
Pulmonary Infarction	syndrome
Collagen-Vascular Diseases	
Rheumatoid arthritis	
Systemic lupus erythematosus	

cause an effusion devoid of tumor cells. The effusion in this case is secondary to lymphatic obstruction by metastatic tumor in the mediastinal lymph nodes or bronchial obstruction by the primary tumor, which causes pneumonia and inflammation in the distal lung and visceral pleura.

POSTMYOCARDIAL INFARCTION SYNDROME (DRESSLER'S SYNDROME)

A syndrome of sterile pleuritis and pericarditis may occur up to 8 weeks after acute myocardial infarction, cardiac resuscitation, or cardiotomy. A pleural effusion develops in 50% of patients, and is generally small in volume and less prominent than the pericardial effusion that also develops. The pleural fluid is a serous or hemorrhagic exudate (Dressler, 1959).

COLLAGEN–VASCULAR DISEASES

Generally, pleural effusions caused by collagen-vascular diseases are not massive and are more a diagnostic than a therapeutic dilemma; consequently, they are not commonly seen by thoracic surgeons. The effusions usually respond to systemic treatment of the underlying disease (Lee et al., 1959).

SUBDIAPHRAGMATIC INFLAMMATION

Pleural effusions often occur in response to sterile or infectious inflammations below the diaphragm (Light and George, 1976). Up to 20% of patients with pancreatitis develop a pleural effusion, which is usually on the left but is occasionally bilateral. The amylase level is higher in the pleural fluid than in a simultaneous peripheral blood sample (Kaye, 1968). Sympathetic pleural effusions resulting from subphrenic abscesses are usually sterile. The effusion becomes a thoracic empyema in only 15 to 20% of patients and is generally secondary to necrosis of the diaphragm (Konjolinka and Olearczyk, 1972). To avoid contamination of the pleural cavity, the chest

should not be entered during surgical drainage of the intra-abdominal collection. If tube thoracostomy is necessary to control the effusion, it should be placed some distance from the abdominal incision.

PULMONARY EMBOLISM

A pleural effusion develops in 50% of patients with a pulmonary embolism with or without a pulmonary infarction. The effusion after an embolism is normally a blood-tinged exudate of small volume that clears spontaneously if no other embolism occurs. If pulmonary infarction develops, the pleural effusion may be greater in volume and take longer to resolve (Bynum and Wilson, 1976).

PULMONARY INFECTION

The most common cause of a pleural exudate is a pulmonary infection. Effusion is seen in 10 to 15% of patients with viral or mycoplasmal pneumonia and in 50% of patients with bacterial pneumonia. Treatment focuses on the underlying infection (Light et al., 1980).

Management of Pleural Effusion

Pleural effusions may be asymptomatic or may cause incapacitating symptoms. Small or asymptomatic effusions do not warrant immediate intervention unless removal is necessary for diagnostic reasons.

An effusion that is not due to malignancy usually responds to treatment of the underlying disease. Most noninfected pleural effusions are due to advanced malignancy, but their treatment may allow months or years of productive life. If the effusion is not controlled, the patient suffers from a decline in pulmonary function secondary to mechanical compression of the lung (Leff et al., 1978).

Treatment of the causative neoplasm with chemotherapy or radiation therapy may resolve the pleural effusion and improve respiratory symptoms. Radiation therapy is effective for effusion secondary to lymphatic obstruction caused by lymphoma or carcinoma of the lung or breast because it removes the cause of the effusion and restores normal pleural fluid dynamics. For life-threatening pleural effusions that interfere with respiratory dynamics, thoracentesis helps control symptoms until a therapeutic response occurs.

THORACENTESIS

This simple procedure is immediately effective and does not require hospitalization. However, in 96% of patients, malignant pleural effusion recurs within 1 month, with an average recurrence time of 4.2 days (Anderson et al., 1974). Repeated thoracentesis, especially with high-protein exudates, can lead to hypoproteinemia, and the resultant decrease in osmotic pressure can lead to more rapid reaccumulation of pleural fluid. Since patients with advanced malignancies are generally in catabolic states, repetitive loss of protein may exacerbate overall debility and malnutrition. Empyema, pneumothorax, bronchopleural fistula, and loculation of fluid are other complications of repeated thoracentesis, and they may prevent pleural apposition during attempts at pleurodesis. Therefore, thoracentesis should be used to evaluate the initial effusion by determining its cause and tendency to reaccumulate and the ability of the underlying lung to reexpand and relieve acute respiratory symptoms.

THORACOSTOMY AND CHEMICAL PLEURODESIS

Symptomatic malignant effusions that do not respond to radiation or chemotherapy require local therapy to relieve symptoms. Treatment consists of removal of the fluid with obliteration of the pleural space to prevent fluid reaccumulation. Obliteration of the pleural space is accomplished by introducing an agent that causes a sterile adhesive pleuritis with subsequent permanent adhesion of the pleural surfaces. This does not affect the systemic disease but may relieve symptoms. Fusion of the pleural surfaces requires reexpansion of the underlying lung and complete removal of pleural fluid so that the parietal and visceral pleural surfaces are in apposition when a sclerosing agent is introduced. Failure to fully reexpand the lung prevents complete pleurodesis and results in fluid reaccumulation.

Intrapleural instillation of chemotherapeutic agents was first performed to destroy local tumor implants. Postmortem studies showed almost complete obliteration of the pleural space by fibrinous adhesions (Thorsrud, 1965) and suggested that the pleural symphysis prevented reaccumulation of the pleural effusion. Various chemotherapeutic agents have been used, including bleomycin, nitrogen mustard, doxorubicin, 5-fluorouracil, and cisplatin (Robinson et al., 1993). Bleomycin, the most popular chemotherapeutic agent for sclerosis of the pleural space, has objective 1-month response rates that average 84% (Hausheer and Yarbro, 1985). However, bleomycin is expensive and can be associated with serious side effects, including leukopenia (Siegel and Schiffman, 1990).

Chemical irritants such as tetracycline and quinacrine are effective and were previously popular as sclerosing agents, but they are no longer commercially available for this purpose. The tetracycline derivative doxycycline has been found to be as effective as tetracycline, with similar side effects including pain and occasional fever. Like tetracycline, doxycycline causes an inflammatory reaction with connective tissue proliferation (Homma et al., 1983). For chemical pleurodesis, a tube is inserted through the sixth or seventh intercostal space in the midaxillary line, and the pleural fluid is drained as completely as possible so that the instilled sclerosing agent is not diluted and the pleural surfaces remain in close contact. A chest film should be obtained to assure that the lung has reexpanded to fill the pleural space. Once drainage has decreased to less than 200 ml/day, the patient is premedicated with a narcotic analgesic. Fifteen milliliters of 1% lidocaine hydrochloride followed by 500

mg of doxycycline dissolved in 30 ml of 0.9% saline solution is injected into the chest tube. The chest tube is flushed with 25 ml of saline and clamped. It was previously felt that position changes were important to distribute the sclerosing agent throughout the pleural space. Studies using radiolabeled tetracycline show that the tetracycline is dispersed throughout the pleural space within seconds, and that patient positioning usually has no effect on its intrapleural distribution. Patient rotation is felt to enhance distribution of the sclerosing agent when the lung is separated substantially from the chest wall, such as with trapped lung (Lorch et al., 1988). After 4 hours, the chest tube is unclamped and connected to suction. Suction can be removed when drainage is less than approximately 100 ml/day.

Iodized talc causes severe reactive pleuritis and is perhaps the most effective sclerosing agent. Success rates as high as 96% have been reported with its use (Hausheer and Yarbro, 1985). Talc can be delivered through a thoracostomy tube in the form of a slurry (Adler and Sayek, 1976; Webb et al., 1992) or under direct visualization using video-assisted thoracoscopy. The video-assisted surgical approach is especially useful in patients with undiagnosed pleural effusions who are found at operation to have malignancy as the cause of their effusions. A mortality rate of 5% has been reported using this procedure in this high-risk, debilitated population (Ohri et al., 1992). Side effects after talc instillation include pain and occasional fever. Talc microemboli, pneumonitis, acute respiratory distress syndrome, and restrictive lung disease have been reported, but are rare (Ohri et al., 1992). Talc pleurodesis is ideal for patients with malignant pleural effusions who are symptomatic and whose advanced disease makes their life expectancy short. It is not recommended for benign disease in young patients or in patients who may require thoracic surgical procedures in the future. Failures of talc pleurodesis are usually the result of incomplete reexpansion of the lung with failure of the pleural surfaces to adhere to one another.

RADIOTHERAPY

External beam radiation can be used to control pleural effusions secondary to lymphatic obstruction (Weick et al., 1973). Improvement is not usually seen before 3 weeks of therapy. As a result, this type of therapy has limited application to acutely symptomatic patients.

SURGICAL PLEURODESIS AND PLEURECTOMY

When previous methods have failed to control a pleural effusion, open pleurectomy or pleural scarification have occasionally been used. These procedures are 95% effective in controlling recurrent effusions, but they require a thoracotomy and have morbidity of 23% and mortality ranging from 6% to 18%, mainly due to the existing pulmonary disease (Austin and Flye, 1979; Hausheer and Yarbro, 1985). When the pleura is thickened or the lung is trapped, a parietal pleurectomy with decortication may be necessary. These procedures should be reserved for patients with an expected long survival.

PLEUROPERITONEAL SHUNT

The Denver pleuroperitoneal shunt (Codman and Shurtleff, Inc.) consists of a valved pumping chamber with attached fenestrated silicone pleural and peritoneal catheters (Fig. 16–18). Manual compression of the pump transfers fluid against the normal abdominal pleural pressure gradient. The method may be useful for patients who have recurrent effusions after chemical pleurodesis or who have cardiac or pulmonary function inadequate to undergo a thoracotomy (Little et al., 1986). Ponn and co-workers (1991) implanted pleuroperitoneal shunts in 17 patients with intractable pleural effusions, of which 15 were malignant. Palliation of dyspnea at rest was achieved in all patients. Occlusion of the shunt device can be a significant problem, but most remain patent for the remainder of the patient's life, which can be only months in patients with malignant disease.

Empyema

Pleural empyema, or empyema thoracis, is an accumulation of pus in the pleural space. Hippocrates first described its symptoms and natural history. Before antibiotics were developed in the 1930s and 1940s, pleural empyema occurred in 10% of patients who survived pneumonia. Antibiotics effectively treated pneumonia and reduced the incidence of postpneumonic empyema. However, as progress in thoracic surgery made the treatment of more intrathoracic diseases possible, the incidence of postoperative empyema increased. Modern antibiotic therapy has made postoperative empyema uncommon, such that many thoracic surgeons have minimal experience recognizing and treating it.

Pathogenesis

The American Thoracic Society (1962) classified empyema into three phases based on the natural history of the disease: (1) The exudative or acute phase is characterized by pleural fluid of low viscosity and low cellular content. The pleural fluid usually has a low white blood cell count and LDH level and a normal pleural fluid glucose and pH. The lung is still expandable. (2) The fibrinopurulent or transitional phase is characterized by more turbid fluid and an increase in polymorphonuclear white blood cells. Fibrin is deposited on both pleural surfaces and forms a limiting peel that prevents extension of the empyema, but also begins to trap the lung. The pleural fluid becomes increasingly turbid and the lung progressively less expandable. Pleural fluid pH and glucose become progressively lower, and the LDH increases. (3) The organizing or chronic phase is characterized by organization of the pleural peel with ingrowth of capillaries and fibroblasts. The pleural fluid is viscous and high in sediment, the pH is often less than 7.0, and the glucose is less than 40 mg/dl.

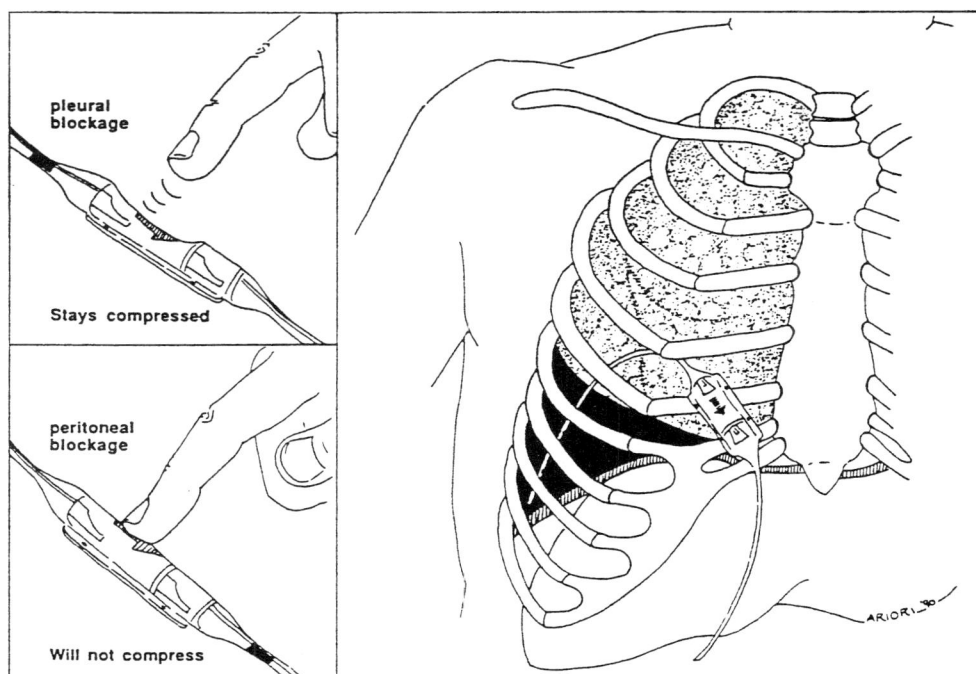

FIGURE 16–18. Diagram showing shunt position and signs of proximal or distal obstruction. (From Ponn, R. B., Blancaflor, J., D'Agostino, R. S., et al.: Pleuroperitoneal shunting for intractable pleural effusions. Reprinted with permission from the Society of Thoracic Surgeons [The Annals of Thoracic Surgery, 1991, Vol. 51, pp. 605–609].)

The organizational phase begins 7 to 10 days after the onset of disease and is generally complete by 4 to 6 weeks.

Half of empyemas are secondary to complications of a primary pneumonic process. Postpneumonic or parapneumonic empyema can be caused by two mechanisms: obstruction of pulmonary lymphatics by inflammatory debris, which contaminates the pleural fluid by lymphatic transport of organisms from the focus of infection in the lungs, and direct extension of the pneumonic process into the pleural space. This occurs with progression of the inflammatory reaction in the lung, causing tissue necrosis and abscess formation around terminal bronchi. The distal airway obstruction that is produced causes air trapping and pneumatocele formation. Subpleural pneumatoceles may rupture spontaneously and deposit organisms in the pleural space. The combination of pleural dead space, a culture medium of pleural fluid, and inoculation of bacteria produces empyema.

The second most common group are patients who have undergone operations on the lung, mediastinum, or esophagus. The operation most frequently implicated is pneumonectomy, which is complicated by empyema 2 to 12% of the time (Light, 1983). Other causes are spontaneous pneumothorax, chest trauma, subphrenic abscesses, foreign bodies retained in the bronchial tree, and spontaneous rupture of the esophagus (Takaro et al., 1977) (Table 16–9).

Before the advent of antibiotic therapy, *Pneumococcus* and *Streptococcus* were the organisms most frequently associated with empyema. Between 1955 and 1965, *Staphylococcus* was the most frequent causative organism and was cultured in 92% of patients under the age of 2 years (Ravitch and Fein, 1961). As culture techniques improved, anaerobic organisms were isolated most frequently (Bartlett and Feingold, 1974; Geha, 1971). Of 83 patients with positive pleural fluid cultures, 35% had only anaerobic organisms, 24% had only aerobic organisms, and 41% had both (Bartlett et al., 1974). The incidence of effusion and its contamination with various organisms are shown in Table 16–10.

Clinical Presentation of Postpneumonic Empyema

The signs and symptoms of empyema are not specific and may be difficult to distinguish from those of the underlying infective process. The clinical presentation depends on the causative organism, the volume of pus in the pleural space, and the patient's circumstances. The patient commonly complains of pleuritic

■ **Table 16–9.** ETIOLOGY OF EMPYEMA

Pneumonia (viral, bacterial, tuberculosis, mycotic)
Lung abscess
Trauma
Postoperative
Extenson of subphrenic abscess
Spontaneous pneumothorax
Generalized sepsis

■ **Table 16–10.** INCIDENCE OF EMPYEMA ACCORDING TO BACTERIAL ORGANISM CAUSING PNEUMONIA

Organism	Incidence of Effusion	Incidence of Infected Effusion (Empyema)
Anaerobic	35	90
Aerobic		
Gram-positive		
Streptococcus pneumoniae	40–60	<5
Staphylococcus aureus (children)	70	80
S. aureus (adults)	40	20
Gram-negative		
Escherichia coli	50	90
Pseudomonas	50	90

chest pain and a heavy sensation on the involved side; is usually febrile, tachypneic, and tachycardic; and may have a cough that produces purulent sputum. Physical examination reveals decreased respiratory excursion, pain on percussion, and a friction rub or distant-to-absent breath sounds on auscultation of the involved side. The chest film suggests the diagnosis. Both posteroanterior and lateral views are necessary to accurately localize the pleural abnormality. The initial film may show pulmonary consolidation with moderate pleural effusion or total opacity of one hemithorax. An airless lung and pleural fluid produce similar densities on chest films. Therefore, when the hemithorax is opacified, it is difficult to distinguish between lung consolidation or atelectasis and pleural fluid. Auscultation of the chest may help make the diagnosis; consolidated lungs transmit bronchial breath sounds, whereas fluid dampens them. Roentgenographic evidence of tracheal and mediastinal shift toward the unaffected side indicates significant pleural fluid, and this shift of the mediastinum can produce cardiopulmonary dysfunction on a mechanical basis (Fig. 16–19). Ultrasound and CT scanning help differentiate consolidation and fluid accumulation in an opacified chest (Fig. 16–20). CT scans are particularly helpful in identifying complex, multiloculated empyemas that may require surgical drainage.

Antibiotic therapy alters the clinical manifestations of empyema. Persistent fever in a patient whose pneumonic process has resolved may be evidence of empyema, which may go undetected until it presents as a subcutaneous abscess and drains spontaneously. This condition, called *empyema necessitatis*, occurs when an undrained empyema erodes through the chest wall, usually near the fifth costochondral junction. Similarly, the empyema can erode into a bronchus to form a bronchopleural fistula, causing a chronic cough with copious, foul-smelling sputum. Excessive drainage may flood the contralateral bronchial tree and cause asphyxia. In this situation, the patient is placed in the lateral decubitus position with the affected side down to prevent leakage into the bronchus until the empyema can be drained (Marks and Eickhoff, 1970). Metastatic abscesses, although

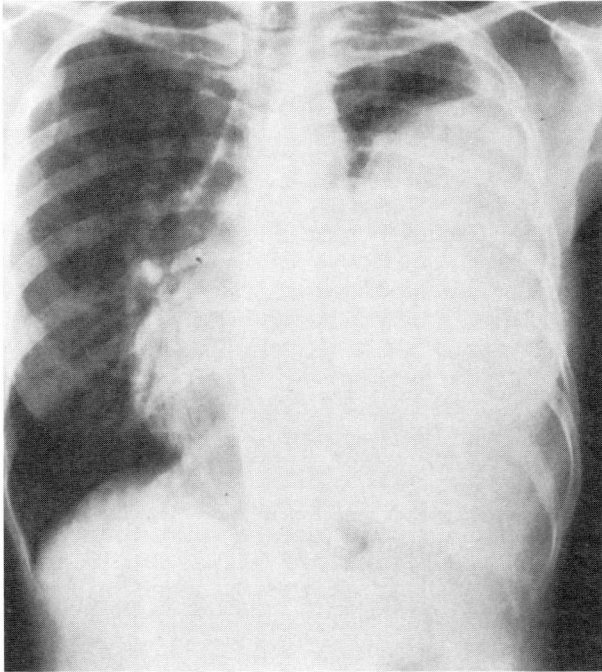

FIGURE 16–19. Upright chest film of a postpneumonic chronic empyema of the left pleural space with compression of the ipsilateral lung and a shift of the mediastinum to the right.

less frequent, can occur in the vertebrae and central nervous system.

An empyema that has been present for 6 weeks or more is in the chronic phase and may restrict movement of the involved hemithorax. Chronic empyema generally results from delay in recognition or inadequate treatment of an acute empyema. The patients are usually debilitated and may be anemic and have early clubbing of the fingers.

Diagnosis of Empyema

Aspiration of pus from the pleural space establishes the diagnosis of empyema. When empyema is sus-

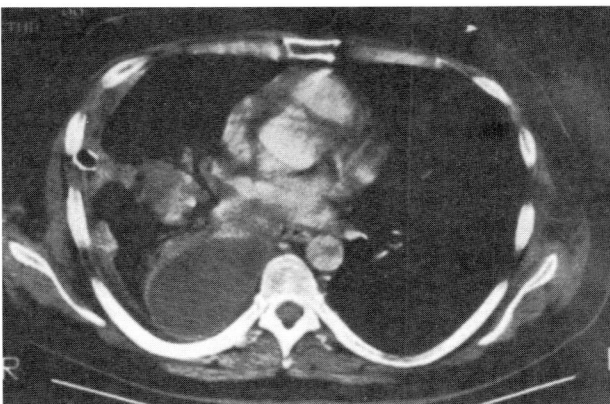

FIGURE 16–20. CT scan of a patient with an empyema in the right costovertebral angle. Note the pleural thickening over the entrapped right lower lobe.

pected, thoracentesis should be performed and fluid sent for appropriate cultures, Gram's stain, pH, cell count with differential, glucose, protein, LDH, and cytology, if there is suspicion of malignancy. With current antibiotic use, the pleural fluid may be only slightly cloudy, and cultures may fail to grow in 50% of patients. Antibiotic therapy or failure to obtain anaerobic cultures may produce negative cultures. A simultaneous sputum culture is helpful because the organism responsible for the pneumonia is frequently the cause of the empyema. Empyema secondary to tuberculosis or fungal infection should be suspected if cultures are repeatedly sterile and the patient fails to improve with therapy. Bronchoscopy may be indicated to exclude the presence of an endotracheal tumor or an inhaled foreign body.

Pleural empyema must be differentiated from an intrapulmonary abscess (Baber et al., 1980). Both are treated with antibiotics and drainage, but inappropriate insertion of a tube into an intraparenchymal abscess can cause empyema, pneumothorax, bronchopleural fistula, and hemorrhage. Peripheral pulmonary abscess can be especially difficult to distinguish from an empyema. The presence of an air fluid level does not help because a loculated empyema may contain air from gas-forming organisms, a previous pneumothorax, a bronchopleural fistula, or an attempted thoracentesis.

Generally, an empyema cavity conforms in shape and extends to the adjacent chest wall. Its vertical and horizontal dimensions are greater than its width. A typical lung abscess is more spherical, does not extend or conform to the chest wall, and is surrounded by the pneumonia from which it developed (Friedman and Hellekani, 1977). CT scanning is valuable in the absence of differentiating criteria on the chest film (Fig. 16–21). It can also show any multiple loculations, the best position for tube insertion to obtain dependent drainage, and the presence of residual collections.

Management

Treatment of an empyema depends on its cause, whether it is acute or chronic, the state of the underlying lung, the presence of a bronchopleural fistula, the ability to obliterate the space, and the patient's clinical condition and nutritional status (Fig. 16–22).

ACUTE AND TRANSITIONAL EMPYEMA

The normal pleural space resists bacterial invasion as long as there is no pleural dead space. Therefore, prevention of dead space and control of the primary pulmonary process are necessary to prevent and eradicate pleural infection. Most surgical procedures are for chronic empyema and focus on managing a persistent pleural space.

Open drainage can be used to decompress the infection. Decortication or thoracoplasty can be used to obliterate the space.

Pleural fluid in acute and transitional empyema

EMPYEMA

LUNG
ABSCESS

Extrapulmonary
fluid
pocket

Intrapulmonary
fluid
pocket

Surrounding
pneumonia

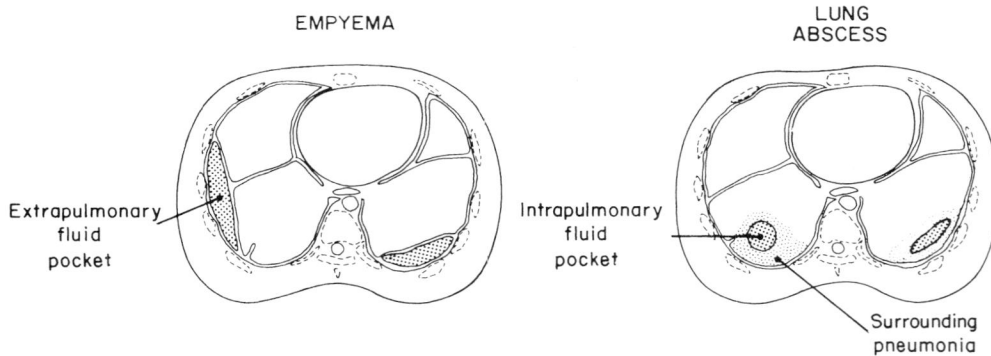

FIGURE 16–21. Schematic drawing of a chest CT scan showing the difference between an empyema and an abscess in the lung. An empyema conforms to the shape of the adjacent chest wall. An abscess in the lung is usually more spherical, does not extend to or conform with the chest wall, and is surrounded by the pneumonia in which it developed.

ranges from serous fluid to bacteria-contaminated cloudy fluid to pus. The last two are diagnostic of an empyema. The objectives of therapy are control of local and systemic infection with specific antibiotic therapy; evacuation of the empyema fluid; and reexpansion of the lung with obliteration of the pleural dead space (Cohn and Blaisdell, 1970).

If the empyema is in the acute phase, the pleural fluid has a low viscosity and may be removed entirely by thoracentesis. In this situation, the combination of thoracentesis and antibiotics can be definitive treatment, particularly in children (Stiles et al., 1970). When thoracentesis produces purulent material, fluid that is positive on Gram's stain, or fluid with a glucose level below 40 mg/dl or a pH below 7, tube thoracostomy is indicated. During the acute phase, the tube evacuates the empyema and reexpands the underlying lung. If it has not been established that the pleural fluid is an empyema, and if it is questionable

whether the lung will reexpand because of an endobronchial tumor or restrictive pneumonitis, a chest tube should not be inserted because it will contaminate the dead space and possibly create empyema.

Tube thoracostomy is performed with a No. 28 to 36 French tube (or a smaller tube in children) placed in a dependent position. If the pleural space is completely drained with improved expansion of the lung, antibiotics are continued and the tube removed approximately 1 week later if drainage has ceased and symptoms of infection have resolved.

In the transitional phase, reexpansion of the lung and drainage of the empyema fluid may be more difficult. Fibrinolytic enzymes have occasionally been used to improve chest tube drainage of thick purulent material (Bergh et al., 1977). Loculated, undrained pockets should be sought by CT scanning and, if possible, drained percutaneously. If CT scanning reveals a complex, multiloculated fluid collection, or

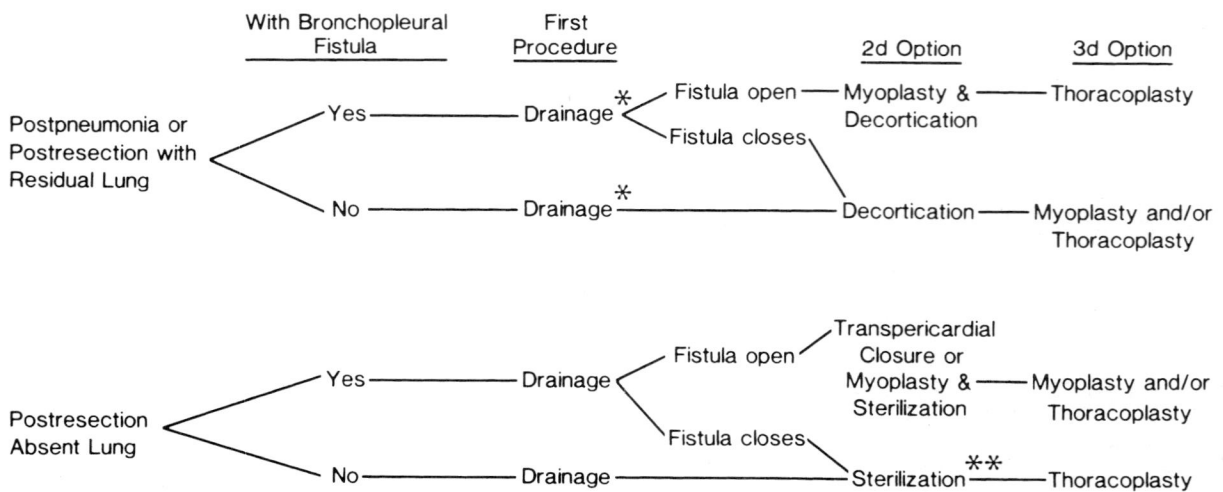

	With Bronchopleural Fistula	First Procedure		2d Option	3d Option
Postpneumonia or Postresection with Residual Lung	Yes	Drainage *	Fistula open	Myoplasty & Decortication	Thoracoplasty
			Fistula closes		
	No	Drainage *		Decortication	Myoplasty and/or Thoracoplasty
Postresection Absent Lung	Yes	Drainage	Fistula open	Transpericardial Closure or Myoplasty & Sterilization	Myoplasty and/or Thoracoplasty
			Fistula closes		
	No	Drainage		Sterilization **	Thoracoplasty

* Convert to open drainage if cavity fails to obliterate with tube drainage alone

** Can be attempted several times

FIGURE 16–22. Algorithm for the management of an empyema.

if loculated pockets cannot adequately be drained percutaneously, then surgical therapy is indicated. This consists of thoracotomy with débridement of the pleural cavity to evacuate its loculations and debris. The wound is closed around a large chest tube that is suctioned to maintain pulmonary reexpansion. If reexpansion of the lung is not immediate, the size of the cavity can be assessed by instilling contrast medium into the tube to judge the progress in healing. The tube is progressively withdrawn over several weeks as the cavity becomes smaller (Fig. 16–23). Persistent toxicity or lack of radiographic evidence that the size of the cavity is being reduced indicates that the empyema is in the chronic stage.

CHRONIC EMPYEMA

Chronic empyema begins approximately 6 weeks after the onset of the acute illness. By then, the wall of the empyema, or the peel, is organized by ingrowth of capillaries and fibroblasts, and expansion of the lung by simple evacuation of the cavity can no longer be expected. When the initial thoracentesis produces pleural fluid with 75% sediment on standing, the empyema is in the chronic phase and open drainage can be safely performed. The chronic phase usually results from delay in seeking medical attention, inadequate antibiotic therapy during the acute phase, persistent conservative management with inadequate drainage, the presence of an endobronchial or intrapleural foreign body, infection of a postresectional space after a segmentectomy or lobectomy, a chronic pulmonary infection such as tuberculosis, or interstitial pulmonary disease that prevents reexpansion of the lung to obliterate the pleural space.

Chronic empyema is treated by open drainage and débridement of the cavity, usually with an open flap procedure (Fig. 16–24). The operation was designed by Eloesser (1935) and usually follows unsuccessful open or closed drainage. The procedure is also used to drain a postpneumonectomy empyema with or without a bronchopleural fistula. The procedure can be difficult when the empyema is located high in the axilla or in the paravertebral area.

The incision for the open flap drainage procedure must be performed carefully. A U-shaped flap of skin is made with a base that is 10 to 12 cm long and parallel to the superior border of the first uninvolved rib above the bottom of the empyema cavity. The full curved end of the flap is 6 to 7 cm long—that is, the length of two ribs and the intervening intercostal space. The rib underlying the base of the flap is resected and the tip of the flap is turned into the chest and tacked to the pleura. The inferior defect in the skin is allowed to heal by secondary intension. The opening should have a valve-like action that makes it more difficult for air to enter than to escape. If properly constructed, the flap can be taken down without difficulty when appropriate.

Open-flap drainage is easier to care for and cleaner than open-tube drainage; the cavity is irrigated and packed at daily or longer intervals, depending on the rate of soilage. *Pseudomonas* colonization frequently develops, and packs soaked in 1% acetic acid control its growth (Samson, 1971).

If the empyema cavity is unusually thick-walled and does not decrease in size satisfactorily, decortication or sterilization can be performed after the inflammatory reaction has subsided. Decortication is successful when the fibroelastic peel that traps the lung leaves the visceral pleura relatively normal and the lung itself expansile so that the empyema space can be obliterated by reexpansion of the lung when the peel is removed. Best results are obtained with decortication in the early chronic phase of an empyema secondary to pneumonia or traumatic hemothorax. Decortication can be combined with pulmonary resection if the underlying lung is grossly diseased (Lopez-Majano and Joshi, 1970; Samson, 1971).

Decortication usually requires that the chest be opened widely through a lateral or standard posterolateral incision. A long-standing empyema causes crowding of the ribs, and a rib resection is usually required. Generally, the chest is entered through the bed of the fifth rib. The decision is made as to whether both parietal and visceral pleural peels or only the visceral peel should be removed. A rigid, thickened parietal pleura that restricts the mobility of the thoracic cage should be excised and usually requires an extrapleural dissection. If both parietal and visceral peels are to be removed, an attempt can be made to excise the entire empyema sac without opening it. This empyemectomy, in theory, should reduce the contamination of the wound and remaining pleural cavity (Samson, 1971). When the parietal wall of the empyema sac is detached from the chest wall by extrapleural dissection (Fig. 16–25), empyemectomy can usually be performed. If the surface of the empyema sac does not show the indentations of the ribs but rather intercostal muscle fibers, the pleural dissection is not in the correct plane. Bleeding may be severe in this part of the operation because infection makes the tissue abnormally vascular, and blood replacement must keep pace with blood loss to avoid sudden hypovolemic collapse. A ridge where the empyema wall meets normal parietal pleura marks the edge of the empyema sac, beyond which a loose areolar plane is entered where the parietal pleura is more easily separated from the chest wall. At this point, the pleural space can be entered by cutting through the parietal pleura, and decortication of the visceral wall of the empyema cavity from the visceral pleura can be initiated.

It is easier to begin detachment of the visceral layer of the empyema sac from an area of minimal adherence to the lung in order to enter the correct plane of cleavage between the lung and the tough membrane. The decortication is performed with a combination of blunt and sharp dissection, using either the finger or a pledget mounted on a clamp (Kitner's) (Fig. 16–26). Gentleness and patience are required to minimize damage to the lung and to reduce postoperative air leak. In places where adherence of the peel is dense, the peel is held up by tissue forceps and the underly-

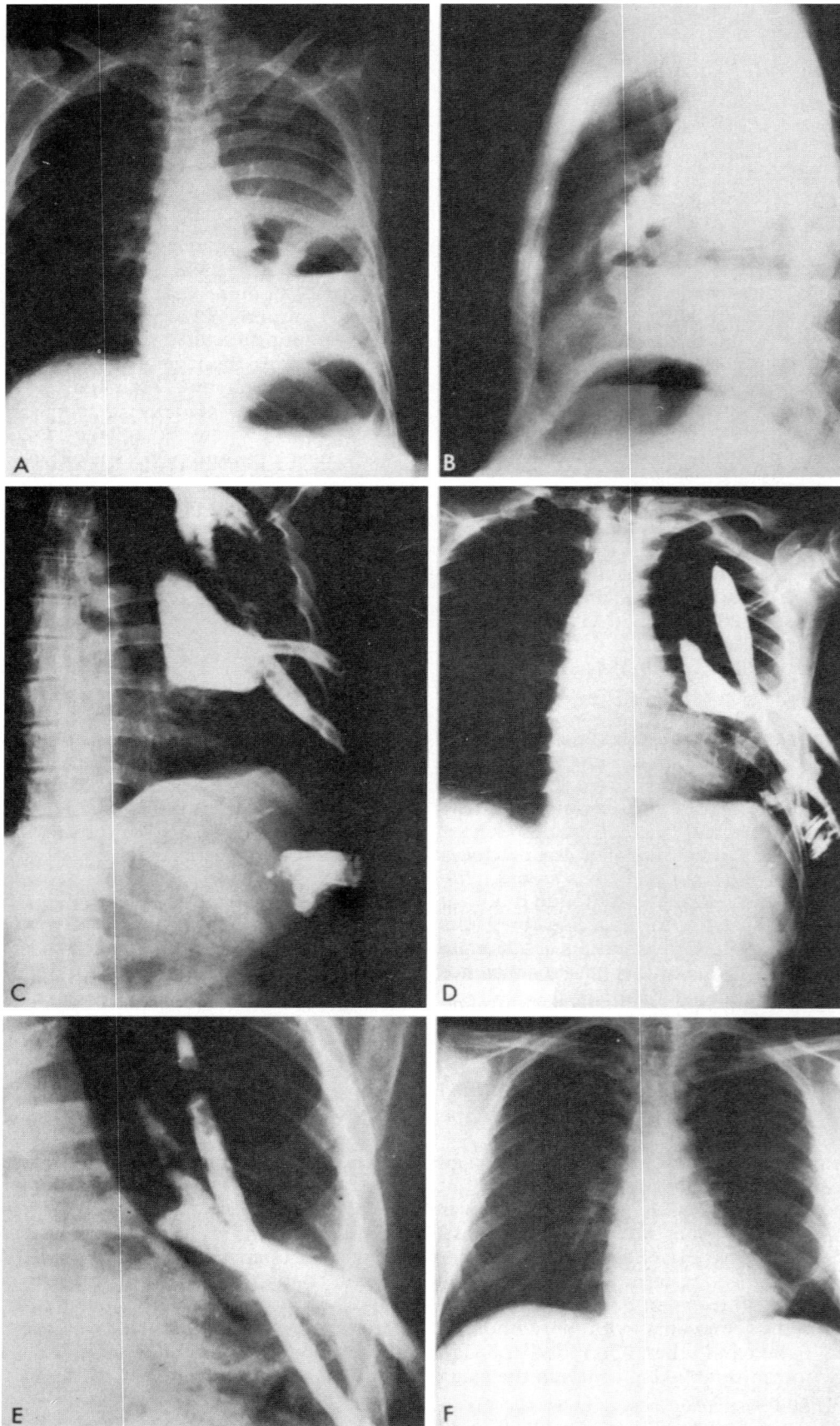

FIGURE 16–23 *See legend on opposite page*

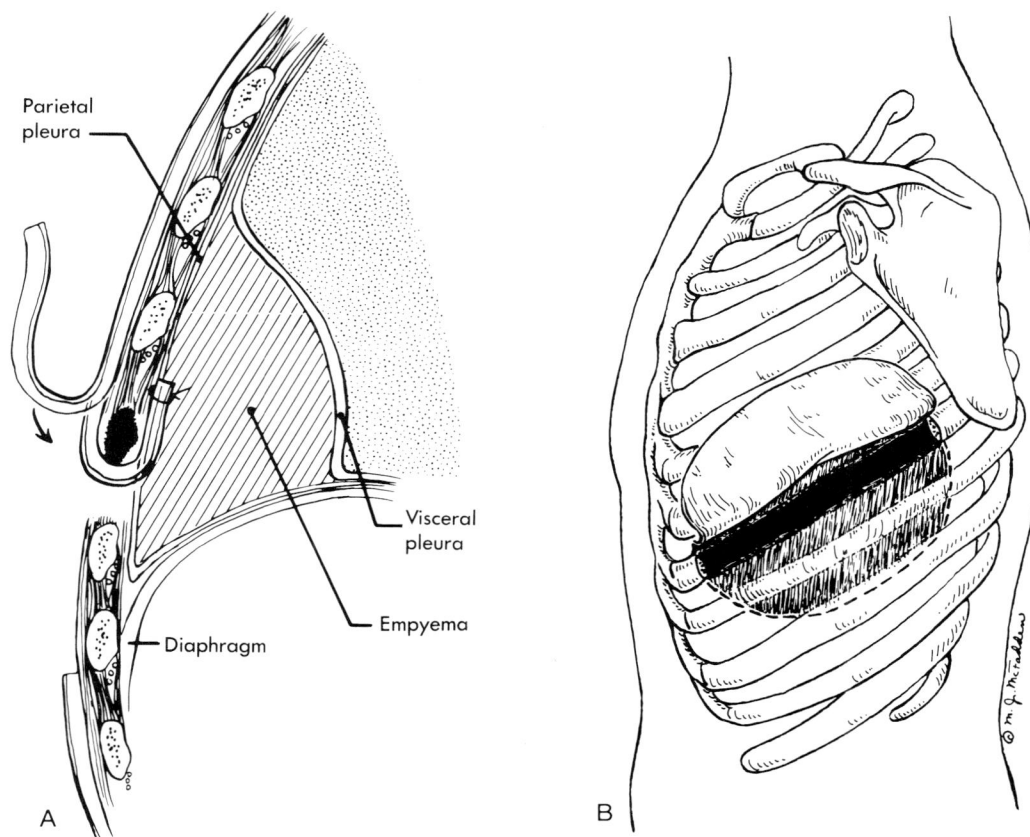

FIGURE 16–24. Schematic drawing showing the technical points in construction of an Eloesser flap. The base of the flap is usually parallel to the superior border of the first rib, freely clear of the bottom of the empyema cavity, and about halfway between the axillary line and the line of the inferior angle of the scapula. The width of the flap is equal to two ribs and their intervening intercostal space. Only the rib at the base of the flap is resected, which allows the flap to be turned in to make a "mailbox-like" opening that gives it a valve-like action. The exposed inferior ribs are partially covered by suturing the edges of the skin together.

ing lung stretched slightly so that the peel can be separated from the lung by sharp dissection with the scalpel. To avoid cutting into the parenchyma of the lung, the blade of the scalpel is held almost parallel to the surface of the lung and cuts are made a fraction of a millimeter from the pigmented lung edge. The process is slow and must be performed meticulously. In areas where visceral peel is fused to the lung, it is best to leave it as an isolated plaque by cutting around it rather than risk injuring the lung.

After decortication is complete, the anesthesiologist applies positive pressure to reinflate the lung, and areas where the lung is folded on itself by adhesions are recognized. Division of these adhesions leads to unfolding the lung until it fills the pleural cavity. The

obliteration of the pleural space prevents further development of pockets of pus, despite any contamination.

All bleeding is controlled before the chest is closed. Apical and basal chest tubes are inserted and connected to two underwater seal bottles. Adequate suction must be applied on the drainage bottles to keep the lung fully expanded and in apposition to the chest wall.

When a pathologic process in the underlying lung prevents its expansion, the pleural space cannot be obliterated without combining the decortication with a space-reducing operation. The space can be obliterated by filling the cavity with a muscle transposition, obliterating the cavity with a thoracoplasty, or a combination of both (Andrews, 1965).

FIGURE 16–23. A series of chest films showing the management of a transitional-phase empyema with thoracostomy tube drainage. The initial posteroanterior *(A)* and lateral *(B)* chest films show a left posterolateral empyema cavity with an air fluid level and a contaminated loculated effusion in the left major fissure. The first sinogram *(C)* was taken 6 weeks after initiation of tube drainage of both spaces. The second sinogram *(D)*, taken at 9 weeks, shows a reduction in the size of the cavities, which have contracted down to the size of the tubes, signaling the initiation of their gradual withdrawal *(E)*. Follow-up chest film *(F)* was obtained 11 months after diagnosis and 7 months after removal of the thoracostomy tubes.

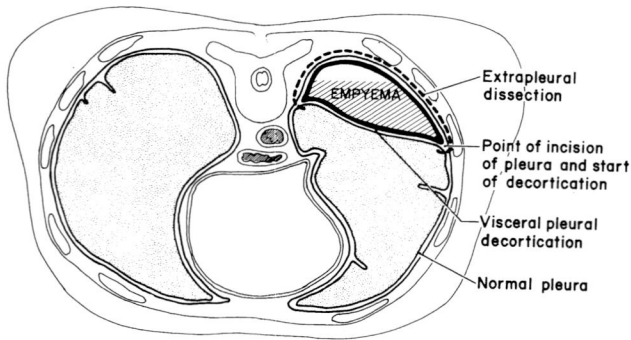

FIGURE 16–25. Schematic drawing of a cross-section of the thorax showing where an extrapleural dissection and decortication dissection are performed during an empyemectomy.

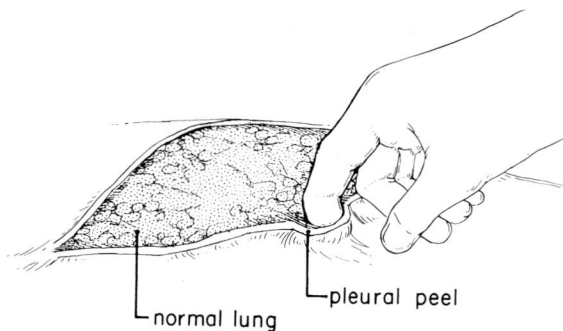

FIGURE 16–27. Schematic drawing showing the bottle and tubing hookup for balanced drainage. This arrangement provides a means of draining a contaminated pneumonectomy cavity when the mediastinum is unstable. It allows fluid drainage and air replacement without changing intrapleural pressures.

POSTPNEUMONECTOMY EMPYEMA

Empyema that involves the entire pleural space is a rare but serious complication after pneumonectomy. The incidence of empyema after pneumonectomy has decreased as a result of antibiotic therapy and improved surgical technique. It usually occurs early in the postoperative period but is occasionally seen months or even years after pneumonectomy. *Staphylococcus aureus* is the organism most commonly cultured from the infected space. Growth of multiple organisms suggests an enteropleural fistula.

In the absence of a bronchopleural fistula, an empyema can be difficult to recognize but should be suspected in the presence of spiking fever, malaise, and roentgenographic evidence of loculations of intrapleural air. Late postpneumonectomy empyemas are frequently overlooked until empyema necessitatis occurs. Symptoms can be confused with recurrence of tumor in patients who have had a previous resection for cancer. If a postpneumonectomy empyema goes undrained, it may erode the bronchus and create a life-threatening condition by flooding the contralateral lung.

Initial treatment of early postpneumonectomy empyema consists of closed-tube balanced drainage (Fig. 16–27). This is maintained until the mediastinum is fixed and stable, after which open drainage of the

empyema cavity can be performed (Miller et al., 1975). This is accomplished by creating an Eloesser flap using the anterior end of the thoracotomy incision in the midaxillary line. This higher level is adequate for drainage because the ipsilateral diaphragm rises after pneumonectomy. Care should be taken not to make the incision too far anteriorly, where less muscle and fascia are available for closure (see Fig. 16–24). The cavity is then sterilized as described by Clagett, by packing for 4 to 8 weeks with a gauze bandage soaked with Dakin's solution (0.5% aqueous sodium hypochlorite) (Clagett and Geraci, 1963; Stafford and Clagett, 1972). When the cavity is clean and cultures are negative, the patient is hospitalized and given frequent irrigations with Dakin's solution. After several days, the Eloesser flap is taken down, the cavity filled with an antibiotic solution, and a tight-layered closure of the thoracic wall opening is performed. Because *Staphylococcus* and *Pseudomonas* are frequently cultured from empyema cavities, the antibiotic solution should consist of 250 mg neomycin, 25,000 units of bacitracin, and 150 mg colistin (Colimycin), all in a 100-ml normal saline solution (Samson, 1971). Neomycin solution should not be used for irrigation before closure because ototoxicity has been reported (Myerson et al., 1970). This sterilization procedure has been used in postpneumonectomy empyema with a success rate of 25 to 77%. If the procedure fails, the Eloesser closure is reopened and the cleansing process is repeated; the second sterilization has the same success rate as the first. Recurrence can occur up to 6 years after closure (Fig. 16–28).

Repeated closed-tube irrigations of an infected pneumonectomy space with a large volume of antibiotic or antiseptic solution have been reported (Karkola et al., 1976; Provan, 1971). Success with this regimen has been variable, although some authors report results similar to those of open drainage (Rosenfeldt et al., 1981). Most surgeons recommend two to four attempts with sterilization before obliterating

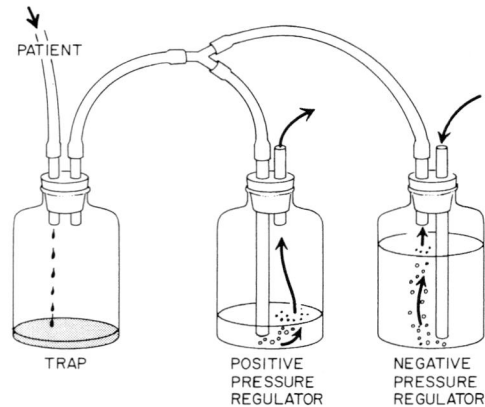

FIGURE 16–26. Schematic drawing showing the position of the finger during a decortication by finger dissection. Pressure and movement of the finger should always be exerted against the peel to avoid inadvertent entry into the soft pulmonary tissue.

Postpneumonectomy Empyema

18 Patients

Sterilization and Closure

11 Patients
Remained Closed 4 mo.–6 yrs.
Median 3 yrs.

7 Patients
Reoccurred

| 4 Early = >1 mo. |
| 3 Late = 7 mo,1 yr, 6 yrs. |

61%
Success

2 Patients
Remained Open

5 Patients

Resterilization and Closure

3 Patients
Remained Closed 4–9 yrs.

2 Patients
Reoccurred

60%
Success

Resterilization and Closure

2 Patients   0
Remained Closed 7–15 mo.

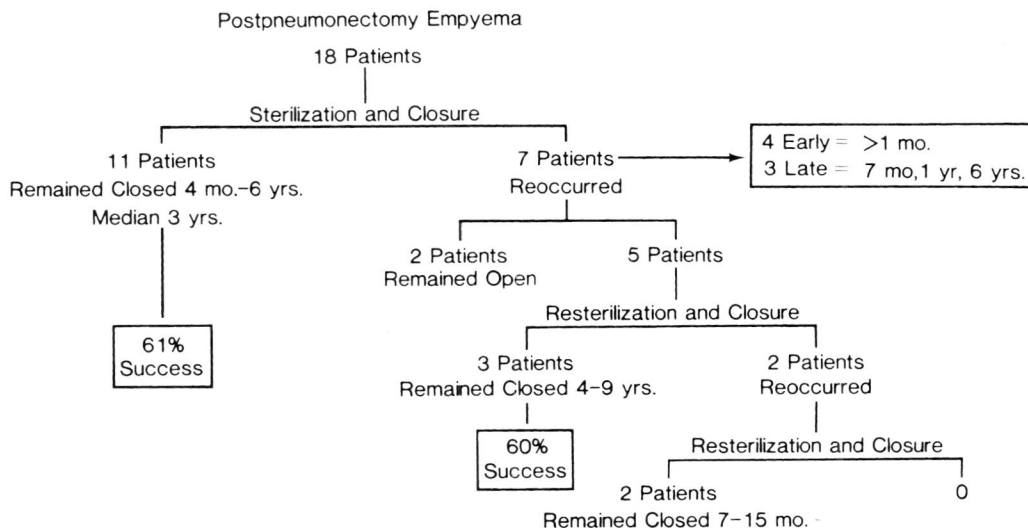

FIGURE 16–28. Expected success of a sterilization procedure for a postpneumonectomy empyema. The success of a second attempt is almost equal to that of the first. Late recurrences can take place up to 6 years. (Based on data from Stafford, E. G., and Clagett, O. T.: Postpneumonectomy empyema: Neomycin instillation and definitive closure. J. Thorac. Cardiovasc. Surg., 63:771, 1972.)

the cavity with transthoracic muscle flaps or a thoracoplasty, or both. Miller and associates (1984) reported a technique to fill the postpneumonectomy space using omentum and transposed muscles with good results. Occasionally, there may be insufficient bulk to fill the space, so thoracoplasty also may be needed. Some patients have been known to do well with permanent open drainage with an Eloesser flap.

Thoracoplasty consists of the resection of a sufficient number of ribs to allow the chest wall to collapse and obliterate the pneumonectomy space. Contact between the collapsed chest wall and the residual lung or mediastinal pleura is necessary to obliterate the space by secondary healing. A number of thoracoplasty techniques have been described (Kergin, 1953; Roberts, 1935; Schede, 1890). Thoracoplasty normally is done in two stages to avoid paradoxic movement of the chest wall. All of the techniques result in chest wall deformity and eventually scoliosis. A single-stage procedure that preserves thoracic cage integrity, *osteoplastic flap thoracoplasty* (Bjork, 1954), retains the first rib to reduce the degree of scoliosis (Bjork, 1954; Gregoire et al., 1987). Knowledge of local anatomy and adherence to the following principles of single-stage thoracoplasty will ensure obliteration of the space with a satisfactory cosmetic result.

1. The operation is performed through the original pneumonectomy incision, which is extended posteriorly and paravertebrally onto the base of the neck. A double-lumen endobronchial tube is used.

2. The technique of rib resection is critical. For closure of a pneumonectomy cavity, the second to the seventh or eighth ribs are removed. A sloping resection of their anterior portion (resection of progressively less anterior rib) preserves the normal configuration of the anterior thoracic wall. Removal of additional lower ribs does not contribute to collapse of the space, but accentuates the deformity. Structural integrity of the neck, shoulder girdle, and upper thorax is maintained by preserving the first rib. To maximize paravertebral collapse, the ribs are divided as posteriorly as possible so that the resected specimen includes the costovertebral joints and part of the vertebral transverse processes. The length of ribs resected becomes shorter as one moves superiorly: 5 fingerbreadths for the fifth rib, 4 fingerbreadths for the fourth rib, and 3 fingerbreadths for the third rib. The second rib is divided at the costochondral junction and is shortened at a later stage to make it as straight as possible (Fig. 16–29). Apicolysis of the pleura is performed to the aortic arch on the left side or the azygos vein on the right. The ribs are bent down on their costochondral junction and the ends of the third to fifth ribs are attached to the sixth rib with strong nylon sutures (Fig. 16–29). Further resection of the ribs may be needed to obtain a better fit. The second rib is tailored so that its straightest portion lies as close as possible to the mediastinum when its posterior end is fixed to the costotransverse ligament of the sixth rib.

3. Preservation of the first rib and apicolysis are performed by incising the periosteum along the outer ridge of the first rib with the cautery and removing it with a periosteal elevator. The subclavian vein and the neurovascular structures along the inner margin of the first rib are protected as the periosteum is stripped off the undersurface of the first rib back toward the mediastinum. By this extrapleural dissection, the apex is dropped.

4. Adequate intrapleural and extrapleural drainage is mandatory to obtain tissue apposition and space obliteration.

POST–TRAUMATIC EMPYEMA

An empyema in a severely injured patient is a potentially lethal complication that results from con-

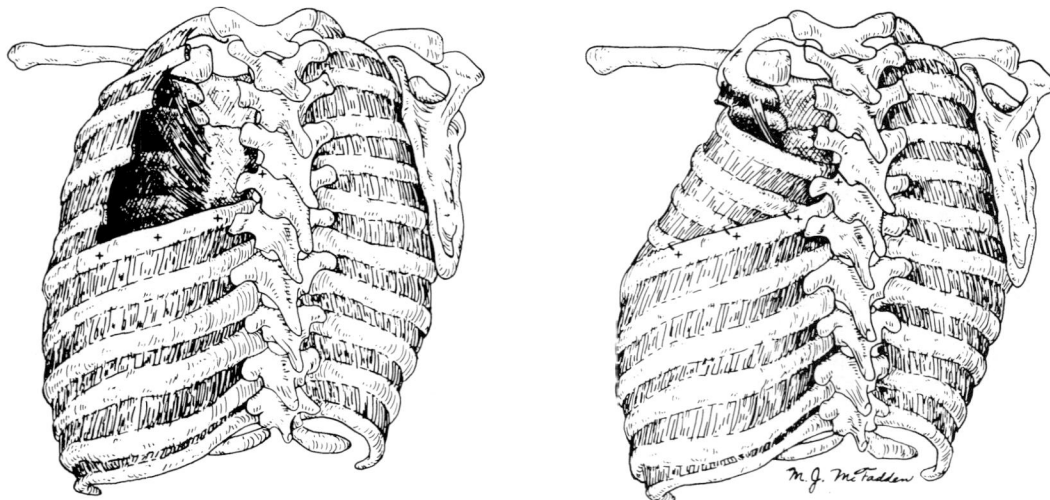

FIGURE 16–29. Posterior view of a Bjork thoracoplasty. The procedure is most applicable to close an empyema space after resection of the upper lobe. Increasing lengths of the posterior portions of the second to fifth ribs are resected along with their intercostal musculature. The remaining portions of the ribs are turned down and sutured to the intact sixth rib.

tamination of blood in the pleural space by a penetrating wound, unrecognized diaphragmatic rupture, emergency insertion of chest tubes, or a continuous air leak. The clotted hemothorax, if incompletely evacuated, is an excellent culture medium and incomplete drainage creates a 5 to 15% incidence of infection. Complete evacuation with full reexpansion of the lung avoids this complication.

When drainage is incomplete, particularly if fever or air fluid levels are present, a thoracotomy should be performed early after the injury before a fibrin peel is established. Treatment of a post-traumatic empyema is similar to that of other types of empyemas (Arom et al., 1977; Coselli et al., 1984).

Bronchopleural Fistula

A bronchopleural fistula is a sinus tract between a bronchus and the pleural space (Woodruff, 1941). In contrast, a pneumothorax is a communication between ruptured blebs or alveolar ducts in the periphery of the lung and the pleural space. Clinically, the former develops from infection of the lung or pleura, whereas the latter usually occurs spontaneously. Both may result from trauma.

A bronchopleural fistula can result as a complication of necrotizing pneumonia, an empyema, pulmonary infarction, and fungal infection. Traumatic causes range from penetrating wounds of the chest to inadvertent lung injury during transbronchial biopsy, pleural biopsy, insertion of a thoracostomy tube, or thoracentesis. The most common cause is breakdown of the bronchial closure after partial or complete resection of the lung. In a series of 3050 pulmonary resections (1122 pneumonectomies, 1622 lobectomies, and 306 segmental resections), bronchopleural fistula occurred in 86 patients, an incidence of 3%. Of these, 64% occurred after pneumonectomy, 28% after lobectomies, and 8% after segmental resections (Williams

and Lewis, 1976). Risk factors for bronchopleural fistula after pulmonary resection are malnutrition, diabetes mellitus, radiation therapy, inflammatory involvement of the bronchial stump, devascularization of the stump, and residual tumor at the bronchial closure. Because of the serious nature of bronchopleural fistula after pneumonectomy, the bronchial stump should be covered with viable tissues such as pericardium, pleura, or intercostal muscle for added protection. In a study of bronchial stump healing, at least 50% of the suture or staple lines separated and healed by secondary intention (Smith et al., 1963). The integrity of peribronchial tissue was more important than the technique by which the stump was closed.

A bronchopleural fistula can occur at any time after operation, but usually occurs in the first 2 weeks. Clinical manifestations include fever and sudden onset of continuous cough with serosanguinous or purulent sputum. Acute respiratory distress may occur if a large fistula leaks sufficient fluid to flood the contralateral lung or if, on rare occasion, a tension pneumothorax develops.

Roentgenographic evidence of a postpneumonectomy bronchopleural fistula includes a drop of 2 cm or more in the air fluid level on the operated side. A smaller drop can be insignificant. By the third week after operation, the air space above the fluid level in a pneumonectomy cavity should be the same as or smaller than on previous chest films and is generally associated with a mediastinal shift toward the operated side. When a fluid drop of more than 2 cm occurs, and the mediastinum shifts away from the operated side or remains stationary, a bronchopleural fistula should be suspected. With a late bronchopleural fistula, a new air fluid level appears in a previously opacified hemithorax. Occasionally, after lobectomy or segmental resection, it is difficult to determine whether an air fluid level is in the parenchyma of the lung or in the pleural space. The air fluid level can be localized better with a CT scan (see "Diagnosis of Empyema," earlier in this chapter).

MANAGEMENT

Acute Bronchopleural Fistula. During acute onset of a postpneumonectomy bronchopleural fistula, the patient should be turned onto the operated side to prevent aspiration of pleural fluid into the contralateral lung until adequate thoracostomy drainage is achieved. When a leak occurs 24 to 48 hours after pulmonary resection, the bronchus should be resutured, provided there is no residual tumor or bronchial infection at the resection line and an empyema is not present. The bronchial stump should be shortened as much as possible, closed, and reinforced by pleura, pericardium, or intercostal muscle. Intercostal muscle is prepared before the large rib retractor is inserted, because pressure from the spreader might jeopardize its blood supply. A rib is resected and the chest is entered through the middle of the periosteal bed of the removed rib, which forms the superior border of the muscle flap. The inferior border of the flap is cut with electrocautery along the superior edge of the rib below. The anterior end of the muscle flap is divided, making a long pedicle graft based posteriorly on the intercostal vessels. The muscle graft is turned back and wrapped in wet gauze until needed, and the chest is opened further with the retractor. After the bronchus has been closed, the muscle graft is brought down to the bronchial stump and fixed to the bronchus; then the chest cavity is closed. For an acute bronchopleural fistula after segmentectomy or lobectomy, an additional pulmonary resection may be necessary.

If the fistula develops weeks after a surgical procedure, an empyema is usually present. Drainage can be open or closed, depending on the stability of the mediastinum. Open drainage and mechanical cleansing of the empyema cavity should be started as soon as possible. With this therapy, 20% of fistulas will heal provided the bronchial margins are free of infection, necrotic tissue, or tumor. The cavity can then be sterilized as described for empyema (Malove et al., 1971). Patients with recurrent malignant disease or poor cardiopulmonary reserve can be treated with open-flap drainage without sterilization and closure (Eloesser, 1935).

Persistent air leak and a chronic productive cough indicate failure of drainage, and operation is necessary. Before operation, all underlying parenchymal and endobronchial infection must be cleared and the wall of the empyema cleansed by repeated packing. If the patient is ventilator-dependent, the fistula must be closed as part of the procedure. This requires dissecting the sinus tract down to normal bronchial cartilage, closing the bronchus, and filling the space with muscle flaps, as described in the next section. If the patient is breathing spontaneously, suture closure of the fistula may not be necessary. Débridement of the cavity is necessary before inserting the muscle flap to avoid disintegration of the pedicle muscle grafts by infection.

Chronic Bronchopleural Fistula. A long-standing bronchopleural fistula is more difficult to manage than an acute one because the empyema cavity is thick-walled and there is extensive fibrosis of the mediastinum around the fistulous opening. A large fistula is generally associated with aphonia and marked breathlessness. These patients are among the most difficult to treat, particularly if they have had radiation therapy. Direct closure of the bronchial opening is almost always impossible. Rather, meticulous dissection of the fistula tract down to normal bronchial cartilage is required, and a muscle flap must be placed over the bronchial closure. Infected debris from the wall of the empyema space is removed by curettage and irrigation until healthy, bleeding granulation tissue lines the cavity. A pedicle muscle graft is used to fill all interstices of the cavity.

Miller and co-workers provided an excellent description of obliterating an empyema space with extrathoracic muscle (Miller et al., 1984). The latissimus dorsi is most commonly used, followed by the serratus anterior, pectoralis major, and rectus abdominis. The muscle flaps are based on their major blood supply (Fig. 16–30), and a combination of two or more muscles may be required to fill the empyema space. Whereas the serratus anterior can be brought into the pleural space via the primary chest incision, transposition of the latissimus dorsi or pectoralis major re-

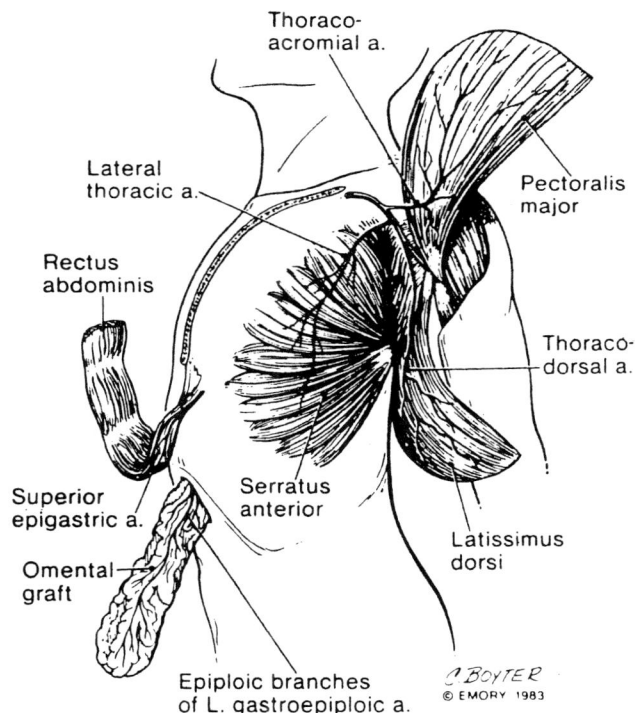

FIGURE 16–30. Extrathoracic muscle flaps that can be used in closure of a postpneumonectomy empyema cavity. a = artery. (From Shields, T. W.: Primary tumors of the pleura. *In* Shields, T. W. [ed]: General Thoracic Surgery. Philadelphia, Lea & Febiger, 1989, p. 642.)

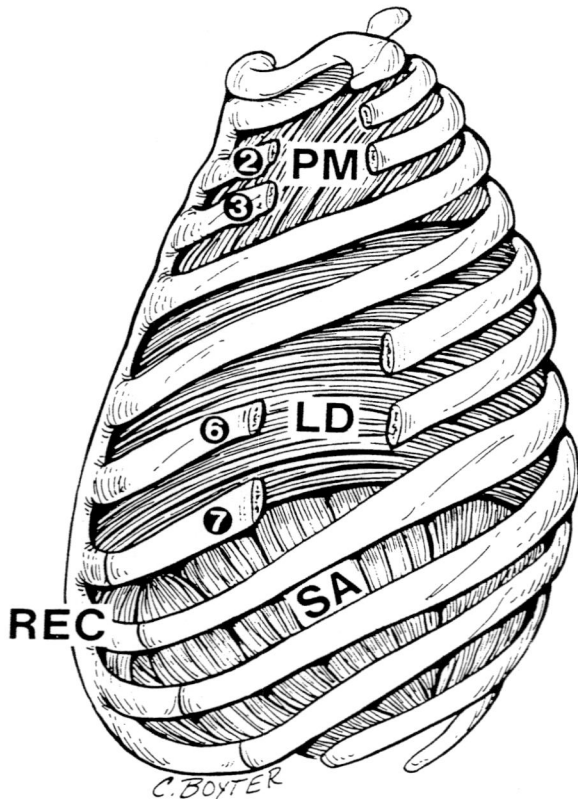

FIGURE 16–31. Usual sites of rib resection for entrance of the pectoralis major (PM) and latissimus dorsi (LD) flaps into the pleural spaces. REC = rectus abdominis; SA = serratus anterior. (From Shields, T. W.: Primary tumors of the pleura. *In* Shields, T. W. [ed]: General Thoracic Surgery. Philadelphia, Lea & Febiger, 1989, p. 643.)

quires a limited rib resection so that the blood supply of the muscle flap is not compromised (Fig. 16–31). In order for muscle flap closure of an empyema to be successful, the entire space must be filled. Occasionally, a limited thoracoplasty may be necessary to assure obliteration of the space.

Omentoplasty for bronchopleural fistula can also been performed with acceptable results (Virkkula, 1989). With this procedure, the omentum is exposed through a short upper midline abdominal incision. It is dissected free from the stomach, transverse colon, and mesocolon without injuring the gastroepiploic vessels. If the pedicle is to be prepared for the right pleural space, the left gastroepiploic artery is divided. The right gastroepiploic artery is divided if the pedicle is to be used in the left pleural space. The omental pedicle is brought through an opening in the diaphragm after the empyema cavity has been débrided via a thoracotomy incision. The pedicle is then fixed to the edges of the bronchial fistula or near it and onto the walls of the cavity. Drainage tubes are placed and the wounds closed (Virkkula, 1989). This procedure effectively closes the fistula and may significantly fill the empyema cavity. It avoids the dissection required of muscle flaps. A partial thoracoplasty may be required with both muscle flaps and omental pedi-

cles when the volume of the tissue to be placed in the empyema cavity does not adequately fill the space.

Transpericardial closure of the mainstem bronchus has been performed in some postpneumonectomy patients with long-standing bronchopleural fistula (Baldwin and Mark, 1985; Perelman et al., 1987) (Fig. 16–32). For patients to be candidates for this procedure, the remaining bronchial stump must be relatively long (Fig. 16–33). The operation is performed through a median sternotomy and the pleura on either side is pushed laterally by swab dissection. The pericardium is opened from its highest point on the aorta to the diaphragm. The right mainstem bronchus is reached by retracting the ascending aorta to the left and the superior vena cava to the right (Fig. 16–34). The right pulmonary artery runs transversely through the posterior aspect of this space and is dissected free on either side. The proximal part of the artery can be doubly ligated behind the ascending aorta or closed with a vascular stapler. After division, the two ends of the artery retract and open up the retropericardial approach to the origin of the right mainstem bronchus. The tracheobronchial angle can be felt by palpation, and the pericardium is divided upward toward this angle to enlarge the access to the right mainstem bronchus.

The bronchial sheath is opened to expose all aspects of the right mainstem bronchus, the carina, and the lower lateral end of the trachea, taking care not to injure the azygos vein. The bronchial stump is stapled or sutured flush with the trachea, and the distal bronchus is removed. The proximal divided end of the bronchus is covered with adjacent tissue.

Operative exposure of the left mainstem bronchus is facilitated by tilting the operating table 35 degrees to the right. The left pulmonary artery is located in the upper left corner of the pericardial cavity superior to the left atrial appendage. It is isolated by dividing the pericardial reflections between the aorta and the left pulmonary artery and extending this incision laterally and superior to the left pulmonary artery. Dur-

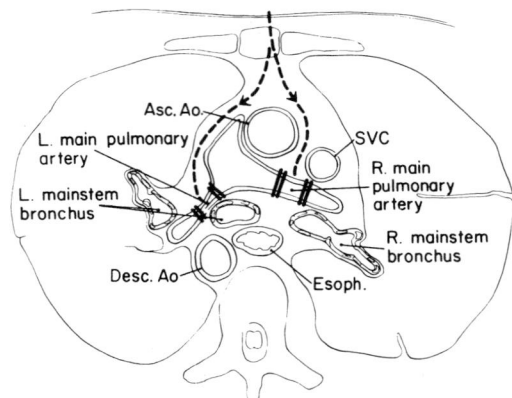

FIGURE 16–32. Schematic drawing showing the transpericardial approach *(dashed lines)* to the right or left mainstem bronchus. The approach necessitates intermittent retraction of the heart and proximal redivision of the respective pulmonary artery. SVC = superior vena cava; Esoph. = esophagus.

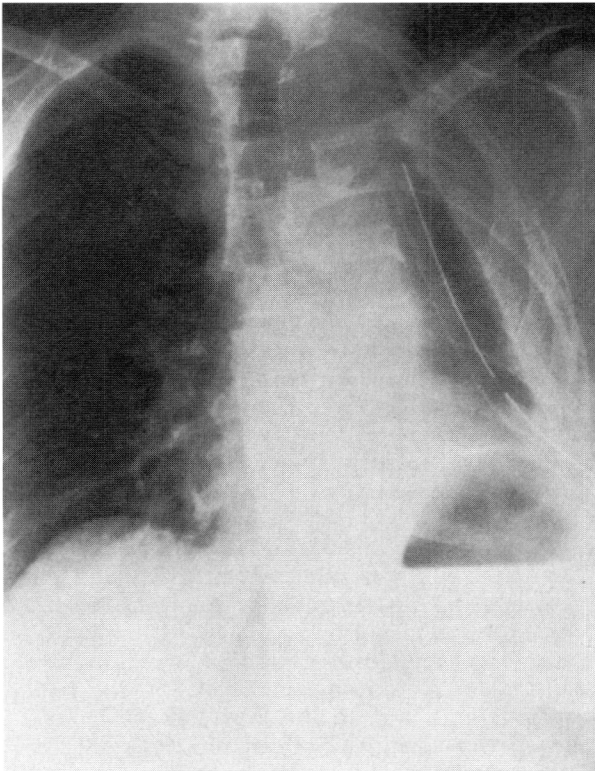

FIGURE 16–33. Chest film of a patient with a chronic bronchopleural fistula and empyema of 8 years' duration after a pneumonectomy for bronchiectasis Note the extensive fibrosis over the mediastinum and chest wall. The long left bronchial stump would allow reclosure by the transpericardial approach.

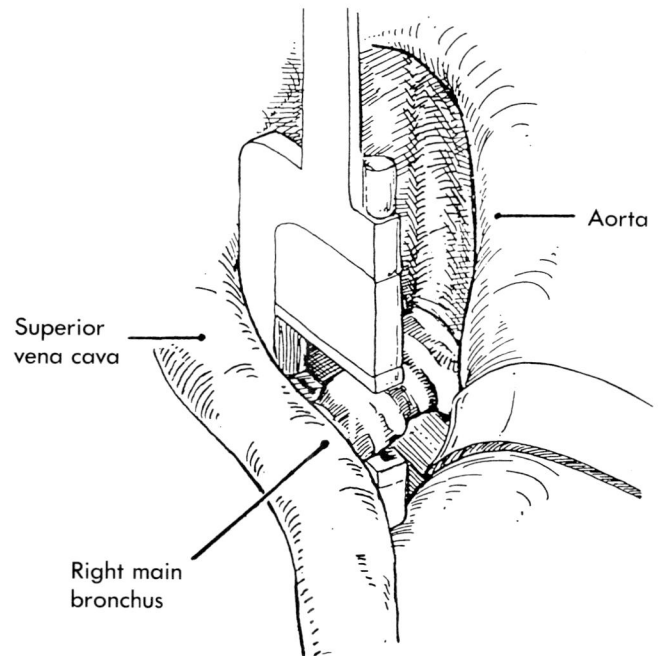

FIGURE 16–34. Schematic drawing showing the exposure of the right mainstem bronchus between the intrapericardial superior vena cava and the aorta after the right pulmonary artery has been redivided more proximally.

ing this and the ensuing maneuvers, the assistant must retract the heart manually to the right. This displacement is not tolerated well by the patient, so the heart must be allowed to return to its normal position at the end of each manipulation.

Finger dissection above and behind the vessel frees it posteriorly, and the tip of the finger can then demonstrate the posterior pericardial wall below the pulmonary artery. An incision into the pericardium parallel to and below the artery allows introduction of the acutely curved vascular clamp or stapler. The divided ends of the pulmonary artery tend to retract and leave a space through which the left mainstem bronchus and the left tracheobronchial angle can be palpated. The superior pulmonary vein is transected similarly and improves access to the origin of the left mainstem bronchus. The pericardial reflections around the vein must be divided before it is safe to encircle this vessel with an instrument.

The bronchus and the lower part of the trachea are exposed by dividing the posterior pericardial wall and by opening the bronchial sheath (Fig. 16–35). The arch of the aorta is retracted superiorly with a suitable retractor. A rubber sling passed around the bronchus makes it possible to pull the bronchial stump into the operative field. To prevent contamination of the posterior mediastinum or pericardial cavity, any bronchial secretions are suctioned and inadvertent open-

ings into the septic pleural cavity are closed. The bronchus is stapled flush with the trachea and covered with adjacent tissue, and the distal bronchus is removed or the mucosa cauterized.

Fibrothorax

Fibrothorax is the pathologic obliteration of the pleural space in which the two layers of pleura become adherent and the lung is covered by a thick layer of nonexpandable fibrous tissue. Organization

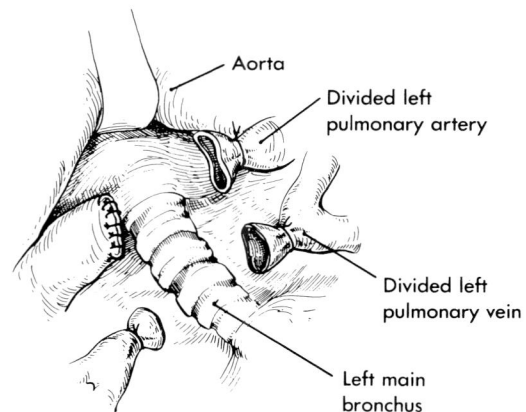

FIGURE 16–35. Schematic drawing showing the exposure of the left mainstem bronchus under the intrapericardial aorta after the left pulmonary artery and the superior pulmonary vein have been redivided more proximally and distally.

of a traumatic or spontaneous hemothorax, a chronic tuberculous effusion, and bacterial empyema are the most common causes. Clinically, fibrothorax is characterized by rigidity of the affected hemothorax with almost total absence of breath sounds on that side. When advanced, the condition is recognized easily on a chest film, but pulmonary function can be significantly altered by a fibrothorax with minor radiologic changes.

When fibrothorax is a complication of trauma, the underlying lung may be normal. When it is caused by tuberculosis or an empyema, the clinical picture may be complicated by parenchymal pulmonary disease. Decortication does not functionally improve the lung if extensive parenchymal disease is present. The lung parenchyma on the involved side can be evaluated by CT scanning.

Fibrothorax causes more interference with pulmonary function on the involved side than might be expected. In fact, pleural fibrosis can have a more severe effect on pulmonary function than many parenchymal lesions (Autio, 1959). Removal of the layer of thick fibrous tissue from the involved lung may improve pulmonary function considerably (Petty et al., 1961). This improvement is usually manifested as an increase in vital capacity, maximal midexpiratory flow rate, maximal breathing capacity, and resting oxygen uptake of the involved lung (Dark and Chatterjee, 1959; Falk et al., 1952; Savage and Fleming, 1955; Siebens et al., 1956). Although the increase in maximal ventilatory capacity measured postoperatively may be modest, the oxygen uptake may be greatly increased.

Severe fibrothorax with restriction of pulmonary function is unusual today because of improved results with early treatment of traumatic hemothorax and the success of antimicrobials for tuberculous and bacterial infections. Obliteration of the pleural space by adhesions still occurs, but a thick pleural peel rarely develops.

Technique for Freeing a Densely Adherent Lung

The approach to freeing the lung is to find the regions in the pleural space that are free from adhesions, work toward the zones where the pleural space is obliterated, and separate the two pleural layers by intrapleural dissection or, if this is impossible, mobilize the lung by extrapleural stripping. Usually, the mediastinal surface of the lung is relatively free from adhesions and is a good starting point.

Extrapleural mobilization is relatively easy when performed in the correct plane. It can be accompanied by considerable blood loss from points on the vascular endothoracic fascia, particularly in long-standing inflammatory processes. In certain regions, damage to underlying structures is possible. Extrapleural dissection anteriorly can injure the internal mammary vessels; in the area of the right paravertebral gutter, dissection can tear the intercostal vessels, or on the left side, it can avulse the descending aorta from the intercostal vessels. When freeing the lung by intrapleural dissection, it is essential to keep in mind the underlying anatomic structures. Posteriorly, the esophagus can be identified in the midst of fibrosis by the passage of a large esophageal bougie by the anesthesiologist. Above the arch of the aorta, on the lateral surface of the esophagus, the thoracic duct is vulnerable. Anteriorly, especially on the left, the lung tends to attach to the pericardial fat, and detachment can cause unnoticed bleeding or damage the phrenic nerve. The mediastinal aspect of the lung is usually less adherent. This applies to the pericardium anterior and posterior to the hilum of the lung, as well as the large vessels superior to the root of the lung—the azygos vein and superior vena cava on the right and aortic arch and subclavian artery on the left. These are routes of access for mobilization of the adherent upper and lower lobes.

The adhesions to the upper lobe are marked in the region of the paravertebral gutter and the apex in the concavity of the first and second ribs. A convenient way to free the upper lobe is to identify the posterior part of the arch of the azygos vein on the right or the posterior end of the aortic arch on the left and then free the adherent anterior edge of the lung to expose the pericardium. It is often possible to tunnel between these two points along the respective "vascular arch" with the index finger and open up a passage. Sometimes, this tunnel can be opened by sliding a curved clamp in from the back along the azygos vein or the aortic arch and by guiding it to the front with the left index finger. This passage is then enlarged with a mounted swab or manually, and an attempt is made to free the mediastinal surface of the upper lobe toward the apex intrapleurally or extrapleurally by stripping the mediastinal pleura off the trachea and esophagus on the right or the subclavian artery and esophagus on the left. Because the costal surface of the upper lobe, the adhesions at the back in the paravertebral gutter, and the adhesions in front along the anterior edge of the lung have already been freed, only the adherent apex remains. It is often possible to continue the extrapleural stripping to the top of the lung and bring the apex down by traction, followed by further detachment of the mediastinal pleura from the underlying structures. Otherwise, the hand may be passed upward toward the apex along the mediastinal aspect, while the other hand is passed upward over the outer costal surface of the lung. Gentle traction combined with a pinching action between the fingers of the two hands often loosens the attachments of the apex. This maneuver is usually successful and is less hazardous than sharp dissection within the concavity of the first rib, where the first thoracic nerve, subclavian vessels, origin of the internal mammary artery, and innominate vein may be injured.

Mobilization of an adherent lower lobe is more difficult because the parietal pleura is fused with the pericardium and the dome of the diaphragm, and extrapleural mobilization in these regions is not possible. Adhesions over the lower lobe tend to be dense in the region of the paravertebral gutter and along the costodiaphragmatic sinus. In mobilizing an adherent lower lobe, the aim is to free, if possible, the basal surface of the lung over the dome of the diaphragm and then to dissect outward toward the costodiaphragmatic sinus. The best approach is to expose the pericardium anteriorly. Any adhesions over the anterior edge of the middle lobe or lingula must be divided so that the lung can be retracted backward to bring the pericardium into view. The lower tip of the middle lobe or lingula, depending on the side of the operation, is probably adherent to the pericardial fat; detachment causes bleeding from hidden vessels within the fat, and these vessels have to be coagulated. In this area, the phrenic nerve can be injured inadvertently. It may then be possible to strip the lung away from the pericardium easily because the lung usually adheres loosely to the pericardium. The lung is freed inferiorly to the pericardiophrenic junction, outward over the diaphragm, and if possible, posteriorly down to the inferior pulmonary ligament below the hilum of the lung. Alternatively, dissection of the lung from the diaphragm is started in front, where the diaphragm is higher and more accessible. After the lung is separated from the pericardial fat, further dissection and retraction of the lung to the back reveal the fleshly muscle fibers of the diaphragm. The lung is detached from the diaphragm toward the back by blunt or sharp dissection with scissors, with care taken to avoid the phrenic nerve on each side and the inferior vena cava on the right.

Extrapleural dissection to mobilize the lower lobe is started from the costal surface of the incision and extended posteriorly toward the mediastinum; the ascending azygos vein and the esophagus may be in jeopardy on the right and the descending aorta and the esophagus are vulnerable on the left. As the dissection is extended posteriorly in the paravertebral gutter and interiorly in the costodiaphragmatic sinus, the risk of detaching the diaphragm from the chest wall is great. Extrapleural mobilization should be discontinued at about the level of the ninth rib posteriorly. Entry into the pleural cavity may be regained by dividing the inferior pulmonary ligament; a two-sided approach from the front and back is preferable. The ligament is lateral to and slightly in front of the esophagus and below the inferior pulmonary vein, so exposure of the esophagus leads to the posterior aspect of the ligament. At the same time, because the lung has been separated from the pericardium, the index finger of the left hand, introduced from the front, can identify the lower limit of the hilum and inferior pulmonary vein and show the ligament posteriorly by exerting pressure from the front. It should now be possible to incise the ligament posteriorly over the anteriorly placed finger and divide it along its full length; the inferior pulmonary vein is at its upper end and the inferior vena cava is close to the front of its lower end on the right side. Blood vessels in the pulmonary ligament bleed when they are divided. Electrocoagulation of the bleeding points is satisfactory if they are determined accurately and the

diathermy does not cause necrosis of the nearby esophageal wall.

The lung is now freed by dividing the remaining adhesions toward the periphery of the diaphragm. It may be helpful for the surgeon to change position and stand in front of the patient when operating in the lateral position to obtain a better view of the lower and posterior parts of the inner chest wall and the posterior costodiaphragmatic sinus.

Post-Thoracotomy Pleural Space

Persistent dead space after thoracotomy, whether it is air, fluid, or foreign body, is a hazard for infection or reduced pulmonary function. After a pneumonectomy, the pleural space gradually fills with serosanguineous fluid until the hemithorax is full and the air is absorbed. The average time required for fluid to opacify the pleural space on a chest film is 3.9 months (O'Meara and Slade, 1974). The size of this space decreases gradually by shifting of the mediastinal structures toward the side of the resection and by elevation of the ipsilateral diaphragm. Total obliteration of the space eventually occurs in one-third of patients. The space contains fluid indefinitely in approximately two-thirds of patients. Late infection is unusual (Suarez et al., 1969) and is often related to seeding from a respiratory or urinary tract infection.

For other types of pulmonary resections, management of the postresectional space depends on the extent and nature of the pulmonary resection, the state of the underlying lung, and whether air or fluid fills the space. If the intersegmental planes or incomplete lobar fissures were dissected, small bronchi may have been injured and air space problems are more likely. Injury to or partial resection of areas such as the superior segment of the lower lobe, especially after an upper lobectomy, may result in incomplete postoperative expansion of the remaining lung (Findlay, 1956). Old tuberculosis, pneumonitis, or interstitial fibrosis can prevent maximal expansion of the underlying lung. Persistent dead air space can be managed conservatively if it shows slow improvement, has not resulted from entrapment of the lung, and is not large enough to restrict the pulmonary function. Absorption of air may be slow. If a persistent air fluid level exists, it is important to determine whether the fluid is blood, has a high protein content (i.e., is able to lay down a fibrinous peel and entrap an otherwise expandable lung), or is infected. Drainage and decortication may be necessary in order to reexpand the lung.

As in the management of empyema, three options are available for managing a chronic residual air space that has become infected. The first is to establish satisfactory drainage and accept that as the end-point. This may be the proper choice for aged, debilitated patients, but is rarely acceptable for a relatively young individual. This approach involves the discomfort of frequent dressing changes, chronic protein loss, repeated superimposed infection, and development of amyloid disease. The second option is sterilization of the space, and the third is thoracoplasty. Of the three options, sterilization of the space is most commonly employed.

Failure of the lung to reexpand fully in the early postoperative period is not the result of pleural complications but of an endobronchial obstruction. This is usually caused by thick mucous secretions and in some situations, notably in the middle lobe, bronchial distortion. Repeated endobronchial suction is imperative, and flexible bronchoscopy may be necessary to remove secretions.

DISEASES OF THE PLEURA

Diagnostic Evaluation of Pleural Pathology

Common causes of pleural pathology in patients who enter the hospital with undiagnosed pleural disease are listed in Figure 16–36 (Scerbo et al., 1971). Unusual causes include congestive heart failure, pancreatitis, and trauma. To assist in the diagnosis, the thoracic surgeon must be knowledgeable in the clinical assessment of pleural pathology and skilled in the use of modern diagnostic equipment.

CLINICAL EVALUATION

Pleuritic chest pain is the most common symptom associated with inflammation of the visceral pleura. The pain is a sharp, stabbing sensation that is often absent or minimal during quiet respiration and intensifies with full inspiration. The major feature is aggravation by respiratory motion. When severe, it impedes respiration and can be confused with an acute thoracic or abdominal emergency.

When the parietal pleura is involved by a tumor or inflammation, a constant, dull pain independent of respiration is present and is aggravated by activity involving the thoracic muscles. This pain can radiate along an intercostal nerve. When the parietal pleura

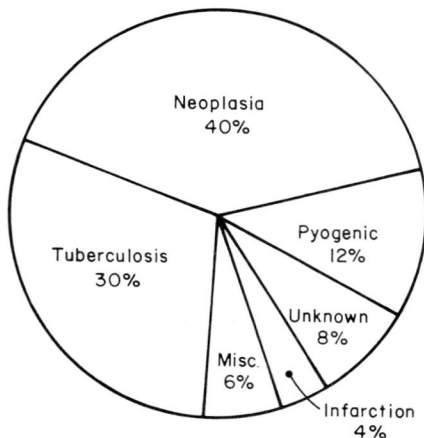

FIGURE 16–36. The spectrum of causes of pleural pathology in patients who enter the hospital with undiagnosed pleural disease.

of the diaphragm is involved, the pain may radiate to the abdomen or shoulder.

Palpable tenderness of the chest wall over the affected site often accompanies parietal pleural pathology. A pleural friction rub can be heard with visceral pleural inflammation if there is little or no effusion. The sound has a squeaking quality and is loudest on inspiration but may be audible on expiration. If inflammation is the cause, fever is usually present.

ROENTGENOGRAPHIC EVALUATION

Pleural abnormalities are generally visible on a chest film. Pleural effusion, thickening, a localized mass, and rib erosion are the most common roentgenographic findings. When pleural adhesions are present, pleural fluid may be loculated rather than free in the pleural cavity (see "Pleural Effusion," earlier in this chapter, and "Pleural Plaques and Calcifications" and "Pleural Tumors," later in this chapter).

ULTRASOUND EXAMINATION OF THE THORAX

Ultrasound of the thorax helps to define the extent of pleural disease and differentiate pleural fluid from other conditions that produce peripheral opacity on chest films. Fluid collections as small as 2 cm can be detected. These are differentiated from a solid mass by their movement with changes in body position. Longitudinal scans localize the fluid collection to above or below the diaphragm. Ultrasound is also useful as a guide for needle aspiration of pleural fluid (Gryminski et al., 1976).

Although ultrasound is helpful for detecting pleural thickening and calcification, it is less useful for identifying the origin of solid pleural abnormalities. In addition, associated bony changes cannot be visualized (Sample, 1977). In most situations, ultrasound has been replaced by CT scanning for detecting and characterizing pleural lesions.

CT SCANNING OF THE THORAX

The high degree of contrast at the pleura-lung interface makes CT scanning extremely useful for detecting small pleural abnormalities. Many of these abnormalities are benign and result from variation of pleural fat deposits. Small calcifications within pleural plaques can be detected and are an early sign of asbestosis.

The transaxial view allows visualization of the retrosternal and paravertebral areas, which are difficult to evaluate with conventional chest films. Hemorrhage, including the phases of coagulation, clot retraction, and liquefaction, can be discriminated from serous pleural effusions. Because all of the chest wall layers can be examined with CT scanning, the extrapleural or pleural origin of a peripheral abnormality can be determined, and subtle bony destruction can be detected.

CT scanning can also be a guide for aspiration of loculated fluid, but the flexibility of ultrasound examination favors its use for this purpose. Since only transverse CT scans are available, subpulmonic and subdiaphragmatic fluid cannot always be differentiated (Kreel, 1978).

CLOSED PLEURAL BIOPSY

Percutaneous biopsy of the parietal pleura helps diagnose two common causes of parietal pleural pathology: tuberculosis and neoplasia (Von Hoff and LiVolsi, 1975). The Cope or Abrams needle can be used even in the absence of an effusion. The biopsies are small and multiple specimens should be obtained. The diagnostic yield for tuberculosis is 60 to 80% and is higher than the 40 to 60% for malignant disease of the pleura because the inflammation is more diffuse (Von Hoff and LiVolsi, 1975). The yield for tuberculosis is increased to 80% by obtaining a culture of the biopsy specimen. Cytologic examination of the pleural fluid at the time of biopsy increases the diagnostic yield for malignancy to 90% (Von Hoff and LiVolsi, 1975). The morbidity of the procedure is low and the biopsy can be repeated. If the second attempt is not conclusive, pleuroscopy or open pleural biopsy is indicated.

VIDEO–ASSISTED PLEUROSCOPY

If the pleural space is not obliterated, pleuroscopy provides a complete endoscopic examination of the visceral, parietal, diaphragmatic, and mediastinal pleurae and subjacent organs. With video-assisted thoracoscopy, high-resolution, magnified views of the pleural space are projected on a color video monitor and can be recorded on videotape. Biopsy of various areas of the pleura can be performed under direct vision. The procedure is indicated for patients with undiagnosed pleural thickening, effusions, or tumors and is performed with the patient under general anesthesia using a double-lumen endotracheal tube to collapse the lung on the affected side. The patient is placed in the lateral decubitus position with the affected side up. The anesthesiologist then allows the lung on the operated side to deflate. A 2-cm incision is made in the sixth interspace in the anterior axillary line. After the pleural space is entered with a clamp, a finger is placed into the chest to assure that the lung has collapsed. A 10.5-mm thoracoscopy trocar is then inserted into the chest, followed by the video telescope. If a large amount of pleural fluid exists, it is aspirated and collected for examination.

All pleural surfaces are inspected: the parietal pleura over the thoracic wall, diaphragm, mediastinum, and pericardium, and the visceral pleura. Insertion of a second trocar at least 5 cm from the first allows manipulation of the lung and more effective examination of the pleural space. Gross characteristics of the pleura are noted, focal lesions are sought, and any accessible abnormality is biopsied. In the absence of lesions, multiple biopsies of representative pleural tissue are taken. The lower paravertebral area is always included because gravity-affected disease is often found in this location. Fibrinous adhesions are incised to facilitate exposure. Biopsies of fibrinous peels and the underlying pleura are obtained, if possible (DeCamp et al., 1973). Specimens are submitted for histologic examinations and multiple cultures. If a malignant pleural effusion has been diagnosed, talc pleurodesis can be performed. At the completion of the procedure, a single chest tube is placed through one of the trocar sites and the other wounds closed. The tube is usually removed a few hours later, after a postoperative chest film documents expansion of the lung. If a lung biopsy was performed, the tube is removed once any air leak ceases.

Thoracoscopic pleuroscopy is a safe and accurate diagnostic technique for patients who have pleural disease with a relatively free pleural space. In the absence of adhesive pleuritis, visualization of the pleural surfaces with the video telescope is better than with a limited thoracotomy. A thoracotomy should be used only when simple techniques have failed.

Tuberculosis of the Pleura

The major cause of acute pleural inflammation is adjacent pulmonary infection. The patient is usually febrile, has an irritating nonproductive cough, and may have a history of a recent upper respiratory infection. If the symptoms persist or a pleural effusion develops, tuberculosis of the pleura should be considered.

Pathology

Tuberculous pleurisy is the most common inflammatory disease of the pleura and can be diagnosed by pleural biopsy (Bates, 1979). It commonly occurs 3 to 7 months after the primary infection, but may be seen anytime in the course of the disease. The pleura is infected with *Mycobacterium tuberculosis* by rupture of the subpleural focus into the pleural space or shedding of the bacilli into the pleural space from involved lymph nodes. It is tempting to refer to this abnormality as tuberculous empyema, but when the pleura is infected by tuberculosis, various clinical patterns can develop and not all of them produce empyema. The patterns range from a thin, relatively transient effusion to one in which the pleural space is filled with thick fluid contaminated with pyogenic organisms from an associated bronchopleural fistula. Hypersensitivity to the tubercle bacillus seems to influence the clinical pattern observed (Berger and Majia, 1973). Although tuberculous pleurisy is the most common type of extrapulmonary tuberculosis, only 8% of patients who have pulmonary tuberculosis develop pleural disease.

Clinical Features and Diagnosis

The onset of tuberculous pleurisy is abrupt in two-thirds of patients and insidious in the remainder.

Older patients more often develop an insidious onset. The cough is usually nonproductive, chest pain is pleuritic, and night sweats, dyspnea, weakness, and weight loss are common. Patients are usually febrile, and the peripheral white blood cell count is generally normal. The chest film may show a pleural effusion without pulmonary parenchymal lesions or advanced parenchymal disease associated with dense pleural thickening between the lung and the chest wall that is often calcified. The diagnosis is confirmed by one or more of the following findings: acid-fast bacilli on a smear of sputum or gastric contents, tubercle bacilli cultured from the pleural fluid or biopsy, or tuberculous granuloma on pleural biopsy (Langston et al., 1967). Bacterial or viral pneumonia, pulmonary infarction, malignancy of the pleura, systemic lupus erythematosus, and subdiaphragmatic conditions can be confused with tuberculous pleurisy.

The tuberculin skin test is positive in 70 to 80% of patients with tuberculous pleurisy, but an initial nonreactive intermediate-strength tuberculin test should not exclude the diagnosis. If repeated intermediate and second-strength tests are nonreactive after 2 months, tuberculous pleurisy is extremely unlikely (Berger and Majia, 1973).

Cultures of the pleural fluid show tubercle bacilli in 30 to 60% of patients (Bates, 1979). The percentage of positive cultures can be increased by centrifuging large volumes of pleural fluid or by doing multiple cultures. Cultures from the sputum or gastric content yield tubercle bacilli infrequently unless pulmonary tuberculosis visible on a chest film coexists with the pleurisy (Falk, 1965).

Management

In most patients, acute tuberculous pleurisy is a self-limited disease that lasts 6 to 8 weeks and leaves the patient with some degree of pleural fibrosis. The outcome depends on the duration and extent of the pleural inflammatory process, amount of intrapulmonary fibrosis, status of the infection in the pulmonary parenchyma, and presence of pyogenic organisms with or without a bronchopleural fistula. The principal hazards of tuberculous pleurisy are later development of pulmonary or extrapulmonary tuberculosis and recurrent pleural effusion (Levine et al., 1968). Antituberculous and antipyogenic therapy is dictated by culture and sensitivity studies. Medical therapy should be continued and surgical therapy, except for emergency drainage, withheld until the tuberculous disease in the lung has regressed or stabilized, as shown on the chest film or reversal of previously positive bacteriologic cultures.

Thoracentesis relieves symptoms of dyspnea by decreasing the size of the pleural effusion. Because of the risk of a secondary infection, tube drainage is avoided unless required for a bronchopleural fistula or superimposed bacterial infection.

DETERMINING THE NEED FOR SURGICAL THERAPY

After maximal resolution is achieved by antituberculous therapy, the residual disease is evaluated to determine the need for operation (Langston et al., 1967). The lateral chest film and CT scan of the chest are valuable in this assessment. If pleural disease is seen on the posteroanterior projection but not the lateral projection, it can be assumed that the process is diffuse throughout the pleural space and the pleural peel is not very thick. If serial films show clearing of the pleural process and an increase in expansion of the chest wall, complete resolution appears likely and decortication is unnecessary.

If the pleural shadow is seen on the lateral view of the chest film, or the CT scan shows a localized lesion, decortication is likely to be required even if clearing has occurred in other locations. This is particularly true in the posteroinferior gutter, where effusions are expected to be thickest. Such encapsulated pleural processes are not likely to resolve completely unless they are small at the onset.

TIMING OF SURGICAL THERAPY

If the residual disease is limited to the pleura, decortication is indicated when clinical toxicity is no longer evident and further thoracentesis fails to yield fluid, or fluid is obtained but its removal fails to alter the roentgenographic appearance. The pleural involvement should include one-third or one-fourth of the hemithorax. The decision for or against decortication should be made after 6 to 12 months of antituberculous therapy. After this time, there is a constant risk of local exacerbation or perforation of the pleural exudate into the bronchus.

When pleuroparenchymal disease is present, the timing of operation is easier to decide. If the parenchymal disease does not require operation, removal of the pleural disease is considered. When the parenchymal disease requires surgical therapy, all existing pleural disease should be managed in the same operation. Resection, decortication, or pleuropneumonectomy is performed as indicated by anatomic extent of the disease (Sterle, 1957). A pulmonary resection in the presence of active pleural tuberculosis requires complete excision of the involved parietal pleura. If a partial resection of the lung is performed, prompt and full reexpansion of the remaining lung is necessary to prevent postoperative empyema, even when appropriate antibiotics and antituberculous therapy are used. If a pneumonectomy is performed, meticulous excision of the pleural tuberculosis is required to prevent postoperative empyema because no lung remains to obliterate the pleural space. A successful outcome with a resection-decortication or pleuropneumonectomy for an associated parenchymal and pleural disease depends on exchanging an actively infected pleural space for one that is fresh and merely contaminated. Antimicrobial and antituberculosis drugs, tissue and host immunity, and particularly the complete excision of all infected tissue contribute to success.

RESULTS OF SURGICAL THERAPY FOR PLEURAL DISEASE

When operation is required for pleural disease only, mortality is low and serious complications such as empyema or bronchopleural fistula are minimal. Mortality and morbidity rise in proportion to the extent of the disease and the complexity of the surgical procedure required. Empyema and bronchopleural fistula occur most often after pleuropneumonectomy, particularly in patients who had a preoperative empyema or bronchopleural fistula. Thoracoplasty for an empyema at this stage of disease will fail because the opposing infected walls are unable to heal and obliterate the space. The lung is so trapped beneath a thick empyemic peel that adequate dependent drainage or decortication rarely permits obliteration of the space by pulmonary reexpansion, particularly when the walls are heavily calcified. These patients can be helped only by pleuropneumonectomy.

Immediate mortality is high for patients with tuberculosis who require a pleuropneumonectomy because of destroyed lung complicated by empyema or bronchopleural fistula, but the patients who survive the procedure have a good chance for a satisfactory outcome. Pleuropneumonectomy can create primary healing even with preexisting empyema. The complications are mainly pyogenic. High amputation of the bronchial stump and adequate coverage by pleural or pericardial flaps produce a surprisingly low incidence of bronchopleural fistulas, even with a preoperative empyema. Prompt dependent drainage is mandatory for postoperative empyema to further protect against breakdown of the bronchial stump. In the absence of a bronchopleural fistula and after infection in the pleural space has resolved, the cavity can be sterilized as discussed earlier for the treatment of chronic empyema. A postoperative fistula may close spontaneously after a period of drainage, and sterilization of the space may be considered. If closure does not occur, the fistula is managed in the same way as described earlier for bronchopleural fistulas. The presence of tubercle bacilli in the postoperative pleural space indicates the need to change antimicrobial therapy to attack resistant organisms. To open tissue planes widely with poor or absent chemotherapeutic coverage is unwise, and chemotherapeutic control should be regained before further operation. An algorithm summarizing the therapeutic decision in the management of a patient with pleural tuberculosis is shown in Figure 16–37.

Pleural Plaques and Calcifications

Pleural plaques are discrete 1- to 5-mm areas of thickened parietal pleura of unknown cause. They are often bilateral and have a bizarre shape with irregular but sharply defined borders. They are most common on the lower half of the thoracic wall and the tendinous part of the diaphragm. They do not occur in the apex of the chest or on the visceral pleura, and do not produce pleural adhesions.

The pleural surface of these plaques is usually smooth and ivory-white, but they can be nodular and grayish-brown. The plaques are covered by smooth and slightly thickened pleura, and the plaque itself consists of a uniform pattern of densely laminated collagen fibers, usually without inflammatory cells or blood vessels. In older patients, extensive layering of calcification may occur throughout the plaque.

The relationship of pleural plaques to the development of mesotheliomas is uncertain (Hourihane et al., 1966). Because these two lesions can appear similar on a chest film, an accurate histologic diagnosis is imperative. Pleural plaques are a common finding at autopsy and the incidence of concomitant mesothelioma is small.

The roentgenographic appearance of a pleural plaque depends on its thickness and degree of calcification. Because noncalcified plaques cannot be visualized until the fibrous tissue is thick, they go undetected and their prevalence is underestimated. When thick enough, the plaques appear as discrete irregular areas of increased radiodensity. Discrete, localized, noncalcified pleural thickening may occur with localized mesothelioma, metastatic disease, lymphoma, or myeloma and can mimic pleural plaques (Sciammas et al., 1971). A tissue diagnosis is then required. An adequate biopsy can be obtained with pleuroscopy or limited thoracotomy. When a pleural plaque is diagnosed, no further treatment is indicated.

The diagnosis can be made with relative certainty when pleural plaques are calcified and located on the lower half of the chest wall or the dome of the diaphragm. They are rarely found in the apices of the lung, below the eleventh rib in the region of the costophrenic angles, or anteriorly beneath the costal cartilages. They are usually bilateral and symmetric. The calcification is uneven and causes irregular roentgenographic outlines. Inflammatory diseases and traumatic injury to the pleura with hematoma formation can produce calcified lesions that look similar but are usually unilateral and localized. Other rare causes of plaque-like pleural calcifications are radiation, scleroderma, and pneumoconiosis (Hourihane et al., 1966; Roberts, 1971).

Chronic pleuritis also can cause calcification of the pleura. The calcification is usually secondary to an unabsorbed traumatic hemothorax but may occur after pleurisy or empyema of tuberculous or nontuberculous origin. An empyema with calcified walls is not expected to heal with drainage and requires decortication of the lung with or without radical thoracoplasty and pleurectomy. With extensive calcification of the visceral pleura, decortication is often impossible and pulmonary resection is required.

Pleural Tumors

Neoplastic involvement of the pleura may be found in 50% of patients seen for diagnosis and treatment of pleural disease (Levallen and Carr, 1955). Primary pleural neoplasms are rare compared with metastatic lesions. Pleural tumors usually present with pleural effusion, but nodular neoplastic masses without effusion or diffuse pleural thickening do occur. The presence of a bloody pleural effusion suggests a neo-

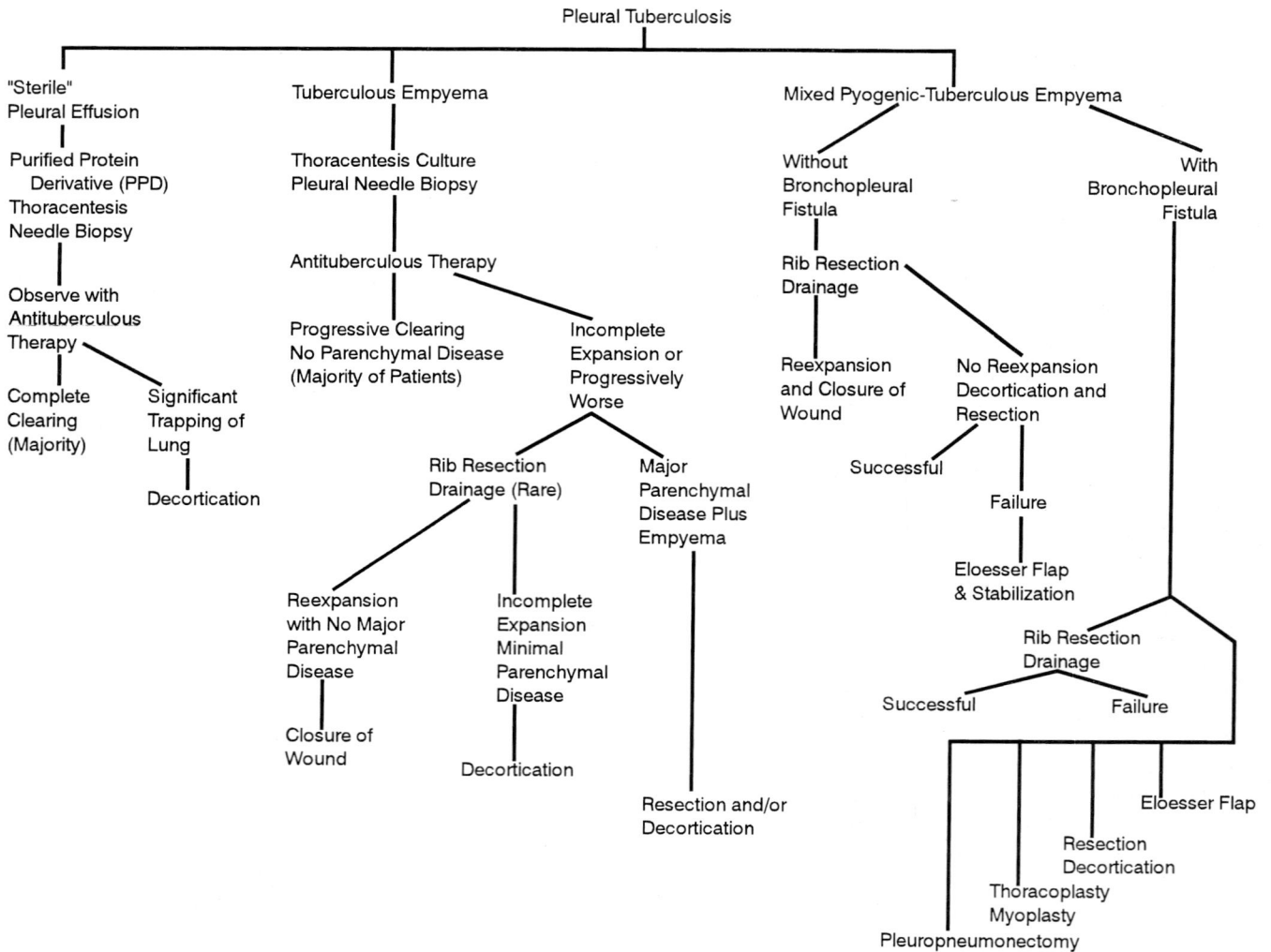

FIGURE 16–37. Algorithm for the management of pleural tuberculosis. (Modified from Hood, R. M. [ed]: Surgical Diseases of the Pleura and Chest Wall. Philadelphia, W. B. Saunders, 1986, p. 117.)

plasm, but in 50% of patients with malignant effusion, the fluid is serous. The pleural fluid is generally an exudate in which lymphocytes and mesothelial cells predominate. Cytologic examination of the pleural fluid for malignant cells is often positive when the tumor invades the pleura; however, hyperplastic mesothelial cells that develop in response to irritants such as inflammation are often clumped and may resemble tumor cells.

Benign Tumors and Cysts of the Pleura

Lipomas, endotheliomas, angiomas, and cysts of the pleura are rare tumors and are usually seen on routine chest films as densities flattened against the chest wall. These lesions are closely associated with the pleura and originate from the subpleural tissues. Lipomas, the most common, are usually well encapsulated, free from the underlying tissue, and firmly fixed to the pleura. Lipomas are treated by surgical excision (LeRoux, 1962). Many can be diagnosed and resected using video-assisted thoracoscopy.

The most common site for pleural cysts is at the pleuropericardial angle. Pleural cysts are generally unilocular and produce a typical water density on chest film. They arise from the parietal pleura, grow slowly, and rarely become symptomatic. Removal is usually indicated on discovery for diagnostic purposes (LeRoux, 1962).

Primary Pleural Mesotheliomas

Primary tumors of the pleura, called mesotheliomas, arise from cells that line the pleural, peritoneal, and pericardial cavities. By definition, mesotheliomas arise from mesothelial cells. However, because all three germ layers are involved in the formation of the pleura, their histologic appearance ranges from an almost pure spindle-cell population that resembles various other mesenchymal tumors to a papillary and tubular pattern that appears epithelial and is difficult to distinguish from metastatic adenocarcinoma. This variation in microscopic appearance has caused controversy about their diagnosis. In addition, the natural history of mesotheliomas differs from that of other sarcomas: Whereas patients with sarcomas generally die of hematogenous disseminated metastasis, those with mesothelioma usually succumb to complications of their primary lesion.

Malignant mesothelioma is an uncommon disease; however, an increased incidence has been associated with long-term exposure to asbestos. This has been observed both in South Africa, in a population containing a large number of asbestos mine workers (Wagner et al., 1960), and in the members of the Asbestos Workers Union in New York and New Jersey (Selikoff et al., 1965). Other studies have reported that 80% of patients with mesothelioma had a history of industrial exposure to asbestos, such as shipyard workers and women in sackware repairing (Whitwell and Rawcliffe, 1971). Pulmonary specimens from patients with histologic asbestosis were found to contain more than 3 million fibers per gram of lung tissue. Patients with mesothelioma and a history of asbestos exposure contained more than 100,000 asbestos fibers per gram of lung tissue, in contrast with less than 20,000 to 50,000 fibers per gram in autopsy specimens from patients without thoracic tumors or a history of industrial asbestos exposure (Whitwell et al., 1977). Studies in animals with intrapleural injection of asbestos fibers demonstrate a carcinogenic role for asbestos. The most harmful form of asbestos fibers are those with the amphibole crystalline structure, including amosite, crocidolite, tremolite, and anthophylite. Crocidolite (blue asbestos) is the most harmful.

Epidemiologic data show that there is a latent period of 20 to 40 years between exposure and emergence of mesothelioma. The younger the age of first exposure, the higher the cumulative lifetime risk (Antman et al., 1986). Cigarette smokers who have been exposed to asbestos have a higher chance of developing bronchogenic carcinoma, which suggests that asbestos may have a synergistic effect with other carcinogens. Among asbestos workers, carcinoma of the lung is still three times as common as mesothelioma. Asbestos may not be the only cause of mesothelioma, since only 7.2% of people who work with asbestos develop the disease, and approximately half of the patients who have the disease have no documented exposure to asbestos. Other factors that may contribute to the development of mesothelioma are chronic severe pulmonary disease, radiation, and zeolite contact (Shields, 1989).

PATHOLOGY

The pathologic diagnosis of mesothelioma remains controversial (McCaughey, 1965). Although malignant mesotheliomas are histologically classified with soft tissue sarcomas, only 20% are purely sarcomatous. Approximately 50% of malignant mesotheliomas have epithelial or tubular papillary histologic findings, and 30% have a mixed epithelial and sarcomatous histology (McCaughey, 1965).

Most pathologists confidently diagnose a mesothelioma only in patients with the sarcomatous or mixed histology. Differentiation of the epithelial variant of mesothelioma from the more common metastatic adenocarcinoma is difficult. The epithelial variant of mesothelioma can be identified with a combination of special stains, newer immunologic techniques, and electron microscopy. Special stains and electron microscopy are not used routinely unless mesothelioma is specifically considered, so an erroneous diagnosis of metastatic adenocarcinoma may be made. Both mesotheliomas and metastatic adenocarcinoma give a positive periodic acid–Schiff reaction, but after digestion of diastase, mesotheliomas become negative and adenocarcinoma remains positive. Colloidal iron or alcian blue stains have been used to demonstrate the presence of hyaluronic acid, which may be produced by malignant mesothelioma cells. Electron microscopy of mesotheliomas shows abundant long, slender microvilli and prominent desmosomes, whereas short, blunt microvilli are found in adenocarcinoma (McCaughey, 1965).

Clinically, there are two forms of mesothelioma: localized and diffusely spreading (Klima et al., 1976). Either form may be benign or malignant. Most localized mesotheliomas are benign and pedunculated; these are called solitary benign mesotheliomas and constitute 10% of all mesotheliomas. Almost all diffuse mesotheliomas are malignant and are called diffuse malignant mesotheliomas.

LOCALIZED BENIGN MESOTHELIOMA

Benign pleural mesotheliomas generally arise from the visceral pleura but have been known to originate from all portions of the parietal pleura, including the mediastinal and diaphragmatic aspects. The tumors are usually on a stalk, but can be sessile, and may be surrounded by lung parenchyma, making them indistinguishable from a primary bronchial lesion. Their size is variable, and can range from small tumors to extremely large masses. They are smooth-walled, may become partially calcified, and can contain fluid-filled cysts. Histologically, three patterns are known to occur: fibrous or acellular, cellular, and mixed.

Localized benign mesotheliomas are growing slowly and are generally asymptomatic. Symptoms may occur if the tumor grows large enough to cause compression of the lung or a major airway (Okike et al., 1978; Shabanah and Sayegh, 1963). Pain is uncommon unless the tumor arises from the parietal pleura. A pleural effusion may occur that can be bloody and must be differentiated from a malignant pleural effusion. Hypertrophic pulmonary osteoarthropathy occurs in 20% of patients and includes joint and bone pain with joint stiffness, arthralgia of long bones, and ankle edema. It is usually associated with benign mesotheliomas larger than 7 cm.

Hypoglycemia can also occur in association with localized benign mesothelioma. Similarly to hypertrophic pulmonary osteoarthropathy, it usually occurs with tumors larger than 7 cm. Various mechanisms for this association have been proposed. Some investigators have suggested a combination of increased use of glucose by the tumor as well as the release of metabolites such as L-tryptophan, which exhibit insulin-like activity (Nelson et al., 1975). When hypoglycemia occurs in conjunction with benign mesothelioma, coma or seizures may result.

The diagnosis of benign solitary mesothelioma is made at operation for a solitary mass seen on chest film. The tumor is generally a lobulated, pedunculated mass that arises from the visceral pleura in 75% of patients (Fig. 16–38). Blood is supplied to the tumor through the pedicle and arises from feeding bronchial, intercostal, or diaphragmatic vessels (Okike et al., 1978; Shabanah and Sayegh, 1963). Therapy consists of complete excision. Although an adequate margin of pulmonary tissue should be removed to assure complete excision of the tumor, lobectomy probably has no benefit over local resection. If the lesion is histologically benign, excision is generally curative. Okike and associates (1978) described 52 patients with benign mesotheliomas who were followed for up to 24 years. Tumor recurred in 2 patients and the survival curve was identical to that for the general population. Surgical therapy completely relieved symptoms of hypertrophic pulmonary osteoarthropathy in 80% of patients, and in almost all patients with hypoglycemia.

LOCALIZED MALIGNANT MESOTHELIOMA

Unlike those patients with localized benign mesothelioma, most patients with localized malignant mesothelioma are symptomatic and may have chest pain, cough, dyspnea, and fever. Osteoarthropathy almost never occurs. Roentgenographic findings are similar to the benign form, although rib erosion may occur secondary to invasion of the chest wall. Grossly, the lesions are firm and encapsulated, but unlike the benign variety, they can be soft and homogeneous with areas of necrosis and hemorrhage. Of eight such tumors described by Okike and associates (1978), none was pedunculated. Four originated in the visceral pleura, three in the parietal pleura, and one was of indeterminate origin.

Differentiation between the malignant and the benign localized mesothelioma is confirmed histologically. Three histologic forms can be identified: tubulopapillary, fibrous, and bimorphic. Some authors believe that almost all fibrous malignant mesotheliomas are fibrosarcomas (Martini et al., 1987).

Survival after resection of localized malignant mesothelioma depends on completeness of resection. Wide excision with adequate margins of pleura, lung, and chest wall, if necessary, should be performed. The specimen should be handled carefully, because recurrences found on the diaphragmatic pleura suggest drop metastasis from manipulation of the tumor at operation. If complete resection is not possible, internal (brachytherapy) and external radiation are indicated (Martini et al., 1987). Whereas long-term survivors have been reported after complete resection, the median survival time after incomplete resection is 7 months (Martini et al., 1987).

DIFFUSE MALIGNANT MESOTHELIOMA

Diffuse malignant mesothelioma can originate in any part of the visceral or parietal pleura. Grossly, the tumor appears as multiple flat nodules or sheets involving the pleural surfaces, including the interlobar pleural surfaces. The lower portions of the pleural space are generally more extensively involved. The tumor may spread to encase the lung as well as surround the pericardium and extend to the contralateral pleural space. On the parietal pleural surface, the lesion may invade the ribs and chest wall. Extension

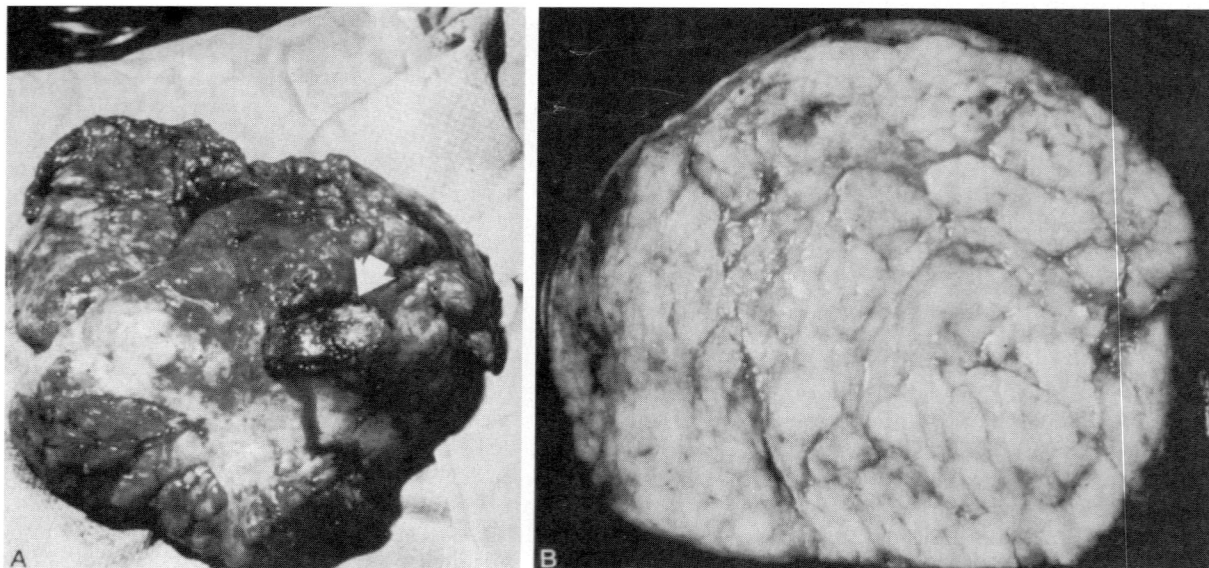

FIGURE 16–38. Surgical specimen of a solitary benign mesothelioma showing (A) the pedicle of the pedunculated lesion (arrow), which was attached to the diaphragm, and (B) the cut surface of the mass, which measured 10.5 cm in diameter.

through the diaphragm into the peritoneal cavity can also occur. Distant metastases probably occur more commonly than was originally thought: Hematogenously disseminated metastasis is seen in approximately 50% and thoracic lymph node metastases are present in as many as 67% of autopsies of patients with the disease (Wanebo et al., 1976).

Diffuse malignant mesothelioma usually occurs in the sixth and seventh decades of life and is three to five times more common in men than women. Insidious onset of pain and shortness of breath are noted in 95% of patients. The pain is nonpleuritic and aching: It is frequently referred to the upper abdomen or shoulders and occasionally leads to an incorrect diagnosis of cardiac, orthopedic, or gallbladder disease (Elmes and Simpson, 1976). With advanced disease, dyspnea is the presenting symptom and is due to interference with respiratory mechanics and inadequate oxygenation. A delay of 4 to 6 months often occurs between the onset of symptoms and an accurate diagnosis. When the patient first seeks medical attention for chest pain, the chest film invariably reveals a unilateral pleural effusion. Other roentgenographic findings include extensive pleural thickening and nodularity (Fig. 16–39). Cytologic studies of pleural fluid and needle biopsy do not yield a definitive diagnosis; more frequently, they prompt a misdiagnosis of adenocarcinoma. Bronchoscopy and cytologic studies of sputum help to exclude bronchogenic carcinoma.

Diagnosis of malignant mesothelioma is best made with a pleural biopsy. Malignant cells in the pleural fluid have been reported to occur in as many as 75% of patients (Ratzer et al., 1967). However, cytologic examination is difficult to interpret in this disease, as are small tissue samples from needle biopsies. Although thoracotomy has sometimes been necessary

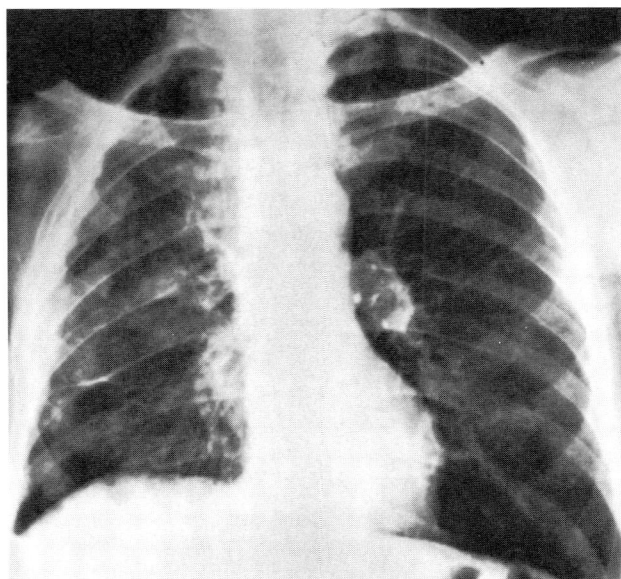

FIGURE 16–40. Chest CT scan of a patient with a diffuse malignant mesothelioma of the right hemithorax. The scan effectively shows that the disease involves all of the right parietal pleura and extends onto the visceral pleura in the region of the major fissure. Caution is needed to distinguish fluid from tumor; this can be done by scanning with the patient in different positions. (From Kreel, L.: Computed tomography in mesothelioma. Semin. Oncol., 8:302, 1981.)

to make a diagnosis, more recently, video-assisted thoracoscopy has been successfully used to obtain tissue for diagnosis and to evaluate the extent of disease.

In patients with malignant mesothelioma, the extent of disease can be determined on CT scans of the chest and abdomen (Fig. 16–40). These correlate well with survival, as measured with a modification of the staging system of Butchart and colleagues (1976) (Table 16–11). Patients with Stages I, II, and III of the disease have a median survival of 16, 9, and 5 months, respectively, after diagnosis. Patients with an epithelial variant have a slightly longer median survival. In contrast to death from other sarcomas that result from blood-borne metastasis, death from mesothelioma generally results from failure to control local disease (Brenner et al., 1982).

Diffuse mesotheliomas have been treated by various approaches, all plagued by high recurrence rates and low survival. Types of therapy have included surgical therapy, brachytherapy, external radiotherapy, intracavitary radioisotopes, chemotherapy, and combinations of these. No approach has given consistently better palliation or survival than others.

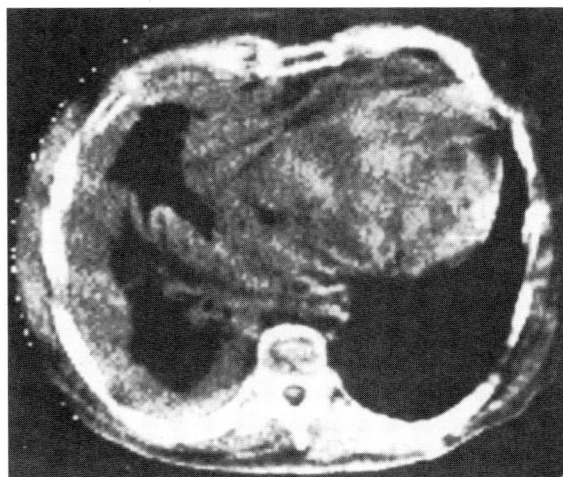

FIGURE 16–39. Chest film of a patient with a diffuse malignant mesothelioma in the right hemithorax showing extensive pleural thickening and nodularity along its surface.

■ **Table 16–11.** STAGING OF MALIGNANT MESOTHELIOMAS

Stage I	Tumor confined to ipsilateral pleura or lung
Stage II	Tumor involving chest wall, mediastinum, pericardium, or contralateral pleura
Stage III	Tumor involving both thorax and abdomen or lymph nodes outside the chest
Stage IV	Distant blood-borne metastases

Based on Butchart, E. G., Ashcroft, T., Barnsley, W. C., and Holoen, M. P.: Pleuroneumonectomy in the management of diffuse malignant mesothelioma of the pleura. Experience with twenty-nine patients. Thorax, 31:15, 1976.

When diffuse malignant mesothelioma encases the lung and obliterates the pleural space, complete excision of the tumor is difficult, so surgeons recommend only supportive therapy. Law and co-workers (1984) found no significant difference in survival between patients treated with decortication, chemotherapy, radiotherapy, or a combination of these, and patients not treated who had a comparable clinical condition at presentation. There was also no difference in survival according to pathology, that is, among epithelial, sarcomatous, or mixed-cell types. Therefore, many authors prefer palliative treatment to pleuropneumonectomy with diaphragmatic resection. At Memorial Sloan-Kettering Cancer Center, a review of patients treated before 1972 did not show any benefit of pulmonary resection in the treatment of these tumors (Wanebo et al., 1976). Since then, patients with these tumors have been treated with pleurectomy without pulmonary resection. This treatment removes the bulk of the disease, preserves pulmonary function, and controls effusion. Pleurectomy is possible in 80% of these patients. Gross residual disease was treated with permanent radioactive ^{125}I; residual diffuse disease was treated by temporary implantation of ^{192}Ir and intrapleural instillation of [32]P. Isotope treatment was followed by external radiotherapy; a dose of 4500 rads in 4.5 weeks was given to the pleural surface with a mixed beam of photons and electrons. Forty-one patients who had such treatment had a survival rate of 65% at 1 year and 40% at 2 years. The median disease-free survival at 1 and 2 years was 11 months, and the disease-free survival at 1 and 2 years was 44 and 13%, respectively (Martini et al., 1987; McCormack et al., 1982).

Radical extrapleural pneumonectomy involves removal en bloc of the parietal pleura, lung, pericardium, and diaphragm. Wörn (1974) reported 62 patients after this procedure. Survival at 2 and 5 years was 37 and 10%, respectively. In a similar group of patients treated conservatively, the survival was 12.5% at 1 year, and there were no survivors at 2 years. Pleuropneumonectomy was associated with 25% operative mortality. More recent reports with this procedure show a decrease in mortality but no change in survival. DaValle and associates (1986) reported 23 patients who had a median survival of 11.2 months after pleurectomy with a mortality of 13%, compared with a median survival of 13.3 months for extrapleural pneumonectomy with a mortality of 9.1%. The Lung Cancer Study Group Trial of extrapleural pneumonectomy for malignant mesothelioma showed that, although overall survival was not affected by operation, recurrence-free survival was significantly longer for patients undergoing extrapleural pneumonectomy as opposed to no therapy or limited resection (Rusch et al., 1991). Radiotherapy alone, using moderate doses for the treatment of diffuse malignant mesothelioma, may help to control pain and pleural effusion, but its effectiveness as primary therapy is limited (Antman et al., 1986). Radiotherapy has been used more effectively in combination with chemotherapy. Trials with single or multiple chemotherapeutic

agents for the treatment of malignant mesothelioma are difficult to interpret because the stage of the disease is often not stated and these agents are often used in combination with other forms of treatment. The most effective agents are cyclophosphamide, doxorubicin, and cisplatin. However, results with chemotherapy alone have been disappointing. Current investigations involve the multimodality approach using various combinations of surgery, chemotherapy, and radiotherapy in hopes of obtaining better results with this deadly disease (Sugarbaker et al., 1993). Sugarbaker and colleagues (1991) reported a survival rate of 70% at 1 year and 48% at 2 years using extrapleural pneumonectomy with postoperative cyclophosphamide, doxorubicin, and cis-platinum chemotherapy with or without radiotherapy.

Diffuse mesothelioma is highly malignant. The usual delay of 6 to 8 months before diagnosis may be responsible for the advanced stage of disease at therapy. The average survival from onset of symptoms is 12 to 15 months and from diagnosis is 8 to 10 months. At present, palliation with pleurectomy to control chest pain and recurrent pleural effusions is the recommended approach (Martini et al., 1987) (Table 16–12). Further trials by large referral centers continue in hopes of obtaining improved survival with multimodality therapy.

Metastatic Tumors of the Pleura

Ninety-five per cent of neoplasms that involve the pleura are metastatic. Metastases occur from neoplasms of almost every primary site. Bronchial carcinoma is the major cause of the metastatic lesions in men, whereas carcinoma of the breast is the major cause in women. Together, they represent 60% of metastatic lesions. An additional 10% arise from lymphomas, especially Hodgkin's disease, lymphosarcoma, and chronic lymphocytic leukemia, and 25% arise from various neoplasms in other primary sites, which include the stomach, pancreas, and colon (Meyer, 1966).

The effusions caused by pleural metastases are usually unilateral; bilateral effusions are often associated with peritoneal involvement. The visceral and parietal pleurae may show multiple small nodular lesions that

■ **Table 16–12.** RESULTS OF SURGICAL RESECTION FOR MESOTHELIOMA

| Study | Year | No. of Patients | Type of Resection | Percentage of Patients Surviving | | |
				1 Yr	2 Yr	5 Yr
Wörn	1974	186	Radical	75	34	9
		62	Pleurectomy	68	37	10
Butchart et al.	1976	29	Radical	30	10	3
Wanebo et al.	1976	33	Pleurectomy	NS	30	15
DeLaria et al.	1978	11	Radical	36	27	0
Antman	1980	10	Pleurectomy	70	30	10

Modified from Antman, K. H.: Malignant mesothelioma. New Engl. J. Med., 303:200, 1980.

Key: Radical = pleuropneumonectomy; NS = not significant.

occasionally spread into thick sheets of tumor cells. The clinical characteristics of a patient with metastatic pleural tumor depend on the primary neoplasm. Pleural metastasis is usually only one site of a generalized metastatic spread. Chest pain, dyspnea, and recurrent massive pleural effusion that requires frequent thoracentesis may dominate the effects of the primary tumor.

BIBLIOGRAPHY

Aaron, B. L., and Doohen, D. J.: Spontaneous hemothorax in the newborn. Ann. Thorac. Surg., 9:258, 1970.

Abolnik, I. Z., Lossos, I. S., Gillis, D., and Breuer, R.: Primary spontaneous pneumothorax in men. Am. J. Med. Sci., 305:297, 1993.

Abyholm, F. E., and Storen, G.: Spontaneous haemopneumothorax. Thorax, 28:376, 1973.

Adkins, P. C., and Smyth, P. C.: Bilateral simultaneous spontaneous pneumothorax. Dis. Chest, 37:702, 1960.

Adler, R. H., and Sayek, I.: Treatment of malignant pleural effusion: A method using tube thoracostomy and talc. Ann. Thorac. Surg., 22:9, 1976.

Agostini, E.: Mechanics of the pleural space. Physiol. Rev., 52:57, 1972.

Agostini, E., Taglietti, A., and Setnikar, A.: Absorption force of the capillaries of the visceral pleura in determination of the intrapleural pressure. Am. J. Physiol., 191:277, 1957.

American Thoracic Society Subcommittee on Surgery: Management of nontuberculosis empyema. Am. Rev. Respir. Dis., 85:935, 1962.

Anderson, C. B., Philpott, G. W., and Ferguson, T. B.: The treatment of malignant pleural effusions. Cancer, 33:916, 1974.

Andrews, B. S., Arora, N. S., Shadforth, M. F., et al.: The role of immune complexes in the pathogenesis of pleural effusions. Am. Rev. Respir. Dis., 124:115, 1981.

Andrews, N. C.: The surgical treatment of chronic empyema. Dis. Chest., 47:533, 1965.

Antman, K. H.: Malignant mesothelioma. N. Engl. J. Med., 303:200, 1980.

Antman, K. H., Shemin, R. J., and Carson, J. M.: Malignant pleural mesothelioma: A combined mortality approach. In Kittle, C. F. (ed): Current Controversies in Thoracic Surgery. Philadelphia, W. B. Saunders, 1986.

Arom, K. U., Grover, F. L., Richardson, J. D., et al.: Post-traumatic empyema. Ann. Thorac. Surg., 23:254, 1977.

Austin, E. H., and Flye, M. W.: The treatment of recurrent malignant pleural effusion. Ann. Thorac. Surg., 28:190, 1979.

Autio, V.: The reduction of respiratory function by parenchymal and pleural lesions: A bronchospirometric study of patients with unilateral involvement. Acta Tuberc. Scand., 37:112, 1959.

Ayres, J. G., Pitcher, D. W., and Rees, P. J.: Pneumothorax associated with primary bronchial carcinoma. Br. J. Dis. Chest, 74:180, 1980.

Baber, C. E., Hedlung, L. W., Oddson, T. A., and Putnam, L. E.: Differentiating empyemas and peripheral pulmonary abscesses. Radiology, 135:755, 1980.

Baldwin, J. C., and Mark, J. B. D.: Treatment of bronchopleural fistula after pneumonectomy. J. Thorac. Cardiovasc. Surg., 90:813, 1985.

Bartlett, J. G., and Finegold, S. M.: Anaerobic infections of the lung and pleural space. Am. Rev. Respir. Dis., 110:56, 1974.

Bartlett, J. G., Gorbach, S. L., Thadepalli, H., et al.: Bacteriology of empyema. Lancet, 1:338, 1974.

Bates, J. H.: Diagnosis of tuberculosis. Chest, 76:757, 1979.

Berger, H. W., and Maher, G. C.: Decreased glucose concentration in malignant pleural effusions. Am. Rev. Respir. Dis., 103:427, 1971.

Berger, H. W., and Majia, E.: Tuberculosis pleurisy. Chest, 63:88, 1973.

Bergh, N. P., Ekroth, R., Larsson, S., and Nagy, P.: Intrapleural streptokinase in the treatment of hemothorax and empyema. Scand. J. Thorac. Cardiovasc. Surg., 11:265, 1977.

Bernstein, A., Wagaruddin, M., and Shah, M.: Management of spontaneous pneumothorax using a Heimlich flutter valve. Thorax, 28:386, 1973.

Bjork, V. O.: Thoracoplasty: A new osteoplastic technique. J. Thorac. Surg., 28:194, 1954.

Boer, H. R., and Andrews, B. F.: Spontaneous pneumothorax in the neonate. South. Med. J., 70:841, 1977.

Borrie, J.: Emergency thoracotomy for massive spontaneous haemopneumothorax. Br. Med. J., 2:16, 1953.

Bower, G. C.: Chyliform pleural effusion in rheumatoid arthritis. Am. Rev. Respir. Dis., 47:455, 1968.

Boyd, A. D.: Pneumothorax and hemothorax. In Hood, R. M., Boyd, A. D., and Culliford, A. T. (eds): Thoracic Trauma. Philadelphia, W. B. Saunders, 1989.

Bradley, S. L., Dines, D. E., Soule, E. H., et al.: Pulmonary lymphangiomatosis. Lung, 158:69, 1980.

Brenner, J., Sordillo, P. P., Magill, G. B., et al.: Malignant mesothelioma of the pleura. Cancer, 49:2431, 1982.

Bresticker, M. A., Oba, J., LoCicero, J., and Green, R.: Optimal pleurodesis: A comparison study. Ann. Thorac. Surg., 55:564, 1993.

Brooks, J. W.: Open thoracotomy in the management of spontaneous pneumothorax. Ann. Surg., 177:798, 1973.

Butchart, E. G., Ashcroft, T., Barnsley, W. C., and Holoen, M. P.: Pleuropneumonectomy in the management of diffuse malignant mesothelioma of the pleura: Experience with twenty-nine patients. Thorax, 31:15, 1976.

Bynum, L. J., and Wilson, J. E., III: Characteristics of pleural effusions associated with pulmonary emboli. Arch. Intern. Med., 136:159, 1976.

Byrnes, T. A., Brevig, J. K., and Yeoh, C. B.: Pneumothorax in patients with acquired immunodeficiency syndrome. J. Thorac. Cardiovasc. Surg., 98:546, 1989.

Calvert, R. D., and Smith, E.: An analytical review of haemopneumothorax. Thorax, 10:64, 1955.

Campbell, G. D., and Webb, W. R.: Eosinophilic pleural effusion. Am. Rev. Respir. Dis., 90:194, 1964.

Carel, R. S., Shapiro, M. S., Shoham, D., et al.: Lupus erythematosus cells in pleural effusion: The initial manifestation of procainamide-induced lupus erythematosus. Chest, 72:670, 1977.

Cevese, P. G., Verchioni, P., D'Amico, D. F., et al.: Postoperative chylothorax. J. Thorac. Cardiovasc. Surg., 69:966, 1978.

Chiles, C., and Ravin, C. E.: Radiographic recognition of pneumothorax in the intensive care unit. Crit. Care Med., 14:677, 1986.

Clagett, O. T., and Geraci, J. E.: A procedure for the management of postpneumonectomy empyema. J. Thorac. Cardiovasc. Surg., 45:141, 1963.

Clark, T. A., Hutchinson, D. E., Deaver, R. M., and Fitchett, V. H.: Spontaneous pneumothorax. Am. J. Surg., 124:728, 1972.

Clyne, A. J., and Hutter, F. H. D.: Spontaneous hemopneumothorax: A surgical emergency. Br. Med. J., 1:1058, 1955.

Cochran, J.: Pancreatic psuedocyst presenting as massive hemothorax. Am. J. Gastroenterol., 69:84, 1978.

Cohn, L. H., and Blaisdell, E. W.: Surgical treatment of nontuberculous empyema. Arch. Surg., 100:376, 1970.

Collins, T. R., and Sahn, S. A.: Thoracentesis: Complications, patient experience, and diagnostic value. Chest, 91:817, 1987.

Coselli, J. S., Mattox, K. L., and Beall, A. C.: Reevaluation of early evacuation of clotted hemothorax. Am. J. Surg., 148:785, 1984.

Crawford, B. K., Galloway, A. C., Boyd, A. D., and Spencer, F. C.: Treatment of AIDS-related bronchopleural fistula by pleurectomy. Ann. Thorac. Surg., 54:212, 1992.

Daniel, T. M., and Wyatt, D. A.: Pneumothorax and bullous disease. In Kaiser, L. R., and Daniel, T. M. (eds): Thoracoscopic Surgery. Boston, Little, Brown, 1993, p. 88.

Dark, J., and Chatterjee, S. S.: Pulmonary decortication. Lancet, 2:950, 1959.

DaValle, M. J., Faber, L. P., Kittle, F., et al.: Extrapleural pneumonectomy for diffuse malignant mesothelioma. Ann. Thorac. Surg., 42:612, 1986.

Davis, H. K.: A statistical study of the thoracic duct in man. Am. J. Anat., 17:211, 1915.

Deaton, W. R., and Johnston, F. R.: Spontaneous hemopneumothorax. J. Thorac. Cardiovasc. Surg., 43:413, 1962.

DeCamp, P., Moseley, P. W., Scott, M. L., et al.: Diagnostic thoracoscopy. Ann. Thorac. Surg., 16:79, 1973.

DeFrance, J., Blewett, J. H., Ricca, J. A., and Patterson, L. T.: Massive hemothorax: Two unusual cases. Chest, 66:82, 1974.

DesLauriers, J., Beaulieu, M., Despres, J. P., et al.: Transaxillary pleurectomy for treatment of spontaneous pneumothorax. Ann. Thorac. Surg., 30:569, 1980.

DeVries, W. C., and Wolfe, W. G.: The management of spontaneous pneumothorax and emphysema. Surg. Clin. North Am., 60:851, 1980.

Dewald, G. W., Hicks, G. A., Dines, D. E., et al.: Cytogenetic diagnosis of malignant pleural effusions: Culture methods to supplement direct preparations in diagnosis. Mayo Clin. Proc., 57:488, 1982.

Dines, D. E., Clagett, O. T., and Good, C. A.: Nontuberculous pulmonary parenchymal conditions predisposing to spontaneous pneumothorax. J. Thorac. Cardiovasc. Surg., 53:726, 1967.

Dines, D. E., Clagett, O. T., and Payne, S. W.: Spontaneous pneumothorax in emphysema. Mayo Clin. Proc., 45:481, 1970.

Dines, D. E., Cortese, D. A., Brennan, M. D., et al.: Malignant pulmonary neoplasms predisposing to spontaneous pneumothorax. Mayo Clin. Proc., 48:451, 1973.

Dressler, W.: A postmyocardial infarction syndrome. Arch. Intern. Med., 103:28, 1959.

Dulchavsky, S. A., Ledgerwood, A. M., and Lucas, C. E.: Management of chylothorax after blunt chest trauma. J. Trauma, 28:1400, 1988.

Elmes, P. C., and Simpson, M.: The clinical aspects of mesothelioma. Q. J. Med., 45:427, 1976.

Eloesser, L.: An operation for tuberculous empyema. Surg. Gynecol. Obstet., 60:1096, 1935.

Faber, E. E.: Spontaneous pneumothorax in 2 siblings. Hospitalstid., 64:573, 1921.

Falk, A.: Tuberculosis pleurisy with effusion: Diagnosis and results of chemotherapy. Postgrad. Med., 38:631, 1965.

Falk, A., Pearson, R. T., and Martin, F. E.: A bronchospirometric study of pulmonary function after decortication in pulmonary tuberculosis. Am. Rev. Tuberc., 66:509, 1952.

Findlay, C. W., Jr.: The management of the pleural space following partial resection of the lung (especially for tuberculosis). J. Thorac. Surg., 31:601, 1956.

Fitzgerald, M. X., Keelan, P. J., Cugell, D. W., and Gaensler, E. A.: Long-term results of surgery for bullous emphysema. J. Thorac. Cardiovasc. Surg., 68:566, 1974.

Friedman, P. J., and Hellekani, C.: Radiologic recognition of bronchopleural fistula. Radiology, 124:289, 1977.

Fromke, V. L., and Schmidt, W. F.: Hemothorax in idiopathic thrombocytopenic purpura (ITP). Thorac. Cariovasc. Surg., 63:962, 1972.

Gaensler, E. A.: Parietal pleurectomy for recurrent spontaneous pneumothorax. Surg. Gynecol. Obstet., 102:293, 1956.

Geha, A. S.: Pleural empyema: Changing etiologic, bacteriologic and therapeutic aspects. J. Thorac. Cardiovasc. Surg., 61:626, 1971.

George, R. B., Herbert, S. J., Shawes, J. M., et al.: Pneumothorax complicating pulmonary emphysema. J. A. M. A., 234:389, 1975.

Gerein, A. N., Brumwell, M. L., Lawson, L. M., et al.: Surgical management of pneumothorax in patients with acquired immunodeficiency syndrome. Arch. Surg., 126:1272, 1991.

Glenert, J.: Sugar levels in pleural effusions of different etiologies. Acta Tuberc. Scand., 42:222, 1962.

Gobbell, W. G., Rhea, W. G., Nelson, I. A., and Daniel, R. A.: Spontaneous pneumothorax. J. Thorac. Cardiovasc. Surg., 46:331, 1963.

Goldman, M., Goldman, G., and Fleischner, F. G.: Pleural fluid amylase in acute pancreatitis. N. Engl. J. Med., 266:715, 1962.

Graham, E. A., and Bell, R. D.: Open pneumothorax: Its relation to the treatment of acute empyema. Am. J. Med. Sci., 156:839, 1918.

Gregoire, R., DesLauriers, J., Beaulieu, M., et al.: Thoracoplasty: Its forgotten role in the management of nontuberculous postpneumonectomy empyema. Can. J. Surg., 30:343, 1987.

Gryminski, J., Krakowka, P., and Lypacewicz, G.: The diagnosis of pleural effusion by ultrasonic and radiologic techniques. Chest, 70:33, 1976.

Gula, G., Nakui, A., Radley-Smith, R., and Yacoub, M.: The spectrum of pulmonary arteriovenous fistulae: Clinicopathological correlations. J. Thorac. Cardiovasc. Surg., 29:51, 1981.

Hamilton, A. A. D., and Archer, G. J.: Treatment of pneumothorax by simple aspiration. Thorax, 38:934, 1983.

Hausheer, R. H. J., and Yarbro, J. W.: Diagnosis and treatment of malignant pleural effusion. Semin. Oncol., 12:54, 1985.

Heimlich, J. H.: Valve drainage of the pleural cavity. Dis. Chest, 53:282, 1968.

Higgins, C. B., and Mulder, D. G.: Chylothorax after surgery for congenital heart diseases. J. Thorac. Cardiovasc. Surg., 61:411, 1971.

Homma, T., Yoneda, S., Komuro, Y., et al.: Pharmacokinetics and pleural reaction of doxycycline after intrapleural administration [English abstract]. Gan To Kagaku Ryoho, 10:1129, 1983.

Hood, R. M.: Surgical Diseases of the Pleura and Chest Wall. Philadelphia, W. B. Saunders, 1986.

Hourihane, D. O. B., Lessof, L., and Richardson, P. C.: Hyaline and calcified pleural plaques as an index of exposure to asbestos: A study of radiological and pathological features of 100 cases with a consideration of epidemiology. Br. Med. J., 1:1069, 1966.

Hucker, J., Bhatnagar, N. K., Al-Jilaihawi, A. N., and Forrester-Wood, C. P.: Thoracoscopy in the diagnosis and management of recurrent pleural effusions. Ann. Thorac. Surg., 52:1145, 1991.

Hyde, P. V. B., Jersky, J., and Gishen, P.: Traumatic chylothorax. S. Afr. J. Surg., 12:57, 1974.

Janetos, G. P., and Ochsner, S. F.: Bilateral pneumothorax in metastatic osteogenic sarcoma. Am. Rev. Respir. Dis., 88:73, 1963.

Johnson, T. R., Comstock, C. H., and Anderson, D. G.: Benign gestational trophoblastic disease metastatic to pleura: Unusual cause of hemothorax. Obstet. Gynecol., 53:509, 1979.

Jones, J. S.: A place for aspiration in the treatment of spontaneous pneumothorax. Thorax, 40:66, 1985.

Karkola, P., Kairaluoma, M. I., and Larmi, T. K. K.: Postpneumonectomy empyema in pulmonary carcinoma patients. J. Thorac. Cardiovasc. Surg., 72:319, 1976.

Kausel, H. W., Reeve, T. S., Stein, A. A., et al.: Anatomic and pathologic studies of the thoracic duct. J. Thorac. Surg., 37:631, 1957.

Kaye, M. D.: Pleuropulmonary complications of pancreatitis. Thorax, 23:297, 1968.

Keagy, B. A., and Wilcox B. R.: Spontaneous pneumothorax. In Grillo, H. C., Austen, W. G., Wilkins, E. W., et al. (eds): Current Therapy in Cardiothoracic Surgery. Philadelphia, B. C. Decker, 1989, p. 112.

Keller, R., Gutersohn, J., and Herzog, H.: The management of persistent pneumothorax by thoracoscopic procedures [English abstract]. Thoraxchirurgie, 22:457, 1974.

Kergin, F. G.: An operation for chronic pleural empyema. J. Thorac. Surg., 26:430, 1953.

Killen, D. A., and Gobbell, W. G., Jr.: Spontaneous pneumothorax. Boston, Little, Brown, 1968.

Kjaergaard, H.: Spontaneous pneumothorax in the apparently healthy. Acta Med. Scand. Suppl., 43, 1932.

Kjaergaard, H.: Pneumothorax simplex: Two cases with autopsy findings. Acta Med. Scand., 80:93, 1933.

Klima, M., Spjut, H. J., and Seybold, W. D.: Diffuse malignant mesothelioma. Am. J. Clin. Pathol., 65:583, 1976.

Konjolinka, C. W., and Olearczyk, A.: Subphrenic abscess. Curr. Probl. Surg., January 1972, pp 1–51.

Kreel, L.: Computed tomography in mesothelioma. Semin. Oncol., 8:302, 1981.

Kreel, L.: Computed tomography of the lung and pleura. Semin. Roentgenol., 13:213, 1978.

Lampson, R. S.: Traumatic chylothorax. J. Thorac. Surg., 17:778, 1948.

Langston, H. T., Barker, W. L., and Graham, A. A.: Pleural tuberculosis. J. Thorac. Cardiovasc. Surg., 54:511, 1967.

Larrieu, A. J., Tyers, F. O., Williams, E. H., et al.: Intrapleural instillation of quinacrine for treatment of recurrent spontaneous pneumothorax. Ann. Thorac. Surg., 28:146, 1979.

Law, M. R., Gregor, A., Hodson, M. E., et al.: Malignant mesothelioma of the pleura: A study of 52 treated and 64 untreated patients. Thorax, 39:255, 1984.

Leach, J. E.: Pneumothorax in young adult males: Descriptive statistics in 126 cases. Arch. Intern. Med., 76:264, 1945.

Lee, P. R., Sox, H. C., North, F. S., and Wood, G. A.: Pleurisy with effusion in rheumatoid arthritis. Arch. Intern. Med., 104:634, 1959.

Leff, A., Hopewell, P. C., and Costello, J.: Pleural effusion from malignancy. Ann. Intern. Med., 83:532, 1978.

LeRoux, B. T.: Pleural tumors. Thorax, 17:111, 1962.

Levallen, E. C., and Carr, D. T.: Pleural effusion. N. Engl. J. Med., 252:79, 1955.

Levine, H., Szanto, P. B., and Cugell, D. W.: Tuberculous pleurisy. Arch. Intern. Med., 122:329, 1968.

Levine, H., Metzger, W., Lacera, D., and Kay, L.: Diagnosis of tuberculous pleurisy by culture of pleural biopsy specimen. Arch. Intern. Med., 126:269, 1970.

Light, R. W.: Parapneumonic effusion and infection of the pleural space. In Light, R. W. (ed): Pleural Diseases. Philadelphia, Lea & Febiger, 1983.

Light, R. W., and George, R. B.: Incidence and significance of pleural effusion after abdominal surgery. Chest, 69:621, 1976.

Light, R. W., Erozan, Y. S., and Ball, W. C.: Cells in pleural fluid. Arch. Intern. Med., 132:854, 1973a.

Light, R. W., Girard, W. M., Jenkinson, S. G., and George, R. B.: Parapneumonic effusions. Am. J. Med., 69:507, 1980.

Light, R. W., MacGregor, M. I., Ball, W. C., Jr., et al.: Diagnostic significance of pleural fluid pH and PCO_2. Chest, 64:591, 1973b.

Light, R. W., MacGregor, M. I., Luchsinger, P. C., and Ball, W. C.: Pleural effusions: The diagnostic separation of transudates and exudates. Ann. Intern. Med., 77:507, 1972.

Lillington, G. A., Mitchell, S. P., and Wood, G. A.: Catamenial pneumothorax. J. A. M. A., 219:1328, 1972.

Lindskog, G. E., and Halasz, N. A.: Spontaneous pneumothorax. Arch. Surg., 75:693, 1957.

Lippert, H. L., Lund, O., Blegvad, S., and Larsen, H. V.: Independent risk factors for cumulative recurrence rate after first spontaneous pneumothorax. Eur. Respir. J., 4:324, 1991.

Little, A. G., Ferguson, M. K., Golomb, H. M., et al.: Pleuroperitoneal shunting for malignant pleural effusions. Cancer, 58:2740, 1986.

Lopez-Majano, V., and Joshi, R. C. H.: Indications for decortication. Respiration, 27:565, 1970.

Lorch, D. G., Gordon, L., Wooten, S., et al.: Effect of patient positioning on distribution of tetracycline in the pleural space during pleurodesis. Chest, 93:527, 1988.

Luck, S. R., Raffensperger, J. G., Sullivan, J. H., and Gibson, L. E.: Management of pneumothorax in children with chronic pulmonary disease. J. Thorac. Cardiovasc. Surg., 74:834, 1977.

Macklin, M. T., and Macklin, C. L.: Malignant interstitial emphysema of the lungs and mediastinum as an important occult complication in many respiratory diseases and other conditions: An interpretation of clinical literature in light of laboratory experiment. Medicine, 23:281, 1944.

Maher, G. C., and Berger, H. W.: Massive pleural effusion: Malignant and nonmalignant causes in 46 patients. Am. Rev. Respir. Dis., 105:458, 1972.

Malove, G., Foster, E. D., Wilson, J. A., and Munro, R. D.: Bronchopleural fistulae: Present study of an old problem. Ann. Thorac. Surg., 11:1, 1971.

Marks, M. I., and Eickhoff, T. C.: Empyema necessitatis. Am. Rev. Respir. Dis., 101:159, 1970.

Martini, N., McCormack, P. M., Bains, M. S., et al.: Pleural mesothelioma. Ann. Thorac. Surg., 43:113, 1987.

Marts, B. C., Naunheim, K. S., Fiore, A. C., and Pennington, D. G.: Conservative versus surgical management of chylothorax. Am. J. Surg., 164:532, 1992.

Maurer, E. R., Schaal, J. A., and Mendez, F. L.: Chronic recurrence of spontaneous pneumothorax due to endometriosis of the diaphragm. J. A. M. A., 168:2013, 1968.

McCaughey, W. T. E.: Criteria for diagnosis of diffuse mesothelial tumors. Ann. N. Y. Acad. Sci., 132:603, 1965.

McClellan, M. D., Miller, S. B., Parsons, P. E., and Cohn, D. L.: Pneumothorax with Pneumocystis carinii pneumonia in AIDS. Chest, 100:1224, 1991.

McCormack, P. M., Nagasaki, F., Hilaris, B. S., et al.: Surgical treatment of pleural mesothelioma. J. Thorac. Cardiovasc. Surg., 84:834, 1982.

Meigs, J. V.: Fibroma of the ovary with ascites and hydrothorax—Meigs' syndrome. Prog. Gynecol., 3:424, 1957.

Melton, L. J., Hepper, N. G. G., and Orford, K. P.: Incidence of spontaneous pneumothorax in Olmsted County, Minnesota: 1950–1974. Am. Rev. Respir. Dis., 120:1379, 1979.

Menzies, R., and Charbonneau, M.: Thoracoscopy for the diagnosis of pleural disease. Ann. Intern. Med., 114:271, 1991.

Mercier, C. P., Page, A., Verdant, A., et al.: Outpatient management of intercostal tube drainage in spontaneous pneumothorax. Ann. Thorac. Surg., 22:163, 1976.

Meyer, P. C.: Metastatic carcinoma of the pleura. Thorax, 21:437, 1966.

Miller, J. I., Fleming, W. H., and Hatcher, C. R.: Balanced drainage of the contaminated pneumonectomy space. Ann. Thorac. Surg., 19:585, 1975.

Miller, J. I., Mansour, K. A., Nahai, F., et al.: Single-stage complete muscle flap closure of the postpneumonectomy empyema space: A new method and possible solution to a disturbing complication. Ann. Thorac. Surg., 38:227, 1984.

Murphy, M. C., Newman, B. M., and Rodgers, B. M.: Pleuroperitoneal shunts in the management of persistent chylothorax. Ann. Thorac. Surg., 48:195, 1989.

Murray, K. D., Matheny, R. G., Howanitz, E. P., and Myerowitz, P. D.: A limited axillary thoracotomy as primary treatment for recurrent spontaneous pneumothorax. Chest, 103:137, 1993.

Myerson, M., Knight, H. F., Gambarini, A. J., and Curran, T. L.: Intrapleural neomycin causing ototoxicity. Ann. Thorac. Surg., 9:483, 1970.

Nandi, P.: Recurrent spontaneous pneumothorax. Chest, 77:493, 1980.

Nathanson, L. K., Shimi, S. M., Wood, R. A., and Cuschieri, A.: Videothoracoscopic ligation of bulla and pleurectomy for spontaneous pneumothorax. Ann. Thorac. Surg., 52:316, 1991.

Nelson, R., Burman, S. O., Kiani, R., et al.: Hypoglycemic coma associated with benign pleural mesothelioma. J. Thorac. Cardiovasc. Surg., 69:306, 1975.

Nix, J. T., Albert, M., Dugas, J. E., and Wendt, D. L.: Chylothorax and chyloascities—A study of 302 selected cases. Am. J. Gastroenterol., 28:40, 1957.

Ohri, S. K., Oswal, S. K., Townsend, E. R., and Fountain, S. W.: Early and late outcome after diagnostic thoracoscopy and talc pleurodesis. Ann. Thorac. Surg., 53:1038, 1992.

Okike, N., Bernatz, P., and Woolner, L. B.: Localized mesothelioma of the pleura: Benign and malignant variants. J. Thorac. Cardiovasc. Surg., 75:363, 1978.

O'Meara, J. B., and Slade, P. R.: Disappearance of fluid from the postpneumonectomy space. J. Thorac. Cardiovasc. Surg., 67:621, 1974.

Pairolero, P. C., Arnold, P. G., and Piehler, J. M.: Intrathoracic transposition of extrathoracic skeletal muscle. J. Thorac. Cardiovasc. Surg., 86:809, 1983.

Patterson, G. A., Todd, T. R. J., Delarue, N. C., et al.: Supradiaphragmatic ligation of the thoracic duct in intractable chylous fistula. Ann. Thorac. Surg., 32:44, 1981.

Paulin, J., and Cheney, F. W., Jr.: Unilateral pulmonary edema in rabbits after reexpansion of collapsed lung. J. Appl. Physiol., 46:31, 1979.

Perelman, M. I., Rymko, L. P., and Ambatiello, G. P.: Bronchopleural fistula: Surgery after pneumonectomy. In Grillo, H., and Eschapasse, H. (eds): International Trends in General Thoracic Surgery. Vol. 2. Philadelphia, W. B. Saunders, 1987, p. 407.

Perlmutt, L. M., Braun, S. D., Newman, G. E., et al.: Timing of chest film follow-up after transthoracic needle aspiration. Am. J. Roentgenol., 146:1049, 1986.

Petty, T. L., Filley, G. F., and Mitchell, R. S.: Objective functional improvement by decortication after twenty years of artificial pneumothorax for pulmonary tuberculosis: Report of a case and review of the literature. Am. Rev. Respir. Dis., 84:572, 1961.

Ponn, R. B., Blancaflor, J., D'Agostino, R. S., et al.: Pleuroperitoneal shunting for intractable pleural effusions. Ann. Thorac. Surg., 51:605, 1991.

Potts, D. E., Levin, D. C., and Sohn, S. A.: Pleural fluid pH in parapneumonic effusions. Chest, 70:328, 1976.

Prakash, V. B. S., and Reiman, H. M.: Comparison of needle biopsy with cytologic analysis for the evaluation of pleural effusion: Analysis of 414 cases. Mayo Clin. Proc., 60:158, 1985.

Pratt, J. H., and Shamblin, W. R.: Spontaneous hemothorax as a direct complication of hemoperitoneum. Ann. Surg., *167*:867, 1968.

Provan, J. L.: The management of postpneumonectomy empyema. J. Thorac. Cardiovasc. Surg., *61*:107, 1971.

Raja, O. G., and Labor, A. J.: Simple aspiration of spontaneous pneumothorax. Br. J. Dis. Chest, *75*:207, 1981.

Randolph, J. G., and Gross, R. E.: Congenital chylothorax. Arch. Surg., *74*:405, 1957.

Rasaretnam, R., Chanmugam, D., and Sivathasan, C.: Spontaneous haemothorax in a mild haemophiliac. Thorax, *31*:601, 1976.

Ratzer, E. R., Pool, J. L., and Melamed, M. R.: Pleural mesotheliomas: Clinical experience with thirty-seven patients. Am. J. Roentgenol., *99*:863, 1967.

Ravitch, M. M., and Fein, R.: The changing picture of pneumonia and empyema in infants and children. J. A. M. A., *175*:1039, 1961.

Rhea, J. T., DeLuca, S. A., and Green, R. E.: Determining the size of pneumothorax in the upright patient. Radiology, *144*:733, 1982.

Rheuban, K. S., Kron, I. L., Carpenter, M. A., et al.: Pleuroperitoneal shunts for refractory chylothorax after operation for congenital heart disease. Ann. Thorac. Surg., *53*:85, 1992.

Roberts, G. H.: The pathology of parietal pleural plaques. J. Clin. Pathol., *24*:348, 1971.

Roberts, J. E. H.: The surgery of pleural and pulmonary infections. Trans. Med. Soc. Lond., *58*:183, 1935.

Robinson, L. A., Fleming, W. H., and Galbraith, T. A.: Intrapleural doxycycline control of malignant pleural effusions. Ann. Thorac. Surg., *55*:1115, 1993.

Rosenfeldt, F. L., McGibney, D., Braimbridge, M. V., and Watson, D. A.: Comparison between irrigation and conventional treatment for empyema and pneumonectomy space infection. Thorax, *36*:272, 1981.

Ross, J. K.: A review of the surgery of the thoracic duct. Thorax, *16*:12, 1961.

Rostand, R. A., Feldman, R. L., and Block, E. R.: Massive hemothorax complicating heparin anticoagulation for pulmonary embolus. South. Med. J., *70*:1128, 1977.

Roy, P. H., Carr, D. T., and Payne, W. S.: The problem of chylothorax. Mayo Clin. Proc., *42*:457, 1967.

Ruckley, C. V., McCormack, R. J. M.: The management of spontaneous pneumothorax. Thorax, *21*:139, 1966.

Rusch, V. W., Piantadosi, S., and Holmes, E. C.: The role of extrapleural pneumonectomy in malignant pleural mesothelioma. A Lung Cancer Study Group trial. J. Thorac. Cardiovasc. Surg., *102*:1, 1991.

Ryan, C. J., Rodgers, R. F., Unni, K. K., and Heppern, G. G.: The outcome of patients with pleural effusion of indeterminate cause at thoracotomy. Mayo Clin. Proc., *56*:145, 1981.

Sahn, S. A.: Pleural fluid analysis: Narrowing the differential diagnosis. Semin. Respir. Med., *9*:22, 1987.

Salyer, W. R., Eggleston, J. C., and Erozan, Y. S.: The efficacy of pleural needle biopsy and pleural fluid cytology in the diagnosis of malignant neoplasm involving the pleura. Chest, *67*:536, 1975.

Sample, W. F.: Ultrasound and computed tomography of the pleura. Semin. Roentgenol., *12*:259, 1977.

Samson, P. C.: Empyema thoracis: Essentials of present-day management. Ann. Thorac. Surg., *11*:210, 1971.

Sattler, A.: Zur Behandlung des Spontanpneumothorax mit besonderer Beřucksicktigung der thorakoskopie. Bietr. Klin. Tuberk., *89*:395, 1937.

Savage, T., and Fleming, H. A.: Decortication of the lung in tuberculous disease: A study in 43 cases. Thorax, *10*:293, 1955.

Scerbo, J., Keltz, H., and Stone, D. J.: A prospective study of closed pleural biopsies. J. A. M. A., *218*:377, 1971.

Schede, M.: Die Behandlung der Empyema. Inn. Med., *9*:41, 1890.

Schoenfeld, A., Ziu, E., Zeelel, Y., and Ouadia, J.: Catamenial pneumothorax—A literature review and report of an unusual case. Obstet. Gynecol. Surv., *41*:20, 1986.

Schulman, P., Cheng, E., Cvitkovic, E., and Golbey, R.: Spontaneous pneumothorax as a result of intensive cytotoxic chemotherapy. Chest, *75*:194, 1979.

Sciammas, F. D., Shetty, S., and Navani, S.: Multiple pleural nodules. Chest, *59*:673, 1971.

Selikoff, I. J., Churgh, J., and Hammond, E. C.: Relation between exposure to asbestos and mesothelioma. N. Engl. J. Med., *272*:560, 1965.

Selle, J. G., Snyder, W. H., and Schreiber, J. T.: Chylothorax: Indications for surgery. Ann. Surg., *177*:245, 1973.

Sepkowitz, K. A., Telzak, E. E., Gold, J. W. M., et al.: Pneumothorax in AIDS. Ann. Intern. Med., *114*:455, 1991.

Serementis, M. G.: The management of spontaneous pneumothorax. Chest, *57*:65, 1970.

Seriff, N. S., Cohen, M. L., Samuel, P., and Schulster, P. L.: Chylothorax diagnosis by lipoprotein electrophoresis of serum and pleural fluid. Thorax, *32*:98, 1977.

Shabanah, F. H., and Sayegh, S. F.: Solitary (localized) pleural mesotheliomas: Report of two cases and review of the literature. Chest, *60*:558, 1963.

Shafiroff, G. P., and Kan, Q. Y.: Cannulation of the human thoracic lymph duct. Surgery, *45*:814, 1959.

Sherr, H. P., Light, R. W., Merson, M. H., et al.: Origin of pleural fluid amylase in esophageal rupture. Ann. Intern. Med., *76*:985, 1972.

Shields, T. W.: Primary tumors of the pleura. *In* Shields, T. W. (ed): General Thoracic Surgery. Philadelphia, Lea & Febiger, 1989, pp. 650–666.

Siebens, A. A., Storey, C. F., Newman, M. M., et al.: The physiological effects of fibrothorax and the functional results of surgical treatment. J. Thorac. Surg., *32*:53, 1956.

Siegel, R. D., and Schiffman, F. J.: Systemic toxicity following intracavitary administration of bleomycin. Chest, *29*:1413, 1990.

Singh, S. U.: Current status of parietal pleurectomy in recurrent pneumothorax. Scand. J. Thorac. Cardiovasc. Surg., *13*:93, 1979.

Smith, D. E., Karish, A. F., Chapman, J. P., and Takaro, T.: Healing of the bronchial stump after pulmonary resection. J. Thorac. Cardiovasc. Surg., *46*:548, 1963.

So, S., and Yu, D.: Catheter drainage of spontaneous pneumothorax: Suction or no suction, early or late removal? Thorax, *37*:46, 1982.

Spear, B. S., Sully, L., and Lewis, C. T.: Pulmonary arteriovenous fistula presenting as spontaneous haemothorax. Thorax, *30*:355, 1975.

Spengler, L.: Zur Chirurgie des pneumothorax. Beitr. Klin. Chir., *49*:80, 1906.

Staats, R. A., Ellefson, R. D., Budahn, L. L., et al.: The lipoprotein profile of chylous and unchylous pleural effusions. Mayo Clin. Proc., *55*:700, 1980.

Stafford, E. G., and Clagett, O. T.: Postpneumonectomy empyema. J. Thorac. Cardiovasc. Surg., *63*:771, 1972.

Steier, M. Ching, N., Roberts, E. B., and Nealm, T. F.: Pneumothorax complicating continuous ventilatory support. J. Thorac. Cardiovasc. Surg., *67*:17, 1974.

Sterle, J. D.: Surgical Management of Pulmonary Tuberculosis. Springfield, IL, Charles C Thomas, 1957.

Stewart, P. B.: The rate of formation and lymphatic removal of fluid in pleural effusions. J. Clin. Invest., *42*:258, 1963.

Stiles, Q. R., Lindesmith, G. G., Tucker, B. L., et al.: Pleural empyema in children. Ann. Thorac. Surg., *10*:37, 1970.

Suarez, J., Clagett, T., and Brown, A. L.: The postpneumonectomy space: Factors influencing its obliteration. J. Thorac. Cardiovasc. Surg., *57*:539, 1969.

Sugarbaker, D. J., Heher, E. C., Lee, T. H., et al.: Extrapleural pneumonectomy, chemotherapy, and radiotherapy in the treatment of diffuse malignant pleural mesothelioma. J. Thorac. Cardiovasc. Surg., *102*:10, 1991.

Sugarbaker, D. J., Mentzer, S. J., DeCamp, M., et al.: Extrapleural pneumonectomy in the setting of a multimodality approach to malignant mesothelioma. Chest, *103*(Suppl.):377S, 1993.

Tanaka, F., Itho, M., Esaki, H., et al.: Secondary spontaneous pneumothorax. Ann. Thorac. Surg., *55*:372, 1993.

Takaro, T., Scott, S. M., Bridgman, A. H., et al.: Suppurative disease of the lungs, pleurae and pericardium. Curr. Probl. Surg., *24*:1, 1977.

Thorsrud, G. K.: Pleural reaction to irritants. Acta Chir. Scand., *355*(Suppl.):1, 1965.

Tocino, I. M., Miller, M. H., and Fairfax, W. R.: Distribution of pneumothorax in the supine and semirecumbent critically ill adult. Am. J. Roentgenol., *144*:901, 1985.

Torre, M. and Belloni, P.: Nd:YAG laser pleurodesis through thoracoscopy: New curative therapy in spontaneous pneumothorax. Ann. Thorac. Surg., 47:887, 1989.

Van Pernis, P. A.: Variations of the thoracic duct. Surgery, 26:806, 1949.

Virkkula, L.: Omentoplasty for bronchopleural fistula. In Current Therapy in Cardiothoracic Surgery. Philadelphia, B. C. Decker, 1989, pp. 103–104.

Vix, V. A.: Roentgenographic recognition of pleural effusion. J. A. M. A., 229:665, 1974.

Vladutiu, A. O., Brason, F. W., and Adler, R. H.: Differential diagnosis of pleural effusions: Clinical usefulness of cell marker quantification. Chest, 79:297, 1981.

Von Hoff, D. D., and LiVolsi, V.: Diagnostic reliability of needle biopsy of the parietal pleura. Am. J. Clin. Pathol., 64:200, 1975.

Vukich, D. J.: Pneumothorax, hemothorax and other abnormalities of the pleural space. Emerg. Med. Clin. North Am., 1:431, 1983.

Wagner, J. C., Sleggs, C. A., and Marchand, P.: Diffuse pleural mesothelioma and asbestos exposure in the North Western Cape Province. Br. J. Ind. Med., 17:260, 1960.

Wakabayashi, A.: Thoracoscopic ablation of blebs in the treatment of recurrent or persistent spontaneous pneumothorax. Ann. Thorac. Surg., 48:651, 1989.

Wakabayashi, A., Brenner, M., Wilson, A. F., et al.: Thoracoscopic treatment of spontaneous pneumothorax using carbon dioxide laser. Ann. Thorac. Surg., 50:786, 1990.

Walker, W. A., Pate, J. W., Amundsen, D., and Kennedy, C.: AIDS-related bronchopleural fistula [Letter]. Ann. Thorac. Surg., 55:1048, 1993.

Wanebo, H. J., Martini, N., Melamed, M. R., et al.: Pleural mesothelioma. Cancer, 38:2481, 1976.

Webb, W. R., Oxmen, V., Moulder, P. V., et al.: Iodized talc pleurodesis for the treatment of pleural effusions. J. Thorac. Cardiovasc. Surg., 103:881, 1992.

Weeden, D., and Smith, G. H.: Surgical experience in the management of spontaneous pneumothorax, 1972–82. Thorax, 38:737, 1983.

Weick, J. K., Kiely, J. M., Harrison, E. G., Jr., et al.: Pleural effusion in lymphoma. Cancer, 31:848, 1973.

Weissberg, D.: Talc pleurodesis: A controversial issue. Poumon-Coeur, 37:291, 1981.

Weissberg, D., Kaufman, M., and Zurkowski, Z.: Pleuroscopy in patients with pleural effusion and pleural masses. Ann. Thorac. Surg., 29:205, 1980.

West, J. B.: Distribution of mechanical stress in the lung: A possible factor in localization of pulmonary disease. Lancet, 1:839, 1971.

Whitwell, F., and Rawcliffe, M. R.: Diffuse malignant pleural mesothelioma and asbestos exposure. Thorax, 26:6, 1971.

Whitwell, F., Scott, J., and Grimshaw, M.: Relationship between occupations and asbestos-fiber content of the lungs in patients with pleural mesothelioma, lung cancer, and other diseases. Thorax, 32:377, 1977.

Williams, K. R., and Burford, T. H.: The management of chylothorax. Ann. Surg., 160:131, 1964.

Williams, N. S., and Lewis, C. T.: Bronchopleural fistula: A review of 86 cases. Br. J. Surg., 63:520, 1976.

Wilson, J. L., Herrod, C. M., Searle, G. L., et al.: The absorption of blood from the pleural space. Surgery, 48:766, 1960.

Wilson, J. W.: Diagnosis of infrapulmonary pleural effusion. J. A. M. A., 158:1423, 1955.

Woodruff, W.: The recognition and management of bronchopleural fistula. Am. J. Surg., 54:236, 1941.

Wörn, H.: Möglichkeiten und Ergebnisse der chirurgischen Behandlung des malignen Pleura mesotheliomas. Thoraxchirurgie, 22:391, 1974.

Youmans, C. R., Jr., Williams, R. D., McMinn, M. R., and Derrick, L. R.: Surgical management of spontaneous pneumothorax by bleb ligation and pleural dry sponge abrasion. Am. J. Surg., 120:644, 1970.

17 The Mediastinum

R. Duane Davis, Jr., H. Newland Oldham, Jr., and David C. Sabiston, Jr.

The mediastinum is an important and complex anatomic division of the thorax, extending from the diaphragm to the thoracic inlet. The mediastinum is the site of many localized disorders and is involved in several systemic diseases. Localized disorders that occur in this region include infection, hemorrhage, emphysema, aneurysms, and many primary tumors and cysts. Systemic diseases include metastatic neoplasms, granulomas, and other generalized inflammatory disorders. Lesions that originate in the esophagus, great vessels, trachea, and heart may present as a mediastinal mass or may cause symptoms related to compression or invasion of adjacent mediastinal structures. Although these lesions are discussed in the sections covering the specific organ system of origin, they are relevant in the differential diagnosis of the various primary mediastinal disease processes. Mediastinal disorders present in a myriad of different clinical settings. Symptoms may be related to local involvement of adjacent structures, tumor-secretory factors, or immunologic factors. In addition, many patients are *asymptomatic* and the tumor must be identified on routine chest films.

HISTORICAL ASPECTS

Before the introduction of endotracheal anesthesia and techniques for closed pleural drainage, few attempts were made to intervene surgically in the mediastinum because of the hazards inherent in entering the pleural cavity, particularly pneumothorax and subsequent respiratory insufficiency. Therefore, the initial procedures involved processes in the anterior mediastinum, which could be exposed through various sternal approaches. In 1893, Bastianelli excised a dermoid cyst from the anterior mediastinum after resecting the manubrium (quoted in Meade, 1961). In 1897, Milton reported the removal of two caseous lymph nodes from the anterior mediastinum of a young Egyptian man with mediastinal tuberculosis. He used a sternal splitting approach, which he developed after working initially on cadavers and subsequently on goats, finding that it provided excellent exposure to the anterior mediastinum without entering the pleural cavities. Because of the involvement of the sternum by the disease process, Milton initially left the wound open, successfully using a delayed primary closure on the second postoperative day.

With the introduction of endotracheal anesthesia, the safe performance of transpleural operations was possible. Harrington in 1929 and Heuer and Andrus

in 1940 reported the first series of patients documenting the safety and efficacy of the transpleural approach to a variety of mediastinal diseases. In 1936, Blalock and co-workers reported the excision of the thymus in a young woman with myasthenia gravis. Subsequently, the patient had a marked amelioration in her symptoms. This success initiated the surgical treatment of myasthenia gravis. Numerous groups have significantly contributed to the treatment of a wide variety of advancement of malignant diseases with chemotherapeutic agents, with significant improvements in survival and cure, particularly in the treatment of lymphomas and germ-cell tumors.

ANATOMY AND EMBRYOLOGY

The mediastinum is defined by the following borders: the thoracic inlet superiorly, the diaphragm infe-

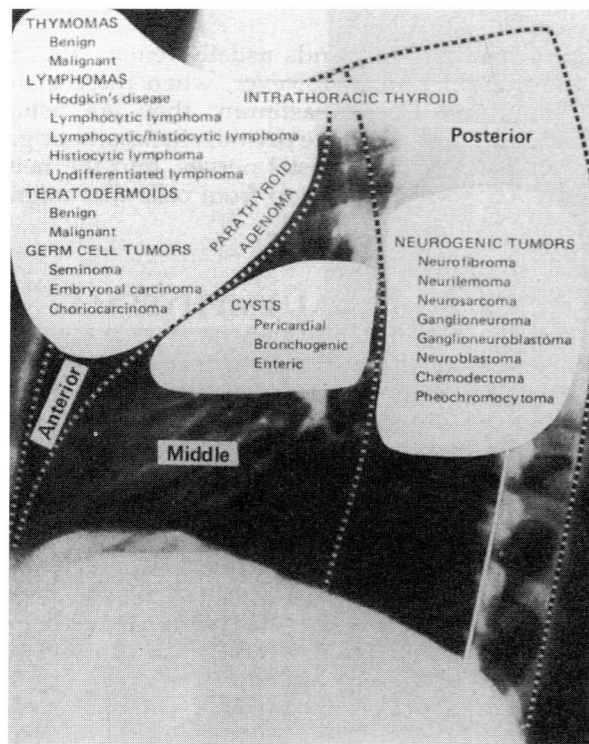

FIGURE 17–1. Lateral chest film divided into three anatomic subdivisions with the most common location of the tumors and cysts. (From Davis, R. D., Jr., and Sabiston, D. C., Jr.: Primary mediastinal cysts and neoplasms. *In* Sabiston, D. C., Jr. [ed]: Essentials of Surgery. Philadelphia, W. B. Saunders, 1987.)

riorly, the sternum anteriorly, the vertebral column posteriorly, and the parietal pleura laterally. Because many mediastinal tumors and cysts occur in characteristic locations, the mediastinum has been subdivided artificially for the convenience of localizing specific types of lesions. Because many anterior mediastinal tumors also frequently occupy the anterior aspect of the mediastinum, and similarly, many posterior mediastinal masses occupy the posterior aspect of the superior mediastinum, the mediastinum has been further subdivided into the anterosuperior, middle, and posterior (Fig. 17–1). The anterior mediastinum is anterior to the pericardium and the pericardial reflection. The middle mediastinum is bordered anteriorly by the anterior pericardial reflection and posteriorly by the posterior pericardial reflection.

The contents of the anterosuperior mediastinum include the thymus gland, the aortic arch and its branches, the great veins, the lymphatics, and the fatty areolar tissue. The middle mediastinal contents include the heart, pericardium, phrenic nerves, tracheal bifurcation and main bronchi, the hila of each lung, and lymph nodes. The posterior mediastinum contains the esophagus, the vagus nerves, sympathetic nervous chain, thoracic duct, descending aorta, azygos and hemiazygos systems, paravertebral lymph nodes, and fatty areolar tissue (Fig. 17–2).

Development of mediastinal structures begins as early as the 5- to 6-mm embryo stage. The pericardial cavity originates from coalescence of mesenchymal spaces in the coelomic cavities on each side of the embryo. The pleural cavities develop from the dorsal parietal recesses. Separation of the body cavity into the thorax and the peritoneal cavities occurs with the development of the diaphragm from the septum transversum and the paired pleuroperitoneal membranes. During this period, the primitive foregut differentiates into the respiratory and upper digestive tracts. The ventral foregut develops into the epithelial lining of the larynx and tracheobronchial tree, as well as the alveolar respiratory epithelium. The dorsal foregut develops into the epithelial lining of the esophagus. The cartilage, smooth muscle, and elastic tissue of the tracheobronchial tree and the fibromuscular tissue of the esophagus arise from mesenchymal tissue surrounding the foregut.

The thymus originates from the ventral aspect of the third branchial pouch, and the dorsal aspect of the third branchial pouch gives rise to the inferior parathyroid glands. The thymus separates from the pharynx and migrates into the anterosuperior mediastinum, whereas the inferior parathyroid glands usually remain attached to the thyroid gland. However, the common embryologic origin explains the frequent finding of the inferior parathyroid glands within the mediastinum closely associated with the thymus.

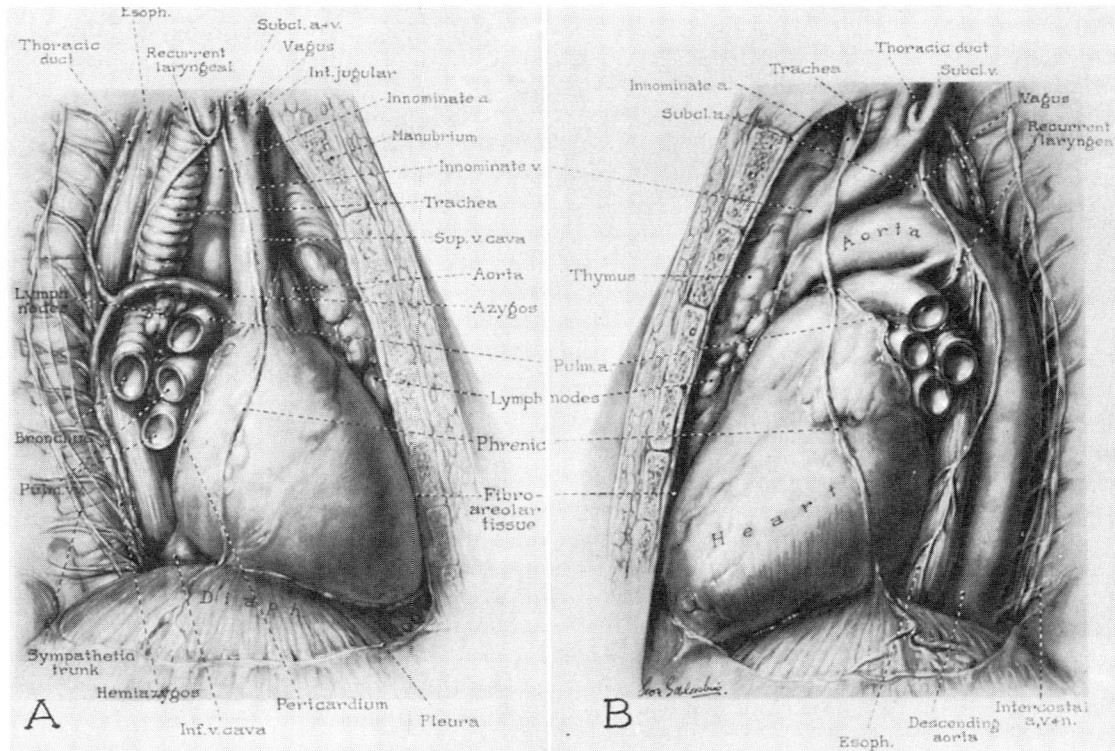

FIGURE 17–2. The anatomic structures of the mediastinum as seen from the right side *(A)* and from the left side *(B)*. *(A* and *B*, From Sabiston, D. C., Jr.: The esophagus and mediastinum. *In* Cooke, R. E., and Levin, S. [eds]: The Biologic Basis of Pediatric Practice. New York, McGraw-Hill, 1968.)

Sympathetic ganglia, paraganglia, intercostal nerves, and the neurilemmal sheath cells originate from the neural crest.

MEDIASTINAL EMPHYSEMA

Air within the mediastinum produces mediastinal emphysema or pneumomediastinum. Air may come from the esophagus, trachea, bronchi, neck, or abdomen. Common causes of pneumomediastinum include penetrating wounds or perforations of these structures, blunt trauma that leads to fractured ribs or vertebrae, and barotrauma caused by either blunt trauma or positive-pressure ventilation. Blunt trauma due to compressive forces on the thorax, especially when the glottis is closed, and ventilation with high pressures, usually in the setting of decreased lung compliance, may create pressures at the intra-alveolar region sufficient to rupture alveoli. Dissection through the visceral pleura causes a pneumothorax. However, dissection of the air along vascular structures into the hilum and mediastinum creates pneumomediastinum. Mediastinal emphysema may also be caused by intra-abdominal air dissecting through the diaphragmatic hiatus.

Spontaneous mediastinal emphysema is usually seen in patients with exacerbation of bronchospastic disease. The pathophysiology of spontaneous pneumomediastinum is thought to involve the rupture of a bleb within the pulmonary parenchyma, creating interstitial emphysema. This occurs in a manner similar to that caused by barotrauma. The air then dissects along vascular or bronchial planes into the mediastinum. The clinical manifestations of this disorder, described initially by Hamman in 1939, include substernal chest pain, which may radiate into the back, and crepitation in the region of the suprasternal notch, chest wall, and neck. With increasing pressure, the air can dissect into the neck, face, chest, arms, abdomen, and retroperitoneum. Frequently, pneumomediastinum and pneumothorax occur simultaneously. The characteristic crunching sound heard over the pericardium, which is accentuated during systole, and is found on auscultation, is called *Hamman's sign*. Only rarely does sufficient pressure develop to cause compression of venous structures so as to impair venous return. With impairment of venous return, clinical manifestations similar to the superior vena caval syndrome occur, including cyanosis, prominence of neck and upper extremity veins, dyspnea, and in severe cases, circulatory failure.

The presence of air within the mediastinum confirms the diagnosis of pneumomediastinum. Air is usually also present in the pectoral muscles, neck, and upper extremities, as visualized on the chest films or *computed tomography* (CT) scans. Contrast studies of the esophagus and bronchoscopy work best to initially evaluate the esophagus, trachea, and major bronchi. Perforations of these structures require urgent surgical treatment. Spontaneous mediastinal emphysema and pneumomediastinum secondary to barotrauma usually respond to conservative measures that treat bronchospasm and minimize further barotrauma without sequelae. Surgical decompression is rarely necessary. In patients with pneumomediastinum and pneumothorax, tube thoracostomy is indicated in the affected pleural space. Patients with pneumomediastinum secondary to barotrauma who require high levels of pressure support may require bilateral tube thoracostomies to prevent development of tension pneumothorax. In patients who are distressed by the inability to open their eyes, 5-mm incisions in the skin folds of the eyelids and neck can be made using local anesthesia. By gently pressing on the surrounding soft tissue, sufficient air can be removed to provide symptomatic relief.

MEDIASTINITIS

Infection of the mediastinal space is a serious and potentially fatal process. Etiologic factors that cause acute mediastinitis include perforation of the esophagus owing to instrumentation, foreign bodies, penetrating or, more rarely, blunt trauma, spontaneous esophageal disruption (Boerhaave's syndrome), leakage from an esophageal anastomosis, tracheobronchial perforation, and mediastinal extension from an infectious process originating in the pulmonary parenchyma, pleura, chest wall, vertebrae, great vessels, or neck. Currently, mediastinitis occurs most frequently following median sternotomy for open heart cardiac operations. Superficial wound infections occur in approximately 4% of patients following cardiac operations; in 1 to 2% of patients, the infection involves the mediastinum. Risk factors for the development of mediastinitis include prolonged operation, lengthy cardiopulmonary bypass, reexploration for postoperative bleeding, dehiscence, external cardiac massage, postoperative cardiogenic shock, and the use of bilateral internal mammary arteries for coronary artery bypass grafting, especially in elderly patients or in patients with diabetes mellitus.

Mediastinitis is manifested clinically by fever, tachycardia, leukocytosis, and pain that may be localized to the chest, back, or neck, although in some patients, the clinical course remains indolent for long periods. When mediastinitis is secondary to esophageal perforation following instrumentation, the pain is most frequently localized to the neck because the most common site of perforation is at the level of the cricopharyngeal muscle. In these patients, subcutaneous emphysema is almost invariably present. Postoperative mediastinitis usually presents between 3 days and 3 weeks following the operation, although delayed manifestations may occur months later. Clinical indications of postoperative mediastinitis include wound erythema, drainage, pain, unstable sternum, spiking fevers, and leukocytosis. The lateral chest film can evaluate air fluid levels, abnormal soft tissue densities, and sternal dehiscence. CT may be useful when mediastinal gas is present to indicate the presence of gas-forming organisms or distinct abscess. CT may also identify associated or contiguous infections, such as an empyema, subphrenic abscess, or cervical soft tissue infection. Water-soluble contrast studies of the esophagus and esophagoscopy are important in evaluating a potential esophageal perforation or disruption. In patients with penetrating or blunt trauma, both procedures have been necessary to minimize the number of overlooked esophageal injuries. Similarly, bronchoscopy is the optimal procedure to evaluate potential tracheobronchial disruption.

Treatment of mediastinitis requires correction of the inciting cause and aggressive supportive therapy. After cultures are obtained, appropriate antimicrobial coverage should be initiated, with modification after culture reports and sensitivities are available. In patients with mediastinal infections in continuity or communication with empyema, subphrenic abscess, or neck abscess, drainage of the empyema with tube thoracostomy or percutaneous drainage of the abscess in conjunction with appropriate antimicrobial therapy is frequently successful. Similarly, mediastinitis associated with catheter sepsis can often be treated with removal of the catheter and antimicrobial therapy. However, in patients who do not respond to these initial measures, or when mediastinitis occurs with most other etiologies, thorough débridement of necrotic and infected tissue is necessary in conjunction with surgical drainage. When costal cartilage is infected, it is necessary to excise the cartilage back to bleeding bone. In patients with descending mediastinitis originating from the oropharynx, cervical drainage and débridement may be adequate to treat infections limited to the superior mediastinum. However, when the involvement is more generalized, transthoracic débridement and drainage are necessary. Delays in making the diagnosis and subsequently initiating therapy, especially when the etiologic factor involves esophageal or tracheobronchial disruption, sharply increase morbidity and mortality.

Postoperative mediastinitis following median sternotomy has been successfully treated with different techniques. The simplest approach involves incision, débridement, and drainage of the involved area in conjunction with local irrigation with antibiotics or antiseptic agents and wound care using dressings soaked in dilute povidone-iodine, Dakin's solution, or acetic acid. Delayed closure is possible, although an unstable sternum is the usual result.

Improved results have been obtained after thoroughly débriding all affected tissue by using closed irrigation systems. Depending on the severity of the infection, the wound can be either closed or left open after the placement of large-bore drainage tubes through which continuous irrigation with antibiotic solution or diluted povidone-iodine is done (approximately 3 1/day for 7 to 14 days). The tubes are removed gradually to minimize residual dead space.

The best results have been obtained by using a variety of tissue flaps to obliterate dead space and to provide immediate coverage of the heart, bypass grafts, and great vessels following effective surgical control of the wound. Débridement of infected and necrotic sternum, cartilage, and soft tissue in conjunction with wound care is often necessary to provide a clean wound. This therapy has further reduced morbidity and mortality, usually produces a good long-term functional result, and has significantly reduced the duration of hospitalization. The pectoralis major and rectus abdominis muscles have been the most commonly used tissue flaps (Fig. 17–3). Because the rectus abdominis flap is based on the superior epigastric artery, this flap is only useful when the internal mammary artery remains viable. In situations in which both internal mammary arteries have been used for bypass conduits or have been sacrificed during débridement, the omentum has been used successfully (Fig. 17–4). Because the omentum is capable of enhancing neovascularization, relieving lymphedema, providing fibroblasts, and providing soft tissue coverage while allowing sternal closure, it is the tissue flap of choice in some centers.

Although chronic mediastinitis may be caused by an indolent bacterial infection, more frequently chronic infections are granulomatous processes that follow tuberculosis or mycotic infections. Active infection requires treatment with antituberculous or antifungal agents. With progressive cases of chronic infection, the granulomatous process within the mediastinal lymph nodes may compress adjacent structures, such as the venae cavae, trachea, bronchi, or esophagus. Of the mycotic infections, histoplasmosis is the most likely to become severely involved with the mediastinal lymph nodes. Active *Histoplasma* infections are treated with itraconazole in the immunocompetent patient and amphotericin B in the immunocompromised patient. Rarely, surgical decompression, excision, or bypass is necessary in addition to medical therapy to treat the resultant obstruction.

HEMORRHAGE

Mediastinal hemorrhage is most frequently caused by blunt or penetrating trauma, thoracic aortic dissection, rupture of aortic aneurysm, or surgical procedures within the thorax. Penetrating trauma to the thorax or cervical region may cause lacerations of major veins or arteries, whereas blunt trauma may cause transection of the aorta or other great vessels. The usual site of aortic transection is immediately distal to the origin of the left subclavian artery, the second most common site occurring prior to the origin of the innominate artery, and the third most common site is distal to the aortic valve annulus. Most mediastinal hemorrhage associated with blunt trauma is due to rupture of small mediastinal veins. However, the possibility of aortic injury should be evaluated with arch aortography in patients with a history of a severe deceleration injury and chest film demonstration of widening of the superior mediastinum, shift of the trachea or nasogastric tube to the right, downward shift of the left main bronchus, or loss of sharpness of the contour of the aortic arch.

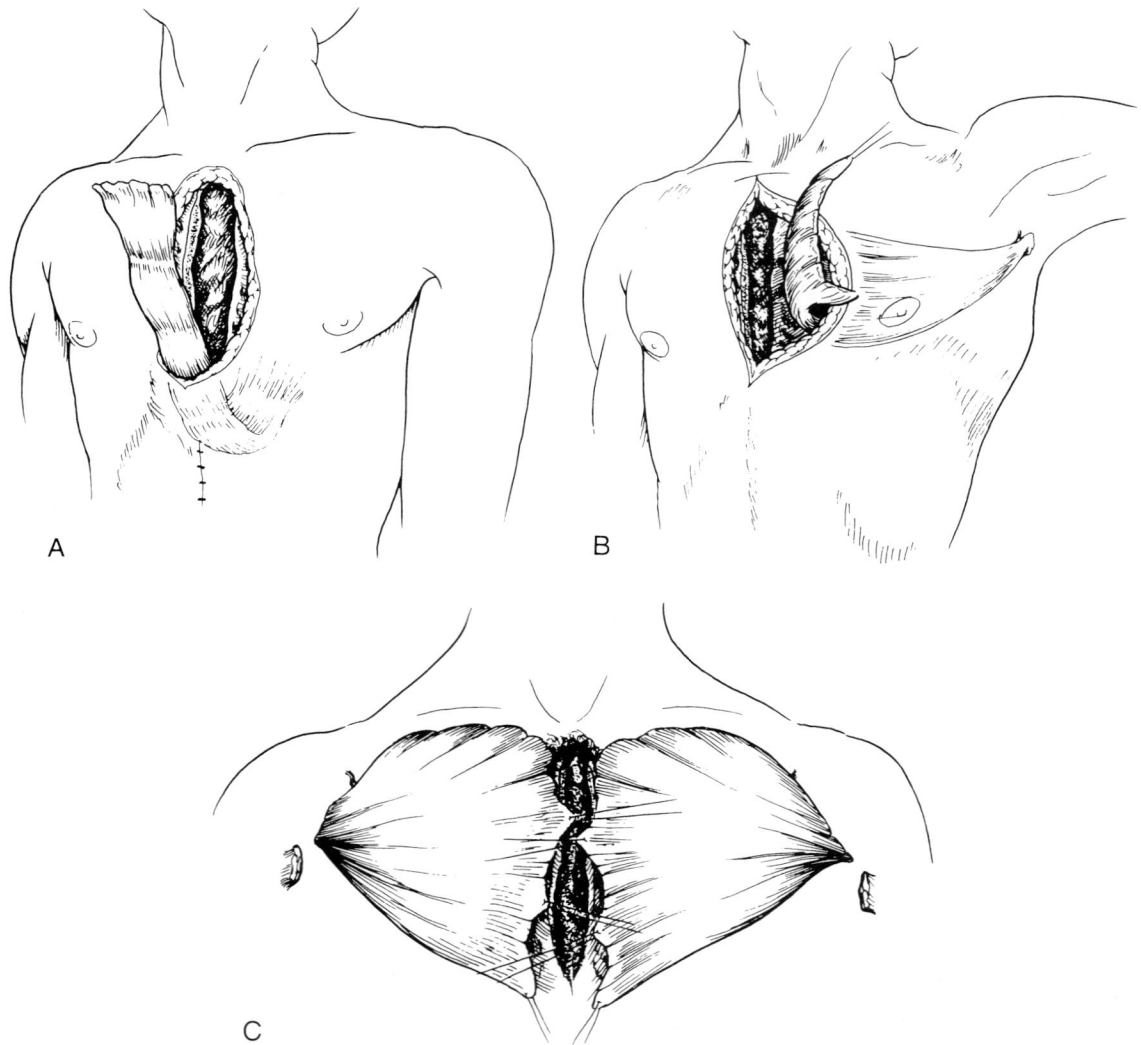

FIGURE 17–3. *A,* The unilateral rectus abdominis muscle flap can be used for a central sternal trough defect when the internal thoracic artery remains intact after débridement. *B,* An upper sternal defect may be filled with a unilateral pectoralis major muscle flap. Usually, however, both muscles are required to adequately fill the defect with healthy tissue. *C,* The humeral insertion of the pectoralis muscle may be divided for mobility, and both pectoralis major muscles may be used for added bulk. *(A–C,* From Seyfer, A. E., Graeber, G. M., and Wind, G. G.: Atlas of Chest Wall Reconstruction. Rockville, MD, Aspen Publishers, 1986.)

Significant hemorrhage may follow thoracic operations, particularly procedures involving the heart and great vessels that require cardiopulmonary bypass. Routine use of large-bore chest tubes for drainage usually prevents mediastinal tamponade. Other iatrogenic causes of mediastinal hemorrhage include laceration of great vessels during angiography, placement of central venous or arterial catheters, erosion of indwelling vascular devices, and erosion of tracheostomy tubes into the great vessels.

Spontaneous mediastinal hemorrhage is a recognized entity with predisposing factors related to the following: (1) complication of a mediastinal mass, of which thymoma, malignant germ-cell tumor, parathyroid adenoma, retrosternal thyroid, and teratoma are the most common; (2) sudden sustained hypertension; (3) altered hemostasis due to anticoagulant therapy,

thrombolytic therapy, uremia, hepatic insufficiency, or hemophilia; and (4) transient, sharp increases in intrathoracic pressure, which occur during coughing or vomiting, an entity initially described by Epstein in 1959 (Epstein and Klassen, 1960). The pathophysiology of this disorder is thought to be associated with rupture of small mediastinal vessels. Usually, the clinical course is benign and the symptoms resolve without long-term sequelae.

The clinical presentation varies with the underlying cause. Retrosternal pain radiating to the back or neck is common. With increased accumulation of blood in the mediastinum, signs and symptoms related to compression of mediastinal structures, primarily the great veins, may develop, including dyspnea, venous distention, cyanosis, and cervical ecchymosis owing to blood dissecting into soft tissue planes. Sufficient

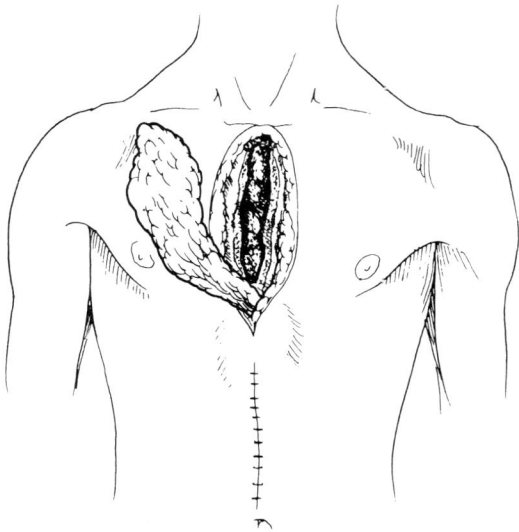

FIGURE 17–4. The omentum provides healthy tissue to fill a large sternal defect when compromise of the internal thoracic arteries makes the rectus muscles unusable. (From Seyfer, A. E., Graeber, G. M., and Wind, G. G.: Atlas of Chest Wall Reconstruction. Rockville, MD, Aspen Publishers, 1986.)

accumulation of blood causes mediastinal tamponade, manifested by tachycardia, hypotension, reduced urinary output, equalization of right- and left-sided cardiac filling pressures, and diastolic collapse of the right ventricle. The development of mediastinal tamponade is more insidious than that of pericardial tamponade because of the larger volume of the mediastinum, and it has a markedly poorer prognosis. Therefore, the goal is to diagnose mediastinal hemorrhage before circulatory compromise. Diagnostic measures include chest films, which may indicate superior mediastinal widening, loss of the normal aortic contour, and soft tissue density in the anterosuperior mediastinum; echocardiography; and CT scanning, which may characterize a mass as containing blood or clot and demonstrate its relationship to vascular structures, particularly if a false lumen is present. Arteriography may be useful in localizing the site of bleeding or intimal disruption. Therapy is directed toward evacuation of the existing clot and repairing the underlying process. In patients who have suffered penetrating trauma with associated profound hypotension, emergency thoracotomy or sternotomy is indicated without initial arteriography. In postoperative patients following cardiac operations, catheter drainage using CT guidance has been successful without significant morbidity (Rousou et al., 1987).

SUPERIOR VENA CAVAL OBSTRUCTION

A number of benign and malignant processes may obstruct the superior vena cava, causing superior vena caval syndrome. The pathophysiology of the syndrome involves increased pressure in the venous system draining into the superior vena cava, leading to the characteristic features of the syndrome—edema of the head, neck, and upper extremities; distended neck veins with dilated collateral veins over the upper extremities and torso; cyanosis; headache; and confusion. These findings are initially noted and remain more prominent when the patient is in a recumbent position. However, they are usually present to some extent even when the patient is upright. With processes that slowly cause obstruction, these features develop insidiously. However, with rapid or sudden occlusion, the clinical presentation is often striking, with rapid development of cerebral edema and intracranial thrombosis that may lead to coma and death.

The pathologic cause of the superior vena caval obstruction varies from compression to invasion as well as thrombosis. The cause may be the primary tumor or mass, often from paratracheal lymph node metastases. Most frequently, the cause is a malignant neoplasm. Bronchogenic carcinoma, most frequently of the right upper lobe, is the most common cause. Malignant germ-cell tumors and thymomas, lymphomas, and primary mediastinal carcinomas as well as metastatic lesions are the common malignant causes. Less than 25% of patients with superior vena caval obstruction have a benign cause. A large number of benign processes have been implicated, including mediastinal granulomatous diseases, particularly histoplasmosis and tuberculosis, idiopathic mediastinal fibrosis, mediastinal goiter, bronchogenic cyst, teratoma, pleural calcification, and thoracic aortic aneurysm. Superior vena caval obstruction secondary to indwelling catheters or trauma to the vessel when placing the catheter has become more common. However, rarely does the superior vena caval syndrome result.

The syndrome is infrequently seen in children. Most superior vena caval obstructions in children occur following cardiac surgery (71%), particularly following Mustard's and, less frequently, Senning's repairs for transposition of the great vessels (Issa et al., 1983; Janin et al., 1982). Other significant causes of childhood superior vena caval syndrome include mediastinal neoplasm (16%; most are non-Hodgkin's lymphomas), ventriculoatrial shunts (5%), and mediastinal fibrosis (3%).

Contrast-enhanced CT scanning or *magnetic resonance imaging* (MRI) is usually adequate to establish the diagnosis of superior vena caval obstruction and to assist in the differential diagnosis of probable cause. Although venous angiography is rarely required to establish the diagnosis, it does provide more accurate anatomic detail regarding the site of obstruction and collateral development, which is necessary if surgical bypass is required.

Because the malignant processes responsible for the superior vena caval syndrome are usually not surgically resectable, the initial attempt to establish a histologic diagnosis is generally a percutaneous needle-biopsy technique. Histologic diagnosis is attempted before the initiation of empiric therapy because such therapy will alter the morphologic appearance. In 42% of patients receiving prebiopsy radiation in one

■ **Table 17–1.** CLASSIFICATION OF PRIMARY
MEDIASTINAL TUMORS AND CYSTS

Neurogenic Tumors	Mesenchymal tumors
Neurofibroma	Fibroma/Fibrosarcoma
Neurilemoma	Lipoma/Liposarcoma
Neurosarcoma	Leiomyoma/Leiomyosarcoma
Ganglioneuroma	Rhabdosarcoma
Neuroblastoma	Xanthogranuloma
Chemodectoma	Myxoma
Paraganglioma	Mesothelioma
	Hemangioma
Thymoma	Hemangioendothelioma
Benign	Hemangiopericytoma
Malignant	Lymphangioma
	Lymphangiomyoma
Lymphoma	Lymphangiopericytoma
Hodgkin's disease	
Lymphoblastic	**Endocrine Tumors**
Large-cell diffuse growth	Intrathoracic thyroid
pattern	Parathyroid adenoma/carcinoma
T-immunoblastic sarcoma	Carcinoid
B-immunoblastic sarcoma	
Sclerosing follicular cell	**Cysts**
	Bronchogenic
Germ-Cell Tumors	Pericardial
Teratodermoid	Enteric
Benign	Thymic
Malignant	Thoracic duct
Seminoma	Nonspecific
Nonseminomas	
Embryonal	**Giant Lymph Node Hyperplasia**
Choriocarcinoma	Castleman's disease
Endodermal	
	Chondroma
Primary Carcinomas	**Extramedullary Hematopoiesis**

series, a histologic diagnosis could not be established
(Loeffler et al., 1986). Open biopsy in patients able to
tolerate anesthesia may be necessary to establish a
diagnosis. However, these patients are at an increased
risk for cardiorespiratory compromise during general
anesthesia. Preoperative screening and intraoperative
management are discussed in a later section.

The most useful types of therapy include radiation,
corticosteroids, and multiagent chemotherapy. The
optimal therapeutic regimen depends on the histologic diagnosis. In patients in whom the syndrome
develops rapidly or when neurologic symptoms are

present, therapy may be necessary on an emergency
basis. Improved success in the treatment of several
malignant causes of the superior vena caval syndrome has evolved, particularly with the lymphomas
and germ-cell tumors. Even when treating obstruction
secondary to bronchogenic carcinoma, at least transient decompression can usually be obtained.

Historically, surgical bypass of obstructing lesions
was associated with poor patency and high morbidity
and mortality. However, improved patency using spiral vein grafts without tumor resection for palliation
has been reported (Doty, 1982). In addition, patency
rates of 92% at 1 year following resection of tumor
and superior vena cava with interposition grafting
using *polytetrafluoroethylene* (PTFE) grafts have been
reported (Dartevelle et al., 1987). Of particular importance for success is the presence of adequate flow
through either of the innominate veins. In conditions
in which long-standing superior vena caval obstruction has been present with collateral development,
the innominate veins are usually thrombosed, making
them unsuitable for revascularization. Although long-
term survival is rarely possible in patients with bronchogenic carcinoma following resection with vascular
reconstruction, in selected patients with primary mediastinal tumors, 5-year survival of 60% is reported
(Dartevelle et al., 1991). The usual approach to these
mediastinal tumors is via a median sternotomy.
Cross-clamping of the superior vena cava is well tolerated if prior intravenous volume loading is performed. Heparin is administered prior to clamping.
An 18- to 20-mm PTFE graft is suitable for superior
vena cava replacement, whereas a stented PTFE graft
between 10 and 14 mm is preferred for replacement
of brachiocephalic vein. Postoperative anticoagulation
for at least 6 months with warfarin sodium (Coumadin) is recommended.

Superior vena caval syndromes that are caused by
benign disease usually respond to medical therapy,
which consists of diuretics, upright positioning, and
fluid restriction until collateral channels develop and
lead to clinical regression.

■ **Table 17–2.** PRIMARY MEDIASTINAL TUMORS AND CYSTS IN 2431 PATIENTS

Type of Tumor	Sabiston and Scott, 1952	Heimburger et al., 1963	Burkell et al., 1969	Fontanelle et al., 1971	Benjamin et al., 1972	Conkle and Adkins, 1972	Rubush et al., 1973
Neurogenic tumor	20	21	13	17	49	8	36
Thymoma	17	10	12	17	34	11	42
Lymphoma	11	9	12	16	32	10	14
Germ-cell neoplasm	9	10	3	7	27	2	14
Primary carcinoma	10	11	0	2	0	10	3
Mesenchymal tumor	1	4	4	0	24	2	10
Endocrine tumor	2	8	4	0	24	0	13
Other	14	0	0	0	0	0	0
Cysts	17	24	13	23	19	0	21
Pericardial	2	4	4	2	3	0	10
Bronchogenic	5	12	9	13	11	0	6
Enteric	2	5	0	4	1	0	2
Other	8	3	0	4	4	0	3
Total	101	97	61	82	209	43	153

PRIMARY NEOPLASMS AND CYSTS

Many different histologic neoplasms and cysts arise from multiple anatomic sites in the mediastinum and present with a myriad of clinical signs and symptoms. The natural history varies from those that are asymptomatic to those with benign slow growth, which cause minimal symptoms, to aggressive, invasive neoplasms that are often widely metastatic and rapidly lead to death. The increased use of chest films and the improved sensitivity of imaging techniques have enabled the diagnosis of a mediastinal mass at an earlier stage of disease, frequently in asymptomatic individuals. In addition, an apparent increase in the number of patients with mediastinal mass has occurred. The ability to cure a large number of patients with a mediastinal mass using surgical excision, chemotherapy, or radiation therapy underscores the importance of establishing a precise histologic diagnosis so that optimal therapy can be initiated. The observation of a mediastinal mass, except in rare circumstances, can seldom be justified when operative morbidity and mortality are less than 10% and 1%, respectively (Davis et al., 1987). A classification of primary mediastinal tumors and cysts is shown in Table 17–1. The relative incidence with which they occur in a series of 2431 patients is shown in Table 17–2. Although some differences in the relative incidence of neoplasms and cysts exist in some series, the most common mediastinal masses are neurogenic tumors (21%), thymomas (19%), primary cysts (21%), lymphomas (13%), and germ-cell tumors (10%).

Mediastinal masses are most frequently located in the anterosuperior mediastinum (54%), with the posterior (26%) and the middle mediastinum (20%) less frequently involved. Many of the mediastinal lesions occur in characteristic sites within the mediastinum. The masses that occur most commonly in each of the three anatomic subdivisions and the relative incidence with which they occurred in a series of 441 patients from the Duke University Medical Center are shown in Table 17–3. In the anterosuperior mediastinum, the most frequent neoplasms are thymoma

(31%), lymphoma (23%), and germ-cell tumor (17%). Posterior mediastinal lesions are usually neurogenic tumors (52%), bronchogenic cysts (22%), and enteric cysts (7%). Middle mediastinal masses are usually pericardial cysts (35%), lymphomas (21%), and bronchogenic cysts (15%). Because of the characteristic location of many mediastinal masses, the site of the mass establishes a useful differential diagnosis that aids the diagnosis and planning for possible operation. In addition, the location of the mass explains some of the typical symptoms related to a mediastinal mass because of compression or invasion of adjacent mediastinal structures. Anterosuperior mediastinal masses are most likely to produce the superior vena caval syndrome; middle mediastinal masses are most

■ **Table 17–3.** ANATOMIC LOCATION OF PRIMARY TUMORS AND CYSTS OF THE MEDIASTINUM

Type of Tumor or Cyst	Percentage
Anterosuperior Mediastinum (n = 245)	
Thymic neoplasms	31
Lymphomas	23
Germ-cell tumors	17
Benign	9
Malignant	8
Carcinoma	13
Cysts	6
Mesenchymal	4
Endocrine	5
Other	1
Middle Mediastinum (n = 83)	
Cysts	61
Lymphomas	20
Mesenchymal	8
Carcinoma	6
Other	5
Posterior Mediastinum (n = 113)	
Neurogenic	52
Benign	40
Malignant	12
Cysts	32
Mesenchymal	10
Endocrine	2
Other	4

■ **Table 17–2.** PRIMARY MEDIASTINAL TUMORS AND CYSTS IN 2431 PATIENTS *(Continued)*

Vidne and Levy, 1973	Ovrum and Birkeland, 1979	Nandi et al., 1980	Adkins et al., 1984	Parish et al., 1984	Duke Medical Center, 1988	Total	Incidence (%)
9	19	27	8	212	61	500	21
9	10	18	4	206	68	458	19
6	11	4	7	107	75	314	13
3	5	7	11	99	44	241	10
2	9	0	5	25	37	114	5
4	4	2	0	60	29	144	6
2	21	6	2	56	13	151	6
1	2	1	1	36	10	65	3
8	10	9	0	196	104	444	18
2	7	2	0	72	37	145	6
2	0	0	0	54	39	151	6
1	0	0	0	29	11	55	2
3	3	7	0	41	17	93	4
44	91	74	38	997	441	2431	100

■ **Table 17–4.** CLINICAL MANIFESTATIONS OF ANATOMIC COMPRESSION OR INVASION BY NEOPLASMS OF THE MEDIASTINUM

Vena caval obstruction	Vocal cord paralysis
Pericardial tamponade	Horner's syndrome
Congestive heart failure	Phrenic nerve paralysis
Dysrhythmias	Chylothorax
Pulmonary artery stenosis	Chylopericardium
Pulmonary vein obstruction	Spinal cord compressive
Tracheal/bronchial	syndrome
compression	Pancoast's syndrome
Esophageal compression	Postobstructive pneumonitis

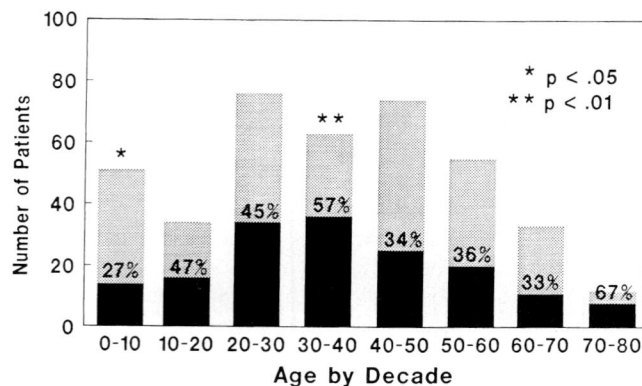

FIGURE 17–5. Age distribution and incidence of malignancy relative to age. The largest number of patients with a mediastinal mass were in the third through fifth decades of life. Those in the fourth decade had a significantly increased proportion of malignant lesions. Those in the first decade of life had a significantly lower proportion of malignant disease. (From Davis, R. D., Oldham, H. N., and Sabiston, D. C., Jr.: Primary cysts and neoplasms of the mediastinum: Recent changes in clinical presentation, methods of diagnosis, management, and results. Reprinted with permission from the Society of Thoracic Surgeons [The Annals of Thoracic Surgery, Vol. 44, 1987, p. 229].)

likely to cause tamponade; posterior mediastinal masses are most likely to cause spinal cord compression syndromes. The common symptoms related to mechanical involvement with mediastinal structures are listed in Table 17–4.

Malignant neoplasms represent 25 to 42% of mediastinal masses. Lymphomas, thymomas, germ-cell tumors, primary carcinomas, and neurogenic tumors are the most common. The relative frequency of mediastinal mass malignancy varies with the anatomic site in the mediastinum. Anterosuperior masses are most likely malignant (59%), relative to middle mediastinal masses (29%) and posterior mediastinal masses (16%). The relative percentage of lesions that are malignant also varies with age (Fig. 17–5). Patients in the second through fourth decades of life have a greater proportion of malignant mediastinal masses. This period corresponds with the peak incidence of lymphomas and germ-cell tumors. In contrast, in the first decade of life, a mediastinal mass is most likely benign (73%).

The incidence of various mediastinal masses varies in infants, children, and adults. In a series of 723 children with mediastinal masses (Table 17–5), neurogenic tumors (35%), lymphomas (25%), germ-cell tumors (10%), and primary cysts (16%) were diagnosed most frequently. The neurogenic tumors in children

most commonly originate from sympathetic ganglion cells, gangliomas, ganglioneuroblastomas, and neuroblastomas. In contrast, neurilemomas and neurofibromas are the most common neurogenic tumors in adults. The childhood lymphomas are usually of a non-Hodgkin variety. The germ-cell tumors are most frequently benign teratomas. Pericardial cysts and thymomas are uncommon in children.

Symptoms

The clinical presentation varies in patients with a mediastinal mass, from those who are asymptomatic

■ **Table 17–5.** PRIMARY MEDIASTINAL TUMORS AND CYSTS IN CHILDREN

Type of Tumor	Haller et al., 1969	Grosfeld et al., 1971	Whittaker and Lynn, 1973	Pokorny and Sherman, 1974	Heimburger and Battersby, 1965	Bower and Kiesewetter, 1977	King et al., 1982	Duke Medical Center, 1988	Total	Incidence (%)
Neurogenic tumor	18	36	37	35	9	41	48	26	250	35
Lymphoma	9	20	9	27	3	12	87	13	180	25
Germ-cell neoplasm	8	5	21	4	4	5	17	11	75	10
Primary carcinoma	10	0	0	6	0	0	0	1	17	2
Mesenchymal tumor	7	1	13	8	6	7	22	5	69	10
Other	0	0	0	0	0	6	4	6	16	2
Cysts	11	6	14	17	10	22	10	26	116	16
Pericardial	1	0	0	0	0	1	0	3	5	1
Bronchogenic	4	0	5	11	8	6	6	14	54	7
Enteric	6	6	7	3	2	11	2	5	42	6
Other	0	0	2	3	0	4	2	4	15	2
Total	63	68	94	97	32	93	188	88	723	100

(the diagnosis is made by routine chest film) to those with symptoms related to mechanical effects of invasion or compression and those who have systemic symptoms. These systemic symptoms may be vague and nonspecific or they may be characteristic for a specific neoplasm, such as the relationship between myasthenia gravis and thymoma.

Of patients with a mediastinal mass, 56 to 65% are symptomatic at presentation. Patients with a benign lesion are more often asymptomatic (54%) than are patients with a malignant neoplasm (15%). The absence of symptoms is associated with a benign histologic diagnosis. In asymptomatic patients with a mediastinal mass at the Duke University Medical Center since the mid-1970s, 76% had a benign lesion. In contrast, 62% of symptomatic patients had a malignant neoplasm during this period. The presenting symptoms in 441 patients are shown in Table 17–6. The most common symptoms were chest pain, cough, and fever. Although myasthenia gravis was present in only 7% of patients from the overall series, of patients with thymoma, 43% had myasthenia gravis. Infants most likely present with symptoms or findings (78%) because of the relatively small space within the mediastinum (King et al., 1982). Paralleling the relative percentages of malignant neoplasms within the different anatomic regions, tumors of the anterosuperior mediastinum are more likely to cause symptoms (75%) than are those of the posterior mediastinum (50%) and the middle mediastinum (45%).

Symptoms related to compression or invasion of mediastinal structures, such as the superior vena caval syndrome, Horner's syndrome, hoarseness, and severe pain usually indicate a malignant histologic diagnosis, although patients with a benign lesion occasionally present in this manner.

Many primary mediastinal lesions produce hormones or antibodies that cause systemic symptoms that may characterize a specific syndrome (Table 17–7), including Cushing's syndrome, caused by ectopic production of *adrenocorticotrophic hormone* (ACTH), most frequently by carcinoid tumors; thyrotoxicosis, caused by a mediastinal goiter; hypertension and a hyperdynamic state caused by pheochromocytoma; and hypercalcemia secondary to increased parathyroid hormone release from a mediastinal parathyroid adenoma.

■ **Table 17–6.** PRESENTING SYMPTOMS IN PATIENTS WITH A MEDIASTINAL MASS

Symptoms	Percentage of Patients (n = 441)
Chest pain	29
Dyspnea	22
Cough	18
Fever	13
Weight loss	9
Superior vena caval syndrome	8
Myasthenia gravis	7
Fatigue	6
Dysphagia	4
Night sweats	3

■ **Table 17–7.** SYSTEMIC SYNDROMES CAUSED BY MEDIASTINAL NEOPLASM HORMONE PRODUCTION

Syndrome	Tumor
Hypertension	Pheochromocytoma, chemodectoma, ganglioneuroma, neuroblastoma
Hypoglycemia	Mesothelioma, teratoma, fibrosarcoma, neurosarcoma
Diarrhea	Ganglioneuroma, neuroblastoma, neurofibroma
Hypercalcemia	Parathyroid adenoma/carcinoma, Hodgkin's disease
Thyrotoxicosis	Thyroid adenoma/carcinoma
Gynecomastia	Nonseminomatous germ-cell tumors
Precocious puberty	Nonseminomatous germ-cell tumors

In other syndromes, the pathophysiology is not as well understood (Table 17–8), such as the association of large mesenchymal tumors with episodic hypoglycemia, which is presumably related to production of circulating factors capable of insulin-like action or of releasing insulin (Doege-Potter syndrome). Autoimmune mechanisms have been implicated in the association of myasthenia gravis and red cell aplasia with thymoma. In other cases, the pathophysiology is less defined: osteoarthropathy and neurogenic tumors, pain after ingestion of alcohol, and the cyclical Pel-Ebstein fevers associated with Hodgkin's disease, the opsomyoclonus syndrome, and neuroblastoma.

Diagnosis

The goal of the diagnostic evaluation in a patient with a mediastinal mass is a precise histologic diagno-

■ **Table 17–8.** SYSTEMIC SYNDROMES ASSOCIATED WITH MEDIASTINAL NEOPLASMS

Tumor	Syndrome
Thymoma	Myasthenia gravis
	Red blood cell aplasia
	White blood cell aplasia
	Aplastic anemia
	Hypogammaglobulinemia
	Progressive system sclerosis
	Hemolytic anemia
	Megaesophagus
	Dermatomyositis
	Systemic lupus erythematosus
	Myocarditis
	Collagen vascular disease
Lymphoma	Anemia, myasthenia gravis
Neurofibroma	von Recklinghausen's disease
Carcinoid	Cushing's syndrome
Carcinoid, thymoma	Multiple endocrine adenomatosis
Thymoma, neurofibroma, neurilemoma, mesothelioma	Osteoarthropathy
Enteric cysts	Vertebral anomalies
Hodgkin's disease	Alcohol-induced pain
	Pel-Ebstein fever
Neuroblastoma	Opsomyoclonus
	Erythrocyte abnormalities
Enteric cysts	Peptic ulcer

sis so that optimal therapy can be performed. The preoperative evaluation of a patient with a mediastinal mass should achieve the following: (1) differentiate a primary mediastinal mass from masses of other causes that have a similar radiographic appearance; (2) recognize associated systemic manifestations that may affect the patient's perioperative course; (3) evaluate the tracheobronchial tree, pulmonary artery, or superior vena cava for possible compression by the mass; (4) ascertain whether the mass extends into the spinal column; (5) determine whether the mass is a nonseminomatous germ-cell tumor; (6) assess the likelihood of resectability; and (7) identify significant factors of medical co-morbidity and optimize overall medical condition.

The initial diagnostic intervention should be a careful history and physical examination. The recognition of associated systemic syndromes with many mediastinal neoplasms is necessary to avoid potentially serious intraoperative and postoperative complications. Although most systemic syndromes listed in Table 17–3 may be of little consequence for planned surgical management, the association of myasthenia gravis, malignant hypertension, hypogammaglobulinemia, hypercalcemia, and thyrotoxicosis with mediastinal neoplasms markedly affects appropriate management.

The posteroanterior and lateral chest films provide important information: location within the mediastinum, size of the lesion, displacement and alteration of anatomic structures in the mediastinum and adjacent regions, and the relative density of the mass with regard to whether the lesion is cystic or solid, whether calcifications are present, and the pattern of the calcifications. Information regarding the anatomic location of the mediastinal mass narrows the differential diagnosis. CT imaging with contrast should be obtained in most patients with a mediastinal mass. In patients with a contraindication to the use of contrast dye or in patients with surgical clips in the anatomic region of interest, MRI is useful. Accurate anatomic information about the relationship of the mass to surrounding structures is provided as well as considerable information about the relative invasiveness and malignant nature of the mediastinal mass. The presence of tumor disruption of fat planes, irregularity of pleural, vascular, or pericardial margins by tumor, and infiltration into muscle or periosteum can differentiate tumor compression from invasion. CT predicts resectability of a neoplasm more accurately than it predicts unresectability. Additional information obtained using CT includes the presence of chest wall invasion, differentiation of multiple masses from a single large mass (useful in distinguishing lymphomas from other common solitary lesions), and possible extension from a posterior mediastinal mass into the spinal column. These posterior mediastinal masses should be further evaluated with CT myelography or MRI.

CT or MRI reliably differentiates mediastinal tumors from mediastinal masses that are of a cardiovascular cause, such as aneurysms, dilatations, and abnormal locations of cardiac or vascular structures, and that may appear on chest film as a mediastinal mass (Table 17–9). Similarly, abnormalities of the spinal column, such as meningoceles, are differentiated from neurogenic tumors and other posterior mediastinal masses. This differentiation is particularly important in patients with neurofibromatosis who are at a greater risk for the development of both meningoceles and neurofibromas. CT or MRI will also differentiate

■ **Table 17–9.** CARDIOVASCULAR ABNORMALITIES THAT MAY APPEAR AS A MEDIASTINAL MASS

Mediastinal Location	Systemic Venous System	Pulmonary Arterial System	Pulmonary Venous System	Systemic Arterial System
Anterior				Aortic stenosis (poststenotic dilatation) Ascending aortic aneurysm
Middle	Superior vena caval aneurysm	Pulmonary valve stenosis	Pulmonary venous varix	Aortic stenosis Right aortic arch
	Partial anomalous pulmonary venous return to the superior vena cava	Idiopathic dilatation of pulmonary trunk Congenital absence of the pulmonary valve Pulmonary embolism	Pulmonary venous confluence	Transverse arch aortic aneurysm Aneurysm/fistula of the coronary artery
	Azygos vein enlargement	Pulmonary arterial hypertension Anomalous left pulmonary artery		
Posterior				Coarctation and pseudocoarctation Descending aortic aneurysm Tortuous innominate artery
Superior	Aneurysms of the innominate veins Persistent left superior vena cava Hemiazygos vein enlargement	Aneurysm of the ductus	Partial anomalous pulmonary venous return to the innominate vein Total anomalous pulmonary venous return (supracardiac)	Cervical aortic arch Coarctation of the aorta Transverse arch aortic aneurysm

other entities that may resemble a mediastinal mass including esophageal lesions, such as esophageal diverticula, tumor, hiatal hernia, and achalasia, diaphragmatic herniations, pancreatic pseudocysts, herniations of peritoneal fat, mediastinitis, and a number of primary pulmonary parenchymal lesions and infections.

Several mediastinal masses can be diagnosed preoperatively using these imaging modalities owing to their characteristic location, appearance, and attenuation values. For example, pericardial cysts usually occur at the cardiophrenic angle; they have smooth, circumscribed borders, and they have near-water attenuation values. Patients with pericardial cysts have been treated using needle aspiration and subsequent follow-up with serial CT scans and chest films to assess recurrence.

Despite the accuracy of CT imaging, emphasis must remain on establishing the precise histologic diagnosis to avoid mistreating a potentially curable neoplasm. Using CT, the correct preoperative diagnosis is made in only approximately 68% of patients (Rendina et al., 1988). Although CT scanning is sensitive in the evaluation of mediastinal masses and lymphadenopathy, it is not specific for tumor involvement. A histologic examination of abnormal mediastinal lymph nodes (>1.5 cm) determined by CT scanning in patients with known malignancies demonstrates that in more than one-third of patients the lymph node was benign (Daly et al., 1987).

Echocardiography may be useful in the evaluation of mediastinal masses, especially tumors that occur in the middle mediastinum, or in patients with tamponade or pulmonary stenosis. In patients with middle mediastinal masses, echocardiography can help differentiate primary masses from intracardiac or pericardial lesions. In patients with acquired pulmonary stenosis, the adjunctive use of color-flow Doppler echocardiography helps to assess the physiologic significance of tumor encasement and compression. Echocardiography delineates the cystic nature of lesions, and it has been used to guide needle biopsy, especially with lesions adjacent to the chest wall. Compared with conventional chest films, echocardiography is more sensitive in evaluating the mediastinum for a mass lesion, particularly in the presence of pericardial or pleural effusion. However, it is not as sensitive as MRI or CT.

Serologic evaluation is indicated in certain patients. Male patients in the second through fifth decades of life with an anterosuperior mediastinal mass should have alpha-fetoprotein (AFP) and human chorionic gonadotropin–beta (HCG-beta) serologies obtained. A positive serology indicates a nonseminomatous germ-cell tumor. Appropriate treatment with cisplatin-based chemotherapy may be initiated without surgical exploration.

Patients with a mediastinal mass and history of significant hypertension or hypermetabolism should have measurement of urinary excretion of vanillylmandelic acid and catecholamines. This enables the initiation of appropriate perioperative adrenergic blockers in patients with hormonally active intrathoracic pheochromocytoma, paraganglioma, and neuroblastoma, limiting perioperative complications secondary to episodic catecholamine release. In these patients, nuclear scans using *meta-iodobenzylguanidine* (MIBG) locate tumors and identify sites of metastatic disease, particularly when located in the middle mediastinum.

Asymptomatic patients with contrast enhancing lesions in the superior mediastinum should be evaluated with an ^{131}I scan. In an *asymptomatic* patient with a positive scan indicating a thyroid lesion and no identifiable active thyroid tissue elsewhere, careful observation without excision using serial CTs to evaluate for growth is indicated.

Increased success has been reported in making a cytologic diagnosis preoperatively by using fine-needle biopsy techniques (No. 22 gauge needle), with low morbidity and almost zero mortality. Fluoroscopic visualization is generally used to guide the biopsy. CT and echocardiography, because of better localization of the mass and improved placement of the needle, have increased the sensitivity of the technique. Although a precise histologic diagnosis is not always possible, a cytologic diagnosis of either benign or malignant can be made in 80 to 90% of patients. Complications related to the procedure include pneumothorax in 20 to 25% of patients, with approximately 5% requiring tube thoracostomy; hemoptysis in 5 to 10%, with rare occurrences of significant hemorrhagic complications; and tumor seeding along the needle tract, a theoretical but extremely rare complication. An increased sensitivity in obtaining a precise histologic diagnosis has been reported using cutting needle techniques (No. 16 gauge needle) without an apparent increase in morbidity (23% incidence of pneumothorax). Needle-biopsy techniques are particularly useful for evaluating patients with small-cell carcinoma or metastatic carcinoma, because they may obviate a thoracotomy or other invasive procedure to establish a histologic diagnosis. Electron microscopy, used to examine the cellular ultrastructure, and immunohistochemical staining have increased the sensitivity of the various needle-biopsy techniques.

Some tumors with marked associated desmoplastic changes, such as nodular-sclerosing Hodgkin's lymphoma, are rarely diagnosed using a needle biopsy. Additionally, needle biopsy rarely provides adequate tissue to do precise immunotyping, which is necessary to determine optimal therapy, particularly with the non-Hodgkin lymphomas. Poorly differentiated malignant tumors of the anterosuperior mediastinum, particularly thymomas, lymphomas, germ-cell tumors, and primary carcinomas, can have remarkably similar cytologic and morphologic appearances. Diagnoses based on examination of frozen sections are therefore frequently incorrect; similarly, therapeutic decisions based on frozen-section examination may be in error. In addition to light microscopy, which uses special staining techniques, immunostaining techniques and electron microscopy of multiple sections of the tumor may be necessary to establish an accurate diagnosis. The characteristic ultrastructural features as evaluated by electron microscopy are shown in Table 17–10. Monoclonal antibodies for surface antigens specific to a cell line of origin and for tumor-secretory products can be useful in establishing a precise diagnosis. Immunotyping of non-Hodgkin's lymphomas has allowed accurate subtyping of these lesions, which has been important in predicting natural history and optimal therapy. Chromosomal analysis of tumor tissue is often useful for differentiating histology (Motzer et al., 1991).

Although surgical excision is not essential for the treatment of a number of malignant neoplasms, the optimal therapeutic regimen often requires precise histologic subclassification. Because needle-biopsy techniques do not usually produce sufficient tissue for this purpose, more invasive procedures are often required, such as mediastinoscopy, mediastinotomy, thoracotomy, and median sternotomy. Mediastinoscopy is a useful technique to evaluate and biopsy lesions of the middle mediastinum, particularly those located in the anterior aspect of the subcarinal space, around the proximal mainstem bronchi, and around the lower trachea. Often, this technique is used to evaluate associated lymphadenopathy in these particular regions. Lesions in the anterosuperior mediastinum that are thought to be unresectable are best biopsied using a limited anterior second or third interspace parasternal mediastinotomy. Similarly, unresectable lesions in the superior mediastinum, hilar, or paratracheal regions can be biopsied through a small lateral thoracotomy in the third or fourth interspace after retracting the apex of the lung inferiorly. Unresectable posterior mediastinal masses may be approached through a limited posterolateral thoracotomy. A representative section of the tissue obtained should be submitted for immediate frozen section to establish adequacy of the biopsy before closing.

It is important that the incision not be made in the portals for potential radiotherapy. Lesions that appear resectable should be excised. Median sternotomy and anterolateral thoracotomy provide optimal exposure for lesions in the anterosuperior mediastinum. A transcervical approach using sternal elevators has been successful in some centers for resection of tumors in the superior aspect of the anterosuperior mediastinum. Middle and posterior mediastinal masses are usually best excised through a posterolateral thoracotomy.

■ **Table 17–10.** ULTRASTRUCTURAL CHARACTERISTICS OF MEDIASTINAL TUMORS

Tumors	Ultrastructure
Carcinoid	Dense core granules, fewer tonofilaments and desmosomes
Lymphoma	Absence of junctional attachments and epithelial features
Thymoma	Well-formed desmosomes, bundles of tonofilaments
Germ-cell	Prominent nucleoli, even chromatin, scant desmosomes, rare tonofilaments
Neuroblastoma	Neurosecretory granules, synaptic endings

Thoracoscopic and thoracoscopically assisted procedures have been used to biopsy and resect a variety of mediastinal lesions in carefully selected patients.

Although most patients undergo surgical procedures safely, a subset of patients, particularly children with large anterosuperior or middle mediastinal masses, has an increased risk of developing severe cardiorespiratory complications during general anesthesia. Exacerbation of superior vena caval obstruction or extrinsic airway compression occurs during general anesthesia because of the loss of negative intrathoracic pressure during respiration, bronchial smooth muscle relaxation that increases the compressibility of the bronchi, and reduced tidal volumes used for ventilation. Patients with posture-related dyspnea and superior vena caval syndrome are at increased risk. Useful techniques for identifying less symptomatic patients who have significant airway compromise include CT imaging, in which a reduction in tracheal cross-sectional area of more than 35% indicates an increased risk with general anesthesia, and pulmonary flow mechanics, in which reductions in peak expiratory flow serve as a sensitive indicator of functional airway compression (Azizkhan et al., 1985; Neuman et al., 1984).

In patients with airway compression or superior vena caval obstruction, the risk of general anesthesia is prohibitive, and attempts to obtain a histologic diagnosis should be limited to needle biopsies or open procedures performed under local anesthesia. If a histologic diagnosis cannot be obtained, treatment with radiation, corticosteroids, and when appropriate, chemotherapy based on a presumptive diagnosis should be used to establish an adequate airway. When such treatment is necessary before biopsy, a histologic diagnosis may not be obtainable in as many as 40% of patients. Most of these lesions are malignant and unresectable; of these, non-Hodgkin's lymphoma, Hodgkin's lymphoma, malignant germ-cell tumors, neuroblastomas, and malignant mesenchymal tumors are the most frequent.

Occasionally, benign tumors, usually benign teratomas in young children and infants, may produce this clinical setting. In patients with large mediastinal masses who have an increased anesthetic risk but for whom a histologic diagnosis is needed before therapy, or for whom complete excision is the preferred treatment, recommendations for anesthetic management include (1) fiberoptic evaluation of the tracheobronchial system for evidence of severe extrinsic compression (Fig. 17–6); (2) induction of anesthesia in a semi-Fowler position, with the ability to change to the lateral or prone positions; (3) use of long endotracheal tubes to advance beyond the site of obstruction; (4) standby rigid bronchoscopy to reestablish an adequate airway; (5) avoidance of muscle relaxants and use of spontaneous ventilation when possible; (6) lower extremity intravenous intubation to provide access to the systemic venous circulation if a sudden superior vena caval obstruction should occur; and (7) standby cardiopulmonary bypass with bilateral groin preparation.

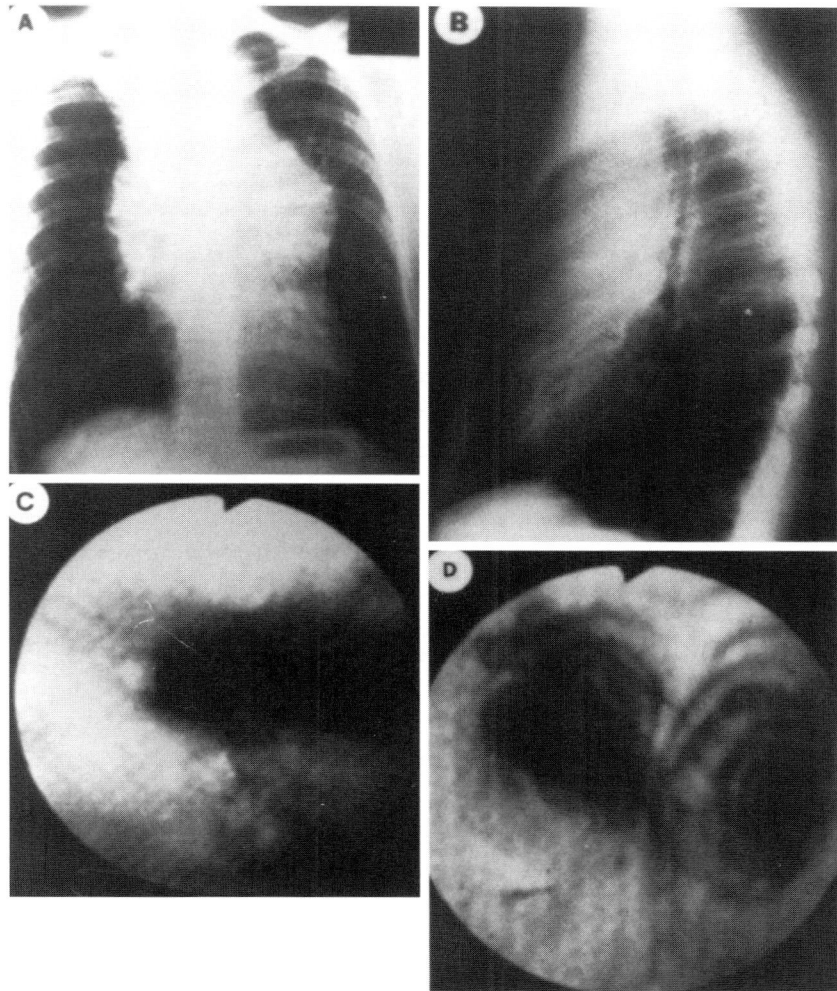

FIGURE 17–6. Posteroanterior (A) and lateral (B) chest films demonstrating a large antero-superior mediastinal mass in a 24-year-old man. C, Fiberoptic bronchoscopic evaluation of the lower trachea with the patient in a supine position, which demonstrates almost total obstruction of the trachea in the anteroposterior plane. D, With the patient in a semi-Fowler position, the lumen appears normal. (A–D, From Prakash, U. B. S., Abel, M. D., and Hubmayr, R. D.: Mediastinal mass and tracheal obstruction during general anesthesia. Mayo Clin. Proc., 63:1004–1011, 1988.)

Neurogenic Tumors

Neurogenic tumors were the most common neoplasm in the collected series of patients, accounting for 21% of all primary tumors and cysts. These tumors are usually located in the posterior mediastinum and originate from the sympathetic ganglia (ganglioma, ganglioneuroblastoma, and neuroblastoma), the intercostal nerves (neurofibroma, neurilemoma, and neurosarcoma), and the paraganglia cells (paraganglioma). Only rarely are these tumors located in the anterosuperior mediastinum. Although the peak incidence occurs in adults, neurogenic tumors represent a proportionally greater percentage of mediastinal masses in children (34%). Whereas the majority of neurogenic tumors in adults are benign, a greater percentage of neurogenic tumors are malignant in children.

Many of these tumors are found in asymptomatic patients on routine chest films. When present, symptoms are usually caused by mechanical factors, such as chest and back pain due to compression or invasion of intercostal nerve, bone, and chest wall; cough and dyspnea due to compression of the tracheobron-

chial tree; Pancoast's syndrome and Horner's syndrome due to involvement of the brachial and cervical sympathetic chain. Approximately 10% of neurogenic tumors have extensions into the spinal column. These are called *dumbbell tumors* because of their characteristic shape, with relatively large paraspinal and intraspinal portions connected by a narrow isthmus of tissue traversing the intervertebral foramen (Fig. 17–7). Although 60% of patients with a dumbbell tumor have neurologic symptoms related to spinal cord compression, the significant proportion of patients without symptoms underscores the importance of evaluating all patients with a posterior mediastinal mass for possible intraspinal extension. CT, MRI, and vertebral tomography are useful for indicating foramen enlargement, bone erosion, and intervertebral widening. If these findings are present, CT with myelography or MRI is indicated to evaluate the presence and extent of the intraspinal component. The recommended surgical approach to dumbbell tumors is a one-stage removal, performed by a team of neurosurgeons and thoracic surgeons. Excision of the intraspinal component is performed before resection of the thoracic component to minimize any spinal column

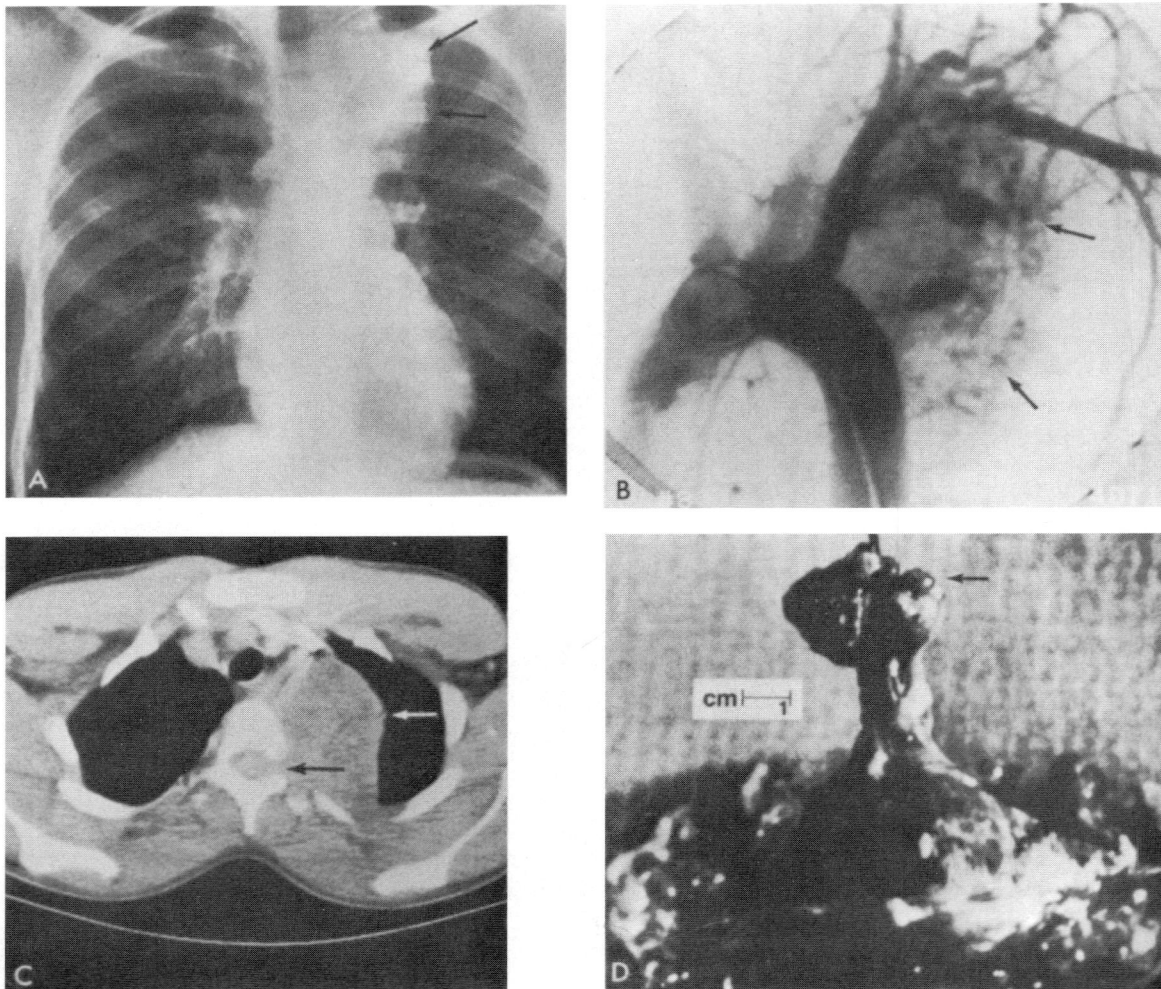

FIGURE 17–7. Chest film showing paraganglioma of the posterior mediastinum *(A)*. Digital subtraction angiogram demonstrates extensive vascularity of the tumor *(B)*. A computed tomography (CT) scan shows the tumor mass *(white arrow)* and the widening of the intervertebral foramen *(black arrow)* caused by "dumbbell" intraspinal extension *(C)*. Gross photograph of the operative specimen shows the intraspinal portion of the tumor above *(arrow)* joined by a narrow neck to the large mediastinal tumor *(D)*. The entire tumor was removed during a one-stage procedure. *(A–D,* Courtesy of Lary A. Robinson, University of Nebraska Medical Center, Omaha, NB.)

hematoma. The incision used for the posterior laminectomy is extended into the appropriate interspace to allow resection of the mediastinal component. Improved results and decreased morbidity have been reported with this approach.

Symptoms may be systemic and related to production of neurohormonal agents. Production of catecholamine by paragangliomas and neuroblastomas causes the constellation of symptoms that is characteristic of pheochromocytomas: hypertension, which is often severe and episodic, sweating, headaches, and palpitations. Production of vasoactive intestinal polypeptide by ganglioneuromas and neuroblastomas causes abdominal distention and profuse watery diarrhea. Secretion of an insulin-like factor or insulin-releasing factor by neurosarcomas causes the Doege-Potter syndrome, characterized by episodic hypoglycemia.

Neuroblastoma

Neuroblastomas originate from the sympathetic nervous system and therefore can occur wherever sympathetic nervous tissue is present. The most common location for a neuroblastoma is in the retroperitoneum; however, 10 to 20% occur primarily in the mediastinum (Fig. 17–8). These are highly invasive neoplasms that frequently have metastasized before diagnosis. Common sites of metastases are the regional lymph nodes, bone, brain, liver, and lung. Most of these tumors occur in children; 75% occur in children under 4 years old. The tumor consists of small, round, immature cells organized in a rosette pattern. On ultrastructural examination, the presence of neurosecretory granules is characteristic. Patients are usually symptomatic, most commonly with cough, dyspnea, dysphagia, back or chest pain, and symptoms related to recurrent pulmonary infections. One series found that paraplegia and other neurologic symptoms related to spinal cord compression were present in one-third of children with mediastinal neuroblastoma (Simpson and Campbell, 1991). Various paraneoplastic syndromes have been reported, including profuse watery diarrhea and abdominal pain related to *vaso-*

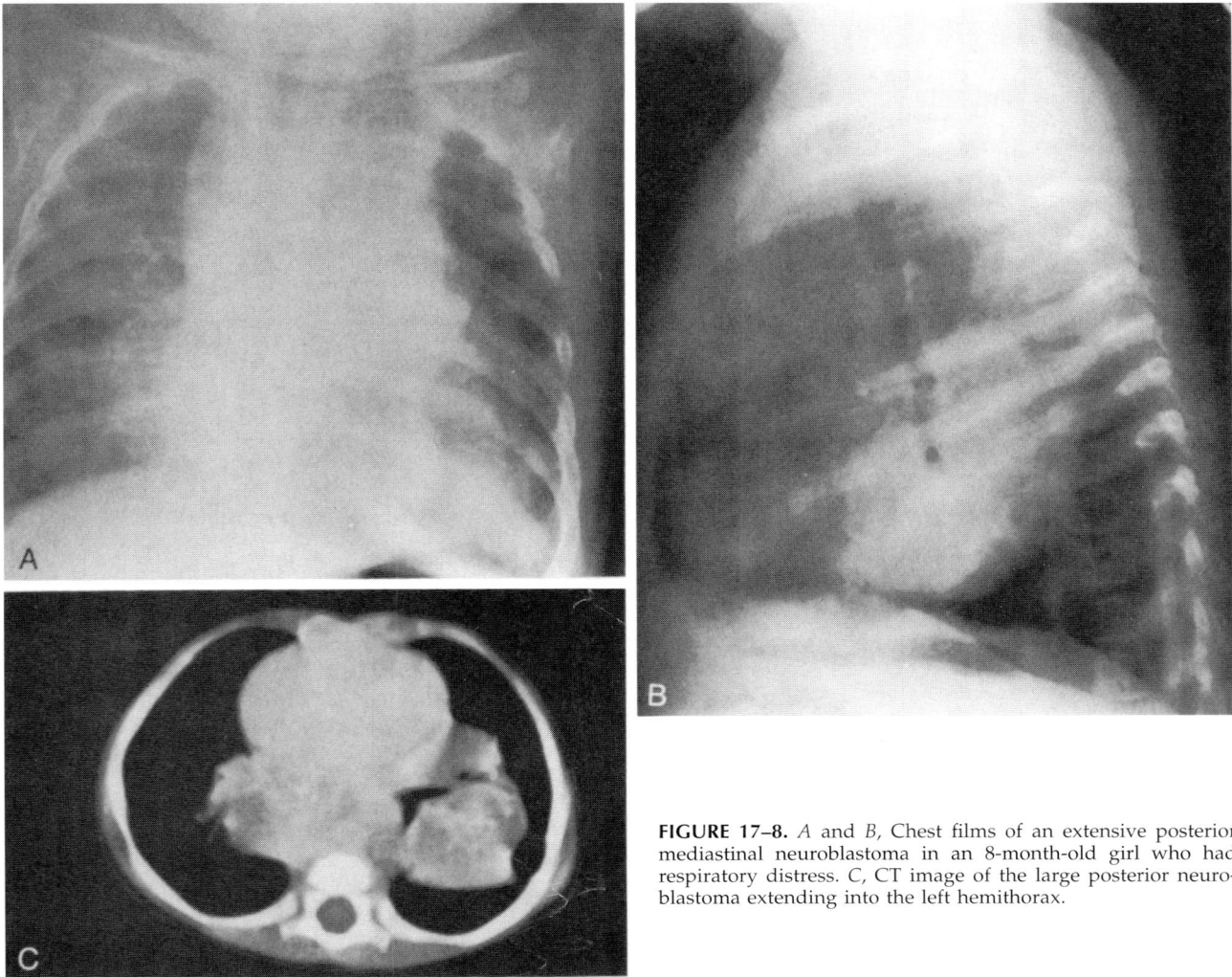

FIGURE 17–8. *A* and *B*, Chest films of an extensive posterior mediastinal neuroblastoma in an 8-month-old girl who had respiratory distress. *C*, CT image of the large posterior neuroblastoma extending into the left hemithorax.

active intestinal polypeptide production; the opsoclonus-polymyoclonus syndrome—an unexplained symptom complex characterized by cerebellar and truncal ataxia with rapid, darting eye movements (dancing eyes) that is possibly related to an autoimmune mechanism; and "pheochromocytoma" syndrome owing to catecholamine secretion. Measurement of 24-hour urine for catecholamines should be obtained in children with a posterior mediastinal mass. In patients with the opsoclonus-polymyoclonus syndrome, successful treatment of the tumor or the use of corticosteroids relieves symptoms.

The immunobiology of neuroblastomas is unique. Well-documented cases of spontaneous regression or maturation of tumor have been reported. Lymphocytes collected from these patients have proved to be cytotoxic T-cells capable of causing tumor lysis in vitro. Patients in whom tumor progression or relapse occurs appear to have suppressor T-cells, as well as circulating antigen-antibody complexes capable of inhibiting tumor regression.

Neuroblastoma and ganglioneuroblastoma are staged as follows—Stage I: well-circumscribed, noninvasive tumor; Stage II: tumor invasion locally without extension across the midline; Stage III: tumor spread across the midline; Stage IV: tumor with metastasis. Therapy is determined by the stage of the disease—Stage I: surgical excision; Stage II: excision and radiation therapy; Stages III and IV: multimodality therapy using surgical debulking, radiation therapy, and multiagent chemotherapy, as well as a second-look exploration to resect residual disease when necessary. The usual chemotherapeutic agents include cisplatin, doxorubicin, cyclophosphamide, and etoposide. Children under 1 year of age have an excellent prognosis even when widespread disease is present. However, with increasing age and extent of involvement, the prognosis worsens. N-myc gene amplification and particularly N-myc protein expression are associated with an unfavorable prognosis (Shamberger et al., 1991). Interestingly, mediastinal neuroblastomas appear to have a better prognosis than tumors occurring elsewhere. In patients with neuroblastomas resistant to therapy or in those who relapse, ablative chemotherapy with autologous bone marrow transplantation has been attempted with some success.

Ganglioneuroblastoma

Ganglioneuroblastomas exhibit an intermediate degree of differentiation between ganglioneuromas and neuroblastomas (see Fig. 17–8). They are composed of mature and immature ganglion cells. Stout defined two histologic patterns that differed in their natural history: composite ganglioneuroblastoma, predominantly mature neuroblasts with focal areas containing primitive neuroblasts, and diffuse ganglioneuroblastoma, a diffuse mixture of well-differentiated and primitive neuroblasts. Composite ganglioneuroblastomas have a much greater incidence of metastasis, with most series reporting an incidence between 65 and 75%. In contrast, less than 5% of patients with the diffuse variety develop metastases.

Younger patients who have a diffuse histologic appearance and a lower-stage tumor have the best prognosis. Five-year survival of 88% has been reported in patients with Stage I or II disease treated solely by excision. Patients with Stage III or IV disease, composite morphology, or age greater than 3 years are treated with multiagent chemotherapy.

Ganglioneuroma

Ganglioneuromas, composed of ganglion cells and nerve fibers, are benign tumors originating from the sympathetic chain. These tumors typically present at an early age and are the most common neurogenic tumors occurring during childhood. The usual location is the paravertebral region. On the chest film, they have an elongated or triangular appearance, with the broader base directed toward the mediastinum. Poorly defined on lateral projection, the inferior and superior margins are often indistinct. These tumors are well encapsulated, and when cross-sectioned, they frequently exhibit areas of cystic degeneration. Surgical excision provides cure.

Neurilemoma and Neurofibromas

The most common neurogenic tumor is the neurilemoma, which originates from the perineural Schwann cells. These tumors are well circumscribed and have a defined capsule. There are two morphologic patterns: Antoni's Type A, which has organized architecture with a cellular pallisading pattern of growth, and Antoni's Type B, which has a loose reticular pattern of growth. The peak incidence of these tumors is in the third through fifth decades of life.

In contrast to neurilemomas, neurofibromas are poorly encapsulated and consist of randomly arranged spindle-shaped cells. These tumors originate as a proliferation of all the elements of the peripheral nerve. Although both neurilemomas and neurofibromas occur as a manifestation of neurofibromatosis (von Recklinghausen's disease), they must be differentiated from the two other common entities in the posterior mediastinum, meningioma and meningocele. With both neurilemoma and neurofibroma, surgical excision results in cure.

Neurosarcoma

Neurosarcomas originate through malignant degeneration of either neurilemomas or neurofibromas, or develop de novo, and they usually occur in adults. However, patients with neurofibromatosis may develop neurosarcomas as children. These rapidly growing tumors frequently invade vital structures, preventing attempts at resection. Microscopically, neurosarcomas are extremely cellular tumors composed of spindle cells. Occasionally, these tumors have been associated with recurrent episodes of hypoglycemia that appear to be related to secretion of an insulin-like product. Control of the tumor has resolved symptoms. Unless tumor excision is possible, the prognosis is extremely poor; adjuvant therapies are unresponsive.

Paraganglioma (Pheochromocytoma)

Mediastinal paragangliomas are rare tumors, representing less than 1% of all mediastinal tumors and less than 2% of all pheochromocytomas. Although most are found in the paravertebral sulcus, an increasing number of middle mediastinal paragangliomas occur in the branchial arch structures, coronary and aortopulmonary paraganglia, the atria, and islands of tissue in the pericardium. Because the clinical behavior of extra-adrenal paragangliomas depends on the site of origin, a division based on anatomic location, histochemical features, and innervation has been created (Glenner and Grimley, 1974): (1) branchiomeric (chemodectoma) paraganglias, which are associated with the arteries and cranial nerves derived from the branchial arches, including intercarotid (carotid body), jugulotympanic (glomus jugulare and glomus tympanic), orbital, laryngeal, subclavian, aortopulmonary, coronary, and pulmonary structures; (2) intravagal paragangliomas; (3) aorticosympathetic paragangliomas, which are associated with the sympathetic chain and retroperitoneal ganglia; and (4) visceral-autonomic paragangliomas, which include the atria, urinary bladder, liver hilum, and mesenteric vessels. The likelihood of functional activity of a paraganglioma is related to the site of origin: adrenal medulla (high likelihood) branchiomeric and intravagal (very low likelihood), aortosympathetic and visceral autonomic (intermediate likelihood). Catecholamine production causes the classic constellation of symptoms associated with pheochromocytomas, including periodic or sustained hypertension, often accompanied by orthostatic hypotension, hypermetabolism manifested by weight loss, hyperhidrosis, palpitations, and headaches. Measurement of elevated levels of urinary catecholamines or their metabolites, the metanephrines and vanillylmandelic acid usually establishes the diagnosis. Although adrenal pheochromocytomas often produce both epinephrine and norepinephrine, extra-adrenal paragangliomas rarely secrete epinephrine.

Tumor localization has improved remarkably through the use of CT and meta-iodobenzylguanidine (^{131}I-MIBG) scintigraphy, particularly when the tumors are hormonally active. Hormonally active tumors may be located with an 85% sensitivity using the ^{131}I-MIBG scan. Owing to the high vascularity of these lesions, enhancement with contrast administration during CT imaging occurs, and in 30% of cases, a tumor blush may be seen during thoracic arteriography. Selective venous angiography with serial sampling for catecholamine levels to observe a step-up is occasionally necessary for preoperative localization. Tumor localization using MRI has been reported.

When appropriate, surgical resection is the optimal therapy. In patients with tumors involving the middle mediastinum, cardiopulmonary bypass may be necessary to allow resection. Differentiation of benign from malignant tumors is determined by the patient's clinical course. Although 50% of tumors appear malignant morphologically, metastatic disease develops in only 3% of patients. In those with metastatic disease, alpha-methyl tyramine, a tyrosine hydroxylase inhibitor that blocks the synthesis of catecholamines, helps control symptoms.

Approximately 10% of patients have multiple paragangliomas. They are more common in patients with *multiple endocrine neoplastic* (MEN) syndrome, a family history of disease, and Carney's syndrome (pulmonary chondroma, gastric leiomyosarcoma, and extraadrenal paraganglioma). In patients who have had excision of an adrenal pheochromocytoma and continue to have symptoms, a search for an extra-adrenal lesion should be undertaken, with careful evaluation of the mediastinum.

Thymoma

Thymoma is the most common neoplasm of the anterosuperior mediastinum and the second most common mediastinal mass (19%; Table 17–2). The peak incidence is in the third through fifth decades of life, but thymomas occur throughout adulthood. They are rare in the first two decades. Roentgenographically, they may appear as a small, well-circumscribed mass or a bulky lobulated mass confluent with adjacent mediastinal structures (Fig. 17–9). Patients are usually symptomatic at presentation, and symptoms may be related to local mass effects causing chest pain, dyspnea, hemoptysis, cough, and the superior vena caval syndrome. However, thymomas are frequently associated with systemic syndromes presumably caused by an immunologic mechanism. The most common syndrome is myasthenia gravis. However, many other syndromes have been associated with thymomas, including red blood cell aplasia, pure white cell aplasia, aplastic anemia, Cushing's syndrome, hypo- and hypergammaglobulinemia, dermatomyositis, systemic lupus erythematosus, progressive systemic sclerosis, hypercoagulopathy with thrombosis, rheumatoid arthritis, megaesophagus, and granulomatous myocarditis.

The etiologic factors involved in these syndromes have not been fully elucidated. Myasthenia gravis is characterized pathologically by destruction of post-synaptic nicotinic receptors. The mechanism is postulated to be an autoimmune process. In most myasthenic patients, antiacetylcholine receptor antibodies are present in high titers. Thymic lymphocytes isolated from myasthenic patients produce significant amounts of antiacetylcholine receptor antibodies, and this production is enhanced by autologous or allogeneic thymic epithelial cells (Safar et al., 1987). The thymic myoid cells bear complete acetylcholine receptors; the thymic epithelial cells and tumor epithelial cell contain acetylcholine receptor–related antigenic determinants, but not the complete acetylcholine receptor. These antigenic determinants are thought to be involved in the autosensitization; the varied antigenic determinants may be related to the heterogeneity of antiacetylcholine receptor antibodies. In patients with myasthenia gravis, there is an intimate relationship between the antigen-producing myoid cells and the interdigitating reticulum cells (potentially antigen-presenting) that are surrounded by T-helper (T3 +) lymphocytes. In these patients, T-lymphocytes reactive to acetylcholine receptors are present, and in the majority, acetylcholine receptor–specific T-lymphocyte cell lines could be established that contain helper and inducer subsets (Melms et al., 1988). Similarly, the various hematologic abnormalities associated with thymomas appear to have an autoimmune basis. Serum from patients with red cell aplasia in the presence of complement, as well as T-lymphocytes isolated from these patients, can suppress erythropoiesis colonies in vitro (Taniguchi et al., 1988). However, the mechanisms that develop and maintain these syndromes have not been completely elucidated. Clinical phenomena related to these syndromes are not well understood. The systemic syndromes often do not improve following successful control of the thymoma. Multiple associated syndromes may be present in a patient with a thymoma, suggesting a possible common etiologic factor. For myasthenia gravis, the number of complete remissions achieved increases with increasing length of follow-up after thymectomy. In addition, the change in the acetylcholine receptor antibody titer following thymectomy does not correlate well with the patient's clinical response.

Myasthenia gravis occurs in 10 to 50% of patients with thymoma and is characterized clinically by weakness and fatigue of the skeletal muscles but sparing the cardiac or smooth musculature. Muscles innervated by cranial nerves are the most frequently involved, particularly the extraocular muscles. However, generalized weakness occurs, and myasthenia crisis may cause respiratory failure. In only 14% of patients does the disease remain localized to the extraocular muscles. In patients in whom the disease becomes generalized, it does so in 87% within the first year after onset of symptoms. Peak severity is reached by 1 year in 55%, by 3 years in 70%, and in 85% by 5 years. Male patients have more rapid progression of disease, fewer remissions, and less improvement with treatment than do females (Berrih-Aknin et al., 1987).

The incidence with which myasthenia gravis occurs

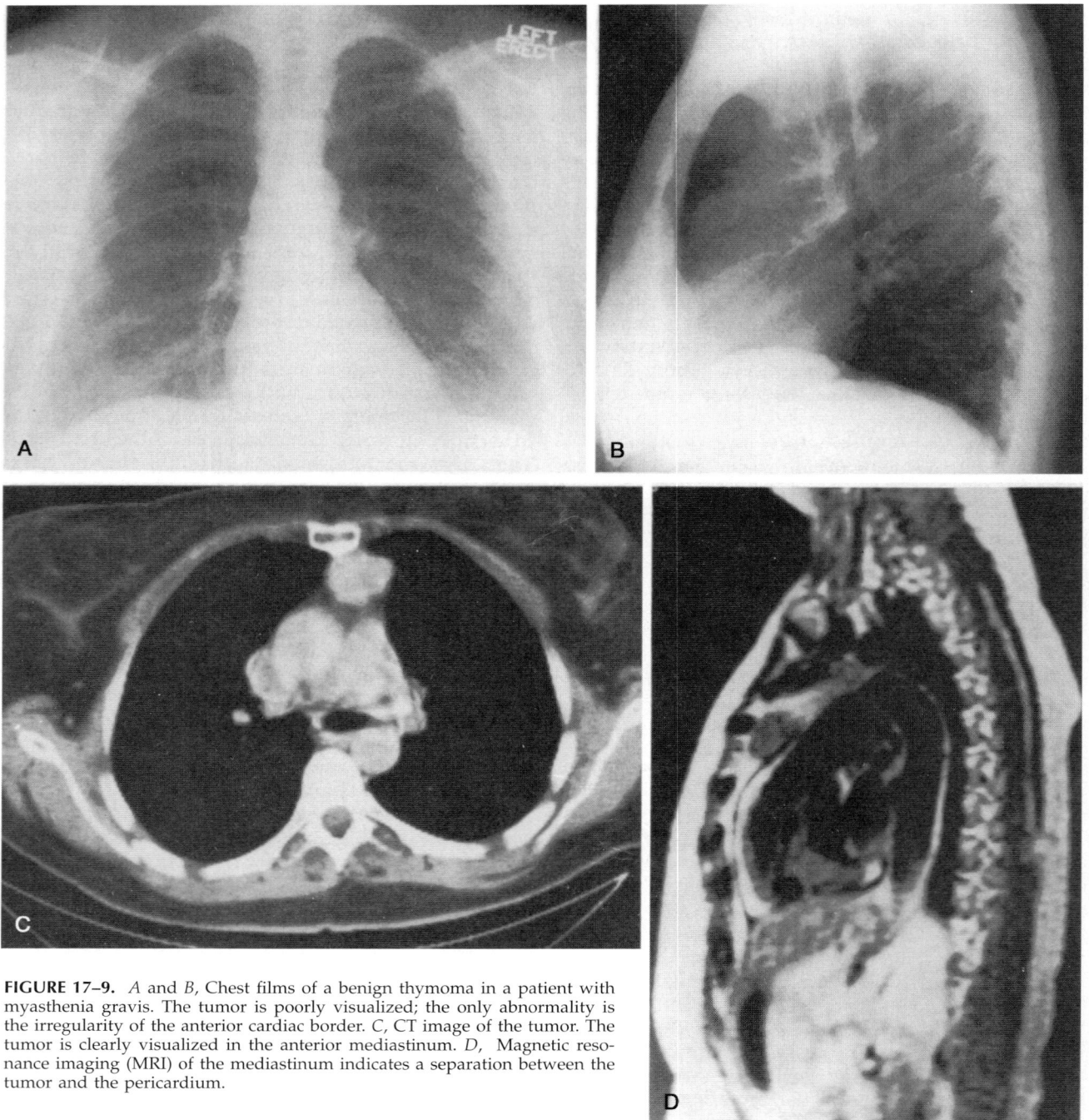

FIGURE 17–9. *A* and *B*, Chest films of a benign thymoma in a patient with myasthenia gravis. The tumor is poorly visualized; the only abnormality is the irregularity of the anterior cardiac border. *C*, CT image of the tumor. The tumor is clearly visualized in the anterior mediastinum. *D*, Magnetic resonance imaging (MRI) of the mediastinum indicates a separation between the tumor and the pericardium.

in patients with thymoma increases with the age of the patient. In men over 50 years and women over 60 years, the incidence appears to be greater than 80%. Most patients with myasthenia gravis do not have thymoma. The incidence is 10 to 42%, depending on the reporting medical center. Male patients with myasthenia gravis are 1.8 to 2 times more likely than females to have a thymoma. Because of the significant association between thymoma and myasthenia gravis, an evaluation of the mediastinum with CT or MRI is recommended for all patients with myasthenia gravis.

The diagnosis of myasthenia gravis is usually con-

firmed by a transient increase in muscle strength following the administration of a short-acting anticholinesterase inhibitor such as edrophonium (Tensilon). Electromyography testing is also used to make the diagnosis and to follow quantitatively the course of the disease. An abnormal loss of muscle contraction strength following multiple stimulations (usually 3 to 5/sec) of the appropriate motor nerve constitutes a positive test.

Since Blalock's pioneering work in 1939, thymectomy has been a significant component in the treatment of myasthenia gravis. The use of median sternotomy to perform extended thymectomy, which includes the removal of all anterior mediastinal fatty-areolar tissue in addition to the thymus gland, has led to improved clinical benefit with fewer recurrences. This technique was developed to extirpate all ectopic foci of thymic tissue and to prevent recurrences, which often followed transcervical thymectomy. In 85 to 96% of patients, clinical improvement, defined as decreased symptoms, decreased use of medications, or remission, occurs following thymectomy (Fischer et al., 1987; Jaretzki et al., 1988). Drug-free remission is achieved in 46 to 63%. Remission rates increase with duration after thymectomy (up to 81% at 89 months). Improved results and earlier remissions are associated with shorter duration of disease before thymectomy, decreased severity of disease, female sex (remission in 82% of females vs. 46% of males) (Fischer et al., 1987), and absence of thymoma (remission rate of 13%, benefit rate 60%) (Jaretzki et al., 1988). Although red blood cell aplasia occurs in only 5% of patients with thymoma, 33 to 50% of adults with red blood cell aplasia have a thymoma.

Thymomas are histologically classified either by the predominance of epithelial or lymphocytic cells (lymphocytic, epithelial, mixed, and spindle) or by the morphologic resemblance to cortical or medullary epithelium. Unfortunately, a wide variance in the cellular composition is often present within the tumor, and a consistent relationship is not present between the microscopic appearance and the biologic behavior, with regard to either tumor invasiveness or association with systemic syndromes. However, one series reported an improved 10-year survival in patients with spindle cell or lymphocyte-rich thymomas (75%), as compared with differentiated (50%) and undifferentiated (0%) epithelial type (Verley and Hollman, 1985). Similarly, the differentiation into medullary and cortical types has been shown to offer no prognostic information in one series (Kornstein et al., 1988), whereas in another series, the presence of cortical morphology was associated with a malignant clinical course (Elert et al., 1988).

The differentiation between benign and malignant disease is determined by the presence of gross invasion of adjacent structures, metastasis, or microscopic evidence of capsular invasion. Morphometric analysis of the nuclei of thymomas shows that invasive thymomas are histologically more malignant than noninvasive thymomas. Of interest, nuclei in noninvasive thymomas from patients with associated myasthenia gravis are larger than those from patients without myasthenia gravis. Fifteen to 65% of thymomas are benign. The relative percentage is partially related to early surgical treatment of myasthenia gravis; if thymectomy is performed early in the course of myasthenia gravis, a greater percentage of thymomas are benign.

Whenever possible, the therapy for thymoma is surgical excision without removing or injuring vital structures. Even with well-encapsulated thymomas, extended thymectomy with eradication of all accessible mediastinal fatty-areolar tissue should be performed to ensure removal of all ectopic thymic tissue. This approach has lowered the number of tumor recurrences. The best operative exposure is obtained using a median sternotomy. Because many thymomas are radiosensitive, the placement of surgical clips to outline the anatomic extent of disease helps determine optimal radiation portals.

In patients with myasthenia gravis, perioperative patient management is extremely important to prevent complications. Discontinuation of anticholinesterase inhibitors decreases the amount of pulmonary secretions and prevents inadvertent cholinergic weakness. This is usually possible with the routine use of plasmapheresis within 72 hours of thymectomy. In most patients, plasmapheresis is very effective in controlling generalized weakness. Also, careful attention to the maintenance of pulmonary function with chest physiotherapy, endotracheal suctioning, and bronchodilators is the mainstay of postoperative management. Decision to extubate is based on evidence of adequate respiratory mechanics (e.g., vital capacity greater than 15 ml/kg and expiratory pressures greater than 40 cm H_2O) rather than evidence of adequate ventilation as determined by analysis of arterial blood gases. Historically, myasthenic patients with thymoma had a poor prognosis. The introduction of plasmapheresis and improvements in anesthesia and medical therapy have eliminated the presence of myasthenia gravis as an adverse prognostic indicator. The prognosis in patients with thymoma depends on the stage of the disease.

Staging of thymoma is as follows: In Stage I, the tumor is well encapsulated without evidence of gross or microscopic capsular invasion; in Stage II, the tumor exhibits pericapsular growth into adjacent mediastinal fat, pleura, or pericardium; in Stage III, the tumor invades adjacent organs or intrathoracic metastasis is present; in Stage IV, extrathoracic metastatic spread can occur uncommonly. The adjunctive use of radiation therapy with a dose of 3500 to 5000 rads is the recommended treatment for Stages II and III disease. In one series with Stage II or III disease following complete resection, the 5-year actuarial mediastinal relapse rate was 53% in those patients not receiving radiation therapy, 0% in those receiving radiation therapy, and 21% in those with biopsy alone and radiation therapy (Curran et al., 1988). In patients with resectable Stage III disease, excellent long-term results can be obtained with radiotherapy: 100% 5-year survival and 95% 10- and 15-year survival (Nakahara et al., 1989). Preoperative radiation therapy is useful when superior vena caval obstruction is present or when extensive invasion is manifested by CT or MRI. Occasionally, tumors not resectable on initial exploration are resectable following therapy. In patients with Stage IV disease or recurrent disease that is unresponsive to prior therapy, multiagent chemotherapy (cyclophosphamide, doxorubicin, vincristine, and prednisone [CHOP] or doxorubicin, cyclophosphamide, and cisplatin [CAP]) has been used. Complete response rates of approximately 40% with 3-

year survival of 34% have been achieved (Goldel et al., 1989). Several groups have advocated aggressive multimodality therapy using radiation, chemotherapy, and surgical resection for aggressive thymomas. The prognosis for patients with thymoma is dependent on clinical stage; 5-year survival is as follows: Stage I, 85 to 100%; Stage II, 60 to 80%; Stage III, 40 to 70%; and Stage IV, 50% (Nakahara et al., 1989; Verley and Hollman, 1985).

Germ-Cell Tumors

Germ-cell tumors are benign and malignant neoplasms thought to originate from primordial germ cells that fail to complete the migration from the urogenital ridge and come to rest in the mediastinum. These tumors are classified as teratomas and teratocarcinomas, seminomas, embryonal cell carcinomas, choriocarcinoma, and endodermal cell (yolk-sac) tumors. Although these lesions are identical histologically to germ-cell tumors originating in the gonads, they are not considered to be metastatic from primary gonadal tumors because mediastinal metastases from primary gonadal tumors are rare and because over 95% of patients with mediastinal germ-cell tumors showed no evidence of tumor in the testes, in contrast to the high incidence of testicular involvement following therapy for apparent primary retroperitoneal tumor. Therapy restricted to the mediastinum only does not cause disease relapse in the testis. In patients with mediastinal germ-cell tumors, the current recommendations for evaluating the testes are careful physical examination and ultrasonography. Biopsy is reserved for positive findings. Blind biopsy or orchiectomy is contraindicated.

Teratomas are neoplasms composed of multiple tissue elements derived from the three primitive embryonic layers foreign to the area in which they occur. The peak incidence is in the second and third decades of life. There is no sex predisposition. These tumors are located most commonly in the anterosuperior mediastinum, although 3 to 8% occur in the posterior mediastinum. Symptoms, when present, are related to mechanical effects and include chest pain, cough, dyspnea, or symptoms of recurrent pneumonitis. If a communication between the tumor and the tracheobronchial tree develops, the pathognomonic finding of a cough productive of hair or sebaceous material may result. Hematogenous infection of the cystic component of the tumor may cause symptoms of hemoptysis and recurrent infections owing to contiguous spread. Unusual presentations include recurrent pericarditis or pericardial tamponade following invasion or rupture into the pericardium. Rupture into the pleural space may cause respiratory distress owing to the markedly irritative nature of the cyst fluid. However, with the greater use of routine chest films, patients are diagnosed more frequently while asymptomatic and with much smaller tumors.

Although rare, the diagnosis of these tumors can be made on routine chest film by the identification of well-formed teeth. CT findings of a predominantly fatty mass with a denser dependent portion containing globular calcifications, bone, or teeth and a solid protuberance into a cystic cavity are considered specific. Despite the mass's occasional characteristic appearances seen through various imaging techniques, the diagnosis usually depends on microscopic examination.

The teratodermoid (dermoid) cyst is the simplest form. It is composed predominantly of derivatives of the epidermal layer, including dermal and epidermal glands, hair, and sebaceous material. However, careful examination of the cyst wall usually reveals endodermal and mesodermal elements (Fig. 17–10) that are generally unilobular, but occasionally multilobular. Teratomas are histologically more complex. The solid component of the tumor contains well-differentiated elements of bone, cartilage, teeth, muscle, connective tissue, fibrous and lymphoid tissue, nerve, thymus, mucous and salivary glands, lung, liver, or pancreas. Pancreatic tissue appears to contain a greater volume of endocrine cells with a predominance of somatostatin-producing delta cells. The presence of primitive or embryonic tissue distinguishes malignant tumors from benign. Therefore, diagnosis and therapy rely on surgical excision. For those benign tumors of such large size or involvement with adjacent mediastinal structures that complete resection is impossible, partial resection has relieved symptoms, frequently without relapse. Late sequelae following excision of a childhood teratoma may include impaired spermatic function and decreased serum levels of testosterone and luteinizing hormone (Lahdenne, 1992).

Malignant Germ-Cell Tumor

Malignant germ-cell tumors also occur predominantly in the anterosuperior mediastinum and represent approximately 4% of the primary tumors and cysts in the collected series. Unlike the benign teratomas, these tumors have a marked male predominance. The peak incidence is in the third and fourth decades of life. Most patients are symptomatic with chest pain, cough, dyspnea, and hemoptysis, and the superior vena caval syndrome occurs commonly. The chest film usually demonstrates a large anterior mediastinal mass that is often multilobulated; frequently, there is evidence of intrathoracic spread of disease. CT or MRI is most helpful in defining the extent of involvement so that response to therapy can be monitored and relapses diagnosed. These imaging modalities also help determine impingement on vital structures that may contraindicate general anesthesia. Serologic measurements of AFP and HCG-beta are useful for differentiating seminomas from nonseminomas, quantitatively assessing response to therapy in hormonally active tumors (plasma half-life of AFP and HCG-beta is 5 days and 12 to 24 hours, respectively), and diagnosing relapse or failure of therapy prior to changes that can be observed in gross disease. Seminomas rarely produce HCG-beta (<7%) and never produce AFP; in contrast, over 90% of nonsemi-

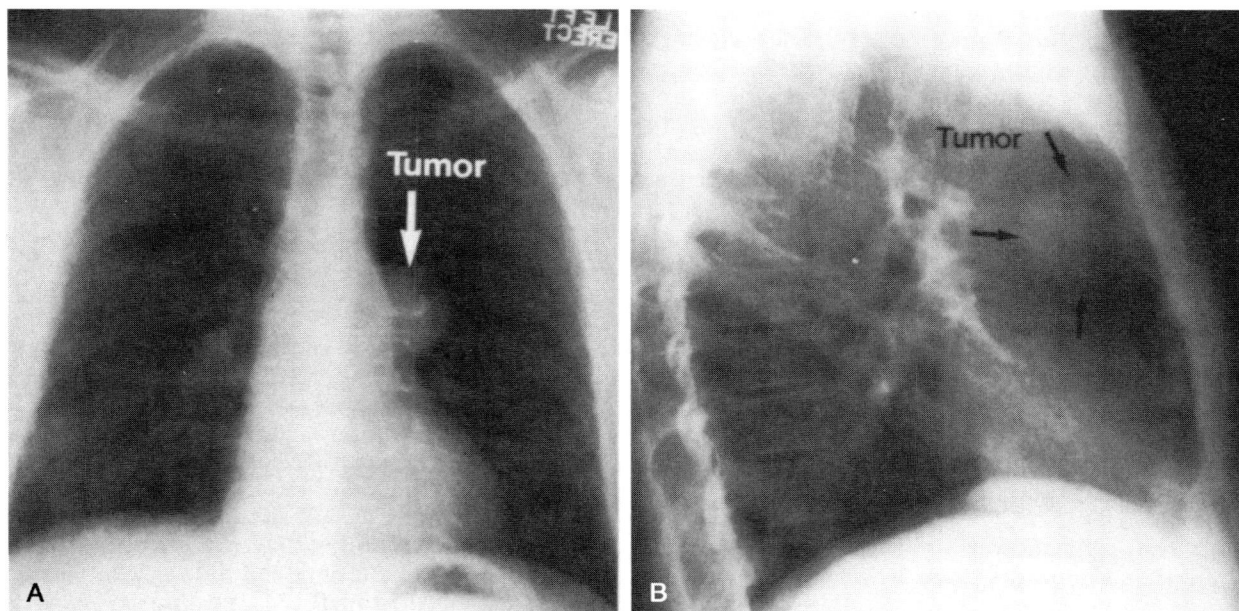

FIGURE 17–10. *A* and *B*, Chest films of a teratoma of the anterior mediastinum.

nomas secrete one or both of these hormones. This differentiation is important owing to the marked radiosensitivity of seminomas and the relative radioinsensitivity of nonseminomas. In a multi-institutional study, 11 of 12 patients with mediastinal seminomas had local control with radiotherapy, whereas none of 13 patients with other germ-cell histologies had local control using radiotherapy (Kersh et al., 1987). Chromosomal analysis of tumor tissue is useful for differentiating germ-cell tumors from other tumors with a similar histologic appearance. A characteristic isochromosome of chromosome 12 has been identified as a karyotypic abnormality of all germ-cell tumors (Motzer et al., 1991).

Seminoma

Seminomas account for 50% of malignant germ-cell tumors and approximately 2 to 4% of all mediastinal masses. These tumors occur predominantly in the anterosuperior mediastinum (Fig. 17–11). Unlike other malignant germ-cell tumors, seminomas usually remain intrathoracic, with local extension to adjacent mediastinal and pulmonary structures. Although metastatic spread occurs first through lymphatics, hematogenous spread with extrathoracic involvement may develop late in the course of disease. Bone and lung are the most common sites of metastatic spread, although liver, brain, spleen, tonsil, and subcutaneous tissue can also be involved. Patients are usually symptomatic owing to the mechanical effects of the tumor on adjacent structures. The most common symptoms are chest pain, cough, lethargy, and weight loss. The superior vena caval syndrome occurs in 10 to 20% of patients. The histologic appearance of this tumor is characterized by large cells with round nuclei, scant cytoplasm, and abundant glycogen.

Therapy is determined by the stage of the disease. Occasionally, excision is possible without injury to vital structures (22%) and is recommended when possible. When complete resection is possible, the use of adjuvant therapy is unnecessary. However, careful follow-up with serial CT examinations is required to diagnose recurrences. When excision is not possible, a biopsy of sufficient size to establish the diagnosis should be obtained. The radiosensitivity of this tumor and the excellent control of local disease with radiation therapy make cytoreductive resection before radiation therapy unnecessary, and contraindicated when vital structures are involved or when the procedure is technically difficult. The basis of therapy is megavoltage radiation to a shaped mediastinal field, including the supraclavicular and neck regions (sites of initial lymphatic spread of disease). When cervical lymph nodes are involved, the field is expanded to incorporate the axilla, the site of subsequent lymphatic spread. A dosage of 4500 to 5000 rads (midplane dosage) is usually given over a 6-week course. In patients with extrathoracic disease, relapse following appropriate therapy, or sufficient intrathoracic disease to preclude the likelihood of a complete response using radiation therapy alone, multiagent chemotherapy has successfully induced remission in a majority of patients using either VBP (vinblastine, bleomycin, and cisplatin, 59%) or VAB-6 (vinblastine, dactinomycin, bleomycin, cisplatin, and cyclophosphamide, 86%). Etoposide and cisplatin may be equally efficacious.

Nonseminoma

Malignant nonseminoma tumors include choriocarcinoma, embryonal cell carcinoma, malignant teratoma, and endodermal cell (yolk-sac) tumors, of

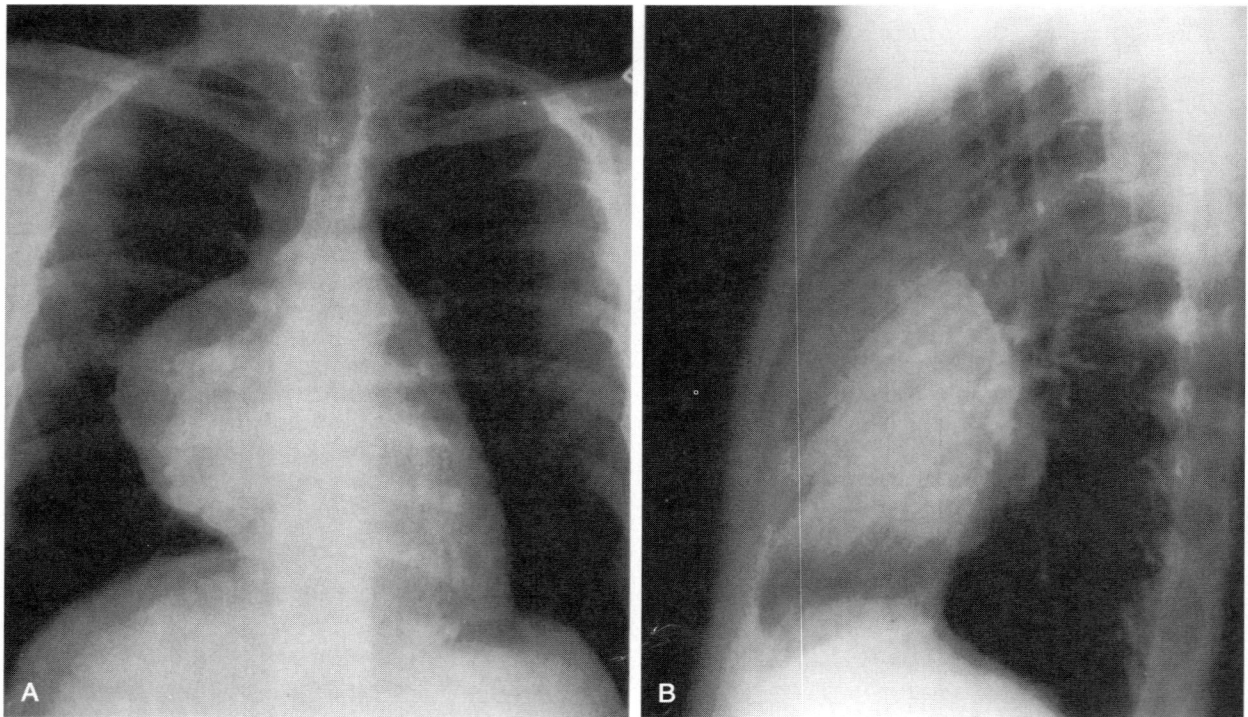

FIGURE 17–11. *A* and *B*, Chest films of a seminoma in an asymptomatic 17-year-old man.

which 40% are a mixture of tissue types. The nonseminomas differ from the seminomas in several aspects: they are more aggressive tumors that are frequently disseminated at the time of diagnosis; they are rarely radiosensitive; and over 90% produce either HCG-beta or AFP. All patients with choriocarcinoma and some patients with embryonal cell tumors have elevated levels of HCG-beta, a hormone secreted by the syncytiotrophoblast. AFP is most commonly elevated in patients with embryonal cell carcinomas and yolk-sac tumors. The presence of a significantly elevated titer of HCG-beta or an elevated titer of AFP indicates a nonseminoma germ-cell component (Fig. 17–12). These tumors follow the natural history of a nonseminoma.

As with seminomas, most patients with these neoplasms are symptomatic with chest pain, dyspnea, weight loss, cough, hemoptysis, fever, chills, and the superior vena caval syndrome (20%). Children with these tumors may present with precocious puberty. Patients are predominantly male and in the third or fourth decades of life. Chest films usually reveal a large anterior mediastinal mass with frequent extension into lung parenchyma and adjacent mediastinal structures. In addition to superior vena caval obstruction, they may cause pulmonary stenosis and coarctation of the aorta. Characteristically, these tumors have extensive intrathoracic involvement and frequently have metastasized outside the thorax. Frequent sites of metastatic disease include brain, lung, liver, bone, and the lymphatic system, particularly the supraclavicular nodes. Chest wall involvement is common.

Numerous chromosomal abnormalities are associated with an increased incidence of germ-cell tumors, including Kleinfelter's syndrome, trisomy 8, and Sq deletion. In one series of patients with germ-cell tumors, the incidence of Kleinfelter's syndrome was 22% (Nichols et al., 1987). These patients were younger (median age of 15 years), and their tumors were nonseminomas. Additionally, mediastinal but not testicular germ-cell tumors are associated with the development of rare hematologic malignancies, such as acute megakaryocytic leukemia, systemic mast cell disease, and malignant histiocytosis, as well as other hematologic abnormalities including the myelodysplastic syndrome and *idiopathic thrombocytopenia* refractory to treatment. One hypothesis for this association is the common derivation from a totipotent germ cell capable of hematopoietic differentiation that depends on the mediastinal environment for development.

The local invasiveness of these tumors and frequent metastases usually preclude surgical resection of all disease at the time of diagnosis. Initially, operative intervention is necessary only to establish the histologic diagnosis in patients without elevations in serum AFP or HCG-beta. Multiagent chemotherapy including cisplatin is the basis of therapy. Other agents to which these tumors respond include vinblastine, bleomycin, methotrexate, etoposide, and doxorubicin. The serum markers AFP and HCG-beta are followed after administration of chemotherapy. When these markers return to normal values, operative exploration should be performed, with removal of as much residual disease as possible without injuring vital structures. In patients in whom serum markers do

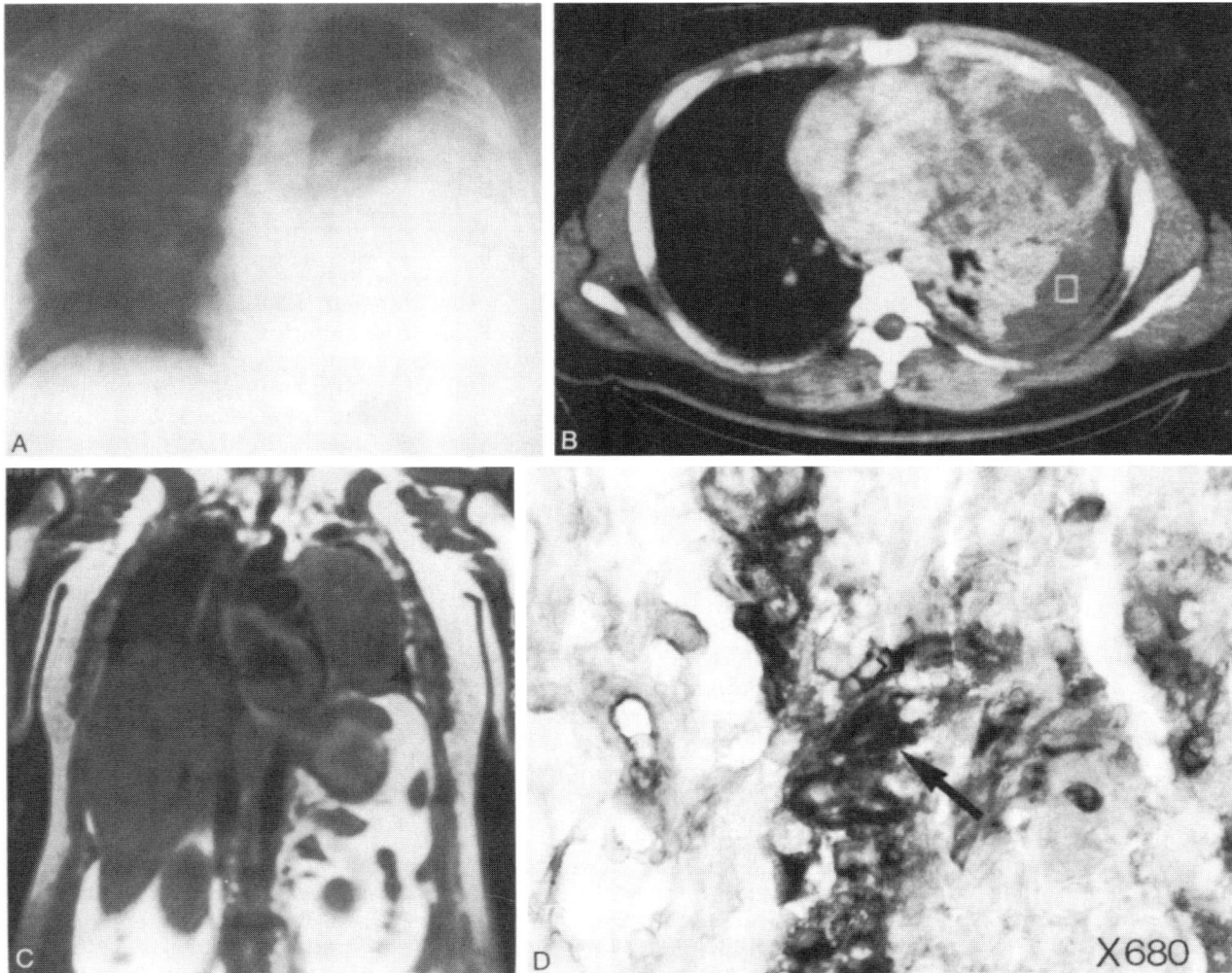

FIGURE 17–12. *A*, Chest film of a 28-year-old man with a malignant germ-cell tumor who had respiratory distress. *B*, CT scan shows a large left anterior mass with lobar collapse and a large pleural effusion. *C*, Coronal MRI delineates pulmonary artery encasement. *D*, Raised serum titer and positive staining for alpha-fetoprotein (dark-stained areas within the cytoplasm) established the diagnosis of a nonseminoma (× 680). (*A–D*, Courtesy of Dr. Thomas B. Clark, Department of Pathology, Duke University Medical Center, Durham, NC 27710.)

not normalize after an initial course of chemotherapy, a second course using a different regimen of agents is indicated. Patients with normalization of AFP and HCG-beta after induction therapy (achievable in up to 60%) have a good long-term prognosis (Kay et al., 1987). The presence of residual disease following reexploration portends an extremely poor prognosis. If viable tumor is present in the postchemotherapy resection specimen, additional chemotherapy is indicated owing to the high relapse rate. A salvage chemotherapeutic regimen is usually employed. The postchemotherapeutic histology is often a mature teratoma, which is associated with a good long-term prognosis. With surgical resection as an adjuvant to multiagent chemotherapy, complete responses of 20 to 80% have been reported. In patients with recurrent or refractory nonseminomatous germ-cell tumors, salvage therapy with high-dose chemotherapy and autologous bone marrow transplant has not been successful (Broun et al., 1991). Endodermal histology is

associated with a worse prognosis than with other germ-cell tumors. Given an aggressive multimodality approach with cisplatin-based chemotherapy, followed by surgical resection of residual disease, 36% of patients were long-term survivors in one series (Dartevelle et al., 1991). However, of patients who relapsed following therapy, no patients were salvaged despite aggressive chemotherapy. Mean survival in these patients was 6 months.

A subset of these tumors also contains malignant tissue that is not germ cell in origin. The histology is adenocarcinoma or sarcoma. Malignant teratomas or other germ-cell tumors with mature differentiated teratoma within the primary are most commonly involved. Non-germ-cell malignant transformation occurred in 29% of patients studied at autopsy (Aliotta et al., 1988). Despite response of the germ-cell component to chemotherapy, there is usually progression of the non-germ-cell component. In these patients, the only effective treatment has been surgical resection, which is rarely possible. The overall prognosis is poor.

Lymphomas

Although the mediastinum is frequently involved in patients with lymphoma sometime during the course of the disease (40 to 70%), it is infrequently the sole site of disease at the time of presentation. Only 5 to 10% of patients with Hodgkin's and non-Hodgkin's lymphomas present with symptoms solely due to local mass effects, such as mediastinal involvement. Patients are usually symptomatic, with chest pain, cough, dyspnea, hoarseness, and the superior vena caval syndrome the most common clinical manifestations. Lymphomas can also cause a clinical pattern compatible with pulmonary stenosis and pulmonary embolism by encasement of the pulmonary artery. Nonspecific systemic symptoms of fever and chills, weight loss, and anorexia are frequently noted and are important in the staging of patients with Hodgkin's lymphoma. Symptoms characteristic of Hodgkin's lymphoma include chest pain after consumption of alcohol and the cyclical fevers that were first described by Pel and Ebstein.

Characteristically, these tumors occur in the antero-superior mediastinum or in the hilar region of the middle mediastinum. CT and MRI are useful in delineating the extent of disease, determining invasiveness into contiguous structures, differentiating the lesions from cardiovascular abnormalities, aiding the selection of radiation portals, and following the response to therapy and diagnosing relapse. Also, differentiation from thymomas and germ-cell tumors, which are usually solitary masses, is possible because lymphomas are usually composed of multiple involved nodes that appear as separate masses on CT.

Hodgkin's Lymphoma

The Hodgkin's lymphomas are subdivided by histologic appearance into nodular sclerosing, lymphocyte predominant, mixed cellularity, and lymphocyte depleted. Mediastinal involvement is most common with nodular sclerosing (55 to 75%) (Fig. 17–13) and lymphocyte predominant (40%). Treatment of Hodgkin's lymphoma is determined by the stage of disease and is based on radiation therapy and chemotherapy (mechlorethamine, vincristine, procarbazine, and prednisone [MOPP] and CHOP). Surgical excision of all disease is rarely possible, and the surgeon's primary role is to provide sufficient tissue for diagnosis and to assist in pathologic staging, a process that frequently requires staging exploratory laparotomy. Although extrathoracic lymph nodes are frequently involved and available for biopsy, when the sole site of involvement is the mediastinum, a needle biopsy is often unsuccessful because larger tissue samples are needed to make a histologic diagnosis, particularly with nodular sclerosing lesions. Thoracotomy, mediastinoscopy, or mediastinotomy may be necessary to obtain sufficient tissue. Although surgical excision, when possible, provides adequate therapy, more often Stages IA and IIA disease, as defined by the Ann Arbor classification, are treated with megavoltage external beam radiation with a total dose of 4500 rads. Ten-year survival greater than 90% has been reported. Patients with Stages IIb, III, and IV disease are usually treated with chemotherapy. Patients with higher-grade tumor, advanced stage of disease, persistence of an abnormal *erythrocyte sedimentation rate*, extensive mediastinal disease, and advanced age (over 50 years) are at an increased risk of disease relapse.

Controversy continues concerning the treatment of patients with extensive mediastinal disease as defined by tumor size greater than 35% of the cardiothoracic diameter. These patients have a higher relapse rate when treated with radiation therapy alone. Although combining chemotherapy with radiation therapy reduces the relapse rate, survival has not necessarily been prolonged because of the efficacy of salvage chemotherapy and the significant risk of secondary malignancies following the use of alkylating chemotherapeutic agents.

Residual abnormalities within the mediastinum are commonly noted radiographically following treatment of Hodgkin's disease (64 to 88%) (Jochelson et al., 1985; Radford et al., 1988). These abnormalities include minimal mediastinal widening in 44% of patients and widening greater than 6 cm in 41%. In 27 to 41% of patients, radiographic abnormalities persist for more than a year. Residual radiographic abnormality is more common in patients with initial bulky mediastinal disease. Residual mediastinal abnormalities were not significantly associated with eventual disease relapse except when treatment was with chemotherapy alone. In addition, benign thymic cysts appear to be more common following radiation therapy for anterior mediastinal neoplasms. Optimal therapy is surgical excision without additional chemotherapy or radiation therapy to determine whether residual disease is present. Gallium-67 scintigraphy has been reported to be useful in those patients with residual mediastinal mass following therapy. In one series of patients treated for Hodgkin's disease, 18 of 21 patients with initially positive gallium scans converted to negative results. The CT scan was negative for a residual mass in 11 of these patients. Seven patients had CT evidence of a persistent mediastinal mass, although biopsy results were negative for residual disease (Weiner et al., 1991).

Non-Hodgkin's Lymphoma

Non-Hodgkin's lymphomas are usually of either lymphoblastic morphology (60%) or large-cell morphology with a diffuse pattern of growth (40%). In 40 to 80% of patients with lymphoblastic lymphoma, the mediastinum is involved. Although all ages may be afflicted, the peak incidence is in the second and third decades of life. Lymphoblastic lymphoma is characterized by the following: (1) advanced stage of disease

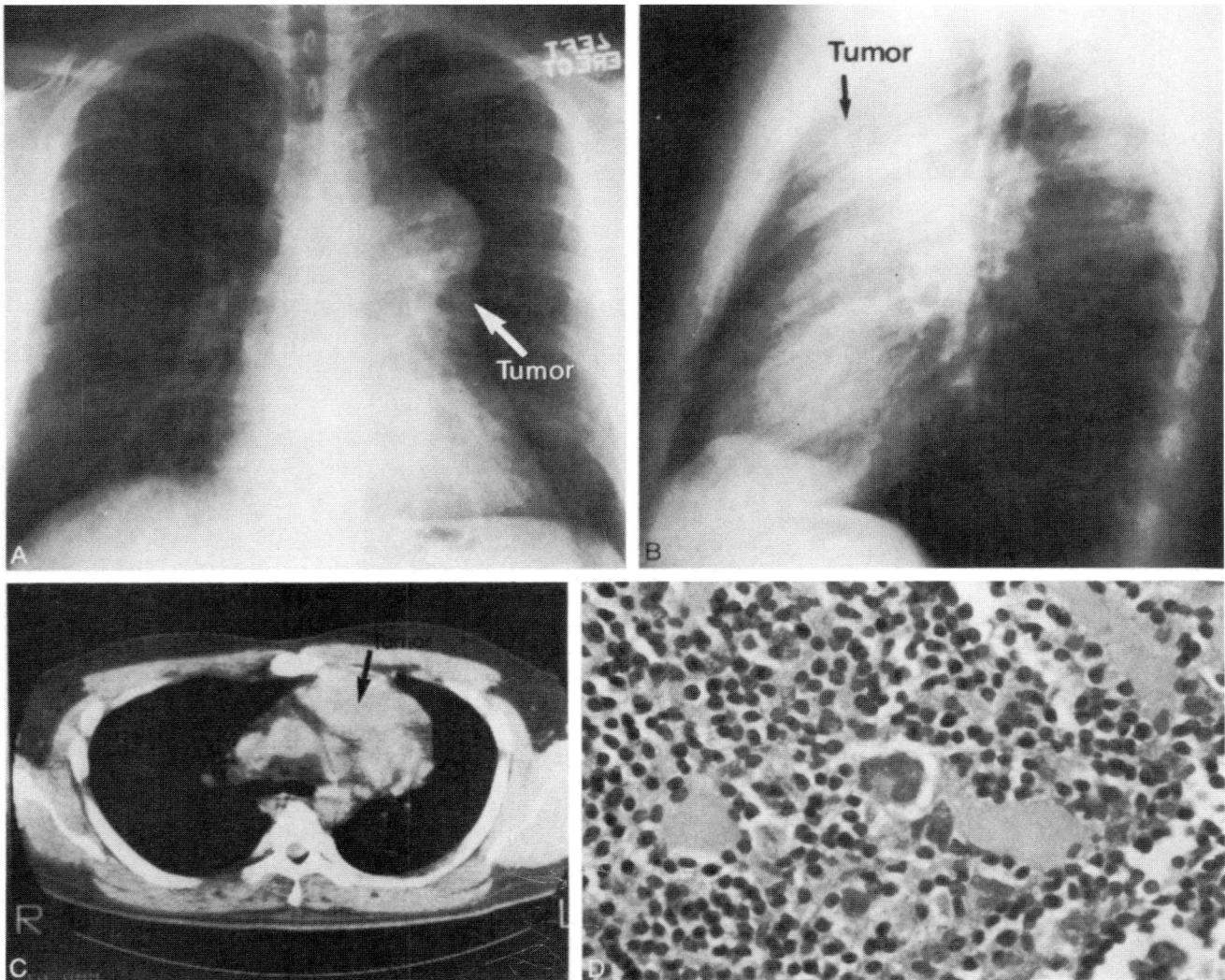

FIGURE 17–13. *A* and *B*, Chest films of an anterior mediastinal Hodgkin tumor. *C*, CT image manifests the invasive nature of the tumor. *D*, The characteristic Reed-Sternberg cell is shown.

at presentation, with 91% of patients having Stage III or IV disease; (2) early bone marrow involvement with frequent development of leukemia; (3) tumor cells that exhibit T-lymphocyte antigens; (4) early metastatic spread to the leptomeninges; and (5) initial responsiveness to radiation therapy, uniformly followed by relapse. Lymphoblastic lymphomas can be divided histologically into convoluted, nonconvoluted, and large-cell, of which the convoluted and nonconvoluted preferentially involve the mediastinum. In the majority of lymphoblastic lymphomas, intermediate (CD1+, CD4+, or CD8+) or mature (CD3+) T-cell differentiation is present (62% and 32%, respectively). Those with an intermediate T-cell differentiation are the subgroup most likely to have a mediastinal mass (Crist et al., 1988). T-cell acute lymphoid leukemia shares morphologic and clinical similarities to lymphoblastic lymphoma, and approximately 70% of patients manifest a mediastinal mass.

Operative intervention is limited to obtaining sufficient tissue to establish the diagnosis and, if necessary, to perform immunologic subtyping. The best results have been obtained using aggressive chemotherapy in conjunction with central nervous system prophylaxis (nearly 100% complete response following induction therapy, with subsequent low rate of relapse). Patients with tumors exhibiting immature T-cell differentiation (CD2+ or CD7+) appear to have higher relapse rates (Azizkhan et al., 1985; Berrih-Aknin et al., 1987).

The large-cell lymphomas of *diffuse growth pattern* (diffuse histiocytic lymphoma [DHL]) are a heterogeneous group differing in cell type of origin, clinical presentation, natural history, and response to therapy. The DHL tumors can be subclassified into at least three diseases: T-immunoblastic sarcoma, B-immunoblastic sarcoma, and sclerosing variants of follicular cell lymphoma. The T-immunoblastic sarcomas are characterized by morphologic appearance similar to that of peripheral T-cell lymphomas; slight female predominance; smaller, more confined masses that usually remain intrathoracic; and a higher incidence of causing the superior vena caval syndrome.

In comparison, the B-immunoblastic and sclerosing follicular cell lymphomas are more aggressive tumors with more extensive intra- and extrathoracic involvement (Fig. 17–14). The peak incidence occurs in the third and fourth decades of life, with no clear gender predisposition. Operative intervention is useful in obtaining tissue for diagnosis, which often requires immunotyping, but is rarely important therapeutically. These tumors may be confused with thymomas, germ-cell tumors, anaplastic carcinoid tumors, and

Hodgkin's lymphoma if the light microscopic appearance alone is used. This is especially true if prior radiation therapy or chemotherapy has been administered. Although needle biopsy frequently does not provide sufficient tumor specimen to establish the diagnosis, extrathoracic tissue is often available for biopsy. Therapy is based on doxorubicin-containing chemotherapeutic protocols, which can induce complete responses in over 90% of patients, with relapse-free survival of 50 to 74% after 2 years.

A subset of patients with primary mediastinal lymphoma has been described with B-cell characteristics (MB2+) (Lavabre-Bertrand et al., 1992). The clinical course in these patients was remarkable for a prolonged phase in which the tumor remained con-

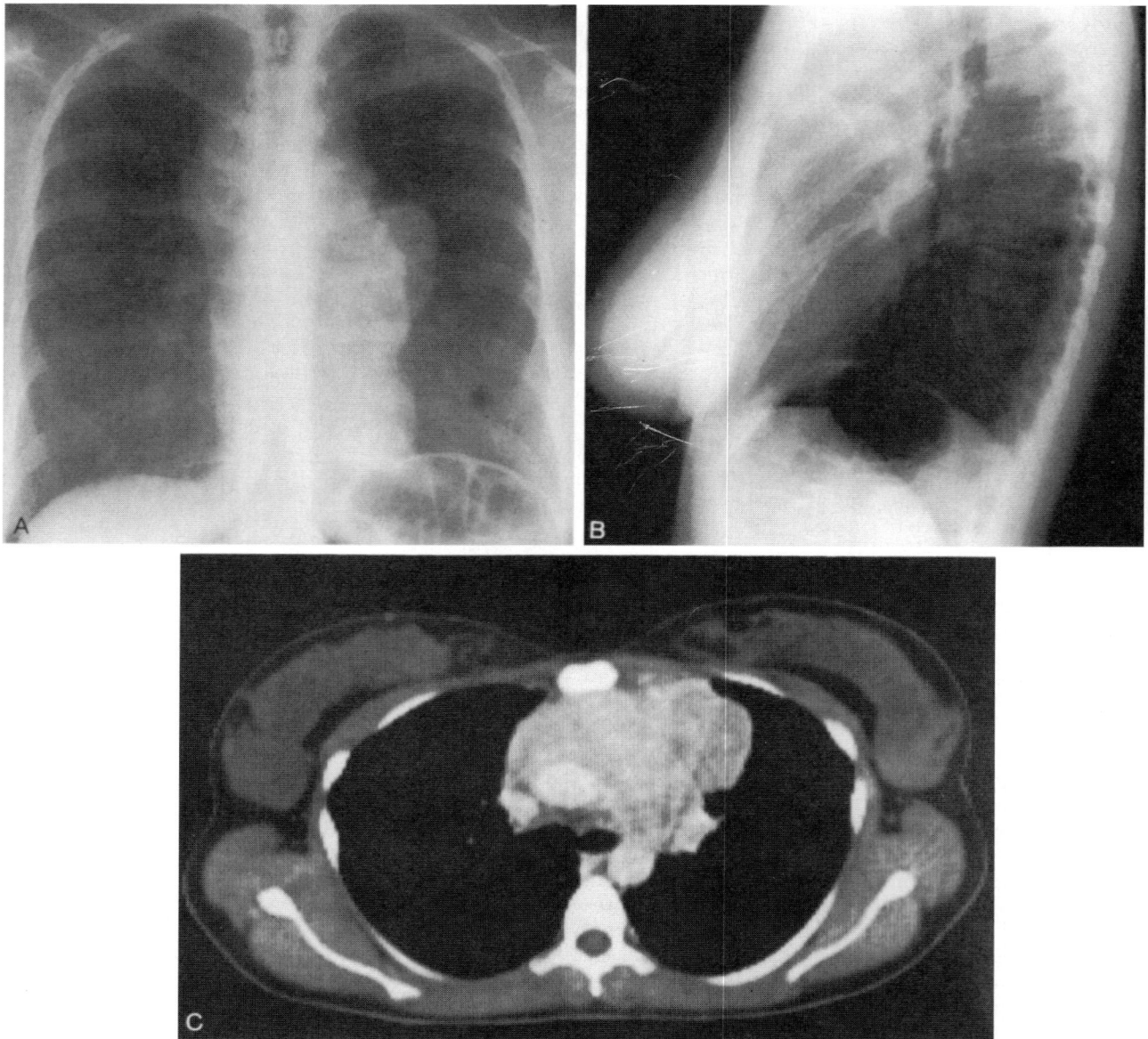

FIGURE 17–14. *A* and *B*, Chest films of a large B-cell non-Hodgkin lymphoma that involves the anterosuperior mediastinum. *C*, CT image shows the involvement of the mediastinal structures by the lymphoma.

fined to the mediastinum and thorax. Histology is remarkable for the amount of fibrosis and necrosis. In only 4 of 15 patients was a complete remission achieved. Although an aggressive chemotherapeutic regimen appears indicated, the prolonged period of strictly local involvement means that surgical resection of residual disease is indicated when technically feasible.

Primary Carcinoma

Primary carcinomas of the mediastinum make up between 3 and 11% of primary mediastinal masses in most series and represent 4% of the mediastinal masses in the collected series. The origin of these tumors is unknown. However, it is important to differentiate them from malignant thymomas, germ-cell tumors, carcinoid tumors, lymphomas, mediastinal extension of bronchogenic carcinomas, and metastatic tumors, which may have a similar light microscopic appearance. Metastatic disease in mediastinal lymph nodes usually derives from bronchogenic or esophageal malignancies and rarely occurs with extrathoracic malignancies. Only 2.3% of 1071 patients with extrathoracic neoplasms developed evidence of hilar or mediastinal lymph node involvement over a 2-year period, as determined by serial chest films. The tumors most likely to metastasize to the mediastinum include those originating in the breast, head and neck, and genitourinary tract, as well as melanomas. Primary carcinomas are usually of the large-cell, undifferentiated morphology, although small-cell and squamous cell carcinomas have been described. Electron microscopic examination of the tumor ultrastructure and the increasing number of immunofluorescent stains for surface antigens and cellular proteins specific for a number of malignancies may better define the origin of some of these primary carcinomas.

These tumors occur with equal frequency in either sex. Most patients are symptomatic owing to the local mass effects of the tumor, which include chest pain, cough, dyspnea, hoarseness, dysphagia, and the superior vena caval syndrome. Extensive involvement within the thorax and often metastatic disease outside the thorax characterize this disease. Surgical excision is rarely possible. Unfortunately, the routine use of radiation therapy and chemotherapy has not prolonged survival. Only 2 of 32 patients treated at the Duke University Medical Center are alive at 6 and 11 years following surgical excision or biopsy and radiation therapy, respectively. Overall, the mean survival is less than 1 year.

Endocrine Tumors

Although substernal extension of a cervical goiter is common, totally intrathoracic thyroid tumors are rare and account for only 1% of all mediastinal masses in the collected series. In a series of 17,000 patients undergoing thyroidectomy, only 135 intrathoracic goi-

ters were encountered. These tumors arise from heterotopic thyroid tissue, which occurs most commonly in the anterosuperior mediastinum but may also occur in the middle mediastinum between the trachea and the esophagus as well as in the posterior mediastinum. Although there may be a demonstrable connection with the cervical gland, usually a fibrous connective tissue band, a true intrathoracic thyroid gland derives its blood supply from thoracic vessels.

The peak incidence is in the sixth and seventh decades of life and females are more commonly affected. When these lesions occur in the anterosuperior or middle mediastinum, symptoms related to tracheal compression are often present—such as dyspnea, cough, wheezing, and stridor. When these tumors occur in the posterior mediastinum, esophageal compression manifested by dysphagia is common. Rarely, symptoms related to thyrotoxicosis may impel a patient to seek medical attention. On chest film, these lesions appear as sharply circumscribed, dense masses, occurring more frequently on the right. Intrathoracic goiters are contrast-enhancing lesions when visualized by CT. The administration of iodinated contrast material causes prolonged enhancement of thyroid tissue. When functioning thyroid tissue is present, the radioactive iodine (^{131}I) scan is generally diagnostic. However, some of these neoplasms are functionally inactive and are not identified by ^{131}I scanning. In asymptomatic patients with anterosuperior or posterosuperior masses, ^{131}I scanning should be performed to document the presence of functioning cervical thyroid tissue, to prevent the removal of the sole functioning thyroid tissue.

Most of these tumors are adenomas, but carcinomas have been reported. If the lesion is identified as the sole functioning thyroid tissue and the patient is asymptomatic, surgical exploration and excision are not indicated. In these patients, frequent follow-up radiographic examinations are indicated to evaluate changes in the size or nature of the lesion. Otherwise, these lesions should be resected because they tend to enlarge and compress adjacent structures. Because of thoracic derivation of the blood supply, intrathoracic thyroid tumors should be approached through the thorax, using either an anterolateral thoracotomy or a median sternotomy for anterior lesions or a posterolateral thoracotomy for posterior lesions. Substernal extensions of a cervical goiter can generally be excised using a cervical approach.

Parathyroid Tumors

Although parathyroid glands may occur in the mediastinum in 10% of patients, they are usually accessible through the cervical incision. A sternotomy incision is necessary to excise a hyperfunctioning parathyroid gland in approximately 2.5% of all patients and in 15% of those with a mediastinal gland (Clark, 1988; Wang et al., 1986). However, in one series of patients with mediastinal parathyroid gland, one-third underwent more than surgical exploration (Conn et al., 1991). Most often, these adenomas are found in the anterosuperior mediastinum embedded in or near the superior pole of the thymus. This anatomic relationship is the result of the common embryogenesis of the inferior parathyroid glands from the third branchial cleft. The superior parathyroid glands and the lateral lobes of the thyroid gland are derived from the fourth branchial pouch. Because they migrate with the lateral lobes of the thyroid gland to a paraesophageal position, they are found in the posterior mediastinum when they migrate farther caudad. Factors contributing to the caudal movement of parathyroid glands into the mediastinum include negative intrathoracic pressure, gravity, and the movement of the pharynx and larynx with deglutition.

The clinical manifestations of a mediastinal parathyroid tumor are similar to those that occur with tumors of the cervical region; symptoms are related to the excess secretion of parathyroid hormone, which causes the hyperparathyroid syndrome. Because of their small size, these neoplasms rarely cause symptoms related to mechanical effects and are not often visualized using conventional roentgenography. Using CT, MRI, thallium/technetium scanning, and selective arteriography, preoperative localization of these tumors can be made in approximately 80% of patients. Venous angiography with selective sampling helps determine the side of the adenoma, but is usually inadequate to define the anatomic location. The utility of localization studies varies between series. In a series reported from the National Institutes of Health, the sensitivity of angiography, CT, and MRI at localizing a mediastinal parathyroid gland was 84%, 35%, and 19%, respectively. Ultrasound and thallium/technetium scans were very insensitive (Doherty et al., 1991).

Most frequently, the mediastinal adenoma may be excised following a negative exploration of the cervical region through the existing cervical incision. Usually, the vascular supply to the adenoma extends from cervical blood vessels. Mediastinal exploration using a median sternotomy is indicated in patients with persistent hyperparathyroidism producing severe biochemical or metabolic disease and following an unsuccessful cervical exploration in which four normal glands have been identified (Wang et al., 1986). A preoperative attempt at anatomic localization is indicated. In patients whose preoperative studies have failed to locate the site of the responsible parathyroid gland, exploration of the mediastinum is often unsuccessful. Approximately 80% of mediastinal parathyroids are located in the anterior mediastinum, with most of the remaining 20% occurring in the posterior mediastinum (Clark, 1988). Almost 75% of the mediastinal parathyroids are found within or adjacent to the thymus. If an adenoma is not found following a systematic exploration of the mediastinum, which may require incision of the pleura and pericardium, the thymus and the parathymic fatty-areolar tissue should be removed. Angioablation of mediastinal parathyroids can be performed with long-term success in 63% of patients (Doherty et al., 1991). In centers with appropriate expertise, angioablation may be indicated as the initial procedure of choice in patients with persistent or recurrent hyperparathyroidism if only one parathyroid gland was removed at the initial operation. In patients in whom two or more parathyroid glands were excised at the initial operation, persistent hypoparathyroidism often results following angioablation. These patients should have surgical exploration and excision with cryopreservation of excised parathyroid tissue.

Parathyroid carcinomas have been reported and are usually hormonally active. Patients differ in clinical presentation in that they often have higher serum calcium levels and manifest more severe symptoms of hyperparathyroidism. When possible, surgical resection is the optimal therapy.

Unlike parathyroid adenomas and carcinomas, parathyroid cysts are usually not hormonally active. These cysts are defined by the presence of parathyroid cells identifiable within the cyst wall. Because these lesions are frequently larger than adenomas, symptoms related to local mass effects are more common, as is visualization on chest film. Surgical excision yields a cure.

Carcinoid Tumors

Mediastinal carcinoid tumors arise from cells of Kulchitsky located in the thymus. Occurring more often in male patients, these tumors usually are located in the anterosuperior mediastinum. Although these tumors originate from the thymus, they are not associated with myasthenia gravis or red blood cell aplasia, nor are they associated with the carcinoid syndrome. However, their origin from amine precursor uptake and decarboxylation (APUD) cells may make these tumors hormonally active, and they may occur as a variant of the *multiple endocrine neoplastic* (MEN) syndromes. Mediastinal carcinoids have been most frequently associated with Cushing's syndrome due to production of ACTH. In a series of 15 patients with mediastinal carcinoid, 5 patients had clinical evidence of Cushing's syndrome, and a 6th patient had elevated ACTH levels without any clinical stigmata (Wick et al., 1982). In addition, 1 of the 15 had Type I MEN syndrome, and 3 others had variants of a MEN syndrome.

In patients with hormonally inactive tumors, symptoms are related to local mass effects and include chest pain, dyspnea, cough, and the superior vena caval syndrome. Hormonally inactive carcinoids tend to be larger and are frequently invasive locally. In addition, metastatic spread to mediastinal and cervical lymph nodes, liver, bone, skin, and lungs occurs in most patients. In the series of 15 patients, 73% developed metastatic disease, with late development of metastases in 3 of the 15 patients (initial metastasis discovered at 5, 6, and 8 years, respectively).

Often, these tumors are difficult to distinguish from other common anterior mediastinal masses, particularly thymomas and germ-cell tumors. However, carcinoids are characterized by the ultrastructural findings of dense-core neurosecretory granules. Positive immunohistochemical staining for ACTH of these granules is also characteristic. Surgical removal when possible is the preferred treatment. When local invasiveness or metastasis precludes the successful use of operative therapy, radiation therapy and multiagent chemotherapy have been tried, although no consistent benefit has been documented.

Mesenchymal Tumors

Mediastinal mesenchymal tumors originate from the connective tissue, striatal and smooth muscle, fat, lymphatic tissue, and blood vessels present within the mediastinum, producing a diverse group of neoplasms. Relative to other sites in the body, these tumors occur less commonly within the mediastinum. Mesenchymal tumors accounted for 7% of the primary masses in the collected series. There is no apparent difference in incidence between sexes. The soft tissue neoplasms include lipomas, liposarcomas, fibrosarcomas, fibromas, xanthogranulomas, leiomyomas, leiomyosarcomas, benign and malignant mesenchymomas, rhabdomyosarcomas, and mesotheliomas. These tumors have a similar histologic appearance and generally follow the same clinical course as the soft tissue tumors found elsewhere in the body. Fifty-five per cent of these tumors are malignant. Surgical resection remains the primary therapy because poor results have been obtained using radiation and chemotherapy.

Similarly, the mesenchymal tumors derived from blood and lymph vessel are common elsewhere in the body but rare in the mediastinum. Although these tumors occur anywhere in the mediastinum, the most frequent location is the anterosuperior mediastinum. These tumors include the capillary, cavernous, and venous hemangiomas, hemangioendotheliomas, hemangiopericytomas, lymphangiomas, and the derivatives of lymphangiomas. Symptoms are related to the size and invasiveness of the lesion. Occasionally, hemorrhage into the lesion may rapidly increase the size. Significant compression and obstruction of mediastinal structures may result, causing a variety of clinical manifestations, of which respiratory failure is the most dramatic. Rupture of hemangiomas into the pleural space may cause exsanguination; rupture into the mediastinum may cause tamponade.

Differentiation between the vascular tumors is based on the morphologic appearance: the size of the vascular space, the relative number and amount of pericytes, smooth muscle, and endothelial cells. Between 10 and 30% of vascular tumors are malignant, although the differentiation may be difficult because the histologic appearance, number of mitotic figures, and even the gross appearance are often similar. Vascular tumors are not well encapsulated, and even benign tumors may exhibit local invasion. However, the incidence of metastatic spread is low, approximately 3%. Hemangiopericytomas have the highest incidence of malignancy, and these tumors usually

occur in older patients. Vascular tumors have a variable roentgenographic appearance from a small discrete lesion to a large multilobulated lesion with ill-defined borders. Because these neoplasms are not supplied by large vessels, tumor opacification does not generally occur during angiographic studies. Excision remains the only effective means of therapy, although radiation therapy has been used with mixed results.

Tumors originating from lymph vessels are differentiated from tumors of blood vessel origin through indirect evidence, such as the absence of red blood cells within the lumen of the tumor vasculature, the extrusion of chylous fluid from the cut edges, and the tumor's relationship to documented lymphatic tissue. Also, these tumors usually occur in the anterior mediastinum, appearing as round or lobulated cystic densities on the chest films. The most common lymphatic tumor is the lymphangioma (also called cystic hygroma, lymphatic cyst, and lymphatogenous cyst), which in most patients occurs in the superior mediastinum as an extension of a cervical lesion. Only 17% of mediastinal lymphangiomas are completely within the mediastinum, whereas 10% of cervical lymphangiomas have a mediastinal extension. Low-lying cervical lymphangiomas are more likely to have a mediastinal component. Lymphangiomas are generally diagnosed in children, and they frequently cause symptoms of obstructed trachea, including stridor, dyspnea, recurrent pulmonary infection, and tachypnea. Lymphangiomas have characteristic appearances on ultrasonography or CT. Growth of these tumors is by proliferation of endothelium-lined buds that spread along tissue planes. The local ingrowth of vessels and fibrous reaction to the endothelial buds prevent easy surgical removal because well-defined tissue planes are lacking. However, because radiation therapy and sclerotherapy have not been successful, operative resection is the optimal treatment. Total excision is not indicated when nerves and vital structures are involved. Multiple procedures may be necessary.

Extramedullary Hematopoiesis

Extramedullary hematopoiesis occurs in all age groups, usually as a result of altered hematopoiesis. In the adult, this is typically caused by massive hemolysis, myelofibrosis, spherocytic anemia, or thalassemia. These lesions appear as bilateral, asymmetric paravertebral masses. They are contrast-enhancing lesions as visualized by CT, a modality that is useful for determining the presence of intraspinal extension. Because these tumors are composed of hematopoietic tissue, they are easily visualized with either radioactive iron (^{59}Fe) or radioisotope-labeled gold scanning. These scanning modalities are useful in differentiating these tumors from other mediastinal lesions in patients with known hematologic abnormalities. Surgical resection is unnecessary unless invasion or compression of mediastinal structures occurs. Radiation therapy can produce rapid shrinkage of these masses.

Giant Lymph Node Hyperplasia (Castleman's Disease)

Giant lymph node hyperplasia was initially described by Castleman in 1956. Although the mediastinum was the site of disease in the initial report and, in most patients, these tumors may develop wherever lymph nodes are present, the retroperitoneum, cervical, axillary, and pelvic regions are the most common nonmediastinal sites. These lesions have been described using different terms, including angiofollicular lymphoid hyperplasia, lymphoid hamartoma, follicular lymphoreticuloma, angiomatosis, and benign giant lymphomas. Although these tumors are usually located in the anterosuperior mediastinum, they also are found in the posterior mediastinum (Fig. 17–15) and at the pericardiophrenic angle, where they may be confused with neurogenic tumors and pericardial cysts, respectively. Two distinct histologic entities exist: hyaline vascular, characterized by small hyaline follicles and interfollicular capillary proliferation, and plasma cell, characterized by large follicles with intervening sheets of plasma cells. The tumors most frequently appear as single, well-demarcated lesions. The hyaline vascular type represents 90% of Castleman's tumors, and these are most often discovered in the asymptomatic patient on routine chest film. Patients with the plasma cell type often exhibit systemic symptoms, including fever, night sweats, anemia, and hypergammaglobulinemia. Surgical excision effects cure, although resection of the hyaline vascular type may be associated with significant hemorrhage owing to extreme vascularity.

Multicentric Castleman's disease is characterized by generalized lymphadenopathy with morphologic features of giant lymph node hyperplasia. Patients are most often symptomatic with fever, chills, weight loss, hepatosplenomegaly and exhibit disordered immunity and autoimmune phenomena. Unlike the benign clinical course of classic Castleman's disease, multicentric disease is a much more malignant disorder, with frequent deaths following infectious complications. It has also been reported in association with human immunodeficiency virus (HIV) infection.

Chondroma

Chondromas are rare tumors that occur in the posterior mediastinum originating from the primitive notochord. Males are affected twice as frequently as females, with the peak age of incidence in the fifth through seventh decades of life. Chest pain, cough, and dyspnea are the most common symptoms. Spinal cord compression may follow extension into the spinal canal. Radical surgical excision is the only effective therapy; however, most patients develop distant metastases. The mean survival is approximately 17.5 months.

Primary Cysts

Primary cysts of the mediastinum make up 20% of the mediastinal masses in the collected series. These cysts can be bronchogenic, pericardial, enteric, or thymic or may be of an unspecified nature. More than 75% of patients are asymptomatic and these tumors rarely cause morbidity. However, owing to the proximity of vital structures within the mediastinum, with increasing size even benign cysts may cause significant morbidity. In addition, these masses need to be differentiated from malignant tumors.

Bronchogenic Cysts

Bronchogenic cysts are the most common primary cysts of the mediastinum, accounting for 6.3% of primary mediastinal masses and 34% of cysts. They originate as sequestrations from the ventral foregut, the antecedent of the tracheobronchial tree. The bronchogenic cyst may lie within the lung parenchyma or the mediastinum. The cyst wall is composed of cartilage, mucous glands, smooth muscle, and fibrous tissue with a pathognomonic inner layer of ciliated respiratory epithelium. When bronchogenic cysts occur in the mediastinum, they are usually located proximal to the trachea or bronchi and may be just posterior to the carina. Rarely, a true communication between the cyst and the tracheobronchial tree exists, and an air fluid level may be observed on the chest film. Two-thirds of patients with bronchogenic cysts are asymptomatic. In infants, these cysts may cause severe respiratory compromise by compressing the trachea or the bronchus; compression of the bronchus may cause bronchial stenosis and recurrent pneumonitis (Fig. 17–16). Since tumors occurring below the carina are sometimes not well visualized with standard roentgenography, the routine use of CT has been recommended to evaluate children with recurrent pulmonary infections for possible bronchogenic cyst. More often, bronchogenic cysts occur in older children and adults, in whom these cysts may cause symptoms of chest pain, dyspnea, cough, and stridor. Bronchogenic cysts appear as a smooth density at the carina level that may compress the esophagus on barium swallow. Differentiation from hilar structures may be difficult. Surgical excision is recommended in all patients to provide definitive histologic diagnosis, alleviate symptoms, and prevent the development of associated complications. Malignant degeneration has been reported, as has the presence of a bronchial adenoma within the cyst wall.

Pericardial Cysts

Pericardial cysts, the second most frequently encountered cysts within the mediastinum, make up 6% of all lesions and 33% of primary cysts (see Table

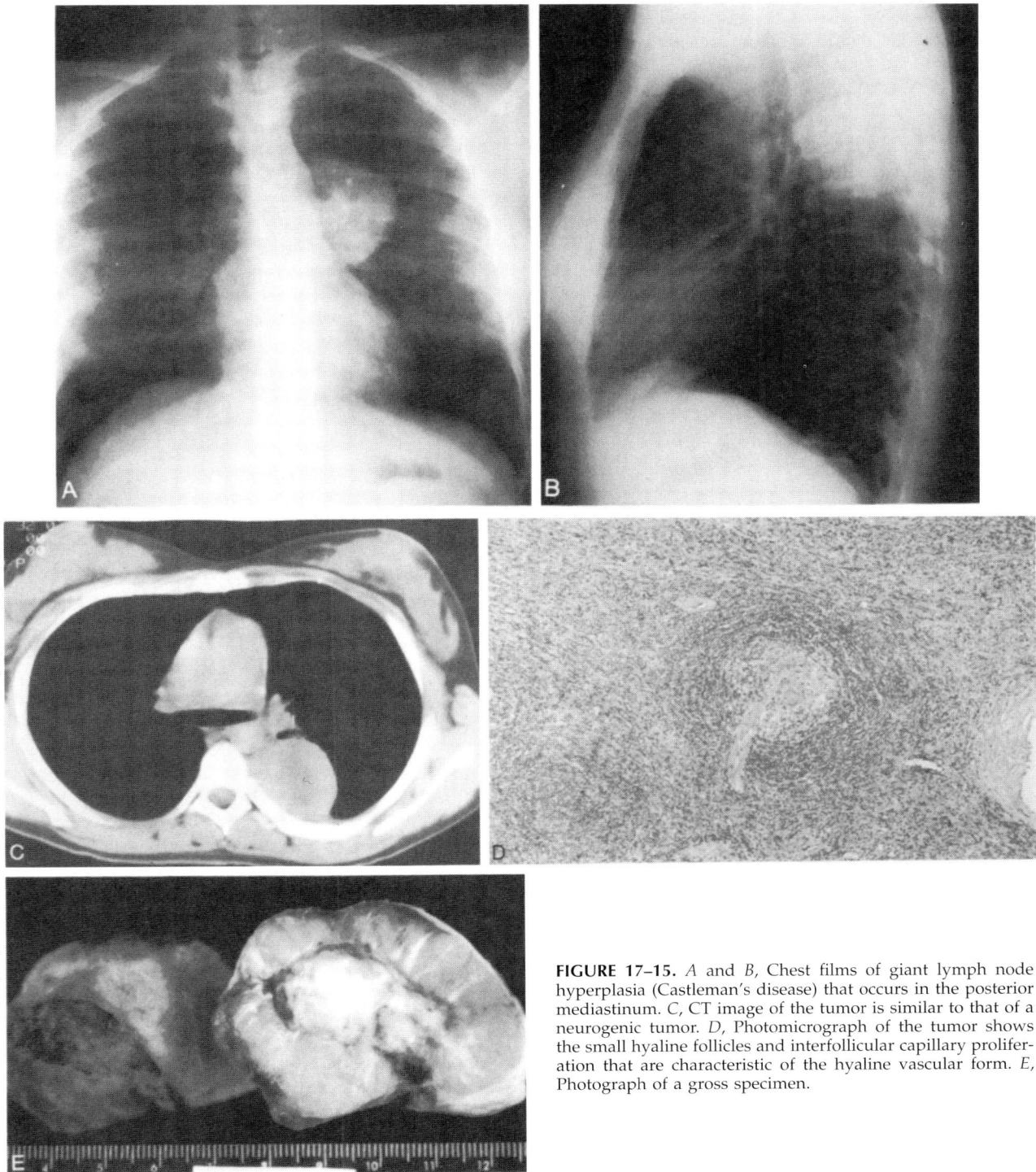

FIGURE 17–15. *A* and *B*, Chest films of giant lymph node hyperplasia (Castleman's disease) that occurs in the posterior mediastinum. *C*, CT image of the tumor is similar to that of a neurogenic tumor. *D*, Photomicrograph of the tumor shows the small hyaline follicles and interfollicular capillary proliferation that are characteristic of the hyaline vascular form. *E*, Photograph of a gross specimen.

17–2). These cysts classically occur in the pericardiophrenic angles (Fig. 17–17), with 70% in the right pericardiophrenic angle, 22% in the left, and the remainder in other sites in the pericardium. The embryogenesis of these cysts is thought to follow failure of fusion of one or more mesenchymal lacunae that coalesce to form the pericardium or a persistent ventral parietal recess of the pericardial coelom. Pericardial cysts may or may not have a communication with the pericardium. Numerous reports have described the characteristic CT appearance of pericardial cysts: pericardiophrenic location, near-water attenuation value, and smooth borders. Patients with lesions and classic CT characteristics for pericardial cysts have been managed with needle aspiration and follow-up with serial CT rather than surgical excision.

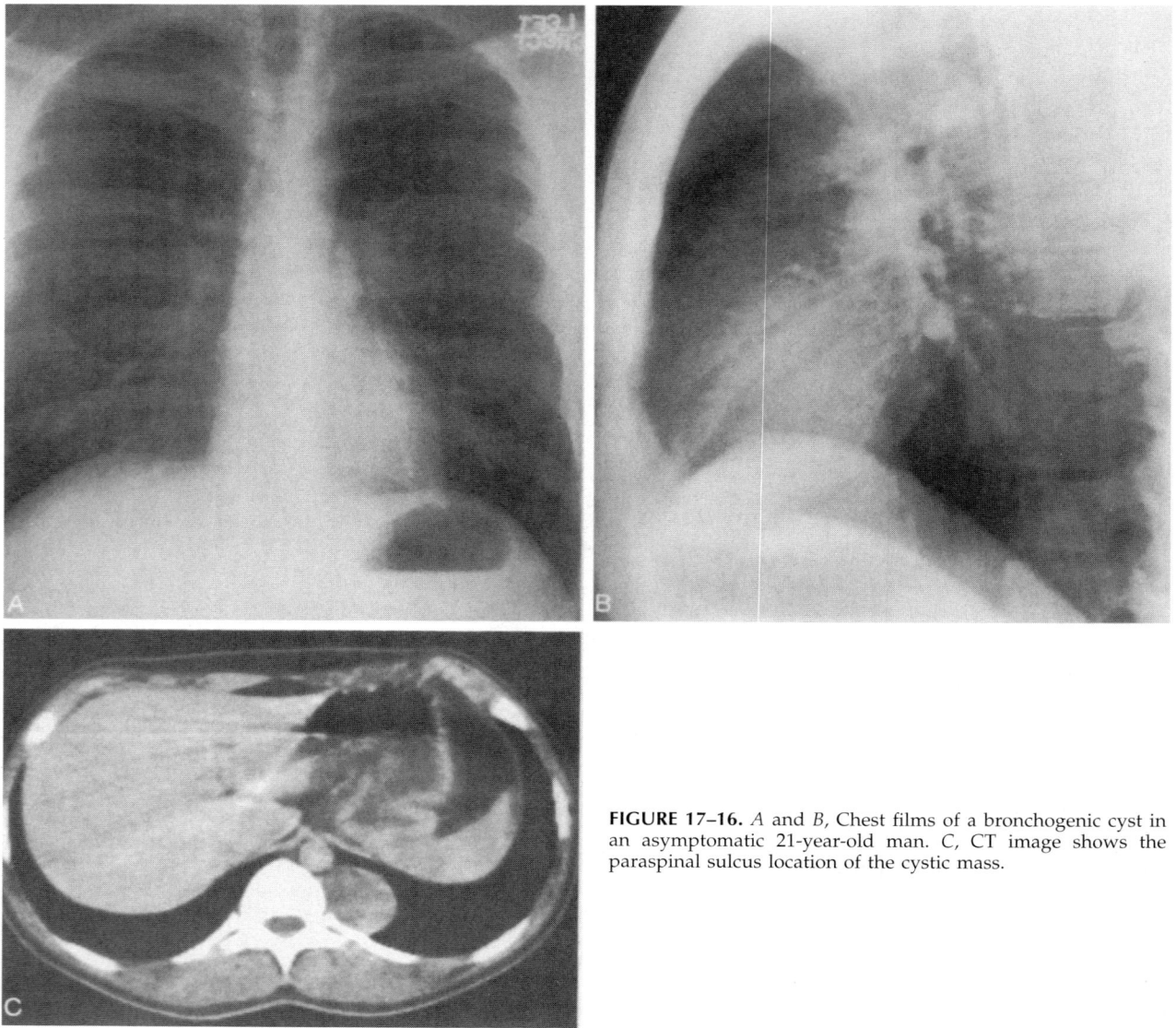

FIGURE 17–16. *A* and *B*, Chest films of a bronchogenic cyst in an asymptomatic 21-year-old man. *C*, CT image shows the paraspinal sulcus location of the cystic mass.

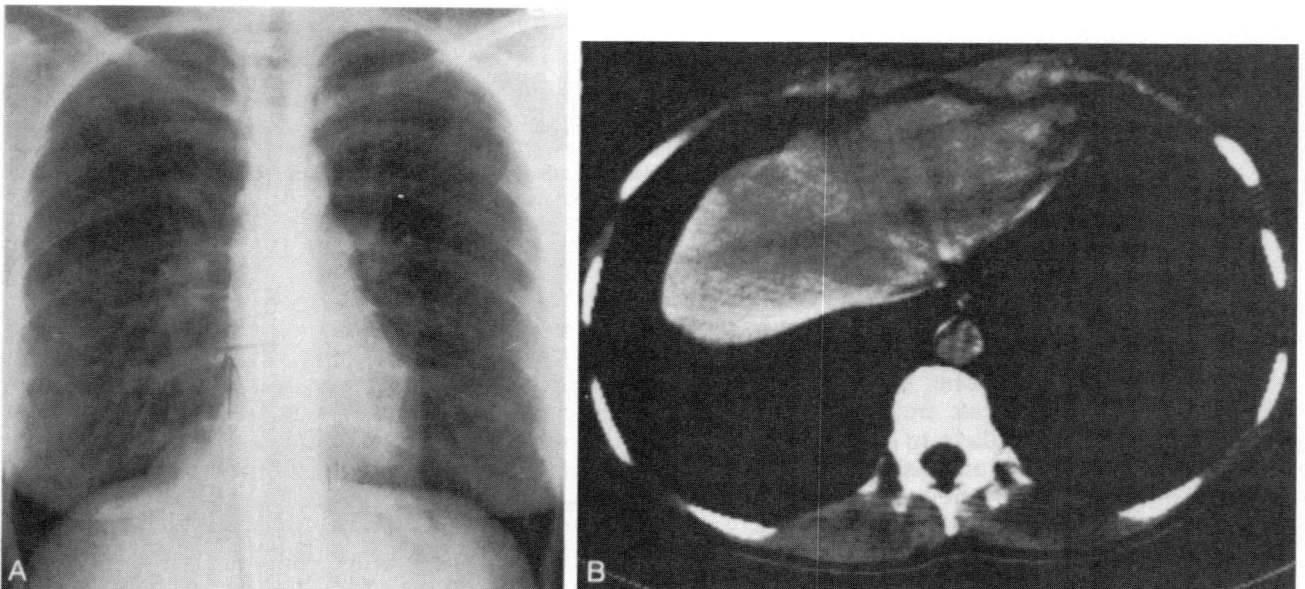

FIGURE 17–17. *A*, Chest film of a pericardial cyst in the right pericardiophrenic angle. *B*, CT image shows the characteristic near-water attenuation of the mass and the typical anatomic location.

Surgical excision of pericardial cysts is indicated primarily for diagnosis and to differentiate these cysts from malignant lesions.

Enteric Cysts

Enteric cysts (duplication cysts) arise from the posterior division of the primitive foregut, which develops into the upper division of the gastrointestinal tract. These cysts are found less frequently than bronchogenic or pericardial cysts and account for 3% of the mediastinal masses in the collected series. They are also known as inclusion cysts, gastric cysts, or enterogenous cysts and are most frequently located in the posterior mediastinum, usually adjacent to the esophagus (Fig. 17–18).

These lesions are composed of smooth muscle with an inner epithelial lining of esophageal, gastric, or intestinal mucosa. When gastric mucosa is present, peptic ulceration with perforation into the esophageal or bronchial lumen may occur, producing hemoptysis or hematemesis. Erosion into the lung parenchyma may cause hemorrhage and lung abscess formation. Gastric mucosa within enteric cysts may be visualized using ^{99}Tc scanning. Usually, enteric cysts have an attachment to the esophagus and may be embedded within the muscularis layer.

Symptoms are usually due to compression of the

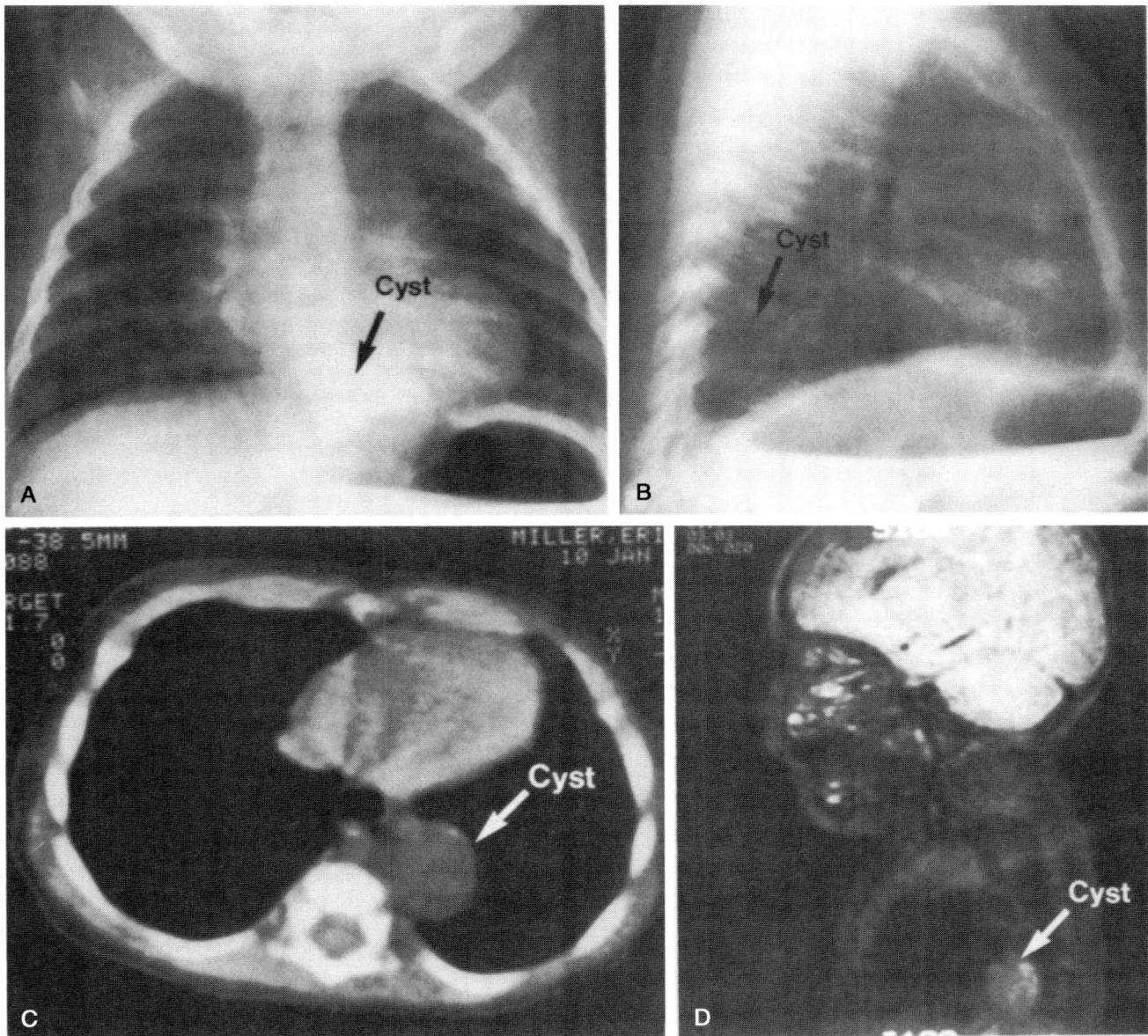

FIGURE 17–18. *A* and *B*, Chest films of an enteric cyst. *C*, CT delineates the anatomic location but does not further differentiate the mass from a neurogenic tumor. *D*, MRI manifests the cystic nature of the mass and its relationship to the esophagus. (*A–D*, From Davis, R. D., and Sabiston, D. C., Jr.: Primary mediastinal cyst and neoplasm. *In* Sabiston D. C., Jr. [ed]: Essentials of Surgery. Philadelphia, W. B. Saunders, 1987.)

esophagus leading to obstruction, commonly presenting as dysphagia. Compromise of the tracheobronchial tree with symptoms of cough, dyspnea, recurrent pulmonary infections, and chest pain may also result. Most enteric cysts are diagnosed in children, who are also more likely to be symptomatic.

When enteric cysts are associated with anomalies of the vertebral column, they are called *neuroenteric cysts*. Such cysts may be connected to the meninges, or less frequently, a direct communication with the dural space may exist. In patients with neuroenteric cysts, preoperative evaluation for potential spinal cord involvement is mandatory. The vertebral anomalies associated with this syndrome include spina bifida, hemivertebrae, and widened neural canal. CT and myelography can delineate the vertebral deformities, extension into the spinal column, and the possibility of a connection with the dural space. The embryogenesis of these tumors appears to be related to the failure of complete separation of the notochord from the primitive gut when these two structures are intimately juxtaposed during development.

Rarely, multiple mediastinal enteric cysts may occur, or there may be an association with a duplication of the abdominal portion of the alimentary tract. In the latter, there may be a transdiaphragmatic connection between abdominal and mediastinal components. Treatment is surgical excision, providing a definite histologic diagnosis as well as alleviating symptoms and preventing potential complications.

Thymic Cysts

Thymic cysts may be inflammatory, neoplastic, or congenital lesions. Congenital cysts are thought to originate from the third branchial arch and are not usually related to thymomas. These cysts are defined by the presence of thymic tissue within the cyst wall. An apparent increase in the incidence of thymic cysts following treatment of malignant anterior mediastinal neoplasms has been reported.

Nonspecific Cysts

Nonspecific cysts include those lesions in which a specific epithelial or mesothelial lining cannot be identified. These lesions may originate in any of the aforementioned cysts by the destruction of the inner epithelial lining by an inflammatory or digestive process. Other causes include postinflammatory cysts and hemorrhagic cysts.

BIBLIOGRAPHY

Adkins, R. B., Maples, M. D., and Hainsworth, J. D.: Primary malignant mediastinal tumors. Ann. Thorac. Surg., 38:648, 1984.
Aliotta, P. J., Castillo, J., Englander, L. S., et al.: Primary mediastinal germ-cell tumors: Histologic patterns of treatment failures at autopsy. Cancer, 62:982, 1988.
Azizkhan, R. G., Dudgeon, D. L., Buck, J. R., et al.: Life-threatening airway obstruction as a complication to the management of mediastinal masses in children. J. Pediatr. Surg., 20:816, 1985.
Bastianelli, R.: Quoted by Meade, R. H.: A History of Thoracic Surgery. Springfield, IL, Charles C Thomas, 1961.
Berrih-Aknin, S., Morel, E., Raimond, F., et al.: The role of the thymus in myasthenia gravis: Immunohistological and immunological studies in 115 cases. Ann. N. Y. Acad. Sci., 505:472, 1987.
Blalock, A., Mason, M. F., Morgon, H. J., and Riven, S. S.: Myasthenia gravis and tumors of the thymic region: Report of a case in which tumor was removed. Ann. Surg., 110:544, 1939.
Broun, E. R., Nichols, C. R., Einhorn, L. H., and Tricot, G. J. K.: Salvage therapy with high-dose chemotherapy and autologous bone marrow support in the treatment of primary nonseminomatous mediastinal germ-cell tumors. Cancer, 68:1513, 1991.
Burkell, C. C., Corss, J. M., Kent, H. P., and Nanson, E. M.: Mass Lesions of the Mediastinum. Chicago, Year Book Medical, 1969.
Castleman, B., Iverson, L., and Menendez, V. P.: Localized mediastinal lymphoid hyperplasia resembling thymoma. Cancer 9:822, 1956.
Clark, O. H.: Mediastinal parathyroid tumors. Arch. Surg., 123:1096, 1988.
Conkle, D. M., and Adkins, R. B.: Primary malignant tumors of the mediastinum. Ann. Thorac. Surg., 14:553, 1972.
Conn, J. M., Goncalves, M. A., Mansour, K. A., and McGarity, W. C.: The mediastinal parathyroid. Am. Surg., 57:62, 1991.
Crist, W. M., Shuster, J. J., Falletta, J., et al.: Clinical features and outcome in childhood T-cell leukemia-lymphoma according to stage of the thymocyte differentiation: A Pediatric Oncology Group Study. Blood, 72:1891, 1988.
Curran, W. J., Kornstein, M. J., Brooks, J. J., and Turrisi, A. T.: Invasive thymoma: The role of mediastinal irradiation following complete or incomplete surgical resection. J. Clin. Oncol., 6:1722, 1988.
Daly, B. D. T., Faling, J., Bite, G., et al.: Mediastinal lymph evaluation by computed tomography in lung cancer: An analysis of 345 patients grouped by TNM staging, tumor size, and tumor location. J. Thorac. Cardiovasc. Surg., 94:664, 1987.
Dartevelle, P. G., Chapelier, A. R., Pastorino, U., et al.: Long-term follow-up after prosthetic replacement of the superior vena cava combined with resection of mediastinal-pulmonary malignant tumors. Thorac. Cardiovasc. Surg., 102:259, 1991.
Dartevelle, P. G., Chapelier, A. R., Navajas, M., et al.: Replacement of the superior vena cava with polytetrafluoroethylene grafts combined with resection of mediastinal-pulmonary malignant tumors. J. Thorac. Cardiovasc. Surg. 94:361, 1987.
Davis, R. D., Oldham, H. N., and Sabiston, D. C.: Primary cysts and neoplasms of the mediastinum: Recent changes in clinical presentation, methods of diagnosis, management, and results. Ann. Thorac. Surg., 44:229, 1987.
Doherty, G. M., Doppman, J. L., Miller, D. L., et al.: Results of a multidisciplinary strategy for management of mediastinal parathyroid adenoma as a cause of persistent primary hyperparathyroidism. Ann. Surg., 215:101, 1991.
Doty, D. B.: Bypass of superior vena cava: Six years experience with spiral vein graft for obstruction of superior vena cava due to benign and malignant disease. J. Thorac. Cardiovasc. Surg., 83:326, 1982.
Elert, O., Buchwald, J., and Wolf, K.: Epithelial thymus tumors—Therapy and prognosis. Thorac. Cardiovasc. Surg., 36:109, 1988.
Epstein, A. M., and Klassen, K. P.: Spontaneous superior mediastinal hemorrhage. J. Thorac. Cardiovasc. Surg., 39:740, 1960.
Fischer, J. E., Grinvalski, H. T., Nussbaum, M. S., et al.: Aggressive surgical approach for drug-free remission from myasthenia gravis. Ann. Surg., 205:496, 1987.
Fontanelle, L. J., Armstrong, R. G., Stanford, W., et al.: Asymptomatic mediastinal mass. Arch. Surg., 102:98, 1971.
Glenner, G. G., and Grimley, P. M.: Tumors of the Extra-adrenal Paraganglion System (Including Chemoreceptors): Atlas of Tumor Pathology. 2nd series; fasci. 9. Washington, DC, Armed Forces Institute of Pathology, 1974.
Goldel, N., Boning, L., Fredrik, A., et al.: Chemotherapy of invasive thymoma. A retrospective study of 22 cases. Cancer, 63:1493, 1989.
Grosfeld, J. L., Weinberg, M., Kilmann, J. W., and Clatworthy, H. W.: Primary mediastinal neoplasms in infants and children. Ann. Thorac. Surg., 12:170, 1971.

Haller, J. A., Mazur, D. O., and Morgan, W. M.: Diagnosis and management of mediastinal masses in children. J. Thorac. Cardiovasc. Surg., 58:385, 1969.

Hamman, L.: Spontaneous mediastinal emphysema. Bull. Johns Hopkins Hosp., 64:1, 1939.

Harrington, S. W.: Surgical treatment of intrathoracic tumors. Arch. Surg., 19:1679, 1929.

Heimburger, I. L., and Battersby, J. S.: Primary mediastinal tumors of childhood. J. Thorac. Cardiovasc. Surg., 50:92, 1965.

Heimburger, I. L., Battersby, J. S., and Vellios, F.: Primary neoplasms of the mediastinum: A fifteen-year experience. Arch. Surg., 86:978, 1963.

Heuer, G. J., and Andrus, W. D.: The surgery of mediastinal tumors. Am. J. Surg., 50:146, 1940.

Issa, P. Y., Brihi, E. R., Janin, Y., and Slim, M. S.: Superior vena cava syndrome in childhood: Report of ten cases and review of the literature. Pediatrics, 71:337, 1983.

Janin, Y., Becker, J., Wise, L., et al.: Superior vena cava syndrome in childhood and adolescence: A review of the literature and report of three cases. J. Pediatr. Surg., 17:290, 1982.

Jaretzki, A., Penn, A. S., Younger, D. S., et al.: Maximal thymectomy for myasthenia gravis. J. Thorac. Cardiovasc. Surg., 95:747, 1988.

Jochelson, M., Mauch, P., Balikian, J., et al.: The significance of the residual mediastinal mass in treated Hodgkin's disease. J. Clin. Oncol., 3:637, 1985.

Kay, P. H., Wells, F. C., and Goldstraw, P.: A multidisciplinary approach to primary nonseminomatous germ-cell tumors of the mediastinum. Ann. Thorac. Surg., 44:578, 1987.

Kersh, C. R., Eisert, D. R., Constable, W. C., et al.: Primary malignant mediastinal germ-cell tumors and the contribution of radiotherapy: A southeastern multi-institutional study. Am. J. Clin. Oncol., 10:302, 1987.

King, R. M., Telander, R. L., Smithson, W. A., et al.: Primary mediastinal tumors in children. J. Pediatr. Surg., 17:512, 1982.

Kornstein, M. J., Curran, W. J., Turrisi, A. T., and Brooks, J. J.: Cortical versus medullary thymomas: A useful morphologic distinction? Hum. Pathol., 19:1335, 1988.

Lahdenne, P.: Late sequelae of gonadal, mediastinal and oral teratomas in childhood. Acta Paediatr., 81:235, 1992.

Lavabre-Bertrand, T., Donadio, D., Fegueux, N., et al.: A study of 15 cases of primary mediastinal lymphoma of B-cell type. Cancer, 69:2561, 1992.

Loeffler, J. S., Leopold, K. A., Recht, A., et al.: Emergency prebiopsy radiation for mediastinal masses: Impact on subsequent pathologic diagnosis and outcome. J. Clin. Oncol., 4:716, 1986.

Melms, A., Schalke, B. C., Kirchner, T., et al.: Thymus in myasthenia gravis: Isolation of T-lymphocyte lines specific for the nicotinic acetylcholine receptors from thymuses of myasthenic patients. J. Clin. Invest., 81:902, 1988.

Milton, H.: Mediastinal surgery. Lancet, 1:872, 1897.

Motzer, R. J., Rodriguez, E., Reuter, V. E., et al.: Genetic analysis as an aid in diagnosis for patients with midline carcinomas of uncertain histologies. J. Natl. Cancer Inst., 83:341, 1991.

Nakahara, K., Ohno, K., Matsumura, A., et al.: Extended operation for lung cancer invading the aortic arch and superior vena cava. J. Thorac. Cardiovasc. Surg., 97:428, 1989.

Nandi, P., Wong, K. C., Mok, C. K., and Ong, G. B.: Primary mediastinal tumors: Review of 74 cases. J. R. Coll. Surg. Edinb., 25:460, 1980.

Neuman, G. G., Weingarten, A. E., Abramowitz, R. M., et al.: The anesthetic management of the patient with an anterior mediastinal mass. Anesthesiology, 60:144, 1984.

Nichols, C. R., Heerema, N. A., Palmer, C., et al.: Klinefelter's syndrome associated with mediastinal germ-cell neoplasms. J. Clin. Oncol., 5:1290, 1987.

Ovrum, E., and Birkeland, S.: Mediastinal tumours and cysts. A review of 91 cases. Scand. J. Thorac. Surg. 13:161, 1979.

Parish, J. M., Rosenow, E. C., and Muhm, J. R.: Mediastinal masses: Clues to interpretation of radiologic studies. Postgrad. Med., 76:173, 1984.

Pokorny, W. J., and Sherman, J. O.: Mediastinal masses in infants and children. J. Thorac. Cardiovasc. Surg., 68:689, 1974.

Radford, J. A., Cowan, R. A., Flanagan, M., et al.: The significance of residual mediastinal abnormality on the chest radiograph following treatment for Hodgkin's disease. J. Clin. Oncol., 6:940, 1988.

Rendina, E. A., Venuta, F., Ceroni, L., et al.: Computed tomographic staging of anterior mediastinal neoplasms. Thorax, 43:441, 1988.

Rousou, J. A., Kirkwood, R., Engelman, R. M., and Breyer, R. H.: Catheter drainage of symptomatic postoperative mediastinal effusion guided by computed tomography. J. Thorac. Cardiovasc. Surg., 93:715, 1987.

Rubush, J. L., Gardner, I. R., Boyd, W. C., and Ehrenhaft, J. L.: Mediastinal tumors: Review of 186 cases. J. Thorac. Cardiovasc. Surg., 65:216, 1973.

Sabiston, D. C., Jr., and Scott, H. W.: Primary neoplasms and cysts of the mediastinum. Ann. Surg., 136:777, 1952.

Safar, D., Berrih, A. S., and Morel, E.: In vitro anti-acetylcholine receptor antibody synthesis by myasthenia gravis patient lymphocytes: Correlations with thymic histology and thymic epithelial-cell interactions. J. Clin. Immunol., 7:225, 1987.

Shamberger, R. C., Allarde-Segundo, A., Kozakewich, H. P., and Grier, H. E.: Surgical management of stage III and IV neuroblastoma: Resection before or after chemotherapy. J. Pediatr. Surg., 26:1113; discussion 1117, 1991.

Simpson, I., and Campbell, P. E.: Mediastinal masses in childhood: A review from a paediatric pathologist's point of view. Prog. Pediatr. Surg., 27:93, 1991.

Taniguchi, S., Shibuya, T., Morioka, E., et al.: Demonstration of three distinct immunological disorders on erythropoiesis in a patient with red cell aplasia and autoimmune haemolytic anaemia associated with thymoma. Br. J. Haematol., 68:473, 1988.

Verley, J. M., and Hollman, K. H.: Thymoma: A comparative study of clinical stages, histologic features and survival in 200 cases. Cancer, 55:1074, 1985.

Vidne, B., and Levy, M. J.: Mediastinal tumors. Surgical treatment in forty-five consecutive cases. Scand. J. Thorac. Cardiovasc. Surg., 7:59, 1973.

Wang, C., Gaz, R. D., and Moncure, A. C.: Mediastinal parathyroid exploration: A clinical and pathologic study of 47 cases. World J. Surg., 10:687, 1986.

Weiner, M., Leventhal, B., Cantor, A., et al.: Gallium-67 scans as an adjunct to computed tomography scans for the assessment of a residual mediastinal mass in pediatric patients with Hodgkin's disease. Cancer, 68:2478, 1991.

Wick, M. R., Bernatz, P. E., Carney, J. A., and Brown, L. R.: Primary mediastinal carcinoid tumors. Am. J. Surg. Pathol., 6:195, 1982.

Whittaker, L. D., Jr., and Lynn, H. B.: Mediastinal tumors and cysts in the pediatric patient. Surg. Clin. North Am., 53:893, 1973.

18 Thoracic Outlet Syndrome

Harold C. Urschel, Jr., and Maruf A. Razzuk

Thoracic outlet syndrome, a term coined by Rob and Standover (1958), refers to compression of the subclavian vessels and brachial plexus at the superior aperture of the chest. It was previously designated according to presumed etiologies as scalenus anticus, costoclavicular, hyperabduction, cervical rib, and first thoracic rib syndromes. The various syndromes are similar, and the compression mechanism is often difficult to identify. Most compressive factors operate against the first rib (Clagett, 1962; Urschel et al., 1968) (Fig. 18–1).

HISTORICAL ASPECTS

Until 1927, the cervical rib was commonly thought to be the cause of symptoms of this syndrome. Galen and Vesalius first described the presence of a cervical rib (Borchardt, 1901). Hunauld, who published an article in 1742, is credited by Keen (1970) as being the first to describe the importance of the cervical rib in causing symptoms. In 1818, Cooper treated symptoms of cervical rib with some success (Adson and Coffey, 1927), and in 1861, Coote did the first cervical rib removal. Halsted (1916) stimulated interest in dilatation of the subclavian artery distal to cervical ribs, and Law (1920) reported the role of adventitious ligaments in the cervical rib syndrome. In 1927, Adson and Coffey suggested the role of the scalenus anticus muscle in cervical rib syndrome. Naffziger and Grant (1938) and Ochsner and associates (1935) popularized section of the scalenus anticus muscle. Falconer and Weddell (1943) and Brintnall and colleagues (1956) incriminated the costoclavicular membrane in the production of neurovascular compression. In 1945, Wright described the hyperabduction syndrome with compression in the costoclavicular area by the tendon of the pectoralis minor. Rosati and Lord (1961) added claviculectomy to anterior exploration, scalenotomy, cervical rib resection, when one was present, and section of the pectoralis minor and subclavian muscles, as well as the costoclavicular membrane. The role of the first rib in causing symptoms of neurovascular compression was recognized by Bramwell in 1903. Murphy (1910) is credited with the first resection of the first rib. Brickner (1927), Brickner and Milch (1925), and Telford and co-workers (1937, 1948) suggested that the first rib was the culprit. Clagett (1962) emphasized the first rib and its resection through the posterior thoracoplasty approach to relieve neurovascular compression. In 1962, Falconer and Li reported the anterior approach for first rib resection, whereas Roos (1966) introduced the transaxillary route for first rib resection and extirpation. Krusen and Caldwell (Caldwell et al., 1971) introduced the method of measuring motor conduction velocities across the thoracic outlet in diagnosing thoracic outlet syndrome. Urschel and associates (1976) popularized reoperation for recurrent thoracic outlet syndrome.

SURGICAL ANATOMY

At the superior aperture of the thorax, the subclavian vessels and the brachial plexus traverse the cervicoaxillary canal to reach the upper extremity. The cervicoaxillary canal is divided by the first rib into two sections: the proximal one, composed of the scalene triangle and the costoclavicular space,* and the distal one, composed of the axilla. The proximal division is the more critical for neurovascular compression. It is bounded superiorly by the clavicle, inferiorly by the first rib, anteromedially by the costoclavicular ligament, and posterolaterally by the scalenus medius muscle and the long thoracic nerve. The scalenus anticus muscle, which inserts on the scalene tubercle of the first rib, divides the costoclavicular space into two compartments: the anteromedial one containing the subclavian vein and the posterolateral one containing the subclavian artery and the brachial plexus (Fig. 18–2). The latter compartment, which is bounded by the scalenus anticus anteriorly, the scalenus medius posteriorly, and the first rib inferiorly, is called the *scalene triangle.*

FUNCTIONAL ANATOMY

The cervicoaxillary canal, particularly its proximal segment, the costoclavicular area, normally has ample space for passage of the neurovascular bundle without compression. Narrowing of this space occurs during functional maneuvers. It narrows during abduction of the arm because the clavicle rotates backward toward the first rib and the insertion of the scalenus anticus muscle. In hyperabduction, the neurovascular bundle is pulled around the pectoralis minor tendon, the coracoid process, and the head of the humerus. During this maneuver, the coracoid process tilts

---

*The term *costoclavicular space* is used here to refer to the space bounded by the clavicle and the first rib.

THORACIC OUTLET SYNDROME

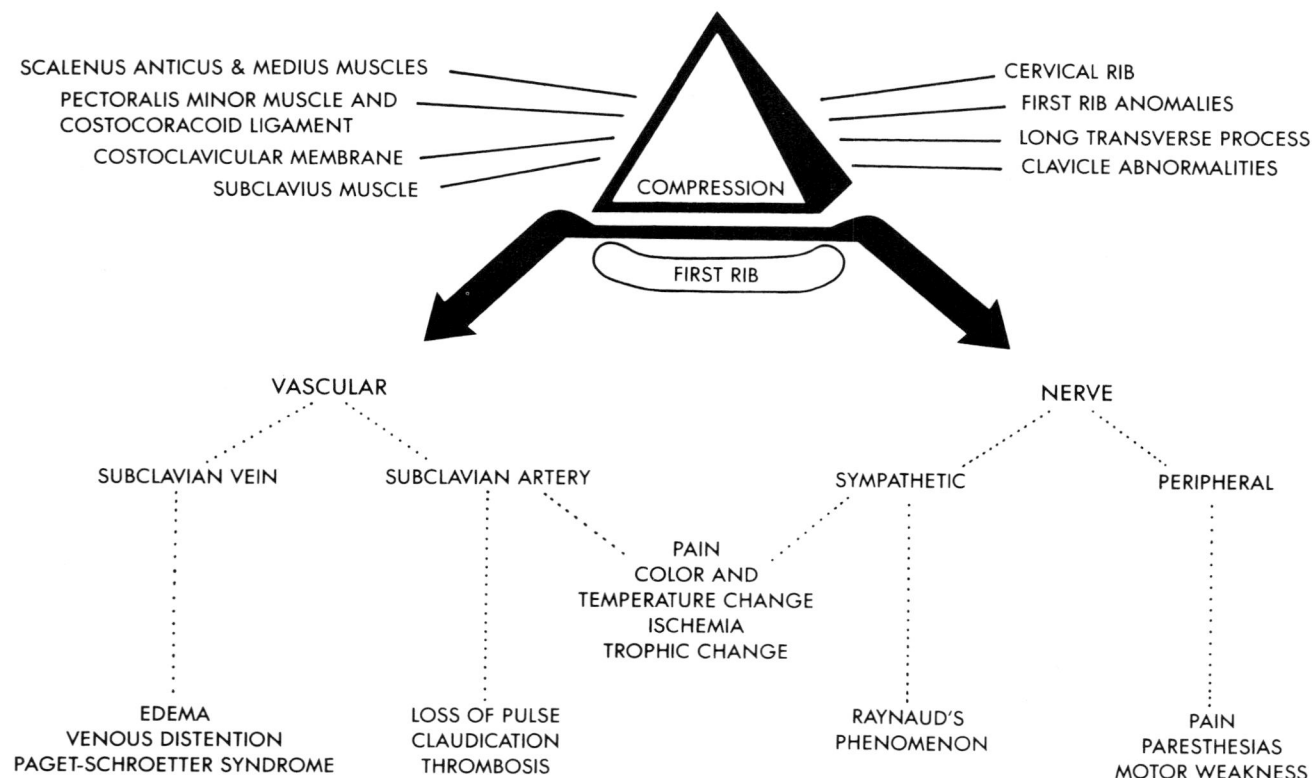

SCALENUS ANTICUS & MEDIUS MUSCLES

PECTORALIS MINOR MUSCLE AND
COSTOCORACOID LIGAMENT

COSTOCLAVICULAR MEMBRANE

SUBCLAVIUS MUSCLE

COMPRESSION

FIRST RIB

CERVICAL RIB

FIRST RIB ANOMALIES

LONG TRANSVERSE PROCESS

CLAVICLE ABNORMALITIES

VASCULAR

NERVE

SUBCLAVIAN VEIN   SUBCLAVIAN ARTERY   SYMPATHETIC   PERIPHERAL

PAIN
COLOR AND
TEMPERATURE CHANGE
ISCHEMIA
TROPHIC CHANGE

EDEMA
VENOUS DISTENTION
PAGET-SCHROETTER SYNDROME

LOSS OF PULSE
CLAUDICATION
THROMBOSIS

RAYNAUD'S
PHENOMENON

PAIN
PARESTHESIAS
MOTOR WEAKNESS

FIGURE 18–1. Schematic diagram showing the relation of muscle, ligament, and bone abnormalities in the thoracic outlet that may compress neurovascular structures against the first rib.

downward and thus exaggerates the tension on the bundle. The sternoclavicular joint, which ordinarily forms an angle of 15 to 20 degrees, forms a smaller angle when the outer end of the clavicle descends (as in drooping of the shoulders in poor posture), and

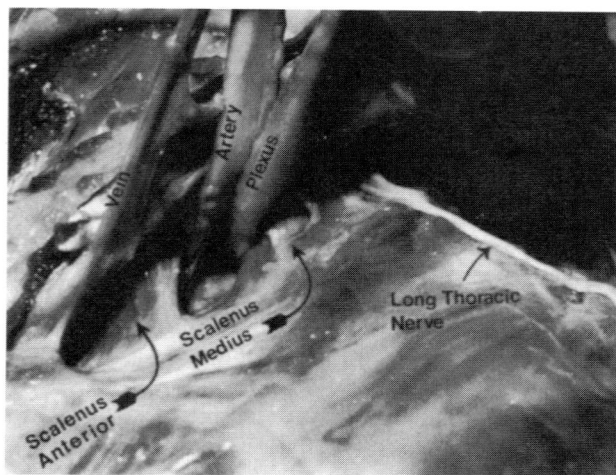

FIGURE 18–2. Anatomic dissection from the transaxillary approach, showing the relation of the neurovascular bundle, the scalenus anterior muscle, and the long thoracic nerve along the posterior border of the scalenus medius muscle.

narrowing of the costoclavicular space may occur (Rosati and Lord, 1961). Normally, during inspiration, the scalenus anticus muscle raises the first rib and thus narrows the costoclavicular space. This muscle may cause an abnormal lift of the first rib, as in cases of severe emphysema or excessive muscular development, which is seen in young adults.

The scalene triangle, which normally occurs between the scalenus anticus anteriorly, the scalenus medius posteriorly, and first rib inferiorly, permits the passage of the subclavian artery and the brachial plexus, which are in direct contact with the first rib. The space of the triangle is 1.2 cm at its base and approximately 6.7 cm in height (Fig. 18–3). There is a close-fitting relationship between the neurovascular bundle and this triangular space. Anatomic variations may narrow the superior angle of the triangle, cause impingement on the upper components of the brachial plexus, and produce the upper type of scalenus anticus syndrome that involves the trunk containing elements of C5 and C6. If the base of the triangle is raised, compression of the subclavian artery and the trunk containing components of C7, C8, and T1 results in the lower type of scalenus anticus syndrome. Both types have been described by Swank and Simeone (1944).

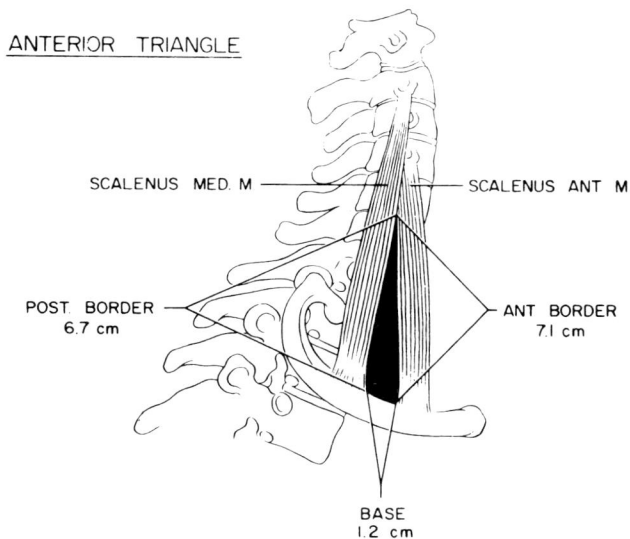

ANTERIOR TRIANGLE

SCALENUS MED. M — SCALENUS ANT. M

POST. BORDER 6.7 cm

ANT. BORDER 7.1 cm

BASE 1.2 cm

FIGURE 18–3. Schematic drawing of the scalene (anterior) triangle showing its measurements and the narrow interval through which the neurovascular bundle passes. (From Rosati, L. M., and Lord, J. W.: Neurovascular Compression Syndromes of the Shoulder Girdle. New York, Grune & Stratton, 1961.)

COMPRESSION FACTORS

Many factors may cause compression of the neurovascular bundle at the thoracic outlet, but the basic factor is deranged anatomy, to which congenital, traumatic, and occasionally, atherosclerotic factors may contribute (Rosati and Lord, 1961) (Table 18–1). Bony abnormalities are present in approximately 30% of patients, either as cervical rib, bifid first rib, fusion of first and second ribs, clavicular deformities, or previous thoracoplasties (Urschel et al., 1968). These abnormalities can be visualized on the plain posteroanterior chest film, but special x-ray views of the lower cervical spine may be required in some cases of cervical ribs.

SYMPTOMS AND SIGNS

The symptoms of thoracic outlet syndrome depend on whether the nerves or blood vessels, or both, are compressed in the cervicoaxillary canal. Neurogenic manifestations are observed more frequently than vascular ones. Symptoms consist of pain and paresthesias, which are present in approximately 95% of cases, and motor weakness and occasionally atrophy of hypothenar and interosseous muscles, which is the ulnar type of atrophy, in approximately 10%. The symptoms occur most commonly in areas supplied by the ulnar nerve, which include the medial aspects of the arm and hand, the fifth finger, and the lateral aspects of the fourth finger. The onset of pain is usually insidious and commonly involves the neck, shoulder, arm, and hand. The pain and paresthesias may be precipitated by strenuous physical exercise or sustained physical effort with the arm in abduction

and the neck in hyperextension. Symptoms may be initiated by sleeping with the arms abducted and the hands clasped behind the neck. In other cases, trauma to the upper extremities or the cervical spine is a precipitating factor. Physical examination may be noncontributory. When present, objective physical findings usually consist of hypesthesia along the medial aspects of the forearm and hand. Atrophy, when evident, is usually described in the hypothenar and interosseous muscles with clawing of the fourth and fifth fingers. In the upper type of thoracic outlet syndrome in which components of C5 and C6 are involved in compression, pain is usually in the deltoid area and the lateral aspects of the arm. The presence of this pain should induce action to exclude a herniated cervical disk (Rosati and Lord, 1961). Entrapment of C7 and C8 components that contribute to the median nerve produces symptoms in the index and sometimes the middle fingers. Components of C5, C6, C7, C8, and T1 can occur at the thoracic outlet by a cervical rib and produce symptoms of various degrees in the distribution of these nerves (Fig. 18–4).

In some patients, the pain is atypical, involving the anterior chest wall or parascapular area, and is termed *pseudoangina* because it simulates angina pectoris. These patients may have normal coronary arteriograms and ulnar nerve conduction velocities decreased to values of 48 m/sec and less, which strongly suggests the diagnosis of thoracic outlet syndrome. The shoulder, arm, and hand symptoms that usually provide the clue for the diagnosis of thoracic outlet syndrome may initially be absent or minimal com-

■ **Table 18–1.** ETIOLOGIC FACTORS OF NEUROVASCULAR COMPRESSION SYNDROMES

Anatomic
Potential sites of neurovascular compression
  Interscalene triangle
  Costoclavicular space
  Subcoracoid area

Congenital
Cervical rib and its fascial remnants
Rudimentary first thoracic rib
Scalene muscles
  Anterior
  Middle
  Minimus
Adventitious fibrous bands
Bifid clavicle
Exostosis of first thoracic rib
Enlarged transverse process of C7
Omohyoid muscle
Anomalous course of transverse cervical artery
Brachial plexus postfixed
Flat clavicle

Traumatic
Fracture of clavicle
Dislocation of head of humerus
Crushing injury to upper thorax
Sudden, unaccustomed muscular efforts involving shoulder
  girdle muscles
Cervical spondylosis and injuries to cervical spine

Atherosclerosis

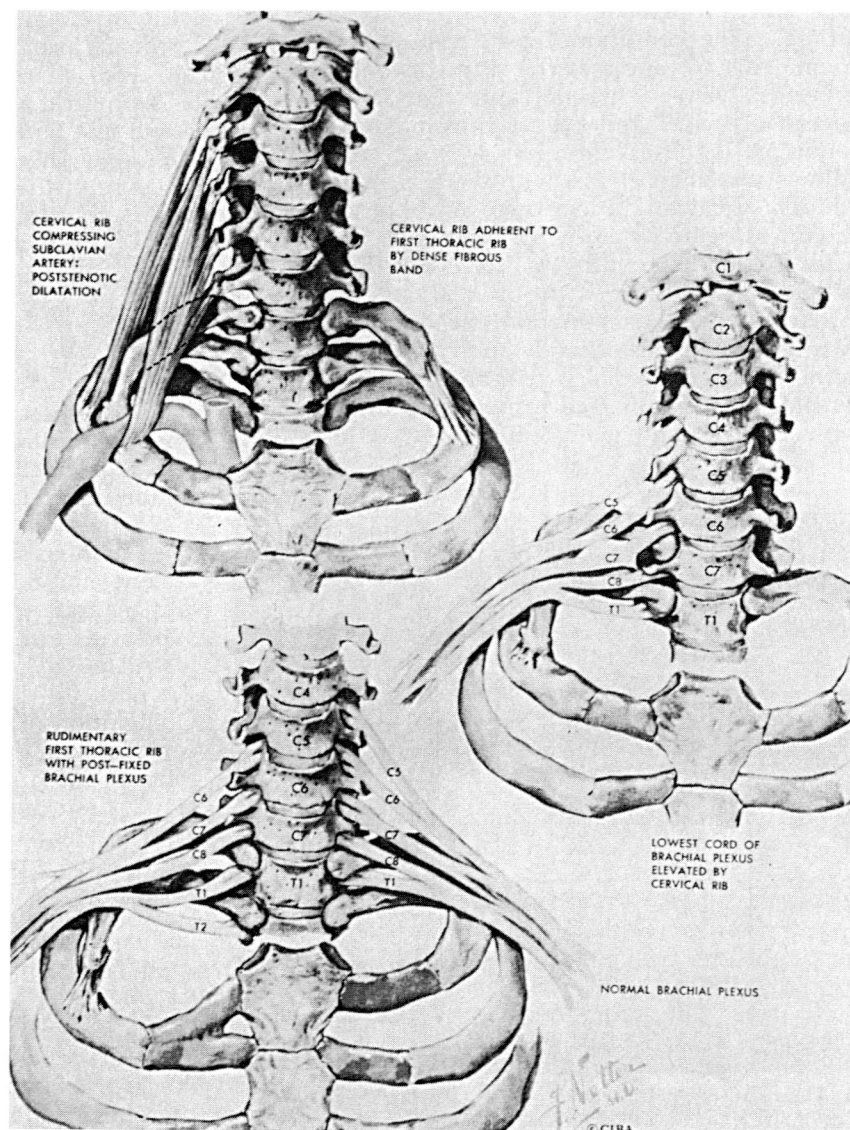

FIGURE 18–4. Compression caused by congenital rib abnormalities. (Copyright 1971. CIBA-GEIGY Corporation. Reproduced with permission from Clinical Symposia by Frank H. Netter, M.D. All rights reserved.)

pared with the severity of the chest pain. The diagnosis of thoracic outlet syndrome is frequently overlooked; many of these patients are committed to becoming "cardiac cripples" without an appropriate diagnosis or develop severe psychologic depression when told that their coronary arteries are normal and that they have no significant cause for their pain (Urschel et al., 1973).

Symptoms of arterial compression include coldness, weakness, easy fatigability of the arm and hand, and pain that is usually diffuse (Urschel et al., 1968; Urschel and Razzuk, 1972). Raynaud's phenomenon is noted in approximately 7.5% of patients with thoracic outlet syndrome (Urschel et al., 1968). Unlike Raynaud's disease, which is usually bilateral and symmetric and elicited by cold or emotion, Raynaud's phenomenon in neurovascular compression is usually unilateral and is more likely to be precipitated by hyperabduction of the involved arm, turning of the head, or carrying of heavy objects. Sensitivity to cold may also be present. Symptoms include sudden onset of cold and blanching of one or more fingers, followed slowly by cyanosis and persistent rubor. Vascular symptoms in neurovascular compression may be precursors of permanent arterial thrombosis (Rosati and Lord, 1961). Arterial occlusion, usually of the subclavian artery, when present, is manifested by persistent coldness, cyanosis or pallor of the fingers, and in some instances, ulceration or gangrene. Palpation in the parascapular area may reveal prominent pulsation, which indicates poststenotic dilatation or aneurysm of the subclavian artery (Rosenberg, 1966) (Fig. 18–5).

Less frequently, the symptoms are those of venous obstruction or occlusion, commonly recognized as *effort thrombosis*, or *Paget-Schroetter syndrome*. The condi-

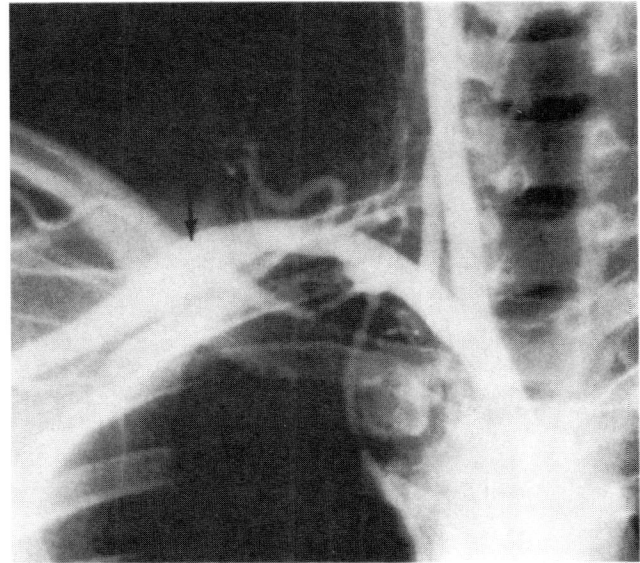

FIGURE 18–5. Arteriogram showing poststenotic dilatation (*arrow*) of the right subclavian artery secondary to thoracic outlet compression.

tion characteristically results in edema, discoloration of the arm, distention of the superficial veins of the limb and shoulder, and some degree of aches and pains. In some patients, the condition is observed on waking; in others, it follows sustained efforts with the arm in abduction. Sudden backward and downward bracing of the shoulders or heavy lifting or strenuous physical activity involving the arm may constrict the vein and initiate venospasm, with or without subsequent thrombosis. On examination, in cases of definite venous thrombosis, there is usually moderate tenderness over the axillary vein and a cord-like structure may be felt that corresponds to the course of the vein. The acute symptoms may subside in a few weeks or days as the collateral circulation develops. Recurrence follows with inadequacy of the collateral circulation (Lord and Urschel, 1988).

Objective physical findings are more common in patients with primarily vascular rather than neural compression. Loss or diminution of radial pulse and reproduction of symptoms can be elicited by the three classic clinical maneuvers—the Adson or scalene test (Adson, 1951), the costoclavicular test, and the hyperabduction test (Urschel and Razzuk, 1973).

DIAGNOSIS

The diagnosis of thoracic outlet syndrome includes history, physical and neurologic examinations, films of the chest and cervical spine, electromyogram, and ulnar nerve conduction velocity (UNCV). In some cases with atypical manifestations, other diagnostic procedures such as cervical myelography, peripheral (Rosenberg, 1966) or coronary arteriography, or phlebography (Adams et al., 1968) should be considered. A detailed history and physical and neurologic examinations can often result in a tentative diagnosis of neurovascular compression. This diagnosis is strengthened when one or more of the classic clinical maneuvers is positive and is confirmed by the finding of decreased UNCV (Urschel and Razzuk, 1972).

Clinical Maneuvers

The clinical evaluation is best based on the physical findings of loss or decrease of radial pulses and reproduction of symptoms that can be elicited by the three classic maneuvers:

1. *Adson or scalene test* (Adson, 1951) (Fig. 18–6). This maneuver tightens the anterior and middle scalene muscles and thus decreases the interspace and magnifies any preexisting compression of the subclavian artery and brachial plexus. The patient is instructed to take and hold a deep breath, extend the neck fully, and turn the head toward the side. Obliteration or decrease of the radial pulse suggests compression (Rosati and Lord, 1961; Urschel and Razzuk, 1973).

2. *Costoclavicular test* (military position) (Fig. 18–7). The shoulders are drawn downward and backward. This maneuver narrows the costoclavicular space by approximating the clavicle to the first rib and thus tends to compress the neurovascular bundle. Changes in the radial pulse with production of symptoms indicate compression (Rosati and Lord, 1961; Urschel and Razzuk, 1973).

3. *Hyperabduction test* (Fig. 18–8). When the arm is hyperabducted to 180 degrees, the components of the neurovascular bundle are pulled around the pectoralis minor tendon, the coracoid process, and the head of the humerus. If the radial pulse is decreased, compression should be suspected (Rosati and Lord, 1961; Urschel and Razzuk, 1973).

Radiographic Findings

Films of the chest and cervical spine are helpful in revealing bony abnormalities, particularly cervical

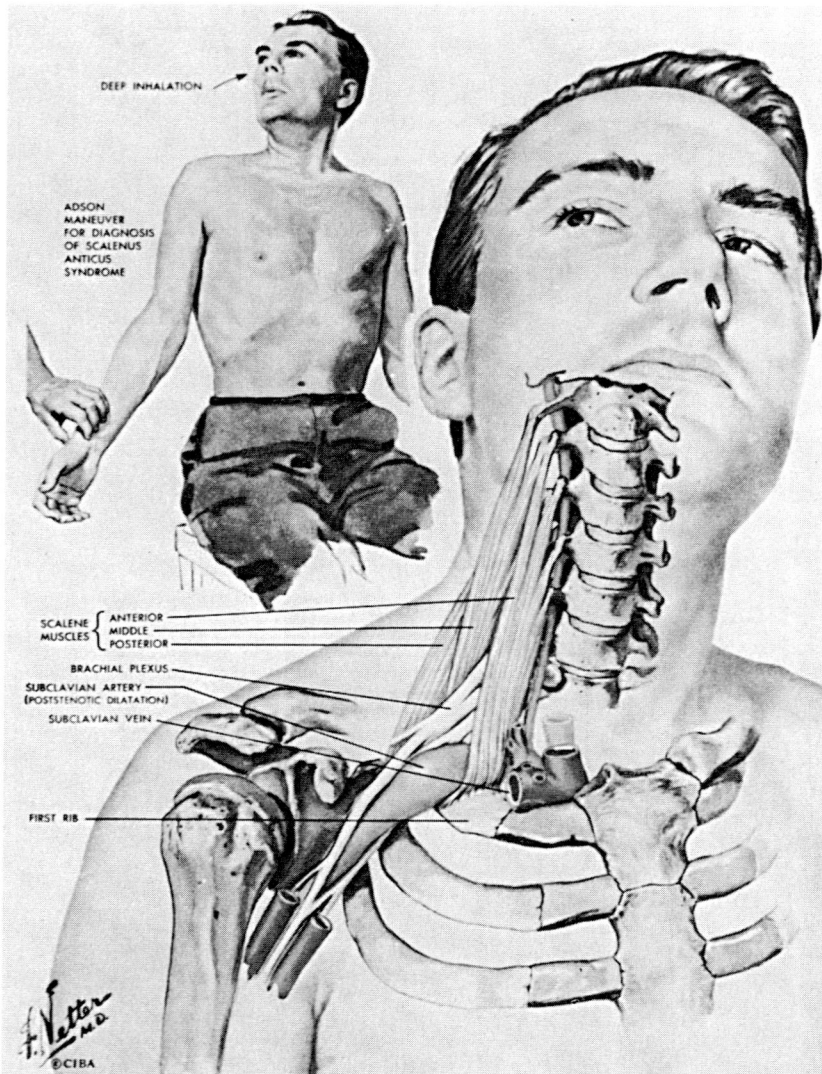

FIGURE 18–6. Adson's maneuver. Relation of the scalene triangle to the neurovascular bundle. (Copyright 1971. CIBA-GEIGY Corporation. Reproduced with permission from Clinical Symposia by Frank H. Netter, M.D. All rights reserved.)

ribs (Fig. 18–9) and bony degenerative changes. If osteophytic changes and intervertebral space narrowing are present on plain cervical films, a cervical computed tomography (CT) scan should be performed to rule out bony encroachment and narrowing of the spinal canal and the intervertebral foramina.

Nerve Conduction Velocity and Electromyography

This test is widely used in differential diagnosis of the causes of arm pain, tingling, and numbness with or without motor weakness of the hand. Such symptoms may result from compression at various sites: in the spine; at the thoracic outlet; around the elbow, where it causes tardy ulnar nerve palsy; or on the flexor aspects of the wrist, where it produces carpal tunnel syndrome. For diagnosis and localization of the site of compression, cathodal stimulation is applied at various points along the course of the nerve. Motor conduction velocities of the ulnar, median, ra-

dial, and musculocutaneous nerves can be measured reliably (Jebsen, 1967). Caldwell and colleagues (1971) have improved the technique of measuring UNCV for evaluation of patients with thoracic outlet compression. Conduction velocities over proximal and distal segments of the ulnar nerve are determined by recording the action potentials generated in the hypothenar or first dorsal interosseous muscles. The points of stimulation are the supraclavicular fossa, middle upper arm, below the elbow, and at the wrist (Urschel and Razzuk, 1972) (Fig. 18–10).

Method of Measuring Conduction Velocities

Equipment

Electromyographic examination of each upper extremity and determination of the conduction velocities are done with the Meditron 201 AD or 312 or the TECA-3 electromyograph; coaxial cable with three needles or surface electrodes are used to record mus-

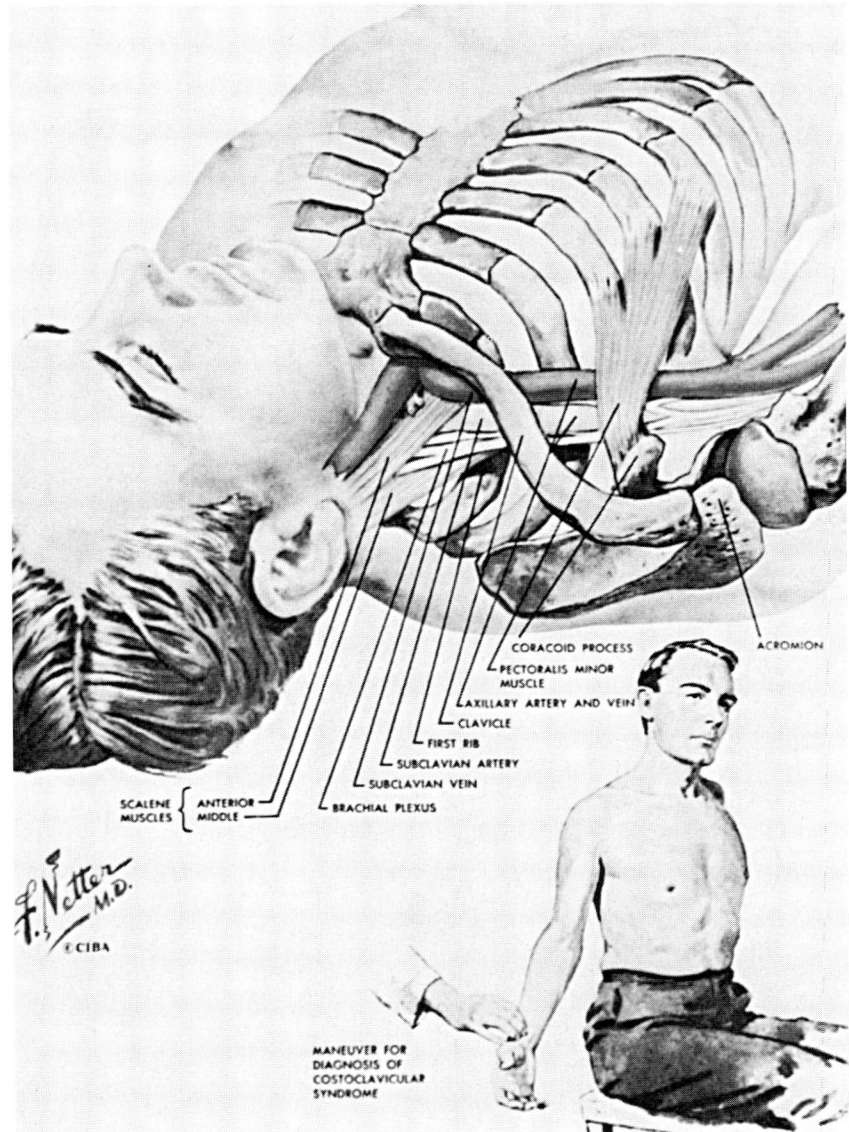

cle potentials, which appear on the fluorescent screen (Fig. 18–11).

Technique

The conduction velocity is determined by the Krusen-Caldwell technique (Caldwell et al., 1971). The patient is placed on the examination table with the arm fully extended at the elbow and in about 20 degrees of abduction at the shoulder to facilitate stimulation over the course of the ulnar nerve.

The ulnar nerve is stimulated at the four points by a special stimulation unit (Fig. 18–12) that imparts an electrical stimulus with a strength of 350 volts with the patient's load, which is approximately equal to 300 volts with the patient's load with a skin resistance of 5000 ohms. Supramaximal stimulation is used at all points to obtain maximal response. The duration

of the stimulation is 0.2 msec, except for muscular individuals, for whom it is 0.5 msec. Time of stimulation, conduction delay, and muscle response appear on the TECA screen; time markers occur each millisecond on the sweep.

The latency period to stimulation from the four points of stimulation to the recording electrode is obtained from the TECA digital recorder or calculated from the tracing on the screen.

Calculation of Velocities

After the latencies, which are expressed in milliseconds, are obtained, the distance in millimeters between two adjacent sites of stimulation is measured with steel tape. The velocities, which are expressed in meters per second, are calculated by subtracting the distal latency from the proximal latency and dividing

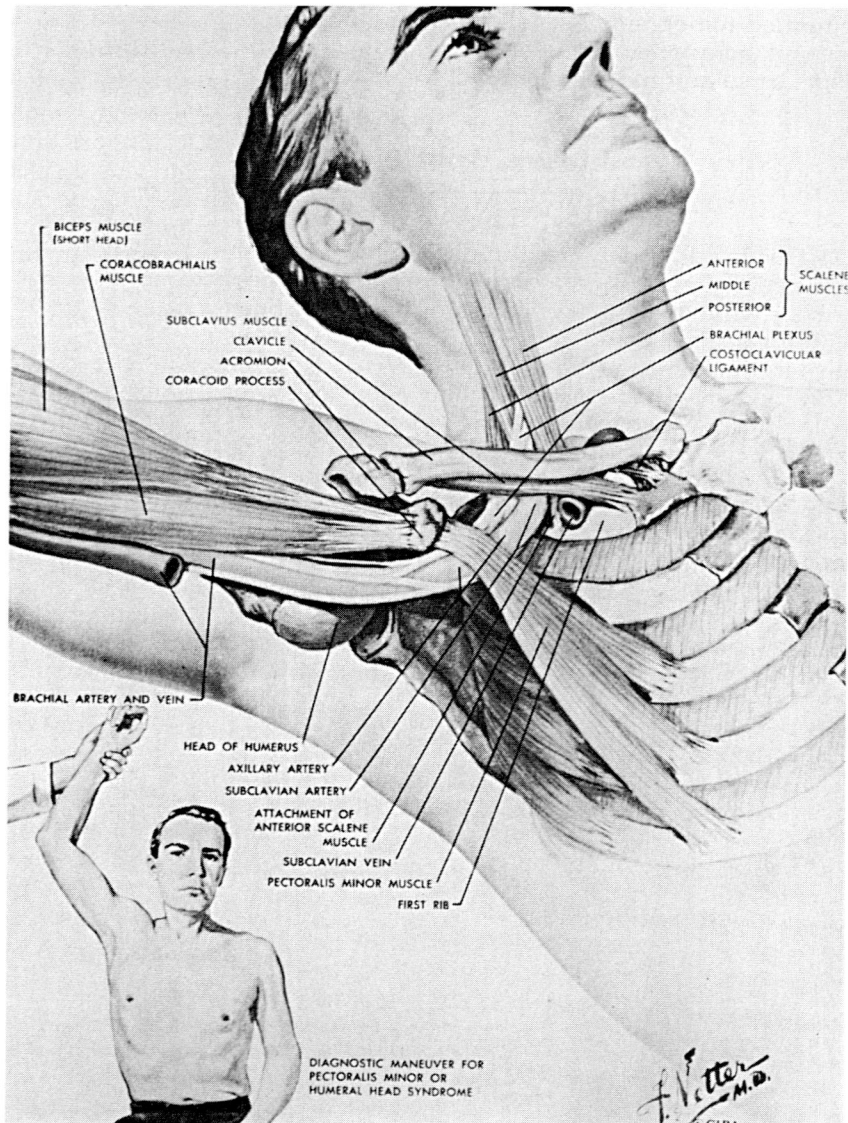

FIGURE 18–8. Hyperabduction maneuver. Relation of the neurovascular bundle to the pectoralis minor tendon, the coracoid process, and the humeral head (pulley effect). (Copyright 1971. CIBA-GEIGY Corporation. Reproduced with permission from Clinical Symposia by Frank H. Netter, M.D. All rights reserved.)

the distance between two points of stimulation by the latency difference (Fig. 18–13) according to the following formula:

Velocity (m/sec) =

$$\frac{\text{distance between two adjacent stimulation points (mm)}}{\text{difference in latency (msec)}}$$

Normal UNCVs

The normal values of the UNCVs according to the Krusen-Caldwell technique (Caldwell et al., 1971) are 72 m/sec or above across the outlet; 55 m/sec or above around the elbow; and 59 m/sec or above in the forearm. Wrist delay is 2.5 to 3.5 msec. Decreased velocity in a segment or increased delay at the wrist indicates either compression, injury, neuropathy, or neurologic disorders. Decreased velocity across the outlet is consistent with thoracic outlet syndrome.

Decreased velocity around the elbow signifies ulnar nerve entrapment or neuropathy. Increased delay at the wrist is encountered in carpal tunnel syndrome.

Grading of Compression

The clinical picture of thoracic outlet syndrome correlates fairly well with the conduction velocity across the outlet. Any value less than 70 m/sec indicates neurovascular compression. The severity is graded according to decrease of velocity across the thoracic outlet: Compression is called slight when the velocity is 66 to 69 m/sec, mild when the velocity is 60 to 65 m/sec, moderate when the velocity is 55 to 59 m/sec, and severe when the velocity is 54 m/sec and below.

Angiography

Simple clinical observations usually suffice to determine the degree of vascular impairment in the upper

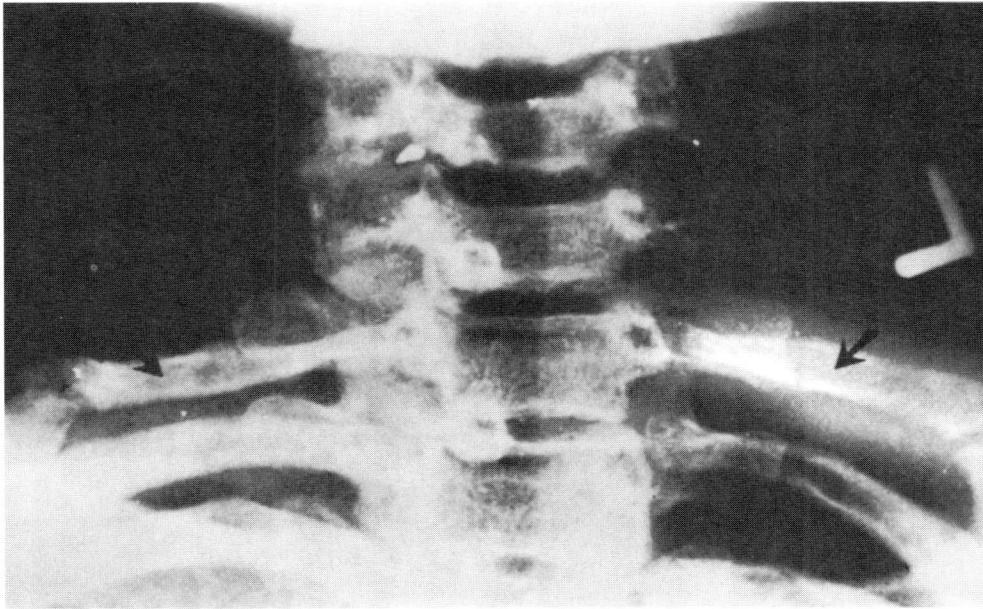

FIGURE 18–9. Film showing bilateral cervical ribs *(arrows)*.

extremity. Peripheral angiography (Lang, 1962; Rosenberg, 1966) is indicated in some cases, as in the presence of a paraclavicular pulsating mass, the absence of radial pulse, or the presence of supracla-

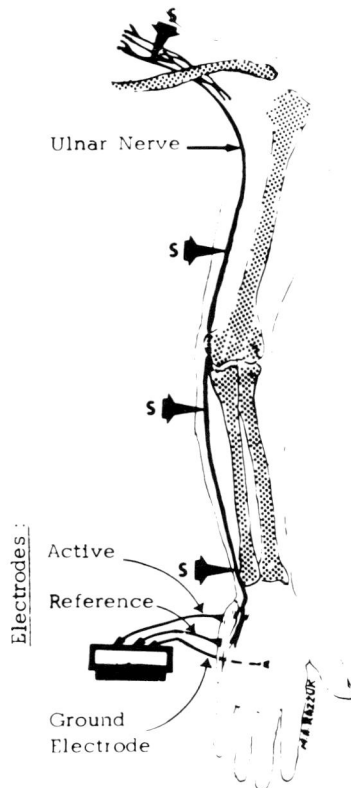

FIGURE 18–10. Ulnar nerve stimulation points (S) in the supraclavicular fossa (over the trunks of the plexus), above the elbow, below the elbow, and at the wrist.

vicular or infraclavicular bruits. Retrograde or antegrade arteriograms of the subclavian and brachial arteries to demonstrate or localize the pathology should be obtained. In cases of venous stenosis or obstruction, as in Paget-Schroetter syndrome, phlebograms are used to determine the extent of thrombosis and the status of the collateral circulation (Fig. 18–14).

DIFFERENTIAL DIAGNOSIS

The thoracic outlet syndrome should be differentiated from various neurologic, vascular, cardiac, pulmonary, and esophageal conditions (Rosati and Lord, 1961; Urschel et al., 1973; Urschel and Razzuk, 1972, 1973) (Table 18–2).

Neurologic causes of pain in the shoulder and arm are more difficult to recognize and may arise from involvement of the nervous system in the spine, the brachial plexus, or the peripheral nerves. A common neurologic cause of pain in the upper extremities is a herniated cervical intervertebral disk. The herniation almost invariably occurs at the interspace between the fifth and the sixth or the sixth and the seventh cervical vertebrae and produces characteristic symptoms. Onset of pain and stiffness of the neck is manifested with varying frequency. The pain radiates along the medial border of the scapula into the shoulder, occasionally into the anterior chest wall, and down the lateral aspect of the arm, at times into the fingers. Numbness and paresthesias in the fingers may be present. The segmental distribution of pain is a prominent feature. A herniated disk between the C5 and the C6 vertebrae, which compresses the C6 nerve root, causes pain or numbness primarily in the thumb and to a lesser extent in the index finger. The biceps

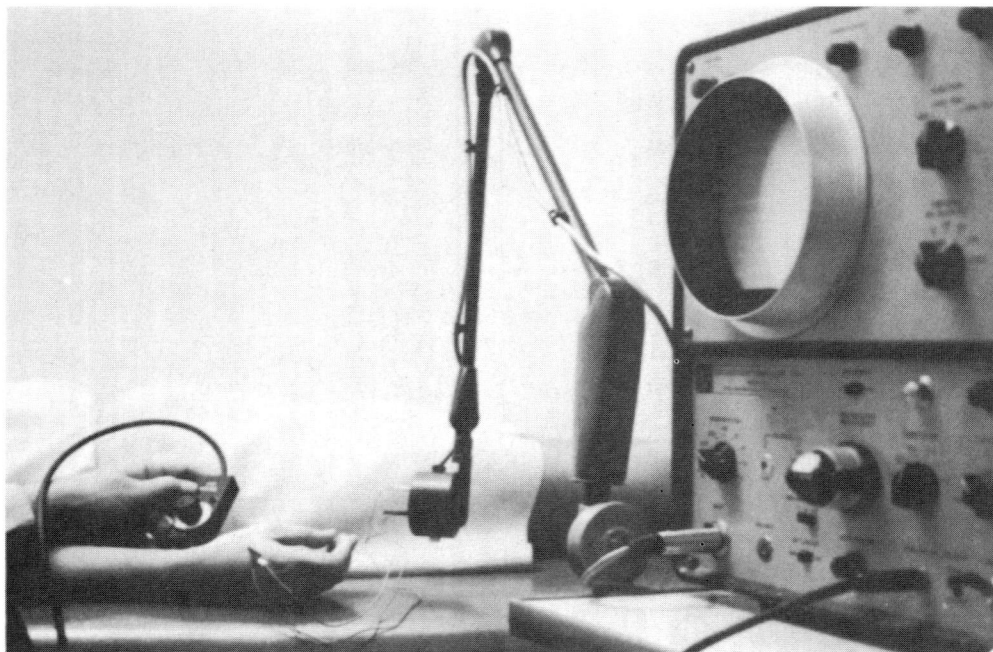

FIGURE 18–11. TECA-3 electromyograph using a coaxial cable and three needles to record generated action potentials.

muscle and the radial wrist extensor are weak, and the reflex of the biceps muscle is reduced or abolished. A herniated disk between the C6 and the C7 vertebrae, which compresses the C7 nerve root, produces pain or numbness in the index finger and weakness of index finger flexion and ulnar wrist extension; the triceps muscle is weak and its reflex is reduced or abolished. Any of these herniated disks may cause numbness along the ulnar border of the arm and hand due to spasm of the scalenus anticus muscle. Rarely, pain and paresthesias in the ulnar distribution

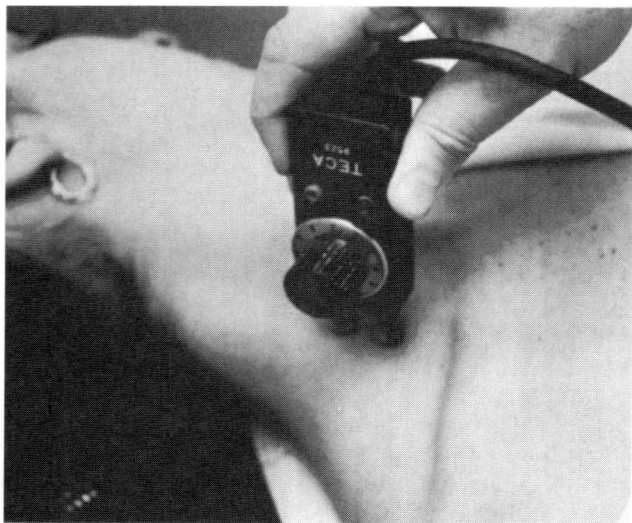

FIGURE 18–12. A stimulating electrode positioned over the cords of the brachial plexus at Erb's point in the supraclavicular fossa posterior to the sternocleidomastoid muscle, which is the stimulation site of the brachial plexus across the outlet.

may be related to herniation between the C7 and the T1 vertebrae, which causes compression of the C8 nerve root. Compression of the latter nerve root produces weakness of intrinsic hand muscles (Krusen, 1968; Rosati and Lord, 1961). Although rupture of the fifth and sixth disks produces hypesthesia in this area, only rupture of the seventh disk produces pain down the medial aspect of the arm (Rosati and Lord, 1961).

The diagnosis of a ruptured cervical disk is based primarily on the history and physical findings; lateral films of the cervical spine reveal loss or reversal of cervical curvature with the apex of the reversal of curvature at the level of the disk involved. Electromyography can localize the site and extent of the nerve root irritation. When a herniated disk is suspected, cervical myelography should be done to confirm the diagnosis (Krusen, 1968; Rosati and Lord, 1961).

Another condition that causes upper extremity pain is cervical spondylosis, a degenerative disease of the intervertebral disk and the adjacent vertebral margin that causes spur formation and the production of ridges into the spinal canal or intervertebral foramina. Films and a CT scan of the cervical spine and electromyography help in making the diagnosis of this condition (Fig. 18–15).

Several arterial and venous conditions can be confused with thoracic outlet syndrome (see Table 18–2); the differentiation can often be made clinically (Rosati and Lord, 1961).

In atypical patients who present with chest pain alone, it is important to suspect the thoracic outlet syndrome in addition to angina pectoris. Exercise stress testing and coronary angiography may exclude coronary artery disease when there is a high index of

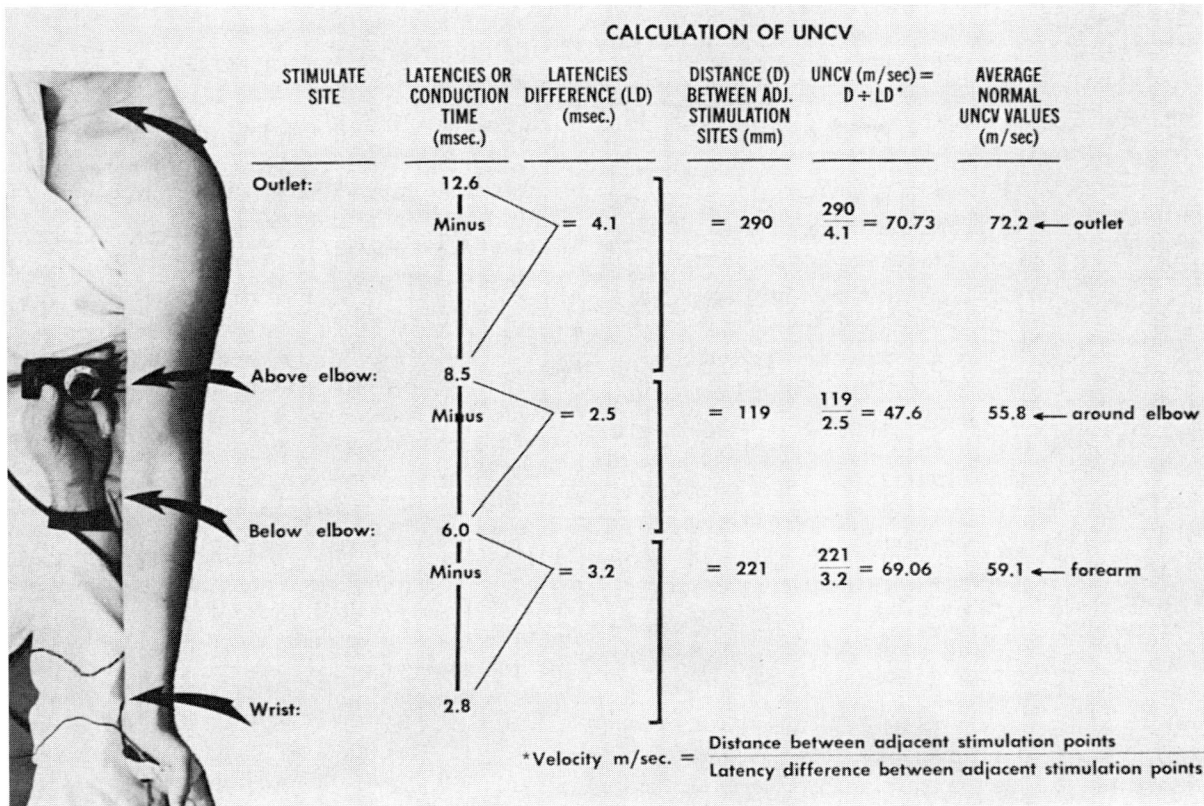

CALCULATION OF UNCV

STIMULATE SITE	LATENCIES OR CONDUCTION TIME (msec.)	LATENCIES DIFFERENCE (LD) (msec.)	DISTANCE (D) BETWEEN ADJ. STIMULATION SITES (mm)	UNCV (m/sec) = D ÷ LD*	AVERAGE NORMAL UNCV VALUES (m/sec)
Outlet:	12.6	= 4.1	= 290	$\frac{290}{4.1} = 70.73$	72.2 ← outlet
	Minus				
Above elbow:	8.5	= 2.5	= 119	$\frac{119}{2.5} = 47.6$	55.8 ← around elbow
	Minus				
Below elbow:	6.0	= 3.2	= 221	$\frac{221}{3.2} = 69.06$	59.1 ← forearm
	Minus				
Wrist:	2.8				

$$*\text{Velocity m/sec.} = \frac{\text{Distance between adjacent stimulation points}}{\text{Latency difference between adjacent stimulation points}}$$

FIGURE 18–13. The sites of stimulation and the formula for calculating velocities.

suspicion of angina pectoris (Urschel et al., 1973; Urschel and Razzuk, 1973).

THERAPY

Patients with thoracic outlet syndrome should be given physiotherapy when the diagnosis is made. Proper physiotherapy includes heat massages, active neck exercises, stretching of the scalenus muscles, strengthening of the upper trapezius muscle, and posture instruction. Because sagging of the shoulder girdle, which is common among the middle-aged, is a major cause in this syndrome, many patients with less severe cases are improved by strengthening the shoulder girdle and by improving posture (Krusen, 1968).

Most patients with thoracic outlet syndrome who have UNCVs of more than 60 m/sec improve with conservative management. If the conduction velocity is below that level, most patients, despite physiotherapy, may remain symptomatic, and surgical resection of the first rib and correction of other bony abnormalities may be needed to provide relief of symptoms (Urschel et al., 1968, 1971; Urschel and Razzuk, 1972).

If symptoms of neurovascular compression continue after physiotherapy, and the conduction velocity shows slight or no improvement or regression, surgical resection of the first rib and cervical rib, when present, should be considered (Urschel et al., 1968,

1971; Urschel and Razzuk, 1972). Clagett (1962) popularized the high posterior thoracoplasty approach for first rib resection; Falconer and Li (1962) emphasized the anterior approach; and Roos (1966) introduced the transaxillary route.

The transaxillary route is an expedient approach

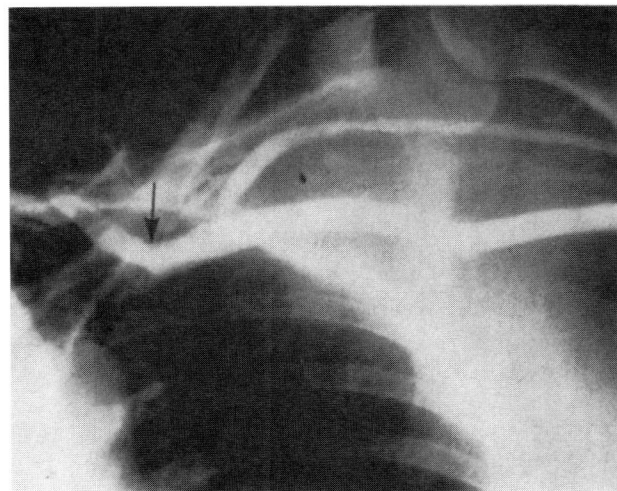

FIGURE 18–14. Phlebogram showing total occlusion *(arrow)* with minimal collateral circulation of the left subclavian vein due to thoracic outlet compression. At operation, no thrombus was present in the vein, and obstruction was relieved by removing the first rib.

■ **Table 18–2.** DIFFERENTIAL DIAGNOSIS OF THORACIC OUTLET SYNDROME NERVE COMPRESSION

Cervical spine	Ruptured intervertebral disk
	Degenerative disease
	Osteoarthritis
	Spinal cord tumors
Brachial plexus	Superior sulcus tumors
	Trauma—postural palsy
Peripheral nerves	Entrapment neuropathy
	Carpal tunnel—median nerve
	Ulnar nerve—elbow
	Radial nerve
	Suprascapular nerve
	Medical neuropathies
	Trauma
	Tumor
Vascular Phenomena	
Arterial	Arteriosclerosis—aneurysm
	occlusive
	Thromboangiitis obliterans
	Embolism
	Functional
	Raynaud's disease
	Reflex vasomotor dystrophy
	Causalgia
	Vasculitis, collagen disease,
	panniculitis
Venous	Thrombophlebitis
	Mediastinal venous obstruction
	Malignant
	Benign
Other Diseases	
Angina pectoris	
Esophageal	
Pulmonary	

for complete removal of the first rib with decompression of the seventh and eighth cervical and first thoracic nerve roots and the lower trunks of the brachial plexus. First rib resection can be performed without the need for major muscle division, as in the posterior approach (Clagett, 1962); the need for retraction of the brachial plexus, as in the anterior supraclavicular approach (Falconer and Li, 1962); and the difficulty of removing the posterior segment of the rib, as in the infraclavicular approach. In addition, first rib resection shortens the postoperative disability and provides better cosmetic results than the anterior and posterior approaches, particularly because 80% of patients are female (Urschel et al., 1968, 1971; Urschel and Razzuk, 1972).

Technique of Transaxillary Resection of the First Rib

The patient is placed in the lateral position with the involved extremity abducted to 90 degrees by traction straps wrapped around the forearm and attached to an overhead pulley. An appropriate weight, usually 3 lb, is used to maintain this position without undue traction (Urschel and Razzuk, 1973) (Fig. 18–16).

A transverse incision is made in the axilla below the hairline between the pectoralis major and the latissimus dorsi muscles and deepened to the external thoracic fascia (Fig. 18–17). Care should be taken to prevent injury to the intercostobrachial cutaneous nerve, which passes from the chest wall to the subcutaneous tissue in the center of the operative field.

The dissection is extended cephalad along the external thoracic fascia up to the first rib. With gentle dissection, the neurovascular bundle and its relation to the first rib and both scalenus muscles are clearly outlined to avoid injury to its components (Fig. 18–18). The insertion of the scalenus anticus muscle is identified, skeletized, and divided (Fig. 18–19). The first rib is dissected subperiosteally with a periosteal elevator and separated carefully from the underlying pleura to avoid pneumothorax. A segment of the middle portion of the rib is resected, followed by subperiosteal dissection and resection of the anterior portion of the rib at the costochondral junction. After the costoclavicular ligament is cut, the posterior segment of the rib is similarly dissected subperiosteally and resected in fragments, including the articulation with the transverse process, the neck, and the head. The scalenus medius muscle should not be cut from its insertion on the second rib but rather stripped with a periosteal elevator to avoid injury to the long thoracic nerve that lies on its posterior margin. The neck and head of the first rib are removed completely with a long, special double-action pituitary rongeur. The eighth cervical and first thoracic nerve roots may be visualized at this point. If a cervical rib is present, its anterior portion, which usually articulates with the first rib, should be resected at a point when the middle portion of the first rib is removed. The remaining segment of the cervical rib should be removed after removal of the posterior segments of the first rib. The wound is drained, and only the subcutaneous tissues and skin require closure, because no large muscles have been divided. The patient is encouraged to use the arm for self-care but to avoid heavy lifting until at least 3 months after operation. Cervical muscle stretching should be started at the end of the first week, and gentle exercising of the arm can be started at the end of the third week after operation.

It is preferable to remove the first rib entirely, including the head and neck, to avoid future irritation of the plexus, because a residual portion, particularly if long, will cause recurrence of symptoms.

EFFORT THROMBOSIS: PAGET–SCHROETTER SYNDROME

"Effort" thrombosis of the axillary-subclavian vein (Paget-Schroetter syndrome) is generally secondary to unusual or excessive use of the arm in addition to the presence of one or more compressive elements in the thoracic outlet (Adams and DeWeese, 1971; Johnston, 1989).

Historically, Paget in 1875 in London and Von Schroetter in 1884 in Vienna described this syndrome

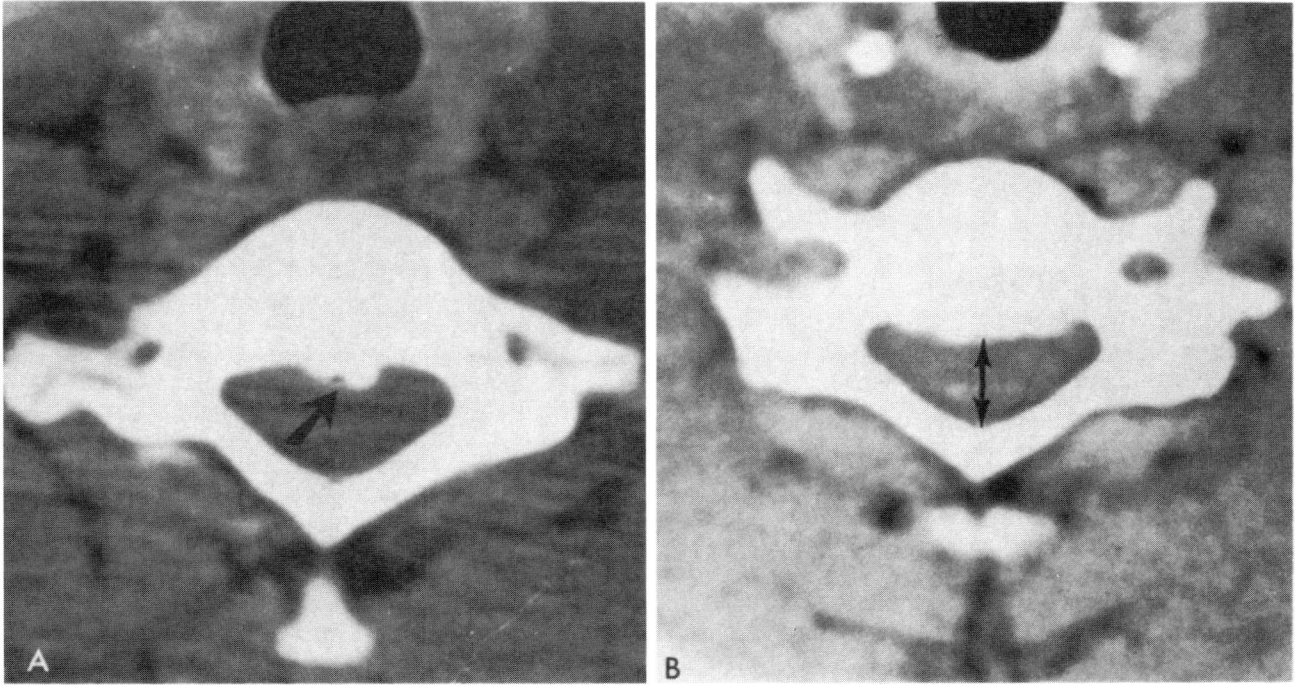

FIGURE 18–15. Computed tomography scans showing osteophytic ingrowth in the spinal canal *(A)* and narrowing of the anteroposterior diameter of the spinal canal *(B)* in a patient with the typical clinical picture of thoracic outlet syndrome.

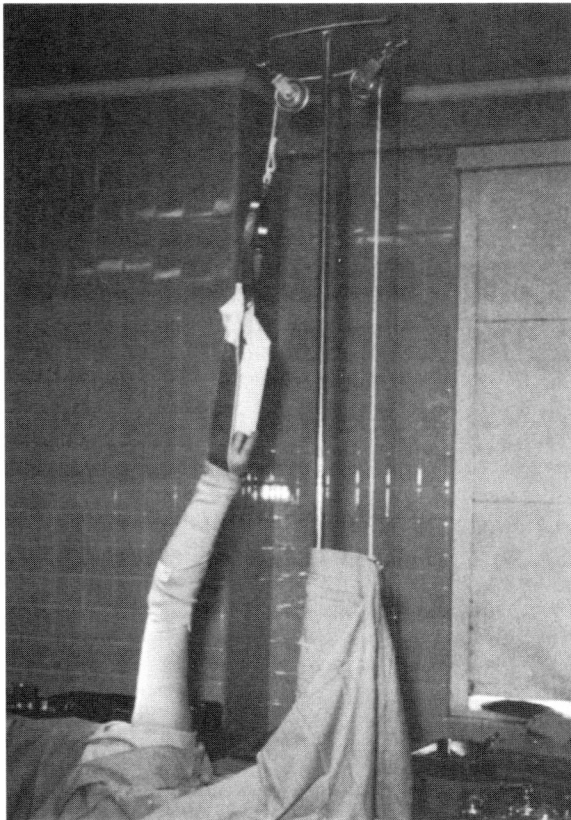

FIGURE 18–16. The arm is abducted to 90 degrees by traction straps on the forearm and is attached to an overhead pulley.

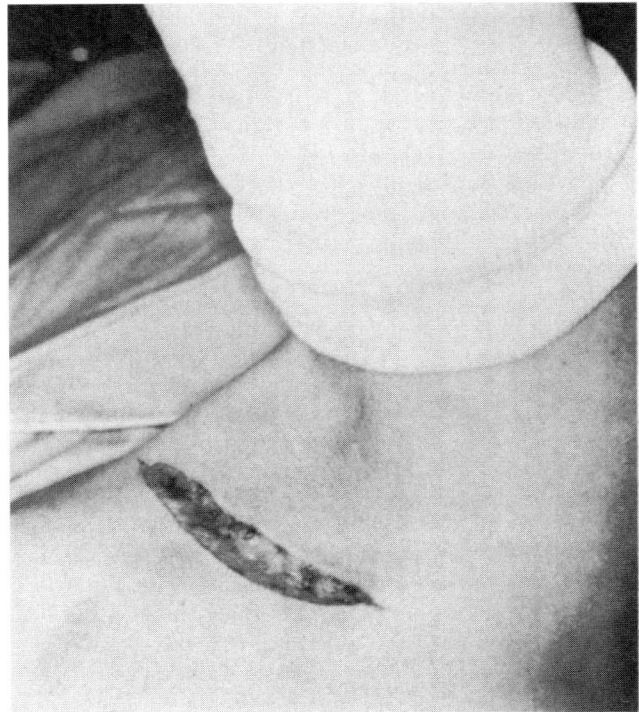

FIGURE 18–17. A transverse incision is made in the axilla below the hairline between the pectoralis major and the latissimus dorsi muscles and is extended to the chest wall.

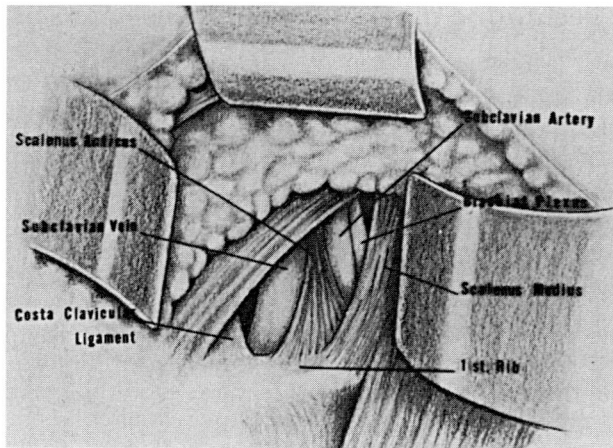

FIGURE 18–18. Schematic drawing showing the relationship of the neurovascular bundle to the scalene muscles, first rib, costoclavicular ligament, and subclavius muscle.

of thrombosis of the axillary-subclavian vein, which bears their names. The word *effort* (Aziz, 1986) was added to *thrombosis* because of the frequent association with exertion producing either direct or indirect compression of the vein. The thrombosis is caused by trauma (Cikrit et al., 1990) or is associated with unusual occupations requiring repetitive muscular activity, as has been observed in professional athletes, Linotype operators, painters, and beauticians. Cold and traumatic factors, such as carrying skis over the shoulder, tend to increase the proclivity for thrombosis (Daskalakis and Bouhoutsos, 1980). Elements of increased thrombogenicity also increase the incidence of the problem and exacerbate its symptoms on a long-term basis.

Adams and colleagues (Adams and DeWeese, 1971; DeWeese et al., 1970) reported long-term results in patients treated conservatively with elevation and warfarin sodium (Coumadin). There was a 12% incidence of pulmonary embolism. Development of occasional venous distention occurred in 18%, and late residual arm symptoms of swelling, pain, and superficial thrombophlebitis were noted in 68% of patients (deep venous thrombosis with postphlebitic syndrome). Phlegmasia cerulea dolens was present in one patient.

For many years, therapy included elevation of the arm and use of anticoagulants, with subsequent return to work. If symptoms recurred, the patient was considered for a first rib resection, with or without thrombectomy (DeWeese et al., 1970), as well as resection of the scalenus anterior muscle and removal of any other compressive element in the thoracic outlet, such as the cervical rib or abnormal bands (Inahara, 1968; Prescott and Tikoff, 1979; Roos, 1989).

Increased availability of thrombolytic agents (Rubenstein and Greger, 1980; Sundqvist et al., 1981; Zimmerman et al., 1981) combined with prompt surgical decompression of the neurovascular compressive elements in the thoracic outlet (Taylor et al., 1985) reduced morbidity and the necessity for thrombectomy

and substantially improved clinical results, including the ability to return to work (Urschel and Razzuk, 1991).

One advantage of urokinase over streptokinase is the direct action of urokinase on the thrombosis distal to the catheter, producing a local thrombolytic effect (Becker et al., 1983; Drury et al., 1984; Eisenbud et al., 1990). Streptokinase produces a systemic effect involving potential complications. Heparin is given postoperatively until the catheter is removed. Another advantage is that the need for thrombectomy decreases after use of the thrombolytic agent followed by aggressive surgical intervention because some of the long-term disability is related to morbidity from thrombectomy as well as recurrent thrombosis (Campbell et al., 1977; Drapanas and Curran, 1966; Painter and Rarpf, 1984).

The natural history of Paget-Schroetter syndrome suggests moderate morbidity (Coon and Willis, 1966; Gloviczki et al., 1986; Tilney et al., 1970) with conservative treatment alone. Bypass with vein or other conduits (Hansen et al., 1985; Hashmonai et al., 1976; Jacobson and Haimov, 1977) has limited application. Causes other than thoracic outlet syndrome must be treated individually (Loring, 1952; Stoney et al., 1976) using the basic principles mentioned. Intermittent obstruction of the subclavian vein (McLaughlin and Popma, 1939) can lead to thrombosis, and decompression should be employed prophylactically (Hashmonai et al., 1976; Jacobson and Haimov, 1977).

DORSAL SYMPATHECTOMY AND THORACIC OUTLET SYNDROME MANAGEMENT WITH VIDEO–ASSISTED THORACIC SURGERY

Dorsal sympathectomy and the management of thoracic outlet syndrome are significantly improved with video assistance through magnification and an improved light system. Video-assisted thoracic surgery (VATS) offers better visualization of anatomic

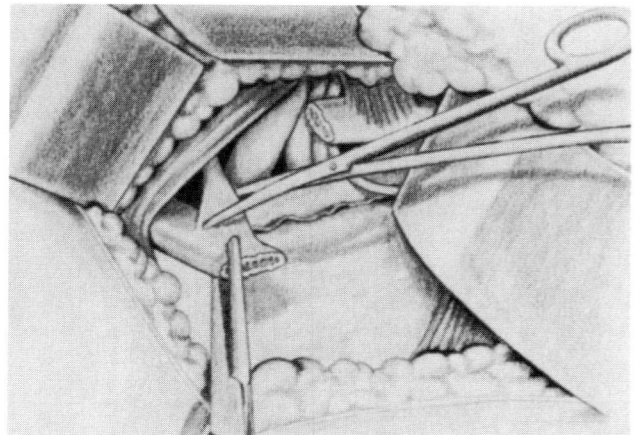

FIGURE 18–19. Schematic drawing showing division of the insertion of the scalenus anterior muscle on the first rib and removal of a segment of the midportion of the first rib.

structures in a "deep hole," with an additional bonus of excellent visualization for other members of the team, particularly surgical residents. In addition, for sympathectomy alone, it offers less pain to the patient and a shorter hospitalization.

Video assistance is employed in two techniques. One involves the sympathectomy through three ports with the standard VATS. The second technique involves a transaxillary incision with removal of the first rib using video-assistance magnification and light; the surgeon operates either directly or secondarily while visualizing the image through the television set. This last technique was popularized by Martinez (1979).

Major indications for dorsal sympathectomy include hyperhidrosis, Raynaud's phenomenon and Raynaud's disease, causalgia, *reflex sympathetic dystrophy* (RSD), and vascular insufficiency of the upper extremity. Except for hyperhidrosis, all of the other indications require the usual diagnostic techniques, including cervical sympathetic block to assess whether the symptoms are relieved by temporary blockade of the sympathetic ganglia. When Raynaud's phenomenon of a minor to moderate degree is associated with thoracic outlet syndrome, the simple removal of the first rib with any cervical rib, in addition to stripping the axillary-subclavian artery (neurectomy), will relieve most symptoms following the initial operation (Urschel et al., 1968).

It is rarely necessary to perform a sympathectomy unless Raynaud's is a very severe type, in which case a dorsal sympathectomy is carried out with first rib resection. In contrast, with recurrent thoracic outlet syndrome and causalgia, it has been found that the dorsal sympathectomy should be performed with the initial reoperation procedure (Urschel et al., 1976; Urschel and Razzuk, 1986a).

Pathophysiology

The principal physiologic effect expected of sympathectomy is the release of vasomotor control and hyperactive tone of the arterioles and smaller arteries that have a muscular element in the vessel wall. Circulation to the skin, peripheral extremity, and bone receives major improvement, but the effect on skeletal muscle of the arm is minimal. The other known function is the control over cutaneous sweating, which is profuse and undesirable. Sympathectomy eliminates perspiration in that quadrant of the body but increases perspiration elsewhere. RSD is associated with pain, neuroesthenia, and cutaneous atrophy (Sudeck-Leriche) and post-traumatic limb. These patients also benefit from a sympathectomy if a diagnostic block is effective. Sympathectomy is not recommended in diabetic neuropathy. Nor should it be performed in any of the vascular vasospastic syndromes until after conservative management, including cessation of tobacco products and institution of beta blockers, peripheral vasodilators, and calcium channel blockers, has been tried (Cooley and Wukasch, 1979).

Preganglionic sympathetic nerves derived from the spinal cord do not follow a corresponding relationship to the accompanying somatic nerves. The cervical ganglia of C1 to C4 are fused into a superior cervical ganglion, C5 and C6 into the middle cervical ganglion, and C7 and C8 into the inferior ganglion, which combines with the ganglion from T1 to the larger stellate ganglion. Cervical ganglionectomy is not used for denervation of the upper extremity, since the preganglionic sympathetic outflow from the spinal cord to the arm is usually from T2 through T9, mostly from T2 through T4. In about 10% of cases, T1 preganglionic fibers also supply the upper extremity. To remove the preganglionic fibers to the upper extremity in most patients, removal of paravertebral ganglia T2 and T3 with the interconnecting chain is sufficient. Postganglionic fibers from these two segments often join and branches then follow the nerves of the brachial plexus. The joined T2 and T3 fibers that bypass the stellate ganglion are known as *the nerve of Kuntz* (Kuntz, 1927). To ensure that all the remaining patients who have a T1 connection through the stellate ganglion obtain adequate sympathetic denervation, the lower third of the stellate ganglion should also be removed, as recommended by Palumbo (1955, 1956).

Patients with RSD or *sympathetic maintained pain syndrome* (SMPS) must complain of pain outside a peripheral nerve distribution (Mackinnon and Dellon, 1988). Although the injury itself may have been minor, the pain appears out of proportion to the injury. We have seen two types of RSD or SMPS; one involves the hand or even a greater majority of the upper extremity and a second is localized to one or more digits. In no instance can the patient's pain be completely accounted for by an injury to a specific nerve, although injury to a specific nerve may cause the more diffuse symptoms. The patient also demonstrates diminished hand function. Several patients have been referred with a diagnosis of SMPS, and on examination, it is quite apparent that, although they may complain of diffuse pain, the hand functions normally with a full range of movement and motor power is demonstrated. These patients, of course, do not have SMPS. The patient must also demonstrate some joint stiffness. The skin and soft tissue trophic changes demonstrate varying amounts of vasomotor instability, depending on the stage of SMPS.

According to Mackinnon (1988), there are early, intermediate, and late stages of SMPS. In the early stages, vasomotor instability is noted, with very dramatic sympathetic overactivity apparent in the hand or digit involved. Instability, with symptoms varying between redness and warmth and cyanosis and sweating, is noted in this early stage. Edema is also a classic finding in the early stage. In the intermediate stage of SMPS, pain is a less dramatic component and is usually elicited by attempts to move the joints. At rest, the patient may be quite comfortable. The edema and vasomotor changes have settled by this time, and the hand has the appearance of a "burned out" dystrophic hand, with marked stiffness and atrophy of the soft tissue noted. The normal wrinkles on the dorsum of the hand are no longer apparent. The fingertips may have a tapered appearance. The nail growth is usually more exaggerated than in the normal hand, and the hand is often cool and pale. The intermediate stage will extend over a number of months. During the late stage, all the superimposed problems of disuse atrophy may take effect. During this stage, problems with the elbow and shoulder are very common, even though the initial SMPS involved only the hand or one or more digits. The degree of pain experienced during the late phase is variable and is often the result of disuse and stiffness. SMPS can affect other areas of the body and has been observed in the foot, face, and penis.

Complications

Horner's Syndrome

If the fibers of C7 and C8 (the upper part of the stellate ganglion) are removed, Horner's syndrome results. This involves miosis, enophthalmos, drooping of the eyelid (ptosis), and flushing of that side of the face, with loss of sweating in that area (Galbraith et al., 1973).

Postsympathetic Neuralgia

The complication of postsympathectomy neuralgia is less common in the upper extremities than in the lower extremities. The pain usually occurs in the shoulder and upper arm on the lateral aspect. Clinical history usually substantiates this diagnosis if the symptoms occur within the first 3 months. The confirmation may be obtained by a test involving skin resistance of pseudomotor activity detection. Tests reveal increased sympathetic activity and suggest a rebound phenomenon from the nonsympathectomized adjacent dermatomes. Rebound may be a regeneration of nerve fibers on an increased response of peripheral nerves to catecholamines. Symptoms are usually resolved in 3 to 6 weeks with conservative management. Phenytoin sodium (Dilantin), carbamazepine (Tegretol), and calcium channel blockers are all used in the medical management of these symptoms (Litwin, 1962).

Recurrent Symptoms

Occasionally following an excellent sympathectomy, with a warm hand and good circulation, recurrent symptoms may present as early as 3 months. These may be secondary to the regeneration or sprouting and rehooking of nerves or failure to strip the sympathetic nerves from the artery itself and the transfer of sympathetic tone through these nerves. Therefore, stripping of the axillary-subclavian artery of its local sympathetic nerves is performed in each case at the initial operation (Urschel, 1993). Also, during the initial procedure cauterization of the bed of

the sympathectomy area produces sympathetic effects that usually last at least 3 years or longer.

Surgical Approaches for Dorsal Sympathectomy

Historically, the anterior cervical approach has been used, with the division of the scalenus-anticus muscle as the approach to the cervical sympathetic chain (White et al., 1952). The stellate ganglion lies on the transverse process of C6, and this approach is used primarily by both neurosurgeons and vascular surgeons. For hypertension, Smithwick (1936) and Urschel and Razzuk (1985) popularized the posterior approach using a longitudinal parasternal incision with the patient in the prone position. A small piece of the first and second ribs is removed and the sympathetic chain is identified in the usual position. This approach has the advantage of allowing bilateral procedures at the same time without changing the patient's surgical position.

The most common approach is the transaxillary transthoracic approach, which is performed through the second or third interspace with the transverse subhairline incision (Atkins, 1949, 1954; Palumbo, 1955, 1956). This is more painful than the other approaches, but with video-assisted thoracoscopy, it can be performed with minimal discomfort. The approach most frequently employed when combined with thoracic outlet syndrome is the transaxillary approach with resection of the first rib, retraction of the pleura caudad, and a dorsal sympathectomy (Urschel et al., 1968, 1971). This combined procedure causes minimal pain and low morbidity. Video assistance is used frequently for this approach as well.

Variations of Dorsal Sympathectomy

Standard sympathectomy involves removal of the sympathetic chain with thoracic ganglia 1, 2, and 3. This involves removing the lower third of the stellate ganglion (Urschel and Razzuk, 1986a) with the second and third ganglia and the interconnecting sympathetic chain. This is the standard approach for hyperhidrosis, Raynaud's phenomena, causalgia, and RSD. It is advantageous that Horner's syndrome does not occur following removal of C8 or the upper two-thirds of the stellate ganglia. Complete dorsal sympathectomy includes the removal of C8 with the total stellate ganglion including 1, 2, and 3 and the cervical chain in between. This procedure is primarily for patients with Raynaud's disease and actual ulceration of the fingers, as well as recurrent problems from the other indications. Newer evidence suggests that removal of only T2 and T3 ganglia, avoiding the stellate ganglia altogether, offers adequate sympathectomy for the standard indications of hyperhidrosis, Raynaud's phenomena, causalgia, and RSD. This is yet to be proved in the authors' experience, since careful attention to anatomy virtually eliminates the possibility of Horner's syndrome; thus, there is no advantage in leaving T1 if it presents potential problems.

Technique

Two approaches are employed. The first is the transaxillary approach with a transthoracic sympathectomy (Ravitch and Steichen, 1988). This involves leaving the first rib, collapsing the lung, and performing the sympathectomy with video-assisted techniques (Urschel, 1993). The second is a transaxillary removal of the first rib and the retraction of the pleura with a dorsal sympathectomy, which was used in the most patients.

Transaxillary Approach with a Transthoracic Sympathectomy

The patient is placed in the lateral thoracotomy position with an axillary roll under the downside arm. The upper arm is suspended at 90 degrees from the chest wall over a pulley system with a 1-pound weight (Atkins, 1954). An arm holder is employed to ensure that no hyperabduction or hyperextension of the shoulder occurs and that relaxation occurs every 3 minutes. Three ports are used between the second and the fourth interspaces. The camera should be placed either anteriorly or in the midaxillary port. A double-lumen endobracheal tube is employed, and the upside lung is collapsed, ventilating only the downside lung (Wood et al., 1972). This shunts blood through the downside lung selectively, and excellent oxygenation usually results.

The lung is retracted and the sympathectomy performed. The mediastinal pleura is cut open and the sympathetic chain identified on the vertebral body near the neck of the ribs. Nerve hooks are employed to elevate the dorsal sympathetic chain, and the nerve connections, including the gray and white rami, are clipped before cutting or cauterization. The stellate ganglion is divided at the junction of the lower third, where it looks like a "cat's claw." The lower third is cut, but it is not photoablated or cauterized because Horner's syndrome may result from either heat or light injury in the adjacent C8 ganglion. The lower ganglia can be cauterized, photoablated with the laser, or cut. Hemostasis is achieved with the cautery. The pleura is left open and the chest tube placed through one of the ports for purposes of drainage. There is a curvature of the sympathetic chain so that in many cases the stellate ganglion lies transversely, rather than vertically, on the transverse process of the vertebral body. Special knowledge of the anatomy is important, especially the location of the thoracic duct, which can simulate the sympathetic chain and be injured if not appropriately identified.

Transaxillary First Rib Resection for Thoracic Outlet Syndrome with Retraction of the Pleura and Sympathectomy

This technique differs slightly from the usual video-assisted thoracoscopy in that an actual incision is made transversely below the axillary hairline and the technique for rib resection is carried out.

A right-angle breast retractor with a light is employed, and a Dever retractor is placed on the other side of the incision. The video camera is a standard thoracoscope, a Wolf scope, or an Olympus flexible operating esophogastroscope.

The pleura is retracted inferiorly using a sponge stick, and the sympathetic chain is identified on the transverse process of the vertebral bodies. It is vertical between T2 and T3 ganglia. However, T1, the lower part of the stellate ganglion, angles anteriorly and lies in almost a transverse position. Clips are placed on all the communicating rami of the sympathetic chain. T2 and T3 ganglia are resected. The stellate ganglion is divided at the junction of its lower third and T1 is removed. This division is carried out with a sharp knife. Cauterization or laser photoablation is not employed in the stellate ganglion. Cautery is used after the removal of the sympathetic chain to prevent sprouting. Hemostasis is secured. A large, round Jackson-Pratt drain is placed and methylprednisolone acetate (Depo-Medrol) is injected over the nerve roots and plexus that have undergone neurolysis. The camera is removed and the wound closed in the usual manner.

Results

In 326 patients, sympathectomy alone or in conjunction with first rib removal for thoracic outlet syndrome has been successful. In only 6 patients has sympathetic activity recurred in less than 6 months. All of these were treated conservatively initially. Three of the 6 required repeat sympathectomy. Post-sympathectomy neuralgia occurred in only 2 of 326 patients. Both of these were managed successfully in a conservative manner. In the patients in whom Horner's syndrome was not created deliberately, 2 patients developed the syndrome. Both resolved spontaneously in several months. Forty-two cases of Raynaud's phenomena were successfully treated with first rib resection alone or with periarterial neurectomy without initial sympathectomy (Urschel, 1993).

REOPERATION FOR RECURRENT THORACIC OUTLET SYNDROME

Extirpation of the first rib relieves symptoms in patients with thoracic outlet syndrome not relieved by physiotherapy. Of the surgically treated patients, 10% develop various degrees of shoulder, arm, and hand pain and paresthesias that are usually mild and short-lasting and that respond well to a brief course of physiotherapy and muscle relaxants. In a few patients (1.6%), symptoms persist, become progressively more severe, and often involve a wider area of distribution because of entrapment of the immediate trunk in addition to the lower trunk and C8 and T1 nerve roots. Symptoms may recur 1 month to 7 years after rib resection; in most patients, they recur within the first 3 months. Symptoms consist of an aching or burning type of pain, often associated with paresthesias, involving the neck, shoulder, parascapular area, anterior chest wall, arm, and hand. Vascular lesions are uncommon and consist of causalgia minor and an occasional injury of the subclavian artery with subsequent false aneurysm formation caused by the sharp edge of a remaining posterior stump of an incompletely resected first rib (Fig. 18–20). Recurrence is diagnosed on the basis of history, physical examination, and decreased nerve conduction velocity across the outlet. Diagnostic evaluation should also include thorough neurologic evaluation, chest and cervical spine films (Fig. 18–21), cervical myelography, subclavian artery angiography, and magnetic resonance imaging of cervical spine and brachial plexus (Rapoport et al., 1988), when indicated.

Two groups of patients who require reoperation can be identified. Pseudorecurrence occurred in patients who did not have relief of symptoms after the initial operation. These patients can be separated etiologically as those in whom the second rib was mistakenly resected instead of the first; the first rib was resected, leaving a cervical rib; a cervical rib was resected, leaving an abnormal first rib; or a second rib was resected, leaving a rudimentary first rib. True recurrence occurred in patients whose symptoms were relieved after the first operation but who retained a significant segment of the first rib or who had complete resection of the first rib but showed excessive scar formation around the brachial plexus.

Physiotherapy should be given to all patients with symptoms of neurovascular compression after first rib

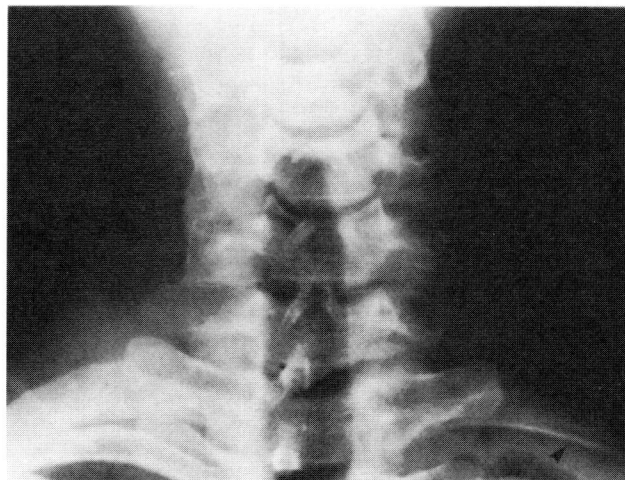

FIGURE 18–21. Cervical film showing a posterior remnant (arrow) of an incompletely resected first rib in a patient who developed recurrent thoracic outlet syndrome.

resection. If the symptoms persist and the conduction velocity remains below normal, reoperation is indicated.

Reoperation for thoracic outlet syndrome is performed with the posterior thoracoplasty approach to provide better exposure of the nerve roots and brachial plexus, which reduces the danger of injury to these structures and provides adequate exposure of the subclavian artery and vein. This incision also provides a wider field for resection of any bony abnormalities or fibrous bands and allows extensive neurolysis of the nerve roots and brachial plexus, which is not always possible with the limited exposure of the transaxillary approach. The anterior or supraclavicular approach is inadequate for reoperation.

The basic elements of reoperation include resection of persistent or recurrent bony remnants of a cervical or first rib, neurolysis of the brachial plexus and nerve roots, and dorsal sympathectomy. Sympathectomy removes T1, T2, and T3 thoracic ganglia. Care is taken to avoid damage to the C8 ganglion (upper aspect of the stellate ganglion), which produces Horner's syndrome. The reoperation provides relief of major and minor causalgia and alleviates the paresthesias in the supraclavicular and infraclavicular areas. The incidence of "postsympathetic" syndrome has been negligible in this group of patients. A nerve stimulator is used to differentiate scar from nerve root to avoid damage with reoperations in these patients.

The technique of the operation includes a high thoracoplasty incision that extends from 3 cm above the angle of the scapula, halfway between the angle of the scapula and the spinous processes, and caudad 5 cm from the angle of the scapula. The trapezius and rhomboid muscles are divided the length of the incision. The scapula is retracted from the chest wall by making a subperiosteal incision over the fourth rib. The posterior superior serratus muscle is divided and the sacrospinalis muscle retracted medially. The first rib remnant and cervical rib remnant, if present, are

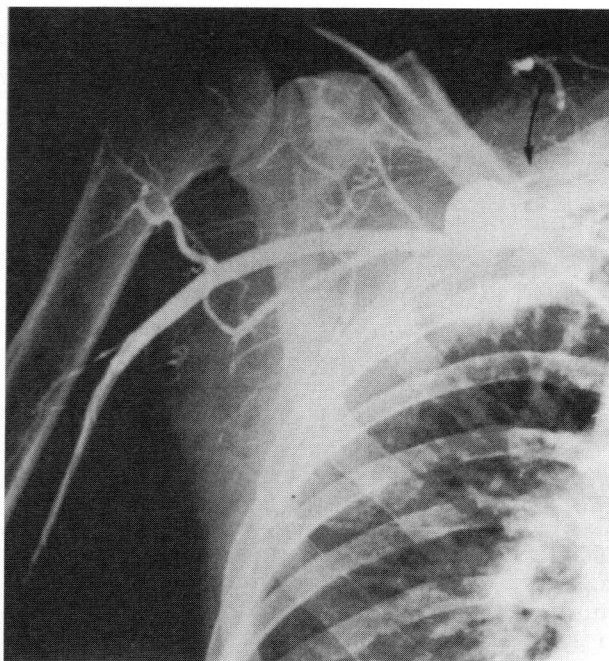

FIGURE 18–20. Arteriogram showing a false aneurysm of the right subclavian artery caused by the pointed end of a posterior stump (arrow) of an incompletely resected first rib.

located and removed subperiosteally. After the rib remnants (Fig. 18–22) have been resected, the regenerated periosteum is removed (Fig. 18–23). In the authors' experience, most regenerated ribs occur from the end of an unresected rib segment rather than from periosteum, although the latter is possible. To reduce the incidence of bony regeneration, it is important in the initial operation to remove the first rib totally in all patients with primarily nerve compression and pain.

After removal of a bony rib remnant, if there is excessive scar it may be prudent to do the sympathectomy initially. A 1-inch segment of the second rib is resected posteriorly to locate the sympathetic ganglion. In that way, the first thoracic nerve may be easier to locate below rather than through the scar.

Neurolysis of the nerve root and brachial plexus is done with a nerve stimulator and is carried down to but not into the nerve sheath. Neurolysis is extended peripherally over the brachial plexus as far as any scarring persists. Excessive neurolysis is not indicated, and opening of the nerve sheath produces more scarring than it relieves. To minimize scarring, the initial operation for thoracic outlet syndrome should include complete extirpation of the first rib, avoidance of hematomas with adequate drainage either by catheter or by opening the pleura, and avoidance of infection.

The subclavian artery and vein are released if symptoms mediate. The scalenus medius muscle is débrided. The dorsal sympathectomy is completed by extrapleural dissection. Meticulous hemostasis is effected, and a large, round Jackson-Pratt catheter drain is placed in the area of, but not touching, the brachial plexus and is brought out through the subscapular space via a stab wound into the axilla. Methylprednisolone acetate (Depo-Medrol; 80 mg) is left in the area of the nerve plexus, but the patient is not given systemic steroids unless keloid formation has occurred. The wound is closed in layers with interrupted heavy Vicryl sutures to provide adequate

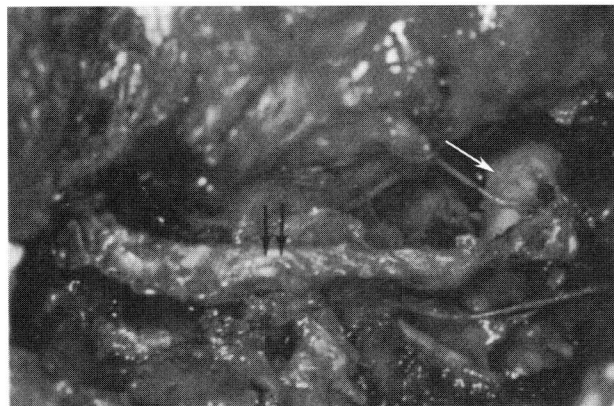

FIGURE 18–23. Fibrocalcific band (*double arrows*) of regenerated periosteum in continuity with a posterior remnant (*single arrow*) of the first rib in a patient with recurrent thoracic outlet syndrome.

strength, and the arm is kept in a sling and used gently for the first 3 months. Range-of-motion exercises are performed to prevent shoulder limitation, but overactivity is avoided to minimize excessive scar formation.

When the problem is vascular and involves false or mycotic aneurysms, special techniques are used for reoperation. A bypass graft is interposed from the innominate or carotid artery proximally, through a separate tunnel distally, to the brachial artery. The graft is usually performed with the saphenous vein, although other conduits may be used. The arteries supplying and leaving the infected aneurysm are ligated. Subsequently, the aneurysm is resected by a transaxillary approach with no fear of bleeding or ischemia of the arm.

Special instruments have been devised to provide adequate resection through the transaxillary or posterior route and include a modified strengthened pituitary rongeur and a modified Leksell double-action rongeur for removal of the first rib without danger to the nerve root.

The sympathectomy relieves chest wall pain that resembles angina pectoris, esophageal disease, or even a tumor in the lung by denervating the deep fibers that accompany the arteries and bone.

The results of reoperation are good if an accurate diagnosis is made and the proper procedure is used (Urschel and Razzuk, 1986a). More than 400 patients have been followed up for 6 months to 15 years. All patients improved initially after reoperation, and in 79%, the improvement was maintained for more than 5 years. In 14% of the patients, symptoms were managed with physiotherapy; 7% required a second reoperation, in every case because of rescarring. There were no deaths, and only 1 patient had an infection that required drainage.

SUMMARY

Thoracic outlet syndrome is recognized in approximately 8% of the population. Its manifestations may

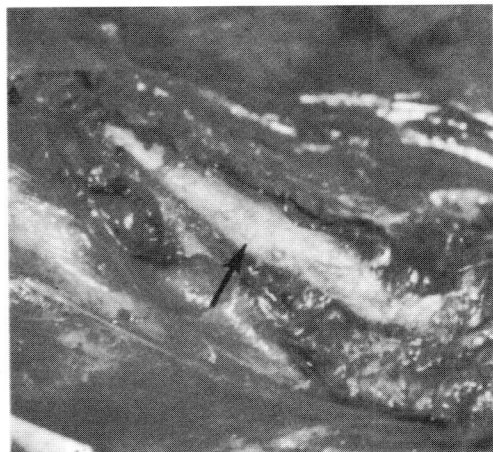

FIGURE 18–22. A long posterior remnant (*arrow*) of an incompletely resected first rib in a patient with recurrent thoracic outlet syndrome.

be neurologic or vascular, or both, depending on the component of the neurovascular bundle predominantly compressed. The diagnosis is suspected from the clinical picture and is usually substantiated by determination of the UNCV. Treatment is initially conservative, but persistence of significant symptoms is an indication for first rib resection and occurs in approximately 5% of patients with diagnosed thoracic outlet syndromes. Primary resection is performed preferably through the transaxillary approach. Symptoms of various degrees may recur after first rib resection in approximately 10% of patients. Most of the patients improve with physiotherapy, and only 1.6% require reoperation. Reoperation for recurrent symptoms is done through a high posterior thoracoplasty incision (Urschel et al., 1976; Urschel and Razzuk, 1986a).

SELECTED BIBLIOGRAPHY

Clagett, O. T.: Presidential address: Research and prosearch. J. Thorac. Cardiovasc. Surg., 44:153, 1962.

This classic reference explains the anatomic and pathophysiologic basis for first rib resection to alleviate neurovascular compression in the thoracic outlet. The incision is the high posterior thoracoplasty approach.

Roos, D. B.: Transaxillary approach for first rib resection to relieve thoracic outlet syndrome. Ann. Surg., 163:354, 1966.

The transaxillary approach to first rib resection was initially described by Atkins and popularized by Roos. The technical aspects of this approach and the pathophysiology are described.

Rosati, L. M., and Lord, J. W.: Neurovascular compression syndromes of the shoulder girdle. Modern Surgical Monographs. New York, Grune & Stratton, 1961.

Frank Netter's drawings appeared first in this classic monograph demonstrating neurovascular compression. It is the "gold standard" for diagnosis and management of neurovascular compression syndromes.

Urschel, H. C., Jr.: Dorsal sympathectomy and management of thoracic outlet syndrome with VATS. Ann. Thorac. Surg., 56:717, 1993.

The relationship of dorsal sympathectomy to thoracic outlet syndrome is described, as are the various techniques, including video-assisted thoracic surgery (VATS), for removing the first rib and performing a sympathectomy. Pathophysiology is emphasized.

Urschel, H. C., Jr., and Razzuk, M. A.: The failed operation for thoracic outlet syndrome: The difficulty of diagnosis and management. Ann. Thorac. Surg., 42:523, 1986.

Recurrent thoracic outlet syndrome is a difficult diagnosis and presents management problems. The techniques of neurolysis and revascularization are described.

Urschel, H. C., Jr., and Razzuk, M. A.: Improved management of the Paget-Schroetter syndrome secondary to thoracic outlet compression. Ann. Thorac. Surg., 52:1217, 1991.

This is the largest series of axillary subclavian vein thromboses describing the current management with urokinase thrombolysis followed by first rib resection.

Urschel, H. C., Jr., Razzuk, M. A., Wood, R. E., and Paulson, D. L.: Objective diagnosis (ulnar nerve conduction velocity) and current therapy of the thoracic outlet syndrome. Ann. Thorac. Surg., 12:608, 1971.

The first positive objective technique for diagnosing neurologic thoracic outlet compression is detailed.

BIBLIOGRAPHY

Adams, J. T., and DeWeese, J. A.: Effort thrombosis of the axillary and subclavian veins. J. Trauma, 11:923, 1971.

Adams, J. T., DeWeese, J. A., Mahoney, E. B., and Rob, C. G.: Intermittent subclavian vein obstruction without thrombosis. Surgery, 63:147, 1968.

Adson, A. W.: Cervical ribs: Symptoms and differential diagnosis for section of the scalenus anticus muscle. J. Int. Coll. Surg., 16:546, 1951.

Adson, A. W., and Coffey, J. R.: Cervical rib: A method of anterior approach for relief of symptoms by division of the scalenus anticus. Ann. Surg., 85:839, 1927.

Atkins, H. J. B.: Peraxillary approach to the stellate and upper thoracic sympathetic ganglia. Lancet, 2:1152, 1949.

Atkins, H. J. B.: Sympathectomy by the axillary approach. Lancet, 1:538, 1954.

Aziz, R., Straenley, C. J., and Whelan, T. J.: Effort-related axillo–subclavian vein thrombosis. Am. J. Surg., 152:57, 1986.

Becker, G. J., Holden, R. W., Robe, F. E., et al.: Local thrombolytic therapy for subclavian and axillary vein thrombosis. Radiology, 149:419, 1983.

Borchardt, M.: Symptomatologie und therapie der Halsrippen. Berl. Klin. Wochenschr., 38:1265, 1901.

Bramwell, E.: Lesion of the first dorsal nerve root. Rev. Neurol. Psychiatr., 1:236, 1903.

Brickner, W. M.: Brachial plexus pressure by the normal first rib. Ann. Surg., 85:858, 1927.

Brickner, W. M., and Milch, H.: First dorsal vertebra simulating cervical rib by maldevelopment or by pressure symptoms. Surg. Gynecol. Obstet., 40:38, 1925.

Brintnall, E. S., Hyndman, O. R., and VanAllen, W. M.: Costoclavicular compression associated with cervical rib. Ann. Surg., 144:921, 1956.

Caldwell, J. W., Crane, C. R., and Krusen, E. M.: Nerve conduction studies in the diagnosis of the thoracic outlet syndrome. South. Med. J., 64:210, 1971.

Campbell, C. B., Chandler, J. G., and Tegtmeyer, C. J.: Axillary, subclavian and brachiocephalic vein obstruction. Surgery, 82:816, 1977.

Cikrit, D. F., Dalsing, M. C., Bryant, B. J., et al.: An experience with upper-extremity vascular trauma. Am. J. Surg., 160:229, 1990.

Clagett, O. T.: Presidential address: Research and prosearch. J. Thorac. Cardiovasc. Surg., 44:153, 1962.

Cooley, D. A., and Wukasch D. C.: Techniques in Vascular Surgery. Philadelphia, W. B. Saunders, 1979, pp. 211–212.

Coon, W. W., and Willis, P. W.: Thrombosis of axillary subclavian veins. Arch. Surg., 94:657, 1966.

Coote, H.: Pressure on the axillary vessels and nerve by an exostosis from a cervical rib; interference with the circulation of the arm; removal of the rib and exostosis; recovery. Med. Times Gaz., 2:108, 1861.

Daskalakis, E., and Bouhoutsos, J.: Subclavian and axillary vein compression of musculoskeletal origin. Br. J. Surg., 67:573, 1980.

DeWeese, J. A., Adams, J. T., and Gaiser, D. I.: Subclavian venous thrombectomy. Circulation, 16(Suppl. 2J):158, 1970.

Drapanas, T., and Curran, W. L.: Thrombectomy in the treatment of "effort" thrombosis of the axillary and subclavian veins. J. Trauma, 6:107, 1966.

Drury, E. M., Trout, H. H., Giordono, J. M., et al.: Lytic therapy in the treatment of axillary and subclavian vein thrombosis. J. Vasc. Surg., 2:821, 1984.

Eisenbud, D. E., Brener, B. J., Shoenfeld, R., et al.: Treatment of acute vascular occlusions with intra-arterial urokinase. Am. J. Surg., 160:160, 1990.

Falconer, M. A., and Li, F. W. P.: Resection of the first rib in costoclavicular compression of the brachial plexus. Lancet, 1:59, 1962.

Falconer, M. A., and Weddell, G.: Costoclavicular compression of the subclavian artery and vein: Relation to scalene syndrome. Lancet, 2:539, 1943.

Galbraith, N. F., Urschel, H. C., Jr., Wood, R. E., et al.: Fracture of first rib associated with laceration of subclavian artery: Report of a case and review of literature. J. Thorac. Cardiovasc. Surg., 65:649, 1973.

Gloviczki, P., Razmier, R. J., and Hollier, L. H.: Axillary-subclavian venous occlusion: The morbidity of a nonlethal disease. J. Vasc. Surg., 4:333, 1986.

Halsted, W. S.: An experimental study of circumscribed dilation of an artery immediately distal to a partially occluding band, and its bearing on the dilation of the subclavian artery observed in certain cases of cervical rib. J. Exp. Med., 24:271, 1916.

Hansen, B., Feins, R. S., and Detmar, D. E.: Simple extra-anatomic jugular vein bypass for subclavian vein thrombosis. J. Vasc. Surg., 2:291, 1985.

Hashmonai, M., Schramek, A., and Farbstein, J.: Cephalic vein cross-over bypass for subclavian vein thrombosis: A case report. Surgery, 80:563, 1976.

Inahara, T.: Surgical treatment of "effort" thrombosis of the axillary and subclavian veins. Am. Surg., 34:479, 1968.

Jebsen, R. H.: Motor conduction velocities in the median and ulnar nerves. Arch. Phys. Med., 48:185, 1967.

Jacobson, J. H., and Haimov, M.: Venous revascularization of the arm: Report of three cases. Surgery, 81:599, 1977.

Johnston, R. W.: Neurovascular conditions involving the upper extremity. In Rutherford, R. B. (ed): Vascular Surgery. 3rd ed. Philadelphia, W. B. Saunders, 1989, pp. 301–898.

Keen, W. W.: The symptomatology, diagnosis and surgical treatment of cervical ribs. Am. J. Sci., 133:173, 1907.

Krusen, E. M.: Cervical pain syndromes. Arch. Phys. Med., 49:376, 1968.

Kuntz, A.: Distribution of the sympathetic rami to the brachial plexus. Arch. Surg., 15:871, 1927.

Lang, E. R.: Roentgenographic diagnosis of the neurovascular compression syndromes. Radiology, 79:58, 1962.

Law, A. A.: Adventitious ligaments simulating cervical ribs. Ann. Surg., 72:497, 1920.

Litwin, M. S.: Postsympathectomy neuralgia. Arch. Surg., 84:591, 1962.

Lord, J. W., and Urschel, H. C.: Total claviculectomy. Surg. Rounds., 11:17, 1988.

Loring, W. E.: Venous thrombosis in the upper extremities as a complication of myocardial failure. Am. J. Med., 12:397, 1952.

Mackinnon, S. E., and Dellon, A. L.: Surgery of the Peripheral Nerve. New York, Thieme Medical, 1988, pp. 210–214.

Martinez, N. S.: Posterior first rib resection for total thoracic outlet sundrome decompression. Contemp. Surg., 15:13, 1979.

McLaughlin, C. W., and Popma, A. M.: Intermittent obstruction of the subclavian vein. J. A. M. A., 113:1960, 1939.

Murphy, T.: Brachial neuritis caused by pressure of first rib. Aust. Med. J., 15:582, 1910.

Naffziger, H. C., and Grant, W. T.: Neuritis of the brachial plexus—Mechanical in origin: The scalenus syndrome. Surg. Gynecol. Obstet., 67:722, 1938.

Ochsner, A., Gage, M., and DeBakey, M.: Scalenous anticus (Naffziger) syndrome. Am. J. Surg., 28:699, 1935.

Paget, J.: Clinical Lectures and Essays. London, Longmans Green, 1875.

Painter, T. D., and Rarpf, M.: Deep venous thrombosis of the upper extremity: 5 years' experience at a university hospital. Angiology, 35:743, 1984.

Palumbo, L. T.: Anterior transthoracic approach for upper extremity thoracic sympathectomy. Arch. Surg., 72:659, 1956.

Palumbo, L. T.: Upper dorsal sympathectomy without Horner's syndrome. Arch. Surg., 71:743, 1955.

Prescott, S. M., and Tikoff, G.: Deep venous thrombosis of the upper extremity: A reappraisal. Circulation, 59:350, 1979.

Rapoport, S., Blair, D. N., McCarthy, S. M., et al.: Brachial plexus: Correlation of MR imaging and CT pathologic findings. Radiology, 167:161, 1988.

Ravitch, M. M., and Steichen, F. M.: Atlas of General Thoracic Surgery. Philadelphia, W. B. Saunders, 1988, pp. 101–109.

Rob, C. G., and Standover, A.: Arterial occlusion complicating thoracic outlet compression syndrome. Br. Med. J., 2:709, 1958.

Roos, D. B.: Thoracic outlet nerve compression. In Rutherford, R. B. (ed): Vascular Surgery. 3rd ed. Philadelphia, W. B. Saunders, 1989, pp. 858–875.

Roos, D. B.: Transaxillary approach for first rib resection to relieve thoracic outlet syndrome. Ann. Surg., 163:354, 1966.

Roos, D. B., and Owens, J. C.: Thoracic outlet syndrome. Arch. Surg., 93:71, 1966.

Rosati, L. M., and Lord, J. W.: Neurovascular compression syndromes of the shoulder girdle. Modern Surgical Monographs. New York, Grune & Stratton, 1961.

Rosenberg, J. C.: Arteriography demonstrations of compression syndromes of the thoracic outlet. South. Med J., 59:400, 1966.

Rubenstein, N., and Greger, W. P.: Successful streptokinase therapy for catheter-induced subclavian vein thrombosis. Arch. Intern. Med., 140:1370, 1980.

Smithwick, R. H.: Modified dorsal sympathectomy for vascular spasm (Raynaud's disease) of the upper extremity. Ann. Surg., 104:339, 1936.

Stoney, W. S., Addlestone, R. B., Alford, W. C., Jr., et al.: The incidence of venous thrombosis following long-term transvenous pacing. Ann. Thorac. Surg., 22:166, 1976.

Sundqvist, S. B., Hedner, U., Rullenberg, R. H. E., et al.: Deep venous thrombosis of the arm: A study of coagulation and fibrinolysis. Br. Med. J., 283:265, 1981.

Swank, W. L., and Simeone, F. A.: The scalenous anticus syndrome. Arch. Neurol. Psychiatr., 51:432, 1944.

Taylor, L. N., McAllister, W. R., Dennis, D. L., et al.: Thrombolytic therapy followed by first rib resection for spontaneous subclavian vein thrombosis. Am. J. Surg., 149:644, 1985.

Telford, E. D., and Mottershead, S.: Pressure of the cervicobrachial junction. J. Bone Joint Surg. Am., 30:249, 1948.

Telford, E. D., and Stopford, J. S. B.: The vascular complications of the cervical rib. Br. J. Surg., 18:559, 1937.

Tilney, N. L., Griffiths, H. F. G., and Edwards, E. A.: Natural history of major venous thrombosis of the upper extremity. Arch. Surg., 101:792, 1970.

Urschel, H. C., Jr.: Dorsal sympathectomy and management of thoracic outlet syndrome with VATS. Ann. Thorac. Surg., 56:717, 1993.

Urschel, H. C., Jr.: Video-assisted sympathectomy and thoracic outlet syndrome. Chest Surg. Clin. N. Am., 3:299, 1993.

Urschel, H. C., Jr., Paulson, D. L., and McNamara, J. J.: Thoracic outlet syndrome. Ann. Thorac. Surg., 6:1, 1968.

Urschel, H. C., Jr., and Razzuk, M. A.: Current concepts: Management of the thoracic outlet syndrome. N. Engl. J. Med., 286:1140, 1972.

Urschel, H. C., Jr., and Razzuk, M. A.: The failed operation for thoracic outlet syndrome: The difficulty of diagnosis and management. Ann. Thorac. Surg., 42:523, 1986a.

Urschel, H. C., Jr., and Razzuk, M. A.: Improved management of the Paget-Schroetter syndrome secondary to thoracic outlet compression. Ann. Thorac. Surg., 52:1217, 1991.

Urschel, H. C., Jr., and Razzuk, M. A.: Posterior thoracic sympathectomy. In Malt, R. A.: Surgical Techniques Illustrated: A Comparative Atlas. Philadelphia, W. B. Saunders, 1985, pp. 612–615.

Urschel, H. C., Jr., and Razzuk, M. A.: Thoracic outlet syndrome. Surg. Annu., 5:229, 1973.

Urschel, H. C., Jr., and Razzuk, M. A.: Thoracic outlet syndrome. In Grillo, H. C. (ed): International Trends in General Thoracic Surgery. Vol. 2. St. Louis, C. V. Mosby Co., 1986b, pp. 130–134.

Urschel, H. C., Jr., Razzuk, M. A., Albers, J. E., and Paulson, D. L.: Reoperation for recurrent thoracic outlet syndrome. Ann. Thorac. Surg., 21:19, 1976.

Urschel, H. C., Jr., Razzuk, M. A., Hyland, J. W., et al.: Thoracic outlet syndrome masquerading as coronary artery disease. Ann. Thorac. Surg., 16:239, 1973.

Urschel, H. C., Jr., Razzuk, M. A., Wood, R. E., and Paulson, D. L.: Objective diagnosis (ulnar nerve conduction velocity) and current therapy of the thoracic outlet syndrome. Ann. Thorac. Surg., 12:608, 1971.

Von Schroetter, L.: Erkrankungen der Gefossl. In Nathnogel, A. K. (ed): Handbuch der Pathologie und Therapie. Wein, Holder, 1884.

White, J. C., Smithwick, R. H., and Simeone, F. A.: The Autonomic Nervous System: Anatomy, Physiology and Surgical Application. 3rd ed. New York, MacMillan, 1952, pp. 104–108.

Wood, R. E., Campbell, D. C., Razzuk, M. A., et al.: Surgical advantages of selective unilateral ventilation. Ann. Thorac. Surg., 14:2, 1972.

Wright, I. S.: The neurovascular syndrome produced by hyperabduction of the arm. Am. Heart J., 29:1, 1945.

Zimmerman, R., Marl, H., Harenberg, J., et al.: Urokinase therapy of subclavian axillary vein thrombosis. Klin. Wochenschr., 59:851, 1981.

19 Neoplasms of the Lung
■ I Carcinoma of the Lung

Thomas A. D'Amico and David C. Sabiston, Jr.

Lung cancer remains the most common cause of death by malignancy in both men and women (Table 19–1). Moreover, the age-adjusted death rate for lung cancer increased steadily from 1930 to 1990, and the rate of increase does not appear to be abating (Boring et al., 1994). It is estimated that more than 170,000 new cases of lung cancer are diagnosed annually, and cigarette smoking is considered the principal etiologic factor. The role of oncogenes in the pathogenesis and therapy of lung cancer has been described; despite advances in the understanding of the molecular biology of pulmonary malignancy, surgical resection offers the best opportunity for cure of non-small-cell lung carcinoma. Chemotherapy and radiotherapy constitute the principal therapy for patients with small-cell carcinoma of the lung, although a subset of patients may be candidates for surgical resection.

HISTORICAL ASPECTS

The first successful thoracotomy and pulmonary resection was performed by Milton Anthony in 1821 (Brewer, 1982). Without using anesthesia, Anthony removed a portion of the lung and part of two ribs, and the patient survived 1 year. The first pneumonectomy was performed in multiple stages by Sir William Macewen in 1895; he applied thermocoagulation to the chest wall, pleura, and lung in a patient with pleuropulmonary tuberculosis (Meade, 1961). That patient returned to full activity and was seen 45 years later, when he presented for hernia repair. In 1933, Evarts Graham performed the first successful single-stage pneumonectomy in a patient with squamous cell carcinoma (Graham and Singer, 1933). The patient recovered completely and survived 2 decades thereafter to die eventually of an unrelated disease, free of cancer. This case demonstrated not only that total pulmonary excision could be achieved, but also that lung cancer was curable by adequate pulmonary resection. Rienhoff and associates (1942) reported the individual ligation technique for pneumonectomy. Churchill and Belsey (1939) described the segmental anatomy and individual ligation technique for lingular resection. Kent and Blades (1942) subsequently developed the individual ligation technique for resection of the lower lobes, and Allison (1946) demonstrated the safety of intrapericardial pneumonectomy.

PATHOLOGY

Pulmonary neoplasms arise in bronchial epithelium. There are four major pathologic cell types: small-cell carcinoma, adenocarcinoma, squamous cell carcinoma, and large-cell carcinoma. With the differences in therapy and prognosis, lung cancer is frequently categorized into two broad subtypes: small-cell carcinoma and non-small-cell carcinoma. *Small-cell lung cancer* (SCLC) is characterized by more rapid growth, stronger likelihood of metastases at the time of diagnosis, and greater responsiveness to chemotherapy and radiation therapy. The remaining three cell types, together considered *non-small-cell lung cancer* (NSCLC), account for 75 to 80% of all lung carcinomas and are often discussed collectively, because therapeutic approaches to patients with any of these cell types are quite similar.

Carcinomas of the lung show progressive pathologic changes in bronchial epithelium with time, particularly squamous cell carcinoma (Fig. 19–1). Basal cell proliferation, the initial event, is followed by hyperplasia of the mucus-secreting goblet cells, metaplasia of the stratified squamous epithelium, and development of nuclear atypia. Finally, carcinoma in situ develops, which may be followed by invasion through the basement membrane, regional infiltration of lymph nodes, and hematogenous dissemination.

■ **Table 19–1.** ESTIMATED CANCER DEATHS BY SITE AND SEX

Type	Men (%)	Women (%)
Lung	33	23
Breast		18
Prostate	13	
Colon and rectum	10	11
Leukemia/lymphoma	8	8
Ovary		5
Pancreas	4	5
Urinary tract	5	3
Uterus		4
Stomach	3	
Melanoma	2	1
Oral	2	1
All other	20	21

Modified from Boring, C. C., Squires, T. S., Tong, T., and Montgomery, S.: Cancer statistics, 1994. CA Cancer J. Clin., 44:7, 1994.

Basal cell proliferation

↓

Hyperplasia of goblet cells

↓

Metaplastic stratification of squamous epithelium

↓

Atypical metaplasia

↓

Carcinoma in situ

↓

Infiltration of cancer through basement membrane

↓

Spread to regional lymph nodes

↓

Hematogenous dissemination

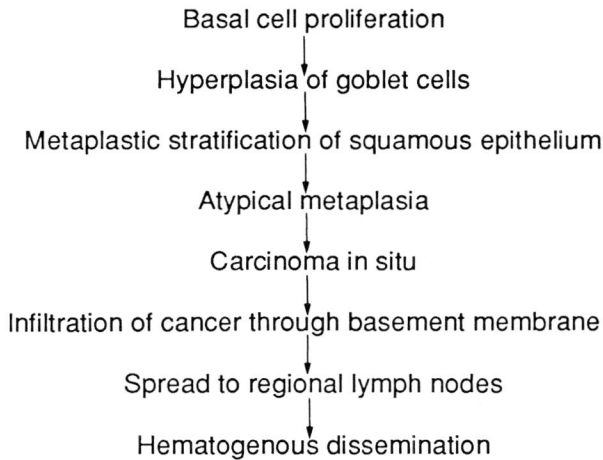

FIGURE 19–1. Histologic progression in the pathogenesis of lung cancer. (From Linnoila, I.: Pathology of non-small-cell lung cancer: New diagnostic approaches. Hematol. Oncol. Clin. North. Am., 4:1027, 1990.)

Non-Small-Cell Lung Cancer

In the World Health Organization classification, the major histologic types of NSCLC are adenocarcinoma, squamous cell carcinoma, and large-cell carcinoma (Kreyburg, 1967). Other histologic types include adenosquamous carcinoma, bronchoalveolar carcinoma (a subset of adenocarcinoma), bronchial carcinoids, and bronchial gland tumors. The incidence of the various histologic types of NSCLC has changed during recent years: Adenocarcinomas have been increasing in frequency, and squamous cell carcinomas have become less common. More than one type of histologic differentiation pattern is present in many pulmonary malignancies, suggesting the possibility of a pluripotential stem cell. In addition, the development of neuroendocrine cell hyperplasia, which may represent precursor lesions of SCLC, may also be responsible for the production of regulatory peptides that influence the development of NSCLC (Linnoila, 1990).

Adenocarcinoma. Adenocarcinoma is the most common cell type, occurring in approximately 50% of patients with lung cancer. These lesions usually are peripheral; they invade the overlying pleura, but may cause bronchial obstruction by local parenchymal or submucosal invasion. Although adenocarcinomas may stain for keratin, they also exhibit mucin production, glandular formation, or papillary structures, varying in differentiation patterns from one microscopic field to another (Linnoila, 1990).

Adenocarcinomas may be subdivided histologically into acinar, papillary, and bronchoalveolar forms. Bronchoalveolar patterns originate from alveolar septa and demonstrate no significant desmoplasia or glandular formation. Bronchoalveolar carcinoma may present in two distinct manners, as a solitary pulmonary nodule or as a diffuse infiltrative process, either localized to a particular segment or generalized (Grover et al., 1989).

Squamous Cell Carcinoma. Squamous cell carcinoma, once the most common cell type, now accounts for approximately 30% of all lung cancers. Squamous cell carcinomas originate centrally, grow toward the mainstem bronchus, and invade bronchial cartilage, pulmonary parenchyma, and lymph nodes. The epithelium in the normal tracheobronchial tree does not contain squamous epithelium; progressive histologic changes occur in the bronchial mucosa in the development of squamous cell carcinoma. The premalignant changes in the epithelium demonstrate that squamous cell carcinoma is a primary tumor, not a metastatic lesion. The characteristic histologic features include intracellular and extracellular keratinization, prominent desmosomes, and bundles of intermediate filaments (Linnoila, 1990).

Large-Cell Carcinoma. Large-cell carcinomas are unrelated to bronchi and are apt to present as peripheral lesions. They rapidly invade the parenchyma and tend to metastasize early. The diagnosis of large-cell carcinoma is that of exclusion of other cell types. These lesions exhibit no evidence of glandular or squamous differentiation; they are distinguished from small-cell carcinoma by the presence of abundant cytoplasm, distinct borders, and enlarged nuclei containing prominent nucleoli. Electron microscopy often shows that many large-cell carcinomas demonstrate aspects of differentiation into adenocarcinoma, squamous cell carcinoma, or small-cell carcinoma (Linnoila, 1990).

Small-Cell Lung Cancer

In SCLC, the histologic features are distinct. The distribution of chromatin within the nucleus is uniform, the nucleoli are unusually small and indistinct, and mitoses are frequent. The cells, which often contain scant cytoplasm, assume a spindle or fusiform shape, arranged in bundles (Goodman and Livingston, 1989). A distinguishing characteristic of small-cell carcinoma is the presence of cytoplasmic neurosecretory granules on electron microscopy (Iglehart et al., 1985). The liver is a frequent site of metastases of small-cell carcinoma, affecting 15 to 30% of patients at the time of diagnosis. Another common site is the bone marrow, where metastatic involvement occurs in 15 to 25% of patients at initial presentation. Other common sites include the brain, cortical bone, and the peritoneum.

Carcinoids

Bronchopulmonary carcinoids, constituting approximately 2% of all lung tumors (World Health Organization, 1982), are low-grade neoplasms characterized by neuroendocrine features: the presence of neurosecretory granules by electron microscopy and the production of peptide hormones. They are characterized by cellular growth in solid sheets or in mixed patterns of sheets, cords, nests, and trabeculae. Atypical carcinoid tumors, which demonstrate cellular pleomorphism, frequent mitoses, hyperchromatic nuclei, and scant cytoplasm, carry a poor prognosis (Linnoila, 1990).

These tumors are not related to race, family history, or smoking history. Although they occur over a wide age range, most patients with bronchial carcinoids are younger than patients with carcinoma of the lung. Most carcinoids are limited to the bronchus or lung, but regional lymph node metastases are present in 10 to 15% of patients at the time of diagnosis (Martini et al., 1994). Bronchial carcinoids have a favorable prognosis after resection: the 5-year survival rate is 95% in patients with Stage I disease (Harpole et al., 1992).

PATHOGENESIS

A full description of the pathogenesis of lung cancer includes assessment of the known environmental factors and the genetic events that transform bronchial epithelial cells to malignant lung cancer cells. Although known etiologic agents include cigarette smoking, exposure to workplace carcinogens, and the presence of chronic obstructive pulmonary disease, most patients with carcinoma of the lung have had considerable exposure to tobacco (Phillips et al., 1988). Thus, reducing this exposure is the predominant goal of preventive programs. Recent investigations of the molecular biology of lung cancer have demonstrated genetic lesions involving activation of dominant oncogenes and inactivation of recessive oncogenes ("tumor suppressor genes").

Etiology

The relationship between occupational exposure and the subsequent development of lung cancer was noted in the sixteenth century among the workers in the mines of Schneeberg, Germany, and Joachimstal, Czechoslovakia. These workers were known to contract serious and ultimately fatal pulmonary disorders over time (Fried, 1958). Uranium and radon gas in these mines are thought to have been primarily responsible for the development of these malignant neoplasms. Today, the most important agent in the pathogenesis of carcinoma of the lung is cigarette smoking.

Cigarette smoking is the most important cause of lung cancer in men and women (Cullen et al., 1986). Indications that cigarette smoking is linked to carcinoma of the lung are abundant. Classic retrospective and prospective studies have established a clear relationship between both the duration and intensity of cigarette use and the incidence of lung cancer. In a landmark postmortem study, Auerbach and associates (1957) examined the entire tracheobronchial tree in 117 men. In this study, 34 died of carcinoma of the lung, and all were smokers. In the remaining 83 patients, four cytologic changes were evaluated in

each histologic section: basal cell hyperplasia, cellular stratification, squamous metaplasia, and carcinoma in situ. In the group of patients who did not die of carcinoma of the lung, the pathologic changes were more frequent among those who smoked. The progressive increases in the severity of cytologic transformation correlated with the amount of tobacco use. In another study, encompassing over 2000 patients with carcinoma of the lung, only 5% were nonsmokers (Kabat and Wynder, 1984). In a large prospective study of British male physicians, 114 cases of SCLC were observed in 155,708 man-years among smokers, compared with only 1 case in 103,383 man-years among nonsmokers (Doll and Peto, 1978). This study also demonstrated a positive dose-response relationship between the number of cigarettes consumed each day and the incidence of SCLC.

Most carcinogens act synergistically with cigarette smoke as etiologic agents in the pathogenesis of carcinoma of the lung. Passive smoking, which accounts for 25% of carcinoma of the lung in nonsmokers, may increase the risk of cancer by 35 to 53% among nonsmokers who live with smokers (Wald et al., 1986). Other carcinogens include arsenic, cadmium, chromium, radon, and workplace chemicals, such as chromoethyl ether. Chronic obstructive pulmonary disease has also been demonstrated to be a predisposing factor in the development of carcinoma of the lung.

CLINICAL MANIFESTATIONS

Symptoms relating to carcinoma of the lung depend on the anatomic location of the tumor, extension into surrounding structures, metastatic spread, and the systemic effects of paraneoplastic syndromes. Most patients found to have lung cancer present with symptomatic disease; only 6% of patients are asymptomatic at the time of diagnosis. By the time the diagnosis of carcinoma of the lung is made, most patients have regional lymph node involvement or distant metastases.

Chest Symptoms

Symptoms referable to the thorax may result from endobronchial growth of the primary tumor, extrinsic growth of the primary tumor, or regional spread of the primary tumor. Centrally located lesions are associated with cough, stridor, wheezing, hemoptysis, dyspnea, and chest pain. The most common symptom is cough, which derives from endobronchial erosion and irritation. Peripheral tumors are associated with chest pain, cough, and dyspnea, owing to pleural and chest wall involvement. Large peripheral tumors may undergo cavitation and present as lung abscesses.

Intrathoracic extension of lung tumors may involve surrounding thoracic structures (Sabiston, 1990). Invasion of the recurrent laryngeal nerve, occurring in up to 8% of patients, may be manifested as hoarseness.

Dysphagia, indicating involvement of the esophagus, occurs in 1 to 5% of patients. Local extension of a tumor at the apex of the lung, involving the eighth cervical and first thoracic nerves, may cause superior sulcus (Pancoast) tumor syndrome, characterized by shoulder and arm pain. Furthermore, paravertebral extension and sympathetic nerve involvement may cause Horner's syndrome, characterized by enophthalmus, ptosis, meiosis, and ipsilateral anhidrosis.

In 60% of patients with adenocarcinoma and 34% of those with squamous cell carcinoma, the pleura is involved (Ihde and Minna, 1991). Malignant pleural effusion often exacerbates symptoms of chest pain and shortness of breath. Recurrence after thoracentesis is a poor prognostic sign.

Metastases to the heart, usually involving the pericardium, occur in 15 to 35% of patients (Strauss et al., 1977). Tumor involving the heart and pericardium may result in effusion, with subsequent pericardial tamponade, arrhythmia, or congestive heart failure.

Superior Vena Caval Syndrome

The superior vena caval syndrome is characterized by plethoric appearance, distention of the venous drainage of the arm and neck, and edema of the face, neck, and arms, often caused by extensive tumor involvement of right mediastinal lymph nodes. This obstruction usually progresses gradually over time, with collateral venous drainage detectable on physical examination. Pericardial effusion and pericardial tamponade may also be present because of the involvement of the heart and pericardium in 15 to 35% of patients with carcinoma of the lung (Strauss et al., 1977).

Paraneoplastic Syndromes

Symptoms and signs that are related to the primary tumor or its metastases by hormonal intermediates may be caused by paraneoplastic syndromes and may accompany carcinoma of the lung. Systemic manifestations of NSCLC include cachexia, parathyroid-like hormone secretion with concomitant hypercalcemia, hypertrophic pulmonary osteoarthropathy, and various neurologic syndromes (Richardson and Johnson, 1992). Weight loss and anorexia occur in as many as one-third of patients. Noncachectic patients may demonstrate increases in protein turnover and glucose production, and muscular catabolism may be demonstrated.

These paraneoplastic syndromes are also associated with SCLC, and are more often present at the time of diagnosis than in patients with NSCLC. In addition to weight loss, anorexia, and neuromyopathies, paraneoplastic syndromes may follow tumor elaboration of antidiuretic hormone, adrenocorticotropin, calcitonin, or parathyroid hormone.

DIAGNOSIS AND STAGING

The diagnosis and staging of lung cancer involve the integration and cooperation of primary physicians, radiologists, and thoracic oncologists. The diagnosis of lung cancer is often suggested by findings on chest film and histologically confirmed by bronchoscopy, by percutaneous biopsy, or at thoracotomy for pulmonary resection. Staging of lung cancer is essential for estimation of prognosis, selection of treatment, and evaluation of protocols (Miller et al., 1992).

Diagnostic Techniques

The principal goal in diagnosing and staging carcinoma of the lung is to identify candidates to undergo thoracotomy for curative pulmonary resection. Following a complete history and physical examination, with particular attention to possible manifestations of the primary tumor—regional invasion, distant metastases, and paraneoplastic syndromes—the current chest films must be reviewed and compared with previous studies.

Chest Films. The classic radiographic presentation of carcinoma of the lung is a solitary pulmonary nodule, which may appear as either a smooth-bordered lesion or an irregular mass. The chest film usually demonstrates a mass arising in the hilum or the lung field, although a pneumonic infiltrate, a pleural effusion, or an elevated diaphragm may also be present. Frequently, gross nodal involvement is evident as well, and collapse of a pulmonary segment or lobe distal to an obstructing endobronchial lesion may be manifested as atelectasis.

For the doubling time of the nodule, the chest film is compared with previous films. If the doubling time is less than 1 month, the etiology of the nodule is likely to be infectious; if the doubling time is greater than 16 months, the nodule is likely to be benign; and if the doubling time is between 1 and 16 months, the nodule is more likely to be malignant (Klingman and DeMeester, 1990).

Computed Tomography. Another useful evaluation of the primary tumor is by *computed tomography* (CT) to assess regional lymph node involvement and to detect satellite nodules or mediastinal metastases. CT should include the apices of the thorax superiorly and extend inferiorly to include the liver and the adrenal glands. When the primary lesion is centrally located or advanced in size, CT is invaluable in assessing margins and dimensions.

CT is useful in assessing involvement of hilar and mediastinal lymph nodes. A maximal diameter of 10 mm indicates that hilar and mediastinal nodes may be uninvolved, suggesting operability. Even lymph nodes determined by CT to be enlarged contain metastatic tumor in only 70% of cases. Thus, suspected inoperability based on positive CT results should be confirmed by direct biopsy, unless evidence of inoperability is overwhelming. Patients without mediastinal lymphadenopathy on CT and who are otherwise operative candidates may proceed to thoracotomy; the false-negative rate in these patients is only 5% (Daly et al., 1987).

Bronchoscopy. An important adjunct in the diagnosis of carcinoma of the lung is flexible fiberoptic bronchoscopy. Bronchial biopsy, brushings, washings, and transbronchial aspiration are used to diagnose malignancy in most cases. Biopsy is more sensitive than bronchial washing and brushing in the diagnosis of carcinoma of the lung, especially in patients with SCLC, owing to its submucosal location. If the tumor is bronchoscopically visible, the yield following washings and brushings is approximately 75%; for biopsy, the yield is approximately 85%, for a total yield of 94%. In contrast, for tumors that are not visualized, bronchoscopy with brushings and washings has a yield of 50%, and bronchoscopy with biopsy has a yield of 60%. The typing accuracy for bronchoscopic biopsy and cytologic analysis is only 66%, with most failures occurring with adenocarcinoma and large-cell carcinoma (Lyubsky and Jacobson, 1991).

Transthoracic Needle Aspiration. *Transthoracic needle aspiration* (TTNA), which may be performed using fluoroscopic, sonographic, or computed tomographic guidance, may be useful in diagnosing lesions that are not visualized by bronchoscopy. TTNA need not be applied to every patient with a solitary pulmonary nodule in order to confirm the diagnosis of malignancy preoperatively. A benign or undetermined histologic diagnosis by TTNA does not definitively exclude the possibility of malignancy, owing to a significant false-negative rate (Lyubsky and Jacobson, 1991). Regardless of the result of TTNA, a candidate for thoracotomy should undergo pulmonary resection for diagnosis and therapy. The indications for TTNA include pulmonary lesions in patients who are poor candidates for thoracotomy yet require definitive diagnosis, a new pulmonary lesion in a patient with a history of prior malignancy, and a lung mass that is suspicious for small-cell carcinoma (Ferguson, 1990). The complications of TTNA include pneumothorax, hemothorax, and infection.

Positron Emission Tomography. *Positron emission tomography* (PET) is a noninvasive imaging method that has demonstrated increased glucose metabolism in malignant cells. Recent studies have demonstrated that PET was accurate in differentiating benign from malignant pulmonary nodules (Dewan et al., 1993). PET may prove especially useful in establishing the diagnosis of malignancy prior to thoracotomy in patients in whom surgery would be a high risk.

Magnetic Resonance Imaging. It is now recognized that *magnetic resonance imaging* (MRI) of the chest differentiates vascular from solid structures and demonstrates parenchymal, hilar, and mediastinal anatomy in both coronal and sagittal planes, without the use of contrast agents or ionizing radiation. Nevertheless, MRI is limited by long scanning times, motion artifacts, and inferior spatial resolution. Comparison of CT and MRI in the evaluation of the primary tumor and nodal involvement demonstrates a slight advantage with CT (Patterson et al., 1987). MRI is

■ **Table 19–2.** INTERNATIONAL TNM STAGING SYSTEM FOR LUNG CANCER

Tumor (T)

TX Occult carcinoma (malignant cells in sputum or bronchial washings but tumor not visualized by imaging studies or bronchoscopy)

T1 Tumor 3 cm or less in greatest diameter, surrounded by lung or visceral pleura, but not proximal to a lobar bronchus

T2 Tumor > 3 cm in diameter, or with involvement of main bronchus at least 2 cm distal to carina, or with visceral pleural invasion, or with associated atelectasis or obstructive pneumonitis extending to the hilar region but not involving the entire lung

T3 Tumor invading chest wall, diaphragm, mediastinal pleura, or parietal pericardium; or tumor in main bronchus within 2 cm of, but not invading, carina; or atelectasis of obstructive pneumonitis of the entire lung

T4 Tumor invading mediastinum, heart, great vessels, trachea, esophagus, vertebral body, or carina; or ipsilateral malignant pleural effusion

Nodes (N)

N0 No regional lymph node metastases
N1 Metastases to ipsilateral peribronchial or hilar nodes
N2 Metastases to ipsilateral mediastinal or subcarinal nodes
N3 Metastases to contralateral mediastinal or hilar, or to any scalene or supraclavicular nodes

Distant Metastases (M)

M0 No distant metastases
M1 Distant metastases

From Mountain, C. F.: A new international staging system for lung cancer. Chest, *89*:225S, 1986.

useful in the staging of carcinoma of the lung for determination of preoperative nodal staging in patients in whom the use of contrast agents is contraindicated and for confirmation of spinal cord involvement in patients with metastatic disease.

Mediastinoscopy. The role of mediastinoscopy in the diagnosis and staging of carcinoma of the lung is controversial. When noninvasive staging demonstrates evidence of mediastinal nodal involvement, mediastinoscopy documents involvement approximately 70% of the time (Patterson et al., 1987). Mediastinoscopy with biopsy is recommended when CT demonstrates mediastinal lymph nodes greater than 10 mm in diameter, to confirm inoperability; however, many nodal groups (posterior subcarinal, pericardial, periesophageal, and para-aortic) are inaccessible by this technique. An alternative approach is to perform mediastinoscopy by a left parasternal approach (Chamberlain procedure). In some patients with carcinoma of the lung, thoracoscopy may be used for biopsy of enlarged nodes in these areas.

Thoracoscopy. Thoracoscopic staging of lung cancer has been demonstrated to be safe and effective in selected patients (Naruke et al., 1993). The most common application is the evaluation of indeterminate pulmonary nodules. However, thoracoscopy also may be used for complete evaluation of suspicious para-aortic, subaortic, tracheobronchial, carinal, para-esophageal, or hilar lymph nodes. Finally, thoracoscopy may help confirm pleural invasion or dissemination (Wain, 1993). Techniques to improve localization and characterization of pulmonary nodules (such as

■ **Table 19–3.** STAGING GROUPS FOR LUNG CANCER

Stage	T	N	M
Occult	TX	N0	M0
Stage I	T1–2	N0	M0
Stage II	T1–2	N1	M0
Stage IIIA	T3	N0–1	M0
	T1–3	N2	M0
Stage IIIB	T4	N0–2	M0
	T1–4	N3	M0
Stage IV	Any T	Any N	M1

From Mountain, C. F.: A new international staging system for lung cancer. Chest, *89*:225S, 1986.

■ **Table 19–4.** FIVE–YEAR SURVIVAL IN NON–SMALL–CELL LUNG CANCER ACCORDING TO STAGE

Stage	Five-Year Survival Rate
Stage I	66.7%
Stage II	43.6%
Stage IIIA	22.4%
Stage IIIB	5.4%
Stage IV	5.9%

From Naruke, T., Goya, T., Tsuchiya, R., et al.: Prognosis and survival in resected lung carcinoma based on the new international staging system for lung cancer. J. Thorac. Cardiovasc. Surg., *96*:440, 1988.

thoracoscopic ultrasonography and preoperative needle localization) will expand the indications for thoracoscopy in the staging of carcinoma of the lung (Shennib, 1993).

Staging of Non-Small-Cell Lung Cancer

The staging of carcinoma of the lung by the TNM approach, devised by the American Joint Committee on Cancer in 1989, provides a consistent, reproducible description of the anatomic extent of disease at the time of diagnosis (Mountain, 1986). In the TNM system, *T* represents the primary tumor, and numeric suffixes describe increasing size or involvement; *N* represents regional lymph nodes, with suffixes to de-

scribe levels of involvement; and *M* designates the presence or absence of distant metastases (Table 19–2). The TNM subsets are then grouped in a series of stages of disease to identify groups of patients with similar prognosis and therapy (Table 19–3; Fig. 19–2). The value of the staging system in estimating prognosis is demonstrated by the 5-year survival statistics, as presented in Table 19–4.

Staging of Small-Cell Lung Cancer

For SCLC, the TNM staging system has not proved to be as prognostically useful, because widespread metastases are often present at the time of initial diagnosis. Even patients who present with small pri-

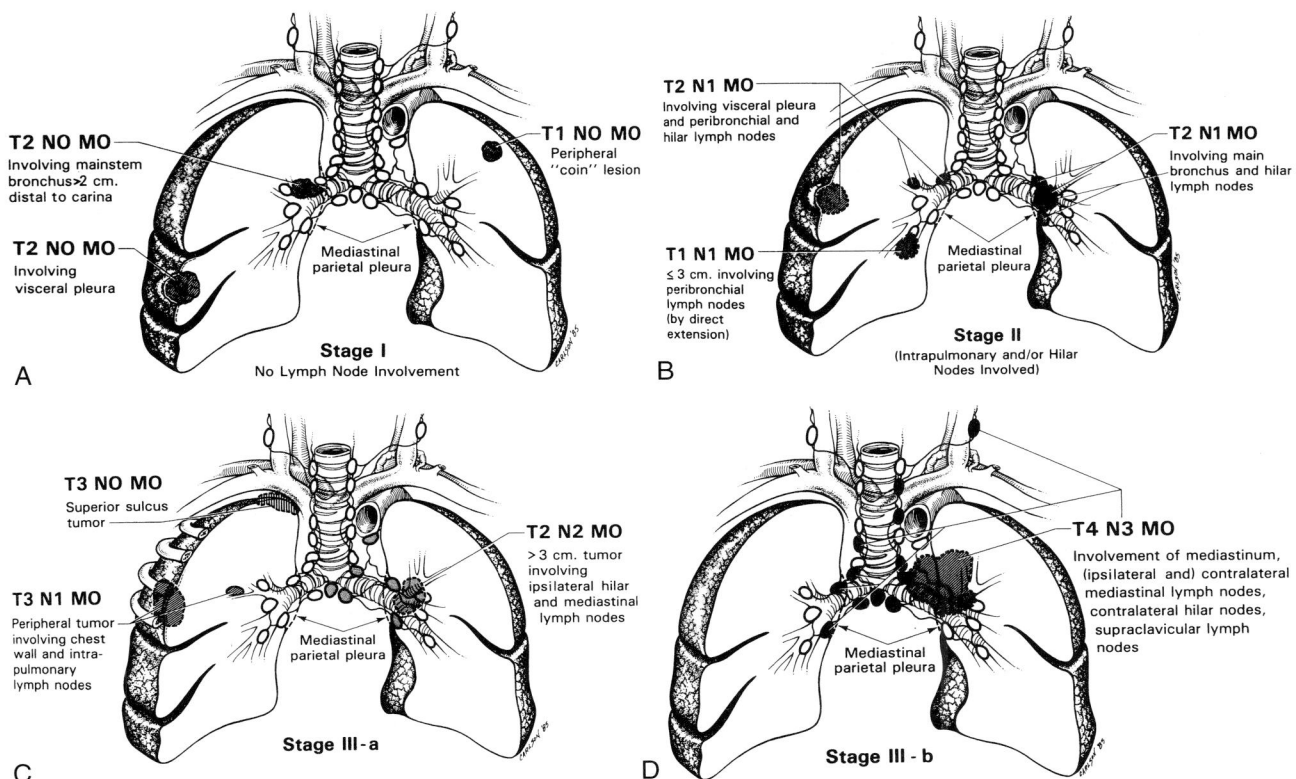

FIGURE 19–2. Lung cancer staging. *A*, Stage I. *B*, Stage II. *C*, Stage III-a. *D*, Stage III-b. (*A–D*, From Mountain, C. F.: A new international staging system for lung cancer. Chest, *89*:225S, 1986.)

mary tumors and no evidence of nodal disease often have distant metastases. Currently, most thoracic oncologists use a staging system that divides patients with SCLC into two major groups: those with *limited* disease and those with *extensive* disease. Disease confined to the hemithorax (with or without ipsilateral hilar or mediastinal lymph nodes) and without detectable distant metastases is considered limited disease. Extensive disease is characterized by involvement of the contralateral thorax or the presence of distant metastases (Cook et al., 1993).

SURGICAL MANAGEMENT OF NON–SMALL–CELL LUNG CANCER

The standard treatment of patients with Stage I or Stage II disease is surgical resection. In addition, a subset of patients with Stage III disease has improved outcome with surgical resection. Every solitary pulmonary nodule should be resected unless the lesion is known to be benign or the patient's medical condition contraindicates surgery. Thorough preoperative evaluation and preparation of a patient with carcinoma of the lung reduces the morbidity and mortality of thoracotomy and pulmonary resection.

Determination of Operability

Operability must be determined by assessment of both the medical risk of thoracotomy and the risk of removal of the requisite pulmonary parenchyma. The degree of cardiopulmonary disease, usually a consequence of tobacco use, is the most significant medical factor in determining operability and the major cause of postoperative morbidity and mortality.

Preoperative Pulmonary Evaluation. Pulmonary function tests and analysis of arterial blood gases help determine the feasibility of pulmonary resection. Postoperative pulmonary function is estimated by calculating the preoperative function and the projected resection of pulmonary parenchyma. Patients are excluded from surgical therapy if estimated postoperative pulmonary function falls below the minimum acceptable values. In particular, when the forced expiratory volume at 1 second (FEV_1) and forced vital capacity are less than 30% of predicted values, thoracotomy is generally contraindicated. If the value of the predicted postoperative FEV_1 is 800 ml or greater, the patient is considered able to tolerate resection. When the results of the preoperative pulmonary function studies are marginal, radionuclide ventilation (xenon-133 radiorespirometry) and perfusion (macroaggregated albumin labeled with technetium-99) scans may be required to determine resectability. Postoperative FEV_1 may be calculated after assessing the contribution of either lung and specific pulmonary segments to overall pulmonary function.

Exercise tolerance and oxygen consumption ($\dot{V}O_2$ max) studies may also be used to determine resectability when pulmonary function test results are borderline. In one study, high mortality was associated with $\dot{V}O_2$ max less than 10 ml/kg/min; when $\dot{V}O_2$ max was greater than 20 ml/kg/min, no deaths occurred (Bechard and Wetstein, 1987).

Medical Contraindications. When a history of angina is elicited or when the preoperative electrocardiogram demonstrates ischemia or arrhythmia, radionuclide evaluation of myocardial perfusion or function is performed. When results of these studies are negative, significant coronary artery disease is reliably excluded; when they are positive, coronary arteriography is indicated. Recent myocardial infarction, uncontrolled congestive heart failure, and uncontrollable arrhythmia preclude thoracotomy for pulmonary resection.

Resectability at Thoracotomy. Final determination of resectability is made at thoracotomy. Contraindications to pulmonary resection at the time of thoracotomy include pleural metastases, extensive mediastinal lymph node involvement (N3 disease), or direct extension of the tumor (T4 disease). In addition, pulmonary resection is aborted when complete resection would render pulmonary reserve inadequate as determined by preoperative pulmonary function studies.

Surgical Procedures

Intraoperative evaluation of tumor extent and the cardiopulmonary status of the patient determine which surgical procedure is employed. If histologic diagnosis has not been confirmed preoperatively, biopsy and frozen section examination are indicated, particularly if the planned resection is more extensive than lobectomy. Complete resection of the tumor and all grossly involved regional bronchial and mediastinal lymph nodes, including en-bloc resection of adjacent structures involved by direct extension of the primary tumor (such as chest wall and pericardium), is undertaken when feasible. Incomplete resection or resection that leaves a patient with an inadequate functional pulmonary reserve should not be performed.

Standard surgical procedures used to manage carcinoma of the lung include pneumonectomy, bilobectomy, lobectomy, segmentectomy, and wedge resection. The course chosen must permit removal of the entire tumor, with adequate margins, while preserving the maximum amount of functional lung tissue. Posterolateral thoracotomy, entering the thorax in the fifth or sixth intercostal space, provides adequate exposure in most cases. Alternatively, anterior thoracotomy through the third intercostal space may be used, particularly in patients with borderline pulmonary function, in order to maximize ventilation of the contralateral lung. At the time of thoracotomy, a systematic lymph node evaluation is undertaken and recorded to ascertain complete pathologic staging. For all pulmonary resections, the automatic stapling device is routinely employed, reducing the incidence of postoperative bronchopleural fistula. After lobectomy or lesser procedures, pleural catheters are placed for the evacuation of air, blood, or fluid until resolution.

Lobectomy. The most commonly performed pulmonary resection for lung cancer is lobectomy. Functional loss after lobectomy usually is greater than predicted immediately after resection; however, over time, pulmonary function improves to the expected level. A sleeve lobectomy may be performed when the primary tumor encroaches upon the lobar orifice, precluding complete resection with margins by standard lobectomy. In the right lung, a bilobectomy may be performed, conserving either the upper or the lower lobe. The indications for bilobectomy include tumor extending across a lobar fissure, absent fissure, endobronchial tumor, or tumor invading bronchus intermedius.

The risk of recurrence after surgical resection according to the magnitude of the resection has been analyzed by the Lung Cancer Study Group (LCSG) (Ginsberg and Rubenstein, 1991). In a prospective, randomized trial involving more than 400 patients with T1N0 lung cancer, lobectomy was compared with segmentectomy and wedge resection. There was no significant difference in morbidity and mortality among the procedures. Furthermore, there was no difference observed in pulmonary function between patients who underwent lobectomy and those who underwent lesser procedures. The rate of locoregional recurrence was significantly lower in patients who underwent lobectomy (5%) than in those who underwent either segmentectomy or wedge resection (15%).

Pneumonectomy. Pneumonectomy is performed when lobectomy does not provide complete resection and when the loss of pulmonary parenchyma will be tolerated. Modifications of the standard pneumonectomy include intrapericardial ligation of the pulmonary vessels, supra-aortic pneumonectomy on the left, and tracheal sleeve pneumonectomy. After pneumonectomy, the ipsilateral pleural cavity is aspirated to prevent contralateral shift of the mediastinum and pulmonary compromise. Alternatively, a pressure-balancing pleural catheter may be placed.

Segmentectomy. Patients with small peripheral lesions may be candidates for segmentectomy. Segmentectomy has been advocated to provide complete resection while preserving more functional parenchyma. A prospective randomized trial by the LCSG revealed a higher local recurrence rate after segmentectomy than after lobectomy; however, actuarial survival at 36 months was not significantly different (Ginsberg and Rubenstein, 1991).

Wedge Resection. Wedge resection may be performed in high-risk patients or in patients with small lesions without lymph node involvement. A retrospective study suggested that wedge resection in properly selected patients yields results similar to those of standard lobectomy (Errett et al., 1985). Data from the LCSG, however, demonstrated a significantly higher recurrence rate with wedge resection compared with either segmentectomy or lobectomy (Ginsberg and Rubenstein, 1991).

Thoracoscopic Procedures. Video-assisted thoraco-scopic resection of carcinoma of the lung has been reported and is being evaluated (Kirby and Rice, 1993). Thoracoscopic management of a solitary pulmonary nodule may achieve specific histologic diagnosis, adequate nodal staging, and complete resection in selected patients. The Video Assisted Thoracic Surgery Study Group collected the results of 1820 thoracoscopic procedures among 40 institutions for analysis (Hazelrigg et al., 1993). The most common procedure performed was wedge resection (49%), and anatomic resection for carcinoma of the lung was achieved in only 38 patients (2%). Of 1820 cases, 439 (24%) were converted to open thoracotomy. When the thoracoscopic approach is used to evaluate and resect primary pulmonary malignancy, complete excision and nodal staging must be ascertained and oncologic principles of thoracic surgery must be observed (Ginsberg, 1993).

Mediastinal Lymph Node Dissection. Regional lymph node stations (Fig. 19–3) should be evaluated at thoracotomy in all patients, regardless of whether curative resection is performed. Mediastinal involvement may be assessed by formal mediastinal lymph node dissection or by systematic sampling of the mediastinal lymph node groups (Bollen et al., 1993). At minimum, the ipsilateral lymph node stations should be sampled routinely, including the subcarinal station. Systematic resection may be accomplished in the right paratracheal compartment, the aorticopulmonary window, and the subcarinal and inferior-posterior compartment on either side. Enlarged nodes anterior to the vena cava, superior to the aorta, or within the superior mediastinum are simply excised. Dissection of the mediastinal lymph nodes improves the accuracy of staging and the survival of patients with N2 disease (Naruke et al., 1988; Watanabe et al., 1991).

Cardiac Surgery and Pulmonary Resection. Patients with resectable lung cancer who require myocardial revascularization may be candidates for concomitant pulmonary resection. Median sternotomy is performed and the pulmonary lesion is assessed. If pulmonary resection can be achieved by lobectomy or a lesser procedure, it is performed after the cardiac procedure is completed and after systemic anticoagulation is reversed. Access to the posterior mediastinum may be limited by this approach, and resection of the left lower lobe is frequently difficult.

Solitary Pulmonary Nodule

A patient with a solitary pulmonary nodule—a single spherical lesion within the lung—presents an important and challenging diagnostic problem in thoracic oncology. A solitary pulmonary nodule is assumed to be primary lung cancer until proved otherwise; the differential diagnosis includes metastatic carcinoma, granuloma, and benign pulmonary tumors. One must consider the relationship of age to the incidence of malignancy when evaluating and managing the solitary pulmonary nodule (Table 19–5). Most solitary pulmonary nodules should be re-

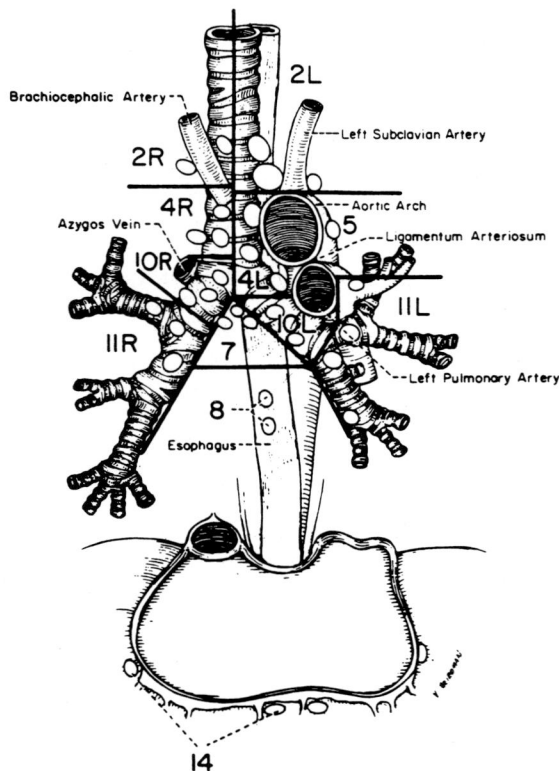

MODIFIED AMERICAN THORACIC SOCIETY DEFINITIONS OF REGIONAL NODAL STATIONS

Nodal Stations	Definitions
X	**Supraclavicular nodes.**
2R	**Right upper paratracheal nodes.** Nodes to the right of the midline of the trachea, between the intersection of the caudal margin of the brachiocephalic artery with the trachea and the apex of the lung or above the level of the aortic arch.
2L	**Left upper paratracheal nodes.** Nodes to the left of the midline of the trachea, between the top of the aortic arch and the apex of the lung.
4R	**Right lower paratracheal nodes.** Nodes to the right of the midline of the trachea, between the cephalic border of the azygos vein and the intersection of the caudal margin of the brachiocephalic artery with the right side of the trachea or the top of the aortic arch.
4L	**Left lower paratracheal nodes.** Nodes to the left of the midline of the trachea, between the top of the aortic arch and the level of the carina, medial to the ligamentum arteriosum.
5	**Aortopulmonary nodes.** Subaortic and paraaortic nodes, lateral to the ligamentum arteriosum or the aorta or left pulmonary artery, proximal to the first branch of the left pulmonary artery.
6	**Anterior mediastinal nodes.** Nodes anterior to the ascending aorta or the innominate artery.
7	**Subcarinal nodes.** Nodes arising caudal to the carina of the trachea but not associated with the lower lobe bronchi or arteries within the lung.
8	**Paraesophageal nodes.** Nodes dorsal to the posterior wall of the trachea and to the right or the left of the midline of the esophagus below the level of the subcarinal region. (Nodes around the descending aorta should also be included.)
9	**Right or left pulmonary ligament nodes.** Nodes within the right or left pulmonary ligament.
10R	**Right tracheobronchial nodes.** Nodes to the right of the midline of the trachea, from the level of the cephalic border of the azygos vein to the origin of the right upper lobe bronchus.
10L	**Left peribronchial nodes.** Nodes to the left of the midline of the trachea, between the carina and the left upper lobe bronchus, medial to ligamentum arteriosum
11	**Intrapulmonary nodes.** Nodes removed in the right or left lung specimen, plus those distal to the mainstem bronchi or secondary carina (includes interiobar, lobar, and segmental nodes).
14	**Superior diaphragmatic nodes.** Nodes adjacent to the pericardium within 2 cm of the diaphragm.

FIGURE 19–3. Definitions of regional nodal stations. (From Miller, J. D., Gorenstein, L. A., and Patterson, G. A.: Staging: The key to rational management. Reprinted with permission from the Society of Thoracic Surgeons [The Annals of Thoracic Surgery, 1992, Vol. 53, p. 170].)

sected after thorough investigation shows that systemic dissemination has not already occurred. Review of previous chest films may help determine the growth pattern of the nodule. A malignant nodule will usually have a doubling time between 30 and 400 days (Lillington and Caskey, 1993). When comparisons of current and prior films demonstrate stability or the calcification is visible, a benign lesion is suggested, and a period of observation may be warranted.

CT of the chest, liver, and adrenals is used to confirm the location of the tumor, to evaluate the mediastinum, and to assess the abdomen for systemic disease. If CT shows no evidence of metastases, the patient should undergo bronchoscopy. Bronchoscopic examination, with brushings and biopsy, may establish the histologic diagnosis and may determine resectability if an endobronchial lesion exists.

Pulmonary function studies are obtained preoperatively to assess the potential for pulmonary resection. Systems are thoroughly reviewed to exclude medical contraindications to thoracotomy. TTNA is not routinely performed and should be reserved for patients with marginal pulmonary function, for whom thoracotomy would only be performed after a malignant histologic diagnosis was verified.

Results of Surgical Resection

Stage I. The treatment of choice, particularly for more centrally located tumors, is lobectomy, although wedge resection or segmentectomy may be performed for small peripheral tumors. A systematic lymph node dissection is performed at thoracotomy to exclude hilar or mediastinal lymph node involvement. Patients with Stage I carcinoma of the lung can expect 3- and 5-year survival rates of approximately 85 and 70%, respectively. The most favorable group of Stage I patients, those with T1N0 disease, experience 5-year survival rates of 80 to 85% (Martini, 1990). Neither chemotherapy nor radiation therapy is recommended following complete resection of Stage I lung cancer.

Stage II. Surgical therapy for Stage II carcinoma includes resection of the primary tumor; en-bloc resection of the hilar, interlobar, lobar, and segmental lymph nodes; and systematic dissection of the mediastinal lymph nodes to exclude mediastinal metastases. Patients with Stage II disease experience 5-year

■ **Table 19–5.** INCIDENCE OF MALIGNANCY IN SOLITARY PULMONARY NODULES RELATED TO AGE

Age (yr)	Malignant (%)
35–44	15
45–49	26
50–59	41
60–69	50
70–79	70

survival rates of 40 to 50% (Martini et al., 1992; Naruke et al., 1988). The rate of recurrence after resection of Stage II disease is greater than 50%, and most recurrences are distant metastases. Postoperative radiation therapy may reduce the incidence of local and regional recurrence but does not affect overall survival (Martini et al., 1992).

Stage IIIA. Carcinoma of the lung that is locally advanced, in which the primary tumor is proximal or has invaded adjacent structures (T3), or in which ipsilateral mediastinal nodes are involved (N2), has a relatively poor prognosis. However, when surgical resection achieves total removal of the primary tumor and involved lymph nodes, there is a reasonable chance for cure.

When the tumor has invaded the chest wall, complete resection of the tumor with involved adjacent tissue is the most effective treatment (Van Raemdonck et al., 1992). Among 111 patients with carcinoma invading the chest wall who were treated surgically, two-thirds underwent complete resection; the 5-year survival rate in this selected group was 40% (Martini, 1990). With N2 disease, the 5-year survival rate after resection was approximately 30%. Although it has improved local control, postoperative irradiation does not appear to improve overall survival (Martini and Ginsberg, 1990).

Invasion of the mediastinal pleura, the diaphragm, or the parietal pericardium also is defined as T3 disease. However, resection for T3 NSCLC with mediastinal invasion is less advantageous than resection for T3 disease with chest-wall invasion. In a series of 225 patients from Memorial Sloan-Kettering, only 22% underwent complete resection, with a subsequent 5-year survival rate of only 9% (Burt et al., 1987).

The resectability of N2 disease is controversial. Several series report 5-year survival rates of 10 to 20% in all patients undergoing thoracotomy and 20 to 30% in patients who have completely resectable disease (Martini and Flehinger, 1987; Naruke et al., 1988; Watanabe et al., 1991). Other series investigating resection of N2 NSCLC have demonstrated 5-year survival rates ranging from 10% (Van Klaveren et al., 1993) to 40% (Daly et al., 1993). Radiologic evidence of N2 disease, concomitant T3 disease, the presence of involved subcarinal nodes, and multiple levels of mediastinal nodes have been identified as negative prognostic factors after resection in patients with N2 disease (Van Raemdonck et al., 1992). Preoperative identification and histologic confirmation of N2 disease usually contraindicates surgical resection; however, when unsuspected N2 disease is encountered, pulmonary resection is performed if complete excision is possible. Multimodality protocols, including neoadjuvant chemotherapy and surgical resection for patients with N2 NSCLC, are currently being evaluated (Kirn et al., 1993; Martini et al., 1993).

Stage IIIB. Resection is generally considered impossible for patients with Stage IIIB NSCLC (T4 or N3 disease). Occasionally, patients with unsuspected T4 disease undergo thoracotomy, and complete resection is attempted. Pneumonectomy with tracheal sleeve resection and direct reanastomosis of the trachea to the contralateral main bronchus has been advocated for proximal lesions, with a 5-year survival rate approaching 20% (Mathisen and Grillo, 1991). Invasion of the vena cava has been treated by resection and graft replacement, with essentially no reported long-term survivors (Burt et al., 1987). In patients with invasion of the myocardium, aorta, esophagus, or vertebral body, complete resection is rarely possible; furthermore, palliative incomplete resection does not aid survival.

Involvement of the contralateral hilar, contralateral mediastinal, scalene, or supraclavicular lymph node groups is considered N3 disease. In most series, there are no 5-year survivors after surgical treatment for N3 disease, which should be considered a definite sign of inoperability.

Superior Sulcus Tumor. The term *superior sulcus tumor* describes a malignancy of the lung of any histologic subtype, arising at the apex of the upper lobes in the superior sulcus, that may invade the pleura, the brachial plexus, the sympathetic chains, adjacent ribs, or vertebral bodies. Patients with superior sulcus tumor receive preoperative radiation therapy to the primary tumor, the mediastinum, and the supraclavicular region. Four weeks later, surgical resection is performed. Besides mediastinal lymph node dissection, the standard resection encompasses en-bloc removal of the involved lobe and chest wall; the entire first rib and the posterior segments of ribs 2, 3, and 4; transverse processes of involved thoracic vertebrae; nerve roots C8 and T1–3; the lower trunk of the brachial plexus; and the dorsal sympathetic chain. Despite the invasiveness of these tumors, a 5-year survival rate of 25 to 30% is expected in patients treated with this regimen (Martini and Ginsberg, 1990).

Multiple Primary Pulmonary Malignancies

Considering the high incidence of carcinoma of the lung in the general population, multiple primary pulmonary malignancies are rare, affecting 1.6 to 3.0% of all patients with lung cancer and 10 to 25% of those who survive more than 3 years. In a series of Stage I patients who underwent resection and were followed by the LCSG, 12% of recurrences were attributed to second primary lung cancer (Feld et al., 1984). Second primary lung carcinomas are categorized as synchronous or metachronous.

Synchronous Primary Carcinoma. The presence of synchronous lung cancer appears to hamper survival. In one series (Deschamps et al., 1990), the 5-year survival rate after complete resection in patients with synchronous lesions was only 16%—significantly lower than such rates in the same series after pulmonary resection of metachronous lesions (34%). Satellite tumor nodules have a poor prognosis as well. When satellite lesions are present, regardless of the size of the primary tumor, the disease is classified as Stage III (Shields, 1993).

Metachronous Primary Carcinoma. The development of a second primary carcinoma of the lung is an increasingly recognized problem in patients after resection for NSCLC. When a second primary carcinoma of the lung develops, limited surgical resection offers the best treatment. In recent series, the 5-year survival rate after resection of a second primary carcinoma of the lung ranged from 62% (Fleisher et al., 1991) to 70% (Rosengart et al., 1991). Often, the second procedures conserve more pulmonary parenchyma than the primary procedures do, allowing resection in patients with borderline lung function. Patients who appear to be disease-free after 5 years may develop second primary lesions; close lifelong follow-up is required for all patients who have undergone resection for carcinoma of the lung.

Patterns of Failure After Surgical Resection

Locoregional Recurrence. The recurrence of lung cancer at the site of resection occurs in 10 to 20% of patients. The risk of locoregional recurrence after pulmonary resection is associated with the magnitude of the resection, according to a prospective, randomized trial conducted by the LCSG (Ginsberg and Rubenstein, 1991). In patients with Stage I lung cancer, the risk of recurrence after lobectomy is 5%, compared with 15% after segmentectomy or wedge resection.

The rate of recurrence by histologic subtypes has been also investigated by the LCSG (Thomas and Piantadosi, 1987). In a study of 572 patients who underwent complete resection of T1N0 NSCLC, postoperative recurrence was observed in 107 (18%). This study demonstrated a significantly higher recurrence rate for nonsquamous than for squamous carcinoma, confirming a previous report by the LCSG (Feld et al., 1984). However, in a study from Memorial Sloan-Kettering, the recurrence rate after resection for Stage II lung cancer was higher in patients with squamous carcinomas (Martini et al., 1992). It is unclear which histologic subtype carries a greater risk for locoregional recurrence after resection.

Metastases. Distant metastases are the first site of recurrence in 80% of patients who undergo resection for NSCLC, with or without locoregional failure (Mountain, 1983). Thus, improved locoregional therapy is unlikely to influence overall survival in patients with NSCLC who are not cured by surgical resection. In addition to lymph nodes, other sites of distant metastases include bone, adrenals, liver, kidneys, heart, lung, and brain. Patients with M1 NSCLC generally are not considered candidates for resection of the primary tumor or the metastasis; however, patients with adenocarcinoma of the lung, a solitary cerebral metastasis, and no other evidence of extrathoracic disease have successfully undergone surgical resection of both the primary lung cancer and brain metastasis, followed by cranial irradiation, with improved survival (Magilligan et al., 1986).

Surgical Morbidity and Mortality

Preoperative optimization of pulmonary status in patients with borderline cardiopulmonary function and meticulous postoperative care reduce morbidity and mortality in patients who undergo pulmonary resection for carcinoma of the lung. Atelectasis, the most common postoperative complication, usually is managed successfully with postural drainage, chest physiotherapy, and bronchodilators. Failure to clear secretions may progress to lobar collapse, requiring therapeutic bronchoscopy.

If air leaks are present after pulmonary resection, they usually resolve spontaneously. Persistence after 7 days may be due to bronchopleural fistula and may require surgical exploration. Infection (pneumonia, empyema, sepsis) after thoracotomy is rare but should be aggressively sought and managed. Other complications after thoracotomy and pulmonary resection include myocardial infarction, atrial arrhythmias, pulmonary embolism, prolonged pulmonary insufficiency, chylothorax, and chronic thoracic pain.

In a series of 2220 pulmonary resections, the LCSG reported an overall 30-day mortality rate of 3.7%. In this series, mortality varied with the extent of resection: 1.4% for wedge resection or segmentectomy, 2.9% for lobectomy, and 6.2% for pneumonectomy (Ginsberg et al., 1983).

ADJUNCTIVE THERAPY IN NON–SMALL–CELL LUNG CANCER

A few patients who present with lung cancer are considered potentially resectable. Systemic dissemination of cancer may be evident at presentation or after a resection for cure. The overall 5-year survival rate for lung cancer is 14% among whites and 11% among nonwhites (Boring et al., 1994). Although resection presents the best opportunity for cure, effective adjunctive therapy benefits many patients for whom complete resection is not possible. Current cooperative trials using adjuvant and neoadjuvant therapy for lung cancer have been summarized in the literature (Rusch and Feins, 1994). Critical evaluation of these trials by thoracic oncologists determines current care of patients with lung cancer and influences the design of future cooperative trials (Benfield, 1994).

Chemotherapy

Distant metastases at the time of initial diagnosis are present in approximately 60% of patients with NSCLC. Among patients with apparently resectable disease, 5% are found at operation to have regional spread; most of the remainder later prove to have systemic disease. Thus, the establishment of effective chemotherapy would dramatically improve survival in patients with NSCLC. In contrast to chemotherapy for SCLC, in which many agents provide response rates up to 80%, chemotherapy in NSCLC induces tumor regression for a minority of patients (Holmes and Ruckdeschel, 1991).

Postoperative Chemotherapy. The LCSG has conducted several prospective randomized trials evaluating adjuvant chemotherapy for NSCLC. The first trial assessed the use of chemotherapy after resection for Stage II or Stage III adenocarcinoma or large-cell undifferentiated carcinoma of the lung (Holmes and Gail, 1986). In this study, patients were randomized postoperatively to receive either a regimen of cyclophosphamide, doxorubicin (Adriamycin), and cisplatin (Platinol) (CAP) or a regimen of immunotherapy with intrapleural bacillus Calmette-Guérin (BCG) and oral levamisole. Disease-free survival was significantly prolonged in the group receiving CAP. After 7 years of follow-up, the difference in time to recurrence and number of cancer deaths remained statistically significant in favor of the group receiving chemotherapy (Holmes, 1993).

The LCSG also evaluated postoperative chemotherapy and radiotherapy in patients with extensive lymph node involvement or with microscopic residual disease after resection (Lad et al., 1988). Patients were randomized to receive CAP and radiotherapy or radiotherapy alone postoperatively. Patients who received chemotherapy and radiotherapy experienced significantly longer disease-free survival than those who received radiotherapy alone. Local recurrences appeared with equal frequency in each group; the difference in disease-free survival is attributed to the significant reduction in systemic recurrences in the group that received both chemotherapy and radiotherapy.

In the third trial, the LCSG evaluated postoperative chemotherapy in patients with high-risk Stage I (T2N0 and T1N1) NSCLC (Holmes, 1993). After resection and lymph node evaluation, patients were randomized to receive either CAP or no further treatment. In this study, there were no significant differences between the control and the treatment groups with regard to survival or disease-free survival.

These trials demonstrate that postoperative chemotherapy may significantly increase disease-free survival in patients with Stage III (and perhaps Stage II) NSCLC. The efficacy of postoperative chemotherapy and radiotherapy in patients with extensive lymph node involvement or positive surgical margins in reducing systemic recurrences and prolonging disease-free survival has also been demonstrated. Adjuvant therapy is not associated with improved overall survival and has not benefitted patients with Stage I NSCLC.

Preoperative Chemotherapy. The ability of preoperative therapy (consisting of chemotherapy alone or chemotherapy with radiation therapy) to improve survival in marginally resectable patients and to allow resection in categorically unresectable patients is being evaluated in numerous studies (Rusch and Feins, 1994). In one series, patients with Stage IIIA (N2) NSCLC were treated with a regimen of mitomycin, vinblastine, and cisplatin preoperatively (Martini et al., 1993). A major response was observed in 66% of patients, and a complete response was observed in 10%. The overall complete resection rate was 65%, with a complete resection rate of 78% in the subset of patients with a major response to chemotherapy. The overall 5-year survival rate was 17%; however, in patients who underwent complete resection, the 5-year survival rate was 26%.

Another study assessed the effect of neoadjuvant chemotherapy on resectability, stage of disease at resection, and patterns of recurrence and survival in patients with Stage IIIA (N2) NSCLC (Kirn et al., 1993). After preoperative chemotherapy with one of various cisplatin-containing regimens, patients underwent thoracotomy, and 75% underwent complete resection. Pathologic analysis demonstrated that 41% of patients were downstaged and that only 19% of patients progressed. In patients with resectable disease, the 2-year survival rate was 67%.

The Southwest Oncology Group reported a series of patients with Stage IIIA or Stage IIIB NSCLC who underwent preoperative chemotherapy (cisplatin and etoposide) and concurrent radiotherapy (Rusch et al., 1993). Complete resection was achieved in 73% of patients, and the 2-year survival rate was 40% for both Stage IIIA and Stage IIIB.

Shepherd (1993) reviewed 15 trials of induction chemotherapy (including 10 with simultaneous radiotherapy) in patients with Stage III NSCLC. Major response was observed in more than 50% of patients, but the complete response rate was less than 15%. Complete resection was achieved in 60% of patients. The overall 3-year survival rate was 25 to 30%. Although neoadjuvant therapy has improved the complete resection rate in patients with Stage III NSCLC, the benefit conferred may be due to patient selection. Furthermore, the morbidity and mortality rates of pneumonectomy after neoadjuvant therapy may be unacceptable (Fowler et al., 1993). Survival is currently significantly better in patients with Stage III NSCLC who receive preoperative chemotherapy and undergo complete resection, as compared with historical control subjects. The evaluation of induction chemotherapy has demonstrated its feasibility; randomized trials are required to prove safety and efficacy.

Palliative Chemotherapy. The management of unresectable NSCLC, often complicated by large tumor burden and poor patient performance status, is largely unsuccessful, owing to poor response rates to chemotherapy. Nevertheless, selected patients should be offered the option of treatment with combination chemotherapy. Candidates for chemotherapy include patients with good performance status, minimal weight loss, and minimal bulk disease (Johnson, 1990).

Radiotherapy

Definitive Radiotherapy. Patients with Stage I or II carcinoma of the lung should undergo thoracotomy for pulmonary resection whenever possible. Thoracic irradiation for cure is reserved for patients with Stage IIIB disease, selected patients with Stage IIIA disease, and patients with medical contraindications to thoracotomy. Special considerations with radiotherapy include tumor extent, volume of normal tissue, and cardiopulmonary reserve (Ihde and Minna, 1991).

Curative radiotherapy is limited to patients in whom the entire tumor volume may be treated with an adequate dosage and with acceptable toxicity. Contraindications to definitive radiotherapy include malignant pleural effusion, distant metastases, inadequate pulmonary reserve, and active pulmonary infection. Present recommendations for definitive irradiation specify conventional fractionation of 200 cGy/day, 5 days per week for 6 weeks, for a total of 6000 cGy. Alternatively, split-course irradiation, which involves a 3-week interruption in the treatment schedule, allows for better patient tolerance and integration of chemotherapy. Regression of the tumor, defined as 50% or greater reduction in tumor mass as assessed by the chest film, is accomplished in 50 to 60% of patients who receive radiotherapy for cure; complete regression is achieved in 20 to 25% of patients.

The survival data for definitive radiotherapy vary with the clinical stage of the disease. Patients with Stage I or II disease who undergo definitive irradiation experience 5-year survival rates of 15 to 20%. For Stage III disease, 5-year survival rates of 3 to 10% have been reported; median survival in most studies ranges from 9 to 12 months (Ihde and Minna, 1991).

Adjuvant Radiotherapy. Radiation therapy is an effective adjuvant treatment in many patients with carcinoma of the lung. Among those with squamous cell carcinoma, the first site of recurrence is frequently local. When applied to patients with completely resected Stage II or Stage III NSCLC, adjuvant radiotherapy has decreased local recurrence but has had no significant effect on survival. Postoperative irradiation may also promote survival in patients who undergo resection and are found to have metastases to hilar or mediastinal lymph nodes. Thus, the purpose of adjuvant radiotherapy is to prevent the recurrence of local tumors, especially when lymph node sampling of the mediastinum at thoracotomy is incomplete.

Palliative Radiotherapy. Radiotherapy in patients with unresectable disease has been reserved for those with symptoms. Few patients with advanced disease, however, are entirely asymptomatic. Symptoms of cough, chest pain, and dyspnea and the clinical signs and symptoms associated with the superior vena caval syndrome can be relieved in most patients (Cox, 1986). At some centers, patients with unresectable disease are offered high-dose radiotherapy, which has produced cure rates of 5 to 10% (Massey and Turrisi, 1991).

Alternative Therapy

Several new modalities are in various stages of evaluation in the management of NSCLC. Interstitial and endobronchial brachytherapy deliver high doses of radiation directly into the tumor, maximizing direct tumor irradiation and minimizing irradiation of surrounding normal tissue (Martinez and Schray, 1991). Photoradiation with the neodymium:yttrium-aluminum-garnet (Nd:YAG) laser may relieve airway obstruction by malignancy and may be used to deliver controlled hyperthermia (Unger, 1991). Photodynamic therapy, which involves the production of cytotoxic oxygen molecules, may ameliorate malignant tracheobronchial obstruction (Pass, 1991). Effective immunotherapy for carcinoma of the lung is currently being developed.

MANAGEMENT OF SMALL–CELL LUNG CANCER

SCLC progresses relentlessly and behaves as a systemic disease. Therapy directed toward the primary tumor is ineffective in prolonging survival, because most patients present with distant metastases or rapidly relapse with metastatic disease. Multimodal therapy, including effective chemotherapy, is therefore required for both locoregional control and systemic treatment of SCLC. The goals of therapy are to prolong survival and to alleviate symptoms while minimizing treatment-associated toxicity. Despite encouraging response rates to aggressive combination chemotherapy, the 2-year survival rate is only 10%.

Chemotherapy

Multiple chemotherapeutic agents effectively treat SCLC. Cyclophosphamide, an alkylating agent, is the most effective single agent and is commonly employed. Cyclophosphamide achieves a major response rate in 40% of patients, and approximately 5% of patients achieve complete remission. Carmustine (BCNU) and lomustine (CCNU), which are nitrosoureas, are also active, achieving response rates of 20 to 30%. Vincristine and vinblastine both have activity as single agents; vinca alkaloids are the class of drugs most frequently included in combination chemotherapy, owing to the minor toxicity profile. Etoposide, doxorubicin, and methotrexate are often used in combination regimens. High-growth fraction, rapid dissemination, and development of resistance to chemotherapy are problems that have not been overcome.

Major response rates can be achieved for 80% of patients with SCLC, regardless of stage. Complete response is produced in up to 50% of patients with limited disease and in 20% of patients with extensive disease. With limited disease, median survival is greater than 12 months, and survival beyond 5 years is attained in 10 to 20% of patients. For patients with extensive disease, median survival is 8 months, and survival beyond 5 years is attained in 3 to 5% (Goodman and Livingston, 1989).

Radiation Therapy

The role of adjuvant radiotherapy in SCLC is being examined in numerous clinical trials. The data indicate that in patients with limited disease, disease-free survival at 2 years improves 5 to 15% when radiation therapy is added to combination chemotherapy. Despite improvement in disease-free survival and complete response rate, there is no clear advantage in overall survival for patients receiving chemotherapy and radiation therapy, as opposed to chemotherapy alone (Goodman and Livingston, 1989).

Surgical Resection

Following conventional management of SCLC by combination chemotherapy and radiation therapy, approximately 20% of patients survive 5 years. With conventional therapy, the local recurrence rate is 30%. Complete resection in patients with limited disease may improve local control. In most surgical series, the rate of recurrence at the primary site is only 10%. Patients being surgically managed for SCLC should undergo complete resection, if possible, followed by postoperative chemotherapy and radiation therapy (Iglehart et al., 1985).

Overview of Small-Cell Lung Cancer

In managing a patient with SCLC, the primary goals are to prolong survival, improve disease-free survival, alleviate symptoms, minimize treatment-associated toxicity, and estimate prognosis. After SCLC has been diagnosed histologically, staging is performed, including thorough neurologic examination and CT of the chest, abdomen, and brain.

With limited-stage disease, treatment is initiated with six cycles of combination chemotherapy (such as cyclophosphamide/doxorubicin/vincristine or cisplatin/etoposide). Radiotherapy to the chest is usually employed after three initial cycles of chemotherapy and is continued for 4 weeks. In patients with limited-stage disease, thoracotomy for pulmonary resection is recommended in the subset of patients with Stage I SCLC; they receive six cycles of adjuvant chemotherapy and radiation therapy postoperatively. Complete responders with limited-stage disease are offered prophylactic cranial irradiation.

For patients with extensive-stage disease, six cycles of chemotherapy are administered. Therapy for local control is not employed; quality-of-life issues are paramount. Complete responders with extensive-stage disease receive prophylactic cranial irradiation (Shepherd et al., 1991).

SUMMARY

Every solitary pulmonary nodule should be resected unless the lesion is known to be benign or operation is medically contraindicated. Accurate preoperative and intraoperative staging is essential in the management of carcinoma of the lung. Surgical resection offers the best chance for cure in patients with Stage I or Stage II NSCLC, provided there are no medical contraindications to thoracotomy. Resection for cure may also be undertaken in selected patients with Stage III disease. Adjuvant therapy for patients with Stage III disease has improved disease-free survival without affecting overall survival. Neoadjuvant protocols are being evaluated in patients with N2 NSCLC. Patients who have undergone resection for cure may nevertheless develop locoregional recurrence, metachronous primary lung cancer, or distant metastases; lifelong surveillance is required for all patients after pulmonary resection for carcinoma of the lung.

SELECTED BIBLIOGRAPHY

Bitran, J. D. (ed): Non-small-cell lung cancer. Hematol. Oncol. Clin. North Am., 4:1023, 1990.

This volume emphasizes a multidisciplinary approach in the treatment of non-small-cell lung cancer. The pathology, staging, and surgical approach to lung cancer are well described. In addition, adjuvant, neoadjuvant, palliative, and supportive modalities are presented.

Cook, R. M., Miller, Y. E., and Bunn, P. A., Jr.: Small cell lung cancer: Etiology, biology, clinical features, staging, and treatment. Curr. Probl. Cancer, 17:74, 1993.

This monograph summarizes the etiology, molecular biology, staging, and treatment of small-cell lung cancer.

Ihde, D. C., and Minna, J. D.: Non-small-cell lung cancer. Curr. Probl. Cancer, 15:65, 1991.

This superb monograph presents the current understanding of the molecular biology of non-small-cell lung cancer.

Pass, H. I. (ed): Adjunctive and alternative treatment of bronchogenic lung cancer. Chest Surg. Clin. North Am., 1:1, 1991.

This review describes the use of adjunctive and alternative modalities in the treatment of bronchogenic lung cancer, including neoadjuvant chemotherapy, neoadjuvant radiation therapy, brachytherapy, photodynamic therapy, and endobronchial laser therapy.

Rusch, V. W., and Feins, R. H.: Summary of ongoing cooperative group clinical trials in thoracic malignancies. Ann. Thorac. Surg., 57:102, 1994.

This summary and analysis of the cooperative trials in thoracic oncology permits critical evaluation of the treatment regimens of lung cancer.

Shields, T. W.: Surgical therapy for carcinoma of the lung. Clin. Chest Med., 14:121, 1993.

Outstanding recent review of the surgical approach to carcinoma of the lung, including preoperative, operative, and postoperative considerations.

BIBLIOGRAPHY

Allison, P. R.: Intrapericardial approach to the lung root in the treatment of bronchial carcinoma by dissection pneumonectomy. J. Thorac. Surg., 15:99, 1946.

Auerbach, O., Gere, J. B., Forman, J. B., et al.: Changes in the bronchial epithelium in relation to smoking and cancer of the lung. N. Engl. J. Med., 256:97, 1957.

Bechard, D., and Wetstein, L.: Assessment of exercise oxygen consumption as preoperative criterion for lung resection. Ann. Thorac. Surg., 44:344, 1987.

Benfield, J. R.: Cooperative trials in thoracic oncology are important. Ann. Thorac. Surg., 57:10, 1994.

Bollen, E. C. M., van Duin, C. J., Theunessen, P. H. M. H., et al.: Mediastinal lymph node dissection in resected lung cancer: Morbidity and accuracy of staging. Ann. Thorac. Surg., 55:961, 1993.

Boring, C. C., Squires, T. S., Tong, T., and Montgomery, S.: Cancer Statistics, 1994. CA Cancer J. Clin., 44:7, 1994.

Brewer, L. A.: Historical notes on lung cancer before and after Graham's successful pneumonectomy in 1933. Am. J. Surg., 143:160, 1982.

Burt, M. E., Pomerantz, A. H., and Bains, M. S.: Results of surgical treatment of Stage III lung cancer invading the mediastinum. Surg. Clin. North Am., 67:987, 1987.

Churchill, E. D., and Belsey, R.: Segmental pneumonectomy in bronchiectasis. The lingula segment of the left upper lobe. Ann. Surg., 109:481, 1939.

Cook, R. M., Miller, Y. E., and Bunn, P. A., Jr.: Small cell lung cancer: Etiology, biology, clinical features, staging, and treatment. Curr. Probl. Cancer, 17:74, 1993.

Cox, J. D.: Non-small-cell lung cancer: The role of radiation therapy. Chest, 89(Suppl. 4):284S, 1986.

Cullen, J., McKenna, J., and Massey, M.: International control of smoking and the U.S. experience. Chest, 89(Suppl. 4):2206S, 1986.

Daly, B. D. T., Faling, L. J., Bite, G. B., et al.: Mediastinal lymph node evaluation by computed tomography in lung cancer. J. Thorac. Cardiovasc. Surg., 94:664, 1987.

Daly, B. D. T., Mueller, J. D., Faling, L. J., et al.: N2 lung cancer outcome in patients with false negative computed tomographic scans of the chest. J. Thorac. Cardiovasc. Surg., 105:904, 1993.

Deschamps, C., Pairolero, P. C., Trastek, V. F., et al.: Multiple primary lung cancer: Results of surgical treatment. J. Thorac. Cardiovasc. Surg., 99:769, 1990.

Dewan, N. A., Gupta, N. C., Redpenning, L. S., et al.: Diagnostic efficacy of PET-FDG imaging in solitary pulmonary nodules. Potential role in evaluation and management. Chest, 104:997, 1993.

Doll, R., and Peto, R.: Cigarette smoking and bronchial carcinoma: Dose and time relationships among regular smokers and lifelong non-smokers. J. Epidemiol. Community Health, 32:303, 1978.

Errett, J. E., Wilson, J., Chiu, R. C., et al.: Wedge resection as an alternate procedure for peripheral bronchogenic carcinoma in poor risk patients. J. Thorac. Cardiovasc. Surg., 90:656, 1985.

Feld, R., Rubenstein, L., and Weisenberger, T. H.: Sites of recurrence in resected Stage I non-small-cell lung cancer: A guide for future studies. J. Clin. Oncol., 2:1352, 1984.

Ferguson, M.: Diagnosis and staging of non-small-cell lung cancer. Hematol. Oncol. Clin. North Am., 4:1053, 1990.

Fleisher, A. G., McElvaney, G., and Robinson, C. L. H.: Multiple primary bronchogenic carcinoma: Treatment and follow-up. Ann. Thorac. Surg., 51:48, 1991.

Fowler, W. C., Langer, C. J., Curran, W. J., and Keller, S. M.: Postoperative complications after combined neoadjuvant treatment of lung cancer. Ann. Thorac. Surg., 55:986, 1993.

Fried, B. M.: Tumors of the Lung and Mediastinum. Philadelphia, Lea & Febiger, 1958.

Ginsberg, R. J.: Thoracoscopy: A cautionary note. Ann. Thorac. Surg., 56:801, 1993.

Ginsberg, R. J., Hill, L. D., Eagan, R. T., et al.: Modern thirty-day operative mortality for surgical resection in lung cancer. J. Thorac. Cardiovasc. Surg., 86:654, 1983.

Ginsberg, R. J., and Rubenstein, L. V.: Patients with T1N0 non-small-cell lung cancer [abstract 304]. Lung Cancer, 7(Suppl.):83, 1991.

Goodman, G. E., and Livingston, R. B.: Small cell lung cancer. Curr. Probl. Cancer, 13:7, 1989.

Graham, E. A., and Singer, J. J.: Successful removal of an entire lung for carcinoma of the bronchus. J. A. M. A., 101:1371, 1933.

Grover, F. L., Piantadosi, S., and The Lung Cancer Study Group.: Recurrence and survival following resection of bronchoalveolar carcinoma of the lung—The Lung Cancer Study Group experience. J. Thorac. Cardiovasc. Surg., 209:779, 1989.

Harpole, D. H., Feldman, J. M., Buchanan, S., et al.: Bronchial carcinoid tumors: A retrospective analysis of 126 patients. Ann. Thorac. Surg., 54:50, 1992.

Hazelrigg, S. R., Nunchuck, S. K., and LoCicero, J.: Video Assisted Thoracic Surgery Study Group data. Ann. Thorac. Surg., 56:1039, 1993.

Holmes, E. C.: Postoperative chemotherapy for non-small-cell lung cancer. Chest, 103:30S, 1993.

Holmes, E. C., and Gail, M.: Surgical adjuvant chemotherapy for Stage II and Stage III adenocarcinoma and large-cell undifferentiated carcinoma. J. Clin. Oncol., 4:710, 1986.

Holmes, E. C., and Ruckdeschel, J. C.: Postoperative chemotherapy for non-small-cell lung cancer. Chest Surg. Clin. North Am., 1:89, 1991.

Iglehart, J. D., Wolfe, W. G., Vernon, W. B., et al.: Electron microscopy in selection of patients with small-cell carcinoma of the lung for medical versus surgical treatment. J. Thorac. Cardiovasc. Surg., 90:355, 1985.

Ihde, D. C., and Minna, J. D.: Non-small-cell lung cancer. Curr. Probl. Cancer, 15:65, 1991.

Johnson, D.: Chemotherapy for unresectable non-small-cell lung cancer. Semin. Oncol., 17(Suppl. 7):20, 1990.

Kabat, G. C., and Wynder, E. L.: Lung cancer in nonsmokers. Cancer, 53:1214, 1984.

Kent, E. M., and Blades, B.: The anatomical approach to pulmonary resection. Ann. Surg., 116:782, 1942.

Kirby, T. J., and Rice, T. W.: Thoracoscopic lobectomy. Ann. Thorac. Surg., 56:784, 1993.

Kirn, D. H., Lynch, T. J., Mentzer, S. J., et al.: Multimodality therapy of patients with Stage IIIA, N2 non-small-cell lung cancer: Impact of preoperative chemotherapy on resectability and downstaging. J. Thorac. Cardiovasc. Surg., 106:696, 1993.

Klingman, R. R., and DeMeester, T. R.: Surgical approach to non-small-cell lung cancer Stage I and II. Hematol. Oncol. Clin. North Am., 4:1079, 1990.

Kreyburg, L.: Histologic typing of lung tumors. In Kreyburg, L. (ed): International Histologic Classification of Tumors. Geneva, World Health Organization, 1967.

Lad, T., Rubenstein, L., Sedeghi, A., et al.: The benefit of adjuvant treatment for resected locally advanced non-small-cell lung cancer. J. Clin. Oncol., 6:125, 1988.

Lillington, G. A., and Caskey, C.: Evaluation and management of solitary and multiple pulmonary nodules. Clin. Chest Med., 14:111, 1993.

Linnoila, I.: Pathology of non-small-cell lung cancer: New diagnostic approaches. Hematol. Oncol. Clin. North Am., 4:1027, 1990.

Lyubsky, S., and Jacobson, M. J.: Lung cancer: Making the diagnosis. Chest, 100:511, 1991.

Magilligan, D. J., Jr., Duvernoy, C., and Malik, G.: Surgical approach to lung cancer with solid cerebral metastasis: Twenty-five years' experience. Ann. Thorac. Surg., 42:360, 1986.

Martinez, A. A., and Schray, M.: Interstitial and endobronchial brachytherapy in lung cancer. Chest Surg. Clin. North Am., 1:109, 1991.

Martini, N.: Surgical treatment of non-small-cell cancer by stage. Semin. Surg. Oncol., 6:248, 1990.

Martini, N., Burt, M. E., Bains, M. S., et al.: Survival after resection of Stage II non-small-cell lung cancer. Ann. Thorac. Surg., 54:460, 1992.

Martini, N., and Flehinger, B. J.: The role of surgery in N2 lung cancer. Surg. Clin. North Am., 67:1037, 1987.

Martini, N., and Ginsberg, R. J.: Surgical approaches to non-small-cell cancer Stage IIIA. Hematol. Oncol. Clin. North Am., 4:1121, 1990.

Martini, N., Kris, M. G., Flehinger, B. J., et al.: Preoperative chemotherapy for Stage IIIA (N2) lung cancer: The Sloan-Kettering experience with 136 patients. Ann. Thorac. Surg., 55:1365, 1993.

Martini, N., Zaman, M. B., Bains, M. S., et al.: Treatment and prognosis in bronchial carcinoids involving regional lymph nodes. J. Thorac. Cardiovasc. Surg., 107:1, 1994.

Massey, V., and Turrisi, A.: Role of primary radiation therapy in the management of non-small-cell lung cancer. Chest Surg. Clin. North Am., 1:99, 1991.

Mathisen, D. J., and Grillo, H. C.: Carinal resection for bronchogenic cancer. J. Thorac. Cardiovasc. Surg., 102:16, 1991.

Meade, R. H.: A History of Thoracic Surgery. Springfield, IL, Charles C Thomas, 1961.

Miller, J. D., Gorenstein, L. A., and Patterson, G. A.: Staging: The key to rational management of lung cancer. Ann. Thorac. Surg., 53:170, 1992.

Mountain, C. F.: A new international staging system for lung cancer. Chest, 89:225S, 1986.

Mountain, C. F.: Therapy of Stage I and Stage II non-small-cell lung cancer. Semin. Oncol., 10:71, 1983.

Naruke, T., Asamura, H., Kondo, H., et al.: Thoracoscopy for the staging of lung cancer. Ann. Thorac. Surg., 56:661, 1993.

Naruke, T., Gcya, T., Tsuchiya, R., et al.: Prognosis and survival in resected lung carcinoma based on the new international staging system for lung cancer. J. Thorac. Cardiovasc. Surg., 96:440, 1988.

Pass, H. I.: Photodynamic therapy for lung cancer. Chest Surg. Clin. North Am., 1:135, 1991.

Patterson, G. A., Ginsberg, R. J., Poon, P. Y., et al.: A prospective evaluation of magnetic resonance imaging, computed tomography, and mediastinoscopy in the preoperative assessment of mediastinal node status in bronchogenic carcinoma. J. Thorac. Cardiovasc. Surg., 94:679, 1987.

Phillips, D., Hewer, A., Martin, C., et al.: Correlation of DNA adduct levels in human lung cigarette smoking. Nature, 336:790, 1988.

Rienhoff, W. F., Jr., Gannon, J., Jr., and Sherman, I.: Closure of the bronchus following pneumonectomy. Ann. Surg., 116:481, 1942.

Richardson, G. E., and Johnson, B. E.: Paraneoplastic syndromes in lung cancer. Curr. Opin. Oncol., 4:323, 1992.

Rosengart, T. K., Martini, N., Ghosu, P., et al.: Multiple primary lung carcinomas: Prognosis and treatment. Ann. Thorac. Surg., 52:773, 1991.

Rusch, V. W., Albain, K. S., Crowley, J. J., et al.: Surgical resection of Stage IIIA and Stage IIIB non-small-cell lung cancer after concurrent induction chemoradiotherapy. J. Thorac. Cardiovasc. Surg., 105:97, 1993.

Rusch, V. W., and Feins, R. H.: Summary of ongoing cooperative group clinical trials in thoracic malignancies. Ann. Thorac. Surg., 57:102, 1994.

Sabiston, D. C., Jr.: Carcinoma of the lung. In Sabiston, D. C., Jr.,

and Spencer, F. C. (eds): Surgery of the Chest. 5th ed. Philadelphia, W. B. Saunders, 1990.

Shennib, H.: Intraoperative localization techniques for pulmonary nodules. Ann. Thorac. Surg., 56:745, 1993.

Shepherd, F. A.: Induction chemotherapy for locally advanced non-small-cell lung cancer. Ann. Thorac. Surg., 55:1585, 1993.

Shepherd, F. A., Ginsberg, R. J., Feld, R., et al.: Surgical treatment for limited small-cell lung cancer. J. Thorac. Cardiovasc. Surg., 101:385, 1991.

Shields, T. W.: Surgical therapy for carcinoma of the lung. Clin. Chest. Med., 14:121, 1993.

Strauss, B. L., Matthews, M. J., Cohen, M. H., et al.: Cardiac metastases in lung cancer. Chest, 71:607, 1977.

Thomas, P. A., and Piantadosi, S.: Postoperative T1N0 non-small-cell lung cancer. J. Thorac. Cardiovasc. Surg., 94:349, 1987.

Unger, M.: Endobronchial Nd:YAG laser treatment. Chest Surg. Clin. North Am., 1:123, 1991.

Van Klaveren, R. J., Festen, J., Otten, H. J. A. M., et al.: Prognosis of unsuspected and completely resectable N2 non-small-cell lung cancer. Ann. Thorac. Surg., 56:300, 1993.

Van Raemdonck, D. E., Schneider, A., and Ginsberg, R. J.: Surgical treatment for higher stage non-small-cell lung cancer. Ann. Thorac. Surg., 54:999, 1992.

Wain, J. C.: Video-assisted thoracoscopy and the staging of lung cancer. Ann. Thorac. Surg., 56:776, 1993.

Wald, N., Nanchahal, K., Thompson, S., et al.: Does breathing other people's tobacco smoke cause lung cancer? Br. Med. J., 293:1217, 1986.

Watanabe, Y., Shimizu, J., Oda, M., et al.: Aggressive surgical intervention in N2 non-small-cell cancer of the lung. Ann. Thorac. Surg., 51:253, 1991.

World Health Organization: The WHO histologic typing of lung tumors, 2nd edition. Am. J. Clin. Pathol., 77:123, 1982.

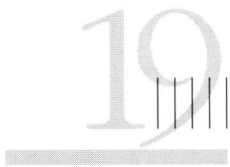

■ II Bronchoplastic Techniques in the Surgical Management of Benign and Malignant Pulmonary Lesions

James E. Lowe, Mark Tedder, and David C. Sabiston, Jr.

Wedge resection, segmentectomy, lobectomy, or pneumonectomy is the appropriate surgical treatment for most pulmonary lesions requiring operation. However, a small but definite number of patients with carcinoma and perhaps most patients with benign endobronchial tumors or neoplasms of low-grade malignant potential in the proximal airways should be considered candidates for conservative resectional procedures. The term *conservative* indicates that normal lung is preserved by these operations. Various names relating to the amount of lung actually removed have been used to describe these procedures, but most commonly they are cited as bronchoplastic procedures (originally suggested by Paulson and Shaw in 1955) or "sleeve" resections. In these operations, a portion of the bronchus is removed, with or without lobectomy, as a sleeve resection, and a primary bronchial reanastomosis is performed to preserve functional pulmonary parenchyma.

Over the past decade, the number of patients reported to have undergone bronchoplastic procedures has increased by almost 4 times. As this chapter describes, bronchoplastic techniques are the ideal surgical therapy for benign endobronchial tumors, for tumors of low-grade malignant potential such as bronchial adenomas, and for repair of traumatic airway injuries and benign strictures. This approach also applies to a select group of patients with carcinoma of the lung whose long-term survival is similar to that achieved through formal pulmonary resections.

HISTORICAL ASPECTS

One of the first bronchoplastic procedures was done in 1932 by Bigger (1935), who performed a bronchotomy to remove a tumor of the left mainstem bronchus in a 14-year-old boy. The patient underwent left-sided pneumonectomy 1 week later because the microscopic pathology was interpreted as showing malignancy. However, following pneumonectomy, the patient developed purulent pericarditis and eventually succumbed. In 1939, Eloesser successfully performed a bronchotomy to remove an adenoma originating at the orifice of the left lower lobe. Eloesser did not actually resect a portion of bronchus, but simply excised the adenoma and fulgurated its base. Taffel, in 1940, and later Daniel, in 1947, showed experimentally in dogs that segments of the mainstem bronchus could be removed and replaced successfully with various types of tissue or synthetic grafts. In 1949, Gebauer was the first person to apply these techniques successfully in patients by using autologous dermal tissue grafts to repair long segments of tuberculous bronchostenosis.

Techniques used today in bronchoplastic surgery were first applied in 1947 by Price-Thomas, who performed the first sleeve resection in a Royal Air Force cadet with a bronchial adenoma that originated in the right mainstem bronchus. A pneumonectomy, the only other surgical alternative at that time, would have prevented the patient from becoming a pilot. Therefore, a sleeve of right mainstem bronchus was removed with a successful primary repair. The patient subsequently recovered and served as a pilot. In 1949, D'Abreu performed a similar operation for an adenoma, and in 1951, Gebauer performed a successful sleeve resection for tuberculous bronchostenosis. Kato and associates, in 1993, reported that 36 patients with tuberculous bronchial stenosis were treated with a variety of different bronchoplastic procedures with excellent long-term results.

Allison performed the first sleeve resection for carcinoma in 1952, and although he never reported the case, he is given credit for it by Price-Thomas, who cited this case as the first successful sleeve lobectomy for carcinoma in a patient who could not have tolerated a pneumonectomy because of limited pulmonary function.

Paulson introduced these techniques in the United States and applied the term *bronchoplastic* to describe these operations. In 1955, he reported with Shaw that 16 patients with traumatic, benign, and malignant conditions were treated successfully with various bronchoplastic procedures, including repair of traumatic airway lacerations, dermal grafting for strictures of the bronchus, simple sleeve resection for bronchial adenomas, and sleeve lobectomies for carcinoma.

In 1959, Johnston and Jones reported the first long-term results of 98 sleeve lobectomies done for carcinoma. In appropriately selected patients, the long-term results equaled those achieved in patients who were treated with conventional lobectomy or pneumonectomy. Since 1959, several authors have reported large series of bronchoplastic procedures, and these reports have confirmed that favorable results can be achieved in appropriately selected patients with carci-

noma as well as in patients with tumors of low-grade malignant potential, such as bronchial adenomas.

INDICATIONS FOR BRONCHOPLASTIC PROCEDURES

Bronchoplastic surgical techniques are the ideal excisional therapy for tumors of low-grade malignant potential and benign endobronchial tumors in the proximal major airways. These procedures apply also to the treatment of areas of bronchostenosis and the repair of traumatic bronchial lacerations. A small but significant number of patients with carcinoma of the lung also are candidates for conservative resectional procedures, a group accounting for some 5 to 8% of all patients with pulmonary carcinoma (Bennett and Smith, 1978; Naruke and Suemasu, 1983; Paulson and Shaw, 1960; Ungar et al., 1981). Lobectomy combined with sleeve resection (sleeve lobectomy) is the most common procedure in this subgroup of patients with carcinoma. In most cases, the procedure serves as a surgical option for patients with central lesions who cannot tolerate pneumonectomy because of inadequate pulmonary reserve. However, Faber and associates (1984) contend that sleeve lobectomy, when technically feasible, is the preferred procedure for bronchogenic carcinoma. In recent years, it has become evident that in appropriately selected patients with carcinoma, the survival rate of sleeve lobectomy is equal to that of standard pneumonectomy (Ayabe et al., 1982; Belli et al., 1985; Bennett and Smith, 1978; Deslauriers et al., 1986; Faber et al., 1984; Firmin et al., 1983; Frist et al., 1987; Huidekoper and Van Ginnekin, 1985; Ishihara et al., 1977; Jensik, 1966; Jensik et al., 1972; Jones, 1959; Keszler, 1986; Mentzer et al., 1993; Naruke et al., 1977, 1983, 1989; Paulson et al., 1970; Paulson and Shaw, 1960; Price-Thomas, 1960; Rees and Paneth, 1970; Robinson et al., 1981; Roder et al., 1987; Sartori et al., 1986; Tedder et al., 1992; Ungar et al., 1981; Van Den Bosch et al., 1981; Van Schil et al., 1991; Vogt-Moykopf et al., 1986; Watanabe et al., 1986, 1990; Weisel et al., 1979). It should be emphasized, however, that at most, only 5 to 8% of all patients with resectable tumors are candidates for bronchoplastic procedures.

PREOPERATIVE EVALUATION

The preoperative evaluation of candidates for a bronchoplastic procedure should include pulmonary function testing, sputum culture, cytologic studies, and careful bronchoscopy to define precisely the limits of the planned bronchial resection. Paulson and associates (1970) and Weisel and colleagues (1979) have routinely used mediastinoscopy in the preoperative evaluation of patients with carcinoma to assess the status of mediastinal lymph nodes. Specific additional studies are obtained, depending on the exact nature of the pathologic process. One of the present undecided issues is the role of preoperative radiation

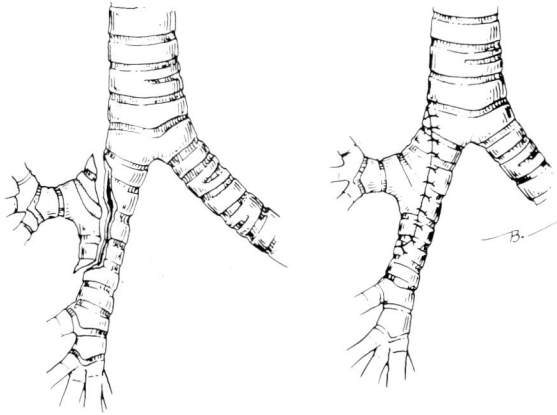

FIGURE 19–4. Bronchoplastic repair of a laceration of the right mainstem bronchus. (From Lowe, J. E., Bridgman, A. H., and Sabiston, D. C., Jr.: The role of bronchoplastic procedures in the surgical management of benign and malignant pulmonary lesions. J. Thorac. Cardiovasc. Surg., 83:227, 1982.)

in patients with carcinoma who are considered candidates for sleeve lobectomy. Routine preoperative radiation therapy has been advocated by Jensik (1966) and Paulson and associates (1960, 1970) with improved results in 5-year survival. Faber and associates (1984) found that preoperative irradiation had no beneficial effect on 5- and 10-year survival. In most patients, however, the presence of significant hilar lymph node involvement or known mediastinal nodal metastases is an absolute contraindication to sleeve lobectomy (Paulson et al., 1970).

Preoperative preparation for bronchoplastic procedures should include measures to improve bronchial hygiene through the use of bronchodilators, nebulized mists, and appropriate antibiotic therapy for tracheobronchitis. The anesthesiologist should be consulted preoperatively about the need for special intraoperative ventilation in these procedures.

SURGICAL MANAGEMENT

Bronchoplastic procedures involve several important technical considerations. A standard posterolateral thoracotomy is generally the preferred incision, although Paulson and associates (1970) and Bennett and Smith (1978) have emphasized the excellent exposure of the hilum achieved by a posterior approach. Because the major airway of the operated side is opened, selective ventilation of the contralateral lung is achieved by use of the Carlens', Robertshaw's, White's, or Magill's endotracheal tube. The choice of the appropriate endotracheal tube depends not only on personal preference but also on the location of the lesion in reference to the carina and on the position of the endotracheal tube in the tracheobronchial tree. Faber and associates (1984) recommend one-lung high-frequency ventilation for bronchoplastic procedures to eliminate the need for double-lumen endotracheal tubes. High-frequency positive-pressure ventilation at a frequency of 1 Hz with a tidal volume of

50 to 250 ml has provided excellent oxygenation during one-lung anesthesia.

The feasibility of a bronchoplastic procedure must be assessed first, and it depends on the size and the extent of the lesion. If the operation is for carcinoma, the status of the lymph nodes beyond the margins of resection should first be determined. Generally, the finding of extensive nodal or bronchial wall involvement or extension of tumor across fissure lines should be considered a contraindication (Paulson et al., 1970; Weisel et al., 1979).

The hilum is dissected as in exposure for pneumonectomy. A tape passed around the pulmonary artery can be used for gentle retraction to expose the proximal mainstem bronchus and carina. For left-sided procedures, it is often advantageous to divide the ligamentum arteriosum in order to gain clear access to the carina and proximal left mainstem bronchus (Boyd et al., 1970). Whether simple bronchotomy, sleeve resection, or sleeve lobectomy is done depends on the location of the lesion and whether it is benign or malignant (Figs. 19–4 through 19–9). The proximal bronchotomy is performed first, followed by the distal bronchotomy. Frozen-section examination of the divided edges may be necessary during the procedure to ensure adequate margins in patients undergoing operations for carcinoma or bronchial adenoma. Adequate distal and proximal margins must be obtained in the case of carcinoma (minimum of 1.5 to 2 cm) (Paulson et al., 1970).

For sleeve resections of the right mainstem bronchus, the proximal division is made just distal to the carina (Fig. 19–6). On the left, the proximal division is made farther from the carina because the left mainstem bronchus is longer and the aortic arch is adjacent to the carina (Fig. 19–7). The distal incision on either side is made flush with the distal bronchi to be preserved. Occasionally, a sleeve of pulmonary artery must also be resected (Belli et al., 1985; Jensik et al., 1972; Maggi et al., 1993; Naruke, 1989; Rendina et al., 1993; Tedder et al., 1992; Vogt-Moykopf et al., 1986).

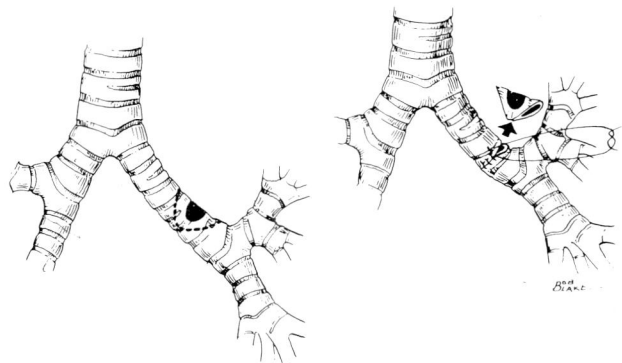

FIGURE 19–5. Partial sleeve resection for excision of a benign tumor of the left mainstem bronchus. This procedure was successfully used to excise an endobronchial hamartoma, as shown in Figure 19–9. (From Lowe, J. E., Bridgman, A. H., and Sabiston, D. C., Jr.: The role of bronchoplastic procedures in the surgical management of benign and malignant pulmonary lesions. J. Thorac. Cardiovasc. Surg., 83:227, 1982.)

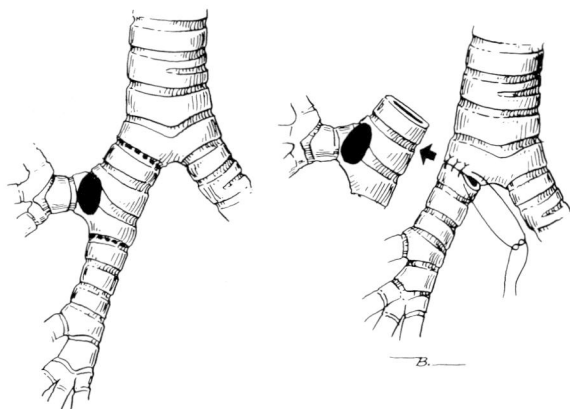

FIGURE 19–6. Right upper sleeve lobectomy. Most commonly, this procedure is done for carcinoma of the upper lobe involving the right mainstem bronchus, although it can also be applied to resect a bronchial adenoma originating in the orifice of the upper lobe and extending into the mainstem bronchus. For sleeve resection of the right mainstem bronchus, the proximal division is made just distal to the carina. After sleeve lobectomy, the bronchus intermedius is reanastomosed to the right mainstem bronchus, as shown. (From Lowe, J. E., Bridgman, A. H., and Sabiston, D. C., Jr.: The role of bronchoplastic procedures in the surgical management of benign and malignant pulmonary lesions. J. Thorac. Cardiovasc. Surg., 83:227, 1982.)

Although bronchoplastic procedures have been applied to upper and lower lobe lesions on both the right and the left, sleeve lobectomy for carcinoma has most often been done in patients with localized squamous cell carcinoma originating in the right upper lobe orifice (Fig. 19–6). A wide sleeve resection of the main bronchus combined with lobectomy and regional lymph node dissection and anastomosis of the intermediate bronchus to the carina achieves the

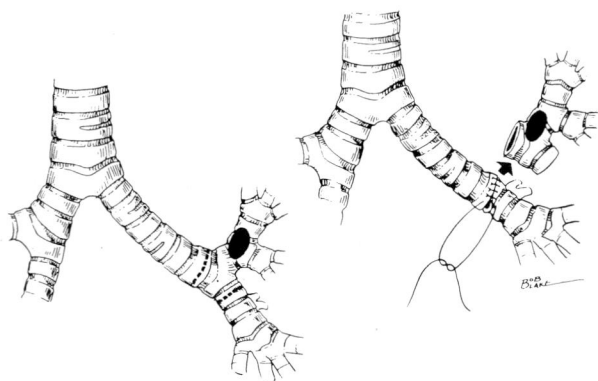

FIGURE 19–7. Left upper sleeve lobectomy. For left-sided procedures, it is often advantageous to divide the ligamentum arteriosum to better expose the proximal mainstem bronchus. Because the left mainstem bronchus is longer than the right mainstem bronchus and because the aortic arch is adjacent to the carina, the proximal division is made farther from the carina for left upper sleeve lobectomy. The distal incision on either side is made flush with the distal bronchi to be preserved. (From Lowe, J. E., Bridgman, A. H., and Sabiston, D. C., Jr.: The role of bronchoplastic procedures in the surgical management of benign and malignant pulmonary lesions. J. Thorac. Cardiovasc. Surg., 83:227, 1982.)

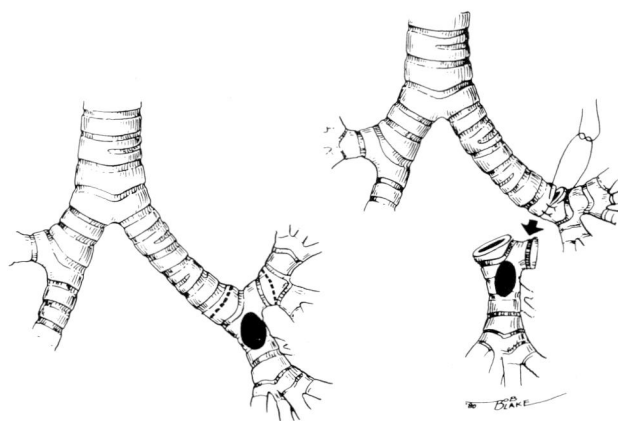

FIGURE 19–8. Left lower sleeve lobectomy for tumors originating in the lower lobe but involving the upper lobe orifice allows preservation of upper lobe function. (From Lowe, J. E., Bridgman, A. H., and Sabiston, D. C., Jr.: The role of bronchoplastic procedures in the surgical management of benign and malignant pulmonary lesions. J. Thorac. Cardiovasc. Surg., 83:227, 1982.)

same surgical margins as a pneumonectomy does but with preservation of the middle and lower lobes.

Bronchial continuity is reestablished by using a single row of through-and-through interrupted sutures applied a few millimeters apart. The incidence of granuloma formation appears to be greater if silk sutures are used; currently, most surgeons use 3-0 or 4-0 soft absorbable sutures such as polyglactin 910 (Vicryl) (Frist et al., 1987). The bronchial blood supply is interrupted only at the line of division, and the cartilaginous portions of the bronchial ends are rejoined first, followed by suturing of the membranous portion. Any difference in luminal size of the rejoined bronchial ends is equalized by uneven spacing of sutures in the membranous portion of the reanastomosis. The risk of one of the most devastating complications, erosion of the bronchial suture line into the pulmonary artery, can be minimized by placing a pleural or pericardial flap around the repair. Pleural drainage is accomplished routinely.

POSTOPERATIVE CARE

Sleeve lobectomy for carcinoma is often selected because of poor pulmonary reserve. For such patients, great care must be taken to maintain maximal pulmonary function postoperatively. Coughing and deep breathing exercises are sufficient in most patients, although some patients may require frequent endotracheal suctioning. Routine postoperative bronchoscopy is not recommended by most authors, but it should be used at an early stage in patients who have difficulty in clearing secretions by conventional methods. Occasionally, tracheostomy may be necessary. Antibiotics are begun preoperatively and continued for a short time postoperatively. The routine postoperative use of steroids is not widely accepted but is advocated by Rendina and associates (1993).

PRESERVATION OF PULMONARY FUNCTION

It has generally been assumed that the loss of pulmonary function after sleeve resection is no greater than such loss after simple lobectomy. Very few studies, however, regard the function of the remaining ipsilateral lung after sleeve resections. Rees and Paneth (1970) compared preoperative and postoperative ratios of forced expiratory volume (1 second) and functional vital capacity in a group of six patients who were treated by sleeve lobectomy. There were no consistent alterations in this ratio, which suggested that sleeve lobectomy did not cause any more physiologic impairment than did simple lobectomy. However, Andrews and Pearson (1973) showed a transient decline in gas exchange after radical hilar stripping with division of the main bronchus in dogs. The exact cause of this observed decline is not known, but it was thought to be the result of division of pulmonary nerves, lymphatics, or bronchial arteries. An elegant study by Wood and associates (1974) compared the effects of right upper lobectomy with right upper sleeve lobectomy in two groups of dogs. There was no change in minute ventilation or functional residual capacity in either group, but there were impressive differences in oxygen uptake and perfusion of the remaining right lung. Significantly less oxygen uptake was measured in animals who were treated by sleeve lobectomy as opposed to simple lobectomy. The fall in oxygen uptake after sleeve lobectomy was maximal at 3 days and required 4 weeks of postoperative recovery to approach values recorded in dogs treated by simple lobectomy. The authors emphasize that the changes in ventilation after sleeve resection do not parallel the defect in oxygen uptake; specifically, the right lung continues to contribute an average of 50% of the ventilation throughout all study intervals after both sleeve resection and simple lobectomy. It was further observed, using ^{133}Xe perfusion, that there was a disproportionate reduction in perfusion of the remaining right lung after sleeve lobectomy compared with simple lobectomy. These data suggest that the transient defect in oxygen uptake after sleeve resection was due to a transient abnormality in perfusion in the remaining ipsilateral lung. The large defect in oxygen uptake corresponded with an increase in physiologic dead space in animals treated by sleeve lobectomy. The exact cause of the transient decline in oxygen uptake and decreased perfusion of the remaining lung in animals treated by sleeve lobectomy is still uncertain, but most likely it is related to surgical division of peribronchial arteries, lymphatics, or nerves.

These studies are pertinent to patients because they show that there is a transient defect in oxygen uptake and perfusion after sleeve resection. Because sleeve lobectomy often is done in patients with marginal pulmonary function, these data suggest that although the goal is to preserve ventilatory function, there may be a transient decline in ventilatory function in the immediate postoperative period when risk of respiratory failure is greatest. These studies further emphasize the absolute necessity of maximizing bronchial hygiene after sleeve lobectomy in the immediate postoperative period. Furthermore, although these data convincingly show a transient decline in oxygen uptake, they suggest that residual long-term pulmonary function following sleeve lobectomy may well be equal to that following simple lobectomy. Deslauriers and associates (1986) reported that sleeve lobectomy in 12 patients with extensive preoperative and postoperative function studies caused no postoperative changes in either ventilation or perfusion of the re-anastomosed lobes.

RESULTS AND COMPLICATIONS

Since 1978, more than 2000 bronchoplastic procedures have been reported in the literature. Approximately 89% of these were performed for malignancy; the remainder were performed for benign lesions and tumors of low-grade malignant potential.

Sleeve Resection for Benign Lesions and Tumors of Low-Grade Malignant Potential

Given the well-documented safety of correctly performed bronchoplastic procedures, sleeve resection for tumors of low-grade malignant potential, such as bronchial adenomas, has been used too rarely. Boyd and associates (1970) noted that sleeve resections rarely are used by many thoracic surgeons because they are unfamiliar with the techniques of exposure of the carina or they fail to realize the safety of the procedures. Because normal lung is conserved by sleeve resection, it appears to be the ideal excisional therapy for benign neoplasms as well as for endobronchial adenomas of low-grade malignant potential. This approach is supported by the initial experience of Price-Thomas (1955) and has been confirmed by numerous authors (Attar et al., 1985; Boyd et al., 1970; Breyer et al., 1980; Hurt, 1984; Jensik et al., 1974; Lima, 1980; Lowe et al., 1982; McCaughan et al., 1985; Okike et al., 1978; Paulson and Shaw, 1955; Ratto et al., 1983; Tedder et al., 1992; Todd et al., 1980; Wilkins et al., 1984).

The results of a literature review for carcinoid tumors treated by sleeve resection are summarized in Table 19–6. For typical carcinoid tumors, the 5- to 20-year survival rate is 96%. These impressive clinical results suggest that sleeve resection is the operation of choice when technically feasible in the patient with a bronchial adenoma.

For benign tumors in the proximal mainstem bronchus, such as endobronchial hamartomas (Fig. 19–9), partial or complete sleeve resection is indicated. For adenomas arising in a lobar orifice, sleeve lobectomy may be required.

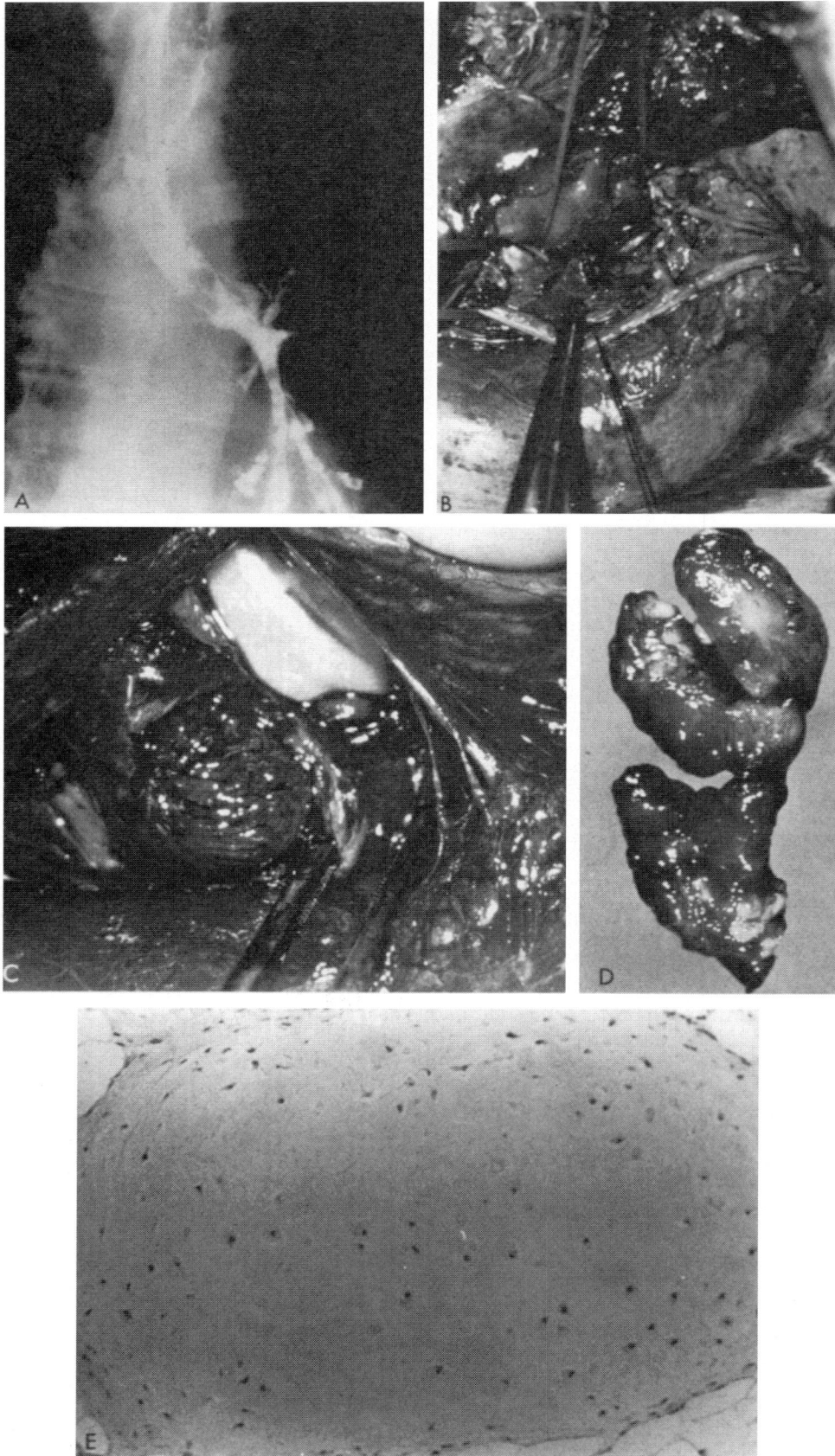

FIGURE 19–9. *See legend on opposite page*

■ **Table 19–6.** RESULTS OF BRONCHOPLASTIC PROCEDURES IN PATIENTS WITH BRONCHIAL CARCINOID TUMORS

Authors	Year Reported	Total No. of Patients	No. Survived 5–20 Years
Price-Thomas	1947*	1	1
D'Abreu	1951	1	1
Linton	1955	1	1
Shaw and Paulson	1959	5	5
Bower	1965	1	1
Peleg et al.	1965	1	1
Batson et al.	1966	1	1
McEvoy	1967	1	1
Donahue et al.	1968	1	1
Boyd et al.	1970	1	1
Jensik et al.	1974	23	20
Okike et al.	1978	16	16
Todd et al.	1980	10	10
Lima	1980	10	10
Hurt	1981	9	8
Lowe et al.	1982	6	6
Ratto et al.	1983	2	2
Wilkins et al.	1984	7	7
McCaughan et al.	1985	5	5
Attar et al.	1985	2	2
Total		**112**	**108 (96%)**

*Year performed; reported in 1955.

Sleeve Resection for Carcinoma

As previously stated, most resections are performed for carcinoma of the lung. Postoperative complications and early mortality are summarized in Tables 19–7 and 19–8. In a review by Tedder and associates (1992), the 30-day mortality rate for 1915 bronchoplastic procedures performed for malignancy was 7.5%. The incidence was 5.5% for sleeve lobectomy and 20.9% for sleeve pneumonectomy (Table 19–9).

The most common cause of early death was respiratory failure (20.9%) (Table 19–8). Cardiac events, consisting of myocardial infarction, congestive heart failure, and malignant ventricular dysrhythmias, constituted 19.8% of the early deaths. In decreasing order of frequency, pneumonia, pulmonary embolism, bronchopleural fistulas, and bronchovascular fistulas were less common causes of early mortality.

The marked disparity between the early mortality rates for sleeve lobectomy (5.5%) and sleeve pneumonectomy (20.9%) suggests that sleeve pneumonectomy be reserved for the surgical candidate with tumor confined or adjacent to the carina (Newton et al., 1991). Sleeve lobectomy usually is employed as an alternative to, and is technically more demanding than, pneumonectomy. The 30-day mortality rate for sleeve lobectomy of 5.5% (Dartevelle et al., 1988; Deslauriers et al., 1989; Jensik et al., 1982; Watanabe et al., 1990) compares favorably with the 6.2% early mortality rate following pneumonectomy reported by the Lung Cancer Study Group (Ginsberg et al., 1983).

The most common postoperative complication is local recurrence (10.3%). The local recurrence rate is higher for sleeve lobectomy (12.5%) than for sleeve pneumonectomy (4.2%). Local recurrence is an unfortunate and devastating problem following both standard pulmonary resections and bronchoplastic procedures. Its effect on long-term survival is appreciated by all thoracic surgeons. Regrettably, most authors do not define local recurrence. Some authors only consider tumor at the suture line as local recurrence, whereas others include subsequent malignancy in intrathoracic lymph nodes and remote pulmonary involvement. Furthermore, both variable follow-up and incomplete initial resection limit the accuracy in reporting recurrence rates (Kittle, 1989; Tedder et al., 1992; Watanabe et al., 1990).

One explanation for suture line recurrence may be lung preservation at the expense of adequate bronchial margins. Paulson and associates (1970) recommend a bronchial margin of 1.5 to 2.0 cm. Frozen sections of the resected specimen are mandatory to

FIGURE 19–9. *A*, Bronchogram from a 63-year-old man with recurrent episodes of shortness of breath and left-sided wheezing. A tumor of the left mainstem bronchus is evident. The tumor appeared pedunculated at bronchoscopy. *B*, Exposure through a left-sided posterolateral thoracotomy. A tape has been passed around the left pulmonary artery, and the vagus nerve is retracted posteriorly to expose the left mainstem bronchus, indicated by the forceps. The ligamentum arteriosum was divided to facilitate exposure of the proximal left mainstem bronchus beneath the aortic arch. *C*, On opening the left mainstem bronchus, the tumor mass was found to be attached to the posterior wall of the bronchus. A wedge of mainstem bronchus was excised to remove the tumor (see Fig. 19–5). *D*, Operative specimen. The tumor mass had a discrete pedicle originating from the posterior bronchial wall. *E*, Microscopic appearance of the tumor showing mature cartilage consistent with a diagnosis of endobronchial hamartoma. (*A–E*, From Lowe, J. E., Bridgman, A. H., and Sabiston, D. C., Jr.: The role of bronchoplastic procedures in the surgical management of benign and malignant pulmonary lesions. J. Thorac. Cardiovasc. Surg., 83:227, 1982.)

■ **Table 19–7.** COMPLICATIONS AND EARLY MORTALITY IN 1915 PATIENTS AFTER BRONCHOPLASTIC PROCEDURES FOR MALIGNANCY

Complication	No. of Patients	Incidence (%)
Local recurrence	110/1064	10.3
Thirty-day mortality	143/1915	7.5
Pneumonia	32/481	6.7
Atelectasis	33/614	5.4
Benign stricture/stenosis	48/966	5.0
Bronchopleural fistula	42/1186	3.5
Empyema	17/599	2.8
Bronchovascular fistula	16/615	2.6
Pulmonary embolism	13/672	1.9

From Tedder, M., Anstadt, M. P., Tedder, S. D., and Lowe, J. E.: Current morbidity, mortality and survival after bronchoplastic procedures for malignancy. Reprinted with permission from the Society of Thoracic Surgeons (The Annals of Thoracic Surgery, 1992, Vol. 54, pp. 387–391).

■ **Table 19–9.** COMPARISON OF COMPLICATIONS AND EARLY MORTALITY AFTER SLEEVE LOBECTOMY VERSUS SLEEVE PNEUMONECTOMY FOR MALIGNANCY

Complication	Sleeve Lobectomy	Sleeve Pneumonectomy
Local recurrence	12.5% (84/673)	4.2% (3/72)
Pneumonia	9.9% (14/141)	16.7% (12/72)
Thirty-day mortality	5.5% (62/1125)	20.9% (29/139)
Atelectasis	5.2% (20/383)	—
Benign stricture/stenosis	4.8% (33/694)	—
Bronchopleural fistula	3.0% (17/565)	10.1% (14/139)
Bronchovascular fistula	2.5% (12/475)	2.9% (1/34)
Pulmonary embolus	2.3% (10/436)	2.1% (2/93)
Empyema	2.0% (6/294)	8.6% (8/93)

From Tedder, M., Anstadt, M. P., Tedder, S. D., and Lowe, J. E.: Current morbidity, mortality and survival after bronchoplastic procedures for malignancy. Reprinted with permission from the Society of Thoracic Surgeons (The Annals of Thoracic Surgery, 1992, Vol. 54, pp, 387–391).

minimize the risk of an incomplete resection. In the absence of extensive nodal or metastatic disease, completion pneumonectomy may be required in patients suffering local recurrence after sleeve lobectomy (Maggi et al., 1993).

Lowe and associates (1982) reported atelectasis to be the most common postoperative complication of bronchoplastic procedures. Unique to these resections, bronchial approximation, lymphatic interruption, local postoperative bronchial edema, and partial or complete denervation of the remaining lung may contribute to postoperative atelectasis. Although Tedder and colleagues (1992) reported an incidence of only 5.4%, the wide range of published rates (2 to 20%) suggests that this complication is reported with varying diligence. Intraoperative creation of an optimal bronchial anastomosis, perioperative attention to pulmonary hygiene, and early ambulation are required to minimize postoperative atelectasis and pneumonia.

Postoperative pneumonia is more likely in patients treated by conservative resections than in patients treated by conventional resections. A compromised bronchial anastomosis, for example, may increase the chance of subsequent pneumonia. This may result from atelectasis or an impaired ability to clear secretions. The incidence of postoperative pneumonia is higher for sleeve pneumonectomy than for sleeve lo-

■ **Table 19–8.** CAUSES OF EARLY MORTALITY AFTER BRONCHOPLASTIC PROCEDURES FOR MALIGNANCY

Cause	No. of Patients	Incidence (%)
Respiratory failure	19/91	20.9
Cardiac event	18/91	19.8
Pneumonia	14/91	15.4
Pulmonary embolus	13/91	14.3
Bronchopleural fistula	8/91	8.8
Bronchovascular fistula	5/91	5.5
Empyema	2/91	2.2

From Tedder, M., Anstadt, M. P., Tedder, S. D., and Lowe, J. E.: Current morbidity, mortality and survival after bronchoplastic procedures for malignancy. Reprinted with permission from the Society of Thoracic Surgeons (The Annals of Thoracic Surgery, 1992, Vol. 54, pp. 387–391).

bectomy (Maeda et al., 1986; Naruke, 1989; Tedder et al., 1992).

Benign stricture or stenosis occurs in 5% of patients and is either technical ("kink" stenosis) or secondary to suture granuloma formation. Benign strictures or stenoses may be treated by bronchoscopic dilatation, bronchoscopic suture excision, or laser excision. Occasionally, early revision of the bronchial anastomosis is necessary; this is preferred to the alternative, a late completion pneumonectomy.

Bronchopleural fistulas occur in 3.5% of patients; the incidence is 3-fold higher following sleeve pneumonectomy than following sleeve lobectomy (10.1% vs. 3.0%). This compares favorably with the 2.7 to 4.3% incidence following conventional pulmonary resections (Hankins et al., 1978; Vester et al., 1991; Williams and Lewis, 1976). Ischemia at the bronchial anastomosis has been postulated as one cause of bronchopleural fistulas. Accordingly, bronchial dissection and orientation for reanastomosis must be performed with minimal disruption of vascular supply. Although pleural flaps do not augment perfusion at the bronchial anastomosis, most surgeons provide tissue coverage for the bronchial anastomosis to minimize the incidence of subsequent bronchopleural and bronchovascular fistulas.

Bronchovascular fistulas following conservative resections are uniformly fatal and present with massive hemoptysis. Tedder and colleagues (1992) reported a 2.6% incidence following bronchoplastic procedures (Table 19–7). Vogt-Moykopf and associates (1986) noted seven patients who died of "acute pulmonary hemorrhage." Ayabe and co-workers (1982) also reported a patient who died of "bleeding" on the first postoperative day. This patient underwent a left-sided upper sleeve lobectomy and a segmental resection of the left pulmonary artery. Two additional deaths were reported by Keszler (1986): In one patient a concomitant pulmonary artery resection was performed; in the other, "reliable tissues" did not separate the pulmonary artery from the anastomosis. These additional deaths might represent bronchovascular fistulas and suggest that the incidence is higher than 2.6%. As previously stated, bronchial anastomotic tissue coverage consisting of either a pleural flap or free pericardium is the most effective means of preventing bronchovascular fistulas.

Distinct from the aforementioned bronchial, parenchymal, and pleural complications is the incidence of pulmonary embolism. The true incidence of pulmonary embolism is difficult to assess; however, it was documented in 13 of 672 patients (1.9%), accounted for 14.3% of early deaths, and was universally fatal (Bennett and Smith, 1978; Keszler, 1986; Roder et al., 1987; Ungar et al., 1981).

The overall 5-year survival rate of 614 patients who underwent sleeve lobectomy for bronchogenic carcinoma was 40% (Tedder et al., 1992). Five-year survival rates for patients with Stage I, II, and III disease were 63%, 37%, and 21%, respectively. The 5-year survival rate for N0 disease was 60%.

In summary, the morbidity and mortality rates for sleeve lobectomy for carcinoma in appropriately selected patients is similar to such rates for pneumonectomy. The major advantage of sleeve lobectomy is to extend surgical therapy and potentially long-term survival for patients with carcinoma who cannot tolerate pneumonectomy because of limited pulmonary function. In addition, the long-term survival of patients treated by sleeve lobectomy compares well with the accepted survival rates for conventional pulmonary resections when stratified by stage.

SELECTED BIBLIOGRAPHY

Bennett, W. F., and Smith, R. R.: A twenty-year analysis of the results of sleeve resection for primary bronchogenic carcinoma. J. Thorac. Cardiovasc. Surg., 76:840, 1978.

This series of 96 patients represents one of the largest groups with bronchogenic carcinoma treated by sleeve resection. Twenty years of detailed follow-up data are summarized. The 5-year survival rate was 34%, which is comparable with that achieved by conventional lobectomy or pneumonectomy.

D'Abreu, A. L., and MacHale, S. J.: Bronchial "adenoma" treated by local resection and reconstruction of the left main bronchus. Br. J. Surg., 39:355, 1951–1952.

This manuscript is the first published report of a sleeve resection. The operation was done on May 23, 1949, in a 48-year-old patient with a 3-year history of recurrent episodes of hemoptysis. The patient recovered uneventfully after resection of a sleeve of left mainstem bronchus. The postoperative bronchoscopy revealed normal mucosa covering the bronchial reanastomosis.

Deslauriers, J., Gaulin, P., Beaulieu, M., et al.: Long-term clinical and functional results of sleeve lobectomy for primary lung cancer. J. Thorac. Cardiovasc. Surg., 92:871, 1986.

Between 1975 and 1985, sleeve lobectomy was performed in 72 patients with bronchogenic carcinoma. For patients without lymph node involvement, the cumulative 5-year survival rate was 67%. Detailed pulmonary function studies that were obtained preoperatively and postoperatively show that reimplanted lobes contribute significantly to the overall remaining pulmonary function.

Faber, L. P., Jensik, R. J., and Kittle, C. F.: Results of sleeve lobectomy for bronchogenic carcinoma in 101 patients. Ann. Thorac. Surg., 37:279, 1984.

From 1961 to 1982, 101 patients underwent sleeve lobectomy for bronchogenic carcinoma of the lung. Life-table analysis of 94 patients shows a 5-year survival rate of 30% and a 10-year survival rate of 22%. Preoperative irradiation was used in 51 patients with 5- and 10-year survival rates of 25 and 16%, respectively. The sleeve lobectomy group that did not undergo radiation therapy had a 5-year survival rate of 36% and a 10-year survival rate of 28%. The operative mortality rate for the entire group was 2%.

Tumor recurred locally in the area of the anastomosis in nine patients. The authors conclude that sleeve lobectomy is a safe procedure and, when technically feasible, is the preferred procedure for bronchogenic carcinoma.

Firmin, R. K., Azariades, M., Lennox, S. C., et al.: Sleeve lobectomy (lobectomy and bronchoplasty) for bronchial carcinoma. Ann. Thorac. Surg., 35:442, 1983.

This is a series of 90 patients who underwent sleeve lobectomy for malignant bronchial tumors at the Brompton Hospital, London, between 1964 and 1974. The operative mortality rate was 1%. Bronchial stenosis occurred in 6% of patients and was caused by recurrent tumor in 4% and by stricture formation in 2%. Most patients had squamous cell carcinomas of the upper lobe (76 of 90). The 5-year survival rate was 71% in patients with hilar lymph nodes free of tumor at the time of operation and 17% when the hilar lymph nodes were involved with tumor. The authors conclude that these 5-year survival rates suggest that tumor-free survival is not significantly compromised by sleeve resection; they strongly recommend that sleeve lobectomy rather than pneumonectomy be the preferred operation for squamous cell carcinomas of the upper lobe orifice involving the main bronchus.

Frist, W. H., Mathisen, D. J., Hilgenberg, A. D., and Grillo, H. C.: Bronchial sleeve resection with and without pulmonary resection. J. Thorac. Cardiovasc. Surg., 93:350, 1987.

The authors emphasize applicability of bronchoplastic techniques for bronchial lesions that do not require concomitant pulmonary resection. Types of disease included a heterogeneous collection of 31 benign tumors, neoplasms of low-grade malignant potential and bronchostenosis, and 33 bronchogenic carcinomas. The actuarial disease-free survival rate for the group with benign lesions was 100% at 5 years. The authors conclude that sleeve resection is an ideal type of excisional therapy for benign endobronchial tumors, bronchostenosis, and tumors of low-grade malignant potential, and for selected patients with carcinoma. The operative technique and the choice of suture materials are discussed in detail.

Jensik, R. J., Faber, L. P., Brown, C. M., and Kittle, C. F.: Bronchoplastic and conservative resectional procedures for bronchial adenoma. J. Thorac. Cardiovasc. Surg., 68:556, 1974.

Long-term results in 33 patients with bronchial adenoma treated by sleeve resections are presented. The recurrence rate in this group was low, and the survival rate, calculated by the life-table method, was 86% at 5 years. This series establishes that sleeve resection techniques are the ideal form of survial therapy for lesions of low-grade malignant potential such as endobronchial adenomas.

Johnston, J. B., and Jones, P. H.: The treatment of bronchial carcinoma by lobectomy and sleeve resection of the main bronchus. Thorax, 14:48, 1959.

This series of 98 patients with bronchogenic carcinoma treated by sleeve resection presents the first follow-up data in a large group of patients using these techniques. The results established that bronchoplastic techniques were applicable to particular patients with carcinoma and that the operative morbidity and mortality as well as survival were equivalent to those achieved in patients treated by conventional resection procedures.

Lowe, J. E., Bridgman, A. H., and Sabiston, D. C., Jr.: The role of bronchoplastic procedures in the surgical management of benign and malignant pulmonary lesions. J. Thorac. Cardiovasc. Surg., 83:227, 1982.

This article describes 28 patients who underwent bronchoplastic procedures for various indications. The details of the preoperative evaluation and surgical management are reviewed. In addition, the results of 565 bronchoplastic procedures previously reported are summarized. The list of references is detailed.

Mentzer, S. J., Myers, D. W., and Sugarbaker, D. J.: Sleeve lobectomy, segmentectomy, and thoracoscopy in the management of carcinoma of the lung. Chest, 103:415S, 1993.

Emphasizing the goal of lung preservation and the need for an adequate resection, these authors review accepted indications for lung-sparing resections, including sleeve lobectomy, segmentectomy, and wedge resection. Caution is emphasized against the liberal use of these procedures when the cancer operation may be compromised.

Paulson, D. L., and Shaw, R. R.: Bronchial anastomosis and bronchoplastic procedures in the interest of preservation of lung tissue. J. Thorac. Surg., 29:238, 1955.

This series describes the operative technique, selection of patients, and results obtained in 16 patients treated by various bronchoplastic techniques for both benign traumatic and malignant airway lesions. This article introduced bronchoplastic techniques to the United States, and the authors have continued to make major contributions to the application of these techniques in the treatment of both malignant and benign airway problems.

Price-Thomas, C.: Conservative resection of the bronchial tree. J. R. Coll. Surg. Edinb., 1–2:169, 1955, 1957.

In a lecture before the Royal College of Surgeons of Edinburgh, Sir Clement Price-Thomas described the first sleeve resecton done in September 1947 on a Royal Air Force cadet with an endobronchial adenoma of the right mainstem bronchus. The only other surgical alternative at the time was right pneumonectomy, which would have prevented the patient from becoming a pilot. A successful sleeve resection of the right mainstem bronchus was performed, and the cadet subsequently was awarded a commission in the Royal Air Force.

Rendina, E. A., Venuta, F., Ciriaco, P., and Ricci, C.: Bronchovascular sleeve resection: Technique, perioperative management, prevention, and treatment of complications. J. Thorac. Cardiovasc. Surg., 106:73; 1993.

A current approach to both simple and complex bronchovascular sleeve resections is explicitly described. The authors prefer a pedicled intercostal flap for bronchial coverage and use of perioperative steroids. They also stress that most postoperative complications can be treated without reoperation. The short-term survival in this cohort is encouraging.

Tedder, M., Anstadt, M. P., Tedder, S. D., and Lowe, J. E.: Current morbidity, mortality, and survival after bronchoplastic procedures for malignancy. Ann. Thorac. Surg., 54:387, 1992.

This review describes the results of bronchoplastic procedures in 1915 patients reported between 1978 and 1990. It highlights the increased frequency with which these procedures are being employed. Within the limits of a retrospective review, it estimates the incidence of postoperative complications. Five-year survival data were available for 614 patients and were comparable to such data for conventional pulmonary resections when adjusted for stage of disease.

Ungar, I., Gyeney, I., Sheer, E., and Szarvas, I.: Sleeve lobectomy: An alternative to pneumonectomy in the treatment of bronchial carcinoma. Thorac. Cardiovasc. Surg., 29:41, 1981.

This series of 261 patients with carcinoma treated by sleeve resection is the largest series reported. In a 20-year period from 1960 to 1979, 3438 resections were performed for carcinoma of the lung; the standard operation was either lobectomy or pneumonectomy in more than 90% of cases. In 261 patients (7.4%), sleeve lobectomy was performed as an alternative to pneumonectomy to conserve pulmonary function. Long-term results are reported for 113 patients who underwent surgery before 1974. Fifty-seven (50%) were alive at least 5 years after resection.

Weisel, R. D., Cooper, J. D., Delarue, N. C., et al.: Sleeve lobectomy for carcinoma of the lung. J. Thorac. Cardiovasc. Surg., 78:839, 1979.

This review describes the operative techniques and results achieved in 70 patients with bronchogenic carcinoma treated by sleeve resections. Twenty-seven patients were considered "compromised" because they had severe pulmonary impairment and would not tolerate pneumonectomy. The remaining 43 patients were "uncompromised" and underwent sleeve resection, even though they could have tolerated conventional pneumonectomy. The results established that sleeve resection can be applied not only to patients with compromised pulmonary function, but also to particular patients with bronchogenic carcinoma and uncompromised pulmonary function whose anatomic findings allow sleeve resection.

BIBLIOGRAPHY

Andrews, M. J., and Pearson, F. G.: The relation of the bronchial arterial circulation and other factors to the transient defect in oxygen uptake following auto transplantation of the canine lung. Can. J. Surg., 16:1, 1973.

Attar, S., Miller, J. E., Hankins, J., et al.: Bronchial adenoma: A review of 51 patients. Ann. Thorac. Surg., 40:126, 1985.

Ayabe, H., Nakamura, Y., Miura, T., et al.: Bronchoplasty for bronchogenic carcinoma. World J. Surg., 6:433, 1982.

Belli, L., Meroni, A., Rondinara, G., and Beati, C. A.: Bronchoplastic procedures and pulmonary artery reconstruction in the treatment of bronchogenic cancer. J. Thorac. Cardiovasc. Surg., 90:167, 1985.

Bennett, W. F., and Smith, R. A.: A twenty-year analysis of the results of sleeve resection for primary bronchogenic carcinoma. J. Thorac. Cardiovasc. Surg., 76:840, 1978.

Bigger, I. A.: The diagnosis and treatment of primary carcinoma of the lung. South. Surg., 4:401, 1935.

Boyd, A. D., Spencer, F. C., and Lind, A.: Why has bronchial resection and anastomosis been reported infrequently for treatment of bronchial adenoma? J. Thorac. Cardiovasc. Surg., 59:359, 1970.

Breyer, R. H., Dainauskas, J. R., Jensik, R. J., and Faber, L. P.: Mucoepidermoid carcinoma of the trachea and bronchus: The case for conservative resection. Ann. Thorac. Surg., 29:197, 1980.

D'Abreu, A. L., and MacHale, S. J.: Bronchial "adenoma" treated by local resection and reconstruction of the left main bronchus. Br. J. Surg., 39:355, 1951–1952.

Daniel, R. A., Jr.: The regeneration of defects of the trachea and bronchi: An experimental study. J. Thorac. Surg., 17:335, 1948.

Dartevelle, P. D., Khalife, J., Chapelier, A., et al.: Tracheal sleeve pneumonectomy for bronchogenic carcinoma: Report of 55 cases. Ann. Thorac. Surg., 46:68, 1988.

Deslauriers, J., Gaulin, P., and Beaulieu, M., et al.: Long term clinical and functional results of sleeve lobectomy for primary lung cancer. J. Thorac. Cardiovasc. Surg., 92:871, 1986.

Deslauriers, J., Beaulieu, M., and McClish, A.: Tracheal sleeve pneumonectomy. In Shields, T. W. (ed): General Thoracic Surgery. 3rd ed. Philadelphia, Lea & Febiger, 1989, pp. 382–387.

Eloesser, L.: Transthoracic bronchotomy for removal of benign tumors of the bronchi. Ann Surg., 112:1067, 1940.

Faber, L. P., Jensik, R. J., and Kittle, C. F.: Results of sleeve lobectomy for bronchogenic carcinoma in 101 patients. Ann. Thorac. Surg., 37:279, 1984.

Firmin, R. K., Azariades, M., and Lennox, S. C., et al.: Sleeve lobectomy (lobectomy and bronchoplasty) for bronchial carcinoma. Ann. Thorac. Surg., 35:442, 1983.

Frist, W. H., Mathisen, D. J., Hilgenberg, A. D., and Grillo, H. C.: Bronchial sleeve resection with and without pulmonary resection. J. Thorac. Cardiovasc. Surg., 93:350, 1987.

Gebauer, P. W.: Plastic reconstruction of tuberculous bronchostenosis with dermal grafts. J. Thorac. Surg., 19:604, 1950.

Gebauer, P. W.: Reconstructive surgery of the trachea and bronchi: Late results with dermal grafts. J. Thorac. Surg., 22:568, 1951.

Ginsberg, R. J., Hill, L. D., Eagan, R. T., et al.: Modern thirty day operative mortality for surgical resections in lung cancer. J. Thorac. Cardiovasc. Surg., 86:654–658, 1983.

Hankins, J. R., Miller, J. E., Attar, S., et al.: Bronchopleural fistula: Thirteen-year experience with 77 cases. J. Thorac. Cardiovasc. Surg., 76:755, 1978.

Huidekoper, J. J., and van Ginneken, P. J. J.: Sleeve resection. Respiration, 47:303, 1985.

Hurt, R.: Benign tumours of the bronchus and trachea. Ann. R. Coll. Surg. Engl., 66:22, 1984.

Ishihara, T., Ikeda, T., Inoue, H., and Fukai, S.: Resection of cancer of lung and carina. J. Thorac. Cardiovasc. Surg., 73:936, 1977.

Jensik, R. J.: Preoperative irradiation and bronchopulmonary sleeve resection for lung cancer. Surg. Clin. North Am., 46:145, 1966.

Jensik, R. J., Faber, L. P., Brown, C. M., and Kittle, C. F.: Bronchoplastic and conservative resectional procedures for bronchial adenoma. J. Thorac. Cardiovasc. Surg., 68:556, 1974.

Jensik, R. J., Faber, L. P., Milloy, F. J., and Amato, J. J.: Sleeve lobectomy for carcinoma. J. Thorac. Cardiovasc. Surg., 64:400, 1972.

Jensik, R. J., Faber, L. P., Kittle, C. F., et al.: Survival in patients undergoing tracheal sleeve pneumonectomy for bronchogenic carcinoma. Thorac. Cardiovasc. Surg., 84:489, 1982.

Johnston, J. B., and Jones, P. H.: The treatment of bronchial carcinoma by lobectomy and sleeve resection of the main bronchus. Thorax, 14:48, 1959.

Jones, P. H.: Lobectomy and bronchial anastomosis in the surgery of bronchial carcinoma. Ann. R. Coll. Surg. Engl., 25:20, 1959.

Kato, R., Kakizaki, T., Hangai, N., et al.: Bronchoplastic procedures for tuberculous bronchial stenosis. J. Thorac. Cardiovasc. Surg., 106:1118–1121, 1993.

Keszler, P.: Sleeve resection and other bronchoplasties in the surgery of bronchogenic tumors. Int. Surg., 71:229, 1986.

Kittle, C. F.: Atypical resections of the lung: Bronchoplasties, sleeve resections, and segmentectomies—Their evolution and present status. Curr. Probl. Surg., 26:57, 1989.

Lima, R.: Bronchial adenoma: Clinicopathologic study and results of treatment. Chest, 77:81, 1980.

Lowe, J. E., Bridgman, A. H., and Sabiston, D. C., Jr.: The role of bronchoplastic procedures in the surgical management of benign and malignant pulmonary lesions. J. Thorac. Cardiovasc. Surg., 83:227, 1982.

Maeda, M., Nanjo, S., Nakamura, K., and Nakamoto, K.: Tracheo-bronchoplasty for lung cancer. Int. Surg., 71:221, 1986.

Maggi, G., Casadio, C., Pischedda, F., et al.: Bronchoplastic and angioplastic techniques in the treatment of bronchogenic carcinoma. Ann. Thorac. Surg., 55:1501, 1993.

McCaughan, B. C., Martini, N., and Bains, M. S.: Bronchial carcinoids. J. Thorac. Cardiovasc. Surg., 89:8, 1985.

Mentzer, S. J., Myers, D. W., and Sugarbaker, D. J.: Sleeve lobectomy, segmentectomy, and thoracoscopy in the management of carcinoma of the lung. Chest, 103:415S, 1993.

Naruke, T.: Bronchoplastic and bronchovascular procedures of the tracheobronchial tree in the management of primary lung cancer. Chest, 96:53S, 1989.

Naruke, T., and Suemasu, K.: Bronchoplastic surgery for lung cancer and the results. Jpn. J. Surg., 13:165, 1983.

Naruke, T., Yoneyama, T., Ogata, T., and Suemasu, K.: Bronchoplastic procedures for lung cancer. J. Thorac. Cardiovasc. Surg., 73:927, 1977.

Newton, J. R., Grillo, H. C., Mathisen, D. J.: Main bronchial sleeve resection with pulmonary conservation. Ann. Thorac. Surg., 52:1272, 1991.

Okike, J., Bernatz, P. E., Payne, W. S., et al.: Bronchoplastic procedures in the treatment of carcinoid tumors of the tracheobronchial tree. J. Thorac. Cardiovasc. Surg., 76:281, 1978.

Paulson, D. L., and Shaw, R. R.: Bronchial anastomosis and bronchoplastic procedures in the interest of preservation of lung tissue. J. Thorac. Cardiovasc. Surg., 29:238, 1955.

Paulson, D. L., and Shaw, R. R.: Results of bronchoplastic procedures for bronchogenic carcinoma. Ann. Surg., 151:729, 1960.

Paulson, D. L., Urschel, H. C., Jr., McNamara, J. J., and Shaw, R. R.: Bronchoplastic procedures for bronchogenic carcinoma. J. Thorac. Cardiovasc. Surg., 59:38, 1970.

Price-Thomas, C.: Conservative resection of the bronchial tree. J. R. Coll. Surg. Edinb., 1–2:169, 1955, 1957.

Price-Thomas, C.: Lobectomy with sleeve resection. Thorax, 15:9, 1960.

Ratto, G. B., Mereu, C., and Scordamaglia, A., et al.: The surgical treatment of bronchial carcinoid adenoma: A personal experience. Ital. J. Surg. Sci., 13:289, 1983.

Rees, G. M., and Paneth, M.: Lobectomy with sleeve resection in the treatment of bronchial tumors. Thorax, 25:160, 1970.

Rendina, E. A., Venuta, F., Ciriaco, P., and Ricci, C.: Bronchovascular sleeve resection: Technique, perioperative management, prevention, and treatment of complications. J. Thorac. Cardiovasc. Surg., 106:73, 1993.

Robinson, C. L. N., Holmes, D., Jamieson, W. R. E.: Lobectomy and bronchoplasty for cancer. Can. J. Surg., 24:196–197, 1981.

Roder, O. C., Christensen, J. B., and Andersen, C., et al.: Bronchoplastic procedures for bronchial carcinoma. Scand. J. Thorac. Cardiovasc. Surg., 21:109, 1987.

Sartori, F., Binda, R., and Spreafico, G., et al.: Sleeve lobectomy in the treatment of bronchogenic carcinoma. Int. Surg., 71:233, 1986.

Taffel, M.: The repair of tracheal and bronchial defects with free fascia grafts. Surgery, 8:56, 1940.

Tedder, M., Anstadt, M. P., Tedder, S. D., and Lowe, J. E.: Current morbidity, mortality, and survival after bronchoplastic procedures for malignancy. Ann. Thorac. Surg., 54:387, 1992.

Todd, T. R., Cooper, J. D., and Weissberg, D., et al.: Bronchial carcinoid tumors. J. Thorac. Cardiovasc. Surg., 79:532, 1980.

Ungar, I., Gyeney, I., Sherer, E., and Szarvas, I.: Sleeve lobectomy: An alternative to pneumonectomy in the treatment of bronchial carcinoma. Thorac. Cardiovasc. Surg., 29:41, 1981.

Van Den Bosch, J. M. M., Bergstein, P. G. M., and Laros, C. D., et al.: Lobectomy with sleeve resection in the treatment of tumors of the bronchus. Chest, 80:154, 1981.

Van Schil, P. E., de la Riviere, A. B., Knaepen, P. J., et al.: TNM staging and long-term follow-up after sleeve resection for bronchogenic tumors. Ann. Thorac. Surg., 52:1096, 1991.

Vester, S. R., Faber, L. P., Kittle, C. F., et al.: Bronchopleural fistula after stapled closure of the bronchus. Ann. Thorac. Surg., 52:1253, 1991.

Vogt-Moykopf, I., Fritz, T., and Meyer, G.: Bronchoplastic and angioplastic operation in bronchial carcinoma: Long-term results of a retrospective analysis from 1973 to 1983. Int. Surg., 71:211, 1986.

Watanabe, T., Kobayashi, H., and Murakami, S., et al.: Bilateral sleeve lobectomy for metachronous multiple primary lung cancer. Jpn. J. Surg., 16:56, 1986.

Watanabe, Y., Shimizu, J., and Oda, M., et al.: Results in 104 patients undergoing bronchoplastic procedures for bronchial lesions. Ann. Thorac. Surg., 50:607, 1990.

Weisel, R. D., Cooper, J. D., and Delarue, N. C., et al.: Sleeve lobectomy for carcinoma of the lung. J. Thorac. Cardiovasc. Surg., 78:839, 1979.

Wilkins, E. W., Grillo, H. C., Moncure, A. C., and Scannell, J. G.: Changing times in surgical management of bronchopulmonary carcinoid tumor. Ann. Thorac. Surg., 38:339, 1984.

Williams, N. S., and Lewis, C. T.: Bronchopleural fistula: A review of 86 cases. Br. J. Surg., 63:520, 1976.

Wood, P. B., Gilday, M. D., Ilves, M. A., and Pearson, F. G.: A comparison of gas exchange after simple lobectomy and lobectomy with sleeve resection in dogs. J. Thorac. Cardiovasc. Surg., 68:646, 1974.

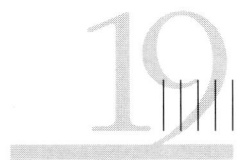

■ III Benign Tumors of the Lung and Bronchial Adenomas

Thomas A. D'Amico and David C. Sabiston, Jr.

BENIGN TUMORS OF THE LUNG

Benign tumors of the lung may arise from the bronchus, the pulmonary parenchyma, or the visceral pleura. These lesions are uncommon, representing only 2% of all pulmonary neoplasms (MacKay et al., 1991) and 8 to 15% of solitary pulmonary nodules (Steele, 1963). The classification of benign tumors of the lung has evolved since the advent of electron microscopy, which has clarified the cell of origin for a number of lesions. Currently, benign pulmonary lesions are organized according to the embryonic tissue of origin (Table 19–10). Bronchial adenomas, which possess malignant potential, are classified elsewhere and discussed individually.

Benign pulmonary lesions are symptomatic in only 40% of patients (Arrigoni et al., 1970). Patients may complain of cough, chest pain, or symptoms of bronchial obstruction, such as wheezing. When bronchial obstruction occurs, patients may demonstrate a history of recurrent pneumonia, bronchiectasis, or lung abscess. Hemoptysis occurs rarely and is associated with endobronchial and endotracheal lesions.

Benign tumors of the lung, usually asymptomatic, are detected on routine chest films. Most lesions are peripheral, with well-defined margins or slight lobulations. Review of previous chest films may help determine the growth pattern of the nodule and the potential for malignancy. A benign pulmonary tumor usually has a doubling time of more than 400 days (Lillington and Caskey, 1993). Stability as demonstrated by comparisons of current and previous films or visible calcification suggests a benign lesion, and a period of observation may be warranted.

In most cases, solitary pulmonary nodules should be resected and examined histologically to exclude malignancy. The treatment of most benign lesions is conservative pulmonary resection, which establishes the pathologic diagnosis. Some lesions, however, may be treated with endobronchial removal.

Epithelial Tumors

Papilloma

Papillomas have been classified into five subtypes: solitary benign papillomas, multiple benign papillomas, benign combined bronchial mucous gland and surface papillary tumors, papillary bronchial carcinoma in situ, and bronchiolar papillomas (Spencer et al., 1980). Papillomas occur most commonly in childhood and are often multiple and recurrent. The etiology of bronchial papillomas is unknown, but the

administration of noncellular extracts of human laryngeal papillomas has produced similar lesions in dogs, suggesting an infective (viral) etiology (Schaff and Thomson, 1955).

Papillomas appear as sessile lesions growing into the bronchial lumen, although proximal lesions may possess a stalk. These lesions contain a core of vascular connective tissue, which is covered by squamous or columnar epithelium.

Bronchoscopic resection has been advocated in the management of patients with papilloma, but the recurrence rate is high, and there is risk of malignant transformation. The strategy of close surveillance and multiple bronchoscopic resections is usually successful; however, large lesions require open resection.

Polyp

The etiology of benign bronchial polyps is probably related to pulmonary infections, and the incidence is decreasing owing to better antimicrobial management. Histologically, these lesions resemble inflammatory polyps and may demonstrate a lining of squamous cell metaplasia or ciliated epithelium with granulation tissue. Bronchoscopic resection is the treatment of choice, and the incidence of recurrence is low (Greenfield and Stirling, 1990).

Mesodermal Tumors

Vascular Tumors

Angioma. Pulmonary angiomas (including hemangiomas, lymphangiomas, and hemangioendotheliomas) are benign tumors of mesodermal origin with vascular characteristics. Hemangiomas consist of a collection of thin-walled vessels with scant supporting stroma. These lesions are multiple in one-third of cases, bilateral in 8% of cases, and supplied by a systemic artery in 4% of cases (Miller and Hatcher, 1991). Pulmonary hemangiomas are a manifestation of hereditary telangiectasia syndrome (Rendu-Osler-Weber disease) in 60% of cases.

Hemangiomas characteristically are found in the upper trachea or subglottic larynx in infants and can produce airway obstruction. The diagnosis is established bronchoscopically. Most lesions respond to radiation therapy, although tracheostomy may be required to relieve airway obstruction before treatment. For endobronchial lesions, laser therapy followed by radiation therapy is the treatment of choice.

Tracheal lymphangiomas may also present with airway obstruction in the infant and require surgical resection. These lesions are often associated with cervical lymphangiomas.

Hemangioendothelioma is a solid tumor of vascular origin that is found exclusively in the lung. This lesion has been described in the newborn, is associated with congenital heart defects, and is usually fatal over a short period. Hemangioendothelioma also may present as a polypoid bronchial lesion.

■ **Table 19–10.** CLASSIFICATION OF BENIGN TUMORS OF THE LUNG

Epithelial Tumors	Neurogenic Tumors
Papilloma	
Polyps	**Developmental Tumors or Tumors of Unknown Origin**
	Hamartoma
Mesodermal Tumors	Teratoma
Vascular tumors	Chemodectoma
Angiomas	Clear cell tumor
Hemangioma	Thymoma
Lymphangioma	
Hemangioendothelioma	**Inflammatory and Other Pseudotumors**
Lymphangiomyomatosis	Plasma cell granuloma
Arteriovenous fistula	Pseudolymphoma
Sclerosing hemangioma	Xanthoma
Bronchial tumors	Amyloid
Fibroma	Tracheobronchopathia
Chondroma	osteoplastica
Lipoma	
Leiomyoma	
Granular cell myoblastoma	

Lymphangiomyomatosis. Lymphangiomyomatosis is characterized by the proliferation of fine multinodular lesions at the base of the lungs that produces honeycombing, loss of parenchyma, and progressive pulmonary insufficiency. Smooth muscle proliferation in the bronchioles and venules has been demonstrated histologically. Complications of lymphangiomyomatosis include pneumothorax, chylothorax, and hemoptysis. Conservative resection is undertaken when possible; however, these lesions are often large and require extensive anatomic resection. Lymphangiomyomatosis has also been treated successfully with pulmonary transplantation (Sleiman et al., 1992).

Arteriovenous Fistula. The failure of arterial and venous septa to completely fuse is responsible for the development of the pulmonary arteriovenous fistula (also called arteriovenous malformation). These lesions are most often found in the lower lobes and are associated with hereditary telangiectasia syndrome (Rendu-Osler-Weber disease), as are pulmonary hemangiomas. Arteriovenous malformations act as right-to-left shunts and may produce cyanosis, polycythemia, pulmonary hypertrophic osteoarthropathy, and systemic embolization.

Radiographically, a pulmonary arteriovenous fistula characteristically appears as a circumscribed mass. Under fluoroscopy, an increase in size with Müller's maneuver and decrease in size with Valsalva's maneuver may be observed. Computed tomography (CT) of the chest with contrast may demonstrate the arterial and venous components supplying the malformation. Although accurate diagnosis may be established by CT, pulmonary arteriography delineates vascular anatomy and excludes the presence of multiple fistulas. Also, arteriography with embolization is effective in some patients who are not candidates for thoracotomy and pulmonary resection.

Sclerosing Hemangioma. Sclerosing hemangiomas are benign pulmonary tumors that arise from epithelial cells, perhaps Type II pneumocytes (Nagata et al., 1985). These lesions appear as solitary nodules in the lower lobes and may also be associated with hereditary telangiectasia.

Bronchial Tumors

Fibroma. Fibromas, although the most common pulmonary nodule of *mesenchymal* origin, are actually rare. These lesions are usually found in the tracheobronchial tree but may also arise in the pulmonary parenchyma. Histologically, fibromas are characterized by varying patterns of spindle cells or myxomatous arrangements. Fibromas may be removed bronchoscopically when visualized, particularly when a stalk is present. Pulmonary resection may be required for distal or sessile lesions.

Chondroma. Chondromas are second in incidence to fibromas among benign pulmonary tumors of mesenchymal origin. Chondromas arise in the major bronchi, are firm and translucent, and may become ossified. They are distinguished from hamartomas in that they consist of mesodermal elements exclusively.

Pulmonary chondromas are one of the manifestations of Carney's syndrome, which also includes extra-adrenal paragangliomas and gastric leiomyosarcomas.

Lipoma. Pulmonary lipomas are rare lesions that arise in the fat cells of the bronchial submucosa, affecting men much more commonly than women. These avascular lesions appear within the bronchus, usually within an intact epithelium. Pulmonary lipomas grow slowly but may eventually produce bronchial obstruction. Small lesions are removed bronchoscopically; larger lesions require thoracotomy and bronchotomy.

Leiomyoma. Pulmonary leiomyomas may appear as endobronchial lesions or peripheral nodules. Endobronchial leiomyomas are submucosal lesions that may produce cough, hemoptysis, or bronchial obstruction. Pulmonary leiomyomas arise from bronchial smooth muscle, and histologic analysis demonstrates the characteristic spindle-shaped cells. Conservative resection is the treatment of choice, although large lesions may require lobectomy.

Granular Cell Tumor. Formerly known as myoblastomas, granular cell tumors are believed to originate from histiocytes or Schwann cells (Sobel et al., 1971). When they occur endobronchially, granular cell tumors may produce obstruction. Granular cell tumors consist of ovoid or polygonal cells with abundant eosinophilic cytoplasm. Removal of granular tumors is most effectively achieved by pulmonary resection; bronchoscopic removal is associated with recurrence.

Neurogenic Tumors

Pulmonary tumors of neurogenic origin are rare and include neuromas, neurofibromas, and neurilemomas. Neuromas arise in the bronchus and may be treated by lobectomy or by endoscopic resection. Neurilemomas occur in the trachea, bronchus, or periphery; surgical resection is advocated because bronchoscopic resection is associated with recurrence.

Developmental Tumors or Tumors of Unknown Origin

Hamartoma

Hamartomas, occurring in 0.25% of the general population (McDonald et al., 1945), are the most common benign neoplasm of the lung, responsible for 75% of benign tumors of the lung (Arrigoni et al., 1970) and 8% of solitary pulmonary nodules (Jones and Cleve, 1954). Ninety per cent of hamartomas occur in the peripheral parenchyma, and 10% are endobronchial. Hamartomas may be parenchymal, pleural, or extralobar (Oldham et al., 1967); they are believed to arise in the bronchiolar parenchyma, compressing adjacent tissue with growth. Histologically, this lesion is described as the disorganized arrangement of tissues that are normally present in the lung. Cartilage often predominates, but it is not associated with the normal cartilage of the tracheobronchial tree. Although hamartomas are considered benign, malignant epithelial transformation has been described (Poulsen et al., 1979).

Most hamartomas are asymptomatic and are discovered on routine chest films as a solitary pulmonary nodule. Hamartomas may appear round or lobulated, usually with a smooth and well-defined border. These lesions are often calcified; the presence of popcorn calcification is pathognomonic for pulmonary hamartomas. To differentiate hamartomas from carcinoma of the lung, as with most solitary pulmonary nodules, resection is undertaken. Conservative resection is sufficient, because recurrence is rare.

Chondromatous Hamartoma. Chondromatous hamartomas, the most common subtype, consist of cartilage, fat, smooth muscle, fibrous connective tissue, and cuboidal epithelium. These lesions are usually discovered as solitary pulmonary nodules on routine chest film, in men more commonly than in women. They may, however, present as an endobronchial lesion, with or without bronchial obstruction. As with most solitary pulmonary nodules, therapy consists of resection to exclude the presence of malignancy. Chondromatous hamartomas may be resected with bronchoplastic techniques when lesions are particularly large or located proximally in the tracheobronchial tree.

Adenomatous Hamartoma. Adenomatous hamartoma of infancy, also called cystic adenomatoid malformation, is a rare lesion, characterized by cystic changes, undifferentiated cells, bronchial elements, and fetal lung tissue. The lesion itself may involve a single lobe or an entire lung. Even when limited to a single lobe, air trapping within the cystic cavities overinflates that lobe and compresses the normal lung. Adenomatous hamartomas may be classified as microcystic or macrocystic. Resection of the involved pulmonary parenchyma is required, and early recognition of the lesion and operative intervention is essential.

Blastoma. Pulmonary blastoma is a rare lesion that develops from embryonal tissue and is considered a low-grade malignancy. Histologically, pulmonary blastoma resembles carcinosarcoma and may metastasize (Spencer, 1985). Surgical resection of the pulmonary blastoma is associated with long-term survival.

Teratoma

Pulmonary teratomas demonstrate undifferentiated tissues of all germ layers and may be benign or malignant. Most teratomas are benign and are in the left upper lobe (Gawtam, 1969). On chest film, teratomas may demonstrate calcification and an eccentric cavity within the tumor. These lesions are rare and must be differentiated from pulmonary metastases from testicular carcinoma or direct extension from mediastinal teratomas.

Chemodectoma

Pulmonary chemodectomas are nonchromaffin paragangliomas, a proliferation of chemoreceptor tissue found adjacent to pulmonary veins, supplied by a dense nerve plexus. Histologically, chemodectomas consist of ovoid or round cells arranged in sheets or nests and divided by connective tissue and dilated vascular channels (Spencer, 1985). Chemodectomas of the lung tend to be solitary and become large. These lesions may be benign or malignant, and large pulmonary chemodectomas may resemble pulmonary carcinoids. Pulmonary resection is usually undertaken; lobectomy may be required in lesions that grow particularly large.

Clear Cell Tumor

The cells of a pulmonary clear cell tumor, resembling renal cell carcinoma, are characterized by large cytoplasm, abundant cytosolic glycogen, and membrane-bound neurosecretory granules. Despite the presence of neurosecretory granules, there is no evidence that the lesion is related to the amine precursor uptake and decarboxylation (APUD) tumors. Conservative resection is usually curative.

Thymoma

Intrapulmonary thymomas may develop from ectopic thymic tissue and are found at the hilum and the periphery. These tumors may be associated with myasthenia gravis (Kung et al., 1985). Conservative pulmonary resection is associated with long-term survival.

Inflammatory and Other Pseudotumors

Plasma Cell Granuloma

Plasma cell granuloma, also called histiocytoma or plasma cell pseudotumor, is characterized by a dense infiltrate of lymphocytes and plasma cells and vascular granulation tissue with whorls of fibroblasts and collagen. These tumors are rare and tend to affect younger patients. Plasma cell granulomas may present as solitary pulmonary nodules or may be associated with systemic manifestations, plasma protein imbalance, or nonspecific local inflammatory responses. Rarely, the plasma cell granuloma is associated with multiple myeloma or other malignancies. Surgical excision is curative in most cases.

Pseudolymphoma

Pseudolymphoma of the lung is a rare tumor that presents as a solitary pulmonary nodule, resembling carcinoma of the lung. These lesions are usually benign, but malignant transformation has been reported (Fisher et al., 1980). Although it presents as a solitary nodule, pulmonary pseudolymphoma histologically resembles lymphoid interstitial pneumonitis. These lesions are composed of a mixture of lymphoid cells (including plasma cells) and well-defined germinal centers, arranged peribronchially. In contrast to malignant lymphoma, the bronchial cartilage is spared and the mucosa is intact. Conservative resection may be performed with minimal risk of recurrence. Although progression to malignancy is rare, long-term follow-up is recommended.

Xanthoma

Pulmonary xanthoma is a rare, benign tumor that is usually found within the parenchyma. Xanthomas are considered postinflammatory lesions, composed of foam cells, spindle cells, and lymphocytes. Conservative resection excludes malignancy.

Amyloid

Pulmonary amyloidosis may present in a number of ways: localized deposits in the bronchus, multiple or diffuse bronchial deposits, localized or multiple parenchymal deposits, and diffuse parenchymal infiltration of the alveoli and pulmonary vasculature (Spencer, 1985). When amyloid is deposited focally in the bronchial submucosa, the lesion may appear as a solitary pulmonary nodule. Pulmonary resection is usually recommended to exclude malignancy.

Tracheobronchopathia Osteoplastica

Tracheobronchopathia osteoplastica is an unusual lesion characterized by cartilaginous projection in the trachea. The lesion represents submucosal growth arising from the tracheal cartilage. Multiple tumors may be present and produce ossification of the cartilaginous rings of the entire trachea. Upon discovery, lesions may be removed bronchoscopically; however, despite diffuse tracheal involvement, tracheobronchopathia osteoplastica is often asymptomatic and found only at autopsy.

BRONCHIAL ADENOMAS

Bronchial adenomas account for 5% of pulmonary neoplasms. Most bronchial adenomas (85 to 90%) are carcinoids (see Chapter 19, part I); the remainder are bronchial gland tumors, including adenoid cystic carcinomas, mucoepidermoid tumors, mixed tumors, and bronchial mucous gland adenomas. In contrast to the benign tumors of the lung, bronchial gland tumors are slow-growing malignancies with variable metastatic potential.

Adenoid Cystic Carcinoma

The most common bronchial gland tumor is the adenoid cystic carcinoma (also called cylindroma). These tumors usually occur in the trachea or mainstem bronchi. Adenoid cystic carcinomas contain small, dark-staining cells in solid or cystic cords with an adenoid appearance. Patients with this tumor present with cough, hemoptysis, or airway obstruction,

typically in the sixth decade of life. Adenoid cystic carcinomas are easily identified bronchoscopically, appearing as a sessile, translucent mass in the trachea or bronchus. These lesions may be removed bronchoscopically, but recurrence is frequent, owing to extensive submucosal and perineural lymphatic spread. Surgical excision with regional lymph node dissection is recommended, including frozen-section examination of margins. Long-term survival is reported in 50% of patients (Conlan et al., 1978). Bronchoscopic removal and radiotherapy are performed when tumors are not resectable.

Mucoepidermoid Tumor

Mucoepidermoid tumor is a rare bronchial adenoma arising in the trachea, mainstem bronchus, and lobar bronchus. These lesions consist of epidermoid elements, mucus-producing cells, and basal cell components. Compared with low-grade lesions, high-grade mucoepidermoid tumors are characterized by greater cellularity, frequent mitotic figures, and hyperchromatic nuclei. Complete surgical resection is recommended. Patients with low-grade lesions have good prognosis; high-grade lesions have poor prognosis, despite therapy.

Mixed Tumors

Mixed tumors of the tracheobronchial tree are rare lesions that resemble mixed tumors of the salivary glands. Histologically, mixed tumors consist of an epithelial component and a connective tissue component. Local recurrence and metastasis have been reported (Payne et al., 1965); resection of particularly large lesions in the trachea may require tracheal reconstruction.

Bronchial Mucous Gland Adenoma

Bronchial mucous gland adenomas are rare, benign lesions that consist of glandular cysts; they are filled with mucus and lined by bronchial glandular epithelium. Conservative resection is usually successful.

SELECTED BIBLIOGRAPHY

Arrigoni, M. G., Woolner, L. B., Bernatz, P. E., et al.: Benign tumors of the lung. A ten-year surgical experience. J. Thorac. Cardiovasc. Surg., 60:589, 1970.

This review describes the experience with 130 patients over 10 years at the Mayo Clinic.

MacKay, B., Lukeman, J. M., and Ordonez, N. G.: Tumors of the Lung. Philadelphia, W. B. Saunders, 1991.

This is a complete, contemporary reference book of pulmonary pathology.

Oldham, H. N., Jr., Young, W. G., Jr., and Sealy, W. C.: Hamartoma of the lung. J. Thorac. Cardiovasc. Surg., 53:735, 1967.

This review of hamartoma of the lung, the most common benign pulmonary lesion, completely describes diagnosis and therapy.

BIBLIOGRAPHY

Arrigoni, M. G., Woolner, L. B., Bernatz, P. E., et al.: Benign tumors of the lung. A ten-year surgical experience. J. Thorac. Cardiovasc. Surg., 60:589, 1970.

Conlan, A. A., Payne, W. S., Woolner, L. B., and Sanderson, D. R.: Adenoid cystic carcinoma (cylindroma) and mucoepidermoid carcinoma of the bronchus. J. Thorac. Cardiovasc. Surg., 76:369, 1978.

Fisher, C., Grubb, C., Kenning, B., et al.: Pseudolymphoma of the lung: A rare case of a solitary pulmonary nodule. J. Thorac. Cardiovasc. Surg., 80:11, 1980.

Gawtam, H. P.: Intrapulmonary malignant teratoma. Am. Rev. Respir. Dis., 100:863, 1969.

Greenfield, L. J., and Stirling, M. C.: Benign tumors of the lung and bronchial adenomas. In Sabiston, D. C., Jr., and Spencer, F. C. (eds): Surgery of the Chest. 5th ed. Philadelphia, W. B. Saunders, 1990.

Jones, R. C., and Cleve, E. A.: Solitary circumscribed lesions of the lung: Selection of cases for diagnostic thoracotomy. Arch. Intern. Med., 93:842, 1954.

Kung, I. T. M., Loke, S. L., So, S. Y., et al.: Intrapulmonary thymoma: Report of two cases. Thorax, 40:471, 1985.

Lillington, G. A., and Caskey, C.: Evaluation and management of solitary and multiple pulmonary nodules. Clin. Chest Med., 14:111, 1993.

MacKay, B., Lukeman, J. M., and Ordonez, N. G.: Tumors of the Lung. Philadelphia, W. B. Saunders, 1991.

McDonald, J. R., Harrington, S. W., and Clagett, O. T.: Hamartoma (often called chondroma) of the lung. J. Thorac. Surg., 14:128, 1945.

Miller, J. I., and Hatcher, C. R., Jr.: Benign tumors of the lower respiratory tract. In Baue, A. E. (ed): Glenn's Thoracic and Cardiovascular Surgery. 5th ed. Norwalk, CT, Appleton & Lange, 1991.

Nagata, N., Dairaku, M., Ishida, T., et al.: Sclerosing hemangioma of the lung. Cancer, 55:116, 1985.

Oldham, H. N., Jr., Young, W. G., Jr., and Sealy, W. C.: Hamartoma of the lung. J. Thorac. Cardiovasc. Surg., 53:735, 1967.

Payne, W. S., Schier, J., and Woolner, L. B.: Mixed tumors of the bronchus (salivary gland type). J. Thorac. Cardiovasc. Surg., 49:663, 1965.

Poulsen, J. T., Jacobsen, M., and Francis, D.: Probable malignant transformation of a pulmonary hamartoma. Thorax, 34:557, 1979.

Schaff, B., and Thomson, R. V.: Papillomatosis of trachea and bronchi. Am. Rev. Tuberc., 71:429, 1955.

Sleiman, C., Mal, H., Jebrak, G., et al.: Pulmonary lymphangiomyomatosis treated by single lung transplantation. Am. Rev. Respir. Dis., 145:964, 1992.

Sobel, H. J., Marquet, E., Avriu, E., and Schwartz, R.: Granular cell myoblastoma. Am. J. Pathol., 65:59, 1971.

Spencer, H.: Pathology of the Lung. 4th ed. Philadelphia, W. B. Saunders, 1985.

Spencer, H., Dail, D. H., and Arneaud, J.: Noninvasive bronchial epithelial papillary tumors. Cancer, 45:1486, 1980.

Steele, J. D.: The solitary pulmonary nodule: Report of a cooperative study of resected asymptomatic solitary pulmonary nodules in males. J. Thorac. Cardiovasc. Surg., 46:21, 1963.

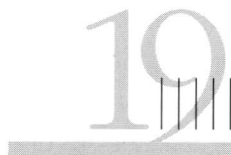

■ IV Immunology and Immunotherapy of Carcinoma of the Lung

Thomas A. D'Amico and David C. Sabiston, Jr.

Investigation of the molecular biology of carcinoma of the lung—the genetic factors responsible for tumor initiation and promotion—has begun to elucidate the pathogenesis and generate novel strategies for the treatment of lung cancer. Mutations in oncogenes are an important stage in the development of pulmonary malignancies, both in *small-cell lung cancer* (SCLC) and in *non-small-cell lung cancer* (NSCLC). Although the precise molecular developments that cause the pathogenesis of carcinoma of the lung have not been completely described, interruption of tumor initiation and promotion may play a role in the treatment and prevention of lung cancer. Current strategies under investigation include administration of adoptive immunotherapy, delivery of monoclonal antibodies, development of antimetastatic immunization, and modulation of oncogene expression.

ONCOGENES

Lung cancer cells exhibit a large number and type of chromosomal lesions, up to 20 genetic lesions per tumor (Whang-Peng et al., 1991). Multiple nonrandom breaks involving chromosomes 1, 3, 7, 15, and 17 have been demonstrated (Mulshine et al., 1993). Genetic transformations involved in the development of carcinoma of the lung—gene amplification, mutation, or deletion—produce activation of dominant proto-oncogenes and the inactivation of recessive oncogenes (Ihde and Minna, 1991).

Dominant Oncogenes

Dominant oncogenes are the mutated forms of the cellular genes (proto-oncogenes) that control cellular proliferation. The involved genes affect growth factors, growth factor receptors, membrane proteins associated with signal transduction, and nuclear proteins involved in transcriptional control and gene expression (Varmus, 1989). Even dominant oncogenes require the cooperation of more than one oncogene to transform normal cells. The involvement of dominant oncogenes has been demonstrated in many malignancies, including carcinoma of the lung.

Point mutations in human lung cancer have been demonstrated in the *ras* family of proto-oncogenes, which includes N-*ras,* K-*ras,* and H-*ras.* The *ras* family of proto-oncogenes encode the membrane-associated *guanosine triphosphate* (GTP)-binding proteins involved in signal transduction, and the mutations induce structural changes within the *ras* gene product to produce an activated protein that constitutively binds GTP (Mulshine et al., 1993). Cytogenic analyses have demonstrated that *ras* family mutations occur in 15 to 35% of patients with NSCLC (Ihde and Minna, 1991; Mitsudomi et al., 1992). These *ras* mutations are found in all histologic types of NSCLC; however, they have not been detected in SCLC. The presence of the *ras* mutation is associated with shorter overall survival and disease-free survival, compared with patients in whom no *ras* mutation has been identified (Slebos et al., 1990).

Another family of oncogenes mutated in human lung cancer is the *erb* B family, which includes *erb* B1 and *erb* B2 (also called Her-2/*neu*). The *erb* B family of proto-oncogenes encode membrane-associated tyrosine kinases that function as growth-factor receptors. The *erb* B1 proto-oncogene is amplified in all histologic variants of NSCLC, including 90% of squamous cell carcinomas and 20 to 75% of adenocarcinomas (Cline and Battifora, 1987). In addition, *erb* B1 is overexpressed in up to 20% of small-cell tumors.

Transcriptional activation of the *myc* family of nuclear proto-oncogenes (c-*myc,* N-*myc,* L-*myc*) also has been demonstrated. The *myc* nuclear proto-oncogenes are activated by overexpression of cellular proto-oncogenes, causing overexpression of the *myc* proteins. The gene products of the *myc* family of oncogenes are nuclear phosphoproteins that are involved in cell-cycle regulation (Cook et al., 1993). The *myc* family of oncogenes is more frequently expressed abnormally in SCLC cells than in NSCLC cells (Little et al., 1983). Small-cell lung tumors with c-*myc* amplified tumors have a poorer prognosis than do other small-cell tumors among patients with advanced-stage SCLC (Wong et al., 1986).

Other dominant oncogenes that are involved in lung cancer include the *raf* family, the *jun* family, and the *src*-related tyrosine kinase oncogenes (Mulshine et al., 1993).

Recessive Oncogenes

The loss, inactivation, or transformation of the genes that suppress cellular proliferation may permit unregulated growth and contribute to the pathogenesis of lung cancer (Marshall, 1991). Such genes are called *recessive oncogenes* (because both genes are deleted or mutated in transformed cells) or *tumor suppressor genes* (because the untransformed genes suppress cellular proliferation).

The retinoblastoma (Rb) gene was the first recessive oncogene to be identified and cloned (Knudson,

1971). The Rb gene has been mapped to the long arm of chromosome 13 (Friend et al., 1986), and the gene product is a phosphoprotein that is involved in cell-cycle regulation (Marshall, 1991). The Rb gene has been demonstrated to be mutated or deleted in up to 60% of SCLC primary tumors and SCLC cell lines (Harbour et al., 1988; Yokota et al., 1988). Furthermore, defective Rb gene product has been discovered in 95% of NSCLC tumors and 20% of NSCLC cell lines (Horowitz et al., 1989).

Mutations of the p53 gene, a tumor suppressor gene that normally codes for a nuclear phosphoprotein required to maintain a transformed (malignant) phenotype, are the most common genetic alteration identified in human cancer (Birrer and Minna, 1988). Recent studies demonstrate that the p53 protein may function by regulation of DNA transcription (Kern et al., 1992). Normal (wild-type) p53 negatively regulates cell growth; mutated forms stimulate cell division and promote malignancy (Finlay et al., 1989). Mutations in p53 have been found in nearly all cell lines from patients with SCLC (D'Amico et al., 1992) and in approximately 50% of cell lines from patients with NSCLC (Chiba et al., 1990). No association has been identified between the presence of p53 mutation and survival (Johnson and Kelley, 1993).

Restrictive fragment length polymorphism analysis has demonstrated 3p, 5q, 9p, 11p, 13q, and 17p allele loss in many cases of carcinoma of the lung (Cook et al., 1993). The most prominent lesion occurs in the 3p21 region, demonstrated in 90% of SCLC cells and up to 79% of NSCLC cells (Brauch et al., 1987; Hibi et al., 1992). The recessive oncogene encoded in the short arm of chromosome 3 has not been definitively identified, but candidates include a beta-retinoic acid receptor gene, the zinc finger-containing genes, and the *PTP*-gamma gene (Croce, 1991). This deletion is found in all histologic types of lung cancer, suggesting either a common requirement for development or an early step in the pathogenesis of lung cancer.

The deletion or mutation of recessive oncogenes is frequently demonstrated in NSCLC and SCLC. The Rb gene abnormalities, p53 gene mutations, and loss of chromosome 3p may be critical occurrences in the transformation on bronchial epithelial cells into lung cancer; they are molecular events in the initiation of the cellular malignant transformation.

GENETIC INTERACTIONS

Evidence is accumulating that some of the genetic changes observed in the development of lung cancer may be inherited. First-degree relatives of lung cancer patients have a strongly increased risk (by 2.4 times) of cancer or other malignant neoplasms (Ihde and Minna, 1991). Furthermore, lung cancer patients, when cured, have a significant risk of second malignancies. Also, patients with other malignancies have an increased risk of carcinoma of the lung.

Investigations have revealed the importance of genetic interrelationships in the expression of the phenotype of lung cancer (Carney, 1992). In a study of 29 human adenocarcinomas of the lung, *erb* B2 was overexpressed in 93% (Bongiorno et al., 1994). Moreover, K-*ras* mutations were detected in 7 tumors (24%), all of which overexpressed *erb* B2; abnormal p53 was demonstrated in 11 tumors (38%), all of which also overexpressed *erb* B2. The presence of the K-*ras* mutations did not correlate with mutation of p53.

Several studies have demonstrated that after long-term culture of lung cancer cell lines, SCLC can transform into any of the NSCLC histologic types. Mabry and colleagues (1991) demonstrated that the cooperation between oncogenes may be necessary in this transition. The transformation of SCLC to NSCLC is accompanied by a change in growth pattern, tumorigenicity, histology, and enzyme content. These findings suggest a common precursor cell in the development of lung cancer, and they support clinical observations of the transformation of small-cell lung cancer to that of another histologic type. The concept of a pluripotential stem cell also explains the finding that many lung tumors demonstrate two or more histologic patterns when multiple sections are examined (Goodman and Livingston, 1989).

THERAPY

Various forms of immunologic modulation have been designed to prevent and treat lung cancer. The strategies for therapeutic intervention at the cellular and molecular levels include administering adoptive immunotherapy, delivering monoclonal antibodies, developing antimetastatic vaccination, and modulating oncogene expression.

Adoptive Immunotherapy

Adoptive immunotherapy with *lymphokine-activated killer* (LAK) cells and high-dose systemic *interleukin-2* (IL-2) has achieved tumor regression in some patients with advanced malignant disease (Rosenberg et al., 1987; West et al., 1988) but has not been effective in patients with NSCLC (Kradin et al., 1987). *Tumor necrosis factor alpha* (TNF) and IL-2 have poor antitumor activity as single agents, yet are synergistic for LAK activation (McIntosh et al., 1988; Owen-Schaub et al., 1988). In a study from the National Cancer Institute, the synergistic activation of LAK, using the combination of low-dose IL-2 and TNF, enhanced oncolytic activity against NSCLC tumor targets when compared with IL-2 alone (Yang et al., 1989). Another study assessed the clinical toxicities and immunomodulatory effects of TNF and IL-2 in 16 patients with advanced NSCLC (Yang et al., 1990). Tumor regression was measurable in 4 patients, and disease was stabilized before progressing in 7 patients. LAK activity was augmented during therapy in all patients. The combination of IL-2 and TNF is biologically more active than either agent alone and may involve long-term stimulation of the immune system.

Monoclonal Antibodies

Generation of monoclonal antibodies using cell-hybridization has been used to produce specific molecular probes in the analysis of tumor cells (Stein and Goldenberg, 1991). Characterization of tumor-associated antigens may provide a new approach to tumor-specific diagnosis and therapy. Tumor-associated antigens are expressed at significantly higher levels in neoplastic cells than in normal cells and may be used for site-directed delivery of therapy, including chemotherapy, radioisotopes, or elements of the antibody-dependent cellular cytotoxicity and complement-mediated toxicity cascades.

Vinca alkaloids have been conjugated to monoclonal antibodies. Application of these conjugates to nude mice bearing human xenografts of adenocarcinoma (Bumol et al., 1989) and squamous cell carcinoma (Johnson et al., 1988) of the lung demonstrated significant growth suppression and tumor regression. The vinca alkaloid conjugates were more efficient than either free drug or free antibodies, whether administered alone or in combination. The use of vinca alkaloid–monoclonal antibody conjugates in humans has thus far been limited by dose-dependent gastrointestinal toxicity and the human antimouse antibody response.

Radioisotopes also have been conjugated to monoclonal antibodies. ^{131}I–monoclonal antibody conjugates delivered to nude mice bearing human adenocarcinoma of the lung demonstrated tumor suppression and tumor regression (Stein and Goldenberg, 1991). However, after cessation of therapy, tumor growth resumed.

Although no totally specific monoclonal antibody against human lung cancer has been developed, the tumor-associated antibodies that have been produced may aid understanding of the molecular biology of lung cancer. A large panel of specific antibodies against lung cancer–associated antigens has been developed; these antibodies may be applied to tumor imaging, conjugation to radioisotopes, or conjugation to chemotherapeutic agents. The development of recombinant human monoclonal antibodies will obviate the limitations of the human antimouse response.

Tumor Immunization

Tumor-bearing animals have been vaccinated by introducing the interferon-gamma (IFN-gamma) gene into tumor cells through retroviral vectors (Porgador et al., 1993). IFN-gamma is an immunomodulatory cytokine that is produced by activated T lymphocytes. IFN-gamma augments the immune response by increasing the cellular antigen-presenting capacity and helps to mediate the inflammatory response by activating macrophages (Nathan and Yoshida, 1988). Direct administration of IFN-gamma to tumor-bearing animals produces antitumor activity (Fidler, 1980). However, adequate IFN-gamma levels—necessary to provide sustained antitumor activity—require constant infusions or repeated administrations (Cantell et al., 1984).

In an experimental study from the Memorial Sloan-Kettering Cancer Center, the insertion (using retroviral vectors) of the IFN-gamma gene into tumor cells of a metastatic, poorly immunogenic murine lung cancer model produced IFN-gamma gene expression and high, sustained serum IFN-gamma levels (Porgador et al., 1993). In this model, immunization of mice carrying an established lung tumor prevented metastatic dissemination. Furthermore, immunization of mice carrying established micrometastases produced significant regression of disease. The use of IFN-gamma transferred tumor cells, by providing high, sustained levels of serum IFN-gamma, may help in the treatment of advanced lung cancer.

Modulation of Oncogene Expression

Modulation of oncogene expression has heretofore been considered an ineffective method of treating carcinoma of the lung, because most lung cancer cells have multiple genetic abnormalities at the time of diagnosis. Recent studies, however, have demonstrated that it may not be necessary to reverse all of the genetic transformations in a lung cancer cell in order to be effective (Roth, 1994).

Several strategies have been described to interfere with the expression of abnormal oncogenes. The antisense technique uses a nucleotide sequence that complements the target mRNA in order to interfere with the translation of the abnormal protein (oncogene product) of the endogenous mRNA. The antisense approach is limited by its reliance on a continuous supply of the appropriate nucleotide sequence in order to interfere with the expression of the abnormal protein. However, if a recombinant construct expressing the antisense sequence becomes part of the cell genome, the antisense mRNA will be continuously produced.

The antisense technique has been investigated in a model of human lung cancer cells (Mukhopadhyay et al., 1991). An antisense K-ras RNA construct was made to interfere with production of abnormal protein (p21) in an NSCLC cell line to determine the contribution of this abnormal gene product to the development of the malignant phenotype. K-ras inhibition reduced the growth rate of malignant cells but did not abolish the growth or alter the malignant phenotype of the cells. These findings suggest that redundancy in the p21 expression by other oncogenic members of the ras family may compensate for the interference of one particular member (K-ras).

Nucleotide sequences that specifically inhibit expression of oncogenes may be delivered by viral vectors. Retroviral vectors have been implemented, which have the advantage of being incorporated in the genome of replicating cells exclusively, favoring integration into cancer-cell DNA. Replication-defective retroviral vectors become integrated into the host genome and produce the protein encoded by the vector but do not replicate the virus. In one study, human lung cancer cells were delivered to immunosuppressed mice (Georges et al., 1993). After the tumors were established, mice were inoculated with retroviral vectors, either with or without the antisense sequence. Tumor growth was suppressed in the group that received retrovirus expressing the antisense K-ras construct. A clinical protocol has been designed to test the efficacy of retroviral antisense K-ras constructs in inhibiting the growth of incompletely resected lung cancer (Roth, 1994).

SUMMARY

Mutations in dominant and recessive oncogenes contribute to the pathogenesis of carcinoma of the lung. Some oncogenic mutations are associated with shorter overall survival and disease-free survival, compared with patients in whom no mutations have been identified. Advances in the understanding of the molecular biology of lung cancer contribute to the development of strategies for cancer prevention and treatment. Strategies that incorporate advances in the immunologic basis of carcinoma of the lung include administration of adoptive immunotherapy, delivery of monoclonal antibodies, development of antimetastatic immunization, and modulation of oncogene expression.

SELECTED BIBLIOGRAPHY

Birrer, M. J., and Minna, J. D.: Molecular genetics of lung cancer. Semin. Oncol., 15:759, 1988.
This concise review summarizes the molecular genetics of carcinoma of the lung.

Carney, D. N.: The biology of lung cancer. Curr. Opin. Oncol., 4:292, 1992.
General overview of the biologic properties of carcinoma of the lung.

Cook, R. M., Miller, Y. E., and Bunn, P. A., Jr.: Small cell lung cancer: Etiology, biology, clinical features, staging, and treatment. Curr. Probl. Cancer, 17:74, 1993.
This monograph encompasses the etiology, molecular biology, staging, and treatment of small-cell lung cancer.

Ihde, D. C., and Minna, J. D.: Non-small-cell lung cancer. Curr. Probl. Cancer, 15:65, 1991.
This superb monograph presents the current understanding of the molecular biology of non-small-cell lung cancer.

Marshall, C. J.: Tumor suppressor genes. Cell, 64:313, 1991.
Comprehensive overview of the role of recessive oncogenes in the pathogenesis of cancer.

Mulshine, J. L., Treston, A. M., Brown, P. H., et al.: Initiators and promoters of lung cancer. Chest, 103:4S, 1993.
A comprehensive review of the molecular biology of lung cancer, the article emphasizes tumor initiation and promotion.

Roth, J. A.: Modulation of oncogene and tumor-suppressor gene expression: A novel strategy for cancer prevention and treatment. Ann. Surg. Oncol., 1:79, 1994.
This review describes the role of the modulation of oncogenes in the prevention and treatment of cancer.

BIBLIOGRAPHY

Birrer, M. J., and Minna, J. D.: Molecular genetics of lung cancer. Semin. Oncol., 15:759, 1988.

Bongiorno, P. F., Whyte, R. I., Lesser, E. J., et al.: Alterations of K-ras, p53, and erb B-2/neu in human lung adenocarcinomas. J. Thorac. Cardiovasc. Surg., 107:590, 1994.

Brauch, H., Johnson, B., Hovis, J., et al.: Molecular analysis of the short arm of chromosome 3 in small cell and non-small cell carcinoma of the lung. N. Engl. J. Med., 317:1109, 1987.

Bumol, T. F., DeHerdt, S. V., Zimmerman, D. L., and Apelgren, L. D.: Monoclonal antibody-oncolytic drug conjugates for site-directed therapy of human adenocarcinomas. Proc. Am. Assoc. Cancer. Res., 30:647, 1989.

Cantell, K., Fiers, W., Hirvonen, S., and Pyhala, L.: Circulating interferon in rabbits after simultaneous intramuscular administration of human alpha and gamma interferons. J. Interferon Res., 4:291, 1984.

Carney, D. N.: The biology of lung cancer. Curr. Opin. Oncol., 4:292, 1992.

Chiba, I., Takahashi, T., Nau, M. M., et al.: Mutations in the p53 gene are frequent in primary, resected non-small cell lung cancer. Oncogene, 5:1603, 1990.

Cline, M. J., and Battifora, H.: Abnormalities of protooncogenes in non-small cell lung cancer: Correlations with tumor type and clinical characteristics. Cancer, 60:2669, 1987.

Cook, R. M., Miller, Y. E., and Bunn, P. A., Jr.: Small cell lung cancer: Etiology, biology, clinical features, staging, and treatment. Curr. Probl. Cancer, 17:74, 1993.

Croce, C. M.: Genetic approaches to the study of the molecular basis of human cancer. Cancer Res., 51(Suppl.):5015s, 1991.

D'Amico, D., Carbone, D., Mitsudomi, T., et al.: High frequency of somatically acquired p53 mutations in small cell lung cancer cell lines and tumors. Oncogene, 7:339, 1992.

Fidler, I. J.: Therapy of spontaneous metastases by intravenous injection of liposomes containing lymphokines. Science, 208:1469, 1980.

Finlay, C. A., Hinds, P. W., and Levine, A. J.: The p53 proto-oncogene can act as a suppressor of transformation. Cell, 57:1083, 1989.

Friend, S. H., Bernards, R., Rogelj, S., et al.: A human DNA segment with properties of the gene that predisposes to retinoblastoma and osteosarcoma. Nature, 323:643, 1986.

Georges, R. N., Mukhopadhyay, T., Zhang, Y. J., et al.: Prevention of orthotopic human lung cancer growth by intratracheal instillation of a retroviral antisense K-ras construct. Cancer Res., 53:1743, 1993.

Goodman, G. E., and Livingston, R. B.: Small cell lung cancer. Curr. Probl. Cancer, 13:7, 1989.

Harbour, J. W., Lai, S. L., Whang-Peng, J., et al.: Abnormalities in structure and expression of the human retinoblastoma gene in SCLC. Science, 241:353, 1988.

Hibi, K., Takahashi, T., Yamakama, K., et al.: Three distinct regions involved in 3p deletion in human lung cancer. Oncogene, 7:445, 1992.

Horowitz, J. M., Park, S. H., Bogenmann, E., et al.: Point mutational inactivation of the retinoblastoma antioncogene. Science, 243:937, 1989.

Ihde, D. C., and Minna, J. D.: Non-small cell lung cancer. Curr. Probl. Cancer, 15:65, 1991.

Johnson, B. E., and Kelley, M. J.: Overview of genetic and molecular events in the pathogenesis of lung cancer. Chest, 103:1S, 1993.

Johnson, D. A., Zimmermann, J. L., Laguzza, B. C., and Eble, J. N.: In vivo antitumor activity demonstrated with squamous carcinoma reactive monoclonal antibody-vinca immunoconjugates. Cancer Immunol. Immunother., 27:241, 1988.

Kern, S. E., Pietenpol, J. A., Thiagalingam, S., et al.: Oncogenic forms of p53 inhibit p53-regulated gene expression. Science, 256:827, 1992.

Knudson, A. G.: Mutation and cancer: Statistical study of retinoblastoma. Proc. Natl. Acad. Sci. U. S. A., 68:820, 1971.

Kradin, R. L., Boyle, L. A., Preffer, F. I., et al.: Tumor-derived interleukin-2 dependent lymphocytes in adoptive immunotherapy of lung cancer. Cancer Immunol. Immunother., 24:76, 1987.

Little, C., Nau, M., Carney, D., et al.: Amplification and expression of the c-myc oncogene in human small cell lung cancer. Nature, 318:69, 1983.

Mabry, M., Nelkin, B. D., Falco, J. P., et al.: Transitions between lung cancer phenotypes: Implications for tumour progression. Cancer Cells, 3:53, 1991.

Marshall, C. J.: Tumor suppressor genes. Cell, 64:313, 1991.

McIntosh, A. K., Mule, J. J., Merino, S. J., and Rosenberg, S. A.: Synergistic antitumor effects of immunotherapy with recombinant interleukin-2 and recombinant tumor necrosis factor-α. Cancer Res., 48:4011, 1988.

Mitsudomi, T., Viallet, J., Linnoila, R. I., et al.: Mutations of the ras genes distinguish a subset of non-small cell lung cancer cell lines from small cell lung cancer cell lines. Oncogene, 6:1353, 1991.

Mukhopadhyay, T., Tainsky, M., Cavender, A. C., et al.: Specific inhibition of K-ras expression and tumorigenicity of lung cancer cells by antisense RNA. Cancer Res., 51:1744, 1991.

Mulshine, J. L., Treston, A. M., Brown, P. H., et al.: Initiators and promoters of lung cancer. Chest, 103:4S, 1993.

Nathan, C., and Yoshida, R.: Cytokines: Interferon-gamma. In Gallin, J. I., Goldstein, I. M., and Snyderman, R. (eds): Inflammation: Basic Principles and Clinical Correlates. New York, Raven Press, 1988.

Owen-Schaub, L. B., Gutterman, J. U., and Grimm, E. A.: Synergy of tumor necrosis factor and interleukin-2 in the activation of human cytotoxic lymphocytes. Cancer Res., 48:788, 1988.

Porgador, A., Bannerji, R., Watanabe, Y., et al.: Antimetastatic vaccination of tumor-bearing mice with two types of IFN-γ gene-inserted tumor cells. J. Immunol., 150:1458, 1993.

Rosenberg, S. A., Lotze, M. T., Muul, L. M., et al.: A progress report on the treatment of 157 patients with advanced cancer using lymphokine-activated killer cells and interleukin-2 or high dose interleukin-2 alone. N. Engl. J. Med., 316:889, 1987.

Roth, J. A.: Modulation of oncogene and tumor-suppressor gene expression: A novel strategy for cancer prevention and treatment. Ann. Surg. Oncol., 1:79, 1994.

Slebos, R. J. C., Kibbelaar, R. E., Dalesio, O., et al.: K-ras oncogene activation as a prognostic marker in adenocarcinoma of the lung. N. Engl. J. Med., 323:561, 1990.

Stein, R., and Goldenberg, D. M.: Prospects for the management of non-small cell carcinoma of the lung with monoclonal antibodies. Chest, 99:1466, 1991.

Varmus, H.: An historical overview of oncogenes. In Weinberg, R. (ed): Oncogenes and the molecular origins of cancer. New York, Cold Spring Harbor Lab Press, 1989.

West, W. H., Tayer, K. W., Yannelli, J. R., et al.: Constant infusion recombinant interleukin-2 in adoptive immunotherapy of advanced cancer. N. Engl. J. Med., 316:898, 1987.

Whang-Peng, J., Knutsen, T., Gazdar, A., et al.: Non-random structural and numerical changes in non-small cell lung cancer. Genes Chromosomes Cancer, 3:168, 1991.

Wong, A. J., Ruppert, J. M., Eggleston, J., et al.: Gene amplification of c-myc and N-myc in small cell carcinoma of the lung. Science, 223:461, 1986.

Yang, S., Owen-Schaub, L., Grimm, E., and Roth, J.: Induction of lymphokine-activated killer (LAK) activity with interleukin-2 and tumor necrosis factor-alpha against fresh primary lung cancer targets. Cancer Immunol. Immunother., 29:193, 1989.

Yang, S. C., Owen-Schaub, L., Mendiguren-Rodriguez, A., et al.: Combination immunotherapy for non-small cell lung cancer. J. Thorac. Cardiovasc. Surg., 99:8, 1990.

Yokota, J., Akiyama, T., Fung, Y., et al.: Altered expression of the retinoblastoma (RB) gene in small cell carcinoma of the lung. Oncogene, 3:471, 1988.

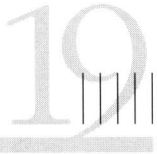

■ V Surgical Management of Pulmonary Metastases

Thomas A. D'Amico and David C. Sabiston, Jr.

The appearance of a solitary pulmonary nodule or multiple pulmonary nodules on the chest film of a patient with a known primary malignancy suggests pulmonary metastatic disease. Autopsy studies have demonstrated that the lungs are the solitary site of metastasis in 20% of patients who die of metastatic pulmonary disease, indicating that surgical resection of pulmonary metastases may prolong life (Farrell, 1935). Many studies have concluded that patients with pulmonary metastases may benefit from complete resection, because systemic therapy for metastatic disease is ineffective.

HISTORICAL ASPECTS

Barney and Churchill (1939) were the first to perform pulmonary resection for metastatic disease, a lobectomy for renal cell carcinoma in a 55-year-old woman. The patient survived for 23 years. Blalock (1944) reported the first pulmonary resection for metastatic adenocarcinoma of the colon. In 1947, Alexander and Haight reported the benefit of surgical resection of solitary pulmonary metastases in patients with primary carcinoma or sarcoma. Martini and associates (1971) reported results in the treatment of patients with metastatic sarcoma, and this successful approach to pulmonary metastases contributed to broadening the indications for pulmonary resection for metastatic disease (McCormack and Martini, 1979). Pulmonary metastases have been resected in a variety of malignant histologies, including primary neoplasms of the breast, kidney, testis, uterus, colon and rectum, muscle, bone, and skin.

PATHOGENESIS

The pathogenesis of metastatic dissemination of a primary malignancy into the lung has not been thoroughly demonstrated. It is known that infiltration of a primary malignancy into contiguous lymphatic channels is responsible for metastases into lymph nodes, and infiltration into local capillary beds leads to blood-borne metastases. Disseminated neoplastic cells may be deposited into the lungs through the pulmonary arteries, yet the nature of the favorable environment for the seeding and growth of metastatic disease is not well understood (McCormack, 1990). Tumor cells are usually deposited in the periphery of the pulmonary parenchyma; however, metastases may also reach the lung via the bronchial circulation and present as endobronchial lesions. A pulmonary metastasis may itself metastasize, through infiltration into lymphatic channels. The resection of pulmonary metastases may prevent further neoplastic dissemination.

DIAGNOSIS

Because most metastatic lesions are asymptomatic, routine chest films are essential in the care of patients with malignancy. After a probable pulmonary metastasis is recognized, *computed tomography* (CT) of the chest confirms the size and number of nodules present. The limit of resolution of CT is approximately 3 mm; however, not all of the nodules identified on CT will prove to be malignant (Cheng et al., 1979). In addition, CT may underestimate the number of malignant foci by 40 to 85% (Swoboda and Tomes, 1986).

Percutaneous biopsy of potential pulmonary metastases may be performed before pulmonary resection. The findings on needle biopsy usually do not alter management, and percutaneous biopsy is recommended only if an alternative method of treatment is available or if the patient is a poor operative risk (McCormack, 1990). As in the management of primary lung cancer, resection of the nodule is preferred if the patient meets the criteria for thoracotomy and resection.

A solitary lesion is more likely to be metastatic if the known primary lesion is sarcoma or melanoma (Johnson et al., 1982). In a patient whose primary tumor is from the breast or the head and neck, a solitary pulmonary lesion is more likely to be primary lung cancer. In a patient with primary tumor of gastrointestinal or genitourinary origin, a solitary pulmonary lesion has an equal chance of being primary or metastatic (Cahan et al., 1974).

CRITERIA FOR RESECTION

The criteria for resection of pulmonary metastases were first described by Ehrenhaft and associates

(1958) and are now well established. To proceed with pulmonary resection of metastases, local control of the primary tumor must be achieved; metastatic disease must be confined to the lung; and the patient must be able to tolerate resection of the requisite pulmonary parenchyma with adequate residual pulmonary function (McCormack and Martini, 1979). Resection should then be undertaken only if complete resection is possible and no superior therapy is available (McCormack, 1990). If the metastatic lesion is discovered in the lung at the same time that a local recurrence is detected, control of the recurrence is usually undertaken first to prevent further metastases. If the primary tumor and the pulmonary metastasis are discovered concurrently, pulmonary resection may be undertaken first in some cases, if local control of the primary tumor will be immediate and the possibility of complete pulmonary resection is uncertain.

Other factors may be considered in selecting patients who are most likely to benefit from pulmonary resection. Although reports vary, analysis of prognostic indicators in patients with pulmonary metastases indicates that survival is enhanced in patients with a longer disease-free interval, longer tumor doubling time, complete resectability, and certain primary histologic pictures. Age and sex are not important prognostic indicators. Analysis of the effect of prognostic indicators among patients with the same histology may more precisely predict the benefit of pulmonary resection for metastatic disease (Putnam and Roth, 1990).

Local Control of the Primary Tumor

Resection of pulmonary metastases should not be performed until the primary neoplasm has been surgically managed. Patients who have undergone limited rather than curative resection of the primary malignancy or who have not undergone the primary resection with clear margins usually are not candidates for resection of pulmonary metastases.

Metastases Confined to the Lung

Tumors must be completely staged according to the histology of the primary tumor before resection of disease metastatic to the lung; the common routes of systemic spread for each histologic subtype are considered and appropriately screened. Virtually all studies have demonstrated that complete resectability is the major factor correlated with improved survival in patients with pulmonary metastases (Putnam and Roth, 1990). Pulmonary metastases may recur in the lungs following resection, and resection of the new pulmonary metastases improves survival compared with patients with unresectable recurrent metastases (Rizzoni et al., 1986).

Disease-Free Interval

Some studies have shown that the disease-free interval—the time from the treatment of the primary tumor to the recognition of the metastasis—correlates with survival, but other reports disagree. A disease-free interval of more than 12 months was a positive prognostic indicator in patients with soft tissue sarcomas in several studies (Jablons et al., 1989; Putnam et al., 1984; Roth et al., 1985). Patients with pulmonary metastases from osteogenic sarcoma demonstrated a survival advantage with a disease-free interval more than 6 months in one study (Putnam et al., 1983), whereas several studies have shown no such advantage (Meyer et al., 1987; Roth et al., 1985). In patients with colorectal carcinoma, a disease-free interval of more than 24 months has been associated with prolonged survival (Brister et al., 1988; Mansel et al., 1986); however, two other studies demonstrated no such survival advantage (Goya et al., 1989; McCormack and Attiyeh, 1979). Disease-free interval, therefore, is an uncertain prognostic indicator in patients with pulmonary metastases. This index may vary in importance according to the histology of the primary malignancy, but it is not used to exclude patients from resection. Further studies are warranted to determine the power of disease-free interval as a prognostic indicator.

Tumor Doubling Time

Tumor doubling time has been suggested as a measure of the aggressiveness of pulmonary metastases. In one study, mean survival was significantly better in patients with tumor doubling time longer than 40 days, compared with patients with tumor doubling times of 20 to 40 days (Joseph et al., 1971). Because multiple metastatic lesions may not grow at the same rate, the fastest-growing nodule is used as the index for tumor doubling time. The use of tumor doubling time as a prognostic indicator usually requires a period of observation before resection, which necessarily delays treatment, albeit for a short time. Tumor doubling time may serve as a prognostic indicator in patients with multiple pulmonary metastases who are under observation for the appearance of new nodules before resection; however, tumor doubling time is not used to deny operation if complete resection is possible.

Number of Pulmonary Metastases

Various authors have investigated the prognostic significance of the number of nodules in patients with pulmonary metastatic disease. Ramming (1980) reported significantly better survival among patients with one or two nodules. Putnam and associates (1983) found that survival was not influenced unless more than four nodules were present. Although studies are divided over whether the number of metastatic lesions influences survival, a report from the National Institutes of Health stated that the number of lesions is not important for estimating outcome among patients with resectable disease (Jablons et al., 1989). However, the timing of surgical intervention is affected in patients in whom the number of pulmonary metastases exceeds five. In this circumstance, it is recommended that the patient be observed for 3 to 6 months. At that time, follow-up CT determines whether additional metastatic disease has developed. If the acknowledged lesions grow in the absence of new metastases, an aggressive surgical approach is indicated (Todd, 1993).

The presence of bilateral lesions, as in the case of multiple unilateral metastases, suggests a greater tumor burden and more advanced stage of metastases. However, if other selection criteria are observed, surgical resection may be beneficial (Putnam et al., 1984). Most authors agree that the completeness of resection is the most important indicator of survival. Regardless of the number of lesions, the resection must include all pulmonary metastases; there is no role for partial resection of metastatic lesions.

Primary Tumor Histology

The pattern of metastatic dissemination and the benefit derived from pulmonary resection is related to the histology of the primary tumor. For example, the clinical course of renal cell carcinoma is characterized by long disease-free intervals and a high incidence of metastatic disease confined to the lung. In contrast, the distant spread of melanoma frequently extends to multiple organs simultaneously, and the chance of finding disease confined to the lung is remote. Among patients with sarcomas, those with osteogenic sarcoma, fibrosarcoma, and chondrosarcoma are often candidates for resection of pulmonary metastases, yet few patients with Ewing's sarcoma, in which the disease frequently showers the lungs bilaterally, are candidates for resection. Patients with the least favorable histologic subtypes should be screened most carefully before resection (Ramming, 1980).

SURGICAL TECHNIQUE

Resection of pulmonary metastases should remove all tumor while sparing the maximum amount of pulmonary parenchyma. In contrast to the resection of primary carcinoma of the lung, wedge resections are accomplished whenever possible for metastatic disease. With subpleural lesions, such as sarcomas, wedge resections are completed with standard stapling devices. For more central lesions, such as carcinomas, resection may involve conization using electrocautery or laser (Casper et al., 1986). Lobectomy or pneumonectomy may be performed if a lesser procedure would not achieve complete resection, and long-term survival has been reported with such procedures

(McCormack et al., 1978). Pulmonary resection with en-bloc resection of the chest wall or other thoracic structures has been reported as well, with long-term survival and minimal morbidity (Putnam et al., 1993).

The entire lung is accessed by standard posterolateral thoracotomy. Thoracoscopy has been suggested in the management of pulmonary metastases. However, thoracoscopic exploration of the chest is currently inferior to manual exploration, and nodules not appreciated preoperatively may be missed. Improved intraoperative localization techniques, such as thoracoscopic ultrasonography, may permit thoracoscopic resection of pulmonary metastases in the future.

In patients with bilateral pulmonary metastases, the procedures may be staged approximately 10 days apart. Alternatively, median sternotomy for bilateral pulmonary resection may be employed, with similar expected morbidity (Roth et al., 1986). Advantages of median sternotomy over staged thoracotomy include the elimination of a second procedure, shorter hospital stay, less postoperative pain, and superior pulmonary function. Exposure to the posterior thorax may be limited through median sternotomy, particularly to the left lower lobe; patients must be selected carefully for this approach.

RESECTION OF PULMONARY METASTASES

Soft Tissue Sarcomas

Soft tissue sarcomas may originate from any anatomic site. Those that arise from an extremity account for more than half of all soft tissue sarcomas and are the most likely to recur initially via distant metastasis (Brennan, 1989). The lung is a common site of metastases from sarcomas, and complete resection offers the best possibility for cure. Despite therapy, only 11% of patients who are candidates for resection of pulmonary metastases survive 3 years (Gadd et al., 1993). Complete resection of pulmonary metastases from soft tissue sarcomas is associated with a 3-year survival rate of 30 to 42% (Casson et al., 1992; Jablons et al., 1989; Putnam et al., 1984; Roth et al., 1985; Verazin et al., 1992). In one study, the 5-year survival rate in patients who underwent pulmonary metastases from soft tissue sarcomas was 25% (Casson et al., 1992). In this study, significant independent prognostic indicators associated with improved survival included doubling time of 40 days or more, unilateral disease, three or fewer nodules, and tumor histology (malignant fibrous histiocytoma superior to all others).

Resection may also be performed for recurrent pulmonary metastases from soft tissue sarcomas. In one study, 89 reexplorations were performed in 43 patients without an operative mortality (Pogrebniak et al., 1991). In this study, 31 patients (72%) were considered free of disease after the second thoracotomy. Median survival from the second thoracotomy among the group of patients who underwent complete resection was 25 months, compared with 10 months among patients whose disease was unresectable. In another study, 37 patients underwent multiple pulmonary resections for recurrent soft tissue sarcoma with no operative mortality and three postoperative complications (Casson et al., 1991). Median survival for those who underwent complete resection at the second thoracotomy was 28 months, compared with 10 months among the patients whose disease was unresectable. Multiple pulmonary resections may be undertaken in patients with recurrent metastases, owing to the absence of other proven therapy. Reexploration is associated with low morbidity and may improve survival.

Combination chemotherapy has produced significant response in patients with metastatic soft tissue sarcoma (Rosenberg et al., 1983), although few patients survive for the long term. In one study, neoadjuvant chemotherapy with doxorubicin, cyclophosphamide, and dacarbazine was administered to 26 patients with pulmonary metastases from adult soft tissue sarcomas; this regimen achieved a complete response in 21% of patients and a partial response in 29% of patients (Lanza et al., 1991). All of the patients who responded completely to the chemotherapy eventually underwent thoracotomy for recurrence of disease in the lung, and all patients with partial or no response to chemotherapy underwent pulmonary resection as well. Among the three groups of patients, there were no significant differences in disease-free or overall survival after thoracotomy. Although chemotherapy may produce complete response in some patients with metastatic soft tissue sarcoma, chemotherapy alone does not achieve long-term disease-free survival, nor does the response to chemotherapy predict postoperative survival. Complete resection and the development of effective adjuvant therapy are essential to improve survival in patients with soft tissue sarcomas and pulmonary metastases.

Osteogenic Sarcomas

Similar to soft tissue sarcomas, osteogenic sarcomas tend to metastasize to the lung. Pulmonary metastases from osteogenic sarcomas are often multiple and recurrent, requiring multiple pulmonary resections for cure. Chemotherapy has been more effective for patients with pulmonary metastases from osteogenic sarcoma than from soft tissue sarcoma, and aggressive regimens of chemotherapy have achieved long-term survival (Mentzer et al., 1993). The 5-year survival rate after pulmonary resection for metastatic osteogenic sarcomas ranges from 20 to 40% (Belli et al., 1989; Mountain et al., 1984; Putnam et al., 1983).

Carcinoma of the Colon and Rectum

Approximately 1000 patients with colorectal adenocarcinoma will develop resectable pulmonary metastases annually (McCormack and Attiyeh, 1979).

McAfee and associates (1992) reported a series of 139 patients who underwent pulmonary resection for metastatic colorectal carcinoma from the Mayo Clinic. Approximately half of the patients were adequately treated by wedge resection, whereas the remainder required lobectomy or pneumonectomy. The number of metastases was a significant predictor of survival: the 5-year survival rate for patients with a single metastasis was 37%, compared with 19% for those with two and 8% for those with more than two metastases. Serum *carcinoembryonic antigen* (CEA) levels also predicted survival. The 5-year survival rate among patients with elevated CEA was 16%, compared with 47% in patients with normal levels.

In another series, the number of pulmonary metastases was an important prognostic indicator among 27 patients who underwent pulmonary resection for metastatic colorectal carcinoma (Yano et al., 1993). Survival did not correlate with disease-free interval, size of metastases, type of pulmonary resection, stage of the primary cancer, or location of the primary tumor. The presence of resectable hepatic metastases was not a contraindication to pulmonary resection in this series, and the cumulative 5-year survival rate for patients with hepatic metastases did not differ from that of the other patients.

Patients with a history of colorectal carcinoma may develop a solitary pulmonary nodule, and preoperative diagnostic evaluation may not be successful in differentiating primary lung cancer from pulmonary metastatic disease. If there is no evidence of extrathoracic metastatic disease and if the patient is otherwise an operative candidate, thoracotomy for pulmonary resection is performed—the appropriate therapy for either malignancy. Pulmonary resection is achieved with minimal morbidity and with the potential for long-term survival.

Renal Cell Carcinoma

Renal cell carcinoma accounts for approximately 4% of all adult malignancies (Boring et al., 1994); half of all patients with renal cell carcinoma will eventually develop pulmonary metastases (Pogrebniak et al., 1992). The 5-year survival rate for patients who have undergone resection of metastases from renal cell carcinoma ranges from 13% (Dineen et al., 1988) to 50% (Mountain et al., 1978). The series from the National Cancer Institute included 23 patients who underwent resection of pulmonary metastases from renal cell carcinoma (Pogrebniak et al., 1992). In this series, 18 of the patients had previously received immunotherapy based on interleukin-2. Patients who underwent complete resection had significantly longer mean survival (49 months) than did patients with incomplete resections (16 months). Survival did not correlate with the number of nodules resected or the disease-free interval. Among the patients who underwent complete resection, there was no significant difference in survival between those whose metastases were synchronous and those whose metastases were metachronous with the primary renal malignancy.

In a series from the Mayo Clinic, 96 patients underwent complete pulmonary resection for metastatic renal cell carcinoma, with no operative deaths (Cerfolio et al., 1994). The 5-year survival rate in patients with single nodules (46%) was significantly greater than that in patients with multiple nodules (27%). In this study, a disease-free interval of 3.5 years or longer was associated with significantly improved survival. Multiple pulmonary resections were performed in 14 patients; the survival rate in this group did not differ from the overall survival rate. No prospective randomized trials address the role of resection of pulmonary metastases from renal cell carcinoma. In the absence of effective chemotherapy, pulmonary resection is recommended in carefully selected patients in whom complete resection is possible.

Carcinoma of the Breast

Breast cancer is the most common solid tumor and second only to lung cancer as a cause of cancer-related deaths among women (Boring et al., 1994). Most patients with breast cancer will develop systemic disease or unresectable metastases. However, approximately 20% will die from isolated, and potentially resectable, metastases to lung (Ramming, 1980).

In a series from the M. D. Anderson Cancer Center, 21 patients underwent pulmonary resection for metastatic breast cancer; the cumulative 5-year survival rate was only 14% (Mountain et al., 1978). In this series, a longer disease-free interval was actually associated with reduced survival. In a series from the Sloan-Kettering Memorial Cancer Center, 34 patients underwent pulmonary resection for metastatic breast cancer (McCormack and Martini, 1979). The median survival was 33 months, and the cumulative 5-year survival rate was 30%.

Lanza and colleagues (1992) reported a series of 44 women who underwent pulmonary resection for metastatic breast cancer. In this series, the median survival was 47 months and the actuarial 5-year survival rate was 49%. Patients with a disease-free interval of more than 12 months had significantly longer median survival time (82 months) than did patients with shorter disease-free intervals (15 months). Survival was not correlated with number of nodules resected, status of the estrogen receptor, or number of axillary lymph nodes. Pulmonary resection for metastatic carcinoma of the breast has been performed with minimal morbidity and may permit long-term survival in carefully selected patients.

Squamous Cell Carcinoma of the Head and Neck

Pulmonary metastases are present in 75% of patients with metastatic squamous cell carcinoma from the head and neck (Papac, 1984). The appearance of a solitary pulmonary nodule on the chest film of a patient with a known primary squamous cell carcinoma of the head and neck must be investigated to determine whether it is a metastatic nodule or a primary lung tumor. Carcinoma in situ in the nodule confirms that the lesion is primary carcinoma of the lung, but a histologic distinction cannot always be made. The current practice is to manage all such lesions as primary lung cancer. In one study, in which 32 patients with squamous cell carcinoma presented with a new pulmonary nodule, 20 patients were found to have primary lung cancer, and 12 patients proved to have metastatic lesions (Judson et al., 1983).

Patients with a history of squamous cell carcinoma of the head and neck may develop a solitary pulmonary nodule, and preoperative diagnostic evaluation may not differentiate primary lung cancer from pulmonary metastatic disease. If there is no evidence of extrathoracic metastatic disease, and if the patient is otherwise an operative candidate, thoracotomy for pulmonary resection is performed with an expected 5-year survival rate of 40 to 50% (Mazer et al., 1988; McCormack, 1990).

Melanoma

Melanoma accounts for 1 to 2% of all cancer-related deaths, and the incidence of melanoma continues to increase (Boring et al., 1994). The lung is the most common initial site of solid organ metastasis (Gromet et al., 1979). Approximately 25% of patients with melanoma will develop pulmonary metastases, but only 5% will be isolated to the lung (Harpole et al., 1992). Nevertheless, selected patients may be candidates for pulmonary resection.

In a series from the M. D. Anderson Cancer Center, 56 patients underwent 65 pulmonary resections for metastatic melanoma with no operative mortality (Gorenstein et al., 1991). Complete resection was achieved in 54 patients (96%), and the 5-year actuarial survival rate was 25%. Survival was not associated with the location of the primary tumor, the histology, the tumor thickness, the Clark level, or the status of regional lymph node metastases. The median survival time among patients in whom the lung was the initial site of recurrence was 30 months, compared with 17 months for patients with regional recurrence.

Harpole and associates (1992) reported the results of a large series from Duke University Medical Center. In this series of 945 patients with pulmonary metastases from melanoma, resection was undertaken in 112 patients, and complete resection was achieved in 98 patients. The median survival time was significantly longer among patients who underwent complete resection (20 months) than among patients who underwent incomplete resection (8 months) or no resection (6 months). The multivariate predictors for improved survival in this study were complete resection, longer disease-free interval, fewer (one or two) pulmonary nodules, and chemotherapy.

After complete metastatic evaluation, patients with

a history of melanoma and a new pulmonary nodule may proceed to thoracotomy and pulmonary resection. Even patients with multiple nodules may benefit from pulmonary resection. Effective chemotherapy is required to improve the outcome of patients in whom resection is not complete.

SUMMARY

Twenty per cent of patients who die of pulmonary metastases are found to have no extrathoracic metastatic disease. Pulmonary resection would have removed life-threatening malignancy in these patients. In addition, resection of pulmonary metastatic disease eliminates a potential source of further metastasis. Resection of pulmonary metastases may be effective in the treatment of many malignancies (Mark, 1993). The overall median survival time in patients after resection of pulmonary metastases is 38 months, compared with 14 months in patients who have unresected pulmonary metastatic disease (McCormack, 1990). The biologic characteristics of pulmonary metastases, which are related to the histology of the primary tumor, may be the most important determinant of patient survival (Moores, 1991). Criteria for the selection of patients for resection of metastases to the lung have been established. Several prognostic indicators are also considered in selecting patients for resection; prognostic indicators, however, differ with tumor histology, and the predictive ability is not constant for all tumors. Although many prognostic indicators correlate with survival, no single criterion should be used to exclude patients from surgical treatment if complete resection is possible.

SELECTED BIBLIOGRAPHY

Casson, A. G., Putnam, J. B., Natarajan, G., et al.: Five-year survival after pulmonary metastasectomy for adult soft tissue sarcoma. Cancer, 69:662, 1992.

Report of a series of patients from the M. D. Anderson Cancer Center who have pulmonary metastases from adult soft tissue sarcoma.

Harpole, D. H., Johnson, C. M., Wolfe, W. G., et al.: Analysis of 945 cases of pulmonary metastatic melanoma. J. Thorac. Cardiovasc. Surg., 103:743, 1992.

The authors present the largest single-institution experience of pulmonary metastatic melanoma. This analysis addresses the risk of pulmonary metastases from cutaneous melanoma, the role of pulmonary resection, and the risk factors for survival.

McCormack, P. M.: Surgical resection of pulmonary metastases. Semin. Surg. Oncol., 6:297, 1990.

This article comprehensively reviews the treatment of pulmonary metastatic disease, including analysis of 415 patients from Memorial Sloan-Kettering Cancer Center.

Mountain, C. F., McMurtrey, M. J., and Hermes, K. E.: Surgery for pulmonary metastases: A 20 year experience. Ann. Thorac. Surg., 38:323, 1984.

Report of a large series of resections for pulmonary metastases from the M. D. Anderson Cancer Center. This study includes an analysis of the outcome of 556 patients and the factors that influence survival.

Putnam, J. B. Jr., and Roth, J. A.: Prognostic indicators in patients with pulmonary metastases. Semin. Surg. Oncol., 6:291, 1990.

This review includes a discussion of the biologic characteristics of pulmo-

nary metastases and a detailed analysis of prognostic indicators in patients with pulmonary metastatic disease.

BIBLIOGRAPHY

Alexander, J., and Haight, C.: Pulmonary resection for solitary metastatic sarcomas and carcinomas. Surg. Gynecol. Obstet., 85:129, 1947.

Barney, J. D., and Churchill, E. J.: Adenocarcinoma of the kidney with metastasis to the lung. J. Urol., 42:269, 1939.

Belli, L., Scholl, A., Livartowski, A., et al.: Resection of pulmonary metastases from osteosarcoma: A retrospective analysis of 44 patients. Cancer, 63:2456, 1989.

Blalock, A.: Recent advances in surgery. N. Engl. J. Med., 231:261, 1944.

Boring, C. C., Squires, T. S., Tong, T., and Montgomery, S.: Cancer statistics, 1994. CA Cancer J. Clin., 44:7, 1994.

Brennan, M. F.: Management of extremity soft tissue sarcoma. Am. J. Surg., 158:71, 1989.

Brister, S. J., DeVarennes, B., Gordon, P. H., et al.: Contemporary operative management of pulmonary metastases of colorectal origin. Dis. Colon Rectum, 31:786, 1988.

Cahan, W. G., Castro, E. B., and Hajdu, S. I.: The significance of a solitary lung shadow in patients with colon carcinoma. Cancer, 33:414, 1974.

Casper, J. D., Perelman, M., Todd, T. R., et al.: Precision cautery excision of pulmonary lesions. Ann. Thorac. Surg., 41:51, 1986.

Casson, A. G., Putnam, J. B., Natarajan, G., et al.: Efficacy of pulmonary metastasectomy for recurrent soft tissue sarcoma. J. Surg. Oncol., 47:1, 1991.

Casson, A. G., Putnam, J. B., Natarajan, G., et al.: Five-year survival after pulmonary metastasectomy for adult soft tissue sarcoma. Cancer, 69:662, 1992.

Cerfolio, R. J., Allen, M. S., Deschamps, C., et al.: Pulmonary resection of metastatic renal cell carcinoma. Ann. Thorac. Surg., 57:339, 1994.

Cheng, A. E., Schaner, E. G., Conkle, D. M., et al.: Evaluation of computed tomography in the detection of pulmonary metastases. Cancer, 43:913, 1979.

Dineen, M. K., Pastore, R. D., Emrich, L. J., and Huben, R. P.: Results of surgical treatment of renal cell carcinoma with solitary metastasis. J. Urol., 140:277, 1988.

Ehrenhaft, J. L., Lawrence, M. S., and Sensenig, D. M.: Pulmonary resection for metastatic lesions. Arch. Surg., 77:606, 1958.

Farrell, J. T.: Pulmonary metastases: Pathological, clinical, roentgenological study based on 78 cases at necropsy. Radiology, 24:444, 1935.

Gadd, M. A., Casper, E. S., Woodruff, J. M., et al.: Development and treatment of pulmonary metastases in adult patients with extremity soft tissue sarcoma. Ann. Surg., 218:705, 1993.

Gorenstein, L. A., Putnam, J. B., Jr., Natarajan, G., et al.: Improved survival after resection of pulmonary metastases from malignant melanoma. Ann. Thorac. Surg., 52:204, 1991.

Goya, T., Miyazawa, N., Kondo, H., et al.: Surgical resection of pulmonary metastases from colorectal cancer: Ten year follow-up. Cancer, 64:1418, 1989.

Gromet, M. A., Ominsky, S. H., Epstein, W. L., and Blois, M. S.: The thorax as the initial site for systemic relapse in malignant melanoma. Cancer, 44:776, 1979.

Harpole, D. H., Johnson, C. M., Wolfe, W. G., et al.: Analysis of 945 cases of pulmonary metastatic melanoma. J. Thorac. Cardiovasc. Surg., 103:743, 1992.

Jablons, D., Steinberg, D. M., and Roth, J. A.: Metastasectomy for soft tissue sarcomas. J. Thorac. Cardiovasc. Surg., 97:695, 1989.

Johnson, H., Fantone, J., and Flye, M. W.: Histologic evaluation of the nodules resected in the treatment of pulmonary metastatic disease. J. Surg. Oncol., 21:1, 1982.

Joseph, W. L., Morton, D. L., and Adkins, P. C.: Prognostic significance of tumor doubling time in evaluating operability in pulmonary metastatic disease. J. Thorac. Cardiovasc. Surg., 61:23, 1971.

Judson, W. F., Harbrecht, P. J., and Fry, D. E.: Associated lung lesions in patients with primary head and neck carcinoma. Am. Surg., 49:487, 1983.

Lanza, L. A., Natarajan, G., Roth, J. A., et al.: Long-term survival after resection of pulmonary metastases from carcinoma of the breast. Ann. Thorac. Surg., 54:244, 1992.

Lanza, L. A., Putnam, J. B., Benjamin, R. S., and Roth, J. A.: Response to chemotherapy does not predict survival after resection of sarcomatous pulmonary metastases. Ann. Thorac. Surg., 51:219, 1991.

Mansel, K. J., Zinsmeister, A. R., Pairolero, P. C., and Jett, J. R.: Pulmonary resection of metastatic colorectal adenocarcinoma. Chest, 91:109, 1986.

Mark, J. B. D.: Surgical treatment of pulmonary metastases: Where do we stand? Ann. Surg., 218:703, 1993.

Martini, N., Huvos, A. G., and Mike, V.: Multiple pulmonary resections in the treatment of osteogenic sarcoma. Ann. Thorac. Surg., 12:271, 1971.

Mazer, T. M., Robbins, K. T., McMurtrey, M. J., et al.: Resection of pulmonary metastases of squamous cell carcinoma of the head and neck. Am. J. Surg., 156:238, 1988.

McAfee, M. K., Allen, M. S., Trastek, V. F., et al.: Colorectal lung metastases: Results of surgical excision. Ann. Thorac. Surg., 53:780, 1992.

McCormack, P. M.: Surgical resection of pulmonary metastases. Semin. Surg. Oncol., 6:297, 1990.

McCormack, P. M., and Attiyeh, F. F.: Resected pulmonary metastases from colorectal cancer. Dis. Colon Rectum, 22:553, 1979.

McCormack, P. M., and Martini, N.: The changing role of surgery for pulmonary metastases. Ann. Thorac. Surg., 28:139, 1979.

McCormack, P. M., Bains, M. S., Beattie, E. J., Jr., et al.: Pulmonary resection in metastatic carcinoma. Chest, 73:163, 1978.

Mentzer, S. J., Antman, K. H., Attinger, C., et al.: Selected benefits of thoracotomy and chemotherapy for sarcoma metastatic to the lung. J. Surg. Oncol., 53:54, 1993.

Meyer, W. H., Schell, M. J., Jumar, P. M., et al.: Thoracotomy for pulmonary metastatic osteosarcoma. An analysis of prognostic indicators. Cancer, 59:374, 1987.

Moores, D. W. O.: Pulmonary metastases revisited. Ann. Thorac. Surg., 52:178, 1991.

Mountain, C. F., Khalil, K. G., Hermes, K. E., and Frazier, O. H.: The contribution of surgery to the management of carcinomatous pulmonary metastases. Cancer, 41:833, 1978.

Mountain, C. F., McMurtrey, M. J., and Hermes, K. E.: Surgery for pulmonary metastases: A 20 year experience. Ann. Thorac. Surg., 38:323, 1984.

Papac, R. J.: Distant metastases from head and neck cancer. Cancer, 53:342, 1984.

Pogrebniak, H. W., Haas, G., Linehan, M., et al.: Renal cell carcinoma: Resection of solitary and multiple metastases. Ann. Thorac. Surg., 54:33, 1992.

Pogrebniak, H. W., Roth, J. A., Steinberg, S. M., et al.: Reoperative pulmonary resection in patients with metastatic soft tissue carcinoma. Ann. Thorac. Surg., 52:197, 1991.

Putnam, J. B., Jr., and Roth, J. A.: Prognostic indicators in patients with pulmonary metastases. Semin. Surg. Oncol., 6:291, 1990.

Putnam, J. B., Jr., Roth, J. A., Wesley, M. N., et al.: Analysis of prognostic factors in patients undergoing resection of pulmonary metastases from soft tissue sarcomas. J. Thorac. Cardiovasc. Surg., 87:260, 1984.

Putnam, J. B., Jr., Roth, J. A., Wesley, M. N., et al.: Survival following aggressive resection of pulmonary metastases from osteogenic sarcoma: Analysis of prognostic factors. Ann. Thorac. Surg., 36:516, 1983.

Putnam, J. B., Jr., Suell, D. M., Natarajan, G., et al.: Extended resection of pulmonary metastases: Is the risk justified. Ann. Thorac. Surg., 55:1440, 1993.

Ramming, K. P.: Surgery for pulmonary metastases. Surg. Clin. North Am., 60:815, 1980.

Rizzoni, W. E., Pass, H. I., Wesley, M. N., et al.: Resection of recurrent pulmonary metastases in patients with soft tissue sarcomas. Arch. Surg., 121:1248, 1986.

Rosenberg, S. A., Tepper, J., Glatstein, E., et al.: Prospective randomized evaluation of adjuvant chemotherapy in adults with soft tissue sarcomas of the extremity. Cancer, 52:424, 1983.

Roth, J. A., Pass, H. I., Wesley, M. N., et al.: Comparison of median sternotomy and thoracotomy for resection of pulmonary metastases in patients with adult soft-tissue sarcomas. Ann. Thorac. Surg., 42:134, 1986.

Roth, J. A., Putnam, J. B., Jr., Wesley, M. N., and Rosenberg, S. A.: Differing determinants of prognosis following resection of pulmonary metastases from osteogenic and soft tissue sarcoma patients. Cancer, 55:1361, 1985.

Swoboda, L., and Tomes, H.: Results of surgical treatment for pulmonary metastases. J. Thorac. Cardiovasc. Surg., 34:149, 1986.

Todd, T. R.: Pulmonary metastasectomy: Current indications for removing lung metastases. Chest, 103(Suppl.):401S, 1993.

Verazin, G. T., Warneke, J. A., Driscoll, D. L., et al.: Resection of lung metastases from soft tissue sarcomas. A multivariate analysis. Arch. Surg., 127:1407, 1992.

Yano, T., Hara, N., Ichinose, Y., et al.: Results of pulmonary resection of metastatic colorectal cancer and its application. J. Thorac. Cardiovasc. Surg., 106:875, 1993.

20

Lung Infections and Diffuse Interstitial Lung Disease

Peter Van Trigt III

This chapter reviews and updates the diagnosis and management of nontuberculous infectious and inflammatory diseases of the chest. Because powerful broad-spectrum antibiotics and effective antifungal agents have been introduced over the last 2 decades, these diseases, like pulmonary tuberculosis, less frequently require intervention by thoracic surgeons. However, in the last few years, fungal and parasitic organisms have become increasingly prevalent in a growing number of immunocompromised patients. The tremendous increase in organ transplantation since the introduction of cyclosporine in the early 1980s has been accompanied by a rising incidence of opportunistic infections in transplant recipients. In addition, aggressive chemotherapy protocols have been initiated and have effectively treated severe lymphoproliferative and neoplastic disease. Finally, the incidence of the *acquired immunodeficiency syndrome* (AIDS) and the wide application of corticosteroids to several collagen-vascular and autoimmune conditions further add to the population of patients at risk for developing these infections, which often are opportunistic (Miller, 1986). Clearly, well-rounded thoracic surgeons must remain familiar with these disorders because they will be required to interact with these patients in several different ways, including providing surgical specimens for diagnosis and definitive therapy for infectious processes that do not respond to medical therapy.

This discussion is necessarily brief because of the diversity of diffuse infiltrative lung diseases. Current concepts of the histopathologic reaction of the lung to these conditions and to the underlying pathophysiology are emphasized.

BRONCHIECTASIS

Bronchiectasis is included in the groups of suppurative diseases of the lungs characterized by dilatation of the bronchi. The condition was first described in 1819 by Laënnec and was especially prevalent in the years before antibiotics became available. Although its overall incidence has declined significantly as a result of effective antimicrobial therapy, bronchiectasis remains an entity with which a thoracic surgeon continues to be involved.

Etiology

The pathogenesis of this disease involves several predisposing factors, both congenital and acquired

(Table 20–1). Although acquired infection of the lungs is commonly the major contributor, congenital factors may also have a role.

Congenital cystic bronchiectasis affects infants and young children (Fig. 20–1). It has been attributed to an arrest in the development of the bronchial tree (Aliabadi and Shafiepoor, 1978), although various congenital immune deficiency states also have played a role. Patients with selective IgA deficiency or with primary hypogammaglobulinemia have been susceptible to bronchiectasis (Chipps et al., 1978; Hilton and Doyle, 1978). Alpha$_1$-antitrypsin deficiency, usually associated with panacinar emphysema, has contributed to the development of bronchiectasis (Varpela et al., 1978).

Acquired infections are the most common cause of bronchiectasis, especially infection acquired in childhood. Pneumonia developing subsequently to measles, pertussis, or influenza was once a prominent cause and is still observed now. Bacterial pneumonia with destruction of alveoli and bronchial walls leads to scarring, and the resultant shrinkage of surrounding lung places traction on the bronchi and causes bronchiectasis (Glenn et al., 1971). Chronic *Pseudomonas aeruginosa* infection also plays a role in

■ **Table 20–1.** ETIOLOGIC FACTORS IN DEVELOPMENT OF BRONCHIECTASIS

Congenital

Congenital cystic bronchiectasis
Selective IgA deficiency
Primary hypogammaglobulinemia
Alpha$_1$-antitrypsin deficiency
Cystic fibrosis
Congenital deficiency of bronchial cartilage
Kartagener's syndrome: situs inversus, sinusitis, and bronchiectasis
Bronchopulmonary sequestration

Acquired

Infection: bacterial, viral
Bronchial obstruction
  Intrinsic: neoplasm, foreign body, mucous plug
  Extrinsic: enlarged lymph nodes
Middle-lobe syndrome
Scarring secondary to tuberculosis
Acquired hypogammaglobulinemia

From Bolman, R. M., and Wolfe, W. G.: Bronchiectasis and bronchopulmonary sequestration. Surg. Clin. North Am., *60*:867, 1980.

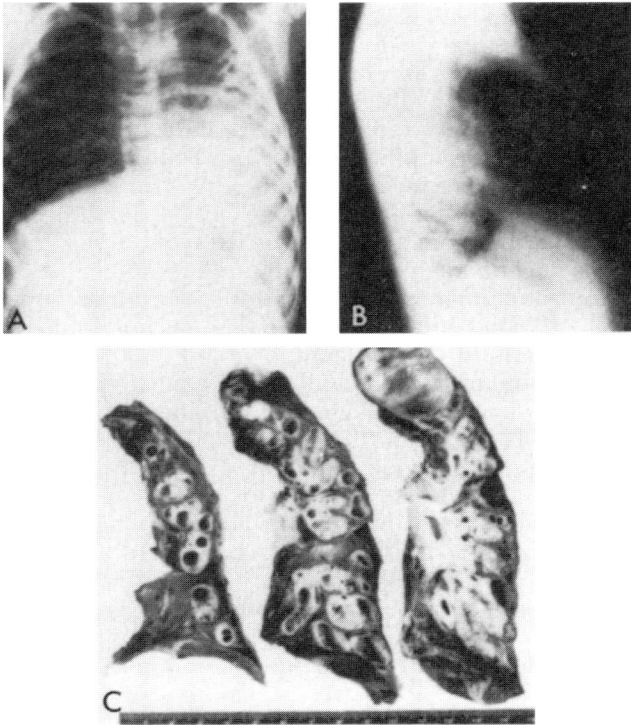

FIGURE 20–1. *A* and *B,* These posteroanterior and lateral chest films of a 5-year-old boy with congenital cystic bronchiectasis show a honeycomb pattern of bronchiectasis. The patient had a history of necrotizing pneumonia at 2 years of age. *C,* Marked cystic and saccular changes are noted throughout the bronchial tree in the left lung of this patient. (*A–C,* From Bolman, R. M., and Wolfe, W. G.: Bronchiectasis and bronchopulmonary sequestration. Surg. Clin. North Am., *60:*867, 1980.)

the development of bronchiectasis in chronic airway diseases (Nagaki et al., 1992).

Endobronchial obstruction with distal infection is considered significant in the development of bronchiectasis, and this obstruction can be either intrabronchial or extrabronchial in origin. Intrinsic causes include retained purulent bronchial secretions, thickened mucous plugs, obstruction from a foreign body, and neoplasm. Extrinsic bronchial obstruction can occur from enlarged hilar nodes (the middle lobe syndrome) (Bradham et al., 1966) and from anomalous great blood vessels, including anomalies of the aortic arch.

Less commonly, bronchiectasis is ascribed to a structural congenital defect. Patients with cystic fibrosis and congenital deficiency of bronchial cartilage are included in this category. There is also an association among situs inversus, sinusitis, and bronchiectasis. These conditions together constitute Kartagener's syndrome, which involves a congenital defect in respiratory cilia (Chipps et al., 1978).

Pathology

Bronchiectasis classically is divided into three groups: cylindrical, with dilated bronchi of regular

outline; varicose, with greater dilatation and irregularity; and saccular or cystic, with bronchial dilatation that increases toward the periphery and creates a balloon-like outline of the bronchi (Reid, 1950). The disease typically involves the distal bronchi (second to fourth order); the proximal bronchi are less affected because they contain more cartilage, are more rigid, and are more resistant to dilatation (Westcott, 1991). The distribution in the lungs corresponds to common sites of necrotizing pneumonia, usually the basal segments of the lower lobes; the superior lobar segments are usually spared. A representative pathologic specimen from a patient with cystic bronchiectasis of the lower lung is shown in Figure 20–2. Bronchiectasis is bilateral in approximately 30% of patients. Once the disease becomes established, between one-third and one-half of patients followed for more than 5 years show worsening of preexisting or development of new radiologic features (Munro et al., 1992).

Clinical Presentation

Bronchiectasis is characterized by recurrent episodes of pulmonary infection associated with persistent purulent secretions. The patient typically presents with a recurrent cough that produces purulent,

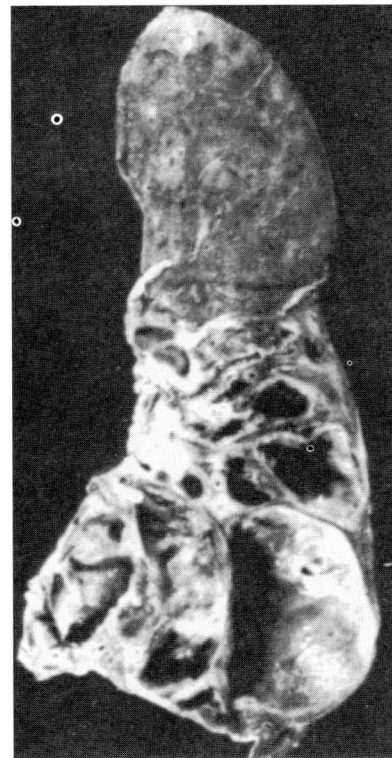

FIGURE 20–2. Resected left lung of a patient with severe cystic bronchiectasis of the left lower lobe and lingular segment of the upper lobe. Multiple cysts of various sizes with destruction of the majority of the pulmonary parenchyma in the lingula and lower lobe. (From Bolman, R. M., and Wolfe, W. G.: Bronchiectasis and bronchopulmonary sequestration. Surg. Clin. North Am., *60:*867, 1980.)

foul-smelling sputum, fever, and hemoptysis. Repeated episodes of pneumonitis in the neighboring parenchyma of the lung are also characteristic of bronchiectasis. During an acute febrile episode, pleuritic pain and an increase in volume and purulent character of sputum are usual. Hemoptysis occurs in approximately half of the adult patients and rarely in pediatric patients. In 10% of patients it is severe, although rarely lethal. Hemoptysis results from bleeding from anastomoses between hypertrophied bronchial arteries and the pulmonary circulation in the diseased segments. Other associated symptoms include anorexia, pleurisy, and arthralgias. These patients can manifest hypertrophic pulmonary osteoarthropathy, including clubbing of the fingers and joint swelling; symptoms usually resolve after surgical resection of the diseased lung. Percussion may reveal dullness over localized areas of involvement. Auscultation during acute phases shows moist or bubbling rales over affected segments of the lung and coarse expiratory rhonchi.

Diagnosis

A history of chronic productive cough, recurrent pneumonic infections, fever, and hemoptysis suggests the diagnosis in most cases. The plain chest film usually shows nonspecific abnormalities, including evidence of pleural thickening, fibrosis, and segmental atelectasis. Increased markings also may present a honeycomb pattern due to areas of destroyed lung

and compensatory overinflation of the remaining normal lung (Snell and Holman, 1972). Bronchography historically has permitted definitive diagnosis as well as information about the distribution of the bronchiectasis. Bronchography is not ordinarily recommended unless surgical therapy for bronchiectasis is seriously considered.

Timing of the study is important. Only one lung is studied at a time, and the patient should be in optimal condition, after postural drainage and antibiotics have controlled any acute exacerbations and secretions are decreased to a minimum. Bronchography should be postponed for 4 to 6 weeks after an acute infectious episode. The radiographic and bronchographic findings in a patient with bronchiectasis are shown in Figure 20–3. In most institutions, bronchography is rarely performed; bronchiectasis is usually diagnosed or confirmed by computed tomography (CT). The radiographic findings are extremely varied and depend on the severity and extent of the bronchiectasis, thickness of the bronchial walls, and contents and status of the lung parenchyma. Thin-cut (2-mm section) high-resolution CT is as sensitive as bronchography and poses no risk to the patient (McGuinness et al., 1993). The usual CT findings of bronchiectasis include lack of bronchial tapering, bronchial dilatation and wall thickening, and visualization of bronchi in the lung periphery (they are usually not seen) (Westcott, 1991). Bronchoscopy helps assess the mucosal surface of the tracheobronchial tree, determine specific segmental localization of purulent secretions, and identify foreign bodies, narrowed bronchi, or

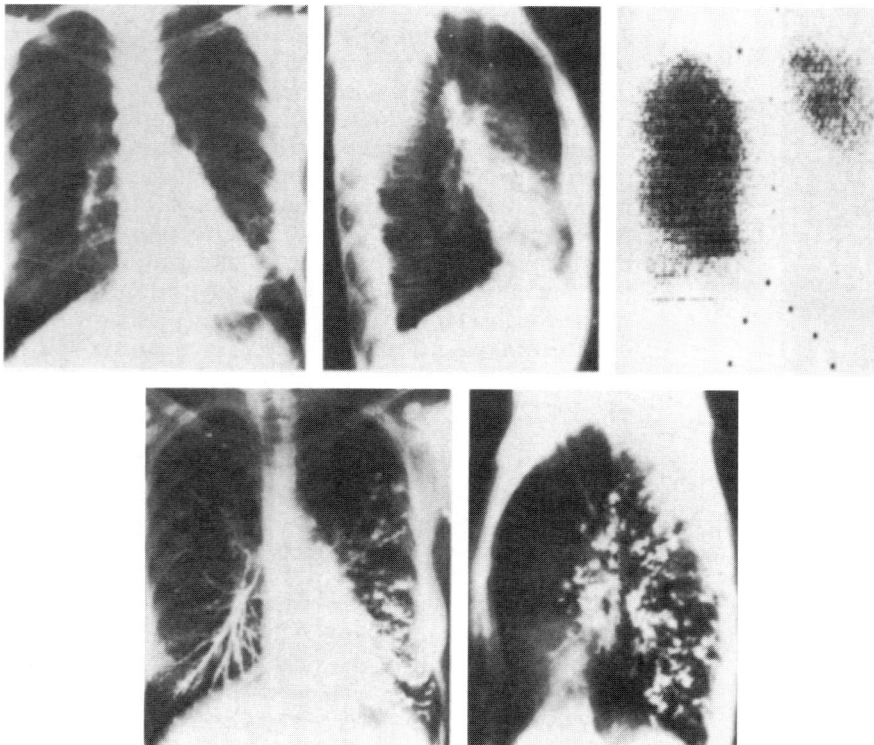

FIGURE 20–3. *Upper row,* Posteroanterior and lateral chest films and a scan of the lung in a patient with chronic saccular bronchiectasis of the left lower lobe. Volume loss and cystic changes are shown in the left lower lobe on chest films as well as diminished perfusion to the area as seen on the scan of the lung at the far right. *Lower row,* Posteroanterior and lateral bronchograms in this patient show saccular dilatation in the bronchi of the left lower lobe and the lingular segment of the left upper lobe. (From Bolman, R. M., and Wolfe, W. G.: Bronchiectasis and bronchopulmonary sequestration. Surg. Clin. North Am., *60:*867, 1980.)

neoplasms. Bronchoscopy also is useful in obtaining uncontaminated secretions for culture, and the procedure may be therapeutic by providing good tracheobronchial toilet.

Treatment

The treatment of bronchiectasis is largely medical and is directed toward prevention and control of infection and mechanical removal of purulent secretions by coughing, postural drainage, and bronchoscopy. A long trial of medical therapy is required to determine the need for surgical intervention. Antibiotics such as tetracycline or ampicillin are usually selected according to culture and sensitivity data, and these drugs should be continued until the production of sputum is minimal. An aggressive regimen of postural drainage and chest physiotherapy should be combined with antimicrobial therapy. Tobacco should be avoided, and all patients should receive pneumococcal vaccine and annual influenza vaccine (Hinshaw and Murray, 1980). Medical therapy is effective in most patients with bronchiectasis. If medical treatment is unsuccessful after several months and significant symptoms remain, with recurrent episodes of pneumonitis, persistent purulent sputum production, or frequent episodes of hemoptysis, surgical therapy should be considered. This is especially true when the disease is localized to one area or segment of a lung. Surgical treatment is less effective in patients in whom the disease is diffuse and multisegmental. The best results are obtained in unilateral disease localized to one lobe, especially if it is the lower lobe in a young patient with adequate pulmonary reserve and without evidence of airway obstruction or sinusitis (Snell and Holman, 1972).

Surgical therapy for bronchiectasis dates to the late 1800s. The mortality rate for the procedure remained high until the 1930s, when Churchill reported 84 cases of bronchiectasis treated by lobectomy with a mortality rate of 4.6%. The current mortality rate after such resections is less than 1%. Sealy and colleagues (1966) reported 140 patients who had bronchiectasis and who required surgical resection, 70 with localized disease and 70 with more diffuse disease. Patients underwent surgery after an intensive period of medical therapy, and preservation of uninvolved lung by careful segmental resection was emphasized. The mortality rate was less than 1%, and follow-up showed that results were good to improved in 95% of patients. Patients who had localized disease fared better after surgical therapy.

Bilateral disease does not contraindicate surgical therapy in selected patients. George and associates (1979) reported 99 patients with bilateral disease who had surgical resection, with an operative mortality rate of 1.4%. The disease occurred primarily in dependent areas of the lungs, specifically the right middle lobe, the lingula of the left upper lobe, and the basal segments of the lower lobes. The side with the most severe disease was resected initially, and the opposite side was staged 2 to 3 months later, if necessary.

Operation must incorporate careful anesthetic management, including the use of selective endotracheal intubation with a double-lumen tube to protect the normal lung from spillage of purulent secretions from the involved side. With proper selection and preparation of patients, careful anesthetic management, and preservation of normal pulmonary parenchyma during resection, surgical therapy has much to offer this group of patients.

LUNG ABSCESS

Lung abscess has always challenged physicians and surgeons because of the long duration of the illness, the significant mortality rate, and the diagnostic and therapeutic problems involved. By definition, a lung abscess is a localized area of suppuration and cavitation in the lung. This discussion concentrates more specifically on the classic primary pyogenic lung abscess, previously called "nonspecific" lung abscess, as well as on the so-called opportunistic lung abscess of more recent origin.

The evolution of effective antibiotic therapy for a primary lung abscess after World War II altered the natural history of the disease and markedly reduced the role of surgical therapy. The course of lung abscess in the era before the advent of antimicrobial agents was one of progressive deterioration. Major forms of medical therapy in these patients included supportive care and postural drainage. Bronchoscopy was used as an adjunctive measure to facilitate drainage and to detect underlying lesions such as a foreign body or carcinoma. The mortality rate in this era was more than 30%, and 30% of patients were left with residual significant symptomatic disease. Patients underwent surgical drainage only in the late stages of illness, when toxemia and general debility were prominent, and the results were often dismal. In the late 1940s, both penicillin therapy and better thoracic surgical techniques significantly improved the prognosis. Mortality was reduced, and the relative merits of surgical and medical therapy were disputed. By the late 1950s, most investigators concluded that a trial of antibiotic therapy was indicated in all patients, and the agents most frequently used were penicillin, tetracycline, or penicillin in combination with streptomycin. The most common indication for surgical intervention was "delayed closure," which was defined as persistence of the cavity after 4 to 6 weeks of medical therapy. Because of the widespread use of penicillin and other antibiotics, most cases of suppurative pneumonia were prevented, and fewer pneumonic processes progressed to form abscesses. Operative intervention became less frequently indicated, and these procedures were usually done electively for chronic illness after medical failure. In the following decades, increasing use of corticosteroids, chemotherapy, and immunosuppressive therapy altered the natural environment of the tracheobronchial tree and introduced the rising incidence of opportunistic lung abscesses—that is, those associated with other diseases or conditions that depress the natural defenses of the body.

Pathogenesis

Aspiration of infectious material is the common etiologic mechanism in the development of pyogenic lung abscess. Aspiration due to dysphagia or compromised consciousness (alcoholism, seizure disorder, cerebrovascular accident, head trauma, general anesthesia) appears to be a common predisposing factor. Poor oral hygiene, dental infections, and gingival disease also are common in these patients. Although lung abscess has occurred in edentulous patients, an occult bronchogenic carcinoma must be suspected. In a review of 50 patients with lung abscess, two of five edentulous patients were found to have underlying bronchogenic carcinoma (Groskin et al., 1991). Most pyogenic lung abscesses thus stem from aspiration of infectious disease from the oropharynx into the lung while the cough reflex is suppressed in a patient with gingivodental disease (Barnett and Herring, 1971; Rubin and Block, 1972). Brock (1952) emphasized the predilection of lung abscesses for the "axillary" segments of the right lung (posterior segment of the upper lobe and superior segment of the lower lobe) by gravitation of the infectious material from the oropharynx into those dependent segments, in which bronchi were in the most direct line of the upper respiratory tract. These two segments are the most common sites of primary nonspecific lung abscesses (Estrera et al., 1980; Shafron and Tate, 1968).

After pyogenic pneumonitis develops in response to the aspirated septic material, liquefaction necrosis can occur secondary to bacterial proliferation and leukocyte invasion to produce an acute abscess. As the liquefied necrotic material empties through the draining bronchus, a necrotic cavity containing an air-fluid level is formed. The microorganisms most commonly responsible for this chain of events are anaerobic bacteria. These bacteria predominate in the upper respiratory tract secretions and are heavily concentrated in areas of dental infection. Secondary involvement of gram-negative organisms may also occur. Quite commonly, the causative organism cannot be isolated from culture because antibiotic therapy was initiated before cultures were obtained. Additionally, expectorated sputum samples are not suitable for anaerobic culture because they are invariably contaminated by the normal oral pharyngeal flora.

Clinical Presentation

The patient typically has a history of upper respiratory tract infection with fever and is often toxic. Chest pain is not uncommon as a result of pleurisy from the peripheral location of the typical lung abscess. Hemoptysis and expectoration of purulent and some-

times putrid sputum commonly follow. The abscess can resolve if the bronchocavitary fistula allows evacuation of contents, expansion of the lung, and collapse of the cavity. A chronic abscess results from inadequate drainage of the cavity, formation of a thick fibrotic wall, and epithelialization of the lining of the abscess cavity. Rarely do the bronchocavitary fistulas develop at the most dependent area of the abscess; in addition, the communications are small and frequently occluded by edema or impaction of debris. This explains the periodic nature of the clinical syndrome: Complaints are relieved each time erosion into anterior bronchiole takes place, allowing partial emptying of the cavity's contents. Sputum is present during the drainage phases, and the cough is relatively nonproductive during the recurrent episodes of increased toxicity.

Primary lung abscesses after the suppurative pneumonias of infancy and childhood due to staphylococci lack the typical indolent periodic course of the more common postaspiration infections. Their onset tends to be sudden and more ominous, producing chills and fever as well as tachycardia, tachypnea, and unremitting production of purulent sputum. Rarely is the sputum malodorous, because there is no indolent course of anaerobic infection.

Diagnosis

The chest film in lung abscess is not pathognomonic in the early stages before communication is established between the abscess cavity and the draining bronchus (bronchocavitary fistula). An area of dense pneumonic consolidation precedes the appearance of the characteristic cavitary air-fluid configuration (Fig. 20–4). This distinguishing radiographic feature of lung abscess, the air-fluid level, is seen only on the upright chest film or in the lateral decubitus position in an immunocompromised patient. Accompanying pleural thickening, atelectasis, or pneumothorax may obscure this picture.

Opportunistic lung abscesses are a more difficult clinical problem. They occur in patients at the extremes of age and in those who have associated conditions, including prior treatment with corticosteroids, chemotherapy, immunosuppression, and incurable malignancy. Under these circumstances, multiple rather than single abscesses often develop, and most of these infections are acquired in the hospital. Bacteriologically, these abscesses also differ from the classic aspiration type of lung abscesses. *Staphylococcus aureus* is a common causative organism, but *Pseudomonas*, *Proteus*, *Escherichia coli*, and *Klebsiella* are all recognized as potential pathogens in the opportunistic form of lung abscess. As in the aspiration type of lung abscess, cavitation is generally apparent on the chest film 10 days to 2 weeks after the onset of cough, fever, and pleuritic chest pain.

Treatment

Because effective broad-spectrum antibiotics such as penicillin are available, primary or nonspecific lung

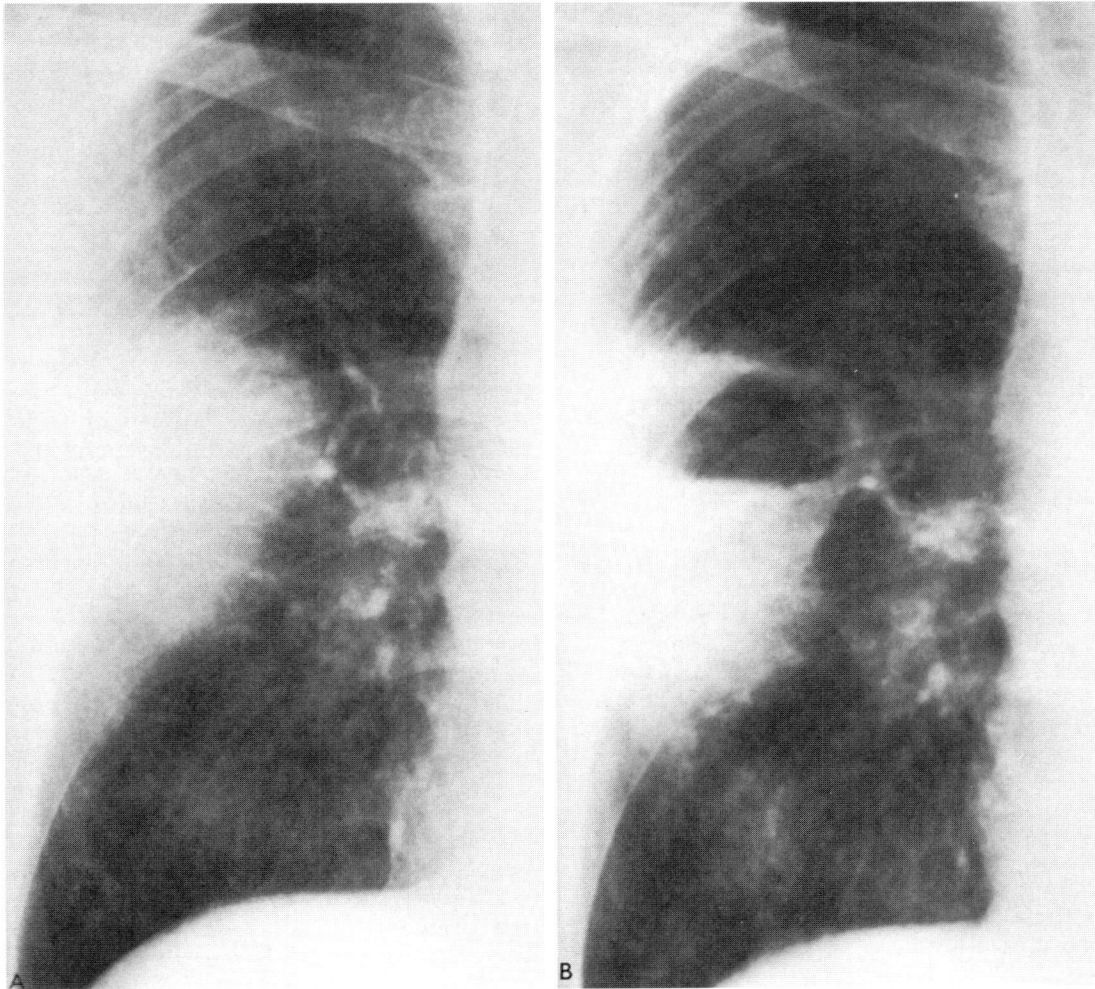

FIGURE 20–4. Acute primary aspiration-type lung abscess. Thoracic films of the right lung show an aspiration pneumonia developing into a lung abscess in a chronic alcoholic patient. *A*, Pneumonic phase of the process that returned mixed bacterial flora on culture. The patient did not respond to broad-spectrum antibiotics. *B*, Cavitation of the lung abscess. After 2 months of antibiotic therapy with inadequate response, the abscess was resected.

abscess often can be aborted in the early stage of suppurative pneumonitis. Accordingly, the incidence of this type of abscess has declined sharply in recent years.

The modern treatment of classic primary aspiration lung abscess is prolonged antimicrobial therapy (Abernathy, 1968). Analysis of the bacteriologic findings in most patients shows that the isolates are usually sensitive to penicillin, because anaerobic bacteria are involved in 60 to 90% of cases (Bartlett, 1991). For patients allergic to penicillin, clindamycin or chloramphenicol is an acceptable alternative. Additional antibiotics are given as indicated by specific bacteriologic cultures. A large-scale prospective study comparing antibiotic regimens for the treatment of anaerobic lung abscess was reported by Levison and colleagues (1983). This study compared the clinical outcome of clindamycin (600 mg every 8 hours) with that of penicillin (6 million units/day administered intravenously). A significant difference favored clindamycin in terms of the number of drug failures, relapses, and

duration of fever. Early bronchoscopy for diagnosis is indicated to obtain material for culture and to exclude the presence of foreign body or neoplasm (Table 20–2). Bronchoscopy can also drain the abscess by aspiration of the appropriate bronchus through the bronchoscope; transbronchial drainage by catheterization of the appropriate bronchus under fluoroscopy has been reported (Conners et al., 1975). In one series of 26

■ **Table 20–2.** PRINCIPLES OF THERAPY FOR LUNG ABSCESS

Identification of etiologic organism
Prolonged antimicrobial therapy
Provision of adequate drainage in the acute stage:
  Physiotherapy—postural drainage, percussion, coughing
    exercises
  Bronchoscopy
    Diagnostic—exclude endobronchial lesion
    Suction drainage
  Emergency surgical treatment
    External drainage (only in specific situations)

Table 20–3. INDICATIONS FOR SURGICAL TREATMENT OF LUNG ABSCESS

Acute Stage (Emergency)
Complications
Bronchopulmonary fistula
Empyema
Chronic Stage (Definitive)
Persistent symptoms and signs
Recurrent complications (hemoptysis)

primary lung abscesses reported over 5 years, surgical therapy was not required, and the outcome of medical therapy for most patients with this condition was successful (Bartlett et al., 1974). If treatment can be initiated in the acute stage of the disease and continued safely, most abscesses will respond to medical treatment alone. Operative treatment is now required in only 10 to 15% of patients; specifically, surgical intervention is indicated for the uncontrolled acute disease and for complications that occur in both the acute and the chronic stages of the disease (Table 20–3).

Surgical treatment is reserved for specific indications that include unsuccessful medical treatment, suspicion of carcinoma, significant hemoptysis, and complications of lung abscess, including empyema and bronchopleural fistula. Successful medical therapy entails resolution of symptoms with no radiographic residual or with only a thin-walled cystic residual cavity of less than 2 cm after 4 to 5 weeks of intensive antibiotic therapy. If a sizable residual cavity remains after 5 weeks of treatment, especially if it is thick-walled or larger than 2 cm in diameter and is associated with persistent symptoms, surgical resection is usually recommended (Fig. 20–5). Otherwise, recurrent infection or hemoptysis may occur, and the long-term prognosis is poor. In asymptomatic patients with small, thin-walled residual cavities after adequate antibiotic therapy, complete healing can be expected in a few weeks or months, and surgical therapy is often unnecessary.

Barnett and Herring (1971) found that the main factors that determine the success of medical therapy are the duration of symptoms before initiation of therapy and the initial size (diameter) of the cavity. In their experience, antibiotic therapy alone was rarely successful if symptoms were present longer than 12 weeks before initiation of antibiotic therapy or if the original diameter of the cavity was 4 cm or more. External drainage may still be necessary occasionally for uncontrolled acute disease, but elective resection is more common in the chronic stage (lobectomy) when medical management has not led to cure (see Table 20–3).

Anesthetic management of the patient during operative resection requires significant planning and care to prevent spillage of the contents of the abscess cavity into the uninvolved portions of the lung. A double-lumen endotracheal tube (Carlen's tube) is preferred in all cases. It is also important to gain prompt control of the involved bronchus as soon as possible after opening the pleural cavity (Garzon, 1972).

Percutaneous tube drainage of complicated lung abscess has been efficacious in selected patients (Rice et al., 1987). In a series of 14 patients with multisystem disease and complicated lung abscesses, many of whom were on mechanical ventilation and were not

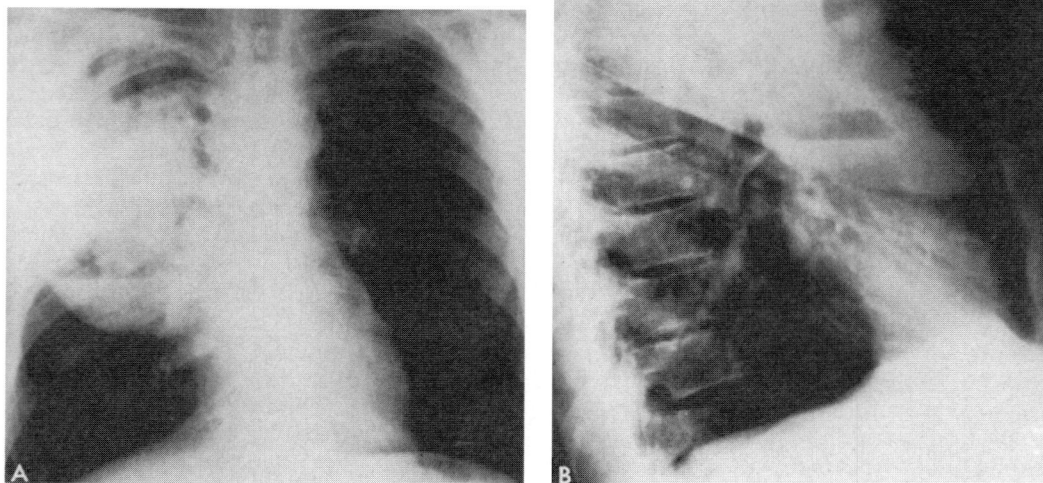

FIGURE 20–5. Chronic lung abscess. Posteroanterior *(A)* and right lateral *(B)* thoracic films of a patient with pyogenic lung abscess due to *Klebsiella pneumoniae* and alpha-streptococci. After 4 weeks of antibiotic therapy, a residual thick-walled cavity 4 cm in diameter was resected with right upper lobectomy. *(A* and *B,* From Takaro, T.: Lung abscess and fungal infections. *In* Sabiston, D. C., Jr. [ed]: Davis-Christopher Textbook of Surgery. 12th ed. Philadelphia, W. B. Saunders, 1981.)

candidates for extensive pulmonary resections, tube drainage effectively decompressed the purulent collection and helped resolve the patients' acute septic conditions. Indications for open drainage were unrelenting sepsis despite antimicrobial therapy, lung abscess under tension as noted by radiographic studies, failure to wean from mechanical ventilation, and contamination of the contralateral lung. Eleven patients were ultimately discharged from the hospital in this group, and 10 were long-term survivors. Although all patients developed bronchopleural fistulas after drainage, these were not significant; in the 9 patients who were on mechanical ventilation, the fistulas did not interfere with respiratory management. Most fistulas closed spontaneously with resolution of the abscess cavity. The authors recommended this approach for acute management of lung abscesses in most patients for whom standard management has failed and for patients who are not candidates for extensive pulmonary resection.

The efficacy of CT-guided percutaneous drainage of lung abscess was reported in a series of 19 patients who had persistent sepsis despite standard medical therapy (Van Sonnenberg et al., 1991). A No. 12 French chest catheter was placed through contiguous abnormal lung and was left to Pleur-Evac drainage with intermittent irrigation for an average duration of 10 days. Within 48 hours, fever and sepsis resolved in 18 of 19 patients, and the abscess was eventually cured in all 19 patients. The authors predict that this technique should obviate major surgery in most patients, because only 3 of the 19 patients required subsequent surgery for decortication. The only significant complication was hemothorax in one patient, in whom the catheter was passed transparenchymally through normal lung.

Hemoptysis, a common complication of lung abscess, has been controlled effectively in some patients who are not surgical candidates by embolization of the bronchial artery on the appropriate side (Bookstein et al., 1977; Remy et al., 1977).

The mortality rate from primary aspiration-type lung abscess is now both significantly lower than it was in earlier years and lower than the mortality rate associated with lung abscesses that occur as a complication of some other serious disease (opportunistic infection). The mortality rate from classic pyogenic lung abscess has declined from approximately 25% in the early 1980s to less than 5% today because of prolonged and adequate antimicrobial therapy. However, the mortality rate for patients with opportunistic lung abscesses is still high and reflects the gravity of the accompanying disease as well as the prognostic significance of the complications of lung abscess.

Actinomycotic and Nocardial Infections

Although *Actinomyces israelii* and the various pathogenic species of *Nocardia* have been classified as bacteria, actinomycosis and nocardiosis are included in this review for historical reasons, because their clinical manifestations resemble those of fungal diseases. Morphologically, these etiologic agents also resemble fungi in that they form hyphae with true branching as well as spores. The distinction must be made between fungal infections and the actinomycetes, because very different therapeutic approaches are taken. Penicillin and sulfonamides are used to treat actinomycosis and nocardiosis, and amphotericin B is the drug of choice for fungal diseases.

Thoracic Actinomycosis

Actinomycosis is a chronic, endogenous infection caused by the anaerobic actinomycete *A. israelii*, which, unlike many fungi, is not found free in nature. When this organism involves the lung, it usually causes a chronic nonhealing infiltrate that may or may not be accompanied by the symptoms of chronic pulmonary infection. Actinomycosis involves a severe inflammatory and granulomatous reaction surrounding the focus of the pulmonary infection. Classically, the disease was characterized by abscess and sinus formation with the purulent drainage containing "sulfur granules" (McQuarrie and Hall, 1968). Thoracic actinomycosis is now more commonly encountered as a disease of parenchyma of the lung; it may mimic bronchogenic carcinoma (Jara et al., 1979; Slade et al., 1973). Actinomycosis can occur clinically in extrathoracic locations. The disease is most common in a cervicofacial form manifested by draining cutaneous sinuses; it occurs less commonly as an abdominal disease that can mimic an ulcerative colonic carcinoma. The thoracic form of the disease derives from bronchopulmonary invasion of infectious material from the oropharynx, where *A. israelii* is usually not pathogenic. Pulmonary parenchymal infection follows a course characteristic of fungal disease, with chronic suppuration surrounded by dense fibrosis in a proliferative granulomatous inflammatory reaction (Fig. 20–6). If left untreated, the disease extends to involve the pleura and can drain through the chest wall (Eastridge et al., 1972).

The bacterium *A. israelii* occurs as a gram-positive coccobacillary body with short branching filaments. In pathologic material, these organisms occur in clusters or microcolonies called granules. Characteristic yellow-brown granules in material draining from abscesses or sinuses are sometimes seen and are referred to as sulfur granules. Material must be obtained from the deepest portion of tissue involvement, because it must be cultured under anaerobic conditions to confirm the diagnosis.

Radiologic signs that are helpful in the diagnosis include chest-wall involvement with the ribs, penetration of interlobar fissures, and vertebral destruction (Slade et al., 1973).

Penicillin is the drug of choice against actinomycosis. Because of the dense fibers and avascular tissues surrounding the colonies of organisms and the dense concentration of the organisms, high doses of antibiotics must be used over a long period. Twenty million

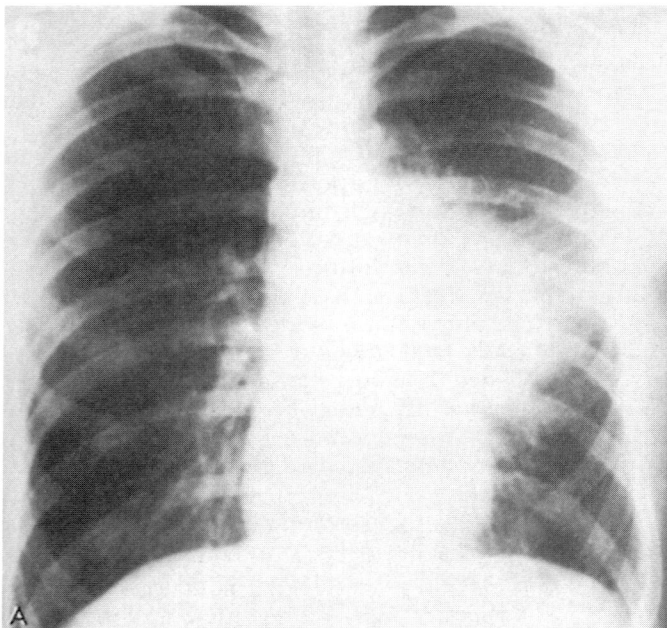

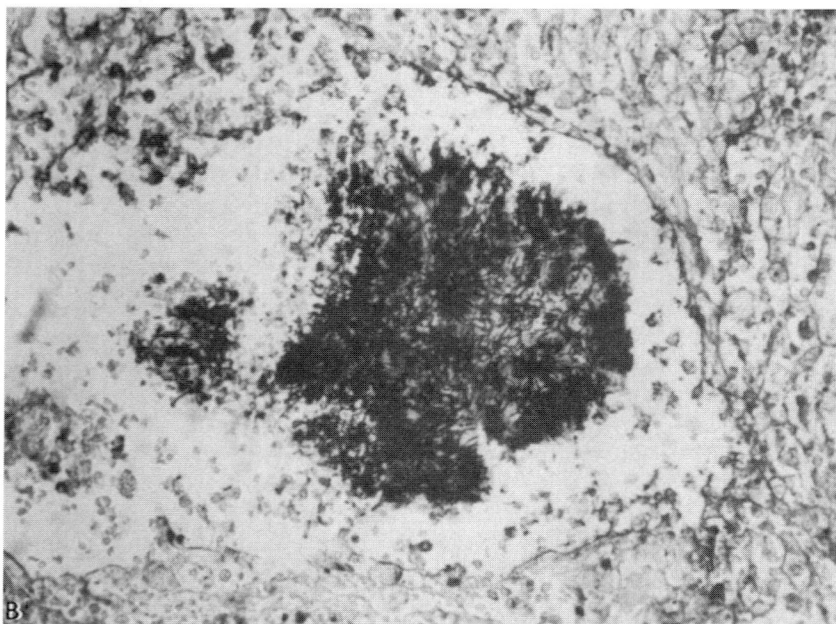

FIGURE 20–6. Actinomycosis. *A,* Thoracic film of a 43-year-old man with hemoptysis, weight loss, and dyspnea. After an extensive work-up that did not yield diagnosis, thoracotomy was done. It showed a firm left hilar mass believed to represent a resectable bronchogenic carcinoma. Multiple operative frozen sections did not confirm the diagnosis; left pneumonectomy was done. An actinomycotic cavity, 2 × 3.5 cm, was found centrally, located in a densely fibrotic area of the lung. *B,* Sulfur granule of actinomyces showing typical hyphae by fungal stains. The patient received a prolonged course of intravenous penicillin therapy and recovered completely (methenamine silver stain, ×250).

units of penicillin G daily for 1 to 3 months is recommended (McQuarrie and Hall, 1968). If resection is to be done, it should be performed under adequate drug coverage. Exploratory thoracotomy is often done when carcinoma of the lung is suspected, and the diagnosis is made on histologic examination. In this situation, adequate and prolonged drug therapy is important to prevent reactivation of disease or development of empyema.

Nocardiosis

Nocardiosis is a chronic bacterial infection caused by the aerobic gram-positive *Nocardia asteroides.* The disease is characterized by primary pulmonary involvement and secondary hematogenous dissemination to other organs, especially the central nervous system. In the past, this disease was rarely encountered. Nocardiosis is being encountered with increasing frequency as an opportunistic disease in patients who have immunologic impairment such as lymphoma, leukemia, or malignancy and in patients receiving corticosteroids or immunosuppressive therapy after organ transplantation (Krick et al., 1975). The disease varies widely in pathology and is usually fatal unless a specific diagnosis can be established and appropriate therapy is initiated. The organism has been confused with *Mycobacterium tuberculosis* because it is characterized by filaments on nonencapsulated bacteria that can accept acid-fast stains.

Unlike actinomycetes, *N. asteroides* is widely disseminated in nature and has been recovered from soil and from several species of animals. No area is known to be endemic for the disease. It is uncommon in the tracheobronchial tree of normal individuals, and if the organism is recovered from the sputum of a patient with abnormal chest film results, nocardiosis is likely.

As with actinomycosis, nocardiosis can be characterized by the formation of soft tissue abscesses and draining sinuses, usually involving the chest wall; purulent material obtained from such areas can contain sulfur granules similar to those observed in actinomycosis. More commonly, nocardiosis is characterized by pyogenic pulmonary lesions that range from subclinical to severe in presentation and can be transitory or chronic. Manifestations of chronic pulmonary disease, including cough, fever, weakness, night sweats, weight loss, pleuritic chest, and hemoptysis, usually are nonspecific. These symptoms suggest pulmonary tuberculosis, and because the radiographic appearance can be similar, these two diseases have sometimes been confused. Empyema can also result from pulmonary nocardiosis. Some reviews show that more than half of patients afflicted with empyema have a predisposing condition with depression of the immune defenses (Palmer et al., 1974).

Signs and symptoms of central nervous system involvement due to brain abscess or meningitis may be an initial manifestation when the primary pulmonary infection is mild and goes unnoticed.

Radiographic findings usually consist of localized pneumonic or infiltrative lesions that can progress to necrosis and cavitation (Bragg and Janis, 1973). In the opportunistic form of the disease, early cavitation and systemic involvement may accelerate the course (Fig. 20–7).

The rapidity and accuracy with which nocardiosis can be diagnosed significantly affects the outcome of therapy. The relatively slow growth of *Nocardia* on typical culture media and a low incidence of isolation from ordinary specimens may delay diagnosis. Sputum is usually a low-yield source in attempts to isolate the pathogen, as in detection of *Pneumocystis carinii* and *Aspergillus*. More aggressive and invasive diagnostic methods are warranted, especially in immunosuppressed patients. Techniques that have speeded diagnosis include bronchoscopy with pulmonary brush biopsy, percutaneous lung aspiration, and open lung biopsy. By Gram's stain, the mycelia of *N. asteroides* typically appear as delicate, gram-positive, irregularly staining, beaded, branching filaments, but they may also fragment into coccobacillary forms.

Over the years, the sulfonamides have remained the single most effective therapy for nocardiosis, and medical treatment has been the primary mode of therapy. Currently used sulfonamides include trimethoprim-sulfamethoxazole (TMP-SMZ) (Septra) and sulfisoxazole (Gantrisin) in doses of 4 to 8 g/day. A minimum of 2 to 3 months of therapy is usually necessary, and antibiotic treatment should probably be continued for as long as 1 year in the presence of underlying immunosuppression (Palmer et al., 1974).

Experience has shown no clinical benefit from resection of lung abscesses, except as they would be managed in other forms or pyogenic abscess, and good healing under medical therapy should be expected. Surgical drainage of empyemas or other complications of pulmonary abscess is indicated.

FUNGAL INFECTIONS OF THE LUNG

Fungal infections of the chest are not rare. It has been estimated that more than 30 million Americans have been infected with the spores of *Histoplasma capsulatum* and that 10 million have been infected by *Coccidioides immitis*. Because of increased clinical surveillance and improved laboratory and microbiologic techniques, disease secondary to *Blastomyces* and *Cryptococcus* organisms is being reported with increasing frequency. Increasing use of chemotherapy for neoplasms, antibiotics for infections, immunosuppressive agents for organ transplantation, and corticosteroids for various conditions has increased opportunistic infections by usually harmless saphrophytes such as *Aspergillus*, *Candida*, and *Mucor*. Under these conditions, the formerly clear differentiation between so-called pathogenic and nonpathogenic fungi has become obscured.

Knowledge of the pathophysiology of fungal infections and of the spectrum of potential clinical involvement has increased considerably over the years. Initially it was thought that major fungal infections, including blastomycosis, histoplasmosis, coccidioidomycosis, and cryptococcosis, were rare and usually fatal diseases. It is now clear that clinically benign and self-limited illnesses may result from infection with these organisms, and that this expression of the disease is more common with eventual spontaneous healing. It has also been clarified that the three major invasive mycotic infections (blastomycosis, coccidioidomycosis, and histoplasmosis) occur in circumscribed geographic areas wherein the infecting agents are found in the soil and can be aerosolized, with the usual portal of entry being the respiratory tract. *Cryptococcus*, *Aspergillus*, and *Mucor* are thought to be ubiquitous and are located in the soil.

Thoracic surgeons are called on to treat mycotic diseases of the chest for three principal reasons. Endoscopy and biopsy are usually required to establish a diagnosis so that appropriate antibiotic therapy can be initiated. Although most fungal diseases do respond to appropriate antimycotic drugs, especially amphotericin B, under certain circumstances surgical therapy does have a role, and a surgeon may be asked to treat patients with pulmonary mycoses that do not respond to medical therapy. Finally, thoracic surgeons may unexpectedly encounter fungal disease while evaluating and staging a possible carcinoma of the lung; proper handling of tissue and culture material is essential for diagnostic accuracy and initiation of appropriate therapy. Careful attention by the surgeon

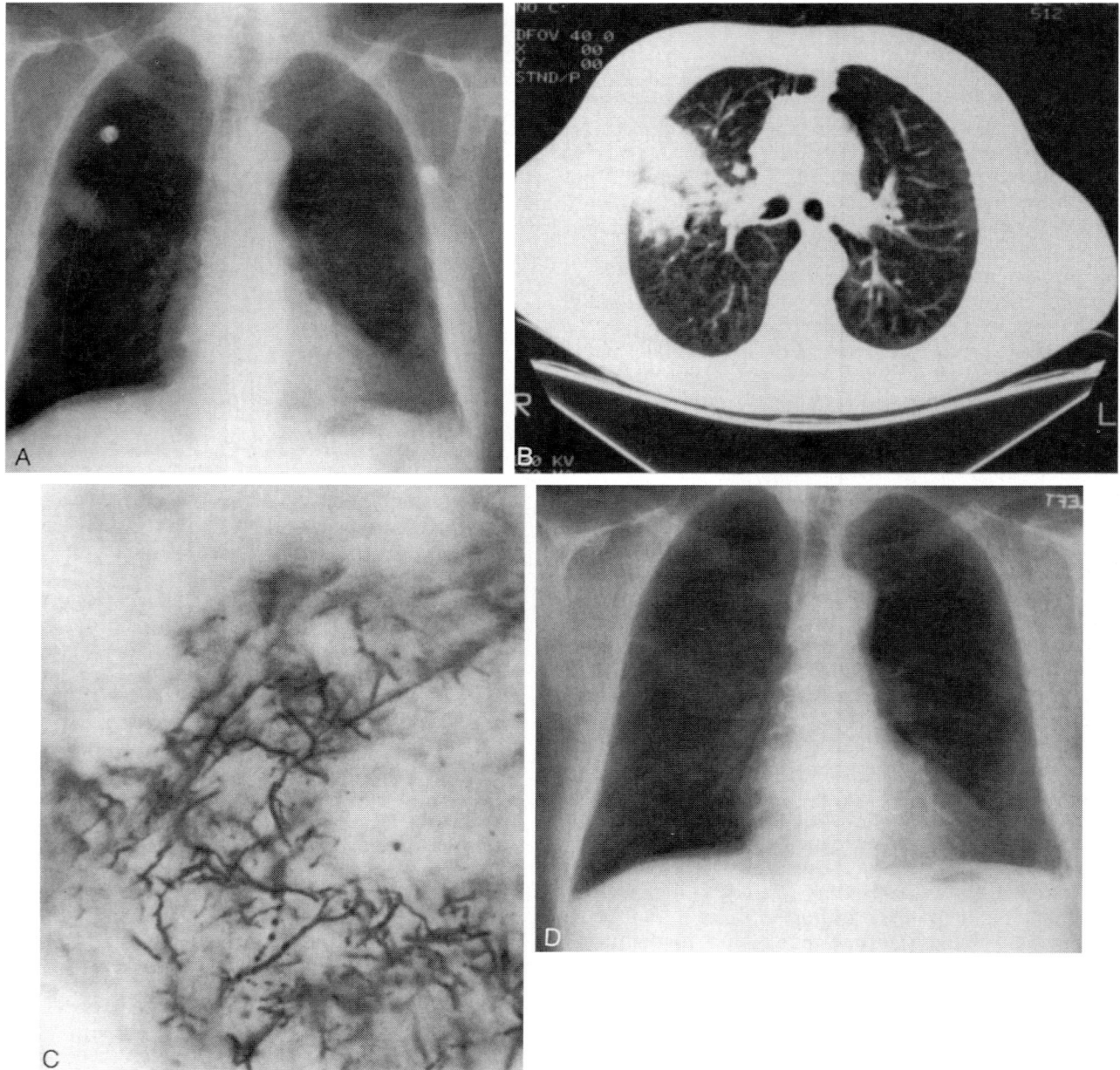

FIGURE 20–7. *A,* Posteroanterior chest film of a 55-year-old patient who presented with a right upper lobe infiltrate 6 months after cardiac transplantation. The lesion was detected on a routine chest film at the time of a scheduled endomyocardial biopsy and was associated with only mild pulmonary symptoms. *B,* Chest tomography of the same patient showing an extensive pleural-based process in the right lung with extension to the right hilum. *C, Nocardia asteroides* was isolated from the sputum. The organisms are acid-fast and have previously been mistaken for tubercle bacilli. *D,* Chest film of the same patient 10 weeks after a course of TMP-SMZ with almost complete resolution of the infiltrate. Because of the high incidence of associated central nervous system involvement with *Nocardia,* a routine brain computed tomography (CT) scan should also be obtained in these patients.

to the proper acquisition and handling of tissue and fluid specimens cannot be overemphasized. Positive identification of the offending organism is important before initiation of therapy, because the major chemotherapeutic agent is amphotericin B, a toxic drug.

In the United States, there are three major mycotic infections in which the fungal agent invades the normal human host and establishes systemic infection. These three infections—blastomycosis, coccidioido-

mycosis, and histoplasmosis—share a number of characteristics. Specific and fairly well-circumscribed geographic areas of endemicity are recognized (Buechner, 1971; Takaro, 1968). The fungal agent in each case is dimorphic; it exists in nature as a mycelium (mold) that bears infectious spores, which later enter the host and develop into a yeast-like phase that is the tissue pathogen. These agents enter the host in an aerosolized form through the respiratory tract; clinical manifestations usually consist of mild pulmonary infection or even an asymptomatic condition. Chronic pulmonary or disseminated infection is actually uncommon. An intact cell-mediated immune response is critical to limitation and control of these diseases. Interference with T cell function correlates with a high risk of disseminated disease. Amphotericin is still the primary therapy for all three fungal infections, although the newer azoles have a role in treating some forms of pulmonary or extrapulmonary disease (Johnson and Sarosi, 1991).

The following section describes in further detail each of the important fungal infections that involve the lungs and thorax and delineates the place of surgical therapy in those diseases.

Histoplasmosis

Histoplasmosis is probably the most common of all the fungal infections and is the most frequently occurring serious systemic fungal disease. It is caused by the dimorphic fungus *Histoplasma capsulatum,* which grows in soil throughout the world, particularly in soil with a high concentration of fecal material of chickens, pigeons, and bats. In the United States, the endemic area is in the eastern central portion of the country within the valleys of the Ohio River and the Mississippi River (Fig. 20–8). Disease occurs when fungus-laden soil is disturbed, which thus creates an aerosol of infectious spores. Although histoplasmosis has long been associated with farming and rural populations, epidemic histoplasmosis has been increasingly reported among urban and suburban populations (Goodwin et al., 1976).

The incidence of primary infection is related to the risk of exposure. Primary histoplasmosis is most commonly observed in farmers, construction workers, and other persons involved in outdoor activities. Most cases of primary histoplasmosis are asymptomatic. Progressive pulmonary disease appears to be predominantly a disease of middle-aged men, because preexisting chronic pulmonary disease is important in the pathogenesis. Disseminated disease occurs most often in elderly patients, infants, and immunosuppressed patients (Wheat et al., 1985).

Histoplasmosis is contracted by the inhalation of *H. capsulatum* spores, which are delivered to the periphery of the lung. Spread to regional lymph nodes and to the bloodstream occurs quickly. One to 3 weeks after the initial infection, a cell-mediated immunity to the agent develops, and a necrotizing granulomatous reaction appears in the mediastinal lymph nodes and lungs (Hague, 1992). As the epithelial cell granulomas age, caseating necrosis develops in the central areas and may calcify as the peripheral portions become fibrotic. Within these lesions, *H. capsulatum* cells are usually found only in the caseous material. They are not well seen with hematoxylin and eosin (H & E) staining, but they are well seen with the methenamine silver stain (Fig. 20–9). The yeast forms of *H. capsulatum* are 2 to 5 μm in size and are often found intracellularly in macrophages (Hague, 1992).

Most patients (60 to 90%) who inhale *H. capsulatum* spores remain asymptomatic or develop a mild illness similar to the common cold. A minority of patients who contract the disease develop a progression of symptoms similar to an acute influenza-like syndrome with cough, pleurisy, shortness of breath, fever, night sweats, myalgias, arthralgias, and weight loss. Radiologically, various findings may be seen with primary histoplasmosis. Patchy areas of bronchopneumonia, diffuse airspace involvement, discrete widely distributed nodules, or a solitary pulmonary nodule may be found. Regional adenopathy is also common. Complete healing usually follows, often with residual scarring and calcification. Scarred or calcified lesions may press against bronchi (middle-lobe syndrome) or may even rupture into the bronchial tree as a broncholith (Cole et al., 1986). The healed pulmonary lesions can present as a solitary

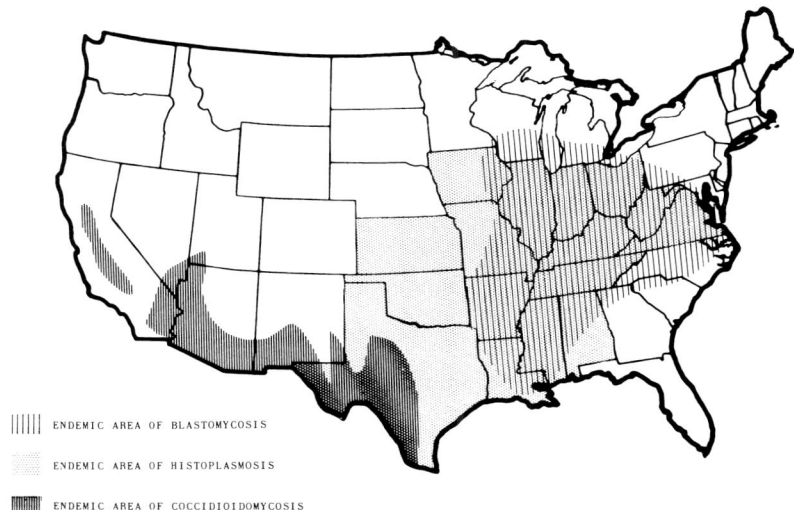

FIGURE 20–8. Map showing the areas in the United States that are recognized as being endemic for North American blastomycosis, histoplasmosis, and coccidioidomycosis. (Courtesy of Veterans Administration Medical Center, Asheville, NC.)

||||| ENDEMIC AREA OF BLASTOMYCOSIS

ENDEMIC AREA OF HISTOPLASMOSIS

ENDEMIC AREA OF COCCIDIOIDOMYCOSIS

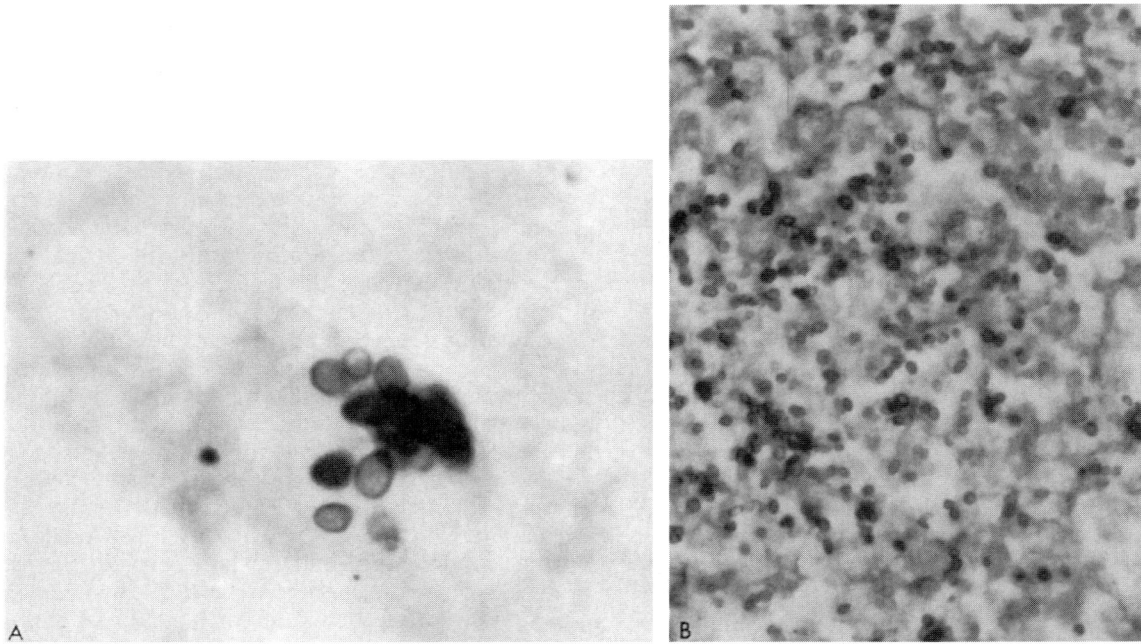

FIGURE 20–9. Forms of *Histoplasma capsulatum* that were found in tissues. *A,* Intracellular organisms (H & E stain, ×2000). *B,* Nonviable capsules of *H. capsulatum* in a necrotic center of a histoplasmoma (methenamine silver stain, ×1000). (*A,* Courtesy of Veterans Administration Hospital, Asheville, NC; *B,* From Takaro, T.: Thoracic actinomycotic and mycotic infections. *In* Ellis, F. H., Jr. [ed]: Thoracic Surgery. Thomaston, CT, Practice of Surgery, 1987.)

nodule and may be confused with carcinoma (Fig. 20–10).

Fewer than 1 in 50,000 patients with primary histoplasmosis develops systemic disseminated disease. Clinically disseminated histoplasmosis may present with multiple organ system involvement; those organs best endowed with reticuloendothelial cells are most commonly involved (liver, spleen, lymph nodes, bone marrow, adrenal glands). Patients with disseminated disease usually have some form of immune disturbance that leads to impaired macrophage destruction of the organisms (Goodwin et al., 1976).

Chronic cavitary pulmonary histoplasmosis usually affects individuals with underlying structural abnormalities of chronic obstructive pulmonary disease. Clinically, the disease is similar to cavitary tuberculo-

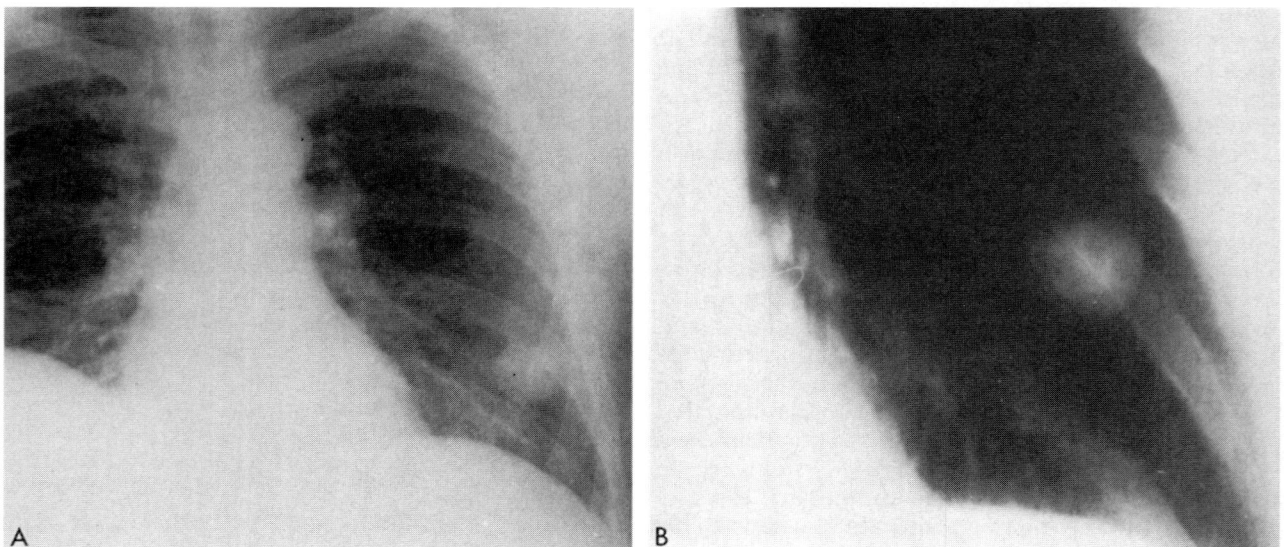

FIGURE 20–10. *A,* Thoracic film of a solitary pulmonary nodule in the left lower lobe. *B,* Tomogram showing a central concentric calcification in a 47-year-old male cigarette smoker. This lesion is typical of chronic granuloma due to histoplasmosis and should not be resected.

sis, accompanied by productive cough, fever, night sweats, fatiguability, weakness, pleurisy, hemoptysis, and dyspnea. It occurs when areas of centrilobular or bullous emphysema become infected with the organism, after which pneumonitis occurs in a localized area, usually the apex of the lung. The area eventually cavitates and becomes thick-walled.

The diagnosis of histoplasmosis depends on isolation of the *H. capsulatum* organism in culture. Serologic techniques are useful adjuncts but are not as reliable as they are in other infectious diseases.

Histoplasmosis in the mediastinum clinically resembles fibrosing mediastinitis and is thought to occur in individuals who react to mediastinal histoplasmosis with exuberant fibrosis (Fig. 20–11). This fibrosis develops either as a reaction to fungal antigen that is released when granulomas rupture or as a result of the host's inability to discontinue further collagen production around a central focus of infection. Although most patients with mediastinal granuloma are asymptomatic, some develop symptoms of chest pain, cough, dysphagia, and dyspnea, as well as signs of superior vena caval obstruction. These symptoms are the result of the intense fibrotic reaction of the patient with subsequent esophageal and tracheal compression, superior vena caval obstruction, and compression of the atria and pulmonary arteries.

Chemotherapy with amphotericin B is the baseline treatment for serious infections with *H. capsulatum*. Most patients with primary disease do not require

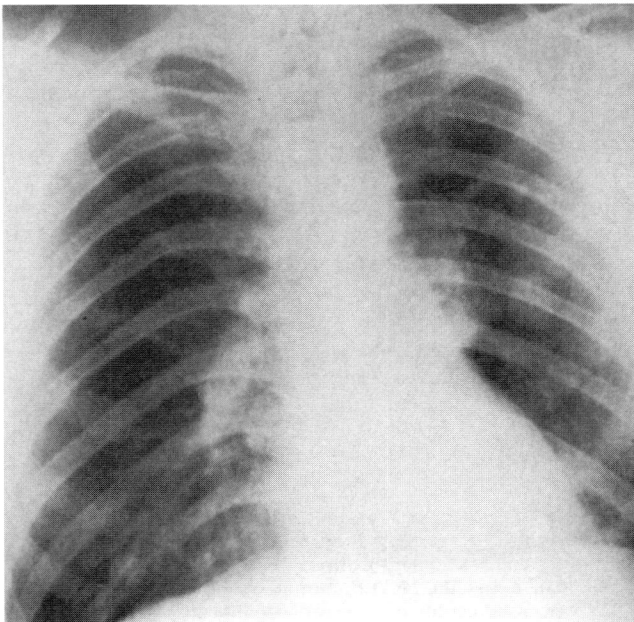

FIGURE 20–11. Thoracic film of a patient with chronic fibrosing mediastinitis due to histoplasmosis. Findings include reduced volume of the left lung, a left hilar mass, and bilateral pulmonary nodules in a 24-year-old white man who presented with hemoptysis and slight hoarseness. A scan showed no perfusion of the left lung. Findings at left thoracotomy included multiple granulomas and a dense fibrosing process involving the left mediastinum and producing thrombosis of the left pulmonary artery. Pathologic specimens were consistent with chronic histoplasmosis.

therapy, but severely ill patients with deterioration of respiratory function can be treated effectively with relatively low doses of amphotericin B. Disseminated disease always requires therapy, and the mortality rate for untreated cases is approximately 90%. Therapy with amphotericin B in a total dose of 30 to 40 mg/kg has reduced the mortality rate in disseminated disease to less than 20%. In a normal host with progressive disseminated histoplasmosis, treatment with ketoconazole can be used if the disease is indolent. A dose of 400 mg daily is given for 6 to 12 months (Johnson and Sarosi, 1991). Surgical resection combined with amphotericin B chemotherapy is indicated in patients with chronic cavitary pulmonary disease. Surgical intervention is indicated when thick-walled cavities persist in a patient with adequate pulmonary reserve after an adequate therapeutic trial with amphotericin (a 2- to 3-g course for 2 to 3 months). Surgical intervention is also indicated for fibrosing mediastinitis with secondary bronchial obstruction (middle-lobe syndrome) or vascular compression. Surgery is necessary to establish a diagnosis if the mediastinal mass is noncalcified and nonspecific. Some authors (Dines et al., 1979) recommended that mediastinal granulomas be excised when the lesions are large to prevent severe sequelae of fibrosis, including superior vena caval obstruction and airway compression. Pericarditis from histoplasmosis with resultant pericardial effusion has occurred more frequently than previously thought and usually responds well to pericardial window drainage. The pathogenesis of this fibrinopurulent pericarditis is thought to be related to direct extension from mediastinal nodes or a hypersensitivity reaction. The prognosis is usually good in these patients once drainage is complete, and amphotericin B therapy is not thought to be indicated (Prager et al., 1980).

Coccidioidomycosis

Coccidioidomycosis is a common disease in the southwestern part of the United States and Mexico, where the causative organism is endemic in the desert soil of this area. In its natural habitat, *Coccidioides immitis* grows as a mold composed of a mesh of hyphae-bearing arthrospores. The arthrospores are readily detached and swept into an aerosol that can be easily inhaled by humans and other mammals. Within the host, the highly infectious arthrospores mature into spherules, which are the tissue pathogens. The spherules enlarge in the lung and become packed with endospores, which ultimately rupture, liberating the tiny endospores and perpetuating the invasive process. In parts of the endemic region, infection is virtually universal: 80% or more of the population is infected within 5 years of initial residence in these areas (Batra, 1992). Infections commonly affect young children, who usually have mild or asymptomatic disease. Adults who are exposed to the agent are at a significantly higher risk of increased severity of the primary disease, as well as of dissemination. In addition to age at first exposure, race and sex appear to influence the risk of dissemination. Approximately 0.5 to 1% of adult white men with primary infection develop disseminated disease; the risk in white women is significantly less. American Indian, Mexican, black, and Filipino populations appear to be more susceptible to the severe form of the disease (Drutz and Catanzaro, 1978).

The severity of the clinical course after inhalation of the endospores is determined mainly by the host's ability to develop cell-mediated immunity against *C. immitis* to control infection. A skin test that shows a reaction to coccidioidin, prepared from the mycelial phase of the organism, is highly correlated with protection and a favorable prognosis. Patients with disseminated disease often lose the measure of cell-mediated immunity, and the persistence of a negative skin test at the completion of therapy is associated with a high rate of relapse.

The pathologic appearance of a tissue reaction to *C. immitis* is similar to the granulomatous reaction in tuberculosis and other systemic mycoses. In active lesions, mature spherules filled with endospores permit positive identification. These spherules may be found directly on wet mount preparations (potassium hydroxide) of specimens of sputum or pus. The endospore-containing spherule is a thick-walled, highly fractile spheric structure, 10 to 80 μm in thickness, and it is diagnostic of infection when identified in tissues or fluid.

The clinical course of *C. immitis* infection depends on whether pulmonary disease or disseminated disease develops; the latter involves the nervous system and genitourinary system. Forty per cent of patients inhaling *C. immitis* arthrospores develop an influenza-like illness 1 to 4 weeks after exposure. Symptoms typically include fever, cough, pleurisy, dyspnea, anorexia, myalgias, headache, and fatigue. The remaining 60% who inhale the fungus remain asymptomatic; their only evidence of infection is positive skin test results. Early in the course, approximately 10% of patients, especially young children, develop a generalized macular erythematous rash prominent in the inguinal folds and on the hands and feet. Approximately 20% of patients have erythema nodosum or erythema multiforme, which is related to development of cell-mediated immunity. The appearance of these skin lesions indicates an excellent prognosis. The combination of pneumonitis, erythema nodosum, and arthralgias is well known in endemic areas as *acute valley fever* (Drutz and Catanzaro, 1978).

In the typical case of acute pneumonitis due to *C. immitis* infection, complete healing occurs even though chest film abnormalities consisting of cavities and cysts may appear transiently during the first few weeks of illness. Only 5% of patients with symptomatic primary pulmonary disease develop irreversible bronchiectasis, pulmonary nodules, pulmonary abscesses, or residual cavities (Fig. 20–12). Chronic pulmonary cavitary lesions are the most frequent long-

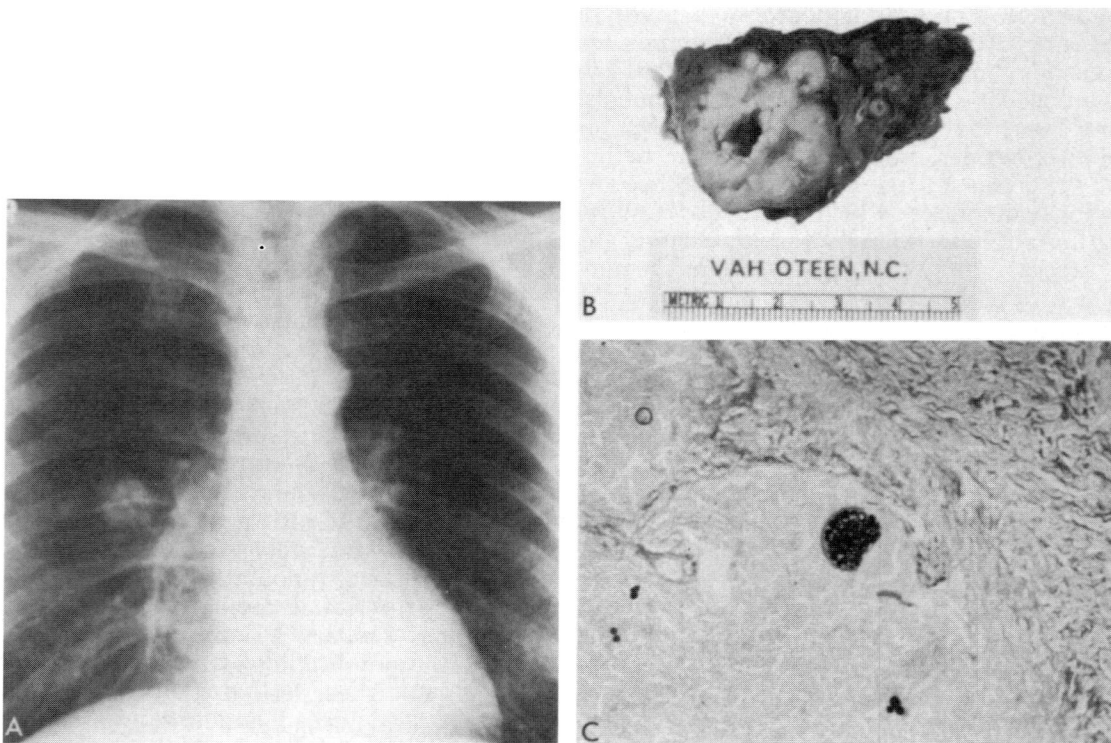

FIGURE 20–12. Coccidioidal granuloma. *A,* Chest film of a 45-year-old asymptomatic man from Texas who was found on routine chest film to have a dense nodule in the superior segment of the right lower lobe. The results of all diagnostic studies were negative. *B,* Chronic granuloma containing central cavitation found in the resected segment. *C,* Fungus stains showing a large spherule with endospores and single large endospores in surrounding necrotic tissue.

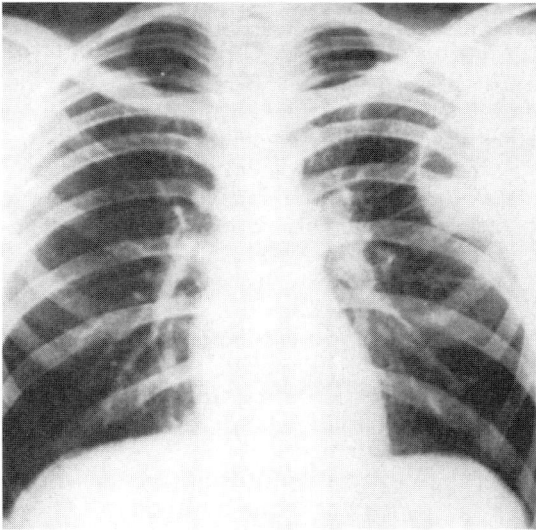

FIGURE 20–13. Cavitary lesion due to coccidioidomycosis. The thin wall of this cavity and its peripheral location are characteristic. (From Hyde, L.: Coccidioidal pulmonary cavitations. Dis. Chest, 54:213, 1968.)

term complication of acute coccidioidomycosis (Fig. 20–13). These lesions are solitary and thin-walled and are associated with a few surrounding inflammatory changes. They are usually peripheral and lie adjacent to the pleura. If the cavities rupture, they cause pleural effusion, bronchopleural fistula, empyema, and pneumothorax. The radiographic appearance of patients who develop localized coin lesions as a result

of the acute primary pulmonary infection is consistent with that of bronchogenic carcinoma (Fig. 20–14).

Dissemination of *C. immitis* infection is usually insidious, and infection appears weeks to months after the initial acute pulmonary syndrome. The most important sites of clinical infection after dissemination are the central nervous system, the skeletal system, and the genitourinary system. The most important extrapulmonary manifestation of coccidioidomycosis is meningitis, which occurs in up to one-third of all cases of disseminated disease. Meningitis from *C. immitis* usually follows a subacute chronic course. Headache is the most common symptom, and meningeal signs are usually absent. After central nervous system involvement, skeletal infection occurs in up to 20% of patients with disseminated disease. The most common sites of involvement are the long bones, the vertebrae, and the skull. On x-ray films, these lesions usually appear lytic with minimal periosteal proliferation, and late sclerosis is present. The radioisotope bone scan delineates the extent of involvement of *C. immitis* in the skeletal system. Finally, *C. immitis* can involve the genitourinary system, more specifically the kidneys rather than the lower urinary tract.

The most effective specific therapy is amphotericin B, but most patients require no therapy. Use of systemic amphotericin B should be considered for specific clinical situations: severe prolonged primary disease, especially if it is associated with rising levels of complement-fixing antibody (although in this situation ketoconazole and fluconazole are now being used); primary disease in which there is risk of dissemination because of pregnancy, racial predisposi-

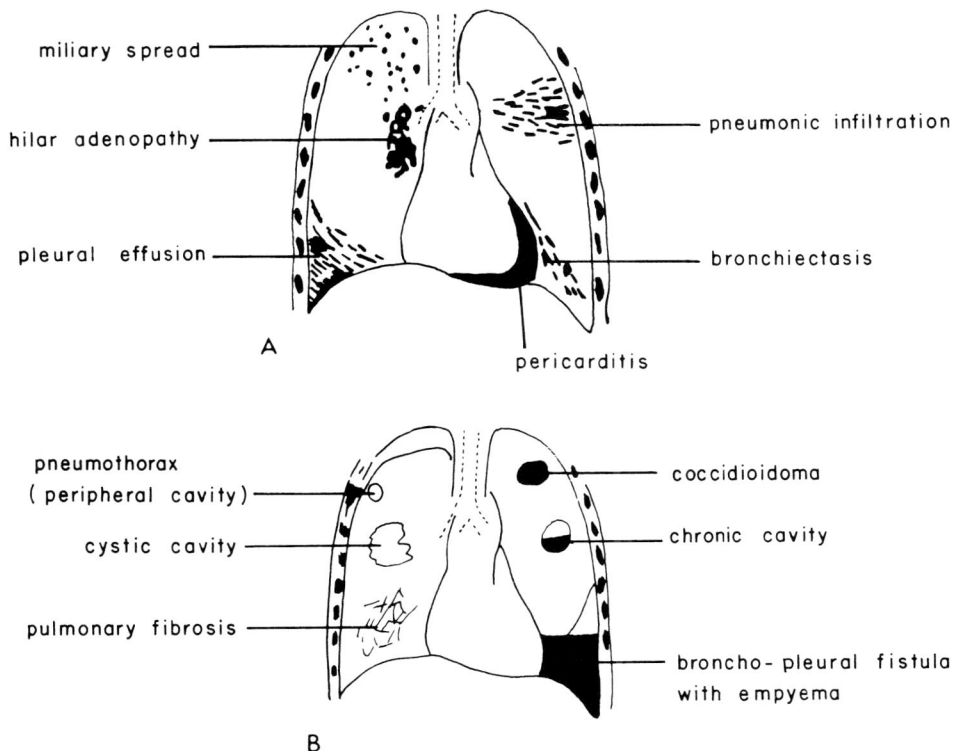

FIGURE 20–14. Pulmonary manifestations of coccidioidomycosis. *A,* Acute stage. *B,* Chronic stage. (*A* and *B,* From Paulsen, G. A.: Pulmonary surgery in coccidioidal infections. *In* Ajello, L. [ed]: Coccidioidomycosis. Tucson, University of Arizona Press, 1967.)

tion, or an immunosuppressed state; chemotherapy used in combination with surgical resection of a known or suspect coccidioidomycotic lesion; and symptomatic chronic cavitary disease. Meningeal involvement is also an absolute indication for intrathecal therapy. The indications for surgical therapy for *C. immitis* include localized granulomatous lesions and cavitary diseases (Nelson, 1974). In an endemic area, a coccidioidal granuloma is resected only if a definitive diagnosis cannot be made and malignancy is suspected (Catanzaro, 1980; Paulsen, 1967). For chronic cavitary disease, the main indications for surgical therapy are the complications of such lesions. Enlarging cavitary lesions may rupture and cause pneumothorax, or they may be the source of hemoptysis or become secondarily infected. In these situations, surgical therapy should remove the cavity as well as the surrounding granulomatous involvement. Perioperative drug therapy with amphotericin B is recommended, but localized resection for this mycotic process still is associated with a 10% incidence of complications, including bronchopleural fistula and empyema (Sarosi et al., 1970). Recurrent cavitation occurs in 10 to 20% of patients after surgical intervention (Salomon et al., 1980).

Blastomycosis

Blastomycosis is a systemic mycotic infection caused by the dimorphic fungus *Blastomyces dermatitidis*. This disease is endemic in the southeastern and south central portions of the United States, with extension northward along the Mississippi and Ohio River valleys. The disease is especially common among young and middle-aged adults, and the incidence is 6 to 10 times greater in men than in women, with a predilection for persons with outdoor vocations (Sarosi and Davies, 1979). The organism exists in moist soil with an acid pH, and primary infection follows inhalation of the fungus, which has been aerosolized at those sites. *B. dermatitidis* is a round, thick-walled, single budding yeast from 8 to 15 μm in diameter. The organism may be seen reasonably well with routine H & E stains, but special fungal stains such as the periodic acid–Schiff and methenamine silver stains usually have many more organisms from smears of cultured sputum or other secretions or tissues. Papanicolaou's stain test is useful in examining pulmonary secretions for this organism. The initial portal of entry is the respiratory tract, and inhaled organisms are deposited in the peripheral airspaces, usually of the lower lobes. The usual cellular immune response controls or eradicates infection in most patients. In a few patients there may be progression of the acute respiratory infection, ranging from mild pulmonary disease with lymphatic spread to regional lymph nodes, to progressive pulmonary suppuration with destruction and cavitation of the lung. Hematogenous dissemination with spread to other sites, particularly the skin, skeletal system, and genitalia, may occur; the disease commonly presents in its chronic

cutaneous form. Between 50 and 70% of patients with chronic blastomycosis have simultaneous multiple organ system involvement. The characteristic lesion in cutaneous blastomycosis is raised, verrucous, and crusted, with an irregular border (Fig. 20–15). The lesion usually is located in the extremities or on the face. Chronically draining fistulas are rare, and erythema nodosum is less common in blastomycosis than in coccidioidomycosis. Biopsy of the skin lesions at the edge is preferable, because it allows a higher yield of organisms for diagnosis.

Pulmonary involvement varies and may be asymptomatic, acute, or chronic. Inhalation of the fungus most frequently causes asymptomatic disease. An acute illness similar to influenza may result and is characterized by fever, cough, pleuritic chest pain, arthralgias, and myalgias. Most symptomatic patients with acute blastomycosis recover 2 to 3 weeks after the onset of symptoms. Less commonly, the disease progresses to chronic pulmonary suppuration and cavitation. Most patients with pulmonary blastomycosis who come to medical attention have chronic pulmonary disease, and the duration of symptoms is usually several weeks to months. These patients show simultaneous involvement of other organs, particularly the skin (Klein et al., 1975).

Radiographic findings in pulmonary blastomycosis vary in the acute and chronic forms of the disease. In acute blastomycosis, the chest film shows airspace consolidation that is patchy and usually located in the lower lobes. Resolution of these abnormalities in acute blastomycosis usually requires up to 3 months. Chronic pulmonary blastomycosis typically involves the upper lobes and is characterized by a fibronodular appearance; smooth-walled cavities are frequently present. A single mass lesion resembling bronchogenic carcinoma can also be seen.

The chronic form of blastomycosis commonly involves the skeletal system; the spine, pelvis, skull, and ribs are the most common sites. Radiographically, the lesions are similar to those from other systemic granulomatous diseases. However, *rib* involvement strongly suggests blastomycosis.

Definitive diagnosis depends on successful growth of the organism in culture or on unequivocal identification of the organism on smear from secretions or tissues. Because culture of the organism may take up to 4 weeks after inoculation on culture plates, identification of the characteristic yeast forms (spherical cells with a thick-walled, refractile, double contour showing *unipolar budding*) is adequate for initiating chemotherapy in the appropriate clinical setting (Fig. 20–16). Immunologic methods for diagnosing blastomycosis have not been reliable (Rubin, 1982).

Treatment of blastomycosis is primarily by drug therapy. Amphotericin B is the treatment of choice, and a total dose of 2 to 2.5 g is administered for 2 to 3 months for patients who have advanced disease with multiorgan involvement. Ketoconazole has been an appropriate alternative agent in immunocompetent patients with moderate to severe disease (Bradsher et al., 1985). A dosage of 400 mg/day for 6

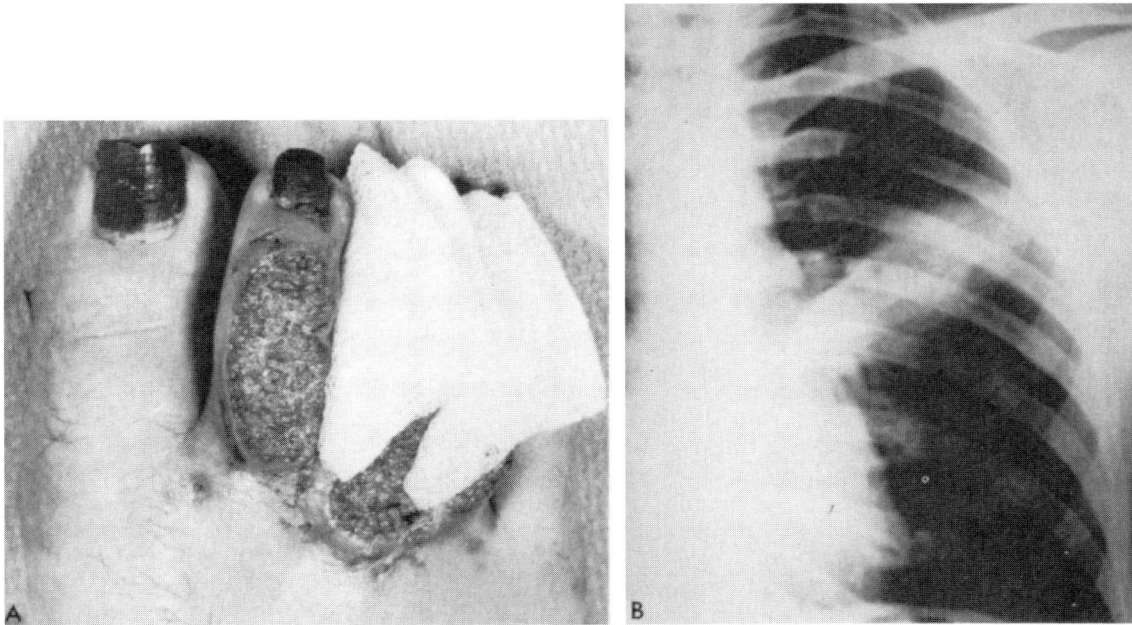

FIGURE 20–15. *A,* Skin lesions of blastomycosis on the dorsum of the toes. Biopsy of the raised edges showed multiple microabscesses containing *Blastomyces dermatitidis. B,* Blastomycotic pneumonic infiltrate. (*A* and *B,* From Takaro, T.: Thoracic actinomycotic and mycotic infections. *In* Ellis, F. H., Jr. [ed]: Thoracic Surgery. Thomaston, CT, Practice of Surgery, 1987.)

months is essentially nontoxic and has an 80% success rate. Long-term follow-up is required regardless of which treatment modality is used, because relapse has been reported several years after an adequate course of treatment.

Surgical treatment is limited to draining large ab-scesses or closing bronchial fistulas. Rarely, in a patient with persistent cavitary disease and residual sputum that demonstrates blastomycosis after medical therapy, resection of the cavity is indicated. When resections are not followed by continued antifungal therapy, the incidence of recurrence is high.

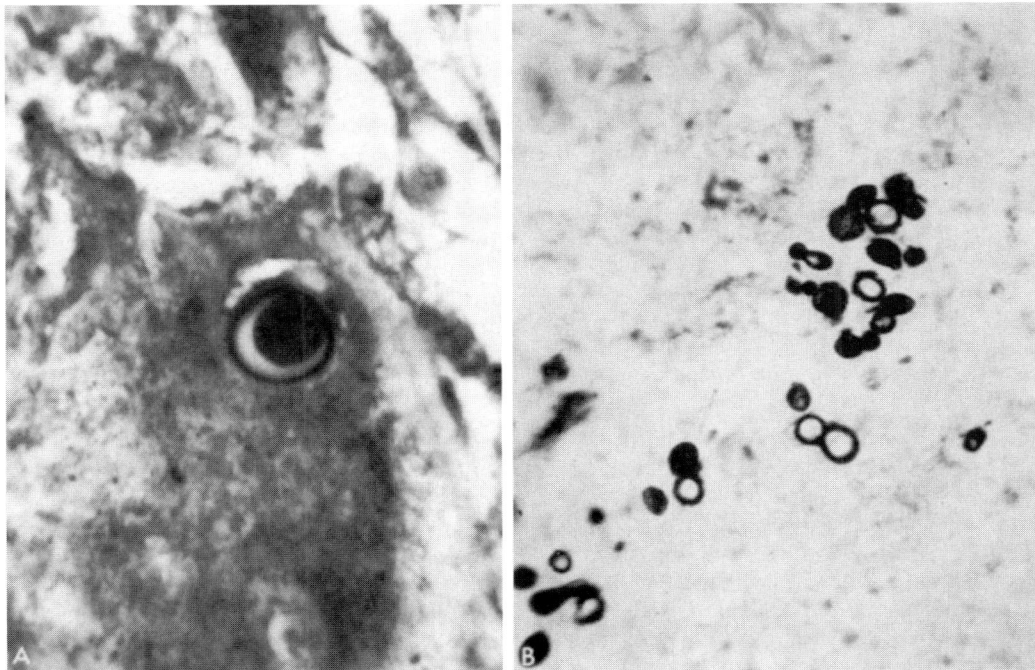

FIGURE 20–16. Organisms of *B. dermatitidis* from resected lung tissue. *A,* A single thick-walled yeast form with refractile cell wall. *B,* Multiple budding yeast forms characteristic of blastomycosis (periodic acid–Schiff stain, ×1100). (*A* and *B,* From Takaro, T.: Thoracic actinomycotic and mycotic infections. *In* Ellis, F. H., Jr. [ed]: Thoracic Surgery. Thomaston, CT, Practice of Surgery, 1987.)

Cryptococcosis

Cryptococcosis (formerly called torulosis) is a chronic infection caused by *Cryptococcus neoformans*. It primarily involves the bronchopulmonary tree but also has a predilection for the meninges, in which case it is in its most lethal form (Littman and Walter, 1968). Although cryptococcosis was previously thought to be a rare and usually fatal infection, a benign form of the disease with pulmonary manifestations actually is more common than the fatal meningeal form. Amphotericin B and 5-fluorocytosine have dramatically reduced the mortality from cryptococcal meningitis. The incidence of opportunistic infection with *C. neoformans* significantly increased during the 1980s, and the disease is commonly encountered in immunosuppressed patients or patients undergoing chemotherapy (Duperval et al., 1977). *C. neoformans* is ubiquitous in soil and dust, especially that contaminated by pigeon droppings, and it is confined to no specific endemic geographic area. The organisms are round, budding yeast cells with a characteristically wide gelatinous capsule and are shown in sputum, bronchial washings, and cerebrospinal fluid by India ink stain or in fixed tissue by mucicarmine stain (Fig. 20–17).

As in the other systemic mycotic infections, the respiratory tract is the portal of entry. Most cases of cryptococcosis occur as isolated pulmonary infections (Hammerman et al., 1973). Pulmonary manifestations are variable and nonspecific, and spontaneous remission occurs in most persons who contract the primary disease. In patients with an abnormal immune response due to underlying illness such as lymphoma or diabetes or to treatment with corticosteroids or immunosuppressive agents, the disease may progress in a disseminated form (Littman and Walter, 1968). The pathologic findings are characterized by a chronic granulomatous reaction in the lungs, which lack an acute inflammatory response. Central necrosis and cavitation are not commonly seen, as in other major pulmonary mycotic infections. Radiographic features of cryptococcosis also are nonspecific, and solitary or multiple lesions may be seen. These lesions often involve the lower lobe and are usually solid. A tumor mass or pneumonitis may be the initial presentation on chest film. Pulmonary cryptococcosis usually is diagnosed from a resected specimen of the lung, although when suspected, the organism can be isolated from respiratory secretions with the appropriate staining techniques. The presence of the organism in sputum can be secondary to colonization in some cases, and the significance of this finding must be interpreted within the total clinical presentation (Hatcher et al., 1971).

Two agents effectively treat cryptococcosis: amphotericin B and 5-fluorocytosine. The latter agent is synergistic with amphotericin B and has fewer side effects, allowing a smaller dose of amphotericin B to be used and minimizing its toxic reactions. In the rare cases of preoperative diagnosis of *C. neoformans* infection, the pulmonary lesion can be resolved completely with amphotericin B. Whenever *C. neoformans* is isolated from either sputum or a surgical specimen, the cerebrospinal fluid should be examined immediately;

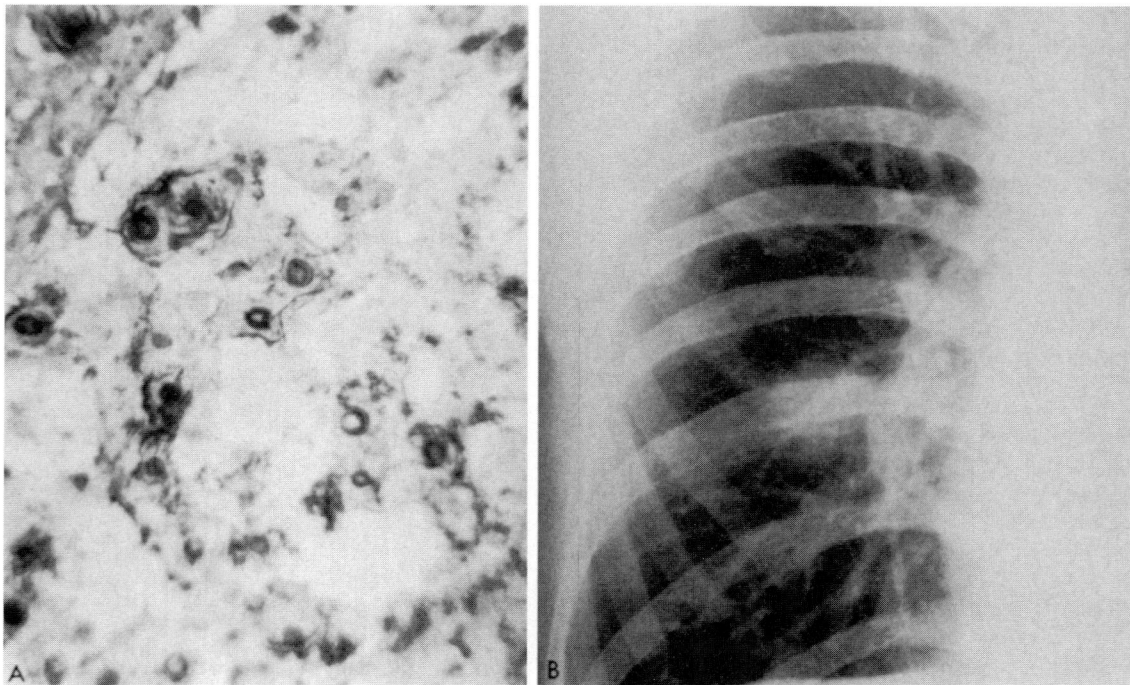

FIGURE 20–17. Cryptococcosis. *A*, Organisms of *Cryptococcus neoformans* in resected pulmonary tissue showing thick capsules surrounding the organisms (mucicarmine, ×950). *B*, Thoracic film showing solitary nodule with ill-defined borders in an asymptomatic man. This was removed by wedge resection of the superior segment of the right lower lobe and proved to be a coccidioidal granuloma. (*A* and *B*, From Takaro, T.: Thoracic actinomycotic and mycotic infections. *In* Ellis, F. H., Jr. [ed]: Thoracic Surgery. Thomaston, CT, Practice of Surgery, 1987.)

the presence of the organism in the cerebrospinal fluid dictates urgent treatment. In most cases of cryptococcosis that involve the thoracic surgeon, the diagnosis is not made until the resected surgical specimen is examined, commonly a solitary pulmonary nodule that is explored for potential malignancy. After demonstration of *Cryptococcus* in the surgical specimen, a spinal tap should be done. If the results are positive, combined amphotericin B and 5-fluorocytosine treatment is indicated. If the central nervous system is uninvolved, a decision must be made regarding the treatment of the patient to avoid dissemination to the central nervous system. Up to 10% of patients with a resected pulmonary lesion develop cryptococcal meningitis after resection (Hatcher et al., 1971). Therefore, if the cryptococcal lesion in the lung is small and inactive, if there is no surrounding infiltrate or pleural reaction, and if the lesion can be resected by leaving a wide margin or normal adjacent pulmonary tissue, usually no chemotherapy is needed. However, if the diseased pulmonary tissue resulting from the cryptococcal infection is extensive and the disease appears to be active at thoracotomy and cannot be completely resected, prophylactic use of amphotericin B is recommended, usually a total dose of 500 mg. Patients who are receiving corticosteroids or who have some alteration in the normal immune response deserve a course of prophylactic amphotericin B when crypto-

coccosis in the lung is discovered or resected (Sen and Louria, 1981).

Aspergillosis

Aspergilli ordinarily are saprophytes widely found in nature. Nevertheless, three recognized distinct clinical entities can be called aspergillosis. The most common manifestation is aspergillar bronchitis, an asthmatic or allergic bronchitis attributed to *Aspergillus*, which is readily isolated from the sputum. The fungus colonizes the airways, which contain abnormally thickened mucus with development of proximal saccular bronchiectasis (Gefter, 1992). The next most common type of *Aspergillus* infection, and one of special interest to thoracic surgeons, is the aspergilloma or fungus ball, in which a mycelial mass lies free in a previously formed cavity or cyst in the lung. The third type is an invasive infection characterized by necrotizing bronchopneumonia, which usually occurs in patients with debilitating disease or who are immunosuppressed (Karas et al., 1976).

Most infections are caused by *Aspergillus fumigatus*, which is a filamentous fungus found in soil and on decaying vegetation. It produces airborne spores. The organisms are present in pathologic material as coarse, fragmented, branching hyphae, either in short strands or in ball-like clusters (Fig. 20–18), which

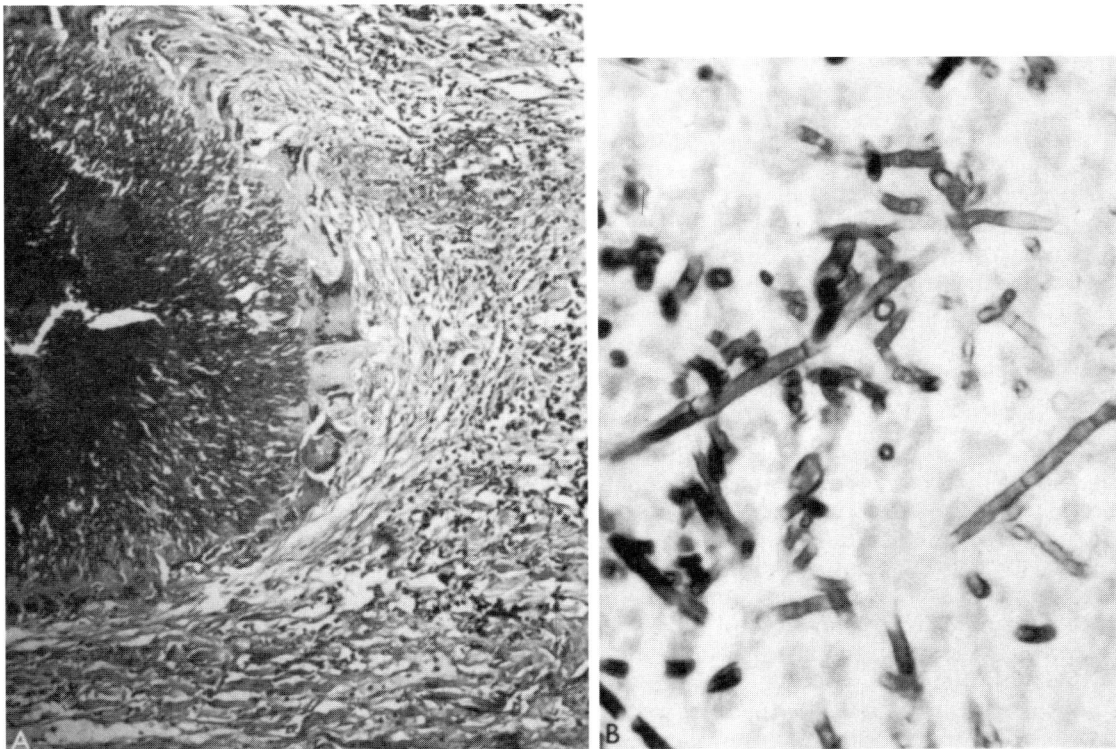

FIGURE 20–18. Organisms of *Aspergillus fumigatus* in tissues. *A,* A colony of aspergilli found in a resected carcinomatous lesion of the lung. Note the mycelia radiating outward from a dark center of the colony (methenamine silver stain, ×250). *B,* High-powered view of coarse, fragmented septate mycelia of *A. fumigatus.* The round bodies are mycelia viewed head on (methenamine silver stain, ×950). (*A* and *B,* From Takaro, T.: Thoracic actinomycotic and mycotic infections. *In* Ellis, F. H., Jr. [ed]: Thoracic Surgery. Thomaston, CT, Practice of Surgery, 1987.)

can be identified unequivocally only by isolation and culture. Most of the surgically resected lesions of aspergillosis are aspergillomas. The fungus ball is a matted sphere of hyphae, fibrin, and inflammatory cells. Its gross appearance is an oval, friable, gray, red-brown, or yellow necrotic-appearing mass, usually in an upper lobe cavity (Fig. 20–19). There is usually evidence of preexisting chronic lung disease, such as tuberculosis, sarcoidosis, bronchiectasis, bronchogenic cyst, chronic pulmonary abscess, or cavitating carcinoma, in the parenchyma surrounding the fungus ball. In a large-scale survey conducted in Great Britain by the British Thoracic and Tuberculosis Association (1970), up to 17% of patients with old tuberculous cavities had aspergillomas.

Aspergillomas are of surgical interest only if symptoms are present. In approximately 50% of these patients, at least one episode of hemoptysis occurs. In up to 10% of patients with aspergillomas, the hemoptysis can be severe and recurrent (Varkey and Rose, 1976). Many aspergillomas remain asymptomatic, however, and some may even resolve spontaneously (Fahey et al., 1981). Invasion and dissemination from an aspergilloma rarely occur (Butz et al., 1985).

Once a patient with an aspergilloma develops hemoptysis, the aspergilloma should be resected if the patient is a candidate for operation. Prophylactic resection in asymptomatic patients is generally not indicated, because there is a significant complication rate after resection in these patients, who usually have significant disease in the parenchyma of the lung surrounding the aspergilloma (Belcher's complex aspergillosis) (Battaglini et al., 1985; Belcher and Plummer, 1960).

Because antifungal drugs (amphotericin B) do not penetrate the poorly perfused cystic cavity containing the aspergilloma, medical therapy is usually unsatisfactory for aspergillosis. In high-risk patients in whom resection cannot be done safely, cavernostomy (Eguchi et al., 1971) or instillation of sodium iodide or amphotericin B through a percutaneous catheter into the cavity has been helpful (Hargis et al., 1980). Amphotericin B given intravenously is useful in the treatment of invasive aspergillosis, which usually occurs in patients with impaired immune responses. Griepp reported a cure rate of 50% in 18 cases of aspergillosis in cardiac transplants by intravenously administering amphotericin B (Henderson et al., 1975). After resection of aspergilloma, long-term therapy with amphotericin B is not necessary. Combined antifungal therapy followed by resection of the involved lung has been used successfully in cardiac transplant recipients with localized, invasive pulmonary aspergillar infections (Mayer et al., 1992).

Selected patients who are poor risks for surgical resection and who have an aspergilloma complicated by hemoptysis can undergo intracavitary infusion of amphotericin B combined with bronchial artery embolization (Magilligan et al., 1981).

The difference in surgical outcome between simple

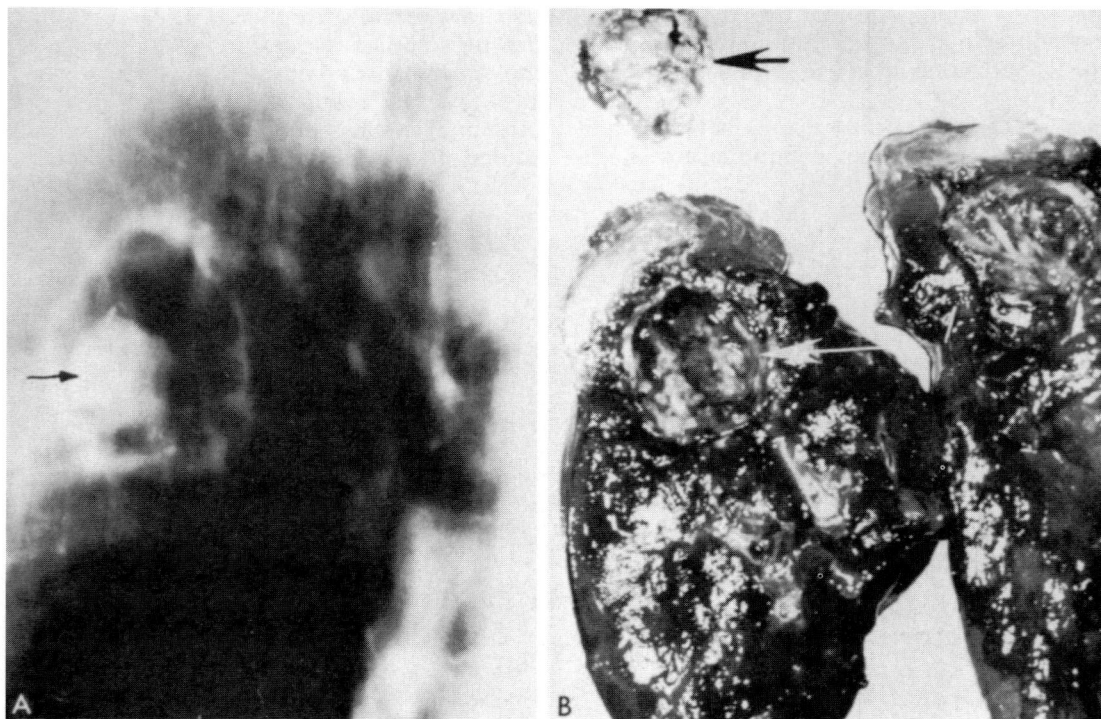

FIGURE 20–19. Aspergilloma. *A*, Tomogram showing the cavitary lesion in the right upper field of the lung containing a fungus ball or aspergilloma (*arrow*) lying free within the cavity. The aspergilloma changes position in the cavity when the patient is moved. *B*, Resected specimen of a right upper lobe showing a smooth-lined chronic cavity (*white arrow*) from which the fungus ball (*black arrow*) was removed. (*A* and *B*, From Takaro, T.: Thoracic actinomycotic and mycotic infections. *In* Ellis, F. H., Jr. [ed]: Thoracic Surgery. Thomaston, CT, Practice of Surgery, 1987.)

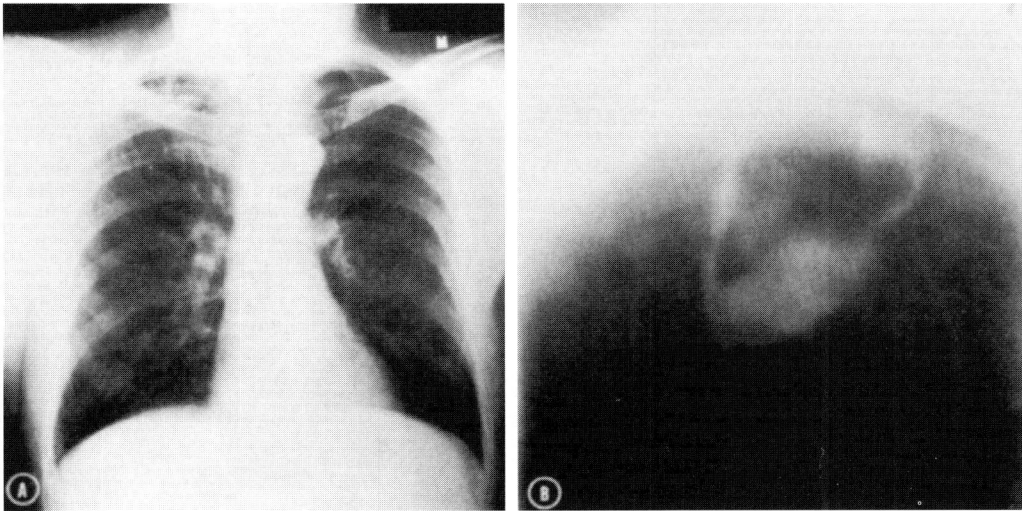

FIGURE 20–20. Example of a simple aspergilloma in the right upper lobe of a 58-year-old man. *A*, Posteroanterior film showing minimal parenchymal disease surrounding the cavitation. *B*, Tomogram of the right apex showing the thin-walled cyst and lack of pulmonary infiltrate. (*A* and *B*, From Daly, R. C., Pairolera, P. C., Piehler, J. M., et al.: Pulmonary aspergilloma: Results of surgical treatment. J. Thorac. Cardiovasc. Surg., *92*:981, 1986.)

aspergillomas and complex aspergillomas is emphasized in a review of 53 patients who underwent thoracotomy for treatment of pulmonary aspergilloma at the Mayo Clinic (Daly et al., 1986). In the series, 31% of patients had simple aspergilloma marked by thin-walled cysts with little surrounding parenchymal pulmonary disease (Fig. 20–20), and 47% had complex aspergilloma characterized by thick-walled cavities, usually larger than 3 mm, with substantial surrounding parenchymal disease or associated infiltrates or both (Fig. 20–21). The operative mortality rate was 5% in patients with simple aspergilloma

and 34% in patients with complex aspergilloma. The postoperative complication rate also was higher in patients who underwent surgery for complex aspergilloma (78% vs. 33%); the specific early complications are shown in Table 20–4. Factors that made pulmonary resection for complex aspergilloma technically difficult included pleural space obliteration, induration of hilar structures, and poor expansion of the remaining lung with residual space problems. However, major pulmonary resection produced good results in survivors of the operation, and 90% of the patients with simple aspergilloma and 67% of patients

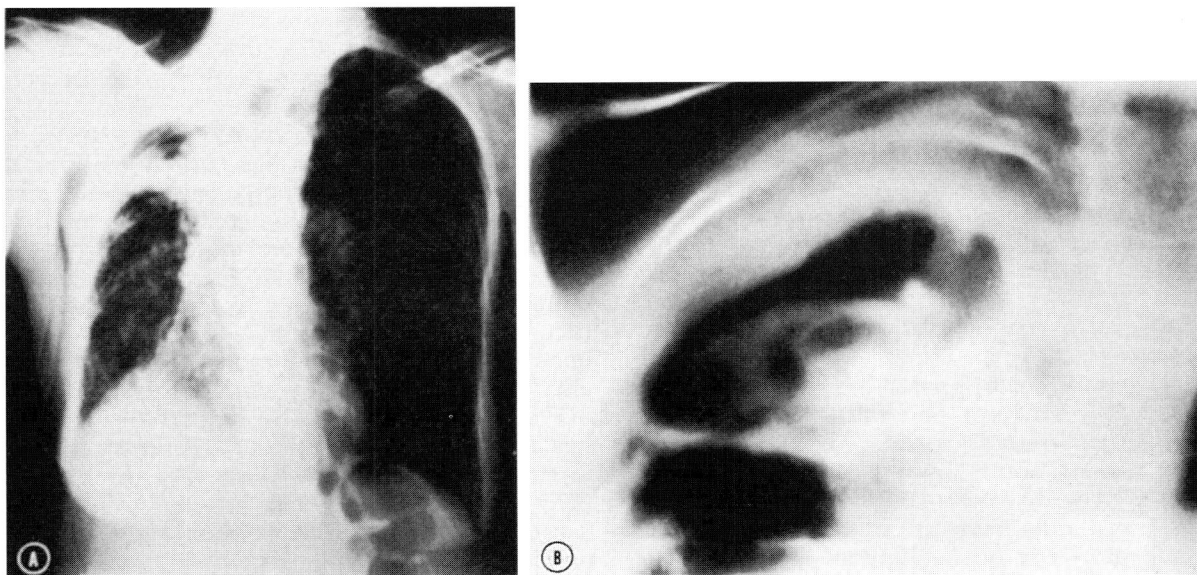

FIGURE 20–21. Example of complex aspergilloma in a 66-year-old woman. *A*, Posteroanterior film showing the apical cavity with extensive pleural and parenchymal reaction. *B*, Tomogram of the right apex showing the thick-walled cavity and extensive pulmonary infiltrate. (*A* and *B*, From Daly, R. C., Pairolera, P. C., Piehler, J. M., et al.: Pulmonary aspergilloma: Results of surgical treatment. J. Thorac. Cardiovasc. Surg., *92*:981, 1986.)

■ **Table 20–4.** EARLY COMPLICATIONS AFTER OPERATION IN 32 PATIENTS WITH ASPERGILLOMAS

Complications	Simple Aspergilloma (7 patients)	Complex Aspergilloma (25 patients)
Empyema	1	11
Prolonged air leak	2	7
Bronchopleural fistula	0	7
Respiratory insufficiency	1	7
Pleural space hemorrhage	2	4
Residual space	1	4
Wound infection	0	4
Bacterial septicemia	0	3
Intrapulmonary bleeding	0	1

From Daly, R. C., Pairolero, P. C., Piehler, J. M., et al.: Pulmonary aspergilloma: Results of surgical treatment. J. Thorac. Cardiovasc. Surg., 92:981, 1986.

with complex aspergilloma were relieved of their symptoms. The authors also discuss the role of cavernostomy and obliteration of the cavity with intrathoracic transposition of extrathoracic skeletal muscle (latissimus dorsi) in selected cases of complex aspergilloma. This technique shows promise for reducing the postoperative complications (air leak, bronchopleural fistula, empyema) that often follow resective therapy of complex lesions. The thoracotomy incision for removal of an aspergilloma should be placed to spare division of the latissimus dorsi so that the muscle may be used later, if necessary, as a transposition flap to cover a bronchopleural fistula or fill in a residual space.

Thoracic Mucormycosis (Phycomycosis)

Mucormycosis is a rare fungal infection caused by fungi belonging to the class *Phycomycetes*. These saprophytic organisms are widespread and are characterized structurally by broad, nonseptate hyphae (Fig. 20–22). The host is entered via inhalation of spores, and involvement of the rhinocerebral sinuses is more common than the pulmonary forms of the disease. Almost all patients who develop mucormycosis have an underlying disease, commonly diabetes or leukemia, or are receiving chemotherapy or corticosteroids, or have other reasons to be chronically debilitated. The organism is usually found adjacent to thrombosed blood vessels and necrotic tissue (pulmonary infarction). The disease usually is rapidly progressive and fatal, because it is rarely diagnosed early enough for therapy to be effective. Treatment has been difficult, because the fungal infection is opportunistic and the drug amphotericin B cannot reach the causative organism because it resides in thrombosed blood vessels and infarcted tissue. Aggressive therapy combining surgical resection of necrotic nonperfused tissue with amphotericin B has led to a few cures (Lehrer et al., 1980).

Sporotrichosis

The dimorphic fungus that causes sporotrichosis, *Sporothrix schenckii*, is a ubiquitous organism that grows well in various soils and decaying vegetation. Infection usually occurs among gardeners, farmers, and florists. The disease is commonly due to subcutaneous inoculation with infectious spores by contaminated thorns or other sharp objects. Less commonly, spores are inhaled and cause a primary pulmonary infection. The incidence of sporotrichosis, especially the pulmonary disseminated form of the disease, is higher among men than among women. Because significant immunologic cross-reactivity has been shown between *S. schenckii* and *Candida albicans*, some experts have suggested that women have an enhanced immune responsiveness to candidal antigens that keeps them relatively resistant to sporotrichosis. *S. schenckii*, in the cutaneous-lymphatic form, produces a verrucous ulceration of the skin and subsequent involvement of the draining lymphatics. The organism occurs as a single or clustered ovoid body called the asteroid body, a central basophilic yeast-like core surrounded by an eosinophilic capsule that stains bright red with periodic acid–Schiff stains (Fig. 20–23).

A few patients with sporotrichosis develop pulmonary infection, which has various manifestations mimicking pulmonary tuberculosis. Patients can present with hilar adenopathy, chronic cavitary disease, and a persistent pulmonary infiltrate. Although dissemination with sporotrichosis may occur after pulmonary infection, this is uncommon. When it does occur, it is insidious in onset and usually involves bones and joints. Less commonly, dissemination also

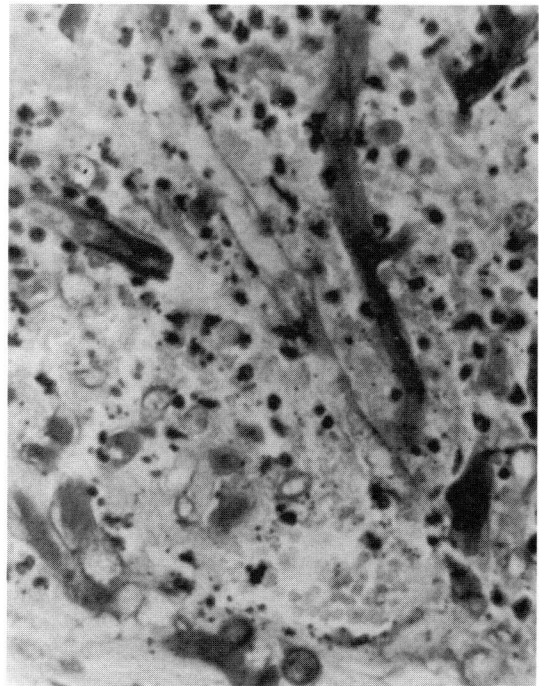

FIGURE 20–22. Mucormycosis (phycomycosis). Broad, nonseptated hyphae of a phycomycete invading a thrombosed pulmonary arterial wall (H & E, ×330). (From Takaro, T.: Thoracic actinomycotic and mycotic infections. *In* Ellis, F. H., Jr. [ed]: Thoracic Surgery. Thomaston, CT, Practice of Surgery, 1987.)

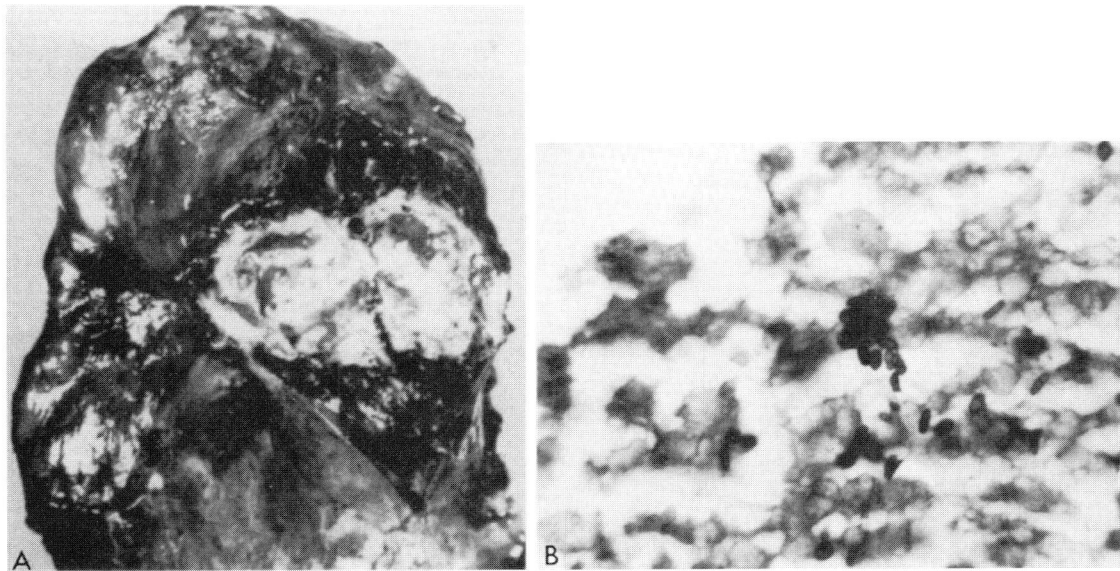

FIGURE 20–23. Sporotrichosis. *A,* Surgical specimen of a resected upper lobe opened to show the cavitary lesions of pulmonary sporotrichosis. *B,* Cigar-shaped organisms of *Sporothrix schenckii* from the resected pulmonary tissue stained with periodic acid–Schiff. (*A* and *B,* From Scott, S. M., Peasley, E. D., and Crymes, T. P.: Pulmonary sporotrichosis: Report of two cases with cavitation. N. Engl. J. Med., *265:*453, 1961.)

affects the skin, oral mucosa, and central nervous system, but in these cases the patient usually has a clear source of immunosuppression, including carcinoma, lymphoproliferative disease, AIDS, diabetes, or alcoholism.

Definitive diagnosis of sporotrichosis depends on isolation of the organism on culture. Microscopic examination of pus or biopsy material usually does not establish the diagnosis because the concentration of fungal cells is low.

Treatment is generally medical, because the cutaneous lymphatic form responds to oral potassium iodide, 3 to 4 mg, three times per day. Pulmonary or disseminated infection requires amphotericin B therapy, usually a total dose of 2 to 2.5 g for 2 to 3 months. Surgical excision should be reserved for patients with residual localized cavitary disease, and the patient should be protected with amphotericin B treatment before and after surgical therapy to prevent relapse.

Miscellaneous Fungal Infections

Candidiasis

Candidiasis, an opportunistic fungal infection, has increased steadily but slowly in incidence since the early 1970s. The causative organism, *Candida albicans,* produces two types of infection: mucocutaneous and systemic. It is usually a superficial fungal infection commonly infecting the oral, bronchial, or vaginal mucosa. Systemic candidiasis is associated with a deep infection involving the lungs, bloodstream, endocardium, meninges, or other organs, and it occurs more commonly in persons with severe underlying disease or immunocompromised conditions. Three

situations lead to endocardial involvement: intravenous drug abuse, insertion of prosthetic valves, and use of indwelling intravenous catheters (Seelig et al., 1973). Among drug abusers, candidal infections usually involve the valves on the left side of the heart, and species other than *C. albicans* are implicated. However, prosthetic endocarditis due to candidal infection is usually caused by *C. albicans* or *C. tropicalis.*

Candidal organisms are widely distributed in the oral pharynx of normal individuals and are ubiquitous contaminants in many hospitals and clinical laboratories. The *Candida* organisms are seen in fresh potassium-hydroxide preparation or on Gram's stain as small, oval, thin-walled budding yeasts that may or may not contain mycelial elements (Fig. 20–24).

Intensive or prolonged broad-spectrum antibiotic therapy may suppress an individual's normal bacterial flora, allowing an overgrowth of the often present saprophytic species of *Candida.* Invasion then can take place through any portal of entry, especially via indwelling catheters used for vascular access or through the gastrointestinal tract. In the presence of altered host immunity, septicemia and generalized infection may result, usually with a fatal outcome. If *C. albicans* is found on culture from blood or from the lung, it cannot be dismissed as a contaminant. Especially in patients who have signs of septicemia, therapy with amphotericin B must be considered if the patient is to have any chance of survival.

Paracoccidioidomycosis (South American Blastomycosis)

Paracoccidioidomycosis is a chronic granulomatous infection endemic in South and Central America. It affects the skin, mucous membranes, lymph nodes,

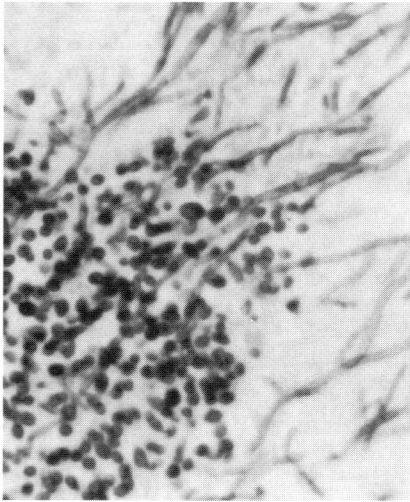

FIGURE 20–24. Organisms of *Candida albicans* showing both yeast and mycelial forms (methenamine silver stain, ×1000). (From Takaro, T.: Thoracic actinomycotic and mycotic infections. *In* Ellis, F. H., Jr. [ed]: Thoracic Surgery. Thomaston, CT, Practice of Surgery, 1987.)

and viscera. Pulmonary lesions resemble those of pulmonary tuberculosis (Emmons et al., 1977). The disease is caused by *Paracoccidioides brasiliensis*, a soil saprophyte that resembles *Blastomyces dermatitidis* or *Cryptococcus neoformans* in tissues. Cavitary pulmonary disease occurs in approximately one-third of patients. The disease is progressive and is fatal unless treated. Amphotericin B therapy has produced the best results, and the role of surgical therapy in this disease is limited, except in providing tissue for diagnosis by lung biopsy (Murray et al., 1974; Restrepo et al., 1980) (Fig. 20–25).

Pulmonary Monosporiosis

Pulmonary monosporiosis is a rare mycotic infection caused by *Monosporium apiospermum*. This organism is an opportunistic invader of previously damaged pulmonary tissue such as a tuberculous cavity or emphysematous bleb. A fungus ball can be formed but is not characteristic of the disease. Localized resections have led to moderate success, but amphotericin B has not been effective. Resection is indicated for good-risk patients with localized cavitary disease or to make a definitive diagnosis when bronchogenic carcinoma is suspected (Jung et al., 1977).

Antifungal Drug Therapy

Amphotericin B is a polyene antibiotic and is the cornerstone of chemotherapy for systemic fungal disease. The agent has a specific affinity for sterols in cell membranes, and its affinity for ergosterol, found in fungal membranes, is 500 times greater than its affinity for cholesterol, the major sterol in human membranes. When amphotericin B binds to the fungal cell membrane, cellular permeability is increased,

causing leakage of essential cellular contents and damage to the cell (Medoff and Kobayashi, 1980). Amphotericin B is highly insoluble and poorly absorbed from the gastrointestinal tract. The drug is always administered intravenously or intrathecally in 5% dextrose and water for 2 to 5 hours and may be combined with small amounts of heparin or hydrocortisone sodium succinate to reduce the incidence of phlebitis. The drug binds rapidly to tissue sites, and only about 10% remains in the plasma, where it is bound to plasma proteins. For most systemic mycoses, a total dose of approximately 2 to 2.5 g is recommended. Patients with severe, rapidly progressing infection should be given an initial 1-mg test dose followed by a therapeutic dosage of 20 to 30 mg/day for 10 weeks. Possible toxic reactions to amphotericin B therapy include immediate systemic reactions (fever, chills, malaise, hypotension), renal toxicity, which is usually the limiting factor in determining the extent of treatment, and hematologic reactions (anemia) (Sarosi et al., 1979).

Newer synthetic, orally active antifungal agents include the azoles (imidazoles, which include ketoconazole, and triazoles, which include itraconazole and fluconazole). The azole antifungal agents all appear to function via a common mechanism of action: inhibitation of a cytochrome P450–dependent enzyme that is needed to synthesize fungal cell membranes. Overall, the azoles have been a major addition to antifungal chemotherapy, displaying less toxicity than am-

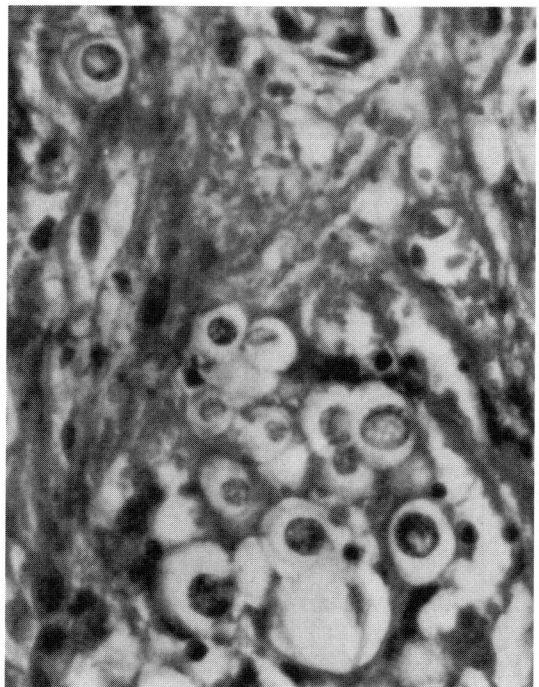

FIGURE 20–25. Paracoccidioidomycosis (South American blastomycosis). Organisms of *Paracoccidioides brasiliensis* in tissue. These lesions resemble the organisms of *Blastomyces dermatitidis*. (From Takaro, T.: Thoracic actinomycotic and mycotic infections. *In* Ellis, F. H., Jr. [ed]: Thoracic Surgery. Thomaston, CT, Practice of Surgery, 1987.)

photericin B, activity against many different fungi, and excellent pharmacokinetic properties (Lyman and Walsh, 1992).

Ketoconazole, an orally administered imidazole antifungal agent, has the potential advantages over amphotericin B of less toxicity, ease of long-term administration for outpatients, and a broad spectrum of activity against various superficial and deep fungal pathogens. Initial clinical results in systemic mycotic infections indicate that this agent is more effective in patients with histoplasmosis and nonmeningeal cryptococcosis than in patients with blastomycosis and coccidioidomycosis (National Institute of Allergy and Infectious Disease Mycosis Study Group, 1985). Effective dosage appears to be 400 to 600 mg/day administered orally for 6 months (Craven et al., 1983). It should not be used to treat disseminated or localized deep visceral candidiasis (Lyman and Walsh, 1992).

Itraconazole, a lipophilic triazole analogue, exhibits excellent activity against most human fungal pathogens. Its advantages over ketoconazole include a broader spectrum of activity (including *Aspergillus*), better pharmacokinetics, and less toxicity. It has been approved by the Food and Drug Administration (FDA) for treatment of blastomycosis and histoplasmosis. Of particular interest is the sensitivity of *Aspergillus* species to itraconazole. In a multicenter study of invasive aspergillosis, itraconazole (400 mg/day following a 4-day loading dose of 600 mg/day) compared favorably with conventional amphotericin B therapy (Lyman and Walsh, 1992).

Fluconazole, a water-soluble fluorine-substituted triazole, has been effective against a variety of fungal infections in both immunocompromised and immunocompetent hosts. It has a greater specificity against inhibition of the fungal cytochrome P450–mediated reactions. Fluconazole has been shown to distribute well into virtually all tissue sites, especially the cerebrospinal fluid (Hay, 1991). Its use has been directed mainly to cryptococcal meningitis (400 mg/day for 2 weeks) and a variety of syndromes due to *Candida* species (many treat infection, candidimia, *Candida* peritonitis).

PARASITIC INFECTIONS

Pneumocystis carinii Pneumonitis

P. carinii is a ubiquitous protozoan that is responsible for an opportunistic infection manifested by a diffuse interstitial pneumonitis occurring in immunodeficient or immunosuppressed patients. With rare exception, the organism is localized to the lungs, even in the most severely immunocompromised host. With the increased medical attention directed toward AIDS and because *P. carinii* pneumonitis is a criterion for the diagnosis of AIDS, this pneumonitis has rapidly gained widespread attention and notoriety, as did legionnaires' disease in the 1970s (Catterall et al., 1985).

P. carinii was first seen in Parisian sewer rats by Delano and Delano (1912) at the Pasteur Institute in Paris. The name *Pneumocystis* was proposed because the cysts characteristic of the organism are found only in the lungs, and the term *carinii* is derived from a previous description by Professor Carini but mistakenly interpreted to be trypanosomes. The first recognition of *P. carinii* pneumonitis in humans was in 1942 by Van der Meer and Brug. In the 1950s, the organism was found to be the cause of interstitial plasma cell pneumonitis in debilitated infants in Europe, where the disease was epidemic in nursing homes. The infection is currently encountered in the United States not in the infantile form but predominantly as a diffuse alveolar disease of adults who are immunocompromised from malignancy, drugs, organ transplantation, and AIDS.

P. carinii is a protozoan, and the primary cyst measures 4 to 6 μm in diameter. This primary cyst contains up to eight pleomorphic intracystic cells, called sporozoites (Fig. 20–26). The cyst is identified with the methenamine silver stain or toluidine blue stain, and the sporozoites are best studied with polychrome stain such as the Giemsa method (Burke and Good, 1973). The organism usually involves Type I pneumocytes that cause desquamation of alveolar lining cells. Proliferation of the trophozoites, formation of cysts, and host response to damaged tissue fill the alveoli with characteristic foamy exudate (Bartlett and Smith, 1991).

P. carinii infection is highly prevalent in humans throughout the world. Serologic surveys of normal individuals in the United States indicate that 75% acquire antibodies to the disease by 4 years of age. In the normal population, most infections are therefore

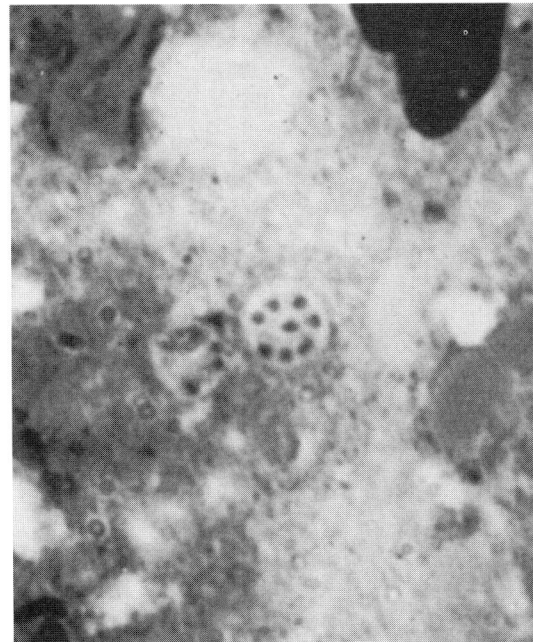

FIGURE 20–26. Typical *Pneumocystis carinii* cysts, showing eight intracystic sporozoites.

asymptomatic or insignificant. Overt pneumonitis represents activation of latent infection in the immunocompromised host and is believed to be the pathogenesis of the disease (Hughes, 1984).

Manifestations of pneumonitis include fever, tachypnea, dry cough, progressive respiratory insufficiency, and cyanosis; if the disease is left untreated, death occurs. The onset is usually abrupt, and the course is one of progressive deterioration. The chest film shows diffuse bilateral alveolar disease, which usually begins in the perihilar areas in the lower fields of the lung. The upper fields of the lung often are not involved until late in the course of the disease (Fig. 20–27).

A definitive diagnosis requires demonstration of *P. carinii* in pulmonary tissue. The most dependable method to obtain this tissue has been the open lung biopsy (Hughes, 1984), but transbronchial biopsy, endobronchial brushings, and percutaneous needle biopsy have been used with various degrees of success (Hodgkin et al., 1973; Ruskin and Hughes, 1983). Immunoserologic tests have been used extensively in *P. carinii* studies; however, these various immunofluorescent, complement fixation, and agglutination methods have little diagnostic worth, because most individuals have detectable antibody before the pneumonitis, and an increase in titer does not occur consistently with the onset of acute reactivation.

The drug of choice for treatment of *P. carinii* pneumonia is TMP-SMZ. Pentamidine isethionate is an alternative agent. The intravenous route of TMP-SMZ administration is more dependable than the oral route, especially for the first few days of treatment. The intravenous dosage is 15 kg of TMP and 75 mg

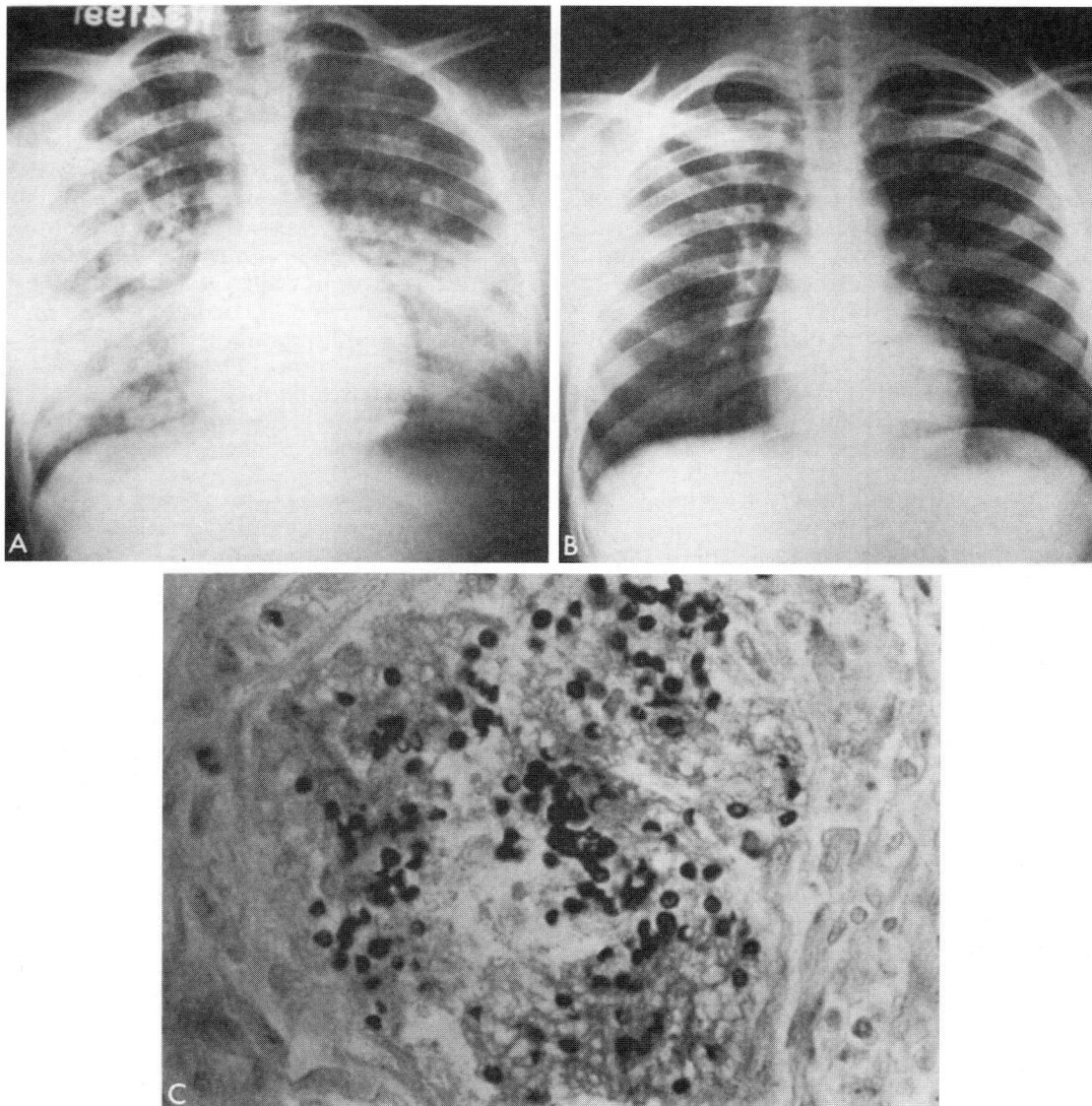

FIGURE 20–27. *P. carinii* pneumonia. *A*, Chest film showing bilateral pneumonic process in a biopsy specimen proved to be *P. carinii*. *B*, Chest film after 1 month of treatment with pentamidine isethionate. *C*, Biopsy specimen showing *Pneumocystis* cysts in an intra-alveolar exudate (Gomori, methenamine silver stain, ×100). (*A–C*, Reprinted with permission from the Society of Thoracic Surgeons [The Annals of Thoracic Surgery, 1972, Vol. 14, p. 335].)

of SMZ/kg/day in four equally divided doses. Side effects include a rash and neutropenia, which are especially common in patients with AIDS. Pentamidine is an alternative drug but is associated with more toxicity, including nephrotoxicity, hypotension, hypoglycemia, hepatic toxicity, anemia, and thrombocytopenia. The usual course required for either TMP-SMZ or pentamidine is 14 days. Recurrence may occur after treatment with either regimen because protective immunity is not achieved. In high-risk patients, prophylaxis can be afforded by low-dose TMP-SMZ given daily (Hughes et al., 1977); or, in patients with sulfa allergy, aerosolized pentamidine is given monthly (Bernard et al., 1992).

Thoracic Amebiasis

Thoracic amebiasis occurs as a secondary process arising from an amebic abscess of the liver, commonly the right lobe. The infection may spread to the thorax by direct erosion through the diaphragm to create an abscess in the lower lobe or middle lobe of the right lung. The infectious agent may also spread by way of lymphatics from an abdominal focus. Rupture of an amebic abscess may produce hepaticobronchial fistula, amebic empyema, effusion, or any complication of these complications.

Patients classically present with symptoms and findings related to the right hemithorax, as well as evidence of abdominal infection, and they expectorate material that resembles chocolate or anchovy paste. The chest film usually shows a right-sided elevation of the hemidiaphragm with right effusion and pneumonic consolidation or abscess formation in the right lower pulmonary field.

Entamoeba histolytica organisms are rarely found in sputum or pleural fluid, and in many patients a pre-sumptive diagnosis must be made, supported by the finding of *E. histolytica* in stools and by positive results on complement fixation tests. Metronidazole is the drug of choice for extraintestinal amebiasis, and indications for surgical therapy are uncommon with effective drug therapy (Cameron, 1978). Amebic empyema is treated effectively with a combination of intercostal tube drainage and metronidazole. With progression of the disease by secondary bacterial infection, surgical drainage by rib resection or decortication may be necessary (Cameron, 1978).

Pulmonary Echinococcosis

Pulmonary echinococcosis is caused by the small tapeworm *Taenia echinococcus,* which commonly produces the hydatid cystic disease of the liver. The organism's ova are inadvertently ingested, and the larvae are carried to the liver in the portal venous circulation. Some larvae escape the liver and lodge in the lungs, where they form one or more hydatid cysts. The cysts may lie dormant for many years and may remain asymptomatic. This disease eventually presents either as an asymptomatic finding on a chest film or with other symptoms (Fig. 20–28). Echinococcosis is rare in North America but is a serious problem in Australia, New Zealand, South America, and the Mediterranean.

As the cyst enlarges, it expands to the pleural surface. In the process, the surrounding lung is compressed, and a layer of atelectasis parenchyma forms around the hydatid cyst that is commonly called the capsule or pericyst. The diagnosis is made by the characteristic radiographic appearance of a round, radiopaque lesion of a homogeneous density with well-demarcated margins and little reaction around the lesion. The hydatid cysts are usually in the mid or lower pulmonary fields.

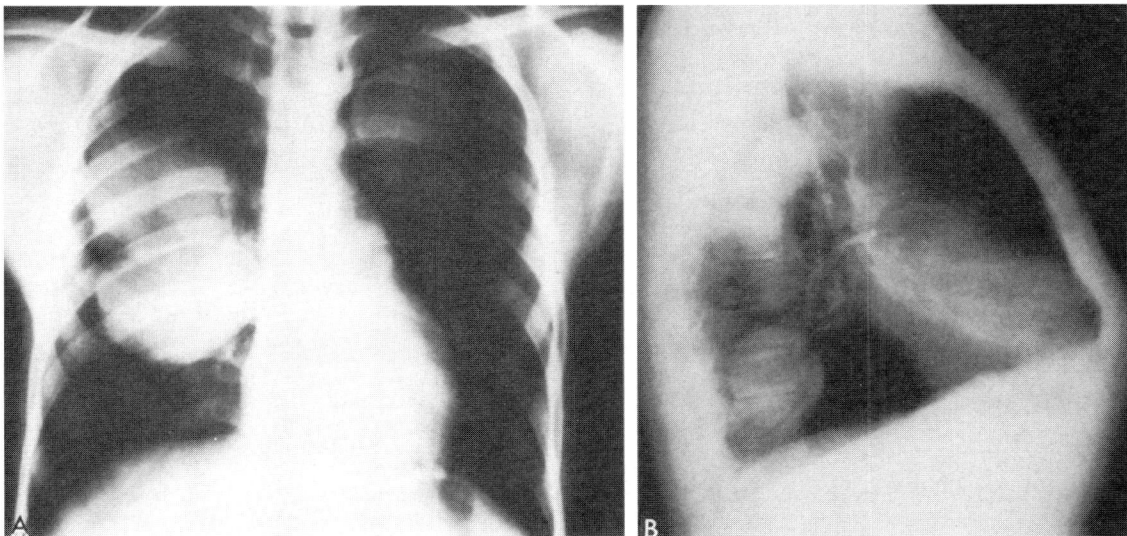

FIGURE 20–28. Pulmonary echinococcus cysts. *A,* Multiple and bilateral cysts. The appearance of large, rounded shadows of homogenous density and well-defined borders is characteristic of the disease. *B,* Solitary cysts lying posteriorly behind the heart. (*A* and *B,* From Wocott, M. W., Harris, S. H., Briggs, J. N., et al.: Hydatid cyst disease of the lung. J. Thorac. Cardiovasc. Surg., *62*:465, 1971.)

An echinococcal cyst is dangerous because rupture can occur at any time and thus extend the disease to surrounding normal parenchyma of the lung. Rupture can also lead to death due to aspiration and asphyxiation or to a hypersensitivity reaction to the contents of the cyst. Secondary infection of a ruptured cyst causes bronchiectasis or lung abscess.

Surgical therapy for an echinococcal cyst consists of enucleation of the intact cyst. Care is taken not to rupture the cyst or to spill the contents into the thoracic cavity (Lichter, 1972). The nonadherent tissue plane between the cyst and pericyst can be carefully opened, with subsequent extrusion of the cyst into a spoon or basin (Fig. 20–29). The remaining space left by the evacuated cyst is obliterated, and if significant areas of destroyed lung remain after the cyst has been removed, adequate segmental resection or lobectomy is needed (Perianayagam et al., 1979). Mebendazole has been used with some success to treat nonresectable lesions (Wilson et al., 1978).

Miscellaneous Parasitic Infections

Dirofilaria immitis, the dog heartworm, has been recognized with increased frequency as the cause of solitary pulmonary nodules that are indistinguishable from suspected bronchogenic carcinoma. These lesions are diagnosed only after thoracotomy and excisional biopsy of the nodule, which is a small pulmonary infarct encompassed by a granulomatous

inflammatory reaction. The nematode usually is found within a pulmonary vessel in an area of necrosis (Merrill et al., 1980).

DIFFUSE INTERSTITIAL DISEASES OF THE LUNG

Since Hamman and Rich initially described diffuse idiopathic interstitial fibrosis in 1935, the number of known causes of diffuse infiltrative pulmonary diseases has dramatically increased. And since Buechner described the differential diagnosis of miliary disease of the lung in 1959, more than 150 known pathologic entities have been found to cause chronic bilateral diffuse interstitial or miliary disease of the lung as seen on chest film. The wide spectrum of pathologic processes that cause diffuse disease of the lung emphasizes the importance of accurate diagnostic techniques, including biopsy, as well as the increasing role of thoracic surgeons in the diagnosis and treatment of diffuse infiltrative disease of the lung (Falk, 1972).

The interstitium of the lung has a limited number of histopathologic responses to a wide variety of disease processes. Granulomatosis, inflammatory cell infiltration, and fibrosis are the more important reactions to infiltrative lung diseases (Falk, 1972). These reactions, occurring alone or in combination, characterize most of the large number of diffuse infiltrative disorders of the lung. Because the differential diagnosis of these conditions is extensive, they are not reviewed

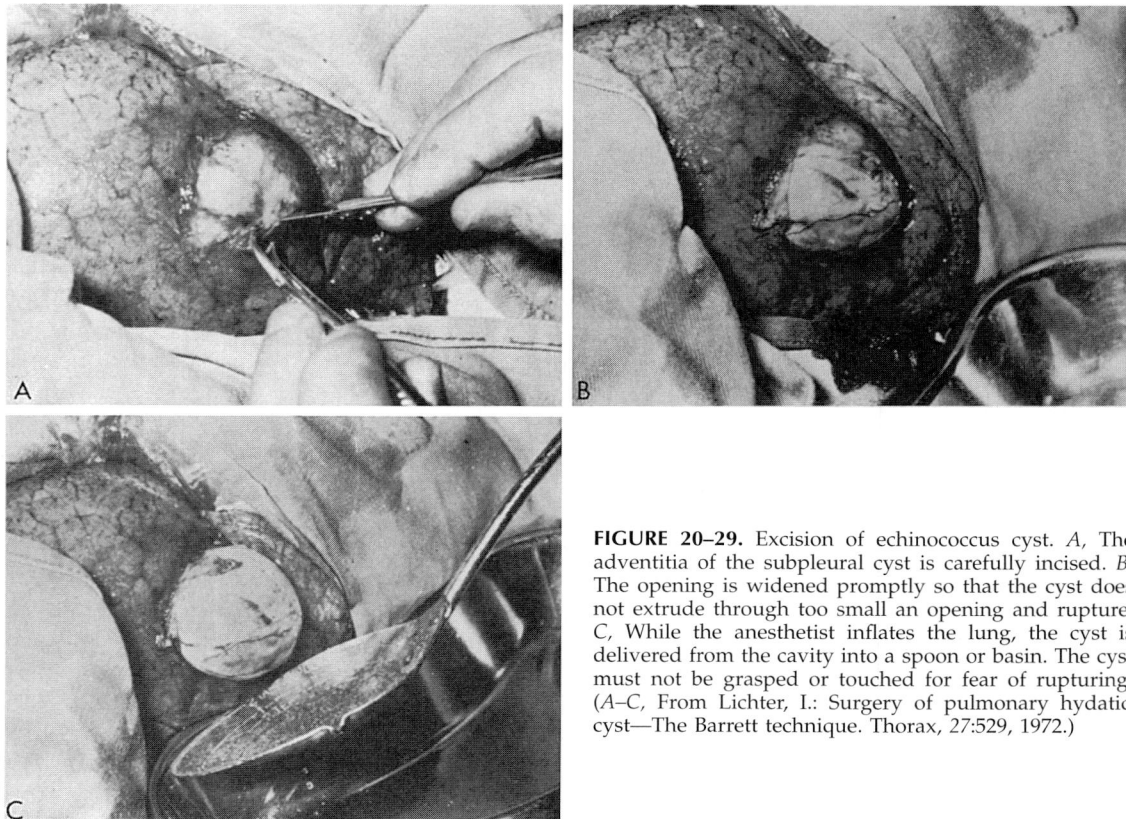

FIGURE 20–29. Excision of echinococcus cyst. *A,* The adventitia of the subpleural cyst is carefully incised. *B,* The opening is widened promptly so that the cyst does not extrude through too small an opening and rupture. *C,* While the anesthetist inflates the lung, the cyst is delivered from the cavity into a spoon or basin. The cyst must not be grasped or touched for fear of rupturing. (*A–C,* From Lichter, I.: Surgery of pulmonary hydatid cyst—The Barrett technique. Thorax, 27:529, 1972.)

comprehensively here. Table 20–5 presents a classification of these diseases according to the different radiographic patterns. Although this classification helps differentiate the pathologic entities, it is limited because different diseases can produce similar chest film patterns, and some diseases (e.g., sarcoidosis) can produce many different patterns.

The chronic diffuse infiltrative pulmonary diseases discussed in this section alter the structure of the lung's elastic tissue and produce stiffening of the lung

■ **Table 20–5.** CLASSIFICATION OF DIFFUSE INFILTRATIVE LUNG DISEASE BY RADIOGRAPHIC PATTERNS

Diffuse Nodular Lesions	Bilateral Perihilar Shadows
Metastatic malignancy	Pulmonary edema
Focal lung abscess	Uremic pneumonitis
Tuberculosis	Alveolar proteinosis
Sarcoidosis	Pulmonary hemosiderosis
Fungal diseases	Collagen-vascular disease
Cysts	Immunologic reaction (graft
Rheumatoid nodular disease	rejection serum sickness)
Mucoid impaction	
Amyloidosis	
Wegener's granulomatosis	**Diffuse Reticular or**
Caplan's syndrome	**Interstitial Edema**
Eosinophilic granuloma	Pulmonary infections
	(bacterial, viral, fungal,
Diffuse Consolidation	protozoal, rickettsial)
	Pneumoconiosis
Bronchoalveolar carcinoma	Aspiration and inhalation
Metastatic carcinoma,	pneumonias
Kaposi's sarcoma	Eosinophilic pneumonia
Tuberculosis	Metastatic malignancy
Atypical mycobacterial	Kaposi's sarcoma
disease	Drug-induced lung disease
Fungal infection	Collagen-vascular disease
Bacterial infection	Sarcoidosis
Viral pneumonitis (varicella,	Histiocytosis X
primary atypical	Idiopathic pulmonary
pneumonia)	fibrosis
Pulmonary infarction	Amyloidosis
Pulmonary edema	Radiation pneumonitis
Vasculitis	Oxygen toxicity
Eosinophilic pneumonia	Mucoid impaction
Necrotizing granulomas	Polycythemia vera
Sarcoidosis	Uremic pneumonitis
Fat embolism	
Aspiration pneumonia	**Honeycomb Lung**
Lipoid pneumonia	
Hypersensitivity	Scleroderma
pneumonitis	Sarcoidosis
Pulmonary hemosiderosis	Pneumoconiosis
Goodpasture's syndrome	Histiocytosis X
Silicosis, dust inhalation	Lipid storage diseases
diseases	Lipoid pneumonia
Respiratory disease of	Rheumatoid arthritis
newborn	Idiopathic pulmonary
ARDS	fibrosis

Bilateral Hilar Enlargement

Tuberculosis
Fungal diseases
Sarcoidosis
Lymphomas (Hodgkin's disease)
Carcinoma (primary, metastatic)
Pneumoconiosis

ARDS = adult respiratory distress syndrome.

and a chest film appearance of diffuse infiltrative changes. These changes are different from the *adult respiratory distress syndrome* (ARDS), which is a form of acute or subacute pulmonary edema resulting from increasing permeability of the pulmonary capillaries within alveolar epithelium. The more acute presentation and rapid clinical progression of ARDS distinguishes this entity from chronic diffuse infiltrative pulmonary disease, although the two categories of disease may share similar clinical characteristics, radiographic findings, and pathophysiologic derangements.

Therapy requires a specific diagnosis in a patient who presents with rather nonspecific clinical features shared by many etiologic processes. The clinical and radiographic presentations of miliary tuberculosis, sarcoidosis, and histoplasmosis may be similar, but the therapy for each disease is specific and significantly different. Miliary tuberculosis is best treated with antituberculous antibiotics, sarcoidosis is treated with corticosteroids, and histoplasmosis is treated with amphotericin B. Therefore, the thoracic surgeon's role in obtaining a specific diagnosis is growing. The thoracic surgeon's close cooperation with the internist and pathologist during diagnostic procedures (bronchoscopy, mediastinoscopy, and open lung biopsy) is important in obtaining a definitive diagnosis, which requires expeditious and proper handling of tissue and body fluids.

Pathophysiology

Interstitial pneumonopathies usually are characterized by thickening of the alveolar-capillary barrier, because inflammatory cells and connective tissue infiltrate this area in response to injury. This is not a uniform process, however, and injury to alveolar epithelium or alveolar capillaries may also be the major focus of disease. Although pulmonary function tests are not diagnostic in this group of disorders, because many dissimilar pathologic entities produce similar physiologic patterns, serial pulmonary function tests are important in following the progression of disease and in assessing the effectiveness of specific therapy, such as the effect of steroids in a patient with sarcoidosis. In general, patients with early diffuse interstitial pulmonary disease present with pulmonary function characterized by normal mechanics of breathing (maximal breathing capacity and FEV_1), normal oxygen saturation with exercise, reduced diffusing capacity for carbon monoxide (DL_{CO}), hypocapnea with a compensated respiratory alkalosis, decreased pulmonary compliance, and increased alveolar-arterial oxygen gradient at rest, which is increased further after exercise. With more severe infiltrative pulmonary disease, a restrictive defect is represented on pulmonary function tests by reduction of pulmonary volumes, including vital capacity and total capacity of the lung associated with resting hypoxemia and pulmonary artery hypertension.

The *basic* pathophysiologic defect in diffuse pulmonary disease of most causes is an increased alveolar-arterial oxygen gradient with a normal oxygen content in the arterial blood on resting, which is reduced after exercise. This pattern was originally called *alveolar-capillary block* by Baldwin and associates (1949). The original hypothesis was that greatly thickened alveolar septa and a reduction in the area of alveolar-capillary interface impaired the adequate diffusion of gas exchange. The actual role of a diffusion block has since been discounted (Gaensler et al., 1972). More sophisticated measurements of pulmonary function have shown that only one-fourth of the diffusing capacity is required for complete equilibration of alveolar with capillary oxygen pressure, and that the histologic lesion noted would not be expected to prevent equilibration across this membrane. Additionally, a diffusion gradient should increase with exercise, whereas in approximately one-half of patients with interstitial pulmonary disease, the gradient decreases with exercise. Finally, the histologic lesions noted in these diseases do not often correspond to the concept of a physical "block" in the alveolar-capillary space. The four major physiologic causes of hypoxemia are alveolar hypoventilation, diffusion defect, *ventilation-perfusion* imbalance, and increased right-to-left shunt (Andrews, 1974). Because it has been shown that the first two causes do not apply in diffuse pulmonary disease, the increased alveolar-arterial oxygen tension gradient and exercise hypoxemia have been attributed mainly to a ventilation-perfusion imbalance throughout the lungs in these patients. The imbalance exists because areas of infiltrated and fibrotic lung have poor ventilation, but with still-normal perfusion producing a physiologic right-to-left shunt. With exercise, increased perfusion exceeds ventilation, and the result is more significant hypoxemia. From the point of view of the thoracic surgeon who is obtaining tissue for a specific diagnosis, the wide range of potential causes of diffuse infiltrative diseases of the lungs can be divided into three types: those that can be diagnosed only by open lung biopsy, those in which a biopsy may confirm the diagnosis, and those that do not usually require a biopsy except as a final procedure after other, less-invasive modalities have failed to yield a diagnosis.

Diseases that require a biopsy of the lung for specific diagnosis include idiopathic diffuse interstitial pneumonias, pulmonary hemosiderosis, eosinophilic granuloma of the lung, pulmonary alveolar proteinosis, and Wegener's granulomatosis. Interstitial pneumonopathies that are difficult to diagnose and that usually require a biopsy of the lung include sarcoidosis, chronic berylliosis, pneumoconiosis, and diffuse neoplastic diseases. The interstitial pulmonary diseases that usually do not require a biopsy include infectious diseases such as miliary tuberculosis, the mycotic infections, rheumatoid disease of the lung, radiation, fibrosis, and scleroderma.

A thorough history is important in establishing the specific diagnosis of diffuse pulmonary disease. In Gaensler and Carrington's series of 381 patients with diffuse or miliary disease of the lung, history alone led to a specific diagnosis in 21% (Gaensler and Carrington, 1980). Thorough questioning must include not only the patient's current job but a list of previous occupations, including details about types of materials handled. In addition, detailed questions about home environment, exposure to animals, and travel should be included. Finally, exposure to infectious agents must be established.

Idiopathic Diffuse Interstitial Pneumonia

Idiopathic diffuse interstitial pneumonia comprises that group of diseases marked by a bilateral reticular nodular infiltrate involving the lower fields of the lung on the chest film. The interstitial tissue progressively thickens so that the lung eventually takes on a honeycomb appearance (Carrington and Gaensler, 1978; Crystal et al., 1984). Within this category of diffuse infiltrative pulmonary disease, the specific disorders are classified as interstitial pneumonia, bronchiolitis obliterans, desquamative interstitial pneumonia, and lymphoid interstitial pneumonia (Gaensler and Carrington, 1972). However, it is often difficult clinically to distinguish among the specific syndromes within this classification (Campbell and Harris, 1981) (Fig. 20–30).

Patients with interstitial pneumonia present with a gradual onset of dyspnea, which is slowly progressive and debilitating. A nonproductive cough may be present, and clubbing and cyanosis may be seen. Hyperventilation is noticeable, first with exercise and then at rest in the later stages of the disease. Pulmonary function tests show changes in oxygen diffusion attributed earlier to the alveolar-capillary block syndrome. Open lung biopsy is usually required for specific diagnosis in these disorders: In a prospective study of 46 patients with infiltrative pulmonary disease, open lung biopsy diagnosed 91%, whereas transbrochial biopsy diagnosed only 36% (Wall et al., 1981).

Histologic examination of the lung specimen shows characteristic thickening of the interstitial tissue. Connective tissue stains emphasize the collagenous contents of the thickened interstitial space. Agents that cause pulmonary fibrosis, such as silica crystals or asbestos crystals, are occasionally identified in the biopsy specimen. Viral causes have been suspected in some cases, and familial tendency has also been reported. Desquamative interstitial pneumonia is characterized histologically by massive filling of distal airspaces with mononuclear cells but with preservation of alveolar walls (Liebow et al., 1965).

Treatment for this group of patients is difficult, because only a few patients respond to corticosteroids with significant symptomatic and radiologic improvement. Desquamative interstitial pneumonitis generally responds to corticosteroid therapy, however, sometimes dramatically (Gaensler et al., 1972). Biopsy of the lung is indicated for identifying patients who have desquamative interstitial pneumonitis and for whom corticosteroids are definitely indicated and for

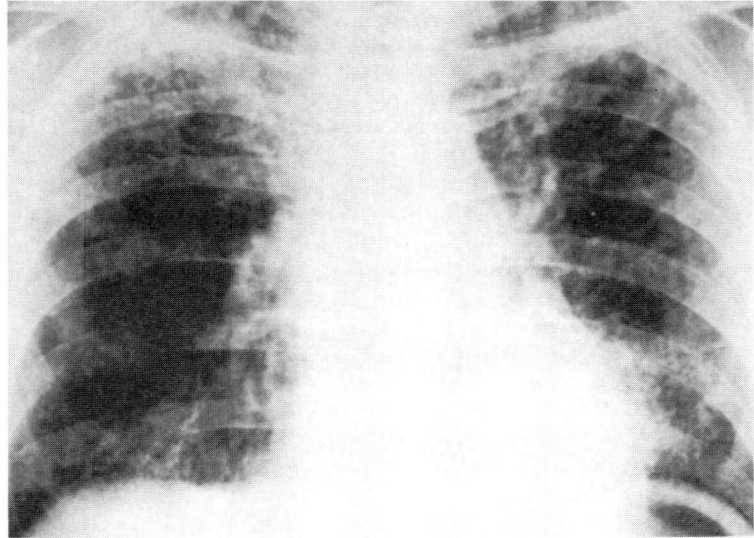

FIGURE 20–30. Usual interstitial pneumonitis. The x-ray film reveals diffuse infiltrative lesions of both lungs and is associated with severe dyspnea. An open lung biopsy for diagnosis was done. It documented diffuse interstitial fibrosis and bronchiolectasis, findings consistent with the diagnosis of usual interstitial pneumonitis.

diagnosing diffuse infiltrative diseases that are associated with a specific etiology amenable to therapy (Fig. 20–31).

Single-lung transplantation has been applied to selected patients with interstitial fibrosis and end-stage pulmonary disease (Cooper et al., 1987; Toronto Lung Transplant Group, 1986). Important in the successful outcome of this procedure, however, is that the patient must be weaned from high-dose steroids before undergoing transplantation. This has been thought to affect the healing of the bronchial anastomoses, the aspect of the procedure responsible for most complications after transplantation. For technical reasons related to the anastomosis of the left atrial cuff of the donor lung, *left-sided* single-lung transplantation is preferred. Thus, patients who have interstitial pulmonary fibrosis should undergo initial open lung biopsy to establish diagnosis on the *right lung* if possible, preserving the left hemithorax from postsurgical pleural adhesions, which could interfere later with a transplant of the left lung.

Sarcoidosis

Sarcoidosis, a systemic granulomatous disease of undetermined cause, not uncommonly comes to the attention of the thoracic surgeon. The disease is characterized by widespread involvement of mediastinal and peripheral lymph nodes, lungs, liver, spleen, skin, eyes, and parotid gland, and is often associated with a depression of cellular immunity (James, 1970, 1973). Hypercalcemia and hyperglobulinemia are common associated findings. The histologic appearance of noncaseating epithelioid tubercules is characteristic but not pathognomonic, inasmuch as fungal infections, berylliosis, and other granulomatous disorders can look similar.

In the United States, sarcoidosis is common among young adults 30 to 40 years of age and is more prevalent among blacks than among whites. Regionally,

there is a higher incidence of sarcoidosis in the South than elsewhere.

Thoracic sarcoidosis evolves with a primary stage of bilateral hilar lymphadenopathy that is reversible. A second stage of diffuse pulmonary involvement follows, and it can also be reversible. Continued progression of the disease leads to a final stage of fibrosis, scarring, and contraction with resultant thin-walled bullae or thicker-walled cavities, which usually is irreversible. Chest films of the primary stage of hilar adenopathy reveal discrete "potato" hilar nodes, which are characteristic of the disease (Kirks et al., 1973). A scalene node or mediastinal node biopsy histologically confirms the disease in this stage.

The diffuse pulmonary involvement of sarcoidosis makes diagnosis more difficult, especially if the enlarged hilar nodes have regressed; a biopsy of the lung may be necessary. Transbronchial biopsy has been recommended by some investigators (Stjernberg et al., 1980), but the technique has obvious disadvantages because of the small amount of tissue retrieved and the risk of pneumothorax. For definitive diagnosis, open lung biopsy is often necessary. In the late stage of fibrosis, parenchymal destruction and formation of cavities can make the diagnosis of sarcoidosis very difficult. Superimposed aspergillomas may develop within a chronic sarcoidal cavity, further obscuring the diagnosis (Israel and Ostrow, 1969).

Prognosis depends on the extent of progression of the pulmonary disease, because sarcoidosis limited to bilateral hilar lymphadenopathy has an excellent prognosis. Most cases of sarcoidosis appear to be self-limited, and many cases may even be asymptomatic. Of those patients with chronically significant sarcoidosis, approximately one-third recover completely, another one-third improve under observation, and the other third continue to worsen (Fig. 20–32). The disease is ultimately fatal in a small percentage of cases. Steroids appear to benefit patients with evidence of ocular, parotid, or renal involvement and patients with progressive pulmonary disease.

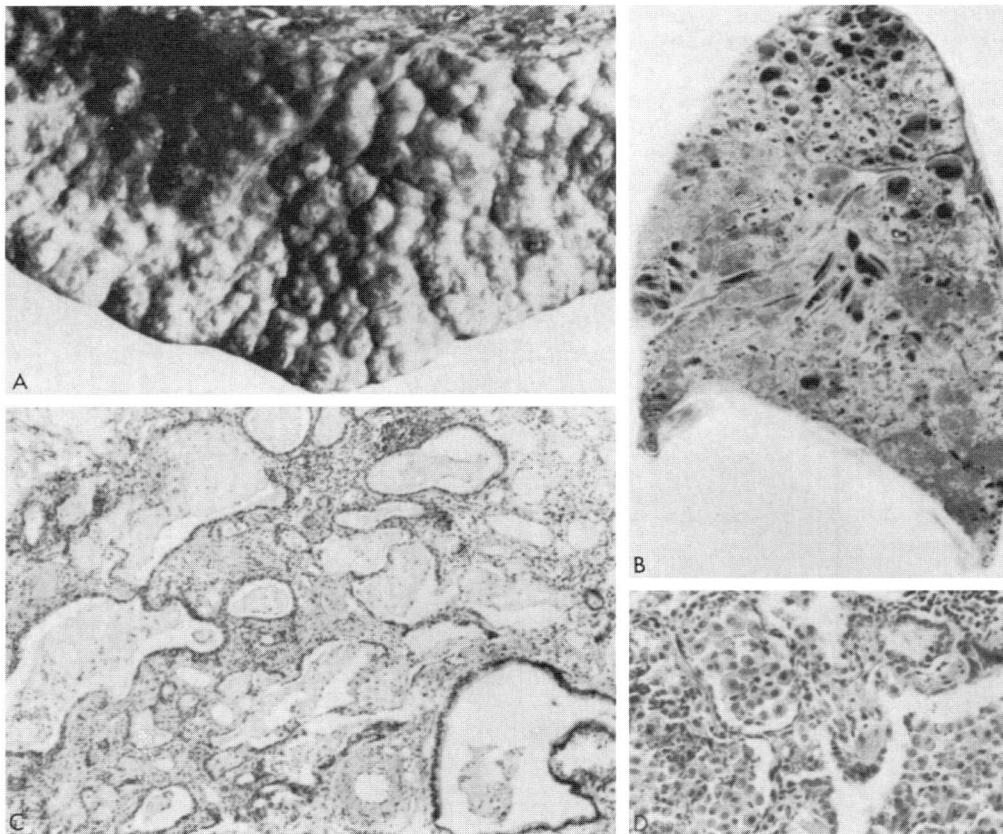

FIGURE 20–31. The late phase of diffuse interstitial fibrosis. *A,* Gross appearance of the pleural surface of the lung, which resembles the pathologic changes in the liver following severe portal cirrhosis. *B,* Cut surface of the lung showing honeycombing, microcyst formation, and bronchiolectasis. *C,* Histologic appearance of severe diffuse interstitial fibrosis. Peripheral microcysts exist with intervening dense scarring of the parenchyma (×120). *D,* Histologic appearance of desquamative interstitial pneumonitis. In contrast to the usual diffuse interstitial pneumonitis, alveolar ducts and alveoli are filled with desquamated alveolar lining cells that simulate sheets of epithelium. There is moderate interstitial thickening but minimal focal fibrosis (H & E, ×350). (*A,* Reprinted by permission from the Southern Medical Journal, Vol. 67, p. 571, 1974; *B* and *C,* From Fraire, A. E., Greenberg, S. D., O'Neal, R. M., et al.: Diffuse interstitial fibrosis of the lung. Am. J. Clin. Pathol., *59*:636, 1973; *D,* From Rosenow, E. C., III, O'Connell, E. C., and Harrison, E. G., Jr.: Desquamative interstitial pneumonia in children. Am. J. Dis. Child., *120*:344, 1970.)

Wegener's Granulomatosis

Wegener's granulomatosis is a serious multisystemic disease. The central pathologic lesion is a granuloma that affects blood vessels, with resultant necrosis of tissue. Lesions appear first in the upper and lower respiratory tract, and progression of the disease leads to a generalized vasculitis that causes severe damage to the kidneys and other end-organs. The highest incidence appears to be in middle adult life; initial involvement is classically in the nose and paranasal sinuses. A localized pulmonary form without renal involvement has a better prognosis (Carrington and Liebow, 1966).

Radiologic features of this disease, which is probably due to a hypersensitivity reaction, include a wide spectrum of findings. Initially, small irregular pulmonary nodules appear bilaterally and can mimic metastatic neoplasms or an infectious granulomatous disease. However, improvement of the lesions in one area with progression of lesions in the other suggests this disease rather than neoplasm (Gohel et al., 1973).

The diagnosis can be suspected clinically but can be confirmed only by histologic examination of involved tissue. Biopsy of the nasal structures or lung shows the characteristic granuloma with a special involvement of arteries and resultant tissue necrosis (Flye et al., 1979).

Steroid therapy generally has been disappointing, and it is now recommended that cytotoxic drugs (cyclophosphamide) be used with or without steroids (Fig. 20–33). If remission is obtained, therapy can sometimes be tapered and discontinued without reappearance of symptoms, but the length of remission cannot be predicted. The usual course of the disease is progressive deterioration, and death is commonly due to renal failure.

Diffuse Infiltrative Disease Due to Inhalation of Dust or Fumes

Pneumoconiosis includes infiltrative diseases of the lungs due to inhalation of dusts of inorganic origin,

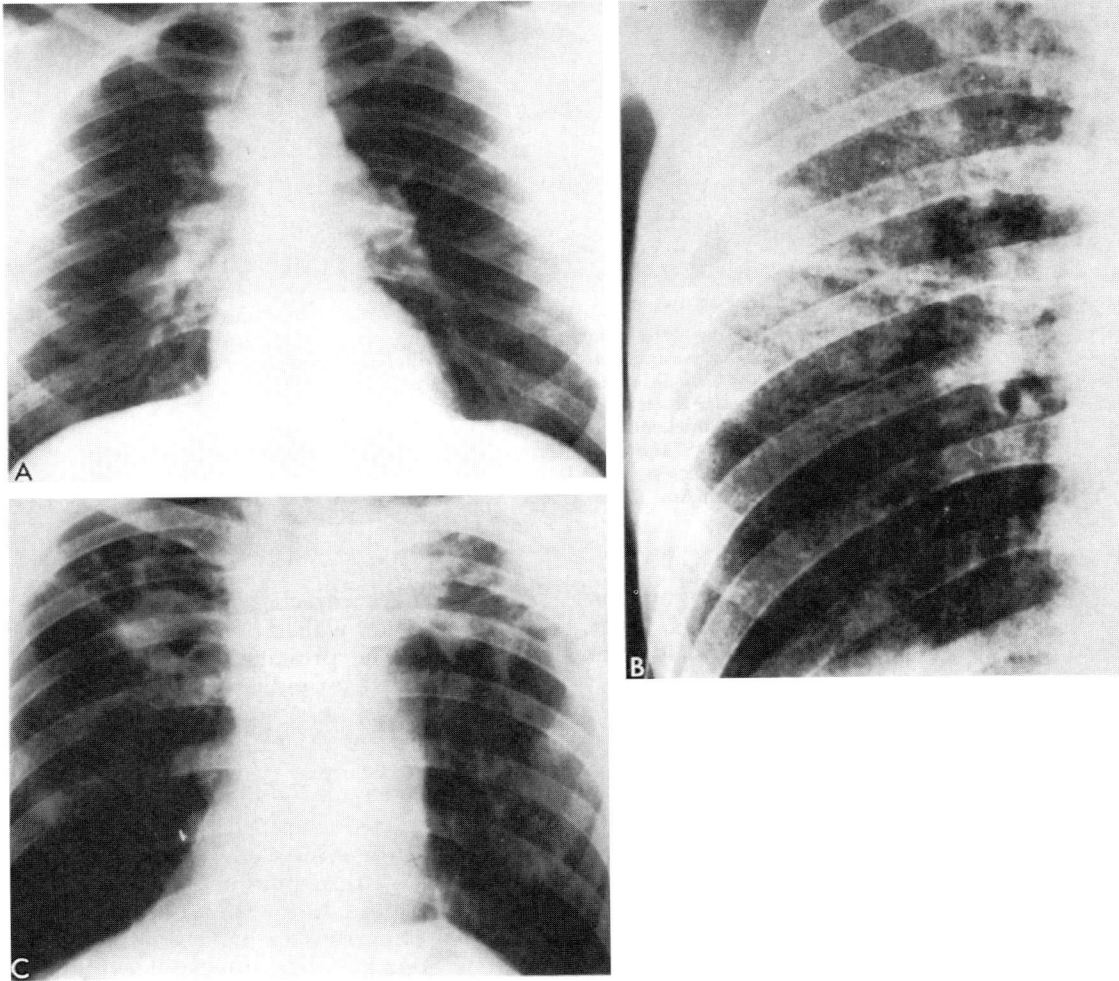

FIGURE 20–32. Sarcoidosis. *A,* The early stages of sarcoidosis showing typical bilateral symmetric hilar lymphadenopathy in a young adult male. The diagnosis was confirmed after mediastinal node biopsy. *B,* Intermediate stage showing disseminated sarcoidosis producing fine miliary lesions seen on a magnified thoracic radiograph. The film in this stage resembles many of the other diffuse infiltrative lesions of the lung. *C,* Late stage of pulmonary sarcoidosis showing chronic fibrosis and volume contraction characteristic of the disease. The interval from the documented early stage of the disease in this individual to the final appearance was 15 years.

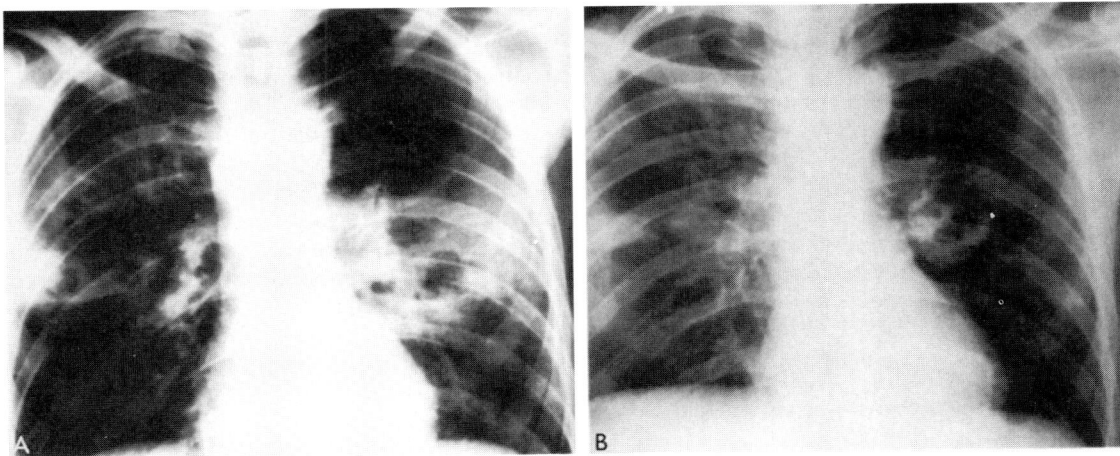

FIGURE 20–33. Wegener's granulomatosis. *A,* Thoracic film in a young adult male revealing bilateral cavitary lesions. Open lung biopsy was done and showed histologic changes consistent with Wegener's granulomatosis. The patient was treated with large doses of corticosteroids. *B,* Chest film 1 week later showing remarkable improvement; clinical improvement was also evident. Two years later, the patient died of an opportunistic infection following renal transplantation. Autopsy showed Wegener's granulomatosis and nocardiosis.

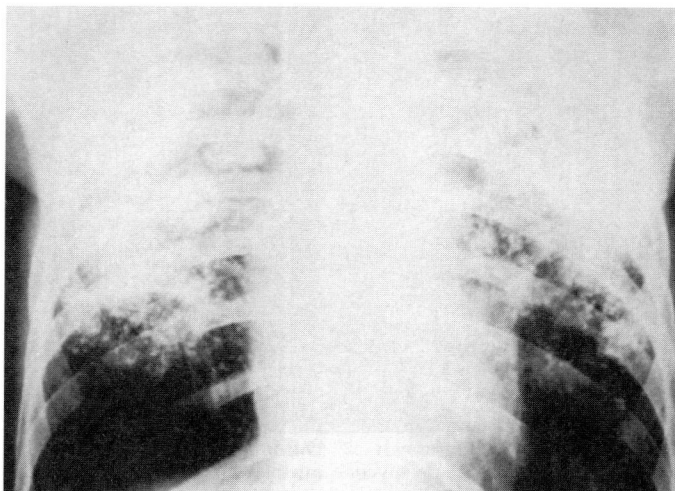

FIGURE 20–34. Pneumoconiosis. The chest film is consistent with the diagnosis of silicosis. The patient's occupation confirmed this diagnosis.

such as silicosis, asbestosis, talcosis, and berylliosis (Fig. 20–34). Inhalation of dusts of organic origin causes byssinosis (cotton or flax) or bagassosis (sugar cane fibers) (Siegesmund et al., 1980). As previously emphasized, a careful occupational history must be obtained from a patient who presents with radiographic findings consistent with these interstitial pneumonitides. Because of the wide spectrum of possibilities, however, thoracic surgeons are often required to provide a diagnosis by open lung biopsy (Fig. 20–35). Special stains, cultures, and electron microscopy are necessary to allow specific diagnoses and to initiate proper therapy (Siegesmund et al., 1980).

Miscellaneous Diffuse Pulmonary Infiltrative Diseases of Unknown Etiology

Patients with pulmonary alveolar proteinosis, Goodpasture's syndrome, eosinophilic granuloma, and lipoid granuloma present with various configurations of interstitial and infiltrative diffuse pulmonary disease that usually require biopsy of the lung for definitive diagnosis.

SURGICAL TECHNIQUES

Biopsy of the Lung

Biopsy of the lung is indicated for diagnosis in localized or diffuse pulmonary disease after initial attempts (sputum studies, bronchoscopic examination, and seroimmunologic studies) have not produced a diagnosis. Techniques available for accomplishing the biopsy include transbronchial biopsy of the lung through the fiberoptic bronchoscope, percutaneous needle biopsy of the lung, usually under fluoroscopic or computed tomographic guidance,

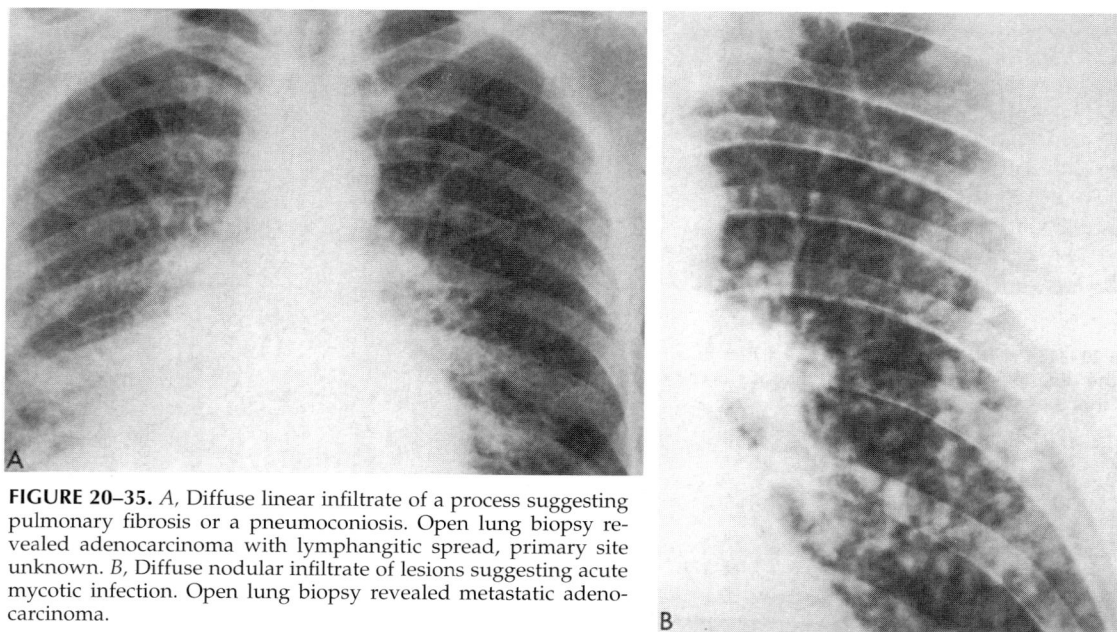

FIGURE 20–35. *A,* Diffuse linear infiltrate of a process suggesting pulmonary fibrosis or a pneumoconiosis. Open lung biopsy revealed adenocarcinoma with lymphangitic spread, primary site unknown. *B,* Diffuse nodular infiltrate of lesions suggesting acute mycotic infection. Open lung biopsy revealed metastatic adenocarcinoma.

thorocoscopic biopsy, and open lung biopsy. Transbronchial biopsy was introduced by Andersen and colleagues in 1965, and it has become popular because it produces low morbidity and obviates the need for general anesthesia (Andersen et al., 1973; Blumenfeld et al., 1984).

Percutaneous needle biopsy of the lung usually is accomplished with a thin-needle aspirate, and cytologic examination and appropriate cultures of the retrieved material are done. The technique has a low complication rate and can have a high yield in experienced hands. A small tissue specimen is obtained. However, it is not informative about the structure of the lung and usually does not help in diffuse infiltrative diseases. The technique is not thought to be suitable for centrally placed lesions, for those smaller than 2 cm in diameter, or for cavitating lesions with air-fluid levels (Berquist et al., 1980).

Open lung biopsy is preferred to needle biopsy for diffuse infiltrative pulmonary disease because of a higher yield for diagnosis and low morbidity and mortality when done by experts (Hiatt et al., 1982; Rossiter et al., 1979). In a review of 502 patients who had *open* lung biopsy for chronic interstitial lung disease, the diagnostic yield was 92%. The incidence of complication was 2.5%, and the mortality rate was 0.3%. In a separate series of 53 patients with diffuse interstitial pulmonary disease, *transbronchial* biopsy was diagnostic in only 38%, whereas open lung biopsy produced a specific diagnosis in 92% of patients (Wall et al., 1981). For diffuse infiltrative pulmonary disease, a small anterior thoracotomy between the fourth and fifth ribs provides adequate access to the involved lung without significantly compromising the mechanics of breathing in patients who usually have serious underlying system disease. The operation is performed with general endotracheal anesthesia and the patient in the supine position. A transverse incision, 4 to 7 cm long, is made over the fourth and fifth interspace, and the pleura is opened carefully. A small Tuffier or Finochietto retractor is placed in the interspace and gently spread. A portion of the left upper lobe (on the left) or a portion of the right middle or lower lobe is allowed to herniate out of the opening under positive-pressure ventilation of the lungs. The lung is grasped carefully by a noncrushing lung clamp in the inflated state. By using the TA-30 stapler or two angled rows of staples placed with the GIA stapler, a 2- to 3-cm-deep portion of the lung is excised expeditiously (Fig. 20–36). It is important to obtain a portion of the lung that contains both normal and abnormal tissue and that is large enough that it can be divided for both histologic and microbiologic study. If necessary, the staple line can be oversewn with an absorbable suture. The pleural cavity is always drained with a catheter after open lung biopsy, and the incision is closed with standard techniques. Postoperative emphasis is on bronchial toilet, encouragement of cough, and early mobilization. With full expansion of the lung confirmed by the chest film the next morning, the chest catheter is removed and ambulation is encouraged.

In general, open lung biopsy should not be unduly delayed by other, less productive diagnostic techniques when a definitive tissue diagnosis can be readily obtained in most cases with low morbidity and mortality (Murray et al., 1984; Pass et al., 1986).

Pulmonary Lobectomy

Right Upper Lobectomy

The chest is opened by a right posterolateral thoracotomy, and the pleural cavity is entered through the

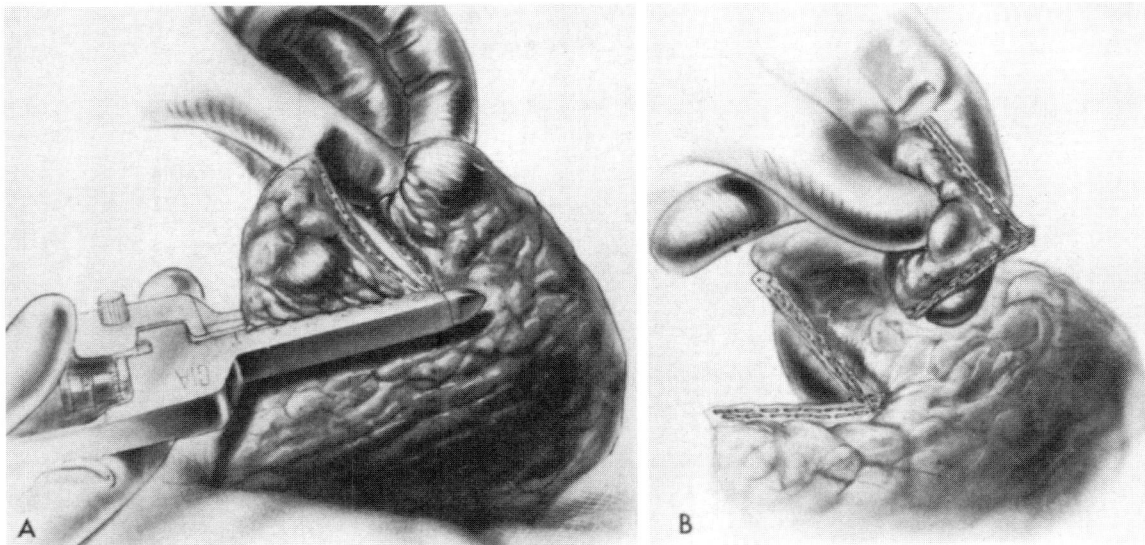

FIGURE 20–36. Open lung biopsy technique. *A,* GIA stapler is used to complete a wedge biopsy of pulmonary tissue containing coin-shaped lesions. Alternatively, a TA-30 stapler may be used to obtain a portion along the edge of the parenchyma of the lung. *B,* The wedge resection has been completed with a double row of staples placed by each application of the stapler. This technique controls air leaks and bleeding from the surface of the lung and rarely needs reinforcement with running suture.

fourth intercostal space. The rib is divided posteriorly (Fig. 20–37). The lung is mobilized if it is not free of adhesions; general exploration is completed, localizing the lesion and determining any possible lymph node involvement. The right hilum is exposed by retracting the lung downward and backward. This displays the arch of the azygos vein above and the hilar vessels in front. The mediastinal pleura is divided parallel to and below the azygos vein, and the division is continued down in front of the edge of the lung. The superior segment of the pulmonary artery is the uppermost structure encountered, and it is dis-

sected together with its two branches, the apical and the anterior. The apical branch of the superior pulmonary vein often crosses at this point and needs retraction, or it can be divided at this stage in order to expose the arterial branches more easily. The most inferior-lying branch of the superior pulmonary vein ordinarily drains the middle lobe, and care must be taken to preserve this vessel. The anterior trunk of the artery is now freed from the right bronchus by blunt dissection in order to facilitate later dissection. The remaining arterial branch of the upper lobe, the posterior ascending segmental artery, is inaccessible

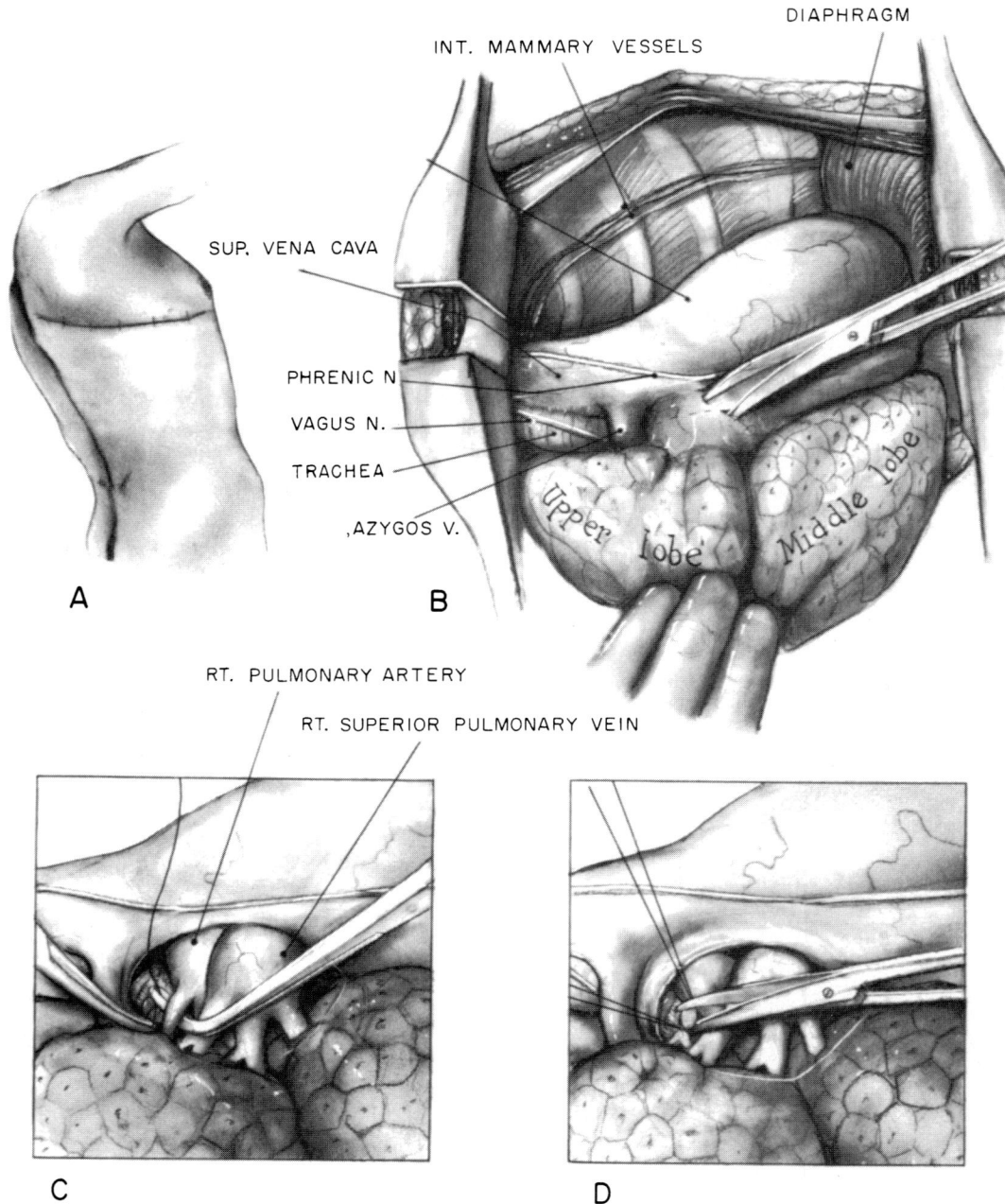

FIGURE 20–37. Technique of right upper lobectomy. *A,* Position of the patient with a right posterolateral thoracotomy incision marked over the fifth rib. *B,* Mediastinal pleura over the right upper lobe hilus is opened. *C* and *D,* Isolation and division of upper lobe pulmonary artery and pulmonary veins.

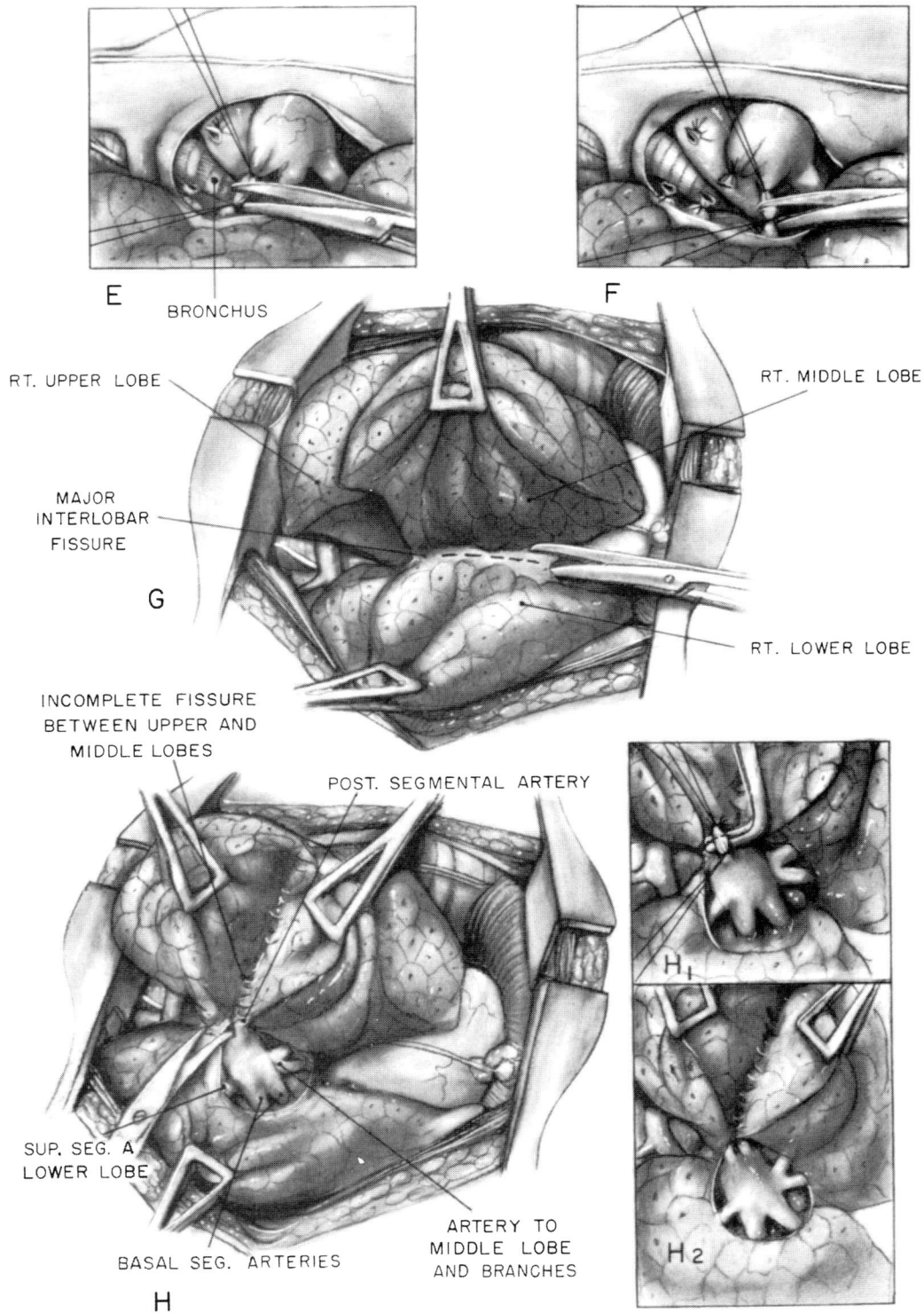

E BRONCHUS

RT. UPPER LOBE

MAJOR
INTERLOBAR
FISSURE

G

INCOMPLETE FISSURE
BETWEEN UPPER AND
MIDDLE LOBES

POST. SEGMENTAL ARTERY

RT. MIDDLE LOBE

RT. LOWER LOBE

H₁

SUP. SEG. A
LOWER LOBE

BASAL SEG. ARTERIES

ARTERY TO
MIDDLE LOBE
AND BRANCHES

H

H₂

FIGURE 20–37. *Continued E* and *F,* Continued isolation and division of the vascular structures to the upper lobe (see text). *G,* The interlobar major fissure is opened, exposing the pulmonary artery and its branches. *H, H₁,* and *H₂,* The posterior ascending artery to the posterior segment of the right upper lobe is identified, ligated, and divided. There may be two arteries in some cases (*H₂*).

Illustration continued on following page

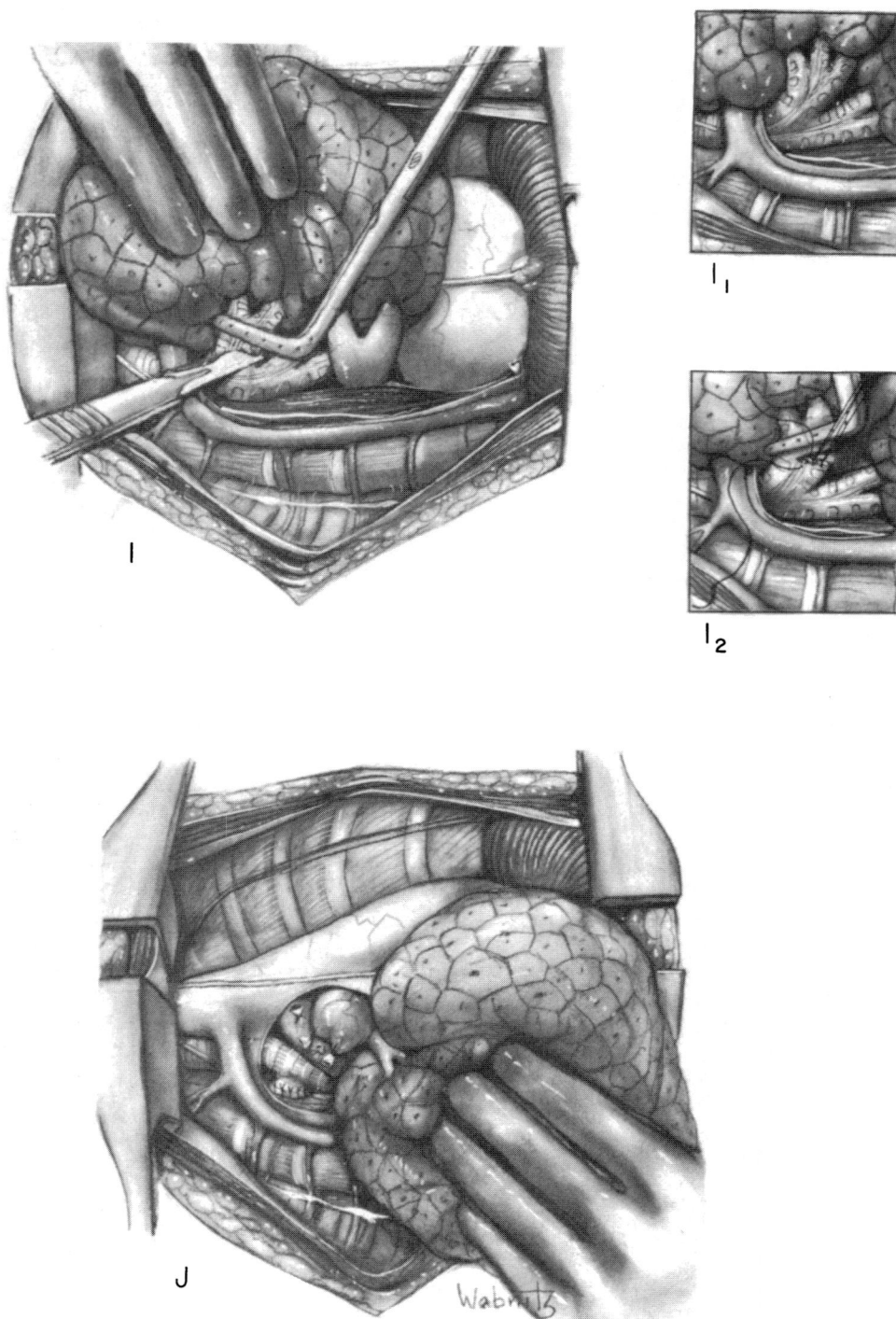

FIGURE 20–37. *Continued I,* Bronchus to the right upper lobe is isolated and partially divided proximal to the clamp. I_1, Exposure of all three segments of right upper lobe. I_2, Closure of partially divided right upper lobe bronchus with interrupted sutures using the "cut and sew" technique. *J,* Right upper lobectomy completed. (*A–J,* From Madden, J. L.: Atlas of Technics in Surgery. East Norwalk, CT, Appleton & Lange, 1964.)

at this stage of the dissection, because it arises in the main fissure from the interlobar portion of the pulmonary artery. Large-caliber arteries, especially if they are short, require the additional safeguard of a suture ligature proximal to the point of division of the vessel, as well as a secure ligature proximal to the suture ligature.

The upper lobe pulmonary veins are managed next. The vein lies anterior to the artery as the latter passes downward into the fissure. It must be separated gently from the artery by blunt dissection, and the tributaries from the middle lobe must be identified and preserved.

Attention then shifts to the oblique fissure between the upper and lower lobes. The interlobar portion of the pulmonary artery is found after dividing the pleura where the lesser and greater fissures join. Dissection along the artery and identification of its branches are important. The origin of the posterior ascending segmental artery that needs division can vary and can also be crossed by anomalous veins. No ligation is done until the anatomy has been clearly defined. After the artery to its posterior segment has been appropriately ligated and divided, one has the option of proceeding with division of the interlobar fissures or moving on to isolation and division of the bronchus to the right upper lobe. These structures may be managed effectively by a mechanical stapling device.

The next step is to isolate the upper lobe bronchus, which is achieved by careful dissection without skeletalizing the bronchus, so that its blood supply is protected. The preferred method of bronchial closure is with the TA-30 stapler, using stainless steel staples, 4.8 mm in length, driven across the walls of the bronchus and crimped into a B shape by the instrument (Fig. 20–38). The spaces in and between each staple are large enough so that circulation to the divided end of the bronchus distal to the staple closure, where healing takes place, is not compromised (Betts and Takaro, 1965). The bronchial stump is tested for air leaks by covering the stump with saline and by asking the anesthesiologist to inflate the remaining lobes to a pressure of 25 to 30 cm H_2O. Closure of the bronchial stump with a pleural flap is optional but is generally recommended when there is adequate adjacent parietal pleura. Any obvious air leaks that need suture on the raw interlobar surfaces are closed with fine atraumatic 5-0 sutures. If the middle lobe is on a narrow pedicle and tends to rotate, it should be fixed to the margin bordering the lower lobe with a few atraumatic absorbable sutures to avoid the risk of torsion in the postoperative period. Apical and basal chest tubes are inserted, and the chest is closed in layers, preferably with interrupted sutures.

Right Middle and Lower Lobectomy

The chest is opened with a posterolateral thoracotomy, and the pleural cavity is entered through the bed of the resected sixth rib. Routine exploration of the chest determines whether only the middle lobe

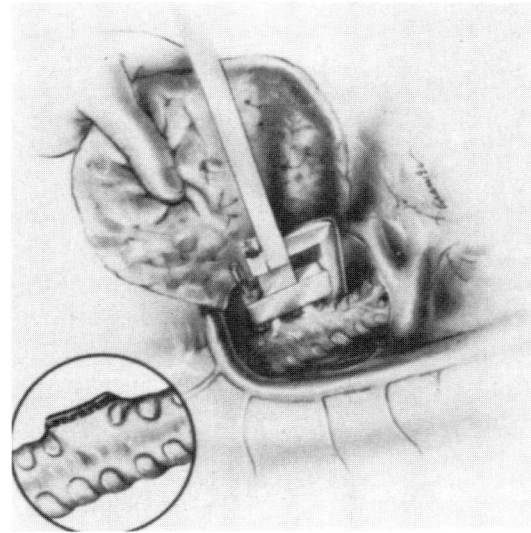

FIGURE 20–38. Technique of bronchial closure using the stapling device. The stapler is applied to the right upper lobe bronchus after ligation and division of all vascular structures. The *inset* shows the staggered double row of staples placed by a single application of the instrument.

needs removal or a bilobectomy is required. Separate excision of the middle lobe was once more common because inflammatory processes tended to involve the lymph nodes around the middle lobe bronchus, causing atelectasis and the so-called middle lobe syndrome, which ultimately caused bronchiectasis. Currently, the middle lobe is more infrequently involved in conjunction with one or another of the adjacent lobes because the underlying disease has spread. After examination of the entire right lung, the lower lobe is mobilized by dividing the inferior pulmonary ligament to improve access to the hilus. The major fissure is exposed; if the fissure is well developed, dissection starts by exposing the interlobar portion of the right pulmonary artery and branches (Fig. 20–39). The arterial supply to the middle lobe varies greatly. In more than half of cases, there are two middle lobe arteries, whereas in the remainder (40%), a single artery supplies the lobe. The posterior ascending artery to the posterior segment of the upper lobe is identified. All of the branches of the pulmonary artery distal to this vessel, which are visible in the fissure, supply the middle and lower lobes, and they should be isolated and divided between ligatures. In exceptional cases, an ascending branch to the posterior segment of the right upper lobe can arise from one of the middle lobe arteries; such a branch, after confirmation, should not be included in the ligature. Division of the minor fissure between the upper and middle lobes is not completed until after division of the bronchus.

Venous drainage of the middle lobe normally enters the superior pulmonary vein, although rarely it enters the left atrium separately or even joins the inferior pulmonary vein. The pulmonary vein from the middle lobe lies anterior to the bronchus. Venous drainage from the middle and lower lobes is approached

Text continued on page 720

MAJOR INTERLOBAR FISSURE

SUP. VENA CAVA

AZYGOS V.

VAGUS N.

TRACHEA

ESOPHAGUS

A

B

MINOR INTERLOBAR FISSURE

POST. SEGMENTAL ARTERY
TO THE UPPER LOBE

SEG. ARTERIES
TO THE
MIDDLE LOBE

LYMPH NODE

D

E

C

SUP. SEGMENTAL A.
TO THE LOWER LOBE

BASAL SEG. ARTERIES
TO THE LOWER LOBE

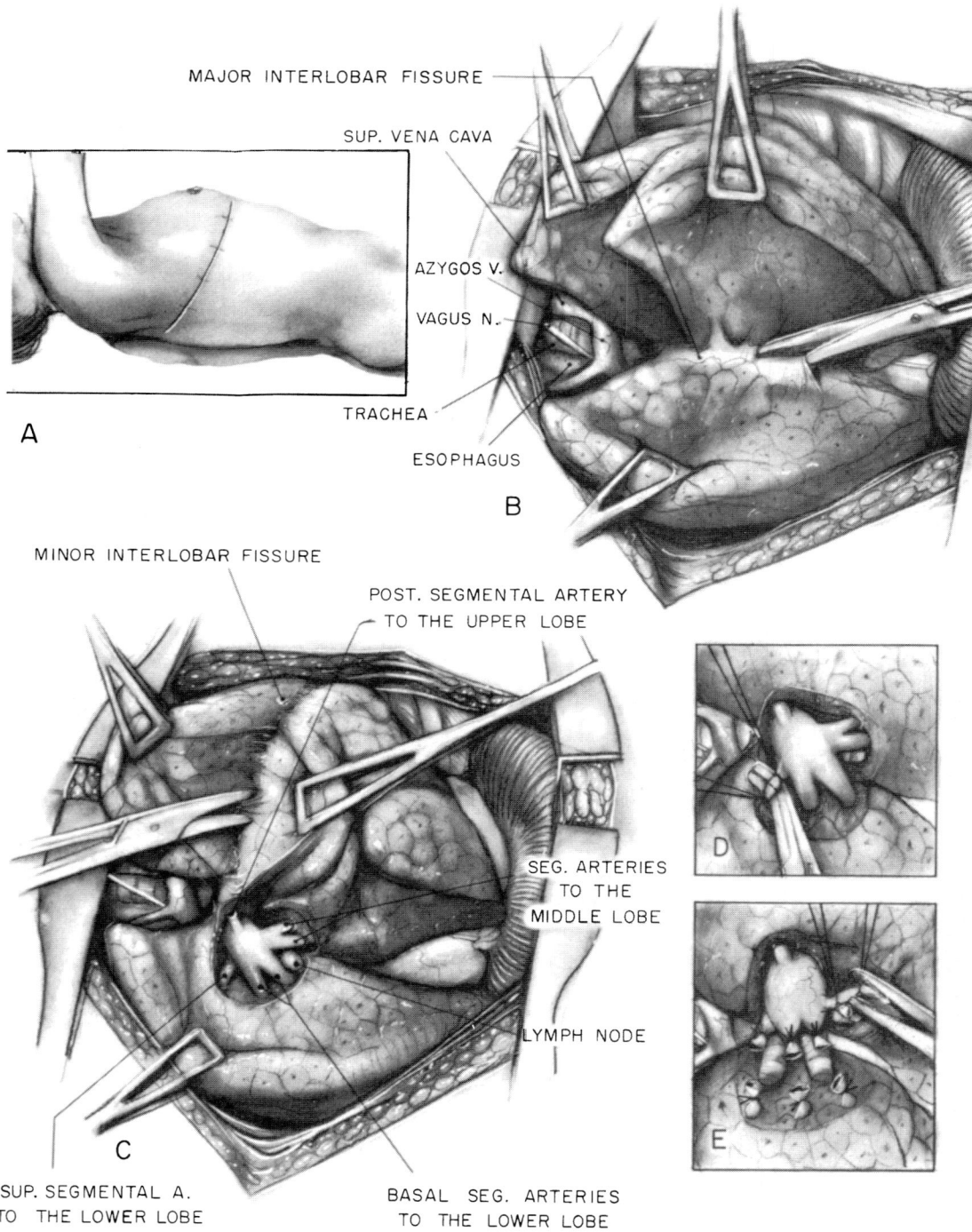

FIGURE 20–39. Technique of right middle and lower lobectomy. *A,* A right posterolateral thoracotomy incision is made over the sixth rib. *B* and *C,* The visceral pleura and the major interlobar fissure are opened and the fissure is developed to expose the pulmonary artery and its branches. *D* and *E,* Isolation, ligation, and division of the arterial branches to the right middle and lower lobes.

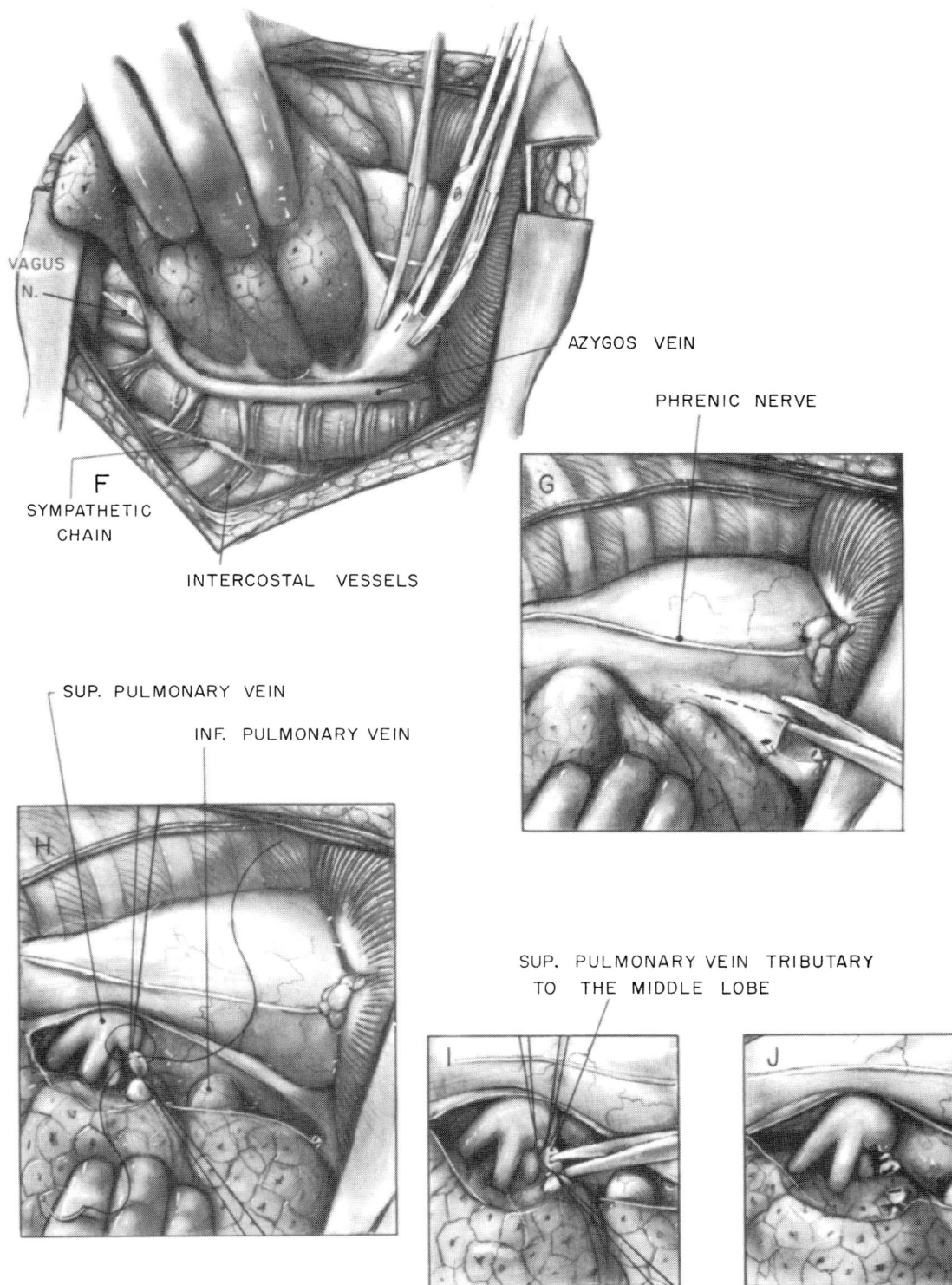

FIGURE 20–39. *Continued F* and *G,* Division of inferior pulmonary ligament inferiorly and anteriorly. *H, I,* and *J,* Isolation and division of branch of superior pulmonary vein to the right middle lobe. Note suture ligature in juxtaposition to ligature on proximal side of venous branch from right middle lobe in *J.* This technique is recommended for all major vascular branches, although not illustrated in most of the diagrams.

Illustration continued on following page

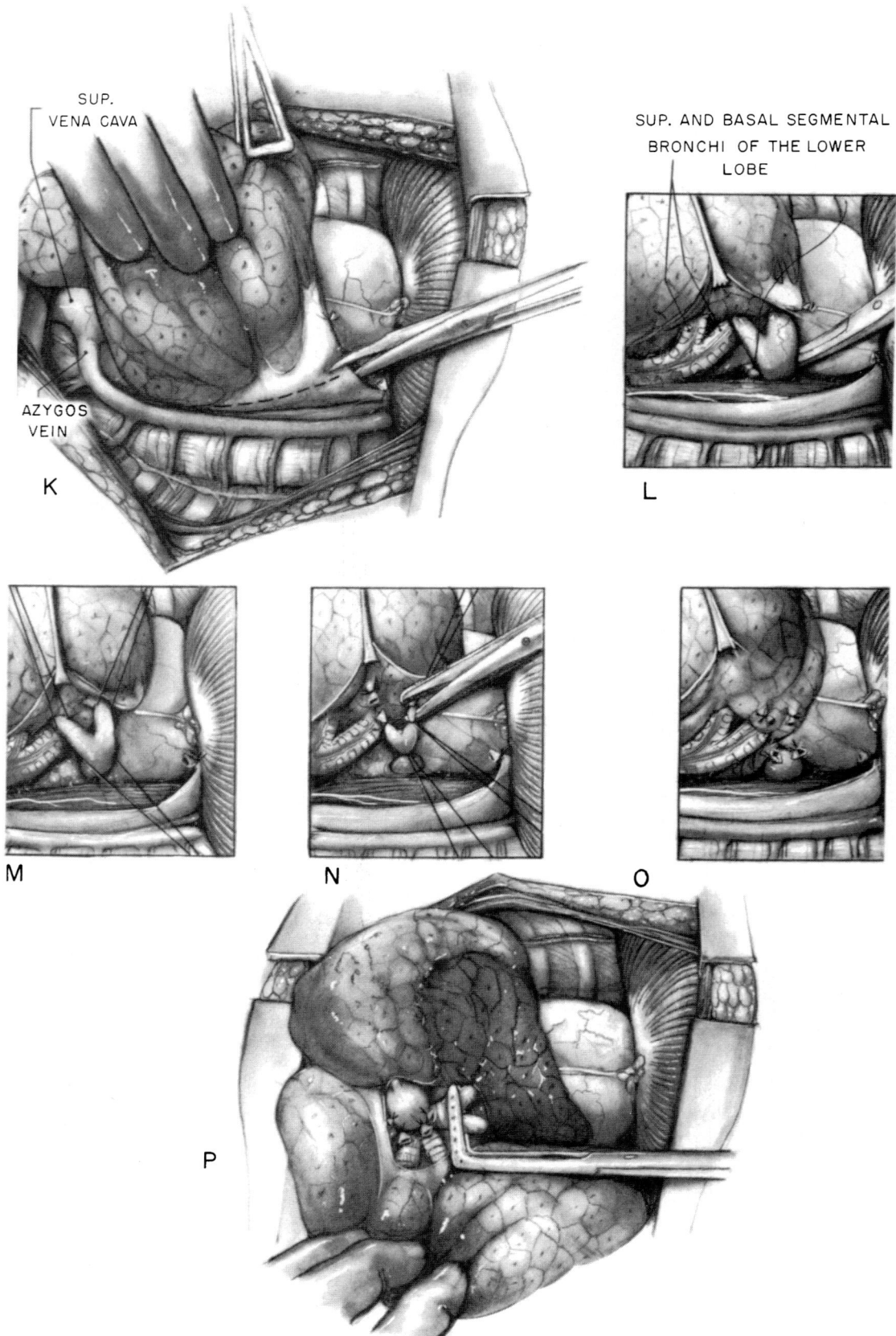

FIGURE 20–39. *Continued K* and *L,* Division of the posterior layer of the inferior pulmonary ligament, exposing inferior pulmonary vein and bronchus to the lower lobe. *M, N,* and *O,* Isolation, ligation, and division of the tributaries of the inferior pulmonary vein. *P,* Isolation of the right middle lobe bronchus in the major fissure. Bronchus has been clamped, and remaining lobes have been inflated to identify the incomplete fissure between the upper and the middle lobes.

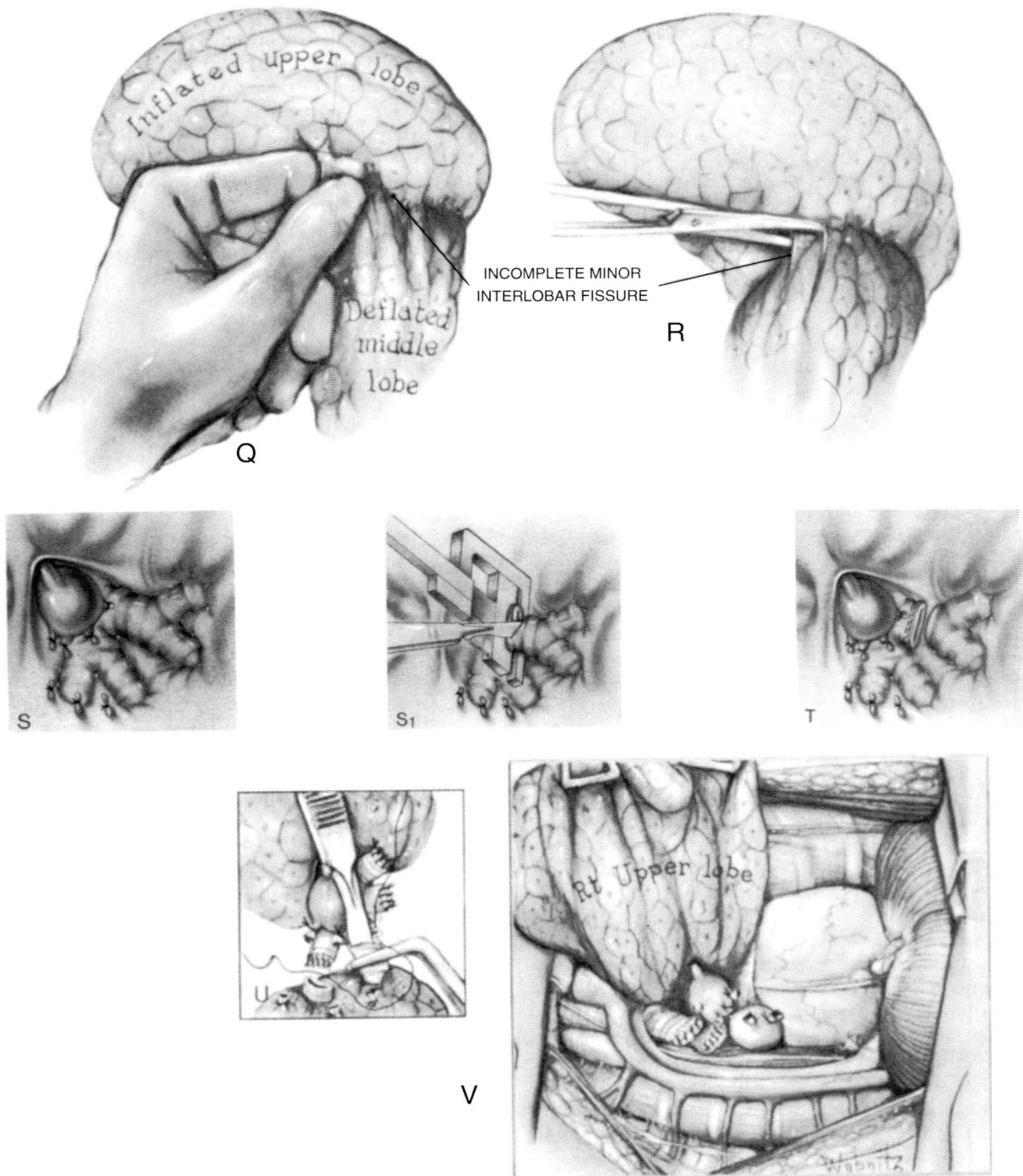

FIGURE 20–39. *Continued Q* and *R*, Division of incomplete fissure between the upper and the middle lobes. *S*, The two divisions of the middle lobe bronchus have been isolated. *S₁*, The divisions are stapled. *T*, The divisions have been divided, and the middle lobe bronchus is divided in its common portion. *U*, Division and closure of lower lobe bronchus. When a middle and a lower lobectomy are done together, it is usually preferable to divide the bronchus intermedius proximal to the middle lobe takeoff, which requires only a single bronchial closure. *V*, Completion of the right and middle lower lobectomy. (*A–V*, From Madden, J. L.: Atlas of Technics in Surgery. East Norwalk, CT, Appleton & Lange, 1964.)

by retracting the lower lobe superiorly and posteriorly. This approach exposes the inferior branch of the superior pulmonary vein that drains the middle lobe, which is doubly ligated and divided. The inferior pulmonary vein, which drains the lower lobe, comes into view as the lower lobe is retracted superiorly and slightly anteriorly. Branches to the lower lobe are isolated, ligated, and divided. At this point, the only remaining connection to the middle and lower lobes is the bronchial structures. Because the bronchus intermedius is accessible and long enough to be divided as a single unit, it is stapled with a TA-30 stapler and divided, or it is separated with a noncrushing clamp, divided, and oversewn with atraumatic sutures. Temporary occlusion of the bronchus to the middle lobe with inflation of the upper lobe helps to identify the minor fissure. The fissure may be divided by peeling the middle lobe away from the upper lobe after dividing the middle lobe bronchus by using the border between the uninflated and inflated lung as a guide. The GIA stapler may be used to complete division of the fissure.

After closure of the bronchus intermedius, the bronchial stump is again tested for air leaks and covered with a pleural flap. The pleural space is drained with an apical and basal chest tube, and the chest is closed in the standard manner.

Left Upper Lobectomy

A left posterolateral thoracotomy is done with entrance into the left pleural cavity through the bed of the subperiosteally resected fifth rib. After full mobilization of the lung, a routine exploration determines the extent of the lesion, possible lymph node involvement, and the state of the fissures. The upper lobe is retracted downward and backward. When difficulty in the arterial dissection is anticipated, it is wise to mobilize the left main pulmonary artery completely at this point and encircle it with a taper (Fig. 20–40). The mediastinal pleura is incised parallel to and below the concavity of the aortic arch in the region of the left vagus nerve. This incision is extended forward and downward between the edge of the lung and the phrenic nerve in front. The left main pulmonary artery becomes visible, and the avascular plane overlying the artery is opened. The upper lobe branches of the pulmonary artery are then dissected. The arteries to the apical and posterior segments are encountered first and are doubly ligated and divided between ligatures. The fissure is then opened along the course of the left pulmonary artery in the proper adventitial plane, and the branches of the anterior lingular segments of the left upper lobe and branches to the lower lobe are exposed.

The artery to the superior segment of the lower lobe lies opposite to and at approximately the same level as the lingular arteries; care must be taken not to injure this vessel.

The surgeon then has a choice of dealing with the bronchus first or ligating and dividing the superior pulmonary vein. In the lateral decubitus position, it is usually safer to ligate the vein first. The lung is therefore retracted backward, and the pleura is incised over the superior vein. The left superior pulmonary and inferior pulmonary veins occasionally unite to form a common vein; also, veins from the lingual segment can join the inferior pulmonary vein. Attention to these potential venous anomalies is important so that drainage of the lower lobe is not compromised. Branches of the superior pulmonary vein are then divided between ligatures. A suture ligature is used for security distal to the free ties of proximal stumps, as with the pulmonary arteries.

The lobe is now suspended only by the bronchus, which usually soon divides into the inferior (lingula) and superior portions. The lingular bronchus may have to be divided and closed separately from the superior division, but it is usually possible to dissect the bronchial divisions proximally to a common left upper lobe stump by gently retracting the left pulmonary artery. The left upper lobe bronchus is then stapled with the TA-30 stapler and divided. This completes resection of the left upper lobe.

Left Lower Lobectomy

Left lower lobectomy is done through a posterolateral thoracotomy incision with entrance into the pleural cavity through the sixth rib bed. The lung is mobilized, and the chest is routinely explored. The resection is best initiated by retracting the left lung superiorly and by dividing the inferior pulmonary ligament to allow better control of the hilum during ensuing dissection. The interlobar fissure is opened (Fig. 20–41). It can be developed by retracting the upper lobe superiorly and the lower lobe inferiorly. The visceral pleura overlying the left pulmonary artery lying in the depth of the fissure is dissected, exposing the artery and staying in the proper avascular adventitial plane. The first arterial branch encountered in the fissure is usually the superior segmental artery to the lower lobe. The arterial supply to this segment is variable, and two or even three branches may arise separately from the main left pulmonary artery. After ligation and division of the vessels to the superior segment, the common basal trunk below the lingular branches is secured. In most cases, it is safer to apply distal ties on the individual basal branches by leaving a long cuff beyond the proximal ligature. An additional transfixing ligature is placed on the proximal side of the main pulmonary artery distal to the lingular branches.

The lung is then retracted forward and upward, and the pulmonary ligament is divided from the diaphragm to the inferior pulmonary vein upward. Small vessels within the pulmonary ligament can be safely coagulated if this is done in an orderly manner. The lymph nodes in the pulmonary ligament are removed, and the inferior pulmonary vein is encircled with blunt dissection. The branches of the vein to the lower lobe are isolated, ligated, and divided between a free suture distally and a transfixing suture proximally. Again, it must be remembered that the superior and

Text continued on page 728

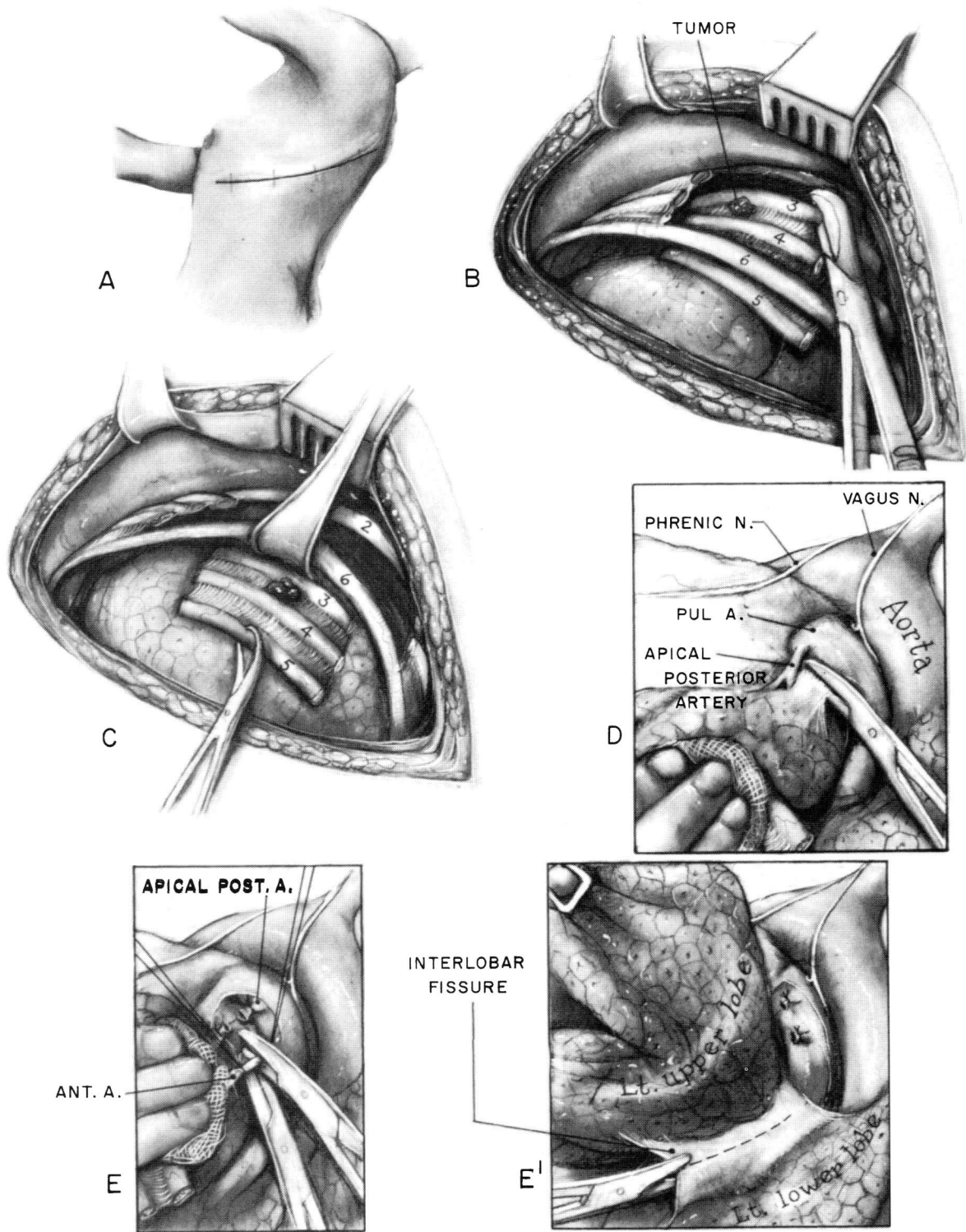

FIGURE 20–40. Technique of left upper lobectomy. *A,* Left posterolateral thoracotomy incision is made overlying the fifth rib. *B* and *C,* Left upper lobectomy for carcinoma involving the chest wall. A portion of the chest wall including ribs 3, 4, and 5 is resected in continuity with the left upper lobe. *D,* Mediastinal pleura is incised between the left pulmonary artery and the inferiorly displaced left upper lobe. *E,* Pulmonary artery branches to the apical-posterior and anterior segments are isolated, ligated, and divided. *E',* The visceral pleura in the interlobar fissure is opened.

Illustration continued on following page

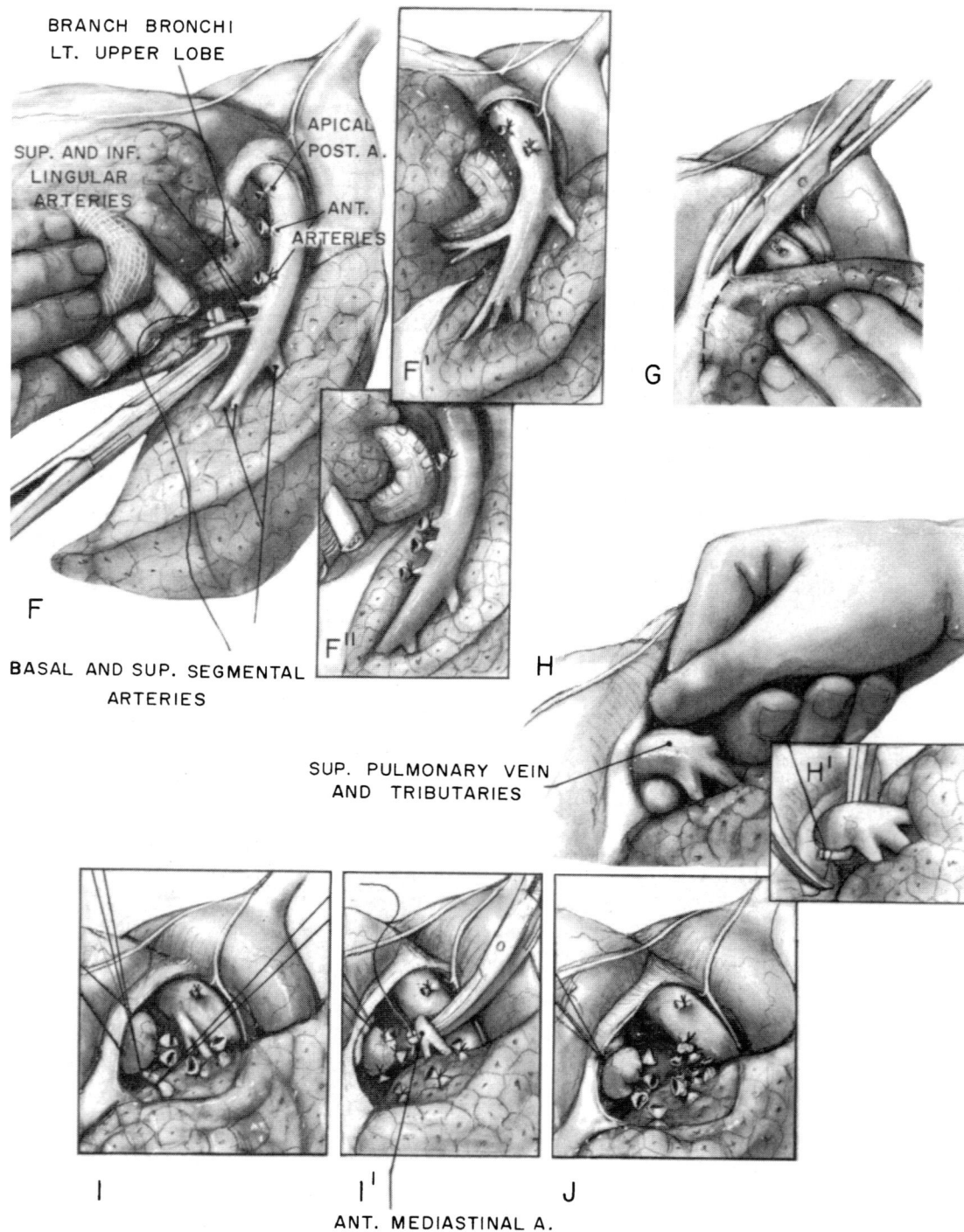

FIGURE 20–40. *Continued F, F', and F'',* The interlobar fissure is developed to expose the left pulmonary artery and its branches. The branches to the lingular segment have been ligated and divided. *G,* Incision of the mediastinal pleura overlying the superior pulmonary vein. *H, H',* and *I,* Isolation, ligation, and division of the branches of the superior pulmonary vein to the left upper lobe. *I'* and *J,* In this case, one additional large artery to the left upper lobe (anterior mediastinal artery) is isolated, ligated, and divided.

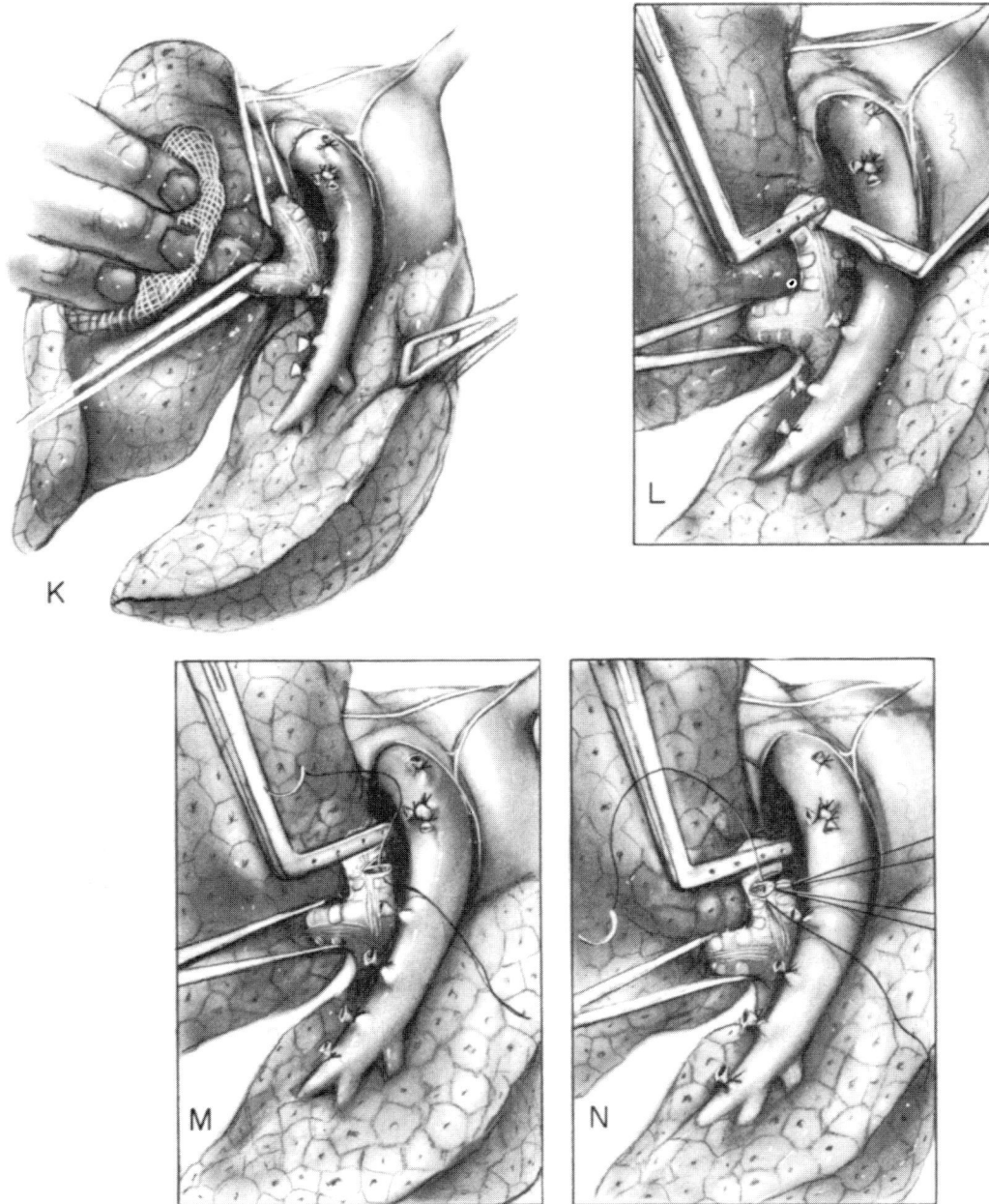

FIGURE 20–40. *Continued K,* The branches of the left upper lobe bronchus are exposed and encircled with tapes. *L, M,* and *N,* Division and closure of the left upper lobe bronchus. The left upper lobe bronchus can usually be divided and closed in its common portion by carrying the dissection slightly more proximally below the main pulmonary artery.

Illustration continued on following page

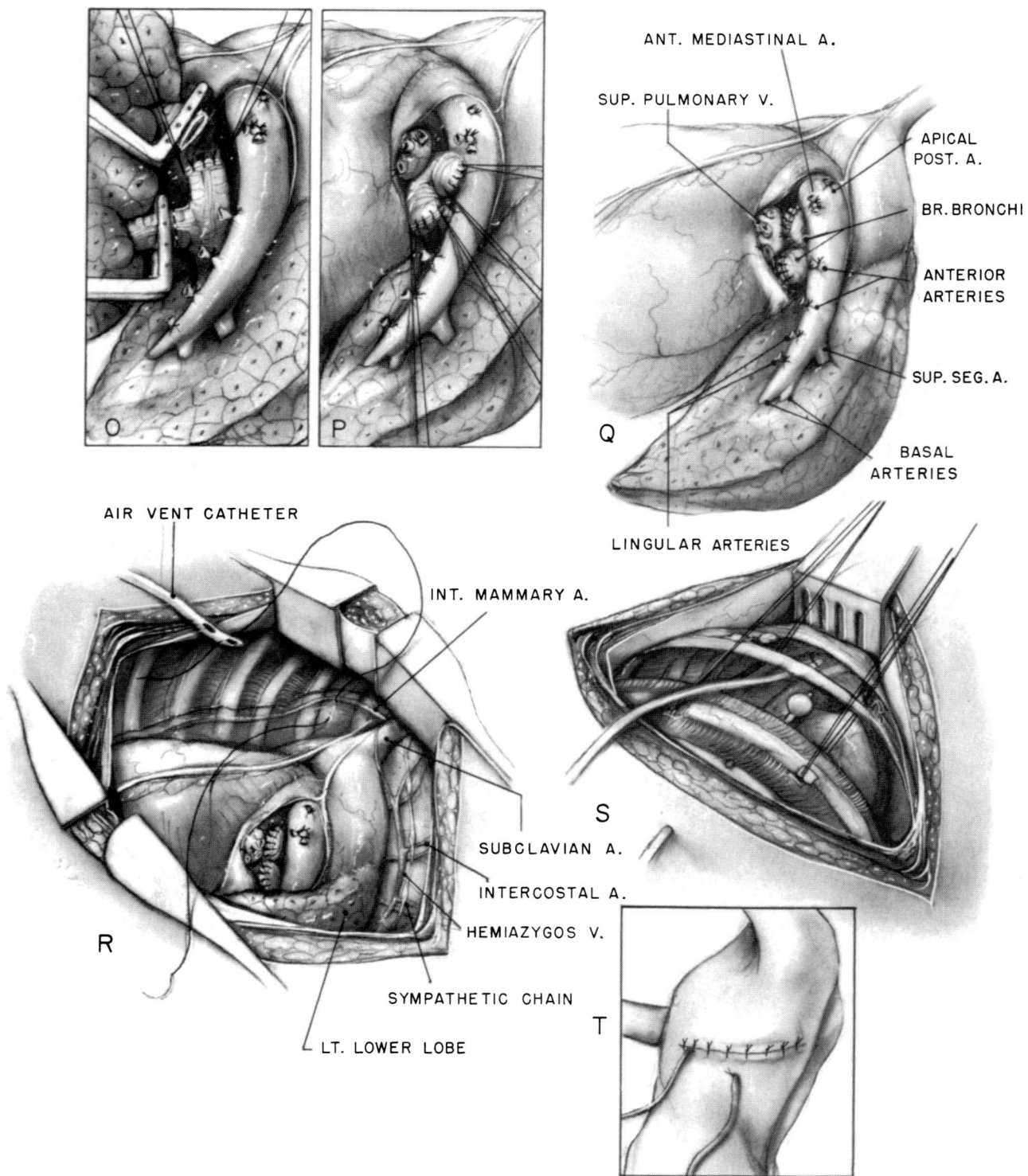

ANT. MEDIASTINAL A.

SUP. PULMONARY V.

APICAL
POST. A.

BR. BRONCHI

ANTERIOR
ARTERIES

SUP. SEG. A.

BASAL
ARTERIES

LINGULAR ARTERIES

AIR VENT CATHETER

INT. MAMMARY A.

SUBCLAVIAN A.

INTERCOSTAL A.

HEMIAZYGOS V.

SYMPATHETIC CHAIN

LT. LOWER LOBE

FIGURE 20–40. *Continued O, P,* and *Q,* Division and closure of the left upper lobe bronchus have been completed, and the resected lobe has been removed. *R, S,* and *T,* Drainage catheters being placed at apex and base for water seal or negative-pressure drainage. Ordinarily, we do not use Foley catheters, and chest tubes are not brought out through the thoracotomy wound but through two separate stab wounds. (*A–T,* From Madden, J. L.: Atlas of Technics in Surgery. East Norwalk, CT, Appleton & Lange, 1964.)

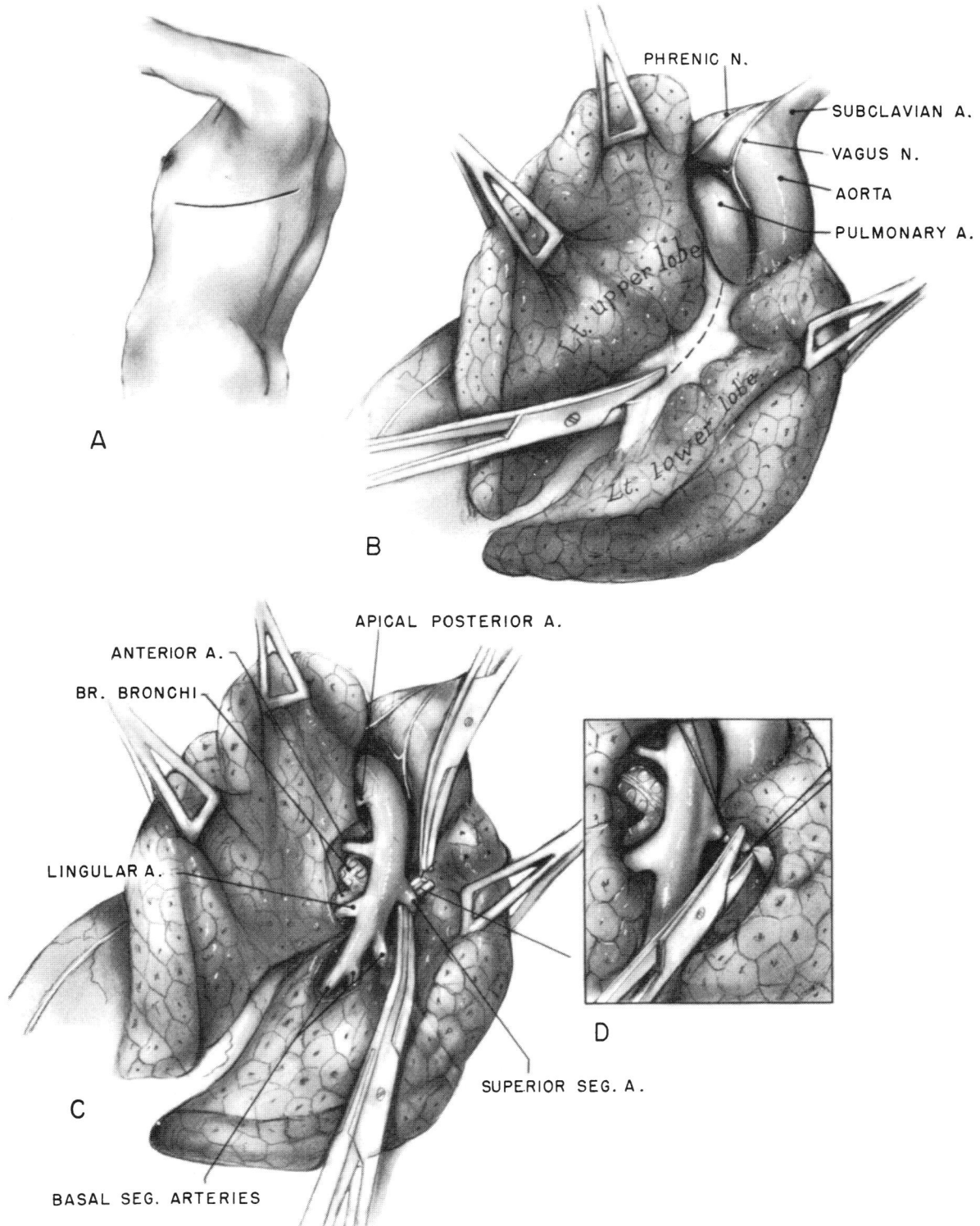

FIGURE 20–41. *A,* Technique of left lower lobectomy. A posterolateral thoracotomy incision is placed over the sixth rib. *B,* This incision of the visceral pleura in the interlobar fissure will be developed to expose the pulmonary artery and its branches. *C* and *D,* Exposure of the branches of the pulmonary artery and isolation and division of those to the lower lobe.

Illustration continued on following page

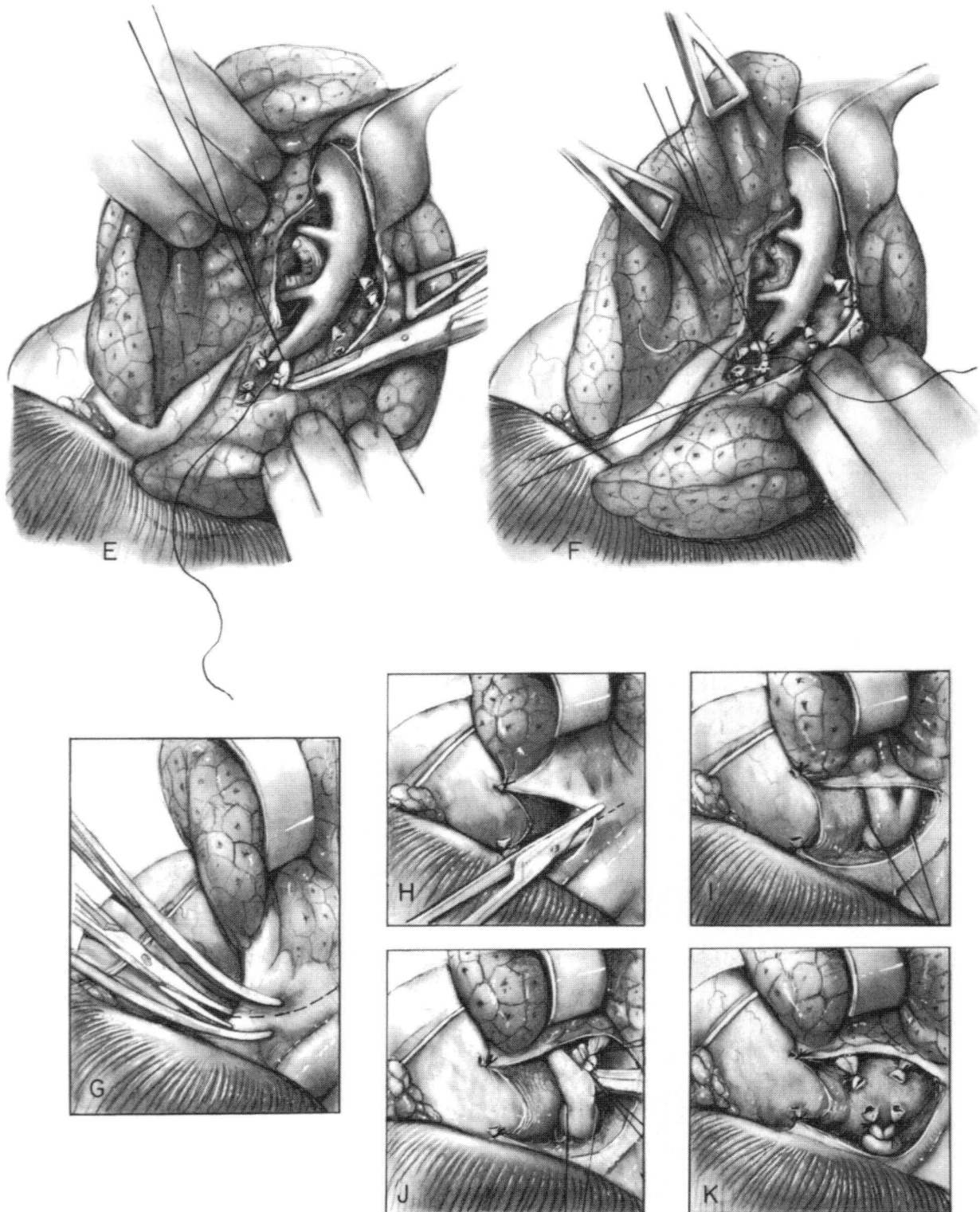

FIGURE 20–41. *Continued E* and *F,* Isolation, ligation, and division of arteries to the lower lobe continue. Branches to the lingular division and the anterior segment of the left upper lobe are carefully preserved. *G* and *H,* Division of the inferior pulmonary ligament to expose the inferior pulmonary vein. *I, J,* and *K,* Ligation and division of the inferior pulmonary vein. A separate suture ligature is placed on the proximal branches of the inferior pulmonary vein in addition to a ligature on the common stem.

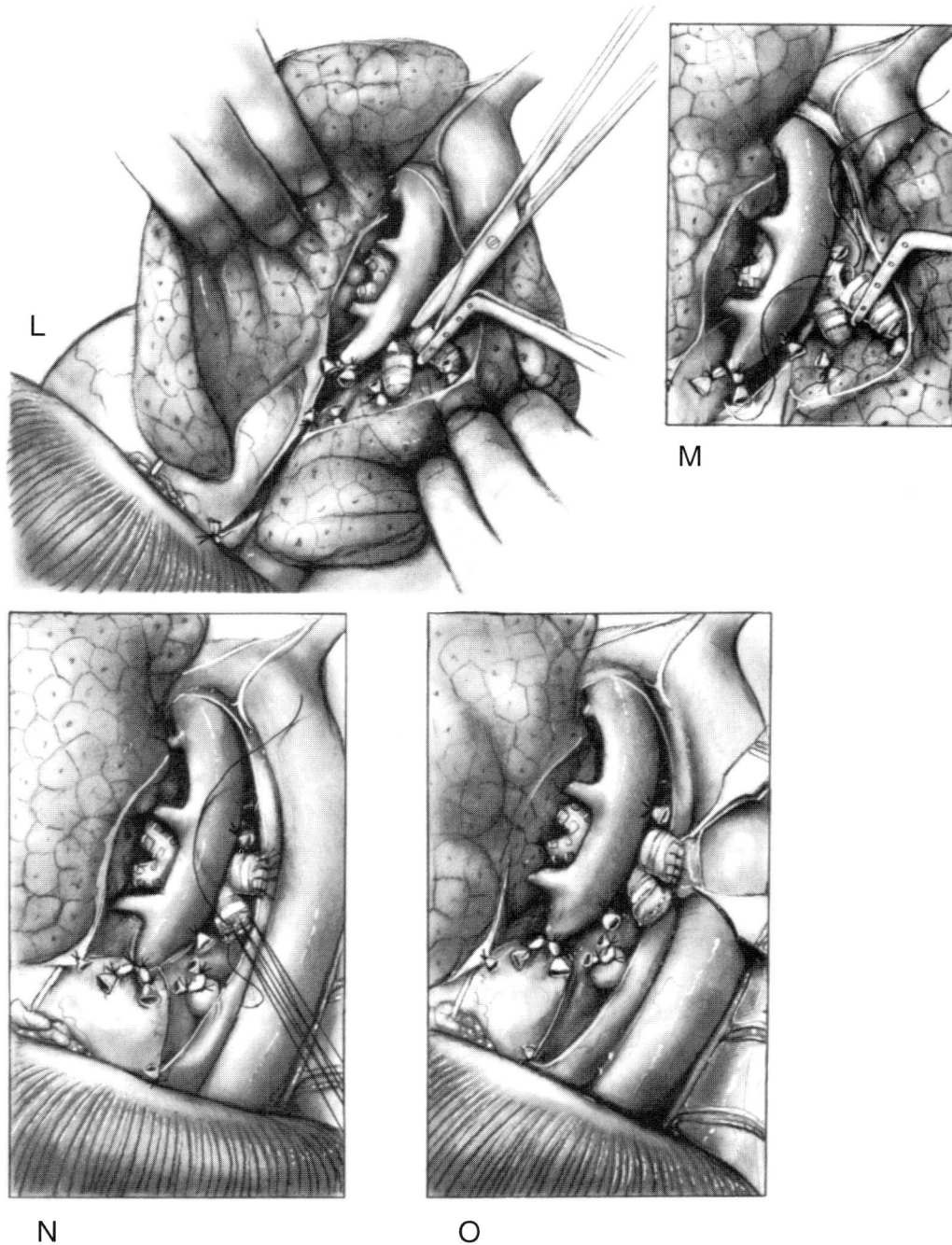

FIGURE 20–41. *Continued L,* Segmental bronchus to the superior segment of the left lower lobe in the interlobar fissure is clamped and partially divided. *M,* The partially severed bronchial stump is closed with interrupted sutures. *N,* The bronchus to the basal segments has been divided and is being sutured. Again, these closures generally are easier with a stapling device. *O,* The bronchial stumps are being covered by pleural flap. (*A–O,* From Madden, J. L.: Atlas of Technics in Surgery. East Norwalk, CT, Appleton & Lange, 1964.)

inferior pulmonary veins sometimes have a common stem outside the pericardium.

Finally, the bronchus is transsected. It can be approached through the fissure, from the back, or from below. The important point is to determine the exact disposition of the superior segmental bronchus of the lower lobe in relation to the origin of the left upper lobe bronchus. If the former arises almost opposite the latter, it is necessary either to staple or to suture the superior segmental bronchus separately from the basal trunk to avoid compromise of the airway to the upper lobe. A pedicle flap of pleura may be carefully lifted off the adjoining aorta and sutured to cover the bronchial stumps. The remainder of the operation is done in a standard manner, with an anterior and posterior pleural catheter being placed for drainage and standard closure of the chest wall.

SELECTED BIBLIOGRAPHY

Bolman, R. M., and Wolfe, W. G.: Bronchiectasis and bronchopulmonary sequestration. Surg. Clin. North Am., 60:867, 1980.

> This chapter in a monograph focusing on noncardiothoracic surgery reviews the etiology, pathology, and clinical presentation of bronchiectasis. The indications and outcome of surgery resection in selected patients are summarized in the review of several surgical series.

Catterall, J. R., Potasman, I., and Remington, J. S.: *Pneumocystis carinii* pneumonia in the patient with AIDS. Chest, 88:758, 1985.

> This review of the clinical and radiologic features of patients with acquired immunodeficiency syndrome and *P. carinii* pneumonia includes the preferred diagnostic modalities and choice of antipneumocystic drugs.

Daly, R. C., Pairolero, P. C., Piehler, J. M., et al.: Pulmonary aspergilloma: results of surgical treatment. J. Thorac. Cardiovasc. Surg., 92:981, 1986.

> This article reviews a series of 53 patients who underwent thoracotomy for treatment of pulmonary aspergilloma at the Mayo Clinic. Patients were classified according to their presentation with either simple aspergilloma (thin-walled mycetoma with minimal surrounding pulmonary infiltration) or complex aspergilloma (thick-walled cavity with extensive infiltrate). Operation in patients with simple aspergilloma was performed with low risk and good long-term outcome. Operative mortality in patients with complex aspergilloma was high, but 67% of survivors had a good long-term clinical result.

Delarue, N. C., Pearson, F. G., Nelems, J. M., et al.: Lung abscess—Surgical implications. Can. J. Surg., 23:297, 1980.

> A 50-year experience at the Toronto General Hospital including 415 patients with lung abscess is reviewed. The pathogenesis of lung abscess and important principles in the management of the patient with lung abscess are described. Indications for surgical treatment of lung abscess also are clearly given.

Gaensler, E. A., and Carrington, C. B.: Open biopsy for chronic diffuse infiltrative lung disease: Clinical, roentgenographic and physiological correlations in 502 patients. Ann. Thorac. Surg., 30:411, 1980.

> Clinical, physiologic, radiographic, and histologic data regarding 502 patients who underwent open lung biopsy for chronic interstitial pulmonary disease are reviewed. The preferred technique of open lung biopsy is described, and emphasis is placed on obtaining a section of average lung to more likely show an active and recognizable process.

Gefter, W. B.: The spectrum of pulmonary aspergillosis. J. Thorac. Imag., 7(4):56, 1992.

> Excellent review of the clinical manifestations of pulmonary aspergillosis. These range from invasive disease in the severely immunosuppressed patient to hypersensitivity in the hyperreactive patient. The radiographic and clinical features of these forms of pulmonary aspergillosis are reviewed with excellent representative chest films.

Medoff, G., and Kobayashi, G. S.: Strategies in the treatment of systemic fungal infections. N. Engl. J. Med., 302:145, 1980.

> This article reviews the pharmacology and clinical indications for use of amphotericin B as well as two more recently introduced agents, ketoconazole and 5-fluorocytosine. The common side effects of these drugs are described, as are principles of combination therapy (synergistic effect of amphotericin B and 5-fluorocytosine against *Cryptococcus neoformans*).

Prager, R. L., Burney, D. P., Waterhouse, G., and Bender, H. W., Jr.: Pulmonary mediastinal and cardiac presentations of histoplasmosis. Ann. Thorac. Surg., 30:385, 1980.

> The authors review 61 patients with histoplasmosis categorized by disease presentation into pulmonary, mediastinal, pericardial, and cardiac. Indications for surgical intervention in each category are reviewed. Most of the pulmonary cavitary lesions were treated by lobectomy, and the single operative death in the series was a patient who required pneumonectomy for mediastinal histoplasmosis.

Van Sonnenberg, E., D'Agostino, N. B., Casola, G., et al.: Lung abscess: CT-guided drainage. Radiology, 178:347, 1991.

> Lung abscesses were drained by means of catheters guided by computed tomography in 19 patients who had persistent sepsis despite standard medical therapy. The abscess was cured in all 19, and fever resolved within 48 hours in 18 of 19 patients. Three patients eventually required surgery for decortication after evacuation of the lung abscess.

BIBLIOGRAPHY

Abernathy, R. S.: Antibiotic therapy of lung abscess: Effectiveness of penicillin. Dis. Chest, 53:592, 1968.

Aliabadi, P., and Shafiepoor, H.: Bronchography in the recognition of congenital cystic bronchiectasis. Am. J. Roentgenol., 131:255, 1978.

Andersen, H. A., Fontana, R. S., and Harrison, E. G., Jr.: Transbronchoscopic lung biopsy in diffuse pulmonary disease. Dis. Chest, 48:187, 1965.

Andersen, H. A., Miller, W. E., and Bernatz, P. E.: Lung biopsy: Transbronchoscopic, percutaneous, open. Surg. Clin. North Am., 53:785, 1973.

Andrews, J. L., Jr.: Physiology and treatment of hypoxia. Clin. Notes Respir. Dis., 13:3, 1974.

Baldwin, E. deF., Cournand, A., and Richards, D. W., Jr.: Pulmonary insufficiency. II: A study of 39 cases of pulmonary fibrosis. Medicine, 28:1, 1949.

Barnett, T. B., and Herring, C. L.: Lung abscess: Initial and late results of medical therapy. Arch. Intern. Med., 127:217, 1971.

Bartlett, J. G.: Antibiotics in lung abscess. Semin. Respir. Infect., 6(2):103, 1991.

Bartlett, J. G., Gorbach, S. L., Tally, F. P., and Finegold, S. M.: Bacteriology and treatment of primary lung abscess. Am. Rev. Respir. Dis., 109:510, 1974.

Bartlett, M. S., and Smith, J. W.: *Pneumocystis carinii*, an opportunist in immunocompromised patients. Clin. Microbiol. Rev., 4(2):137, 1991.

Batra, P.: Pulmonary coccidioidomycosis. J. Thorac. Imag., 7(4):29, 1992.

Battaglini, J. W., Murray, G. F., Keagy, B. A., et al.: Surgical management of symptomatic pulmonary aspergilloma. Ann. Thorac. Surg., 39:512, 1985.

Belcher, J. R., and Plummer, N. S.: Surgery in broncho-pulmonary aspergillosis. Br. J. Dis. Chest, 54:335, 1960.

Bernard, E. M., Sepkowitz, K. A., Telzak, E. E., and Armstrong, D.: Pneumocystosis. Med. Clin. North Am., 76(1):107, 1992.

Berquist, T. H., Bailey, P. B., Cortese, D. A., and Miller, W. E.: Transthoracic needle biopsy: Accuracy and complications in relation to location and type of lesion. Mayo Clin. Proc., 55:475, 1980.

Betts, R. H., and Takaro, T.: Use of a lung stapler in pulmonary resection. Ann. Thorac. Surg., 1:197, 1965.

Blumenfeld, W., Wagar, E., and Hadley, W. K.: Use of the transbronchial biopsy for diagnosis of opportunistic pulmonary infections. Am. J. Clin. Pathol., 81:1, 1984.

Bolman, R. M., and Wolfe, W. G.: Bronchiectasis and bronchopulmonary sequestration. Surg. Clin. North Am., 60:867, 1980.

Bookstein, J. J., Moser, K. M., Kalafer, M. E., et al.: Role of bronchial arteriography and therapeutic embolization hemoptysis. Chest, 72:658, 1977.

Bradham, R. R., Sealy, W. C., and Young, W. G.: Chronic middle lobe infection. Ann. Thorac. Surg., 2:612, 1966.

Bradsher, R. W., Rice, D. C., and Abernathy, R. S.: Ketaconazole therapy for endemic blastomycosis. Ann. Intern. Med., 103:872, 1985.

Bragg, D. G., and Janis, B.: Radiographic presentation of pulmonary opportunistic inflammatory disease. Radiol. Clin. North Am., 11:357, 1973.

British Thoracic and Tuberculosis Association: Aspergilloma and residual tuberculous cavities—The results of a resurvey. Tubercle, 51:227, 1970.

Brock, R. C.: Lung Abscess. Oxford, Blackwell Scientific, 1952.

Buechner, H. A.: Management of Fungus Diseases of the Lungs. Springfield, IL, Charles C Thomas, 1971.

Burke, B. A., and Good, R. A.: *Pneumocystis carinii* infection. Medicine, 52:23, 1973.

Butz, R. O., Acetina, J. R., and Leininger, B. J.: Ten-year experience with mycetomas in patients with pulmonary tuberculosis. Chest, 87:356, 1985.

Cameron, E. W. J.: The treatment of pleuropulmonary amebiasis with metronidazole. Chest, 73:647, 1978.

Campbell, E. J., and Harris, B.: Idiopathic pulmonary fibrosis. Arch. Intern. Med., 141:771, 1981.

Carrington, C. B., and Gaensler, E. A.: Clinical-pathologic approach to diffuse infiltrative lung disease. In Thurlbeck, W. W., and Abell, M. R. (eds): The Lung. International Academy of Pathology Monograph No. 19. Baltimore, Williams & Wilkins, 1978.

Carrington, C. B., and Liebow, A. A.: Limited forms of angiitis and granulomatosis of the Wegener's type. Am. J. Med., 41:497, 1966.

Catanzaro, A.: Pulmonary coccidioidomycosis. Med. Clin. North Am., 64:461, 1980.

Catterall, J. R., Potasman, I., and Remington, J. S.: *Pneumocystis carinii* pneumonia in the patient with AIDS. Chest, 88:758, 1985.

Chipps, B. E., Talamo, R. C., and Winkelstein, J. A.: IgA deficiency, recurrent pneumonias and bronchiectasis. Chest, 73:419, 1978.

Cole, F. H., Cole, F. H., Jr., Khandekar, A., and Watson, D. C.: Management of broncholithiasis: Is thoracotomy necessary? Ann. Thorac. Surg., 42:255, 1986.

Conners, J. P., Roper, C. L., and Ferguson, T. B.: Transbronchial catheterization of pulmonary abscesses. Ann. Thorac. Surg., 19:254, 1975.

Cooper, M. D., Pearson, F. G., Patterson, G. A., et al.: Technique of successful lung transplantation in humans. J. Thorac. Cardiovasc. Surg., 93:173, 1987.

Craven, P. C., Graybill, J. R., Jorgensen, J. H., et al.: High-dose ketoconazole for treatment of fungal infections of the central nervous system. Ann. Intern. Med., 98:160, 1983.

Crystal, R. G., Bitterman, P. B., Rennard, S. L., et al.: Interstitial lung diseases of unknown cause: Disorders of the lower respiratory tract. N. Engl. J. Med., 310:154, 235, 1984.

Daly, R. C., Pairolero, P. C., Piehler, J. M., et al.: Pulmonary aspergilloma: Results of surgical treatment. J. Thorac. Cardiovasc. Surg., 92:981, 1986.

Delano, P., and Delano, M.: Sur les rapports des kystes de carinii du poumon des rats avec le *Trypanosoma lewisii*. Comptes Rendus Acad. Sci., 155:658, 1912.

Dines, D. E., Payne, W. S., Bernatz, P. E., et al.: Mediastinal granuloma and fibrosing mediastinitis. Chest, 75:320, 1979.

Dismukes, W. E., Stamm, A. M., Graybill, J. R., et al.: Treatment of systemic mycoses with ketoconazole: Emphasis on toxicity and clinical response in 52 patients. Ann. Intern. Med., 86:13, 1983.

Drutz, D. J., and Catanzaro, A.: Coccidioidomycosis. Am. Rev. Respir. Dis., 117:559, 1978.

Duperval, R., Hermans, P. E., Brewer, N. S., and Roberts, G. D.: Cryptococcosis with emphasis on the significance of isolation of *Cryptococcus neoformans* from the respiratory tract. Chest, 72:13, 1977.

Eastridge, C. E., Prather, M. R., Hughes, F. A., Jr., et al.: Actinomycosis: A 24-year experience. South. Med. J., 65:839, 1972.

Eguchi, S., Endo, S., Sakashita, I., et al.: Surgery in the treatment of pulmonary aspergillosis. Br. J. Dis. Chest, 65:111, 1971.

Emmons, C. W., Binford, C. H., Utz, J. P., et al.: Medical Mycology. 3rd ed. Philadelphia, Lea & Febiger, 1977.

Estrera, A. S., Platt, M. R., Mills, L. H., et al.: Primary lung abscess. J. Thorac. Cardiovasc. Surg., 79:275, 1980.

Fahey, P. J., Utell, M. H., and Hyde, R. W.: Spontaneous lysis of mycetomas after acute cavitating lung disease. Am. Rev. Respir. Dis., 123:336, 1981.

Falk, G. A.: Diffuse infiltrative disorders of unknown etiology. In Holman, C. W., and Muschenheim, C. (eds): Bronchopulmonary Diseases and Related Disorders. New York, Harper & Row, 1972.

Flye, M. W., Mundinger, G. H., Jr., and Fauci, A. S.: Diagnostic and therapeutic aspects of the surgical approach to Wegener's granulomatosis. J. Thorac. Cardiovasc. Surg., 77:331, 1979.

Gaensler, E. A., and Carrington, C. B.: Open biopsy for chronic diffuse infiltrative lung disease: Clinical, roentgenographic and physiological correlations in 502 patients. Ann. Thorac. Surg., 30:411, 1980.

Gaensler, E. A., Carrington, C. B., and Coutu, R. E.: Chronic interstitial pneumonias. Clin. Notes Respir. Dis., 10:1, 1972.

Garzon, A. A.: Discussion of Thoms, N. W., Wilson, R. F., Puro, H. E., and Arbulu, E.: Life-threatening hemoptysis in primary lung abscess. Ann. Thorac. Surg., 14:347, 1972.

Gefter, W. B.: The spectrum of pulmonary aspergillosis. J. Thorac. Imag., 7:56, 1992.

George, S. A., Leonardi, H. K., and Overhold, R. A.: Bilateral pulmonary resection for bronchiectasis: A 40-year experience Ann. Thorac. Surg., 28:48, 1979.

Glenn, W. W. L., Liebow, A. A., and Linkskog, G. E.: Thoracic and Cardiovascular Surgery with Related Pathology. Norwalk, CT, Appleton & Lange, 1971.

Gohel, V. K., Dalinka, M. K., Israel, H. L., et al.: The radiological manifestations of Wegener's granulomatosis. Br. J. Radiol., 46:427, 1973.

Goodwin, R. A., Jr., Owens, F. T., Snell, J. D., et al.: Chronic pulmonary histoplasmosis. Medicine, 55:413, 1976.

Groskin, S. A., Panicek, M. D., Ewing, D. K., et al.: Bacterial lung abscess—A review of the radiographic and clinical features of 50 cases. J. Thorac. Imag., 6(3):62, 1991.

Hague, A. K.: Pathology of common pulmonary fungal infections. J. Thorac. Imag., 7:1, 1992.

Hamman, L., and Rich, A. R.: Fulminating diffuse interstitial fibrosis of lungs. Trans. Am. Clin. Climatol. Assoc., 51:154, 1935.

Hammerman, K. J., Powell, K. E., Christianson, C. S., et al.: Pulmonary cryptococcosis: Clinical forms and treatment. Am. Rev. Respir. Dis., 108:1116, 1973.

Hargis, J. L., Bone, R. C., Stewart, J., et al.: Intracavitary amphotericin B in the treatment of symptomatic pulmonary aspergillomas. Am. J. Med., 68:389, 1980.

Hatcher, C. R., Jr., Sehdeva, J., Waters, W. C., III, et al.: Primary pulmonary cryptococcosis. J. Thorac. Cardiovasc. Surg., 61:39, 1971.

Hay, R. J.: Antifungal therapy and the new azole compounds. J. Antimicrob. Chemother., 28:35, 1991.

Henderson, R. D., et al.: Surgery in pulmonary aspergillosis. J. Thorac. Cardiovasc. Surg., 70:1093, 1975.

Hiatt, J. R., Gong, H., Mulder, D. G., and Ramming, K. P.: The value of open lung biopsy in the immunosuppressed patient. Surgery, 92:285, 1982.

Hilton, A. M., and Doyle, L.: Immunological abnormalities in bronchiectasis with chronic bronchial suppuration. Br. J. Dis. Chest, 72:207, 1978.

Hinshaw, H. C., and Murray, J. F.: Diseases of the Chest. 4th ed. Philadelphia, W. B. Saunders, 1980.

Hodgkin, J. E., Anderson, H. A., and Rosenow, E. C.: Diagnosis of *Pneumocystis carinii* pneumonia by transbronchoscopic lung biopsy. Chest, 64:551, 1973.

Hughes, W. T.: *Pneumocystis carinii* pneumonitis. Chest, 85:810, 1984.

Hughes, W. T., Kuhn, S., Feldman, S., et al.: Successful chemoprophylaxis for *Pneumocystis carinii* pneumonitis. N. Engl. J. Med., 297:1419, 1977.

Israel, H. L., and Ostrow, A.: Sarcoidosis and aspergilloma. Am. J. Med., 47:243, 1969.

James, D. G.: Modern concepts of sarcoidosis [Editorial]. Chest, 64:675, 1973.

James, D. G.: Sarcoidosis. Disease-A-Month, February 1970, p. 43.

Jara, F. M., Toledo-Perreyra, L. H., and Magilligan, D. J.: Surgical implications of pulmonary actinomycosis. J. Thorac. Cardiovasc. Surg., 78:600, 1979.

Johnson, P., and Sarosi, G.: Current therapy of major fungal diseases of the lung. Infect. Dis. Clin. North Am., 5(3):635, 1991.

Jung, J. Y., Salas, R., Almond, C. H., et al.: The role of surgery in the management of pulmonary monosporosis: A collective review. J. Thorac. Cardiovasc. Surg., 73:1399, 1977.

Karas, A., Hankins, J. R., Attar, S., et al.: Pulmonary aspergillosis: An analysis of 41 patients. Ann. Thorac. Surg., 22:1, 1976.

Kirks, D. R., McCormick, V. D., and Greenspan, R. H.: Pulmonary sarcoidosis. Roentgenologic analysis of 150 patients. Am. J. Roentgenol. Radium Ther. Nucl. Med., 177:777, 1973.

Klein, B. S., Vergeront, J. M., Weeks, R. J., et al.: Isolation of *Blastomyces dermatitidis* in soil associated with a large outbreak of blastomycosis in Wisconsin. N. Engl. J. Med., 82:18, 1975.

Krick, J. A., Stinson, E. B., and Remington, J. S.: *Nocardia* infection in heart transplant patients. Ann. Intern. Med., 82:18, 1975.

Lehrer, R. I., Howard, D. H., Sypherd, P. S., et al.: Mucormycosis. Ann. Intern. Med., 93:93, 1980.

Levison, M. E., Mangura, C. T., Lurber, B.: Clindamycin compared with penicillin for the treatment of anaerobic lung abscess. Ann. Intern. Med., 98:466, 1983.

Lichter, I.: Surgery of pulmonary hydatid cyst—The Barrett technique. Thorax, 27:529, 1972.

Liebow, A. A., Steer, A., and Billingsley, J. G.: Desquamative interstitial pneumonia. Am. J. Med., 39:369, 1965.

Littman, M. L., and Walter, J. W.: Cryptococcosis: Current status. Am. J. Med., 45:922, 1968.

Lyman, C. A., and Walsh, T. J.: Systemically administered antifungal agents. Drugs, 44(1):9, 1992.

Magilligan, D. J., Ravipati, S., Aayat, P., et al.: Massive hemoptysis: Control by transcatheter bronchial artery embolization. Ann. Thorac. Surg., 32:392, 1981.

Mayer, J. M., Nimer, L., and Carroll, K.: Isolated pulmonary aspergillar infection in cardiac transplant recipients. Clin. Infect. Dis., 15:698, 1992.

McGuinness, G., Naidich, D. P., Leitman, B. S., and McCauley, D. I.: Bronchiectasis—CT evaluation. Am. J. Radiol., 160:253, 1993.

McQuarrie, D. G., and Hall, W. H.: Actinomycosis of the lung and chest wall. Surgery, 64:905, 1968.

Medoff, G., and Kobayashi, G. S.: Strategies in the treatment of systemic fungal infections. N. Engl. J. Med., 302:145, 1980.

Merrill, J., Otis, J., Logan, W. D., Jr., et al.: The dog heart worm (*Dirofilaria immitis*) in man: An epidemic pending or in progress? J. A. M. A., 243:1066, 1980.

Miller, J. I.: The thoracic surgical spectrum of acquired immune deficiency syndrome. J. Thorac. Cardiovasc. Surg., 92:977, 1986.

Munro, N. C., Har, L. Y., Currie, D. G., et al.: Radiological evidence of progression of bronchiectasis. Respir. Med., 86:397, 1992.

Murray, H. W., Littman, M. L., and Roberts, R. B.: Disseminated paracoccidioidomycosis (South American blastomycosis) in the United States. Am. J. Med., 56:209, 1974.

Murray, J. F., Felton, C. P., Garay, S. M., et al.: Pulmonary complications of the acquired immune deficiency syndrome. N. Engl. J. Med., 310:1682, 1984.

Nagaki, M., Shimura, S., Tanno, Y., et al.: Role of chronic *Pseudomonas aeruginosa* infection in the development of bronchiectasis. Chest, 102:1464, 1992.

National Institute of Allergy and Infectious Disease Mycosis Study Group: Treatment of blastomycosis and histoplasmosis with ketoconazole: Results of a prospective randomized clinical trial. Ann. Intern. Med., 103:861, 1985.

Nelson, A. R.: The surgical treatment of pulmonary coccidioidomycosis. Curr. Probl. Surg., October 1974, pp. 1–48.

Palmer, D. L., Harvey, R. L., and Wheeler, J. K.: Diagnostic and therapeutic considerations in *Nocardia asteroids* infection. Medicine, 53:391, 1974.

Pass, H. I., Potter, D., Shelhammer, J., et al.: Indications for and diagnostic efficacy of open-lung biopsy in the patient with acquired immunodeficiency syndrome (AIDS). Ann. Thorac. Surg., 41:307, 1986.

Paulsen, G. A.: Pulmonary surgery in coccidioidal infections. *In* Ajello L. (ed): Coccidioidomycosis. Tucson, University of Arizona, 1967.

Perianayagam, W. J., Freitas, E., Sharma, S. S., et al.: Pulmonary hydatid cyst: A 25-year experience. Aust. N. Z. J. Surg., 49:450, 1979.

Prager, R. L., Burney, D. P., Waterhouse, G., and Bender, H. W., Jr.: Pulmonary mediastinal, and cardiac presentations of histoplasmosis. Ann. Thorac. Surg., 30:385, 1980.

Reid, L.: Reduction in bronchial subdivision in bronchiectasis. Thorax, 5:233, 1950.

Remy, J., Arnaud, A., Fardou, H., et al.: Treatment of hemoptysis by embolization of bronchial arteries. Radiology, 122:33, 1977.

Restrepo, A., Stevens, D. A., Leiderman, E., et al.: Ketoconazole in paracoccidioidomycosis: Efficacy of prolonged oral therapy. Mycopathologica, 72:35, 1980.

Rice, T. W., Ginsburg, R. J., and Todd, T. R.: Tube drainage of lung abscesses. Ann. Thorac. Surg., 44:356, 1987.

Rossiter, S. J., Miller, D. C., Churg, A. M., et al.: Open lung biopsy in the immunosuppressed patient. Is it really beneficial? J. Thorac. Cardiovasc. Surg., 77:338, 1979.

Rubin, P. E., and Block, A. J.: Nonspecific lung abscess: A perspective. Geriatrics, 27:125, 1972.

Rubin, R. H.: Mycotic infections. *In* Rubenstein, E., Federman, D. D. (eds): Scientific American Medicine. New York, Scientific American, 1982.

Ruskin, J., and Hughes, W. T.: *Pneumocystis carinii. In* Remington, J. S., and Kline, J. O. (eds): Infectious Diseases of the Fetus and Newborn Infant. Philadelphia, W. B. Saunders, 1983.

Salomon, N. W., Osborne, R., and Copeland, J. G.: Surgical manifestations and results of treatment of pulmonary coccidioidomycosis. Ann. Thorac. Surg., 30:433, 1980.

Sarosi, G. A., Armstrong, D., Barbee, R. A., et al.: Treatment of fungal diseases. Am. Rev. Respir. Dis., 120:1393, 1979.

Sarosi, G. A., and Davies, S. F.: Blastomycosis. Am. Rev. Respir. Dis., 120:911, 1979.

Sarosi, G. A., Parker, J. D., Doto, I. L., et al.: Chronic pulmonary coccidioidomycosis. N. Engl. J. Med., 283:325, 1970.

Sealy, W. C., Bradham, R. R., and Young, W. G.: The surgical treatment of multisegmental and localized bronchiectasis. Surg. Gynecol. Obstet., 123:80, 1966.

Seelig, M. S., Speth, C. P., Kozinn, P. J., and Toni, E. F.: *Candida* endocarditis after cardiac surgery: Clues to earlier detection. J. Thorac. Cardiovasc. Surg., 65:583, 1973.

Sen, P., and Louria, D. B.: Fungal infections in the compromised host. D. M., 27:1, 1981.

Shafron, R. D., and Tate, C. F., Jr.: Lung abscesses: A 5-year evaluation. Dis. Chest, 53:12, 1968.

Siegesmund, K. A., Funahashi, A., Pintar, K., et al.: Elemental content in alveolar septa in various pneumoconioses. Chicago, Scanning Electron Microscopy/II, 1980.

Slade, P. R., Slesser, B. V., and Southgate, J.: Thoracic actinomycosis. Thorax, 28:73, 1973.

Snell, J. D., and Holman, C. W.: Supportive lung disease: Lung abscess and bronchiectasis. *In* Holman, C. W., and Muschenheim, C. (eds): Bronchopulmonary Disorders. New York, Harper & Row, 1972.

Stjernberg, N., Bjornstad-Pettersen, H. J., and Truesdsson, H.: Flexible fiberoptic bronchoscopy in sarcoidosis. Acta Med. Scand., 208:397, 1980.

Takaro, T.: Thoracic actinomycetic and mycotic infections. *In* Goldsmith, H. S., Ellis, F. H., Jr. (eds): Goldsmith's Practice of Surgery. New York, Harper & Row, 1968.

Toronto Lung Transplant Group: Unilateral transplantation for pulmonary fibrosis. N. Engl. J. Med., 314:1140, 1986.

Van Sonnenberg, E., D'Agostino, N. B., Casola, G., et al.: Lung abscess: CT-guided drainage. Radiology, 178:347, 1991.

Varkey, B., and Rose, H. D.: Pulmonary aspergilloma: A rational approach to treatment. Am. J. Med., 61:626, 1976.

Varpela, E., Koistinen, J., Korhola, O., et al.: Deficiency of alpha$_1$ antitrypsin and bronchiectasis. Ann. Clin. Res., 10:79, 1978.

Wall, C. P., Gaensler, E. A., Carrington, C. B., and Hayes, J. A.: Comparison of transbronchial and open biopsies in chronic infiltrative lung diseases. Am. Rev. Respir. Dis., 123:280, 1981.

Westcott, J. L.: Bronchiectasis. Radiol. Clin. North Am., 29(5):1031, 1991.

Wheat, L. J., Slama, T. G., and Zecker, M. L.: Histoplasmosis in the acquired immune deficiency syndrome. Am. J. Med., 78:203, 1985.

Wilson, J. B., Davidson, M., and Rausch, R. L.: A clinical trial of mebendazole in the treatment of alveolar hydatid disease. Am. Rev. Respir. Dis., 118:747, 1978.

21

Thoracic Disorders in the Immunocompromised Host

H. Kim Lyerly, John A. Bartlett, and J. Michael DiMaio

Thoracic surgeons are commonly consulted in the care of immunocompromised patients. For immunocompromised patients with infectious complications, the chest remains the most common site for localized infection. This chapter focuses on the thoracic manifestations of persons infected with the *human immunodeficiency virus* (HIV) and persons who are iatrogenically immunosuppressed from transplantation or chemotherapy. Because of their increasing size, these two populations demand the attention of the thoracic surgeon. The number of persons with HIV is increasing throughout the United States, especially in areas outside of the east and west coast metropolitan centers that were previously recognized as the epicenters of HIV. There are also increasing numbers of persons receiving solid organ and bone marrow transplantations with concurrent immunosuppressive drugs, including heart and lung transplants, which directly involve the thoracic surgeon. The role of the thoracic surgeon may include diagnostic procedures such as bronchoscopy with *bronchoalveolar lavage* (BAL) or *transbronchial biopsy* (TBB), lung biopsy by an open or thoracoscopic approach, and pleural biopsy or endoscopy, as well as therapeutic interventions. As a member of the team involved in heart or lung transplants, the thoracic surgeon is directly involved in the care of immunosuppressed patients. The thoracic surgeon needs a pathophysiologic understanding of the underlying immunosuppression to properly construct differential diagnoses and choose the appropriate diagnostic procedure. The differential diagnoses may be quite numerous, so empiric therapy may be difficult to choose. Establishing a definitive diagnosis may yield critical information—for example, in selecting the most appropriate and least toxic antimicrobial therapy. Finally, the thoracic surgeon may need to perform therapeutic interventions in the immunocompromised host, such as chest tube placement in HIV-infected patients with *Pneumocystis carinii pneumonia* (PCP), valve replacements in HIV-infected patients with endocarditis, and resection of pulmonary mucormycosis in a patient after organ transplantation.

THORACIC MANIFESTATIONS OF HUMAN IMMUNODEFICIENCY VIRUS INFECTION

In 1981, previously healthy young homosexual men were first described with PCP and *Kaposi's sarcoma* (KS). This original description of an unprecedented and unexplained immunosuppressive illness eventually led to the recognition of the *acquired immunodeficiency syndrome* (AIDS). The hallmark of AIDS is profound compromise of the cellular immune system, causing a marked predisposition to opportunistic infections and neoplasms (Gottlieb et al., 1981; Hymes et al., 1981; Masur et al., 1981; Siegal et al., 1981). Eventually, AIDS was recognized as the end-stage of progressive infection with HIV. The natural history of HIV infection has become more clearly elucidated, from a mononucleosis-like syndrome that may be associated with acute HIV infection, through a prolonged asymptomatic period that involves progressive immunologic impairment, and finally to full-blown AIDS. It is during the later stages of HIV infection that thoracic surgeons are most commonly consulted; this chapter concentrates on manifestations in the thorax associated with progressive disease.

HUMAN IMMUNODEFICIENCY VIRUS

HIV is a human retrovirus that was first isolated by Montagnier and associates at the Pasteur Institute in 1983 and was shown conclusively to be the etiologic agent of AIDS by Gallo and associates at the National Institutes of Health in 1984 (Barre-Sinoussi et al., 1983; Gallo et al., 1984; Popovic et al., 1984; Sarngadharan et al., 1984). Both share credit for the discovery of the causative agent of AIDS, initially called *human T-lymphotropic virus Type III* (HTLV-III) or *lymphadenopathy-associated virus* (LAV), now called HIV.

Epidemiology

Since the initial reports of AIDS in 1981, more than 340,000 cases have been reported in the United States, with more than 200,000 deaths (Centers for Disease Control, 1993). The rate of rise in the number of reported persons with AIDS temporarily stabilized during the early 1990s. It is estimated that more than 1,000,000 Americans are infected with HIV. High-risk groups continue to include homosexual men, intravenous drug abusers, heterosexual partners of HIV-infected individuals, recipients of blood and blood-product transfusion, and children of infected mothers.

731

However, during the past 5 years, the risk behaviors of persons reported with AIDS have more often been drug use through injection and heterosexual contact with a person at risk. It has been estimated that more than 75% of all HIV infections are spread through sexual contact. Increasing numbers of women and minorities are being reported with AIDS, forcing clinicians to address the issues of perinatal transmission, families with HIV infection, and the complicating circumstances of socioeconomic deprivation. Encouraging seroprevalence data from populations of homosexual men suggest dramatic decreases in seroconversions, which may suggest that education is helping to reduce risk.

Transmission and Risk to Health Care Workers

HIV infection can be acquired through five routes: sexual contact (either homosexual or heterosexual), needlesticks, contact with infected blood, perinatally, or through breast feeding. Careful investigations have failed to identify HIV transmission outside of these five routes.

Health care workers exposed to the blood or bodily fluids of an HIV-infected patient have a small but definite risk of acquiring HIV infection (Baker et al., 1987; Friedland and Klein, 1987). Major prospective evaluations of health care workers who received percutaneous inoculations of blood from HIV-infected individuals showed only rare cases of documented seroconversion after needlestick injury, and the risk of parenteral or mucous membrane exposure leading to infection is approximately 0.4% (1 in 250) (Centers for Disease Control, 1993). In sharp contrast is an approximately 15 to 20% incidence of infection associated with parenteral exposure to blood or body fluids from an infectious hepatitis B carrier (Lettau et al., 1986). Nearly all health care workers who have acquired HIV infection in the workplace have been exposed to infected blood; a single circumstance of HIV infection following exposure to bloody pleural fluid has been reported. These observations correlate with the amount of virus cultured from bodily fluids and suggest that the risk of exposure is greatest with blood, fluids contaminated with blood, cerebrospinal fluid, and semen (Busch et al., 1991). In addition, the method of exposure may correlate with subsequent infectious risk. Increased risk of HIV acquisition has been associated with the severity of exposure (such as deep intramuscular needlesticks or larger lacerations from sharp instruments) and exposure to concentrated virus in facilities that perform HIV culture. The results of animal studies are discouraging, and suggest that the use of antiretroviral agents may not prevent *simian immunodeficiency virus* (SIV) transmission (Schinazi et al., 1990). Numerous studies have explored the use of postexposure treatment with *zidovudine* (previously called AZT) to further decrease the risk of HIV acquisition in exposed health care workers (Henderson and Gerberding, 1989; Lafon et al.,

1990). Clinical failures of zidovudine given immediately post exposure to health care workers have been reported (Durand et al., 1991; Lange et al., 1990; Looke and Grove, 1990). Health care workers do not tolerate zidovudine easily, and nearly two-thirds require dose reduction because of severe nausea and fatigue when begun on 1200 mg daily (Tokars et al., 1993).

Such results reinforce the need for health care workers to adhere strictly to universal blood and body fluid precautions and to handle and dispose of sharp instruments meticulously. When accidental percutaneous exposures to HIV-infected blood or bodily fluids do occur, the area should be immediately cleansed and the incident reported to an appropriate occupational health or infection control reviewer. The exposed health care worker should be carefully counseled and reassured that the risk of HIV transmission is approximately 0.4%. HIV serologic tests should be performed immediately and at 3 and 6 months; testing beyond 6 months is unnecessary because of the absence of late seroconversions among health care workers. The role of zidovudine in preventing HIV acquisition is unproven and is not generally recommended in this low-risk situation.

A major concern to surgeons is the risk of iatrogenic or nosocomial infection with HIV, especially the risk of AIDS from blood transfusions, although transfusion-associated AIDS accounts for less than 1% of all cases of AIDS. After the initiation of routine serologic screening of donated blood, the risk of acquiring HIV after blood or blood-product transfusion has been drastically reduced and is currently estimated to be 1 in 61,000 (Busch et al., 1991). HIV can also be transmitted by artificially inseminated sperm and by solid organ transplantation; thus, these donors are also tested before donation.

Pathogenesis

HIV is a single strand plus sense RNA virus approximately 100 nm in diameter. This virus has a characteristic cylindrical nucleoid core containing core proteins, genomic RNA, and the sine qua non of retroviruses, the RNA-dependent DNA polymerase, *reverse transcriptase*, surrounded by a lipid envelope. The viral envelope is derived from the membrane of the host cell and is studded by the viral envelope glycoproteins GP 120 and GP 41 (Gonda et al., 1986; Ratner et al., 1985).

The life cycle of HIV begins by the binding of the cell-free virion to the target cell through a specific interaction between the viral envelope and the host-cell membrane. The specificity of this recognition is due to the high-affinity interaction between the GP 120 studded in the viral envelope and the target cell CD4 molecule (Dalgleish et al., 1984; Klatzmann et al., 1984; Lasky et al., 1987; Lyerly et al., 1987; McDougal et al., 1986). After virus adsorption, the viral and cellular membranes fuse, leading to internalization of the viral core components. Reverse transcription of the viral RNA genome, a unique process requiring the enzyme reverse transcriptase, leads to a double-stranded DNA copy of the viral genome that can be incorporated into the host DNA. Expression of the viral DNA is controlled by viral and host-regulatory elements and leads to the production of virus-specific proteins that are assembled into infectious progeny (Baltimore, 1970; Temin and Mitzutani, 1970).

HIV has a unique tropism for the CD4 molecule found in T-helper cells (also known as CD4 lymphocytes), macrophages, and monocytes, and it infects these cells preferentially, although various other cells can be infected. In progressive HIV infection, the amount of recoverable virus increases and the absolute number of CD4 lymphocytes decreases. The CD4 lymphocyte is important in the host cellular immune system because it orchestrates the proliferation of natural-killer cells and cytolytic T lymphocytes that defend the host from infection by various viruses, fungi, and protozoa and are thought to protect against solid tumors; therefore, any disturbance in CD4 lymphocyte cell number or function has dire consequences for the host. In vitro HIV infection of CD4 lymphocytes usually causes rapid death of the cells, and this cytolytic effect is thought to contribute to the depletion of the CD4 lymphocytes in vivo and to lead to the global defects in host cellular immunity (Biggar et al., 1984; Fahey et al., 1984; Lane et al., 1985). However, the pathogenesis of the immune defects in patients with HIV infection is not completely understood and may involve additional mechanisms of CD4 lymphocyte depletion. In addition to the characteristic defects in cellular immunity of persons with late-stage HIV infection, deficits in humoral immunity and reticuloendothelial clearance may become clinically manifest.

Natural History

Advances in basic science investigations have greatly contributed to our understanding of the pathogenesis and natural history of HIV infection. Clinically, HIV infection can be divided into three phases: a period of acute infection that follows the initial acquisition of HIV, a prolonged period of asymptomatic HIV infection during which progressive immunologic dysregulation and subsequent damage occurs, and the final period of late HIV infection, dominated by the clinical manifestations of severe immunosuppression (Fig. 21–1). The median period from the acquisition of HIV infection to the development of AIDS is 11 years (Liu et al., 1988), and the median period of survival with AIDS is 2.1 years (Moore et al., 1991). CD4 lymphocytes are an important target for HIV infection, and the measurement of CD4 lymphocytes in the peripheral blood generally correlates with the clinical manifestations of HIV infection. The absolute CD4 lymphocyte count remains the most useful surrogate marker for assessing the immunosuppression of progressive HIV infection.

Acute infection with HIV may produce a mononucleosis-like syndrome, typically occurring 2 to 4 weeks after the initial acquisition of HIV. During this period, large amounts of HIV can be detected in pe-

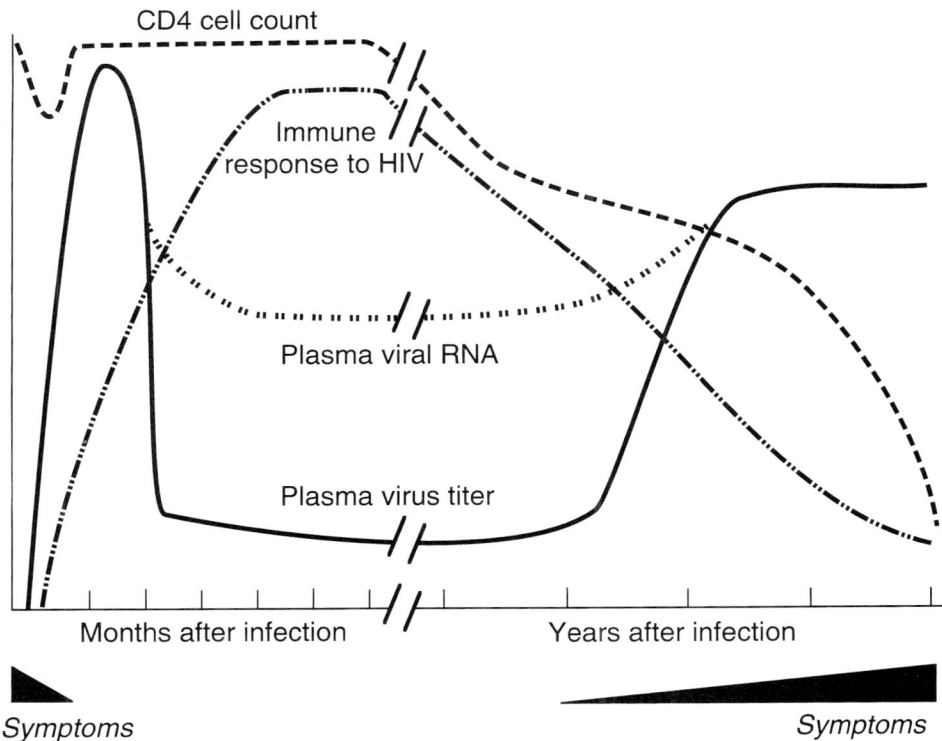

FIGURE 21–1. Course of HIV infection.

■ **Table 21–1.** CENTERS FOR DISEASE CONTROL REVISED CLASSIFICATION SYSTEM FOR HIV INFECTION IN ADOLESCENTS AND ADULTS

CD4+ Cell Categories	Clinical Categories		
	A Asymptomatic	B Symptomatic, Not A or C	C AIDS–Indicator Conditions
≥500/mm³	A1	B1	C1
200–499/mm³	A2	B2	C2
<200/mm³	A3	B3	C3

ripheral blood of patients through the measurement of p24 antigenemia, quantitative virus culture of plasma or mononuclear cells, or quantitative polymerase chain reaction for viral RNA (Clark et al., 1991; Daar et al., 1991). When an individual initially acquires HIV infection, a single virus strain that is tropic for monocyte/macrophages usually is transmitted (Zhu et al., 1993). HIV rapidly disseminates to involve many lymphoid organs, including lymph nodes, spleen, tonsils, adenoids, thymus, and small intestine, and tissue macrophages in the bone marrow, liver, lungs, and skin (Embretson et al., 1993; Pantaleo et al., 1993). Soon thereafter, the amount of easily detectable virus in peripheral blood decreases, perhaps reflecting the impact of virus-specific immune responses. Serologic responses, including neutralizing antibodies, can be detected within 4 to 12 weeks after initial infection but do not appear to correlate with the decrease in measurable virus in the peripheral blood. Reports suggest that cytotoxic T lymphocytes may be the predominant host immunologic mechanism that limits the initial phase of high-level viremia (Zhu et al., 1993).

Within 4 weeks of acute HIV infection, most symptoms resolve, and patients enter a prolonged asymptomatic period. Clinically, the asymptomatic period may be characterized only by the presence of diffuse lymphadenopathy. The amount of measurable virus in the peripheral blood is relatively low. However, active viral replication can be detected within lymphoid organs and is an important reservoir of virus production. Vigorous host immune responses against HIV can be measured during the asymptomatic period, including neutralizing antibodies, cytotoxic T lymphocytes, antibody-directed cellular cytotoxicity, and cell-mediated cytotoxicities. These responses may be important in prolonging this period and are the subject of intense investigation. During asymptomatic HIV infection, CD4 lymphocyte numbers may progressively decrease. The mechanism of CD4 lymphocyte depletion is incompletely understood but may reflect such processes as direct viral infection and destruction, autoimmunity, and apoptosis (Golding et al., 1989; Meyaard et al., 1992). As CD4 lymphocytes decrease, the clinical manifestations of early immunosuppression may occur. These manifestations can include recurrent oral or vaginal candidiasis, herpes zoster, oral hairy leukoplakia, pneumococcal infections, cervical dysplasia in

women, unexplained weight loss, fevers, and diarrhea. When the absolute CD4 lymphocyte count reaches 200/mm³ or less, an important biologic threshold has been reached and the frequency of complicating opportunistic infections and neoplasms greatly increases. This final phase of HIV infection is known as AIDS when the CD4 lymphocyte count is less than 200/mm³ or when specified AIDS indicator conditions have occurred. The Centers for Disease Control (CDC) have revised their staging system to include both the presence of clinical symptoms or AIDS indicator conditions and the determination of absolute CD4 lymphocyte numbers in classifying HIV infection (Table 21–1).

Diagnosis

The two fundamental methods of determining whether HIV infection exists are *directly*, by the detection of HIV or HIV-specific antigens, and *indirectly*, by the identification of the host immune response to the virus by detection of anti–HIV-specific antibodies.

Figure 21–1 is an idealized diagram of the virologic and immunologic events after exposure to HIV. Most clinical testing for HIV infection relies on indirect methods that assay for HIV-specific antibodies (Table 21–2).

■ **Table 21–2.** TESTS FOR HUMAN ANTIBODY TO HIV THAT MEASURE PREVIOUS EXPOSURE

Western Blot

Comment: Nearly 100% positive in patients with HIV infection, and very specific. Virus proteins are separated by electrophoresis, transferred to a membrane, and then incubated with human sera. The antigen-antibody complex is identified by a radioactively labeled protein with a high affinity for these complexes (*Staphylococcus* protein A). This test identifies sets of antibodies to individual viral proteins. Largely qualitative; valuable after disease progression.

Enzyme-linked Immunosorbent Assay (ELISA)

Comment: Highly sensitive, but specificity depends on population being tested. Most commonly employed screening test for HIV. Recombinant viral proteins are absorbed to wells in plastic dishes. These react with HIV antibodies in a patient's serum. Antihuman globulin with attached enzyme is added. A colorimetric reagent is the final step. If the human serum is bound to virus, subsequent reagents bind, and the color develops to show positive results. Largely qualitative.

Radioimmunoassay

Comment: Measures the response only to a single viral antigen. Uses purified radiolabeled viral protein. Antibody is made in an animal species. The labeled reaction can be competed for by human antibody.

Immunofluorescent Assay

Comment: This test is good for antigens on the cell membranes of live cells. A human target cell infected with HIV, live or fixed, is made to react with human serum. Binding is recognized by a fluorescein-labeled antihuman globulin.

Such serologic studies have achieved outstanding sensitivity and specificity when both enzyme-linked immunosorbent assay (ELISA) and western blot assays are employed. False-negative HIV antibody test results may occur during acute HIV infection before the development of host serologic responses or rarely during late HIV infection when immunologic competence is severely compromised. The utility of HIV antibody testing in the screening of blood donations has recently been confirmed in a large study of 76,000 donors, and the risk of falsely negative results is estimated at 1/61,000 donations. Methods for the direct detection of HIV include the detection of specific nucleic acid sequences through the polymerase chain reaction, the identification of HIV-specific antigens in body fluids, and the isolation of HIV through culture. The relative merits of these methods are summarized in Table 21–3. Direct viral detection is principally used in patients with clinical signs or symptoms of HIV infection whose antibody test results are negative, especially when acute HIV infection is suspected.

Antiretroviral Therapy

Antiretroviral therapy for persons with HIV infection can significantly improve quantity and quality of

■ **Table 21–3.** CLINICAL TESTS FOR HIV OR HIV ANTIGENS

Measure of Infectious Virus

• Culture of peripheral blood mononuclear cells: assay for reverse transcriptase or cell-free viral antigen
• Culture of plasma: assay for reverse transcriptase or cell-free viral antigen
  Comment: May be quantitative; specialized laboratory needed; expensive; main value in examining suspected seronegative patients or assessing efficacy of experimental antiviral therapy.

Tests for Viral Antigens

• ELISA or radioimmunoassay antigen assays for measurement of antigens present in serum, plasma, or lymphocytes. Acid dissociation of antigen-antibody complexes may increase sensitivity
  Comment: Qualitative, depends on clinical stage of disease; questionable sensitivity; use competitive radioimmunoassay or antigen-capture technologies.

Test for Viral Nucleic Acid

• Polymerase chain reaction for viral DNA or RNA
  Comment: Nucleic acid probes amplify sequences to detectable levels. Viral DNA may be detected throughout the course of HIV infection and therefore may be useful for diagnosis, especially during acute HIV infection before antibodies can be measured. Viral RNA fluctuates with increases during periods of higher viral activity and thus may be a sensitive quantitative marker for viral activity.
• Southern blot
  Comment: Detects proviral sequences in DNA; good if RNA or antigen is not expressed but requires cloned virus probes and adequate cells; not routinely available.
• In-situ hybridization
  Comments: Cumbersome because of low frequency of virus-infected peripheral cells.

■ **Table 21–4.** ANTIRETROVIRAL THERAPY

Agent	Mechanism of Action
FDA-Approved	
Zidovudine (AZT)	Reverse transcriptase inhibitor
Didanosine (DDI)	Reverse transcriptase inhibitor
Zalcitabine (DDC)	Reverse transcriptase inhibitor
Investigational	
Stavudine (D4T)	Reverse transcriptase inhibitor
Lamivudine (3TC)	Reverse transcriptase inhibitor
Nevirapine	Non-nucleoside reverse transcriptase inhibitor
Ateviridine	Non-nucleoside reverse transcriptase inhibitor
Merck 524	Protease inhibitor
Abbott 538	Protease inhibitor

life. All currently available antiretroviral agents inhibit the enzyme reverse transcriptase, which catalyzes the conversion of viral RNA to DNA. Three drugs have received Food and Drug Administration approval: zidovudine (previously known as AZT), didanosine (previously known as DDI), and zalcitabine (previously known as DDC) (Table 21–4). Zidovudine is the agent of first choice in the initial treatment of HIV-infected persons if they do not exhibit severe hematologic toxicities. Zidovudine can prolong survival in patients with AIDS-related complex (ARC) and AIDS (Fischl et al., 1987), decrease the frequency of complicating opportunistic infections, improve HIV-associated dementia (Schmitt et al., 1988), and transiently delay progression to full-blown AIDS among persons with asymptomatic HIV infection (Volberding et al., 1990). It is indicated for HIV-infected persons with less than 500 CD4 lymphocytes/mm^3. Patients who deteriorate despite zidovudine therapy may have evolved HIV strains with in vitro resistance to zidovudine (Larder et al., 1989; Larder and Kemp, 1989; Richman et al., 1990). The emergence of resistance is associated with four nucleotide mutations in the HIV gene that encodes reverse transcriptase (Larder et al., 1989); the appearance of these mutations correlates with the duration of zidovudine therapy and the relatively high viral burdens of later HIV infection. Fortunately, zidovudine-resistant virus remains sensitive to didanosine and zalcitabine, so changing to these agents may clinically benefit patients who do not respond to zidovudine (Kahn et al., 1992). The principal toxicities of didanosine and zalcitabine include peripheral neuropathy, pancreatitis, and esophageal ulcerations (zalcitabine). Unfortunately, HIV can also evolve resistance to these agents in association with clinical progression. Preliminary trials of combination therapies have suggested more prolonged benefits (Meng et al., 1992), and the optimal use of combination strategies should be better defined by clinical trials in progress. In summary, current antiretroviral therapy can provide meaningful but transient clinical benefit to patients through the inhibition of reverse transcription.

The development of therapeutic agents that inhibit other stages in the virus life cycle are a clear priority in present scientific and clinical research (Table 21–5). The HIV protease, which cleaves polyprotein precursors into functional HIV proteins, is an attractive target, and specific inhibitors of this enzyme have been developed. Preliminary clinical studies of HIV protease inhibitors have suggested antiviral activity. Immune-based therapies are under study as ways to augment those components of the host immune response that may control virus replication. Such strategies have included passive immunotherapy through the administration of HIV-immune globulins or monoclonal antibodies; adoptive immunotherapy with lymphokine-activated killer cells, CD8 lymphocytes, or HIV-specific cytotoxic T lymphocytes; active immunization with HIV-derived immunogens; and cytokine manipulation with the administration of alpha-interferon, interleukin-2, or inhibitors of tumor necrosis factor. Ultimately, improved medical management of HIV infection will probably require multiple drugs that can inhibit different stages of the virus life cycle and restore or maintain the immunologic competence of the infected patient.

INFECTIOUS DISEASES

Most of the morbidity and mortality seen in HIV-infected individuals is related to overwhelming infection. Common clinical syndromes include wasting, pneumonia, diarrhea, central nervous system infections, and esophagitis. The opportunistic infections most commonly seen in HIV-infected individuals are listed in Table 21–6.

Pneumocystis Carinii

P. carinii is a ubiquitous protozoan that can cause diffuse interstitial pneumonitis. *P. carinii* was first ob-

■ **Table 21–5.** NOVEL APPROACHES TO HIV THERAPY

Protease Inhibitors

Immune-Based Therapies

Passive immunotherapy
  HIV immunoglobulin
  Monoclonal antibodies
Active immunotherapy
  HIV immunization
Adoptive immunotherapy
  Lymphokine activated killer (LAK) cells
  HIV-specific cytotoxic T lymphocytes
Cytokine therapy
  Alpha-interferon
  Interleukin-2
  Tumor necrosis factor inhibition

Gene Therapies

Ribozymes
Rev response element decoys
TAR decoys
Rev transdominant mutants

■ **Table 21–6.** OPPORTUNISTIC INFECTIONS IN HIV-INFECTED PATIENTS IN THE UNITED STATES

Organism	Clinical Manifestations
Pneumocystis carinii	Pneumonia; infrequently dissemination
Toxoplasma	Encephalitis; retinochoroiditis; infrequently pneumonia
Cryptosporidium	Enteritis; infrequently bronchopleural
Isospora belli	Enteritis
Candida	Stomatitis, esophagitis; infrequently dissemination
Cryptococcus neoformans	Meningitis, pneumonitis, dissemination
Histoplasma capsulatum	Dissemination
Coccidioides immitis	Dissemination
Mycobacterium tuberculosis	Pneumonia, dissemination; infrequently meningitis
Mycobacterium avium complex	Dissemination
Mycobacterium kansasii	Pneumonia; dissemination
Streptococcus pneumoniae	Pneumonia; sepsis
Haemophilus influenzae	Pneumonia; sepsis
Cytomegalovirus	Retinitis; esophagitis; colitis; adrenal necrosis; pneumonia
Herpes simplex	Mucocutaneous
Herpes zoster	Dermatomal; infrequently dissemination
Epstein-Barr	Hairy leukoplakia; lymphoma

served in Parisian sewer rats by Delano and Delano at the Pasteur Institute (Delano and Delano, 1912). The first recognition of *P. carinii* was in 1942 by van der Meer and Brug. *P. carinii* was the cause of interstitial plasma cell pneumonitis in debilitated infants in Europe in the 1950s.

The *P. carinii* primary cyst form measures 4 to 6 μm in diameter, which in turn contains as many as eight pleomorphic intracystic cells called sporozoites. This type is highly prevalent throughout the world; in the United States, serologic surveys indicate that 75% of the population acquire antibodies by 4 years of age. Overt pneumonitis is thought to represent activation of latent infection in the immunocompromised host.

PCP is a commonly recognized form of life-threatening opportunistic infection in HIV-infected patients (Kovacs et al., 1988; Phair et al., 1990). Following the widespread use of preventive strategies against PCP, it has become a less frequent complication of AIDS (Hoover et al., 1993). Patients with PCP usually have some combination of fever, chest tightness, exercise intolerance, dyspnea, cough, or chest film abnormality. However, early clinical symptoms, signs, and chest film findings are nonspecific. Although chest films, gallium scans, pulmonary function tests, and computed tomography (CT) can each show abnormalities of pulmonary function or structure, the diagnosis of PCP requires the demonstration of organisms within the respiratory tract. Because the differential diagnosis of pneumonitis in HIV-infected persons is extensive, most clinicians seek a definitive diagnosis and avoid empiric therapy.

Sputum can be induced from AIDS patients with PCP in many cases. Evaluation of sputum with Giemsa or methenamine silver staining techniques can show organisms in 50 to 60% of patients (Pitchenik et al., 1986). The efficiency can be approximately 90% if immunofluorescent monoclonal antibodies against *P. carinii* are used (Kovacs et al., 1988; Kovacs and Masur, 1989). Bronchoalveolar lavage and transbronchial biopsy should demonstrate organisms in more than 95% of cases (Murray et al., 1984) (Fig. 21–2). The diagnosis of PCP in patients receiving prophylaxis may be more difficult because there are fewer organisms (Jules-Elysee et al., 1990).

Intravenously or orally administered *trimethoprim-sulfamethoxazole* (TMP/SMX) remains the treatment of choice for PCP. Alternative oral regimens include dapsone and trimethoprim, atovaquone, or clindamycin plus primaquine. Intravenous pentamidine may be administered intravenously to patients who cannot tolerate oral medications or intravenously administered TMP/SMX. Clinical and radiographic findings may worsen for 3 to 4 days after the initiation of therapy, but usually improve after 7 to 10 days. For patients with widened alveolar-arterial gradients, adjuvant steroids may decrease the risk of progression to respiratory failure requiring mechanical ventilation (Bozzette et al., 1990). Current recommendations suggest the use of steroids when the arterial oxygen tension falls below 70 mm Hg on room air. Eighty to 90% of patients with a first episode of PCP are expected to survive with standard therapy, and 60 to

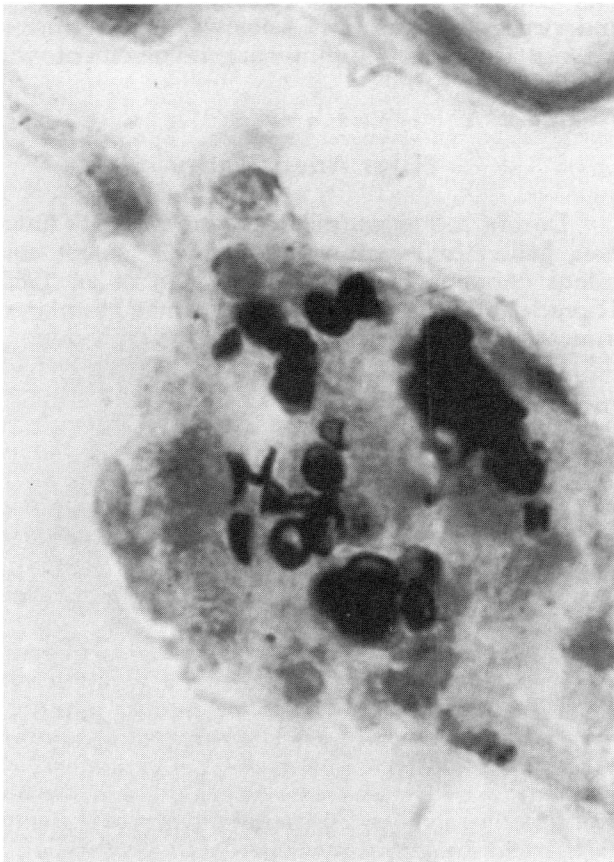

FIGURE 21–2. *Pneumocystis carinii* organisms in bronchoalveolar lavage fluid, methenamine silver stain.

70% of all patients with PCP are expected to survive (Brenner et al., 1987; Murray et al., 1987). The major difficulty with standard therapy is the frequency of adverse effects such as rash and fever (Kovacs et al., 1988).

The risk of PCP is clearly associated with absolute CD4 lymphocyte counts below $200/mm^3$ or CD4 lymphocyte percentages below 20% (Phair et al., 1990). In addition, the 1-year relapse rate for patients recovering from their first episode of PCP approaches 60% (Fischl et al., 1990). As a result, PCP prophylaxis is strongly recommended for these populations. Options for prophylaxis include TMP/SMX, dapsone, and aerosolized pentamidine. TMP/SMX is superior to aerosolized pentamidine in preventing PCP (Hardy et al., 1992; Schneider et al., 1992); direct comparative trials with dapsone are being analyzed. *Pneumocystis* infections may occur in patients on aerosol pentamidine and can be associated with extrapulmonary disease or unusual radiographic presentations such as upper lobe disease, nodules, or cavitating lesions (Jules-Elysee et al., 1990).

Thoracic surgeons may be called on following spontaneous pneumothoraces in patients with HIV infection. Pneumothorax is associated with PCP (Sepkowitz et al., 1991), perhaps reflecting alveolar destruction by the organism. A spontaneous pneumothorax in a patient with HIV infection should prompt careful consideration of PCP; pneumothoraces are frequently impossible to resolve until PCP has been treated.

Mycobacterium Tuberculosis

Since the early 1980s, the number of persons reported with tuberculosis in the United States has shown a reversal of a stable downward trend, and the number of recognized cases is increasing (Bloom and Murray, 1992). The re-emergence of tuberculosis in the United States is associated with failures to implement control measures, especially in crowded conditions; inadequate and incomplete therapy; worsening socioeconomic circumstances, particularly for the homeless; and co-evolution with the HIV epidemic. The large numbers of persons co-infected with HIV and *Mycobacterium tuberculosis* have offered new insights into the pathogenesis of tuberculosis. The appearance of multidrug-resistant strains, their transmission to contacts including health care workers, and the lull in the development of new antituberculous therapies have prompted a concerned response from health care professionals and the general public.

Among the 1,000,000 HIV-infected persons in the United States, it has been estimated that 100,000 are co-infected with *M. tuberculosis* (Centers for Disease Control, 1993). The largest numbers of reported persons with tuberculosis and HIV infection reside in New York City, Florida, Texas, and California. Outbreaks of *multidrug-resistant tuberculosis* (MDR TB) have been reported in New York City and Miami (Edlin et al., 1992; Fischl et al., 1992). In New York

City, at least 40% of the MDR TB cases occur in persons with HIV infection (Frieden et al., 1993). Approximately 8% of co-infected patients will develop active tuberculosis each year (Selwyn et al., 1989); thus, co-infected persons constitute a group of persons at extraordinarily high risk. Isoniazid prophylaxis for HIV-infected persons with positive PPD skin test results can prevent the later development of tuberculosis; the CDC currently recommend screening all HIV-infected persons with PPD skin testing followed by 1 year of isoniazid prophylaxis for persons with induration of at least 5 mm.

Tuberculosis is most commonly an early complication of AIDS, and it occurs when CD4 lymphocytes number less than 300/mm³. The development of active tuberculosis in HIV-infected persons may reflect either reactivation of long-standing infection or primary infection. Interestingly, HIV-infected patients who have recently recovered from active tuberculosis have been re-infected with distinct strains of *M. tuberculosis* and developed primary pulmonary infection (Small et al., 1993). Therefore, this immunosuppressed population is not immune from reinfection. HIV-infected persons with tuberculosis frequently develop extrapulmonary disease and large burdens of microorganisms involving multiple organ systems. Pulmonary disease may vary in presentation from typical upper lobe disease, miliary patterns, pulmonary nodules, and patchy infiltrates in any lung field. It is critical to consider the diagnosis of tuberculosis in any HIV-infected person with pneumonia and to initiate appropriate infection control measures pending the results of sputum acid-fast smears.

Current treatment of tuberculosis includes four drugs: isoniazid, rifampin, ethambutol, and pyrizinamide. Four drugs are recommended as initial therapy because of increasing problems with multi-drug-resistant strains. After drug susceptibilities are available, antituberculous therapy may continue with at least two active agents for a minimum of 1 year (Barnes and Barrows, 1993). Careful consideration should be given to *directly observed therapy* (DOT) to ensure compliance and to minimize the risk of relapse with a drug-resistant strain.

Mycobacterium avium *Complex*

Mycobacterium avium complex (MAC) may cause disseminated disease in persons with AIDS, especially those with late-stage immunosuppression (CD4 count ≤ 100/mm³). Disseminated MAC infection may be recognized in more than 50% of patients before their deaths (Masur et al., 1993). MAC is commonly isolated from a variety of environmental sources including tap water; although the pathogenesis of disseminated MAC infection in persons with AIDS is not clearly understood, it may involve an initial gastrointestinal focus of infection before dissemination. The diagnosis is most commonly established by culture of blood, and usually there has been widespread dissemination to many organ systems, including bone marrow, liver, spleen, adrenals, and the respiratory and

gastrointestinal tracts. Recent advances in treatment have improved the quantity and quality of life for patients. Multiple-drug regimens, including a newer macrolide such as clarithromycin or azithromycin in combination with at least one other agent, have led to bacteriologic and clinical successes (Dautzenberg et al., 1991). High-risk patients (CD4 count ≤ 100/mm³) may now be offered preventive treatment with rifabutin to decrease the short-term risk of disseminated disease (Nightingale et al., 1993).

Cytomegalovirus

Cytomegalovirus (CMV) is a common persistent viral infection. It is transmitted by contact with blood and bodily fluids, and an estimated 45 to 80% of the United States population is infected with CMV. CMV may reactivate and cause disease in HIV-infected persons, usually in those with late-stage disease and CD4 lymphocyte count below 100/mm³. Disseminated CMV disease is found at autopsy in approximately 30% of patients with AIDS. CMV infections are usually clinically manifested in the retina, gastrointestinal tract including the esophagus, adrenals, and central nervous system. The role of CMV in the respiratory tract of persons with AIDS remains controversial, but usually CMV does not cause clinically significant pneumonitis. The diagnosis of CMV disease is most commonly established by the characteristic fundoscopic appearance of perivascular exudative retinitis and by histopathologic confirmation in gastrointestinal tract samples following biopsy of mucosal ulcerations. CMV infection is treated with either intravenously administered ganciclovir or foscarnet, both inhibitors of the viral DNA polymerase. Patients with AIDS-associated CMV disease require maintenance therapy with either ganciclovir or foscarnet to avoid recurrences. Unfortunately, CMV resistance to either agent or both agents has been reported during prolonged therapy, so newer strategies of alternating or combination therapy are being evaluated.

PLEUROPULMONARY DISEASE IN THE PATIENT WITH AIDS

The differential diagnosis of pleuropulmonary disease in the patient with AIDS is given with an outline of the relevant diagnostic procedures (Fig. 21–3). The causes of pneumonitis in patients with AIDS are shown in Table 21–7.

When HIV-infected patients have pulmonary symptoms, their immunologic status is a major clue to the likelihood that they have an opportunistic infection. In early to middle HIV infection, patients may develop more typical community-acquired pneumonias, especially with *Streptococcus pneumoniae* and *Haemophilus influenzae*. As HIV infection progresses, patients may develop pulmonary tuberculosis. Finally, as the CD4 lymphocyte count falls below 200/mm³ and full-blown AIDS is diagnosed, patients may develop

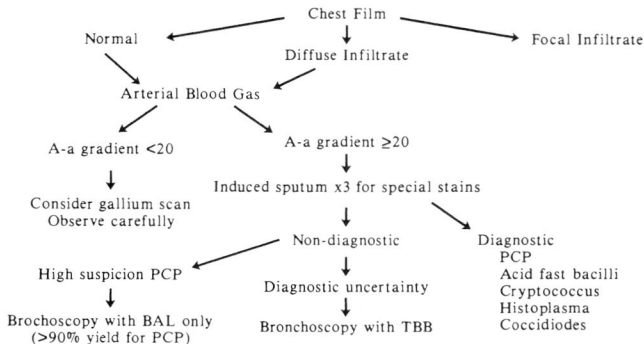

FIGURE 21–3. Differential diagnosis in an HIV-infected patient with CD4 count less than 250 mm and respiratory symptoms.

■ **Table 21–8.** PLEUROPULMONARY DISEASE IN THE PATIENT WITH AIDS

Infectious Etiologies	Noninfectious Etiologies
Focal Infiltrates	
Bacteria	Kaposi's sarcoma
Mycobacteria	Lymphoma
Fungi	
Pneumocystis	
Diffuse Infiltrates	
Pneumocystis	Adults: interstitial pneumonitis
Fungi	Children: lymphoid interstitial pneumonitis
Mycobacteria	Kaposi's sarcoma
Cytomegalovirus	
Pleural Effusions	
Bacteria	Kaposi's sarcoma
Fungi	Lymphoma
Mycobacteria	
Hilar Adenopathy	
HIV	Kaposi's sarcoma
Mycobacteria	Lymphoma
Fungi	

pneumonia with opportunistic pathogens such as *Pneumocystis carinii, Cryptococcus neoformans, Histoplasma capsulatum,* and *Coccidioides immitis.* These patients are also susceptible to pulmonary involvement with KS or lymphoma. Given the increasing variety and severity of potential causes of pneumonia during progressive HIV infection, it is more urgent to proceed to sputum evaluation, bronchoscopy, or open lung biopsy with patients who have an absolute CD4 lymphocyte count of less than $250/mm^3$.

Four patterns of pleuropulmonary involvement are discussed: focal infiltrates, diffuse infiltrates, pleural effusions, and hilar adenopathy (Table 21–8).

Focal Infiltrates

Focal infiltrates in the patient with AIDS may derive from a broad spectrum of infectious organisms. Patients with AIDS are clearly at risk for infection with encapsulated organisms, especially *Pneumococcus,* and are less at risk for *Haemophilus influenzae* (Chaisson, 1988). Other bacterial pneumonias seem to be uncommon in patients with AIDS.

Mycobacterial pneumonia due to typical or atypical organisms occurs relatively commonly. *Mycobacterium*

■ **Table 21–7.** ETIOLOGY OF 232 EPISODES OF PNEUMONITIS IN 174 AIDS PATIENTS AT NATIONAL INSTITUTES OF HEALTH, 1982–1987, DETERMINED BY BRONCHOSCOPY OR OPEN LUNG BIOPSY

Etiology	Episodes (%)
Pneumocystis ($n = 94$)	40.5
Nonspecific pneumonitis ($n = 75$)	32.3
Cytomegalovirus ($n = 7$)	3.0
Mycobacterium avium-intracellulare ($n = 4$)	1.7
Kaposi's sarcoma ($n = 12$)	5.2
Bacteria ($n = 6$)	2.6
Cryptococcus ($n = 1$)	1.3
Legionella ($n = 1$)	<1.0
Lymphoma ($n = 1$)	<1.0
No diagnosis ($n = 24$)	10.3

From Kovacs, J. A., and Masur, H.: Opportunistic infections. *In* DeVita, V. T., Jr., Hellman, S., and Rosenberg, S. A.: AIDS. Etiology, Diagnosis, Treatment, and Prevention. 2nd ed. Philadelphia, J. B. Lippincott, 1988.

tuberculosis pneumonia may occur outside of the classic upper-lobe distribution (Chaisson and Slutkin, 1989).

Atypical mycobacteria, especially MAC but also *M. kansasii* and *M. xenopi,* can cause focal pulmonary infiltrates. MAC typically disseminates widely outside of the chest and is frequently detected through the culture of blood, bone marrow, or stool (Macher et al., 1983).

Fungal pneumonias, including those caused by *Cryptococcus neoformans, Histoplasma capsulatum, Coccidioides immitis,* and *Aspergillus* species have been reported (Brady et al., 1984; Bronnimann et al., 1986; Gal et al., 1986; Huang et al., 1987; Mandell et al., 1986; Zuger et al., 1986). The prevalence of *Cryptococcus, Histoplasma,* and *Coccidioides* depends greatly on geographic factors. *Aspergillus* pneumonia appears to be rare.

Although the radiographic involvement of PCP typically is either absent or diffuse, PCP occasionally presents as a focal infiltrate. This focal presentation may become more common because of the widespread use of aerosolized pentamidine as prophylaxis for PCP (Bernard et al., 1987; Montgomery et al., 1987). Aerosolized pentamidine may not disperse adequately throughout both lungs and may leave localized areas of lung susceptible to focal infection with *Pneumocystis.*

Finally, neoplastic disease may present as a focal pulmonary infiltrate. The most common tumors that involve the lung are lymphoma and KS (Hamm et al., 1987).

Diffuse Infiltrates

PCP is the most common cause of diffuse infiltrates in adult patients with AIDS. Almost 80% of patients

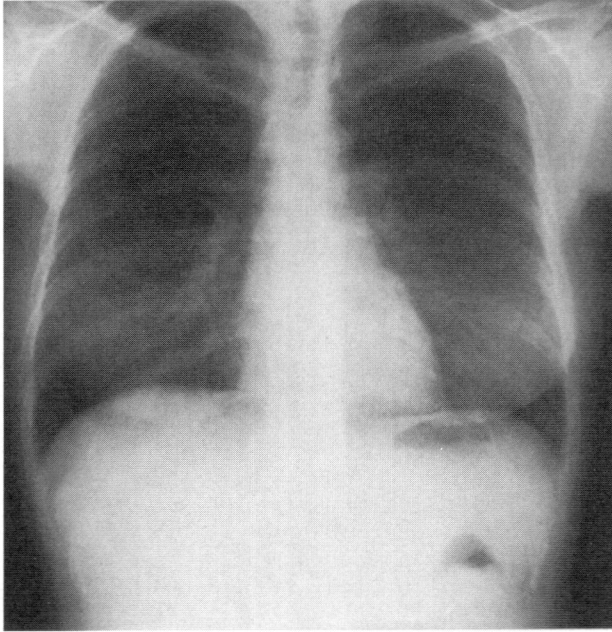

FIGURE 21–4. Normal chest radiograph in a patient with early *Pneumocystis carinii* pneumonia (PCP).

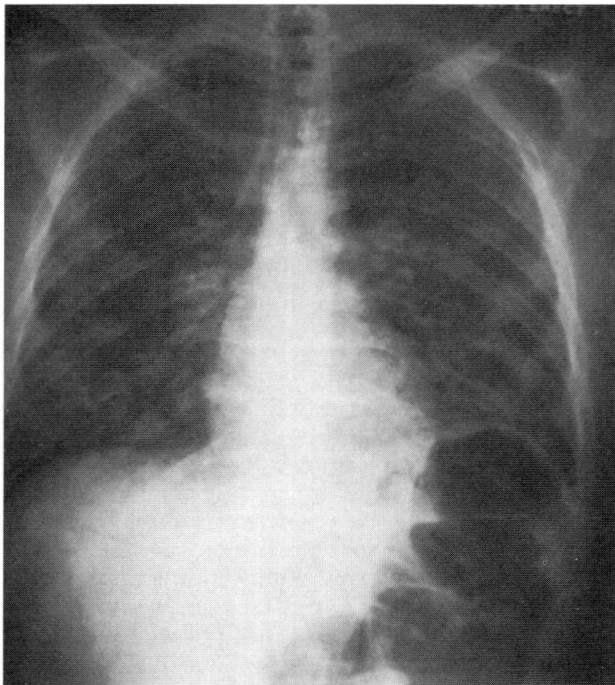

FIGURE 21–6. Chest radiograph showing interstitial infiltrates in a patient with pulmonary cryptococcosis.

with AIDS develop at least one episode of PCP (Kovacs et al., 1988). Although the appearance of PCP on chest film usually is normal (Fig. 21–4), it frequently presents with patchy interstitial and alveolar infiltrates (Fig. 21–5). Hypoxemia is frequently associated.

Fungal organisms, including *Cryptococcus, Histoplasma capsulatum,* and *Coccidioides,* may cause bilat-

eral disease (Fig. 21–6). Mycobacterial disease with typical or atypical organisms may also cause bilateral disease (Fig. 21–7).

CMV disease commonly causes diffuse pneumonitis, but the radiographic manifestations are usually subtle, and patients with AIDS are rarely symptomatic from CMV pneumonitis. In children with AIDS,

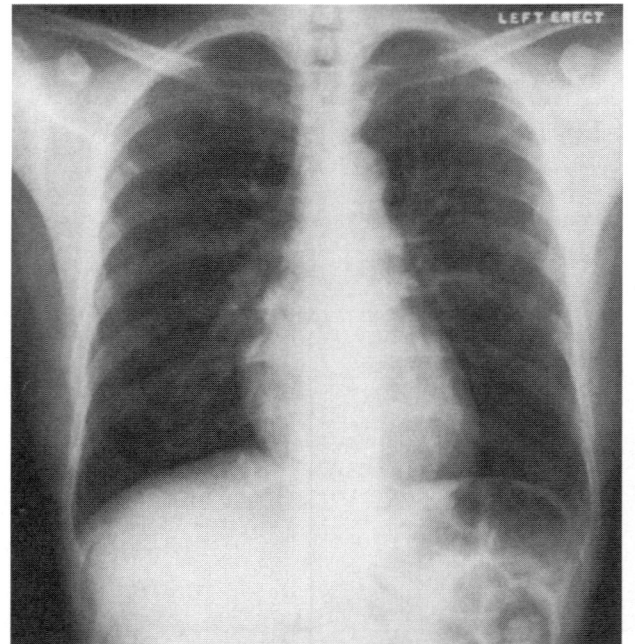

FIGURE 21–5. Chest radiograph showing interstitial and alveolar infiltrates in a patient with progressive PCP.

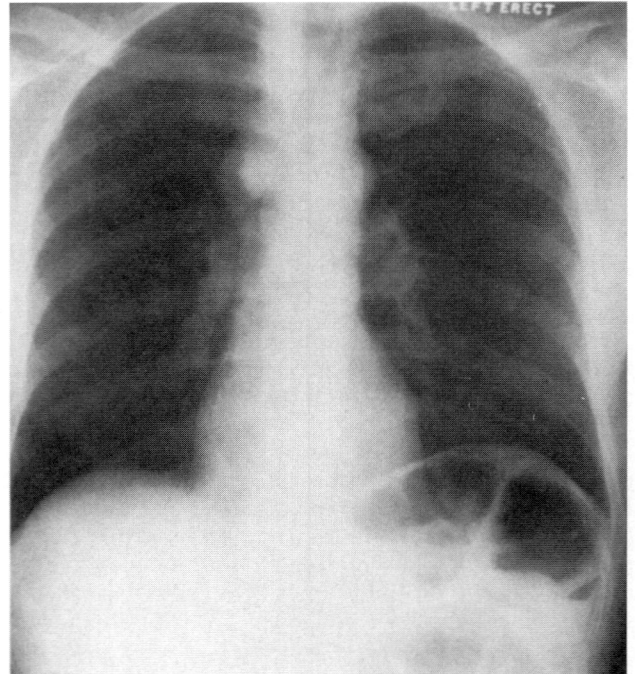

FIGURE 21–7. Chest radiograph in a patient with miliary tuberculosis.

the most common form of pulmonary involvement is lymphoid interstitial pneumonitis, a diffuse pneumonitis that is probably associated with Epstein-Barr virus infection (Joshi and Oleske, 1986; Rubinstein et al., 1986).

Finally, some adult patients with AIDS develop interstitial pulmonary disease without any recognized causative organism (Suffredini et al., 1987). These patients may have symptoms that cannot be distinguished from those of patients with PCP. Chest films show interstitial pulmonary disease, and gallium scans may show diffuse pulmonary uptake. Arterial hypoxemia is common. The pathogenesis of this entity is poorly understood, and no treatment is currently available.

Pleural Effusions

The differential diagnosis of pleural fluid in the patient with AIDS is broad (Joseph et al., 1993). Useful information may be gained from the chest film (see Table 21–9) and sputum. Fungal causes include *Cryptococcus* and *Aspergillus*. Both typical and atypical mycobacteria may involve the pleura. Pleural involvement by *Pneumocystis carinii* and viruses such as CMV is rare. Pleural effusions are not unusual in pulmonary involvement with KS.

Hilar Adenopathy

During the asymptomatic period of HIV infection, generalized lymphadenopathy is almost ubiquitous (Abrams et al., 1984; Fishbein et al., 1985). Thoracic and intraabdominal nodes may be enlarged in association with the generalized lymphadenopathy. However, when thoracic nodal involvement appears to be disproportionate to the extrathoracic nodes, a second diagnosis must be considered. Potential causes include infections such as *Mycobacterium tuberculosis*, atypical mycobacteria, *Cryptococcus, Histoplasma,* and *Coccidioides.* Neoplastic causes include lymphoma and KS (Levine et al., 1985; Ziegler et al., 1984).

ESOPHAGEAL DISEASE IN THE PATIENT WITH AIDS

Esophagitis is not uncommon in the patient with AIDS. Three infectious causes of esophagitis should be considered: *Candida albicans,* herpes simplex virus, and CMV. Each of these entities requires different therapy; thus, establishing a specific diagnosis is critical. Noninfectious causes include medication-associated esophagitis due to zalcitabine and idiopathic aphthous ulcerations.

When a patient with AIDS has esophageal pain, the physical examination can be useful in differentiating the diagnostic possibilities. If oral thrush is present, then *Candida* esophagitis becomes the most likely diagnosis. If the oral lesions appear as shallow ulcer-

ations, herpes simplex esophagitis becomes more likely. CMV esophagitis is more difficult to diagnose on physical examination unless the patient has evidence of CMV infection in other organ systems, especially the retina.

Empiric therapy without initial endoscopy is the clinical practice of most clinicians. If *Candida* esophagitis is suspected, empiric fluconazole, 100 to 200 mg/day, or ketoconazole, 400 mg/day, may be prescribed for 1 week. If the condition improves, an additional 2 weeks of therapy is given. If no improvement occurs after 1 week of empiric therapy, endoscopy and direct visualization and biopsy of the lesion should be seriously considered. When patients are given ketoconazole, concomitant H_2 antagonists or antacids should be avoided, because gastric acidity is essential for absorption.

Empiric therapy for presumed herpetic esophagitis consists of acyclovir (400 mg by mouth 5 times daily). Again, a 1-week course is given, and the dosage is lowered to 200 mg by mouth, 5 times a day for an additional 2 weeks if the condition has improved. If no improvement has occurred, the patient should undergo endoscopy.

Empiric therapy is usually not given for CMV esophagitis without strong supporting evidence. The only available therapies, ganciclovir and foscarnet, must be administered parenterally. CMV esophagitis usually responds well to treatment and may require chronic suppressive therapy with either agent.

When diagnosis is made by endoscopy, a biopsy should accompany direct visualization of the lesion. Owing to the necrotic nature of these ulcerations, biopsy samples taken from the periphery of the lesion may increase the diagnostic yield. Specimens should be sent to the laboratory for fungal and viral cultures, and the pathologist should be aware of the need for viral and fungal immunofluorescent stains on biopsy samples.

NEOPLASMS

Infectious complications are prominent thoracic manifestations of AIDS; so are chest neoplasms. The neoplasms commonly associated with AIDS and their thoracic manifestations follow.

Kaposi's Sarcoma

KS was first described in 1872 by Moritz Kaposi. Classic KS usually occurs in older individuals of European or Jewish origin (Kaposi, cited in Braun, 1982; Kaposi, 1872). It commonly involves asymptomatic brown-red to purple or blue patches, plaques, or nodular lesions that are located most frequently on the lower extremities, especially on the ankles and soles of the feet. These lesions tend to increase slowly, starting initially as a single or a few discrete nodules that may coalesce to form larger plaques or nodules. Although the lesions appear to be highly vascular, they rarely bleed excessively when cut or traumatized. After prolonged periods, untreated lesions may increase in size, fungate, and become ulcerated. Chronic venous stasis and lymphedema of the involved extremities are frequently complications of long-standing disease (Reynolds et al., 1965).

Epidemic KS, usually seen in patients with AIDS, is characterized by the sudden onset and often widespread appearance of lesions that involve not only the skin, but also oral mucosa, lymph nodes, and visceral organs. The lung, as well as the gastrointestinal tract, liver, and spleen, may be involved (Hamm et al., 1987; Ognibene et al., 1985). Two other types of KS not related to AIDS are African KS and renal-transplant-associated KS (Bayley, 1984; Bayley et al., 1985; Biggar et al., 1984; Stribling et al., 1978). The clinical features of each of these types are listed in Table 21–9.

Histologically, the lesions appear to be similar regardless of the differences in clinical behavior of the various populations studied (Fig. 21–8). *Early* lesions show an increase in the number of bizarre-shaped dilated vascular spaces lined with thin endothelial cells, and in the dermis there is a sparse infiltrate. Plaque lesions are characterized by increased numbers of grouped spindle-shaped cells located between the collagen bundles, with a few extravasated erythrocytes between the spindle cells. More advanced *nodular* lesions reveal few, thin, endothelium-lined vascular slits surrounded and compressed by dense bundles of spindle-shaped cells. The inflammatory cells are absent at this stage.

Approximately 96% of men with epidemic KS in the United States are homosexual or bisexual. Approximately 26% of all homosexual men with AIDS have or eventually develop KS during their illness. Only 3% of intravenous drug abusers with AIDS and 9% of Haitians with AIDS develop KS. As the risk behaviors associated with AIDS evolve to include fewer gay or bisexual men, the proportion of persons with AIDS developing KS is decreasing. These observations suggest a potentially transmissible cause of KS, although no agent has yet been identified.

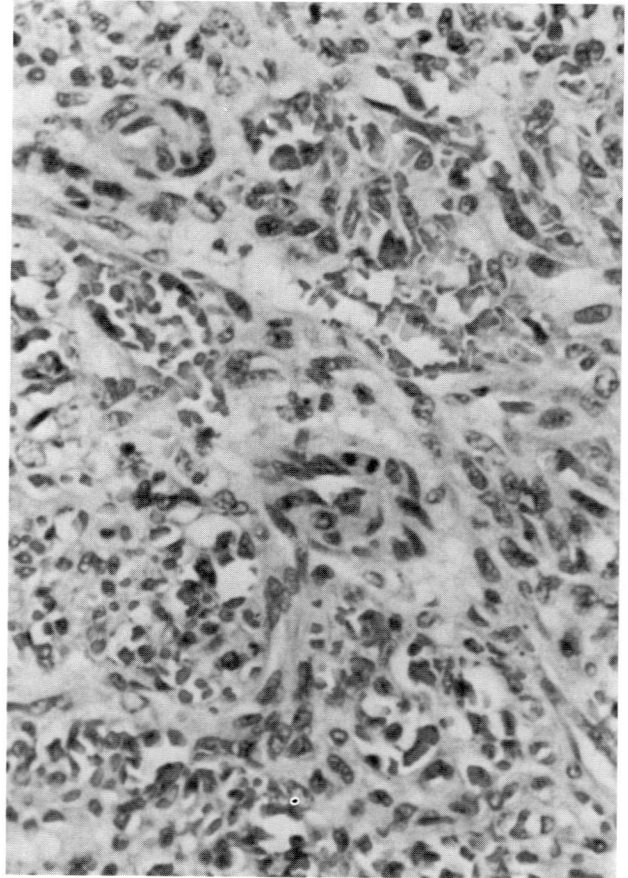

FIGURE 21–8. Histopathology of Kaposi's sarcoma (KS) showing abundance of vascular endothelium and spindle cells.

The sites of disease at presentation are more varied with epidemic KS than with classic KS. In an early report of 49 patients with epidemic KS, most patients had skin disease (90%), although 35% had fewer than five skin lesions or none (Krigel et al., 1983). KS can involve lymph nodes or the gastrointestinal tract before cutaneous lesions appear. Although epidemic KS involves the lung in 10% of patients at the time of

■ **Table 21–9.** CLINICAL FEATURES OF KAPOSI'S SARCOMA VARIANTS

Variant	Population	Features	Course
Classic	Older men of Jewish or Italian heritage	Usually confined to the lower extremities, often with venous stasis and lymphedema; late widespread cutaneous and visceral involvement	Indolent; survival 10–15 years
Epidemic	Patients with AIDS; primarily homosexual men; few Haitians, intravenous drug users, Africans	Disseminated mucocutaneous lesions, often involving lymph nodes and visceral organs, especially gastrointestinal tract and lungs	Fulminant; 2-year survival rate is less than 20% if associated with opportunistic infections
African	Young adult black men in Central Africa	Localized nodular lesions; large, aggressive tumors that are exophytic or that invade underlying bone	Indolent if nodular; otherwise slow; progessive and fatal within 5–8 years
Renal transplant	Iatrogenically immuno-compromised patients; usually of Jewish or Mediterranean heritage	May be localized to skin or widespread with systemic involvement	Indolent or rapidly progressive; may regress when immuno-suppressive therapy is discontinued; fatal in 30% of cases

presentation, pleuropulmonary disease is more often a late finding and is usually an ominous sign. Autopsy studies of patients with KS show pulmonary involvement in more than 50% (Welch et al., 1984).

A staging classification has been proposed that includes all the clinical variants of KS (Table 21–10). Stage I represents classic KS. Stage II represents typical African KS when locally invasive. Stages III and IV stratify the disseminated and systemic KS observed in patients with AIDS. Each stage is further subtyped according to the absence or presence of systemic symptoms (A or B, respectively). Survival is related to stage; Stage I patients live up to 2 years after diagnosis, whereas those with generalized tumor lesions without symptoms have an estimated survival rate of 60% at 28 months (Krigel, 1984). Patients with disseminated disease with symptoms have a median survival time of 15 months. Patients with a concomitant or previous opportunistic infection have a median survival time of 7 months. However, there is no universally accepted classification of epidemic KS. Prognosis may be related to distinct laboratory parameters as well as clinical factors.

Treatment of KS is difficult to evaluate because the natural course among the various types is so variable. It has not yet been shown that local or systemic therapy alters the ultimate course of the disease. Treatment may eliminate or reduce the size of specific lesions and may control symptoms from visceral lesions (Muggia, 1984).

Small localized lesions of KS may be treated satisfactorily by electrodesiccation and curettage or by surgical excision. However, KS tumors generally respond to local radiation therapy, and palliation has been excellent with doses of 2000 cGy (Chak et al., 1988; Hill, 1987; Nobler et al., 1987). Intralesional injections of vinblastine may also be used for the treatment of isolated lesions. For patients with progressive cutaneous disease, single-agent chemotherapy (usually vincristine and vinblastine) or alpha-interferon may be effective clinically. Alpha-interferon offers best results when employed in patients with higher CD4 lymphocyte counts. Visceral disease may be palliated via combination chemotherapy with dox-

■ **Table 21–11.** TREATMENT STAGING SYSTEM OF KAPOSI'S SARCOMA

Condition	Treatment
Localized	Observation radiation therapy or intralesional vinblastine
Progressive cutaneous	Alpha-interferon or single-agent chemotherapy
Visceral involvement	Combination chemotherapy

orubicin, bleomycin, and vinblastine. Current recommendations for the treatment of KS are listed in Table 21–11.

Malignant Lymphomas

Lymphoma was not considered a part of the spectrum of AIDS until 1985, when the case definition criteria of AIDS were expanded to include high-grade B-cell lymphomas in seropositive individuals. Lymphoma may be the first manifestation of AIDS, but many patients have opportunistic infection or KS before the diagnosis of lymphoma. AIDS-related lymphomas have B-cell tumors of high-grade pathologic type (62 to 81%). This phenomenon is distinct from the incidence of high-grade lymphomas occurring in the general population (3.5 to 7.9%) (Lukes et al., 1978).

Most patients have systemic B symptoms, including fever, night sweats, and weight loss (Kaplan et al., 1987). Another distinctive feature is the frequency of extranodal disease. Up to 63% may have Stage IV disease. Nine per cent have pulmonary disease, and 9% have cardiac involvement. A study by Levine and associates showed that all patients with involvement of the myocardium had extensive disease in other extranodal sites: Several patients had chest pain that could not be distinguished from acute myocardial infarction on an electrocardiogram (Levine et al., 1985).

The therapy of choice for AIDS-related lymphoma is unknown. Patients usually have high-grade disease that requires intensive multiagent chemotherapy. However, because of the underlying HIV-induced immunosuppression, multiagent chemotherapy may increase to immunocompromise and susceptibility to infection. The median survival time of patients with AIDS-related lymphoma is less than 1 year.

PLEUROPULMONARY INFECTIONS IN PATIENTS WHO UNDERGO TRANSPLANTATION

Various acquired immune defects can predispose to opportunistic infections in adults. However, a more common type of immunodeficiency is secondary to the lifelong immunosuppression necessary to prevent rejection of transplanted organs. Infection remains a critical problem of transplantation, because two-thirds

■ **Table 21–10.** STAGING SYSTEM OF KAPOSI'S SARCOMA

Stage	Characteristics
I	Classic; cutaneous, locally indolent
II	African, locally aggressive; cutaneous, locally aggressive or without regional lymph nodes
III	African lymphadenopathic and epidemic; generalized cutaneous or lymph node involvement
IV	Epidemic; visceral
Subtypes	
A	No systemic symptoms or signs
B	Systemic signs: 10% weight loss, fever > 100°F lasting for more than 2 weeks without source of infection

of recipients are infected at least once in the first 6 months, and most deaths are caused by infection (Bieber et al., 1982; Dummer et al., 1983; Gentry and Zeluff, 1986; Hofflin et al., 1987; Maurer et al., 1992; Rhenman et al., 1989). The thoracic infectious complications following solid organ transplantation, with an emphasis on cardiac and pulmonary transplantation, are now discussed in detail.

Infectious Diseases

The advent of *cyclosporine* (CsA) into the immunosuppressive regimen has altered the incidence and type of infections dramatically. Reports from several centers, including a comparative study from Stanford, have found that patients treated with CsA had a lower incidence of and mortality rate due to infectious complications than did patients who received conventional immunosuppression. Bacteria remain the most common organisms (30 to 60%), followed by viruses (25 to 50%), fungi (15 to 25%), and protozoa (5%) (Cooper et al., 1983; Emery et al., 1986; Hofflin et al., 1987; Wagener and Yu, 1992).

A timetable of infections in the organ-transplant recipient is a useful approach. Different infections may occur at different points following transplantation because the risk for individual infections depends on the previous operative events and on the degree and length of immunosuppression (Rubin et al., 1981). Cardiac, pulmonary, renal, and liver transplants all have similar timetables, which are shown in Figure 21–9 and can be categorized as the three distinct periods described by Rubin and associates.

First Month

Infections occurring in the first month following transplantation can be classified as *continuing* infections that were present in the recipient before the transplant, infections *acquired with the allograft,* and *routine postoperative* infections of the surgical incision, intravenous and urinary catheters, lungs, and mediastinum.

To decrease morbidity and mortality after a transplant the surgeon must eradicate any active infections in the recipient before initiating immunosuppressive therapy. Besides bacterial infections, particular attention must be paid to mycobacterial, fungal, and parasitic infections, including *Strongyloides stercoralis* infections (Stone and Schaffner, 1990).

The organ itself may be a source of infection because of long-standing infections that predate the transplantation, such as mycobacteria, fungus, hepatitis B, CMV, and HIV (Erice et al., 1991; Rubin, 1993). Another source may be acute infections in the donor due to indwelling catheters, tubes, or lines. To avoid such infections, persons with a documented infection such as sepsis, viral encephalitis, or systemic viral infection and those at high risk for occult infection such as drowning or burn victims and patients on respiratory support with indwelling lines should not

be used as donors (Ciulli et al., 1993; Klein, 1993). All donors are now screened for the presence of HIV antibody.

The most common type of infection that can be treated in the early period is wound infection. In patients who undergo thoracic transplantation, wound infections range as high as 62.5% and are particularly common in patients re-explored for bleeding (Maurer et al., 1992). The most important factor in preventing a wound infection is the technical quality of the surgery. The prolonged presence of chest tubes in the pleural spaces may increase susceptibility to wound infection. A high index of suspicion is required to diagnose wound infection because of the reduced immune response of these patients. Unexplained fever in the first month after the transplantation usually requires sterile needle aspiration of the wound and either computed tomographic scanning or ultrasonography to evaluate other sites as possible sources of infection.

Meticulous care and changing of central venous and arterial lines every 72 hours can limit the incidence and severity of bacteremia associated with invasive hemodynamic monitoring. Indwelling bladder catheters should be removed as soon as possible.

Postoperative pneumonia remains a difficult problem in the post-transplantation population because of prolonged endotracheal intubation. The morbidity and mortality rates of hospital-acquired postoperative pneumonia are high; the mortality rate is almost 50% (Anderson and Jordan, 1990; Dummer et al., 1983; Mermel and Maki, 1990). Patients undergoing cardiac and pulmonary transplantation are at especially high risk because of the frequency of underlying pulmonary disease.

1 to 6 Months

Risk of infection is greatest in this period for two reasons: First, host defenses have become depressed because of the duration of immunosuppression. Second, the immunosuppressive regimen has led to viral infection. Viruses such as CMV, EBV, and non-A, non-B (NANB) hepatitis may have a role in the high incidence of opportunistic infections seen in this period. Symptomatic infections may occur with these viruses as well as with herpes simplex and varicella zoster viruses or with other pathogens, including *C. neoformans, Listeria monocytogenes,* and *P. carinii* (Tolkoff-Rubin and Rubin, 1992).

Cytomegalovirus. More than two-thirds of cardiac, pulmonary, renal, and liver transplantation recipients show evidence of active CMV infection. Three major patterns are seen: primary infection, reactivation infection, and superinfection (Rubin, 1990; Wreghitt, 1989). In a primary infection, a seronegative recipient acquires infection from a seropositive donor from either the transplanted organ (80 to 95%) or from leukocytes contained within transfused blood products. In reactivation infection, the recipient has a latent infection and undergoes reactivation of endogenous latent virus following transplantation when immunosup-

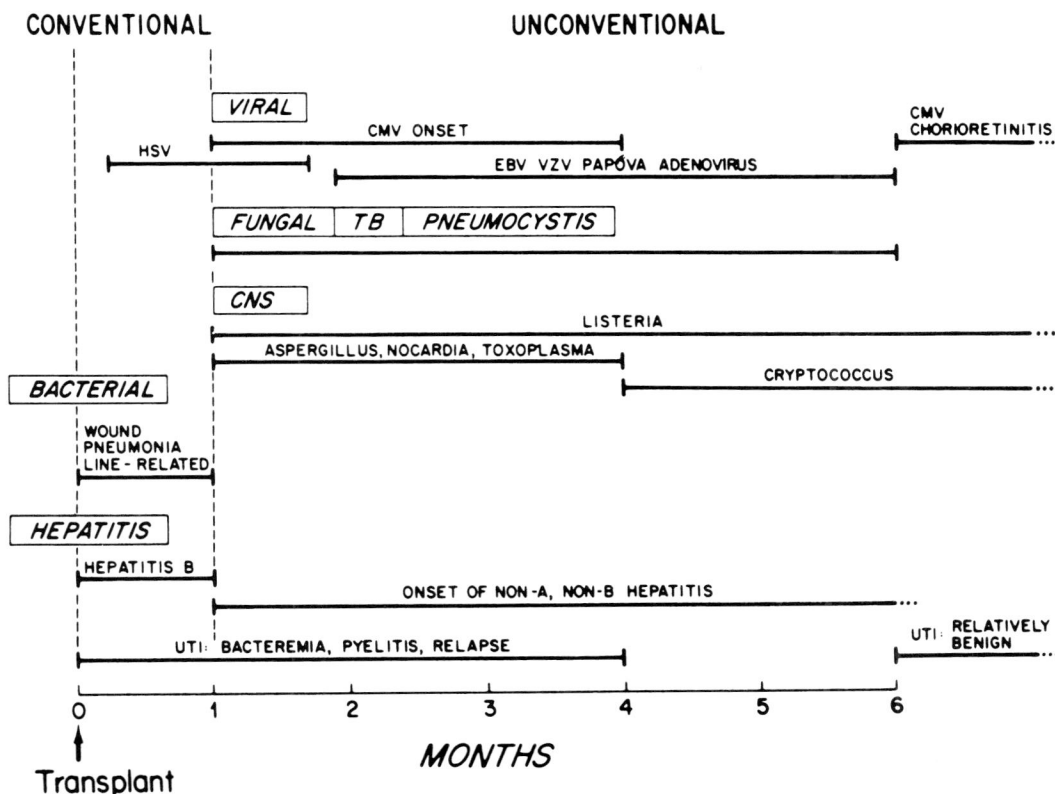

FIGURE 21–9. Timeline of common infectious process occurring in transplant recipients after transplantation and initiation of immunosuppression. (From Rubin, R. H.: Infection in cardiac and other organ transplant recipients. *In* Root, R. K., Trunkey, D. D., and Sande, M. A. [eds]: New Surgical and Medical Approaches in Infectious Diseases. New York, Churchill Livingstone, 1987. Modified from Rubin, R. H., Wolfson, J. S., Cosimi, A. B., and Tolkoff-Rubin, N. E.: Infection in the renal transplant patient. Am. J. Med., *70*:405, 1981.)

pressed. In superinfection, CMV infection transmitted from a seropositive donor to a seropositive recipient becomes superinfected from a slightly different strain, as demonstrated by molecular techniques (Tegtmeier, 1989).

Primary CMV infection has a much greater impact than either reactivation or superinfection. Ninety per cent of primary infections, as compared with only 20% of reactivation infections, are symptomatic (Rubin, 1990; Snydman et al., 1993). The major factor influencing the severity and clinical significance of CMV infection is the intensity and type of immunosuppression. A prospective study to determine the risk factors for CMV disease was done in patients receiving renal transplants. In the CMV-seropositive patient, administration of OKT3 was the most important predictor of CMV disease, increasing the risk by five times (Hibberd et al., 1992).

The most common early manifestation of CMV infection is a mononucleosis type of syndrome that causes anorexia, fever, malaise, myalgia, and arthralgia. Pneumonitis may develop in one-third of individuals with a febrile illness secondary to CMV infection. A dry, nonproductive cough is evident, and chest films may reveal a variety of findings, including bilateral symmetric peribronchovascular infiltrates predominantly in the lower lobes, or, less commonly, a focal infiltrate or a solitary nodule.

Involvement of other systems with hepatitis, ulcerative gastroenteritis, hemorrhagic colitis, or retinitis may signal pulmonary disease. Leukopenia, thrombocytopenia, and atypical lymphocytes are common. CMV infection can cause further depression of the host immune response, including severe leukopenia and suppression of cell-mediated immunity (Costanzo et al., 1992; Duncan et al., 1991; Smyth et al., 1991).

Strategies against CMV infections have taken three routes: the prevention of transplanting antibody-positive donor organs into antibody-negative recipients; avoidance of antibody-positive blood transfusions; and treatment with CMV hyperimmunoglobulin (Snydman et al., 1993). Although CMV infection is difficult to treat, new therapies, including anti-CMV antisera and ganciclovir, may prove to be effective (Cerrina et al., 1991). Prevention of primary infection by avoiding transfusion of CMV-seropositive blood products in CMV-seronegative recipients is also critical. Table 21–12 shows the protocol for prophylaxis used in solid organ transplantation at Duke University Medical Center.

Epstein-Barr Virus. Reactivation of EBV infection may be evident in as many as two-thirds of transplant recipients, but the clinical consequences are less clear than with CMV (Anderson and Jordan, 1990; Rostaing et al., 1993; Wreghitt et al., 1989). Starzl first reported

■ **Table 21–12.** PROPHYLAXIS FOR SOLID ORGAN TRANSPLANTATION AT DUKE UNIVERSITY MEDICAL CENTER

Cytomegalovirus (CMV) and Herpes Simplex Virus (HSV)		
Donor/Recipient CMV Exposure Status	*Immunosuppression Without OKT3/ATG/ALG*	*Immunosuppression with OKT3/ATG/ALG*
Low Risk Donor(−)/recipient(−)		
If HSV negative	No prophylaxis	No prophylaxis
If HSV positive	Acyclovir 200 mg tid	Acyclovir 200 mg tid
Intermediate Risk Donor(−)/recipient(+) or Donor(+)/recipient(+)	Acyclovir 800 mg tid	Ganciclovir 5 mg/kg (14 days), then acyclovir 800 mg tid
High Risk Donor(+)/recipient(−)	Ganciclovir 5 mg/kg (14 days), then acyclovir 800 mg qid	Ganciclovir 5 mg/kg (14 days), then acyclovir 800 mg qid

Pneumocystis carinii

Trimethoprim/sulfamethoxazole (Septra, Bactrim), double-strength, 3 days a week for 1 year. Also provides urinary tract infection prophylaxis for kidney transplant recipients.

Candida

Mycostatin troche 10 mg qid or nystatin 5 ml swish and swallow qid for 2–6 months.

an increased incidence of reticulum cell sarcoma in immunosuppressed organ transplant recipients (Starzl, 1968). Matas and co-workers recognized the association between EBV and these tumors (Matas et al., 1975). An overwhelming body of evidence points to EBV as a causative agent in both B-lymphocytic lymphomas and T-cell tumors (Hanto et al., 1981a, 1981b; Penn, 1990; Penn and Bronson, 1988; Starzl et al., 1984). These are grouped under the heading of *post-transplantation lymphoproliferative disorders* (PTLDs). Armitage and associates noted PTLD in 15 heart (3.4%) and 5 lung transplant (7.9%) recipients from 1980 to 1989 (Armitage et al., 1991).

Other Viruses. Two other members of the herpes family, *herpes simplex virus* (HSV) and *varicella-zoster virus* (VZV), can be found in the transplantation patient through primary infection or reactivation. Acyclovir is quite effective in treating mucocutaneous HSV infection. Reactivation VZV rarely disseminates, in contrast with the malignant course primary VZV can take.

More Than 6 Months

Patients who have late graft survival requiring long-term immunosuppression usually can be subdivided into risk groups that depend on the degree of immunosuppression. Low-risk patients have minimal rejection activity that does not require alterations in their immunosuppressive therapy. These patients are at minimal risk for opportunistic infections. The small group of patients at high risk—those who have received multiple courses of immunosuppressive therapy for acute rejection and who require profound immunosuppression to prevent chronic rejection—are at highest risk of life-threatening infections, particularly those due to *Cryptococcus neoformans* (Rubin et

al., 1981). A third group consists of patients with the chronic effects of an infection acquired earlier. Examples include patients with chronic NANB hepatitis and progressive chorioretinitis due to CMV.

A group at Oregon reported their infection rates for heart recipients more than 1 year after transplantation. There were 15 infections in 54 patients. Bacterial infections made up the largest group at 9 patients (60%), followed by infections in 4 (27%) and fungal and parasitic infections in one each (Hosenpud et al., 1991).

PLEUROPULMONARY INFECTIONS IN PATIENTS RECEIVING CHEMOTHERAPY

Compared with AIDS patients or transplant recipients, the predominant immunologic defect in patients who receive chemotherapy for the treatment of malignant disease is a reduction in the number and function of *neutrophils*. The incidence of infections is directly related to the granulocyte count. A number of organisms can cause pleuropulmonary disease, mainly bacteria and fungi (Table 21–13). However, the general principle that diagnostic certainty is essential because of the broad spectrum of possible causes remains true for patients receiving chemotherapy for pleuropulmonary disease. The clinician's critical decision is whether to perform invasive procedures such as fiberoptic bronchoscopy (with or without lavage), transbronchial biopsy, transthoracic aspiration, or lung biopsy through an open or thoracoscopic approach (Chauncey et al., 1990).

Focal Infiltrates

The differential diagnosis of focal pulmonary disease includes both infectious and noninfectious

■ **Table 21–13.** PLEUROPULMONARY DISEASE IN PATIENTS RECEIVING CHEMOTHERAPY

Infectious Etiologies	Noninfectious Etiologies
Focal Infiltrates	
Bacteria	Pulmonary emboli
Fungi	Radiation pneumonitis
Mycobacteria	Malignancy
Diffuse Infiltrates	
Pneumocystis	Drug reactions
Cytomegalovirus	Radiation pneumonitis
Fungi	Graft-versus-host disease
Mycobacteria	Congestive heart failure
	Malignancy
Pleural Effusions	
Bacteria	Pulmonary emboli
Fungi	Malignancy
Mycobacteria	
Hilar Adenopathy	
Mycobacteria	Malignancy
Fungi	

causes. Potential infections are bacterial pneumonias, especially those due to gram-negative rods, *Staphylococcus, Legionella,* and *Streptococcus pneumoniae;* fungal pneumonias, especially those due to *Aspergillus, Mucor, Nocardia,* and *Candida;* and mycobacterial pneumonias, both typical and atypical. *Aspergillus* pneumonias typically occur peripherally after a period of prolonged granulocytopenia. Both *Aspergillus* and *Mucor* invade vasculature, and patients may have signs and symptoms that suggest pulmonary infarction. Noninfectious causes of focal disease include pulmonary emboli with infarction, radiation pneumonitis, and malignancy.

Diffuse Interstitial Disease

Diffuse interstitial disease may also be due to infectious and noninfectious causes. Infectious etiologic agents are *P. carinii,* CMV, fungi, and mycobacteria. CMV pneumonitis, especially in recipients of bone marrow transplants, has a mortality rate exceeding 80%. Noninfectious causes include drug reactions (especially to bleomycin, busulfan, methotrexate, nitrosourea compounds, cyclophosphamide, and chlorambucil), graft-versus-host disease, radiation pneumonitis, congestive heart failure, and malignancy (Rubin and Greene, 1988).

Pleural Effusions

The differential diagnosis of pleural effusions includes bacterial infections, fungal infections, mycobacterial infections, malignancy, and pulmonary infarction.

Hilar Adenopathy

Diagnostic considerations must include malignancy, mycobacterial infections, and occasionally fungal infections.

Diagnostic Management

Overall, establishing a diagnosis in patients receiving chemotherapy with pleuropulmonary disease is more difficult than in AIDS patients or organ transplant recipients. The diagnostic yield of sputum induction is lower, perhaps because of a lower number of infecting organisms and the lack of neutrophils available for bronchial and alveolar inflammatory responses (Chauncey et al., 1990). Transbronchial biopsy may be useful; bronchial alveolar lavage without transbronchial biopsy can be done if PCP or CMV pneumonitis is strongly suspected. Definitive diagnosis may require open or thoracoscopic lung biopsy (Martin et al., 1987). Patients with mucormycosis involving the parenchyma of the lung deserve special attention, because they usually require surgical débridement or lobectomy as well as medical management. The diagnosis of pleural disease may require thoracentesis, closed-needle biopsy of the pleura, or pleural biopsy by an open or thoracoscopic approach. Hilar adenopathy may be evaluated by mediastinoscopy or open biopsy.

Esophagitis in patients requiring chemotherapy may be caused by *Candida,* HSV, CMV, reflux, or malignancy. *Candida* and HSV are occasionally diagnosed noninvasively by the observation of oral thrush or herpetic ulcerations that have spread contiguously down the esophagus. Diagnostic endoscopy with esophageal biopsy is necessary in other patients.

SUMMARY

With the increasing numbers of AIDS patients and organ transplant recipients, the thoracic surgeon will have a more important role in the care of immunocompromised patients with pleuropulmonary or esophageal disease. Diagnostic certainty may provide the immunocompromised patient with the best chance for survival with the institution of early specific therapy and the avoidance of potentially incorrect and toxic therapy. Bronchoscopy, thoracentesis, lung or pleural biopsy by open or thoracoscopic procedures, and endoscopy may all be useful diagnostic procedures within the proper context. An understanding of the pathophysiologic differences between the immunocompromised states and the likely etiologies allows the thoracic surgeon to choose the most appropriate procedure with the best diagnostic yield and choice of therapy.

BIBLIOGRAPHY

Abrams, D. I., Lewis, B. J., Beckstead, J. F., et al.: Persistent diffuse lymphadenopathy in homosexual men: Endpoint or prodrome? Ann. Intern. Med., *100*:801, 1984.

Anderson, D. J., and Jordan, M. C.: Viral pneumonia in recipients of solid organ transplants. Semin. Respir. Infect., 5:38, 1990.

Armitage, J. M., Kormos, R. L., Stuart, R. S., et al.: Posttransplant lymphoproliferative disease in thoracic organ transplant patients: Ten years of cyclosporine-based immunosuppression. J. Heart Lung Transplant, 10:877,1991.

Baker, J. L., Kelen, G. D., Sivertson, K. T., and Quinn, T. C.: Unsuspected human immunodeficiency virus infection in critically ill emergency patients. J. A. M. A., 257:2609, 1987.

Baltimore, D.: RNA-dependent DNA polymerase in virions of RNA tumor viruses. Nature, 226:1209, 1970.

Barnes, P. F., and Barrows, S. A.: Tuberculosis in the 1990s. Ann. Intern. Med., 119:398–410, 1993.

Barre-Sinoussi, F., Chermann, J. C., Rey, F., et al.: Isolation of a T cell lymphotropic virus from a patient at risk for acquired immunodeficiency syndrome (AIDS). Science, 220:868, 1983.

Bayley, A. C.: Aggressive Kaposi's sarcoma in Zambia, 1983. Lancet, 1:1318, 1984.

Bayley, A. C., Downing, R. G., Cheingsong-Popov, R., et al.: HTLV-III distinguishes atypical and endemic Kaposi's sarcoma in Africa. Lancet, 1:359, 1985.

Bernard, E. M., Pagel, L., Schmitt, H. J., et al.: Clinical trials with aerosol pentamidine for prevention of Pneumocystis carinii pneumonia. Clin. Res., 35:468A, 1987.

Bieber, C. P., Hunt, S. A., Schwinn, D. A., et al.: Complications in long term survivors of cardiac transplantation. Transplant Proc., 13:207, 1982.

Biggar, R. J., Melbye, M., Ebbesen, P., et al.: Low T-lymphocyte ratios in homosexual men. J. A. M. A., 251:1441, 1984.

Bloom, B. R., and Murray, C. J.: Tuberculosis: Commentary on a reemergent killer. Science, 257:1055–1064, 1992.

Bozzette, S. A., Sattler, F. R., Chiu, J., et al.: A controlled trial of early adjunctive treatment with corticosteroids for Pneumocystis carinii pneumonia in the acquired immunodeficiency syndrome. N. Engl. J. Med., 323:1451–1457, 1990.

Brady, E. M., Margolis, M. L., and Korzeniowski, O. M.: Pulmonary cryptosporidiosis in acquired immunodeficiency syndrome. J. A. M. A., 252:89, 1984.

Braun, M.: Classics in Oncology: Idiopathic multiple pigmented sarcoma of the skin by Kaposi. Cancer, 32:342, 1982.

Brenner, M., Ognibene, F. P., Lack, E. E., et al.: Prognostic factors and life expectancy of acquired immune deficiency syndrome patients with Pneumocystis carinii pneumonia. Am. Rev. Respir. Dis., 139:1199, 1987.

Bronnimann, D. A., Adam, R. D., Galgiani, J. N., et al.: Coccidioidomycosis in the acquired immunodeficiency syndrome. Ann. Intern. Med., 106:372, 1986.

Busch, M. P., Eble, B. E., Khayan-Bashi, H., et al.: Evaluation of screened blood donations for human immunodeficiency virus type 1 infection by culture and DNA amplification of pooled cells. N. Engl. J. Med., 325:1–5, 1991.

Centers for Disease Control: HIV/AIDS Surveillance Report, October 1993.

Cerrina, J., Bavoux, E., Le-Roy-Ladurie, F., et al.: Ganciclovir treatment of cytomegalovirus infection in heart-lung and double-lung transplant recipients. Transplant. Proc., 23:1174, 1991.

Chaisson, R. E.: Infections due to encapsulated bacteria, Salmonella, Shigella and Campylobacter in medical management of AIDS. Infect. Dis. Clin. North Am., 2:475, 1988.

Chaisson, R. E., and Slutkin, G.: Tuberculosis and human immunodeficiency virus infection. J. Infect. Dis., 159:96, 1989.

Chak, L. Y., Gill, P. S., Levine, A. M., et al.: Radiation therapy for acquired immunodeficiency syndrome-related Kaposi's sarcoma. J. Clin. Oncol., 6:863, 1988.

Chauncey, J. B., Lynch, J. P., III, Hyzy, R. C., and Toews, G. B.: Invasive techniques in the diagnosis of bacterial pneumonia in the intensive care unit. Semin. Respir. Infect., 5:215, 1990.

Ciulli, F., Tamm, M., Dennis, C., et al.: Donor-transmitted bacterial infection in heart-lung transplantation. Transplant. Proc., 25:155, 1993.

Clark, S. J., Saag, M. S., Decker, W. D., et al.: High titers of cytopathic virus in plasma of patients with symptomatic primary HIV-1 infection. N. Engl. J. Med., 324:954–960, 1991.

Cooper, D. K. C., Lanza, R. P., Oliver, S. P., et al.: Infectious complications following heterotopic heart transplantation. Thorax, 38:822, 1983.

Costanzo, N. M. R., Swinnen, L. J., Fisher, S. G., et al.: Cytomegalovirus infections in heart transplant recipients: Relationship to immunosuppression. J. Heart Lung Transplant., 11:837, 1992.

Daar, E. S., Moudgil, T., Meyer, R. D., and Ho, D. D.: Transient high levels of viremia in patients with primary human immunodeficiency virus type 1 infection. N. Engl. J. Med., 324:961–964, 1991.

Dalgleish, A. G., Beverly, P. C. L., Clapham, P. R., et al.: The CD4 (T4) antigen is an essential component of the receptor for the AIDS retrovirus. Nature, 312:763, 1984.

Dautzenberg, B., Truffot, C., Legris, S., et al.: Activity of clarithromycin against Mycobacterium avium infection in patients with the acquired immunodeficiency syndrome: A controlled clinical trial. Am. Rev. Respir. Dis., 144:564–569, 1991.

Delano, P., and Delano, M.: Sur les rapports des kystes de carini du poumon des rats avec le Trypanosoma lewisii. C. R. Acad. Sci., 155:658, 1912.

Dummer, J. S., Bahnson, H. T., Griffith, B. P., et al.: Infections in patients on cyclosporine and prednisone following cardiac transplantation. Transplant. Proc., 15(Suppl. 1–2):2779, 1983.

Duncan, A. J., Dummer, J. S., Paradis, I. L., et al.: Cytomegalovirus infection and survival in lung transplant recipients. J. Heart Lung Transplant., 10:638, 1991.

Durand, E., LeJunne, C., Hugues, F. C.: Failure of prophylactic zidovudine after suicidal self-inoculation of HIV-infected blood. N. Engl. J. Med., 324:1062, 1991.

Edlin, B. R., Tokars, J. I., Grieco, M. R., et al.: An outbreak of multidrug resistance tuberculosis among hospitalized patients with the acquired immunodeficiency syndrome. N. Engl. J. Med., 326:1514–1521, 1992.

Embretson, J., Zupancic, M., Ribas, J. L., et al.: Massive covert infection of helper T lymphocytes and macrophages by HIV during the incubation period of AIDS. Nature, 362:359–362, 1993.

Emery, R. W., Cork, R., Christiansen, R., et al.: Cardiac transplant patients at one year. Chest, 90:29, 1986.

Erice, A., Rhame, F. S., Heussner, R. C., et al.: Human immunodeficiency virus infection in patients with solid-organ transplants: Report of five cases and review. Rev. Infect. Dis., 13:537, 1991.

Fahey, J. L., Prince, H., Weaver, M., et al.: Quantitative changes in T helper or T suppressor/cytotoxic lymphocyte subsets that distinguish acquired immune deficiency syndrome from other immune subset disorders. Am. J. Med., 76:95, 1984.

Fischl, M. A., Parker, C. B., Pettinelli, C., et al.: A randomized controlled trial of a reduced daily dose of zidovudine in patients with the acquired immunodeficiency syndrome. N. Engl. J. Med., 323:1009–1014, 1990.

Fischl, M. A., Richman, D. D., Grieco, M. H., et al.: The efficacy of azidothymidine (AZT) in the treatment of patients with AIDS and AIDS-related complex. N. Engl. J. Med., 317:185, 1987.

Fischl, M. A., Utlamchandani, R. B., Daikos, G. L., et al.: An outbreak of tuberculosis caused by multi-drug resistant bacilli among patients with HIV infection. Ann. Intern. Med., 117:177–183, 1992.

Fishbein, D. B., Kaplan, J. E., Spira, T. J., et al.: Unexplained lymphadenopathy in homosexual men: A longitudinal study. J. A. M. A., 254:930, 1985.

Frieden, T. R., Sterling, J., Pablos-Mendez, A., et al.: The emergence of drug-resistant tuberculosis in New York City. N. Engl. J. Med., 328:521–526, 1993.

Friedland, G. W., and Klein, R. S.: Transmission of the human immunodeficiency virus. N. Engl. J. Med., 317:1125, 1987.

Gal, A. A., Koss, M. N., Hawkins, J., et al.: The pathology of pulmonary cryptococcal infections in the acquired immunodeficiency syndrome. Arch. Pathol. Lab. Med., 110:502, 1986.

Gallo, R. C., Salahuddin, S. Z., Popovic, M., et al.: Frequent detection and isolation of cytopathic retroviruses (HTLV-III) from patients with AIDS and at risk for AIDS. Science, 224:500, 1984.

Gentry, L. O., and Zeluff, B. J.: Diagnosis and treatment of infection in cardiac transplant patients. Surg. Clin. North Am., 66:459, 1986.

Golding, H., Sheaver, G. M., Hillman, K., et al.: Common epitote in human immunodeficiency virus (HIV) I-gp41 and HLA class II elicits immunosuppressive autoantibodies capable of contributing to immune dysfunction in HIV-1 infected individuals. J. Clin. Invest., 83:1430–1435, 1989.

Gonda, M. A., Braun, M. J., Clements, J. E., et al.: Human T-cell lymphotropic virus type III shares sequence homology with a family of pathogenic lentiviruses. Proc. Natl. Acad. Sci. U. S. A., 83:4007, 1986.

Gottlieb, M. S., Schroff, R., Schanker, H. M., et al.: *Pneumocystis carinii* pneumonia and mucosal candidiasis in previously healthy homosexual men: Evidence of a new acquired immunodeficiency. N. Engl. J. Med., 305:1425, 1981.

Hamm, P. G., Judson, M. A., and Aranda, C. P.: Diagnosis of pulmonary Kaposi's sarcoma with fiberoptic bronchoscopy and endobronchial biopsy: A report of five cases. Cancer, 59:807, 1987.

Hanto, D. W., Frizzera, G., Purtilo, D., et al.: Clinical spectrum of lymphoproliferative disorders in renal transplant recipients, and evidence for the role of Epstein-Barr virus. Cancer Res., 41:4253, 1981a.

Hanto, D. W., Sakamoto, K., Purtilo, D. T., et al.: The Epstein-Barr virus in the pathogenesis of post-transplant lymphoproliferative disorders. Surgery, 90:204, 1981b.

Hardy, W. D., Feinberg, J., Finkelstein, D. M., et al.: A controlled trial of trimethoprim-sulfamethoxazole or aerosolized pentamidine for secondary prophylaxis of *Pneumocystis carinii* pneumonia in patients with the acquired immunodeficiency syndrome. N. Engl. J. Med., 327:1842–1848, 1992.

Henderson, D. K., and Gerberding, J. L.: Prophylactic zidovudine after occupational exposure to the human immunodeficiency virus: An interim analysis. J. Infect. Dis., 160:321–327, 1989.

Hibberd, P. L., Tolkoff, R. N. E., Cosimi, A. B., et al.: Symptomatic cytomegalovirus disease in the cytomegalovirus antibody seropositive renal transplant recipient treated with OKT3. Transplantation, 53:68, 1992.

Hill, D. R.: The role of radiotherapy for epidemic Kaposi's sarcoma. Semin. Oncol., 14(Suppl. 3):19, 1987.

Hofflin, J. M., Potasman, I., Baldwin, J. C., et al.: Infectious complications in heart transplant recipients receiving cyclosporine and corticosteroids. Ann. Intern. Med., 106:209, 1987.

Hoover, D. R., Saah, A. J., Bacellar, H., et al.: Clinical manifestations of AIDS in the era of pneumocystis prophylaxis. N. Engl. J. Med., 329:1922–1926, 1993.

Hosenpud, J. D., Hershberger, R. E., Pantely, G. A., et al.: Late infection in cardiac allograft recipients: Profiles, incidence, and outcome. J. Heart Lung Transplant., 10:380, 1991.

Huang, C. T., McGarry, T., Cooper, S., et al.: Disseminated histoplasmosis in the acquired immunodeficiency syndrome: Report of five cases from a nonendemic area. Arch. Intern. Med., 147:1181, 1987.

Hymes, K. B., Cheung, T., Greene, J. B., et al.: Kaposi's sarcoma in homosexual men: A report of eight cases. Lancet, 2:598, 1981.

Joseph, J., Strange, C., and Sahn, S. A.: Pleural effusions in hospitalized patients with AIDS. Ann. Intern. Med., 118:856–859, 1993.

Joshi, V. V., and Oleske, J. M.: Pulmonary lesions in children with acquired immunodeficiency syndrome: A reappraisal based on data in additional cases and follow-up study of previously reported cases. Hum. Pathol., 17:641, 1986.

Jules-Elysee, K. M., Stover, D. E., Zaman, M. B., et al.: Aerosolized pentamidine: Effect on diagnosis and presentation of Pneumocystis carinii pneumonia. Ann. Intern. Med., 112:750–757, 1990.

Kahn, J. O., Lagakos, S. W., Richman, D. D., et al.: A controlled trial comparing continued zidovudine with didanosine in human immunodeficiency virus infection. N. Engl. J. Med., 327:581–587, 1992.

Kaplan, M. H., Susin, M., Pahwa, S. G., et al.: Neoplastic complications of HTLV-III infection: Lymphomas and solid tumors. Am. J. Med., 82:389, 1987.

Kaposi, M.: Idiopathiches multiples pigment sarcom der Haut. Arch. Dermatol. Syphil., 4:465, 1872.

Klatzmann, D., Champagne, E., Chamaret, S., et al.: T-lymphocyte T4 molecule behaves as the receptor for human retrovirus LAV. Nature, 312:767, 1984.

Klein, H. G.: Transfusion in transplant patients: The good, the bad, and the ugly. J. Heart Lung Transplant., 12:S7, 1993.

Kovacs, J. A., and Masur, H.: *Pneumocystis carinii* pneumonia: Therapy and prophylaxis. J. Infect. Dis., 158:254, 1988.

Kovacs, J. A., Ng, V. L., Masur, H., et al.: Diagnosis of *Pneumocystis carinii* pneumonia: Improved detection in sputum with use of monoclonal antibodies. N. Engl. J. Med., 318:589, 1988.

Krigel, R. L.: The treatment and natural history of epidemic Kaposi's sarcoma. *In* Selikoff, I. J., Tierstein, A. S., and Hirschman, S. Z. (eds): Annals of the New York Academy of Sciences. New York, New York Academy of Sciences, 1984.

Krigel, R., Laubenstein, L. J., and Muggia, F.: Kaposi's sarcoma: A new staging classification. Cancer Treat. Rep., 67:531, 1983.

Lafon, S. W., Mooney, B. D., McMullen, J. P., et al.: A double blind, placebo controlled study of the safety of Retrovir. Abstract 489. Interscience Conference on Antimicrobial Agents and Chemotherapy. Atlanta, 1990.

Lane, H. C., Masur, H., Gelmann, E. P., et al.: Correlation between immunologic function and clinical subpopulations of patients with the acquired immune deficiency syndrome. Am. J. Med., 78:417, 1985.

Lange, J., Boucher, C., Hollak, C., et al.: Failure of zidovudine prophylaxis after accidental exposure to HIV-1. N. Engl. J. Med., 322:1375–1377, 1990.

Larder, B. A., Darby, G., and Richman, D. D.: HIV with reduced sensitivity to zidovudine (AZT) isolated during prolonged therapy. Science, 243:1731–1734, 1989.

Larder, B. A., and Kemp, S. D.: Multiple mutations in HIV-1 reverse transcriptase confer high-level resistance to zidovudine (AZT). Science, 246:1155–1158, 1989.

Lasky, L. A., Nakamura, G., Smith, D. H., et al.: Delineation of a region of the human immunodeficiency virus type 1 gp120 glycoprotein critical for interaction with the CD4 receptor. Cell, 50:975, 1987.

Lettau, L. A., Smith, J. D., Williams, D., et al.: Transmission of hepatitis B with resultant restriction of surgical practice. J. A. M. A., 255:934, 1986.

Levine, A. M., Gill, P. S., Meyer, P. R., et al.: Retrovirus and malignant lymphoma in homosexual men. J. A. M. A., 254:1921, 1985.

Liu, K. J., Darrow, W. W., and Rutherford, G. W.: A model-based estimate for the mean incubation period for AIDS in homosexual men. Science, 240:1333, 1988.

Looke, D. F., and Grove, D. I.: Failed prophylactic zidovudine after needlestick injury. Lancet, 1:1280, 1990.

Lukes, R. J., Parker, I. W., Taylor, C. R., et al.: Immunologic approach to non-Hodgkin's lymphomas and related leukemias: Analysis of the results of multiparameter studies of 425 cases. Semin. Hematol., 15:322, 1978.

Lyerly, H. K., Matthews, T. I., Langlois, A. J., et al.: HTLV-IIIb glycoprotein (GP 120) bound to CD4 determinants on normal lymphocytes and expressed by infected cells serves as target for immune attack. Proc. Natl. Acad. Sci. U. S. A., 84:4601, 1987.

Macher, A. M., Kovacs, I. A., Gill, V., et al.: Bacteremia due to *Mycobacterium avium-intracellulare* in the acquired immunodeficiency syndrome. Ann. Intern. Med., 99:782, 1983.

Mandell, W., Goldberg, D. M., and Neu, H. C.: Histoplasmosis in patients with the acquired immunodeficiency syndrome. Am. J. Med., 81:974, 1986.

Martin, W. J., Smith, T. F., Sanderson, D. R., et al.: Role of bronchoalveolar lavage in the assessment of opportunistic pulmonary infections: Utility and complications. Mayo Clin. Proc., 62:549, 1987.

Masur, H., and the Public Health Service Task Force on Prophylaxis and Therapy for *Mycobacterium avium* Complex: Recommendations on prophylaxis and therapy for disseminated *Mycobacterium avium* complex disease in patients infected with the human immunodeficiency virus. N. Engl. J. Med., 329:898–904, 1993.

Masur, H., Michelis, M. A., Greene, J. B., et al.: An outbreak of community acquired *Pneumocystis carinii* pneumonia: Initial manifestations of cellular dysfunction. N. Engl. J. Med., 305:1431, 1981.

Matas, A. J., Simmons, R. L., and Najarian, J. S.: Hypothesis: Chronic antigen stimulation, herpesvirus infection, and cancer in transplant recipients. Lancet, 1:1277, 1975.

Maurer, J. R., Tullis, D. E., Grossman, R. F., et al.: Infectious complications following isolated lung transplantation. Chest, 101:105, 1992.

McDougal, J. S., Kennedy, M. S., Sligh, J. M., et al.: Binding of HTLV-III/LAV to T4 + T cells by a complex of the 110K viral protein and the T4 molecule. Science, 231:382, 1986.

Meng, T. C., Fischl, M. A., Boota, A. M., et al.: Combination therapy with zidovudine and dideoxycytidine in patients with advanced human immunodeficiency virus infection: A phase I/II study. Ann. Intern. Med., 116:13–20, 1992.

Mermel, L. A., and Maki, D. G.: Bacterial pneumonia in solid organ transplantation. Semin. Respir. Infect., 5:10, 1990.

Meyaard, L., Otto, S. A., Jonker, R. R., et al.: Programmed death of T cells in HIV-1 infection. Science, 257:217–219, 1992.

Montgomery, A. B., Luce, J. M., Turner, J., et al.: Aerosolized pentamidine as sole therapy for Pneumocystis carinii pneumonia in patients with acquired immunodeficiency syndrome. Lancet, 11:480, 1987.

Moore, R. D., Hidalgo, J., Sugland, B. W., and Chaisson, R. E.: Zidovudine and the natural history of the acquired immune deficiency syndrome. N. Engl. J. Med., 324:1412–1416, 1991.

Muggia, F. M.: Treatment of classical Kaposi's sarcoma: A new look. In Friedman-Kien, A. E., and Laubenstein, L. J. (eds): AIDS: The Epidemic of Kaposi's Sarcoma and Opportunistic Infections. New York, Masson, 1984, p. 57.

Murray, J. F., Felton, C. P., Garay, S. M., et al.: Pulmonary complications of the acquired immune deficiency syndrome. N. Engl. J. Med., 310:1682, 1984.

Murray, J. F., Garay, S. M., Hopewell, P. C., et al.: Pulmonary complications of the acquired immune deficiency syndrome: An update. Am. Rev. Respir. Dis., 135:509, 1987.

Nightingale, S. D., Cameron, D. W., Gordin, F. M., et al.: Two controlled trials of rifabutin prophylaxis against Mycobacterium avium complex in AIDS. N. Engl. J. Med., 329:828–833, 1993.

Nobler, M. P., Leddy, M. E., and Huh, S. H.: The impact of palliative irradiation on the management of patients with acquired immune deficiency syndrome. J. Clin. Oncol., 5:107, 1987.

Ognibene, F. P., Steis, R. G., Macher, A. M., et al.: Kaposi's sarcoma causing pulmonary infiltrates and respiratory failure in the acquired immunodeficiency syndrome. Ann. Intern. Med., 102:471, 1985.

Pantaleo, G., Graziosi, C., Demarest, J. K., et al.: HIV infection is active and progressive in lymphoid tissue during the clinically latent stage of disease. Nature, 362:355–358, 1993.

Penn, I.: Cancers complicating organ transplantation. N. Engl. J. Med., 323:1767, 1990.

Penn, I., and Brunson, M. E.: Cancers after cyclosporine therapy. Transplant. Proc., 20:885, 1988.

Phair, J., Munoz, A., Detels, R., et al.: The risk of Pneumocystis carinii pneumonia among men infected with human immunodeficiency virus type 1. N. Engl. J. Med., 322:161–165, 1990.

Pitchenik, A. E., Ganjei, P., Torres, A., et al.: Sputum examination for the diagnosis of Pneumocystis carinii pneumonia in the acquired immune deficiency syndrome. Am. Rev. Respir. Dis., 133:226, 1986.

Popovic, M., Sarngadharan, M. G., Reed, E., and Gallo, R. C.: Detection, isolation, and continuous production of cytopathic retroviruses (HTLV-III) from patients with AIDS and pre-AIDS. Science, 224:497, 1984.

Ratner, L., Haseltine, W., Patarca, R., et al.: Complete nucleotide sequence of the AIDS virus, HTLV-III. Nature, 313:217, 1985.

Reynolds, W. A., Winkelmann, R. K., and Soule, E. H.: Kaposi's sarcoma: A clinicopathological study with particular reference to its relationship to the reticuloendothelial system. Medicine, 44:419, 1965.

Rhenman, B., Rhenman, M. J., Icenogle, T. B., et al.: Heart-lung transplantation: The initial Arizona experience. J. Thorac. Cardiovasc. Surg., 98:922, 1989.

Richman, D. D., Grimes, J. M., and Lagakos, S. W.: Effect of stage of disease and drug dose on zidovudine susceptibilities of isolates of human immunodeficiency virus. J. AIDS, 3:743–746, 1990.

Rostaing, L., Icart, J., Durand, D., et al.: Clinical outcome of Epstein-Barr viremia in transplant patients. Transplant. Proc., 25:2286, 1993.

Rubin, R. H.: Fungal and bacterial infections in the immunocompromised host. Eur. J. Clin. Microbiol. Infect. Dis., 12(Suppl. 1):S42, 1993.

Rubin, R. H.: Impact of cytomegalovirus infection on organ transplant recipients. Rev. Infect. Dis., 7:S754, 1990.

Rubin, R. H., and Greene, R.: Etiology and management of the compromised patient with fever and pulmonary infiltrates. In Rubin, R. H., and Young, L. S. (eds): Clinical Approach to Infection in the Immunocompromised Host. New York, Plenum, 1988, pp. 131–164.

Rubin, R. H., Wolfson, J. S., Cosimi, A. B., and Tolkoff-Rubin, N. E.: Infection in the renal transplant patient. Am. J. Med., 70:405, 1981.

Rubinstein, A., Morecki, R., Silverman, B., et al.: Pulmonary disease in children with acquired immune deficiency syndrome and AIDS-related complex. J. Pediatr., 108:498, 1986.

Sarngadharan, M. G., Popovic, M., Bruch, L., et al.: Antibodies reactive with human T-lymphotropic viruses (HTLV-III) in the serum of patients with AIDS. Science, 224:506, 1984.

Schinazi, R. F., Anderson, D. C., Fultz, P., and McClure, H. M.: Prophylaxis with antiretroviral agents in rhesus macaques inoculated with simian immunodeficiency virus. [Abstract 962]. Interscience Conference on Antimicrobial Agents and Chemotherapy. Atlanta, 1990.

Schmitt, F. A., Bigley, J. W., McKinnis, R., et al.: Neuropsychological outcome of zidovudine (AZT) treatment of patients with AIDS and AIDS related complex. N. Engl. J. Med., 319:1573–1578, 1988.

Schneider, M. E., Hoepelman, A. M., Schattenkerk, J., et al.: A controlled trial of aerosolized pentamidine or trimethoprim-sulfamethoxazole as primary prophylaxis against Pneumocystis carinii pneumonia in patients with human immunodeficiency virus infection. N. Engl. J. Med., 327:1836–1840, 1992.

Selwyn, P. A., Hartel, D., Lewis, V. A., et al.: A prospective study of the risk of tuberculosis among intravenous drug users with human immunodeficiency virus infection. N. Engl. J. Med., 320:545–550, 1989.

Sepkowitz, K. A., Telzak, E. E., Gold, J. W., et al.: Pneumothorax in AIDS. Ann. Intern. Med., 114:455–459, 1991.

Siegal, F. P., Lopez, C., Hammer, G. S., et al.: Severe acquired immunodeficiency in male homosexuals, manifested by chronic perianal ulcerative herpes simplex lesions. N. Engl. J. Med., 305:1439, 1981.

Small, P. M., Shafer, R. W., Hopewell, P. C., et al.: Exogenous reinfection with multidrug resistant Mycobacterium tuberculosis in patients with advanced HIV infection. N. Engl. J. Med., 328:1137–1144, 1993.

Smyth, R. L., Scott, J. P., Borysiewicz, L. K., et al.: Cytomegalovirus infection in heart-lung transplant recipients: Risk factors, clinical associations, and response to treatment. J. Infect. Dis., 164:1045, 1991.

Snydman, D. R., Rubin, R. H., and Werner, B. G.: New developments in cytomegalovirus prevention and management. Am. J. Kidney Dis., 21:217, 1993.

Starzl, T. E.: Five years' experience in renal transplantation with immunosuppressive drugs: Survival, function, complications, and the role of lymphocyte depletion by thoracic duct fistula. Ann. Surg., 168:416, 1968.

Starzl, T. E., Porter, K. A., Iwatsuki, S., et al.: Reversibility of lymphomas and lymphoproliferative lesions developing under cyclosporin-steroid therapy. Lancet, 1:583, 1984.

Stone, W. J., Schaffner, W.: Strongyloides infections in transplant recipients. Semin. Respir. Infect., 5:58, 1990.

Stribling, J., Wertzner, S., and Smith, G. V.: Kaposi's sarcoma in renal allograft recipients. Cancer, 42:442, 1978.

Suffredini, A. F., Ognibene, F. P., Lack, E. E., et al.: Nonspecific interstitial pneumonitis: A common cause of pulmonary disease in the acquired immune deficiency syndrome. Ann. Intern. Med., 107:7, 1987.

Tegtmeier, G. E.: Posttransfusion cytomegalovirus infections. Arch. Pathol. Lab. Med., 113:236, 1989.

Temin, H. M., and Mitzutani, S.: RNA-directed DNA polymerase in virions of Rous sarcoma virus. Nature, 226:1211, 1970.

Tolkoff-Rubin, N. E., and Rubin, R. H.: Clinical approach to viral and fungal infections in the renal transplant patient. Semin. Nephrol., 12:364, 1992.

Tokars, J. I., Marcus, R., Culver, D. H., et al.: Surveillance of HIV infection and zidovudine use among health care workers after occupational exposure to HIV-infected blood. Ann. Intern. Med., 118:913–919, 1993.

Volberding, P. A., Lagakos, S. W., Koch, M. A., et al.: Zidovudine in asymptomatic human immunodeficiency virus infection: A controlled trial in patients with fewer than 500 CD4-positive cells per cubic millimeter. N. Engl. J. Med., *322*:941–949, 1990.

Wagener, M. M., and Yu, V. L.: Bacteremia in transplant recipients: A prospective study of demographics, etiologic agents, risk factors, and outcomes. Am. J. Infect. Control., *20*:239, 1992.

Welch, K., Finkbeiner, W., Alpers, C. E., et al.: Autopsy findings in the acquired immune deficiency syndrome. J. A. M. A. *252*:1152, 1984.

Wreghitt, T.: Cytomegalovirus infections in heart and heart lung transplant recipients. J. Antimicrob. Chemother., *23*:49, 1989.

Wreghitt, T. G., Sargaison, M., Sutehall, G., et al.: A study of Epstein-Barr infections in heart and heart and lung transplant recipients. Transplant. Proc., *21*:2502, 1989.

Zhu, T., Mo, H., Wang, N., et al.: Genotypic and phenotypic characterization of HIV-1 in patients with primary infection. Science, *261*:1179–1181, 1993.

Ziegler, J. L., Beckstead, J. A., Volberding, P. A., et al.: Non-Hodgkin's lymphoma in 90 homosexual men: Relationship to generalized lymphadenopathy and acquired immunodeficiency syndrome (AIDS). N. Engl. J. Med., *311*:565, 1984.

Zuger, A., Louie, E., Holzman, R. S., et al.: Cryptococcal disease in patients with the acquired immunodeficiency syndrome: Diagnostic features, and outcome of treatment. Ann. Intern. Med., *104*:234, 1986.

22

Surgical Treatment of Pulmonary Tuberculosis

Jon F. Moran

Thoracic surgery emerged as a separate surgical specialty during the first half of the 20th century, and the basic techniques developed during that period focused primarily on the treatment of pulmonary tuberculosis. The efforts of the surgeons of the 1930s and 1940s culminated in the perfection of pulmonary resectional techniques as currently practiced. Surgical treatment of suppurative diseases of the lung, although required less frequently today, is largely unchanged since 1950.

Pulmonary tuberculosis remains the leading infectious killer in the world, causing at least 3 million deaths annually. In the 1990s, tuberculosis occurs most frequently in South America, Africa, and Asia. Five million new cases of active pulmonary tuberculosis occur worldwide each year, but active tuberculosis has become relatively uncommon in North America and Europe. Even before the introduction of effective chemotherapy, the incidence of mycobacterial infection declined in Western Europe and the United States as a result of improved nutrition and better living conditions (Fig. 22–1). With the development of effective chemotherapy for tuberculosis in the mid-20th century, the incidence of tuberculosis and the death rate from tuberculosis decreased dramatically. Mortal-

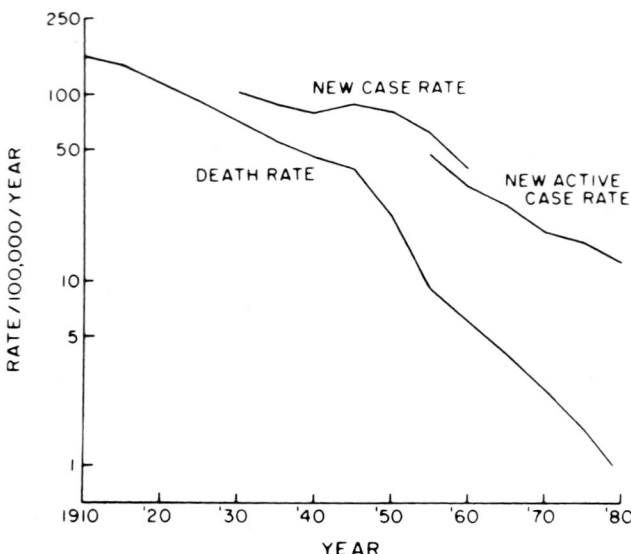

ity per 100,000 population in the United States fell from 200 cases per year in 1900 to 1 case in 1980. However, beginning in 1985, the steady (approximately 5% per year) decline in the reported incidence of tuberculosis cases in the United States leveled off, and since 1988, the number of cases has increased slightly each year (Fig. 22–2). This reversal of the declining incidence of tuberculosis in the United States and Europe has been most noticeable in urban areas and has been associated with the epidemic of human immunodeficiency virus (HIV) infection (Horsburgh, 1992). The total number of reported cases of tuberculosis in the United States in 1987 was approximately 22,500, but nearly 28,000 cases of tuberculosis were reported in 1992. An even sharper increase in the incidence of mycobacterial infections other than tuberculosis has been associated with the acquired immunodeficiency syndrome (AIDS) epidemic.

Pulmonary tuberculosis represents 85% (Bloch et al., 1989) of all cases of tuberculosis today. Despite antituberculous chemotherapy, approximately 2% of pulmonary mycobacterial infections require surgical treatment. Because an increasing number of patients with pulmonary mycobacterial infection have drug-resistant organisms or are immunocompromised (Iseman and Madsen, 1989; Rieder et al., 1989), the frequency of surgical intervention for these infections will probably increase gradually.

HISTORICAL ASPECTS

Tuberculosis was a scourge of early humanity, as is shown by its discovery in the lungs of Egyptian mummies and the spine of an Incan mummy. Hippocrates (c. 470 to 376 B.C.) wrote extensively about clinical tuberculosis, or *phthisis*, as it was termed by the Greeks. *Phthisis* meant "a disease characterized by progressive weight loss and wasting." The Latin synonym was *consumption*—because the disease seemed to consume its victims. Tubercles (Fig. 22–3) in the lung were described as a hallmark of the disease by the Greeks, and in 1839, Schonlein was the first to use the term *tuberculosis* to describe the pathologic changes seen in the lungs at autopsy.

An epidemic of tuberculosis in Western Europe began in England in the 18th century and spread across Europe to peak in the 19th century. A similar epidemic spread through the urbanized parts of the United States from 1800 to 1920. Tuberculosis is

FIGURE 22–1. Tuberculosis death rate and new case rates in the United States, 1910–1980. (From Comstock, G. W.: Epidemiology of tuberculosis. Am. Rev. Respir. Dis., *125*[Suppl.]:9, 1982.)

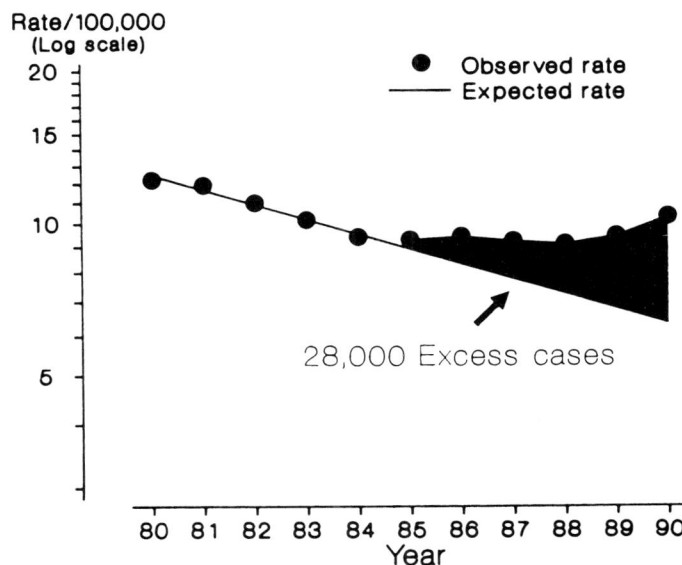

FIGURE 22–2. Observed and expected tuberculosis case rates in the United States by year from 1980 to 1990. Expected rates are based on a 5% average annual decline observed before 1985. Between 1985 and 1990, at least 28,000 more cases than expected were reported. This upward trend since 1985 has continued. (Data from Centers for Disease Control and Prevention, Atlanta, Georgia.)

thought to have caused approximately 20% of all deaths in Europe during the 18th and 19th centuries. In the United States in the 1920s, tuberculosis was still the second leading cause of death, and most of its victims were young adults.

Clustering of cases and the common predisposing factors of poverty, overcrowded living conditions, poor nutrition, and poor overall health were noted before the 19th century and several key observations were made during the 19th century. Rokitansky (1804 to 1878) observed that, in 30,000 autopsies, more than 90% of those who had *not* died of tuberculosis had

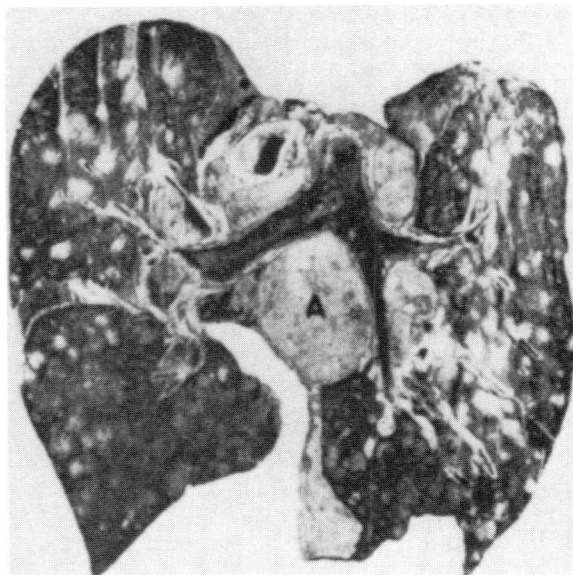

FIGURE 22–3. Large necrotic tubercles from generalized spread of tuberculosis with particular enlargement of the hilar lymph node (A). Tubercles or nodules such as these were the gross pathologic hallmark of phthisis or consumption. (From Auerbach, O.: The natural history of the tuberculous pulmonary lesion. Med. Clin. North Am., 43:242, 1959.)

evidence of tuberculous infection in their lungs. In 1826, Laënnec, on the basis of similar autopsy studies, recognized that tuberculosis, whether acute or chronic, pulmonary or extrapulmonary, was a single disease entity. Laënnec's unified view was initially disputed widely. In 1865, Villeman, a French military surgeon, demonstrated that tuberculosis could be transmitted to guinea pigs or rabbits by injection of infected material from either humans or cows. Villeman suggested that a "virus" was the causative agent.

A landmark breakthrough in understanding the cause of tuberculosis was made by Robert Koch, a German general practitioner confronted daily with clinical tuberculosis. Koch had turned to the newly emerging science of bacteriology and developed methods for plate cultivation that allowed isolation of individual strains of bacteria. Koch's announcement on March 24, 1882, of his isolation of the tubercle bacillus (Koch, 1932) marked the beginning of a medical crusade against tuberculosis that led to control of the disease in developed countries within 100 years. At the same time, Koch showed that it was more difficult to infect previously exposed animals than nonexposed animals (Koch's phenomenon). Simultaneously, he enunciated his postulates for proving bacterial causation of disease, which became the standard for establishing the infectious cause of a disease: "To prove that tuberculosis . . . is caused by invasion of bacilli and . . . the growth and multiplication of the bacilli, it was necessary to isolate the bacteria from the body; to grow them in pure culture . . . ; and by administering the isolated bacilli to animals to reproduce the same morbid condition."

Later Koch attempted to use "old tuberculin," a sterile filtrate of the cultured tubercle bacilli, as therapy for tuberculosis (Hanson and Reichman, 1989). Although his efforts failed therapeutically, tuberculin skin testing evolved from these efforts and, in combination with the newly discovered chest roentgenogram, made mass screening for tuberculosis possible by 1940. Earlier case identification led to earlier treatment, usually in a sanatorium, since antituberculous chemotherapy was not yet available. Meanwhile, it had been established that transmission of tuberculosis was almost exclusively by airborne bacilli, and this led to isolation of tuberculosis patients, which reduced the spread of tuberculosis. The Nobel Prize–winning discovery of streptomycin in 1946 by Waksmann and the release of isoniazid (INH) in 1952 provided effective chemotherapy for tuberculosis. For the first time, pulmonary tuberculosis was easily curable in most patients.

Understanding of the bacteriology and pathophysiology of tuberculosis increased during this period (1875 to 1950), and simultaneously, the clinical treatment of pulmonary tuberculosis evolved rapidly. The first sanatorium specializing in the treatment of tuberculosis opened in 1854 in Gorbersdorf, Germany. By 1952, there were over 100,000 sanatorium beds in the United States for the treatment of tuberculosis. The regimental routine of the sanatoria, stressing bedrest, diet, and fresh mountain air, seemed to help many patients with early cases of pulmonary tuberculosis, but was probably rarely effective in patients with advanced cavitary disease. Collapse therapy for pulmonary tuberculosis (Alexander, 1925) was first advocated by Carson in 1821 and was tried sporadically in the last two decades of the 19th century. Therapeutic pneumothorax, phrenic nerve division, and pneumoperitoneum were all employed widely in the early decades of the 20th century to produce collapse of infected portions of the lung. Thoracoplasty was used by Simon in 1869 but was not perfected or used widely until after 1910. Sauerbruch in Germany popularized extrapleural paravertebral thoracoplasty as treatment of pulmonary tuberculosis (Sauerbruch and Schumacher, 1911). John Alexander popularized thoracoplasty in the United States, and it became a standard treatment for cavitary pulmonary tuberculosis by the 1930s. It is noteworthy that even before effective chemotherapy existed, the yearly death rate from tuberculosis in the United States fell from 300 per 100,000 in 1880 to only 69 per 100,000 in 1935. This improvement can be attributed to improved case screening, isolation, sanatorium care, and the introduction of various forms of collapse therapy.

The first actual pulmonary resection for pulmonary tuberculosis was done by Block in 1882; however, the patient died. In 1891, Tuffier performed the first successful partial lung resection for tuberculosis, resecting the apex of the right lung of a 25-year-old man. Resectional pulmonary surgery for tuberculosis remained rare until the 1930s. The first successful formal lobectomy for tuberculosis was performed in Cleveland by Freelander in 1934, and this revived interest in resection as a treatment option for tuberculosis. Prior to effective antituberculous chemotherapy, resectional surgery had a nearly prohibitive mortality rate from active tuberculous infection. The discovery of streptomycin, para-aminosalicylic acid, and INH made resectional surgery much safer; but almost si-

multaneously, these agents decreased the need for surgical treatment of pulmonary tuberculosis. The use of resectional surgery peaked in the 1950s and declined rapidly in the 1960s, as improved chemotherapy decreased both the incidence and the severity of pulmonary tuberculosis in the developed areas of the world.

BACTERIOLOGY

The genus *Mycobacterium* includes the two bacterial species that cause two of the most dreaded human diseases, tuberculosis and leprosy. The name *Mycobacterium* was chosen for this genus by Lehmann and Neumann in 1896 because of the mold-like appearance of the bacterial colonies when growing on nutrient broth. Despite the name, mycobacteria are no more related to fungi than are other bacteria. Mycobacterial cell walls have a high lipid content that prevents permeation by aniline dyes, but when a dye binds, decolorization is difficult. Mycobacteria are gram-positive rods but do not stain well with Gram's stain. Koch was the first to discover the peculiar "acid-fast" staining property of mycobacteria, and his original staining technique was modified slightly by Ehrlich. The modern acid-fast staining technique, which bears the names of Ziehl and Neelsen, is relatively unchanged from Ehrlich's original method. The Ziehl-Neelsen staining procedure employs heat to enable the carbolfuchsin stain to penetrate the mycobacterial cell wall. Acid-fast organisms stain red against a methylene blue counterstain. The species isolated by Koch, *Mycobacterium tuberculosis*, is responsible for most clinically significant cases of pulmonary mycobacterial disease. *M. tuberculosis* is an obligate parasite, and humans provide its only reservoir. Primates and domestic animals in close contact with humans can develop infection. *M. tuberculosis* is an aerobic, nonmotile, slow-growing bacillus; and when cultured, colonies are buff-colored, rough, and friable and become visible only after 4 to 6 weeks of growth.

Many other species of mycobacteria were isolated during the first half of the 20th century (Grange, 1988). Species of mycobacteria other than *M. tuberculosis* were generally ignored as potential sources of pulmonary infection initially because of the overwhelming number of cases of tuberculosis. Gradually, it was recognized that several other species of mycobacteria could occasionally cause pulmonary disease. The species of mycobacteria other than *M. tuberculosis*, *M. bovis*, and *M. leprae* are referred to as *atypical mycobacteria*. Atypical mycobacteria are frequently resistant to antituberculous drugs (Contreras et al., 1988; Davidson, 1989), and approximately 50% of patients referred for surgical therapy of mycobacterial disease have atypical mycobacterial pulmonary infections. Mycobacterial lung infections are classified precisely by the species of the infecting organism. Before precise specification was available, the mycobacteria were divided by Runyon (1959) into four groups according to differences in growth rate and pigment production by the growing colonies (Table 22–1). Runyon Group I, the photochromogens, grow slowly and form a yellow or orange pigment only after exposure to light. Group II organisms, the scotochromogens, grow slowly and produce an orange or red pigment both when grown in the dark and when grown in the light. Group III, the nonchromogens, grow slowly and form cream-colored colonies even when exposed to light. *M. tuberculosis* and *M. bovis* have both growth and pigment production characteristics similar to those of the nonchromogens. Group IV organisms grow rapidly and show visible colonies within a few days. The rapid growers generally do not produce pigment. *M. leprae,* the causative organism of leprosy, cannot be grown using standard culture techniques.

Mycobacterium avium–intracellulare and *M. kansasii* are the atypical organisms that most frequently cause clinical pulmonary infection (O'Brien, 1989a). *M. avium* and *M. intracellulare* can be distinguished by sophisticated serologic testing, but they are so similar that they are generally considered collectively. *M. avium–intracellulare* is found worldwide and is isolated from soil, water, and birds. In the United States, pulmonary infection with *M. avium–intracellulare* was most commonly found in the Southeast prior to the epidemic spread of HIV infection. *M. avium–intracellulare* was originally called the Battey bacillus after Battey State Hospital, a sanatorium in Rome, Georgia. Now it is a particularly common cause of disease in patients with AIDS and, as a result, is found much more commonly throughout the world than it was in the early 1980s. Although patients with AIDS very commonly develop *M. avium–intracellulare* infection, it is rarely localized in these patients; therefore, surgical treatment is rarely indicated in this patient group (Goodman, 1990; Sathe and Raichman,

1989). *M. avium–intracellulare* is usually resistant to most antituberculous drugs in vitro. *M. kansasii* is found worldwide, but in the United States it occurs most frequently in the Midwest and Southwest. Unlike *M. avium–intracellulare,* it has not become a common pathogen in individuals with AIDS. In contrast to *M. avium–intracellulare, M. kansasii* more often shows in vitro susceptibility to antimycobacterial drugs; as a result, patients with *M. kansasii* pulmonary disease require surgical treatment less frequently (Horsburgh et al., 1987).

Drug susceptibility testing is very important in the treatment of pulmonary mycobacterial infection (Davidson and Le, 1992; Horsburgh et al., 1987; Tsukamura, 1988). Since most mycobacteria grow slowly, 3 to 4 weeks are often required to isolate the infecting organism and another 3 to 4 weeks are needed to assess the organism's sensitivity to various antimycobacterial drugs. Bacteria are considered resistant if more than 1% of the population grows on media containing the standard drug concentration. This definition of drug resistance correlates well with clinical responsiveness. Because of the inevitable delay in precise speciation and susceptibility testing, therapy is often begun empirically while awaiting the test results.

PATHOLOGY

The pathologic responses within the lung to the various common mycobacteria are identical (Auerbach and Dail, 1988). *M. tuberculosis* is a virulent organism requiring a very small inoculum for infection to occur even in normal lung tissue. The atypical mycobacteria are less virulent and more frequently cause infection either in previously damaged lung tissue or in immunocompromised individuals (Haque, 1990). There are several pathologic patterns of response to pulmonary mycobacterial infection. Mycobacteria gain entry to the body by inhalation of droplet nuclei less than 5 μm in diameter; such a droplet probably contains only one to three bacteria. A first infection in an unsensitized host causes a localized necrotizing pneumonia, most commonly in the middle or lower lobes. Mycobacteria spread from the pneumonic focus through the lymphatics to the hilar lymph nodes. Organisms may pass into the venous blood and thereby be disseminated widely. The peripheral pneumonic process is characterized by "caseous" necrosis with formation of a granuloma containing mycobacteria, polymorphonuclear granulocytes, and fibrin with a rim of granulation tissue (Fig. 22–4). Epithelioid histiocytes or Langhans' giant cells are commonly seen, and the lesion develops a pseudocapsule. The histologic hallmark of mycobacterial infection is the caseating granuloma. *Caseous* describes the gross appearance of the lesion with a yellow-white, semisoft cheese–like material filling the thin capsule. Microscopically, the hilar lymph nodes show a necrotizing inflammatory reaction similar to that of the pulmonary lesion. The peripheral lung

■ **Table 22–1.** CLASSIFICATION OF MYCOBACTERIAL SPECIES*

Mycobacteria and Runyon Groups	Speed of Growth	Pigment Production	
		Dark	Light
M. tuberculosis	Slow	−	−
M. bovis	Slow	−	−
Group I: Photochromogens			
M. kansasii	Slow	−	+
M. marinum	Slow	−	+
Group II: Scotochromogens			
M. scrofulaceum	Slow	+	+
M. szulgai	Slow	+	+
Group III: Nonchromogens			
M. avium–intracellulare complex	Slow	−	−
M. xenopi	Slow	+	−
Group IV: Rapid growers			
M. fortuitum	Rapid	−	−
M. chelonae	Rapid	−	−

Adapted from Boyars, M. C.: The microbiology, chemotherapy, and surgical treatment of tuberculosis. J. Thorac. Imaging, 5:1, 1990.

*Species listed are those that have been documented as pulmonary pathogens in humans.

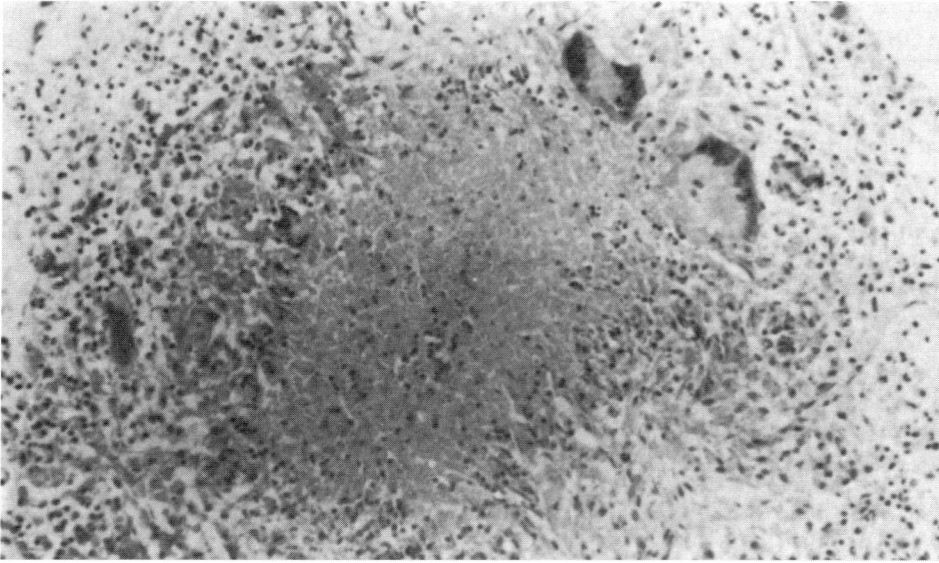

FIGURE 22–4. Typical tuberculous granuloma with central caseation and surrounding epithelioid and Langhans' giant cells. H & E, ×250. (From Dunnill, M. S.: Pulmonary Pathology, 2nd ed. Edinburgh, Churchill Livingstone, 1987, p. 447.)

lesion accompanied by hilar nodal enlargement is called the *primary Ghon complex,* which is most often 1 to 2 cm in diameter and solitary (Fig. 22–5). Generally, the infection is contained at this stage by the body's immune responses. Any hematogenous spread that has occurred usually becomes inactive as the host's immune response mounts.

Primary tuberculosis refers to the initial infection with *M. tuberculosis* in a previously unsensitized host; it progresses locally or by wide hematogenous dissemination. In the past, this form of disease most frequently occurred in children and was referred to as *childhood tuberculosis.* With the declining prevalence of tuberculosis infection over the past few decades, the incidence of primary tuberculosis in adults has risen. Primary tuberculosis may present as a large,

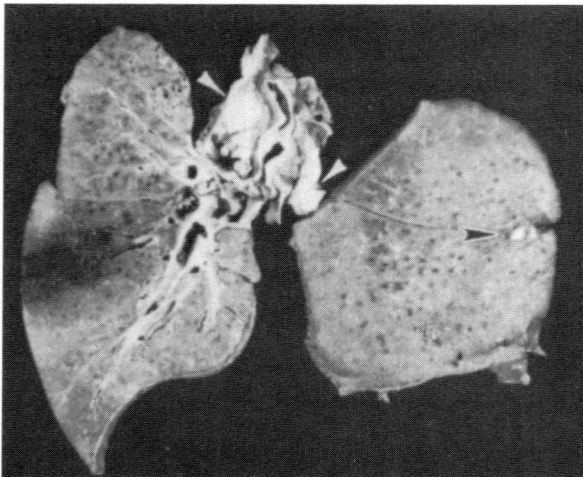

FIGURE 22–5. Lungs and lower tracheobronchial tree showing a calcified subpleural lesion in the left lower lobe (Ghon focus, *black arrowhead*) and several hilar and paratracheal lymph nodes with caseous necrosis and calcification (Ghon complex, *white arrowheads*). (From Haque, A. K.: The pathology and pathophysiology of mycobacterial infections. J. Thorac. Imaging, 5:11, 1990.)

necrotizing pneumonia that progresses to cavitation with transbronchial spread. The areas of pneumonic infiltrate in primary tuberculosis tend to be in the lower lobes. When hematogenous spread is not stopped by cell-mediated immunity, the disease spreads most commonly to the lung apices, the kidneys, the epiphyses of long bones, or the brain. These locations are favored by the strict aerobic growth requirement of mycobacteria. Occasionally, hematogenous spread leads to miliary tuberculosis, which involves massive hematogenous spread, giving rise to thousands of 1- to 2-mm (millet seed–sized) tubercles throughout the body (Fig. 22–6). Currently, most miliary tuberculosis occurs in elderly or severely immunocompromised patients.

The most common pattern of mycobacterial infection is *reinfection* or *postprimary* tuberculosis. In the past, this was termed *adult* tuberculosis, in contrast to *childhood* (primary) tuberculosis. Postprimary tuberculosis begins as a segmental pneumonia in the apical or posterior segment of an upper lobe or the superior segment of a lower lobe (Fig. 22–7). It continues to be debated whether this pattern of infection is caused by reactivation of a dormant prior focus or infection from a new exogenous exposure. Bilateral lung involvement is relatively common in postprimary tuberculosis. Histologically, the acute necrotizing pneumonia resembles primary tuberculosis. The pneumonic infiltrate progresses to caseous necrosis, and cavity formation occurs when the area of liquefaction erodes into an adjacent bronchus. Drainage into a bronchus leads to expectoration of debris from the cavity, including destroyed lung tissue elements and viable mycobacteria. Endobronchial spread can affect an entire lobe or an entire lung in this manner. The size of the cavities formed varies from 2 to 10 cm and depends on the amount of lung destroyed before spontaneous drainage occurs (Fig. 22–8). Small cavities may fuse to form larger cavities, the walls of which consist of granulation tissue with organizing reaction in a rim

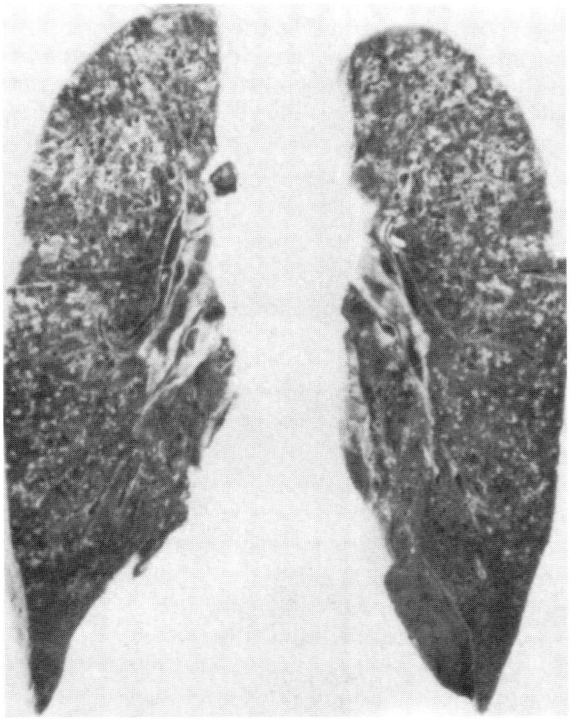

FIGURE 22–6. Gross pathologic appearance of miliary tuberculosis in the lungs. Similar 1- to 2-mm foci of mycobacterial infection are disseminated throughout the body. (From Dunnill, M. S.: Pulmonary Pathology. 2nd ed. Edinburgh, Churchill Livingstone, 1987, p. 446.)

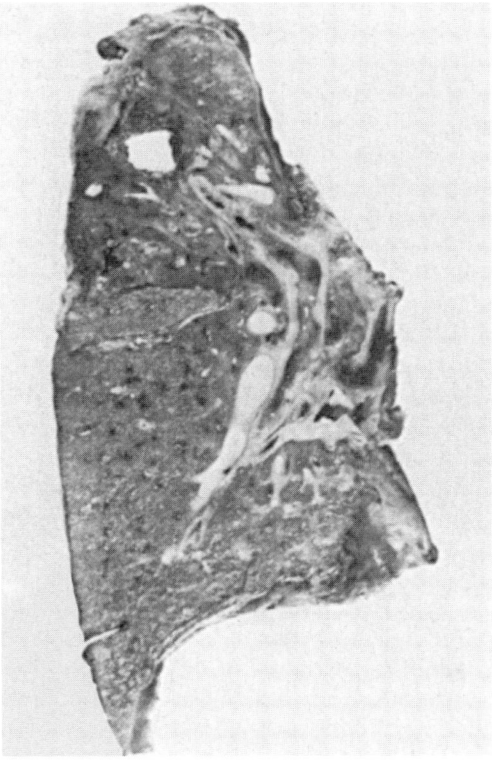

FIGURE 22–7. Cut surface of the right lung showing upper lobe infiltration and cavitation, a typical pattern of adult pulmonary tuberculosis. (From Dunnill, M. S.: Pulmonary Pathology. 2nd ed. Edinburgh, Churchill Livingstone, 1987, p. 449.)

of surrounding lung tissue (Fig. 22–9). Erosion of a cavity into a bronchial vessel may cause severe hemoptysis. A Rasmussen aneurysm—an aneurysm of a pulmonary artery or arteriole within or adjacent to a cavity—is found in about 4% of advanced cavitary disease. These aneurysms may rupture, causing massive hemoptysis and asphyxiation.

An intense inflammatory reaction in the rim of lung around tuberculous cavities is characteristic of postprimary tuberculosis. When cavities are peripheral in the lung, as they usually are, this reaction extends to the pleural surface of the lung. The overlying visceral pleura tends to contract and decrease the volume of the involved portion of the lung. The visceral and parietal pleurae are both affected by this intense reaction. The overlying pleural space is often completely obliterated with dense fusion of the visceral and parietal pleurae over these cavities. This intense pleural reaction makes operative separation of the two pleural surfaces overlying the diseased portions of the lung essentially impossible.

Antituberculous chemotherapy may interrupt the necrotizing pneumonic process and allow healing prior to cavitation. Patients infected with resistant organisms or patients not receiving chemotherapy early in the course of their infections are more likely to progress to cavitation and its complications, which do not respond well to chemotherapy alone. Therefore, the complications that ensue from cavitation,

such as hemoptysis or bronchopleural fistula, will likely require surgical intervention.

Erosion of the cavity into an airway permits infection of the proximal bronchial mucosa, which frequently leads to necrotizing inflammation and ulceration. Endobronchial tuberculosis may cause bronchial stenosis with distal superimposed nontuberculous infection (bacterial or fungal) even after healing of the mycobacterial process (Chan et al., 1990). Cavities can rupture into the pleural space and create a tuberculous

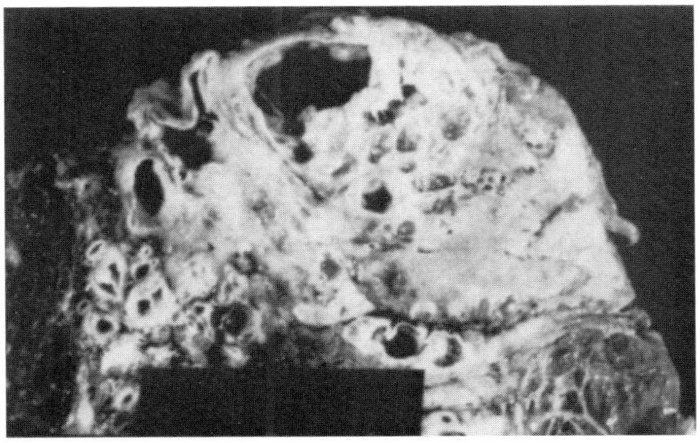

FIGURE 22–8. Section of the right lung with one large and numerous smaller tuberculous cavities. The adjacent lung shows pneumonic consolidation with areas of caseous necrosis. (From Haque, A. K.: The pathology and pathophysiology of mycobacterial infections. J. Thorac. Imaging, 5:13, 1990.)

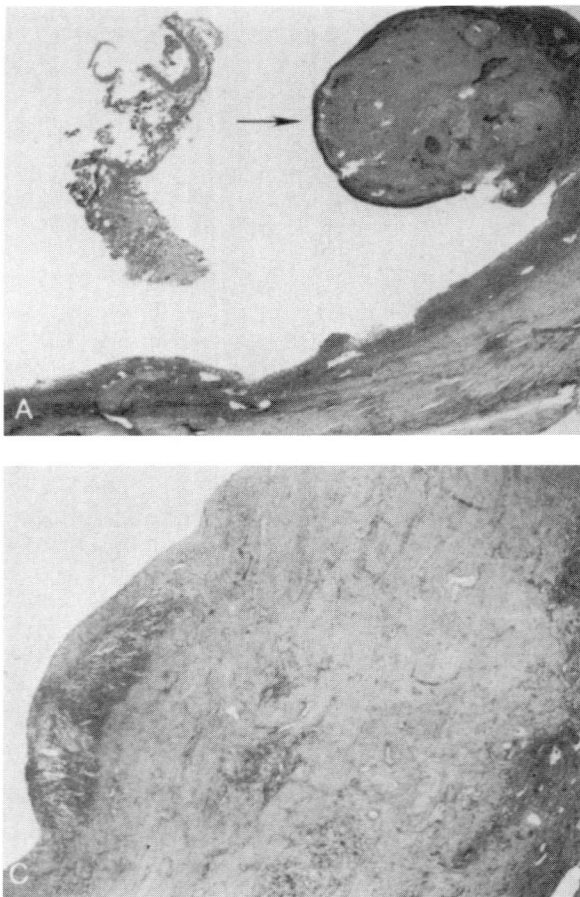

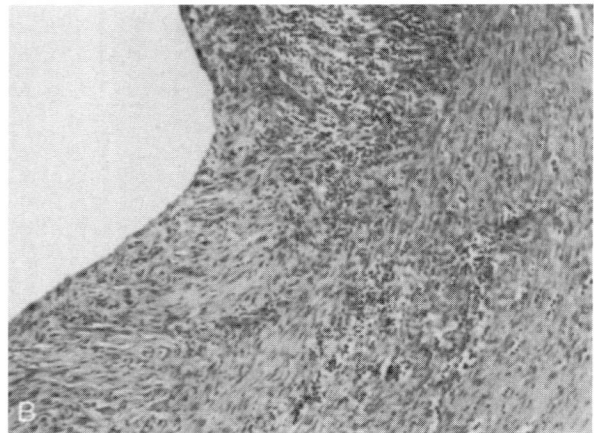

FIGURE 22–9. Photomicrographs of the lining of tuberculous cavities illustrating (A) the inner membrane (arrow; original magnification, ×25), (B) the middle zone (original magnification, ×100), and (C) the outer zone, showing an organizing exudative reaction in the adjacent lung (original magnification, ×25). (A–C, From Haque, A. K.: The pathology and pathophysiology of mycobacterial infections. J. Thorac. Imaging, 5:13, 1990.)

or mixed tuberculous and bacterial empyema. Subsequent cavity erosion into an airway produces a bronchopleural fistula. Tuberculous empyema can also occur secondary to hematogenous or lymphatic seeding of the pleural space. Pure tuberculous effusions are usually serofibrinous, whereas mixed effusions resemble a conventional bacterial empyema. Many pleural effusions associated with tuberculosis are the result of a hypersensitivity reaction in the pleural space and do not represent actual infection of the pleural space. Pure tuberculous effusions or effusions secondary to a hypersensitivity reaction tend to resolve very quickly with effective chemotherapy.

Mycobacterial infection, with the intense inflammatory response that it incites in the lung, usually progresses to fibrosis. Healing and cavity closure may occur spontaneously even as the infection spreads to other areas of the lung. After apparent healing has occurred, reactivation and further spread are fairly common. The fibrosis that accompanies healing in postprimary tuberculosis contracts the surrounding lung (usually the upper portions of the lung) and elevates the hilar structures toward the apex on the affected side.

DIAGNOSIS

There is an important distinction between mycobacterial infection and mycobacterial disease. Infection implies entry of a mycobacterial organism into the body without symptoms or overt clinical evidence of disease. The diagnosis of mycobacterial pulmonary disease depends on the confirmation of active disease by appropriate radiographic and bacteriologic studies (Crawford et al., 1989). Only 5 to 15% of individuals infected with M. tuberculosis develop clinically significant disease. The American Thoracic Society's classification of tuberculosis infection recognizes four categories: Category 0, no tuberculosis exposure (no exposure history, negative tuberculin skin test); Category I, tuberculosis exposure without infection (history of exposure, negative tuberculin skin test); Category II, tuberculosis infection without disease (positive tuberculin skin test without clinical disease); and Category III, tuberculosis disease proved by symptoms, roentgenographic studies, and bacteriologic studies.

The symptoms of pulmonary mycobacterial disease are often subtle; they include chronic productive cough, persistent "chest cold," easy fatigability, weight loss, chest pain, and fever. Hemoptysis and night sweats are the classic specific symptoms of tuberculosis. A history of exposure to tuberculosis or membership in a high-risk group should increase the index of suspicion for mycobacterial disease. Pulmonary mycobacterial infection is more common in the immunosuppressed patient (secondary to corticosteroids, cancer chemotherapy, transplant immunosuppression, or AIDS); in diabetics; after gastrectomy; in the elderly; and in individuals with silicosis, pneumoconiosis, or reticuloendothelial malignancies (Contreras et al., 1988; Horsburgh, 1992; Rieder et al., 1989; Sathe and Raichman, 1989).

Mycobacterial disease of the lung can cause a variety of roentgenographic abnormalities (Buckner and Walker, 1990). The most common findings in pulmonary tuberculosis are apical upper lobe infiltrates, often bilateral, with frequent cavitation (Figs. 22–10 and 22–11). The superior segments of the lower lobes are also frequently affected by infiltrates. Pleural effusions, solitary parenchymal nodules, lower lung field infiltrates, and lymphadenopathy are some of the other roentgenographic abnormalities that can be seen with mycobacterial disease. The roentgenographic findings in atypical mycobacterial disease are indistinguishable from the changes seen with tuberculosis

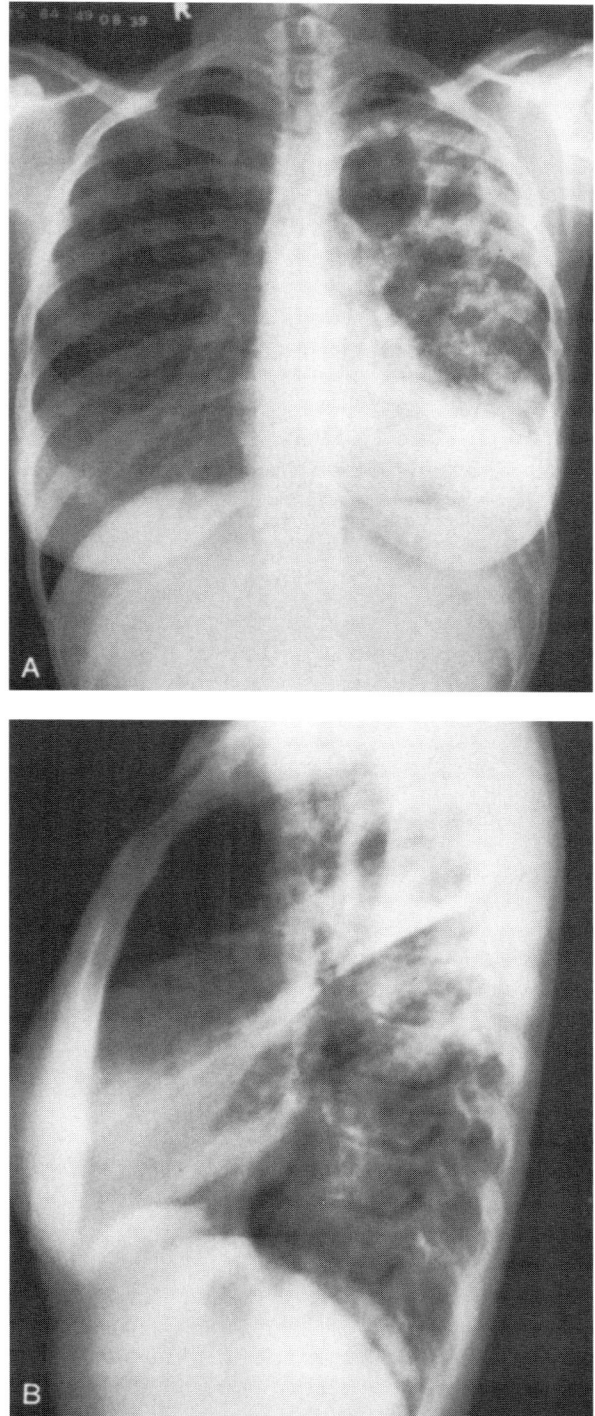

FIGURE 22–10. Posteroanterior (A) and lateral (B) chest radiographs showing typical appearance of postprimary tuberculosis. The patient presented with a 2-month history of malaise, fever, chills, and productive cough. Extensive air space disease is evident in the left upper and lower lobes with multiple cavities. (A and B, From Buckner, C. B., Walker, C. W.: Radiologic manifestations of adult tuberculosis. J. Thorac. Imaging, 5:35, 1990.)

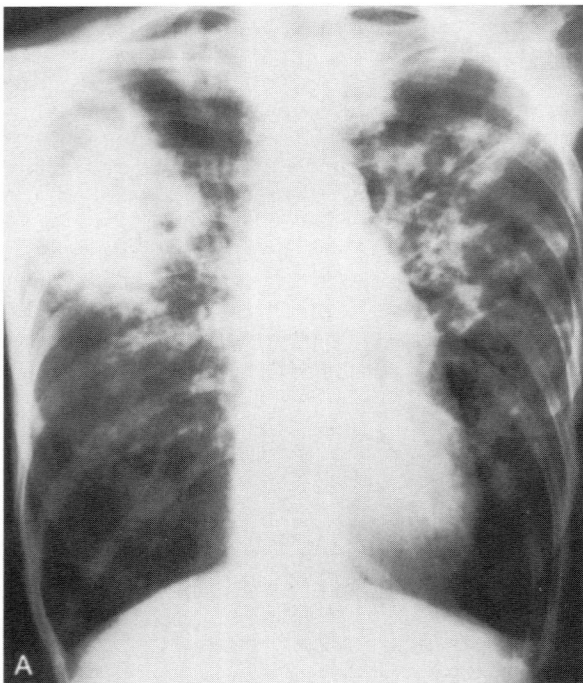

Figure 22–11. posteroanterior chest radiographs of a 68-year-old woman with postprimary tuberculosis localized to the apical and posterior segments of the upper lobes. *A,* Fibroexudative changes with cavitation are present bilaterally at the time of presentation. *B,* After 4 months of antituberculous chemotherapy, multiple mass-like lesions are present in both upper lobes, but the patient has improved radiographically and clinically. *C,* After 2 more months of antituberculous chemotherapy, a tuberculoma in the right upper lobe and residual bilateral fibrocystic changes in the upper lobe remain. (*A–C,* From Winer-Muram, H. T., Rubin, S. A.: Thoracic complications of tuberculosis. J. Thorac. Imaging, *5:*48, 1990.)

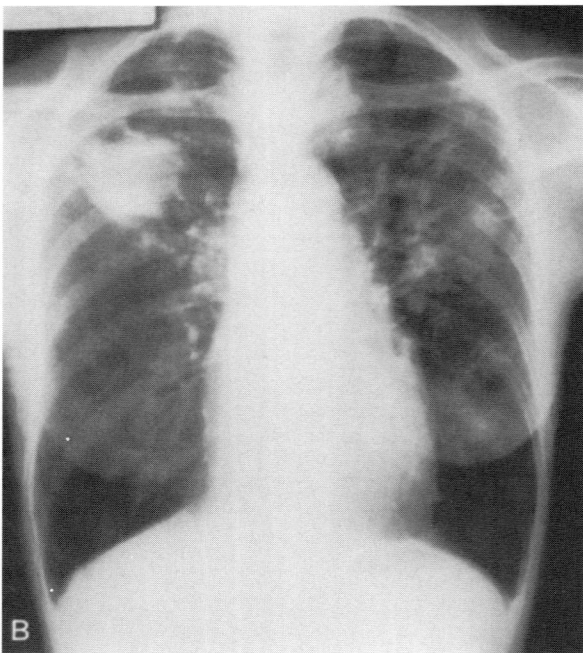

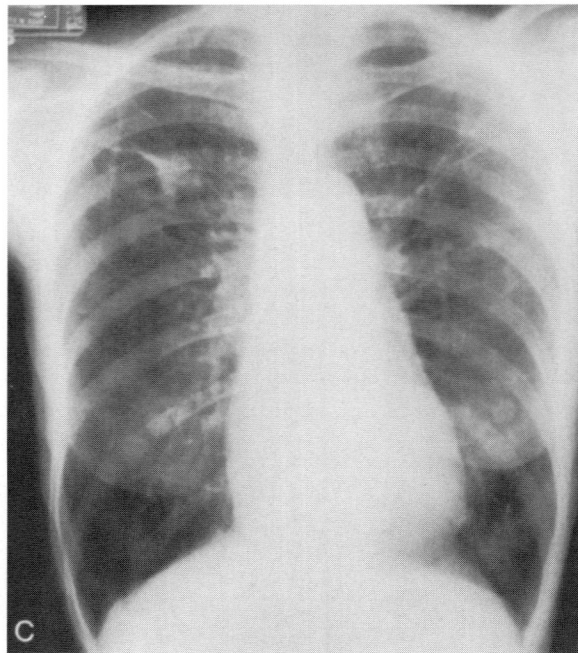

(Woodring and Vandiviere, 1990) (Fig. 22–12). Originally, pulmonary mycobacterial disease was classified on the basis of chest films as minimal, moderately advanced, or far advanced. *Minimal* disease was defined as a unilateral infiltrate with no cavities or dense areas of confluent disease. *Moderately advanced* disease was defined as infiltrates of slight to moderate density extending throughout a total volume less than that of one lung, dense confluent disease involving less than one-third of one lung, or cavitary disease with a total diameter less than 4 cm. *Far advanced* disease de-

scribed any lesions more extensive than the criteria for moderately advanced disease.

Skin Testing

Koch discovered that the subcutaneous injection of heat-killed tubercle bacilli caused an intense local reaction in patients with tuberculosis. Skin testing was refined by Florence Siebert after she isolated the purified protein derivative (PPD) from *M. tuberculosis*

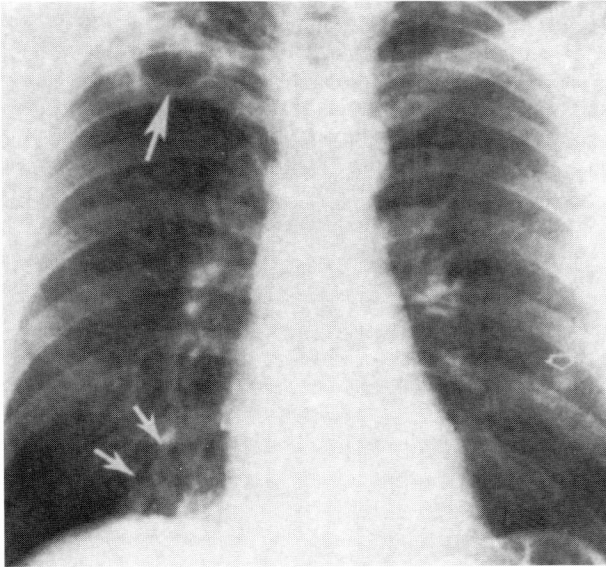

FIGURE 22–12. Large cavity in the apex of right lung *(large arrow)* with surrounding infiltrate in a patient with *Mycobacterium kansasii* pulmonary disease. Right lower lobe densities *(smaller arrows)* are from endobronchial spread. A Ghon lesion *(open arrow)* can be seen in lower left lung. (From Woodring, J. E., Vandiviere, H. M., Melvin, I. G., and Dillon, M. L.: Roentgenographic features of pulmonary disease caused by atypical mycobacteria. South. Med. J., *80*:1493, 1987.)

organisms in 1939 (Hanson and Reichman, 1989). Tuberculins prepared from other mycobacterial species were developed later. Skin testing was widely adopted as a screening test for mycobacterial infection. Most patients are sensitized to the protein fraction of the tubercle bacilli within several weeks after the onset of infection. Current standard tuberculosis skin testing involves the intracutaneous injection of 5 tuberculin units (TU) of PPD stabilized with Tween 80 on the volar aspect of the forearm. This is termed an *intermediate PPD,* and the extent of local reaction is evaluated after 48 to 72 hours. A width of induration greater than 10 mm defines a positive test. Tuberculin reactions may be blunted in the elderly or in seriously ill individuals, producing a false-negative skin test. A second intermediate PPD applied 1 week after the first minimizes the likelihood of false-negative tests. The intermediate PPD is positive in at least 90% of cases of tuberculosis infection. First-strength (1 TU) PPD and second-strength (250 TU) PPD skin tests are rarely used to confirm tuberculosis infection. PPD prepared from atypical mycobacteria can show the specific cause of mycobacterial disease weeks before culture results are available and can provide a basis for early specific chemotherapy (Woodring and Vandiviere, 1990).

Smear and Culture

The isolation of mycobacterial organisms from sputum or lung tissue is required to confirm the diagnosis of pulmonary mycobacterial disease. Early-morning sputum specimens or washings obtained by fiberoptic bronchoscopy can be especially helpful in establishing a diagnosis. The presence of acid-fast organisms on a smear allows a rapid presumptive diagnosis, but *Nocardia* are also acid-fast, and the exact infecting organism must be identified by culture and biochemical analysis. Growth of mycobacterial cultures may take 3 to 6 weeks, and it is often necessary to obtain multiple sputum samples before a positive smear or culture is obtained. Microscopic examination of a sputum smear is not particularly sensitive, since approximately 10,000 organisms per milliliter of sputum are required for smear positivity. When the clinical pattern supports the diagnosis of pulmonary mycobacterial disease, antimycobacterial chemotherapy is often begun as a 1- to 2-month therapeutic trial during the wait for sputum cultures. Because patients referred for surgical therapy frequently are infected with organisms resistant to many antimycobacterial drugs, culture results with accurate sensitivity testing for all available antimycobacterial agents are particularly important in patients being considered for surgical intervention.

CHEMOTHERAPY

The vast majority of patients with pulmonary mycobacterial disease can be cured with appropriate chemotherapy. Many antimycobacterial drugs have been developed since the early 1940s (Davidson and Le, 1992; Cynamon and Klemens, 1989). Chemotherapy for tuberculosis has become so effective that tuberculosis sanatoria and older surgical techniques for treating mycobacterial pulmonary disease have become obsolete. Effective antimycobacterial drugs have made surgical treatment of these diseases, and resectional therapy in particular, relatively safe procedures when they are required.

Treatment of pulmonary mycobacterial disease is often begun before the infecting organism is precisely identified and before the drug sensitivity pattern of the infecting organism is known. Generally, it is presumed that the infecting organism is *M. tuberculosis,* which is usually sensitive to most antimycobacterial drugs. Two or three antimycobacterial drugs should be administered initially to avoid the emergence of drug-resistant organisms (O'Brien, 1989b; Perez-Stable and Hopewell, 1989). Compliance with a prescribed chemotherapy regimen is essential to a successful outcome, and patients must be monitored closely to avoid drug toxicity. Mycobacterial organisms within the lung react differently to antimycobacterial drugs, depending on whether the organisms are extracellular or intracellular. Extracellular organisms tend to multiply rapidly in the hyperoxic neutral pH environment of the pulmonary cavity. Organisms within activated macrophages are in an acidic environment that suppresses growth. An effective treatment program halts mycobacterial growth, both intracellularly and extracellularly, converting the patient to a sputum-negative status within 6 weeks. An appropriate treatment regimen must also prevent the emergence of drug-resistant organisms, and a wide choice of antimycobacterial agents is available. Fifteen of the most commonly used antimycobacterial drugs, dosage recommendations, and the most frequently observed side effects are shown in Table 22–2.

Until recently, the standard pharmacologic regimen for the treatment of pulmonary mycobacterial infection required 18 to 24 months of continuous therapy. Two or three drugs were administered throughout the treatment period. So-called short-course therapy (6 to 9 months) has now been shown to be equally effective. The two currently recommended regimens for treatment of pulmonary tuberculosis are (1) a 6-month course with INH, rifampin, and pyrazinamide for 2 months and then INH and rifampin for 4 months or

(2) a 9-month course of INH and rifampin (Perez-Stable and Hopewell, 1989). With either regimen, ethambutol should be added for individuals with epidemiologic characteristics suggesting a greater likelihood of drug resistance (Iseman and Madsen, 1989). In this way, ethambutol is administered until sensitivity testing is completed and the drug regimen can be adjusted appropriately. Both INH and rifampin are bactericidal to extracellular and intracellular mycobacteria. If INH or rifampin cannot be tolerated, streptomycin and pyrazinamide may be substituted. Streptomycin is bactericidal to extracellular acid-fast organisms in tuberculous cavities, and pyrazinamide kills intracellular mycobacteria. If resistance to INH is documented, a 12-month course of rifampin and ethambutol, supplemented with pyrazinamide for the

■ **Table 22–2.** ANTIMYCOBACTERIAL DRUGS

Drug	Daily Dosage		Common Side Effects	Comments
	Children	*Adults*		
Isoniazid	10–20 mg/kg PO or IM	5 mg/kg PO or IM	Hepatitis; peripheral neuritis	Bactericidal to both intracellular and extracellular organisms; pyridoxine 10 mg/day as prophylaxis for neuritis
Rifampin	10–20 mg/kg PO	10 mg/kg PO	Hepatitis; febrile reaction	Bactericidal to both intracellular and extracellular organisms; colors urine orange; inhibits the effect of oral contraceptives and warfarin sodium (Coumadin)
Pyrazinamide	15–20 mg/kg PO	15–30 mg/kg PO	Hepatotoxicity; hyperuricemia; arthralgia	Bactericidal to intracellular organisms
Streptomycin	20–40 mg/kg IM	15 mg/kg IM	Eighth cranial nerve damage; nephrotoxicity	Bactericidal to extracellular organisms within cavities; limit dose to 10 mg/kg in elderly patients
Ethambutol	15–25 mg/kg PO	15–25 mg/kg PO	Optic neuritis (reversible); skin rash	Bacteriostatic for both intracellular and extracellular organisms
Ethionamide	15–20 mg/kg PO	15–20 mg/kg PO	Gastrointestinal intolerance; hepatotoxicity	Bacteriostatic to both intracellular and extracellular organisms; divided or bedtime dosage may decrease gastrointestinal intolerance
Para-aminosalicylic acid	150 mg/kg PO	150 mg/kg PO	Gastrointestinal intolerance; hepatotoxicity	Bacteriostatic to extracellular organisms only; greater than 50% incidence of gastrointestinal intolerance
Kanamycin	15–30 mg/kg IM	15–30 mg/kg IM	Eighth cranial nerve damage; nephrotoxicity	Bactericidal to extracellular organisms in cavities
Capreomycin	15–30 mg/kg IM	15–30 mg/kg IM	Eighth cranial nerve damage; nephrotoxicity	Bactericidal to extracellular organisms in cavities
Cycloserine	15–20 mg/kg PO	15–20 mg/kg PO	Psychosis; depression; seizures	Bacteriostatic to both intracellular and extracellular organisms; rarely tolerated; pyridoxine 50 mg/day may block side effects
Rifabutin	5–7 mg/kg PO	5–7 mg/kg PO	Neutropenia; nausea; diarrhea	Bactericidal; transiently colors body fluids and skin brownish-orange; rarely may cause thrombocytopenia or hepatitis
Thiocetazone	NI	2 mg/kg PO	Nausea; skin rash; bone marrow depression	Bacteriostatic; effective substitute for para-aminosalicylic acid
Ciprofloxacin	NI	15–20 mg/kg PO	Nausea; headache	Bactericidal; active against majority of mycobacteria; generally well tolerated
Ofloxacin	NI	10 mg/kg PO	Nausea; diarrhea	Bactericidal; usually well tolerated
Clofazimine	NI	1.5–2 mg/kg PO	Nausea; diarrhea; mild skin pigmentation changes	Bactericidal; usually well tolerated at dosage of 1.5 mg/kg/day

Key: PO = orally; IM = intramuscularly; NI = not indicated.

first 3 months, is recommended. Streptomycin is often also included for the first 1 to 3 months.

The primary drug-resistance rate for *M. tuberculosis* in the United States varies geographically and among ethnic groups, but is generally about 10%. In some specific groups, the rate is higher than 50% (Iseman and Madsen, 1989). Worldwide, the prevalence of primary drug resistance in *M. tuberculosis* is generally higher than that found in the United States. Areas with the highest incidence of active tuberculosis tend also to have the highest rates of *M. tuberculosis* with primary drug resistance. The primary drug-resistance rate for tuberculosis is estimated to be 20% in China and India and 30% to 35% in Pakistan and the Philippines. The increasing frequency of primary drug-resistant tuberculosis and of atypical mycobacterial pulmonary disease make accurate sensitivity testing to a wide spectrum of chemotherapeutic agents critical to optimize the drug regimen. Although atypical mycobacteria are frequently resistant in vitro to many or all of the common antimycobacterial drugs, chemotherapy regimens utilizing four and five drugs simultaneously may continue to be moderately effective (Tsukamura, 1988). Efficacy of any drug regimen is increased by selection of drugs to which the particular mycobacterial organism is susceptible (Horsburgh et al., 1987). Because pulmonary mycobacterial disease caused by drug-resistant organisms is selectively referred for surgical intervention, accurate drug-susceptibility testing and familiarity with the use of a wide variety of antimycobacterial drugs are important for the thoracic surgeon.

Coordination of chemotherapy and surgical intervention requires careful planning. Patients who have been converted to sputum-negative status preoperatively have fewer complications of resectional surgery (Moran et al., 1983; Pomerantz et al., 1991). Optimal pulmonary toilet, careful selection of chemotherapy, and the addition of one or two new antimycobacterial drugs during the perioperative period are useful in reducing perioperative morbidity. Whenever possible, the patient should receive 1 to 2 months of appropriate chemotherapy prior to operation. In treating multiple drug–resistant organisms (either *M. tuberculosis* or atypical mycobacteria), two or three drugs to which the infecting organism is sensitive should be given perioperatively and for 6 to 9 months postoperatively. In the case of organisms that exhibit resistance to all antimycobacterial drugs, the administration of INH and rifampin and an aminoglycoside perioperatively and INH and rifampin for a period of 9 to 12 months postoperatively is still recommended.

COLLAPSE THERAPY

During the 19th century, it was noted that, when a pneumothorax occurred in a patient with pulmonary tuberculosis, the patient's symptoms often seemed to improve, popularizing the concept that collapsing the affected portion of lung allowed the diseased area to rest and recover. It is likely that the efficacy of collapse therapy derived from the lowering of oxygen tensions in the collapsed portions of the lung. *M. tuberculosis* is a strict aerobe, and an anaerobic environment effectively inhibits mycobacterial growth. Artificially induced pneumothorax gained popularity at the beginning of the 20th century, although it required repetitive instillations of gas into the pleural space at 2- to 3-week intervals. Various other techniques to induce collapse of the infected portions of the lung were developed subsequently. Unilateral phrenic nerve division, pneumoperitoneum, thoracoplasty, extrapleural pneumonolysis, and extraperiosteal thoracoplasty with plombage were employed with varying degrees of success. Surgical division of the phrenic nerve and pneumoperitoneum tended to collapse the lower lobes as a result of elevation of one or both hemidiaphragms and to compress the apex only slightly. Extrapleural pneumonolysis separated both pleurae and the lung from the overlying chest wall and filled the space that was created with paraffin, fat, air, or another foreign material. The lung and overlying pleurae were taken down from the rib cage in the extrapleural plane, creating an apical space adjacent to the diseased portion of the lung. When air was used as a space filler, frequent refills were required, just as with artificially induced pneumothorax. Plombage thoracoplasty was a variant of extrapleural pneumonolysis using a foreign material such as paraffin or lucite spheres to fill the extrapleural space created within the rib cage. Perforation or erosion of the filling material into the lung, which created a bronchial fistula into the extrapleural space, was a serious potential complication. Extraperiosteal thoracoplasty with plombage involved stripping the periosteum and intercostal muscles away from the ribs so that they could collapse inward with both pleural layers. In this procedure, the plombage material was separated from the lung by the thickness of the chest-wall muscles as well as both layers of pleura, reducing the frequency of erosion of the filling material into the lung parenchyma. These procedures collapsed the diseased upper lobe of the lung without significantly impairing ventilation of the middle or lower lobes. Collapse of the apex of the lung was desirable in most patients because this was the portion of the lung most frequently involved by tuberculosis. Plombage thoracoplasty was a relatively nondeforming operation, because the shape of the overlying chest wall remained unchanged. Plombage thoracoplasty interfered less with chest-wall function and stability than did standard thoracoplasty.

The various forms of collapse therapy achieved sputum conversion without chemotherapy surprisingly in 30% to 60% of patients. Nevertheless, complications such as erosion of the plombage material into the lung were common, and collapse therapy in its various forms is now obsolete. However, patients who have been treated with these forms of collapse therapy may be referred to a thoracic surgeon for late complications of their original operations. Therefore, thoracic surgeons need to be familiar with these out-dated procedures.

THORACOPLASTY

In the 50 years preceding the discovery of effective chemotherapy for tuberculosis in 1946, extrapleural paravertebral thoracoplasty was the most frequently employed surgical procedure for the treatment of pulmonary tuberculosis. The procedure was developed in the German university clinics and refined in the United States by John Alexander. Thoracoplasty achieved closure of tuberculous cavities in more than 80% of patients without chemotherapy and with an operative mortality of approximately 10%. Today, thoracoplasty is rarely, if ever, indicated as primary treatment for pulmonary tuberculosis (Hopkins et al., 1985). Paravertebral thoracoplasty remains a reasonable operation for the treatment of selected tuberculous bronchopleural fistulas and empyemas and for bronchopleural fistulas complicating surgical resections in other settings. The resurgence of tuberculosis and atypical mycobacterial disease in immunocompromised patients, especially those with AIDS, has created a clinical setting similar to that in the era prior to effective antimycobacterial chemotherapy. Many of these patients develop bronchopleural fistulas and empyemas related to mycobacterial infections. They respond poorly to chemotherapy and are often too debilitated to be candidates for aggressive resectional surgery. Thoracoplasty and other "outdated" surgical procedures from the prechemotherapy era may need to be employed with increasing frequency in this subgroup of patients.

Thoracoplasty should be considered when the virulence of the infecting organism or the poor overall condition of the patient makes resectional surgery hazardous.

A modified or "tailoring" thoracoplasty, removing only four to five ribs, is indicated as a secondary procedure to obliterate an infected apical space and the accompanying bronchopleural fistula that may complicate a lung resection. A modified thoracoplasty may be indicated at the time of a primary resection for suppurative pulmonary disease when the extensive pleural reaction inhibits full expansion of the remaining lung and makes it obvious that a large apical space will persist. Under such circumstances, any parenchymal air leaks in the remaining lung seal much more quickly if a modified thoracoplasty is performed. The pleural reaction caused by tuberculosis inhibits shift of the mediastinum and upward movement of the diaphragm, predisposing to postoperative "space problems" following pulmonary resections. Such space problems increase the likelihood of a postresectional bronchopleural fistula following lung resection for suppurative disease.

Operative Procedure

Thoracoplasty is a deforming operation that radically alters the shape of the patient's chest wall. In planning a thoracoplasty, it is important to remember that the operation causes an irreversible loss of ventilatory capacity on the operated side. The patient's pulmonary function must be assessed to be certain that this loss can be tolerated. An appropriately planned thoracoplasty removes enough of the chest wall to collapse the cavitated part of the lung or obliterate the residual pleural space problem. The number of ribs that must be removed can be judged from the posteroanterior chest film by tracing the projection of each upper rib on the lung posteriorly and anteriorly. Originally, it was recommended that no more than three to five ribs be removed at any one stage to avoid excessive chest-wall instability. With the availability of ventilators, more ribs can be resected at one time without excessive postoperative complications. General anesthesia is routinely used, although the operation was originally performed with the patient under regional anesthesia. The patient is placed in the full lateral position or slightly toward the prone position from the lateral. A high parascapular incision is made extending from 5 to 6 cm below the upper edge of the trapezius along the posterior border of the scapula and turning anteriorly just below the tip of the scapula (Fig. 22–13). The trapezius and rhomboid muscles are divided and the scapula is elevated off the chest wall. The insertions of the serratus onto the upper ribs are divided and the entire second rib and the posterior two-thirds of the third rib are resected subperiosteally. The first rib is approached inferiorly and its periosteum is stripped off its inferior surface. The periosteum is stripped off the superior surface of the first rib, working from within the periosteal sheath, which aids in avoidance of damage to the subclavian vessels and the brachial plexus. The first rib is divided posteriorly with rib shears, with care taken to avoid any trauma to the subclavian vessels or the brachial plexus. Downward traction on the divided first rib allows exposure of the bands of Sebileau, which must be divided to allow collapse of the apex of the thorax (Fig. 22–14). Traction on the posterior portion of the first rib allows exposure and division of the anterior costochondral junction. At the same time, or occasionally at a second-stage operation 2 weeks later, progressively shorter segments of the fourth through sixth or seventh ribs are removed through the same incision with a slight anterior extension. The fourth rib is resected as far as the anterior axillary line, and at each successive lower rib, less is resected anteriorly. A five-rib thoracoplasty reduces the size of the thoracic cavity by 25 to 30% but does not allow the scapula to collapse medially against the mediastinum. If a five-rib thoracoplasty is performed, the scapular tip should be resected to avoid pressure on the edge of the sixth or seventh rib and to avoid possible entrapment of the scapular tip inside the sixth rib, which is an aggravating complication that limits shoulder mobility and can be very annoying. A seven-rib thoracoplasty is required to achieve a severe degree of collapse of the thorax and the underlying lung. The thoracoplasty incision is closed in layers without drainage.

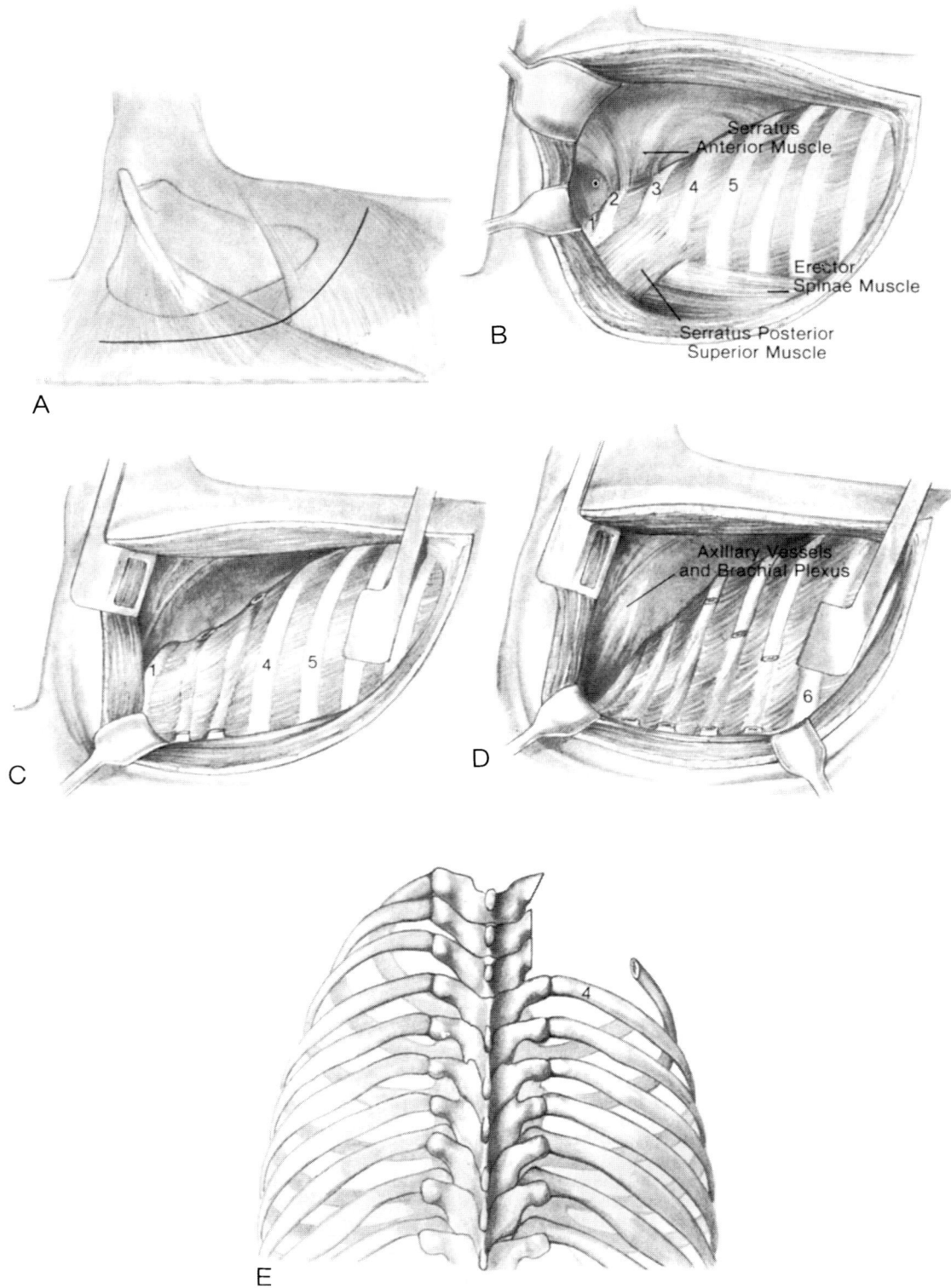

FIGURE 22–13. Technique of extrapleural paravertebral thoracoplasty. *A,* With a patient in the lateral position, the extent of the skin and muscle incision is shown. *B,* Exposure after elevation of the scapula from the chest wall. *C,* The second and third ribs are excised subperiosteally before first rib resection. *D,* Progressively less rib is resected anteriorly proceeding inferiorly. *E,* Appearance of the rib cage "squared off" superiorly, fashioned by leaving the anterior portions of the lower ribs. (*A–E,* From Hood, R. M.: Techniques in General Thoracic Surgery. Philadelphia, W. B. Saunders, 1985, p. 187.)

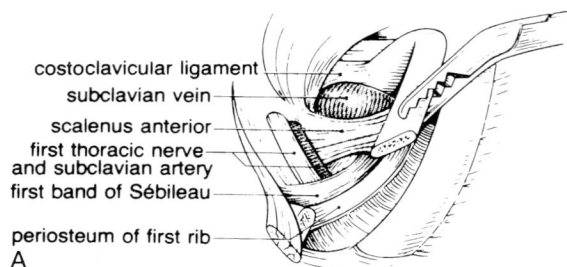

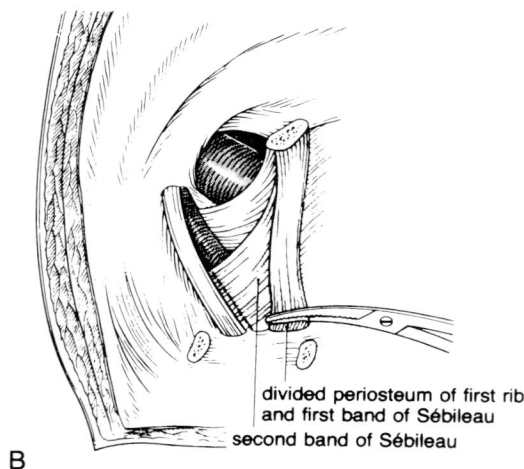

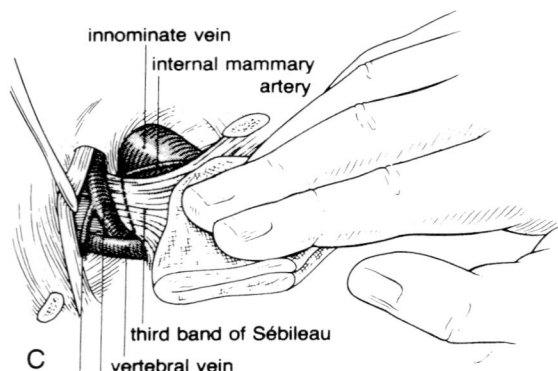

FIGURE 22–14. Operative technique of excision of the first rib and division of bands of Sebileau during thoracoplasty. After the first rib is divided posteriorly, downward traction on the first rib facilitates exposure of the neurovascular structures, the anterior scalene muscle, the first band of Sebileau, and the costoclavicular ligament anteriorly. After dividing the first rib far anteriorly, full mobilization and collapse of the apex of the pleural space require division of the periosteum of the first rib and the fascia (the first band of Sebileau) over the first thoracic nerve. The second band (the fascia over the artery) is divided next. Division of the third band, anterior to the artery, completes the extrafascial apicolysis. (*A–C*, Reprinted with permission from Nohl-Oser, H. C., Nissen, R., and Schreiber, H. W.: Surgery of the Lung, p. 150. 1981, copyright Thieme Medical Publishers, Inc.)

Postoperative Care

Postoperative care after thoracoplasty includes intensive pulmonary toilet, nutritional support, and physiotherapy for generalized conditioning and to minimize scoliosis. Some degree of scoliosis is ensured by removal of the first rib, but this can be lessened by postoperative exercises. Lying on the operated side with a roll or sandbag positioned in the axilla improves posture, accentuates the collapsing effect, and discourages development of fluid collections in the deeper layers of the incision. Any such fluid collections may become infected and require drainage.

PULMONARY RESECTION FOR MYCOBACTERIAL DISEASE

Operative treatment of pulmonary mycobacterial disease is rarely necessary. When an operation is required, resection of the diseased or destroyed portion of the lung is the procedure of choice. Prior to the availability of effective chemotherapy, pulmonary resection for tuberculosis had an operative mortality of 20 to 40%. Once effective chemotherapy for pulmonary tuberculosis became available, pulmonary resection rapidly replaced thoracoplasty as the surgical treatment of choice. Compared with thoracoplasty, pulmonary resection has the advantage of achieving prompt conversion to sputum-negative status in a single stage without creating any chest-wall deformity or severe limitation of ventilatory capacity. Elective pulmonary resection for mycobacterial disease now carries a low mortality and morbidity (Moran et al., 1983; Pomerantz et al., 1991).

Indications for Resection

The efficacy of modern antimycobacterial chemotherapy has reduced the commonly accepted indications for surgical intervention and pulmonary resection to the following:

1. **Persistently positive sputum cultures with cavitation after 5 to 6 months of continuous optimal chemotherapy with two or more drugs.** The chemotherapy should include INH and rifampin, and the organism must be shown to be susceptible to both drugs. Otherwise, a change in the chemotherapy regimen is indicated. Relative indications for surgical intervention such as severe cavitation, bronchiectasis, or bronchial stenosis may contribute to the failure of chemotherapy in some individuals. In such circumstances, these complications of mycobacterial disease become relative indications for surgical treatment.

2. **Localized pulmonary disease caused by *M. avium–intracellulare* (or another atypical mycobacterium with a similar broad resistance to chemotherapy).** Localized pulmonary disease due to drug-resistant *M. tuberculosis* is also an indication for pulmonary resection. *Localized* disease is any disease that can be encompassed by one or two pulmonary resections (Fig. 22–15).

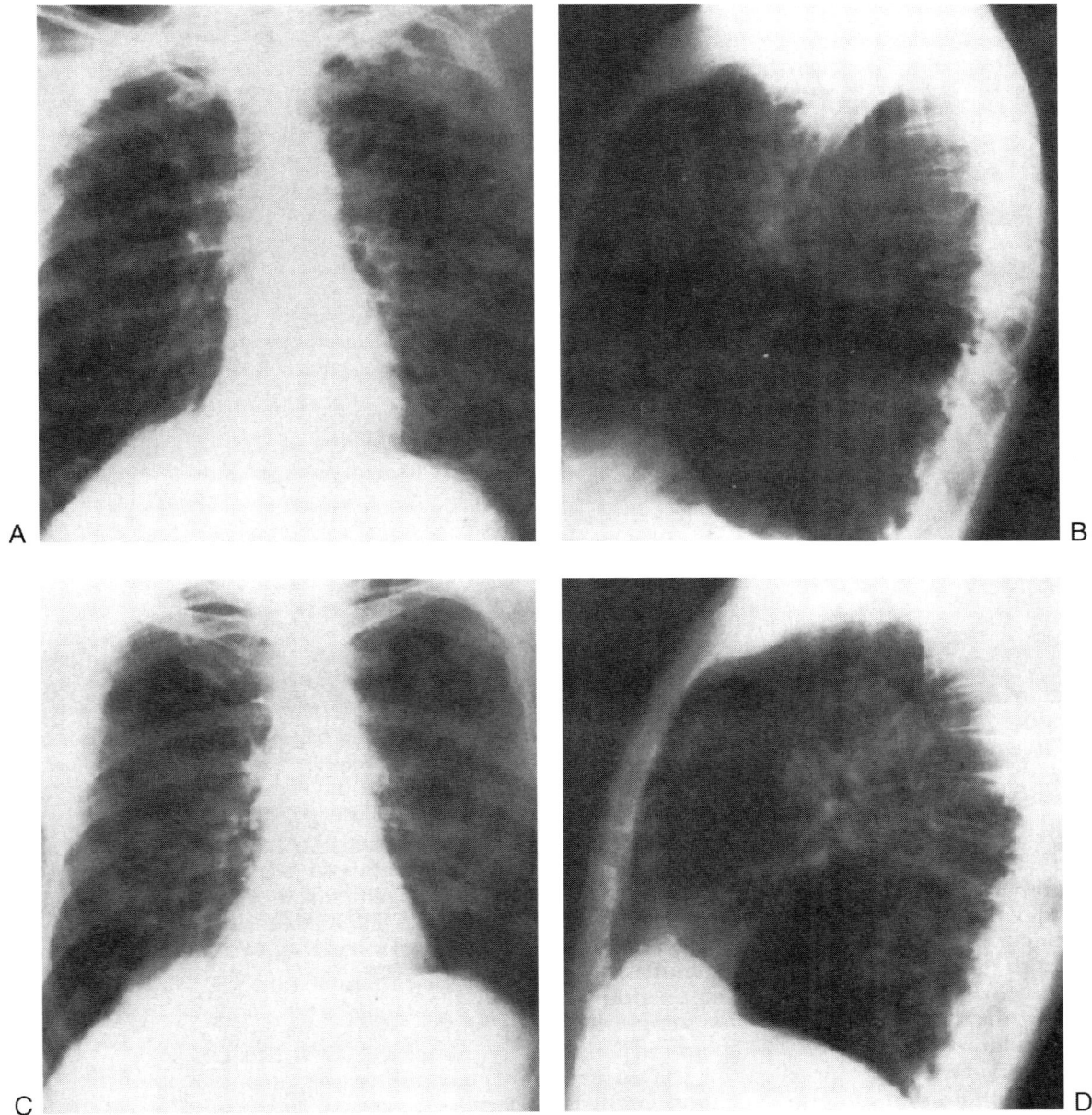

FIGURE 22–15. Preoperative posteroanterior *(A)* and lateral *(B)* chest radiographs of a 64-year-old man with extensive infiltration of both upper lobes by *M. avium–intracellulare* infection, and postoperative posteroanterior *(C)* and lateral *(D)* chest radiographs of the same patient following staged bilateral upper lobectomies. *(A–D,* From Moran, J. F., Alexander, L. G., Staub, E. W., et al.: Long-term results of pulmonary resection for atypical mycobacterial disease. Ann. Thorac. Surg., *35:*602, 1983.)

3. **A mass lesion of the lung in an area of tuberculous involvement.** Resection is done for simultaneous diagnosis of the lesion and treatment of the mycobacterial disease. In the 1990s, this is undoubtedly the most common indication for surgical resection of pulmonary mycobacterial disease (Whyte et al., 1989).

4. **Massive life-threatening hemoptysis or recurrent severe hemoptysis.** This is an indication for resection of the portion of the lung that is the source of the hemorrhage. Pulmonary hemorrhage is a rare but frequently fatal complication of pulmonary mycobacterial disease. Massive hemoptysis is defined as greater than 600 ml/24 hr, whereas severe hemoptysis is defined as greater than 200 ml/24 hr. Tuberculosis continues to be the most common cause of massive hemoptysis. Asphyxiation, rather than hypovolemia, is the usual cause of death from hemoptysis. The site of bleeding in severe hemoptysis is almost invariably a cavitary lesion (Fig. 22–16). The bleeding arises from the abundant bronchial arterial circulation to the cavitated portion of the lung. Mild or moderate hemorrhage usually ceases with sedation, bedrest, and careful control of the patient's blood pressure. Bronchoscopy is performed to determine the lobe from

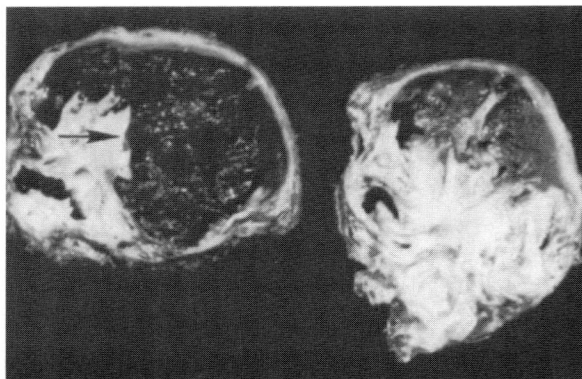

FIGURE 22–16. Right upper lobectomy specimen showing a large tuberculous cavity *(arrow)* filled with clotted blood adjacent to an area of fibrosis with smaller chronic cavities. The patient presented with massive hemoptysis. (From Haque, A. K.: The pathology and pathophysiology of mycobacterial infections. J. Thorac. Imaging, 5:14, 1990.)

which the bleeding arises. Frequently, these patients have bilateral cavitary changes radiographically. The source of bleeding should be resected on an urgent basis after an episode of massive or recurrent severe hemoptysis, because mortality is high when resection is not done (Corey and Hla, 1987). Prior to resection, the area of hemorrhage can be controlled by using a double-lumen endotracheal tube or selective mainstem bronchus blockade with a balloon catheter placed at the time of bronchoscopy. Severe hemoptysis is very unpredictable, and fatal hemorrhage can occur suddenly in seemingly stable patients who are awaiting endoscopy or operation.

5. **A bronchopleural fistula secondary to mycobacterial infection that does not respond to tube thoracostomy.** Usually, this requires surgical treatment and may require pulmonary resection. Simple tuberculous effusions almost always resolve spontaneously or respond promptly to chemotherapy. The mixed tuberculous and pyogenic empyema that occurs when a bronchopleural fistula develops in a lung severely damaged by mycobacterial disease rarely responds to antimicrobial therapy alone. The efficacy of tube thoracostomy is limited in such cases by the dense pleural reaction that inhibits full reexpansion of the lung and prevents complete reapposition of the pleural surfaces. Formal decortication can lead to full reexpansion of the underlying lung with excellent recovery of pulmonary function, and localized areas of infection can be resected simultaneously. Often, the pleural reaction is so intense and extends so far into the substance of the lung that decortication is impossible. Open drainage of the pleural space by creation of an Eloesser flap (Eloesser, 1969) is an excellent alternative procedure for such cases, especially if the patient's overall condition is marginal. When an entire lung is destroyed by mycobacterial disease and there is a surrounding empyema, pleuropneumonectomy can be a dramatically effective treatment in carefully selected patients.

Special Circumstances

Several special situations occasionally call for surgical treatment of pulmonary mycobacterial disease. In general, surgical intervention is indicated when the expected operative morbidity and mortality are small compared with the natural history of the disease, the prospect for control of the disease is excellent, and the period of disability as a result of the surgical intervention is likely to be brief. Patients severely symptomatic from a destroyed lobe or bronchiectatic area of the lung may benefit from resection. Patients may have persistent low-grade hemoptysis or recurrent episodes of bacterial infection in such areas. Patients with thick-walled cavities who have reactivated mycobacterial disease or who cannot comply with prolonged chemotherapy may benefit from resection of the diseased area. A patient with a "trapped lung" with severely decreased ventilatory capacity after a tuberculous empyema may benefit from decortication with or without partial resection in order to allow full expansion of the underlying lung and restoration of the patient's ventilatory capacity. There are a few specific contraindications to pulmonary resection for mycobacterial disease. Widespread pulmonary or endobronchial disease is generally a contraindication to resection. Children with mycobacterial disease rarely require lung resection (Smith, 1989; Starke et al., 1992). Mycobacterial disease in children often progresses to lobar tuberculous pneumonia with massive lymph node enlargement, but cavitation is rare (Stansberry, 1990). The enlarged hilar lymph nodes often obstruct the lobar bronchus completely in children (Fig. 22–17). Although these radiologic findings may persist for months, chemotherapy is almost invariably curative even in advanced mycobacterial disease in children. The advanced radiographic findings generally resolve completely in children with excellent recovery of pulmonary function.

In planning an operation for mycobacterial disease, as in other pulmonary surgery, it is important that the patient's cardiopulmonary reserve be adequate to sustain the patient through the contemplated procedure. The patient's likely 1-second forced vital capacity (FEV_1) after operation can be predicted from pulmonary function tests and a careful examination of the patient's chest films. Adults with a postoperative FEV_1 of less than 1000 ml have severe difficulty clearing pulmonary secretions and are at high risk for postoperative complications. Every effort should be made to convert the patient to sputum-negative status prior to operation, including the administration of additional antimycobacterial drugs perioperatively. Nutritional support and physical therapy to encourage overall physical conditioning and optimal pulmonary toilet are beneficial preoperatively. Preoperative bronchoscopy should be performed on all patients considered for pulmonary resection to exclude active proximal endobronchial disease. Active endobronchial disease contraindicates resection because it interferes with the healing of the bronchial stump. Gener-

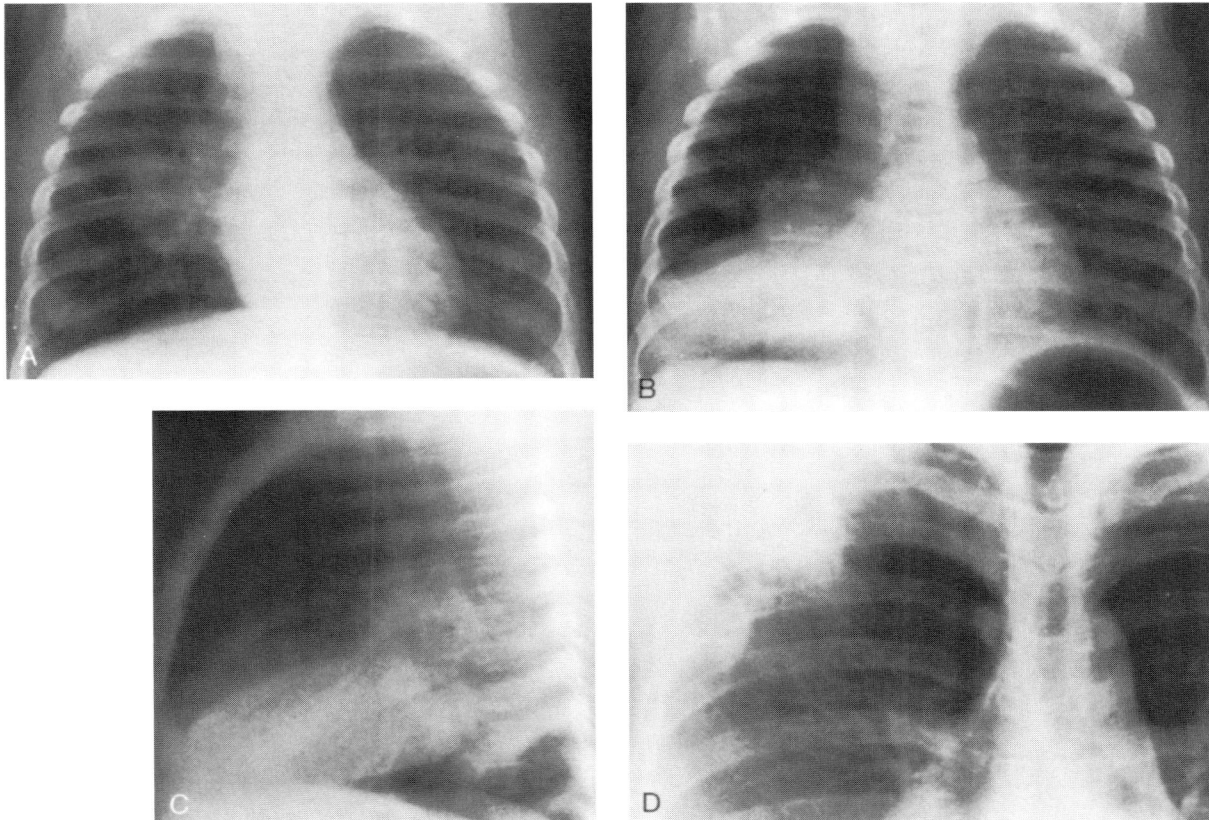

FIGURE 22–17. Chest radiographs of a 5-month-old girl with a family history of active tuberculosis. The initial film *(A)* shows prominent right hilar and right paratracheal adenopathy. One month later *(B* and *C)*, right middle lobe atelectasis has occurred. The patient's mother *(D)* had right upper lobe tuberculosis. *(A–D,* From Stansberry, S. D.: Tuberculosis in infants and children. J. Thorac. Imaging, 5:22, 1990.)

ally, proximal endobronchial disease can be cleared by chemotherapy prior to pulmonary resection.

OPERATIVE MANAGEMENT

Use of a double-lumen endotracheal tube makes resection for tuberculosis technically easier and safer. The dependent lung can be protected from contamination by secretions from the infected upper lung while the patient is in the lateral position. With severe hemoptysis, a double-lumen tube partially protects the dependent lung during the resection of the bleeding portion of the upper lung.

The extent of pulmonary resection depends on the extent of the mycobacterial disease and is guided by the principle that all gross evidence of disease should be resected. The extent of pulmonary involvement can be determined by careful examination of preoperative chest films or computed tomograms (Kuhlman et al., 1990), and quantitative ventilation-perfusion scans can be very useful in planning the extent of pulmonary resection (Pomerantz et al., 1991). Conservation of pulmonary tissue and pulmonary function is desirable; however, wedge resection and segmentectomy are not often applicable for the control of pulmonary mycobacterial disease. A generous wedge resection using staplers can be applied in the setting of a mass

lesion that is being excised to exclude the presence of carcinoma or, in the case of hemoptysis, secondary to a localized peripheral cavity. The dense pleural reaction characteristic of mycobacterial disease makes separation of the segments in the upper lobes difficult. For active mycobacterial disease, a lobectomy or pneumonectomy is usually required, and it is occasionally necessary to combine an upper lobectomy with wedge excision of the superior segment of the lower lobe to remove all gross disease (Moran et al., 1983). Pneumonectomy is required only in the setting of a totally destroyed lung. Patients can tolerate bilateral staged upper lobectomies, even if the superior segment or right middle lobe has been resected in combination with the upper lobe on the same side.

The operative techniques of lobectomy and pneumonectomy as presented elsewhere in this text do not need to be altered for the patient with tuberculosis. Because mycobacterial disease is a peripheral process with overlying dense pleural reaction, it is frequently necessary to mobilize portions of the lung in the *extrapleural* plane. Liberal use of the electrocautery in dissecting the extrapleural plane reduces blood loss. Blood loss during these procedures is often relatively large. Great care must be taken to avoid damage to neural and vascular structures at the apex of the pleural space when developing the extrapleural plane over the apex of the lung. Full reexpansion of the remaining lung tissue is important to avoid the complications of atelectasis, hemothorax, and apical space problems. Two large chest tubes should be inserted in the apex of the pleural space and placed on suction postoperatively. Postoperative bronchoscopy may be required at the end of the procedure to clear infected secretions or blood from the airway, even when a double-lumen endotracheal tube has been used. Bedside bronchoscopy with the patient under topical anesthesia may be required during the first several postoperative days to optimize pulmonary toilet and to avoid segmental or lobar atelectasis. These patients tend to have very thick, tenacious secretions.

When extensive pulmonary parenchymal mycobacterial disease is complicated by a chronic empyema, an extrapleural pneumonectomy may be required. This is a difficult procedure that carries a significant morbidity and mortality. The preoperative preparation and anesthetic management should be the same as those described earlier for other patients with pulmonary tuberculosis. With the patient in a full lateral position, a standard posterolateral thoracotomy incision is made, resecting the fifth rib subperiosteally. The goal is to resect the entire reactive pleura, the underlying empyema cavity, and the lung without entering the empyema cavity itself (Fig. 22–18). A plane of dissection along the extrapleural space is developed superiorly and inferiorly from the fifth rib incision. This plane is developed further anteriorly and posteriorly until the entire empyema cavity, still enclosed by its overlying peel, has been mobilized from the chest wall. Once the mediastinal surface of the lung is reached, the adhesions tend to be less dense and more easily divided. As the hilum of the lung is approached, the dissection can be taken back inside the pleura or can remain extrapleural and even be taken within the pericardium. The most hazardous part of this procedure is mobilization of the apex of the lung. Damage to the subclavian vessels and brachial plexus must be avoided as the apex of the lung is mobilized, and care must be taken posteriorly to avoid damage to the esophagus. Placement of a nasogastric tube or a bougie within the esophagus at the start of the procedure facilitates identification of the esophagus. Once the entire lung has been mobilized to the hilum, the hilar structures are separated in the standard manner. The bronchus, pulmonary artery, and both pulmonary veins are divided and secured by standard techniques. After a careful check for hemostasis, the pleural space is irrigated copiously and the incision is closed by standard techniques with or without drainage of the pleural space.

Complications of Resection

Administration of effective antimycobacterial drugs, judicious timing of operation, careful operative technique, and attentive postoperative care are the critically important factors in avoiding serious complications from pulmonary resection for mycobacterial disease (Moran et al., 1983; Pomerantz et al., 1991).

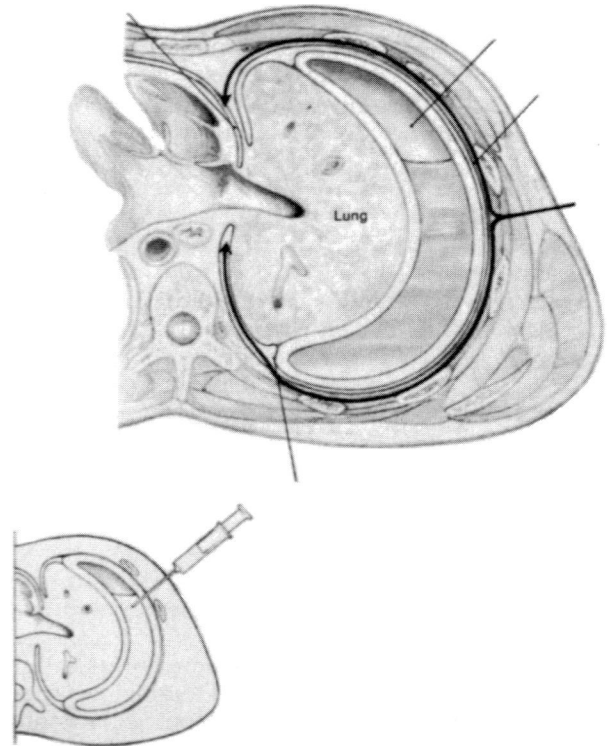

FIGURE 22–18. Technique of extrapleural pneumonectomy. *A,* The plane of dissection is developed in the extrapleural space and is carried beyond the empyema sac to the mediastinal surface of the lung. *B,* With a large empyema sac, aspiration is useful to allow more room within the chest for dissection. Aspiration also reduces the likelihood of endobronchial spillage during dissection and manipulation. (*A* and *B,* From Hood, R. M., Antman, K., Boyd, A., et al.: Surgical Diseases of the Pleura and Chest Wall. Philadelphia, W. B. Saunders, 1986, p. 126.)

Patients referred for operation generally have problems that predispose them to perioperative complications (Reed et al., 1989). Good pulmonary toilet and careful attention to the pleural drainage system are necessary to ensure full reexpansion of the remaining lung and to avoid apical space problems. Two specific complications of resection for mycobacterial disease are particularly worrisome: *empyema,* with or without bronchopleural fistula, and *bronchogenic* spread of the mycobacterial disease. These complications occur more frequently when the patient is sputum-positive at the time of operation. The incidence of bronchopleural fistula after resection for mycobacterial disease is approximately 3%, clearly higher than in pulmonary resections for other reasons. An apical space problem occurs after approximately 20% of resections for mycobacterial disease, but only 10 to 15% of these patients develop a bronchopleural fistula or empyema. Judicious use of thoracoplasty or liberal use of muscle flaps in patients with positive sputa at the time of operation can minimize the incidence of bronchopleural fistulas and apical space problems (Pomerantz et al., 1991). Appropriate treatment of empyema in this setting is tube thoracostomy with later conversion to open drainage if a lung remnant remains. Subsequent thoracoplasty may be required. Bronchogenic spread of mycobacterial infection perioperatively is a serious but uncommon complication. Appropriate chemotherapy, double-lumen endotracheal tubes, and good pulmonary toilet perioperatively have essentially eliminated this complication.

Mortality and Long-Term Results

Careful patient selection, improved anesthetic techniques, the use of stapling devices, and better chemotherapy have contributed to the steadily decreasing morbidity and mortality associated with resectional surgery for pulmonary mycobacterial disease. Resectional surgery is now employed in a highly selected group of patients who have failed chemotherapy or who have suffered complications such as massive hemoptysis or bronchopleural fistula. Mortality for pulmonary resection is low with minimal morbidity when surgical intervention is elective. When resection is performed as an emergency procedure, mortality is significant and perioperative morbidity quite common. Pneumonectomy and especially extrapleural pneumonectomy carry significantly higher risks. Despite perioperative complication rates for pulmonary resection for mycobacterial disease that range from 20 to 45%, the incidence of major complications is generally less than 15%. Long-term prognosis after successful resection is excellent, with 85 to 95% of patients who undergo operation for active mycobacterial disease surviving and free of disease 5 to 8 years after operation.

SELECTED BIBLIOGRAPHY

Alexander, J.: The Collapse Therapy of Pulmonary Tuberculosis. Springfield, IL, Charles C Thomas, 1937.

This text is the classic in the surgical treatment of pulmonary tuberculosis. The history of surgical treatment is covered and all forms of collapse therapy, including thoracoplasty, are described in detail.

Bates, B.: Bargaining For Life: A Social History of Tuberculosis, 1876–1938. Philadelphia, University of Pennsylvania Press, 1992.

This volume is a well-written account of the social impact and medical treatment of tuberculosis prior to effective chemotherapy.

Caldwell, M.: The Last Crusade: The War on Consumption 1862–1954. Riverside, NJ, Atheneum, 1988.

This cultural history of the battle against tuberculosis focuses on sanatorium treatment in the United States.

Davidson, P. T., and Le, H. Q.: Drug Treatment of Tuberculosis—1992. Drugs, 43:651, 1992.

Exhaustive summary of current chemotherapy for tuberculosis, including rationale of treatment strategies and pharmacologic recommendations about all currently available antituberculous drugs.

Grange, J. M.: Mycobacteria and Human Disease. London, Edward Arnold, 1988.

A detailed review of the bacteriology of mycobacteria and the diseases caused by the various mycobacteria.

Iseman, M. D., and Gobal, M.: Treatment of tuberculosis. Adv. Intern. Med., 33:253, 1988.

This article outlines alternative medical therapies for pulmonary mycobacterial infections.

Pomerantz, M., Madsen, L., Goble, M., and Iseman, M.: Surgical management of resistant mycobacterial tuberculosis and other mycobacterial pulmonary infections. Ann. Thorac. Surg., 52:1108, 1991.

A recent large series of lung resections for drug resistant M. tuberculosis infection and other mycobacterial infections is reported in detail. Current guidelines for surgical intervention for pulmonary mycobacterial infections are given.

Rieder, H. L., Cauthen, G. M., Comstock, G. W., and Snider, D. E., Jr.: Epidemiology of tuberculosis in the United States. Epidemiol. Rev., 11:79, 1989.

This article carefully analyzes the changing epidemiology of tuberculosis in the United States.

Rubin, S. A.: Tuberculosis 1990. J. Thorac. Imaging, 5:1, 1990.

This symposium reviews the microbiology, pathophysiology, and treatment of pulmonary mycobacterial infections with particular emphasis on the radiologic manifestations of these diseases and their complications.

Snider, D. E., Jr.: Mycobacterial diseases. Clin. Chest Med., 10:297, 1989.

This volume presents recent reviews of the epidemiology of tuberculosis and atypical mycobacterial diseases. Recent advances in short-course chemotherapy and the most current mycobacterial diagnostic techniques are presented.

BIBLIOGRAPHY

Alexander, J.: The Surgery of Pulmonary Tuberculosis. Philadelphia and New York, Lea & Febiger, 1925.
Auerbach, O., and Dail, D. H.: Mycobacterial infections. In Dail, D. H., and Hammer, S. P. (eds): Pulmonary Pathology. New York, Springer-Verlag, 1988.
Bloch, A. B., Rieder, H. L., Kelly, G. D., et al.: The epidemiology of tuberculosis in the United States. Semin. Respir. Infect., 4:157, 1989.
Boyars, M. C.: The microbiology, chemotherapy, and surgical treatment of tuberculosis. J. Thorac. Imaging, 5:1, 1990.
Buckner, C. B., and Walker, C. W.: Radiologic manifestations of adult tuberculosis. J. Thorac. Imaging, 5:28, 1990.
Chan, H. S., Sun, A., and Hoheisel, G. B.: Endobronchial tuberculosis—Is corticosteroid treatment useful? A report of 8 cases and review of the literature. Postgrad. Med. J., 66:822, 1990.
Contreras, M. A., Cheung, O. T., Sanders, D. E., and Goldstein, R. S.: Pulmonary infection with nontuberculous mycobacteria. Am. Rev. Respir. Dis., 137:149, 1988.
Corey, R., and Hla, K. M.: Major and massive hemoptysis: Reassessment of conservative management. Am. J. Med. Sci., 294:301, 1987.
Crawford, J. T., Eisenach, K. D., and Bates, J. H.: Diagnosis of tuberculosis: Present and future. Semin. Respir. Infect., 4:171, 1989.
Cynamon, M. H., and Klemens, S. P.: New antimycobacterial agents. Clin. Chest Med., 10:355, 1989.
Davidson, P. T.: The diagnosis and management of disease caused by M. avium complex, M. kansasii, and other Mycobacteria. Clin. Chest Med., 10:431, 1989.
Davidson, P. T., and Le, H. Q.: Drug treatment of tuberculosis in 1992. Drugs, 43:651, 1992.
Eloesser, L.: Of an operation for tuberculous empyema. Ann. Thorac. Surg., 8:355, 1969.
Goodman, P. C.: Pulmonary tuberculosis in patients with acquired immunodeficiency syndrome. J. Thorac. Imaging, 5:38, 1990.
Grange, J. M.: Mycobacteria and Human Disease. London, Edward Arnold, 1988.
Hanson, C. A., and Reichman, L. B.: Tuberculosis skin testing and preventive therapy. Semin. Respir. Infect., 4:182, 1989.
Haque, A. K.: The pathology and pathophysiology of mycobacterial infections. J. Thorac. Imaging, 5:8, 1990.
Hopkins, R. A., Ungerleider, R. M., Staub, E. W., and Young, W. G., Jr.: The modern use of thoracoplasty. Ann. Thorac. Surg., 40:181, 1985.
Horsburgh, C. R., Jr.: Epidemiology of mycobacterial diseases in AIDS. Res. Microbiol., 143:372, 1992.
Horsburgh, C. R., Jr., Mason, U. G., III, Heifets, L. B., et al.: Response to therapy of pulmonary Mycobacterium avium–

intracellulare infection correlates with results of in-vitro susceptibility testing. Am. Rev. Respir. Dis., *135*:418, 1987.

Iseman, M. D., and Madsen, L. A.: Drug-resistant tuberculosis.
Clin. Chest Med., *10*:341, 1989.

Koch, R.: Die Aetiologie der Tuberculose, a translation by B. Pinner
and M. Pinner. Am. Rev. Tuberc., *25*:285, 1932.

Kuhlman, J. E., Deutsch, J. H., Fishman, E. K., and Siegelman, S. S.:
CT features of thoracic mycobacterial disease. Radiographics,
10:413, 1990.

Moran, J. F., Alexander, L. G., Staub, E. W., et al.: Long-term results
of pulmonary resection for atypical mycobacterial disease.
Ann. Thorac. Surg., *35*:597, 1983.

O'Brien, R. J.: The epidemiology of nontuberculous mycobacterial
disease. Clin. Chest Med., *10*:407, 1989a.

O'Brien, R. J.: Present chemotherapy of tuberculosis. Semin. Respir.
Infect., *4*:216, 1989b.

Perez-Stable, E. J., and Hopewell, P. C.: Current tuberculosis treatment regimens. Choosing the right one for your patient. Clin.
Chest Med., *10*:323, 1989.

Pomerantz, M., Madsen, L., Goble, M., and Iseman, M.: Surgical
management of resistant mycobacterial tuberculosis and other
mycobacterial pulmonary infections. Ann. Thorac. Surg.,
52:1108, 1991.

Reed, C. E., Parker, E. F., and Crawford, F. A.: Surgical resection
for complications of pulmonary tuberculosis. Ann. Thorac.
Surg., *48*:165, 1989.

Rieder, H. L., Cauthen, G. M., Comstock, G. W., and Snider, D. E.,
Jr.: Epidemiology of tuberculosis in the United States. Epidemiol. Rev., *11*:79, 1989.

Runyon, E. H.: Anonymous mycobacteria and pulmonary disease.
Med. Clin. North Am., *43*:273, 1959.

Sathe, S. S., and Raichman, L. B.: Mycobacterial disease in patients
infected with the human immunodeficiency virus. Clin. Chest
Med., *10*:445, 1989.

Sauerbruch, F., and Schumacher, E. D.: Technik der Thoraxchirurgie. Berlin, Springer-Verlag, 1911.

Smith, M. H.: Tuberculosis in children and adolescents. Clin. Chest
Med., *10*:381, 1989.

Stansberry, S. D.: Tuberculosis in infants and children. J. Thorac.
Imaging, *5*:17, 1990.

Starke, J. R., Jacobs R. F., and Jereb, J.: Resurgence of tuberculosis
in children. J. Pediatr., *120*:839, 1992.

Tsukamura, M.: Evidence that antituberculosis drugs are really
effective in the treatment of pulmonary infection caused by
Mycobacterium avium complex. Am. Rev. Respir. Dis., *137*:144,
1988.

Whyte, R. I., Deegan, S. P., Kaplan, D. K., et al.: Recent surgical
experience for pulmonary tuberculosis. Respir. Med., *83*:357,
1989.

Winer-Muram, H. T., and Rubin, S. A.: Thoracic complications of
tuberculosis. J. Thorac. Imaging, *5*:46, 1990.

Woodring, J. H., and Vandiviere, H. M.: Pulmonary disease caused
by nontuberculous mycobacteria. J. Thorac. Imaging, *5*:64,
1990.

23 Pulmonary Embolism
▪ I Acute Pulmonary Embolism

Gregory P. Fontana and David C. Sabiston, Jr.

Despite an improved understanding of its pathogenesis, diagnosis, and management, *pulmonary embolism* (PE) remains a frequent and sometimes fatal disorder. The true incidence of PE is unknown; however, it has been estimated that more than 500,000 people in this country suffer acute PE, with approximately 10% of patients dying within 1 hour of the onset of symptoms. Although PE is a well-recognized complication of many surgical procedures, most patients with this disorder are *nonsurgical* and develop PE secondary to a serious medical disorder, such as congestive heart failure, cerebrovascular accidents, chronic pulmonary disease, systemic infection, and carcinomatosis.

HISTORICAL ASPECTS

The 175-year history of the evaluation and treatment of thromboembolic disease involves three major periods: the understanding of the pathophysiology of thromboembolism, the evolution of imaging techniques (radiography, nuclear medicine, and ultrasound) that allow for reliable diagnosis, and the development of a rationale for the therapeutic management of the disease (Newman, 1989).

Pathologists have long known that thrombi may be found in the pulmonary arteries at autopsy, but in the past, they regarded these thrombi as arising as a primary process. In 1819, Laënnec described the clinical and pathologic characteristics of PE as *pulmonary apoplexy* in his *De L'Auscultation Médiate*, a treatise on the diagnosis of diseases of the lung and heart. The term *apoplexy* was used because it applied not only to cerebral hemorrhage but also to bleeding in any organ. Laënnec differentiated the lesion caused by PE from other pulmonary disorders that cause hemoptysis (e.g., tuberculosis and carcinoma):

The lesion consists of an induration, which is partial, and never occupies a larger portion of the lung; its usual size is 1 to 4 cubic inches. The surrounding parenchyma is entirely normal—the swollen part is very dark red. The cut surface shows granularity like the hepatized lung; but, otherwise, these two conditions are entirely different from each other. One encounters two or three such engorgements in one lung, and, rather frequently, both lungs are similarly affected.
Laënnec, 1819

In 1829, Cruveilhier meticulously described thrombi not only in the central and peripheral veins but also in the pulmonary arteries. He believed that pulmonary arterial thromboses developed in situ, but he did not identify their embolic origins (Fig. 23–1). Although Laënnec and Cruveilhier did not draw the relationship between peripheral thrombosis and pulmonary emboli (PEs), they observed that these pulmonary changes occurred in patients with cardiac disease that led to pulmonary congestion, and they emphasized the noninflammatory nature of this condition.

In 1842, Rokitansky confirmed Laënnec's findings and introduced the term *hemorrhagic infarct*. Although he did not initially recognize the etiologic basis for these infarcts, he later stated: "They are caused by fragments of clots in the veins or in the right heart. They are associated with thrombosis of the major branches of the pulmonary artery." He also recognized the supporting significance of pulmonary venous congestion and described in much detail the association of the condition with severe mitral stenosis.

The acknowledged father of modern pathology, Rudolph Virchow, introduced the *embolic* concept of this disorder. In 1858, in an extraordinary discourse, he stated:

In the peripheral veins the danger proceeds chiefly from the small branches. By no means rarely do these become quite filled with masses of coagulum. As long, however, as the thrombus is confined to the branch itself, so long as the body is not exposed to any particular . . . only the greater number of the thrombi in the small branches do not content themselves with advancing up to the level of the main trunk, but pretty constantly new masses of coagulum deposit themselves from the blood upon the end of the thrombus layer after layer; the thrombus is prolonged beyond the mouth of the branch into the trunk in the direction of the current of blood, shoots out in the form of a thick cylinder farther and farther, and becomes continually larger and larger. Soon this prolonged thrombus [Fig. 23–2] no longer bears any proportion to the original (autochthonous) thrombus from which it proceeded. The prolonged thrombus may have the thickness of a thumb, the original one that of a knitting-needle. From a lumbar vein, for example, a plug may extend into the vena cava as thick as the last phalanx of the thumb.

It is these prolonged plugs that constitute the source of real danger; it is in them that ensues the crumbling away which leads to secondary occlusion in remote vessels.

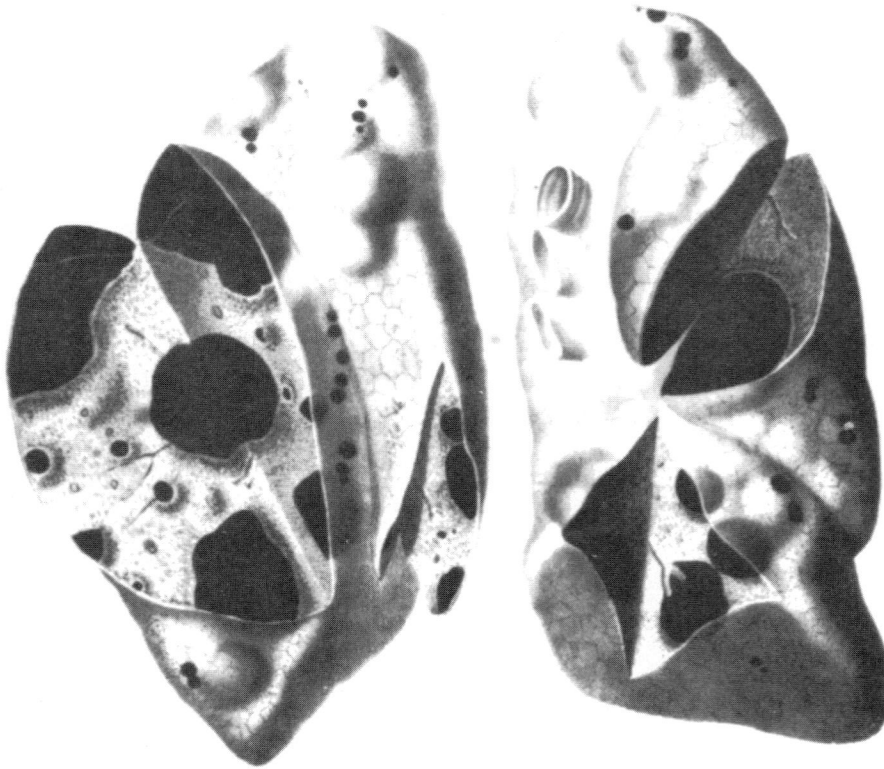

FIGURE 23–1. Illustration from Cruveilhier's atlas showing a patient diagnosed as having "pulmonary apoplexy." Cruveilhier described abnormal areas of lung, discrete from healthy tissue, with arterial branches leading to these sites filled with thrombi. However, Cruveilhier believed that thrombi form in situ in pulmonary arteries, and he did not understand their embolic origin. (From Cruveilhier, J.: Anatomie pathologique du corps humain. Paris, J. B. Baillière, 1829 to 1842. From The Trent Historic Collection, Duke University Medical Library.)

Virchow also observed two types of thrombus in the pulmonary arteries in such patients: first, the *embolus* that arises as a thrombus in a systemic vein and, after being dislodged from its site of origin, is swept into the venous return and then through the heart in the pulmonary arteries; and second, the thrombus that occurs in situ into the pulmonary artery distal to the occluding embolus as a result of stagnant blood flow in that segment (Fig. 23–3).

Responding to critics of his newly announced pathogenesis of PE, and in a desire to prove the embolic doctrine, Virchow inserted pieces of rubber or venous thrombi recovered from humans at autopsy into the jugular veins of dogs. When the animals were sacrificed, the emboli were found in the pulmonary arteries. An essential part of Virchow's studies concerned the identification of the assumed embolic particle with the apparent structure from which it had been detached. Embolism alone did not explain the development of the hemorrhagic infarct, and because occluding emboli in pulmonary branches *without* infarct were frequently found, Virchow considered the problem of *infarction* of pulmonary tissue difficult to explain. He postulated that it was related to the protective nutrient blood flow from the systemic bronchial arteries. It was not until 1932 that Berry

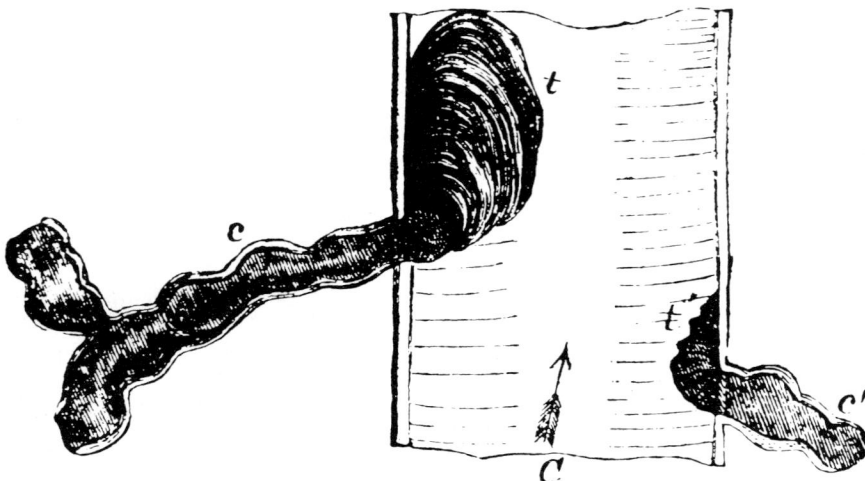

FIGURE 23–2. This illustration shows mechanisms of thrombus propagation in veins. Small venous channels (c,c') are occluded with thrombi (t,t'), which extend into a larger proximal vein. Extension of the thrombi into the current of blood flow (C) initiates further fibrin and platelet deposition in the proximal vein. (From Virchow, R.: Die Cellularpathologie. Berlin, A. Hirschwald, 1858.)

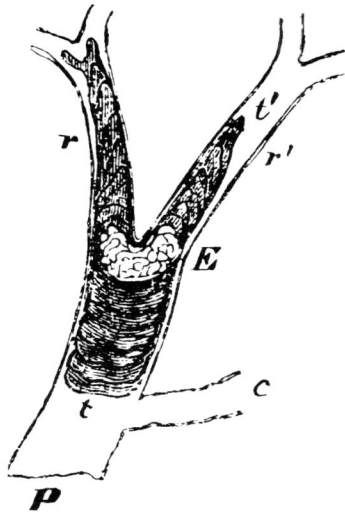

FIGURE 23–3. Illustration from Virchow's text showing differential emboli of venous origin from in situ thrombi forming about the embolus in the pulmonary artery (P) and a bifurcating vessel (C). An embolus (E) is lodged at a distal bifurcation, and in situ thrombosis (t) has occurred proximal and distal to the occluding lesion. (From Virchow, R.: Die Cellularpathologie. Berlin, A. Hirschwald, 1858.)

and Daly described bronchial artery enlargement after pulmonary obstruction.

In 1872, Cohnheim described the importance of *pulmonary congestion* and *left ventricular failure* in the development of *hemorrhagic* infarction and proved that clinical evidence of congestive heart failure is associated with the hemorrhagic death of pulmonary tissue.

White (1935) described the concept of *acute cor pulmonale.* His observations led to the first recognition of PE by its hemodynamic and other physiologic features. It became apparent that PE was not exclusively a postoperative surgical complication but also an occurrence found frequently in cardiac patients and as

a part of various chronic illnesses. The diagnosis of embolism was often missed by the clinician and also, to a lesser degree, by the pathologist.

While knowledge of the development of thrombosis evolved, scant attention was directed toward the basic pathogenesis of venous thrombosis. The first known description of thrombophlebitis appeared in the 13th century (Dexter and Folch-Pi, 1974) (Fig. 23–4). Virchow was attentive to basic pathogenesis, and his conclusions are still important today. He concluded that primary thrombosis in the systemic veins resulted from three factors now termed Virchow's triad: stasis of blood flow, injury to the vein, and a state of hypercoagulability (Virchow, 1856).

Once the concepts of the pathophysiology of venous thrombosis and PE were developed, the need for an accurate diagnosis and therapy became obvious. Radiographic imaging dates back to 1895 when Roentgen first described x-rays; however, the development of angiography was delayed until the discovery of nontoxic contrast agents. Lipiodol, strontium bromide, and sodium iodide (all noxious agents) were used as contrast agents in the 1920s. The first organic iodide was introduced in 1929. In the 1940s, iodopyracet (Diodrast) became the most widely used angiographic agent before the introduction of diatrizoate sodium (Renografin) in the mid-1950s (Newman, 1989).

The first central catheterization was performed by Werner Forssman in 1929. In 1931, Moniz reported the first pulmonary angiogram. Further technical refinements of pulmonary angiography, including branch and segmental, were described by Jonsson and Bolt, respectively. PE was rarely described in these early publications, because at that time most angiograms were performed for pulmonary hypertension, cor pulmonale, tuberculosis, fibrothorax, or carcinoma of the lung. In 1963 and 1964, publications began to identify the utility and importance of angiography in the diagnosis of PE (Newman, 1989).

Dos Santos first reported venography in 1938, al-

FIGURE 23–4. Painting from the Bibliothèque Nationale in Paris documenting the first known description of venous thrombosis. (From Dexter, L., and Folch-Pi, W.: Venous thrombosis. An account of the first documented case. J. A. M. A., *228*:195, 1974. Copyright 1974, American Medical Association.)

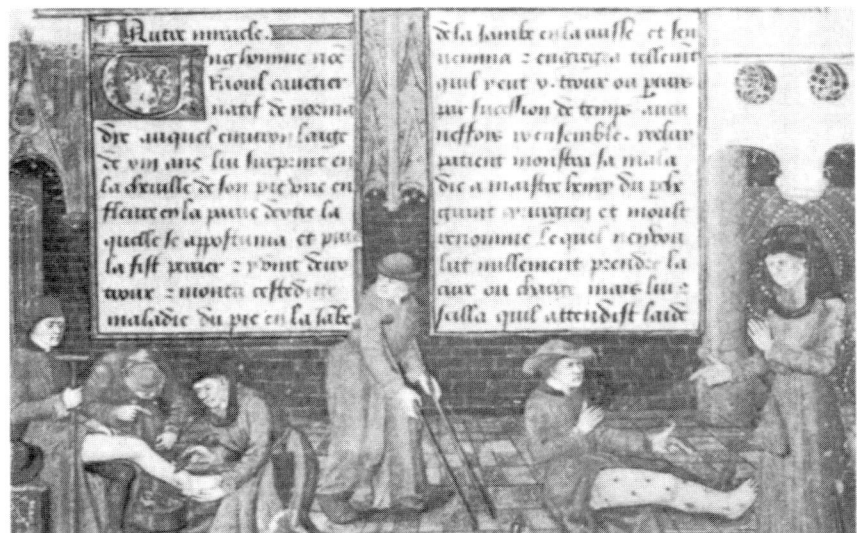

though Bauer was the first to use the technique to identify venous thrombosis in the lower extremities. He used venography to study the natural history of untreated and treated (heparin) venous thrombosis (Bauer, 1959).

Radionuclide imaging was not feasible until both imaging equipment and radiopharmaceuticals were developed. Cassen's group developed the first scanning instrument in 1951. Ventilation imaging began in 1955 when Knipping described a technique for the noninvasive assessment of ventilation with a nonabsorbable noble gas. In 1958, Ernst described a noninvasive technique that demonstrated distribution of pulmonary perfusion using a nonbiodegradable radiopharmaceutical (Newman, 1989). In 1964, Wagner and co-workers first reported the diagnosis of PE in humans by radioisotope scanning. By 1970, the clinical value of ventilation and perfusion images and chest radiographs for the diagnosis of acute PE was well established (DeNardo et al., 1970).

The first treatment of PE was surgical. In 1908, Trendelenburg attempted the first pulmonary embolectomy with the immediate opening of the pulmonary artery and removal of the embolus. In his original report, Trendelenburg described three patients on whom embolectomy was performed. The longest survivor lived for 37 hours and ultimately died of hemorrhage from an internal mammary artery. Trendelenburg's approach was cumbersome and required resection of three ribs. In 1924, his student Kirschner was first to perform a pulmonary embolectomy successfully with long-term survival. Steenburg and colleagues performed the first successful embolectomy in the United States in 1957 (Steenburg et al., 1958), and in 1961, Sharp was first to perform pulmonary embolectomy using cardiopulmonary bypass (Sharp, 1962).

Medical therapy awaited the discovery of anticoagulants. In 1916, while he was still a medical student, McLean discovered heparin. The value of this agent in the management of venous thrombosis was not shown until 1937 by Murray and associates. Crafoord and Jorpes (1941) were the first to demonstrate the effectiveness of heparin as a prophylactic agent against venous thrombosis in the postoperative period. Considerable credit is due to Bauer (1959) and to Barritt and Jordan (1960) for showing the life-saving potential of heparin in the management of acute PE.

The syndrome of chronic PE in patients with progressive respiratory insufficiency who at postmortem examination had multiple unresolved PEs, dilated proximal pulmonary arteries, and increased right ventricular size was first described by Ljungdahl in 1928. Much attention has been given to the surgical management of chronic PE (Daily et al., 1990; Jamieson et al., 1993; Moor and Sabiston, 1970; Sabiston et al., 1977). This subject is considered in a separate section.

PATHOGENESIS OF VENOUS THROMBOSIS

The three primary factors of thrombogenesis cited by Virchow more than a century ago and now recognized as his *triad* include stasis or reduction of blood flow in the veins, injury to the intimal surface predisposing to the thrombosis, and a state of hypercoagulability. These factors, either singly or in combination, are important in the formation of thrombi in the systemic veins. When these thrombi become detached from the venous wall, they are swept into the circulation and pass through the heart and into the lungs.

The most important factor in thrombus formation in the systemic veins is *stasis*. Radiopaque contrast medium injected into the deep veins of the leg may take a long time to clear when the patient remains in the horizontal position (McLachlin et al., 1960), especially in the postoperative period, when movement is often painful. Moreover, Allison (1967) showed that, in postoperative patients, radiopaque dye may remain in the calf veins for as long as 25 minutes after injection. Similarly, patients ill for any reason are less likely to move the extremities, and this also predisposes to intravenous thrombosis.

The sinuses of the venous valves are especially vulnerable to stasis and thrombosis. Here, local stasis permits the accumulation of sufficient clotting factors to initiate the primary thrombus (Fig. 23–5). Platelets adhere to the pockets created by the valves and a thrombus develops. The thrombus grows by successive deposition of aggregated platelets, leukocytes,

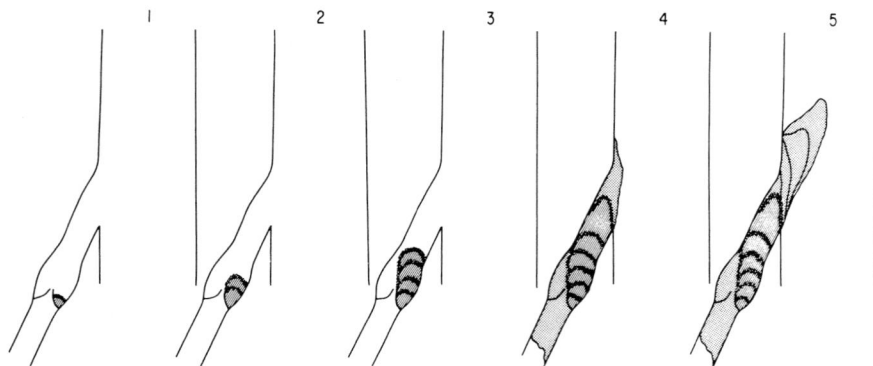

FIGURE 23–5. Illustration showing propagation of a deep thrombus arising in a valvular pocket with deposition of successive layers and ultimate extension of the nonadherent red thrombus into the lumen of a larger parent vein. (From Cox, J. L., and Sabiston, D. C., Jr.: Phlebitis, thrombosis, and pulmonary embolism. *In* Condon, R. E., and DeCosse, J. J. [eds]: Surgical Care: A Physiologic Approach to Problems in the First Fifteen Postoperative Days. Philadelphia, Lea & Febiger, 1980.)

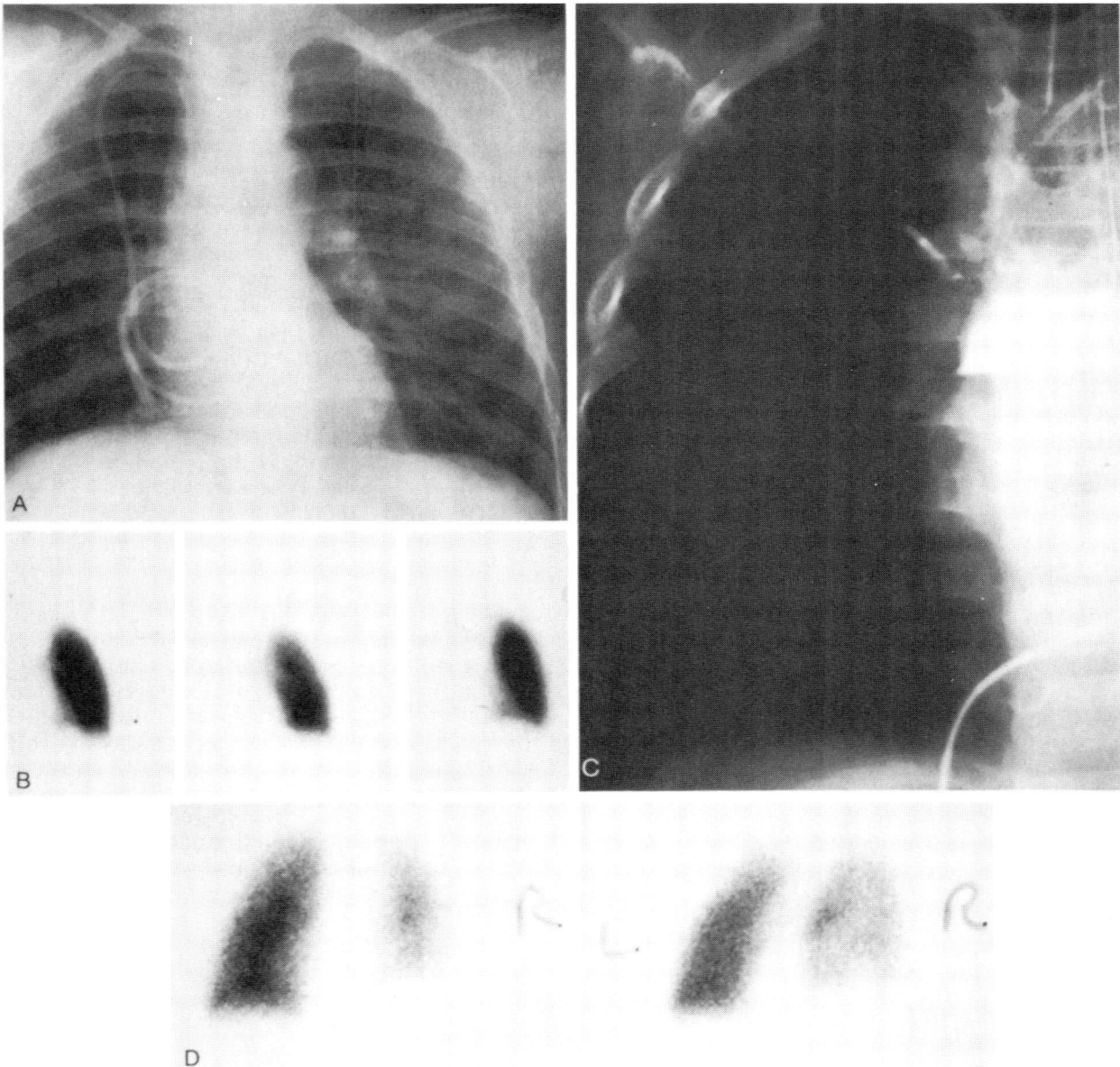

FIGURE 23–6. *A,* Plain chest film of a child with a chronically implanted hyperalimentation catheter in the right atrium. Note the marked *hypovascularity* of the right lung compared with that of the left lung (Westermark's sign). *B,* Pulmonary radioactive scan showing no perfusion of the right lung. *C,* Pulmonary arteriogram confirming occlusion of the right main pulmonary artery. *D,* Pulmonary scan after intravenous streptokinase therapy showing great improvement in pulmonary arterial blood flow to the right lung.

and fibrin. Propagation of the thrombus may occur upstream, or the process may spread retrograde as proximal obstruction develops (Cox and Sabiston, 1980).

Soft tissue *injury* either by blunt trauma or through an operative procedure is known to be associated with an increased incidence of venous thrombosis.

Hypercoagulability has been defined as the existence of an excessive amount or activity of one or more procoagulant substances or a decrease in anticoagulant factors (Coon and Coller, 1959). For example, during pregnancy, the concentrations of fibrinogen, prothrombin, Factor VII, Stuart's factor, Christmas factor, and antihemophilic factor are elevated (Alex-

ander et al., 1956), so the risk of venous thrombosis is increased.

Another important embolic source is thrombosed intravascular foreign bodies. For example, a massive embolus to the right pulmonary artery from an indwelling catheter in the right atrium occurred in a child receiving total intravenous hyperalimentation for short gut syndrome. In the plain chest film (Fig. 23–6A), there is marked oligemia of the entire right lung (Westermark's sign), and the pulmonary radioactive scan shows no perfusion of the right lung (Fig. 23–6B). The pulmonary arteriogram shows total occlusion of the right main pulmonary artery with an embolus (Fig. 23–6C). After 24 hours of intravenous streptokinase therapy, the pulmonary scan returned to normal (Fig. 23–6D).

PATHOPHYSIOLOGY

Clinical diagnosis of PE is frequently difficult to establish, and its presence is often recognized for the first time at autopsy (Fig. 23–7). The importance of routine autopsies for the diagnosis of PE is emphasized by a study showing evidence of old or fresh PEs discovered at autopsy in 64% of persons over the age of 40 years (Freiman, 1965). As far as the physiologic changes after embolism are concerned, *mechanical* factors of arterial occlusion are considerably more important than *reflex* responses. These features are well demonstrated in the classic pathologic studies by Gorham (1961a, 1961b). Of 100 consecutive patients with fatal PEs, 85 had both occlusion involving one pulmonary artery and emboli in the opposite lung. Of the 100 patients, only 15 had emboli restricted solely to one lung, and 12 of these patients were more than 54 years of age (an age group with an appreciable incidence of underlying cardiac and respiratory disease). Also, it is usual to find emboli in more than one pulmonary artery in patients with massive PE in whom embolectomy is performed (Baker, 1963; Sabiston, 1968; Sabiston and Wagner, 1965). This evidence supports the importance of *mechanical* occlusion in the cardiodynamic sequelae of massive PE. In addition, these data agree with similar observations on reduction of pulmonary blood flow by other causes, including arterial ligature, intravascular balloons, pulmonary resection, and various

forms of emboli (Brofman et al., 1957; Burnett et al., 1949; Sloan et al., 1955). After injection of experimental PEs, reduced function of the embolized lung occurs immediately, and pulmonary function returns almost to normal within several weeks (Marshall et al., 1963; Sabiston and Wolfe, 1968). Similarly, marked histologic changes occur in these thrombi, including intravascular resolution and ultimate disappearance. Such resolution can be confirmed by serial pulmonary radioactive scans, arteriograms, pulmonary function studies, and gross and microscopic evaluation (Fig. 23–8). Also, the resolution of large PEs, with or without the use of anticoagulants or fibrinolysins, is recognized as a common clinical phenomenon (Fig. 23–9). These observations have shown convincingly that the natural history of PE in most cases is one of spontaneous resolution (Dalen and Alpert, 1975; Fred et al., 1966; Sabiston and Wolfe, 1968; Sautter et al., 1964). This concept has become increasingly significant in a more complete understanding of the principles of diagnosis and management.

Emboli that are found at postmortem examination are generally 1 to 1.5 cm in diameter, apparently having arisen in sizable veins. Their length ranges up to 50 cm or more (Hume et al., 1970), and after they arrive in the lungs, they often break into multiple small portions and occlude multiple branches of the pulmonary arteries. Generally, the right pulmonary artery and its branches are more commonly involved than the left pulmonary artery, and the lower lobes are usually involved bilaterally.

PEs originate primarily in the systemic venous circulation, and the prevailing evidence indicates that most emboli arise from the *iliac* and *femoral veins*

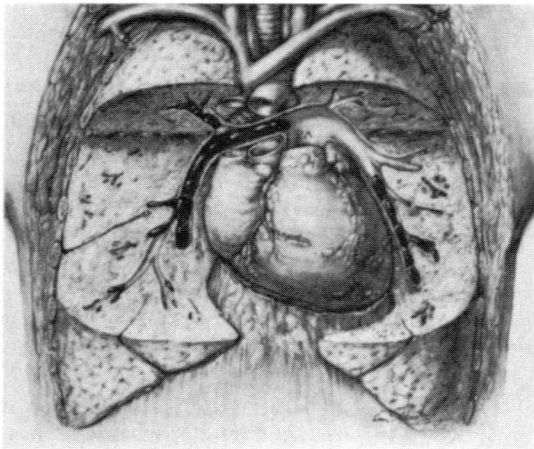

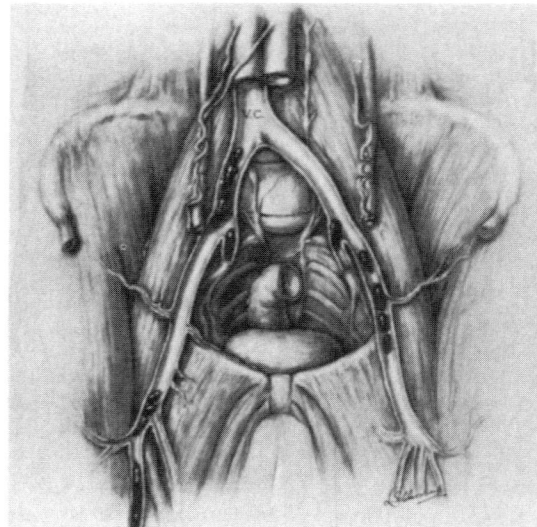

FIGURE 23–7. Findings in a patient with massive pulmonary embolism at the time of postmortem examination. Multiple thrombi were present in the iliofemoral system. The right pulmonary artery and its branches are totally occluded by emboli. The left lower lobar pulmonary artery is also occluded. Under these circumstances, the entire output of the right ventricle must pass through the left lower lobe, which greatly increases pulmonary resistance and right ventricular work. The sudden development of this degree of pulmonary arterial occlusion produces a clinical state of severe shock because the left ventricle receives a diminished amount of blood to supply the systemic arterial circulation. In otherwise normal patients, 50% or more of the pulmonary arterial circulation must be occluded before serious cardiovascular manifestations are produced. (From Sabiston, D. C., Jr.: Pathophysiology, diagnosis and management of pulmonary embolism. Adv. Surg., 3:351, 1968.)

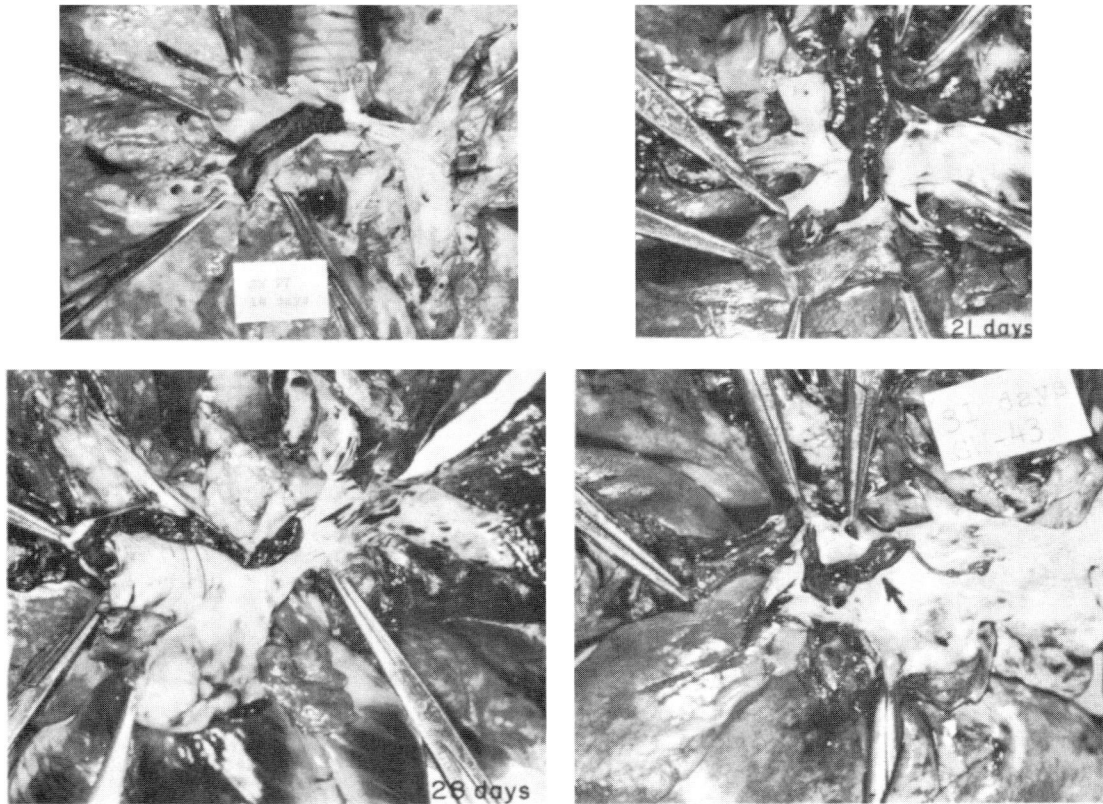

FIGURE 23–8. Progressive changes in experimental pulmonary emboli from the 14th to the 31st day. The attachments are demonstrated at the tip of the *arrow* at 21 days *(top right)*. The diameter of the embolus is definitely smaller by the 28th day. The embolus at 31 days demonstrates the variation in resolution in different parts of the thrombus. One end of the thrombus has been reduced to a small fragment, whereas the remaining part is larger. (From Sabiston, D. C., Jr., and Wolfe, W. G.: Experimental and clinical observations on the natural history of pulmonary embolism. Ann. Surg., *168*:1, 1968.)

(Table 23–1). Approximately 50% of iliofemoral thromboses will embolize if untreated (Hull et al., 1985). Calf vein thromboses are thought to embolize rarely, but this remains controversial (Mohr et al., 1988; Moser and LeMoine, 1981). Although the smaller leg veins (such as those of the calf) may be involved, they are not as likely to cause serious clinical manifestations of PE. However, 5 to 20% of patients with small vein thrombosis will have subsequent clot propagation to the larger deep veins of the thighs and pelvis, which then do represent a source of significant emboli (Kakkar et al., 1969).

The iliofemoral and pelvic veins are the most common sites of thrombi; other possible sources include the inferior vena cava, the subclavian, axillary, and internal jugular veins, and the cavernous sinuses of the skull. Some physicians have emphasized that as many as one-fifth of PEs arise from sources other than veins drained by the inferior vena cava (Gurewich et al., 1966). *Tumor emboli* should also be considered in the differential diagnosis. For example, renal cell carcinoma is recognized for its ability to metastasize early in the course of the disease (Daughtry et al., 1977; Winterbauer et al., 1968). Involvement of the renal vein and inferior vena cava by direct extension from a renal cell carcinoma with fragmentation caus-

■ **Table 23–1.** SITE OF ORIGIN OF VENOUS THROMBI

Reference	% of Cases with Thrombosis at Necropsy	% of Cases with Thrombi in				
		Iliac Veins	*Femoral Veins*	*Popliteal Veins*	*Soleal Veins*	*Any Deep Calf Vein*
Rossle (1937)	94		49			92
Neumann (1938)	100		22			87
McLachlin and Paterson (1951)	34	9	82			41
Gibbs (1957)	149		42			65
Sevitt and Gallagher (1961)	81		70	33	67	74
Roberts (1963)	58	14	43	41	86	95

Reprinted with permission of the publishers from Venous Thrombosis and Pulmonary Embolism by Michael Hume, Simon Sevitt, and Duncan P. Thomas, Cambridge, Mass.: Harvard University Press © 1970 by the President and Fellows of Harvard College.

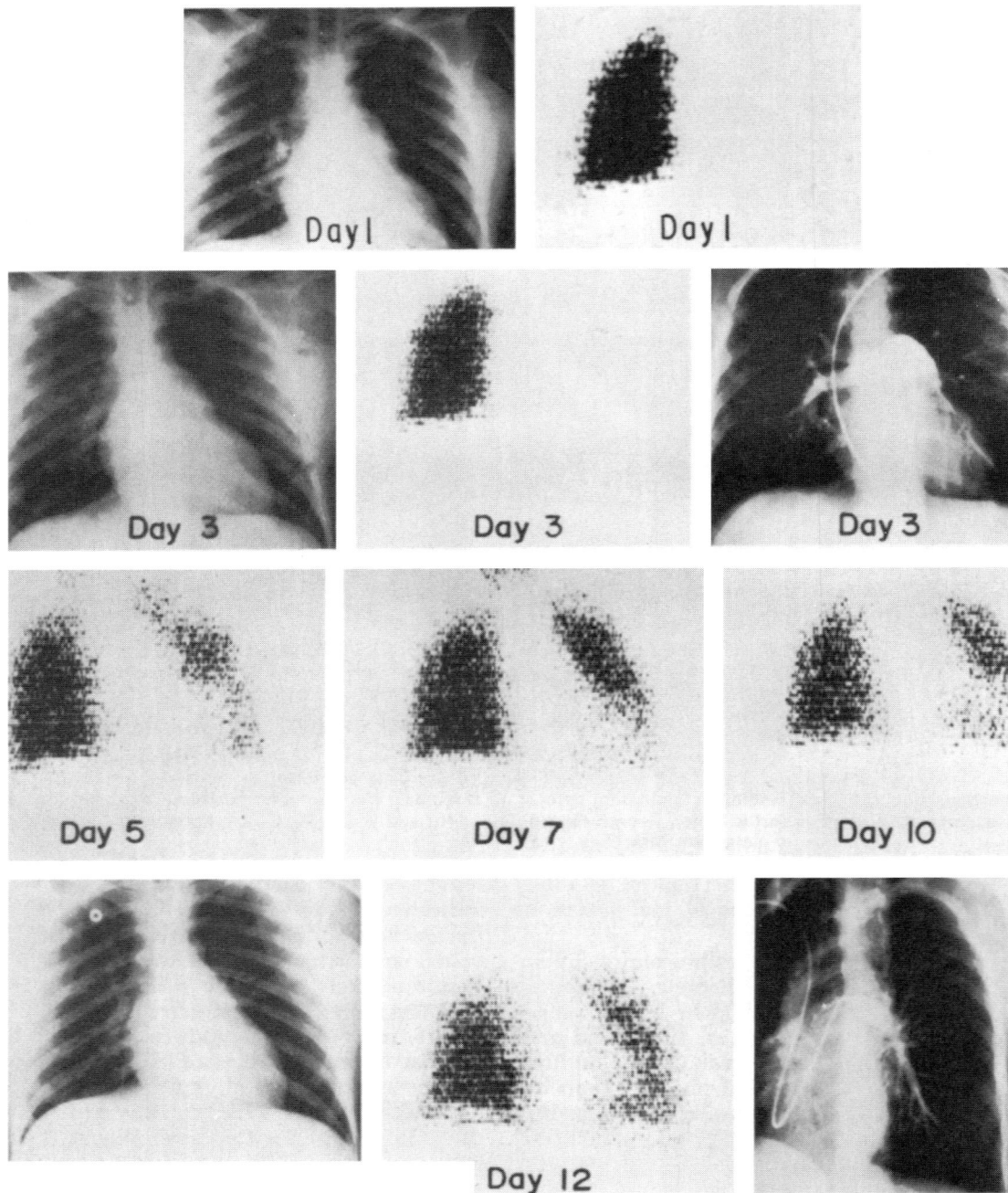

FIGURE 23–9. Serial chest films and scans after a massive pulmonary embolus to the left pulmonary artery in a 25-year-old woman after a pelvic operation. On the 5th postoperative day, discomfort was noted in the left chest with dyspnea. A plain chest film taken on this day (Day 1) showed diminished vascular markings (Westermark's sign). A radioactive pulmonary scan showed no evidence of pulmonary flow to the entire left lobe. Beginning on the 3rd day after the embolus, both the scan and the arteriogram showed evidence of flow to the left lung. In scans and pulmonary arteriograms, the thrombus resolved with progressively increasing amounts of flow by the 12th day. (From Sabiston, D. C., Jr.: Pulmonary embolism. *In* Sabiston, D. C., Jr. [ed]: Textbook of Surgery. 13th ed. Philadelphia, W. B. Saunders, 1986.)

ing PE has been variously reported to occur in 9.5 to 54% of patients with this disorder (Arkless, 1965; Coman, 1953; Svane, 1969). Moreover, primary pulmonary neoplasms can mimic PE (Myerson et al., 1976; Sethi et al., 1972). In addition, cardiac tumors arising in the right atrium and right ventricle also can produce extensive PEs (Hansen et al., 1969; Talley et al., 1970). Finally, PEs may result from missiles, and several reports in the literature describe *bullet embolization* of the pulmonary arteries (Stephenson et al., 1976). Missiles lodging in the pulmonary arteries usually manifest themselves through ensuing complications, including erosion of the vessel, infarction of the distal lung, sepsis, and pulmonary vascular thrombosis. Among 18 cases collected from the world literature, there were 7 deaths (37%), and deaths occurred in all patients who did *not* undergo removal of the missiles from the pulmonary arteries. Therefore, if a missile embolus is present in the pulmonary vascular system, surgical removal is indicated.

A clear differentiation should be made between PE and pulmonary infarction. PE is common, whereas pulmonary infarction occurs less frequently. Pathologically, an infarct is a circumscribed area less than 5 cm in diameter of local hemorrhage and demonstrates *necrosis* of the lung parenchyma. In most instances, infarction from emboli occurs in patients with preexisting congestive heart failure or pulmonary infection. In one series, the proportion of infarcts to emboli was 1:10 (Smith et al., 1965).

The fact that *asymptomatic PE* occurs frequently in postoperative patients is emphasized in a study of 158 patients having surgical procedures in whom ventilation and perfusion lung scans were obtained preoperatively and at weekly intervals postoperatively. Pulmonary arteriograms were obtained in 21 of 33 patients with perfusion scan patterns that strongly suggested PE. PE was shown in 19 of the 21 arteriograms. From autopsy and clinical data, 36 patients were diagnosed as having an embolism while under study, and 12 patients were suspected of having had an embolism during their illness before entry into the study. Only 4 of these 48 patients had symptoms that suggested PE. The study thus indicated that asymptomatic PE is a common event of surgical patients postoperatively (Williams et al., 1982).

Paradoxic embolism is the passage of a thrombus through an intracardiac opening (patent foramen ovale, atrial septal defect, or ventricular septal defect) with embolization of a systemic organ (Silver and Gleysteen, 1970). This condition is more likely to occur when right ventricular and right atrial hypertension are present. A number of these paradoxic emboli have been diagnosed during life (Laughlin and Mandel, 1977).

Although PE usually occurs in adults, it has also been reported in children. In one study of children examined at autopsy, the incidence was approximately 1%. PE is usually a secondary manifestation of serious illness, such as respiratory infection, phlebitis, systemic infection, congenital heart disease, or rheumatic heart disease (Jones and Sabiston, 1966). PE in children is rarely diagnosed before death, and its clinical manifestations are similar to those in adults.

PREDISPOSING FACTORS

A British study reports that PE is responsible for 110 deaths per million in women, compared with 77 deaths per million in men (Registrar-General's Statistical Review of England and Wales, 1966). More recently, Lilienfield and co-workers (1990b) reported that the age-specific incidence for men was higher than that for women in all age groups except those under 45 years. Mortality rates for PE were the same for men and women. Besides sex, age is an important factor in the incidence of PE: the disorder primarily affects the middle-aged and elderly (Coon et al., 1973; Coon and Coller, 1959; Lilienfield et al., 1990b). Reports show a decreasing incidence of PE in the United States; however, the case mortality remains constant (Gillum, 1987; Lilienfield et al., 1990a). The suggested reasons for the declining incidence are the widespread use of preventive measures, the use of anticoagulants (such as aspirin), and the reduction of cardiovascular risk factors such as serum cholesterol and cigarette smoking.

Bedrest and lack of exercise in general are well-established antecedent causes of PE, and they produce a twofold or greater incidence (Barker et al., 1941). However, a recent prospective study evaluating the frequency of PE in patients with pelvic vein thrombosis shows that, while on heparin and wearing compression stockings, patients restricted to bedrest are no more at risk for PE than are those on the same therapy who exercise (Partsch et al., 1992).

Heart disease, especially congestive heart failure or atrial fibrillation, is particularly conducive to the development of PE. After acute myocardial infarction, 34 to 37% of patients have developed deep venous thrombosis (Mauer et al., 1971; Murray et al., 1970), and after cerebrovascular accidents, the incidence may be as high as 60% (Vossschulte, 1965). Cancer, particularly carcinoma of the pancreas and prostate and carcinomatosis, is associated with a high incidence of PE (Coon and Coller, 1959).

The fact that PE is often a complication of surgical procedures has long been recognized. Scanning of the lower extremities after intravenous injection of radioactive fibrinogen (a simple technique that allows the identification of thrombosis in the extremities) has shown deep venous thrombosis in 54% of patients with hip fractures, 50% of those having prostatectomy, and 28% of general surgical patients over the age of 40 years (Kakkar, 1972).

Pregnancy clearly increases the risk of PE. In a study of 2475 maternal deaths, PE was thought to be the cause of death in 11% (Kaunitz et al., 1985). Another study found the maternal death rate in Massachusetts between 1982 and 1985 to be 10 per 100,000, with PE the second most common cause (Sacks et al., 1987). Several risk factors during pregnancy have been identified, including the retardation of venous flow from the limbs and pelvis owing to pressure from the gravid uterus and the alteration in the levels and function of clotting factors (Demers and Ginsberg, 1992; Ikard et al., 1971; Stirling et al., 1984). Infection in the postpartum patient may also cause septic thrombophlebitis and embolism. There is a clear increased risk for the development of deep venous thrombosis in pregnant patients; however, it remains unclear whether pregnant women have a higher risk of embolization than nonpregnant women who have deep venous thrombosis (Demers and Ginsberg, 1992).

Oral contraceptives have a positive association with the occurrence of PE, according to studies in both the United States and Britain. British studies (Medical Research Council Subcommittee, 1967; Vessey and

Doll, 1968) showed that the risk of venous thrombosis or PE was increased threefold in women who received oral contraceptives and about sixfold in women who were pregnant or in the puerperium.

Underlying primary clotting disorders also predispose toward PE. Examples of these abnormalities include antithrombin III deficiency, the presence of a lupus anticoagulant, and congenital deficiencies of protein C and its cofactor, protein S. Because only a few patients have PE as a result of these abnormalities, routine investigation for these abnormalities may not be cost-effective (Gray and Firoozan, 1992). Coagulation profile studies are indicated, however, in the young, in patients with recurrent emboli of undetermined cause, and in those with a known family history of thromboembolism.

PHYSIOLOGIC RESPONSES

When considering the physiologic responses to PE, one must recognize that in the normal individual the output of the left and right sides of the heart is equal. A characteristic feature of the pulmonary circulation is its low vascular resistance, which enables flow in the pulmonary vascular bed to be increased severalfold with minimal elevation of pulmonary arterial pressure. Despite numerous experimental and clinical studies, opinion is divided concerning the relative importance of *reflex* versus *mechanical* effects in PE. The occasional finding of a small PE in a patient after sudden death has been cited as evidence that occlusion of a relatively small pulmonary artery can produce death, presumably as a result of reflex mechanisms. Currently, such an explanation would be accepted only in very unusual circumstances.

In experimental PE, the physiologic changes appear to be related to the size of the emboli and can be divided into those that produce *microembolism* (obstruction of terminal small arteries and arterioles) and those that produce *macroembolism* (occlusion of the larger pulmonary vessels). Considerable reduction in the diameter of the main pulmonary artery or of the primary branches is required to reduce pulmonary blood flow significantly or to produce pulmonary hypertension proximal to the obstruction. Large experimental thrombi produced in the inferior vena cava and transferred to either the right or the left pulmonary artery produce minimal cardiovascular and respiratory responses 10 to 14 days later. Specifically, occlusion of one pulmonary artery produces only minimal and generally insignificant changes in the central venous pressure, the right ventricular pressure, the pulmonary artery pressure, the aortic pressure, the cardiac output, the total oxygen consumption, and the electrocardiogram, despite occlusion of half of the pulmonary arterial circulation (Marshall et al., 1963). Therefore, this type of embolism produces few circulatory effects that can be attributed specifically to reflex action.

Pneumonectomy is relatively well tolerated if the opposite lung is normal or almost normal. Tidal volume and oxygen consumption at rest after resection of a lung change only a small degree (Burnett et al., 1949). Resection of less than one lung is followed by only minor changes in the pulmonary arterial pressure, whereas removal of greater amounts of pulmonary tissue elevates pulmonary arterial pressure (Weideranders et al., 1964). Similarly, occlusion of one pulmonary artery by ligature or an intraluminal balloon is accompanied by few cardiodynamic changes. Patients have tolerated balloon occlusion well for up to 2 hours (Brofman et al., 1957). Even during exercise with similar occlusion, pulmonary arterial pressure is increased only 12 to 50%, whereas cardiac output may increase as much as threefold. Arterial occlusion of this type closely simulates the obstruction produced by large PEs. These studies have been conducted in otherwise normal subjects.

The presence of underlying cardiac or respiratory insufficiency is likely to alter this response appreciably. For example, in patients with heart disease, exercise during temporary unilateral occlusion of the right or left pulmonary artery by a balloon catheter sharply elevates pulmonary arterial pressure (Sloan et al., 1955). Cardiac output does not increase significantly with exercise, although arteriovenous oxygen difference does increase. The hemodynamic effect of PE is not confined to the right side of the heart. Obstruction of pulmonary arterial blood flow causes a reduction in the filling of the left side of the heart and in the dilatation of a failing right ventricle, which displaces the interventricular septum into the left ventricle, further impairing the filling of the left ventricle and reducing end-diastolic volume (Belenkie et al., 1988; Jardin et al., 1987). These factors explain why the dyspnea of patients with acute severe PE is eased by maneuvers that increase systemic venous return, such as having the patient lie flat, placing the patient in the Trendelenburg position, and infusing the patient with volume.

Although mechanical factors are most important in determining the cardiodynamic effects of PE, reflex effects, including tachypnea, pulmonary hypertension, and systemic hypotension, can follow the embolization with small particles (100 μm or less). However, *microembolism* of the lung is infrequently encountered as a clinical problem (although it does occur after massive blood transfusions, during which platelet, leukocyte, and fibrin emboli may occlude the pulmonary microcirculation) (Dawidson et al., 1975). As a precaution, transfusion filters should be used at all times. Embolization with larger particles requires considerably more blockage of the pulmonary arterial system to produce significant effects. In general, arterial emboli produce pulmonary hypertension by *mechanical* obstruction, whereas arteriolar embolism produces bronchoconstriction and vasoconstriction by *reflex* changes (Dexter, 1965). Thus, clinical manifestations of PE are produced primarily by occlusion of the larger pulmonary arteries, a concept supported by both clinical and pathologic studies.

One of the primary findings in severe PE is the presence of *cyanosis*. The cause of reduced oxygen tension in the arterial blood has elicited considerable discussion. Possible causes include alveolar hypoventilation, ventilation-perfusion abnormality, decreased diffusing capacity of the lungs, pulmonary edema, venoarterial shunting, and rapid transit of blood through the capillary bed without adequate time for oxygenation. A combination of these factors may cause cyanosis (Kovacs et al., 1966).

Reflex bronchoconstriction has aroused considerable interest (Boyer and Curry, 1944). Pulmonary function studies after injection of intravenous heparin show a prompt improvement in the maximal expiratory flow rate or a reduction in pulmonary resistance (Gurewich et al., 1965). These observations are cited as evidence of a *humoral* factor. Humoral factors mediated by platelets may be important in the genesis of cardiopulmonary disturbances in patients with PE. It is known that platelets are a concentrated source of biologically active amines. Experimental studies have demonstrated that 5-hydroxytryptamine (serotonin) and thromboxane A_2 are liberated from platelets in the process of blood coagulation and produce bronchoconstriction (Comroe et al., 1953; Manny, 1985).

Hypoxia also causes pulmonary vasoconstriction (Fishman, 1976). This response is considered a self-regulatory mechanism by which pulmonary capillary blood flow is automatically adjusted to alveolar ventilation. Such a response is classically seen in acute hypoxia as well as in the chronic hypoxia of high altitude, which has also been associated with pulmonary vasoconstriction (Blount and Vogel, 1967; Moret et al., 1972). This physiologic feature should be remembered in the interpretation of the pulmonary hypertension that is often found with both acute and chronic PE.

Therefore, both experimental and clinical evidence suggest that various factors contribute to the changes that occur after embolism. Most evidence favors a primary *mechanical* basis for the physiologic changes, with the belief that the blockage produced by the emboli causes the most serious changes. Clearly, pre-embolic status significantly affects the clinical manifestations, and the presence of preexisting cardiac or respiratory insufficiency is important. If such preexisting disease is present, lesser degrees of PE cause greater clinical responses. Reflex changes occur as well, although, in general, these are of secondary importance. The vasoactive amines, probably arising from the emboli themselves, appear to exert a significant influence in the pathogenesis of bronchospasm.

INCIDENCE

A carefully performed study demonstrated that some 630,000 patients are subject to PE annually in the United States alone, and of these, approximately 200,000 succumb each year (Dalen and Alpert, 1975). Approximately 11% of these patients die within the first hour, and the remaining 89% survive 1 hour or longer. In 71% of those surviving 1 hour or longer, the diagnosis is not made, and among these patients,

there is a 30% mortality rate. Among the 29% of those who survive for more than 1 hour, and in whom a diagnosis *is* made and appropriate therapy is started, the mortality is only 8%.

The risk of death from PE after surgical procedures from a collected series was 0.11% (DeBakey, 1954). The incidence of death from PE and infarction in the United States had increased until the early 1980s (Hume, 1975; Lilienfield et al., 1990b). Factors responsible for the increase include the rise in the number of older members of the population, larger numbers and greater magnitude of operative procedures, increased recognition, and use of hormonal agents for birth control. There is evidence that the incidence of PE has peaked or possibly declined, perhaps because of routine use of preventive measures, use of anticoagulants (such as aspirin), and reduction of cardiovascular disease risk factors (Lilienfield et al., 1990b).

DIAGNOSIS

Clinical Manifestations

It may be difficult to establish a *clinical* diagnosis of PE, because it is similar to other cardiorespiratory disorders, including myocardial infarction, pneumonia, congestive heart failure, aortic dissection, pleuritis asthma, chronic obstructive pulmonary disease (COPD), and intrathoracic cancer. Symptoms of dyspnea, chest pain, hemoptysis, and hypotension may be present in the classic example, but these are not sufficiently specific to permit a definite diagnosis. The following points should be emphasized: Many patients have underlying cardiac or pulmonary disease; dyspnea and tachypnea are the most common clinical findings; pleuritic pain, tachycardia, rales, and accentuation of the pulmonary second sound are common, whereas the more classic signs of hemoptysis, pleural friction rub, gallop rhythm, cyanosis, and chest splinting are present in only one-quarter or less of patients; and clinical evidence of venous thrombosis is the exception and occurs in only one-quarter to one-third of patients (Sasahara, 1965; Stein et al., 1991). The symptoms in 1000 consecutive patients diagnosed with PE at the Duke University Medical Center are shown in Table 23–2. The symptoms and physical signs of PE are frequently insufficient to establish an accurate diagnosis.

Special Examinations

In many patients with PE, the findings on the initial plain chest film are within normal limits; however, over 90% may reveal some abnormality within a few days, including plate-like atelectasis, pleural effusions, parenchymal infiltrates, elevated hemidiaphragm, and prominence of the pulmonary artery (Moses et al., 1974; Ryu and Rosenow, 1992). Although the plain chest radiograph has been an essential part of work-ups, the findings are of limited value

■ **Table 23–2.** CLINICAL MANIFESTATIONS IN 1000 PATIENTS WITH PULMONARY EMBOLISM AT THE DUKE UNIVERSITY MEDICAL CENTER

Symptoms	%
Dyspnea	77
Chest pain	63
Hemoptysis	26
Altered mental status	23
Dyspnea, chest pain, hemoptysis	14
Signs	
Tachycardia	59
Recent fever	43
Rales	42
Tachypnea	38
Leg edema and tenderness	23
Elevated venous pressure	18
Shock	11
Accentuated P_2	11
Cyanosis	9
Pleural friction rub	8

in establishing a diagnosis (Greenspan et al., 1982). Chest radiographs are probably most important in excluding other diagnoses that may mimic PE, such as pneumothorax. Diminished pulmonary vascular markings at the site of the embolus may be present, such as Westermark's sign (Westermark, 1938), but this has been an inconstant and frequently equivocal sign occurring in less than 10% of cases (Stein et al., 1991; Torrance, 1963).

Although formerly considered diagnostically important, specific serum enzyme changes are seldom conclusive and rarely necessary. The triad of elevated serum *lactate dehydrogenase* activity, increased serum bilirubin, and normal *serum glutamic-oxaloacetic transaminase* activity is often present in patients with PE (Wacker and Snodgrass, 1960).

The *electrocardiogram* (ECG) is abnormal in most patients, even if they have no history of cardiac or pulmonary disease (Stein et al., 1991). The ECG is most helpful in establishing the presence or absence of other clinical conditions that present similarly to PE. In the Urokinase and Streptokinase Pulmonary Embolism Trials, 23% of patients with submassive PE had a normal ECG. In the event of a massive PE, essentially all patients will exhibit an abnormal ECG (Bell et al., 1977). In most cases the ECG is nonspecific, demonstrating only sinus tachycardia, or nonspecific ST-T wave changes. In patients with acute cor pulmonale as a consequence of massive PE, the ECG may demonstrate P-pulmonale, right axis deviation, right bundle-branch block, or other signs of right ventricular strain (Worsley et al., 1993).

Arterial blood gases have long been included in the evaluation of PE. However, hypoxemia is not a sensitive indicator, since 10 to 26% of cases of documented PE have a normal Pa_{CO_2}. Measurement of the increased $P(A-a)_{CO_2}$ gradient and hypocapnia improves the sensitivity of arterial blood gas analysis to 98%, if both are present. Therefore, a normal $P(A-a)_{CO_2}$ gradient and a normal Pa_{CO_2} obtained from a patient breathing room air can be used as evidence

against the presence of a PE (Cvitanic and Marino, 1989).

Among 171 patients who had abdominal and pelvic operative procedures, ^{111}In platelet imaging was performed. Fifteen had inadequate circulating blood pools of ^{111}In platelets, which made their study nondiagnostic. Of 156 patients with technically satisfactory images, 46 (29.5%) had images consistent with deep venous thrombosis or PEs. The incidence, time of occurrence, and location of thromboemboli were similar to those of other reports of postoperative groups of patients studied by ^{125}I fibrinogen uptake testing. Eighty patients had normal ^{111}In scans, and 30 patients had diffusely distributed indium platelets found in the operative field, which suggested accumulation in a postoperative hematoma. None of these results was confused with a diagnosis of deep venous thrombosis. When compared with another accurate diagnostic test in 23 patients, ^{111}In platelet imaging had a sensitivity of 100% and specificity of 90%. This imaging technique is easily performed and has the advantage of allowing surveillance of the legs, pelvis, abdomen, and chest by a single method, making it appropriate for the identification of postoperative thromboemboli (Clarke-Pearson et al., 1985).

Impedance plethysmography is an accurate noninvasive method for assessing the presence of proximal venous thrombosis, but it is mostly insensitive to calf vein thrombi. In a study of patients with clinically suspected deep vein thrombosis, normal impedance plethysmographic findings were randomly assigned to either serial impedance plethysmography alone or impedance plethysmography and radioactive leg scanning combined (which has been essentially as sensitive as venography). The long-term outcomes were compared. During the initial surveillance, deep venous thrombosis was detected in 6 of 311 patients (1.9%) who were tested by serial impedance plethysmography alone and in 30 of 323 patients (9.3%, most with calf vein thrombi) who were tested by the combined approach ($p < .001$). During long-term follow-up, no patient died of PE, but 6 patients tested by serial impedance plethysmography developed deep venous thrombosis, compared with 7 patients tested by the combined approach. These data indicate that serial impedance plethysmography used alone is an effective method in evaluating these symptomatic patients (Hull et al., 1985).

Pulmonary function testing is nonspecific and may show abnormal parameters, but is of some benefit in assessing functional recovery after PE (Prediletto et al., 1990). The physiologic dead space increases, with the ratio of dead space to tidal volume reaching greater than 40% (Burki, 1986). Occlusion of a major pulmonary arterial branch decreases gas exchange in the corresponding segment of the lung, while alveolar ventilation continues. In a ventilated but underperfused segment of lung, the composition of the alveolar air tends to approach that of inspired air, with a low partial pressure of carbon dioxide. This air is mixed with the air from the normal areas of the lung during expiration, but reduces the mean alveolar carbon dioxide tension to a degree that can be detected in the expired air. Arterial carbon dioxide tension remains at a nearly normal level because of the presence of normal pulmonary tissue. Knowledge of the difference between the arterial and the alveolar carbon dioxide tensions, therefore, may help in the diagnosis of PE.

Wagner and co-workers (1964) introduced *radioisotope pulmonary scanning*. It is still the technique most frequently employed for the objective diagnosis of PE. The method measures macromolecules of human serum albumin (10 to 100μm in diameter) labeled with ^{131}I, ^{51}Cr, or ^{99m}Tc, which are intravenously injected and subsequently become lodged in the pulmonary capillary bed. This measurement allows the assessment of the distribution of pulmonary arterial blood flow, and thus reveals areas of decreased perfusion. Lesions present on the plain chest film (such as pneumonitis, atelectasis, hemothorax, pleural effusion, emphysematous bullae, or neoplasm) uniformly show scanning defects; therefore, these areas must be excluded from consideration. It is essential, therefore, that the chest film be reviewed simultaneously with the scanning. Radioisotope pulmonary scanning has been particularly useful in patients with massive PE, especially if the plain chest film is essentially normal. *Inhalation scanning* with ^{133}Xe has also helped in the interpretation of the perfusion pulmonary scan. Inhalation scanning shows the differentiation of underperfused and underventilated areas in the lungs. PE produces bronchoconstriction, thus reducing the amount of air delivered to the embolized portion of the lung, and areas of the lung without PE show bronchoconstriction with reduced ventilation. This and other pathologic processes may cause a ventilation-perfusion mismatch, which produces an abnormal scan (Table 23–3). Approximately 5% of the normal population will have a ventilation-perfusion scan read as abnormal (Ryu and Rosenow, 1992).

The ventilation-perfusion lung scan is a safe, noninvasive technique that has undergone a great deal of study and refinement. Some controversy remains regarding the true accuracy of the technique; however, several large trials have defined its utility and limitations. The National Institutes of Health–sponsored study Prospective Investigation of Pulmonary Embolism Diagnosis (PIOPED) was a multicenter effort to estimate the sensitivity and specificity of the ventilation-perfusion lung scan. In PIOPED, 98% of patients with clinically important PE had lung scans that fell into one of three categories: high, intermediate (indeterminate), or low probability. If all three abnormal categories were combined, the lung scan was sensitive enough to serve as a screening tool. However, the specificity was limited. The high-probability scan lacked sensitivity, failing to identify 59% of patients with angiographically documented PE. If the clinical evaluation was combined with the ventilation-perfusion scan, the predictive value improved substantially. When there was a discrepancy between the clinical and the scan category, the angiographic correlation was less predictable (Nyman,

■ **Table 23–3.** VENTILATION–PERFUSION MISMATCH

1. Pulmonary embolism (acute or chronic)
2. Pneumonia
3. Bronchogenic carcinoma
4. Radiation therapy
5. Tuberculosis/histoplasmosis
6. Metastasis
7. Obstructive lung disease
8. Collagen vascular disease/vasculitis
9. Sarcoidosis
10. Systemic arterial supply
11. Vascular compression
12. Lymphangitic carcinomatosis
13. Dog heartworm
14. Air/fat embolism
15. Pulmonary hypertension
16. Mitral valve disease
17. Sickle cell disease
18. Congenital pulmonary vascular abnormalities (agenesis/stenosis)
19. Pulmonary arteriovenous malformation
20. Traumatic pulmonary artery pseudoaneurysm
21. Pulmonary artery sarcoma
22. Pulmonary veno-occlusive disease
23. Hemangioendotheliomatosis
24. Hiatal hernia
25. Wedged Swan-Ganz catheter

From Nyman, U.: Diagnostic studies in acute pulmonary embolism. Haemostasis, 23(Suppl.):220, 1993. By permission of S. Karger AG, Basel.

1993; PIOPED Investigators, 1990; Worsley et al., 1993) (Fig. 23–10).

In a prospective study by Hull and colleagues (1989), 874 patients with suspected PE were enrolled in an effort to ascertain if anticoagulation could be withheld in patients with a *non*–high probability ventilation-perfusion scan, adequate cardiorespiratory reserve, and absent proximal vein thrombosis, as determined by impedance plethysmography. In such patients, only 2.7% had evidence of thromboembolism at interval follow-up. Unfortunately, this study's use of unconventional criteria to categorize the ventila-

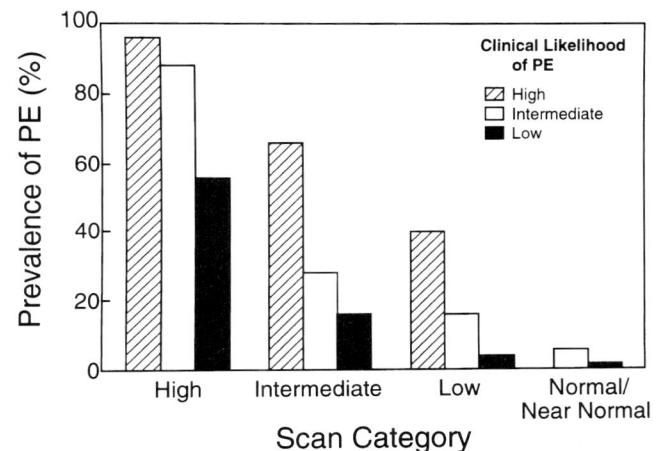

FIGURE 23–10. Value of correlating $\dot{V}/\dot{Q}$ scan category with the clinical likelihood of pulmonary embolism (PE). (Modified from Worsley, D. F., Alavi, A., and Palevsky, H. I.: Role of radionuclide imaging in patients with suspected pulmonary embolism. Radiol. Clin. North Am., *31*:849, 1993.)

tion-perfusion scans made the comparison of its results with those of PIOPED and other studies impossible.

Because treatment for patients with deep venous thrombosis is similar whether or not there is clinical suspicion of PE, some authors advocate an approach that eliminates a ventilation-perfusion scan from the evaluation process in patients who are *stable* after suspected PE. Others believe all derivable information important, and *all* agree to proceed with the ventilation-perfusion scan in the unusual, the difficult to diagnose, and the critically ill (Kruit et al., 1991; Nyman, 1993).

Thus, the ventilation-perfusion scan is used routinely to evaluate patients suspected to have PE. When the clinical suspicion correlates with the scan as either high or low probability, a highly accurate diagnosis can be made. When the clinical diagnosis disagrees with the ventilation-perfusion scan results, further studies must be performed to accurately conclude the presence of PE.

Fifty-two per cent of asymptomatic patients with documented deep venous thrombosis have perfusion defects on lung scans, and many will develop clinical symptoms subsequently (Moser and LeMoine, 1981). In another study, patients with a diagnosis of venous thrombosis were treated with heparin, and a baseline lung perfusion scan was obtained. Forty-three had abnormal scans, and 17% of those with high-probability scans developed acute signs of PE on heparin. A repeat scan in these patients did not disclose new perfusion defects. In the absence of a baseline perfusion study, these scans may be interpreted as demonstrating PE during treatment, and this misinterpretation may lead to unnecessary vena caval interruption or filter placement for failed heparin therapy (Monreal et al., 1989). This study supports routine lung perfusion scans for patients with deep venous thrombosis and no symptoms of acute PE.

Venograms are useful in establishing a definitive diagnosis of deep venous thrombosis, particularly in the legs. The use of venograms is especially significant if the diagnosis is in doubt or if interruption of the vena cava is being considered. Radioiodinated fibrinogen, although sensitive in detecting the development of new thrombi in the extremities, is less accurate in detecting thrombi in the *iliofemoral* region, owing to poor penetration of ^{125}I and to the background of radioactivity in the urinary bladder.

Two-dimensional transthoracic and transesophageal echocardiography can reveal direct and indirect signs of PE, but only in the main and central portions of the left and right pulmonary arteries. Intravascular ultrasound has been successful in evaluating large central as well as smaller, more peripheral pulmonary arteries. An indwelling intravascular ultrasonic probe may be used to monitor thrombolytic therapy (Görge et al., 1991).

Pulmonary arteriography is the most definitive method in the diagnosis of PE. The results of the angiogram are, however, indeterminate in 3 to 15% of patients (Hull et al., 1985; PIOPED Investigators,

1990). It is important to recognize the appearance of a normal pulmonary angiogram, so that morphologic and physiologic changes can be interpreted properly (Simon and Sasahara, 1965; Stein et al., 1967). The arteries in the lower areas of the lung are normally larger than those in the upper portions, because they serve a larger volume of pulmonary tissue. Major branches are readily identifiable by comparison with normal anatomic charts of the pulmonary arteries. These vessels usually follow the branching pattern of the bronchi.

Total obstruction of the main pulmonary artery is associated with the most profound symptoms, and is usually followed by sudden death. In most patients who survive the initial attack, the obstruction in the pulmonary arteries involves lobar or segmental branches (Fig. 23–11). Stein and associates (1967) evaluated the angiographic signs of PE and concluded that an intraluminal filling defect and vessel cut-off with a trailing edge were the only two primary angiographic criteria that were reliable. The filling defect may be sharply delineated, usually manifested as a convex shadow with a blunt end or an irregular taper. For an accurate diagnosis, the defect should remain constant on several successive films in the series, and the flow may be sluggish, which is shown by a small pool of contrast medium that may persist in the artery above the obstruction well into the venous phase of the angiogram. When pulmonary arteriography is done later in the course of embolism, contrast medium may pass around the obstruction, causing delayed opacification of the artery distally. In some areas, the pattern may show avascular segments that represent the result of unresolved thromboembolism. Oblique views of the pulmonary arteriogram allow maximal visualization and more accurate diagnosis (Gomes et al., 1977).

Diagnosis of PE in patients with *chronic obstructive pulmonary disease* (COPD) is often difficult, because the presentation of an acute embolic event may closely mimic the symptoms of acute airway obstruction. Lesser and associates (1992) evaluated 108 patients with COPD and suspected PE. In most patients, the ventilation-perfusion scan diagnosis was indeterminate, and such patients required more investigational studies. In the few patients with a high-probability scan, PE was confirmed by angiography. If the scan was of low probability or near-normal to normal, the negative predictive value was not lower than that of the general hospital population.

MANAGEMENT

The goal of therapy is to avoid mortality or recurrence and reduce morbidity (including pulmonary hypertension and postphlebitic syndrome) from acute PE. The single most important feature to be established before starting therapy for PE is an unequivocal diagnosis. The two most important and reliable means of diagnosis are pulmonary *scanning* and *arteri-*

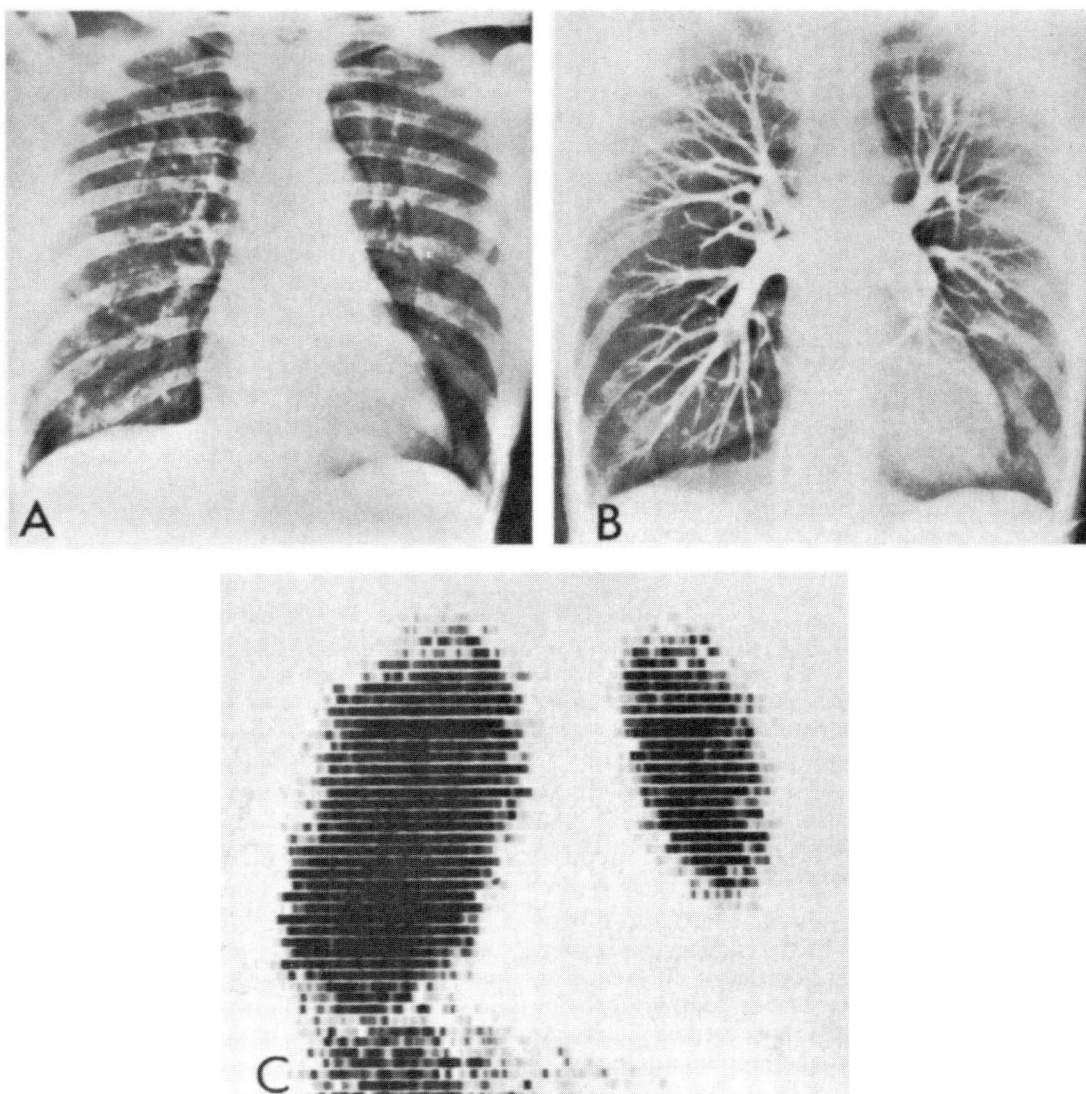

FIGURE 23–11. Films from a patient with pulmonary embolism involving the left lower lobar pulmonary artery. *A*, Slight diminution of the vascular markings to the left lower lobe is noted in comparison with those in the right lower lobe of the plain chest film (Westermark's sign). *B*, Pulmonary arteriogram showing occlusion of the right lower lobar pulmonary artery. *C*, Pulmonary scan showing absence of perfusion of the left lower lobe. (*A–C*, From Sabiston, D. C., Jr., and Wagner, H. N., Jr.: The diagnosis of pulmonary embolism by radioisotope scanning. Ann. Surg., *160*:585, 1964.)

ography. Because scanning is a simple, safe, and reliable technique, it is generally preferred. It causes the patient little inconvenience and has no appreciable risk. If the pulmonary scan is to be used for definitive diagnosis, a concomitant plain chest film must show a normal pulmonary appearance in the area in which the scan is positive for pulmonary arterial occlusion.

Medical Management

Prevention

One of the most important aspects of the entire spectrum of PE is its *prophylaxis*, especially in postoperative patients, in whom its incidence can be predicted. However, no proven method or combination of methods currently exists for total prevention of thromboembolism. Two major risk factors have been identified: *venous stasis* secondary to immobility, venous obstruction, or congestive heart failure; and *trauma*, which includes operation and childbirth.

Several prophylactic treatment regimens that modify thrombogenesis have been studied. These include drugs that inhibit blood coagulation (such as heparin and the coumarins), drugs that inhibit platelet function (such as aspirin and dextran), and techniques to counteract venous stasis (such as leg elevation [Fig. 23–12], compression stockings, pneumatic compression devices, and perioperative calf muscle stimulation) (Hyers et al., 1989).

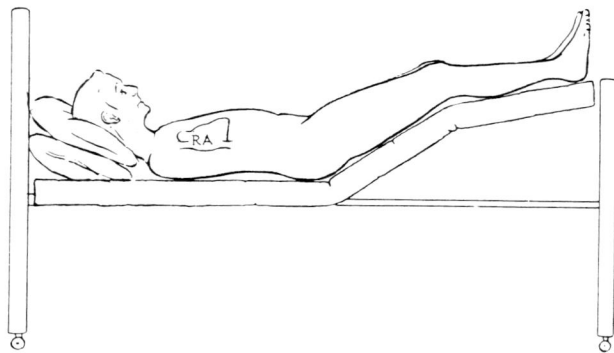

FIGURE 23–12. Correct position for the lower extremities in prophylaxis of pulmonary embolism. Note the additional break at the knees. It is important that the level of the veins in the lower extremities be above the mean level of the right atrium (RA). (From Sabiston, D. C., Jr.: Pulmonary embolism. *In* Sabiston, D. C., Jr. [ed]: Textbook of Surgery. 13th ed. Philadelphia, W. B. Saunders, 1986.)

Early ambulation and resumption of physical activity after operation or bedrest for other illness have long been recommended. In a classic study performed to evaluate the role of exercise as prophylaxis, postmortem vein dissections showed that thrombi were found in only 18% of patients who had exercised before death, compared with 53% in controls (nonexercised and nonambulatory) (Hunter et al., 1945). Other studies have been less confirmatory, including one in which the ^{125}I-labeled fibrinogen method for detection of leg vein thrombi was used. The patients in this study had an intensive regimen, including vigorous leg exercises both before and after operation, elevation of the foot of the bed, and the continuous use of elastic stockings. Despite these intensive efforts, thrombosis was detected in 25% of the patients on the regimen, compared with 35% in controls. In older patients undergoing major surgical procedures, the incidence was 24%, compared with 61% in the controls. Therefore, this regimen has a significant prophylactic effect for the elderly.

Certain groups of patients have shown proven benefit by prophylactic anticoagulation, especially those who have experienced trauma and those undergoing orthopedic (predominantly hip and knee procedures) or genitourinary tract operations (Hull et al., 1986a; Hume et al., 1970; Hyers et al., 1989; Sevitt and Gallagher, 1961).

In 1966, the concept of *low-dose heparin* as a prophylactic measure was introduced (Sharnoff, 1966). With one exception, many trials with low-dose heparin administered to surgical patients postoperatively have shown a decrease in deep venous thrombosis in those patients treated compared with those untreated (Fratantoni and Wessler, 1975; Hull et al., 1986a; Hyers et al., 1989; Wessler, 1976). These trials included ^{125}I-labeled fibrinogen leg scanning or venography, or both, for demonstration of venous thrombosis. The most important of these studies is included in a multicenter clinical trial involving more than 4000 patients (International Multicentre Trial, 1975).

Although the dosage and duration of the administration of heparin have varied among authors, a dose of 5000 units subcutaneously every 12 hours until the patient is fully ambulatory is recommended (Hull et al., 1986a). The routine coagulation tests are prolonged minimally, if at all, and have a low risk of bleeding. The protection offered by this regimen may be in its potentiation of a naturally occurring plasmin inhibitor of activated Factor X (Kakkar et al., 1971).

Dextran is a branched polysaccharide produced by bacteria, which interferes with both platelet and coagulation protein function. In several large studies, dextran has been as effective as low-dose heparin in moderate-risk patients and superior in high-risk patients. The major drawback of dextran therapy is its potential contribution to volume overload in patients with poor cardiac reserve. Dextran rarely causes an allergic reaction (Hyers et al., 1989).

Aspirin has failed in multiple trials to decrease the incidence of venous thromboembolism. There are a few reports of its efficacy in high-risk hip surgery patients (Hyers et al., 1989).

Combination therapy with low-dose heparin and dihydroergotamine has been comparable to dextran and associated with greater safety for patients undergoing emergency or elective abdominal or thoracic surgery (Sasahara et al., 1986).

Mechanical means of preventing venous thrombosis appear to be the most promising in high-risk and neurosurgical patients, in whom even a minimal amount of bleeding can be serious. Perioperative electrical stimulation of the calf muscles is effective, but this is not tolerated in awake patients (Rosenberg et al., 1975). Intermittent external pneumatic compression has relatively few complications and is extremely useful in patients undergoing orthopedic, urologic, or neurologic procedures (Hyers et al., 1989).

Anticoagulants

For most patients with venous thrombosis and PE, anticoagulants constitute the primary basis of therapy. The scanning and arteriographic features of an appropriate patient for treatment with anticoagulants are shown in Figure 23–9. Heparin is generally used initially, and its effect when administered intravenously is immediate. Heparin is derived from bovine lung or porcine intestinal mucosa and acts primarily by enhancing the effect of antithrombin III by 1000-fold. Antithrombin III inactivates a number of serine proteases, the most sensitive of which are Factors IIa (thrombin), IXa, and Xa. Therefore, heparin inhibits both the *intrinsic* and the *extrinsic* coagulation mechanisms. In high doses, heparin prevents the action of thrombin on platelets. Heparin is degraded by the liver (heparinase) and excreted mainly in the urine. Its therapy prevents both extension of the thrombus in the venous system and the formation of distal in situ thrombi in the pulmonary arteries.

Heparin should be administered in a concentration designed to maintain the clotting time at two to three times normal (20 to 35 minutes, assuming a normal clotting time of 8 to 12 minutes) or to prolong the *activated partial thromboplastin time* (APTT) to approximately twice the value of the patient's preheparin time (Hyers et al., 1989; Ryu and Rosenow, 1992). The amount required varies. Ten thousand units are given intravenously as the initial dose, followed by an infusion of 1000 units per hour via a central venous catheter. The continuous intravenous infusion, versus intermittent bolus, provides a more stabilized level of anticoagulation and a reduced incidence of hemorrhage (Salzman et al., 1975). The APTT should be checked frequently the first 24 hours (two to four times), and once or twice per day therafter. The risk of recurrent thromboembolism is significantly increased if the APTT is not elevated to 1.5 times or greater than control within the first 24 hours (Hull et al., 1986b). In addition, heparin clearance from the circulation is increased in patients with PE or massive venous thrombosis; therefore, these patients require higher doses (Hirsch et al., 1976).

The optimal duration of initial heparin therapy is not known. Traditionally, 8 to 10 days of heparin with extension of the APTT 1.5 to 2 times normal is recommended, because this approximates the time necessary for the venous thrombi to become firmly adherent to the vessel wall. Oral anticoagulation is initiated on the fourth or fifth day, leading to an overlap of both drugs for 3 to 5 days. During this period, a moderate amount of thrombolysis also occurs. A recent study concludes that first-day warfarin introduced in patients with submassive PE is as effective as fourth- or fifth-day introduction; therefore, hospital length of stay and costs can be reduced by introducing warfarin earlier (Gallus et al., 1986).

Postoperative delayed hemorrhage may occur in patients receiving heparin therapy for PEs, particularly those with prosthetic arterial grafts. There may be a continuous lysis and resorption of old thrombus, with replacement by new thrombus at arterial prosthesis suture lines, until the suture line is sealed by regeneration of new intima. Thus, patients have had serious hemorrhages for as long as 1 month after the placement of aortic arterial grafts, when maintained on heparin therapy for treatment of venous thromboembolism (Ariyan and Stansel, 1976).

Oral anticoagulation in the form of warfarin sodium is customarily begun several days before cessation of heparin therapy to allow adequate prolongation of the *prothrombin time*. Warfarin sodium (Coumadin, Panwarfarin, Sofarin) inhibits vitamin K–dependent carboxylation of Factors II, VII, IX, and X and proteins C and S. Warfarin is rapidly absorbed from the gastrointestinal tract, and approximately 97% becomes albumin-bound. Warfarin is concentrated primarily in the liver, where it is metabolized into inactive products, secreted into bile, reabsorbed, and excreted in urine. The loading dose on the first and second days is 10 to 20 mg. The maximal effect usually is reached in 1.5 to 2 days, and the average daily maintenance dose is between 5 and 10 mg (range from 2 to 20 mg). The half-life is 36 to 72 hours (average, 42 hours). The recovery time required after maximal effect is 2 to 5 days. Administration of par-

enteral vitamin K counteracts the effect of the warfarin and should be used if bleeding complications occur. Many important drug interactions alter the bioavailability of warfarin, including drugs that reduce the anticoagulant effect by increasing hepatic clearance (e.g., phenobarbital) and drugs that enhance the effect by displacing it from albumin binding (e.g., trimethoprim-sulfamethoxazole) (Hyers et al., 1989). The optimal duration of warfarin therapy is controversial; however, the local responses and subsequent course of the patient are the primary indications for continuing anticoagulation.

The Research Committee of the British Thoracic Society (1992) performed a multicenter analysis of 4 weeks versus 3 months of anticoagulation in patients admitted with PE, deep venous thrombosis, or both. Four weeks of anticoagulation was adequate if a venous thromboembolism occurred after surgery. In patients with a new deep venous thrombosis or PE, or both, who did not have a persistent underlying risk factor, anticoagulation for at least 3 months was advantageous. After recurrent thromboembolic events, at least 1 year of anticoagulation therapy is recommended. If three or more thromboembolic episodes occur, anticoagulation should be continued indefinitely (Hirsch and Hull, 1986; Hyers et al., 1989). Patients with antithrombin III or protein C or S deficiency also should be continued on indefinite anticoagulant therapy.

In a study to determine the effects of the duration of warfarin anticoagulant therapy and the probabilities of recurrent thromboembolism and hemorrhage, the medical records of 2422 patients hospitalized with PE or thrombophlebitis, or both, were reviewed. Among 370 patients who had positive venography or pulmonary angiography, or who had a pulmonary scan showing a high probability of PE and no history of the disease, warfarin therapy for more than 6 weeks was not associated with a lower risk of recurrent thromboembolism when compared with warfarin therapy for 1 to 6 weeks. The longer the time of warfarin therapy, the higher the risk of medically important complications. From 1 week to 5 years, the probability of major hemorrhage increased almost linearly: 10% at 12 weeks, 18% at 1 year, 26% at 2 years, and 41% at 5 years. This study suggests that intensive, long-term warfarin anticoagulation in patients with a first episode of venous thromboembolism and no predisposing factors was associated more with toxicity than efficacy and should be abandoned (Petitti et al., 1986).

Thrombolytic Agents

Since the early 1960s, much effort has been directed toward finding suitable thrombolytic agents for use in the treatment of venous thrombosis and PE. In the body, *plasminogen* is the inactive precursor of *plasmin,* the active fibrinolytic enzyme. Under normal circumstances, plasminogen is present in the blood and tissues. Exercise, stress, and shock cause plasminogen to be activated to plasmin through a labile activator present in many tissues, especially in venous endothelium. Plasmin activity in the bloodstream is prevented by inhibitors (antiactivators and antiplasmins). Several thrombolytic agents that act by converting plasminogen to plasmin have been studied, including streptokinase, urokinase, and *recombinant tissue plasminogen activator* (rTPA).

Streptokinase is a soluble product of the metabolism of *Streptococcus pyogenes* (Lancefield Group A) and is available in a highly purified form. Patients who have had previous streptococcal infections may be allergic to streptokinase; therefore, it can produce toxic reactions (pyrexia, dyspnea, tachycardia, and anaphylaxis). Urokinase is a strong thrombolytic agent found in human urine. In an effort to document its effects, the National Heart and Lung Institute conducted a national cooperative study with urokinase. The results showed that urokinase combined with heparin therapy, compared with heparin therapy alone, significantly accelerated the resolution of pulmonary thromboemboli at 24 hours, as shown by pulmonary arteriograms, pulmonary scans, and right-sided heart pressure measurements. However, no significant differences were noted between heparin and urokinase therapy in recurrence rate of PE or in the 2-week mortality (9% versus 7%, respectively). Bleeding complications were prominent in both groups and occurred in 45% of the patients receiving urokinase, compared with 27% of those given heparin alone. Most bleeding complications were at the angiogram catheterization sites. It was concluded that, because the urokinase regimen did not usually achieve complete or almost complete thrombolysis, and especially because of its hemorrhagic potential, further studies with urokinase were necessary before specific therapeutic recommendations could be made (Urokinase Pulmonary Embolism Trial Study Group, 1970).

Subsequently, the Urokinase Streptokinase Pulmonary Embolism Trial was performed, randomizing 167 patients with angiographically proven PE to receive either urokinase (12 or 24 hours) or streptokinase (24 hours). No difference was detected in mortality rate, resolution of clot, or bleeding complications (Urokinase Streptokinase Pulmonary Embolism Trial Study Group, 1974).

Goldhaber and co-workers (1988) performed a series of clinical trials evaluating rTPA in the treatment of PE compared with urokinase therapy. In one study, rTPA was superior in improving perfusion at 24 hours versus urokinase. Also, there was more bleeding in the urokinase group.

Levine and colleagues (1990) compared bolus rTPA followed by heparin with placebo bolus plus heparin in a double-blind study. Resolution of the perfusion defect by lung scan at 24 hours was significantly improved in the rTPA/heparin group versus the placebo/heparin group; however, by 7 days, there was no difference in the two groups. No major bleeding complications appeared in either group. Minor bleeding complications were more common in the rTPA group.

In a study designed to determine the long-term effects of thrombolytic treatment in patients with acute and massive embolism, seven patients with this condition had pulmonary angiography and pressure measurements before and after treatment with intrapulmonary infusions of urokinase (average dose, 1724 units/kg/hr) and heparin (average dose, 17 units/kg/hr). Treatment was guided by daily measurements of pulmonary arterial pressure and was continued until the pressure had normalized (an average of 6 days later). Each patient returned for pulmonary angiographic examination and right-sided heart catheterization at rest and during bicycle exercise, as well as phlebography of the deep veins of both legs. The pulmonary angiograms showed massive obstructions before therapy, with improvement within 6 days after treatment. The mean pulmonary arterial pressure declined from an average of 37 ± 9 to 13 ± 3 mm Hg after 6 days, and to 15 ± 3 mm Hg after 15 months. No recurrence of PE was observed. In six of seven patients at rest and during supine bicycle exercise, mean pulmonary arterial pressure and total pulmonary resistance remained within normal limits. Over the short term, all patients showed clinical signs of deep venous thrombosis. Fifteen months later, four patients had normal deep veins, but three had phlebographic signs of old thrombosis. Thus, after thrombolytic treatment of acute massive PE, normal pulmonary arteriograms were obtained in six of the seven patients studied, and the reserve capacity of the pulmonary vasculature that was assessed during heavy exercise was normal in those patients (Schwarz et al., 1985).

A study of eight centers compared intrapulmonary and intravenous administration of rTPA in 34 patients with acute massive PE (Verstraete et al., 1988). This trial indicates that the pulmonary arterial infusion of rTPA does not offer a significant benefit over the intravenous route, but does suggest that a prolonged infusion of rTPA (100 mg) over 7 hours is superior to a single infusion of 50 mg over 2 hours.

In conclusion, thrombolytic therapy leads to a more rapid resolution of radiographic and hemodynamic abnormalities caused by acute PE than does heparin therapy alone. However, 1 week after therapy, the resolution of perfusion abnormalities is similar. In addition, no differences have been found in mortality rates in thrombolytic therapy versus heparin therapy alone. Many have criticized the aforementioned studies as too small to show possible treatment advantages. Bleeding complications appear to be higher in urokinase and streptokinase and lower in heparin therapy, when compared with rTPA. A shorter infusion or bolus of rTPA has effectively reduced bleeding rates (Levine, 1993).

Therefore, thrombolytic therapy should be reserved for critically ill patients who are hemodynamically compromised and who may benefit from rapid resolution of the embolism. To date, studies of patients in shock after PE have not demonstrated a significant reduction in death rate with thrombolytic therapy (Anderson and Levine, 1992).

Percutaneous Catheter Techniques

A percutaneous technique to fragment proximal clot with distal dispersion has successfully treated acute massive PE (Brady et al., 1991; Schmitz-Rode and Günther, 1991). This technique has also been combined with thrombolytic therapy in small series with encouraging results (Brady et al., 1992; Essop et al., 1992). Transvenous suction devices and spiral embolectomy catheters have also been used to treat PEs (Greenfield et al., 1969, 1971; Günther and Vorwerk, 1990; Starck et al., 1985). Greenfield and associates (1969, 1971) used a transvenous method for pulmonary embolectomy by passing a large catheter into the femoral vein, through the heart, and into the pulmonary arteries. A suction cup was attached to the end of the catheter, and once the cup had engaged the embolus, suction was applied. The catheter and the embolus were then withdrawn and delivered through the femoral incision. Greenfield and others have reported clinical success with this technique; it is clearly innovative, but its ultimate role is not yet established. Finally, a clot-trapper device for transjugular thrombectomy from the inferior vena cava has been described experimentally (Ponomar et al., 1991).

Surgical Management

Anticoagulant therapy for PE most often is successful; however, at times, its use is contraindicated. In these situations, the physician must choose one of the aforementioned percutaneous techniques or choose surgical therapy.

Venous Thrombectomy

Although the direct removal of venous thrombi was previously recommended (DeWeese et al., 1960; Haller, 1962), this procedure is rarely used today because of the high incidence of recurrent thrombosis in the postoperative period (Karp and Wylie, 1966), and because of the possibility of massive PE intraoperatively. Most observers agree, however, that in patients with phlegmasia cerulea dolens, thrombectomy is indicated. Secondary arterial spasm frequently accompanies phlegmasia cerulea dolens, and even though venous thrombosis may recur after thrombectomy, patency of the venous lumen may persist long enough to relieve the arterial spasm and permit the limb to recover from arterial insufficiency. In these cases, systemic heparinization is clearly indicated to prolong the patency of the vein.

Interruption of the Inferior Vena Cava

For many years, interruption of the vena cava has been advocated for selected patients with PE. Some physicians have recommended complete ligation (Ochsner, 1960), whereas others prefer plication (Spencer et al., 1962, 1965), filter or screen methods (Braverman et al., 1992; DeWeese and Hunter, 1963), or plastic clips (Adams and DeWeese, 1969; Miles et al., 1964; Moretz et al., 1959). Evidence of recurrent PE has been reported in as many as 20% of patients after vena caval ligation (Gurewich et al., 1966). Recurrent emboli have been shown to arise from the portion of the inferior vena cava between the ligature and the renal veins and from the veins of the upper extremities and neck. The right atrium and right ventricle have also been sources of recurrent emboli, including emboli arising from chronic indwelling catheters placed for parenteral alimentation and pacemaker leads. It is important to consider all systemic veins and the right side of the heart as potential sources of PEs.

Venous interruptive procedures can prevent recurrent and potentially fatal PEs. These procedures must be considered *adjuvant* approaches, because they do not directly attack the thromboembolic process. Barker and co-workers (1941) carefully documented the natural history of PE for which no specific therapy was administered, on the basis of the large experience of the Mayo Clinic. This study of 1665 patients showed that the likelihood of a second embolus was 30%, and that a fatal second embolus occurred in 18% of the untreated group. After the work of Murray and Best (1938), anticoagulation with heparin evolved as the standard accepted treatment for venous thrombosis and PE, and it continues to be used as the baseline for measurement of all other approaches. The effectiveness of this method was documented by Coon and colleagues (1969), who summarized a 20-year experience. In 639 patients with a single PE treated with anticoagulant therapy, the fatal recurrent PE rate was only 1.3%. In patients with venous thrombosis and no demonstrated embolus, the fatal PE rate was 0.14%. Because the risk associated with most surgical procedures designed to prevent recurrent thromboembolism substantially exceeds the 1.3% mortality reported by Coon and associates, surgical treatment should be reserved for exceptional patients who fail to respond to anticoagulant therapy or for those who have specific contraindications to its institution (Silver and Sabiston, 1975).

The indications for vena caval interruption continue to be controversial. One group of authors recommends the use of inferior vena caval interruption frequently, often after the first attack of PE and not necessarily dependent on the severity of the clinical and radiologic findings (Ochsner et al., 1970). In this series, long-term complications were minimal. An opposite view is given in another series, in which the complications and mortality after vena caval interruption were significant (Piccone et al., 1970). The trend has been away from the use of inferior vena caval interruption, with increased attention given to intensive heparin anticoagulation, including its use in recurrent PE. Among 1000 patients with PE treated at the Duke University Medical Center, only 2% had interruption of the inferior vena cava. Nevertheless, vena caval interruption is occasionally required, and the indications for this procedure include the contraindications for anticoagulation therapy, recurrent PE despite adequate anticoagulation therapy, multiple small PEs creating chronic pulmonary insufficiency, pulmonary hypertension, septic emboli *refractory* to a combination of antibiotic and anticoagulant therapy, and after pulmonary embolectomy.

INFERIOR VENA CAVAL LIGATION

The approach to the inferior vena cava may be through a right flank incision, in which the exposure of the inferior vena cava is extraperitoneal, or through a midline, paramedian, or right subcostal abdominal incision, through which the exposure is intraperitoneal. In general, the right flank approach is most often used for men. The transabdominal route is preferred for women in order to expose and ligate the ovarian veins, a possible source of emboli. In both approaches, the vena cava is interrupted just below the origin of the renal veins (DeWeese, 1976).

USE OF TRANSLUMINAL FILTERS

Several technical procedures designed to simplify caval interruption have been developed with particular emphasis on reducing postoperative morbidity and mortality. In each of these techniques, an intraluminal device is introduced to trap large emboli arising from the branches of the inferior vena cava (Gardner, 1978). In 1968, Eichelter and Schenk advocated the transvenous approach for partial caval occlusion using local anesthesia. Later, several transvenous implantation devices evolved to prevent emboli from passing into the lungs, while avoiding excessive narrowing of the lumen. For example, the *umbrella* described by Mobin-Uddin and colleagues (1969, 1972) has had widespread application (Fig. 23–13). The most serious complication of this umbrella is improper insertion of the device into the iliac or renal vein. Another problem associated with the umbrella

is the possibility of migration, with passage into the right atrium, right ventricle, or pulmonary artery (Isch and Schumacker, 1976). To prevent migration, the diameter of the umbrella was increased, but the problem has continued, and migration has had fatal consequences in some patients. Additional complications reported with these intraluminal devices include misplacement, retroperitoneal hemorrhage, perforation of the duodenum and of the ureter, pericardial tamponade, and development of a thrombus proximal to the umbrella, producing recurrent emboli. Furthermore, the umbrella stimulates distal thrombosis in the vena cava, and occlusion occurs in 60 to 70% of patients in long-term follow-up studies.

A cone-shaped stainless-steel umbrella designed to trap emboli without significant reduction in venous flow has been developed by Greenfield and associates (1973, 1988). Since its introduction in 1972, the Greenfield filter has been placed in over 70,000 patients in the United States. Numerous reports cite operative mortality of less than 1%, recurrent emboli in less than 5%, and postoperative caval patency in 92 to 95% (Braverman et al., 1992). This device may be inserted with the patient under local anesthesia through either the femoral or the jugular vein (Fig. 23–14). Fixation is achieved by hooks that grasp the wall of the inferior vena cava, with care taken not to penetrate the full thickness of the caval wall. This *fishhook* device is designed to prevent proximal migration, with the filter becoming even more securely fixed when emboli become trapped. Distal migration can occur down to the bifurcation of the inferior vena cava, the struts may protrude through the caval wall, and thrombus may form on the filter itself (Wingerd et al., 1978). In one study, 167 patients in whom a Greenfield vena cava filter had been inserted were evaluated. The mean follow-up period of the survivors was 42 months, and the mean survival time of the 48% who died was 9.3 months. The mortality in 50 comparable patients without PE, but who had a

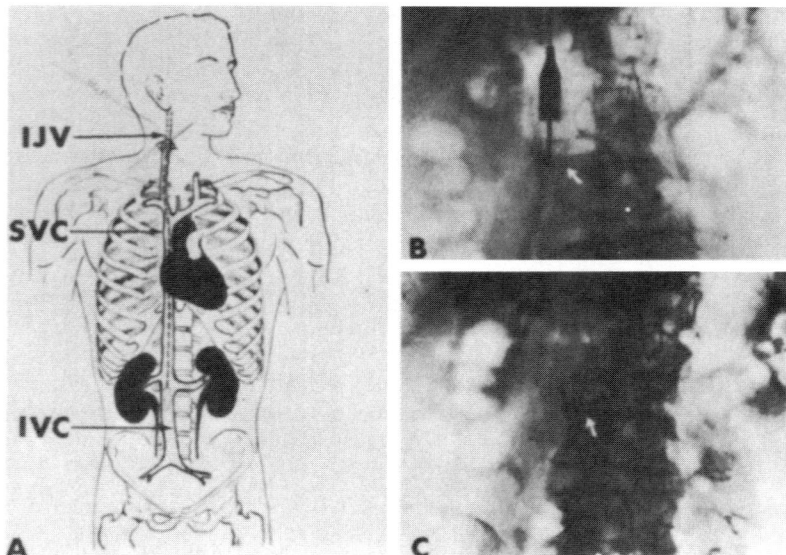

FIGURE 23–13. *A,* Applicator-capsule containing the collapsed umbrella filter inserted via the right internal jugular vein (IJV) and advanced through the superior vena cava (SVC) and the right atrium and into the inferior vena cava (IVC) below the renal veins. *B,* Position of the capsule distal to the renal pelvis in the inferior vena cava. The umbrella filter has been ejected from the capsule. It has sprung open and become fixed in place. *C,* The stylet has been unscrewed from the filter, and the applicator has been withdrawn. (*A–C,* From Mobin-Uddin, K., Callard, G. M., Bolooki, H., et al.: Transvenous caval interruption with umbrella filter. N. Engl. J. Med., *286:*55, 1972.)

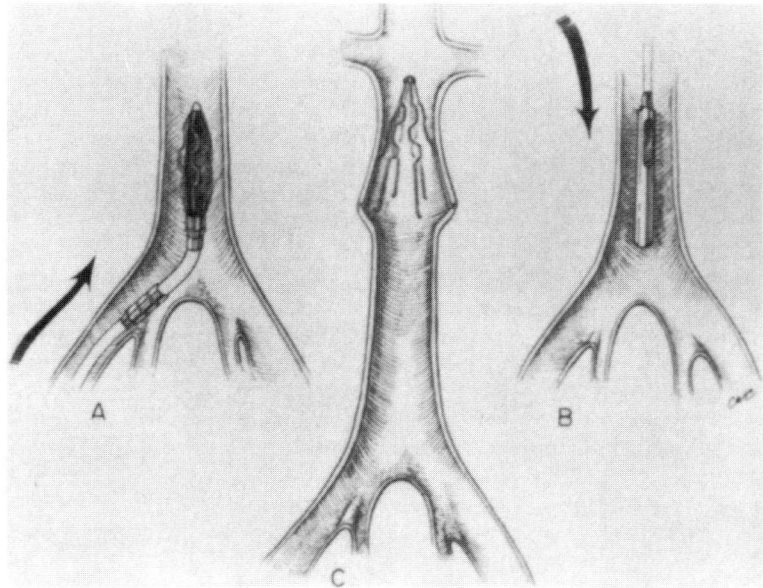

FIGURE 23–14. Insertion of the cone filter is accomplished by a carrier catheter inserted from the femoral vein *(A)* or retrograde from the jugular vein *(B)*. To avoid misplacement into the right renal vein, the jugular inserter should be passed down to the level of the pelvis and then withdrawn to the level of L3 for discharge *(C)*. Fixation is automatic, as the limbs spring open and the recurved hooks engage the wall of the inferior vena cava. *(A–C,* From Greenfield, L. J.: Pulmonary embolism: Diagnosis and management. Curr. Probl. Surg., *13:*1, 1976.)

prophylactic filter inserted, was 52%, with a mean survival time of 9.4 months. The mean follow-up period of the survivors was 28 months. Age, mean pulmonary artery pressure, and severity of the initial embolic episode did *not* predict the increased rate of late mortality. The study concluded that for patients who survive acute PE and have treatment to prevent recurrence, the embolic history of thromboembolism has little impact on late mortality, which instead is determined by preexisting medical conditions (Maxwell and Greenfield, 1987).

Magnant and associates (1992) reported 84 patients who underwent vena caval filters for contraindication to anticoagulation (64%), anticoagulation failure (25%), and prophylaxis (11%). Fifty per cent had documented lower extremity deep vein thrombosis, and 45% had documented PE. Five per cent received prophylactic filters without documented thromboembolism. One procedure-related death occurred (acute inferior vena cava occlusion). At a mean follow-up of 11 months, 50% had died of malignancy (n = 25), multisystem organ failure (MSOF, n = 7), cardiovascular events (n = 4), recurrent PEs (n = 2), cerebrovascular events (n = 4), or unknown causes (n = 1). Twenty-seven per cent (n = 23) died before hospital discharge, 16 of whom died of a malignancy or MSOF.

Of the subgroup of malignancy and MSOF, 43% died before discharge and another 25% died within 1 year. Because of a poor survival rate, the benefit of filter placement in patients with advanced malignancy or MSOF is questionable. Twenty-five per cent of patients who received a filter derived little or no benefit; therefore, careful patient selection is necessary to avoid unnecessary and costly filter placements.

Braverman and co-workers (1992) reported 120 patients who underwent vena caval interruption with either a Greenfield filter (n = 107) or an external vena caval clip (n = 13). They found a 98% success rate for interruption, a 7% complication rate, and no procedure-related major morbidity or mortality. Morbidity and mortality were summarized from several series and are illustrated in Table 23–4. Late follow-up revealed venous stasis ulcer in 1 patient, late caval thrombosis in 2 patients, and recurrent emboli in 1 patient. Sixteen per cent of patients with Greenfield's filters required support stockings.

Transluminal screening procedures are simple compared with other forms of caval interruption, but they are associated with a significant incidence of edema of the extremity and recurrent thrombophlebitis, as well as recurrent embolism. Intraluminal devices may have advantages over caval interruption because they

■ **Table 23–4.** GREENFIELD FILTER

First Author	Patients	Operative Mortality (%)	Recurrent Emboli (%)	Caval Patency (%)
Greenfield, 1988	169	1	4	98
Towne, 1978	33	0	0	95
Cutler, 1989	260	0	4.5	97
Sicard, 1987	90	0	2	97
Talkington, 1986	88	0	3.1	92
Braverman, 1991	107	0	3	98

From Braverman, S. J., Battey, P. M., and Smith, R. B., III: Vena caval interruption. Am. Surg., *58:*188, 1992.

avoid a major abdominal incision, but significant complications continue with their use. There appears to be a trend away from inferior vena caval interruption in favor of intensive anticoagulant therapy. Caval interruption, including that by various types of filters, should be reserved for patients in whom heparin therapy is definitely contraindicated, or in those with recurrent emboli who are unquestionably refractory to heparin therapy.

Pulmonary Embolectomy

In 1908, Trendelenburg performed the first pulmonary embolectomy at the University of Leipzig. He approached the problem in the laboratory by removing a large experimental embolus from the pulmonary artery of a calf. After reviewing the clinical course of nine patients who had succumbed with massive PE, he noted that in seven of the victims, death occurred between 10 and 60 minutes after the onset of symptoms. In only two patients was death sudden, with clinical symptoms of such short duration that treatment was precluded. He therefore proposed that the pulmonary artery be opened rapidly at thoracotomy and that the embolus be removed. In the original report, Trendelenburg described three patients on whom embolectomy was done; the longest survivor lived for 37 hours and ultimately died of hemorrhage from a surgically traumatized internal mammary artery. In 1924, his student Kirschner was the first surgeon to perform pulmonary embolectomy successfully with a long-term survivor. Despite Trendelenburg's logical concept and Kirschner's brilliant feat, it is generally recognized that more patients have succumbed from this approach than have survived. Moreover, among the survivors, significant brain damage due to cerebral hypoxia was common. By 1951, 22 patients managed by Trendelenburg's technique were reported in a collective review (Benichoux, 1951). Most of these patients had postoperative brain damage resulting both from hypoxia before embolectomy and from that occurring after the procedure. Only 3 of the 22 patients were long-term survivors.

The first successful pulmonary embolectomy in the United States was performed by Steenburg in 1957 (Steenburg et al., 1958). At that time, only 12 successful results had been reported in the world literature. Vossschulte (1965) reported 43 Trendelenburg's procedures performed between 1957 and 1963, with 7 survivors—more evidence of the high mortality associated with embolectomy without cardiopulmonary bypass. Because of the high mortality and serious complications in the few survivors, this operation is rarely done today.

In 1960, a significant advance was made by Allison in performing a pulmonary embolectomy on a young athlete with massive PE secondary to traumatic thrombophlebitis. With total-body hypothermia (20° C) and temporary interruption of the circulation, the chest was opened and both venae cavae were occluded. The pulmonary artery was entered, and a massive embolus was removed. With the brain and heart protected by hypothermia, the patient made a good recovery (Allison et al., 1960).

In 1961, Sharp became the first surgeon to perform a pulmonary embolectomy using extracorporeal circulation (Sharp, 1962). Later the same year, Cooley performed a similar procedure (Cooley et al., 1961). This technique is now preferred because it allows the entire body to be perfused with concomitant oxygenation while the emboli are safely and deliberately removed from the pulmonary artery.

Massive PEs may cause sudden death, but it has long been recognized that many patients, even those with massive embolism, survive for a period of minutes or hours. The protocols of 52 patients with fatal PE at the Duke University Medical Center were reviewed, and two groups were identified: those in good general condition before the embolism and those who had serious underlying or terminal illnesses. Among the patients previously in good condition, 55% lived longer than 2 hours and 48% survived for 8 or more hours. However, among those with terminal illnesses, only 32% lived for 2 hours (Flemma and Young, 1964). These data clearly emphasize the significance of a serious underlying illness in the prognosis.

In the selection of patients for pulmonary embolectomy, the classic pathologic and clinical studies by Gorham (1961a, 1961b) should be carefully reviewed. Among the 100 patients in his study who died because of PE, 85 had occlusion involving one pulmonary artery and emboli in the arteries of the opposite lung. Only 15 of the 100 patients had emboli restricted to one lung, and 12 of these patients were more than 54 years of age, a group with an appreciable incidence of underlying cardiac and respiratory disease. Patients with massive PE having embolectomy rarely have emboli restricted to only one of the two major pulmonary arteries. In other words, in these patients, *bilateral* emboli are usually present. This evidence supports the importance of *mechanical blockage* in the symptom complex of massive PE and reinforces the data obtained from the occlusion of the pulmonary circulation by arterial ligature, intraluminal balloon occlusion, pulmonary resection, and various forms of experimental emboli. From each of these experimental studies, it is clear that *extensive* pulmonary arterial occlusion is required to produce serious symptoms. Thus, the most appropriate candidates for pulmonary embolectomy are those with more than half of the pulmonary arterial system occluded with emboli. *An important exception is the patient with preexisting cardiac or respiratory insufficiency.* In this case, a lesser amount of embolism may produce severe symptoms, and embolectomy may be required as a life-saving procedure.

INDICATIONS

At present, the primary indication for pulmonary embolectomy is persistent and refractory hypotension, despite maximal resuscitation for massive embolism unquestionably documented by either a pulmo-

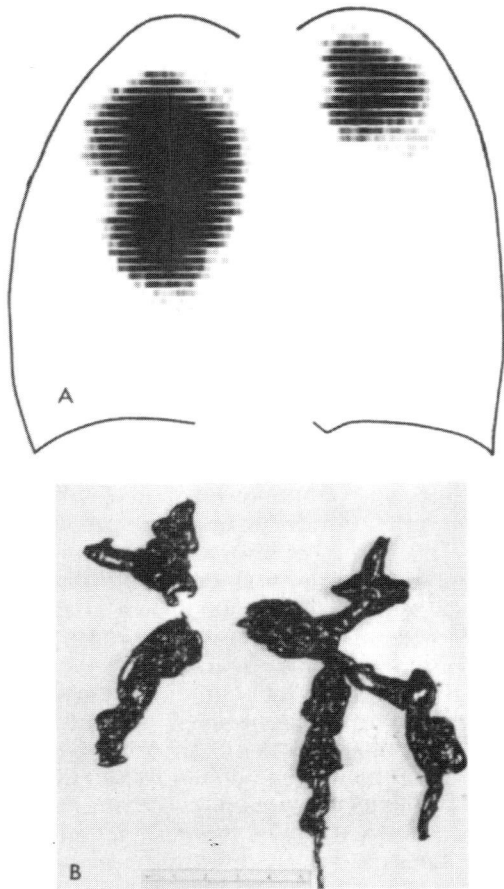

FIGURE 23–15. Illustrations from a patient with massive pulmonary embolism on the 12th day after an orthopedic operation and accompanied by intractable shock. *A,* The pulmonary scan shows massive occlusion of the right lower and middle lobar pulmonary arteries as well as almost all of the pulmonary arterial circulation to the left lung. *B,* Emboli removed from both pulmonary arteries at the time of embolectomy. (*A* and *B,* From Sabiston, D. C., Jr.: Pathophysiology, diagnosis, and management of pulmonary embolism. Adv. Surg., 3:351, 1968.)

patient with massive PE and intractable shock are shown in Figure 23–15. Such a patient is appropriate for the procedure, because all attempts to correct the severe state of hypotension failed and, despite vigorous resuscitative therapy, shock persisted for several hours. The pulmonary scan showed multiple emboli with more than 75% of the pulmonary arterial bed occluded. With such persistent and refractory hypotension unresponsive to the most vigorous regimen available, the patient was placed on extracorporeal circulation, and a massive amount of embolus was removed from the pulmonary arteries.

That small amounts of PE in the presence of preexisting cardiac and pulmonary insufficiency can produce serious cardiovascular manifestations is illustrated by another patient (Fig. 23–16). Admitted for an ophthalmic procedure under local anesthesia, this 72-year-old man had a history of hypertensive cardiovascular disease and chronic respiratory insufficiency due to emphysema. In the postoperative period, he was found in a state of cardiovascular collapse. A pulmonary scan showed evidence of obstruction in the pulmonary artery to the left lower lobe. Under usual circumstances, this relatively small amount of

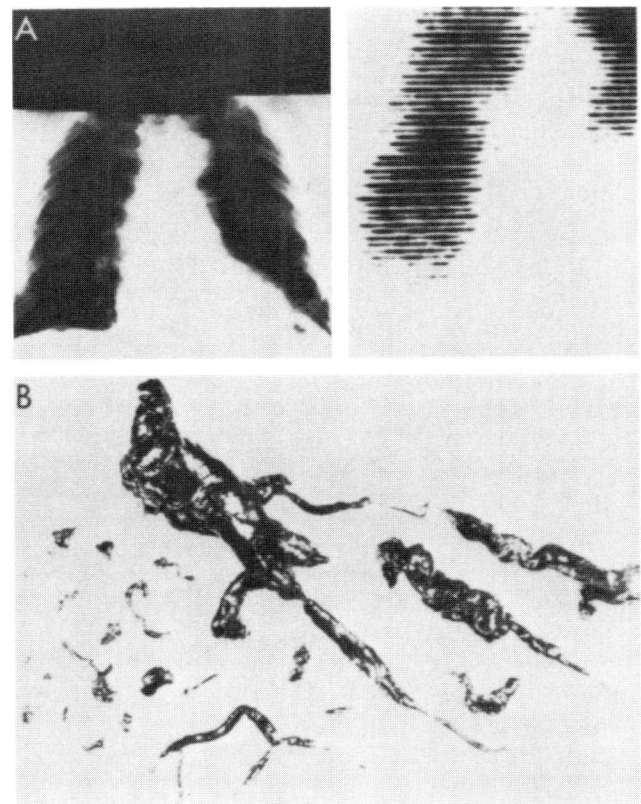

FIGURE 23–16. *A,* Chest film from a postoperative patient with preexisting cardiac and respiratory insufficiency. Pulmonary emboli are present in the left lower lobe. The patient was in severe and refractory shock. *B,* Emboli removed from the left lower lobe pulmonary artery at embolectomy. The result was that the patient's signs and symptoms improved and he made an uneventful recovery. (*A* and *B,* From Sabiston, D. C., Jr., and Wolfe, W. G.: Pulmonary embolectomy. *In* Moser, K. M., and Stein, M. [eds]: Pulmonary Thromboembolism. Chicago, Year Book Medical, 1973.)

nary scan or a pulmonary arteriogram. However, some authors dispute the need for surgery even when this indication is present (Oakley, 1989). The immediate treatment of these patients includes systemic heparinization, the administration of vasopressors and inotropic agents, and fluid and acid-base management. With such management, most patients previously thought to require embolectomy respond favorably, without the need for surgical treatment. If this therapy is effective in maintaining a blood pressure of 60 to 80 mm Hg, as shown by a continuous intra-arterial recording, embolectomy may be deferred, particularly if reasonable renal and cerebral function are maintained. Some have placed considerable emphasis on pressure in the right side of the heart and its prognostic significance (Del Guercio et al., 1964). Others hold that, although these data alone are useful, these pressures should be evaluated in context with other parameters.

The pulmonary scan of the emboli removed from a

embolism would not produce serious cardiopulmonary symptoms. In this patient, however, a persistent state of serious hypotension ensued and could not be corrected by vigorous supportive management. The presence of preexisting cardiac and respiratory insufficiency obviously augmented the effects of obstruction. Ultimately, it was necessary to remove the emboli using cardiopulmonary bypass. All emboli were confined to the left lower lobe pulmonary artery. The patient made an uneventful recovery (Sabiston and Wolfe, 1973).

TECHNIQUE

A median sternotomy provides excellent exposure of the pulmonary artery for pulmonary embolectomy. Once the pericardium is opened, cardiopulmonary bypass is established. The main pulmonary artery is exposed and incised; it is usually free of emboli, although partial obstruction may be present. With the use of a long sponge or gallstone forceps, the emboli are removed from the right and left pulmonary arteries and their major branches. A Fogarty catheter is then passed into the pulmonary arterial branches to remove smaller emboli. Finally, the entire pulmonary arterial tree is irrigated with saline. During this portion of the procedure, gentle compression of both lungs with the hand directs peripheral emboli toward the central arteries for more effective aspiration. The pulmonary artery is then closed, and cardiopulmonary bypass is gradually discontinued. This allows the heart and lungs to resume normal function. The stepwise operative approach for pulmonary embolectomy is shown in Figure 23–17. After closure of the median sternotomy, the inferior vena cava may be interrupted with ligation, plication, or clip to prevent further emboli from entering the lungs. Interruption can also be accomplished by abdominal extension of the median sternotomy incision (Moran, 1978) (Fig. 23–18).

When severe cardiovascular collapse is present, the patient can be supported by partial cardiopulmonary bypass, using the femoral vein to the femoral artery circuit for immediate resuscitation. If extracorporeal circulation is not available, either a right or a left thoracotomy, with exposure of one of the pulmonary arteries, can be performed. In most patients with massive PE, one pulmonary artery is primarily affected. Thus, the side with the predominant amount of embolus, previously determined by scan or arteriography, can be approached without the need for extracorporeal circulation. An anterior thoracotomy in the third interspace is appropriate for exposure of either the right or the left pulmonary artery. The artery can then be dissected to its origin, clamped, and opened distally for the removal of emboli, while circulation and pulmonary function in the opposite lung continue. Successful results with this technique have been described (Bradley et al., 1964; Camishion et al., 1966; Sautter et al., 1962). Nevertheless, cardiopulmonary bypass is preferred when available. One of the complications reported to follow pulmonary embolec-

tomy is massive endobronchial hemorrhage. Successful management of this complication has been achieved by the use of a double-lumen endotracheal tube for selective collapse of the lung and entrapment of the bleeding into a single right or left mainstem bronchus (Lyerly et al., 1986). The immediate institution of positive end-expiratory pressure (20 cm H_2O) may also control bleeding (Rice et al., 1981).

Reperfusion pulmonary edema after pulmonary artery thromboendarterectomy was described by Levinson and colleagues (1986). This complication may be serious enough to require prolonged mechanical ventilation. Retrospectively, these researchers analyzed the course and potential determinants of reperfusion pulmonary edema after thromboendarterectomy in 22 patients, with attention directed toward location of the thrombus, the thrombectomized regions, and the postoperative chest films, as well as preoperative and postoperative hemodynamic data. Reperfusion edema developed within 72 hours after operation in all but 1 patient. The anatomic site of the pulmonary edema corresponded to the anatomic locations distal to the vessels on which thromboendarterectomy had been performed. Those regions of the lung that did not have reperfusion after thromboendarterectomy were spared this form of pulmonary edema. Capillary wedge or left atrial pressures preoperatively and postoperatively were not elevated. It was not possible to predict which patients would develop reperfusion pulmonary edema, and it was thought that this phenomenon was a peculiar, local form of pulmonary edema, the basis of which had yet to be defined. This syndrome is a cause of hypoxemia postoperatively with local pulmonary infiltration, and often requires prolonged mechanical ventilation and increased inspired oxygen concentration for days to weeks.

RESULTS

Some of the early results of pulmonary embolectomy with the use of extracorporeal circulation were reported in a collected series from 28 medical centers in the United States and Canada (Cross and Mowlem, 1967). Of this group, 115 patients had the procedure performed with cardiopulmonary bypass, and 22 were approached without the use of extracorporeal circulation. Emboli were found in both pulmonary arteries in 110 patients. Fifty of the 115 patients (43%) operated on with cardiopulmonary bypass survived, although the ultimate mortality (late deaths) reduced the final survival rate to 32%. Of the 22 patients operated on without the use of extracorporeal circulation, 7 had emboli in one pulmonary artery, requiring unilateral pulmonary embolectomy. All 7 patients survived, but only 2 of the 15 patients with bilateral emboli survived. In 7 patients, the diagnosis was incorrect, and at the time of operation, no emboli were found. All 7 patients succumbed after operation. These findings emphasize strongly the need to establish an objective diagnosis of PE, either by pulmonary scan or by pulmonary arteriography.

Several recent series report improved results after

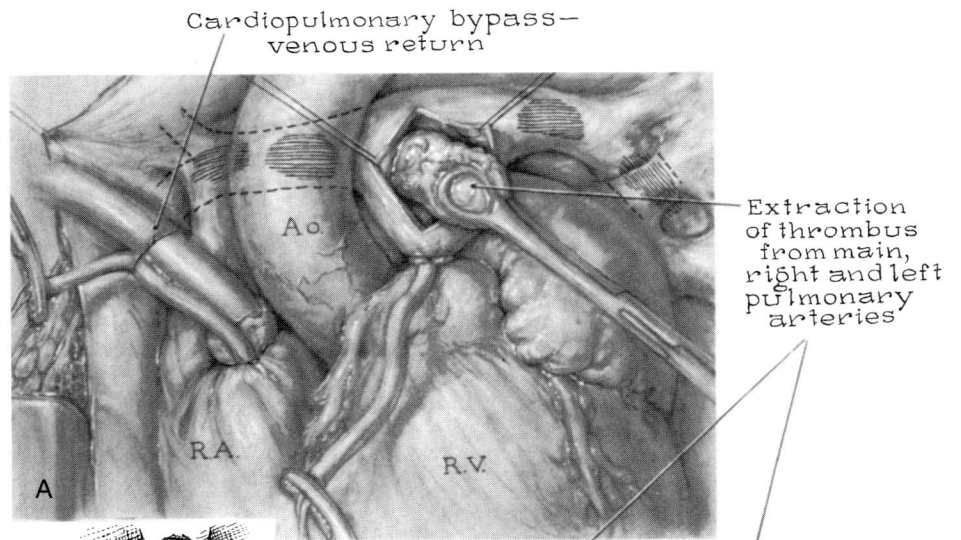

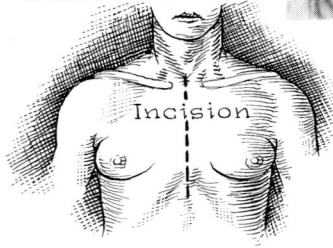

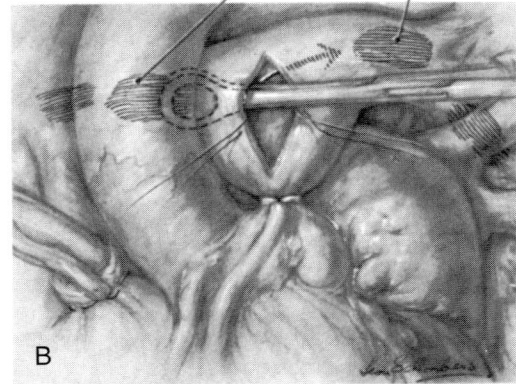

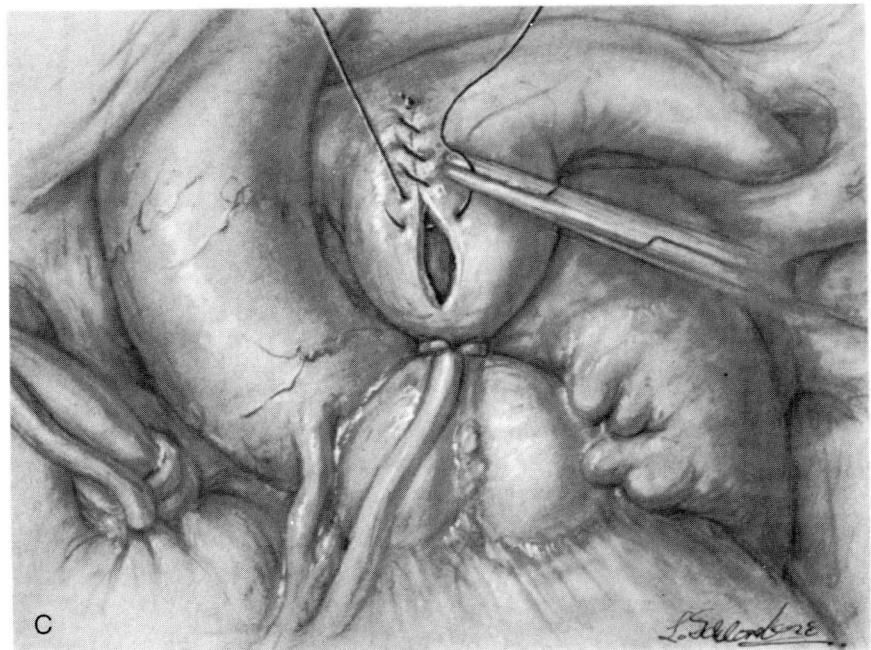

FIGURE 23–17. Acute pulmonary embolectomy. *A,* For an emergency pulmonary embolectomy, a median sternotomy is used. The patient is placed on cardiopulmonary bypass, with the cardiopulmonary venous return cannula in the right atrium and the arterial cannula either in the ascending aorta or in the femoral artery. A tape is passed beneath the proximal pulmonary artery, and after the patient is on full cardiopulmonary bypass, the tape is occluded. The pulmonary artery is opened, and the emboli are extracted. *B,* By use of various forceps, the right and left branches, including their tributaries, are explored thoroughly for removal of emboli. After all obtainable emboli have been extracted, the pulmonary arterial tree is irrigated copiously with saline. *C,* The pulmonary arteriotomy is closed with a continuous suture. (*A–C,* From Wolfe, W. G., and Sabiston, D. C., Jr.: Pulmonary Embolism. Volume 25 of the series Major Problems in Clinical Surgery. Philadelphia, W. B. Saunders, 1980.)

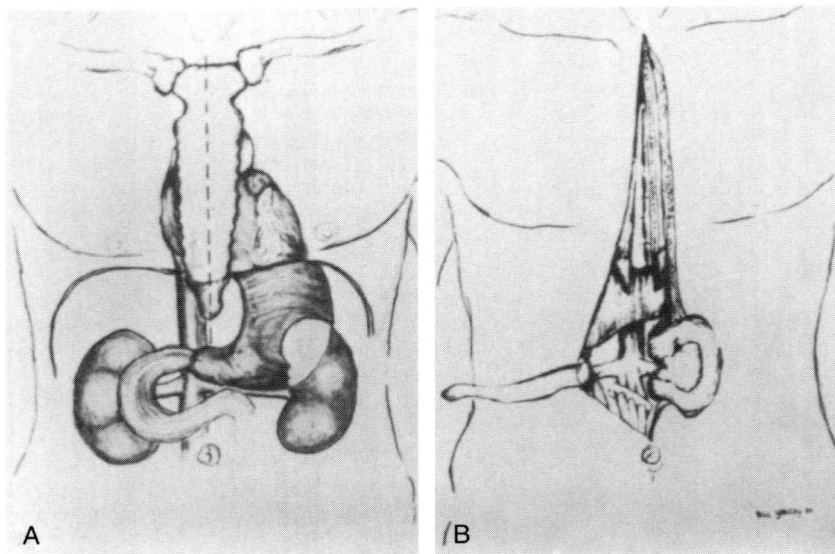

FIGURE 23–18. *A,* The *dotted line* indicates the usual extent of incision for midsternotomy. Note the proximity of the infrarenal cava to the lower end of the incision. *B,* Extension of sternotomy to the umbilicus, performed after completion of definitive cardiac procedure. (*A* and *B,* From Moran, J.: Vena cava interruption after pulmonary embolectomy. Reprinted with permission from the Society of Thoracic Surgeons [The Annals of Thoracic Surgery, 1978, Vol. 25, p. 248].)

pulmonary embolectomy for acute PE. In a report of 24 patients having pulmonary embolectomy with extracorporeal circulation, 17 (71%) had acute PE after a surgical procedure (Tschirkov et al., 1978). The remaining 7 patients (29%) had embolism secondary to a chronic medical disorder. The interval between clinical manifestations of acute PE and the embolectomy was from 8 to 36 hours. A definitive diagnosis of PE was made in all patients by pulmonary arteriography. Each patient was in a state of shock, was acidotic, and had an arterial oxygen tension less than 65 mm Hg. The indication for embolectomy was occlusion of the right or left pulmonary artery. The operative mortality in 17 patients was 23%.

Clarke (1989) reported a series of 35 patients who underwent pulmonary embolectomy for profound hypotension, but who had not proceeded to cardiac arrest, with a 97% early survival rate and only 3 late deaths. If cardiac arrest occurred before embolectomy, the early survival rate was 25%.

Meyer and associates (1981) reported a 20-year experience of pulmonary embolectomy for acute massive PE in 96 patients. All procedures were performed on cardiopulmonary bypass. The operative mortality was 37.5%. Multivariate analysis indicted two independent predictors of postoperative outcome: cardiac arrest and associated cardiopulmonary disease.

Kieny and co-workers (1991) also reported a 20-year experience in 134 patients. One hundred twenty-two procedures were performed on cardiopulmonary bypass. Twenty-three required external cardiac massage before surgery. The overall pulmonary bed was obstructed from 65 to 90% (mean, 79.4%) according to Miller's index. In patients both with and without prior cardiac arrest, the 1-month survival was 84.3%.

Therefore, pulmonary embolectomy can be performed successfully in properly selected patients with contraindication to thrombolysis, when thrombolysis is ineffective, or when severe alterations of hemodynamics do not allow delay for initiating thrombolysis.

One of the more encouraging reports of the results of pulmonary embolectomy is that of Gentsch and colleagues (1969), who reported 10 patients who had emergency pulmonary embolectomy. In 8, the embolism was discovered while the patients were confined to a community hospital. All patients were transferred to a medical center for operation, and 7 of the 10 survived.

Finally, cardiopulmonary support has been used successfully to resuscitate patients requiring external cardiac massage after acute massive PE (Kurose et al., 1993). Subsequent thrombectomy may not be required.

SELECTED BIBLIOGRAPHY

Braverman, S. J., Battey, P. M., and Smith, R. B., III: Vena caval interruption. Am. Surg., *58*:188, 1992.

Gorham, L. W.: A study of pulmonary embolism. Part I. Arch. Intern. Med., *108*:8, 1961a.

Gorham, L. W.: A study of pulmonary embolism. Part II. Arch. Intern. Med., *108*:189, 1961b.

Kieny, R., Charpentier, A., and Kieny, T.: What is the place of pulmonary embolectomy? J. Cardiovasc. Surg., *32*:549, 1991.

Lilienfield, D. E., Chan, E., Ehland, B. A., et al.: Mortality from pulmonary embolism in the United States: 1962–1984. Chest, *98*:1067, 1990a.

Magnant, J. G., Walsh, D. B., Jurasky, L. I., and Cronenwett, J. L.: Current use of vena cava filters. J. Vasc. Surg., *16*:701, 1992.

Meyer, G., Tamisier, D., Sors, H., et al.: Pulmonary embolectomy: A 20-year experience at one center. Ann. Thorac. Surg., *51*:232, 1991.

Nyman, U.: Diagnostic strategies in acute pulmonary embolism. Haemostasis, *23*(Suppl.):220, 1993.

Sabiston, D. C., Jr., and Wolfe, W. G.: Experimental and clinical observations on the natural history of pulmonary embolism. Ann. Surg., *168*:1, 1968.

Stein, P. D., Terrin, M. L., Hales, C. A., et al.: Clinical, laboratory, roentgenographic, and electrocardiographic findings in patients with acute pulmonary embolism and no preexisting cardiac or pulmonary disease. Chest, *100*:598, 1991.

Wagner, H. N., Sabiston, D. C., Jr., McAfee, J. G., et al.: Diagnosis of massive pulmonary embolism in man by radioisotope scanning. N. Engl. J. Med., *271*:377, 1964.

Worsley, F. F., Alavi, A., and Palevsky, H. I.: Role of radionuclide imaging in patients with suspected pulmonary embolism. Radiol. Clin. North Am., *31*:849, 1993.

BIBLIOGRAPHY

Adams, J. T., and DeWeese, J. A.: Partial interruption of the inferior vena cava with a new plastic clip. Surg. Gynecol. Obstet., *170*:559, 1969.

Alexander, B., Meyers, L., Kenny, J., et al.: Blood coagulation in pregnancy. Proconvertin and prothrombin, and the hypercoagulable state. N. Engl. J. Med., *254*:466, 1956.

Allison, P. R.: Pulmonary embolism and thrombophlebitis. Br. J. Surg., *54*:466, 1967.

Allison, P. R., Dunhill, M. S., and Marshall, R.: Pulmonary embolism. Thorax, *15*:273, 1960.

Anderson, D. R., and Levine, M. N.: Thrombolytic therapy for the treatment of acute pulmonary embolism. Can. Med. J., *146*:1317, 1992.

Ariyan, S., and Stansel, H. C., Jr.: Further hazards of heparin therapy in vascular disease. Arch. Surg., *111*:120, 1976.

Arkless, R.: Renal carcinoma: How it metastasizes. Radiology, *84*:496, 1965.

Baker, R. R.: Pulmonary embolism. Surgery, *54*:687, 1963.

Barker, N. W., Nygaard, K. K., Walters, W., and Priestly, J. T.: A statistical study of postoperative venous thrombosis and pulmonary embolism: Predisposing factors. Mayo Clin. Proc., *16*:1, 1941.

Barritt, D. W., and Jordan, S. C.: Anticoagulant drugs in the treatment of pulmonary embolism. A controlled trial. Lancet, *1*:1309, 1960.

Bauer, G.: The introduction of heparin therapy in cases of early thrombosis. Circulation, *19*:108, 1959.

Belenkie, I., Dani, R., Smith, E. R., and Tyberg, J. V.: Ventricular interaction during experimental acute pulmonary embolism. Circulation, *78*:761, 1988.

Bell, W. R., Simon, T. L., and DeMets, D. L.: The clinical features of submassive and massive pulmonary emboli. Am. J. Med., *62*:355, 1977.

Benichoux, R.: The surgical treatment of massive pulmonary embolism: Report of 22 cases of Trendelenburg's operation. J. Int. Chir. *11*:464, 1951.

Berry, J. L., and Daly, I.: The relation between the pulmonary and bronchial vascular systems. Proc. R. Soc. Lond., *59*:319, 1932.

Blount, S. G., Jr., and Vogel, J. H. K.: Altitude and the pulmonary circulation. Adv. Intern. Med., *13*:11, 1967.

Boyer, N. H., and Curry, J. J.: Bronchospasm associated with pulmonary embolism. Arch. Intern. Med., *73*:403, 1944.

Bradley, M. N., Bennett, A. L., III, and Lyons, C.: Successful unilateral pulmonary embolectomy without cardiopulmonary bypass. N. Engl. J. Med., *271*:713, 1964.

Brady, A. J. B., Crake, T., and Oakley, C. M.: Percutaneous catheter fragmentation and distal dispersion of proximal pulmonary embolus. Lancet, *338*:1186, 1991.

Brady, A. J. B., Crake, T., and Oakley, C. M.: Simultaneous mechanical clot fragmentation and pharmacologic thrombolysis in acute massive pulmonary embolism. Am. J. Cardiol., *70*:836, 1992.

Braverman, S. J., Battey, P. M., and Smith, R. B., III: Vena caval interruption. Am. Surg., *58*:188, 1992.

Brofman, B. L., Charms, B. L., Kohn, P. M., et al.: Unilateral pulmonary artery occlusion in man. J. Thorac. Surg., *34*:206, 1957.

Burki, N. K.: The dead space to tidal volume ratio in the diagnosis of pulmonary embolism. Am. Rev. Respir. Dis., *133*:679, 1986.

Burnett, W. E., Long, J. H., Norris, C., et al.: The effect of pneumonectomy on pulmonary function. J. Thorac. Surg., *18*:569, 1949.

Camashion, R. C., Pierucci, L., Jr., Fishman, N. H., et al.: Pulmonary embolectomy without cardiopulmonary bypass. Am. J. Surg., *111*:723, 1966.

Cassen, B.: Instrumentation for ^{131}I use in medical studies. Nucleonics, *9*:46, 1951.

Clarke, D. B.: Pulmonary embolectomy has a well-defined and valuable place. Br. J. Hosp. Med., *41*:468, 1989.

Clarke-Pearson, D. L., Coleman, R. E., Siegel, R., et al.: Indium-111 platelet imaging for the detection of deep venous thrombosis

and pulmonary embolism in patients without symptoms after surgery. Surgery, *98*:98, 1985.

Cohnheim, J. F.: Untersuchugen über die embolischen processe. Berlin, A. Hirschwald, 1872.

Coman, D. R.: Mechanisms responsible for the origin and distribution of bloodbourne tumor metastases: A review. Cancer Res., *13*:397, 1953.

Comroe, J. H., Jr., Van Lingen, B., Stroud, R. C., and Roncoroni, A.: Reflex and direct cardiopulmonary effects of 5-OH-tryptamine (serotonin). Am. J. Physiol., *173*:379, 1953.

Cooley, D. A., Beall, A. C., Jr., and Alexander, J. K.: Acute massive pulmonary embolism: Successful treatment using temporary cardiopulmonary bypass. J. A. M. A., *177*:283, 1961.

Coon, W. W., and Coller, F. A.: Some epidemiologic considerations of thromboembolism. Surg. Gynecol. Obstet., *109*:487, 1959.

Coon, W. W., Willis, P. W., and Keller, J. B.: Venous thromboembolism and other venous disease in the Tecumseh community health study. Circulation, *48*:839, 1973.

Coon, W. W., Willis, P. W., and Synoms, M. J.: Assessment of anticoagulant treatment in venous thromboembolism. Ann. Surg., *170*:559, 1969.

Cox, J. L., and Sabiston, D. C., Jr.: Phlebitis, thrombosis and pulmonary embolism. *In* Condon, R. E., and DeCosse, J. J. (eds): Surgical Care: A Physiologic Approach to Problems in the First Fifteen Postoperative Days. Philadelphia, Lea & Febiger, 1980.

Crafoord, C., and Jorpes, E.: Heparin as a prophylactic against thrombosis. J. A. M. A., *116*:2831, 1941.

Cross, F. S., and Mowlem, A.: A survey of the current status of pulmonary embolectomy for massive pulmonary embolism. Circulation, *35*:I-86, 1967.

Cruveilhier, J.: Anatomie Pathologique de Corps Humain. Paris, J. B. Baillière, 1829, p. 42.

Cvitanic, O., and Marino, P. L.: Improved use of arterial blood gas analysis in suspected pulmonary embolism. Chest, *95*:48, 1989.

Daily, P. O., Dembitsky, W. P., Iversen, S., et al.: Risk factors for pulmonary thromboendarterectomy. J. Thorac. Cardiovasc. Surg., *99*:670, 1990.

Dalen, J. E., and Alpert, J. S.: Natural history of pulmonary embolism. Prog. Cardiovasc. Dis., *17*:259, 1975.

Daughtry, J. D., Stewart, B. H., Golding, L. A. R., and Groves, L. K.: Pulmonary embolus presenting as the initial presentation of a renal cell carcinoma. Ann. Thorac. Surg., *24*:178, 1977.

Dawidson, I., Barrett, J. A., Miller, E., and Litwin, M. S.: Pulmonary microembolism associated with massive transfusion: I. Physiologic effects and comparison in vivo of standard and Dacron wool (Swank) blood transfusion filters in its prevention. Ann. Surg., *181*:51, 1975.

DeBakey, M. E.: A critical evaluation of the problem of thromboembolism [Abstract]. Int. Surg., *98*:1, 1954.

Del Guercio, L. R. M., Coomaraswamy, R. P., Feins, N. R., and State, D.: Bedside hemodynamic diagnosis of acute pulmonary embolism. Surg. Forum, *15*:192, 1964.

Demers, C., and Ginsberg, J. S.: Deep venous thrombosis and pulmonary embolism in pregnancy. Clin. Chest Med., *13*:645, 1992.

DeNardo, G. L., Goodwin, D. A., Ravasini, et al.: The ventilatory lung scan in the diagnosis of pulmonary embolism. N. Engl. J. Med., *282*:1334, 1970.

DeWeese, J. A.: Interruptions of the femoral veins and vena cava. *In* Rob, C., Smith, R., and Dudley, H. (eds): Operative Surgery. 3rd ed. London, Butterworth, 1976.

DeWeese, J. A., and Hunter, D. C., Jr.: A vena caval filter for the prevention of pulmonary embolism: A five-year clinical experience. Arch. Surg., *86*:852, 1963.

DeWeese, J. A., Jones, T. L., Lyon, J., and Dale, W. A.: Evaluation of thrombectomy in the management of ileofemoral venous thrombosis. Surgery, *47*:140, 1960.

Dexter, L.: Cardiovascular responses to experimental pulmonary embolism. *In* Sasahara, A. A., and Stein, M. (eds): Pulmonary Embolic Disease. New York, Grune & Stratton, 1965.

Dexter, L., and Folch-Pi, W.: Venous thrombosis. An account of the first documented case. J. A. M. A., *228*:195, 1974.

Eichelter, P., and Schenk, W. G., Jr.: Prophylaxis of pulmonary embolism: A new experimental approach with initial results. Arch. Surg., *97*:348, 1968.

Essop, M. R., Middlemost, S. Skoulargis, J., and Sareli, P.: Simultaneous mechanical clot fragmentation and pharmacologic thrombolysis in acute massive pulmonary embolism. Am. J. Cardiol., 69:427, 1992.

Fishman, A. P.: Hypoxia on the pulmonary circulation: How and where it acts. Circ. Res., 38:221, 1976.

Flemma, R. J., and Young, W. G., Jr.: Feasibility of pulmonary embolectomy: A case report. Circulation 30:234, 1964.

Fratantoni, J., and Wessler, S.: Prophylactic therapy of deep vein thrombosis and pulmonary embolism. Washington, DC, DHEW Publication No. (NIH) 75–866, 1975.

Fred, H. L., Axelrad, M. A., Lewis, J. M., and Alexander, J. K.: Rapid resolution of pulmonary thromboemboli in man. J. A. M. A., 196:1137, 1966.

Freiman, D. G.: Pathologic observations on experimental and human thromboembolism. In Sasahara, A. A., and Stein, M. (eds): Pulmonary Embolic Disease. New York, Grune & Stratton, 1965.

Gallus, A., Jackaman, J., Tillett, J., et al.: Safety and efficacy of warfarin started early after venous thrombosis or submassive pulmonary embolism. Lancet, 1:1293, 1986.

Gardner, A. M. N.: Inferior vena caval interruption in the prevention of fatal pulmonary embolism. Am. Heart J., 95:679, 1978.

Gentsch, T. O., Larsen, P. B., Daughtry, D. C., et al.: Community-wide availability of pulmonary embolectomy with cardiopulmonary bypass. Ann. Thorac. Surg., 7:97, 1969.

Gibbs, N. M.: Venous thrombosis of the lower limbs with particular reference to bed rest. Br. J. Surg., 45:209, 1957.

Gillum, R. F.: Pulmonary embolism and thrombophlebitis in the United States, 1970–1985. Am. Heart J., 114:1262, 1987.

Goldhaber, S. Z., Kessler, C. M., Heit, J., et al.: Randomized controlled trial of recombinant tissue plasminogen activator versus urokinase in the treatment of acute pulmonary embolism. Lancet, 2:293, 1988.

Gomes, A. S., Grollman, J. H., Jr., and Mink, J.: Pulmonary angiography for pulmonary emboli: Rational selection of oblique views. Am. J Roentgenol., 129:1019, 1977.

Görge, G., Erbel, R., and Schuster, S.: Intravascular ultrasound in the diagnosis of acute pulmonary embolism. Lancet, 337:623, 1991.

Gorham, L. W.: A study of pulmonary embolism. Part I. Arch. Intern. Med., 108:8, 1961a.

Gorham, L. W.: A study of pulmonary embolism. Part II. Arch. Intern. Med., 108:189, 1961b.

Gray, H. H., and Firoozan, S.: Management of pulmonary embolism. Thorax, 47:825, 1992.

Greenfield, L. J., Kimmell, G. O., and McMurdy, W. C., III: Transvenous removal of pulmonary emboli by vacuum-cup catheter technic. J. Surg. Res., 9:347, 1969.

Greenfield, L. J., McCurdy, J. R., Brown, P. P., et al.: A new intracaval filter permitting continued flow and resolution of emboli. Surgery, 73:599, 1973.

Greenfield, L. J., and Michna, B. A.: Twelve-year clinical experience with the Greenfield vena caval filter. Surgery, 104:706, 1988.

Greenfield, L. J., Reif, M. E., and Guenter, C. E.: Hemodynamic and respiratory reponses to transvenous pulmonary embolectomy. J. Thorac. Cardiovasc. Surg., 62:890, 1971.

Greenspan, R. H., Ravin, C. E., Polansky, S. M., and McLoud, T. C.: Accuracy of chest radiograph in diagnosis of pulmonary embolism. Invest. Radiol., 17:539, 1982.

Günther, R. W., and Vorwerk, D.: Aspiration catheter for percutaneous thrombectomy: Clinical results. Radiology, 175:271, 1990.

Gurewich, V., Sasahara, A. A., Wilk, J., et al.: Pulmonary embolism, bronchoconstriction, and response to heparin. In Sasahara, A. A., and Stein, M. (eds): Pulmonary Embolic Disease. New York, Grune & Stratton, 1965.

Gurewich, V., Thomas, D. P., and Rubinov, K. R.: Pulmonary embolism after ligation of the inferior vena cava. N. Engl. J. Med., 274:1350, 1966.

Haller, J. A.: Thrombectomy for deep thrombophlebitis of the leg. N. Engl. J. Med., 267:65, 1962.

Hansen, J. F., Lyngborg, K., Anderson, M., and Wennevold, A.: Right atrial myxoma. Acta Med. Scand., 86:165, 1969.

Hirsch, J., and Hull, R. D.: Treatment of venous thromboembolism. Chest, 89(Suppl.):426S, 1986.

Hirsch, J., van Aken, W. G., and Gallus, A. S.: Heparin kinetics in venous thrombosis and pulmonary embolism. Circulation, 53:691, 1976.

Hull, R. D., Hirsch, J., Carter C. J., et al.: Diagnostic efficacy of impedance plethysmography for clinically suspected deep venous thrombosis. Ann. Intern. Med., 102:21, 1985.

Hull, R. D., Raskob, G. E., Coates, G., et al.: A new innovative management strategy for patients with suspected pulmonary embolism. Arch. Intern. Med., 149:2549, 1989.

Hull, R. D., Raskob, G. E., and Hirsch, J.: Prophylaxis of venous thromboembolism: An overview. Chest, 89(Suppl.):374S, 1986a.

Hull, R. D., Raskob, G. E., Hirsch, J., et al.: Continuous intravenous heparin compared with intermittent subcutaneous heparin in the initial treatment of proximal vein thrombosis. N. Engl. J. Med., 315:1109, 1986b.

Hume, M.: Pulmonary embolism. In Glenn, W. W. L., Liebow, A. A., and Lindskog, G. E. (eds): Thoracic and Cardiovascular Surgery with Related Pathology. 3rd ed. New York, Appleton-Century-Crofts, 1975.

Hume, M., Sevitt, S., and Thomas, D. P.: Venous Thrombosis and Pulmonary Embolism. Cambridge, MA, Harvard University Press, 1970.

Hunter, W. C., Krygier, J. J., Kennedy, J. C., and Sneeden, V.: Etiology and prevention of thrombosis of the deep leg veins. Surgery, 17:178, 1945.

Hyers, T. M., Hull, R. D., and Weg, J. G.: Antithrombotic therapy for venous thromboembolic disease. Chest, 95(Suppl.):37S, 1989.

Ikard, R. W., Ueland, K., and Folse, R.: Lower limb venous dynamics in pregnant women. Surg. Gynecol. Obstet., 132:483, 1971.

International Multicentre Trial: Prevention of fatal postoperative pulmonary embolism by low doses of heparin: An international multicentre trial. Lancet, 2:45, 1975.

Isch, I. H., and Schumacker, H. B., Jr.: Embolization of caval umbrella. Discussion and report of successful removal from the right ventricle. J. Thorac. Cardiovasc. Surg., 72:256, 1976.

Jamieson, S. W., Auger, W. R., Fedullo, P. F., et al.: Experience and results with 150 pulmonary thromboendarterectomy operations over a 29-month period. J. Thorac. Cardiovasc. Surg., 106:116, 1993.

Jardin, F., Dubourg, O., Gueret, P., et al.: Quantitative two-dimensional echocardiography in massive pulmonary embolism: Emphasis on ventricular interdependence and leftward septal displacement. J. Am. Coll. Cardiol., 10:1201, 1987.

Jones, R. H., and Sabiston, D. C., Jr.: Pulmonary embolism in childhood. Monogr. Surg. Sci., 3:35, 1966.

Kakkar, V. V.: The diagnosis of deep vein thrombosis using the ^{125}I-fibrinogen test. Arch. Surg., 104:152, 1972.

Kakkar, V. V., Field, E. S., Nicolaides, A. N., et al.: Low doses of heparin in prevention of deep-vein thrombosis. Lancet, 2:669, 1971.

Kakkar, V. V., Flanc, C., Howe, C. T., et al.: Natural history of postoperative deep vein thrombosis. Lancet, 2:230, 1969.

Karp, R. B., and Wylie, E. J.: Recurrent thrombosis after iliofemoral thrombectomy. Surg. Forum, 17:147, 1966.

Kaunitz, A. M., Hughes, J. M., and Grimes D. A.: Causes of maternal mortality in the United States. Obstet. Gynecol., 65:605, 1985.

Kieny, R., Charpentier, A., and Kieny, T.: What is the place of pulmonary embolectomy? J. Cardiovasc. Surg., 32:549, 1991.

Kirschner, M.: Ein durch die Trendelenburgsche operation geheilter fall von embolie der arterien pulmonalis. Arch. Clin. Chir., 133:312, 1924.

Kovacs, G. S., Hill, J. D., Abert, T., et al.: Pathogenesis of arterial hypoxemia in pulmonary embolism. Arch. Surg., 93:813, 1966.

Kruit, W. H. J., de Boer, A. C., Sing, A. K., and van Roon, F.: The significance of venography in the management of patients with clinically suspected pulmonary embolism. J. Intern. Med., 230:333, 1991.

Kurose, M., Okamoto, K., Sato, T., et al.: Extracorporeal support for patients undergoing prolonged external cardiac massage. Resuscitation, 25:35, 1993.

Laënnec, R. T. H.: De L'auscultation médiate. Paris, Brossen et Chaude, 1819.

Laughlin, R. A., and Mandel, S. R.: Paradoxical embolism. Case report and review of the literature. Arch. Surg., 112:648, 1977.

Lesser, B. A., Leeper, K. V., Stein, P. D., et al.: The diagnosis of acute pulmonary embolism in patients with chronic obstructive pulmonary disease. Chest, 102:17, 1992.

Levine, M. N.: Thrombolytic therapy in acute pulmonary embolism. Can. J. Cardiol., 9:158, 1993.

Levine, M. N., Hirsch, J., Weitz, J., et al.: A randomized trial of a single-bolus dosage regimen of recombinant tissue plasminogen activator in patients with acute pulmonary embolism. Chest, 97:528, 1990.

Levinson, R. M., Shure, D., and Moser, K. M.: Reperfusion pulmonary edema after pulmonary artery thromboendarterectomy. Am. Rev. Respir. Dis., 134:1241, 1986.

Lilienfield, D. E., Chan, E., Ehland, B. A., et al.: Mortality from pulmonary embolism in the United States: 1962–1984. Chest, 98:1067, 1990a.

Lilienfield, D. E., Godbold, J. H., Burke, G. L., et al.: Hospitalization and case fatality for pulmonary embolism in the Twin Cities: 1979–1984. Am. Heart J., 120:392, 1990b.

Ljungdahl, M.: Gibt es eine chronische embolisierung der lungenarterie? Arch. Klin. Med., 160:1, 1928.

Lyerly, H. K., Reves, J. G., and Sabiston, D. C., Jr.: Management of primary sarcomas of the pulmonary artery and reperfusion intrabronchial hemorrhage. Surg. Gynecol. Obstet., 163:291, 1986.

Magnant, J. G., Walsh, D. B., Jurasky, L. I., and Cronenwett, J. L.: Current use of vena cava filters. J. Vasc. Surg., 16:701, 1992.

Manny, J., and Hectman, H. B.: Vasoactive humoral factors. In Goldhaber, S. Z. (ed): Pulmonary embolism and deep venous thrombosis. Philadelphia, W. B. Saunders, 1985, p. 283.

Marshall, R., Sabiston, D. C., Jr., Allison, P. R., and Dunhill, M. S.: Immediate and late effects of pulmonary embolism by large thrombi in dogs. Thorax, 18:1, 1963.

Mauer, B. J., Wray, R., and Shillingford, J. P.: Frequency of venous thrombosis after myocardial infarction. Lancet, 2:1385, 1971.

Maxwell, R. J., and Greenfield, L. J.: Effects of pulmonary embolism on survival of patients with Greenfield vena caval filters. Surgery, 101:389, 1987.

McLachlin, A. D., McLachlin, J. A., Jory, T. A., and Rawling, E. G.: Venous stasis in the lower extremities. Ann. Surg., 152:678, 1960.

McLachlin, J. A., and Paterson, J. C.: Some basic observations on venous thrombosis and pulmonary embolism. Surg. Gynecol. Obstet., 93:1, 1951.

McLean, J.: The thromboplastin action of cephalin. Am. J. Physiol., 41:250, 1916.

Medical Research Council Subcommittee: Risk of thromboembolic disease in women taking oral contraceptives. Br. Med. J., 2:355, 1967.

Meyer, G., Tamisier, D., Sors, H., et al.: Pulmonary embolectomy: A 20-year eperience at one center. Ann. Thorac. Surg., 51:232, 1991.

Miles, R. M., Chappell, F., and Renner, O.: Partially occluding vena caval clip for prevention of pulmonary emboli. Am. Surg., 30:40, 1964.

Mobin-Uddin, K., Bolooki, H., and Jude, J. R.: A new simplified method of caval interruption for the prevention of pulmonary emboli. Circulation, 40-III:149, 1969.

Mobin-Uddin, K., Callard, G. M., Bolooki, H., et al.: Transvenous caval interruption with umbrella filter. N. Engl. J. Med., 286:55, 1972.

Mohr, D. N., Ryu, J. H., Litin, S. C., et al.: Recent advances in the management of venous thromboembolism. Mayo Clin. Proc., 63:281, 1988.

Moniz, E., Carvallio, L., and Limer, H.: Angiopneumographie. Presse Med., 53:996, 1931.

Monreal, M., Rey-Joly Barroso, C., Ruiz Manzano, J., et al.: Asymptomatic pulmonary embolism in patients with deep vein thrombosis. Is it useful to take a lung scan to rule out this condition? J. Cardiovasc. Surg., 30:104, 1989.

Moor, G. F., and Sabiston, D. C., Jr.: Embolectomy for chronic pulmonary embolism and hypertension. Case report and review of the problem. Circulation, 41:701, 1970.

Moran, J.: Vena cava interruption after pulmonary embolectomy. Ann. Thorac. Surg., 25:248, 1978.

Moret, P., Covvarrubias, E., Coudert, J., and Duchosal, F.: Cardiocirculatory adaptation to chronic hypoxia. III. Comparative study of cardiac output, pulmonary and systemic circulation between sea level and high altitude residents. Acta Cardiol. (Brux.), 27:596, 1972.

Moretz, W. H., Rhode, C. M., and Shepherd, M. H.: Prevention of pulmonary emboli by partial occlusion of the inferior vena cava. Am. Surg., 25:617, 1959.

Moser, K. M., and LeMoine, J. R.: Is embolic risk conditioned by deep venous thrombosis? Ann. Intern. Med., 94:439, 1981.

Moses, D. C., Silver, T. M., and Bookstein, J. J.: The complementary roles of chest radiography, lung scanning, and selective pulmonary angiography in the diagnosis of pulmonary embolism. Circulation, 49:179, 1974.

Murray, G. D. W., and Best, C. H.: Use of heparin in thrombosis. Ann. Surg., 108:163, 1938.

Murray, G. D. W., Jacques, L. B., Perrett, T. S., and Best, C. H.: Heparin and thrombosis of the veins following injury. Surgery, 2:163, 1937.

Murray, T. S., Lorimer, A. R., Cox, F. C., and Lawrie, T. D. V.: Leg-vein thrombosis following myocardial infarction. Lancet, 2:272, 1970.

Myerson, P. J., Myerson, D. A., Katz, R., and Lawson, J. P.: Gallium imaging in pulmonary artery sarcoma mimicking pulmonary embolism: Case report. J. Nucl. Med., 17:893, 1976.

Neumann, R.: Ursprungszentren und Entwicklungsformen der Beinthrombose. Virchows Arch. (Pathol. Anat.), 301:708, 1938.

Newman, G. E.: Pulmonary thromboembolism: A historical perspective. J. Thorac. Imaging, 4:1, 1989.

Nyman, U.: Diagnostic strategies in acute pulmonary embolism. Haemostasis, 23(Suppl.):220, 1993.

Oakley, C. M.: There is no place for acute pulmonary embolectomy. Br. J. Hosp. Med., 41:469, 1989.

Ochsner, A.: Indications for and results of inferior vena caval ligation for thromboembolic disease. Postgrad. Med., 27:193, 1960.

Ochsner, A., Ochsner, J. L., and Sanders, H. S.: Prevention of pulmonary embolism by caval ligation. Ann. Surg., 171:923, 1970.

Partsch, H., Oburger, K., Mostbeck, A., et al.: Frequency of pulmonary embolism in ambulant patients with pelvic vein thrombosis: A prospective study. J. Vasc. Surg., 16:715, 1992.

Petitti, D. B., Strom, B. L., and Melmon, K. L.: Duration of warfarin anticoagulant therapy and the probabilities of recurrent thromboembolism and hemorrhage. Am. J. Med., 81:255, 1986.

Piccone, V. A., Jr., Vidal, E., Yarnoz, M., et al.: The late results of caval ligation. Surgery, 68:980, 1970.

PIOPED Investigators: Value of the ventilation/perfusion scan in acute pulmonary embolism: Results of the prospective investigation of pulmonary embolism diagnosis (PIOPED). J. A. M. A., 263:2753, 1990.

Ponomar, E., Carlson, J. E., Kindlund, A., et al.: Clot-trapper device for transjugular thrombectomy from the inferior vena cava. Radiology, 179:279, 1991.

Prediletto, R., Paoletti, P., Fornai, E., et al.: Natural course of treated pulmonary embolism. Evaluation by perfusion lung scintigraphy, gas exchange, and chest roentgenogram. Chest, 97:554, 1990.

Registrar-General's Statistical Review of England and Wales. London, H. M. S. O., 1966.

Research Committee of the British Thoracic Society: Optimum duration of anticoagulation for deep-vein thrombosis and pulmonary embolism. Lancet, 340:873, 1992.

Rice, P. L., Pifarre, R., El-Etr, A., et al.: Management of endobronchial hemorrhage during cardiopulmonary bypass. J. Thorac. Cardiovasc. Surg., 81:800, 1981.

Roberts, G. H.: Venous thrombosis in hospital patients. A postmortem study. Scott. Med. J., 8:11, 1963.

Rokitansky, C.: Handbuch der pathologischen anatomie, Handbuch der speciellen pathologischen anatomie, Wien, 1842–1846.

Rosenberg, I. L., Evans, M., and Pollok, A. V.: Prophylaxis of postoperative leg vein thrombosis by low-dose subcutaneous heparin or perioperative calf muscle stimulation. Br. Med. J., 1:649, 1975.

Rossle, R.: Über die Bedeutung und die Entstehung der Wadenvenenthrombosen. Virchows Arch. (Pathol. Anat.), 30:180, 1937.

Ryu, J. H., and Rosenow, E. C.: Acute pulmonary embolism. Cardiovasc. Clin., 22:103, 1992.

Sabiston, D. C., Jr.: Pathophysiology, diagnosis, and management of pulmonary embolism. Adv. Surg., 3:351, 1968.

Sabiston, D. C., Jr., and Wagner, H. N., Jr.: The pathophysiology of pulmonary embolism: Relationships to accurate diagnosis and choice of therapy. J. Thorac. Cardiovasc. Surg., 50:339, 1965.

Sabiston, D. C., Jr., and Wolfe, W. G.: Experimental and clinical observations on the natural history of pulmonary embolism. Ann. Surg., 168:1, 1968.

Sabiston, D. C., Jr., and Wolfe, W. G.: Pulmonary embolectomy. In Moser, K. M., and Stein, M. (eds): Pulmonary Thromboembolism. Chicago, Year Book Medical, 1973.

Sabiston, D. C., Jr., Wolfe, W. G., Oldham, H. N., et al.: Surgical management of chronic pulmonary embolism. Ann. Surg., 185:699, 1977.

Sacks, B. P., Brown, D. A. J., Driscoll, S. G., et al.: Maternal mortality in Massachusetts. Trends and prevention. N. Engl. J. Med., 31:667, 1987.

Salzman, E. W., Deykin D., Shapiro, R. M., and Rosenberg, R.: Management of heparin therapy: A controlled prospective trial. N. Engl. J. Med., 292:1046, 1975.

Sasahara, A. A.: Clinical studies in pulmonary thromboembolism. In Sasahara, A. A., and Stein, M. (eds): Pulmonary Embolic Disease. New York, Grune & Stratton, 1965.

Sasahara, A. A., Koppenhagen, K., Haring, R., et al.: Low molecular weight heparin plus hihydroergotamine for prophylaxis of postoperative deep vein thrombosis. Br J. Surg., 73:697, 1986.

Sautter, R. D., Fletcher, F. W., Emanuel, D. A., et al.: Complete resolution of massive pulmonary thromboembolism. J. A. M. A., 189:948, 1964.

Sautter, R. D., Lawton, B. R., Magnin, G. E., and Burns, J. L.: Pulmonary embolectomy: A simplified technique. Wis. Med. J., 61:309, 1962.

Schmitz-Rode, T., and Günther, R. W.: New device for percutaneous fragmentation of pulmonary emboli. Radiology, 180:135, 1991.

Schwartz, F., Stehr, H., Zimmerman, R., et al.: Sustained improvement of pulmonary hemodynamics in patients at rest and during exercise after thrombolytic treatment of massive pulmonary embolism. Circulation, 71:117, 1985.

Sethi, G. K., Slaven, J. E., Kepes, J. J., et al.: Primary sarcoma of the pulmonary artery. J. Thorac. Cardiovasc. Surg., 63:587, 1972.

Sevitt, S., and Gallagher, N. G.: Venous thrombosis and pulmonary embolism in injured patients: A trial of anticoagulant prophylaxis with phenindione, in middle-aged and elderly patients with fractured neck of femur. Lancet, 2:981, 1961.

Sharnoff, J. G.: Results in the prophylaxis of postoperative thromboembolism. Surg. Gynecol. Obstet., 123:303, 1966.

Sharp, E. H.: Pulmonary embolectomy: Successful removal of a massive pulmonary embolus with the support of cardiopulmonary bypass: A case report. Ann. Surg., 156:1, 1962.

Silver, D., and Gleysteen, J. J.: Paradoxical arterial embolism. Am. Surg., 36:47, 1970.

Silver, D., and Sabiston, D. C., Jr.: The role of vena caval interruption in the management of pulmonary embolism. Surgery, 77:1, 1975.

Simon, M., and Sasahara, A. A.: Observations on the angiographic changes in pulmonary thromboembolism. In Sasahara, A. A., and Stein M. (eds): Pulmonary Embolic Disease. New York, Grune & Stratton, 1965.

Sloan, H., Morris, J. D., Figley, M., and Lee, R.: Temporary unilateral occlusion of the pulmonary artery in the preoperative evaluation of thoracic patients. J. Thorac. Surg., 30:591, 1955.

Smith, G. T., Dexter, L., and Dammin, G. J.: Postmortem quantitative studies in pulmonary embolism. In Sasahara, A. A., and Stein, M. (eds): Pulmonary Embolic Disease. New York, Grune and Stratton, 1965.

Spencer, F. C., Jude, J., Reinhoff, W. F., III, and Stonesifer, G.: Plication of the inferior vena cava for pulmonary embolism: Long-term results in 39 cases. Ann. Surg., 161:788, 1965.

Spencer, F. C., Quattlebaum, J. K., Quattlebaum, J. K., Jr., et al.: Plication of the inferior vena cava for pulmonary embolism: A report of 20 cases. Ann. Surg., 155:827, 1962.

Starck, E. E., McDermott, J. C., Crummy, A. B., et al.: Percutaneous aspiration thromboembolectomy. Intervent. Radiol., 156:61, 1985.

Steenburg, R. W., Warren, R., Wilson, R. E., and Rudolf, L. E.: A new look at pulmonary embolectomy. Surg. Gynecol. Obstet., 107:214, 1958.

Stein, P. D., O'Connor, J. F., Dalen, J. E., et al.: The angiographic diagnosis of acute pulmonary embolism: Evaluation of criteria. Am. Heart J., 73:730, 1967.

Stein, P. D., Terrin, M. L., Hales, C. A., et al.: Clinical, laboratory, roentgenographic, and electrocardiographic findings in patients with acute pulmonary embolism and no preexisting cardiac or pulmonary disease. Chest, 100:598, 1991.

Stephenson, L. W., Worman, R. B., Aldrete, J. S., and Karp, R. B.: Bullet emboli to the pulmonary artery. Ann. Thorac. Surg., 21:333, 1976.

Stirling, Y., Woolf, L., North, W. R. S., et al.: Haemostasis in normal pregnancy. Thromb. Heamost., 52:176, 1984.

Svane, S.: Tumor thrombus of the inferior vena cava resulting from renal carcinoma. A report on 12 autopsied cases. Scand. J. Urol. Nephrol., 3:245, 1969.

Talley, R. C., Baldwin, B. J., Symbas, P. N., and Nutter, D. O.: Right atrial myxoma. Unusual presentation with cyanosis and clubbing. Am. J. Med., 48:256, 1970.

Torrance, D. J.: The chest film in massive pulmonary embolism. Springfield, IL, Charles C Thomas, 1963.

Trendelenburg, F.: Uber die operative behandlung der embolie der lungenarterie. Arch. Klin. Chir., 86:686, 1908.

Tschirkov, A., Krause, E., Elert, O., and Satter, P.: Surgical management of massive pulmonary embolism. J. Thorac. Cardiovasc. Surg., 75:730, 1978.

Urokinase Pulmonary Embolism Trial Study Group: Urokinase Pulmonary Embolism Trial: Phase I trial results. J. A. M. A., 214:2163, 1970.

Urokinase Streptokinase Pulmonary Embolism Trial (USPET) Study Group: Urokinase Streptokinase Pulmonary Embolism Trial (USPET): Phase 2 results. J. A. M. A., 229:1606, 1974.

Verstraete, M., Miller, G. A. H., Bounameaux, H., et al.: Intravenous and intrapulmonary recombinant tissue-type plasminogen activator in the treatment of acute massive pulmonary embolism. Circulation, 77:353, 1988.

Vessey, M. P., and Doll, R.: Investigation of relation between the use of oral contraceptives and thromboembolic disease. Br. Med. J., 2:199, 1968.

Virchow, R.: Die cellularpathologie in ihrer begrudung auf physiologische und pathologische gewebelehre. Berlin, A. Hirschwald, 1858.

Virchow, R.: Gesammelte Abhandlungen zur wissenschaftlichen medizin. Frankfurt, Meidinger, 1856, p. 219.

Vossschulte, K.: The surgical treatment of pulmonary embolism. J. Cardiovasc. Surg., 6(Suppl.):197, 1965.

Wacker, W. E. C., and Snodgrass, P. J.: Serum LDH activity in pulmonary embolism diagnosis. J. A. M. A., 174:2142, 1960.

Wagner, H. N., Sabiston, D. C., Jr., and McAfee, J. G., et al.: Diagnosis of massive pulmonary embolism in man by radioisotope scanning. N. Engl. J. Med., 271:377, 1964.

Weideranders, R. E., White, S. M., and Saichek, H. B.: The effect of pulmonary resection on pulmonary artery pressures. Ann. Surg., 160:889, 1964.

Wessler, S.: Prevention of venous thromboembolism by low-dose heparin. A 1976 status report. Mod. Concepts Cardiovasc. Dis., 45:105, 1976.

Westermark, N.: On the roentgen diagnosis of lung embolism. Acta Radiol., 19:357, 1938.

White, P.D.: The acute cor pulmonale. Ann. Intern. Med., 9:115, 1935.

Williams, J. W., Eikman, E. A., and Greenberg, S.: Asymptomatic pulmonary embolism: A common event in high-risk patients. Ann. Surg., 195:323, 1982.

Wingerd, M., Bernhard, V. M., Maddison, F., et al.: Comparison of vena caval filters in the management of venous thromboembolism. Arch. Surg., 113:1264, 1978.

Winterbauer, R. H., Elfenbein, I. B., and Ball, W. C., Jr.: Incidence and clinical significance of tumor embolization to the lungs. Am. J. Med., 45:271, 1968.

Worsley, F. F., Alavi, A., and Palevsky, H. I.: Role of radionuclide imaging in patients with suspected pulmonary embolism. Radiol. Clin. North Am., 31:849, 1993.

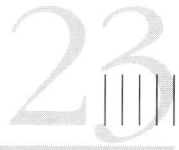

23 ■ II Chronic Pulmonary Embolism

Mark W. Sebastian and David C. Sabiston, Jr.

Although pulmonary embolism usually presents as an *acute* clinical problem, it can also be a *chronic* disorder. Most pulmonary emboli undergo spontaneous resolution as a result of naturally occurring fibrinolytic systems in the bloodstream (Dalen et al., 1969; Dalen and Alpert, 1975). However, in chronic pulmonary embolism, defective fibrinolysis begins a cycle of incomplete lysis of emboli, partial recanalization within the pulmonary vasculature, organization, and proximal thrombotic extension causing a gradual accumulation of emboli in the pulmonary arterial system. These emboli may ultimately produce pulmonary hypertension and cause symptoms of progressive respiratory insufficiency, hypoxemia, and right ventricular failure (Dalen and Alpert, 1975; Kapitan et al., 1989; Owen et al., 1953; Sabiston et al., 1977; Tilkian et al., 1976). In most patients, medical management is unsatisfactory, with studies revealing a poor prognosis (McIntyre et al., 1971; Riedel et al., 1982; Sutton et al., 1977; Wilhelmsen et al., 1972). The syndrome of chronic pulmonary embolism is distinct from that of primary pulmonary hypertension, which consists of distal pulmonary arterial and arteriolar occlusion with no evidence of a primary source of emboli. The treatment in this group of patients is therapy with appropriate pharmacologic agents. Although the number of patients with chronic pulmonary embolism remains comparatively small, the knowledge obtained from an understanding of this disease has been dependent on a knowledge of pulmonary physiology, pulmonary and cardiac surgery, coagulation, arteriography, and critical care.

In patients with chronic embolic disease of the main, lobar, or segmental pulmonary arteries, the presence of elevated pulmonary arterial pressures is the most important clinical consideration, because it has been shown that the natural history of this syndrome is related to the magnitude of the pulmonary arterial hypertension. If the mean pulmonary artery pressure is more than 30 mm Hg, survival at 5 years is only 30%. In those patients with mean pressure greater than 50 mm Hg, only 10% are alive at 5 years (Fig. 23–19). Fortunately, it is now established that pulmonary embolectomy in patients with proximal pulmonary arterial obstruction is likely to produce a reduction in pulmonary hypertension with decreased respiratory insufficiency and improvement in right-sided heart failure.

HISTORICAL ASPECTS

The number of patients with documented chronic pulmonary emboli has increased in recent years, and the number of patients identified and treated arises from improved diagnostic techniques and recognition that surgical therapy can cause dramatic clinical improvement in properly selected patients.

Chronic pulmonary emboli were suspected by Hart in 1916 and Moller in 1920. In 1928, Ljungdahl described two patients, one aged 38 years and the other aged 51 years, who had suffered for several years with symptoms of dyspnea, cyanosis, and palpitation. Both ultimately died of right-sided heart failure, and chronic pulmonary arterial obstruction was noted at autopsy, with marked dilatation of the proximal pulmonary artery. The bronchial circulation was increased and the lungs were free of infarction. Ljungdahl emphasized that it was likely that the obstruction was due to pulmonary emboli, compared with the previously held concept that in patients with cor pulmonale, the process was caused by primary thrombosis of the pulmonary artery. Several years later, Brenner (1935) reported a systematic study of the pulmonary vasculature and attributed numerous

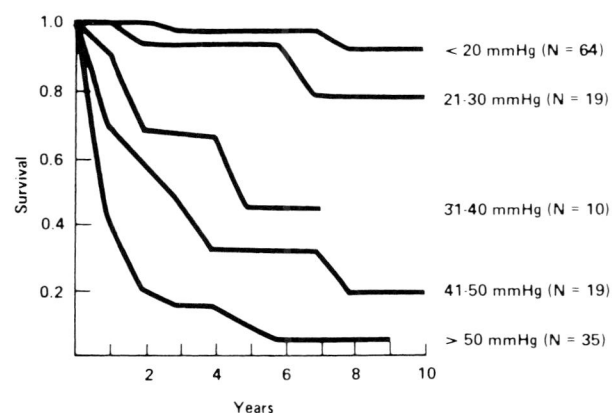

FIGURE 23–19. Survival in patients with pulmonary hypertension resulting from chronic recurrent emboli. Groups of patients are compared at different mean pulmonary artery pressures. (Modified from Riedel, M., Stanek, V., Widimsky, J., et al.: Long-term follow-up of patients with pulmonary thromboembolism. Chest, *81:*151, 1982.)

changes in the pulmonary vessels to pulmonary embolism.

In the last century, Virchow (1847) suspected that pulmonary infarction did not occur in most patients after pulmonary embolism, because bronchial collateral circulation was adequate. In 1948, Blalock confirmed these early observations by detecting bright red arterial perfusion of pulmonary vessels distal to chronic emboli, and collateral perfusion by bronchial arteries was shown angiographically by Viamonte in 1964.

Carroll (1950) described the clinical features of chronic pulmonary emboli and made a diagnosis of the syndrome prior to the death of a 30-year-old patient with progressive dyspnea, cardiac failure, and absence of vascular markings in the left lung field. Right heart catheterization demonstrated complete absence of perfusion of the left lung. The diagnosis in this patient was established at thoracotomy when an atretic left pulmonary artery was opened and found to contain chronic emboli confirmed by the histology of the excised specimen. Although several early attempts at surgical therapy were made, the first successful embolectomy for recurrent pulmonary emboli was reported by Allison in 1960.

In 1967, Fleishner reviewed the clinical and diagnostic aspects of chronic recurrent pulmonary emboli and emphasized the radiolucency of the vascular markings that were sometimes apparent on chest films. Chitwood and colleagues (1985) emphasized the importance of bronchial arteriography and the need for identifying obstructing lesions in the proximal pulmonary arterial system. Cabrol and co-workers (1978) recommended lateral thoracotomy to easily approach the distal pulmonary arterial branches. Daily and associates (1987) reported bilateral thromboendarterectomy by a median sternotomy and extrapericardial dissection of the pulmonary arteries. Cardiopulmonary bypass was used with deep hypothermia and intermittent circulatory arrest while a pulmonary thromboendarterectomy was performed. Daily and colleagues (1989) reported the first series of over 100 consecutive patients treated in this manner.

CLINICAL PRESENTATION

Patients with the syndrome of chronic pulmonary embolism have a history of exertional dyspnea progressing to severe respiratory insufficiency over months to years. They may also complain of recurrent episodes of thrombophlebitis, chest pain, and hemoptysis owing to the presence of large bronchial collaterals (Table 23–5). Physical findings include signs of severe pulmonary hypertension, often combined with evidence of right ventricular failure. These signs may include an increased pulmonary second sound, a systolic murmur, hepatomegaly, and an S3 or S4 gallop. Other physical findings are pulmonary rales, jugular venous distention, cyanosis, and clubbing of the fingers (Table 23–6).

■ **Table 23–5.** SYMPTOMS OF PATIENTS WITH CHRONIC PULMONARY EMBOLI (n = 48)

Symptom	% Afflicted
Dyspnea—exertion (44)	92
Thrombophlebitis (26)	54
Dyspnea—progressive (39)	81
Hemoptysis (13)	28
Chest pain (12)	25
Fatigue (12)	25

NATURAL HISTORY

The natural history of chronic pulmonary embolism has been studied by Moser and associates in a 1990 review of 250 consecutive patients, of whom 195 underwent surgical correction. A careful history usually reveals an acute event in most patients, often characterized by swelling of the leg, pneumonia, and dyspnea, and the patients have been given a diagnosis of primary pulmonary hypertension. After the initial embolic event, improvement ensues with increased functional ability largely independent of anticoagulation. It is during this period that the right ventricle hypertrophies in response to increased pulmonary vascular resistance. Experimental data indicate that noninvolved as well as occluded pulmonary vascular beds show pathologic changes. Deterioration is exacerbated by proximal extension of thromboemboli. Right ventricular failure, hypoxemia, opening of the foramen ovale, and development of pulmonary arteriovenous fistulas ensue, with eventual death.

CLINICAL FINDINGS

The chest film shows a dilated pulmonary artery with oligemic pulmonary fields in approximately half of the patients. A typical preoperative chest film is shown in Figure 23–20. Although some patients with chronic pulmonary emboli have been described as having a normal chest film, this is unusual. In Sabiston's series, all plain films showed abnormalities, including cardiomegaly (85%), right-sided heart enlargement (58%), enlargement of the pulmonary artery (42%), azygos vein enlargement (27%), chronic volume loss (25%), atelectasis (23%) or effusion (17%), and pleural thickening (12%) (Woodruff et al., 1985).

■ **Table 23–6.** PHYSICAL FINDINGS IN PATIENTS WITH CHRONIC PULMONARY EMBOLISM (n = 48)

Physical Finding	% Afflicted
Increased P$_2$ (28)	59
Cardiac murmur (22)	45
Hepatomegaly (13)	27
S3 or S4 gallop (12)	25
Pulmonary rales (12)	25
Jugular venous distention (10)	21
Cyanosis (2)	4
Clubbing (1)	2

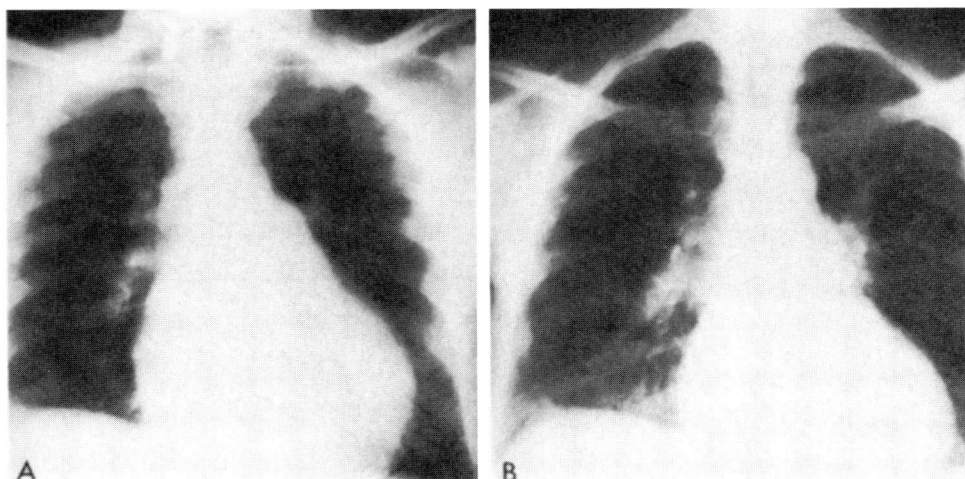

FIGURE 23–20. The anteroposterior chest film is shown before (A) and after (B) embolectomy of the right lower lobe pulmonary artery for chronic pulmonary emboli. Note an increase in parenchymal flow to the right lower lobe after operation. Also note the decrease in the size of both the right main pulmonary artery and the cardiac silhouette after embolectomy. (A and B, From Chitwood, W. R., Jr., Lyerly, H. K., and Sabiston, D. C., Jr.: Surgical management of chronic pulmonary embolism. Ann. Surg., 201:11, 1985.)

(Table 23–7). Embolic involvement of the right lung was present in 96% of patients, and of the left lung in 80%; bilateral emboli were present in 82% of patients. Arterial blood gases at room air revealed evidence of severe respiratory insufficiency, with hypoxemia and arterial oxygen tension (Pa_{O_2}) values ranging from 55 to 60 mm Hg and an arterial carbon dioxide tension (Pa_{CO_2}) of approximately 30 mm Hg (Table 23–8). The pH showed a mild respiratory alkalosis (pH = 7.5).

Electrocardiographic findings usually show the presence of chronic cor pulmonale with right-axis deviation and right ventricular hypertrophy. ST segment and T wave changes are present in approximately a third of patients, and somewhat fewer have right bundle-branch block.

Peripheral *venography* usually indicates the source of the emboli. Magnetic resonance imaging is now often used to demonstrate thrombi in the pelvic vein and is a reliable and noninvasive technique. Right ventricular function may be assessed by first-pass radionuclide angiography and shows severe chronic pulmonary arterial obstruction with a significant delay in arrival of the tracer. The mean resting ejection fraction for patients in the series was 23.5 + 2.2 at rest and 28.0 + 4.0 with exercise.

Ventilation and perfusion radionuclide scans are consistent with pulmonary emboli, and perfusion defects correspond to the oligemic regions on the plain film and arteriogram (Wolfe and Sabiston, 1980). Perfusion defects are usually noted bilaterally. Typical preoperative and postoperative perfusion scans show definite improvement in pulmonary flow (Fig. 23–21).

Pulmonary arteriography usually shows emboli in both lungs, with between 55 and 75% of the total pulmonary blood flow being obstructed (Fig. 23–22). Pulmonary hypertension was present in all 48 patients with chronic pulmonary emboli evaluated at the Duke University Medical Center. The systolic pulmonary arterial pressure was 75.0 + 8.0 mm Hg, the diastolic pressure 26.0 + 3.0 mm Hg, and the mean pressure 42.0 + 5.0 mm Hg (Table 23–9).

PREOPERATIVE EVALUATION

A thorough preoperative evaluation is necessary before the suitability of an operation for each patient can be determined. The most appropriate candidates for pulmonary embolectomy are those with severe respiratory insufficiency and a low Pa_{O_2} and those who demonstrate enlarged bronchial vessels by arteriography. Some patients with the syndrome are unsuitable for embolectomy, and the most common contra-

■ Table 23–7. CHEST FILM FINDINGS IN PATIENTS WITH CHRONIC PULMONARY EMBOLISM (n = 48)

Finding	% Afflicted
Cardiomegaly (41)	85
Right-sided heart enlargement (26)	58
Enlargement of pulmonary artery (20)	42
Azygos vein enlargement (13)	27
Chronic volume loss (12)	25
Atelectasis (11)	23
Effusion (8)	17
Pleural thickening (6)	12

■ Table 23–8. LABORATORY DATA IN PATIENTS WITH CHRONIC PULMONARY EMBOLI (n = 47)

Laboratory Test	Findings		
Arterial blood gas	Pa_{O_2}	Pa_{CO_2}	pH
Average value	55 mm Hg	30 mm Hg	7.5
Electrocardiogram	Right ventricular hypertrophy	Right-axis deviation	ST-T wave changes
% Afflicted	86%	50%	33%

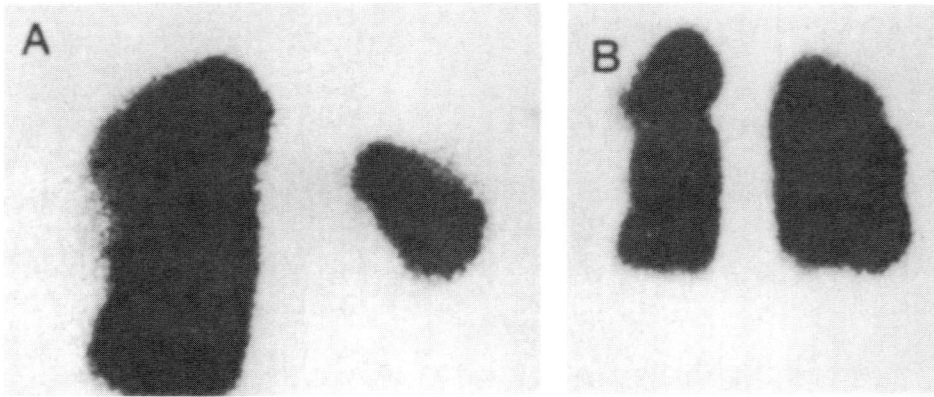

FIGURE 23–21. The posterior view of a pulmonary perfusion scan before *(A)* and after *(B)* embolectomy for a right lower lobe chronic pulmonary embolism. *B* shows the scan 3 months after embolectomy and shows the reestablishment of flow to the right lower lobe. *(A* and *B,* From Chitwood, W. R., Jr., Lyerly, H. K., and Sabiston, D. C., Jr.: Surgical management of chronic pulmonary embolism. Ann. Surg., *201:*11, 1985.)

indication is *distal* pulmonary emboli that diffusely involve the small pulmonary arteries and are not amenable to surgical removal (Chitwood et al., 1985) (Figs. 23–23 to 23–25). Other contraindications include severe cardiac failure and massive obesity. Most of these patients are disabled and New York Heart Association (NYHA) Class IV.

Pulmonary arteriography is critical in any patient being considered for surgical intervention. Auger and colleagues (1992) reviewed 250 patients being considered for embolectomy and identified five major arteriographic findings considered highly suggestive for chronic pulmonary embolism amenable to surgical correction, including:

1. Pouching or concave configuration of pulmonary arterial occlusion;

2. Pulmonary arterial webs or bands defined as decreased opacity lines traversing a pulmonary vessel at the level of lobar or segmental vessels;

3. Intimal irregularity;

4. Abrupt narrowing of major pulmonary vessels secondary to recanalization, concentric narrowing, or reactive arterial contraction; and

5. Lobar vascular obstruction.

These characteristic findings are distinct from the sharply defined intraluminal defects of acute pulmonary embolism.

Other preoperative studies include thoracic aortography or selective bronchial arteriography to show dilated and tortuous bronchial vessels (Figs. 23–26 and 23–27). The bronchial circulation is often considerably augmented and communicates by collateral

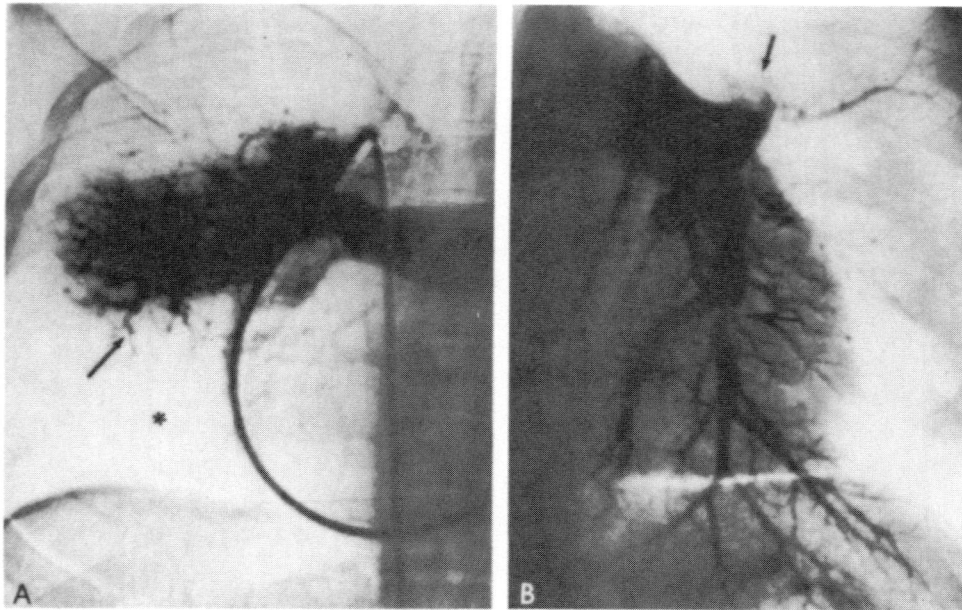

FIGURE 23–22. Preoperative angiograms of the same patient depicted in Figure 23–21. These angiograms represent the classic arteriographic findings of chronic pulmonary emboli. *A,* Tapered arterial defects are visible in the distal pulmonary arteries *(arrow),* indicating chronic pulmonary emboli. Note the total obstruction of the right lower lobe pulmonary artery leading to oligemia *(asterisk).* Moreover, segmental occlusion to the right upper lobe is also present. *B,* Proximal dilatation of the main pulmonary artery is noted. A plaque is visible in the left upper lobe pulmonary artery *(small arrow).* In the left lower lobe pulmonary artery, a residual web is evident *(large arrow).* This represents a partially resolved chronic pulmonary embolus. *(A* and *B,* From Chitwood, W. R., Jr., Lyerly, H. K., and Sabiston, D. C., Jr.: Surgical management of chronic pulmonary embolism. Ann. Surg., *201:*11, 1985.)

■ Table 23–9. ANGIOGRAPHIC AND HEMODYNAMIC DATA FROM 22 PATIENTS UNDERGOING EMBOLECTOMY FOR CHRONIC PULMONARY EMBOLI

Patient	Leg Venogram	Vena Cavogram	Magnetic Resonance	Bronchial Angiogram	Major Occlusions	% Occlusion	Preoperative			Postoperative		
							PAS	PAD	$\overline{PA}$	PAS	PAD	$\overline{PA}$
1	+	–	None	None	RLL, left main (total)	65	75	20	32	35	14	20
2	+	+	None	None	RUL, RML, RLL, LLL (total)	60	48	18	30	37*	14*	21*
3	+	–	None	Large bronchial, large intercostal, L. lung only	RLL, left main (total)	55	43	23	27	36*	17*	21*
4	+	None	None	None	RUL, RLL, lung, LLL (total)	55	44	18	28	38	12	21
5	–	–	None	None	RUL, RLL, (total), lung, LLL	55	85	22	40	53	18	30
6	None	None	None	None	RUL, left main (total)	65	100	30	45	100	20	46
7	+	–	None	Large bronchial R > L	RLL (total), RML, LLL	60	65	30	42	None	None	None
8	–	–	None	Large bronchial L > R	RLL (diffuse), lung, LLL (total)	65	50	20	30	50	14	24
9	+	None	None	Large bronchial R > L	RUL, RML, RLL, lung	65	75	25	45	None	10*	None
10	+	None	None	Moderately dilated bronchial—no flow	RUL, RML, RLL (diffuse), LLL (total)	60	95	30	54	54*	14*	27*
11	+	None	None	Large bronchial R > L	RUL (total), RLL (total) LLL	70	130	55	82	65*	15*	32*
12	–	None	None	Large bronchial left supplying right	RLL (total), RML, LLL (total), LUL	70	78	20	45	80	24	36
13	+	None	None	Large bronchial left lung only	RUL, RML (total), LUL (total), LLL	60	58	17	32	None	10*	None
14	None	None	None	Large bronchial right lung only	Right main (total), LUL (diffuse)	65	80	36	50	74*	12*	32*
15	–	None	None	Large bronchial left lung only	Left main	55	80	45	30	None	14*	None
16	+	None	+	None	RLL, RML, LUL	60	100	65	45	55	19	31
17	–	None	None	Moderately dilated bronchial	Left main	55	100	60	40	None	None	None
18	None	None	–	Large bronchial left lung only	Left main	55	43	28	17	None	7*	None
19	None	None	None	Large bronchial left lung only	Left main, RUL	75	75	52	40	70	40	50
20	None	None	None	Large bronchial right lung only	RML, RLL	50	75	55	25	65	20	35
21	None	None	None	Large bronchial right lung only	RLL, RUL, LLL	70	70	42	22	24	12	16
22	None	None	None	Large bronchial right lung only	RLL, RUL	55	76	46	26	46	20	28

*Indicates data obtained using Swan-Ganz pulmonary arterial catheters. Other postoperative data were obtained from cardiac catheterizations.
Key: PAS = pulmonary artery systole; PAD = pulmonary artery diastole; $\overline{PA}$ = mean pulmonary artery pressure; R = right; L = left; UL = upper lobe; ML = middle lobe; LL = lower lobe.

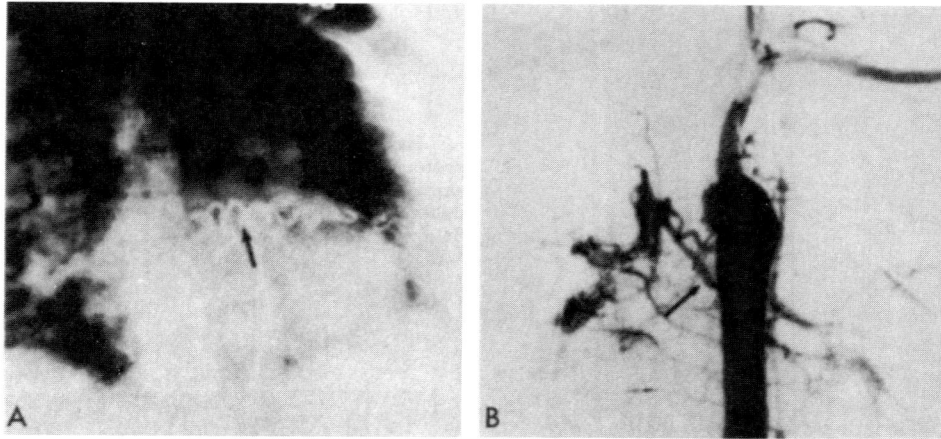

FIGURE 23–23. *A,* A tortuous dilated intercostal artery *(arrow)* from which collateral vessels arose to supply underperfused lung in a patient with left lower arterial obstruction. *B,* Aortogram in a patient with chronic obstruction of the right upper lobe pulmonary artery. Note the large intercostobronchial artery *(arrow)* that arises from the aorta to supply the distal pulmonary parenchyma. In the left lower lobe, several pulmonary artery channels fill in a retrograde manner from collateral vessels. (*A* and *B,* From Chitwood, W. R., Jr., Lyerly, H. K., and Sabiston, D. C., Jr.: Surgical management of chronic pulmonary embolism. Ann. Surg., *201:*11, 1985.)

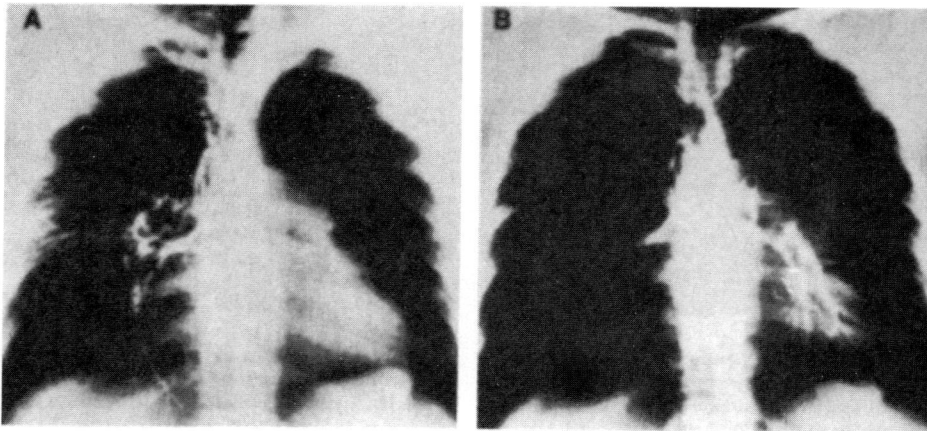

FIGURE 23–24. *A,* A selective bronchial arterial injection showing dilated bronchial collaterals on the right supplying the distal pulmonary parenchyma. *B,* A later phase of the same injection. Collaterals from the right side supply the distal pulmonary parenchyma in the left lower lobe. The left lower lobe pulmonary artery was noted to have a total proximal obstruction on the pulmonary arteriogram. (*A* and *B,* From Chitwood, W. R., Jr., Lyerly, H. K., and Sabiston, D. C., Jr.: Surgical management of chronic pulmonary embolism. Ann. Surg., *201:*11, 1985.)

FIGURE 23–25. Systolic, diastolic, and mean preoperative and postoperative pulmonary artery pressures are compared. After embolectomy, these pressures improved significantly; $p < .05$ denotes a statistically significant value (Student's t-test for paired data).

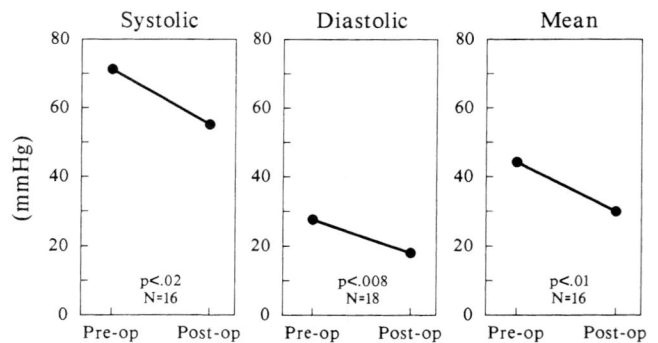

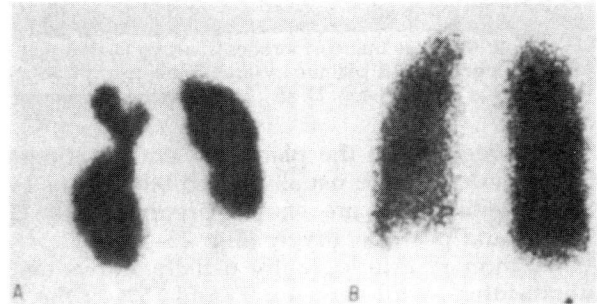

FIGURE 23–26. *A,* A perfusion scan from a patient who had multiple distal perfusion defects and who was not a candidate for operation. *B,* A ventilation scan from the same patient as in *A.* No sizable ventilation defects were evident. (*A* and *B,* From Chitwood, W. R., Jr., Lyerly, H. K., and Sabiston, D. C., Jr.: Surgical management of chronic pulmonary embolism. Ann. Surg., *201:*11, 1985.)

vessels with the distal pulmonary arteries. In patients in whom selective bronchial arteriograms were performed, patency of the distal pulmonary arteries is quite common (Viamonte et al., 1965). Moreover, when the *distal* pulmonary arteries are patent, the prognosis is favorable because thrombectomy will be followed by pulmonary arterial blood flow.

SURGICAL MANAGEMENT

Pulmonary embolectomy may be performed on one or both pulmonary arteries. In a number of patients, the pulmonary artery is occluded unilaterally and there are few, if any, proximal emboli in the contralateral lung. These patients usually improve dramatically after embolectomy. In those with primarily unilateral involvement, either a right or a left anterior

thoracotomy can be used when there is proximal occlusion of the vessel (Fig. 23–28). In patients with bilateral pulmonary emboli or in those with involvement of the main pulmonary artery, median sternotomy with extracorporeal circulation is indicated.

Involvement of the main pulmonary artery and the left pulmonary artery and its branches is shown in Figure 23–29. Meticulous dissection is necessary, with removal of all distal emboli, to achieve optimal postoperative results (Fig. 23–30). The procedure is a true endarterectomy, as the thromboemboli are well organized and densely adherent to the wall of the pulmonary artery. Great care must be taken in the dissection. All distal emboli should be removed until adequate backbleeding of bright red blood is shown. Even with circulatory arrest, backbleeding obscures the operative field. Daily and co-workers (1991) described a thromboendarterectomy dissector designed to allow

FIGURE 23–27. A pulmonary arteriogram from the same patient shown in Figure 23–26 demonstrates multiple peripheral filling defects. Organized emboli can be seen within the proximal right pulmonary arteries (*A, arrowheads*). In the left lower lobe, a calcified embolus is present (*B, arrow* and *inset*). (*A* and *B,* From Chitwood, W. R., Jr., Lyerly, H. K., and Sabiston, D. C., Jr.: Surgical management of chronic pulmonary embolism. Ann. Surg. *201:*11, 1985.)

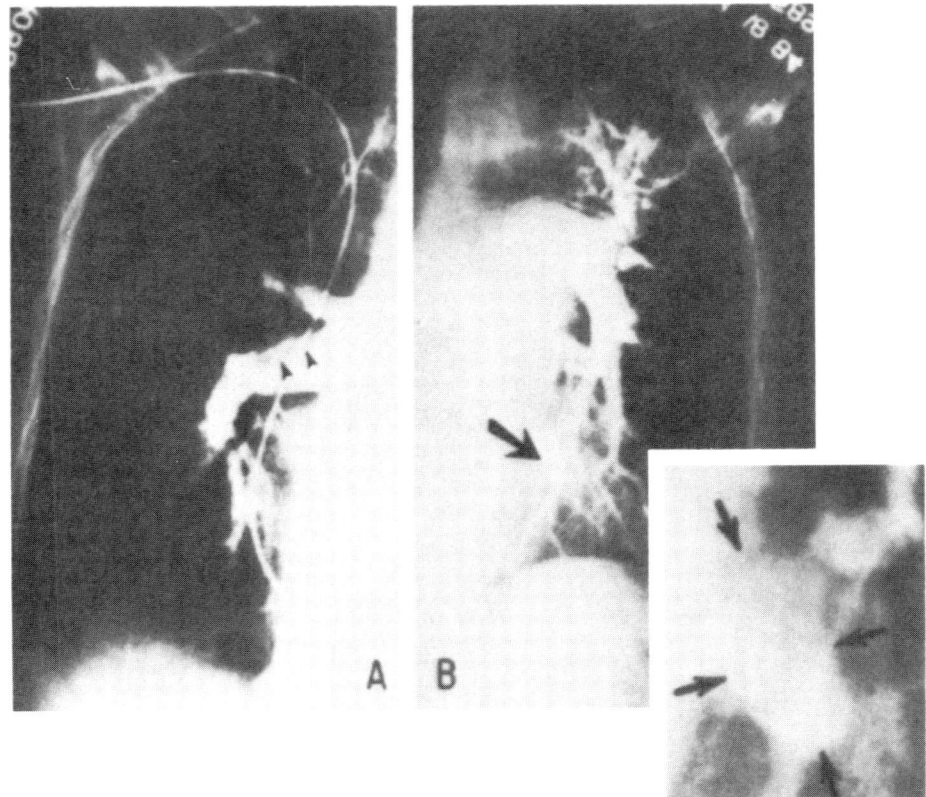

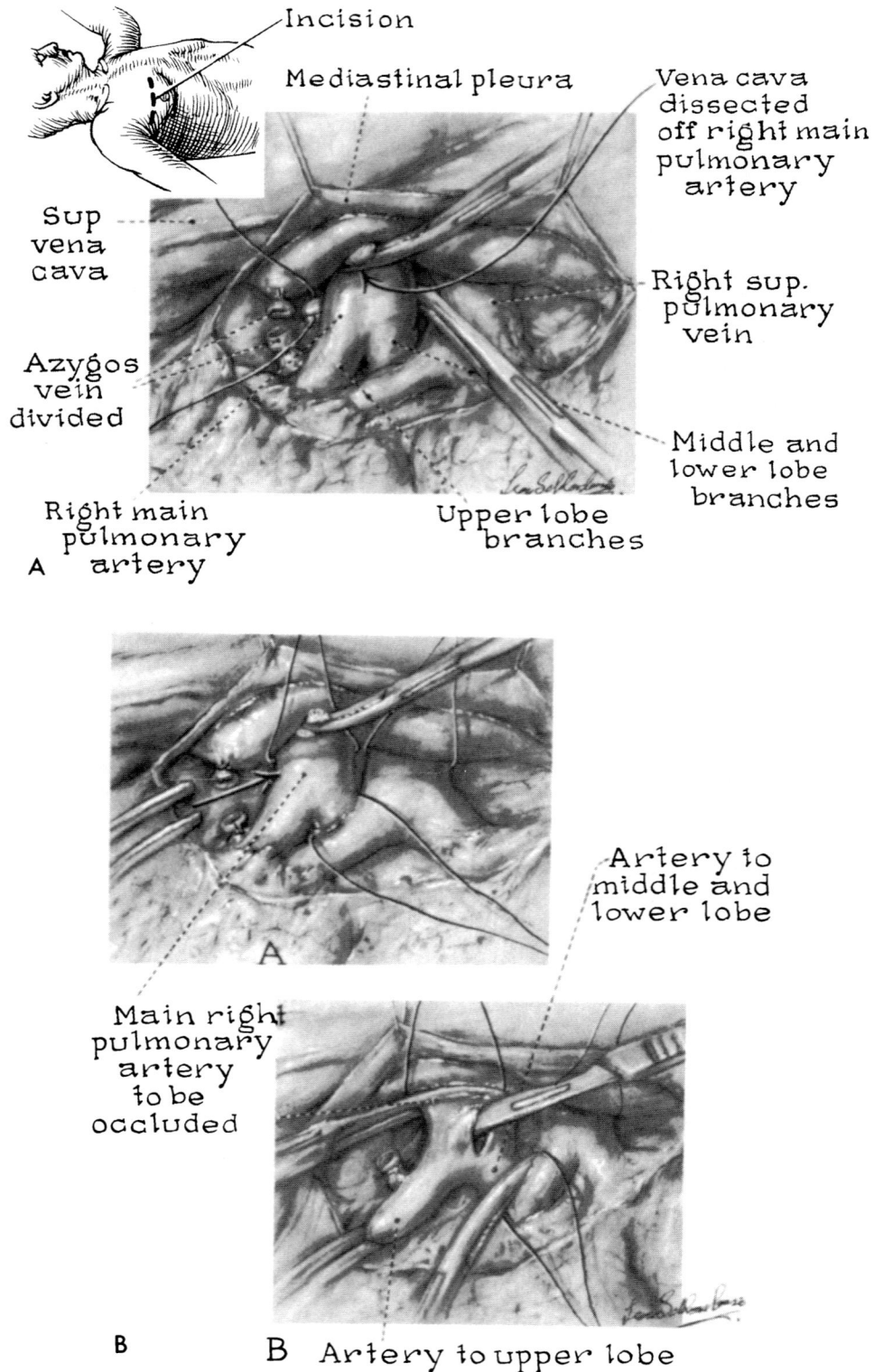

FIGURE 23–28. Technique of unilateral pulmonary embolectomy (without the necessity for extracorporeal circulation). *A,* The incision is made in the right anterior chest with division of the pectoral muscles and entry into the pleural cavity in the third intercostal space. The lung is retracted, and the anterior mediastinum is opened posterior to the phrenic nerve. The azygos vein is ligated and divided for ideal exposure of the right pulmonary artery. *B,* A ligature is passed loosely around the right main pulmonary artery as well as around its distal branches. (A) The proximal right pulmonary artery is occluded with a vascular clamp, as are the distal branches. An arteriotomy is made on the anterior surface of the right pulmonary artery for exposure of the embolus (B).

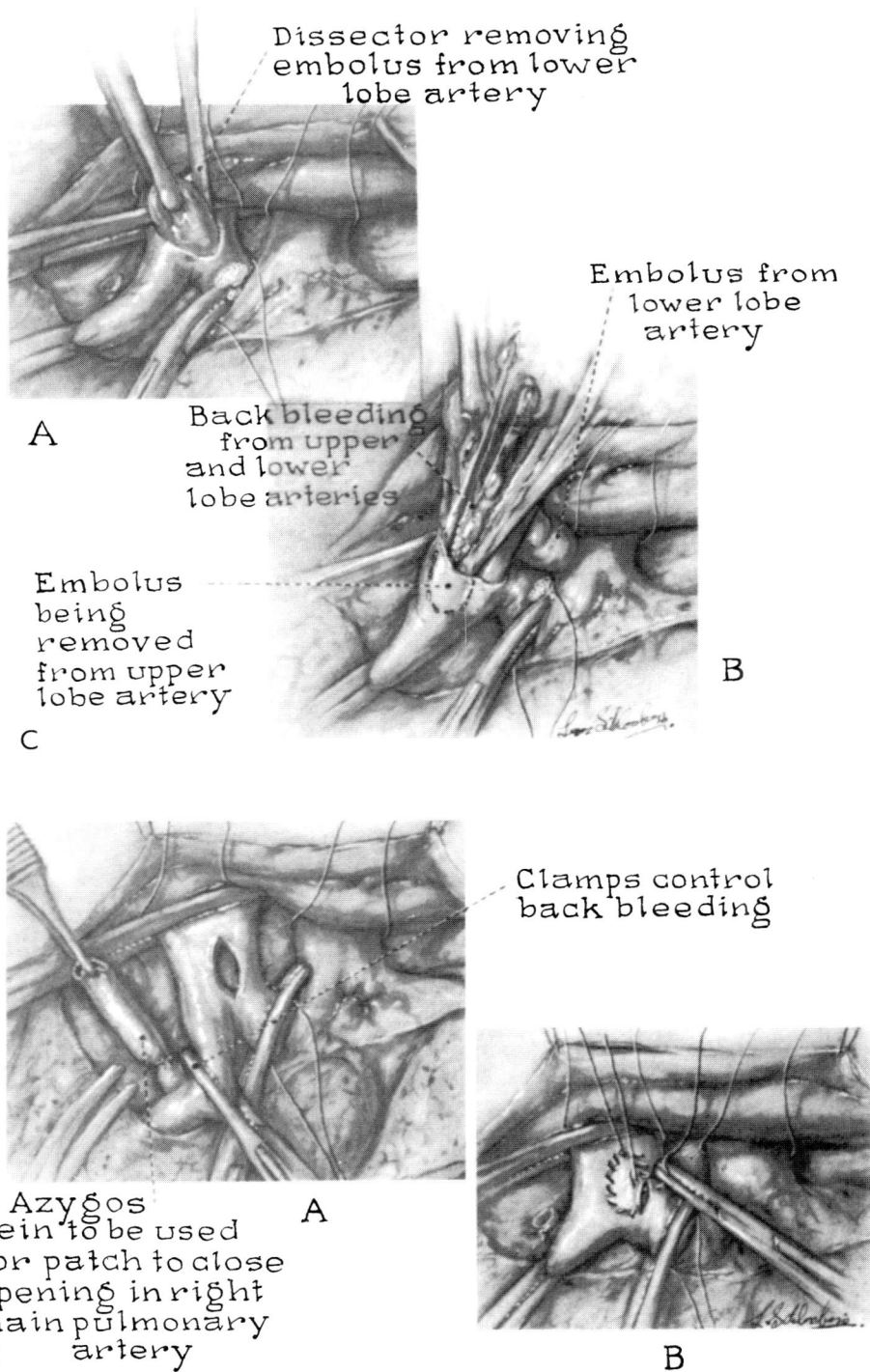

Dissector removing
embolus from lower
lobe artery

A

Back bleeding
from upper
and lower
lobe arteries

Embolus from
lower lobe
artery

B

Embolus
being
removed
from upper
lobe artery

C

Clamps control
back bleeding

Azygos
vein to be used
for patch to close
opening in right
main pulmonary
artery

D

A

B

FIGURE 23–28 *Continued C* The embolus is removed with forceps (A). In patients with chronic pulmonary emboli, it may be necessary to dissect the embolus away from the arterial wall (B). If the embolus is chronic, prominent arterial backbleeding of bright red arterial blood should ensue when the embolectomy is complete. *D,* The arteriotomy in the right main pulmonary artery may be closed directly with a continuous suture, or a vein patch may be used if it is thought that the primary closure would significantly reduce the lumen of the pulmonary artery. The venous graft may be easily obtained from the nearby azygos vein.

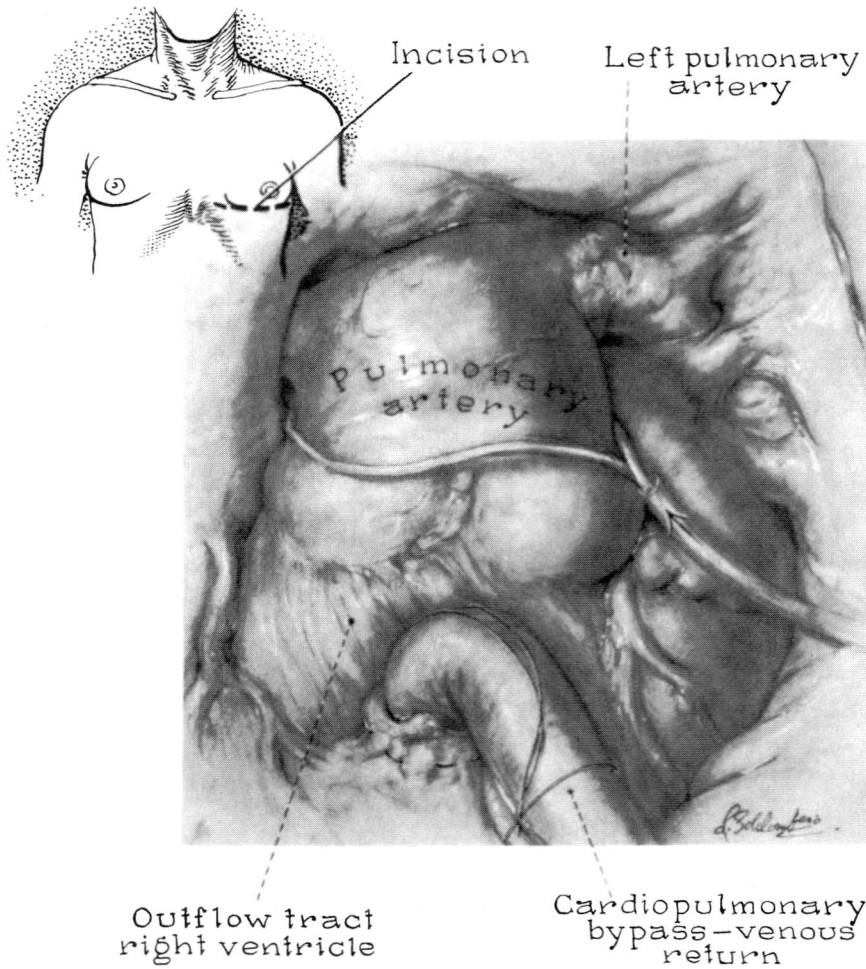

Incision   Left pulmonary artery

Pulmonary artery

Outflow tract right ventricle   Cardiopulmonary bypass—venous return

FIGURE 23–29. A left anterolateral thoracotomy is made, with the pleural cavity entered through the third intercostal space. This is the approach for the main pulmonary artery and for the left pulmonary artery. The venous outflow cannula may be placed in the outflow tract of the right ventricle through a purse-string suture as shown, and the arterial cannula is placed in the femoral artery. The main pulmonary artery is massively enlarged with significant pulmonary hypertension. A tape is passed around the proximal pulmonary artery for control. If the right pulmonary artery requires exposure for embolectomy, the sternum can be transected and the incision can be extended into the right third intercostal space with entry into the right chest. In that case, the venous return cannula may be placed in the right atrium and the aorta can be used as the side for the arterial inflow cannula. (From Wolfe, W. G., and Sabiston, D. C., Jr.: Pulmonary Embolism. Major Problems in Clinical Surgery, Volume 25 of the series. Philadelphia, W. B. Saunders, 1980.)

FIGURE 23–30. A, After occlusion of the proximal pulmonary artery by the tape when the patient is on cardiopulmonary bypass, an incision is made into the main pulmonary artery for removal of the chronic embolus. B, The thrombus is densely adherent to the wall of the pulmonary artery and requires exacting and tedious dissection. As much of the thrombus as possible is removed through this incision preparatory to a counterincision in the distal left pulmonary artery. (A and B, From Wolfe, W. G., and Sabiston, D. C., Jr.: Pulmonary Embolism. Major Problems in Clinical Surgery. Volume 25 of the series. Philadelphia, W. B. Saunders, 1980.)

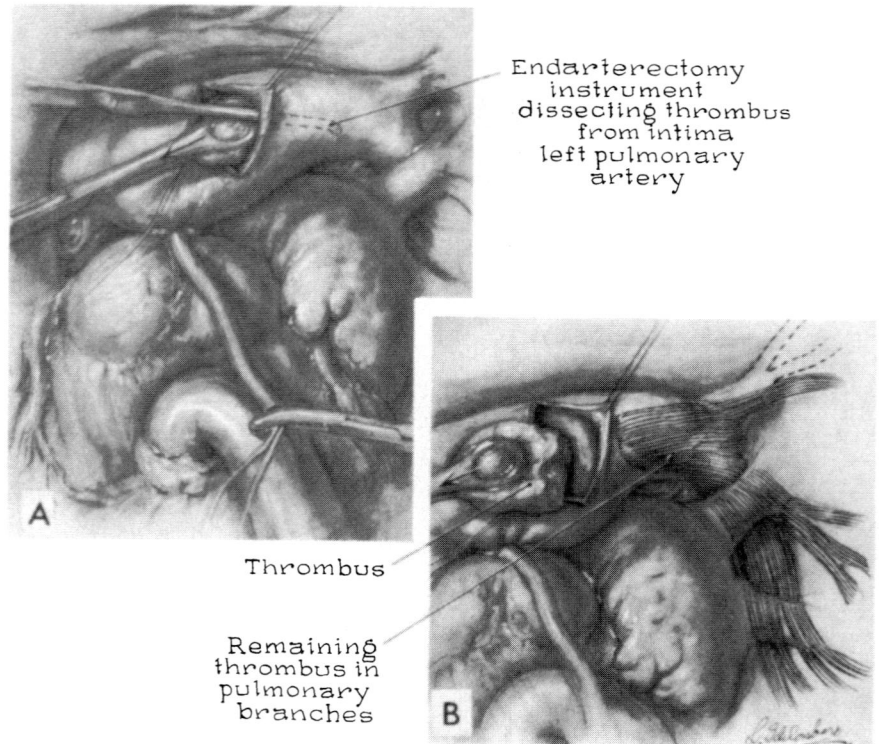

Endarterectomy instrument dissecting thrombus from intima left pulmonary artery

Thrombus

Remaining thrombus in pulmonary branches

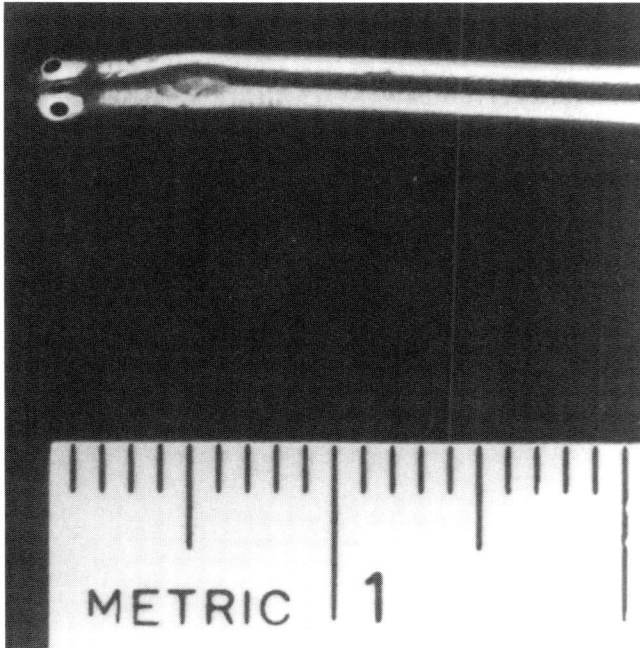

FIGURE 23–31. Thromboendarterectomy dissectors. These instruments are specifically designed for simultaneous dissection and suction required in the true endarterectomy necessary for removal of chronic pulmonary emboli. (From Daily, P. O., Dembitsky, W. P., and Daily, R. P.: Dissectors for pulmonary thromboendarterectomy. Reprinted with permission from the Society of Thoracic Surgeons [The Annals of Thoracic Surgery, 1991, Vol. 51, p. 842].)

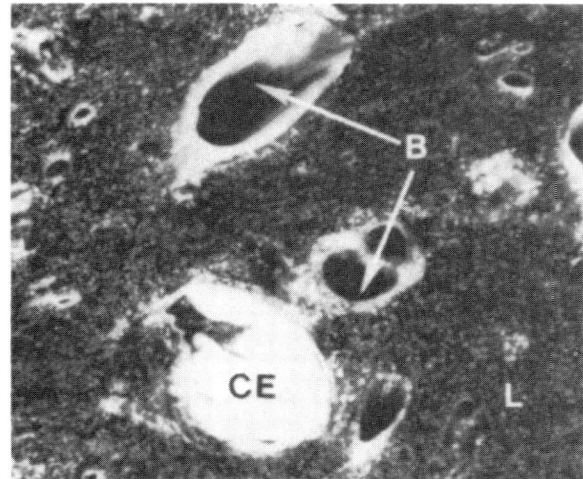

FIGURE 23–33. A gross pathologic specimen of lung tissue. B = medium-sized bronchi; L = lung parenchyma; CE = an organized fibrotic chronic embolus within a distal pulmonary arterial branch. (From Chitwood, W. R., Jr., Lyerly, H. K., and Sabiston, D. C., Jr.: Surgical management of chronic pulmonary embolism. Ann. Surg., 201:11, 1985.)

simultaneous dissection and suction of blood from the operative field (Fig. 23–31). It may be preferable to close the arteriotomy with a pericardial patch to prevent constriction of the lumen. It is usually neces-

sary to make a counterincision on the distal pulmonary artery to completely remove the adherent emboli in the secondary and tertiary branches of the pulmonary arteries (Figs. 23–32 to 23–35). Typical specimens removed at operation are shown in Figure 23–36.

Satisfactory distal backbleeding can usually be predicted in advance from the information gained by the thoracic aortogram with selective injection of the

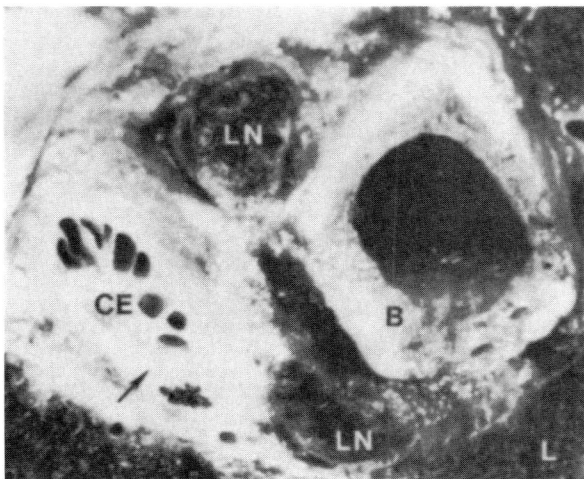

FIGURE 23–32. A recanalized chronic embolus (CE) is shown within a lobar pulmonary artery. The *arrow* indicates the juncture between the organized embolus and the pulmonary artery wall. Very little separation exists between the embolus and the thickened pulmonary artery wall. B = lobar bronchus; LN = peribronchial lymph nodes; L = lung parenchyma. (From Chitwood, W. R., Jr., Lyerly, H. K., and Sabiston, D. C., Jr.: Surgical management of chronic pulmonary embolism. Ann. Surg., 201:11, 1985.)

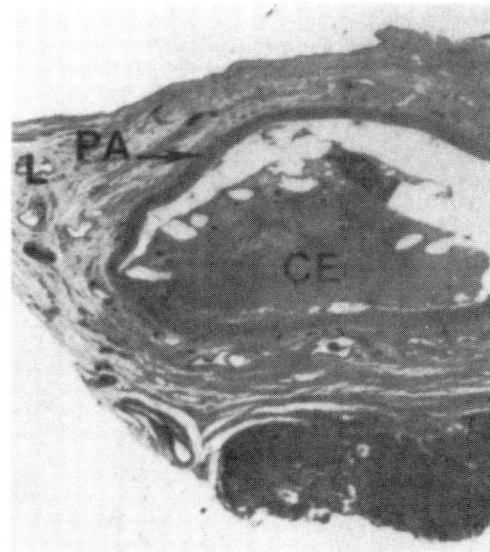

FIGURE 23–34. A whole mount cross-section of a medium-sized pulmonary artery. The chronic embolus (CE) is tightly adherent to the pulmonary arterial wall along the inferior aspect. Note recanalization of the chronic embolus. PA = pulmonary artery; L = lung parenchyma. (From Chitwood, W. R., Jr., Lyerly, H. K., and Sabiston, D. C., Jr.: Surgical management of chronic pulmonary embolism. Ann. Surg., 201:11, 1985.)

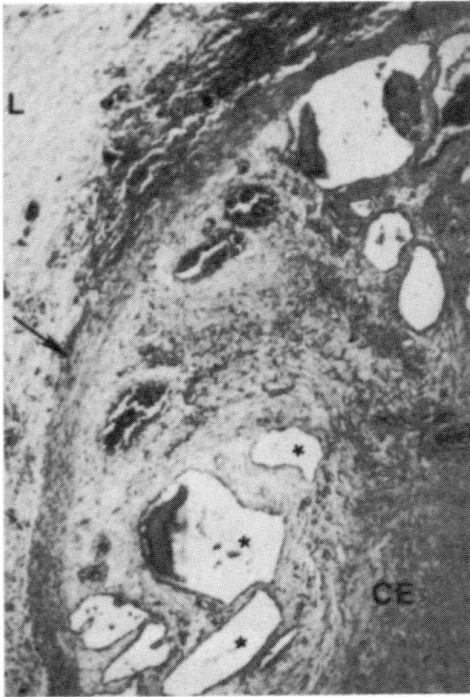

FIGURE 23–35. Photomicrograph of an organized chronic embolus within a large pulmonary artery. Note that the pulmonary artery closely adheres to the fibrotic embolic material (CE). L = lung parenchyma; *arrow* = medial elements of pulmonary artery; *asterisks* = endothelial-lined channels indicating recanalization. (From Chitwood, W. R., Jr., Lyerly, H. K., and Sabiston, D. C., Jr.: Surgical management of chronic pulmonary embolism. Ann. Surg., *201*:11, 1985.)

bronchial arteries. These arteries are often dilated and tortuous and fill the distal pulmonary arterial circuit retrograde.

POSTOPERATIVE COMPLICATIONS

Postoperative complications include severe right ventricular failure in patients with long-standing cor pulmonale and pulmonary hypertension and hemorrhagic lung syndrome. One patient in Sabiston's series died of right ventricular failure 3 days after operation despite removal of the chronic pulmonary emboli. After embolectomy and after reestablishment of pulmonary blood flow, massive parenchymal and intrabronchial hemorrhage may occur during or after cardiopulmonary bypass. Successful management of this complication can be achieved by the use of a Carlens (Broncho-Cath) catheter for tracheal intubation (Lyerly et al., 1986). A Fogarty catheter is inserted transbronchially to occlude the right and left mainstem bronchus and tamponade the blood within the lumen until appropriate blood coagulation can be achieved (Fig. 23–37). The bleeding usually ceases when pro-

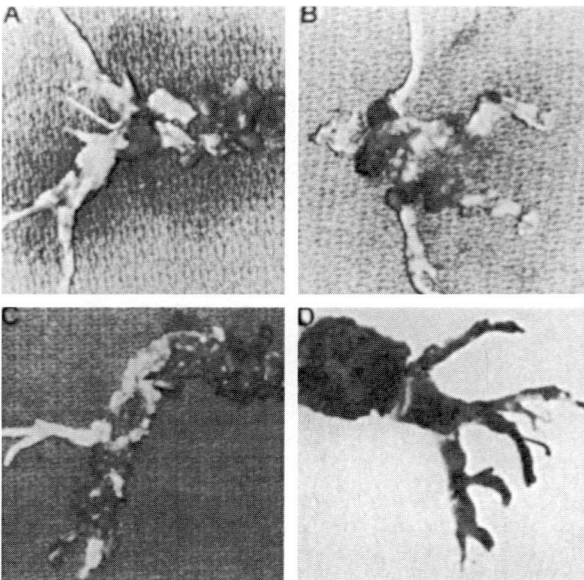

FIGURE 23–36. Chronic emboli removed from four patients undergoing pulmonary embolectomy. Patients (specimens shown in *A–C*) underwent embolectomy via thoracotomy and localized lobar pulmonary artery occlusion. One patient (specimen shown in *D*) required cardiopulmonary bypass because of very proximal pulmonary artery involvement. Note that the tenacious fibrotic material has extended into the segmental vessels. In most patients, distal branches could be embolectomized. (*A–D*, From Chitwood, W. R., Jr., Lyerly, H. K., and Sabiston, D. C., Jr.: Surgical management of chronic pulmonary embolism. Ann. Surg., *201*:11, 1985.)

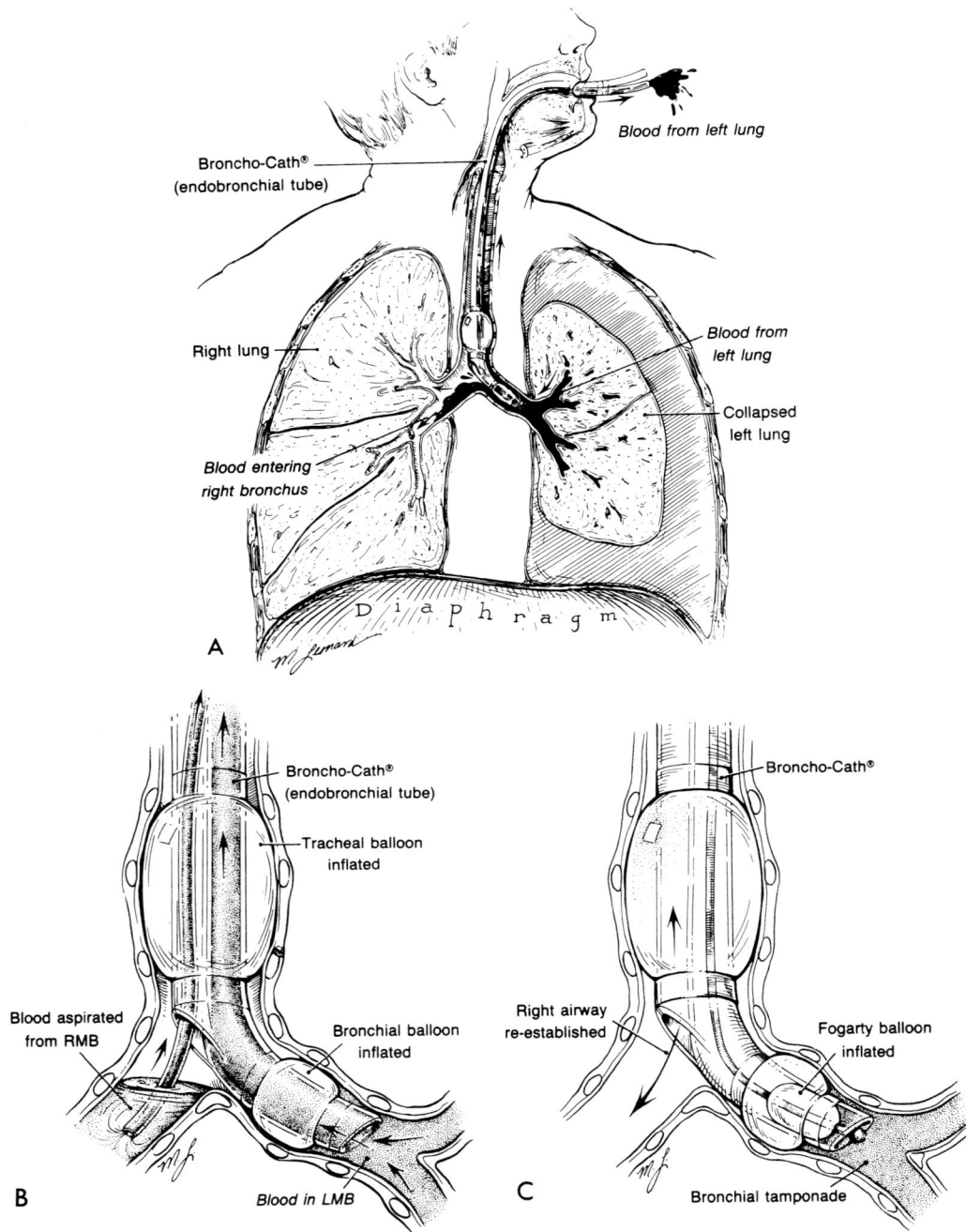

FIGURE 23–37. Method to control reperfusion intrabronchial hemorrhage. *A,* The Broncho-Cath endobronchial tube is shown in place with reperfusion intrabronchial hemorrhage from the left lung, resulting in massive blood loss to the right lung and out the Broncho-Cath tube. *B,* A detailed view of the inflation of the bronchial balloon and aspiration of blood from the right main bronchus. *C,* A detailed view of the insertion of a Fogarty catheter into the endobronchial tube and inflation of the balloon to provide bronchial tamponade of the left main bronchus. Tamponade is provided until the patient's coagulation factors return to normal, at which time the intrabronchial reperfusion hemorrhage should cease. (*A–C,* From Lyerly, H. K., and Sabiston, D. C., Jr.: Diagnosis and management of chronic pulmonary embolism. *In* Sabiston, D. C., Jr. [ed]: Textbook of Surgery. 13th ed. Philadelphia, W. B. Saunders, 1986.)

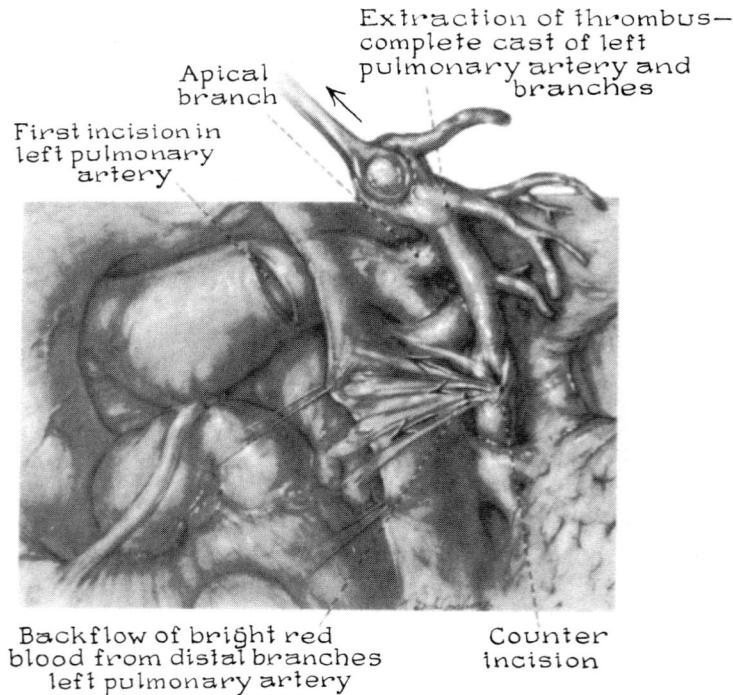

Extraction of thrombus—
complete cast of left
pulmonary artery and
branches

Apical
branch

First incision in
left pulmonary
artery

Backflow of bright red
blood from distal branches
left pulmonary artery

Counter
incision

FIGURE 23–38. Through a counterincision in the distal left pulmonary artery, the branches of the chronic embolus are removed (as shown). Actually, the chronic embolus has formed a cast of the pulmonary arterial tree. After the cast has been removed, a large amount of backbleeding occurs. The retrograde blood flow is bright red, which indicates that its source from the bronchial circulation is supplied by the aorta. The arteriotomies are closed. (From Wolfe, W. G., and Sabiston, D. C., Jr.: Pulmonary Embolism. Volume 25 in the series Major Problems in Clinical Surgery. Philadelphia, W. B. Saunders, 1980.)

tamine is administered to counteract the heparin used during cardiopulmonary bypass.

POSTOPERATIVE RESULTS

After embolectomy for chronic pulmonary embolism, a decrease in pulmonary artery pressures occurs (Fig. 23–38). An increase in Pa_{O_2} and a return of Pa_{CO_2} to normal are expected reactions (Fig. 23–39). Long-term follow-up data show that the NYHA functional class of most patients changes dramatically, moving from Class III or IV to Class I in most cases and in others to Class II (Fig. 23–40). These data, combined with other similar series in the literature, indicate the

favorable results (Fig. 23–41). A long-term follow-up arteriogram is shown in Figure 23–42. In contrast, those patients found unsuitable for embolectomy have a poor prognosis. In this medically managed group, many succumb and most of the survivors are disabled.

DISCUSSION

In most patients, a naturally active fibrinolytic system is responsible for the rapid resolution of pulmonary emboli, and most pulmonary emboli are, therefore, acute clinical problems. Animal studies have shown that by 21 days after embolism, major perfu-

Arterial Blood Gases (N=17)

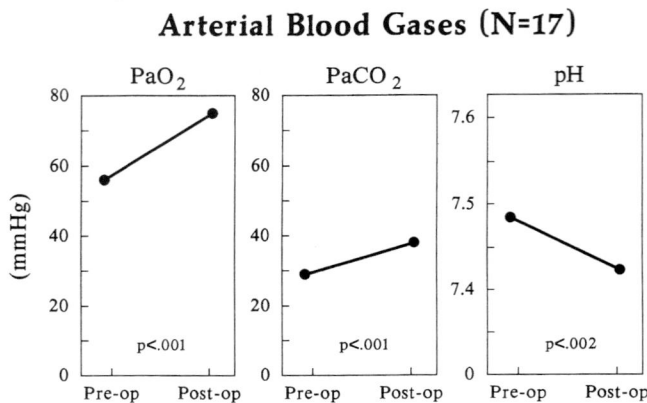

FIGURE 23–39. In the present series, arterial blood gases are shown before and after embolectomy. All values were statistically significant ($p < .05$).

Post-Operative Functional Class

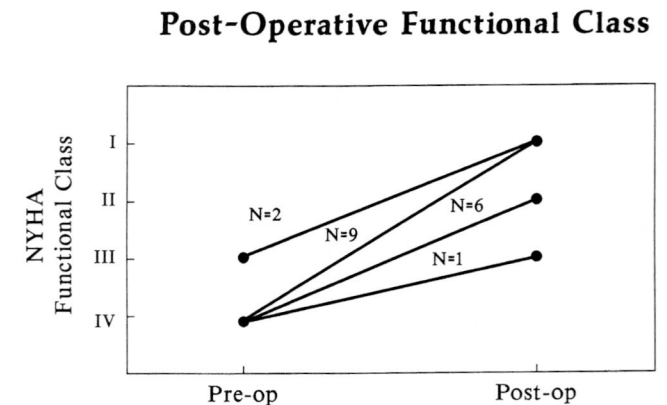

FIGURE 23–40. Preoperative and postoperative functional class of 12 patients having successful pulmonary embolectomy. NYHA = New York Heart Association.

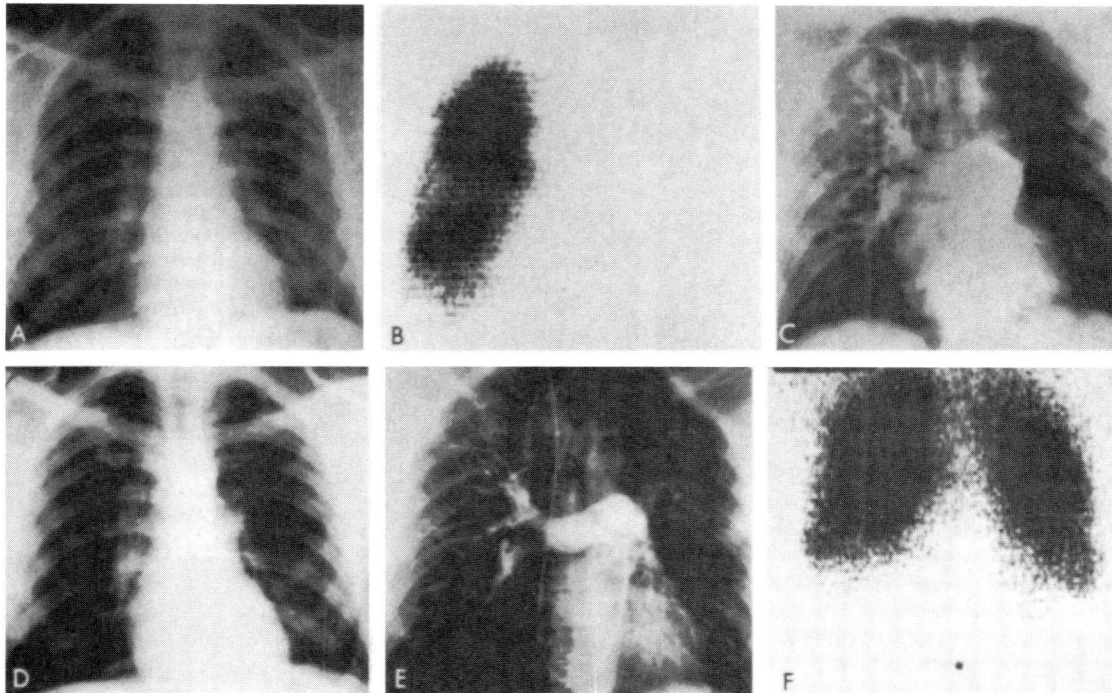

FIGURE 23-41. Findings in a patient with chronic pulmonary emboli and hypertension. *A,* Plain chest film that appears essentially normal. *B,* Pulmonary arterial scan showing no pulmonary arterial circulation to the left lung. *C,* Pulmonary arteriogram showing total absence of pulmonary flow to the left lung and to a portion of the right lower lobe. *D,* Postoperative film after embolectomy. *E,* Postoperative arteriogram showing return of pulmonary arterial flow to the left lung. *F,* Pulmonary arterial scan, performed postoperatively, showing excellent flow to the left lung. *G,* Specimen removed from the left pulmonary artery and its branches. Microscopically, the specimen was shown to be a well-organized thrombus. (*A–G,* From Moor, G. F., and Sabiston, D. C., Jr.: Embolectomy for chronic pulmonary embolism and hypertension: Case report and review of the problem. Circulation, *41:*701, 1970. By permission of the American Heart Association, Inc.)

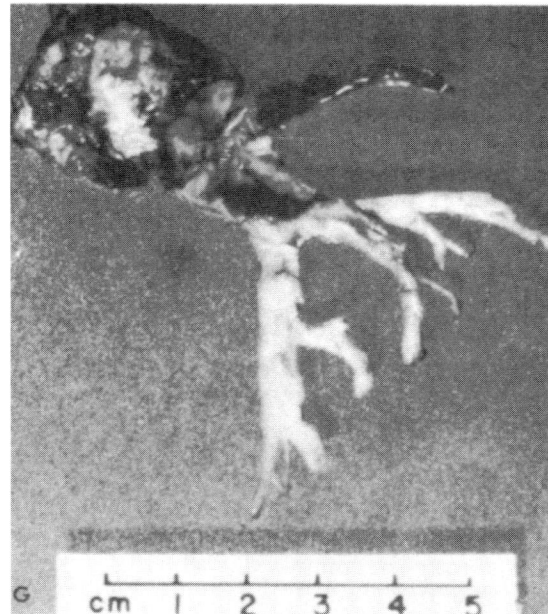

sion defects are usually resolved almost completely (Wolfe and Sabiston, 1968). Clinical studies using pulmonary scans and arteriograms have shown that complete resolution of pulmonary emboli may occur as early as 8 to 14 days after the clinical event, although in some patients this response may be delayed for several months and may uncommonly persist for months or years, especially in the presence of congestive heart failure (Dalen et al., 1969; Sasahara and Hyers, 1973; Tow and Wagner, 1967; Wagenvoort and Wagenvoort, 1977).

A small but definite cohort of patients develops recurrent pulmonary emboli. As many as 16% of patients with pulmonary emboli have been shown to have continued pathologic evidence of emboli as a long-term phenomenon, although most of these chronic changes do not produce pulmonary hypertension or clinical manifestations (Freiman et al., 1965). In one series, 22% of patients had findings of unresolved emboli and only 2% actually developed chronic cor pulmonale (Paraskos et al., 1973). Nevertheless, in this small number of patients, recurrent attacks of

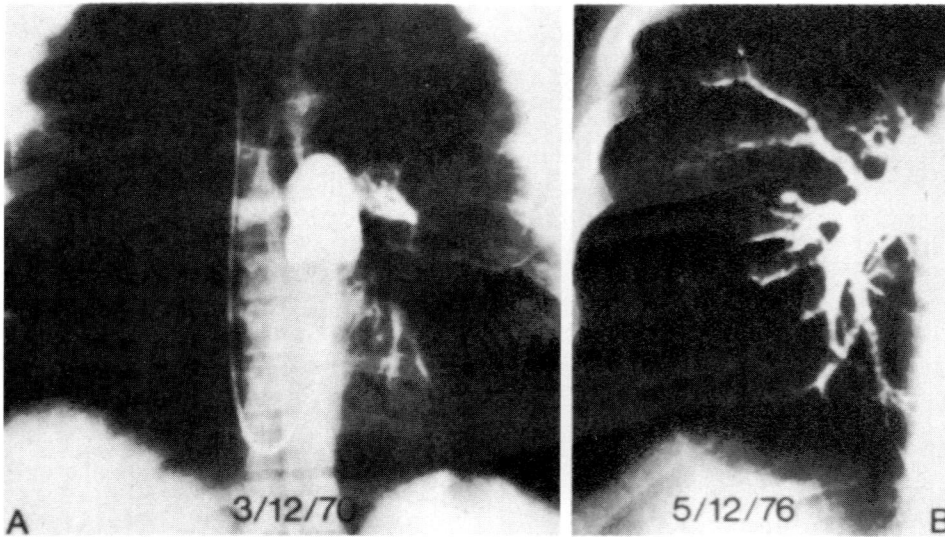

FIGURE 23–42. *A,* Pulmonary arteriogram in a patient before embolectomy. *B,* Six years after right lower lobe embolectomy. Note the continued perfusion of the right lower lobe after embolectomy. (*A* and *B,* From Chitwood, W. R., Jr., Lyerly, H. K., and Sabiston, D. C., Jr.: Surgical management of chronic pulmonary embolism. Ann. Surg., *201*:11, 1985.)

pulmonary emboli without resolution led to a syndrome of chronic pulmonary hypertension and ensuing complications.

The failure of the emboli to resolve is thought to be due to inadequate fibrinolysis. Congenital abnormalities of fibrinolysis include plasminogen deficiency, endothelial deficiencies of plasminogen activation, and abnormal fibrinogens. Diminished fibrinolysis has been described in coronary artery disease, cerebrovascular disease, systemic lupus erythematosus, and thrombotic thrombocytopenic purpura, and with use of oral contraceptives. Deficiencies of coagulation inhibitors may lead to an inability to regulate intravascular clot formation (Francis, 1989). Antithrombin III (ATT III), a protein essential for coagulation hemostasis, is released during coagulation and inactivates thrombin and other serine proteases (Cosgriff et al., 1983). Patients with deficiencies of ATT III have a hypercoagulable state clinically manifested by recurrent thrombosis and pulmonary emboli. Deficiencies of activated protein C, which inhibits Factors V and IV, and protein S (which serves as a cofactor for activated factor C) have also been reported to lead to an increased incidence of thromboembolism (Comp et al., 1984; Griffin et al., 1983). Besides inadequate fibrinolysis, embolization of previously organized thrombi that are resistant to resolution may be another cause of chronic pulmonary emboli, but this has not been proved.

Adequate anticoagulation in patients with chronic emboli decreases the number of recurrent episodes of pulmonary emboli. Despite anticoagulation, a few patients continue to have showers of emboli in the absence of significant resolution, which may proceed to major pulmonary arterial obstruction (deSoyza and Murphy, 1972; Hollister and Cull, 1956; Tilkian et al., 1976).

In patients with chronic pulmonary embolism, a major determinant of appropriateness as a surgical candidate is the response of the bronchial artery circulation. The adaptation of the bronchial circulation was demonstrated by Sherrier and associates in 1989 with a model of hypertrophy in the bronchial vessels in response to chronic pulmonary embolism with vascular casts of normal lungs and lungs with chronic pulmonary embolism (Figs. 23–43 to 23–45). Other studies of the endothelium of the pulmonary vasculature have shown that permutations of the normal endothelium can create a procoagulant environment that could lead to the development of thrombus in situ at the level of the large or smaller pulmonary vessels. Some patients develop proximal pulmonary thromboemboli, which may cause retrograde propagation of the thrombi after the initial pulmonary embolism. Other patients present with unexplained pulmonary hypertension secondary to thrombotic occlusion of the pulmonary microvasculature. A perfusion pulmonary scan shows abnormalities that should suggest the correct clinical diagnosis. However, the perfusion scan may underestimate the true pathophysiology. Kapitan and colleagues (1989) examined the mechanism of hypoxemia in chronic pulmonary embolism. Through inert gas elimination analysis, the mechanism was shown to be a combination of ventilation-perfusion mismatching and a low mixed venous PO_2. The level of inert gas dead space in these patients was less than expected because areas of complete obstruction were removed from the dead-space volume through anastomotic connection with bronchial arteries. The authors emphasized that the magnitude of hemodynamic compromise correlates only roughly with radionuclide scanning and does not correlate with direct angiographic estimates of vascular obstruction. Although the ventilation-perfusion scan suggests the diagnosis, pulmonary arteriography is critical in patients with chronic pulmonary embolism.

Medical management of chronic pulmonary emboli includes vasodilators in patients with obstruction at the arteriolar level. Patients with proximal and patients with arteriolar chronic pulmonary embolism should be treated with chronic warfarin anticoagulant

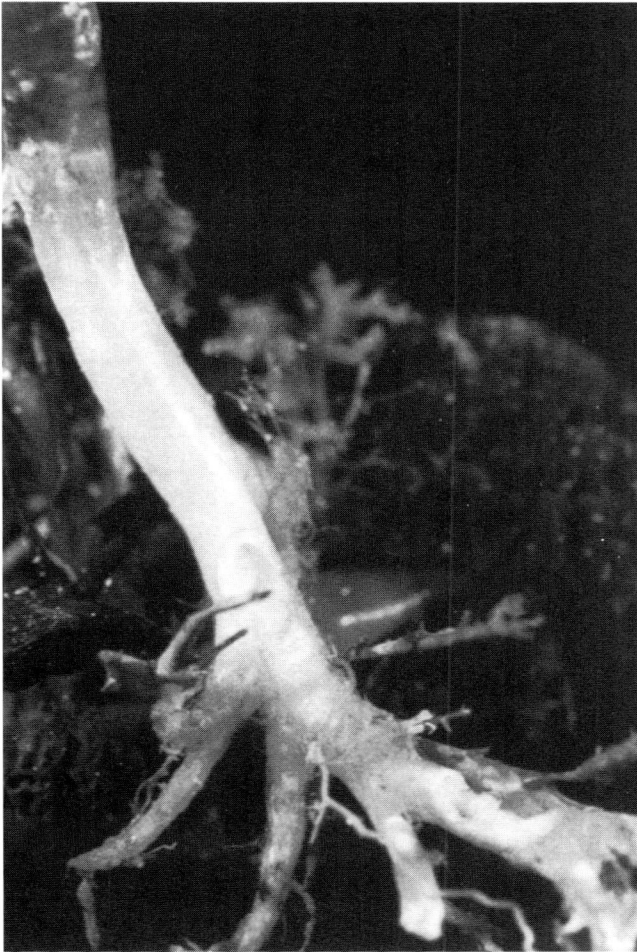

FIGURE 23–43. Normal bronchial vessels. Batson's solution vascular casts. (From Sherrier, R. H., Chiles, C., and Newman, G. E.: Chronic multiple pulmonary emboli. Regional response of the bronchial circulation. Invest. Radiol., *24:437, 1989.*)

therapy to protect against progression of thromboembolism. Medical management also includes a number of fibrinolytic and vasodilating agents, although these are usually ineffective (Dash et al., 1980; Olukotun, 1980; Rubin and Peter, 1980; Ruskin and Hutter, 1979). Plasminogen activation has been shown to provide local thrombolysis of relatively old thrombi in peripheral veins and may lead to the future resolution of chronic pulmonary emboli (Weimar et al., 1981). However, the organized emboli with ingrowth of fibroblasts may be resistant to any form of thrombolytic therapy. Surgical management is the most successful therapy in appropriate patients.

Daily and associates (1987) described 41 patients who had pulmonary embolectomy for chronic pulmonary emboli. In Group A ($n = 16$), myocardial protection consisted of single-dose crystalloid cardioplegia followed by pericardial irrigation with cold saline. Extrapericardial dissection of the pulmonary arteries was performed. In Group B ($n = 7$), the treatment was the same as for Group A except for the substitution of saline slush contained in a laparotomy pad for iced saline. In Group C ($n = 18$), myocardial protection was single-dose blood cardioplegia followed by the application of a specially designed cooling jacket to the right and left ventricles. Another modification was the use of intrapericardial dissection of the pulmonary arteries with extension of the dissection into the hilar tissues *without* entrance into either pleural cavity. The hospital mortality rates of Groups A, B, and C were 18.7%, 14.3%, and 5.5%, respectively (not statistically significantly different). However, other significant differences ($p < .05$) among the groups were observed. Phrenic nerve paresis occurred in 5 of 7 (71%) Group B patients but none in Group A or C. Patients in Group B required ventilatory support for 32.2 days, compared with 8.4 days for Group A and 6.2 days for Group C. The time spent in the intensive care unit was 36 days for patients in Group B compared with 13 days for patients in Group A and 10.3 days for patients in Group C. Pulmonary vascular resistance decreased 59% (649 versus 259) intraoperatively in 13 patients in Group C. It is believed that simultaneous bilateral pulmonary thromboendarter-

FIGURE 23–44. Bronchial vessel response to chronic pulmonary emboli. The *arrow* points to the vascular cast of a normal left bronchial artery. The *arrowhead* points to the vascular cast of an experimentally induced hypertrophied right pulmonary artery. (From Sherrier, R. H., Chiles, C., and Newman, G. E.: Chronic multiple pulmonary emboli. Regional response of the bronchial circulation. Invest. Radiol., *24:437, 1989.*)

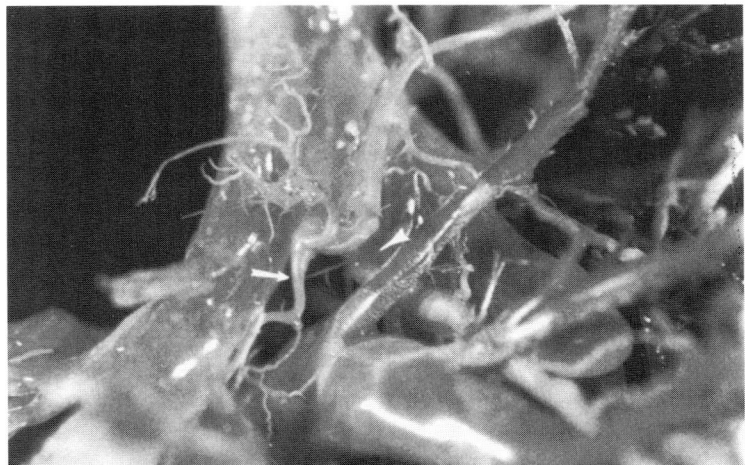

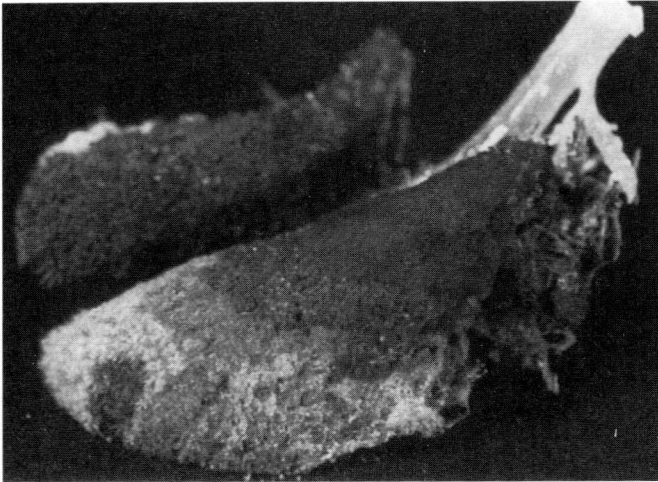

FIGURE 23–45. Bronchial vessel response to chronic pulmonary emboli. The vascular cast reveals distal pulmonary perfusion via the bronchial arteries. This is shown in the color change from proximal to distal. The *light areas* indicate complete reliance on perfusion by bronchial collaterals.

ectomy through a medial sternotomy, cardiopulmonary bypass, deep hypothermia with circulatory arrest, and modified methods of myocardial preservation and intrapericardial dissection of the pulmonary arteries constitutes the optimal surgical procedure, with the most recent series from this group of 127 consecutive patients having a mortality of 12.6% and significant defined risks for prolonged ventilator dependence and mortality. The statistically significant risks for prolonged ventilator dependence were identified as ascites and transfusion of four or more units of packed red blood cells. The significant predictor of mortality was a failure to achieve 50% reduction in pulmonary vascular resistance (Daily et al., 1991).

In summary, selected patients with symptoms of severe respiratory insufficiency, hypoxemia, and pulmonary hypertension with proximal pulmonary arterial occlusion and adequate bronchial collateral circulation with minimally impaired right ventricular function are appropriate candidates for surgical embolectomy. However, patients who additionally have distal pulmonary emboli in the small arterial branches with patent proximal vessels, as well as patients with severe right ventricular failure and massive obesity, are generally unsuitable for surgical management. Long-term follow-ups of patients with operable pulmonary emboli show favorable respiratory and cardiodynamic changes. These patients have relief of incapacitating symptoms and maintain clinical improvement for prolonged periods.

SELECTED BIBLIOGRAPHY

Cabrol, C., Cabrol, A., Acar, J., et al.: Surgical correction of chronic postembolic obstructions of the pulmonary arteries. J. Thorac. Cardiovasc. Surg., 76:620, 1978.

A report of a relatively large series of patients with chronic pulmonary embolism managed by embolectomy. Discussion is directed toward diagnosis, details of surgical management, and results.

Chitwood, W. R., Jr., Lyerly, H. K., and Sabiston, D. C., Jr.: Surgical management of chronic pulmonary embolism. Ann. Surg., 201:11, 1985.

A report of the experience of a large series of patients with surgical

management of chronic pulmonary embolism. The clinical manifestations, management, and results are evaluated.

Daily, P. O., Dembitsky, W. P., and Iversen, S.: Technique of pulmonary thromboendarterectomy for chronic pulmonary embolism. J. Card. Surg., 4:10, 1989.

This is the first reported series of over 100 consecutive patients with a diagnosis of chronic pulmonary embolism treated with median sternotomy, cardiopulmonary bypass, deep hypothermia, and circulatory arrest. The surgical technique is described in detail.

Goldhaber, S. Z. (ed): Pulmonary Embolism and Deep Venous Thrombosis. Philadelphia, W. B. Saunders, 1985.

This is a monograph by a number of authorities in the field. It is a valuable updated resource for all forms of pulmonary embolism and contains an excellent discussion of the hypercoagulable state in the management of massive pulmonary embolism and pulmonary thromboendarterectomy. It is a resource for details of all aspects of pulmonary embolism.

BIBLIOGRAPHY

Auger, W. R., Fedullo, P. F., Moser, K., et al.: Chronic major-vessel thromboembolic pulmonary artery obstruction: Appearance at angiography. Radiology, 182:393, 1992.

Brenner, O.: Pathology of the pulmonary circulation. Arch. Intern. Med., 56:1189, 1935.

Cabrol, C., Cabrol, A., Acar, J., et al.: Surgical correction of chronic postembolic obstructions of the pulmonary arteries. J. Thorac. Cardiovasc. Surg., 76:620, 1978.

Carroll, D.: Chronic obstruction of major pulmonary arteries. Am. J. Med., 9:175, 1950.

Chitwood, W. R., Jr., Lyerly, H. K., and Sabiston, D. C., Jr.: Surgical management of chronic pulmonary embolism. Ann. Surg., 201:11, 1985.

Comp, P. C., and Esmon, C. T.: Recurrent venous thromboembolism in patients with a partial deficiency of protein S. N. Engl. J. Med., 311:1525, 1984.

Cosgriff, T. M., Bishop, D. T., Hershgold, E. J., et al.: Familial antithrombin III deficiency: Its natural history, genetics, diagnosis and treatment. Medicine, 62:209, 1983.

Daily, P. O., Dembitsky, W. P., and Daily, R. P.: Dissectors for pulmonary thromboendarterectomy. Ann. Thorac. Surg., 51:842, 1991.

Daily, P. O., Dembitsky, W. P., and Iversen, S.: Technique of pulmonary thromboendarterectomy for chronic pulmonary embolism. J. Card. Surg., 4:10, 1989.

Daily, P. O., Dembitsky, W. P., Peterson, K. L., and Moser, K. M.: Modifications of techniques and early results of pulmonary thromboendarterectomy for chronic pulmonary embolism. J. Thorac. Cardiovasc. Surg., 93:221, 1987.

Dalen, J. E., and Alpert, J. S.: Natural history of pulmonary embolism. Prog. Cardiovasc. Dis., 17:259, 1975.

Dalen, J. E., Banas, J. S., Jr., Brooks, H. L., et al.: Resolution rate of acute pulmonary embolism in man. N. Engl. J. Med., 280:1194, 1969.

Dash, H., Ballentine, N., and Zelis, R.: Vasodilators ineffective in secondary pulmonary hypertension. N. Engl. J. Med., 303:1062, 1980.

deSoyza, W. D., and Murphy, M. L.: Persistent post-embolic pulmonary hypertension. Chest, 62:665, 1972.

Fleishner, F. G.: Recurrent pulmonary embolism and cor pulmonale. N. Engl. J. Med., 276:1213, 1967.

Francis, R. B.: Clinical disorders of fibrinolysis: A critical review. Blut, 59:1, 1989.

Freiman, D. G., Suyemoto, J., and Wessler, S.: Frequency of pulmonary thromboembolism in man. N. Engl. J. Med., 272:1278, 1965.

Griffin, J. H., Bezeaud, A., Evatt, B., and Mosher, D.: Functional and immunologic studies of protein C in thromboembolic disease. Blood, 62:1, 1983.

Hollister, L. E., and Cull, V. L.: The syndrome of chronic thrombosis of the major pulmonary arteries. Am. J. Med., 21:312, 1956.

Kapitan, K. S., Buchbinder, M., Wagner, P. D., and Moser, K.: Mechanisms of hypoxemia in chronic thromboembolic pulmonary hypertension. Am. Rev. Respir. Dis., 139:1149, 1989.

Ljungdahl, M.: Bibt es eine chronische embolistierung der lungen arterie? Deutsches Arch. Klin. Med., 120:1, 1928.

Lyerly, H. K., Reeves, J. G., and Sabiston, D. C., Jr.: Primary sarcomas of the pulmonary artery and management of intrabronchial hemorrhage. Surg. Gynecol. Obstet., 163:291, 1986.

McIntyre, K. M., and Sasahara, A. A.: The hemodynamic response to pulmonary embolism in patients without prior cardiopulmonary disease. Am. J. Cardiol., 28:288, 1971.

Moser, K. M., Auger, W. R., and Fedullo, P. F.: Chronic major-vessel thromboembolic pulmonary hypertension. Circulation, 81:1735, 1990.

Olukotun, A. Y.: Vasodilator therapy for pulmonary hypertension [Letter]. N. Engl. J. Med., 302:1261, 1980.

Owen, W. R., Thomas, W. A., Castleman, B., and Bland, E. F.: Unrecognized emboli to the lungs with subsequent cor pulmonale. N. Engl. J. Med., 249:919, 1953.

Paraskos, J. A., Adelstein, S. J., Smith, R. E., et al.: Late prognosis of acute pulmonary embolism. N. Engl. J. Med., 289:55, 1973.

Riedel, M., Stanek, V., Widimsky, J., and Prerovsky, I.: Long-term follow-up of patients with pulmonary thromboembolism: Late prognosis and evaluation of hemodynamic and respiratory data. Chest, 81:151, 1982.

Rubin, L. J., and Peter, R. H.: Oral hydralazine therapy for primary pulmonary hypertension. N. Engl. J. Med., 302:69, 1980.

Ruskin, J. N., and Hutter, A. M.: Primary pulmonary hypertension treated with oral phentolamine. Ann. Intern. Med., 90:772, 1979.

Sabiston, D. C., Jr., Wolfe, W. G., Oldham, H. N., et al.: Surgical management of chronic pulmonary embolism. Ann. Surg., 185:699, 1977.

Sasahara, A. A., and Hyers, T. M.: Urokinase pulmonary embolism trial: A national cooperative study. Circulation, 47:38, 1973.

Sherrier, R. H., Chiles, C., and Newman, G. E.: Chronic pulmonary emboli. Regional response of the bronchial circulation. Invest. Radiol., 24:437, 1989.

Sutton, G. C., Hall, R. J. C., and Kerr, I. H.: Clinical course and late prognosis of subacute massive, acute minor, and chronic pulmonary thromboembolism. Br. Heart J., 39:1135, 1977.

Tilkian, A. G., Schroeder, J. S., and Robin, E. D.: Chronic thromboembolic occlusion of main pulmonary artery or primary branches: Case report and review of the literature. Am. J. Med., 60:563, 1976.

Tow, D. E., and Wagner, H. N., Jr.: Recovery of pulmonary arterial blood flow in patients with pulmonary embolism. N. Engl. J. Med., 276:1053, 1976.

Viamonte, M.: Selective bronchial arteriography in man. Radiology, 83:830, 1964.

Viamonte, M., Parks, R. E., and Smoak, W. M., III: Guided catheterization of the bronchial arteries. Radiology, 85:205, 1965.

Virchow, R.: Uber die standpunkte in der wissenschaftlichen medizin. Virchows Arch. (Pathol. Anat.), 1:1, 1847.

Wagenvoort, C. A., and Wagenvoort, N.: Pathology of Pulmonary Hypertension. New York, John Wiley & Sons, 1977, p. 143.

Weimar, W., Stibbe, J., Van Seyen, A. J., et al.: Specific lysis of an ileofemoral thrombus by administration of extrinsic (tissue type) plasminogen activator. Lancet, 7:1018, 1981.

Wilhelmsen, L., Hagman, M., and Werko, L.: Recurrent pulmonary embolism: Incidence, predisposing factors, and prognosis. Acta Med. Scand., 192:565, 1972.

Wolfe, W. G., and Sabiston, D. C., Jr.: Pulmonary Embolism: Major Problems in Clinical Surgery. Philadelphia, W. B. Saunders, 1980.

Wolfe, W. G., and Sabiston, D. C., Jr.: Radioactive ventilation scanning in the diagnosis of pulmonary embolism. J. Thorac. Cardiovasc. Surg., 55:149, 1968.

Woodruff, W. W., III, Hoeck, B. E., Chitwood, W. R., Jr., et al.: Radiographic findings in pulmonary hypertension from unresolved embolism. AJR 144:681, 1985.

24 Congenital Lesions of the Lung and Emphysema

T. Bruce Ferguson, Jr., and Thomas B. Ferguson

Congenital lesions of the lung encompass a wide array of fascinating pulmonary, tracheal, and foregut anomalies that present clinically in infancy, childhood, and young adulthood. Precisely because they are relatively rare in the spectrum of surgical pulmonary disease, these lesions require a high index of suspicion and careful diagnosis for optimal therapeutic intervention, which can save the life of the neonate or infant. This diagnostic capability has improved considerably in the past several years because of radiologic advances in *computed tomography* (CT) and *magnetic resonance imaging* (MRI). Perhaps the most important advance in this area is the reliable prenatal diagnosis of a number of these lesions using ultrasound technology, thus increasing the efficiency of emergent intervention in the neonate.

At the other end of the chronologic spectrum, the surgical treatment of elderly patients with emphysematous lung disease requires the same precision of diagnosis and treatment. Most importantly, lung transplantation has become a viable therapeutic modality for end-stage emphysema, both for *chronic obstructive pulmonary disease* (COPD) and for homozygous *alpha₁ - antiprotease* (A-1-AP) deficiency. Advances in genetic engineering, including identifying the gene defects responsible for A-1-AP deficiency and cystic fibrosis and correcting them in transgenic experimental models, will almost certainly improve our ability to treat these disease processes.

HISTORICAL ASPECTS

Pathologic recognition of congenital lesions of the lung began in the middle of the last century, when extralobar sequestration was referred to as a Rokitansky lobe. In the early part of this century, conceptualization of the developmental aspects and the wide spectrum of these lesions was complicated by prevalence of infectious diseases. Gladstone and Cockayne in 1917 first proposed the theory that sequestrations (or accessory lobes, as they were referred to at that time) were derived from displaced rests of embryonic tissue of the pulmonary groove or one of the primitive lung buds; this was one of many pathophysiologic classification schemes developed during this time. The first review of "congenital cystic disease of the lung" was published in 1925 by Koontz; it included bronchiectasis, sequestrations, and bronchogenic cysts. The demonstrated benefit of surgical in-

tervention began in 1933 with Rienhoff's local excision of a chronically infected pulmonary cyst in a 3-year-old child. Several pioneers in the fields of pediatric, congenital heart, and thoracic surgery advanced surgical treatment of congenital lung abnormalities: Potts performed successful lobectomy in a 5-day-old infant in 1949; Gross performed successful lobectomy on a 4-year-old girl with infantile lobar emphysema in 1943; and Lewis reported on the anatomic dangers of attempted lobectomy for sequestration based on his experience with a 5-year-old child who exsanguinated after inadvertent severing of the systemic arterial supply. As surgical techniques for adult pulmonary disease were developed, they were applied to the infant and pediatric populations with life-threatening congenital anomalies with gratifying results, thus setting the standards for therapy today.

DEVELOPMENTAL ANATOMY

There is no unifying concept for the development of these congenital lesions; all classification schemes are by definition arbitrary. Nevertheless, a knowledge of normal developmental anatomy facilitates the classification and understanding of the various congenital lesions of the lung that develop in the neonate, infant, or child.

Growth and development of the lung can be divided into intrauterine and postnatal stages, with birth representing one point in the continuum (Fraser et al., 1988). The intrauterine stage can be divided into an embryonic, pseudoglandular, canalicular, and terminal sac stages. Between the ninth and thirteenth postovulatory days, the precursor of the epithelium of the respiratory tract, called the embryonic endoderm, develops in the yolk sac. This tissue gives rise to the primitive foregut. At 22 days, the medial pharyngeal groove appears on the foregut (Table 24–1), and at about 26 days of embryonic life (3-mm embryo) the lung begins to develop as a ventral outpouching or diverticulum of the foregut lined by endodermal epithelium and invested by splanchnic mesenchyme. The respiratory portion of the gut becomes separated from the esophageal portion by lateral ingrowths of surrounding mesoderm that progressively meet to form the tracheoesophageal septum. An alternative theory has been suggested by O'Rahilly and Muller (1984)—that a mesenchymal septum lies between the lung bud and the esophagus during their entire devel-

■ **Table 24–1.** NORMAL EMBRYOLOGIC DEVELOPMENT OF THE LOWER RESPIRATORY TRACT

Estimated Ovulatory Age	Developmental Stage or Size	Embryologic Development
	Embryonic Period	
22 days	7 somites	Median pharyngeal groove appears on foregut
24–26 days	20 somites (3 mm)	Lung bud appears and soon bifurcates
	Pseudoglandular Period	
5–6 weeks	8–10 mm	Lung sac acquires lobar buds
7th week	11 mm	Mesoderm forms bronchial muscle
		Pulmonary capillary plexus develops
		Truncus arteriosus separates into aorta and main pulmonary artery
		Pulmonary plexus and the sixth pharyngeal arches fuse
8th week		Distinct lobar architecture
8–16 weeks		Bronchial divisions are established and proliferate rapidly
	Canalicular Period	
4–6 months		Respiratory bronchioles and alveoli develop
		Mature alveolar cells appear
	Terminal Sac Period	
6 months to birth		Alveolar walls become progressively thinner as alveoli mature

Adapted from Luck, J. R., Reynolds, R., and Raffensberger, J.: Congenital bronchopulmonary malformations. Curr. Probl. Surg., 23:245–314, 1986.

opment, and thus the separation point between the trachea and the esophagus, which eventually becomes the larynx, remains stationary throughout development.

By 28 days, the two buds have developed, with the left bud directed more transversely than the right. By days 32 to 34, the five lobar bronchi have appeared as outgrowths of the primary bronchi. This development at the end of the fifth week marks the end of the embryonic period. The pseudoglandular period extends from the fifth to the sixteenth week of gestation. During this time, the bronchial tree develops from the five lobar bronchi by rapid, irregularly dichotomous branching. By the sixteenth week, all conducting airways are present, lined by columnar or cuboidal epithelium, and cartilage and tracheobronchial gland development have begun (Fig. 24–1).

The sixteenth to the twenty-fifth weeks of gestation mark the canalicular period; the appearance of primitive canaliculi represents early stages of the acinar airways. The mesenchyme adjacent to the canaliculi becomes vascularized through capillary ingrowth. By the twenty-fifth week, saccules, thin-walled terminal spaces with flattened epithelium, become apparent at the end of the canalicular stage. During this terminal sac, or alveolar, period, which lasts until birth, saccular proliferation, progressive vascularization, and organization of the surrounding mesenchyme occur (Langston et al., 1984). At any one time, the pseudoglandular, canalicular, and terminal sac stages can be present in different portions of the developing lung.

Alveolar development begins between 30 and 36 weeks. Histologically, the respiratory epithelium progressively decreases in height during the canalicular period, so that the entire acinar pathway is lined by flattened or cuboidal epithelium. Differentiation into Type I and Type II alveolar epithelial cells begins at about 28 weeks, when Type II osmophilic granules can be identified. At birth, the structures recognized as precursor components of the typical acinar unit are

present: three generations of respiratory bronchioles, one of transitional ducts, and three of saccules ending in a terminal saccule. Whereas the airways are nearly fully developed in utero, alveolar development occurs postnatally. At birth, the gas-exchange portions of the lung are made up of some 20 million large, thick-walled cellular terminal air sacs. In the early postnatal period, acinar length increases, and its components are remodeled as true alveoli form. Most alveoli appear during early childhood, ages 2 to 4 years (Thurlbeck, 1982). Multiplication of alveoli occurs until at least the eighth year, when the adult number of approximately 300 million alveoli is reached. From age 10 to adulthood, the changes are those of alveolar enlargement, not growth. Pulmonary tissue accounts for 10% of the weight of the inflated adult lung; another 10% is accounted for by blood and 80% by air; in the newborn, tissue accounts for 30% of lung volume. The air-tissue interface area increases from 3 to 4 m^2 at birth to greater than 75 m^2 in the adult. In children up to age 5, distal airway diameter increases disproportionately to proximal airway diameter, but after this age, peripheral airway conductance increases significantly.

Normal postnatal growth changes the trachea from a funnel-shaped tube, wider at the laryngeal end than the carinal end, to the cylindrical tube seen in the mature mediastinum (Wailoo and Emery, 1982). Most of this remodeling occurs between 1 month and 4 years of age. As the lung grows within the primitive cavity of the embryo, it carries before it a layer of mesenchymal tissue derived from the splanchnic mesoderm. The mesoderm adapts over the surface of the developing lobe with differentiation into the connective and mesothelial tissues that constitute the visceral pleura. The internal surface of the primitive body cavity is also lined with mesenchymal tissue that ultimately differentiates into the parietal pleura.

A diffuse plexus of endothelial tubes in the mesenchyme forms the earliest embryonic blood vessels in

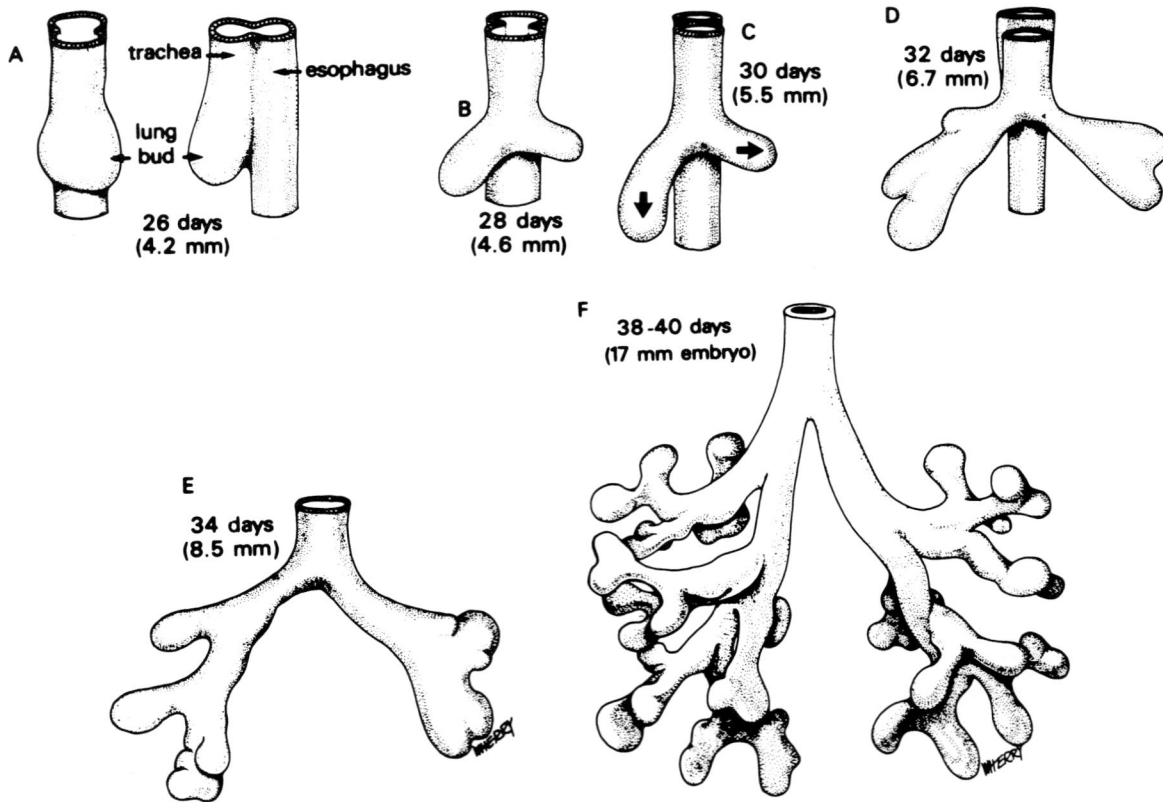

FIGURE 24–1. *A–F,* Development of the human lung in the embryonic and pseudoglandular periods. *A* is shown from the side; all others are shown from the front only. (*A–F,* From Fraser, R. G., Pare, J. A. P., Pare, P. D., et al.: Diagnosis of Diseases of the Chest. 3rd ed. Philadelphia, W. B. Saunders, 1988.)

the developing foregut; a portion of this plexus divides into the pulmonary and esophageal components. By 7 weeks, the upper portion of the truncus arteriosus has already separated into the aorta and main pulmonary artery (see Table 24–1); during the latter part of the seventh week, the pulmonary plexus and the sixth pharyngeal arch fuse to become the definitive pulmonary arteries. Branches from both arches grow toward the developing lung buds and become incorporated with them in the future hila (Fig. 24–2). The portion of the right arch beyond the lung bud disappears; the branch to the left lung bud persists as the ductus arteriosus. During the pseudoglandular period, pulmonary arteries develop at approximately the same rate and manner as the airways; by the sixteenth week, most of preacinar branches are present (Reid, 1984). Vessel diameter and length increase during the latter part of fetal life, and this continues in the postnatal stage with the development of conventional branches until about age 18 months. Each pulmonary artery becomes closely related to the stem bronchi, dividing and following the course of the branching air passages. The artery gives off many more branches than its airway counterpart, however. Between age 18 months and 8 years, the supernumerary branches that form the intra-acinar arteries increase significantly in parallel with alveolar growth.

Histologically, the extrapulmonary arterial wall of

the fetus closely resembles the aorta in thickness and structure, with multiple, thick, medial elastic laminae. The muscular arteries are morphologically mature by the end of the canalicular period, but their lumina are small and their media are thick, presumably because of the high pulmonary pressures in utero. As pulmonary pressure reverses by the second or third day after birth, diameter increases significantly; subsequently, wall thickness slowly decreases and the laminae decrease in number until the adult configuration is reached at about 2 years of age (Reid, 1986).

The pulmonary veins appear to originate from the vascular plexus overlying the lung bud. During early fetal life, the pulmonary venous blood drains via the splanchnic plexus into the primordia of the systemic venous system (Hislop and Reid, 1973). Subsequently, the primitive (or common) pulmonary vein extends as an outpouching of the sinoatrial region of the heart toward that portion of the splanchnic plexus draining the lungs (Fig. 24–3). This common pathway vein is eventually incorporated into the left atrial wall as the splanchnic-pulmonary connections are obliterated, leaving four independent pulmonary veins entering the left atrium. These veins are identifiable in the 25-week embryo. The extra-acinar venous drainage pattern is complete by the midpoint of fetal life, whereas the intra-acinar portion develops during childhood. In size, number of veins, and branching,

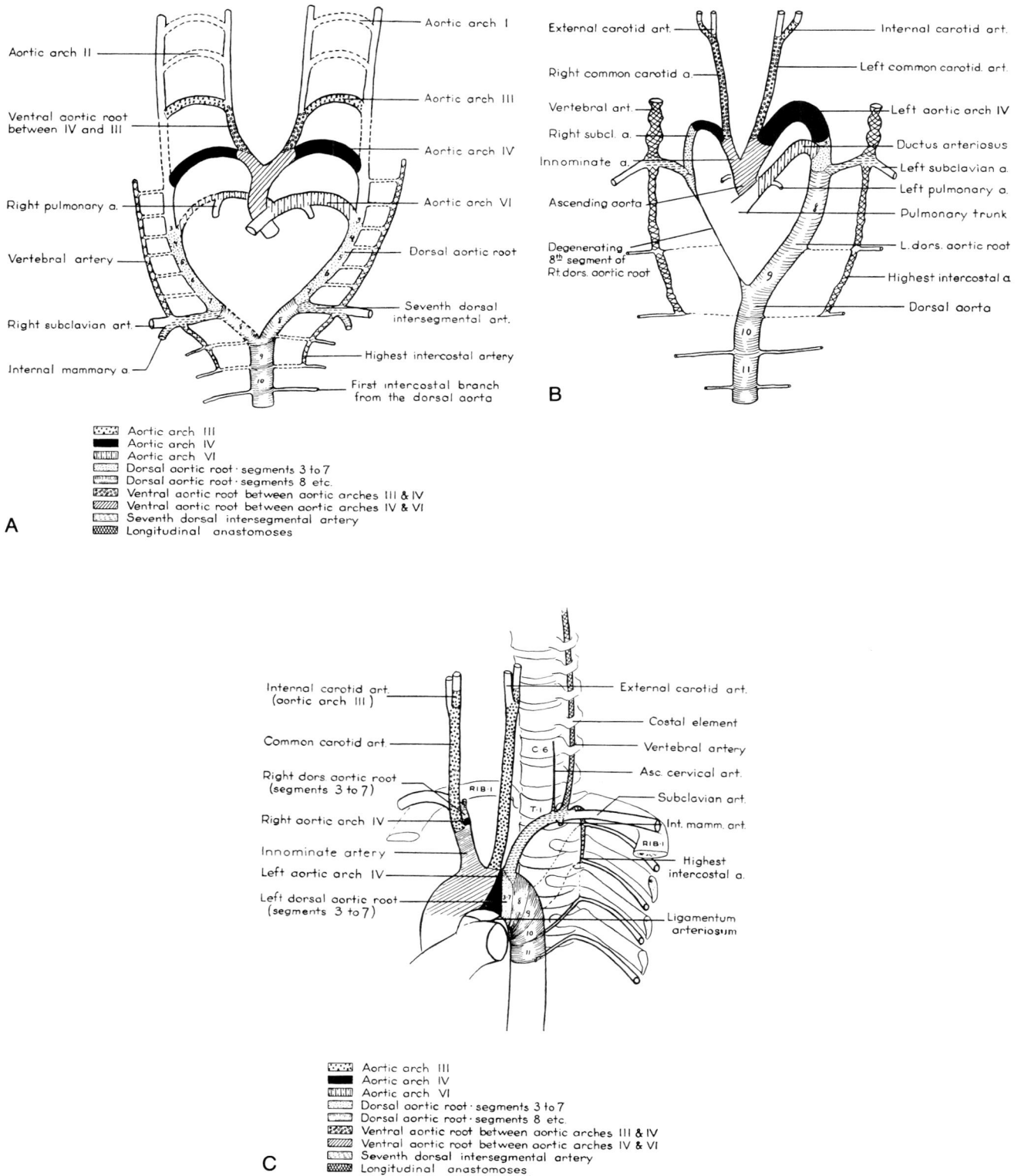

FIGURE 24–2. Development of the aortic arch system. The components that do not normally persist in the adult are indicated by *dashed lines.* Arabic numbers indicate the segments of each dorsal root and the dorsal aortas. *A,* Embryonic arch complex in the human embryo. *B,* Aortic arch complex in a human embryo of 15-mm crown-rump length. *C,* Adult configuration. (*A–C,* From Barry, A.: The aortic derivatives in the human adult. Anat. Rec., *111*:221, 1951.)

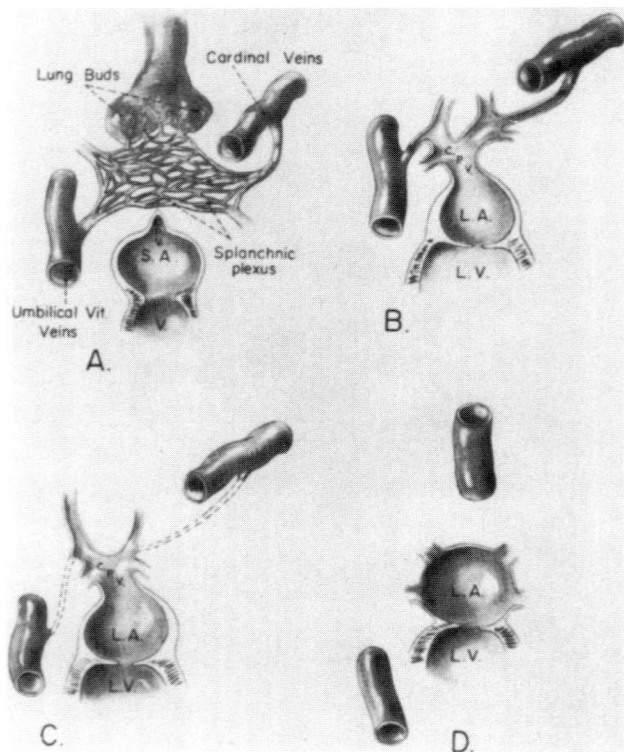

FIGURE 24–3. Normal development of the pulmonary venous system. A, Early; the splanchnic plexus drains the lung buds. This primitive pulmonary vascular bed has no direct connection with the heart and shares the routes of drainage of the splanchnic plexus, the cardinal venous system, and the umbilicovitelline system. B, The common pulmonary vein (CPV) originates as an evagination from the left atrial (LA) side of the common atrium and joins with the splanchnic plexus. Pulmonary venous blood may now drain to the left atrium or indirectly to the heart via primitive venous connections. C, No longer necessary, the primitive pulmonary venous connections disappear. D, Finally, by differential growth of the left atrium, the individual pulmonary veins are incorporated into the left atrium, and the common pulmonary vein no longer exists as an anatomic structure. (LV = left ventricle.) (A–D, From Lucas, R. V., Anderson, R. C., Amplatz, K., et al.: Congenital causes of pulmonary venous obstruction. Pediatr. Clin. North Am., 10:781, 1963.)

the pattern of growth of the veins is similar to that of the arteries. Histologically, however, fetal veins are less muscular than those of the adult.

The bronchial arteries develop from a series of segmental vessels arising from the ventral side of the dorsal paired aortas. The systemic blood supply to the lung shifts from these earlier cervical vessels to the bronchial arteries arising from the proximal aorta, subclavian artery, and eventually the thoracic artery as the lung shifts in position relative to the rest of the body (Tobin, 1952).

The multiple normal and abnormal factors that affect lung development are not completely understood. Local mesenchymal-epithelial interactions, as well as neural and hormonal influences, appear to be of some importance. In vitro culture studies of developing lung buds after removal from an animal fetus demonstrate continuation of the branching process, but only in the presence of adjacent specific mesenchyme. Cell surface interactions and production of locally active soluble factors may be involved in this process. The central nervous system may also be important to normal development, as illustrated by studies that demonstrate that intrauterine cervical or phrenic nerve injury is associated with pulmonary hypoplasia in animals (Fraser et al., 1988). Hormonal influences on growth and development are poorly understood but undoubtedly are important. Finally, because lung development continues well into the childhood years, bronchopulmonary or systemic diseases acquired in childhood, such as viral infection, starvation, and hypoxia, can influence lung growth.

Thus, normal anatomic development clearly is a complex process, and it is surprising that more developmental abnormalities do not occur. Conflicting embryologic theories are supported because they may best explain a certain defect or small group of defects. Although a certain skepticism toward embryologic-clinical correlations is warranted, a discussion of bronchopulmonary foregut malformations by Fowler and associates (1988) provides a framework on which many of these lesions can be conceptualized. The assumption is that the pathogenesis of these anomalies can be attributed to a regional mesenchymal disturbance that disrupts the orderly division of the foregut. This concept is illustrated in Figures 24–4 and 24–5.

In the mature lung, a scanning electron micrograph discloses that the lung parenchyma consists of alveoli that are closely packed and separated only by thin alveolar septa (Fig. 24–6). Most of the septa are occupied by blood contained in a single network of capillaries, such that the blood is exposed to air on two sides across a barrier that consists of two layers—an alveolar epithelium and a capillary endothelium—and across an intercalated interstitial layer containing the supportive fibers. The interstitial space always contains some free fluid, and the space accessible to this fluid is bounded by the basement membranes of epithelial and endothelial cells. As Figure 24–7 shows, on those parts of the air-blood barrier in which there are no connective tissue fibers or cells (about half the alveolar surface), the basement membranes are fused. Interstitial fluid in the alveolar septa is rapidly drained along the septal fiber strand into the interacinar septa, which contain the lymphatic capillaries and

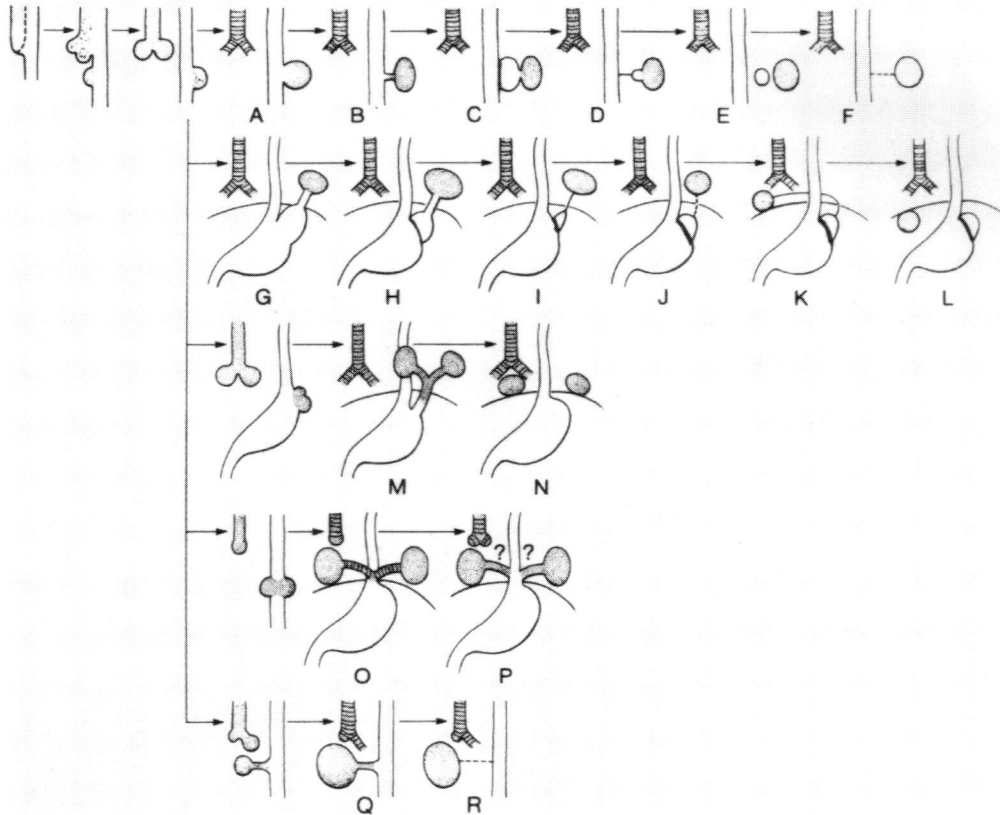

FIGURE 24–4. Abnormal division of primitive foregut leaves respiratory rest tissue *(stippled area)* on gastrointestinal (GI) tract *(unmarked area)* and produces various types of anomalies. Letters indicate reported malformations; proposed intermediate developmental stages are unlabeled. When possible, cases are sequenced from left to right as progressive stages of obliteration of abnormal cysts and tracts. *A,* Esophageal diverticulum ending blindly in left sequestration + pancreatic rest. *B,* Patent tract between esophagus and left or right sequestration. *C,* Right sequestration communicating with esophageal cyst. *D,* Left sequestration and partially patent tract with pancreatic rest. *E,* Separate left or right sequestration and bronchogenic cyst or cystic adenomatoid malformation. *F,* Left or right sequestration + obliterated fibrous tract to esophagus. *G,* Left sequestration to patent gastric diverticulum. *H,* Left sequestration to noncommunicating gastric duplication cyst. *I,* Left sequestration with partially patent tract to noncommunicating gastric duplication cyst. *J,* Left sequestration and separate noncommunicating gastric duplication cyst. *K,* Right sequestration with fibrous tract to noncommunicating gastric duplication cyst. *L,* Right subdiaphragmatic sequestration and separate gastric duplication cyst. *M,* Bilateral sequestrations with patent common bronchus to gastric fundus. *N,* Bilateral supradiaphragmatic sequestrations. *O,* Tracheal agenesis and bilateral sequestration with patent common bronchus to gastroesophageal junction. *P,* Bronchial agenesis and bilateral total lung sequestrations, unknown type of communication to GI tract. *Q,* Right bronchial agenesis and total right lung sequestration with patent tract to esophagus. *R,* Right bronchial agenesis and right-sided total lung sequestration. (*A–R,* From Fowler, C. L., Podorny, W. J., Wagner, M. L., and Kessler, M. S.: Review of bronchopulmonary foregut malformations. J. Pediatr. Surg., *23:*793–797, 1988.)

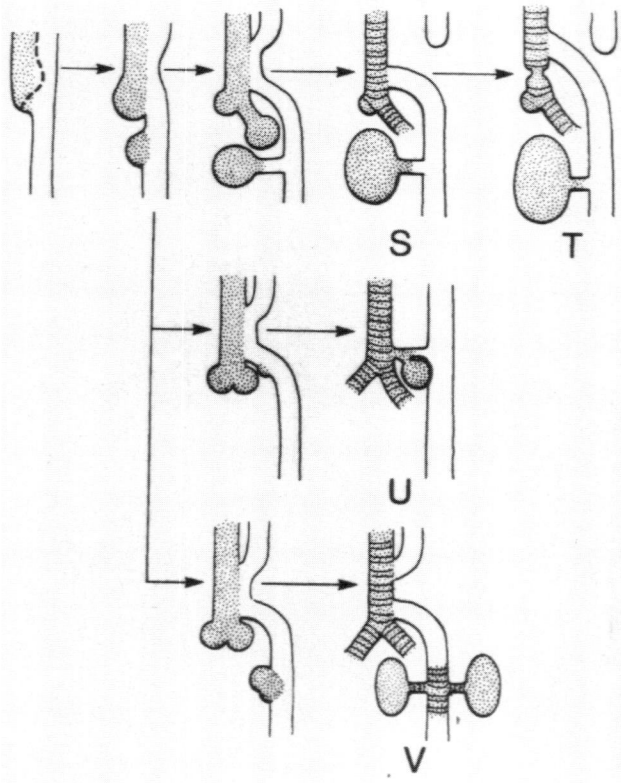

FIGURE 24–5. A slightly different distorted division plane of the primitive foregut will lead to other types of bronchopulmonary foregut malformations containing esophageal atresia plus tracheo-esophageal (TE) fistulas. S, Esophageal atresia, distal TE fistula, right bronchial agenesis, and right total lung sequestration with patent tract to esophagus. T, Same abnormality as shown in S, but with tracheal stenosis. U, Left sequestration patent at site of H-type TE fistula. V, Esophageal atresia, proximal and distal TE fistulas, and bilateral sequestrations communicating with common bronchial segment replacing distal esophagus. (S–V, From Fowler, C. L., Podorny, W. J., Wagner, M. L., and Kessler, M. S.: Review of bronchopulmonary foregut malformations. J. Pediatr. Surg., 23:793–797, 1988.)

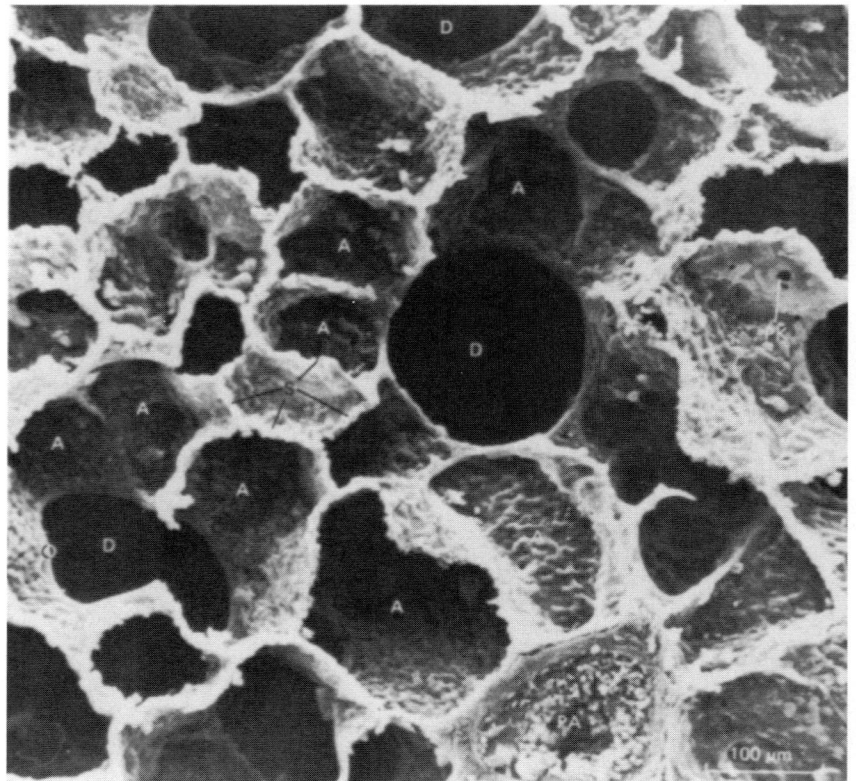

FIGURE 24–6. Scanning electron micrograph of human lung parenchyma. Alveolar ducts (D) are surrounded by alveoli (A), which are separated by thin septa (S). Note small branch of pulmonary artery (PA). (PK = interalveolar pore of Kohn.) (From Weibel, E. R.: Design and structure of the human lung. In Fishman, A. P. [ed]: Assessment of Pulmonary Function. New York, McGraw-Hill, 1980, pp. 18–65.)

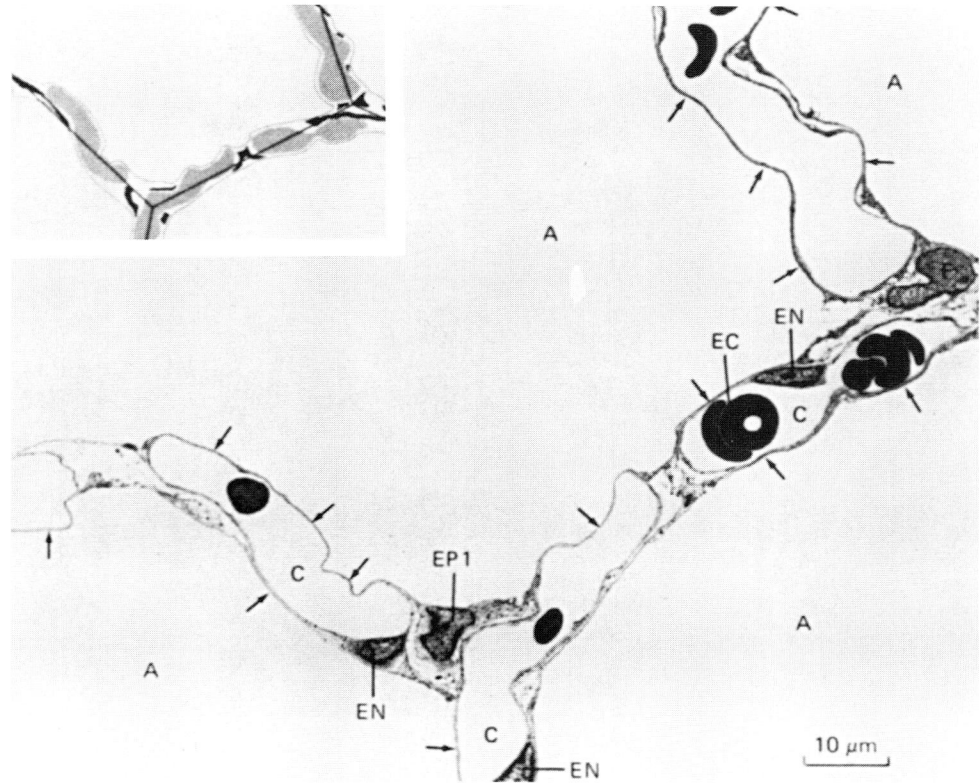

FIGURE 24–7. Thin section of alveolar septa from human lung. The major part is occupied by capillaries (C), which form the thinnest barrier to air on alternating sides of the septum (arrows). Note distribution of connective tissue fibers (black spots on inset). (A = alveolus; EC = erythrocyte; EN = endothelium; EP1 = Type I epithelial cell; F = fibroblast.) (From Weibel, E. R.: Design and structure of the human lung. In Fishman, A. P. [ed]: Assessment of Pulmonary Function. New York, McGraw-Hill, 1980, pp. 18–65.)

cells of the lung defense systems—histiocytes, mast cells, and lymphoid cells.

The capillary endothelium is typically a single-cell layer (Weibel, 1980). The cytoplasm is poor in organelles of any kind, and in some regions the two plasma membranes are separated only by a very thin layer of cytoplasmic matrix. Many of the nonrespiratory metabolic functions of the lung, including transformation of certain bioactive substances, are performed in endothelial cells.

The alveolar epithelium is a mosaic of several cell types (Fig. 24–8). Most of the surface (97%) is covered by hyperextended epithelial cells called Type I cells; like capillary endothelial cells, these Type I cells contain few organelles and form extensive branches and multiple cytoplasmic extensions that line the alveolar surface on all sides of the alveolar septum. Small discontinuities in the alveolar epithelium, known as pores of Kohn, are present in most mammals. The size of the aperture usually ranges from 2 to 10 μm. In vascular perfused tissue, the pore is frequently occluded by a thin film of material continuous with and identical to alveolar surfactant, casting some doubt on the significance of alveolar pores as a means of collateral ventilation (Takaro et al., 1979). They probably represent an interacinar pathway for the spread of fluid, with or without pathogenic microorganisms.

The other major cell type is the Type II alveolar cell, also called the granular pneumocyte. These cells are smaller but bulkier cuboidal cells interspersed into the predominantly squamous Type I cell lining.

Macklin (1954) recognized the need for a substance to regulate surface tension in the alveoli and surmised that it was secreted by the Type II cell. Pulmonary surfactant is the complex surface active material synthesized and secreted from alveolar Type II cells (Lewis and Jobe, 1993). The major components of surfactant are phospholipids, neutral lipids, and at least three different surfactant-specific proteins designated SP-A, SP-B, and SP-C. SP-A, a hydrophilic multimeric protein and the major surfactant protein, is synthesized and secreted by Type II cells into the airspace; this protein binds phosphatidylcholine and is felt to promote formation of tubular myelin-like structures from newly secreted phospholipids; SP-A also regulates the metabolic pathways of secretion and uptake of surfactant between the Type II pneumocyte and alveolar space. In contrast, SP-B and SP-C are low-molecular-weight hydrophobic proteins that accelerate the adsorption and spreading of surfactant phospholipids at the air-liquid interface. Phospholipids make up about 85% of natural pulmonary surfactant; saturated phosphatidylcholine is the main surface active component.

Briefly, surfactant phosphatidylcholine is synthesized in the endoplasmic reticulum of the Type II cell and transferred to lamellar bodies, which are in turn secreted into the alveolus. The tightly packed lamellar bodies then unravel to form tubular myelin structures composed of dipalmitoylphosphatidylcholine, unsaturated phosphatidylcholine, phosphatidylglycerol, and other surfactant lipids that are essential for surface adsorption and spreading of surfactant in order

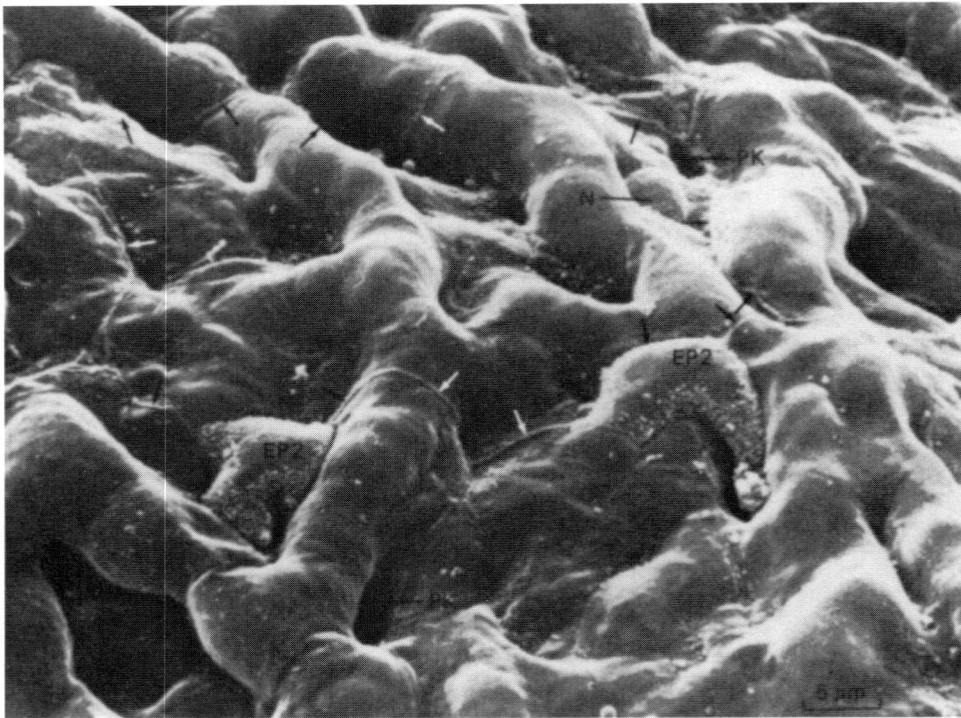

FIGURE 24–8. Surface view of alveolar epithelium made predominantly of Type I cells; the terminal bar surrounding one of them is outlined by *small arrows*; its nucleus (N) is located eccentrically. Two Type II epithelial cells (EP2) are interspersed into lining. The terminal bars of epithelial cells extend into interalveolar pores (PK). (From Weibel, E. R.: Design and structure of the human lung. *In* Fishman, A. P. [ed]: Assessment of Pulmonary Function. New York, McGraw-Hill, 1980, pp. 18–65.)

to achieve rapid film formation. This acellular layer covering the alveolar surface thus consists of a film of highly surface-active phospholipids facing the alveolar air space and a layer containing surface-active phospholipids linked to proteins deep to the film. As this film is formed, the protein and lipid components appear to be squeezed out with preferential retention of dipalmitoylphosphatidylcholine (Wright and Clements, 1987). The surface film is therefore dynamic, with new surfactant continuously entering, followed by surface refinement and film collapse to form smaller vesicular structures.

The surface area changes that result from the respiratory cycle likely modulate this continual turnover of surfactant at the alveolar surface (Puskas et al., 1992). Although the metabolic degradation of the surfactant components remains incompletely understood, most of the surfactant film appears to be taken up by the Type II cell and either catabolized or cleared from the lungs by unknown mechanisms (Wright, 1990). The overall synthesis, storage, and secretion of surfactant is under complex neural, hormonal, and chemical control. Surfactant has a very rapid rate of turnover, between 14 hours and 2 days in normal adults. The concentration of surfactant is higher in the neonate than in the adult, and the rate of synthesis reaches a peak at term, declining rapidly to normal adult levels shortly thereafter. About 90% of surfactant phosphatidylcholine cleared from the alveoli of developing lungs is recycled, as compared with 50% in the mature lung. Avery (1969) emphasizes that surfactant must be present at birth to allow for creation of a functional residual capacity. Although the Type II pneumocyte begins synthesis of surfactant at

about 7 months of interuterine life, there is a burst in phospholipid synthesis just before birth with the appearance of phosphatidylglycerol and an increase above 2.0 in the lecithin/sphingomyelin ratio, both measured on amniocentesis. These measurements have proved invaluable in the assessment of fetal lung maturation and the likelihood of developing *neonatal respiratory distress syndrome* (NRDS), which is now recognized to be primarily a surfactant-deficient state (Jobe and Ikegami, 1987).

Surfactant is necessary for mechanical stability of the alveoli (King, 1982). Because it can spread along the air-liquid interface and lower surface tension, surfactant allows collapsed alveoli to open at lower inspiratory pressures and to maintain alveolar size once inflated. Surfactant also decreases the work of breathing and prevents the adherence of alveolar walls. The compliance of lung tissue deficient in surfactant is considerably reduced, and the pressures necessary to achieve tidal ventilation are increased; intrapulmonary shunting is increased in these circumstances as well. The decrease in surface tension imparted by surfactant may counteract the tendency for fluid to be sucked into alveolar spaces from the capillary lumen. Surfactant may also contain a protective factor that inhibits the lysis of alveolar macrophages, thus enhancing host lung defenses, and may aid alveolar macrophage migration in acute lung injury. Finally, several in vitro studies suggest that the surfactant present in the alveolar space down-regulates the host immune responses (Richman et al., 1990).

Disorders of surfactant metabolism are important in a number of disease states, including NRDS, *adult respiratory distress syndrome* (ARDS), alveolar pro-

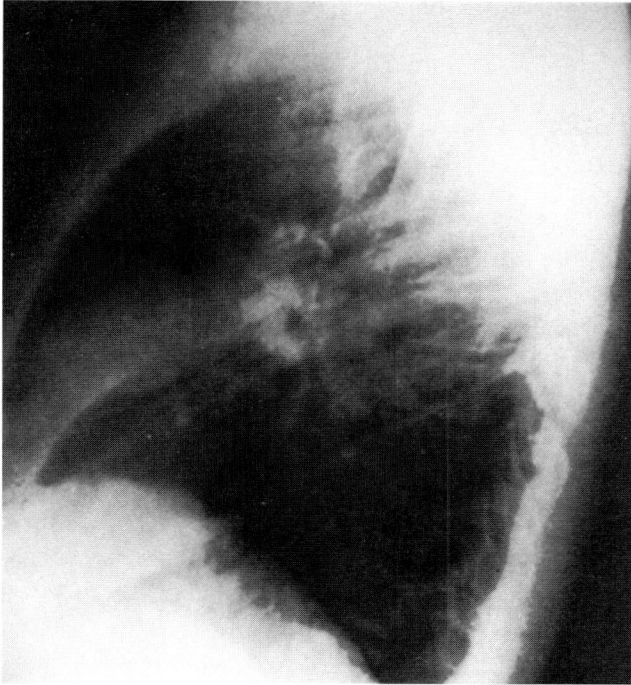

FIGURE 24–9. Fascial band from the right posterior chest wall to the diaphragm, partially dividing the right lower lobe. This anomaly was encountered during right middle lobectomy for bronchiectasis.

teinosis, oxygen toxicity, and atelectasis. Alveolar proteinosis is related to an overproduction of phospholipid, exceeding the capacity of the lung to remove it (Singh et al., 1983). Primary surfactant deficiency is the major cause of respiratory failure in neonates with NRDS. Elastolytic damage and barotrauma may both contribute to acute pulmonary injury in the early stages of NRDS as well, in part mediated by neutrophil elastase (Speer et al., 1993). Neonates with NRDS who are treated with exogenous surfactant have improved dramatically in a number of clinical trials

(Gortner, 1992). Because of the parallels between NRDS and ARDS, clinical trials of exogenous surfactant in ARDS are under way (Lewis and Jobe, 1993).

ANATOMIC VARIATIONS

Before discussing specific congenital lesions, certain anatomic variations should be noted. These aberrations mostly cause no clinical difficulty, but the thoracic surgeon must be able to recognize them on the chest film or at operation.

There is a wide range of normal variation in the completeness or incompleteness of the fissures between the lobes. The superior segment of the lower lobe may be delineated by a fissure; occasionally, more unusual types of fascial bands or pleural investments that subdivide the normal lung tissue are encountered (Mehta et al., 1983) (Fig. 24–9). A medial accessory left lower lobe and an azygos lobe can be demonstrated radiographically. Felson (1955) found an azygos lobe on 0.5% of routine chest film examinations. In this entity, the azygos vein lies within the substance of the right upper lobe, and the anomalous part is isolated from the remainder of the lobe by a double fold of visceral pleura that is the mesentery of the azygos vein. The characteristic "inverted comma" is produced on the chest film. The lobe may be the seat of tuberculous or neoplastic disease, whereas the remaining portion of the right upper lobe is uninvolved (Fig. 24–10).

Lung herniation occurs in conjunction with developmental defects of the chest wall. In infancy, lung protrusions through Sibson's fascia at the apex of the thorax may be confused with laryngoceles or pharyngoceles (Grunebaum and Griscom, 1978).

Total developmental derangements can occur where the lung tissue itself is relatively unaffected. Instances of bilateral bilobation and trilobation have been described, but these are quite rare. Situs inversus is produced by an abnormal rotation of the viscera

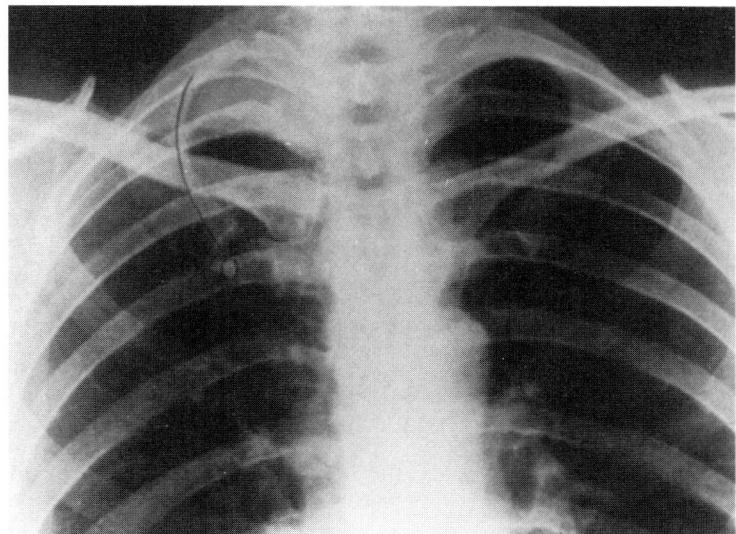

FIGURE 24–10. Azygos lobe. In this case, the azygos lobe contained a metastatic lymphosarcoma. The jejunum is the primary site.

during the tenth to fifteenth days of gestation. The organs are perfectly reversed in a mirror-image manner, involving the thoracic viscera alone (situs inversus thoracis) or the thoracic and abdominal viscera (situs inversus totalis). The incidence of the totalis form is 1 in 8000, and most such patients have no other abnormalities, congenital or otherwise. Kartagener (1933) called attention to the association of situs inversus with bronchiectasis and pansinusitis—the three component lesions of Kartagener's syndrome (KS) (Fig. 24–11). This is part of the immotile cilia syndrome (ICS) (Bianchi et al., 1992; Rubin, 1988). ICS is caused by ciliary dysfunction due to a variety of genetically determined ciliary defects (Greenstone et al., 1988); it is an autosomal recessive disease of the microtubules of ciliated cells, spermatozoa, and possibly neutrophil leukocytes. Symptoms related to the immotile cilia include male sterility, chronic or recurrent respiratory tract infections, and bronchiectasis due to absence of mucociliary clearance. In 50% of patients, situs inversus totalis occurs, and hence KS is present. In a clinical review of KS by Kinney and De Luca (1991), bronchopulmonary symptoms included chronic rhinitis in childhood and lower airway tract symptoms in young adulthood. Bronchiectasis was present in 56% of patients. In general, most patients have mild symptoms; with adequate medical supervision, a full life span should be expected. Surgery may be required for pansinusitis or bronchiectasis in isolated cases.

More serious congenital abnormalities include cases of right isomerism (asplenia syndrome) and left isomerism (polysplenia syndrome) (Marcelletti et al., 1983) (Fig. 24–12). These two syndromes have many com-

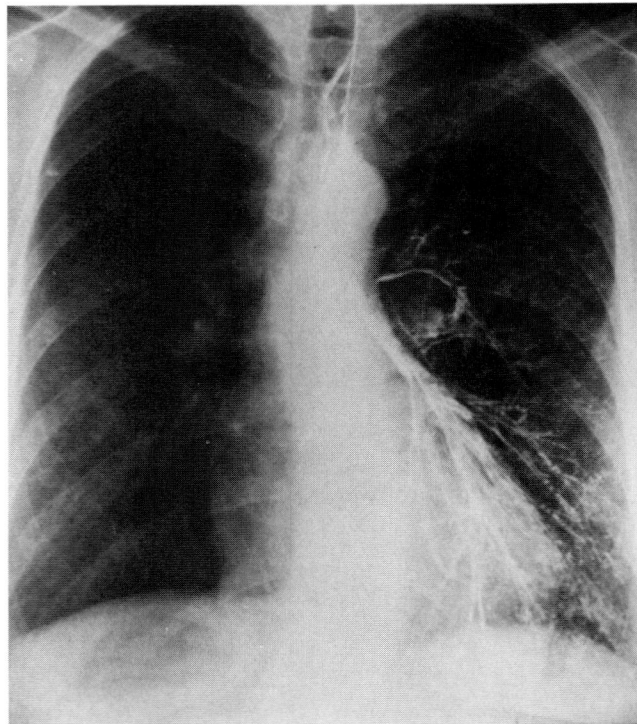

FIGURE 24–12. Asplenia syndrome in a severely cyanotic 30-year-old woman. Lipiodol bronchogram shows the right lung in the left side of the chest, a stomach gas bubble on the right, and levocardia. At autopsy, transposition of the great vessels, valvular pulmonic stenosis, and atrial and ventricular septal defects were found. No splenic tissue could be identified.

mon characteristics, namely, situs inversus or situs ambiguus of various visceral organs, severe cardiovascular anomalies, and a generally dismal prognosis. Rose and colleagues (1975) reviewed the clinical features of these syndromes, and surgical palliation of the congenital cardiac defects has been described (Di Donato et al., 1987).

TRACHEOBRONCHIAL TREE

Complete tracheal agenesis is an extremely rare and almost uniformly fatal anomaly in which the trachea is absent from the larynx to the carina, and the distal trachea or stem bronchi communicate directly with the esophagus (Holinger et al., 1987). An association between tracheal agenesis and the vertebral, anal, cardiac, tracheal, esophageal, renal, and limb (VACTERL) complex has been established (Milstein et al., 1985). The structures affected in this syndrome (vertebral defects, imperforate anus, tracheoesophageal fistula, radial and renal dysplasia) undergo organogenesis during the fourth to seventh postovulatory weeks, concomitant with tracheal development; a mesodermal defect occurring before the thirty-fifth day of embryonic development could result in these developmental abnormalities. The diagnosis of tracheal agenesis should be suspected in any newborn with respiratory distress and an absent cry who is difficult

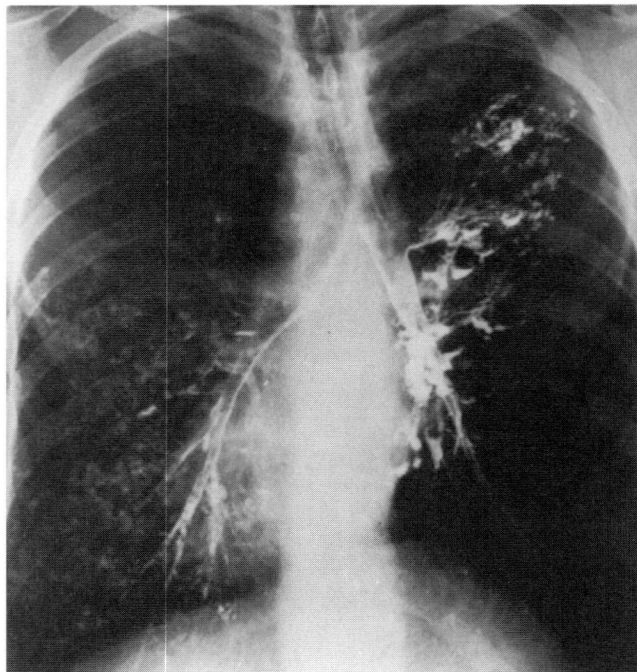

FIGURE 24–11. Case of Kartagener's syndrome. The patient had only mild symptoms of bronchiectasis. Sinusitis was also present.

to intubate. In these cases, the larynx is normal but the trachea is completely absent. Bronchi communicate with the distal esophagus separately or through a trachea-like fistulous communication; cartilage usually is found in the esophageal wall at the site of the communication. Many of these infants are premature, and the incidence of maternal polyhydramnios and additional congenital defects determined at autopsy is high; no suitable surgical treatment is possible.

Tracheal stenosis can be either congenital or acquired. Congenital tracheal stenosis is a rare lesion that may produce only mild symptoms but more commonly is fatal early in infancy. Cantrell and Guild (1964) classified this lesion as (1) stenosis involving the entire length of the trachea, (2) a funnel stenosis involving either the upper, the lower, or the entire portion of the trachea, or (3) segmental stenosis usually located in the lower trachea. Types 2 and 3 may be associated with an erratically localized bronchus or, more often, with an aberrant left pulmonary artery or vascular "sling." In all three types of stenoses there may be completely circular "O" rings of cartilage. Embryologically, segmental stenosis results from abnormal distribution of tissue between the foregut and trachea; hypoplasia and funnel stenosis represent failure of normal tracheal growth. Diagnostically, CT can delineate the extent of the involved stenotic segment for appropriate surgical correction, particularly when complete bronchoscopic examination could not be performed because of the stenosis (Hernandez and Tucker, 1987).

Determination of whether the problem is tracheal or vascular in origin is essential to proper management (see "Vascular Abnormalities," later in this chapter). In the neonatal age group, aggressive surgical intervention is indicated because of the high incidence of sudden death (DeLorimer et al., 1990). Most surgeons believe that up to 50% of the infant trachea can be resected with primary anastomosis. Repair is more difficult if the lesion is near or includes the carina or involves more than 50% of the trachea; most of these infants require tracheal reconstruction with costochondral grafts, pericardium, and esophagus (Walker et al., 1992). Grillo (1983) has noted, however, that the juvenile human trachea does not seem to tolerate tension as well as the adult trachea. Messineo and co-workers (1992) have demonstrated experimentally that cryopreserved cartilaginous allografts can function as tracheal stents for tracheoplasty; this method of stabilizing the repaired trachea may prove superior to existing techniques. Walker and associates (1992) have used *extracorporeal membrane oxygenation* (ECMO) for perioperative support during congenital tracheal stenosis repair, and Ziemer and associates (1992), as well as others, have reported a one-stage repair of pulmonary artery sling and tracheal stenosis using cardiopulmonary bypass and deep hypothermic arrest. For the premature infant with congenital tracheal stenosis, Messineo and co-workers (1992b) have attempted balloon dilatation to split the posterior aspect of the tracheal rings, with some success,

because no reconstructive techniques are available in this subset of patients.

Acquired tracheal stenosis in infants and children may occur following intubation and/or tracheostomy. Resection and primary reanastomosis has been successfully performed in infants (Salzer et al., 1987) and children with postoperative demonstration of normal tracheal growth. Additional therapeutic modalities, including bronchoscopic curettage, laser photoresection, and cryotherapy, have been reported with varying results (Rodgers et al., 1983). Successful balloon dilatation therapy has been reported for tracheobronchial stenosis in infants with both congenital and acquired lesions (Brown et al., 1987). Benign bronchial stenosis in infants and stenosis following lung transplant have been treated with stenting techniques (Huddleston, 1993; Tsang and Goldstraw, 1992).

Tracheomalacia and tracheobronchomalacia are rare congenital malformations in which the supporting cartilaginous rings permit expiratory collapse of the airway. Tracheal narrowing occurs with expiration causing stridor, cyanosis, and respiratory distress in the infant. Symptoms are not present at birth but appear insidiously after the first weeks of life and are made worse by respiratory tract infections and agitation. Cyanosis and apnea with or immediately following feedings are not uncommon. A mild form of the primary anomaly usually requires only supportive treatment until the infant outgrows the lesion, usually by age 2. However, in severe forms of tracheomalacia, mortality rates may be as high as 80%.

The primary or congenital form of the disease is believed to be due to immaturity of the tracheobronchial cartilage and may be associated with tracheoesophageal fistula, both Type III and the H type (Frey et al., 1987). Greenholz and associates (1986) have described diffuse, proximal, and distal forms of the congenital lesion. Pulsatile collapse of the trachea by normal vascular structures should be included in the differential diagnosis, along with mediastinal or tracheal tumors and bronchial webs. Bronchoscopy demonstrates a marked fluctuation in the size of the tracheal lumen on inspiration and expiration, with indistinct tracheal rings. In addition, newer diagnostic modalities, including cine-CT scanning and MRI, have been used to evaluate airway obstruction in infants and children (Fig. 24–13).

The incidence of subsequent complications was high when tracheostomy alone was utilized as therapy for the severe form of the anomaly (Greenholz et al., 1986). Intraoperative bronchoscopy and aortopexy with or without tracheal stenting or reconstruction has been employed with some success for severe forms of the primary disease (Blair et al., 1986). In secondary tracheomalacia, previously normal tracheal cartilages degenerate in association with inflammatory processes, extrinsic vascular compression or bronchial neoplasms, pectus excavatum, and bronchopulmonary dysplasia (Miller et al., 1987). For distal secondary tracheomalacia, current therapeutic recommendations include intraoperative bronchoscopy and aortopexy; stenting of the airway by tracheostomy in

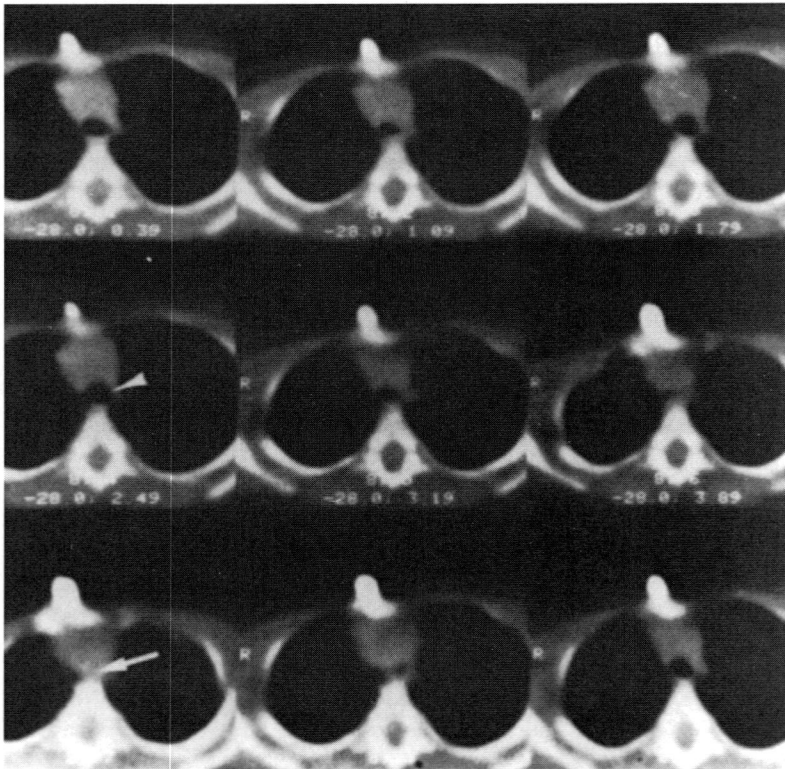

FIGURE 24–13. Tracheomalacia. (Read images from left to right.) Cine computed tomography (CT) airway examination of 16-month-old patient with previously repaired tracheoesophageal fistula and esophageal atresia shows complete expiratory collapse of trachea *(arrow)* several centimeters above carina. Trachea remains widely patent during inspiration *(arrowhead)*. Endoscopy confirmed complete tracheal collapse during expiration at site of previously ligated tracheoesophageal fistula. (From Frey, E. E., Smith, W. L., Grandgeorge, S., et al.: Chronic airway obstruction in children: Evaluation with cine-CT. A. J. R, Vol. *148*. pp 347–352, 1987. Copyright by Williams & Wilkins Company.)

localized proximal disease or by T tube stenting in diffuse tracheomalacia may still be necessary in certain cases (Nashef et al., 1992; Tocewicz et al., 1993). The surgical techniques developed for stenosis may also be applicable to certain cases of tracheomalacia (Vinograd et al., 1987).

Airway branching abnormalities are rarely symptomatic, although Atwell (1967) reported a 10% incidence of tracheobronchial abnormalities in patients undergoing bronchography. Patients in whom an anomalous airway originates from one mainstem bronchus and crosses the mediastinum to supply the opposite lung have been reported. Tracheal bronchus is an aberrant bronchus that results from additional tracheal outgrowth early in embryonic life. Anomalies of tracheal budding must occur at approximately the twenty-sixth day when the lung bud bifurcates. McLaughlin and co-workers (1985) have classified these lesions as *displaced* when a normal bronchus arises from an abnormal site and as *supernumerary* when the anomalous bronchus is additional to a normal bronchus on that side. The bronchus can supply the apical segment of the upper lobe or be a true lobar bronchus. Most occur on the right side, and they may end blindly, form cystic structures, supply accessory pulmonary tissue, or communicate with normal lung (Fig. 24–14). In many cases the bronchus is morphologically normal, but the lesion may be associated with other bronchopulmonary anomalies. Clinical symptoms result from associated stenosis of the bronchus or the other lesion, and can include stridor, wheezing, recurrent infection (bronchiectasis

and/or pneumonia), and hemoptysis. Resection should cure patients with recurrent symptoms and tracheal bronchus (Fig. 24–15). Resection of an asymptomatic tracheal bronchus and lobe is not necessary, however.

Isolated reports of tracheal or bronchial diverticula have appeared. They occur near the junction of the trachea and the right mainstem bronchus and usually are an incidental finding on bronchogram or at autopsy (Atwell, 1967). Diverticula resembling a bronchus can originate from the cervical trachea and end blindly or in a rudimentary lung; such diverticula may regress before birth (Bremer, 1932). Bronchial atresia is characterized by a bronchocele resulting from a mucus-filled, blindly terminating segmental or lobar bronchus, with hyperinflation of the obstructed segment of lung. It is the second most common tracheobronchial malformation after tracheoesophageal fistula. Though the condition was first reported by Ramsay in 1953, it was not until 1963 that Simon and Reid described three cases at the segmental level and established the criteria for diagnosis. Jederlinic and co-workers reviewed the literature in 1987 and reported on 86 total cases. The lesion occurs most frequently in young adult males who present for evaluation of abnormal radiographic results. In older patients, symptoms at presentation are rare; neonates and infants, however, usually present with respiratory distress due to the obstruction of flow of secretions and air from the distal lung to the tracheobronchial tree. The lesion can simulate emphysema or a mediastinal mass.

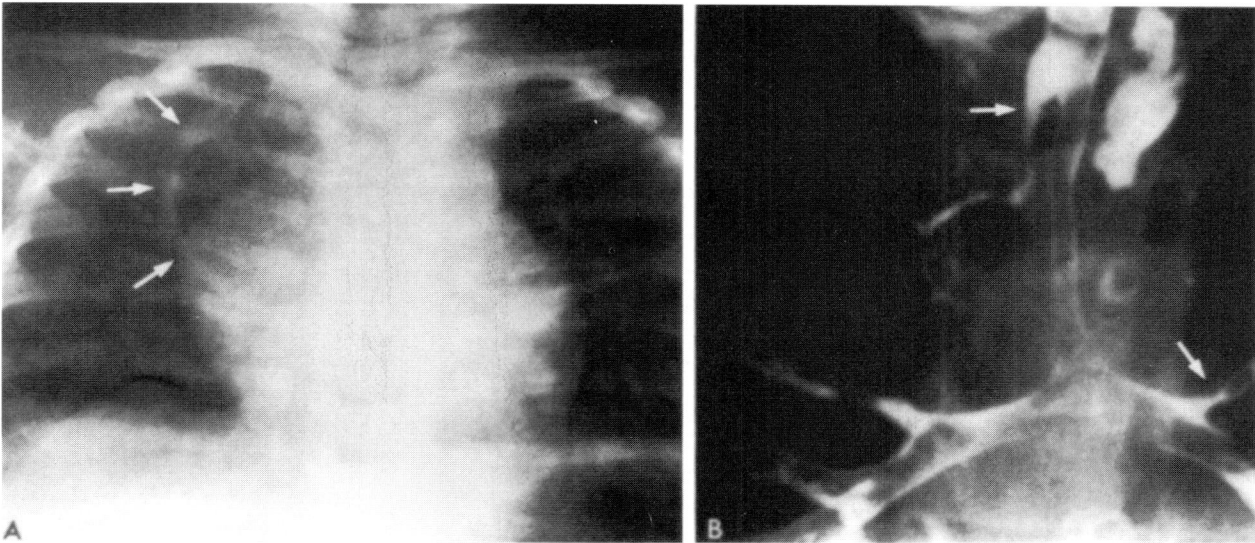

FIGURE 24–14. *A,* Ten-month-old infant with dextroposition of the heart and a thick-walled cyst in the right upper lobe *(arrows). B,* Tracheobronchogram at 6 years of age shows an anomalous tracheal bronchus that arises 6 cm above the carina *(upper arrow).* The trachea is hypoplastic beyond this point, and focal stenosis of each upper lobe bronchus is present *(lower arrow). (A* and *B,* From Siegel, M. J., Shackelford, G. D., Francis, R. S., and McAlister, W. H.: Tracheal bronchus. Radiology, *130:*353–355, 1979.)

The typical radiographic picture, often present for many years, is one of localized transradiance (Fig. 24–16). The lung tissue distal to the atresia becomes emphysematous as air entering across the pores of Kohn, through the bronchoalveolar channels of Lambert, and via interbronchiolar channels is trapped in the segment. This collateral ventilation produces hyperinflation of segmental or lobar distribution on the chest film; and the blind, dilated bronchus becomes a mucocele, seen as a circular or oval density interposed between the emphysematous area and the hilum. The most frequent location is in the left upper lobe, followed by the left lower and right upper lobes, respectively. Almost invariably, only a segment, not the entire lobe, is involved. The alveoli are enlarged, but absolute alveolar hypoplasia is present. Two theories for the embryologic derivation of this anomaly have been proposed. The first is that the tip of the primitive bronchial bud separates from the bud and continues to develop, producing a normal distal bronchial branching pattern that does not communicate with the central airway (Shady et al., 1992). Williams and Schuster (1985) have suggested that a vascular insult

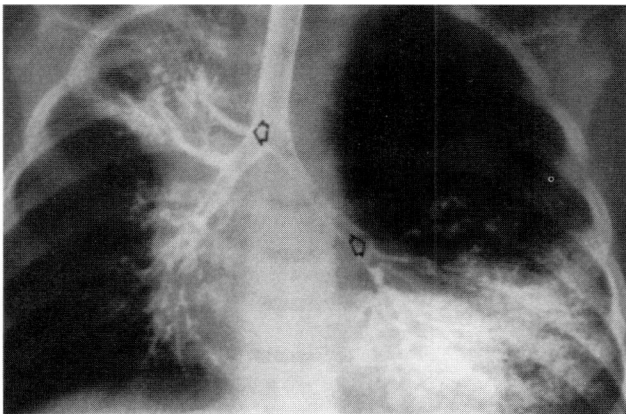

FIGURE 24–15. Aberrant bronchi in a 3-year-old girl with chronic wheezing. Bronchogram shows a right apical tracheal bronchus and the obstructed left upper lobe apical bronchus with emphysema of the left upper lobe. Left upper lobectomy was performed, and the patient has remained well. (From Raffensperger, J. G. [ed]: Swenson's Pediatric Surgery. 4th ed. New York, Appleton-Century-Crofts, 1980, p. 700.)

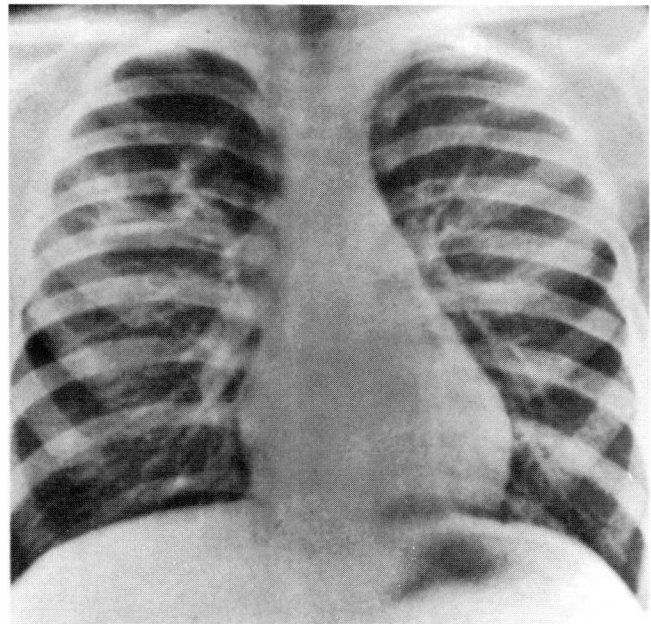

FIGURE 24–16. Chest film of a 14-year-old boy showing hyperlucency of the right upper lobe and an oval density nearer the hilum. (From Williams, L. E., Murray, G. F., and Wilcox, B. R.: Congenital atresia of the bronchus. J. Thorac. Cardiovasc. Surg., *68:*957, 1974.)

is responsible, and that the simultaneous occurrence of bronchial atresia and a bronchogenic cyst indicates that the insult occurred in the early phase of lung budding (fourth to sixth weeks of gestation). In contrast, McAlister and colleagues (1987) have reported on the intrauterine sonographic diagnosis of mainstem bronchial atresia and suggest that the vascular insult occurs after the fifteenth menstrual week, when bronchial branching is complete.

Bronchography was formerly used to confirm the clinical diagnosis. As this technique has become a lost art, CT has become the diagnostic modality of choice (Fig. 24–17). It permits mapping of the bronchocele with highlighting of the regional hypertransradiance. Other CT findings include multiple tubular areas of soft tissue attenuation, representing small abnormal bronchi distal to the central mucoid impaction, and displacement of the surrounding normal parenchyma (Fig. 24–18). With contrast enhancement, a vascular abnormality can be excluded (Jederlinic et al., 1987). The differential diagnosis includes conditions that

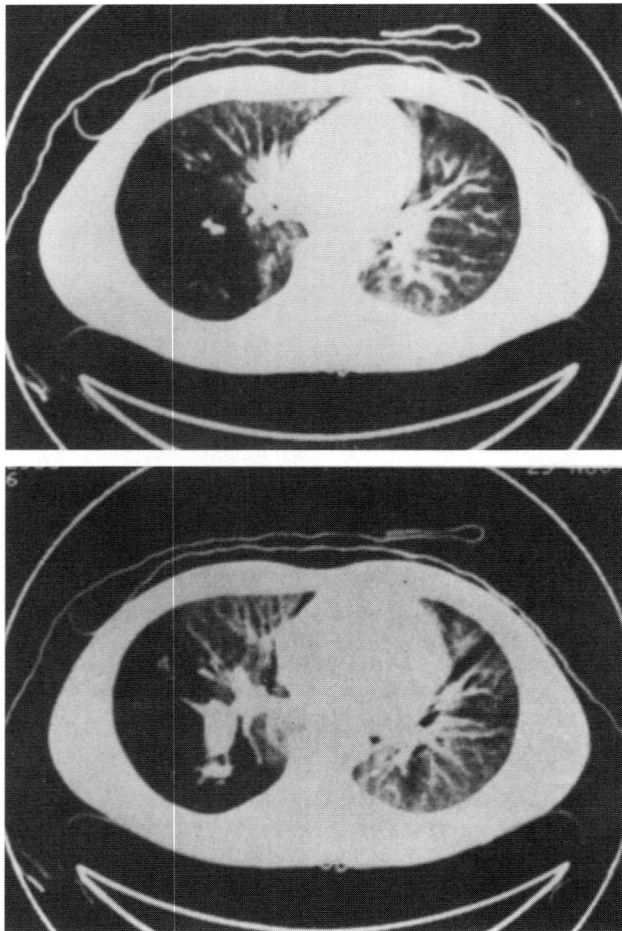

FIGURE 24–17. CT scans show a rounded, nonenhancing density in the medial aspect of the right lower lobe. The serial sections show the branching configuration of the mass associated with distal hyperinflation. (From Jederlinic, P. J., Sicilian, L. S., Baigelman, W., and Gaensler, E. A.: Congenital bronchial atresia. Medicine, Vol 66, pp. 13–83. Copyright by Williams & Wilkins, 1987.)

show peripheral hyperlucency with a proximal mass lesion—namely, bronchial adenoma, mucoid impaction of the bronchus (most commonly due to allergic bronchopulmonary aspergillosis), vascular compression, sequestration, Swyer-James (Macleod) syndrome, and occasionally atypical bronchogenic cysts (Lillington, 1986).

In the past, surgical resection was often performed in asymptomatic patients to establish a diagnosis. With the increased diagnostic accuracy of CT, operative intervention should probably be limited to specific indications. Most commonly, this is pulmonary infection, which in some cases can be serious (Luck et al., 1986). A documented increase in the size of the emphysematous segment may also be an indication (Haller et al., 1980). Segmental resection, if technically possible, is preferable.

A failure of the mesenchyme to develop into cartilage and muscle about the endodermal bronchus is thought to cause congenital bronchiectasis. The segmental bronchi are normal to the second or third divisions, but the distal bronchi have insufficient cartilage and are soft and cystic (Mitchell and Bury, 1975). Typically, a chronic moist cough and bouts of pneumonia are present in the history. Infiltrates and sometimes cystic spaces are seen on chest film, and CT and sometimes bronchography are required to define the extent of the disease process. Lobectomy or pneumonectomy is usually well tolerated, but the prognosis depends on the number of involved lobes. Pathologically, the bronchi that terminated in cystic spaces have closely resembled those seen in the 17-mm stage of development.

Tracheobronchomegaly is a rare disorder of the lower respiratory tract characterized by marked dilatation of the trachea and bronchi (Woodring et al., 1991). Described as a clinicopathologic entity by Mounier-Kuhn in 1932, tracheobronchomegaly is due to a congenital tissue defect resulting in a primary atrophy of the elastic and smooth muscle of the trachea and major bronchi. It occurs rarely in siblings and is associated with the Ehlers-Danlos syndrome and cutis laxa. This anomaly most commonly presents in older children and adults (Fig. 24–19); in these circumstances, recurrent lower respiratory tract infection supervenes, leading ultimately to death from respiratory insufficiency. Neonatal tracheobronchomegaly has been reported (Engle et al., 1987); barotrauma was thought to be the primary pathophysiologic factor in these cases. All patients were premature with NRDS and required prolonged, intensive ventilatory support. Plain chest films will demonstrate the ectasia of the trachea and the mainstem bronchi. Bronchography will confirm the diagnosis if necessary and differentiate this lesion from acquired bronchiectasis (Fig. 24–20).

The most common congenital abnormality of the trachea involves a fistulous connection to the gastrointestinal tract and thus embryologically is distinct from pure tracheal anomalies in its involvement with the foregut. Incomplete differentiation of the lung bud from the primitive gut results in persistent com-

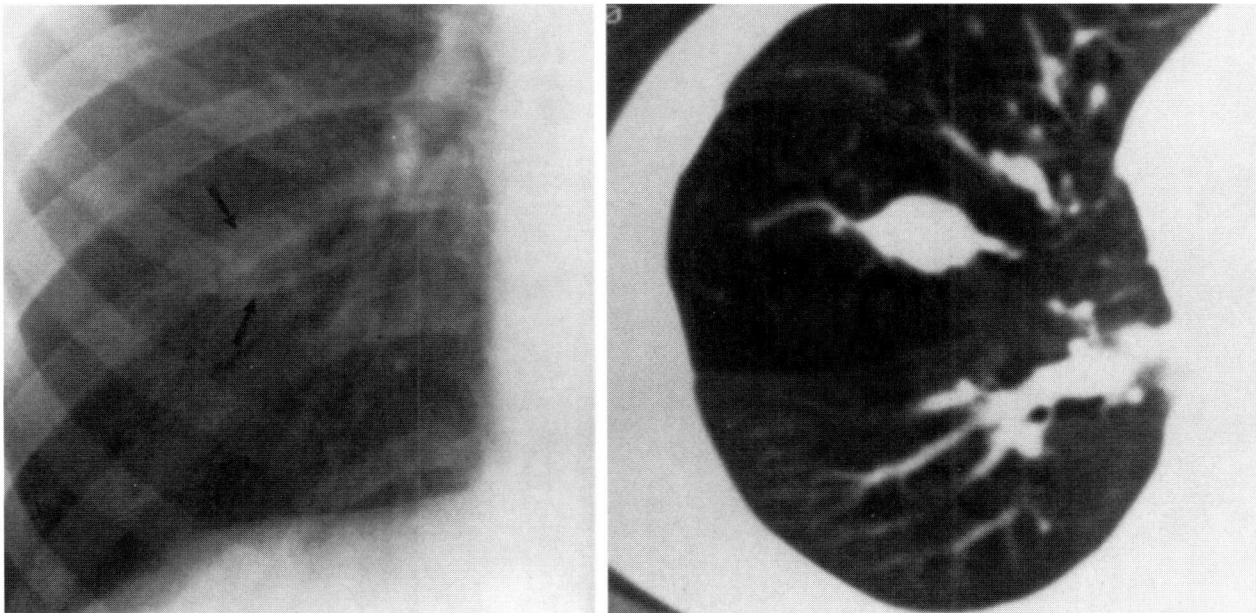

FIGURE 24–18. Bronchial atresia in a 13-year-old boy with wheezing. *Left,* Posteroanterior chest film shows a nodule *(arrows)* in the right middle lobe. *Right,* CT scan shows an ovoid soft tissue nodule in the middle lobe. Overinflation of the lung distally is also noted. The overinflation was not apparent on plain films. Bronchial atresia with mucoid impaction proximal to the atresia was confirmed at surgery. (From Shady, K., Siegel, M., and Glazer, H. S. CT of focal pulmonary masses in childhood. RadioGraphics, *12*:505–514, 1992.)

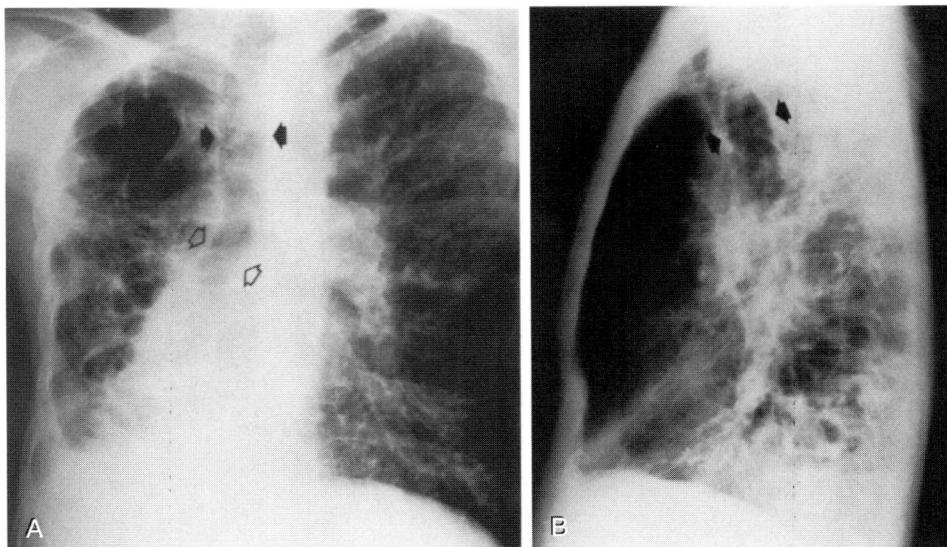

FIGURE 24–19. *A,* Posteroanterior and *B,* lateral chest radiographs of 26-year-old man with Mounier-Kuhn syndrome demonstrating tracheobronchomegaly, severe cystic bronchiectasis in the right lung with multiple air-fluid levels in bronchiectatic cysts, diffuse cylindrical and mild cystic bronchiectasis in the left lung, and massive enlargement of the left pulmonary artery from cor pulmonale. The transverse diameter of the trachea measures 26 mm *(solid arrows* in *A),* the sagittal diameter of the trachea measures 29 mm *(solid arrows* in *B),* and the right main bronchus measures 23 mm in transverse diameter *(open arrows* in *A).* (*A* and *B* from Woodring, J. H., Howard, R. S., and Rehm, S. R.: Congenital tracheobronchomegaly [Mounier-Kuhn syndrome]: A report of 10 cases and review of the literature. J. Thorac. Imag., *6*:1–10, 1991.)

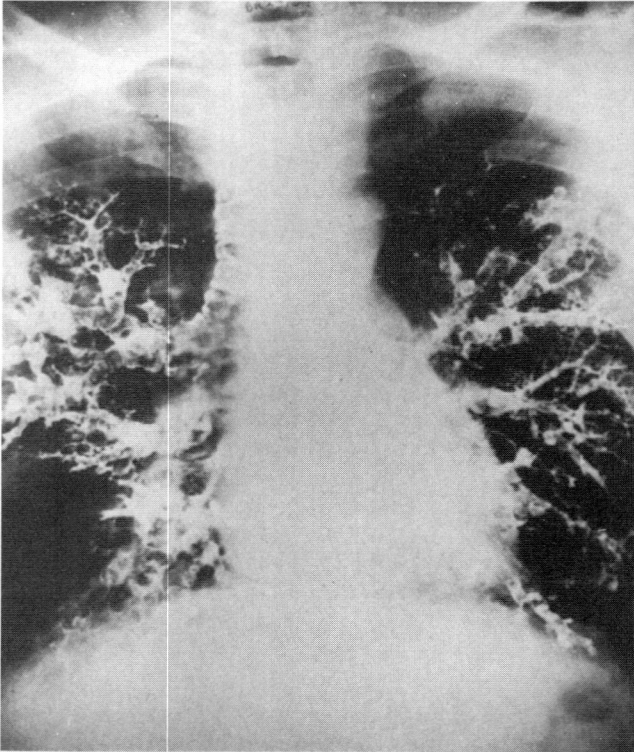

FIGURE 24–20. Bronchogram of a 31-year-old black man with tracheobronchomegaly. The patient also had classic features of Ehlers-Danlos syndrome. (Courtesy of Blake, H. A., Col. M. C.)

FIGURE 24–21. Upper illustrations show the embryologic division of the primitive foregut containing cells with respiratory and GI potential. A normal division produces a trachea with lung buds and a separate GI tract by 4 weeks of development. An abnormal division may lead to esophageal atresia with proximal and distal tracheoesophageal *(t-e)* fistulas *(lower illustrations).* (From Fowler, C. L., Podorny, W. J., Wagner, M. L., and Kessler, M. S.: Review of bronchopulmonary foregut malformations. J. Pediatr. Surg., 23:793–797, 1988.)

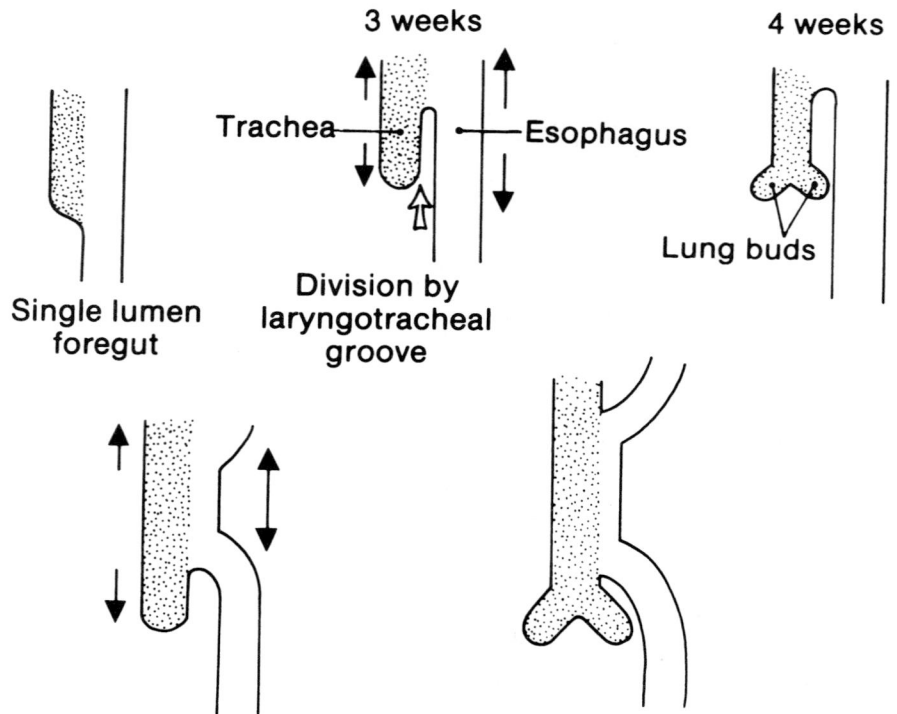

munication or communications below the level of the pharynx (Fig. 24–21). Although most cases of tracheo-esophageal fistula are associated with esophageal atresia, an H type fistula occurs with a "normal" tracheobronchial tree and a "normal" esophagus in 5 to 7% of patients in most series (Newman and Randolph, 1990). This H type anomalous connection is usually small and situated in the cervical region and thus may be difficult to detect clinically. Feeding difficulties, attacks of cyanosis, and recurrent episodes of infections signal the possibility of fistula. Infants with cervical fistulas are air swallowers, and air in the esophagus or a large volume of gas in the stomach or small bowel may be noted on radiologic studies. The diagnosis is established by having the infant swallow a thin contrast medium with demonstration of the fistulous connection by cinefluoroscopy (Fig. 24–22). With positive pressure ventilation at esophagoscopy, air bubbles may emanate through the fistula. Surgical division and closure of the fistula results in complete cure. For the H type tracheoesophageal connections, the approach is best made through the cervical region on the right side, thereby avoiding the thoracic duct. The sternocleidomastoid muscle is divided and a plane is developed between the carotid

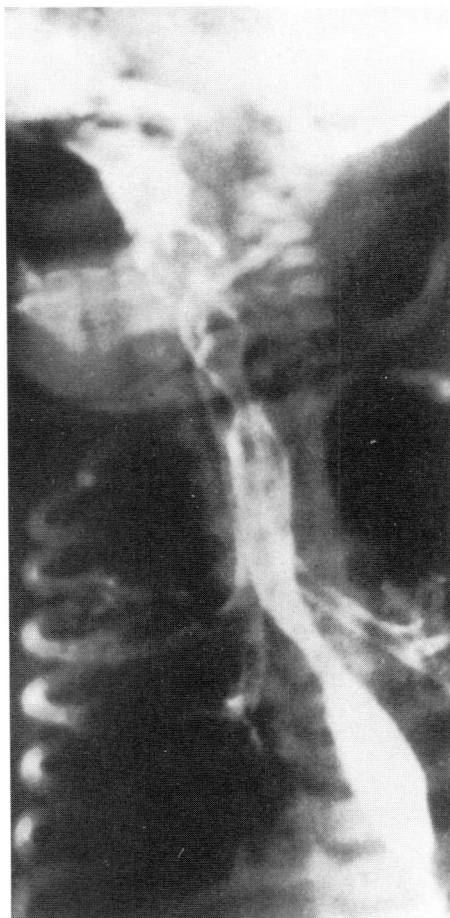

FIGURE 24–22. H-type tracheoesophageal fistula without esophageal atresia in a 1-week-old infant. Contrast material placed in the esophagus flows readily into the tracheobronchial tree.

sheath and the trachea and esophagus, which are retracted medially. The recurrent laryngeal nerve should be recognized and spared. After isolation, the fistula should be divided and each end should be oversewn with a nonabsorbable suture. Placement of an interposition tissue flap of muscle is preferred to decrease the incidence of recurrence, which can be high.

As demonstrated in Figures 24–4 and 24–5, connections between the bronchi and other foregut derivatives can occur. The origin of lobar or segmental bronchi from either the right or the left side of the esophagus has been reported, involving either the upper or the lower lobes (Fowler et al., 1988). The vascular supply to the anomalous lung tissue varies but can be normal. Two cases of an anomalous right mainstem bronchus arising from the distal esophagus were reported by Luck and co-workers (1986). Progressive respiratory distress led to an esophagram, which allowed the correct diagnosis. Surgical treatment should be individualized, but most infants require resection via thoracotomy because of mediastinal shift from the normally inflated contralateral lung.

LUNG PARENCHYMAL ABNORMALITIES: AGENESIS, APLASIA, AND HYPOPLASIA

First described by Morgagni in 1762, underdevelopment of lung tissue was classified by Schneider (1900) into three groups. Agenesis of the lung refers to complete absence of the carina, the main bronchus, the lung, and the pulmonary vasculature of the affected side. Aplasia occurs when the carina and a rudimentary main bronchus are present, but the pulmonary vessels and the alveolar tissue are absent. Hypoplasia occurs when an ill-formed bronchus is capped by poorly developed alveolar tissue forming a fleshy, but unlobulated, structure lying in the mediastinum.

Congenital bilateral pulmonary agenesis follows failure of the primitive lung buds to develop and is uniformly fatal. The trachea ends blindly or in primitive lung buds, suggesting that the arrest in development must occur prior to the 4-mm embryo stage. There are no pulmonary vessels and a high incidence of associated cardiovascular abnormalities. All but two reported cases have been associated with other congenital anomalies, including the hydrolethalus, VACTERL, and tracheal agenesis syndromes (Toriello and Bauserman, 1985). These associations suggest that bilateral pulmonary agenesis may be an extreme expression of the same developmental field defect that more often leads to abnormal lobulation or hypoplasia.

Unilateral pulmonary agenesis is a rare anomaly, occurring once in every 10,000 to 15,000 autopsies. Recent evidence suggests that the defect may be related to a basic chromosomal abnormality (Campanella and Odell, 1987). The average life expectancy with this lesion is shortened to 6 years for right-sided and to 16 years for left-sided agenesis (Mardini and Nyhan, 1985), largely as a result of associated congen-

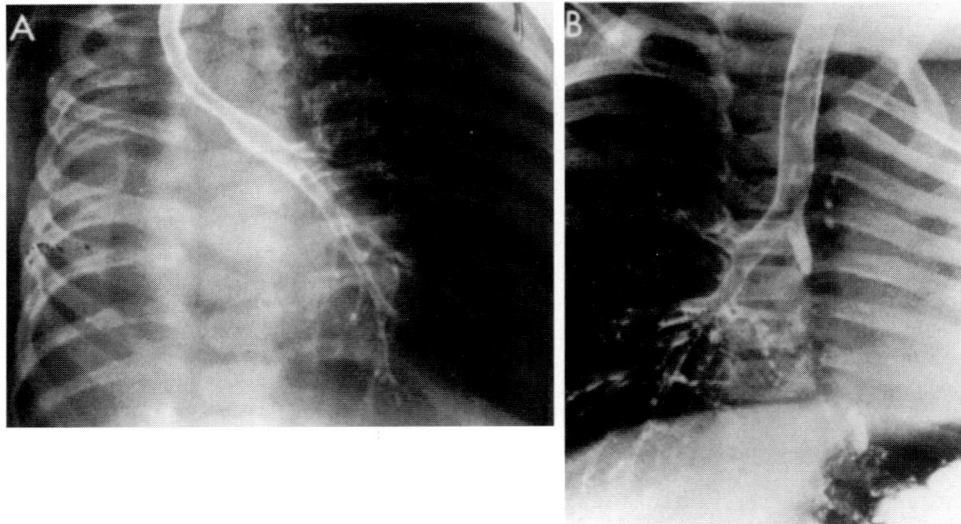

FIGURE 24–23. *A,* Pulmonary agenesis. Physical examination of this tachypneic newborn showed decreased breath sounds on the right and a right shift of the heart tones and cardiac impulse. Further evaluation failed to demonstrate a cardiovascular anomaly. Long-term survival is expected. Bronchogram demonstrates the absence of a carina. The trachea leads directly into a deviated mainstem bronchus. *B,* Pulmonary aplasia. A blind bronchial stump is formed. Early clinical course is identical with that of agenesis, but pulmonary infection can develop at any age from retained secretions in the bronchial stump. The atretic bronchus of this infant was resected. (*A,* from Raffensperger, J. G. [ed]: Swenson's Pediatric Surgery. 4th ed. New York, Appleton-Century-Crofts, 1980, p. 705. *B,* from Swenson, O. [ed]: Pediatric Surgery. 3rd ed. New York, Appleton-Century-Crofts, 1969, p. 298.)

ital anomalies that occur in more than 50% of patients with unilateral pulmonary agenesis. In the absence of cardiac disease, however, infants who survive 5 years can expect an almost normal life span (Luck et al., 1986). Such agenesis is distributed equally between the right and left sides and is more common in males.

The existence of embryonic pulmonary tissue is important for the growth and vascularization of the pulmonary artery, because agenesis and aplasia are, for practical and developmental purposes, the same; there is no lung tissue or ipsilateral pulmonary artery. Cyanosis or respiratory distress in the infant usually

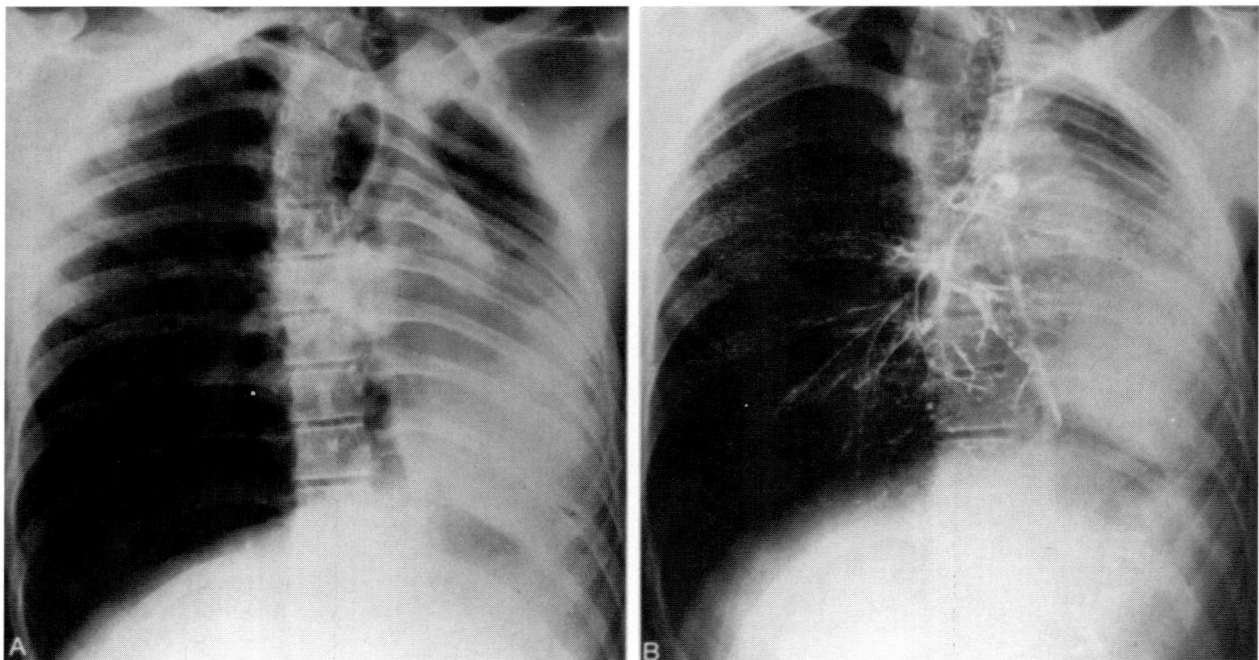

FIGURE 24–24. *A,* Pulmonary aplasia of the left lung in a 17-year-old male with no pulmonary symptoms. The lesion was discovered during investigation of postural deformity. *B,* Bronchogram shows absent left lung and marked displacement of the mediastinum to the right. Note that the contrast is pooled in the left tracheal remnant and that the solitary right lung shows no evidence of emphysematous change.

indicates a co-existing congenital cardiac lesion. In the absence of cardiac disease, the clinical picture in agenesis and aplasia may vary from no symptoms to severe respiratory distress, usually precipitated by infection. The associated mediastinal shift, impairment of the normal bellows mechanism, and deficit in total pulmonary tissue determine the degree of ventilatory deficit; these findings can be demonstrated on physical examination. The appearance of the chest is usually normal, however, because in utero the single lung expands to fill the entire chest, leading to normal chest wall development, and there is no associated diaphragmatic elevation or narrowing of the intercostal spaces (Fig. 24–23).

CT and an esophogram can distinguish total lung sequestration or other foregut anomalies from these lesions, and echocardiography can determine whether there are associated cardiac lesions. In asymptomatic infants, an arteriogram to document anatomy is unnecessary. Ultrasonographic antenatal diagnosis of this condition and its differentiation from congenital diaphragmatic hernia has been described (Yancey and Richards, 1993). No specific surgical therapy is necessary for agenesis unless there are associated cardiac or chest wall abnormalities. Recognition of the true nature of the lesion is important in asymptomatic patients, however, so that nothing meddlesome will be done (Campanella and Odell, 1987) (Fig. 24–24). In pulmonary aplasia, surgical involvement is limited to removal of the documented source of recurrent infection, because the rudimentary bronchial stump on the involved side can be an infectious source.

The concurrence of pulmonary agenesis with

Table 24–2. PULMONARY HYPOPLASIA

Type	Associated Conditions
I. Primary	Idiopathic
	Fetal stress
II. Secondary	Oligohydramnios
	Potter's syndrome (bilateral renal agenesis)
	Renal dysplasias
	Amniotic fluid leak
	Bone dysplasias with a small or rigid chest wall
	Achondroplasia
	Chondrodystrophia fetalis calcificans
	Spondyloepiphyseal dysplasia
	Osteogenesis imperfecta
	Thanatophoric dwarfism
	Neonatal hypophosphatemia
	Decreased fetal respiratory movements
	Congenital arthrogryposis multiplex congenita
	Camptodactyly and multiple ankylosis syndrome
	Congenital myotonic dystrophy
	Asphyxiating thoracic dystrophy
	Diaphragmatic elevation
	Membranous diaphragm
	Abdominal mass or ascites
	Phrenic nerve agenesis
	Intrathoracic space-occupying lesions
	Congenital diaphragmatic hernia
	Congenital cystic adenomatoid malformation
	Mediastinal neoplasms and cystic hygroma
	Enteric cysts (esophageal duplication)
	Pulmonary vascular anomalies
	Pulmonary artery agenesis/atresia
	Scimitar syndrome
	Miscellaneous
	Omphalocele
	Down syndrome
	Rhesus isoimmunization of the fetus

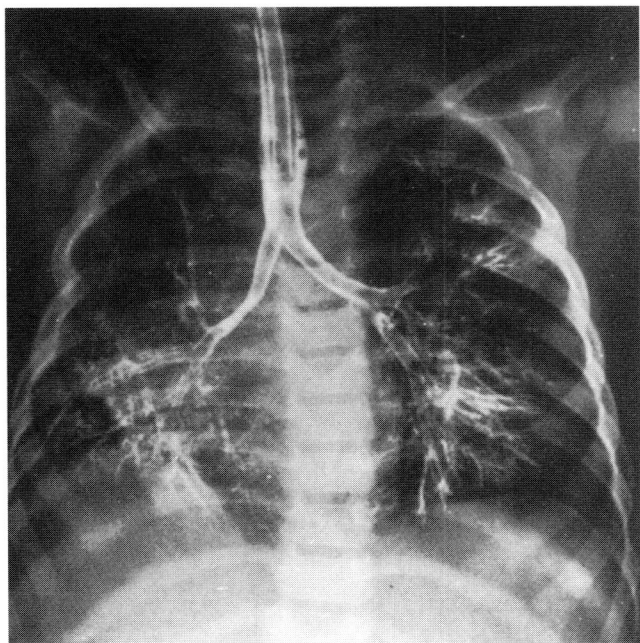

FIGURE 24–25. Infant with lobar agenesis of the right middle and right upper lobe. The right lower lobe fills the entire hemithorax. On bronchoscopy, no nubbin of right upper or middle lobe bronchus was seen. The child also had a Type III tracheoesophageal fistula, which was corrected.

esophageal atresia and tracheoesophageal fistula has been reported, with dismal survival. The importance of tracheomalacia associated with esophageal atresia in worsening the pulmonary status of the infants has been emphasized. Palliation with delayed intervention, thus giving time for the function of the solitary lung to improve, seems to be the most promising approach (Takayanagi et al., 1987). Cases of lobar agenesis have been described but are much rarer than the instances in which the whole lung fails to develop (Fig. 24–25). Congenital hypoplasia of the lung may be primary or secondary (Table 24–2). The radial alveolar count and the lung weight/body weight ratio greater than one standard deviation from mean for gestational year provide the best measurement for identifying pulmonary hypoplasia (Page and Stocker, 1982).

Primary hypoplasia is rare and often fatal. Hypertrophy in pulmonary arterial smooth muscle has been demonstrated at autopsy in infants dying with primary hypoplasia; this was attributed to prolonged fetal stress and development of systemic and pulmonary hypertension (Luck et al., 1986). It has been hypothesized that normal postnatal regression of pulmonary arterial muscle does not occur, and that the pericytes and intermediate cells mature into additional smooth muscle cells. At birth, the infants are in respiratory distress in the delivery room. The chest film demonstrates clear but small lung fields. Persistence of a fetal circulation pattern results from the sustained pulmonary vasoconstriction superimposed on the hypoplastic lungs. No specific corrective therapy is available.

There are multiple causes of secondary pulmonary hypoplasia, including oligohydramnios, bone dysplasias creating a small or rigid chest wall, decreased fetal respiratory movement due to muscular dystrophy or camptodactyly, diaphragmatic elevation, intrathoracic space-occupying lesions, pulmonary vascular anomalies, and prematurity with development of NRDS (Luck et al., 1986). In the case of compression, hypoplasia probably results from interference with the developing alveolar system during the period of rapid growth in the last 2 months of gestation. Hypoplasia may be associated with pulmonary and bronchovascular abnormalities that occur as an isolated lesion or as part of a syndrome complex (Currarino and Williams, 1985). Pulmonary hypoplasia, along with other anomalies resulting from conditions that cause oligohydramnios, has been documented (Prouty and Meyers, 1987) (Fig. 24–26). Unilateral hypoplasia is a feature of the scimitar syndrome (see "Vascular Abnormalities," later in this chapter).

Functionally, the lung or lungs fail to develop to the usual size but contain the essential anatomic components for respiration; the severity of the hypoplasia determines the degree of compromise in ventilation. The microscopic pattern in hypoplasia is characteristic, with a disproportionate number of bronchi but a reduced number of alveolar ducts and alveoli. A lining membrane of cuboidal cells extends as far as the alveolar ducts, and ingrowing capillary buds are less numerous. The arterioles often demonstrate medial

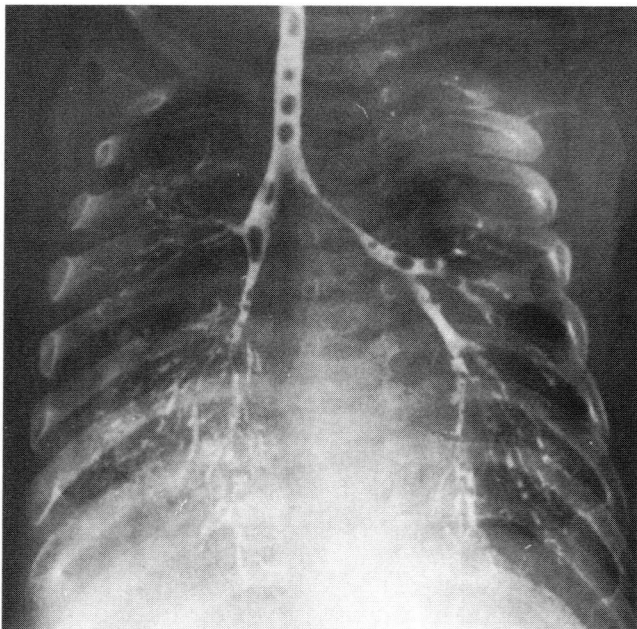

FIGURE 24–26. Bronchogram of an infant with achondroplasia. Note the limited volume of the thoracic cage, the prominence of bronchi, and the paucity of parenchyma.

muscular hypertrophy (Margraf et al., 1991). The findings indicate that the major abnormality in hypoplasia is a decrease in the number of generations of airway and pulmonary artery branchings.

Some degree of pulmonary hypoplasia is invariably present in *congenital diaphragmatic hernia* (CDH) and along with pulmonary hypertension is a major determinant of survival (Nakayama et al., 1992). Infants with this entity who decompensate immediately after birth have the most severe form of hypoplasia. Despite advances in neonatology, the mortality rate for critically ill infants who experience severe respiratory distress within 24 hours of birth remains 40 to 50% (Butt et al., 1992). Treatment is first directed toward the underlying cause of decompensation, namely, the increased pulmonary vascular resistance in the face of hypoplasia. Sedation, paralysis, high-frequency ventilation, induction of respiratory alkalosis, and pulmonary vasodilators to alter prostanoid synthesis are mainstays of therapy. Bartlett and co-workers (1987) successfully used ECMO in congenital diaphragmatic hernia and other neonatal conditions that result in severe respiratory failure. Currently, many centers delay CDH repair, using ECMO for stabilization and, if necessary, maintaining patients on ECMO during repair; survival rates of 65% have been achieved in this high-risk subset (Lally et al., 1992; West et al., 1992). A study by Beals and co-workers (1992) demonstrated significant lung growth and postnatal vascular remodeling that produced larger and less muscular arteries after CDH repair, indirectly supporting this delayed approach. ECMO is not without complications, however, and these have been well delineated (Nagaraj et al., 1992; Weber et al., 1992). Breaux and colleagues (1992) have devised a prognostic and management classification for this congenital defect.

The hypoplastic lung should not be surgically removed at the time of hernia repair. Neither should vigorous efforts to inflate the lung be attempted at this time, since this will only produce interstitial emphysema and further compromise ventilation. In long-term follow-up of survivors following CDH repair, a significant decrease in airflow resistance, a persistent decrease in pulmonary blood flow to the lung on the side of the defect, and persistent elevation of pulmonary vascular resistance indicates the presence of continued hypoplasia despite varying results as to pulmonary function (Luck et al., 1986). However, abnormal muscle extension and medial hypertrophy in the pulmonary vessels persist following repair (Reid, 1986). In contrast, Saifuddin and Arthur (1993) noted that the postoperative radiographic features of patients with CDH who presented late and underwent correction were characteristic of complete expansion and no pulmonary vascular hypoplasia.

Although not a surgical condition, NRDS is one of the causes of acute respiratory failure in the neonatal period and must be distinguished from surgical lesions (Avery et al., 1981). The typical circumstance is that of an infant born 2 to 4 months early by cesarean section; prenatal or postnatal asphyxia may complicate the delivery. NRDS is also seen in full-term infants born to diabetic mothers. The chest film shows a ground-glass appearance with diffuse atelectasis and air bronchograms (DeLorimer, 1986) (Fig. 24–27). (The relationship between NRDS and pulmonary surfactant was discussed earlier—see "Developmental Anatomy.") Diminished surfactant leads to hypoxemia, pulmonary shunt, pulmonary edema, and the formation of the alveolar hyaline membranes. Microscopically, there is engorgement of capillaries and filling of the alveolar ducts and respiratory bronchioles with the acidophilic membrane. Exogenous surfactant replacement has decreased the intensity of mechanical ventilation and reduced the inspired oxygen concentration necessary for adequate systemic oxygenation (Gortner, 1992). Overall outcome has been improved, including increased survival and decreased incidence of bronchopulmonary dysplasia (BPD) (Abbasi et al., 1993). Approximately 45% of infants with NRDS will require careful respiratory care but not ventilatory support; the remainder will require some form of prolonged assisted ventilation, either by *continuous positive airway pressure* (CPAP) or by endotracheal intubation. *Interstitial pulmonary emphysema* (IPE) occurs as a complication of assisted ventilation and high ventilator pressures, and is discussed below in the section on (see "Parenchymal Cystic Disease: Lung Bud Anomalies" later in this chapter). Despite these advances, however, more than 15% of patients succumb to NRDS.

Survival after prolonged intubation and ventilatory support for NRDS has led to the recognition of BPD as a clinical entity. Between 15 and 38% of infants under 1500 g who require mechanical ventilation for NRDS will develop BPD. The etiology is multifactorial and includes oxygen toxicity, barotrauma, patent ductus arteriosus, fluid overload, associated pulmonary disease, and prematurity. Strange and associates (1990) demonstrated that expression of at least three antioxidant enzymes in premature infants was similar to that in adults; however, the level of expression of these antioxidants (superoxide dismutases) may not be high enough to effectively detoxify the increased levels of reactive oxygen species that result from continuous oxygen therapy. Bruce and co-workers (1992) identified risk factors for the degradation of lung elastic fibers in the ventilated neonate; elastic fibers are believed to provide the structural support for alveolar septal development, and this study demonstrated that proteolytic degradation of these fibers was associated with prolonged ventilatory support and poor clinical outcome once BPD was established. Margraf and colleagues (1991) demonstrated that, in fatal BPD, marked impairment of lung development with alveolar hypoplasia, bronchiolar smooth muscle hypertrophy, and bronchial gland hyperplasia all contributed to airflow limitation. Neurodevelopmental outcome has been demonstrated to be worse following BPD in comparable very-low-birth-weight infants (Teberg et al., 1991). However, although the symptoms of pulmonary dysfunction following BPD last for years, the condition of these infants improves significantly by age 2 in long-term survivors. Lung function continued to improve between 7 and 10 years of age in patients with and without normal lung function who had BPD as infants (Blayney et al., 1991). Long-term treatment of symptoms includes therapy for bronchospasm and pulmonary edema.

PARENCHYMAL CYSTIC DISEASE: LUNG BUD ANOMALIES

Lesions involving local aberrations of parenchymal tissue development have been arbitrarily classified as "lung-bud anomalies." The lesions in this category that are discussed here include *infantile lobar emphysema* (ILE), congenital cysts of the lung, *congenital cystic adenomatoid malformation* (CCAM), and interstitial pulmonary emphysema. In some classifications, bronchogenic cysts are included with lung bud anomalies, because these four surgically curable lesions are responsible for acute respiratory distress in the newborn infant and are therefore potential surgical emergencies. In this discussion, however, bronchogenic cysts are discussed later under the heading "Bronchopulmonary Foregut Malformations."

ILE accounts for approximately 50% of congenital lung malformations (Berlinger et al., 1987). Many terms have been used to describe this lesion (congenital lobar emphysema, congenital lobar overinflation, congenital segmental bronchomalacia, and emphysema of infancy or childhood), reflecting the diverse congenital causes of the check-valve mechanism that produces the symptom complex. In ILE, the term *emphysema* refers to overexpansion of the air spaces of a segment or lobe of the lung; in contrast to the emphysematous processes seen in adult pulmonary disease, there is no significant parenchymal destruction.

Although ILE was once thought to be a progressive process, in fact many affected infants may develop a

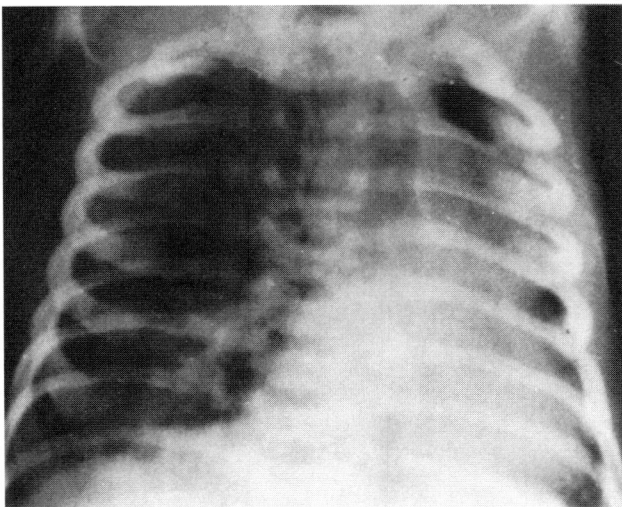

FIGURE 24–27. Neonatal respiratory distress syndrome in a newborn premature infant. The child did not survive.

stable overexpanded lobe with minimal encroachment on adjacent lung tissue and have mild symptoms that do not progress. Typically, infants with ILE appear normal at birth. In half of cases, symptoms appear within several days and consist of tachypnea, cough, dyspnea, inspiratory and expiratory wheezing, and possibly cyanosis (DeLorimer, 1986). Physical findings include hyperresonance and decreased breath sounds in the involved area of the chest. Diagnosis in most neonatal cases is suggested from the chest film, which shows a marred radiolucency in the region of the involved lobe with mediastinal shift to the opposite side (Fig. 24–28). In extreme cases, the emphysematous segment may herniate into the opposite side anterior to the heart and great vessels. Care must be taken not to misinterpret the film by presuming the area of compressed normal lung to be atelectatic and the emphysematous lobe merely compensatory. The diaphragm on the affected side is usually depressed. In a review by Hendren and McKee (1966), the location of lung involvement was the left upper lobe in 42%, right upper lobe in 21%, right middle lobe in 35%, and right and left lower lobes in less than 1% of patients. Bilateral involvement has been reported, usually in the right middle and left upper lobes. The male/female ratio is 3:1. In the remaining infants the onset of respiratory distress is more gradual, but 80% are symptomatic by age 6 months. In general, the earlier the onset of symptoms, the more likely they are to progress. Cardiac anomalies are present in 14% of these infants, and associated noncardiac lesions include anomalies of the ribs or thoracic cage.

The causes of ILE are diverse (DeLorimer, 1986). In Gross' original surgical cure, the lobar bronchus was devoid of cartilage (Gross and Lewis, 1945). Bronchial obstruction can be implicated in about 25% of cases (Table 24–3). Whatever the cause, air trapping results in overexpansion of the lung and breakdown of the

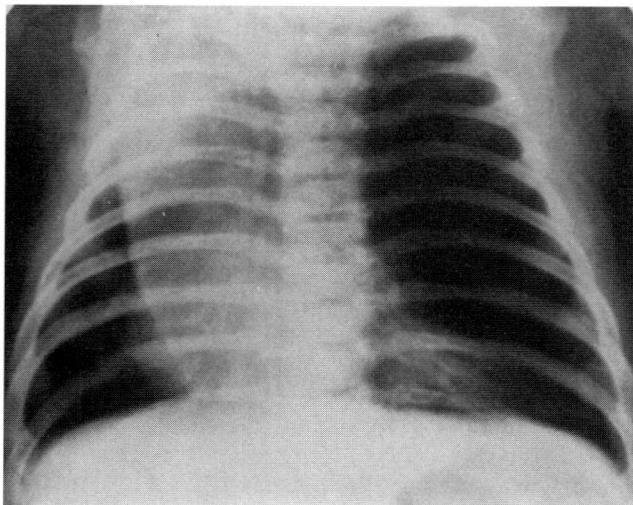

FIGURE 24–28. Infantile lobar emphysema. Marked emphysema of the left upper lobe with mediastinal shift to the right and compression of the right lung. The infant was cured by left upper lobectomy.

■ **Table 24–3.** CAUSES OF BRONCHIAL OBSTRUCTION

Intrinsic

Hypoplastic, deficient, or dysplastic bronchial cartilages
Redundant bronchial mucosal folds
Inspissated mucous plugs or inflammatory exudates
Bronchial atresia or stenosis
Kinked bronchus
Bronchial granulations

Extrinsic

Cardiovascular
  Patent ductus arteriosus
  Pulmonary artery sling
  Hypertensive, dilated pulmonary arteries
  Pulmonic stenosis
  Tetralogy of Fallot with absent pulmonic valve
  Dilated superior vena cava in anomalous pulmonary venous
    return
Others
  Bronchogenic cyst
  Esophageal duplication cyst
  Mediastinal adenopathy
  Mediastinal teratoma or neuroblastoma
  Accessory diaphragm

Modified from Berlinger, N. T., Porto, D. P., and Thompson, T. R.: Infantile lobar emphysema. Ann. Otol. Rhinol. Laryngol., 96:106, 1987.

alveolar septa; other alveolar or interstitial involvement is minimal, although alveolar fibrosis may be present. ILE has also been described in certain forms of pulmonary hypoplasia wherein the number of alveoli for each acinus is normal but the total number of alveoli is greatly diminished. Despite air-trapping and overdistention in these cases, no mediastinal shift or compression occurs, because the lung is hypoplastic. Finally, ILE can result from hyperplasia of alveoli or the polyalveolar lobe (Tapper et al., 1980). The number of bronchial branches is normal, but each acinus contains an abnormally increased number of alveoli; the individual alveoli appear normal. The polyalveolar lobe may become greatly overexpanded and hyperlucent and produce severe respiratory distress. These cases tend to present earlier in infancy, but this type of ILE is indistinguishable from the other types on clinical grounds. Overall, however, the etiology remains unclear in up to 50% of cases.

The indication for treatment in ILE is life-threatening progressive pulmonary insufficiency from compression of adjacent normal lung. In addition to the plain film, CT may yield valuable information about the cause of ILE in certain cases (Fig. 24–29). MRI can be helpful as well (Cohen et al., 1987) (Fig. 24–30). Diagnostic bronchoscopy is of little value in infants and in fact may be harmful in the presence of acute respiratory distress. Therapeutic bronchoscopy for mucous plugs or aspirated foreign bodies may be curative and should be considered in older children capable of aspirating a foreign body. When indicated, however, endoscopy should be performed under the same anesthetic as is used for the thoracotomy. Bronchography rarely is indicated but will show severe compression of the affected lung (Fig. 24–31). With

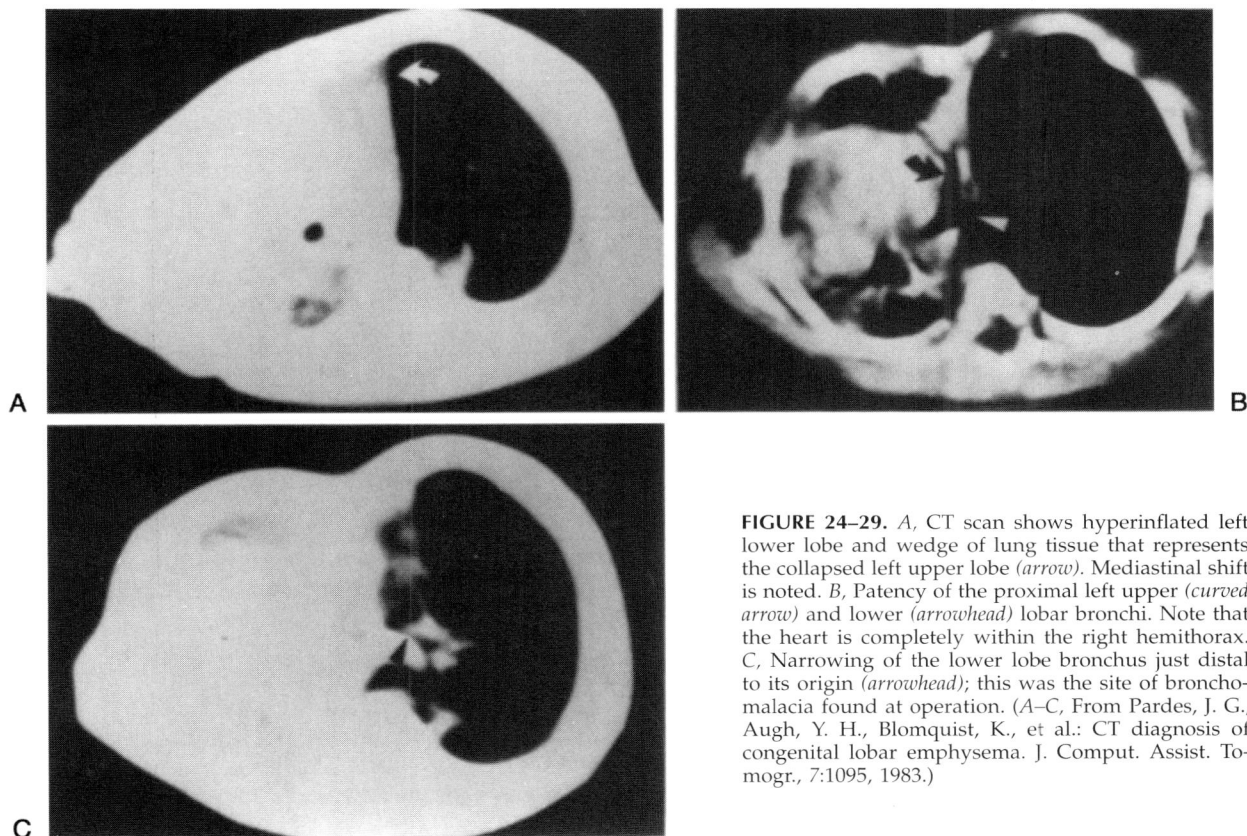

FIGURE 24–29. *A*, CT scan shows hyperinflated left lower lobe and wedge of lung tissue that represents the collapsed left upper lobe *(arrow)*. Mediastinal shift is noted. *B*, Patency of the proximal left upper *(curved arrow)* and lower *(arrowhead)* lobar bronchi. Note that the heart is completely within the right hemithorax. *C*, Narrowing of the lower lobe bronchus just distal to its origin *(arrowhead)*; this was the site of bronchomalacia found at operation. *(A–C,* From Pardes, J. G., Augh, Y. H., Blomquist, K., et al.: CT diagnosis of congenital lobar emphysema. J. Comput. Assist. Tomogr., *7*:1095, 1983.)

FIGURE 24–30. Congenital lobar emphysema. The chest film *(A)* shows hyperexpansion of the left upper lung field with herniation of lung across the midline and displacement of the mediastinal structures from left to right. *B*, A coronal magnetic resonance image, TE = 30 msec and TR = 1000 msec. Obtained through the anterior chest, this image shows marked hyperexpansion of the left upper lung field with significant displacement of heart and mediastinum. The appearance corresponds to that of the chest film. A more posterior image *(C)* obtained at the level of the descending aorta delineates the abnormality. The left upper lobe is hyperinflated and of much lower signal intensity than the right lung. The partially collapsed left lower lobe has a slightly higher intensity than the normal right lung. There is a very sharp interface between the upper and lower lobes owing to the left oblique fissure. The magnetic resonance image localizes the abnormality more clearly than does the chest film. *(A–C,* From Cohen, M. D., Scales, R. L., Eigen, H., et al.: Evaluation of pulmonary parenchymal disease by magnetic resonance imaging. Br. J. Radiol., *60*:223, 1987.)

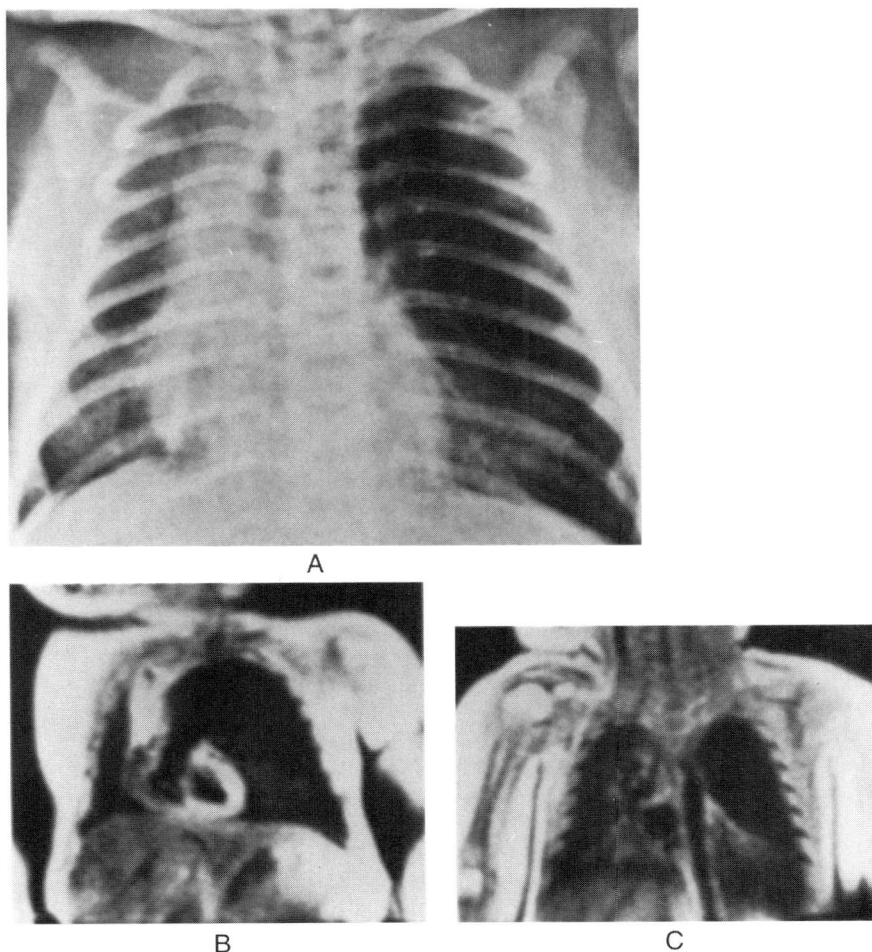

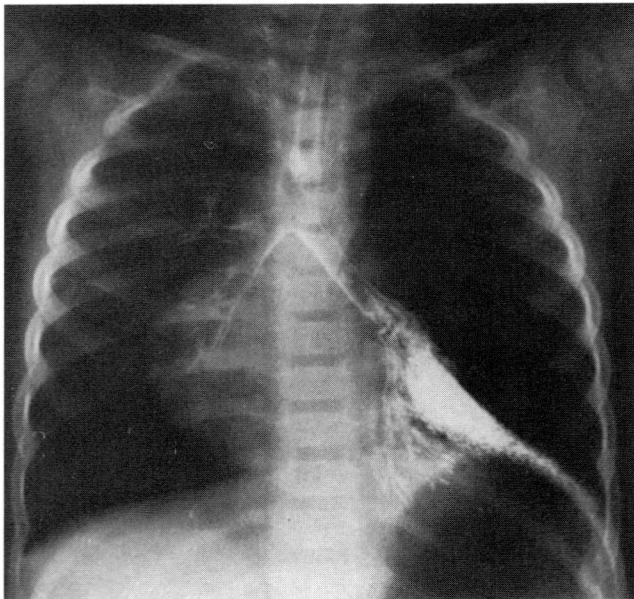

FIGURE 24–31. Bronchogram of an infant with infantile lobar emphysema of the left upper lobe shows severe compression of the left lower lobe and nonfilling of the involved lobe.

progressive symptoms, prompt surgical excision of the involved lobe is warranted and may be lifesaving (Hendren and McKee, 1966). In the critically ill infant, thoracotomy must be performed immediately after intubation, because the artificial ventilation required can produce sudden, exaggerated expansion of the affected lung with compression of the normal lung and mediastinal structures. Goto and associates (1987) have reported the successful use of high-frequency jet ventilation to manage an infant with ILE during resection. The diseased lobe is apparent by its noncollapsible, overdistended state and has the consistency of sponge rubber; it springs back into shape after it is compressed. Although the edges of the lobe are rounded and not well defined, surgical resection is accomplished quite easily because the hilar anatomy is normal. Surrounding atelectatic lung tissue should be spared because it will re-expand with time. Conversely, all emphysematous lung tissue should be resected, because recurrence has been documented (Haller et al., 1980). Simultaneously, any extrinsic cause of compression should be removed. Microscopically, the alveoli and alveolar ducts are overdistended, and the alveolar walls are fragmented and ruptured to a varying degree (Fig. 24–32). Cystic degeneration does not occur, and there is no evidence of infection. Deficient and/or deformed bronchial cartilage is found in 25 to 40% of pathologic specimens.

Lobectomy usually produces complete cure. In long-term follow-up of patients after lobectomy for ILE, Frenckner and Freyschuss (1982) demonstrated some compensatory growth of remaining lung tissue; pulmonary functional impairment due to the loss of lung tissue or residual disease could not be demonstrated. Development was normal, and patients were largely asymptomatic. Others have reported that

many children continue to have mild wheezing following lobectomy, especially during respiratory infections (Luck et al., 1986). Asymptomatic infants who do not need resection have late pulmonary function results equivalent to those of surgically treated patients. When ILE is diagnosed in infants over 1 year of age, observation is warranted, because pulmonary function is likely to remain stable over time.

Congenital parenchymal cystic lesions of the lung are a poorly understood group of defects that present a variety of clinical and pathologic features. Controversy exists over the embryology, pathology, etiology, and nomenclature of the various cysts (Seiber, 1986). Distinct from bronchogenic cysts, ILE, CCAM, and cysts associated with systemic disease, congenital pulmonary cysts are thought to originate by entrapment of a portion of the developing lung bud. The site of origin of the cyst determines the composition of the cyst wall; cysts arising from bronchial structures proximal to the alveolar duct have bronchial glands, smooth muscle, and occasionally cartilage, with cuboidal or ciliated columnar epithelium; lesions arising distal to the duct create thin-walled alveolar cysts or pneumatocele-like cysts. It was once believed that all cysts of infancy and childhood were congenital;

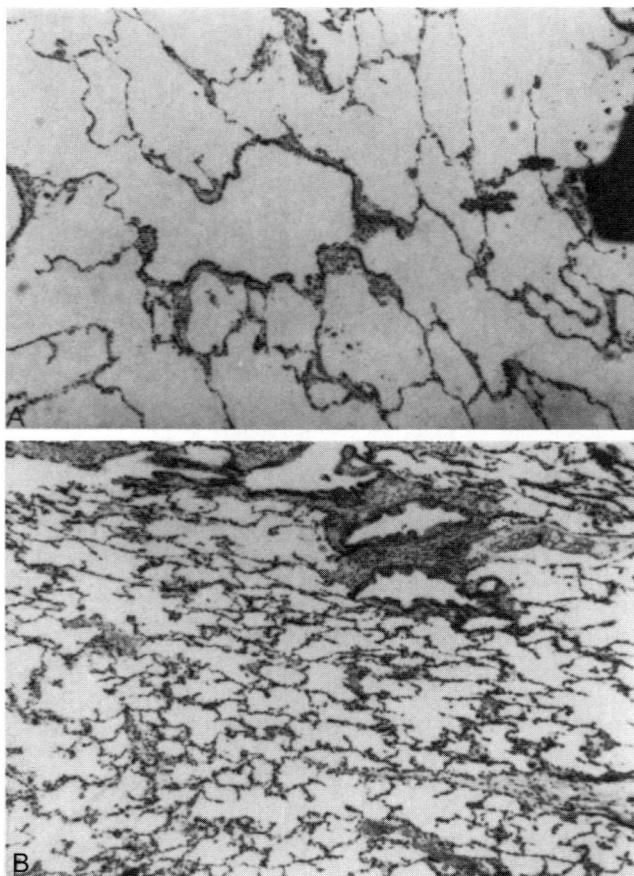

FIGURE 24–32. A, Photomicrograph of infantile lobar emphysema showing overdistention of alveoli ($\times$ 90). B, Photomicrograph of normal lung at same magnification for comparison with A. (A and B, From Katzenstein, A., and Askin, F. B.: Surgical Pathology of Non-Neoplastic Lung Disease. Philadelphia, W. B. Saunders, 1982.)

however, the rarity of cysts in the fetus and newborn in comparison with their incidence in older infants and children often suggests an acquired origin.

Most congenital cysts are unilocular and solitary, usually confined to one side and more frequently involving the lower lobe. Symptoms may be produced by extremely rapid expansion requiring emergency thoracotomy or by infection with fever, cough, and sepsis (Fig. 24–33). Alternatively, safe observation for months or years in the absence of expansion or infection may be possible. However, the persistence of one of these lesions for more than a year indicates that resolution is unlikely. Furthermore, squamous metaplasia may occur in recurrently infected cysts, and cancer has occurred within lung cysts of presumably congenital origin (Womack and Graham, 1941). The diagnosis of congenital lung cyst is usually suggested by radiologic examination, although congenital diaphragmatic hernia and multiple pneumatoceles may be difficult to differentiate by plain films alone. Bronchography may be necessary for definitive diagnosis. CT has also helped to diagnose these lesions (Putman et al., 1984).

Treatment of isolated parenchymal congenital cysts involves surgical removal. Lobectomy may be necessary, but cystectomy can yield good results on occasion and should always be considered in an effort to conserve pulmonary tissue. If the cyst is infected, systemic antibiotics should be administered, and lobectomy should be performed during an aquiescent interval. Pneumonectomy is rarely necessary. Persistent solitary congenital cysts that are secondarily infected are difficult to differentiate from pyogenic lung abscess if infection has destroyed the epithelial lining membrane of the cyst (Fig. 24–34). As with abscesses, lobectomy is the surgical procedure of choice in these instances.

Tension cysts usually occur in infancy or early childhood as a complication of cystic disease and are associated with rapid onset of symptoms, including respiratory stridor, dyspnea, and cyanosis (Fig. 24–35). Differentiation from pneumothorax may be difficult, except that lung cysts do not collapse with external drainage. The common sequela of placing a chest tube into a cyst is empyema, which can also result from ill-advised attempts to aspirate the cysts. Lobectomy is usually required for tension cysts because smaller cysts and areas of emphysematous lung are always present around the tension cyst. Pathologically, the lesion is characterized by a very thin wall and a smooth glistening lining membrane, although secondary infection markedly alters this picture (Fig. 24–35B).

Multiple congenital parenchymal cysts occur rarely in the neonate; most fetuses have other congenital lesions and are stillborn. An acquired or metabolic etiology should be sought when multiple cysts are present. Staphylococcal pneumonia with pneumatocele production is the most frequent acquired cause of multiple cystic lesions in infants and children (McGarry et al., 1987). They develop rapidly and often fluctuate in size. Confirmation that a cystic lesion is a pneumatocele depends primarily on establishing its association with staphylococal pneumonia. Surgical intervention in these patients with chest tube drainage or thoracotomy is contraindicated, because the pneumatoceles resolve as the pneumonia subsides.

Multiple pulmonary cysts due to a developmental metabolic cause are seen in *cystic fibrosis* (CF) (Alton

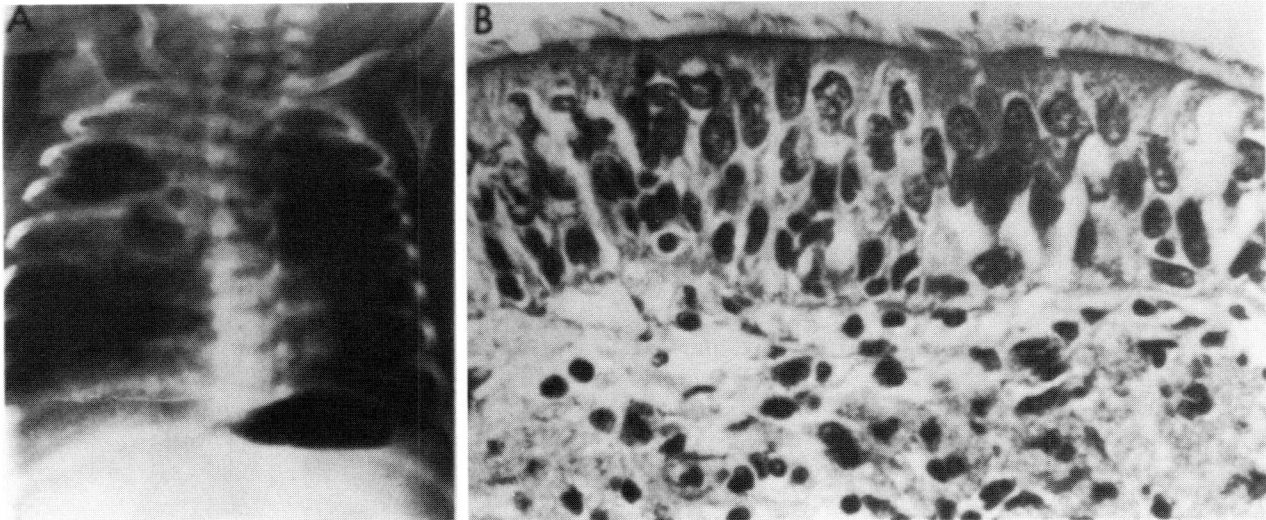

FIGURE 24–33. Congenital cystic disease of the lung. Infection in a 13-week-old infant with a 3-week history of cough. At operation, cysts were found to involve the upper lobe, to which the middle lobe was fused; both were removed. A, Preoperative chest film showing a number of separate air sacs in the opacified right upper lobe. B, Photomicrograph of the cyst lining, which consisted of tall columnar ciliated bronchial epithelium. There were a few mucous glands in the cyst wall and a thin layer of smooth muscle between the basement membrane and the fibrous wall of the cyst; in some areas, there was acute inflammation. (A and B, From Seiber, W. K.: Lung cysts, sequestration, and bronchopulmonary dysplasia. *In* Welch, K. H., Randolph, J. G., Ravitch, M. M., et al. [eds]: Pediatric Surgery. 4th ed. Vol. 1. Chicago, Year Book Medical, 1986, p. 645.)

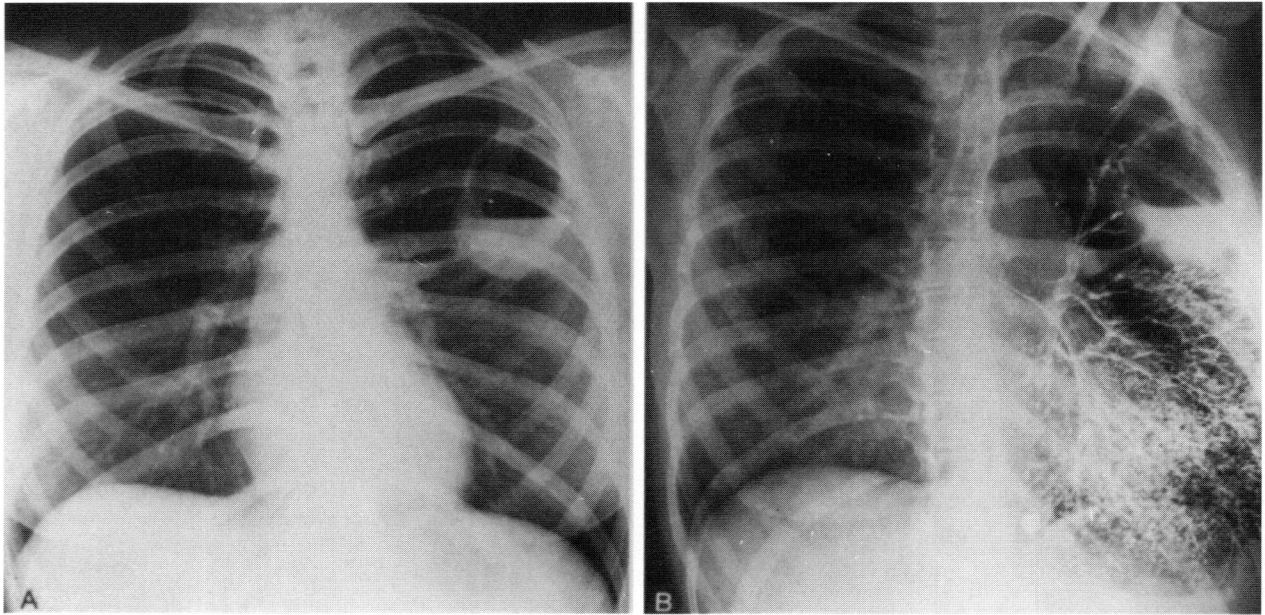

FIGURE 24–34. *A,* Cystic lesion in the left upper lobe in a 25-year-old woman with a history of respiratory infection since 8 years of age. Left upper lobectomy cured the condition. The pathologist could not determine whether the cyst was congenital or acquired. *B,* Bronchogram of the same patient.

et al., 1992). The advances in the treatment of this disease process since 1985 are among the most dramatic in all of medicine (Super, 1992). Pulmonary disease, the most debilitating and life-threatening aspect of CF, includes obstruction of the bronchi by thick, tenacious secretions leading to inspissation, focal atelectasis, obstructive emphysema (Fig. 24–36), and recurrent respiratory infection complicated by bronchiectasis. The basic problem underlying the clinical manifestations is a defect in the chloride permeability at the luminal surface of epithelial cells; an inadequate response to cyclic adenosine monophosphate (cAMP) stimulation prevents the normal secretion of chloride and allows excess reabsorption of sodium from the airway lumen into the cytoplasm. This combines to reduce the water content and increase the viscosity and tenacity of airway secretions (Weinberger, 1993). The defective gene responsible for CF was identified in 1989, and the gene product, cystic fibrosis transmembrane conductance regulator, is probably the chloride channel itself (Sferra and Collins, 1993). This genetic development has led the

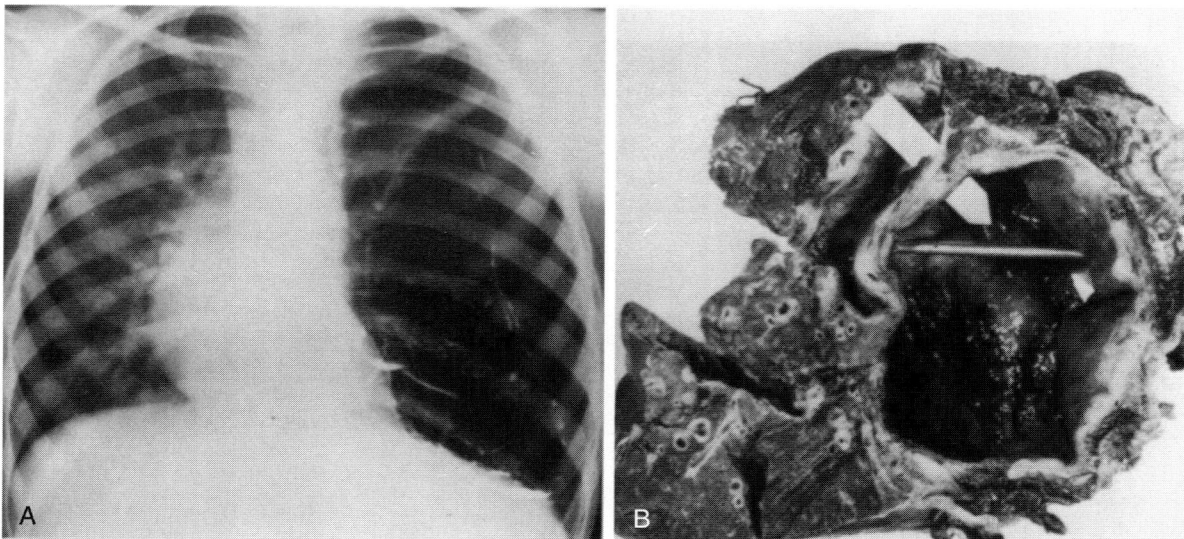

FIGURE 24–35. *A,* Large tension cyst on the left lung with associated pneumothorax. Note the marked shift of the mediastinum to the right. Bronchographic contrast material outlines the limits of the cyst. *B,* Gross specimen of infected tension cysts. Several cysts communicate, as indicated by the pointers. A marked fibrous tissue reaction is present in the cyst wall.

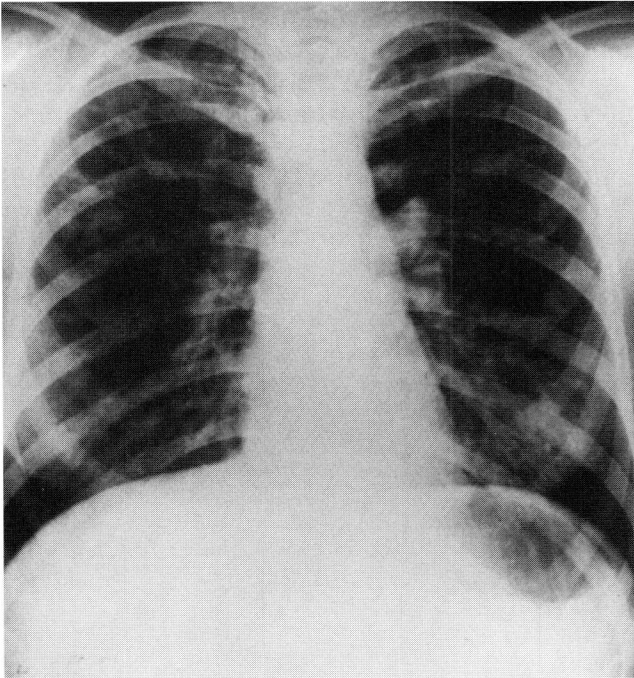

FIGURE 24–36. Cystic fibrosis in a 19-year-old man. The patient was maintained on pancreatic extract. He had severe recurrent pulmonary infections and occasionally required bronchoscopy for removal of inspissated mucus.

way for a number of therapies, including the real possibility of genetic alteration of the respiratory tract epithelial cells of CF patients (Gibaldi, 1993; Harris and Argent, 1993). Correction of the ion transport defect in CF transgenic mice by gene therapy has been reported (Hyde et al., 1993).

Recurrent pulmonary infection is always part of the clinical picture, creating pathologic cystic and fibrotic changes in the lung tissue (Rosenfeld and Ramsey, 1992). In the past, surgical intervention was almost always contraindicated except for tube thoracostomy for pneumothorax. Since 1990, the role of bilateral sequential lung transplantation for end-stage cystic disease has become well established in adults (Kaiser et al., 1991b) as well as children (Spray and Huddleston, 1992). Bilateral transplantation for CF is necessary because of the risk of infection from a contralateral native lung and is technically difficult (Armitage et al., 1993). Transplantation techniques are discussed in more detail in Chapter 57, Part III.

Congenital cystic adenomatoid malformation (CCAM) was first described by Ch'in and Tang in 1949. It accounts for 25% of congenital lung malformations, is usually symptomatic in the first days of life, and occasionally presents as a life-threatening emergency in the delivery suite. The essential feature of the predominantly unilateral lesion is an excessive overgrowth of terminal bronchiolar-type structures with a lack of mature alveoli. CCAM has many of the criteria of hamartoma, but cartilage is not present. Grossly, it resembles a large rubbery mass that can enlarge rapidly by air trapping in the cystic areas, causing acute

respiratory distress in the newborn period. Three morphologically distinct types have been described, all of which share histologic features.

There are two classifications. Bale (1979) has described three clinical presentations (Table 24–4). The term newborn or older infant presents with recurrent pulmonary infections; the lesion is primarily cystic, associated anomalies are rare, and the prognosis with surgical intervention is good. The near-term infant presenting with severe respiratory distress at birth usually has a mixed solid-cystic lesion, and surgical intervention frequently is necessary as an emergency. Other anomalies are rare as well. The premature infant with a predominantly solid mass does not survive after birth or is stillborn; other malformations are common.

According to the pathologic classification of Stocker and associates (1977), Type I lesions are characterized by multiple large cysts or occasionally a single large cyst surrounded by multiple smaller cysts (Fig. 24–37). A smooth, glistening membrane lines the cysts, which may be filled with air or fluid. Smooth muscle and connective tissue compose the wall, and the lining mucosa is columnar or pseudostratified and ciliated. The Type I lesion may occupy a portion of one lobe or more than one lobe. The degree of symptoms depends on the amount of lung involved, the size of the cysts, and the extent of bronchial-cyst communication. Mediastinal shift occurs in 75% of cases, and tachypnea, cyanosis, grunting, and sternal retractions can occur immediately after birth or can be delayed for weeks to months. When the onset of symptoms is delayed, the infant has difficulty feeding and repeated infections.

The Type II lesion is composed of multiple, evenly spaced cysts that rarely exceed 1.2 cm in diameter, filled with air and lined by a smooth to wrinkled, glistening membrane. The entire lesion may measure less than 1 cm in diameter, occupy an entire lobe, or rarely, occupy an entire lung. Mediastinal shift is unusual (12%). Microscopically, the cysts resemble dilated terminal bronchioles lined by ciliated columnar epithelium. There is a high incidence of stillbirths, fetal congenital anomalies, and early death with this type of CCAM.

The Type III lesion is a bulky, firm mass that usually encompasses an entire lobe, rarely with cysts larger than 0.5 cm in diameter. The size and weight of the lesion produce mediastinal shift in all cases. Well delineated from surrounding normal lung, the lesion is composed of lobules of adenomatoid hyperplasia or bronchial structures lined by tall epithelium. This type occurs most frequently in the left lower lobe, but it may occur in any lobe of the lung. Severe respiratory distress is apparent shortly after birth, with death from inadequate ventilation usually occurring within 1 to 5 hours. The arterial supply and venous drainage of all types of CCAM are usually via the normal pulmonary artery and vein to the involved lobe, although multiple cases with abnormal arterial and venous connections have been reported (Stocker et al., 1978).

■ Table 24–4. CLASSIFICATION OF CONGENITAL CYSTIC ADENOMATOID MALFORMATIONS*

Clinical Presentation (Bale)	Cystic Lesion	Intermediate Lesion	Solid (Adenomatoid) Lesion
Age	Term newborn or older	Infant	Stillborn or premature
Fetal anasarca/ascites			
Maternal polyhydramnios	None	±	Occasional
Other anomalies	Rare	Rare	Common
Gross appearance	Cystic; sometimes solid areas	Either or both	Solid; sometimes cystic areas
Histopathology			
Bronchiolar proliferation	+	Varying degrees	+ + +
Alveolar appearance	Mature; separating bronchiolar-type cysts		Immature
Mucoid epithelium/ cartilage	Occasional	Occasional	Common
Prognosis	Good	Good	Poor

Clinical Presentation (Stocker)	Type I Lesion	Type II Lesion	Type III Lesion
Age	Term, occasional stillborn	Stillborn or Premature	
Fetal anasarca/maternal polyhydramnios	Rare	Common	Common
Other anomalies	Rare	Common	None reported
Gross appearance	Single or multiple large cysts 2 cm diameter	Multiple, evenly spaced cysts; 1 cm diameter	Large mass, no or tiny cysts
Histopathology			
Bronchiolar proliferation	+	+ +	+ + +
Mucoid epithelium/ cartilage	Mucoid cells in 1/3 of cases; rare cartilage prominent bands of smooth muscle and elastic tissue	None	None
Cyst wall		Striated muscle in 5/16 of cases	
Prognosis	Good	Poor	Poor

* + to + + + indicates increasing proportion.
From Luck, S. R., Reynolds, M., and Raffensperger, J. G.: Congenital bronchopulmonary malformations. Curr. Probl. Surg., 23:245–314, 1986.

Most infants present with respiratory distress at birth or before 1 month of age. CCAM occurs as often in premature as in term infants, and antenatal diagnosis of CCAM by ultrasonography (Clark et al., 1987) permits efficient neonatal therapy when indicated, particularly in Bales' Group II patients. Radiographically, the Type I lesions vary from a unilateral, large, dilated cystic lesion to a solid, homogeneous mass. Mediastinal shift, pulmonary herniation, and inferior displacement of the hemidiaphragm with multiple spherical spaces of varying size are present. The cystic space may be filled with air or fluid; a partially or completely fluid-filled lesion can be seen as an air-fluid level or a homogeneous density, respectively, on chest film (Fig. 24–38). The Type II lesions demonstrate smaller cystic spaces in a nonhomogeneous mass, and the Type III lesions demonstrate a homogeneous mass filling the hemithorax. Both types vary as to degrees of mediastinal shift (Figs. 24–39 and 24–40).

The differential diagnosis includes ILE, multiple congenital cysts, and particularly congenital diaphragmatic hernia, because the multicystic lesion mimics gas-filled loops of bowel within the thorax. A barium swallow will differentiate these two. CT can be useful (Fig. 24–41) in differentiating among CCAM and ILE, bronchogenic cysts, and infectious conditions including bronchopleural fistula, particularly in children presenting beyond infancy (Shackelford and

Siegel, 1989). The MRI characteristics of CCAM in infants also have been described (Cohen et al., 1987).

Radiologic demonstration of this malformation is an indication for surgical removal. The appearance at surgery varies, and the lesion may grossly mimic ILE or a bronchogenic cyst. Classically, lobectomy is performed, and occasionally pneumonectomy is required (Fig. 24–42). Becker and associates (1987) have performed enucleation and segmental resection, and local resection for the Type III lesions has been described. However, because of the increased incidence of neoplasia associated with these lesions (Luck et al., 1986), lobectomy with complete resection of the entire lesion is advisable. If the diagnosis is not delayed, an excellent long-term result should be expected.

IPE is an acquired lesion characterized by gas in the interstitial tissue surrounding bronchovascular bundles and along interlobular septa. The incidence of IPE along with the accompanying complications of pneumothorax, pneumomediastinum, and ventilatory compromise has been reported to be 20% in infants with NRDS treated with intermittent positive pressure breathing and 40% in patients treated with positive end-expiratory pressure.

The incidence of IPE has increased with improvement in the survival of premature infants with NRDS, and the variable features of this disease have been described (Stocker and Madewell, 1977). Acute inter-

TYPE I   TYPE II   TYPE III

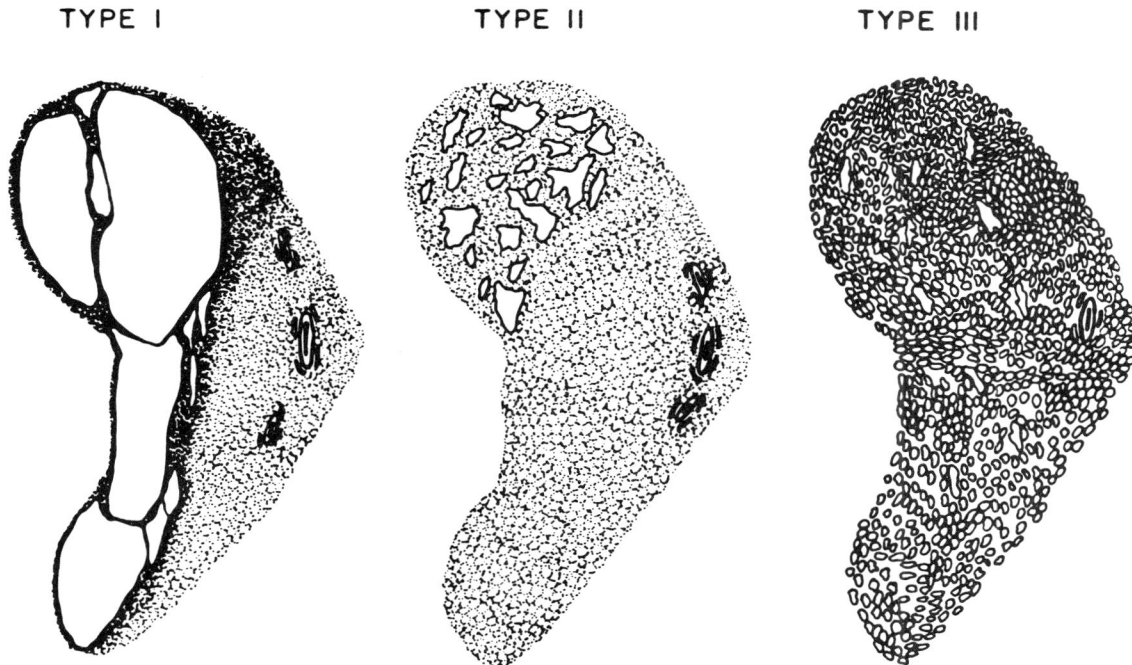

FIGURE 24–37. Classification of congenital cystic adenomatoid malformation (CCAM) Type I is composed of a small number of large cysts with thick smooth muscle and elastic tissue walls. Relatively normal alveoli are seen between and adjacent to these cysts. Mucous glands may be present. Type II contains numerous smaller cysts (<1 cm in diameter) with a thin muscular coat beneath the ciliated columnar epithelium. The area between the cysts is occupied by large alveolus-like structures. The lesion blends with the normal parenchyma. Type III occupies the entire lobe or lobes and consists of regularly spaced bronchiole-like structures separated by masses of cuboidal epithelium-lined alveolus-like structures. (From Stocker, J. T., Madewell, J. E., and Drake, R. M.: Congenital cystic adenomatoid malformation of the lung, classification and morphologic spectrum. Hum. Pathol., 8:155, 1977.)

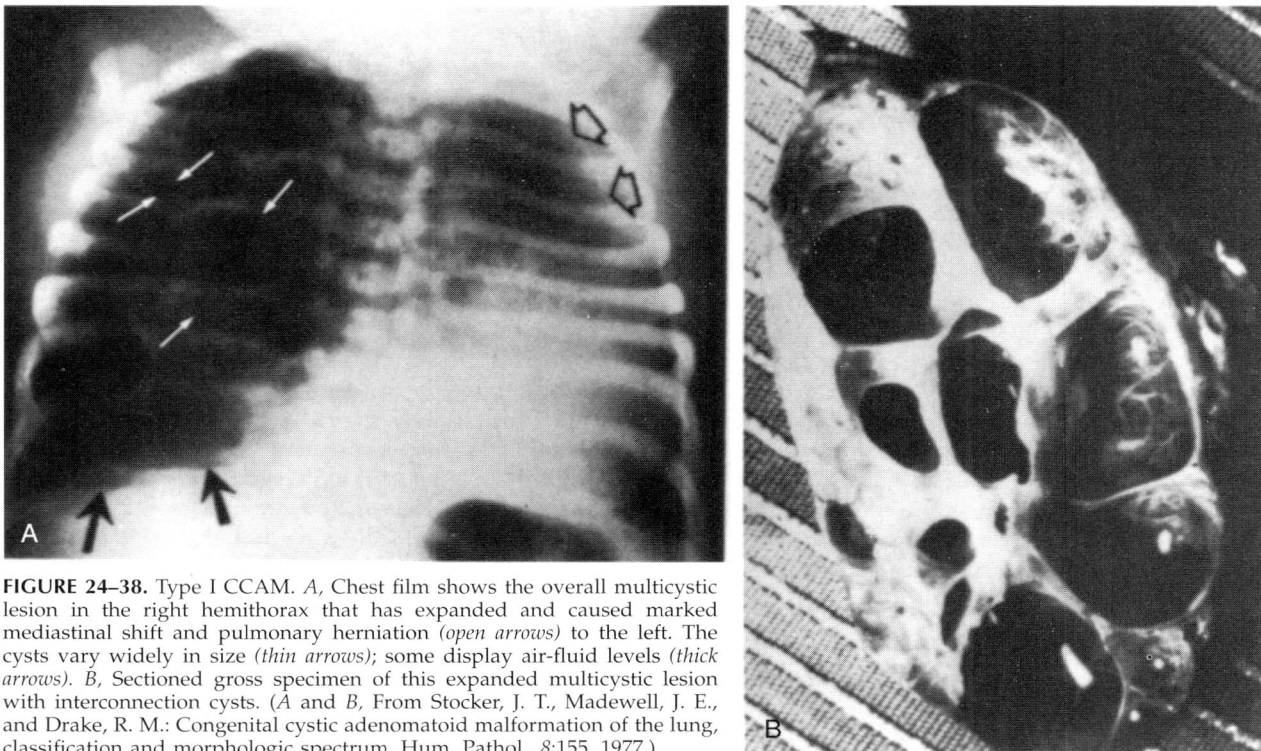

FIGURE 24–38. Type I CCAM. *A,* Chest film shows the overall multicystic lesion in the right hemithorax that has expanded and caused marked mediastinal shift and pulmonary herniation *(open arrows)* to the left. The cysts vary widely in size *(thin arrows)*; some display air-fluid levels *(thick arrows). B,* Sectioned gross specimen of this expanded multicystic lesion with interconnection cysts. *(A* and *B,* From Stocker, J. T., Madewell, J. E., and Drake, R. M.: Congenital cystic adenomatoid malformation of the lung, classification and morphologic spectrum. Hum. Pathol., 8:155, 1977.)

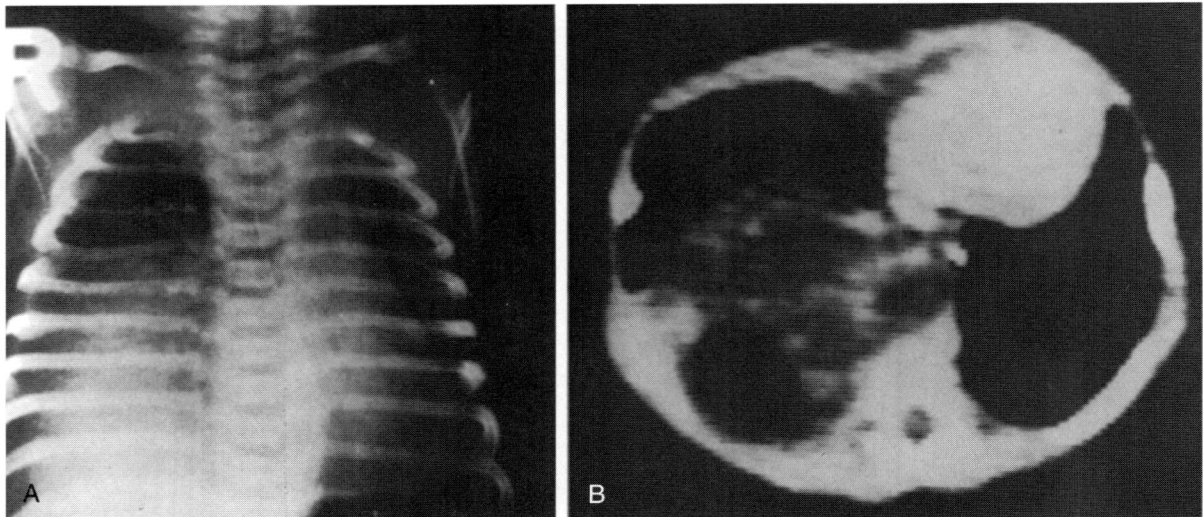

FIGURE 24–39. Type II CCAM. *A,* Chest film shows nearly homogeneous shadowing over 5 to 6 cm of the right middle and lower pulmonary fields. *B,* CT scan shows a nearly homogeneous multicystic lesion in the right hemithorax with some displacement of the mediastinum. A successful right middle and lower lobectomy was done. (*A* and *B,* From Becker, M. R., Schindera, F., and Maier, W. A.: Congenital cystic adenomatoid malformation of the lung. Prog. Pediatr. Surg., *21:*113, 1987.)

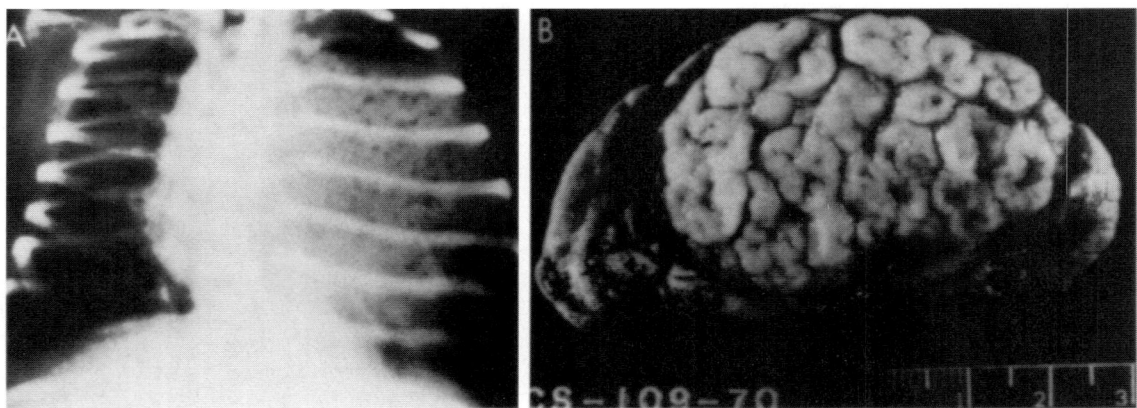

FIGURE 24–40. Type III CCAM. *A,* Chest film of a newborn male infant with respiratory distress. *B,* Gross specimen of transsected left upper lobe of lung removed as an emergency procedure. The lobulated tissue characteristic of Type III CCAM is sharply demarcated from normal lung. A similar smaller lesion was removed from the left lower lobe. (*A* and *B,* From Miller, R. K., Seiber, W. K., and Yunis, E. J.: Congenital adenomatoid malformation of the lung: A report of 17 cases and review of the literature. Pathol. Ann., *15:*387, 1980.)

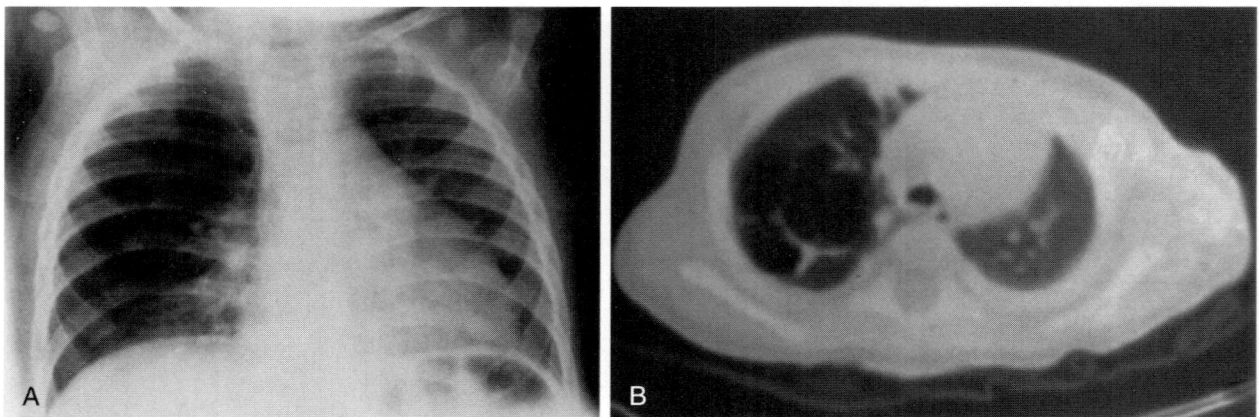

FIGURE 24–41. Cystic adenomatoid malformation of the right upper lobe in a 5-month-old girl. *A,* Anteroposterior chest film demonstrates a hyperinflated right upper lobe with large cystic areas. *B,* CT scan through the upper chest confirms the presence of a hyperinflated right upper lobe with large cysts separated by thin, well-defined walls. (*A* and *B,* From Shackelford, G. D., and Siegel, M. J.: CT appearance of cystic adenomatoid malformations. J. Comput. Assist. Tomogr., *13:*612–616, 1989.)

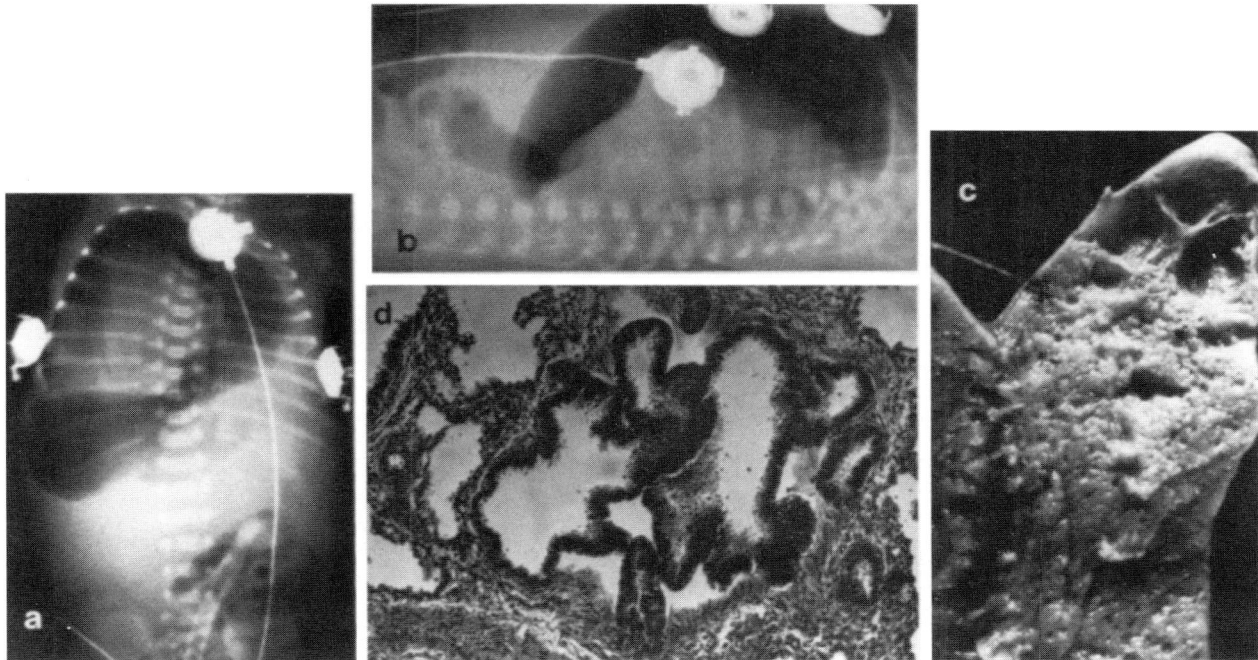

FIGURE 24–42. *a,* Anteroposterior supine chest film at 1 hour of life shows a dense homogeneous mass occupying the right lung, tracheal and mediastinal shift to the left where no aerated lung parenchyma is recognizable, a right tension pneumothorax extending almost to the left thoracic wall, and downward displacement of the right diaphragm. *b,* Cross-table lateral view shows extension of pneumothorax and downward displacement of the mass. *c,* Gross specimen cut surface shows abnormal, polymorphous lung tissue with solid and spongy areas. *d,* Microscopy shows cysts to be lined by ciliated columnar epithelium and interspersed alveolar-like structures. Some ciliated tall epithelial buds are present (CCAM Type II, H & E stain, × 125). (*a–d,* From Beluffi, Brokensha, C., Koslowski, K., et al.: Congenital cystic adenomatoid malformation of the lung. Fortschr. Rontgenstr., *150*:523–530, 1989.)

stitial pulmonary emphysema is seen in the first few days of life in infants with NRDS, pulmonary hypoplasia, diaphragmatic hernia, or anencephaly. The risk of pneumothorax is moderate, which may be beneficial inasmuch as the chest tube provides rapid evacuation of the pulmonary and parenchymal air. Symptoms may appear acutely or gradually, depending on the amount of entrapped interstitial air, which comes from rupture of the bases of overdistended alveoli. The development of IPE in infants with NRDS markedly worsens the prognosis of NRDS.

This acute type may persist and create localized small or large (3-cm) interstitial cysts with reactive giant cells along their walls. The cysts follow interlobular septa as far as the pleura, and the left upper lobe is most commonly involved. Most of these infants have a history of typical NRDS treated briefly with oxygen therapy and artificial ventilation, but they have little or no BPD. The radiographic features of localized persistent IPE may resemble those of CCAM and consist of an expanded multicystic lesion confined to one or more lobes, with mediastinal shift and depression of the hemidiaphragm. Diffuse persistent IPE that involves all lobes of both lungs may also occur, and the pathologic and clinical features of this form are often indistinguishable from those of BPD. All infants have had prolonged treatment with oxygen and ventilatory support for NRDS. Pneumothorax occurs in most of these patients, but mediastinal shift is unusual. The radiographic features include

diffuse multicystic changes within all lobes and stippling or streaking due to perivascular air (Unger et al., 1989).

In the babies who survive, the interstitial air will slowly be resorbed. Schneider and colleagues (1985) determined that persistent localized IPE was now the most common indication for pulmonary resection in the newborn period, ahead of ILE and CCAM, although less than 2% of infants with IPE in this series required operation. Indications for resection included the development of large discrete cystic areas that decreased effective lung volume and produced atelectasis, recurrent infections, or ventilator dependence (Fig. 24–43). The long-term outcome in these patients was generally good. Selective bronchial intubation has been useful as an alternative to surgical excision of the affected lobe in infants with localized acute ILE (Chan et al., 1992) and persistent IPE (Glenski et al., 1986). This technique did not help correct ILE or treat patients with histologic evidence of bronchopulmonary dysplasia.

BRONCHOPULMONARY FOREGUT MALFORMATIONS

Abnormalities in ventral foregut budding assume a wide variety of anatomic forms; although many classification schemes have been proposed, the terminology remains confusing. For the purposes of this

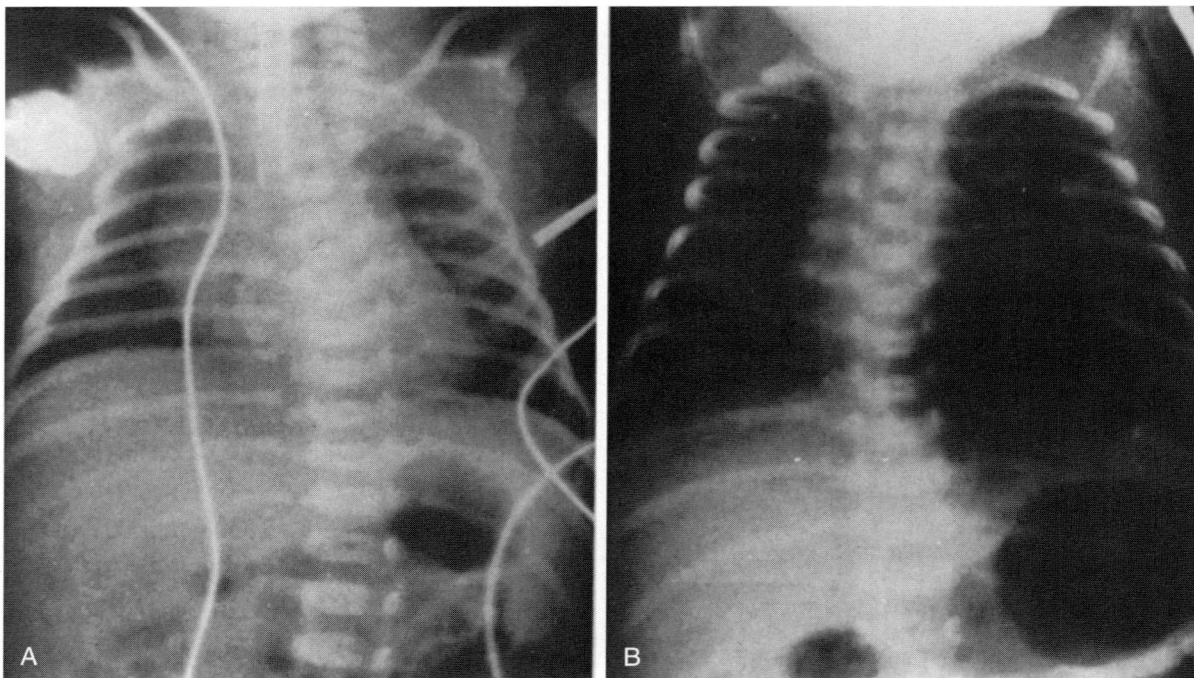

FIGURE 24–43. Pulmonary interstitial emphysema. *A,* Chest film taken shortly after admission is typical of respiratory distress syndrome. *B,* One month later, the chest film shows a large cyst with adjacent atelectasis of the left lower lobe. The child was successfully extubated but had multiple episodes of pneumonia and atelectasis. (*A* and *B,* From Schneider, J. R., St. Cyr, J. A., Thompson, T. R., et al.: The changing spectrum of cystic pulmonary lesions requiring surgical resection in infants. J. Thorac. Cardiovasc. Surg., *89*:332, 1985.)

discussion, the term *bronchopulmonary foregut malformation* (BPFM), originally proposed by Gerle and coworkers (1968), is used to group the following lesions together: *intralobar pulmonary sequestration* (ILS), *extralobar pulmonary sequestration* (ELS), bronchogenic cysts, and *communicating bronchopulmonary foregut malformation* (CBPFM).

No completely encompassing theory of embryogenesis can explain all the congenital lesions that have been reported (Fowler, 1988). Rodgers and associates (1986) have described these lesions as abnormalities of ventral foregut budding directly involving the pulmonary parenchyma and originating from either the tracheobronchial tree or the gastrointestinal tract. Embryogenesis of the pulmonary arterial supply as it replaces the primitive blood supply from the dorsal aorta, the degree of involution of the original communication to the foregut, and the timing of the occurrence of the malformation as the determinant of the presence of a separate pleural envelope would then be the three major developmental variables that determine the ultimate anatomic outcome of the malformations. This analysis modifies the unifying theory proposed by Heithoff and colleagues (1976). They suggested that bronchopulmonary foregut malformations occur when independent collections of cells with respiratory potential arise from the primitive esophagus caudal to the normal lung bud or when part of the lung bud originates from the dorsal esophagus instead of the ventral laryngotracheal tube. These cells evaginate into adjacent normally developed pulmonary tissue, initially connected to the parent viscus

by a pedicle. Involution of the pedicle occurs because of blood supply outgrowth, and a simple malformation occurs. If the pedicle fails to involute, the accessory lung freely communicates with the gastrointestinal tract, producing a CBPFM, usually between the distal esophagus and lung. If the accessory lung tissue arises before pleural development, it becomes invested in adjacent normal lung, producing an ILS. Later development, after the pleura has formed, produces a bud that grows separate from the adjacent lung and is invested in its own pleura—an ELS (Leithiser et al., 1986).

In contrast to this theory, Gebauer and Mason (1954) proposed that ILS is an acquired lesion, resulting from a primary pathologic process with coexisting hypertrophy of bronchial and mediastinal arteries. In support of Gebauer and Mason's theory, Stocker and Malczak (1984) hypothesized that in the presence of recurring bronchial obstruction and distal infection, pulmonary ligament arteries develop as collateral vessels to the infected segment as it becomes sequestered from the adjacent normal lung tissue, and that ILS is, at least in most cases, an acquired disease process (Stocker, 1986). An additional theory is that of Sade and associates (1974), who in a collective review proposed a sequestration spectrum, extending from normal lung with an anomalous vascular supply to abnormal lung with normal vascularity. Marks and Marks (1987) included bronchogenic cysts in this grouping, noting the presence of an abnormal systemic vascular supply to the cysts in their series. This grouping will be used in this discussion (Table 24–5).

Harris and Lewis (1940) first brought sequestrations to the attention of the thoracic surgeon when they reported fatal hemorrhage from the anomalous vessel during pulmonary resection. The clinical characteristics of ILS and ELS provide the most useful means of description. Table 24–5 describes the most common manifestations of sequestration lesions, although multiple variations have been reported.

ILS is defined as a segment of parenchyma, situated within the normal pleural investment but not connected to the tracheobronchial tree, that is supplied by the systemic circulation. In a review of 540 published cases of sequestration, Savic and associates (1979) found that ILS accounted for between 0.15 and 1.7% of all congenital anomalies. The lesion is slightly more common in males, and left-sided lesions predominate. Most important, in this series, the intrathoracic location was the lower lobe in 97.75% of the 400 cases of ILS. Most of these are located in the medial and posterior basilar segments. Associated congenital anomalies occur infrequently. ILS most often presents with symptoms in the adolescent or young adult, rarely in children, and virtually never in neonates. However, a recent report describes the prenatal diagnosis of an ILS lesion confirmed at thoracotomy on day 5 of extrauterine life (Maulik et al., 1987).

The clinical hallmark of ILS is repeated bouts of pulmonary infection with cough, sputum production, hemoptysis, and low-grade fever; infection is due to communication between the sequestered tissue and the bronchus that is either present initially or is later established from adjacent normal lung parenchyma. In virtually all cases of ILS, the histologic picture consists of a monocystic or polycystic area of parenchyma with extensive fibrosis, chronic inflammation, and vascular sclerosis. Gustafson and associates (1989) have emphasized the propensity for missing

this diagnosis in patients with repeated bouts of lower lobar pneumonia (Fig. 24–44).

The vascular supply in ILS is via a systemic artery. In the series of Savic and associates, this artery came off the thoracic aorta in 74%, off the abdominal aorta in 18.7%, and from the intercostals in 3.2% of cases. As mentioned, pulmonary ligament arteries have been identified as possible candidates for this aberrant arterial supply. Multiple arteries are present in up to 20% of cases, and vessels up to 2.5 cm in diameter have been reported, although most are less than 1 cm. Six cases of bilateral ILS have been reported, all of which had anomalous arteries supplying each side (Juettner et al., 1987). The venous return is usually via the pulmonary veins, although systemic drainage to the hemiazygos, azygos, cavae, and intercostal veins has been reported in 5% of cases (Alivizatos et al., 1985). Right-sided lesions may be associated with more severe anomalies of venous drainage; Collin and associates (1987) found an association between right-sided ILS and the scimitar syndrome, and they recommended that all patients with right-sided ILS undergo pulmonary arteriography to define the venous return before surgery.

The chest film in ILS usually demonstrates a mass or infiltrate in the lower lobe, usually in the medial or posterior basilar segment (Fig. 24–45). A cystic structure may be present with or without an air-fluid level. Bronchoscopy is of little benefit except to obtain aspirate for culture, and although a bronchial communication may exist, it seldom fills on bronchographic examination. Whether or not to perform routine aortography depends on the individual patient. CT with contrast enhancement has become the procedure of choice for diagnosis (Fig. 24–46). Multiple or anomalous vessels supplying or draining the sequestrum may be difficult to resolve by CT alone, however.

■ **Table 24–5.** BRONCHOPULMONARY FOREGUT MALFORMATIONS

Characteristics	ELS	ILS	CBPFM	Bronchogenic Cyst
Incidence	Rare	Uncommon	Rare	Uncommon
Sex predominance	4:1 M:F	1.5:1 M:F	1:1.5 M:F	1:1 M:F
Laterality	L > R	L > R	R > L	L = R
Pleural investment	Yes	No	Yes or no	No
Arterial supply	Systemic; rare pulmonary	Systemic	Systemic or pulmonary	Involuted
Venous drainage	Systemic	Pulmonary	Pulmonary or systemic	Involuted
Communication				
Bronchial	No	Yes	No	Possible
Foregut	No	No	Yes	Rare
Associated anomalies	> 50%	Rare	> 50%	Rare
Diaphragmatic hernia	30%	Isolated	18%	Isolated
Clinical aspects				
Age	Neonate	Adolescent, young adult	Infant	Infants; adolescent
Symptoms	Respiratory distress	Cough, fever	Cough, fever	Respiratory distress; fever
Radiograph	Triangular mass lesion	Lower lobe abscess	Increased density	Spherical mass; lucent or radiopaque
Pathology	Spongy, cystic	Abscess cavity	Varied; fistula tract epithelial lining	Varied; respiratory

Modified from Stocker, J. T., Drake, R. M., and Madewell, J. E.: Cystic and congenital lung disease in the newborn. Perspect. Pediatr. Radiol., 4:93, 1978.
M = male; F = female; L = left; R = right; ELS = extralobar sequestration; ILS = intralobar sequestration; CBPFM = communicating bronchopulmonary foregut malformation.

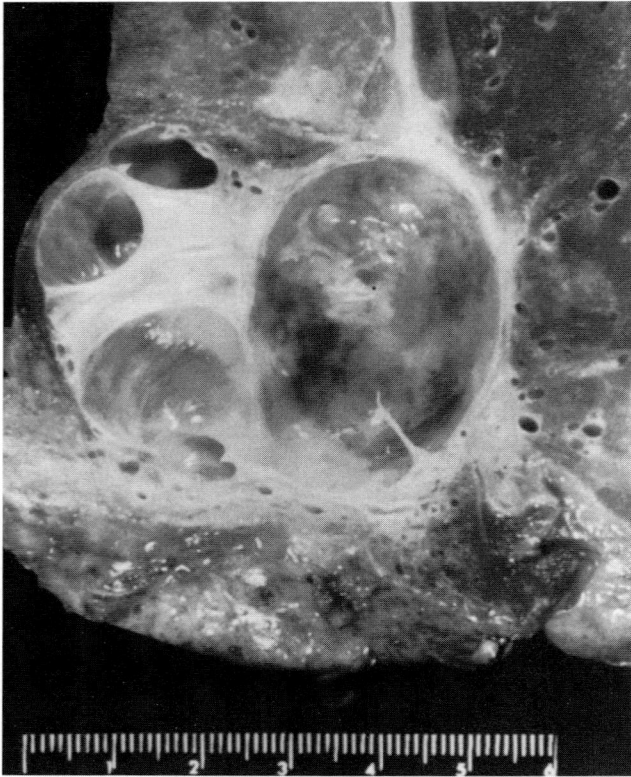

FIGURE 24–44. An intralobar sequestration is a multicystic mass of nonfunctioning lung tissue that is partly surrounded by normal lung and contained within the visceral pleura. Mucous secretion in obstructed bronchioles and alveolar tissue results in multiple cysts, which compress surrounding lung, causing atelectasis. (From Gustafson, R. A., Murray, E. F., Warden, H. E., et al.: Intralobar sequestration: A missed diagnosis. Ann. Thorac. Surg., 47:841–847, 1989. Reprinted with permission from the Society of Thoracic Surgeons [The Annals of Thoracic Surgery, 1989, Vol. 47, 841–849].)

MRI has been demonstrated to delineate intralobar sequestration with systemic arterial supply in a number of cases and has the advantage of not requiring contrast dye (Cohen et al., 1987) (Fig. 24–47). Most authors have advocated radiographic evaluation of the upper gastrointestinal tract in patients with ILS to rule out the possibility of communication with the esophagus or stomach (Haller et al., 1979).

Surgical treatment of ILS is recommended in all cases. In symptomatic patients, lobectomy is the procedure of choice because of the accompanying inflammatory response (see Fig. 24–44). When performing any type of resection for inflammatory disease in a child or young adult, surgeons must consider the possibility of ILS as well as potential communication with the gastrointestinal tract. The operation should be done in the quiescent stage with appropriate antibiotic coverage. In patients not infected, early planned surgical resection is the treatment of choice, and usually a more conservative (segmental) resection can be performed. Simple ligation of the arterial supply has been attempted with limited success. Appropriate caution with respect to additional congenital anomalies should accompany resection in young children. Accidental transection of the

anomalous artery can be disastrous, because it can lead to retraction to an inaccessible point within the mediastinum or below the diaphragm. White and associates (1974) first called attention to the possibility of heart failure resulting from a large left-to-right shunt through the sequestrum in a patient with an ILS, and surgical therapy was curative. Finally, resection has been recommended to prevent the long-term infectious and neoplastic changes that may occur in these lesions. Superinfection with tuberculosis and aspergillosis, as well as bronchial carcinoid and bronchogenic squamous cell carcinoma, have been reported to occur in an ILS (Juettner et al., 1985). Excellent results in children and adults can be expected with proper management (Bailey et al., 1990; Gustafson et al., 1989).

ELS is a segment of lung tissue with a distinct pleural investment and complete anatomic and physiologic separation from the normal lung. It is clearly a congenital lesion (Stocker, 1986). This form of sequestration occurs one-third to one-sixth as commonly as the intralobar form (Stocker and Malczak, 1984). In the review by Savic and co-workers (1979), 77.4% of the 133 cases of ELS collected were located between the diaphragm and the lower lobe. By virtue of its complete pleural investment, the extralobar form resides as a separate lobe within the pleural cavity, often attached to parts of the mediastinum or the diaphragm by a stalk that contains the bundle of vessels, nerves, and blindly ending bronchi. ELS occurs at least twice as often in the left thorax as in the right, and it predominates in males. In contrast with

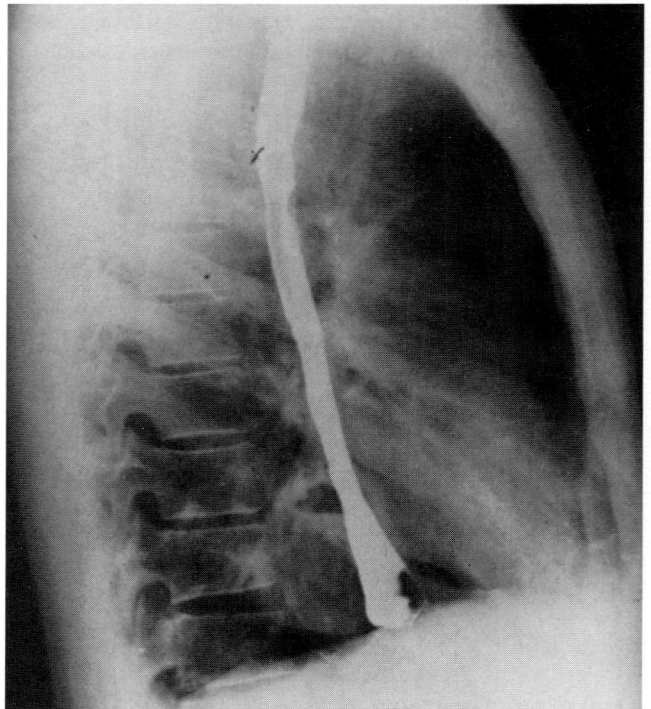

FIGURE 24–45. Intralobar pulmonary sequestration (ILS). The lesion was retrocardiac in the right lower lobe and barely discernible on the posteroanterior x-ray projection. The patient had protracted symptoms typical of lung abscess.

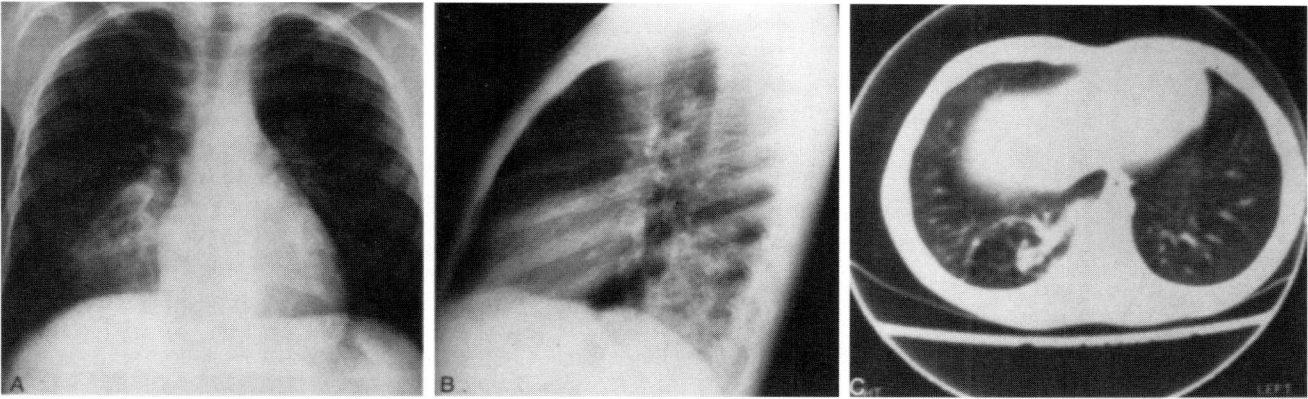

FIGURE 24–46. ILS diagnosed by CT scanning. *A* and *B,* Posteroanterior and lateral views of the chest show inflammation in the right posterior basilar segment. *C,* CT scan shows anomalous vessel that arises from the mediastinum and courses posteriorly into the right lower lobe.

ILS, other congenital abnormalities are present in over 50% of patients with ELS, including congenital diaphragmatic hernia (30%), other diaphragmatic lesions, other lung anomalies, and congenital heart defects.

In the series of Savic and colleagues, the arterial supply to the ELS was most often from the thoracic or abdominal aorta. The sequestration was supplied by a branch of the pulmonary artery in 5.5% of their cases, however, and in several isolated cases from subdiaphragmatic systemic vessels. In general, the artery enters the pulmonary parenchyrna near the draining vein and is much smaller than in ILS, ranging from 1 to 12 mm in diameter. Venous drainage usually is systemic to the azygous or hemiazygous systems, but in approximately 20% of cases drainage is to the pulmonary veins (Stocker et al., 1978).

The clinical presentation of patients with ELS is quite different from that of the intralobar form. Most cases are seen within the first few months of the patient's life, because large sequestered segments cause respiratory distress in the neonate or infant (Leijala and Louhimo, 1987). ELS is commonly found in newborn infants at the time of repair of diaphrag-

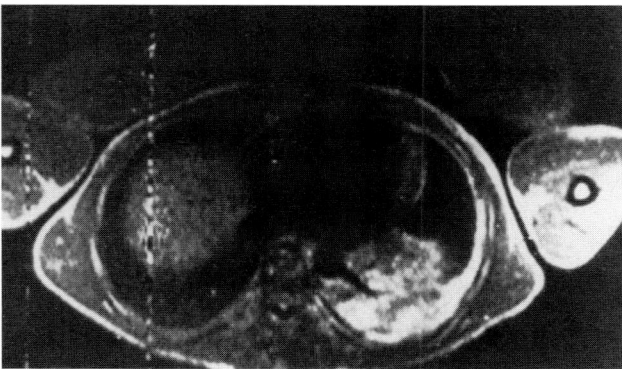

FIGURE 24–47. Magnetic resonance imaging (MRI) scan of the chest in an axial plane shows the origin of the ILS's arterial supply from the descending aorta. (From Oliphant, L., McFadden, R. G., Carr, T. J., and MacKenzie, D. A.: Magnetic resonance imaging to diagnose intralobar pulmonary sequestration. Chest, *87*:500, 1987.)

matic hernia (Fig. 24–48). Fifteen per cent of patients are asymptomatic, however, in these cases, detection is by chest film. Symptoms may also be related to the associated congenital anomalies. Congestive heart failure as a presenting symptom in infants in the absence of congenital cardiac disease has been reported (Levine et al., 1982).

On chest film, ELS presents as a homogeneous radiodense mass of lung tissue with no connection to the tracheobronchial tree. It is characteristically triangular, with the apex of the wedge pointing toward the hilum (Fig. 24–49). Loculated effusion and empyema are easily ruled out by clinical evaluation and, if necessary, thoracentesis. Bronchoscopy and bronochography are usually not helpful; CT can localize the lesion in the hemithorax, but often the supplying vessels are too small to warrant contrast injection or aortography. Most authors feel that other diagnostic procedures are not required, because the lesion is an undiagnosed mass within the chest, and surgical removal should be recommended. Some authors are comfortable with observation in asymptomatic younger patients, provided that radiologic and biochemical examination definitely rule out neuroblastoma (Luck et al., 1986).

During surgery, the entire sequestered lobe, along with its pleural investment, should be removed (Collin et al., 1987). Care must be taken to look for the characteristically small stalk of the sequestrum and securely ligate the anomalous vascular supply. Although infection is uncommon, tuberculous changes have been reported in the pulmonary parenchyma of resected specimens, along with one case of a keratinizing squamous cell carcinoma (Savic et al., 1979). On gross examination, the lesion is a mass of loose, spongy-to-solid tissue with numerous cystic spaces (Fig. 24–50). There is no communication with the normal bronchial tree. Histologic examination shows normal lung elements in an abnormal and disorderly arrangement; dilated bronchioles and alveolar ducts compose the bulk of the lesion. Numerous small cysts contain clear fluid.

As mentioned, bronchogenic cysts have been in-

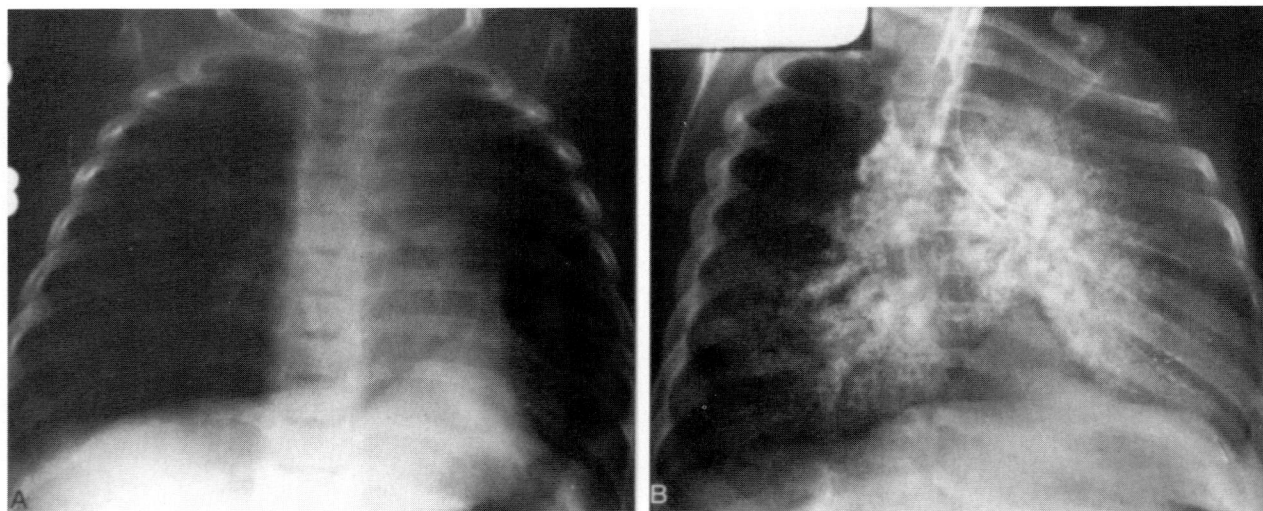

FIGURE 24–48. *A,* Extralobar sequestration (ELS) associated with congenital diaphragmatic hernia. The lesion was triangular, with a feeder vessel from the aorta below the diaphragm. There was a diaphragmatic defect in the posterolateral quadrant with colon present in the lower chest. *B,* Oblique view after instillation of contrast material in tracheobronchial tree. Note the delineation of sequestration.

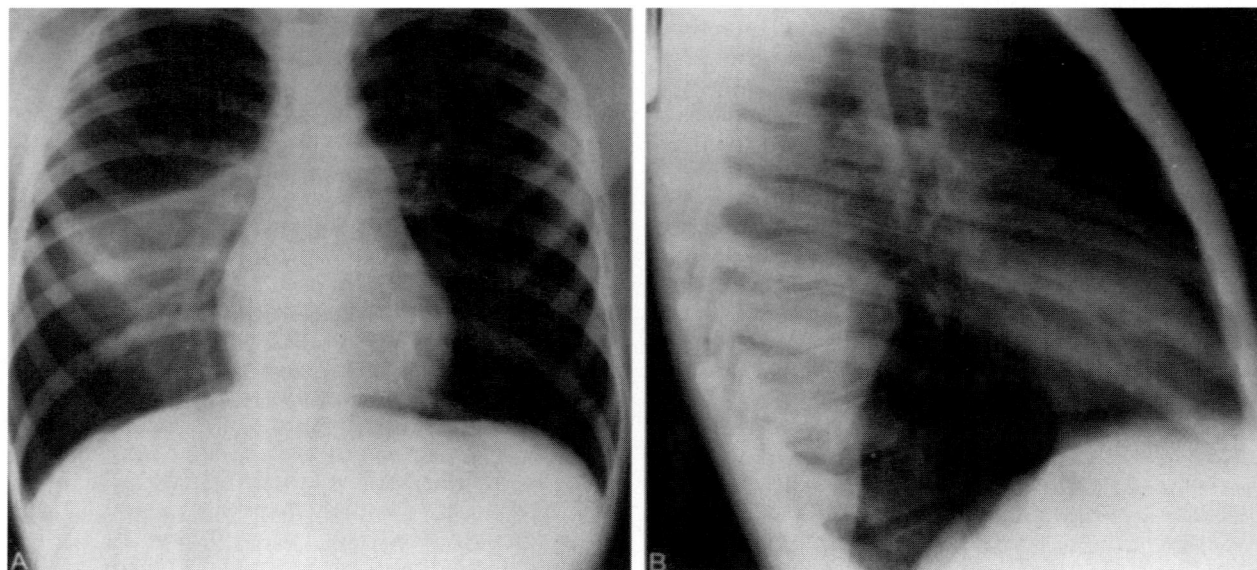

FIGURE 24–49. *A,* ELS in an asymptomatic 8-year-old boy. The only attachment was through a small stalk at the hilum of the lobe. *B,* Lateral view. The resected pathologic specimen of this lesion is seen in Figure 24–50.

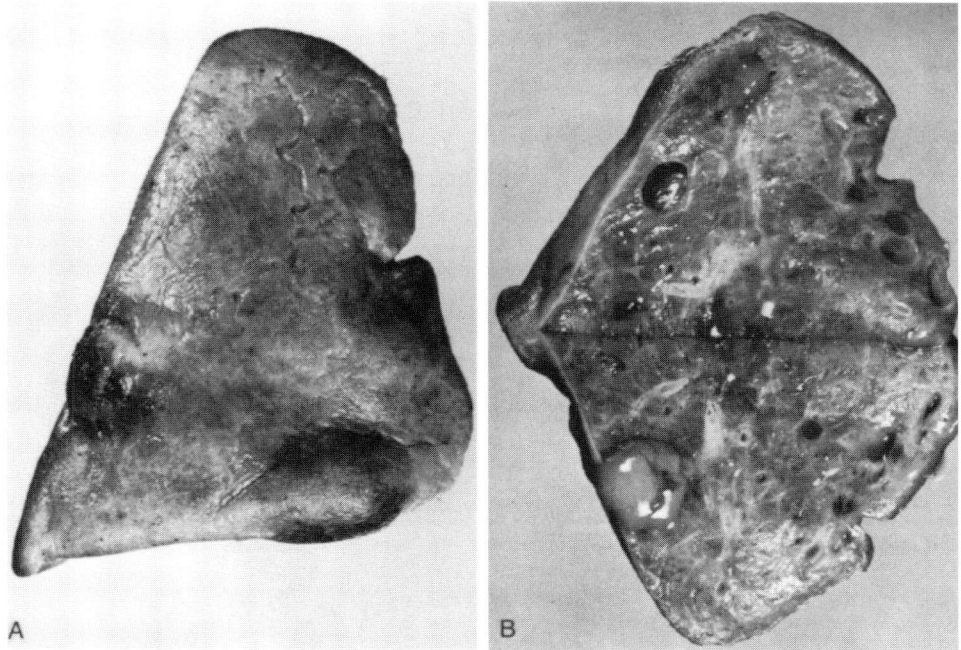

FIGURE 24–50. *A,* Gross specimen of the ELS seen in Figure 24–49. *B,* Cut surface of the lobe.

cluded in the spectrum of bronchopulmonary foregut malformations (Rodgers et al., 1986) as well as of lung bud anomalies (Haller et al., 1979). These cysts are thought to result from aberrant budding from the primitive foregut or budding off the tracheobronchical tree after it has arisen as a diverticulum from the foregut (DuMontia et al., 1985). Maier successfully resected a bronchogenic cyst in 1948 and classified them by location in the thorax and mediastinum: *paratracheal,* especially on the right side, attached to the tracheal wall above the carina; *carinal,* attached to the carina and often to the anterior esophageal wall; *hilar,* attached to one of the main lobar bronchi and thus intrapulmonary; and *paraesophageal,* without attachment to the bronchial tree but possibly attached to or communicating with the esophagus. They have also been reported within the diaphragm, presternal tissues, pericardium, skin, and subcutaneous tissues, extending from the mediastinum through the diaphragm into the abdomen, and below the diaphragm (Coselli et al., 1987). The cysts are generally round or oval, between 2 and 10 cm in diameter, and unilocular. Wall thickness of the single cavity varies from thin to moderately thick, composed of fibrous tissue interspersed with normal bronchial elements—that is, smooth muscle, elastic tissue, and cartilage (Fig. 24–51). The lining is generally smooth and most often composed of pseudostratified ciliated columnar epithelium. Although they are closely attached to major airways or the esophagus by dense fibrous tissue, the cysts usually demonstrate no patent communication with the airway. The typical noninfected cyst contains clear mucus; occasionally the fluid is whitish or contains blood. If communication with the bronchus is present, the cyst may become infected; the finding of smooth muscle and cartilaginous elements in the cyst

wall differentiates an infected cyst from pyogenic lung abscess.

The clinical presentation depends on the location of the cyst. The most common symptoms of bronchogenic cyst in the newborn are periodic episodes of progressive dyspnea, wheezing, stridor, and cyanosis. It is thought that obstructive symptoms occur most often in infants less than 1 year of age when the tracheobronchial tree is easily compressible. Cysts in the paratracheal, carinal, and hilar regions tend to be asymptomatic. The right side is more often affected than the left, and cysts are more common in males. If the patient is asymptomatic, the diagnosis is usually made by finding a solitary lung shadow on chest film (Fig. 24–52). Communicating cysts are almost always symptomatic, although cough, fever, sputum production, and hemoptysis may be present. The chest film shows a cystic structure with an air-fluid level (Fig. 24–53). There may be pericystic pneumonitis.

Other symptoms, especially in older children and adults, may be present. Worsnop and co-workers (1993) reported unilateral pulmonary artery obstruction due to a mediastinal cyst, and Volpi and associates (1988) reported a patient with paroxysmal atrial fibrillation due to left atrial compression by a mediastinal cyst.

The usual radiographic finding in a bronchogenic cyst is of a homogeneous water-density mass with borders that are sharply delineated unless obscured by other mediastinal structures. Barium swallow and bronchography may be useful, especially in cysts with open communications. CT has become the diagnostic modality of choice, delineating the density and anatomic relationships of the mass (Rodgers et al., 1986) (Fig. 24–54). Most bronchogenic cysts have a low CT number (0 to 20 Hounsfield units), but occasionally

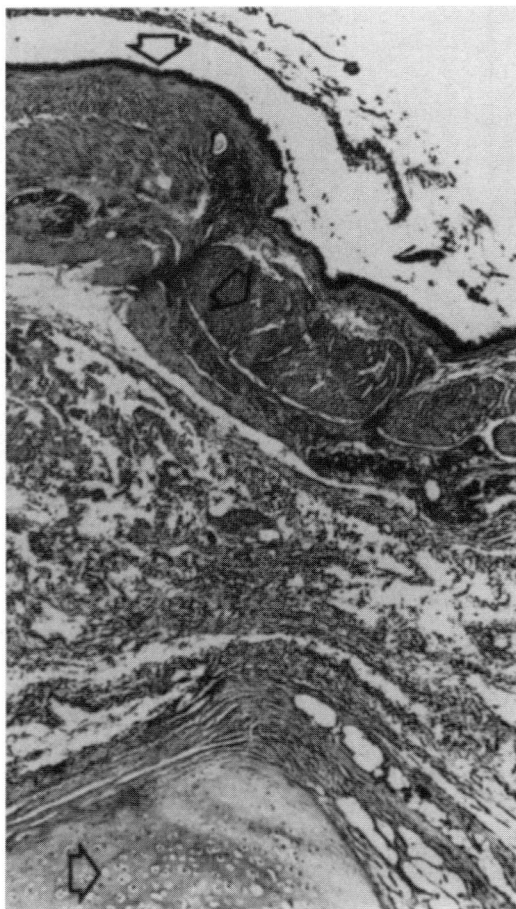

FIGURE 24–51. Photomicrograph of the wall of a bronchogenic cyst showing respiratory epithelium *(vertical arrow)*, smooth muscle *(oblique arrow)*, and cartilage *(horizontal arrow)*. (H & E, × 30.) (From Dhamash, N. S., Chen, J. T. T., Ravin, C. E., et al.: Unusual radiologic manifestations of bronchogenic cysts. Reprinted by permission from the Southern Medical Journal. Vol. 77, pp. 762–764, 1984.)

the cysts contain turbid mucoid fluid resulting in high CT numbers and may appear solid. Others have reported on the MRI characteristics of bronchogenic cysts and other intrathoracic pediatric abnormalities (Marin et al., 1991; Nakata et al., 1993).

The differential diagnosis includes lymphadenopathy from infectious or neoplastic causes, cysts of foregut or pericardial origin, pulmonary sequestration, and various tumors: teratoma, hemangioma, lipoma, hamartoma, and neurogenic tumors. In a compilation of 706 mediastinal lesions in children, 8% were bronchogenic cysts (Davis et al., 1990). Ravitch (1986) has classified mediastinal cysts of foregut origin into three groups: bronchogenic (55 to 65%), enteric (15 to 30%), and esophageal (10 to 15%). Enteric cysts, also called enterogenous cysts or esophageal duplications, occur in the posterior mediastinum and are closely associated with the esophagus. They ordinarily do not communicate with the alimentary tract but enlarge with fluid secreted from the lining secretory epithelium and cause symptoms in infancy or early childhood.

Enteric cysts occur twice as often on the right side, and peptic ulceration can occur in those lined by gastric mucosa. Esophageal cysts are frequently intramural but contain a ciliated epithelial lining, cartilage in the wall, and no intestinal mucosa.

The proper therapy for bronchogenic cysts is surgical excision. Complete extirpation with ligation of the point of attachment to the parent bronchus is usually possible. If cysts have adhered to intrathoracic structures, partial excision or segmentectomy may be necessary (Sirivella et al., 1985). Removal of the asymptomatic cyst is justified to establish the diagnosis and to avoid the possible complications of secondary bronchial communication, hemorrhage, or perforation into the pleural space. In addition, there are reports of carcinomas and fibrosarcomas arising in benign-appearing bronchogenic cysts (Wesley et al., 1986). Secondarily infected cysts should be treated as pulmonary abscesses are. In infants with respiratory compromise, surgical resection of the cyst may be lifesaving. The prognosis following surgical excision is excellent in all age groups (Coselli et al., 1987).

Other, less invasive surgical techniques have been attempted. Asymptomatic subcarinal bronchogenic cysts have been diagnosed and treated using transbronchial needle aspiration (Schwartz et al., 1986). More recently, use of *video-assisted thoracoscopic surgery* (VATS) for management of bronchogenic cysts has been advocated (Rogers et al., 1993) (Fig. 24–55).

Three large series of bronchogenic cysts are of interest. Suen and associates (1993) reported on a 30-year experience involving 42 patients; MRI was able to provide specific diagnostic information in more recent cases. Complete excision was recommended in most instances to prevent complications, confirm the diagnosis, and relieve symptoms. In the pediatric series reported by Di Lorenzo and co-workers (1989), most cysts were in the mediastinum near the trachea, esophagus, or pericardium. Finally, the clinical spectrum of bronchogenic cysts in adults was emphasized by St.-Georges and colleagues (1991). Of their 86 patients, 82% had a cyst that was symptomatic or complicated or both; in the symptomatic adult patient, surgical resection is more difficult because of complicating anatomic factors.

Communicating bronchopulmonary foregut malformations are defined by Stocker and associates (1978) as segments of extralobar or intralobar sequestered tissue that communicate with the alimentary tract. A patent fistula between the foregut and extralobar sequestrations occurs in about 10% of cases (fewer in intralobar sequestrations); these most often communicate with the distal esophagus or stomach, but they can occur anywhere. Location, pleural investment, and blood supply are not consistent in these communicating anomalies. Approximately 30% of these lesions arise from evagination of pulmonary tissue into the right hemithorax and are associated with agenesis or hypoplasia of the right lung; another third are formed by evagination into the left lower lobe. The timing of evagination determines whether the lesion is enveloped by its own separate pleura.

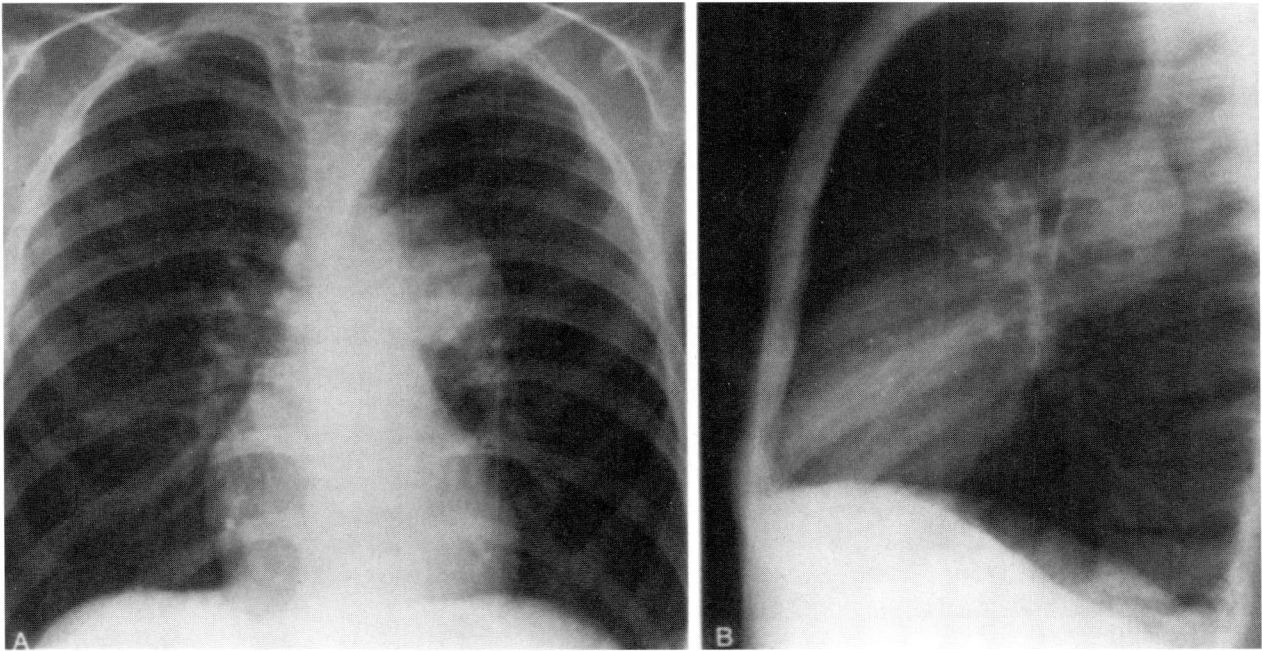

FIGURE 24–52. *A,* Bronchogenic cyst in an asymptomatic 13-year-old boy. The cyst was attached to the left mainstem bronchus but did not communicate. *B,* Lateral view of lesion.

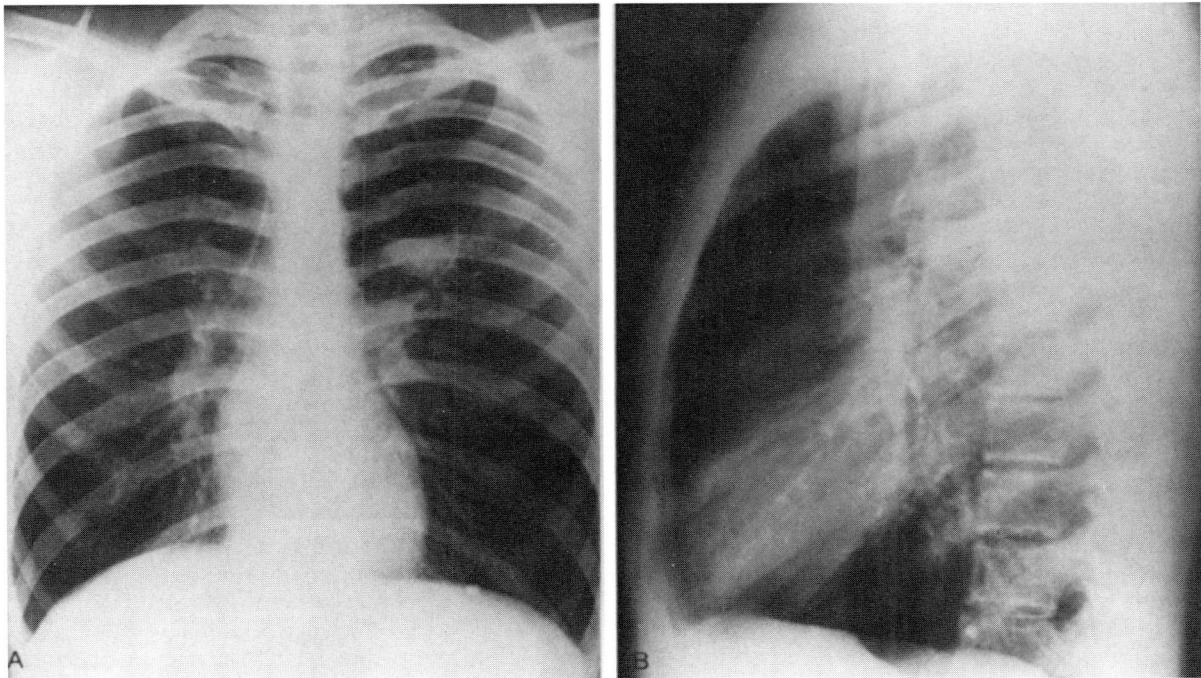

FIGURE 24–53. *A,* Infected bronchogenic cyst. The patient had recurrent fever and productive cough. Operation revealed a communication between the cyst and the left mainstem bronchus. *B,* Lateral view of lesion.

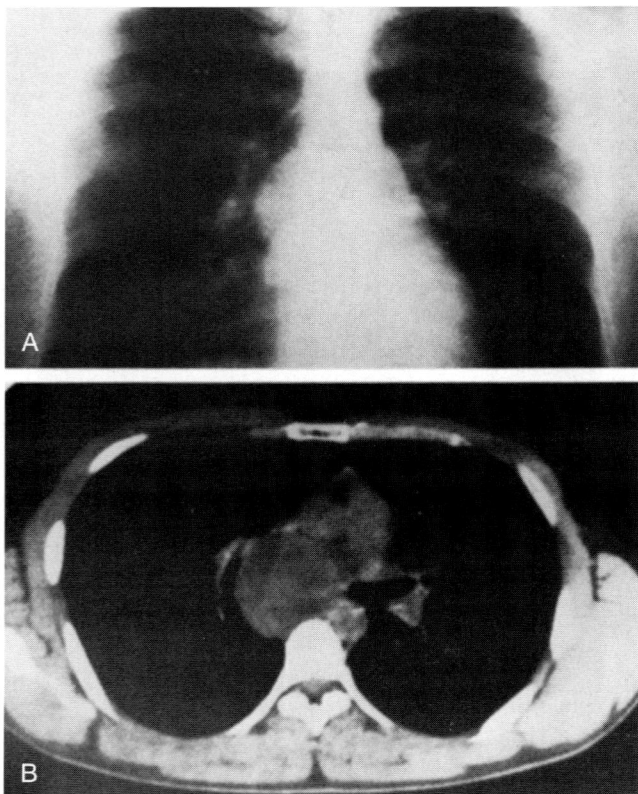

FIGURE 24-54. Chest film *(A)* and CT scan *(B)* of a fluid-density subcarinal bronchogenic cyst displacing and compressing the right mainstem bronchus and intermediate bronchus. *(A* and *B,* From Schwartz, A. R., Fishman, E. K., and Wang, K. P.: Diagnosis and treatment of a bronchogenic cyst using transbronchial needle aspiration. Thorax, *41*:326, 1986.)

Most lesions are supplied by a systemic arterial source, but pulmonary arterial supply can occur. Venous drainage can be either pulmonary or systemic (Leithiser et al., 1986). Twenty to 40% of children with a CBPFM have associated anomalies of the ribs and vertebrae; additional associated anomalies include diaphragmatic hernia, duodenal stenosis or atresia, congenital cardiac lesions, and genitourinary lesions.

The gross appearance of CBPFM depends on whether the involved lung tissue is extralobar or intralobar. Communication with the foregut is usually tubular, resembling a bronchus and containing creamy mucoid material (Stocker et al., 1978). The fistula tract often shows transition of esophageal to bronchial mucosa; rarely, gastric mucosa is present. In the absence of infection, the parenchyma resembles normal atelectatic lung or ELS; if infection has occurred, signs of chronic inflammation are present.

The clinical presentation of most infants with CBPFM is respiratory distress, exacerbated during feedings (Leithiser et al., 1986). Presentation before 8 months of age is common, and the lesion is more common in females. In the older child, chronic and recurrent pneumonia, cough, and hemoptysis can occur. Radiographic findings on plain film may include persistent alveolar densities, hypoplasia, or atelectasis. A "soap-bubble" pattern of cystic or tubular lucencies within the lung, representing air in the fistula tract, may be seen. Additional diagnostic studies include a contrast study of the esophagus with barium or bronchographic contrast medium; most authors consider this study necessary whenever a diagnosis

of generic bronchopulmonary foregut malformation is entertained (Heithoff et al., 1976). Bronchography and aortography may be necessary for diagnosis (Fig. 24-56).

Hruban and associates (1989) have emphasized the broad clinical, radiologic, and pathologic spectra of these lesions (Fig. 24-57). Bronchogenic cysts in abnormal locations can also communicate with the foregut, emphasizing their embryologic derivation (Braffman et al., 1988). The treatment of choice is surgical removal of the involved lung tissue, depending on the type of pulmonary involvement, and closure/removal of the fistulous communication (Hruban et al., 1989). A careful surgical approach, similar to that used for intralobar and extralobar sequestrations without foregut communication, is needed for these lesions.

VASCULAR ABNORMALITIES

Despite the complex embryology of the pulmonary arterial and venous systems, congenital vascular abnormalities are relatively rare. They may be grouped into abnormalities of arterial structures, venous structures, or both; the lesions may or may not involve the pulmonary parenchyma (Clements and Warner, 1987).

Proximal and distal pulmonary artery stenosis or atresia falls within the spectrum of congenital heart disease, and is discussed in Chapter 41. Unilateral absence of a main pulmonary artery is a rare anomaly as an isolated lesion; more often, it occurs in associa-

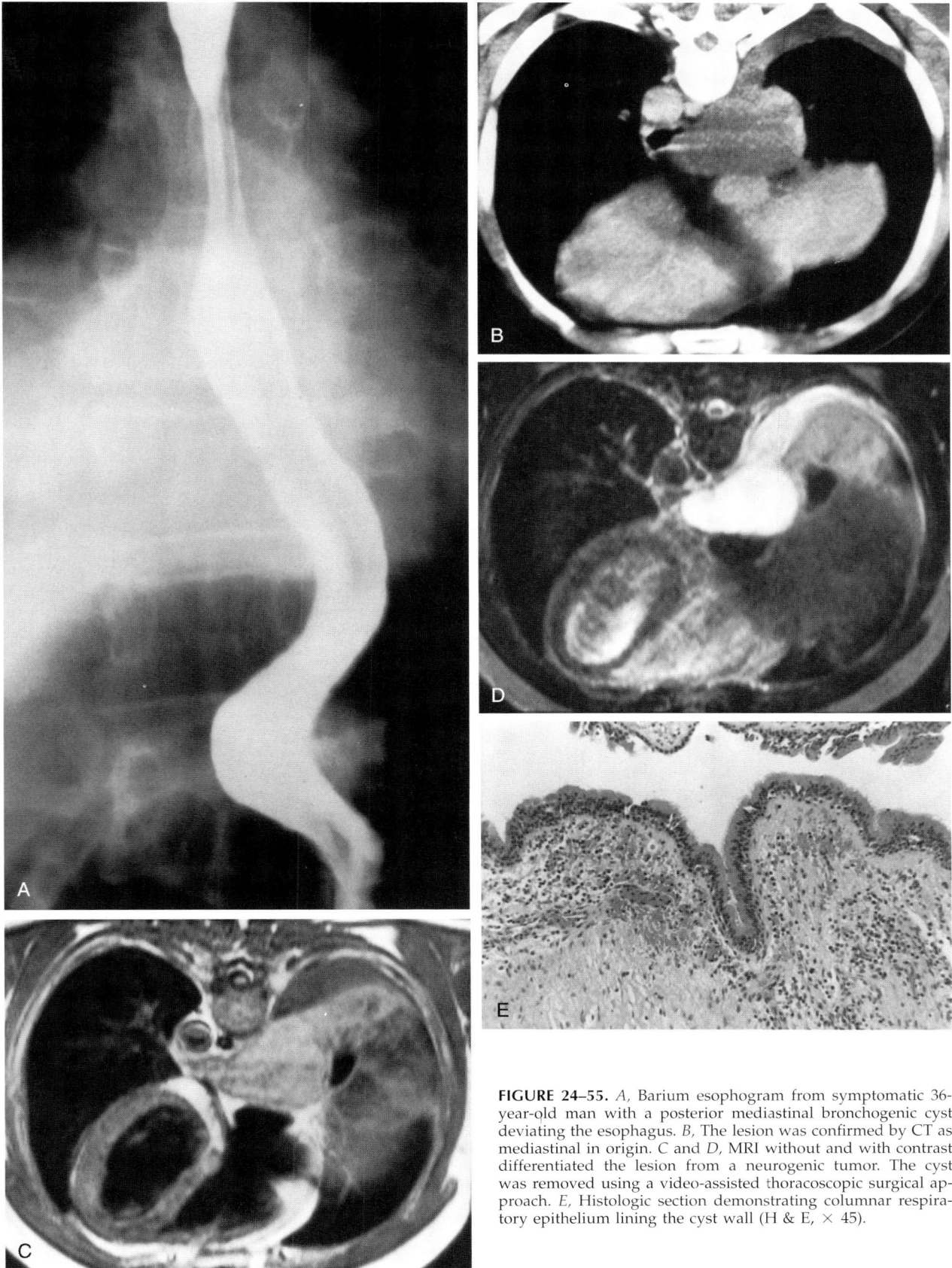

FIGURE 24–55. *A*, Barium esophogram from symptomatic 36-year-old man with a posterior mediastinal bronchogenic cyst deviating the esophagus. *B*, The lesion was confirmed by CT as mediastinal in origin. *C* and *D*, MRI without and with contrast differentiated the lesion from a neurogenic tumor. The cyst was removed using a video-assisted thoracoscopic surgical approach. *E*, Histologic section demonstrating columnar respiratory epithelium lining the cyst wall (H & E, × 45).

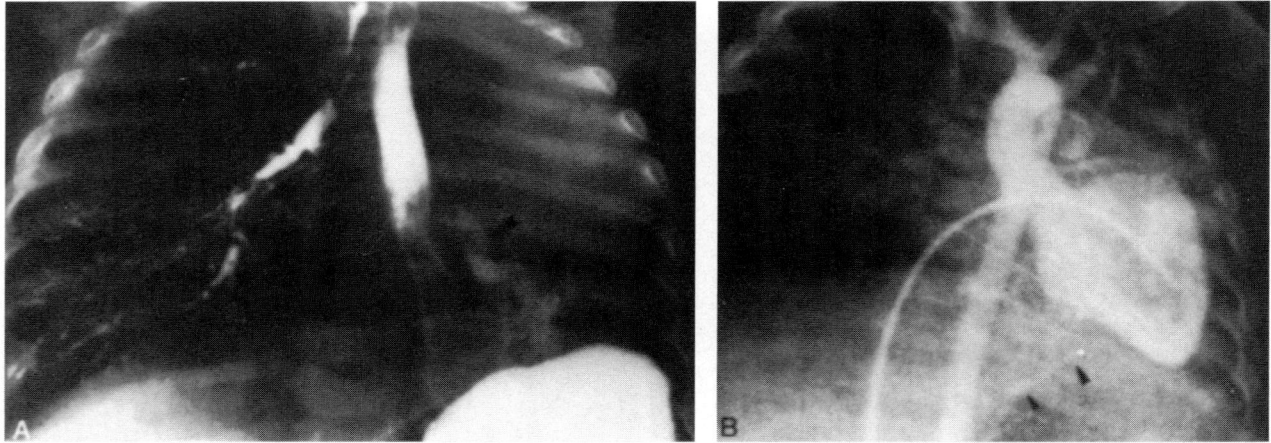

FIGURE 24–56. Communicating bronchopulmonary foregut malformation. *A,* Simultaneous esophagram and bronchogram. Left main bronchus *(arrowhead)* arises from the esophagus and not from the trachea. *B,* Left ventriculogram shows aberrant artery arising from aorta *(arrowheads)* to supply the "left lung." (*A* and *B,* From Leithiser, R. E., Capitanio, M. A., Macpherson, R. I., and Wood, B. P.: "Communicating" bronchopulmonary foregut malformations. A. J. R., Vol *146.* pp. 227–231, 1986. Copyright by Williams & Wilkins Company.)

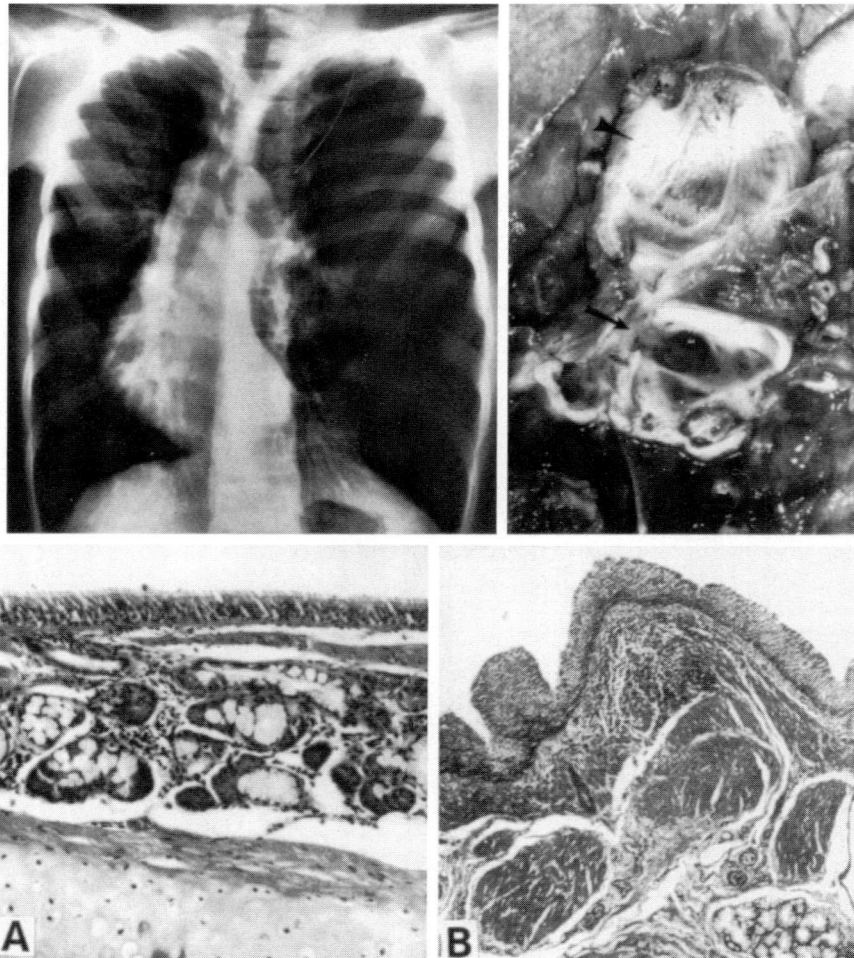

FIGURE 24–57. *Upper Left,* PA chest film shows significant hyperinflation of the left upper lobe, atelectasis of the left lower lobe, and a shift of the heart and mediastinum to the right. *Upper right,* Examination of the resected specimen in case 1 revealed a cystic mass *(arrow)* within the parenchyma of the emphysematous lobe. The cystic mass was lined by cartilage and communicated with a small tubular segment *(arrowhead).* The gross appearance of the tubular segment was similar to that of the esophagus. Histologically, the cystic mass was lined by cartilage covered with respiratory epithelium *(A),* whereas the tubular structure *(B)* was lined by smooth muscle covered with squamous epithelium. (*A,* H & E, × 170; *B,* H & E, × 65.) (*Top* and *A* and *B,* From Hruban, R. H., Shumway, S. J., Orel, S. B., et al.: Congenital bronchopulmonary foregut malformation. Am. J. Clin. Pathol., *91:*403–409, 1989.)

tion with congenital cardiac disease. The findings on chest film may be diagnostic: cardiac and mediastinal displacement, absence of the pulmonary arterial shadow, smaller hemithorax, and elevation of the hemidiaphragm, all on the affected side. On the opposite side, there may be hyperinflation and herniation of the lung across the midline. There is no predilection for the left or right side, although right-sided lesions are less frequently associated with cardiac abnormalities. In most cases, only the proximal part of the affected artery is atretic, often over a short distance. The peripheral branches are usually patent and fed by a systemic collateral supply from enlarged bronchial, mediastinal, and intercostal vessels (Harris et al., 1992).

The lesion may present in infancy or remain asymptomatic until adulthood. Symptoms (when present) include hemoptysis, history of recurrent pulmonary infection, pain in the chest, dyspnea on exertion, and cyanosis (Werber et al., 1983). Physical examination reveals decreased breath sounds on the affected side, and screening laboratory, bronchoscopic, and bronchographic results are normal. The diagnosis may be confirmed by ventilation-perfusion nuclear medicine scan, pulmonary arteriography, or digital subtraction angiography (Fig. 24–58). Dynamic CT has been used to confirm the diagnosis and avoid more invasive procedures (Harris et al., 1992) (Fig. 24–59).

Physiologically, oxygen exchange in the abnormally perfused lung is negligible, and even asymptomatic patients show decreased diffusing capacity on pulmonary function testing. Nutrition to the abnormally vascularized lung is well preserved by bronchial arteries. Normally, only mild pulmonary arterial hypertension develops in these patients; those who become hypertensive do so at an early age and die of right-sided heart failure. Resection is performed only for the development of hemoptysis or bronchiectasis (Luck et al., 1986).

Idiopathic hyperlucent lung (Swyer-James or Macleod's syndrome) is caused by chronic pulmonary infection, usually bronchiectasis, with resultant pulmonary vascular changes. The chest film shows hyperlucency of the involved lung, and the bronchogram shows extensive destruction and alteration of the normal architecture (Gottlieb and Turner, 1976). On pulmonary arteriogram, the vessels are markedly diminished in caliber, accounting for the hyperlucency (Fig. 24–60). The compensatory shift in pulmonary blood flow from the affected side to the good lung restores ventilation-perfusion relationships—in other words, an autopneumonectomy.

Pulmonary artery sling (anomalous origin of the left pulmonary artery) is a recognized cause of respiratory obstruction in infants. In this anomaly the pulmonary trunk arises normally from the right ventricle,

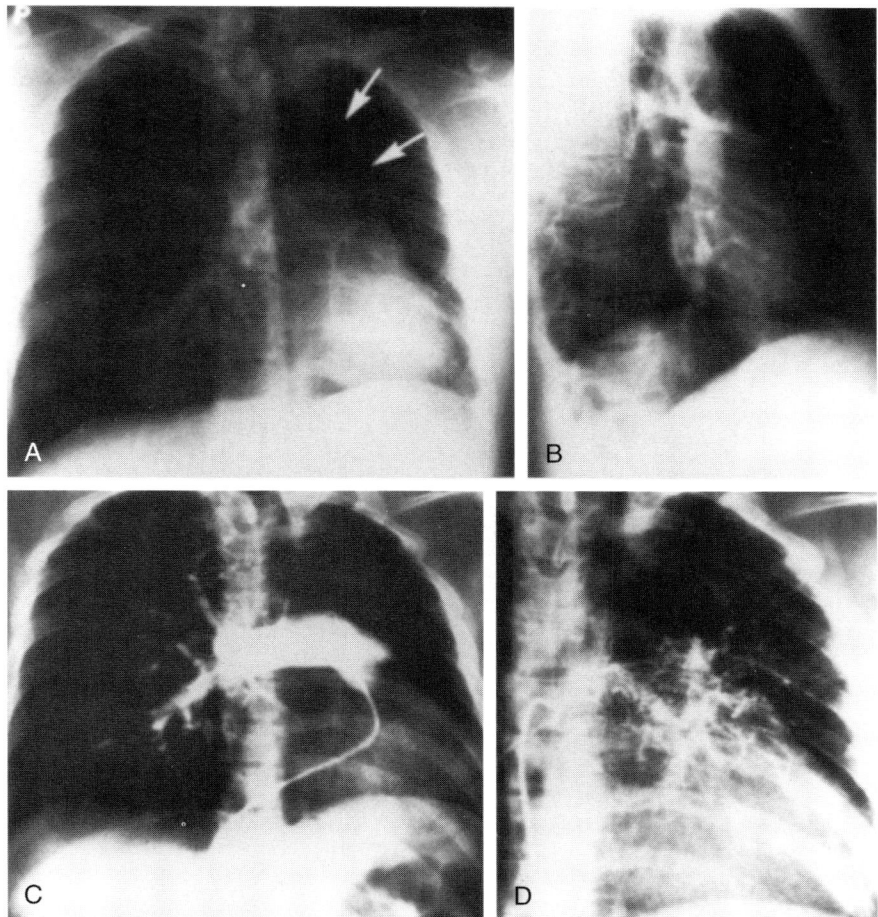

FIGURE 24–58. Unilateral absence of a pulmonary artery. A and B, Hypoplastic left lung. Note the marked shift to the left of the mediastinum. The left pulmonary artery and its branches are not visualized. Compensatory emphysema is noted on the right. Anterior junctional line (arrows in A) extends into the mid-left thorax. C, Hypoplastic left lung. Pulmonary angiogram demonstrates opacification of the pulmonary arterial system and complete absence of filling of left pulmonary artery. D, Hypoplastic left lung. Thoracic aortogram reveals hypertrophy of the bronchial arteries. (A–D, From Mehta, A. C., Ahmad, M., Golish, J. A., and Buonocore, E.: Congenital anomalies of the lung in the adult. Cleveland Clin. Q., 50:401, 1983.)

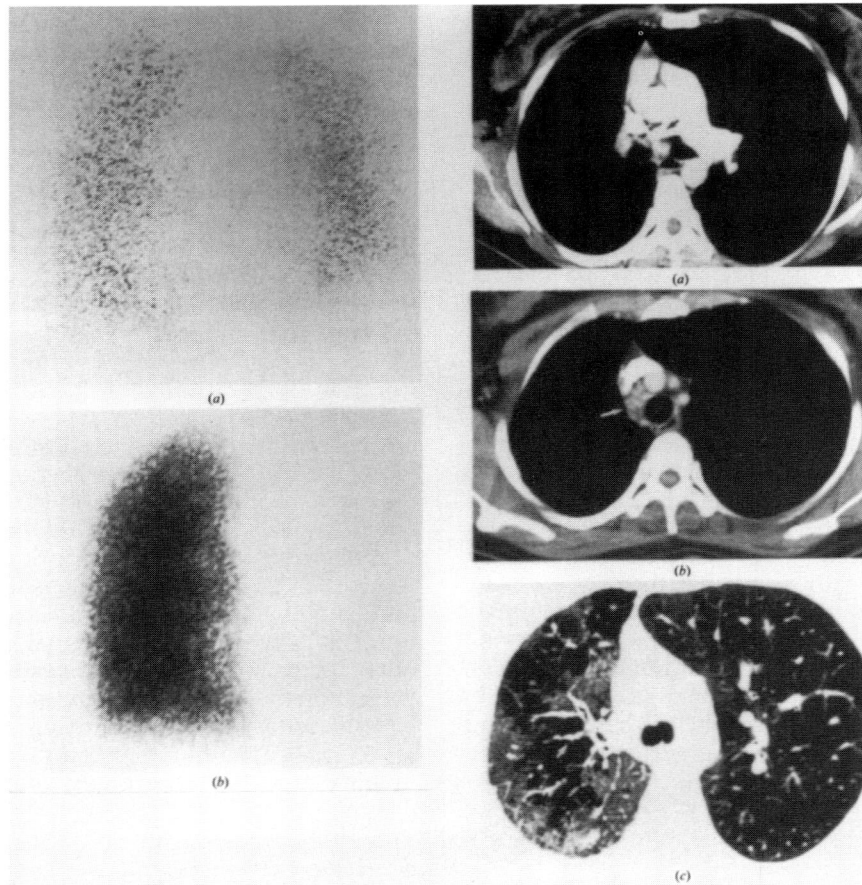

FIGURE 24–59. *Left,* Radionuclide ventilation/perfusion scan in right-sided pulmonary artery atresia. *(a),* Xe-133 ventilation scan, posterior projection. Reduced by homogeneous ventilation to the right lung. *(b),* Corresponding perfusion scan shows completely absent perfusion to the right lung. *Right:* *(a),* Contrast-enhanced CT demonstrates absence of the right pulmonary artery apart from a small diverticulum *(arrow;* WW 250H. WL + 50H). *(b),* At a higher level, abnormal vessels representing a collateral supply are visible within the superior mediastinum *(arrow;* WW 400H, WL + 40H). *(c),* Patchy areas of ground-glass density are present within the parenchyma of the affected lung (WW 800H, WL − 700H). Some of the vessels have a beaded appearance *(arrows).* (From Harris, D. M., Lloyd, D. C. F., Morrissey, B., and Adams, H.: The computed tomographic appearances in pulmonary artery atresia. Clin. Radiol., *45:*382–386, 1992.)

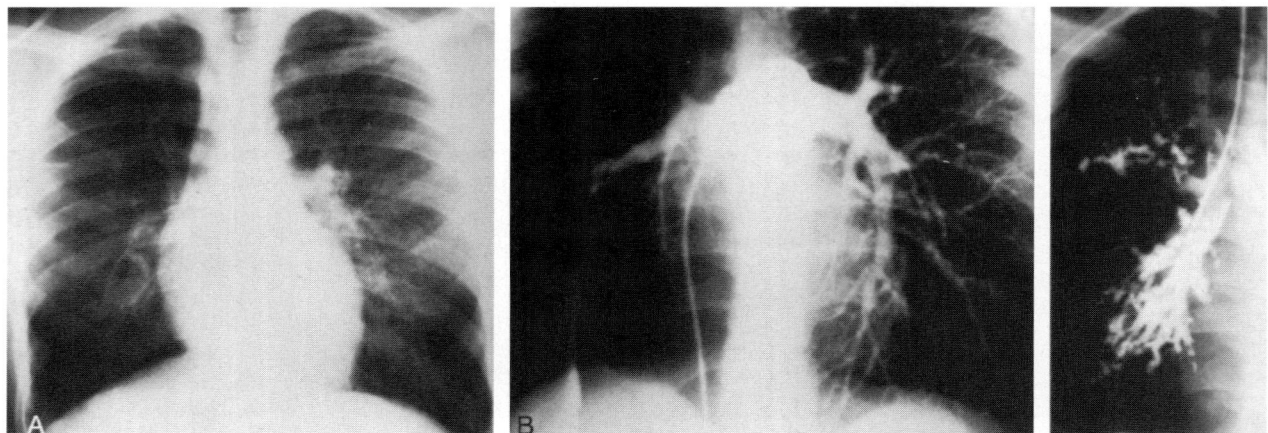

FIGURE 24–60. Classic features of Swyer-James syndrome (Macleod's syndrome). *A,* Chest film shows hyperlucency of the right lung. *B, Left,* Pulmonary angiogram shows sharp decrease in blood flow to the entire right lung. *Right,* Bronchogram shows severe bronchiectasis of the right lung.

passing upward and to the right first as the main pulmonary artery and then as the right pulmonary artery. In the vicinity of the carina it then lies anterior and to the right of the trachea. The aberrant left pulmonary artery arises from the trunk at this point, passing over the right mainstem bronchus and between the trachea and esophagus to reach the hilus of the left lung (Fig. 24–61). The precise course and size of the anomalous artery, and the presence or absence of associated tracheal disease, determine the severity of symptoms. In a review by Koopot and associates (1975), over 90% of infants had serious difficulty at presentation, including wheezing, stridor, choking spells, and apnea associated with cyanosis.

The diagnostic work-up of patients with congenital vascular rings and slings has been discussed by Bertolini and co-workers (1987). In pulmonary artery sling, the chest film usually shows obstructive hyperinflation of the right or occasionally the left lung. On the lateral film, the anomalous vessel can be seen end-on, lying between the back of the trachea and the front of the esophagus and causing posterior indentation of the trachea. Barium esophagram demonstrates anterior indentation of the esophagus, and tracheobronchography or pulmonary angiography can confirm distal tracheal indentation and compression of the right mainstem bronchus (Fig. 24–62). Echocardiography has been used following screening barium esophagram to confirm the diagnosis, clarify anatomy, and exclude other major intracardiac pathology before operation (Lillehei and Colan, 1992). It has become clear, however, that tracheobronchial narrowing in this condition may also stem from congenital tracheal stenosis distant from the site of the crossing vessel. Siegel and associates (1982) have demonstrated the efficacy of tracheobronchography in identifying patients with both anomalies. In patients with both lesions, repeated bouts of infection, wheezing, stridor, and problems with intubation suggest primary tracheal pathology. Instead of right-sided hyperaeration on the chest film, symmetric hyperaeration or even a normal-appearing film may be present. Berdon and co-workers (1984) called this association the *ring-sling complex,* and noted that CT scanning might be useful in illustrating both anomalies.

In patients with isolated pulmonary artery sling, early operative intervention can completely cure. The infant is explored through the left chest, and the anomalous artery is isolated as far into the right mediastinum as possible and divided near its origin. The end of the divided vessel is then anastomosed to the pulmonary arterial trunk where the normal left pulmonary artery would have originated. If necessary, the ductal remnant is divided. The experience over the past 23 years at Great Ormond Street using microsurgical techniques was recently reported; of 18 patients undergoing surgical resection, 4 had congenital tracheal stenosis that was repaired on cardiopulmonary bypass at the time of anterior reimplantation of the left pulmonary artery anterior to the trachea. There was 1 late death, 3 patients have residual tracheobronchial problems, and the remainder show normal pulmonary and constitutive growth and development (Pawade et al., 1992).

In contrast, the surgical mortality rate with the ring-sling group of patients has exceeded 50% when only the sling was taken down (Sade et al., 1975). Surgical results in patients with both lesions depend on the degree of tracheal stenosis and whether any pars membranacea offsets the tracheal tissue (Dunn et al., 1979; Pawade et al., 1992). Newer techniques for repair of tracheal stenosis are discussed in the earlier section, "Tracheobronchial Tree."

Isolated pulmonary artery aneurysm in the absence of associated congenital heart disease is rare and has been reviewed by Ungaro and associates (1976). The most common abnormalities of pulmonary venous drainage are the scimitar syndrome, a rare but well-described constellation of cardiopulmonary abnormalities, pulmonary varix, and azygous lobe, which are described in the earlier section, "Anatomic Variations."

The scimitar syndrome was described by Neill and colleagues in 1960 and consists of hypoplasia of the right lung, dextroposition of the heart, hypoplasia and malformation of the right pulmonary arterial and bronchial trees, anomalous systemic arterial supply to the lower lobe of the right lung, and venous drainage of one or all three lobes of the right lung into the inferior vena cava, azygos system, or right atrium. Diagnosis is often made on plain film, which demonstrates a curved shadow along the right sternal border of the heart (Fig. 24–63). CT is useful in establishing

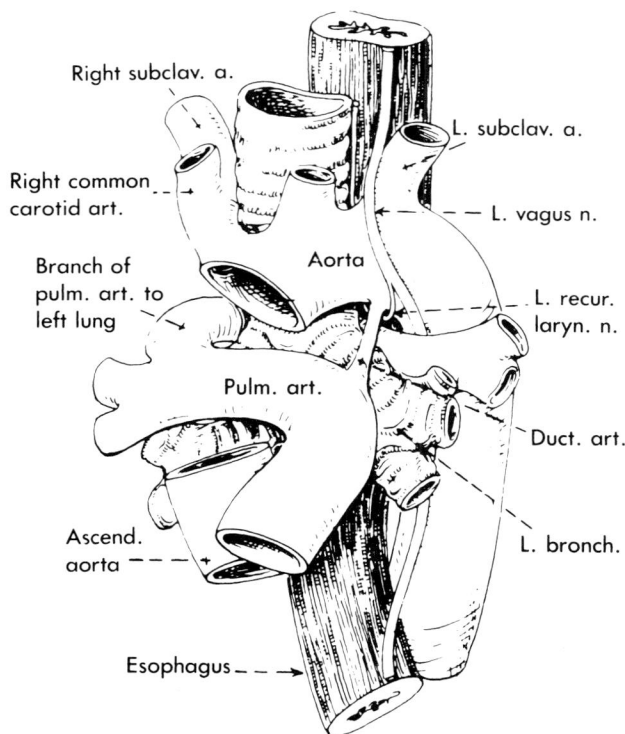

FIGURE 24–61. Anatomy of a pulmonary artery sling. (From Nikaidoh, H., Riker, W. L., and Idriss, F. S.: Surgical management of "vascular rings." Arch. Surg., *105*:327–333, 1972. Copyright 1972, American Medical Association.)

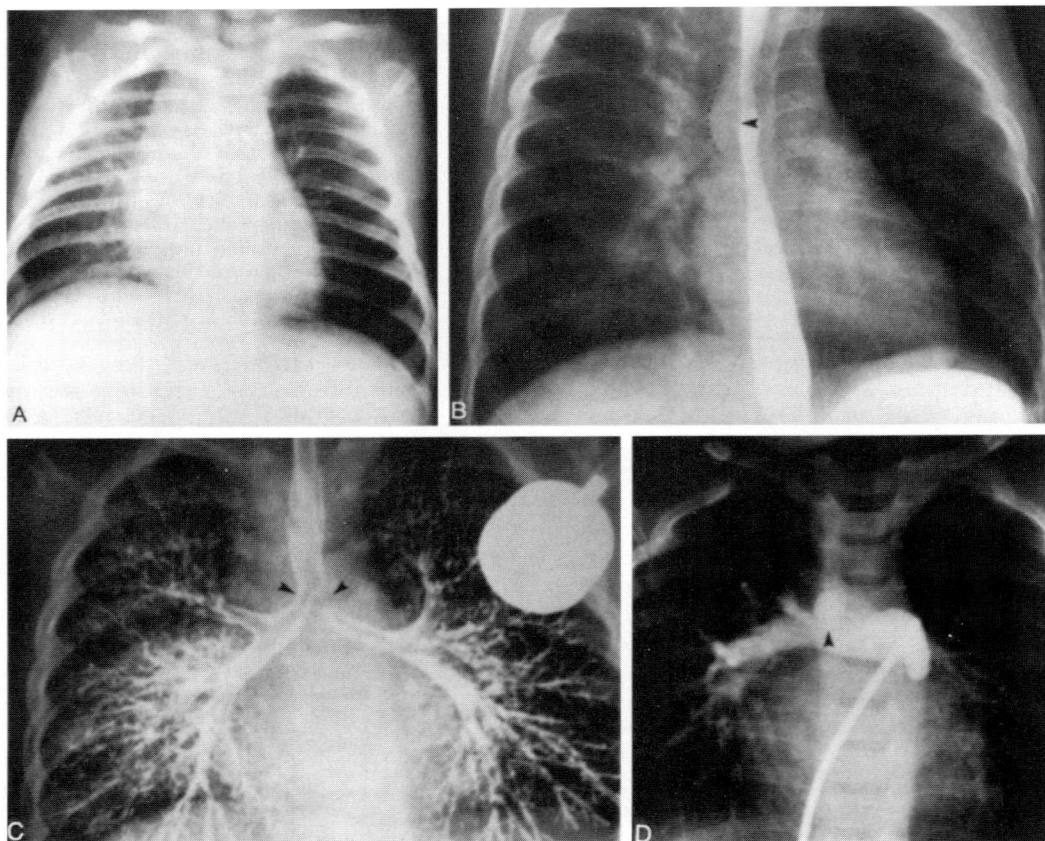

FIGURE 24–62. Radiologic findings in a 1-year-old boy with pulmonary artery sling. *A,* Obstructive hyperinflation of the left lung. *B,* Oblique view shows the aberrant left pulmonary artery crossing between the trachea and the esophagus. *C,* Bronchogram shows the indentation in the right lateral wall of the trachea and the near-total obstruction of the left mainstem bronchus, the cause of the obstructive hyperinflation seen in *A. D,* Pulmonary angiogram shows the origin of the left pulmonary artery from the right pulmonary trunk and the arching of the vessel around the trachea to reach the left lung. The child was cured by transposing the origin of the left pulmonary artery to the left side of pulmonary trunk, approximately at the point where the tip of the cardiac catheter lies.

the diagnosis. Canter and associates (1986), in a series of 15 patients, noted considerable variability in each of the pulmonary arterial, venous, and parenchymal components of the syndrome. When diagnosed in

infancy, approximately 40% of patients with the scimitar syndrome have a variety of congenital heart defects; these infants are markedly symptomatic with cyanosis, failure to thrive, and pulmonary hyperten-

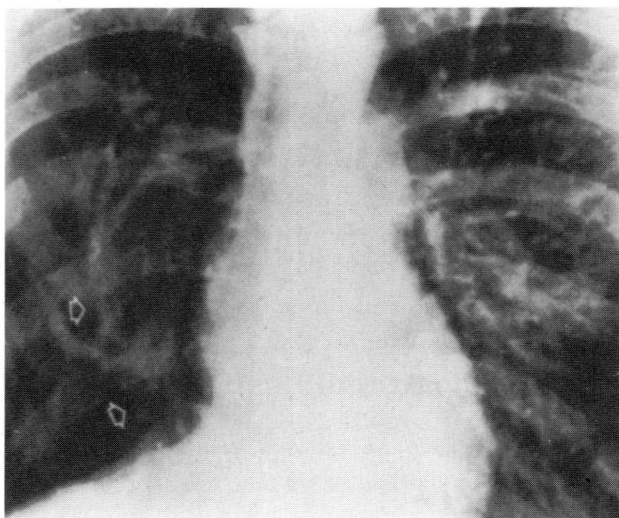

FIGURE 24–63. Scimitar syndrome. Chest film shows the curvilinear venous pathway *(arrows)* that resembles a Turkish scimitar. (From Eisenberg, R. L.: Diagnostic Imaging in Surgery. New York, McGraw-Hill, 1987, p. 171.)

sion associated with the heart defects. The details of anatomy are obtained with cardiac catheterization and selective angiography; bronchoscopy usually is not required. Operative management is difficult and mortality is high, principally in patients with pulmonary hypertension accompanying congenital cardiac conditions (Honey, 1977). Surgical treatment should be directed toward ligation of systemic arterial supply to the right lung, diversion of venous return to the left atrium with an intracardiac baffle, or direct anastomosis and repair of associated intracardiac anomalies, possibly as a two-stage procedure. In contrast, older children present with a heart murmur, recurrent infections, or abnormal chest film results; these patients have no pulmonary hypertension and a benign prognosis. Right pneumonectomy should be reserved for older patients with recurrent infection or hemoptysis, patients with clotted shunts, or patients with marked hypoplasia of the right lung (Canter et al., 1986).

Pulmonary varix is a rare venous malformation that has recently been reviewed by Mehta and co-workers (1983).

Pulmonary arteriovenous malformations (PAVMs) are probably the most common congenital abnormality of the pulmonary circulation. The term *PAVM* describes the spectrum of direct connections between branches of the pulmonary artery and pulmonary vein, extending from single arteriovenous aneurysmal lesions (PAVA) to multiple microscopic communications that are too small to visualize radiographically. Churton, in 1897, first described PAVM, and Shenstone in 1940 performed the first successful operation, a case that required pneumonectomy for extirpation. More recently, surgical intervention for this lesion has been supplanted by balloon catheter occlusion techniques (Kaufman, 1987).

PAVM may occur as an isolated entity but is commonly associated with the syndrome of *hereditary hemorrhagic telangiectasia* (HHT), also known as Osler-Weber-Rendu disease. This disease is an autosomal dominant disorder characterized by mucocutaneous and visceral telangiectasis associated with recurrent episodes of epistaxis and gastrointestinal hemorrhage (Peery, 1987). The incidence of PAVM in HHT ranges from 7 to 15%, whereas HHT is an associated finding in approximately 35% of patients with PAVM. PAVM may also be an acquired lesion, occurring with trauma, schistosomiasis, long-standing hepatic cirrhosis, metastatic carcinoma, and actinomycosis. The female/male ratio is 1.5:1, and although PAVM is a congenital lesion, the mean age at presentation is approximately 40 years (range 3 to 73 years) (Dines et al., 1983).

The embryology, anatomic variation, and classification of PAVA were described by Anabtawi and associates (1965) and have been reviewed by Lyerly and Sabiston (1990). The pathologic characteristic of the arteriovenous connection is a persistence of one or more sizable communications that bypass the pulmonary capillary bed; 4% of cases are associated with a systemic arterial supply or anomalous venous drain-

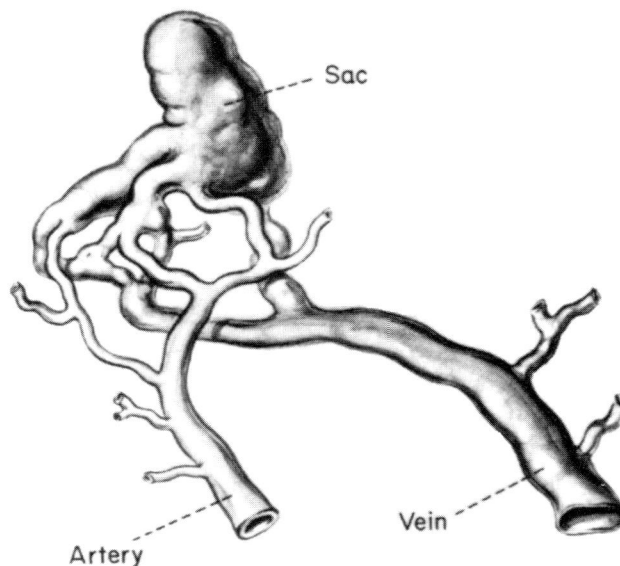

FIGURE 24–64. Anatomy of a typical arteriovenous fistula of the lung.

age (Fig. 24–64). Histologically, single or multiple thin-walled saccular channels lined with endothelium are present, and there is no reaction in the surrounding lung tissue. The majority of lesions occur in the lower lobes, usually subpleurally such that some part of the vascular abnormality is visible on the pleural surface (Fig. 24–65). They occur as single lesions in 60 to 75% of patients, but multiple lesions may occur in one or both lungs. Unlike its systemic counterpart, PAVA usually manifests normal hemodynamics. Because the vascular resistance both in the pulmonary capillary bed and in the malformation is negligible, the volume of blood transferred from the right ventricle through the PAVM to the left atrium is approximately the same as the volume that flows

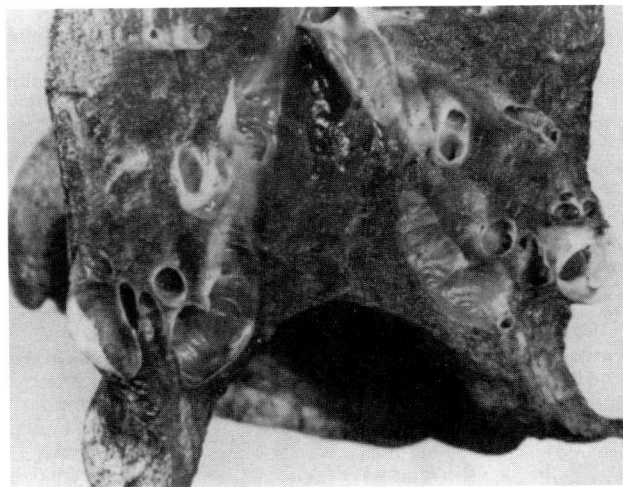

FIGURE 24–65. Pulmonary arteriovenous malformation (PAVM). Cut section of resected lobe. Note subpleural location of several sacs, thinness of the vascular walls, and lack of tissue reaction in the surrounding lung.

through normal lung, and cardiac dynamics are unaffected. Associated pulmonary hypertension is distinctly unusual. The essential defect is a right-to-left shunt from pulmonary artery to vein, which may be sizable. Diffuse lesions with many small communications are more common in infants, who may present with cyanosis and congestive heart failure (White et al., 1986).

The proportion of asymptomatic patients varies from 13 to 56% in reported series (Burke et al., 1986). Larger shunts, which occur in 20% of patients, give rise to the classic clinical triad of dyspnea on inspiratory effort, cyanosis, and clubbing, but the age at presentation varies. Other symptoms may include hemorrhage, hemoptysis, palpitations, and chest pain. Epistaxis, hematuria, or neurologic symptoms (vertigo, headache, numbness, paresis, syncope, confusion, and dysphagia) should alert the physician to the possibility of HHT. It is clear that the stigmata of either PAVM or HHT should raise the suspicion of the other disease process.

Physical findings are abnormal in 75% of patients with PAVA, including cyanosis, clubbing, pulmonary vascular bruits, and systolic murmurs. In one-third of patients, mucocutaneous telangiectasia is associated with HHT. The pulmonary bruit is increased by the Müller maneuver (forced inspiration against a closed glottis after full expiration) and decreased by the Valsalva maneuver. Laboratory studies will show arterial desaturation, elevated hematocrit, and secondary polycythemia. Unlike the case with systemic arteriovenous fistulas, however, blood volume is not markedly increased.

The characteristic chest radiographic findings are of a single circumscribed noncalcified lobular opacity; connecting blood vessels between the lesion and the hilum of the lung may be seen. Serial studies may document enlargement of the lesion, especially in patients with HHT. Chest radiography and arterial blood-gas studies in the sitting or standing position are recommended as screening tests in family members of patients with HHT or PAVM. Orthodeoxia (desaturation in the upright position) is present in patients with basal PAVAs, probably caused by a combination of gravity-induced redistribution of blood flow to the malformation and the increase in lung volume with the change from the supine to the upright posture (Terry et al., 1983). Contrast echocardiography and radionuclide angiocardiography indicate a right-to-left shunt. They are not specific for PAVA, but a negative study result effectively excludes the diagnosis. Pulmonary angiography remains the diagnostic gold standard for PAVM. In therapeutic candidates, angiography is mandatory to establish the number, extent, and location of the malformations, delineate the arterial supply and venous drainage, and define the angioarchitecture prior to therapy (Fig. 24–66).

Complications of PAVM are attributable either to the malformation or to the accompanying polycythemia. Pleurisy over the PAVM may occur, as well as fatal hemothorax following rupture of the subpleural PAVA. Significant neurologic complications, including headache, dizziness, tinnitus, convulsions, and hemiplegia, occur in about 30% of patients, whereas 5 to 10% of patients have the more serious complications of cerebral thrombosis, brain abscess, and paradoxical embolus. Dines and co-workers (1983) reported an 11% mortality and 26% morbidity rate in untreated patients followed for a mean of 6 years.

Until recently, surgical resection has been the treatment of choice. Local excision, segmental resection, or lobectomy have been used to treat solitary lesions. The rich collateral blood supply and danger of systemic arterial embolus make simple ligation of the individual feeder vessels to the PAVA ill advised. Proximal vessel control must be obtained before mobilizing peripheral adhesions to the chest wall or dia-

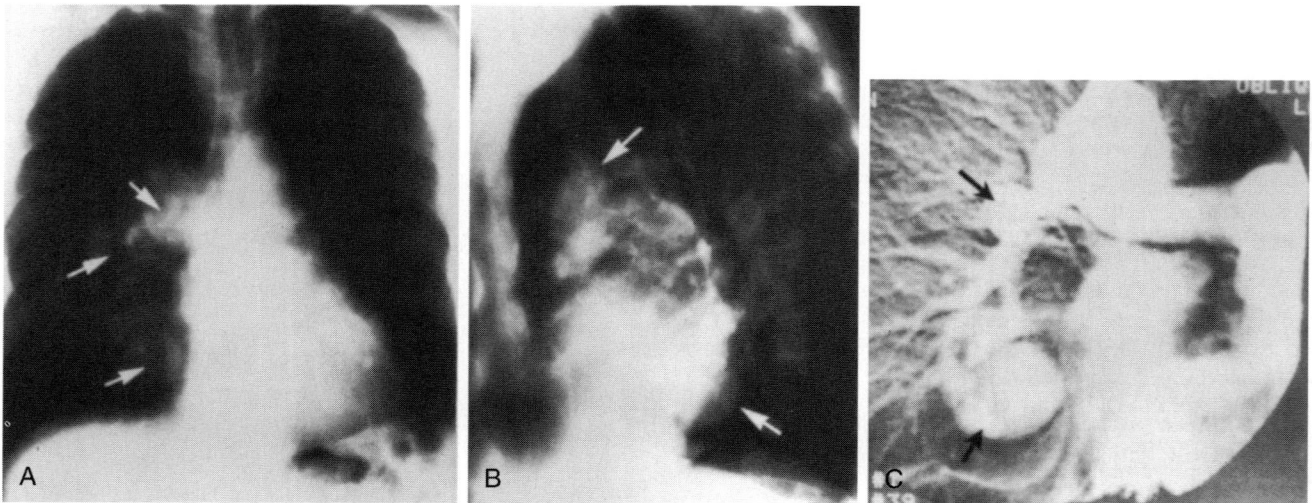

FIGURE 24–66. PAVM in a patient with hereditary hemorrhagic telangiectasia. A and B, Chest films show multiple large, well-circumscribed nodular densities (arrows). C, Digital subtraction angiogram. Nodules (arrows) opacify after injection of contrast material through a peripheral vein. (A–C, From Mehta, A. C., Ahmad, M., Golish, J. A., and Buonocore, E.: Congenital anomalies of the lung in the adult. Cleveland Clin. Q., 50:401, 1983.)

phragm, because alarming hemorrhage can occur from a tear in the thin-walled subpleural sacs. Resection in the acutely cyanotic infant can be life-saving. Conservative local resection is indicated in multiple lesions, and staged bilateral thoracotomies have been used (Brown et al., 1982). Surgical mortality rates of approximately 5% or less have been reported, with minimal morbidity and a very small incidence of recurrence after surgery (Burke et al., 1986).

In 1980, successful balloon embolotherapy for multiple PAVAs was reported; the place of this technique as the treatment of choice in PAVA has been reviewed by Reidy and associates (1985). Careful selective angiography is required before treatment, because approximately 80% of lesions have a single feeding vessel and nonseptated aneurysmal sac, whereas the remaining 20% have multiple feeding arteries associated with a septated arteriovenous communication. Arterial occlusion of simple PAVM is easier but is associated with a higher risk of distal paradoxic embolism; occlusion of all feeding vessels to a complex lesion is more time consuming, but the septations in the sac prevent distal embolization (Fig. 24–67). After 8 years of experience, Flower reported no deaths or serious complications with this technique (Flower, 1987). In patients with massive, multiple PAVMs, bilateral transplantation has been successful (Armitage et al., 1993).

Currently, most authors recommend that when lesions are symptomatic and enlarging or associated with complications, they should be treated. Treatment of asymptomatic patients is more controversial but probably is warranted, especially in patients with HHT, because of the high rate of complications in untreated patients. Balloon embolotherapy appears preferable to surgical excision in patients with single and multiple lesions, except in unusual circumstances. However, this technique must be performed by radiologists with considerable skill and experience, and it should probably be undertaken in only a few centers. In the absence of this modality, surgical resection should be performed.

EMPHYSEMA AND ASSOCIATED CONDITIONS

As agreed on by the World Health Organization and the American Thoracic Society, pulmonary emphysema is characterized by an increase beyond normal in the size of air spaces distal to the terminal nonrespiratory bronchiole, arising from destruction of their walls (Fletcher and Pride, 1984). This definition includes the two major anatomic features of emphysema—dilatation and tissue destruction—but does not specify the extent and distribution of each. Pathologic quantification of the amount of emphysema is possible, but correlation of the pathologic findings with adequate clinical descriptions of the pulmonary disease processes has not yet been achieved. The term *chronic obstructive pulmonary disease* (COPD) has come into wide use because it is difficult, with the usual

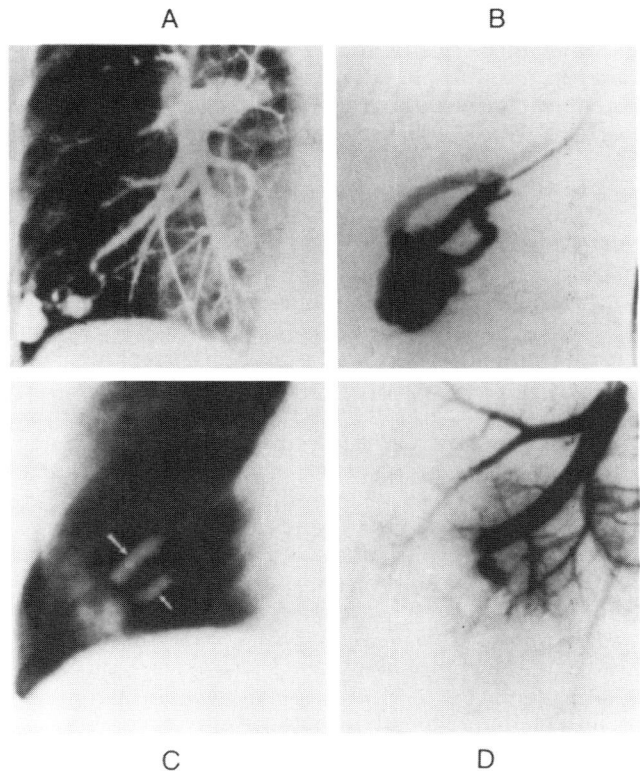

FIGURE 24–67. Complex-type PAVM. *A*, Selective right pulmonary arteriogram shows that the PAVM in the right lower lobe has at least two feeding arterial branches. *B*, Selective digital arteriogram of the proximal arterial branch supplying the PAVM. Two arterial branches feed the PAVM. *C*, A balloon *(small arrow)* has been detached in the lower feeding artery. A second balloon *(large arrow)* has been inflated but not detached in the second feeding arterial branch. *D*, Digital arteriogram shows occlusion of the PAVM. (*A–D*, From Kaufman, S. L.: Intrathoracic interventional vascular techniques in congenital cardiovascular disease. Reprinted from Journal of Thoracic Imaging, Vol. 2, No. 2, p. 3, with permission of Aspen Publishers, Inc., copyright April 1987.)

clinical and epidemiologic tools, to diagnose emphysema accurately and to determine the relative roles of emphysema and bronchiolitis in causing airway obstruction. Further confusion is produced by the overlap in etiology and symptoms between the two major components of COPD, chronic bronchitis and emphysema; these entities may occur with or without airway obstruction. It is airway obstruction, however, that causes impairment of lung function, disability, and death (Snider, 1989).

It is clear that these diseases are prevalent in the United States. An estimated two-thirds of adults have some degree of emphysema at autopsy; about 10% of these have severe clinical disease. About 4.5 million of the 55 million cigarette smokers have significant chronic airflow obstruction associated with chronic bronchitis. Finally, about 7 million persons suffer from asthma (Snider, 1985). The presence of these diseases must be taken into account in planning surgical therapy for any problem within the thorax in patients over the age of 45 and considered in any patient over 50 undergoing any major surgical procedure. Risk factors for COPD (and therefore for emphysema), including age, education level, sex, tobacco smoking, homozygous alpha$_1$-protease inhibitor (A-1-PI) deficiency, air pollution, and occupation, are established as increasing the risk and severity of COPD (Snider, 1989).

The pathogenesis of emphysema has not been fully elucidated. Earlier studies dealt with infectious, degenerative, and obstructive mechanical factors that might predispose to disruption or degeneration of connective tissue fibers. In recent years, focus has shifted to enzymatic mechanisms of tissue destruction. The most widely held explanation for the development of emphysema is the protease pathogenesis hypothesis (Sifers et al., 1992). This protease-antiprotease theory, which hypothesizes that progressive destruction of the interstitium is due to an excess of proteolytic enzymes related to the availability of proteolytic inhibitors, was suggested by two signal observations. Laurell and Eriksson (1963) recognized that selected cases of early-onset familial emphysema were associated with heritable A-1-PI deficiency, whereas Gross and co-workers (1964) showed that intrapulmonary instillation of elastolytic proteases produced anatomic derangements in experimental animals characteristic of human emphysema. Because the major endogenous sources of elastases in the lung are the polymorphonuclear neutrophil (PMN) leukocytes and the alveolar macrophage (AM), much research has focused on the effects of phagocyte-derived elastases and their inhibitors in regulating the degradation of lung elastin (Hoidal and Niewoehner, 1983). Newer studies have pointed to several mechanisms by which mononuclear phagocytes can affect the homeostatic balance between elastolytic enzymes and their inhibitors in lung tissue. Hoidal and associates (1981) demonstrated that AM cells of cigarette smokers generated increased amounts of oxygen radicals and peroxide. Alpha-$_1$ AP is the major antiprotease in the normal human lower respiratory tract. Exposure to cigarette smoke produces oxidative inactivation of alpha-$_1$ AP, either as a direct result of oxidants in smoke or secondarily by active oxygen species liberated by lung phagocytes recruited to the lung by cigarette smoke exposure. This inactivation causes a relative elastase excess, coupled with a recruitment of elastase-producing neutrophils to the lung as a result of the cigarette smoke insult (Weinberger, 1993). Bronchoalveolar lavage yields 4 to 5 times more cells from the lungs of smokers than from nonsmokers; the proportion of neutrophils, a rich source of elastase, is unchanged, but the absolute number of neutrophils is increased. The increased elastolytic activity seen in smokers has also been seen in other diseases such as CF.

The role of oxidants and antioxidants in mediating this inactivation has been investigated. The mechanism of injury may involve free-radical oxidation (see Table 24–5). Oxidants are abundantly present in cigarette smoke (Burns, 1991); free radicals generated by the neutrophil myeloperoxidase in the presence of hydrogen peroxide are able to inactivate A-1-PI. The

mechanism for this is oxidation of a critical methionine residue that renders the molecule incapable of inactivating elastase (Snider, 1989; Gadek and Pacht, 1990). Data suggest that there is a decreased amount of functionally active A-1-PI in the lungs of smokers. Under normal conditions, the serum concentration of alpha$_1$ AP ranges from 150 to 350 mg/ml, which is apparently sufficient to provide a protease-antiprotease balance in the lung that protects the elastin fibers from degradation. In patients with severe COPD, serum concentrations are below 35%. Direct evidence for this hypothesis is provided by Damiano and associates (1986), who demonstrated immuno-ultrastructurally that neutrophil elastase is bound to elastic fibers in the lungs of smokers and that the amount of elastase is proportional to the amount of emphysema.

Free radicals can impair connective tissue repair as well, and attention has focused on the role of impairment of connective tissue synthesis or resynthesis following injury (Snider, 1989). Cigarette smoke exposure reduces elastin resynthesis after elastolytic destruction of lung tissue in experimental animals, possibly by impairing lysil oxidase activity, which is critical for elastin synthesis. This impairment of elastase synthesis may be qualitative (disorganized resynthesis) or quantitative (inadequate resynthesis). Emphysema may thus result from the destruction of lung parenchyma while the lung is unable to repair itself adequately. Whether infectious processes and malnutrition play a role in this is still unclear.

A-1-PI can inhibit a wide variety of serine proteases (Sifers et al., 1992). It is synthesized in the liver, but a primary site of its physiologic action is in the alveolar structure of the lung, acting by inhibiting PMN elastase and protecting the elastic fibers from hydrolysis. In individuals with the genetic deficiency of the enzyme, the risk of degenerative lung disease is 20 to 30 times that of the general population. It has been estimated that over 40,000 persons in the United States have A-1-PI deficiency, accounting for only 1 to 2% of patients with emphysema. The severity of the pulmonary disease is directly influenced by environmental factors such as industrial pollutants and cigarette smoke. In addition, approximately 14% of deficient individuals will develop severe liver cirrhosis during infancy, which is frequently fatal, and cirrhosis and primary liver cancer have been reported in adults with the disease (Weinberger, 1993).

Synthesis of A-1-PI in the liver is controlled by an autosomal and allelic gene system. Over 30 different phenotypes of the protein have been classified; most individuals are homozygous for PiM and show the normal phenotype. Individuals with the PiZ phenotype suffer from a severe deficiency of the enzyme, and individuals homozygous for this abnormal phenotype have plasma levels that are 10 to 15% of normal. Other phenotypes are associated with relatively normal levels of serum enzyme. The genetic deficiency involving the PiZ phenotype is inherited through an autosomal recessive trait. The phenotype of adults can be readily defined by conventional Pi-typing of plasma A-1-PI after the diagnosis is suspected clinically and by serum protein electrophoresis. Prenatal diagnosis has been made for a number of years by analysis of the A-1-PI gene in amniotic cells to diagnose siblings with liver disease.

Anatomically, four types of emphysema are recognized, classified by the way the disease involves the acinus (Thurlbeck, 1983). Proximal acinar emphysema, also called centrilobular emphysema, selectively involves the respiratory bronchioles, which are enlarged and destroyed both in series and in parallel. This type is almost invariably associated with cigarette smoking and inflammation of the distal airways, and it is the form of emphysema most commonly encountered in patients with symptomatic chronic airflow obstruction. It is localized more frequently in the upper zones of the lung, and is distributed unevenly, with some lobules uninvolved. Panacinar or panlobular emphysema involves the entire acinus more or less uniformly. This type is classically associated with homozygous (PiZ) A-1-PI deficiency and other forms of Pi-associated emphysema, and it is characteristically worse in the lower lung zones. Proximal acinar emphysema may be superimposed on panacinar disease in smokers with the familial deficiency. Whether these two forms of emphysema are distinctly different diseases is controversial, and theoretical explanations for the characteristic distribution of each type based on regional ventilation and perfusion differences in the lung have been proposed. Distal acinar or paraseptal emphysema involves the distal part of the acinus, ducts, and alveolar sacs and is often associated with fibrosis. The subpleural location leads to the characteristic association of this form of emphysema with spontaneous pneumothorax and bullous disease (Thurlbeck, 1984). Irregular emphysema affects the acinus in an irregular manner. It is for practical purposes always associated with scarring and fibrosis and probably occurs to some degree in all lungs.

More clinically useful than this pathologic grouping is a classification that divides pulmonary overinflation into three types: compensatory "emphysema," diffuse obstructive emphysema, and bullous emphysema. Certain basic abnormalities are common to all types, including enlarged air spaces with hyperinflation of the chest, increased residual lung volume, narrowing of the air passages, impaired breathing capacity, and an increased expenditure for breathing (Dijkman, 1986).

Compensatory "emphysema" is not truly an emphysematous process, because actual destruction of the acinus does not occur; unfortunately, classifications of lesions associated with this process have retained the terminology. These include ILE, localized emphysema occurring with infection, bronchial tumor or aspirated foreign body, and the compensatory changes following pulmonary resection. These postoperative changes do not lead to parenchymal disruption and emphysema in patients following pneumonectomy, and age-related changes in the remaining lung progress at the same rate as in normal lungs.

Diffuse obstructive emphysema constitutes the major component of the clinical entity known as COPD (Snider, 1985, 1989). Two major forms are described, depending on whether sputum is produced (i.e., infection from chronic bronchitis). Type A, also called dry emphysema, is associated with some cough, but patients mainly complain of dyspnea. They have distant breath sounds and the typical "barrel" chest. The chest film shows diffuse overinflation with little or no fibrosis, flat diaphragms, and an apparent decrease in pulmonary vasculature (Fig. 24–68). Pathologically, the destruction is of the panacinar type—all elements of the secondary lobules are dilated. The prognosis for longevity in dry emphysema is reasonably good. Symptoms of chronic bronchitis may develop after the onset of dyspnea. Type B, or wet emphysema, does not produce the characteristic physical and radiographic signs of emphysema so obvious in the other group. The patients are decidedly symptomatic with severe cough and copious sputum production, rales, and wheezing, and cyanosis is often present. Dyspnea is a later symptom. The chest film is characterized by moderate degrees of hyperinflation, pronounced fibrosis, particularly in the lower lobes, and an increase in central pulmonary vascularity with rapid tapering of the vessels toward the periphery. The pathologic changes are centrilobular, with the architectural destruction localized around the respiratory bronchioles (Fig. 24–69). The prognosis for longevity in Type B is poor.

The distinctive features of these two types of obstructive emphysema are compared in Table 24–6. Medical management consists primarily of prevention of infection and control of obstructive symptoms, the mainstays of which are bronchodilator therapy, antiinflammatory therapy, and oxygen. These are coupled with multidisciplinary pulmonary rehabilitation in many circumstances.

Attempts to surgically treat diffuse emphysema either have not documented clinical improvement or have been associated with prohibitively high mortality rates (Delarue, 1977), and it is doubtful that surgical therapy in any form will ever help any large number of patients suffering from diffuse obstructive emphysema. Surgical procedures are of great help in managing the complications of this disease, however. Spontaneous pneumothorax is the most common complication of Type A emphysema. The most common complication of the B type is retention of secretions and respiratory failure. Tracheostomy was originally recommended to treat exacerbations of Type B emphysema (Gaensler et al., 1983). The disadvantages of tracheostomy, including loss of cough reflexes and pulmonary superinfection, have prevented widespread acceptance of the technique. Fenestrated tracheostomy tubes or tubeless tracheal vents have been advocated, but without prolonged success. In acute respiratory failure due to excessive secretions in Type B patients, aggressive pulmonary treatment with endotracheal or nasotracheal intubation and ventilatory support should be undertaken. If prolonged support appears to be necessary, then tracheostomy or cricothyroidotomy can be performed.

The term *bullous emphysema* encompasses a wide

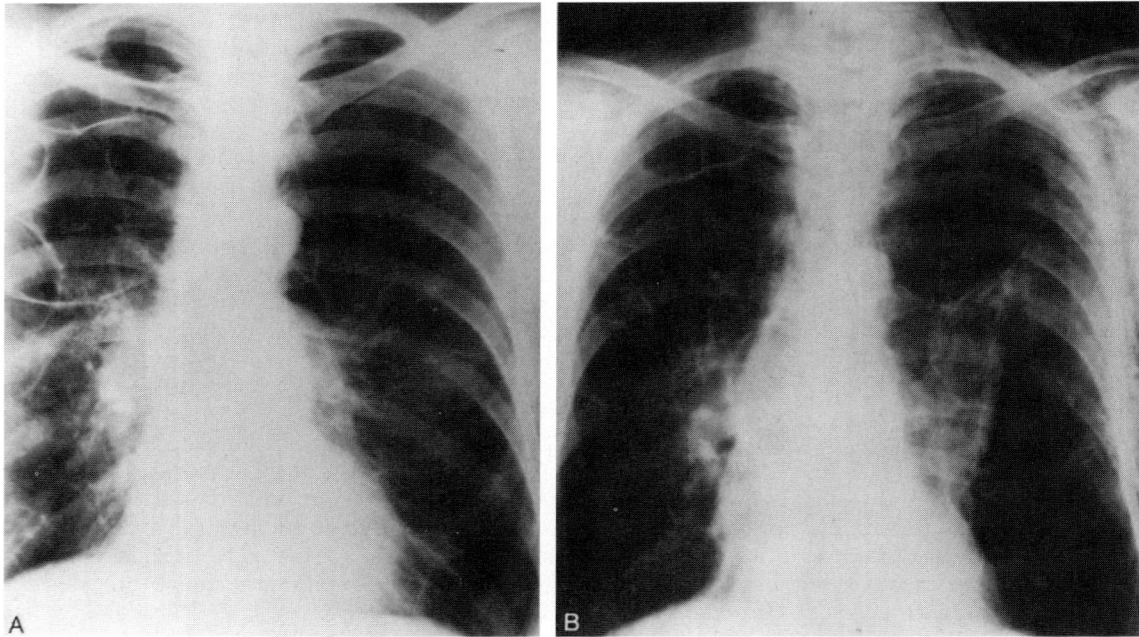

FIGURE 24–68. *A,* Far advanced emphysema with later development of a left pneumothorax. *B,* This condition was treated successfully by intercostal water-seal decompression.

range of pathologic entities; undoubtedly, many patients reported in the literature as benefiting from surgical resection did not have bullous emphysema but rather some form of congenital cyst or bleb; certain types of cystic disease in children with otherwise normal lungs and some forms of emphysematous blebs in adults with emphysema have been compared by Soosay and associates (1992). A bleb is an intrapleural air space separated from alveoli by a thin pleural covering. Because the pleural covering is so thinned, spontaneous rupture is not uncommon. A bulla is a subpleural air space usually larger than a bleb that results from destruction of lung tissue (Pratt, 1988). Bullous emphysema should refer only to thin-

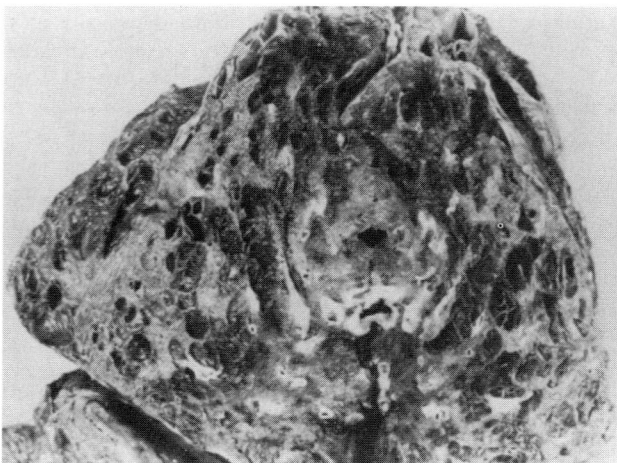

FIGURE 24–69. Cut section of lung from a patient who died of wet emphysema. The destruction is centrilobular in type. Note the marked inflammatory changes in and around the bronchi.

walled air sacs under tension that cause compressive atelectasis of normal lung tissue. Such sacs may develop singly or be multiple, and may attain enormous size (Fig. 24–70).

Sudden idiopathic formation of a pneumothorax was described in 1809 by Itard, and in 1819 Laënnec suggested that emphysematous blebs were the most frequent cause. Pneumothorax is the cause of 1 in every 1000 admissions to a general hospital, and approximately 85% of spontaneous pneumothoraces occur in patients under 40 years of age. Most pneumothoraces are idiopathic and thus primary, but etiologic considerations at the time of diagnosis must include inflammatory processes (tuberculosis, pneumonia, bronchiectasis, lung abscess), emphysematous causes (bullae or blebs), trauma, and connective tissue or immunologic causes (scleroderma, eosinophilic granuloma); neoplasms can cause secondary spontaneous pneumothoraces (Tanaka et al., 1993). Familial spontaneous pneumothorax also has been linked with human leukocyte antigen (HLA) and alpha$_1$ AP phenotypes. Almost all patients present with acute pleuritic chest pain, and most complain of dyspnea. Examination reveals decreased tactile fremitus, hyperresonant percussion, and decreased breath sounds on the affected side (Fig. 24–71).

Most pneumothoraces (75%) are larger than 25% of thoracic volume. Tube thoracostomy has become the standard form of treatment, yielding a decreased rate of recurrence and shorter hospital stay than nonoperative or needle-aspiration therapy. Pneumothoraces smaller than 20% of thoracic volume may be treated conservatively with success. Pleural scarifying agents such as tetracycline with xylocaine may be injected through the tube to promote symphysis of the visceral

■ **Table 24–6.** DIFFUSE OBSTRUCTIVE EMPHYSEMA

Characteristics (Parameter)	Type A	Type B
Synonyms	Dry emphysema; "pink puffer"	Wet emphysema; "blue bloater"
Subjective		
Dyspnea	Severe	Usually severe
Cough	Occasional	Severe
Wheeze	Absent usually	Severe
Sputum	Scant, mucoid	Copious, often purulent
Physical		
Breath sounds	Distant	Rales and wheezes
Cyanosis	None	Frequent
Radiographic findings	Diffuse hyperinflation	Pulmonary fibrosis
	Bullae	
Airway resistance and work of breathing	Severely increased	Severely increased
Maximal breathing capacity and FEV_1	Severely reduced	Severely reduced
Pulmonary volumes		
Vital capacity	Slightly reduced	Severely reduced
Residual volume	Severely increased	Moderately increased
Total lung capacity	Increased	Normal
Blood gases		
Po_2	Slightly reduced	Severely reduced
Pco_2	Slightly reduced	Elevated
Diffusion capacity	Severely reduced	Slightly reduced
Polycythemia	Rare	Frequent
Cor pulmonale	Rare	Frequent
Prognosis for longevity	Fairly good	Quite poor
Pathologic appearance	Usually panacinar	Usually centriacinar

Adapted from Knudson, R. J., and Gaensler, E. A.: Surgery for emphysema—Collective review. Ann. Thorac. Surg., 1:332, 1965.

and parietal pleurae; insufflation of talcum through the thoracoscope has also been advocated in the past. Tanaka and associates (1993) have endorsed this conservative approach for cases of secondary spontaneous pneumothorax due to the underlying disease processes. Surgical intervention consisting of a lateral thoracotomy, pleurodesis, and stapling or oversewing of blebs should be carefully individualized. A 50 to 80% recurrence rate has been reported following a second ipsilateral spontaneous pneumothorax, and

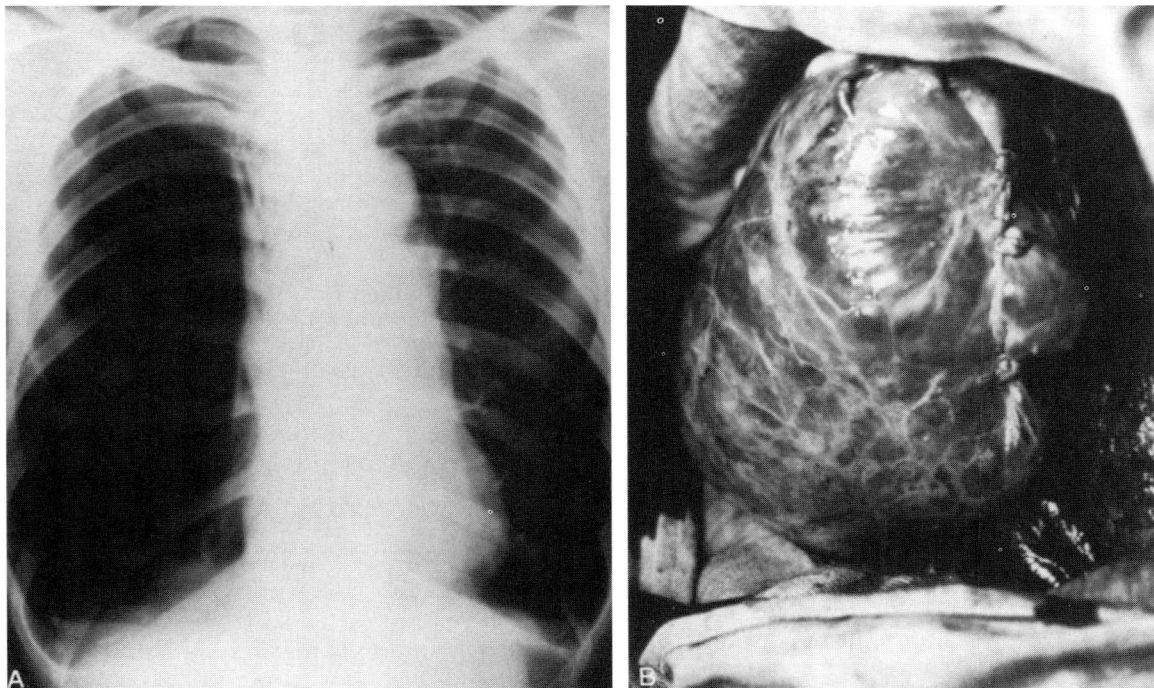

FIGURE 24–70. *A,* Large bulla of the right upper lobe occupies the entire right side of the chest, with compression of the lower and middle lobes. *B,* Bulla at the time of operation. Note the essentially normal lower and middle lobes to the right of the cyst.

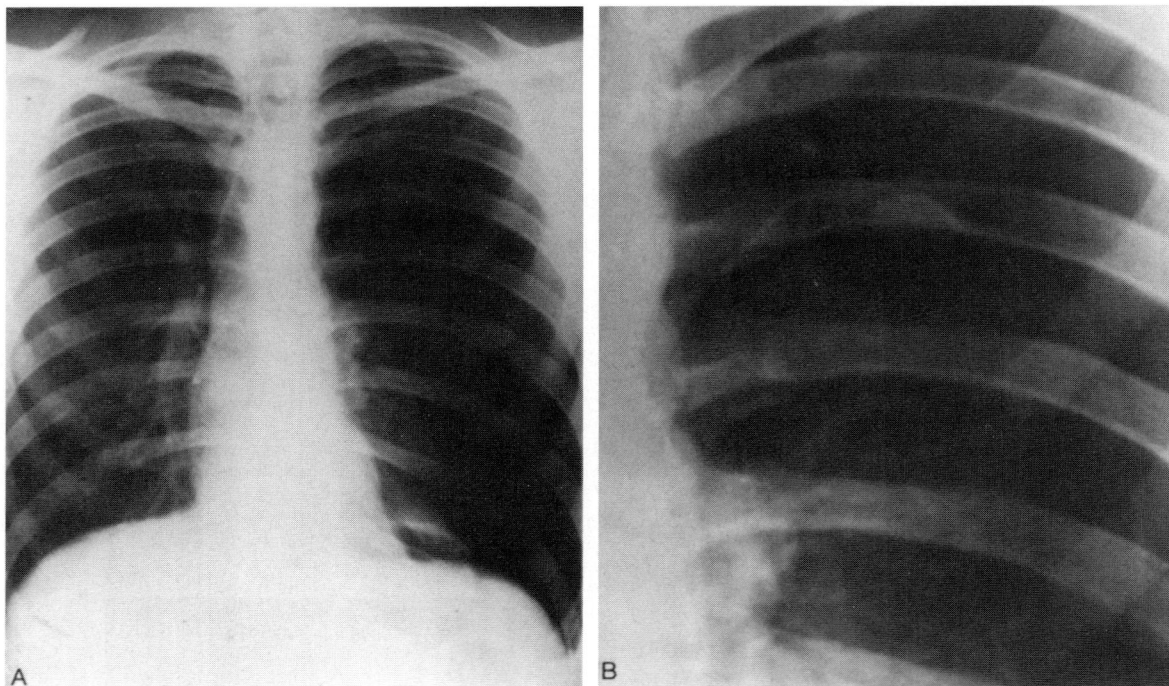

FIGURE 24–71. *A,* Spontaneous pneumothorax on the left side in a patient with minimal emphysema. *B,* The film shows a small apical bleb.

most authors would intervene surgically at this juncture. Other indications for thoractomy include simultaneous bilateral pneumothoraces, life-threatening spontaneous pneumothorax, hemopneumothorax, CF, high-risk occupation, and bullous disease. In advanced Type A obstructive emphysema, management of pneumothorax may be difficult (see Fig. 24–68). The air leak is large, and there is tendency toward loculation of air and fluid. Symphysis between the parietal pleura and emphysematous lung occurs slowly, and patience is required by both the patient and surgeon. Multiple chest tubes and vigorous suction may be necessary. Most cases of pneumothorax secondary to diffuse emphysema can be managed without thoracotomy; in patients with marginal pulmonary function, frank respiratory failure usually resolves with treatment of the pneumothorax.

Bullae can form with all pathologic forms of emphysema (Thurlbeck, 1984). Periacinar emphysema is probably quite common in patients with bullae who are referred for surgery. The coalescing of several subpleural bullae into one or several giant bullae produces collapse of the relatively normal lung that is now separated from its visceral pleura (Fig. 24–72). The net result is a large, poorly ventilated area that is not perfused. Despite free communication between the bullae and the tracheobronchial tree, the bullae infrequently fill with fluid or become infected.

The selection of patients for surgical resection can be a simple or a very difficult task, and the decision must be based on clinical, radiologic, and physiologic data (Gaensler et al., 1983; Morgan et al., 1989). The goal of this evaluation is to compare the quantity of symptoms that are related to the bullae (which can

be removed) with those related to the underlying generalized pulmonary disease (which is a contraindication to surgery). Dyspnea is the most common symptom associated with bullous disease, and when isolated, dyspnea may suggest a good surgical result. The classic case is a younger patient with a large tension bulla and normal-appearing lungs who complains of dyspnea as the bulla enlarges. A long history of chronic cough suggests a poor surgical result. Cor pulmonale and right-sided heart failure are not contraindications to operation because the increased vascular resistance may be largely the result of relaxation or compression of normal adjacent lung. Spectacular successes have been recorded in such cases. Pulmonary function testing may or may not be helpful; with small bullae, spirometry will be unaffected, whereas in patients with bullae superimposed on severe emphysematous disease, results of function testing will be uniformly poor and can rule out surgical intervention. Gaensler and colleagues (1983) suggested that a discrepancy between functional residual capacity determined by body plethysmography as compared with helium rebreathing reflects the amount of trapped gas in the bulla; a large discrepancy is an indication for surgery. Other authors have emphasized a normal diffusing capacity of carbon monoxide as an indication of normal underlying lung function. Expiration radiographic studies and review of old chest films to document growth of the bulla may be useful. Bronchography may show clumping suggestive of compression but may cause bronchitis. Perfusion scans may be used to estimate split lung function. Pulmonary arteriography may show crowding of the pulmonary arterial branches in areas of normal

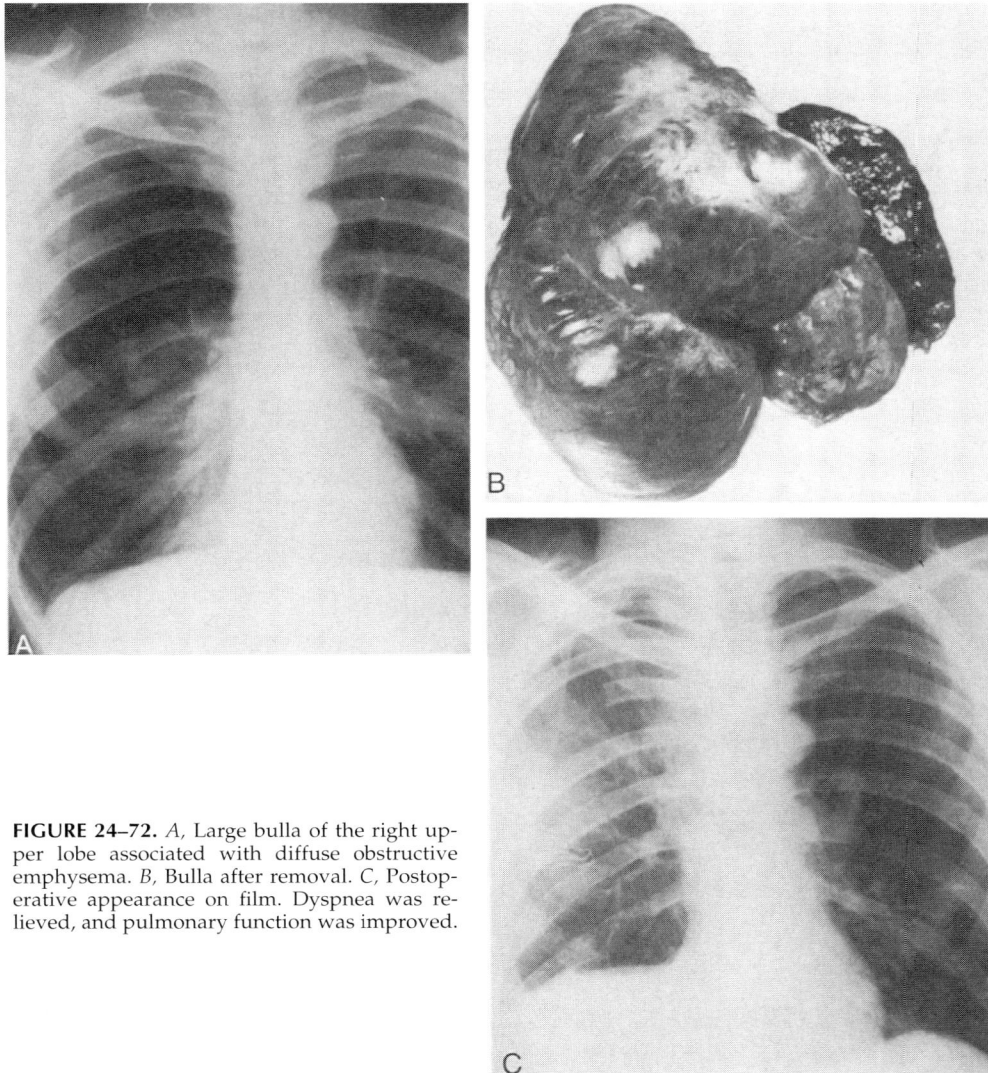

FIGURE 24–72. *A,* Large bulla of the right upper lobe associated with diffuse obstructive emphysema. *B,* Bulla after removal. *C,* Postoperative appearance on film. Dyspnea was relieved, and pulmonary function was improved.

lung compressed by the bullae. Tenholder and associates (1980) recommended the use of progressive incremental exercise pulmonary function testing in the selection and follow-up of patients being considered for operation. Morgan and co-workers (1986) have advocated CT in selecting patients with bullous lung disease for surgery.

No single test determines which patients with bullous emphysema will benefit from an operation. Each case requires careful study, and surgeons must remind themselves that they will at times be surprised at the degree of improvement that follows resection, at other times disappointed that the improvement is not greater.

The surgical objective in bullous disease is to remove as little functioning lung tissue as possible. Upon inspection, these bullae have a thin outer surface resembling a fish bladder. The base blends imperceptibly into the adjacent lung, with many small air pockets and trabeculations in the transition zone; innumerable bronchial communications of various sizes lead into the sac. Classically, the thin wall is trimmed away, and all bronchial communications in the base are carefully closed with continuous and interrupted catgut sutures and meticulous surgical technique. The pleural surfaces are approximated, unless this compromises the function of the adjacent lung, in which case the raw surface is left exposed to abut against the parietal pleura. Smaller bullae will invariably be present, particularly along the margin of the lobes; these should always be obliterated, for they can become bullae of significant size. Some bullae with narrow pedicles may be ligated. The surgical stapling devices provide a more secure and airtight closure of the structurally delicate parenchyma than can be provided by a closure with sutures and should be used when possible. Persistent parenchymal air leaks and residual pneumothorax are the most frequent complications of these surgical procedures, and adequate intercostal chest drainage with multiple tubes is mandatory.

More recently, thoracoscopic bullectomy has been

achieved, and its use is expanding; identification of the true extent of the bulla and its boundary with normal lung may be difficult, however (Rice, 1993). Current stapling devices are still inadequate for the entire spectrum of this disease. Thoracoscopic laser ablation has also been attempted but should still be considered an experimental approach (Barker et al., 1993; Wakabayashi et al., 1991).

The operative mortality rate in the surgical management of bullous disease has been reported to be between 10 and 22%, closely related to the severity of diffuse obstructive disease (Delarue et al., 1977). With better patient selection and preoperative preparation, O'Brien and associates (1986) reported no mortality and minimal morbidity in a series of 20 patients undergoing resection for bullous disease. For bilateral disease, Cooper and associates (1978) reported that median sternotomy was associated with less postoperative morbidity and more rapid recovery of lung function than lateral thoracotomy in patients with bilateral disease. In patients considered too ill for formal thoracotomy, intracavitary (Monaldi) suction may be used. MacArthur and Fountain (1977) treated 31 patients with this technique, with two operative deaths and radiographic improvement in all but 1 patient; Morgan and associates (1986) reported suc-

cessful use of this technique in 7 of 12 patients with preoperative FEV$_1$ less than 1 l.

Long-term results of operation are quite good. Gaensler and associates (1983) reported sustained improvement in all patients with large localized lesions following resection for at least 5 years, with some functional decline and in some cases return to preoperative values within 7 to 12 years. For patients with bilateral or severe disease, the average decline in FEV$_1$ over a 10-year follow-up period was 101 ml/year, versus an annual decline of 80 ml/year for patients with COPD and 28 ml/yr in normal subjects. These findings were corroborated by others. Further improvement can be documented in patients who quit smoking following surgery (Hughes et al., 1984). Documented improvement in ventilatory capacity with exercise as compared with preoperative evaluation has been demonstrated by Vigneswaran and associates (1992).

Onset of disease in patients with A-1-PI deficiency usually is before age 40, and there is a higher incidence in women. The family history is important. The pulmonary films show that the emphysematous changes are most marked in the lower half of the chest (Fig. 24–73), consistent with the panacinar type of emphysema seen in these patients. Pulmonary an-

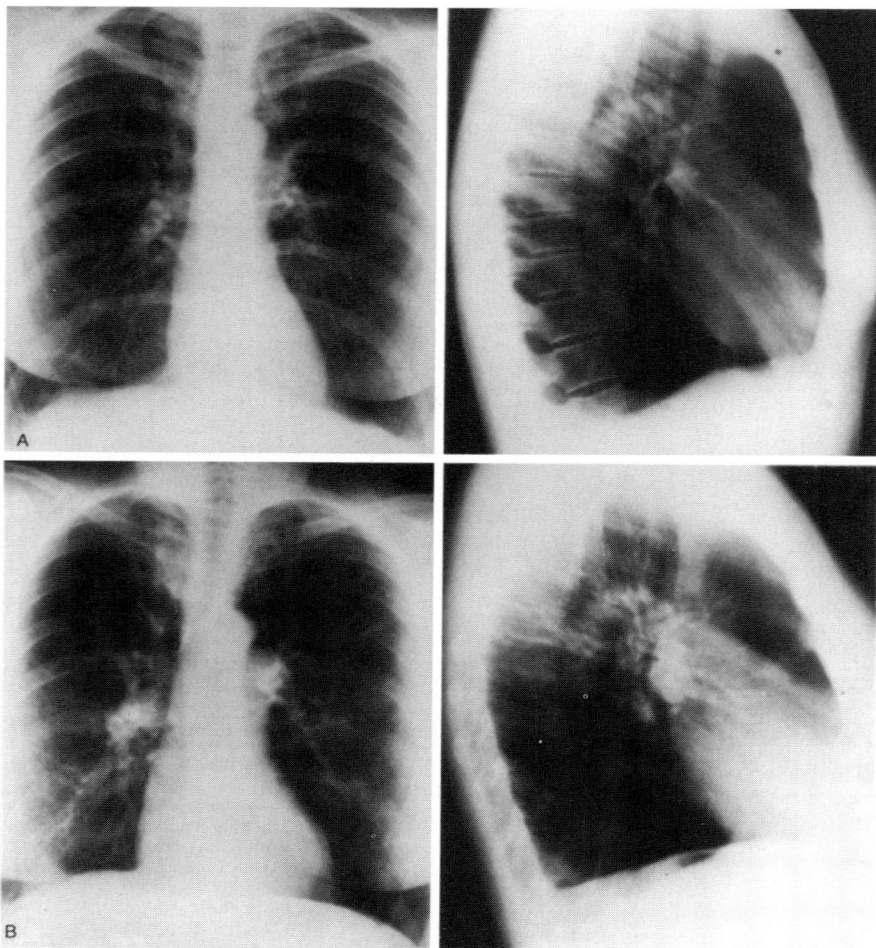

FIGURE 24–73. Pattern of emphysema in a patient (female) with alpha$_1$-antiprotease deficiency (PiZ phenotype). In 1964, at age 38, she was dyspneic (FEV$_1$ 30% of normal). *A* and *B* show the relentless progression over 9 years despite excellent medical treatment. Note the involvement of the lower lobes, particularly striking on the lateral views.

giograms and scintigrams show a greater perfusion in the upper lobes than the bases, whereas ventilation scans show basal air trapping. Smoking has an important role in the disease, both increasing the severity of the disease and decreasing the age at onset. Pharmacologic treatment has been directed at augmentation therapy using human $alpha_1$ AT prepared from pooled plasma from normal donors. The preparation is treated with heat to destroy viral pathogens such as the human immunodeficiency virus (HIV) and hepatitis viruses (Weinberger, 1993). Both weekly and monthly replacement therapeutic regimens appear to be effective (Hubbard et al., 1988; Wewers et al., 1987). Aerosolized preparations using recombinant technology are in development, and gene therapy using a replication-deficient adenovirus vector to transfer a recombinant human $alpha_1$ antitrypsin gene to airway epithelial cells in an animal model has been successfully demonstrated (Rosenfeld et al., 1991).

Pharmacologic therapy for symptomatic emphysema in the setting of COPD may hold promise for the future as well. Anthonisen (1991) reviewed the design of a clinical trial to test a treatment of emphysema with inhibitors of human neutrophil elastase.

Before 1986, no definitive therapy for end-stage emphysematous disease of either iatrogenic or genetic origin was available. Following the pioneering work of the Toronto Lung Transplant Group, the potential role of lung transplantation in the treatment of this disease process has been demonstrated (Patterson and Cooper, 1993). Initially, bilateral lung transplantation was thought to be necessary because of concern that unilateral transplantation for COPD would be complicated by hyperexpansion and air trapping in the native lung, shifting the mediastinum, and restricting ventilation to the transplanted lung (Wildevuur and Benfield, 1970). Other groups have attempted combined heart-lung transplantation for emphysema for the same reasons (Khaghani et al., 1991). Experimental studies (Margulies et al., 1992) demonstrated in dogs that the static volume distribution between emphysematous and nonemphysematous lungs is determined only by differences in lung recoil and compliance. Single-lung transplantation for emphysema was cautiously tried by Kaiser and associates (1991a) with good results; only 1 of 11 patients had significant air trapping, and pulmonary function improved significantly by 6 postoperative weeks. Other groups (Mal et al., 1989; Marinelli et al., 1992) have achieved similar results. Novick and co-workers (1991) have even successfully resected the contralateral emphysematous lung following single-lung transplantation for emphysema. Low and associates (1992) compared bilateral with single-lung transplantation for emphysema in 32 consecutive patients; patients undergoing bilateral lung transplantation were at greater risk for postoperative complications, but significantly higher FEV_1, single breath diffusing capacity, and arterial oxygen tension values were obtained in the bilateral group. The final role of single- versus double-lung transplantation in emphysematous disease continues to evolve. Excellent results have been obtained in both groups of patients with end-stage disease accom-

panied by extreme degrees of prelethal morbidity, however (Borst and Schafers, 1993).

SELECTED BIBLIOGRAPHY

Alton, E., Caplen N., Geddes, D., and Williamson, R.: New treatments for cystic fibrosis. Br. Med. Bull., *48*:785–804, 1992.

Excellent discussion of the medical therapeutic advances for CF.

Breaux, C. W., Rouse, T. M., Cain, W. S., and Georgeson, K. E.: Congenital diaphragmatic hernia in an era of delayed repair after medical and/or extracorporeal membrane oxygenation stabilization: A prognostic and management classification. J. Pediatr. Surg., 27:1192–1196, 1992.

A prognostic classification based on a large clinical experience.

Burns, D. M.: Cigarettes and cigarette smoking. Clin. Chest Med., *12*:631–642, 1991.

Discussion of the known epidemiologic data connecting cigarette smoke and pulmonary disease that focuses on reactive intermediate species produced in or as a result of cigarette smoke.

Di Lorenzo, M., Collin, P. P., Vaillancourt, R., and Duranceau, A.: Bronchogenic cysts. J. Pediatr. Surg., 24:988–991, 1989.

Report of a large, single-institution experience with this lesion in the pediatric population; for adult experience from the same institution, see later reference to St.-Georges et al., 1991.

Fowler, C. L., Podorny, W. J., Wagner, M. L., and Kessler, M. S.: Review of bronchopulmonary foregut malformations. J. Pediatr. Surg., 23:793–797, 1988.

Thorough review of the potential variations in embryogenesis that can result in these lesions.

Gadek, J. E., and Pacht, E. R.: The protease-antiprotease balance within the human lung: Implications for the pathogenesis of emphysema. Lung, *168*(Suppl):552–564, 1990.

Complete presentation of the data supporting this pathogenic mechanism for at least some types of pulmonary emphysema.

Hruban, R. H., Shumway, S. J., Orel, S. B., et al.: Congenital bronchopulmonary foregut malformation. Am. J. Clin. Pathol., *91*:403–409, 1989.

An excellent clinicopathologic correlation discussion of these lesions is included in this article from the University of Minnesota.

Hyde, S. C., Gill, D. R., Higgins, C. F., et al.: Correction of the ion transport defect in cystic fibrosis transgenic mice by gene therapy. Nature, *362*:250–255, 1993.

This tremendously exciting study describing "cure" of the biochemical defect in CF lays the foundation for similar types of therapy in humans in the not-too-distant future.

Jederlinic, P. J., Sicilian, L. S., Baigelman, W., and Gaensler, E. A.: Congenital bronchial atresia. Medicine, *66*:73, 1987.

Excellent review of this topic, with a review of the world's literature to date (86 cases).

Lewis, J. F., and Jobe, A. H.: Surfactant and the adult respiratory distress syndrome. Am. Rev. Respir. Dis., *147*:218–233, 1993.

The authors expand on the pathologic mechanisms responsible for NRDS to the clinical and pathologic mechanisms responsible for ARDS.

Luck, S. R., Reynolds, M., and Raffensperger, J. G.: Congenital bronchopulmonary malformations. Curr. Probl. Surg., 23:245–314, 1986.

Outstanding review of this topic by surgeons at the University of Chicago with a long-standing interest in this field.

Newman, K. D., and Randolph, J.: Surgical problems of the esophagus in infants and children. *In* Sabiston, D. C., and Spencer, F. C.: Surgery of the Chest. 5th ed. Chapter 25. Philadelphia, W.B. Saunders, 1990, pp. 815–846.

Excellent reference source for tracheoesophageal fistulas and other esophageal anomalies in infants and children.

Patterson, G. A., and Cooper, J. D. (eds): Lung transplantation. Chest. Clin. North Am., *3*:1–178, 1993.

Monograph on the current status of adult and pediatric lung transplantation.

Pawade, A., de Leval, M. R., Elliott, M. J., and Stark, J.: Pulmonary artery sling. Ann. Thorac. Surg., 54:967–970, 1992.

The experience at the Great Ormond Street Hospital with this lesion over the past 25 years is described in this article. The importance of accompanying tracheomalacia is emphasized.

Sferra, T. J., and Collins, F. S.: The molecular biology of cystic fibrosis. Ann. Rev. Med., 44:133–144, 1993.

Excellent summation of the current understanding of this disease process.

Shady, K., Siegel, M., and Glazer, H. S.: CT of focal pulmonary masses in childhood. RadioGraphics, 12:505–514, 1992.

Good description of the application of newer CT and MRI modalities to the diagnosis of congenital lesions of the lung.

Sifers, R. N., Finegold, M. J., and Woo, S. L. C.: Molecular biology and genetics of alpha-1 antitrypsin deficiency. Semin. Liver Dis., 12:301–310, 1992.

Brief description of the molecular biologic basis of this pulmonary and hepatic disease process.

Snider, G. L.: Chronic obstructive pulmonary disease: Risk factors, pathophysiology and pathogenesis. Ann. Rev. Med., 40:411–429, 1989.

Excellent review of the current state of understanding about COPD, including emphysema, chronic bronchitis, and asthma.

St.-Georges, R., Deslauriers, J., Duranceau, A., et al.: Clinical spectrum of bronchogenic cysts of the mediastinum and lung in the adult. Ann. Thorac. Surg., 52:6–13, 1991.

Adult experience with this lesion; for pediatric experience, refer to earlier citation (Di Lorenzo et al., 1989).

Vigneswaran, W. T., Townsend, E. R., and Fountain, S. W.: Surgery for bullous disease of the lung. Eur. J. Cardiothorac. Surg., 6:427–430, 1992.

Recent experience with a large series of patients undergoing surgery for this entity.

Weinberger, S. E.: Recent advances in pulmonary medicine. N. Engl. J. Med., 328:1389–1397, 1462–1470, 1993.

Outstanding description of the current status of several aspects of pulmonary medicine.

Wright, J. R.: Clearance and recycling of pulmonary surfactant. Am. J. Physiol., 259:1–12, 1990.

This excellent article describes what is known and unknown about surfactant in pulmonary disease, both congenital and adult types.

Woodring, J. H., Howard, R. S., and Rehm, S. R.: Congenital tracheobronchomegaly (Mounier-Kuhn syndrome): A report of 10 cases and review of the literature. J. Thorac. Imag., 6:1–10, 1991.

Excellent review of this rare but fascinating disease process.

BIBLIOGRAPHY

Abbasi, S., Bhutani, V. K., and Gerdes, J. S.: Long-term pulmonary consequences of respiratory distress syndrome in preterm infants treated with exogenous surfactant. J. Pediatr., 122:446–452, 1993.

Alivizatos, P., Cheatle, T., De Leval, M., and Stark, J.: Pulmonary sequestration complicated by anomalies of pulmonary venous return. J. Pediatr. Surg., 20:76, 1985.

Alton, E., Caplen, N., Geddes, D., and Williamson, R.: New treatments for cystic fibrosis. Br. Med. Bull., 48:785–804, 1992.

Anabtawi, I. N., Ellison, R. G., and Ellison, L. T.: Pulmonary arteriovenous aneurysms and fistulas: Anatomical variations, embryology, and classification. Ann. Thorac. Surg., 1:277, 1965.

Anthonisen, N.: Design of a clinical trial to test a treatment of the underlying cause of emphysema. New York Academy of Sciences trial for emphysema. Ann. N. Y. Acad. Sci., 624(Suppl):31–34, 1991.

Armitage, I. M., Fricker, F. J., Kurland, G., et al.: Pediatric lung transplantation. J. Thorac. Cardiovasc. Surg., 105:337–346, 1993.

Atwell, S. W.: Major anomalies of the tracheobronchial tree with a list of minor anomalies. Dis. Chest., 52:611, 1967.

Avery, M. E.: The J. Burns Amberson Lecture. In pursuit of understanding the first breath. Am. Rev. Respir. Dis., 100:295, 1969.

Avery, M. E., Fletcher, B. D., and Williams, R. G.: The Lung and Its Disorders in the Newborn Infant. 4th ed. Philadelphia, W. B. Saunders, 1981, pp. 228–237.

Bailey, P. V., Tracy, T., Connors, R. H., et al.: Congenital bronchopulmonary malformations. J. Thorac. Cardiovasc. Surg., 99:597–603, 1990.

Bale, P. M.: Congenital cystic malformation of the lung. Am. J. Clin. Pathol., 71:411–420, 1979.

Barker, S. J., Clarke, C., Trivedi, N., et al.: Anesthesia for thoracoscopic laser ablation of bullous emphysema. Anesthesiology, 78:44–50, 1993.

Bartlett, R. H., Toomasian, J., Roloff, D., et al.: Extracorporeal membrane oxygenation (ECMO) in neonatal respiratory failure. Ann. Surg., 204:236, 1987.

Beals, D. A., Schloo, B. L., Vacanti, J. P., et al.: Pulmonary growth and remodeling in infants with high-risk congenital diaphragmatic hernia. J. Pediatr. Surg., 27:997–1002, 1992.

Becker, M. R., Schindera, F., and Maier, W. A.: Congenital cystic adenomatoid malformation of the lung. Prog. Pediatr. Surg., 21:113, 1987.

Berdon, W. E., Baker, D. H., Wung, J., et al.: Complete cartilage-ring tracheal stenosis associated with anomalous left pulmonary artery: The ring-sling complex. Radiology, 152:S7, 1984.

Berlinger, N. T., Porto, D. P., and Thompson, T. R.: Infantile lobar emphysema. Ann. Otol. Rhinol. Laryngol., 96:106, 1987.

Bertolini, A., Peliza, A., Panizon, G., et al.: Vascular rings and slings. J. Cardiovasc. Surg., 28:301, 1987.

Bianchi, E., Saviasta, S., Calligaro, A., et al.: HLA haplotype segregation and ultrastructural study in familial immotile-cilia syndrome. Hum. Genet., 89:270–274, 1992.

Blair, G. K., Cohen, R., and Filler, R. M.: Treatment of tracheomalacia: Eight years' experience. J. Pediatr. Surg., 21:781, 1986.

Blayney, M., Kerem, E., Whyte, J., and O'Brodovich, H.: Bronchopulmonary dysplasia: Improvement in lung function between 7 and 10 years of age. J. Pediatr., 118:201–216, 1991.

Borst, H. G., and Schafers, H. J.: Lung transplantation. Clin. Invest., 71:98–101, 1993.

Braffman, B., Keller, R., Gendal, E. S., and Finkel, S. I.: Subdiaphragmatic bronchogenic cyst with gastric communication. Gastrointest. Radiol., 13:309–311, 1988.

Breaux, C. W., Rouse, T. M., Cain, W. S., and Georgeson, K. E.: Congenital diaphragmatic hernia in an era of delayed repair after medical and/or extracorporeal membrane oxygenation stabilization: A prognostic and management classification. J. Pediatr. Surg., 27:1192–1196, 1992.

Bremer, I. L.: Accessory bronchi in embryos: Their occurrence and probable fate. Anat. Rec., 54:361–374, 1932.

Brown, S. B., Hedlund, G. L., Glasier, C. M., et al.: Tracheobronchial stenosis in infants: Successful balloon dilation therapy. Radiology, 164:475, 1987.

Brown, S. E., Wright, P. W., Renner, J. W., and Riker, J. B.: Staged bilateral thoracotomies for multiple pulmonary arteriovenous malformations complicating hereditary hemorrhagic telangiectasia. J. Thorac. Cardiovasc. Surg., 83:285, 1982.

Bruce, M. C., Schuyler, M., Martin, R. J., et al.: Risk factors for the degradation of lung elastic fibers in the ventilated neonate. Am. Rev. Respir. Dis., 146:204–212, 1992.

Burke, C. M., Safai, C., Nelson, D. P., and Raffin, T. A.: Pulmonary arteriovenous malformations: A critical update. Am. Rev. Respir. Dis., 134:334, 1986.

Burns, D. M.: Cigarettes and cigarette smoking. Clin. Chest. Med., 12:631–642, 1991.

Butt, W., Taylor, B., and Shann, F.: Mortality prediction in infants with congenital diaphragmatic hernia: Potential criteria for ECMO. Anaesth. Intens. Care., 20:439–442, 1992.

Campanella, C., and Odell, J. A.: Unilateral pulmonary agenesis. S. Afr. Med. J., 71:785–787, 1987.

Canter, C. E., Maltin, T. C., Spray, T. L., et al.: Scimitar syndrome in childhood. Am. J. Cardiol., 58:652, 1986.

Cantrell, J. P., Guild, H. G.: Congenital stenosis of the trachea. Am. J. Surg., 108:297, 1964.

Chan, V., and Greenough, A.: Severe localized pulmonary interstitial emphysema—Decompression by selective bronchial intubation. J. Perinatol. Med., 20:313–316, 1992.

Ch'in, K. Y., and Tang, M. Y.: Congenital adenomatoid malformation of one lobe of a lung with general anasarca. Arch. Pathol., 48:221, 1949.

Clark, S. L., Vitale, D. J., Minton, S. D., et al.: Successful fetal therapy for cystic adenomatoid malformation associated with second-trimester hydrops. Am. J. Obstet. Gynecol., 157:294, 1987.

Clements, B. S., and Warner, J. O.: Pulmonary sequestration and related congenital bronchopulmonary-vascular malformations: Nomenclature and classification based upon anatomical and embryological considerations. Thorax, 42:401, 1987.

Cockcroft, D. W., and Home, S. L.: Localization of emphysema within the lung. Chest, 82:483, 1982.

Cohen, M. D., Scales, R. L., Eigen, H., et al.: Evaluation of pulmonary parenchymal disease by magnetic resonance imaging. Br. J. Radiol., 60:223, 1987.

Collin, P.-P., Desjardins, J. G., Kahn, A. H.: Pulmonary sequestration. J. Pediatr. Surg., 22:760, 1987.

Cooper, J. D., Nelems, J. M., and Pearson, F. G.: Extended indications for median sternotomy in patient requiring pulmonary resection. Ann. Thorac. Surg., 26:413, 1978.

Coselli, M. P., de Ipolyi, P., Bloss, R. S., et al.: Bronchogenic cysts above and below the diaphragm: Report of eight cases. Ann. Thorac. Surg., 44:491, 1987.

Currarino, G., and Williams, B.: Causes of unilateral pulmonary hypoplasia: A study of 33 cases. Pediatr. Radiol., 15:15, 1985.

Damiano, V. V., Tsang, A., Kucuch, U., et al.: Immunolocalization of elastase in human emphysematous lungs. J. Clin. Invest., 78:482–493, 1986.

Davis, D. D., Oldham, N. H., and Sabiston, D. C.: The mediastinum. In Sabiston, D. C., and Spencer, F. C.: Surgery of the Chest. 5th ed. Chapter 17. Philadelphia, W. B. Saunders, 1990, pp. 498–535.

Delarue, N. C., Woolf, C. R., Sanders, D. E., et al.: Surgical treatment for pulmonary emphysema. Can. J. Surg., 20:222, 1977.

DeLorimer, A. A.: Congenital malformations and neonatal problems of the respiratory tract. In Welch, K. J., Randolph, J. G., Ravitch, M. M., et al. (eds): Pediatric Surgery. 4th ed. Vol. 1. Chicago, Year Book, 1986, p. 631.

DeLorimer, A. A., Harrison, M. R., Hardy, K., et al.: Tracheobronchial obstructions in infants and children. Ann. Surg., 212:277–289, 1990.

Di Donato, R., Di Carlo, D., Squitieri, C., et al.: Palliation of cardiac malformations associated with right isomerism (asplenia syndrome) in infancy. Ann. Thorac. Surg., 44:35, 1987.

Di Lorenzo, M., Collin, P. P., Vaillancourt, R., and Duranceau, A.: Bronchogenic cysts. J. Pediatr. Surg., 24:988–991, 1989.

Dijkman, J. H.: Morphological aspects, classification and epidemiology of emphysema. Bull. Eur. Physiopathol. Respir., 22:241, 1986.

Dines, D. E., Seward, I. B., and Bernatz, P. E.: Pulmonary arteriovenous fistulas. Mayo Clin. Proc., 58:176, 1983.

DuMontier, C., Graviss, E. R., Silberstein, M. J., and McAlister, W. H.: Bronchogenic cysts in children. Clin. Radiol., 36:431, 1985.

Dunn, J. M., Gordon, I., Chrispin, A. R., et al.: Early and late results of surgical correction of pulmonary artery sling. Ann. Thorac. Surg., 28:230, 1979.

Engle, W. A., Cohen, M. D., McAlister, W. H., et al.: Neonatal tracheobronchomegaly. Am. J. Perinatol., 4:81, 1987.

Felson, B.: The lobes and interlobar pleura: Fundamental roentgen considerations. Am. J. Med. Sci., 230:572, 1955.

Fletcher, C. M., and Pride, N. B.: Definitions of emphysema, chronic bronchitis, asthma and airflow obstruction: 25 years on from the Ciba symposium. Thorax, 39:81, 1984.

Flower, C. D. R.: Imaging pulmonary arteriovenous malformations. Br. Med. J., 294:1633, 1987.

Fowler, C. L., Podomy, W. J., Wagner, M. L., and Kessler, M. S.: Review of bronchopulmonary foregut malformations. J. Pediatr. Surg., 23:793–797, 1988.

Fraser, R. G., Pare, J. A. P., Pare, P. D., et al.: Diagnosis of Diseases of the Chest. 3rd ed. Philadelphia, W. B. Saunders, 1988.

Frenckner, B., and Freyschuss, U.: Pulmonary function after lobectomy for congenital lobar emphysema and congenital cystic adenomatoid malformation. Scand. J. Thorac. Cardiovasc. Surg., 16:293, 1982.

Frey, E. E., Smith, W. L., Grandgeorge, S., et al.: Chronic airway obstruction in children: Evaluation with cine-CT. A. J. R., 148:347, 1987.

Gadek, J. E., and Pacht, E. R.: The protease-antiprotease balance within the human lung: Implications for the pathogenesis of emphysema. Lung, 168(Suppl.):552–564, 1990.

Gaensler, E. A., Cugell, D. W., Knudson, R. J., and FitzGerald, M. X.: Surgical management of emphysema. Clin. Chest. Med., 4:443, 1983.

Gebauer, P. W., and Mason, C. B.: Intralobar pulmonary sequestration associated with anomalous pulmonary vessels: A nonentity. Chest, 35:282, 1954.

Gerle, R. D., Jaretzki, A., Ashley, C. A., and Berne, A. S.: Congenital bronchopulmonary foregut malformation: Pulmonary sequestration communicating with the gastrointestinal tract. N. Engl. J. Med., 278:1413, 1968.

Gibaldi, M.: Human gene therapy. Pharmacotherapy, 13:79–87, 1993.

Glenski, J. A., Thibeault, D. W., Hall, F. K., et al.: Selective bronchial intubation in infants with lobar emphysema: Indications, complications, and long-term outcome. Am. J. Perinatol., 3:199, 1986.

Gortner, L.: Natural surfactant for neonatal respiratory distress syndrome in very premature infants: A 1992 update. J. Perinatol. Med., 20:409–419, 1992.

Goto, H., Boozalis, S. T., Benson, K. T., et al.: High-frequency jet ventilation for resection of congenital lobar emphysema. Anesth. Analg., 66:684, 1987.

Gottlieb, L. S., and Turner, A. F.: Swyer-James (Macleod's) syndrome: Variations in pulmonary-bronchial arterial blood flow. Chest, 69:62, 1976.

Greenholz, S. K., Karrer, F. M., and Lilly, J. R.: Contemporary surgery of tracheomalacia. J. Pediatr. Surg., 21:511, 1986.

Greenstone, M., Rutman, A., Dewar, A., et al.: Primary ciliary dyskinesia: Cytological and clinical features. Q. J. Med., 67:405–423, 1988.

Grillo, H. C.: Tracheal surgery. Scand. J. Thorac. Cardiovasc. Surg., 17:67, 1983.

Gross, R. E., and Lewis, J. E.: Defect of the anterior mediastinum: Successful surgical repair. Surg. Gynecol. Obstet., 80:549–554, 1945.

Gross, P., Babjak, M. A., Tolker, E., and Kaschak, M.: Enzymatically produced pulmonary emphysema: A preliminary report. J. Occup. Med., 6:481, 1964.

Grunebaum, M., and Griscom, N. T.: Protrusion of the lung apex through Sibson's fascia in infancy. Thorax, 33:290, 1978.

Gustafson, R. A., Murray, E. F., Warden, H. E., et al.: Intralobar sequestration: A missed diagnosis. Ann. Thorac. Surg., 47:841–847, 1989.

Haller, J. A., Golladay, E. S., Pichard, L. R., et al.: Surgical management of lung bud anomalies: Lobar emphysema, bronchogenic cyst, cystic adenomatoid malformation, and intralobar pulmonary sequestration. Ann. Thorac. Surg., 28:33, 1979.

Haller, J. A., Golladay, E. S., Pickard, L. R., et al.: The natural history of bronchial atresia: Serial observations of a case from birth to operative correction. J. Thorac. Cardiovasc. Surg., 79:868, 1980.

Harris, A., and Argent, B. E.: The cystic fibrosis gene and its product CFTR. Cell. Biol., 4:37–44, 1993.

Harris, H. A., and Lewis, I.: Anomalies of the lungs with special reference to the danger of abnormal vessels in lobectomy. J. Thorac. Surg., 9:666, 1940.

Harris, D. M., Lloyd, D. C. F., Morrissey, B., and Adams, H.: The computed tomographic appearances in pulmonary artery atresia. Clin. Radiol., 45:382–386, 1992.

Heithoff, K. B., Sane, S. M., Williams, H. J., et al.: Bronchopulmonary foregut malformations: A unifying etiologic concept. Embryology, 126:46, 1976.

Hendren, W. H., and McKee, D. M.: Lobar emphysema of infancy. J. Pediatr. Surg., 1:24, 1966.

Hernandez, R. J., and Tucker, G. F.: Congenital tracheal stenosis: Role of CT and high KV films. Pediatr. Radiol., 17:192, 1987.

Hislop, A., and Reid, L.: Fetal and childhood development of the intrapulmonary veins in man: Branching pattern and structure. Thorax, 28:313, 1973.

Hoidal, J. R., Fox, R. B., LeMarbe, P. A., et al.: Altered oxidative metabolic responses in vitro of alveolar macrophages from asymptomatic cigarette smokers. Am. Rev. Respir. Dis., 123:85, 1981.

Hoidal, J. R., and Niewoehner, D. E.: The role of tissue repair and leukocytes in the pathogenesis of emphysema. Chest, 83(Suppl. 5):58S, 1983.

Holinger, L. D., Volk, M. S., and Tucker, G. F.: Congenital laryngeal anomalies associated with tracheal agenesis. Ann. Otol. Rhinol. Laryngol., 96:505, 1987.

Honey, M.: Anomalous pulmonary venous drainage of right lung to inferior vena cava (scimitar syndrome). Clinical spectrum in older patients and role of surgery. Q. J. Med., 46:463, 1977.

Hruban, R. H., Shumway, S. J., Orel, S. B., et al.: Congenital bronchopulmonary foregut malformation. Am. J. Clin. Pathol., 91:403–409, 1989.

Hubbard, R. C., Sellers, S., Czerski, D., et al.: Biochemical efficacy and safety of monthly augmentation therapy for alpha-1 antitrypsin deficiency. J. A. M. A., 260:1259–1264, 1988.

Huddleston, C. R.: Use of reduced-sized lungs for transplant in children. In Kron, I., and Kean, J. (eds): Pediatric Lung Transplantation. Austin, TX, Medical Intelligence Unit, RG Landes, 1993, pp. 4–23.

Hughes, J. A., MacArthur, A. M., Hutchinson, D. C. S., and Hugh-Jones, P.: Long term changes in lung function after surgical treatment of bullous emphysema in smokers and ex-smokers. Thorax, 39:140, 1984.

Hyde, S. C., Gill, D. R., Higgins, C. F., et al.: Correction of the ion transport defect in cystic fibrosis transgenic mice by gene therapy. Nature, 362:250–255, 1993.

Jederlinic, P. J., Sicilian, L. S., Baigelman, W., and Gaensler, E. A.: Congenital bronchial atresia. Medicine, 66:73, 1987.

Jobe, A., and Ikegami, M.: Surfactant for the treatment of respiratory distress syndrome. Am. Rev. Respir. Dis., 136:1256–1275, 1987.

Juettner, F. M., Pinter, H. H., Friehs, G. B., and Hoefler, H.: Bronchial carcinoid arising in intralobar bronchopulmonary sequestration with vascular supply from the left gastric artery. J. Thorac. Cardiovasc. Surg., 90:25, 1985.

Juettner, F. M., Pinter, H. H., Lammer, G., et al.: Bilateral intralobar pulmonary sequestration: Therapeutic implications. Ann. Thorac. Surg., 43:660, 1987.

Kaiser, L. R., Cooper, J. D., Trulock, E. P., et al.: The evolution of single lung transplantation for emphysema. J. Thorac. Cardiovasc. Surg., 102:333–341, 1991a.

Kaiser, L. R., Pasque, M. K., Trulock, E. P., et al.: Bilateral sequential lung transplantation: The procedure of choice for double lung replacement. Ann. Thorac. Surg., 52:438–446, 1991b.

Kartagener, M.: Zur Pathogenese der Bronchiektasien. I. Bronchiektasien bei Situs Viscerum Inversus. Bietr. Klin. Tuberk., 83:489, 1933.

Kaufman, S. L.: Intrathoracic interventional vascular techniques in congenital cardiovascular disease. J. Thorac. Imag., 2:1, 1987.

Khaghani, A., Banner, N., Pzdogan, E., et al.: Medium-term results of combined heart and lung transplantation for emphysema. J. Heart Lung Transplant., 10:15–21, 1991.

King, R. J.: Pulmonary surfactant. J. Appl. Physiol., 53:1, 1982.

Kinney, T. B., and De Luca, S. A.: Kartagener's syndrome. Am. Fam. Physician, 44:133–134, 1991.

Koopot, R., Nikaidoh, H., and Idriss, F. S.: Surgical management of anomalous left pulmonary artery causing tracheobronchial obstruction: Pulmonary artery sling. J. Thorac. Cardiovasc. Surg., 69:239, 1975.

Lally, K. P., Paranka, M. S., Roden, J., et al.: Congenital diaphragmatic hernia. Stabilization and repair on ECMO. Ann. Surg., 216:569–573, 1992.

Langston, C., Kida, K., Reed, M., et al.: Human lung growth in late gestation and in the neonate. Am. Rev. Respir. Dis., 129:607, 1984.

Laurell, C. B., and Eriksson, S.: The electrophoretic alpha-1 globulin pattern of serum in alpha-1 antitrypsin deficiency. Scand. J. Clin. Lab. Invest., 15:132, 1963.

Leijala, M., and Louhimo, I.: Extralobar sequestration of the lung in children. Prog. Pediatr. Surg., 21:99–106, 1987.

Leithiser, R. E., Capitanio, M. A., Macpherson, R. I., and Wood, B. P.: "Communicating" bronchopulmonary foregut malformations. A. J. R., 146:227, 1986.

Levine, M. M., Nudel, D. B., Gootman, N., et al.: Pulmonary sequestration causing congestive heart failure in infancy: A report of two cases and review of the literature. Ann. Thorac. Surg., 34:581, 1982.

Lewis, J. F., and Jobe, A. H.: Surfactant and the adult respiratory distress syndrome. Am. Rev. Respir. Dis., 147:218–233, 1993.

Lillehei, C. W., and Colan, S.: Echocardiography in the preoperative evaluation of vascular rings. J. Pediatr. Surg., 27:1118–1121, 1992.

Lillington, G. A.: Unilateral hyperlucency. In Lillington, G. A.: A Diagnostic Approach to Chest Diseases. Baltimore, Williams & Wilkins, 1986.

Low, D. E., Trulock, E. P., Kaiser, L. R., et al.: Morbidity, mortality and early results of single versus bilateral lung transplantation for emphysema. J. Thorac. Cardiovasc. Surg., 103:1119–1126, 1992.

Luck, S. R., Reynolds, M., and Raffensperger, J. G.: Congenital bronchopulmonary malformations. Curr. Probl. Surg., 23:245–314, 1986.

Lyerly, K., and Sabiston, D. C.: Pulmonary arteriovenous malformations. In Sabiston, D. C., and Spencer, F. C. (eds): Surgery of the Chest. 5th ed. Chapter 26. Philadelphia, W. B. Saunders, 1990, pp. 840–846.

MacArthur, A. M., and Fountain, S. W.: Intracavitary suction and drainage in the treatment of emphysematous bullae. Thorax, 32:668, 1977.

Macklin, C. C.: The pulmonary alveolar mucoid film and pneumocytes. Lancet, 1:1099, 1954.

Maier, J. D.: Bronchogenic cysts of the mediastinum. Ann. Surg., 127:424, 1948.

Mal, H., Andreassian, B., Pamela, F., et al.: Unilateral lung transplantation in end-stage pulmonary emphysema. Am. Rev. Respir. Dis., 140:797–802, 1989.

Marcelletti, C., Di Donato, R., Nijveld, A., et al.: Right and left isomerism: The cardiac surgeon's view. Ann. Thorac. Surg., 35:400, 1983.

Mardini, M. K., and Nyhan, W. L.: Agenesis of the lung. Report of four patients with unusual anomalies. Chest, 87:522, 1985.

Margraf, L. R., Tomashefski, J. F., Bruce, M. C., and Dahms, B. B.: Morphometric analysis of the lung in bronchopulmonary dysplasia. Am. Rev. Respir. Dis., 143:391–400, 1991.

Margulies, S. S., Schriner, R. W., Schroeder, M. A., and Hubmayr, R. D.: Static lung-lung interactions in unilateral emphysema. J. Appl. Physiol., 73:545–551, 1992.

Marin, M. L., Romney, B. M., Franco, K., et al.: Bronchogenic cyst: A case report emphasizing the role of magnetic resonance imaging. J. Thorac. Imag., 6:43–46, 1991.

Marinelli, W. A., Hertz, M. I., Shumway, S. J., et al.: Single lung transplantation for severe emphysema. J. Heart Lung Transplant., 11:577–583, 1992.

Markowitz, R. I., Frederick, W., Rosenfield, N. S., et al.: Single, mediastinal, unilobar lung—A rare form of subtotal pulmonary agenesis. Pediatr. Radiol., 17:269, 1987.

Marks, C., and Marks, P.: The embryologic basis of tracheobronchopulmonary maldevelopment. Int. Surg., 72:109, 1987.

Maulik, D., Robinson, L., Kaily, D. K., et al.: Prenatal sonographic depiction of intralobar pulmonary sequestration. J. Ultrasound Med., 6:703–706, 1987.

McAlister, W. H., Wright, J. R., and Crane, J. P.: Mainstem bronchial atresia: Intrauterine sonographic diagnosis. A. J. R., 148:364, 1987.

McGarry, T., Giosa, R., Rohman, M., and Huang, C. T.: Pneumatocele formation in adult pneumonia. Chest, 92:717, 1987.

McLaughlin, F. J., Streider, D. J., Harris, G. B. C., et al.: Tracheal bronchus: Association with respiratory morbidity in childhood. J. Pediatr., 106:751, 1985.

Mehta, A. C., Ahmad, M., Golish, J. A., and Buonocore, E.: Congenital abnormalities of the lung in the adult. Cleve. Clin. Q., 50:401, 1983.

Messineo, A., Filler, R. M., Bahoric, A., and Smith, C. R.: Repair of long tracheal stenosis with cryopreserved cartilaginous allografts. J. Pediatr. Surg., 27:1131–1135, 1992a.

Messineo, A., Forte, V., Joseph, T., et al.: The balloon posterior tracheal split: A technique for managing tracheal stenosis in the premature infant. J. Pediatr. Surg., 27:1142–1144, 1992b.

Miller, R. W., Woo, P., Kellman, R. K., et al.: Tracheobronchial abnormalities in infants with bronchopulmonary dysplasia. J. Pediatr., 111:779, 1987.

Milstein, J. M., Lau, M., and Bickers, R. G.: Tracheal agenesis in infants with VATER syndrome. Am. J. Dis. Child., 139:77, 1985.

Mitchell, R. E., and Bury, R. G.: Congenital bronchiectasis due to deficiency of bronchial cartilage. J. Pediatr., 87:230–234, 1975.

Morgan, M. D. L., Denison, D. M., and Strickland, B.: Value of computed tomography for selecting patients with bullous lung disease for surgery. Thorax, 41:855, 1986.

Morgan, M. D. L., Edwards, C. W., Morris, J., and Matthews, H. R.: Origin and behaviour of emphysematous bullae. Thorax, 44:533–538, 1989.

Nagaraj, H. S., Mitchell, K. A., Fallat, M. E., et al.: Surgical complications and procedures in neonates on extracorporeal membrane oxygenation. J. Pediatr. Surg., 27:1106–1110, 1992.

Nakata, H., Egashira, K., Watanabe, H., et al.: MRI of bronchogenic cysts. J. Comput. Assist. Tomogr., 17:267–270, 1993.

Nakayama, D. K., Motoyama, E. K., Evand, R., and Hannakan, C.: Relation between arterial hypoxemia and plasma eicosanoids in neonates with congenital diaphragmatic hernia. J. Surg. Res., 53:615–620, 1992.

Nashef, S. A. M., Dromer, C., Velly, J., et al.: Expanding wire stents in benign tracheobronchial disease: Indications and complications. Ann. Thorac. Surg., 54:937–940, 1992.

Neill, E. A., Ferenez, C., Sabiston, D. C., et al.: The familial occurrence of hypoplastic right lung with systemic arterial supply and venous drainage, "scimitar syndrome." Johns Hopkins Med. J., 107:1–20, 1960.

Newman, K. D., Randolph, J.: Surgical problems of the esophagus in infants and children. In Sabiston, D. C., and Spencer, F. C.: Surgery of the Chest. 5th ed. Chapter 25. Philadelphia, W. B. Saunders, 1990, pp. 815–846.

Novick, R. J., Menkis, A. H., Sandler, D., et al.: Contralateral pneumonectomy after single-lung transplantation for emphysema. Ann. Thorac. Surg., 52:1317–1319, 1991.

O'Brien, C. J., Hughes, C. F., and Gianoutsos, P.: Surgical treatment of bullous emphysema. Aust. N. Z. J. Surg., 56:241, 1986.

O'Rahilly, R., and Muller, F.: Respiratory and alimentary relations in staged human embryos. New embryological data and congenital anomalies. Ann. Otol. Rhinol. Laryngol., 93:421–429, 1984.

Page, D. V., and Stocker, J. T.: Anomalies associated with pulmonary hypoplasia. Am. Rev. Respir. Dis., 125:861–870, 1982.

Patterson, G. A., Cooper, J. D. (eds): Lung transplantation. Chest Clin. North Am., 3:1–178, 1993.

Pawade, A., de Leval, M. R., Elliott, M. J., and Stark, J.: Pulmonary artery sling. Ann. Thorac. Surg., 54:967–970, 1992.

Peery, W. H.: Clinical spectrum of hereditary hemorrhagic telangiectasis. Am. J. Med., 82:989, 1987.

Pratt, P. C.: Emphysema and chronic airways disease. In Dail, D. H., Hammar, S. P., (eds): Pulmonary Pathology. New York, Springer-Verlag, 1988, pp. 653–658.

Prouty, L. A., and Myers, T. L.: Oligohydramnios sequence (Potter's Syndrome). South Med. J., 80:585, 1987.

Puskas, J. D., Hirai, T., Christie, N., et al.: Reliable thirty-hour lung preservation by donor lung hyperinflation. J. Thorac. Cardiovasc. Surg., 104:1075–1083, 1992.

Putman, C. E., Godwin, J. D., et al.: CT of localized lucent lung lesions. Semin. Roentgenol., 19:173, 1984.

Ravitch, M. M.: Mediastinal cysts and tumors. In Welch, K. J., Randolph, J. G., Ravitch, M. M., et al. (eds): Pediatric Surgery. 4th ed, Vol. 1. Chicago, Year Book, 1986, p. 602.

Reid, L.: Lung growth in health and disease. Br. J. Dis. Chest, 78:113, 1984.

Reid, L.: Structure and function in pulmonary hypertension. Chest, 89:279, 1986.

Reidy, J. F., Jones, O. D. H., Tynan, M. J., et al.: Embolisation procedures in congenital heart disease. Br. Heart J., 54:184, 1985.

Rice, T. W.: The role of thoracoscopy in the surgery of emphysema. Chest Surg. Clin. North Am., 3:241–247, 1993.

Richman, P. S., Batcher, S., and Catanzaro, A.: Pulmonary surfactant suppresses the immune lung injury response to inhaled antigen in guinea pigs. J. Lab. Clin. Med., 116:18–26, 1990.

Rodgers, B. M., Harnam, P. K., and Johnson, A. M.: Bronchopulmonary foregut malformations. Ann. Surg., 203:517, 1986.

Rodgers, B. M., Moazam, F., and Talbert, J. L.: Endotracheal cryotherapy in the treatment of refractory airway strictures. Ann. Thorac. Surg., 35:52, 1983.

Rogers, D. A., Lobe, T. E., and Schropp, K. P.: Video-assisted thoracoscopic surgery in the pediatric patient. Chest Surg. Clin. North Am., 3:325–336, 1993.

Rosenfeld, M. A., Siegfried, W., Yoshimura, K., et al.: Adenovirus-mediated transfer of a recombinant alpha-1 antitrypsin gene to the lung epithelium in vivo. Science, 252:431–434, 1991.

Rosenfeld, M., and Ramsey, B.: Evolution of airway microbiology in the infant with cystic fibrosis: Role of nonpseudomonal and pseudomonal pathogens. Semin. Respir. Infect., 7:158–167, 1992.

Rubin, B. K.: Immotile cilia syndrome (primary ciliary dyskinesia) and inflammatory lung disease. Clin. Chest Med., 9:657–668, 1988.

Sade, R. M., Clouse, M., and Ellis, F. H.: The spectrum of pulmonary sequestration. Ann. Thorac. Surg., 18:644, 1974.

Sade, R. M., Rosenthal, A., Fellows, K., and Castañeda, A. R.: Pulmonary artery sling. J. Thorac. Cardiovasc. Surg., 69:335, 1975.

Saifuddin, A., and Arthur, R. J.: Congenital diaphragmatic hernia—A review of pre- and postoperative chest radiology. Clin. Radiol., 47:104–110, 1993.

Salzer, G. M., Hartl, H., and Wurnig, P.: Treatment of tracheal stenoses by resection in infancy and early childhood. Prog. Pediatr. Surg., 21:72, 1987.

Savic, B., Birtel, F. J., Tholen, W., et al.: Lung sequestration: Report of seven cases and review of 540 published cases. Thorax, 34:96, 1979.

Schneider, J. R., St.-Cyr, J. A., Thompson, T. R., et al.: The changing spectrum of cystic pulmonary lesions requiring surgical resection in infants. J. Thorac. Cardiovasc. Surg., 89:332, 1985.

Schneider, P.: Die Missbildungen der atmungsorgane. In Schwalbe, E. (ed): Die Morphologie der Missbindungen des Menschen und der Tiere. Vol. 3. Jena, Gustav Fisher, 1900–1913, pp. 817–822.

Schwartz, A. R., Fishman, E. K., and Wang, K. P.: Diagnosis and treatment of a bronchogenic cyst using transbronchial needle aspiration. Thorax, 41:326, 1986.

Seiber, W. K.: Lung cysts, sequestration, and bronchopulmonary dysplasia. In Welch, K. J., Randolph, J. G., Ravitch, M. M., et al. (eds): Pediatric Surgery. 4th ed. Vol. 1. Chicago, Year Book, 1986, p. 645.

Sferra, T. J., and Collins, F. S.: The molecular biology of cystic fibrosis. Ann. Rev. Med., 44:133–144, 1993.

Shackelford, G. D., and Siegel, M. J.: CT appearance of cystic adenomatoid malformations. J. Comput. Assist. Tomogr., 13:612–616, 1989.

Shady, K., Siegel, M., and Glazer, H. S.: CT of focal pulmonary masses in childhood. RadioGraphics, 12:505–514, 1992.

Sifers, R. N., Finegold, M. J., Woo, S. L. C.: Molecular biology and genetics of alpha-1 antitrypsin deficiency. Semin. Liver Dis., 12:301–310, 1992.

Siegel, M. J., Shackelford, G. D., McAlister, W. H.: Tracheobronchography in the evaluation of anomalous left pulmonary artery. Pediatr. Radiol., 12:235, 1982.

Simon, G., and Reid, L.: Atresia of an apical bronchus of the left upper lobe—Report of three cases. Br. J. Dis. Chest, 57:126, 1963.

Singh, G., Katyal, S. L., Bedrossian, C. W., et al.: Pulmonary alveolar proteinosis. Staining for surfactant apoprotein in alveolar proteinosis and in conditions simulating it. Chest, 83:82, 1983.

Sirivella, S., Ford, W. B., Zikria, E. A., et al.: Foregut cysts of the mediastinum. J. Thorac. Cardiovasc. Surg., 90:776, 1985.

Snider, G. L.: Chronic obstructive pulmonary disease: Risk factors, pathophysiology and pathogenesis. Ann. Rev. Med., 40:411–429, 1989.

Snider, G. L.: Distinguishing among asthma, chronic bronchitis, and emphysema. Chest, 87(Suppl. 1):35S, 1985.

Soosay, G. N., Baudouin, S. V., Hanson, P. J. V., et al.: Symptomatic cysts in otherwise normal lungs of children and adults. Histopathology, 20:517–522, 1992.

Speer, C. P., Ruess, D., Harms, K., et al.: Neutrophil elastase and acute pulmonary damage in neonates with severe respiratory distress syndrome. Pediatrics, 91:794–799, 1993.

Spray, T. L., and Huddleston, C. B.: Pediatric lung transplantation. In Patterson, G. A., and Cooper, J. D.: Lung transplantation. Chest Surg. Clin. North Am., 3:123–144, 1993.

St.-Georges, R., Deslauriers, J., Duranceau, A., et al.: Clinical spectrum of bronchogenic cysts of the mediastinum and lung in the adult. Ann. Thorac. Surg., 52:6–13, 1991.

Stocker, J. T.: Sequestrations of the lung. Semin. Diagn. Pathol., 3:106–121, 1986.

Stocker, J. T., Drake, R. M., and Madewell, J. E.: Cystic and congenital lung disease in the newborn. Perspect. Pediatr. Radiol., 4:93, 1978.

Stocker, J. T., and Madewell, J. E.: Persistent interstitial pulmonary emphysema: Another complication of the respiratory distress syndrome. Pediatrics, 59:847, 1977.

Stocker, J. T., Madewell, J. E., and Drake, R. M.: Congenital cystic adenomatoid malformation of the lung, classification and morphologic spectrum. Hum. Pathol., 8:155, 1977.

Stocker, J. T., and Malczak, H. T.: A study of pulmonary ligament arteries. Chest, 86:611, 1984.

Strange, R. C., Cotton, W., Fryer, A. A., et al.: Lipid peroxidation and expression of copper-zinc and manganese superoxide dismutase in lungs of premature infants with hyaline membrane disease and bronchopulmonary dysplasia. J. Clin. Lab. Med., 116:666–673, 1990.

Suen, H. C., Mathisen, D. J., Grillo, G. C., et al.: Surgical management and radiological characteristics of bronchogenic cysts. Ann. Thorac. Surg., 55:476–481, 1993.

Super, M.: Milestones in cystic fibrosis. Br. Med. Bull., 48:717–737, 1992.

Takaro, T., Price, H. P., and Parra, S. C.: Ultrastructural studies of apertures in the interalveolar septum of the adult human lung. Am. Rev. Respir. Dis., 119:425, 1979.

Takayanagi, K., Brochowska, E., Abu-El Nas, S.: Pulmonary agenesis with esophageal atresia and tracheoesophageal fistula. J. Pediatr. Surg., 22:125, 1987.

Tanaka, F., Itoh, M., Esaki, H., et al.: Secondary spontaneous pneumothorax. Ann. Thorac. Surg., 55:372–376, 1993.

Tapper, D., Schuster, S., McBride, J., et al.: Polyalveolar lobe: Anatomic and physiologic parameters and their relationship to congenital lobar emphysema. J. Pediatr. Surg., 15:931, 1980.

Teberg, A. J., Pena, I., Finello, K., et al.: Prediction of neurodevelopmental outcome in infants with and without bronchopulmonary dysplasia. Am. J. Med. Sci., 301:369–374, 1991.

Tenholder, M. F., Jones, P. A., Matthews, J. I., and Hooper, R. G.: Bullous emphysema: Progressive incremental exercise testing to evaluate candidates for bullectomy. Chest, 77:802, 1980.

Terry, P. B., White, R. I., Barth, K. H., et al.: Pulmonary arteriovenous malformations. N. Engl. J. Med., 308:1197, 1983.

Thurlbeck, W. M.: Overview of the pathology of pulmonary emphysema in the human. Clin. Chest Med., 4:337, 1983.

Thurlbeck, W. M.: Postnatal human lung growth. Thorax, 37:564, 1982.

Thurlbeck, W. M.: The pathobiology and epidemiology of human emphysema. J. Toxicol. Environ. Health, 13:323, 1984.

Tobin, C. E.: The bronchial arteries and their connections with other vessels in the human lung. Surg. Gynecol. Obstet., 95:741–750, 1952.

Tocewicz, K., Wren, C., Warren, S., and Dark, J. H.: Extensive patch tracheoplasty with a silicon "T" tube stent in a 7-month-old infant. Eur. J. Cardiothorac. Surg., 7:101–103, 1993.

Toriello, H. V., and Bauserman, S. C.: Bilateral pulmonary agenesis. Am. J. Med. Genet., 21:93, 1985.

Tsang, V., and Goldstraw, P.: Self-expanding metal stent for tracheobronchial strictures. Eur. J. Cardiothorac. Surg., 6:555–560, 1992.

Ungaro, R., et al.: Solitary peripheral pulmonary artery aneurysms: Pathogenesis and surgical treatment. J. Thorac. Cardiovasc. Surg., 71:566, 1976.

Unger, J. M., England, D. M., and Bogust, G. A.: Interstitial emphysema in adults: Recognition and prognostic implications. J. Thorac. Imag., 4:86–94, 1989.

Vigneswaran, W. T., Townsend, E. R., and Fountain, S. W.: Surgery for bullous disease of the lung. Eur. J. Cardiothorac. Surg., 6:427–430, 1992.

Vinograd, I., Filler, R. M., and Bahoric, A.: Long-term functional results of prosthetic airway splinting in tracheomalacia and bronchomalacia. J. Pediatr. Surg., 22:38, 1987.

Volpi, A., Cavalli, A., Maggioni, A. P., and Pieri-Nierli, F.: Left atrial compression by a mediastinal bronchogenic cyst presenting with paroxysmal atrial fibrillation. Thorax, 43:216–217, 1988.

Wailoo, M. P., and Emery, J. L.: Normal growth and development of the trachea. Thorax, 7:584, 1982.

Wakabayashi, A.: Expanded applications of diagnostic and therapeutic thoroscopy. J. Thorac. Cardiovasc. Surg., 102:721–723, 1991.

Walker, L. K., Wetzel, R. C., and Haller, J. A.: Extracorporeal membrane oxygenation for perioperative support during congenital tracheal stenosis and repair. Anesth. Analg., 75:825–829, 1992.

Weber, T. R., Tracy, R. F., Connors, R., et al.: Prolonged extracorporeal support for non-neonatal respiratory failure. J. Pediatr. Surg., 27:1100–1105, 1992.

Weibel, E. R.: Design and structure of the human lung. In Fishman, A. P. (ed): Assessment of Pulmonary Function. New York, McGraw-Hill, 1980, pp. 18–65.

Weinberger, S. E.: Recent advances in pulmonary medicine. N. Engl. J. Med., 328:1389–1397, 1462–1470, 1993.

Werber, J., Ramilo, J. L., London, R., and Harris, V. J.: Unilateral absence of a pulmonary artery. Chest, 84:729, 1983.

Wesley, J. R., Heidelberger, K. P., DiPietro, M. A., et al.: Diagnosis and management of congenital cystic disease of the lung in children. J. Pediatr. Surg., 21:202, 1986.

West, K. W., Bengston, K., Rescorla, F. J., et al.: Delayed surgical repair and ECMO improves survival in congenital diaphragmatic hernia. Ann. Surg., 216:454–462, 1992.

Wewers, M. D., Casolaro, M. A., Sellers, S. E., et al.: Replacement therapy for alpha-1 antitrypsin deficiency associated with emphysema. N. Engl. J. Med., 316:1055–1062, 1987.

White, J. J., Donahoo, J. S., Ostrow, P. T., et al.: Cardiovascular and respiratory manifestations of pulmonary sequestration in childhood. Ann. Thorac. Surg., 18:286, 1974.

White, R. I., Mitchell, S. E., and Kan, J.: Interventional procedures in congenital heart disease. Cardiovasc. Intervent. Radiol., 9:286, 1986.

Wildevuur, D. R. H., and Benfield, J. R.: A review of 23 human lung transplantations by 20 surgeons. Ann. Thorac. Surg., 9:489–515, 1970.

Williams, A. J., and Schuster, S. R.: Bronchial atresia associated with a bronchogenic cyst. Chest, 87:396, 1985.

Wright, J. R., and Clements, J. A.: Metabolism and turnover of lung surfactant. Am. Rev. Respir. Dis., 135:426–444, 1987.

Wright, J. R.: Clearance and recycling of pulmonary surfactant. Am. J. Physiol., 259:1–12, 1990.

Wohl, M. E. B., Griscom, N. T., Streider, D. J., et al.: The lung following repair of congenital diaphragmatic hernia. J. Pediatr., 90:405, 1977.

Womack, N. A., and Graham, E. A.: Epithelial metaplasia in congenital cystic disease of the lung. Am. J. Pathol., 17:645–653, 1941.

Woodring, J. H., Howard, R. S., and Rehm, S. R.: Congenital tracheobronchomegaly (Mounier-Kuhn syndrome): A report of 10 cases and review of the literature. J. Thorac. Imag., 6:1–10, 1991.

Worsnop, C. J., Teichtahl, H., and Clarke, C. P.: Bronchogenic cyst: A cause of pulmonary artery obstruction and breathlessness. Ann. Thorac. Surg., 55:1254–1255, 1993.

Yancey, M. K., and Richards, D. S.: Antenatal sonographic findings associated with unilateral pulmonary agenesis. Obstet. Gynecol., 81:847–849, 1993.

Zeimer, G., Heinemann, M., Kaulitz, R., et al.: Pulmonary artery sling with tracheal stenosis: Primary one-stage repair in infancy. Ann. Thorac. Surg., 54:971–973, 1992.

25

Surgery of the Esophagus in Infants and Children

Kurt D. Newman and Judson Randolph

ESOPHAGEAL ATRESIA AND RELATED ANOMALIES

Historical Aspects

Esophageal atresia and tracheoesophageal fistula were first described in the late 1600s. In 1939, Ladd (1944) in Boston and Leven (1941) in Minneapolis successfully managed two infants with this heretofore lethal lesion. Both surgeons performed a gastrostomy, followed later by ligation of the fistula and end-cervical esophagostomy. This staging permitted the children to survive and ultimately undergo esophageal reconstruction with an antethoracic skin tube (Fig. 25–1). These two historic patients were the first babies to survive with esophageal atresia. Ironically, Ladd's patient was treated for a squamous cell carcinoma, which developed in the skin conduit 44 years after its construction (LaQuaglia et al., 1987).

The early 20th century was notable for many at-

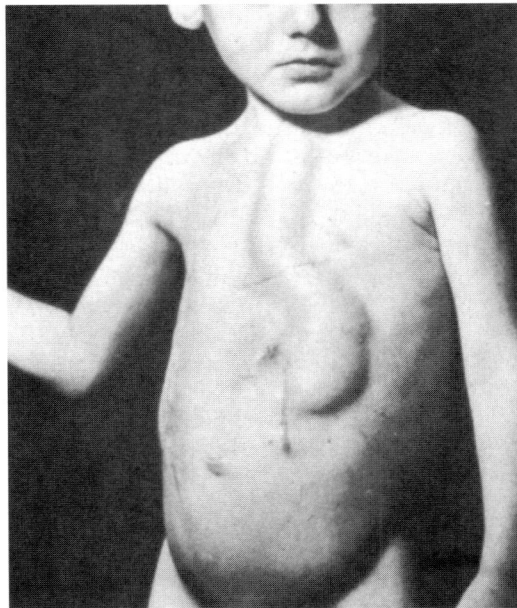

FIGURE 25–1. Photograph of an early survivor who was born with esophageal atresia and tracheal esophageal fistula. He was originally treated with division of the fistula, gastrostomy, and esophagostomy. An antethoracic skin tube was then created. Approximately 10 years later, a coloesophagoplasty was successful. (From Gross, R. E.: The Surgery of Infancy and Childhood. Philadelphia, W. B. Saunders, 1953, p. 76.)

tempts at staging the repair of this congenital lesion, but none of the infants survived. In 1936, Lanman performed the first primary extrapleural esophageal anastomosis in a newborn with atresia of the esophagus, but the infant died. In Lanman's report of his experience in 1940, he recounted 32 consecutive patients without a single survivor. This forthright essay was the stimulus for pediatricians and surgeons to focus on this unsolved problem, and in 1941, Haight achieved the first survival of an infant by using a primary surgical anastomosis for esophageal atresia.

The impact of Haight's success in the early 1940s cannot be overestimated. For the first time, an infant born with esophageal atresia and tracheoesophageal fistula could lead a potentially normal life with eating and swallowing. This accomplishment initiated clinical studies that have led to refined and improved care of infants born with this anomaly. Many of the advances are derived from progress in the supportive care of the newborn, such as total parenteral nutrition, anesthetic techniques, ventilator management, antibiotics, and diagnostic imaging. These improvements permit survival rates in excess of 90%, despite the fact that the basic surgical principles of repair have not changed appreciably since the early 1940s.

Embryology

The esophagus and trachea arise from the same primitive foregut tissue. The separation into discrete structures is completed at 7 to 8 weeks' gestation. The process by which division occurs is incompletely understood but relates to elongation of the esophagus and invagination of the lateral walls (DeLorimier and Harrison, 1985) (Fig. 25–2). Imperfect separation of the esophagus and trachea in the fourth week of gestation leads to esophageal atresia and tracheoesophageal fistula (Smith, 1957). The association of anomalies such as vertebral, anorectal, tracheoesophageal, cardiac, radial, and renal (VATER) conditions in some children represents a spectrum of defects in other organs whose development may be altered at the same time (Ein et al., 1989; Weaver et al., 1986). Embryologic studies seem to indicate that interruption in the fourth week of gestation in the elongation and partitioning of the esophageal and tracheal tubes is a causative factor in the persistence of fistulas and clefts between the two channels and in the develop-

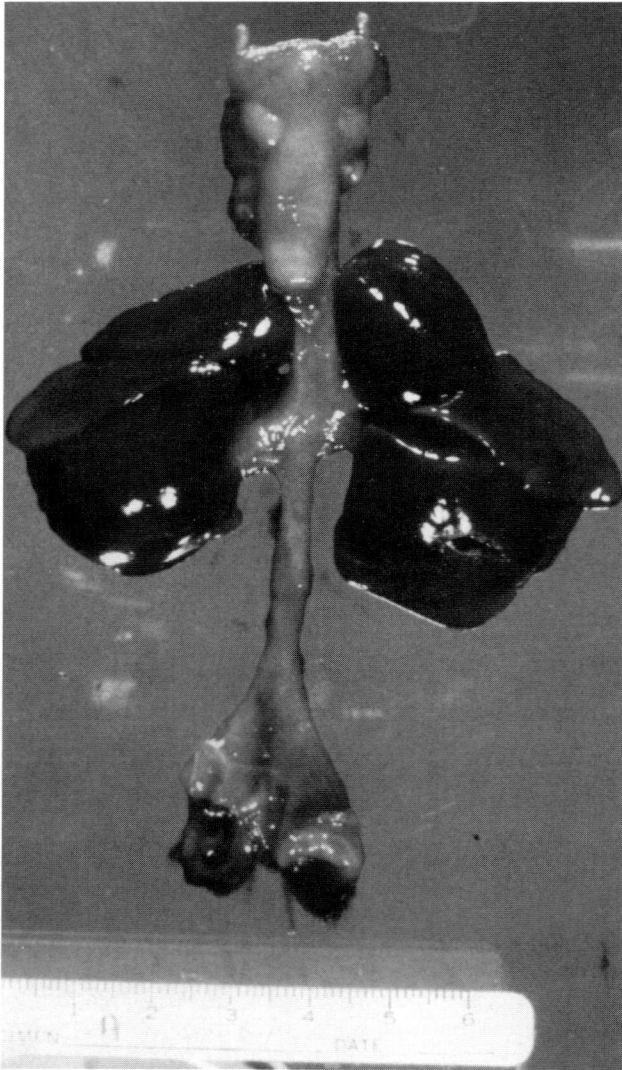

FIGURE 25–2. A pathologic specimen from the posterior perspective showing the proximal esophageal pouch and the fistula, which is connected to the carina. The photograph demonstrates the failure of division of the trachea and esophagus into separate structures.

ment of atresia of the esophagus (Hopkins, 1972; Kluth, 1976).

Incidence

The most common anomalies associated with the trachea and esophagus, in order of frequency, are (Holder et al., 1993) (Fig. 25–3):

1. Esophageal atresia with distal tracheoesophageal fistula, 86%.
2. Esophageal atresia without tracheoesophageal fistula, 5%.
3. Tracheoesophageal fistula without esophageal atresia ("H-type"), 3%.
4. Esophageal atresia with fistula between the upper esophageal pouch and the trachea, 1%.

5. Esophageal atresia with fistula to both pouches, 3%.

Large series of patients (Louhimo and Lindahl, 1983; Manning et al., 1986) generally support this distribution of anomalies; differences are related to variation in diagnostic methods. For this group of anomalies as a whole, the incidence is approximately 1 per 4500 births (Myers, 1974).

ESOPHAGEAL ATRESIA WITH LOWER–SEGMENT TRACHEOESOPHAGEAL FISTULA

Anatomy

Atresia with associated tracheoesophageal fistula constitutes the overwhelming majority of congenital malformations of the esophagus. The blind-ending upper esophageal segment usually extends only into the upper portion of the thorax. Typically, the proximal end of the lower portion of the esophagus is connected to the trachea, usually at or just above the tracheal bifurcation. This connection is usually 3 to 5 mm in cross-sectional diameter and easily admits inspired air or, in a retrograde fashion, the acidic gastric juice from the stomach.

Associated anomalies are common and are often the most significant factor in survival. Major chromosomal abnormalities are found in 4.6% of patients. In almost 20% of infants born with esophageal atresia, some variant of congenital heart disease is present, and imperforate anus occurs in approximately 10%. Some combination of the vertebral defects, imperforate anus, tracheoesophageal fistula, and radial and renal dysplasia comprising the VATER association of anomalies was found in 17.5% of patients (Manning et al., 1986).

Clinical Signs

With the advent and widespread application of prenatal ultrasonography, it is not uncommon for the diagnosis of esophageal atresia to be made before birth. The mother frequently exhibits polyhydramnios because the fetus is unable to swallow amniotic fluid owing to the esophageal obstruction. Failure to visualize a fetal fluid-filled esophagus or stomach suggests esophageal atresia (Pretorius et al., 1987). Other related anomalies such as cardiac defects can also be identified prenatally. The value of prenatal diagnosis lies in the enhanced ability to make appropriate arrangements for care immediately after birth, such as transport, operative care, and family counseling.

The earliest and most obvious clinical sign of esophageal atresia is regurgitation. This may consist of saliva bubbling out of the mouth or aspiration of the first feeding. Aspiration of a feeding is often followed by choking and coughing. Abdominal distention frequently occurs because inspired air is trans-

FIGURE 25–3. *A–F,* Classic diagram showing types of esophageal anomalies and related tracheal malformation. (Originally described by Vogt and used by Gross). (*A–F,* From Gross, R. E.: The Surgery of Infancy and Childhood. Philadelphia, W. B. Saunders, 1953, p. 76.)

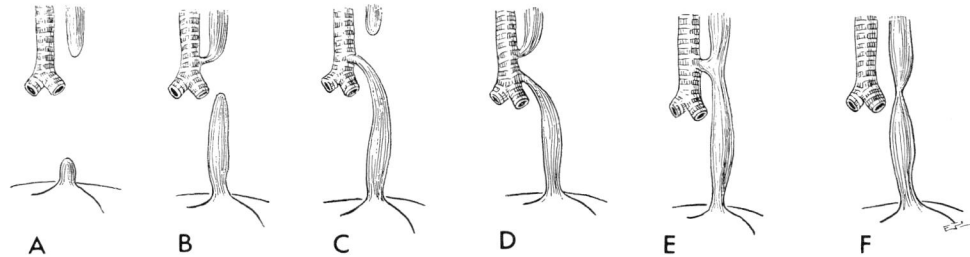

A B C D E F

mitted through the fistula and distal esophagus into the stomach. Regurgitated gastric juice passes through the fistula and into the trachea and lungs, causing a chemical pneumonia. The pulmonary problems may be compounded by atelectasis, which results from diaphragmatic elevation secondary to gastric distention.

The diagnosis may not be obvious at the initial examination unless an attempt is made to pass a tube into the stomach. Members of the nursing staff who are feeding the baby often observe the accumulation of mucus or saliva, which suggests the diagnosis. If esophageal atresia is suspected, the diagnosis can be confirmed by passing a catheter through the nose or mouth. For this maneuver, tiny flexible feeding catheters should be avoided because they may coil up and give the false impression that they have passed into the stomach. A larger catheter, slowly advanced, will meet the obstruction.

Some surgeons rely solely on a plain chest film showing an air-filled upper esophageal pouch to make a diagnosis. However, an x-ray study with 1 or 2 ml of contrast confirms the diagnosis and gives specific information about the level of the obstructed upper pouch (Fig. 25–4). Upper-pouch fistulas or clefts may also be identified preoperatively. If air is seen in the bowel, the presence of a tracheoesophageal communication can be inferred, since the air must have entered the stomach via the fistula. If no bowel gas is identified, the surgeon should suspect pure esophageal atresia without a fistula.

The condition of the lungs with respect to the existence of pneumonia and atelectasis is also essential information. Preliminary endoscopy has been advocated to identify preoperative anatomic variants (Filston et al., 1984), particularly unsuspected upper-pouch fistulas or laryngotracheoesophageal clefts (Fig. 25–5). In addition, Kosloske found that preoperative identification of a carinal fistula with bronchoscopy was helpful in planning technical measures to deal with a potential long gap between pouches (McKinnon and Kosloske, 1990).

When a heart murmur is identified, cardiac echocardiography is used to characterize the cardiac anomaly. This study also identifies the location of the aortic arch. If the arch is on the right side, a surgical approach to the esophagus via a right thoracotomy may prove difficult, and a left-sided approach is recommended.

Management

With the diagnosis of esophageal atresia and tracheoesophageal fistula confirmed, the following measures should be initiated immediately: (1) use of an infant warmer to prevent hypothermia, (2) 30-degree head-up position to diminish the potential for aspiration, (3) route for intravenous therapy to maintain hydration, (4) antibiotic treatment (even if pneumonia is not yet clinically manifest), and (5) sump catheter suction in the upper esophageal pouch (Replogle, 1963).

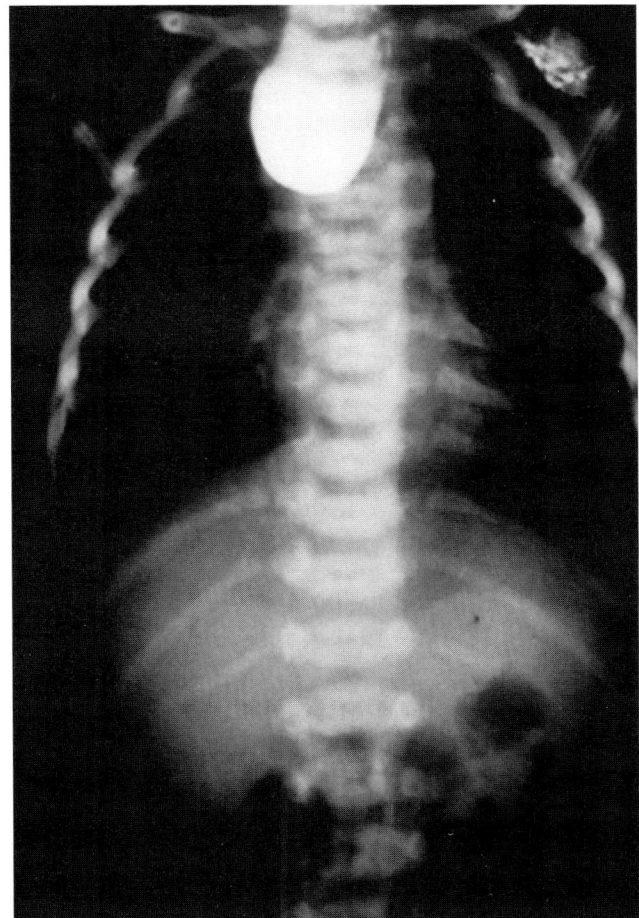

FIGURE 25–4. Chest radiograph with barium in the upper pouch. Air in the gastrointestinal tract demonstrates the presence of a tracheoesophageal fistula.

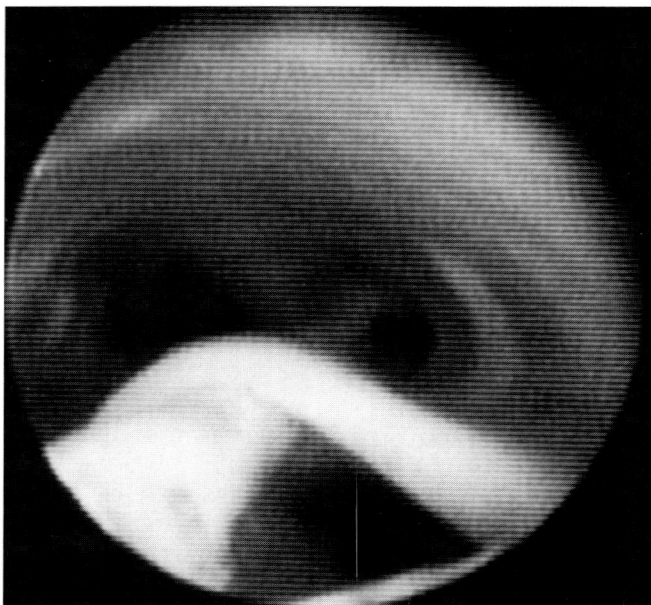

FIGURE 25–5. Endoscopic photograph showing the tracheoesophageal fistula with a catheter in it. The carina is visualized as a double opening just beyond the fistula.

Once stabilized, most infants can be safely managed with a primary repair, including division of the fistula and anastomosis of the esophagus. In 1962, Waterston and associates developed risk categories for infants with esophageal atresia and tracheoesophageal fistula, and classified the infants as follows:

Category A
  Birth weight more than 5½ lb and otherwise well
Category B
  1. Birth weight of 4 to 5½ lb and well *or*
  2. Higher birth weight and moderate pneumonia and other congenital anomaly
Category C
  1. Birth weight under 4 lb *or*
  2. Higher birth weight and severe pneumonia and severe congenital anomaly

This classification was the mainstay of clinical appraisal for 25 years and served as the basis for selection of a surgical management plan. With the rapid progress in neonatal supportive care, low birth weight and pulmonary problems are no longer clearly independent risk factors. Therefore, the Waterston classification is less frequently employed in the choice of surgical strategy, although it is still useful for comparison of institutional results. In recent years, the physiologic status of the infant has become the primary determinant of the surgical treatment plan (Randolph et al., 1989). Infants who are stable undergo either prompt total surgical correction or short-term delay with subsequent primary repair. For unstable infants, particularly those with severe cardiac or genetic anomalies, a plan incorporating a long-term delay with staged repair may be wise. If the infant is stable and shows no other major congenital anomalies, primary repair is undertaken promptly.

Operative Technique for Primary Repair

The operation for primary repair of esophageal atresia and tracheoesophageal fistula (Fig. 25–6) has changed very little since its description by Haight and Towsley (1943), although most surgeons now perform a single-layer anastomosis, as opposed to the "classic" two-layer Haight anastomosis. A retropleural approach as originally advocated by Lanman (1940) is most frequently used, although some surgeons believe that a transpleural approach is just as safe and much more expeditious (Bishop et al., 1985). Surgical exposure with the retropleural method is adequate, and the protection of the lung afforded by maintaining its pleural envelope has a salutary postoperative effect. More important, an anastomotic leak will not communicate with the pleural cavity and can be drained directly from the mediastinum posteriorly with decreased morbidity or mortality.

A standard posterolateral approach through the fourth intercostal space is used, without removing the rib. After the intercostal muscle bundles are divided, the pleura is teased gently from the undersurface of the fourth and fifth ribs and retracted anteriorly as the posterior mediastinal dissection continues. The azygos vein is encountered as it turns anteriorly across the mediastinum; it is ligated and divided between fine ligatures. The tracheoesophageal fistula most commonly lies just beneath the divided azygos vein. The dissection is then extended further into the mediastinum until the posterior wall of the trachea is seen. The vagus nerve, in the groove just behind the trachea, should be protected. Attention is then turned to the lower esophageal segment, and a tape is passed circumferentially around this structure. With gentle traction on the tape, the area of the tracheoesophageal fistula is better defined. The fistula is transected, and a cuff of approximately 3 mm is left at the site of attachment to the trachea. This remaining cuff ensures that the tracheal fistula can be closed without compromising the tracheal lumen. Although some surgeons advocate simple ligation of the tracheal fistula, three or four interrupted sutures are recommended to provide more secure closure. The adequacy of the closure is tested by covering the suture line with warm saline solution and then observing for bubbles when the anesthesiologist gently hand-bags the infant with a sustained inspiration.

The tip of the fistula is excised from the thin-walled lower esophageal segment, which is prepared for anastomosis. The blood supply to the lower esophagus is segmental from the aorta. Extensive mobilization must be avoided because of the risk of devascularization. Dissection cephalad discloses the blind upper pouch of the esophagus. This dissection is enhanced if the anesthesiologist gently pushes down on a small catheter that has been previously positioned in the upper pouch. The blood supply to the upper pouch is derived from cervical vessels and travels in the submucosal layers; therefore, the pouch can be dissected extensively in a circumferential manner so

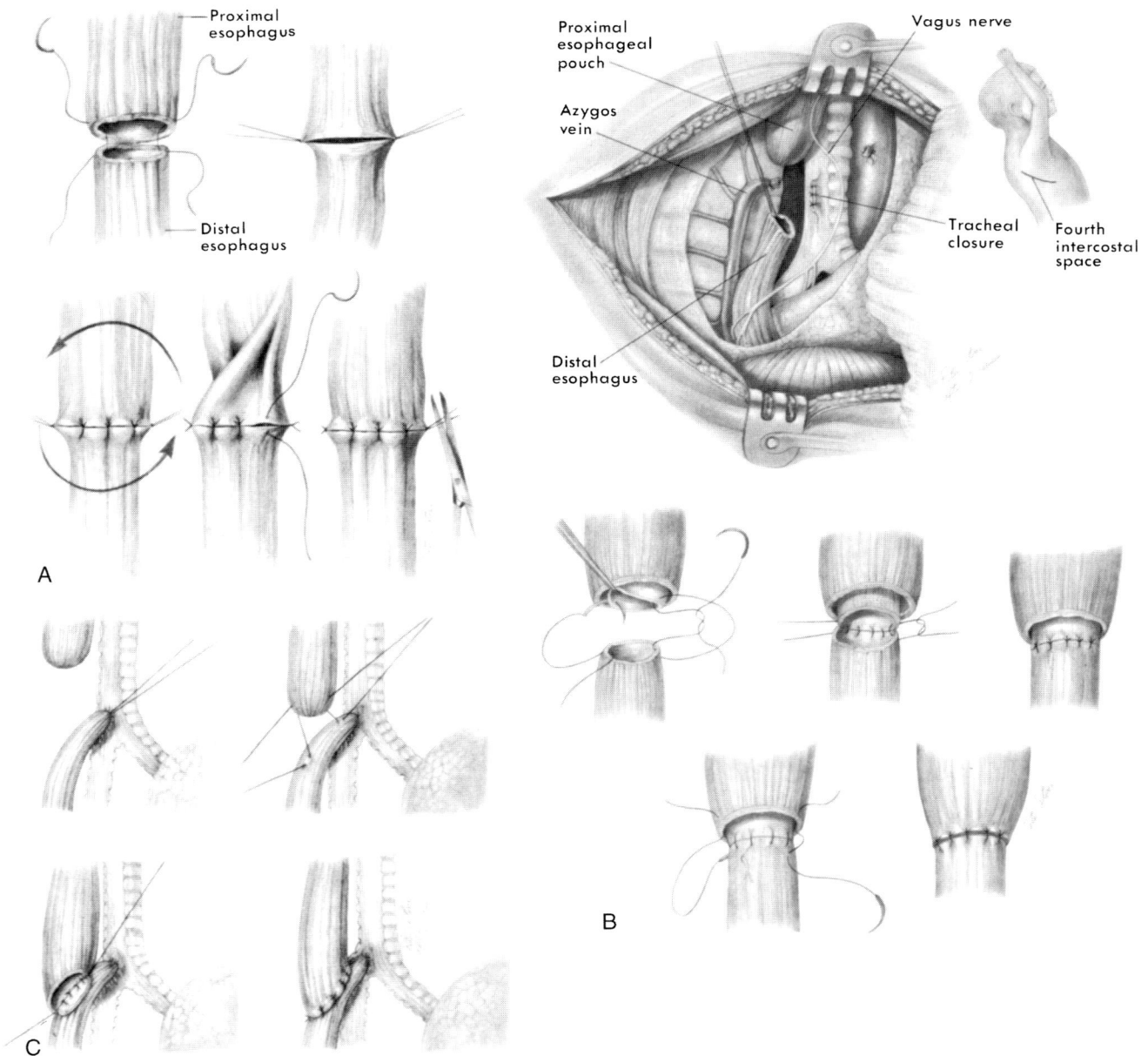

FIGURE 25–6. Different types of esophageal anastomosis in patients with esophageal atresia and associated tracheoesophageal fistula. *A,* A simple end-to-end anastomosis has the advantages of simplicity and speed. Corner sutures are placed to draw the ends of the esophageal segments together. A single row of simple sutures completes the front-presenting portions of the anastomosis, with the knots on the outside. One of the corner sutures is passed behind the esophagus, which is then rotated 180 degrees. The anastomosis is completed with simple sutures in the presenting posterior surface, which has been rotated into view. *B,* The "Haight" anastomosis takes advantage of the thick, strong musculature of the upper pouch. The first layer of sutures incorporates the mucosa of the upper pouch in the entire wall of the thinner lower esophagus. The muscular coat of the upper pouch is drawn down as a protective sleeve over the inner layer of sutures. Only six or eight sutures should be used in this outer layer to avoid injuring the blood supply to the end of the lower esophagus segment. *C,* With a "Beardmore"-type repair, the fistula is closed by a compressing (but not tightly tied) ligature. The upper pouch is brought into apposition with the presenting surface of the lower esophageal segment, which remains attached to the trachea. An opening is made in the lower segment, and an end-to-end anastomosis is constructed with a single layer of sutures.

that it may be drawn downward into the thorax for the anastomosis.

The tip of the upper pouch is cut across to expose the lumen of the pouch. The ends are then approximated with a single-layer technique with sutures passing through the full thickness of both the lower and the upper segments, tying the knots on the outside (see Fig. 25–6A). Corner sutures are placed, and the anterior row is completed first. The corner sutures are then used to turn the esophagus 180 degrees, and the presenting posterior surface is closed with interrupted sutures. Although this method has a slightly higher incidence of postoperative leak than a two-layer anastomosis, the incidence of stricture is significantly less. Spitz and co-workers (1987) reported a lower leak and stricture rate when Prolene or polyglycolic sutures are used instead of silk sutures.

For the classic Haight two-layer anastomosis, the mucosa of the upper pouch is separated from its muscular coats for a distance of approximately 6 to 8 mm by blunt dissection (see Fig. 25–6B). Corner sutures are then placed, with only the mucosal layer of the upper pouch brought into approximation with the entire thickness of the lower esophageal segment. Interrupted sutures are then placed circumferentially to complete the inside layer. The suture line is rotated to facilitate suturing the back wall. Next, the sleeve of muscle of the upper pouch is drawn down over this anastomosis and secured with interrupted sutures placed in the wall of the lower segment of the esophagus and the muscular wall of the upper pouch. Usually, seven or eight sutures are sufficient to telescope this outer sleeve down over the internal mucosal anastomosis.

An alternative approach for esophageal repair was developed by Sulamaa and colleagues (1951) and championed by Beardmore (Ty et al., 1967) in North America (see Fig. 25–6C). With a single large ligature, the fistula is ligated adjacent to the trachea. The lower esophageal segment is not detached from the trachea; rather, the upper pouch is brought down to the presenting side of the lower esophageal segment that is incised. An end-to-side union is created with sutures placed through the full thickness of both upper-pouch and lower-esophageal segments. There have been reports that the ligature on the fistula has penetrated and produced recurrent tracheoesophageal fistula, and that the mortality was higher when this technique was used (Poenaru et al., 1991). However, Touloukian (1992) studied patients who had this repair and reported excellent esophageal function with minimal postoperative stenosis.

One of the primary determinants of outcome is the amount of tension on the esophageal suture line (Fig. 25–7). Occasionally, there is too wide a gap between the two esophageal ends to produce a safe anastomosis. Livaditis (1973) introduced a technique for increasing the length of the upper pouch, thereby expanding the number of infants who could have primary repair without undue tension. A circular incision is made through all layers of the esophagus except the mucosa. The myotomy is placed 1 to 2 cm

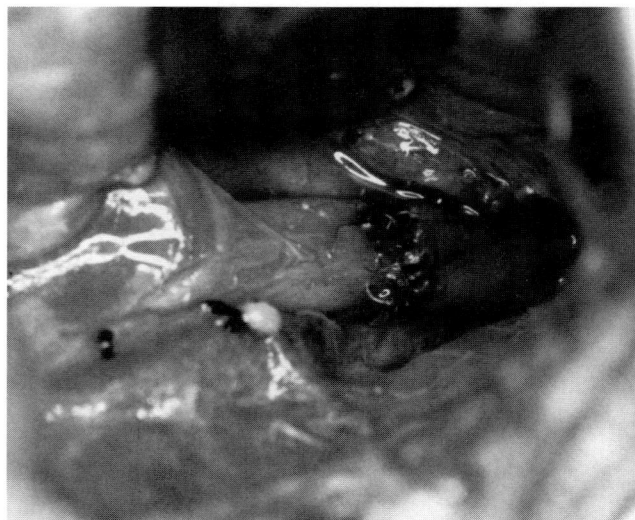

FIGURE 25–7. This operative photograph demonstrates a completed single-layer anastomosis with good approximation of both ends without tension.

above the distal end of the upper pouch, permitting significant lengthening of the pouch. This lengthening procedure does not jeopardize the blood supply to the distal portion of the upper esophageal pouch because the main arterial supply is located in the submucosal layer, but care must be taken to avoid entering the esophageal lumen.

Short-Term Delay

If the infant is initially unstable or has a medical problem that is easily correctable, the operation may be deferred for a short time. In these patients, a gastrostomy was once routine, yet now most are managed without a gastrostomy (Shaul et al., 1989). Safe management includes upper-pouch suction, head-up position, antibiotics, parenteral nutrition, and when necessary, gastrostomy drainage (Fig. 25–8). Time is thus provided for stabilization and medical management of pulmonary, cardiac, or gastrointestinal difficulties. This method of management is useful for only a limited period, because reflux into the tracheobronchial tree via the tracheoesophageal fistula may occur. Primary repair is performed as soon as the infant's condition is stable and the risk of operation has been reduced to a satisfactory level.

Unstable Patients

For infants with serious coexisting anomalies or severe prematurity, survival is limited. The possibility of decreasing the mortality in compromised infants by staging the operative procedure has received much attention. The first stage consists of gastrostomy placement and retropleural division of the fistula. This permits time for growth with evaluation and correction of life-threatening anomalies while avoiding the dangers of persistent reflux and aspiration. Later, the esophageal anastomosis is performed

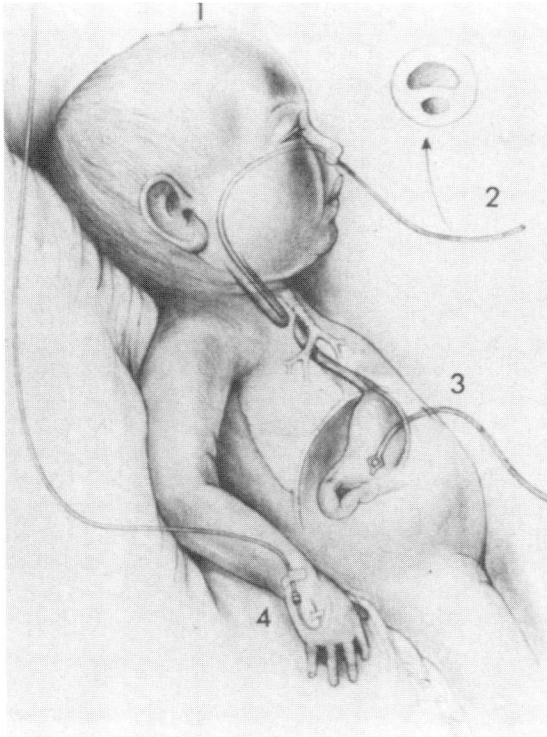

FIGURE 25–8. Elements of care in delayed operation: 1, Head-up position. 2, Upper pouch suction. 3, Gastrostomy for drainage, which is required only if there is a long delay. 4, Intravenous route for parenteral nutrition.

electively through a second thoracotomy. Although staged repair is much less frequent than a delayed primary repair, this approach has merit in selected patients. Improved survival in high-risk infants when the surgical treatment has been staged was reported by Holder and associates (1962) and Wise and co-workers (1987). These investigators advocated early retropleural fistula division, gastrostomy feedings, and continuous sump suction of the upper pouch. This clinical arrangement requires constant intensive nursing care, but it can be successful and the esophageal anastomosis can be accomplished. For infants with severe life-threatening respiratory distress, particularly premature infants with noncompliant lungs, Templeton and colleagues (1985) advocate primary

ligation of the fistula to improve ventilation, followed by gastrostomy and esophageal anastomosis.

With long-term nutritional support combined with suction of the upper pouch and gastrostomy drainage, infants with esophageal atresia and tracheoesophageal fistula can be maintained indefinitely while growth and weight gain are achieved, pulmonary status is cleared, and other congenital anomalies are studied and corrected. This approach is an alternative to the extensive surgical maneuvers necessary for staging the surgical correction, but is not appropriate if aspiration is a persistent problem.

Complications

The best results are achieved with a multidisciplinary approach by a team committed to long-term follow-up of these patients and families. Complications are frequent and the presenting symptoms may be difficult to distinguish. For example, tracheomalacia, recurrent fistula, reflux, and stricture all may present as intermittent respiratory distress. A careful, methodical approach is required to delineate the source of problems.

Although once considered a fatal lesion, a leak at the anastomosis can usually be managed satisfactorily, particularly if the pleural envelope has been maintained and drainage has been accomplished from the mediastinum by the retropleural route (Chittmittrapap et al., 1992). Improved management of infection, nutrition, and respiratory support in infants has contributed to success in managing this complication. The seriousness of a leak from the esophageal suture line should not be minimized. However, with the support mechanisms now available for infants, only 1 death attributable to a leaking anastomosis has occurred in the 21 patients at Children's Hospital in Washington, District of Columbia, who developed a leak.

The mediastinal infection seen with esophageal disruption may cause recurrence of the tracheoesophageal fistula. This complication is particularly distressing because it necessitates another major operation to divide the tracheoesophageal fistula. Coran advocates the use of an interposition pericardial flap at the time of reoperation for a recurrent fistula (Wheatley and Coran, 1992) (Figs. 25–9 and 25–10).

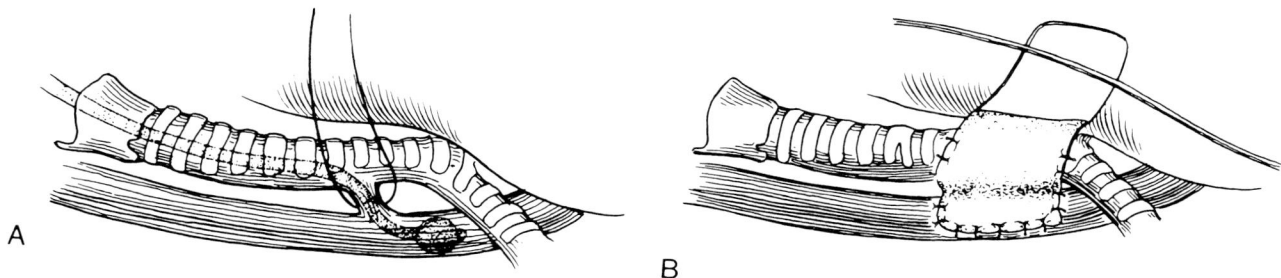

A

B

FIGURE 25–9. A and B, Diagram of a technique in which a pericardial pedicle flap is interposed between the tracheal and the esophageal suture lines to provide definitive management of a recurrent tracheoesophageal fistula. (A and B, From Wheatley, M. J., and Coran, A. G.: Pericardial flap interposition for the definitive management of recurrent tracheoesophageal fistula. J. Pediatr. Surg., 27:1122, 1992.)

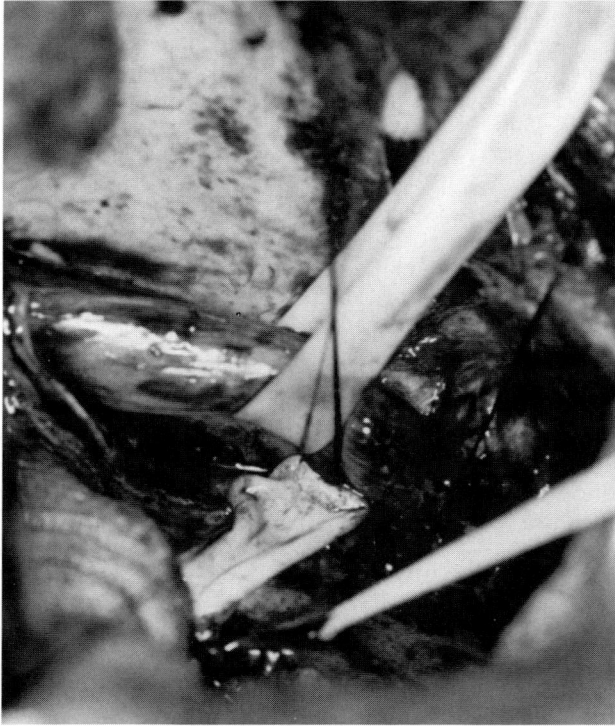

FIGURE 25–10. Operative photograph of a vascularized pericardial flap being interposed between the esophagus (surrounded by a Penrose drain) and the trachea, which is in the foreground.

Strictures are a common problem postoperatively, occurring in approximately 20% of patients in some series. The stricture is usually caused by scarring at the anastomosis, but may be related to reflux injury or may be secondary to a tiny leak. Most strictures respond to dilatation; however, if gastroesophageal reflux is causing the stricture, an antireflux procedure must be considered. In rare situations, resection of a persistent stricture is required to reestablish an adequate esophageal lumen.

It has become apparent that the mobilization and denervation necessary to complete the esophageal anastomosis has, in many patients, altered the anatomy and motility of the gastroesophageal junction and led to gastroesophageal reflux (Shono et al., 1993). The clinical manifestations of this reflux are identical to those seen in infants with primary gastroesophageal reflux. They vomit frequently or incessantly, fail to thrive, show recurrent aspiration, have esophagitis, or develop a severe stricture. The incidence of significant gastroesophageal reflux is between 20 and 40% in infants operated on for esophageal atresia (Manning et al., 1986). Many infants have required an antireflux procedure because of the severity of symptoms (Ashcraft et al., 1977; Orringer et al., 1977). Recurrent reflux and dysphagia may complicate the course following antireflux surgery (Lindahl et al., 1989; Wheatley et al., 1993).

Tracheomalacia may be a significant problem following repair and is manifested by varying grades of respiratory compromise. Diagnosis is by bronchoscopy or with ultrafast computed tomography (CT) scanning (Kao et al., l990) (Fig. 25–11). Tracheomalacia has occurred in 10 to 16% of patients reported by several centers; in some patients, relief has been obtained by aortopexy (Kimura et al., 1990; Schwartz and Filler, 1980).

Results

Almost all infants born with esophageal atresia and tracheoesophageal fistula survive. Deaths are most frequently related to fatal genetic or cardiac anomalies. Even in the smallest and sickest infants, survival rates of 90% have been achieved (Ein et al., 1989; Goh and Brereton, 1991). Another significant trend has been the use of immediate primary repair for infants who traditionally underwent a staged approach. Good results have been achieved with this approach (Randolph et al., 1989; Pohlson et al., 1988).

ISOLATED ESOPHAGEAL ATRESIA

Approximately 8% of infants with esophageal anomalies present with isolated esophageal atresia.

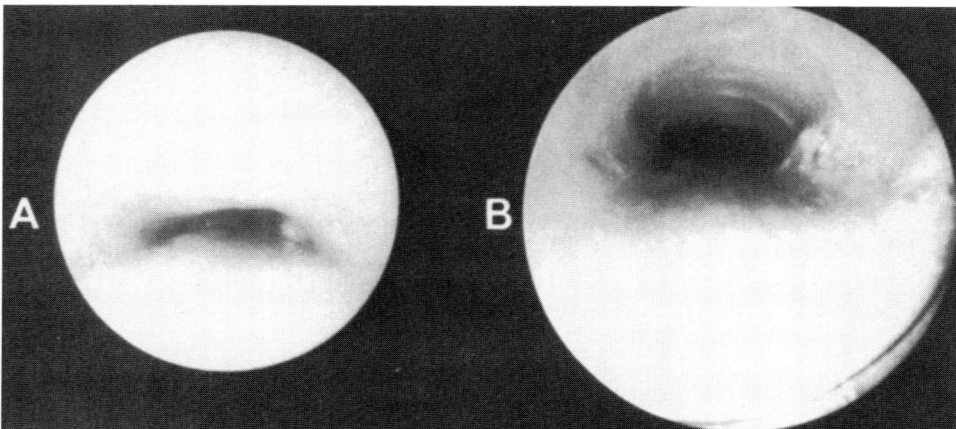

FIGURE 25–11. *A,* Endoscopic view of a child with a collapsed trachea from tracheomalacia following repair of esophageal atresia. *B,* Endoscopic view of the same child following aortopexy, with which the trachea was suspended, to provide a patent airway. (*A* and *B,* Courtesy of Dr. M. Z. Schwartz.)

With this variation, no fistula to the respiratory tract is present. In these infants, the short nubbin of lower esophagus barely protrudes above the diaphragm. Foreknowledge of this anatomy is important because it prevents an early, fruitless exploratory thoracotomy in the hope that the two ends will reach.

Signs and Symptoms

As in other forms of esophageal atresia, these infants cannot handle their saliva or feedings. Babies with isolated esophageal atresia show a scaphoid abdomen because the gastrointestinal tract is devoid of air. Radiographic findings of a blind upper pouch (Fig. 25–12) and absence of air below the diaphragm are pathognomonic of isolated esophageal atresia without fistula.

Management

Prompt esophagostomy with the upper esophageal pouch brought to the skin of the left side of the neck allows drainage of saliva and prevents aspiration. The left side of the neck is chosen so that esophageal replacement can be performed through the left side of the chest. Gastrostomy serves for feeding until esophageal replacement can be safely undertaken,

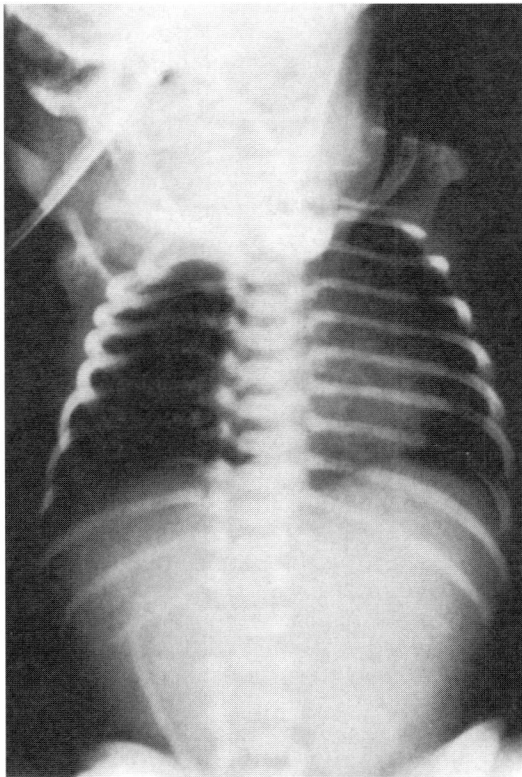

FIGURE 25–12. Chest radiograph of a child with esophageal atresia without tracheoesophageal fistula. Note the high pouch outlined by dye. No air is present below the diaphragm; this is diagnostic for "pure" esophageal atresia.

usually at approximately 1 year of age. The gastrostomy should be placed along the lesser curvature of the stomach to allow the later option of a reversed gastric tube as an esophageal replacement.

Using a different approach, Mahour and associates (1974) and Howard and Myers (1965) showed that daily bougienage of the upper pouch permits enough elongation that the two ends may ultimately be brought together for a primary anastomosis. The babies are treated initially with gastrostomy and upper-pouch suction. Usually, 2 or 3 months of elongation are required before operative correction can be accomplished, although Raffensperger (1990) advocates abandoning this approach if no progress is made in the first 2 weeks. Because of the traction required in the operative repair, leak, stenosis, and gastroesophageal reflux have been observed frequently, and this approach has not been universally adopted. In an effort to obtain additional length to span the gap in isolated atresia, DeLorimier and Harrison (1980) used Livaditis' muscular incision at two or even three levels of the upper pouch. More recently, some surgeons have simply waited for the upper pouch to elongate with natural growth, and in 3 to 6 months, they accomplished end-to-end union (Puri et al., 1992).

ISOLATED (H–TYPE) TRACHEOESOPHAGEAL FISTULA

Isolated (H-type) tracheoesophageal fistula without an atresia occurs in approximately 4% of esophageal anomalies. Although congenital tracheoesophageal communication may be found at any level, most fistulas occur in the upper third of the trachea and esophagus. Of the cases in which the level of the fistula has been carefully determined, at least 70% of the reported H-type fistulas occurred at or above the level of the second thoracic vertebra (Yazbeck and Dubuck, 1983). The important surgical implication is that the fistula can usually be reached by an incision in the neck. The fistula occurs in the posterior membranous portion of the trachea. Because of the proximity of the adjacent esophagus, the fistula is necessarily short, although it may be broad in external diameter (Fig. 25–13).

Signs and Symptoms

In the infant or young child with congenital isolated tracheoesophageal fistula, choking and coughing with feeding are almost always present; liquids cause greater difficulty than semisolids. Prompt relief is achieved by gavage feeding. Coughing or crying causes air to escape through the fistula into the esophagus and into the stomach. The resultant intermittent abdominal distention is a recognizable clinical finding. Pneumonitis develops in the early days of life and recurs frequently as patchy bronchopneumonia. Continued aspiration via the fistula creates a constant state of bronchopneumonia with all the manifesta-

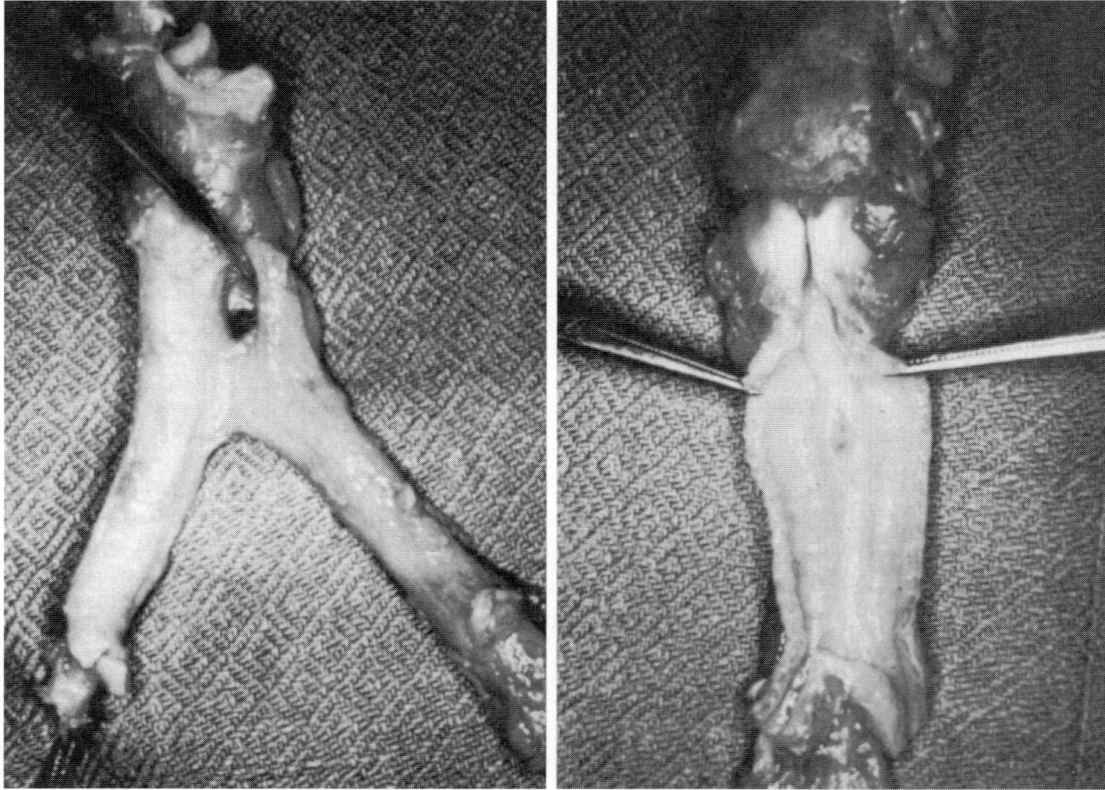

FIGURE 25–13. Pathology specimen from a 5-month-old infant who died with an unrecognized (H-type) tracheoesophageal fistula. Note the level of the fistula with respect to the larynx in the photograph of the opened trachea. (From the slide collection of Dr. W. H. Hendren.)

tions of chronic infection. Thus, in a child with recurrent pneumonia that may be the result of an H-type fistula, other disease entities must be considered in the differential diagnosis, including gastroesophageal reflux, esophageal stenosis, vascular ring, neurogenic dysfunction of the esophagus, and generalized diseases such as immune dysfunction and cystic fibrosis.

Diagnosis

A child with a congenital fistula that connects the esophagus and trachea shows signs of aspiration pneumonitis on the routine chest film. In some cases, increased pulmonary markings and hilar adenopathy appear as signs of chronic pneumonitis. Gastric distention may be appreciated even on the chest film. An esophageal swallow, with a dilute contrast medium and careful positioning of the patient, may reveal the fistula. Tamponade of the distal esophagus by a balloon catheter has been helpful during barium swallow. This allows distention of the esophagus with the column of radiopaque dye, which improves the chance of demonstrating the fistula. Tracheography (combined with tracheobronchoscopy) has also shown this lesion. Esophagoscopy is a less reliable method of demonstrating the fistula, although a drop of methylene blue dye instilled through the endotracheal tube may appear in the esophagus and confirm

the presence of an abnormal communication (Moncrief and Randolph, 1966).

Operative Correction

Cervical Fistula

Even though the esophagus lies slightly to the left of the midline at the thoracic inlet, the position of the fistula requires a right-sided approach. A curving incision in the skin line low in the neck is made from the midline and is extended laterally beyond the sternocleidomastoid muscle (Fig. 25–14). The sternocleidomastoid muscle is dissected free and retracted laterally or divided as necessary. The carotid sheath is also retracted laterally. With proper traction to separate the esophagus and the trachea, a plane between these two structures is developed until the fistula is encountered. The fistula usually lies at the level of the clavicle. Dissection is continued until an adequate length of the esophagus and trachea can be cleared below the fistula. When the fistula has been clearly defined, division can be performed safely. Division of this short, wide structure is best accomplished by severing the fistula almost flush on the esophageal side. The additional length achieved by leaving some of the fistula wall on the tracheal side ensures a secure closure without compromising the tracheal lumen. The trachea is closed with a single layer of mattress

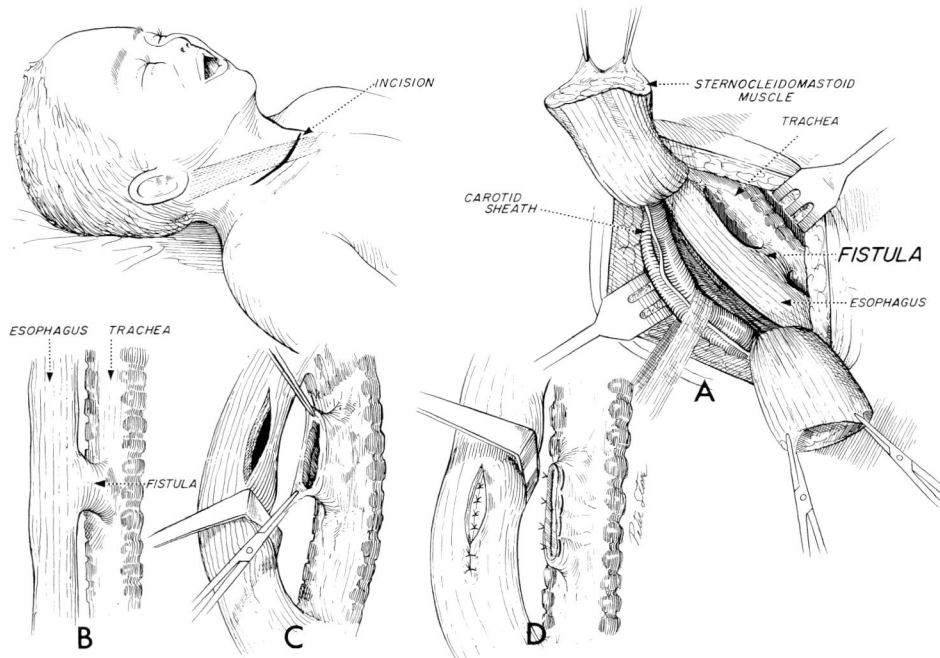

FIGURE 25–14. *A–C,* Isolated (H-type) tracheoesophageal fistula in the typical cervical location. An incision is made in the neck. The sternocleidomastoid is retracted or severed. The fistula is divided, flush with the esophagus, to ensure closure of the trachea without narrowing the lumen.

sutures; the esophagus is closed with two layers of interrupted sutures.

Thoracic Fistula

When the fistula is located within the thorax, right-sided thoracotomy should be performed in the third interspace. A standard transthoracic approach is recommended. The fistula is divided as described earlier. Double fistulas connecting the trachea and esophagus are rare; separate cervical and thoracic incisions may be necessary in such cases.

Esophageal Atresia with Upper-Pouch or Double Fistulas

Atresia of the esophagus with tracheal fistula to both the upper and the lower pouches is rare, but small upper-pouch fistulas in association with lower tracheoesophageal fistula may be more common than was previously recognized (Dudgeon et al., 1972). Esophageal atresia with a short, blind lower segment and only the upper pouch entering the trachea through a fistula is a very rare anomaly. When saliva and liquids pass directly into the lungs through the upper-pouch fistula, there is increased pulmonary hazard. The surgical considerations are similar to those described earlier, but the mortality is higher because of the greater insult to the lungs.

LARYNGOTRACHEAL CLEFT

A laryngotracheal cleft is an abnormal communication between the esophagus and the trachea. The defect may be confined to the larynx or may extend to the bifurcation of the trachea, and the lesion may coexist with esophageal atresia and tracheoesophageal fistula (Donahoe and Gee, 1984). The infants are usually seen early in life with severe respiratory distress. The diagnosis is made by endoscopy with visualization of the cleft and assessment of its extension below the vocal cords. Clefts have been surgically repaired in a few patients (DuBois et al., 1990; Ryan et al., 1991). The authors have successfully repaired clefts in four patients, three of whom had associated esophageal atresia and tracheoesophageal fistula, a common association (Newman, 1988).

The operative approach must be individualized, but a staged approach that includes early tracheostomy, an antireflux procedure, and gastrostomy reduces mortality. Operative exposure for repair can be achieved through an anterior midline approach via the larynx or a lateral incision in the pharynx and esophagus (Myer et al., 1990). The posterior wall of the larynx and trachea is closed by using a longitudinal flap of the esophagus. Donahoe and Hendren (1972) advocate an interposition of the strap muscles to protect against recurrence. Management of these children requires meticulous anesthetic and endotracheal tube care and intensive postoperative occupational and speech therapy.

CONGENITAL STENOSIS AND WEBS

Congenital stenosis is a rare malformation of the esophagus. A variant of congenital narrowing of the esophagus occurs as a persistent web that stretches across most of the esophageal lumen and has a small opening. The opening in the web is usually adequate for liquids, and symptoms characteristically occur when the infant begins to eat solid food. In some children, the diagnosis is not made until they reach 2 or 3 years, when recurrent aspiration pneumonia and dysphagia bring attention to the lesion. Another source of stenosis is persistence of cartilaginous bronchial remnants in the esophagus (Ibrahim and Sandry, 1981; Scherer and Grosfeld, 1986).

Esophageal stenosis or web is usually obvious on barium swallow (Fig. 25–15) and is easily visualized by esophagoscopy. In rare patients, esophageal dilatation is feasible and provides a cure. However, in most children with congenital esophageal stenosis, the opening is so small or the web so unyielding that dilatation is unsatisfactory. Thoracotomy with exploration of the esophagus and excision of the web or sleeve resection of the stenotic segment is usually required.

NEUROMUSCULAR DISORDERS OF THE ESOPHAGUS

Children with neuromuscular derangement of the esophagus usually show a failure to thrive, dysphagia, regurgitation, or respiratory symptoms. Diffuse esophageal spasm, scleroderma, and achalasia are differentiated on the basis of manometry, contrast studies, pH probe, and endoscopy (Hill, 1986). Diffuse

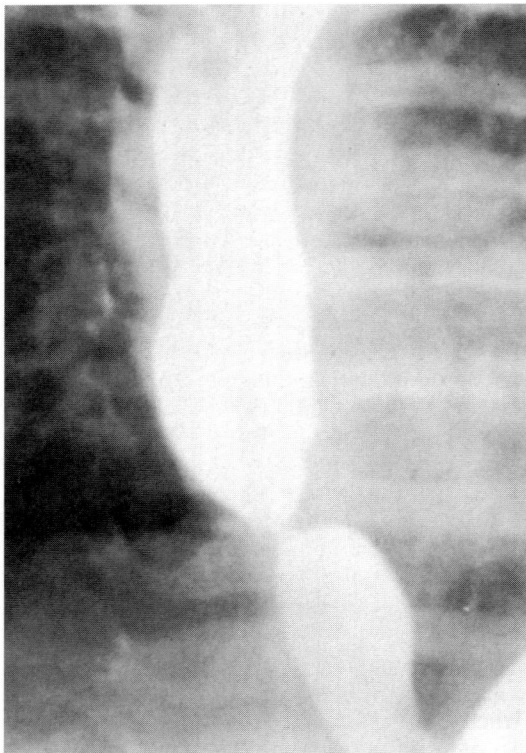

FIGURE 25–15. Barium swallow demonstrating an esophageal web in a 9-month-old infant with progressive dysphagia to solid foods. The diagnosis was made by observing the notch that indicated the location of the web's attachment. This was confirmed at esophagoscopy. Surgical cure involved thoracotomy, esophagomyotomy, and resection of the web.

esophageal spasm causes coexisting pressure peaks in the distal esophagus, with a relaxed lower sphincter and appearance of a "corkscrew" esophagus on the chest film. Vigorous achalasia shows some contractions, but the sphincter does not relax. Scleroderma can involve esophageal dysmotility and the esophagus becomes weak, loses tone, and is prone to damage from reflux. The cause and pathophysiology of these disorders are controversial and are subjects of active research (Hollwarth and Uray, 1985). Consequently, treatment must be individualized and consists of bougienage, pharmacologic agents, dilatation, and esophagomyotomy. A new group of infants with diffuse esophageal dilatation and reflux has been described by Stolar and co-workers (1988); these neonates have survived diaphragmatic hernia repair with the use of extracorporeal membrane oxygenation.

ACHALASIA

Achalasia of the esophagus is a failure of the gastroesophageal junction to relax during swallowing. This condition is relatively rare in adults and extremely uncommon in children. In children, the symptoms of achalasia may resemble those of esophageal stricture, congenital stenosis, or gastroesophageal reflux. The triad of regurgitation, failure to thrive, and aspiration-related respiratory symptoms is seen with both reflux and achalasia.

Achalasia is diagnosed by barium swallow, which shows a dilated esophagus that tapers smoothly into a tight esophagogastric junction (Fig. 25–16). Irregular or ineffectual peristalsis of the esophagus and failure of the lower sphincter to relax during swallowing are seen at fluoroscopy and can be documented by motility studies (Willich, 1973). Manometry shows poor relaxation of the esophageal sphincter and weak or absent peristalsis after swallowing. Esophagoscopy is not essential for diagnosis but may be helpful, especially when esophagitis or stricture cannot be excluded.

The treatment of achalasia is controversial. Although dilatation has been recommended, ordinary bougienage provides only temporary relief. Mechanical dilators are available, but these devices are dangerous and their use is beset with complications. Permanent relief requires forceful disruption of the lower esophageal muscle with mechanical, pneumatic, or hydrostatic pressure by placing a balloon across the gastroesophageal junction under fluoroscopic control and inflating it under measured pressure.

Nakayama and colleagues (1987) reported good results with pneumatic dilatation in a group of 15 children, and considered the procedure safe and effective as a first step. The risk of esophageal rupture by pneumatic dilatation is a significant consideration.

Despite dilatation, some children go on to require a Heller myotomy. Successful operative therapy for achalasia was introduced in 1913 by Heller, who described a transthoracic anterior and posterior esophagomyotomy. Since gastroesophageal reflux may fol-

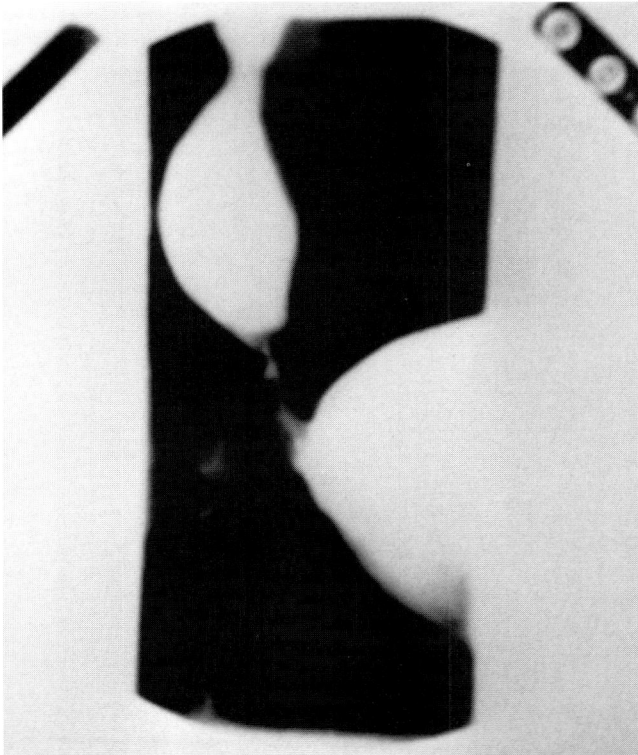

FIGURE 25–16. A barium swallow demonstrating the typical appearance of a child with achalasia. Note the tiny, narrow channel. A Heller myotomy was curative.

low the myotomy because of the obligatory dissection of the esophageal hiatus, the extramucosal muscle-splitting procedure should be combined with a reconstruction of the hiatus or a formal antireflux operation (Buick and Spitz, 1985; Vane et al., 1988). Azizkhan and associates (1980) recommended Heller's procedure for children under the age of 9 years, and the use of dilatation for older children. Lemmer and co-workers (1985) and Nihoul-Fekete and colleagues (1989) achieved good long-term results in a large group of children combining a Heller myotomy and an antireflux procedure. Recent application of minimal-access surgery to children may permit this operation to be performed thoracoscopically.

GASTROESOPHAGEAL REFLUX

Neuhauser and Berenberg (1947) described a group of infants who vomited excessively and were shown to have unimpeded gastroesophageal reflux. The term *chalasia* ("relaxation" at the cardia) was widely accepted, and the upright position that these investigators advocated became the standard therapy. Spontaneous recovery from reflux occurred in most infants as they grew up and assumed an upright position. Other groups studied the anatomic derangements seen in some infants and young children and described hiatal hernia with and without stricture formation (Forshall, 1955). It became apparent that in a

certain percentage of infants, the symptoms were not controlled by the upright positioning technique. It was recognized that persistent gastroesophageal reflux had the potential to negatively affect growth and development (Filler et al., 1964) as well as cause complications in the respiratory tract (Lilly and Randolph, 1968). As more attention was focused on the consequences of gastroesophageal reflux, surgical experience with the correction of gastroesophageal reflux in infants was gained in a number of centers (Bettex and Kuffer, 1969; Carcassonne et al., 1973; Randolph et al., 1974).

Clinical Presentation

Infants

A history of repeated or protracted vomiting in an infant is the clearest indication of gastroesophageal reflux. Anatomic obstruction at or beyond the pylorus must be excluded. When the vomiting is associated with failure to thrive or respiratory symptoms, suspicion of gastroesophageal reflux is increased.

A contrast esophagogram shows reflux in many infants and children who are affected and is necessary to exclude obstructive problems below the pylorus. However, a barium swallow is an imperfect method for diagnosis and fails to demonstrate known symptomatic reflux in 20 to 40% of infants studied. In addition, an esophagogram that shows massive reflux is not specific and cannot be used alone to determine whether the reflux is clinically significant because it provides information only at the time of the study.

Miniaturized equipment allows constant monitoring of the esophageal pH, even in infants. Analysis of these recordings shows the frequency and character of the reflux episodes with accuracy and has provided sequential quantitative data for pH values in infants (Euler and Ament, 1977; Friesen et al., 1992; Jolley et al., 1978). Using these refined techniques, Jolley and associates (1979) showed various patterns of abnormal reflux. Probe monitoring of pH has demonstrated alkaline reflux in a small percentage of children (Malthaner et al., 1991), and this reflux may be responsible for symptoms in children with otherwise "normal" pH tracings.

Esophagoscopy with biopsy is necessary to assess the presence and extent of esophagitis (Leape et al., 1981) and to diagnose Barrett's esophagus (Cheu et al., 1992). Esophagoscopy is most often performed just before the definitive operation for gastroesophageal reflux or to assess the impact of medical therapy. Gastroesophageal scintiscanning and esophageal manometry may in some instances be helpful in diagnosing and managing reflux (Euler and Ament, 1977; Jona et al., 1981).

Older Children

A smaller group of patients than those seen in the first year of life are the older children with persistent reflux who have various symptoms such as chronic pulmonary disease, esophagitis, or frank stricture. These symptoms occur sporadically after the first year of life. In addition, some adolescents show the same symptoms of gastroesophageal reflux as adult patients and, unlike infants, often have an associated hiatal hernia. In these patients, diagnosis and treatment decisions are identical to those for adult patients. Another subgroup of patients have neurologic impairment and may require gastrostomy for long-term feeding. These patients may have preexisting reflux, and gastrostomy alone may exacerbate the reflux (Canal et al., 1987; Wesley et al., 1981). The role of routine antireflux procedures in patients with neurologic impairment undergoing gastrostomy has become controversial because of the high incidence of complications and recurrence (Martinez et al., 1992; Smith et al., 1992).

Therapy

Simple measures such as upright positioning and thickening of feedings are effective in eliminating the symptoms in most infants. Alterations in feeding frequency or viscosity may reduce reflux. Antacids, metoclopramide, and H_2 receptor blockers are also used to alleviate reflux symptoms. If there is no change in nutritional or respiratory symptoms, despite medical therapy for several months, most infants benefit from operative correction. Older children profit from more individualized decisions regarding the success or failure of medical treatment. Careful clinical judgment is required in deciding whether to end medical therapy or to extend medical trial (Herbst, 1986).

With medical therapy, 80 to 90% of patients should improve. For children with the following conditions, a lower threshold for surgical intervention is required:

1. Life-threatening apneic spells related to the reflux
2. Congenital displacement of a major portion of the stomach in the chest (Fig. 25–17)
   3. Significant esophagitis
   4. Established stricture
   5. Chronic pulmonary changes

Failure to grow properly is the primary symptom in half of the infants selected for operation; one-third will have respiratory symptoms as the primary indication for surgery. In contrast, in children older than 1 year, vomiting, aspiration, stricture, pain, failure to thrive, and esophagitis are the chief determinants of surgery (Randolph, 1983).

Operative Considerations

The most prevalent operation with the longest period of follow-up in children is the fundoplication described by Nissen and Rossettiu (1959). This entails a complete 360-degree wrap of the fundus around the gastroesophageal junction. The surgical correction is

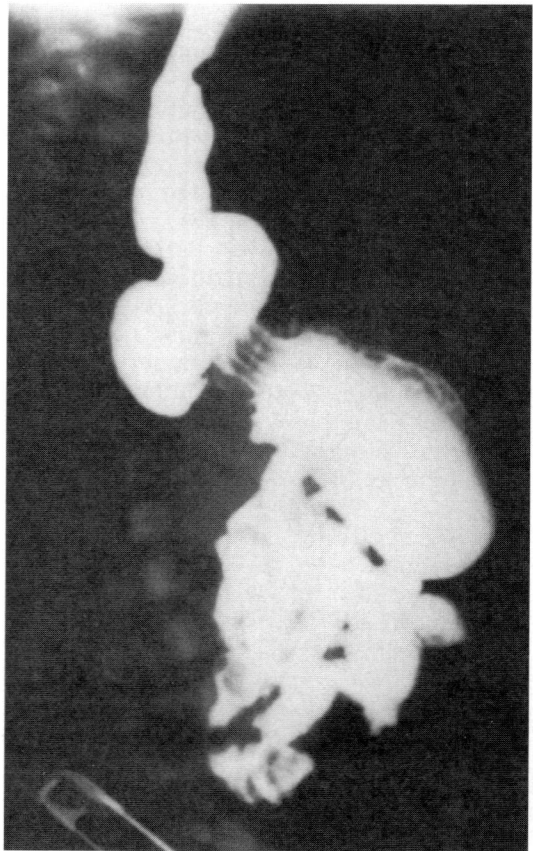

FIGURE 25–17. X-ray of a 3-day-old infant with major translocation of the stomach in the thorax and unrestricted reflux. Prompt surgical correction is recommended.

performed over a No. 24 to 36 bougie, depending on the age and size of the patient. After dissection of the hiatus, sutures are placed in the crura to reduce the hiatus. The short gastric vessels are freed to allow the fundus to be brought around the gastroesophageal junction. Sutures are placed in the esophagus as well as both presenting surfaces of the fundus to secure the circular wrap in the appropriate position. Tacking sutures to ensure that the repair is placed against the diaphragm are included. Many patients have evidence of delayed gastric emptying with nuclear scintigraphy and benefit from gastric antroplasty (Fonkalsrud et al., 1989; Randolph et al., 1974) (Fig. 25–18). Schropp and colleagues (1993) reported success with a laparoscopic approach to fundoplication, although long-term results are not available (Fig. 25–19).

An alternative to the Nissen fundoplication is Thal's anterior fundoplication, in which a 270-degree anterior wrap is done. Using this approach, Ashcraft and associates (1984) reported excellent results with a low morbidity in a large number of patients.

Results

The long-term results of Nissen fundoplication have been excellent in several large series. Randolph

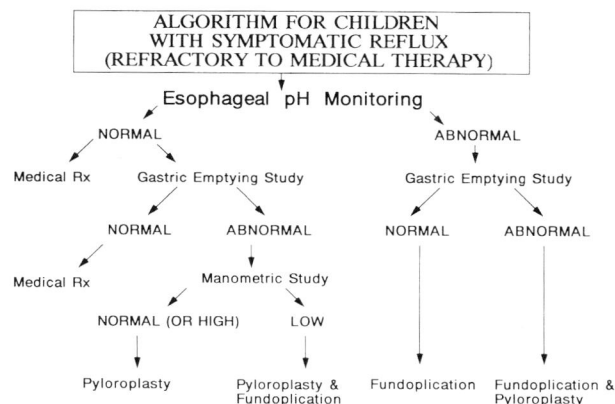

FIGURE 25–18. Algorithm proposed by Dr. E. W. Fonkalsrud for evaluation of children with symptomatic gastroesophageal reflux to determine when fundoplication, pyloroplasty, or both procedures are recommended. (From Fonkalsrud, E. W., Foglia, R. P., Ament, M. E., et al.: Operative treatment for the gastroesophageal reflux syndrome in children. J. Pediatr. Surg., 24:528, 1989.)

reported excellent results in 170 of 199 infants and children with the initial operation; 16 patients required a second operation because of recurrence of symptoms, and 11 of these were successful. These results have been corroborated in large series by Boix-Ochoa (1981), Spitz and Kirtane (1985), and Johnson (1986). Turnage and co-workers (1989) reported a 74% success rate at 5 years in a large series, but also noted that 45% of patients had at least one postoperative complication. Small-bowel obstruction is a serious complication with a high mortality following fundoplication (Jolley et al., 1986). Recurrence of reflux is a significant problem and is related to technical factors such as slippage of the wrap, as well as underlying neurologic or pulmonary disease.

FOREGUT DUPLICATION

A congenital duplication may occur in any part of the alimentary tract (Bower et al., 1978). Most esophageal duplication cysts are smooth, cystic masses that are distinct from the esophagus but are attached to it by a common wall (Superina et al., 1984). Most duplications do not communicate with the esophageal lumen. Respiratory symptoms are frequent and newborn infants may develop severe respiratory distress. Dysphagia is a common symptom and is related to compression of the esophagus. The cyst may be asymptomatic and may be recognized on a routine chest film. Neurenteric cysts arise from an incomplete separation of the notochord and foregut. These cysts lie in the posterior mediastinum and are associated with vertebral anomalies.

The diagnostic work-up of these mass lesions includes a chest x-ray, barium esophagogram, CT scan (Fig. 25–20), and possibly magnetic resonance imaging (MRI) or myelography if spinal involvement is suspected. Thoracotomy with surgical excision is curative and can usually be performed without difficulty. Resection of a sleeve of esophagus or stripping of the mucosa of the cyst may be necessary when the duplication is intimately related to the esophageal wall.

FOREIGN BODIES IN THE ESOPHAGUS

It is not unusual for a toddler to swallow a foreign object such as a coin or safety pin and have it lodge

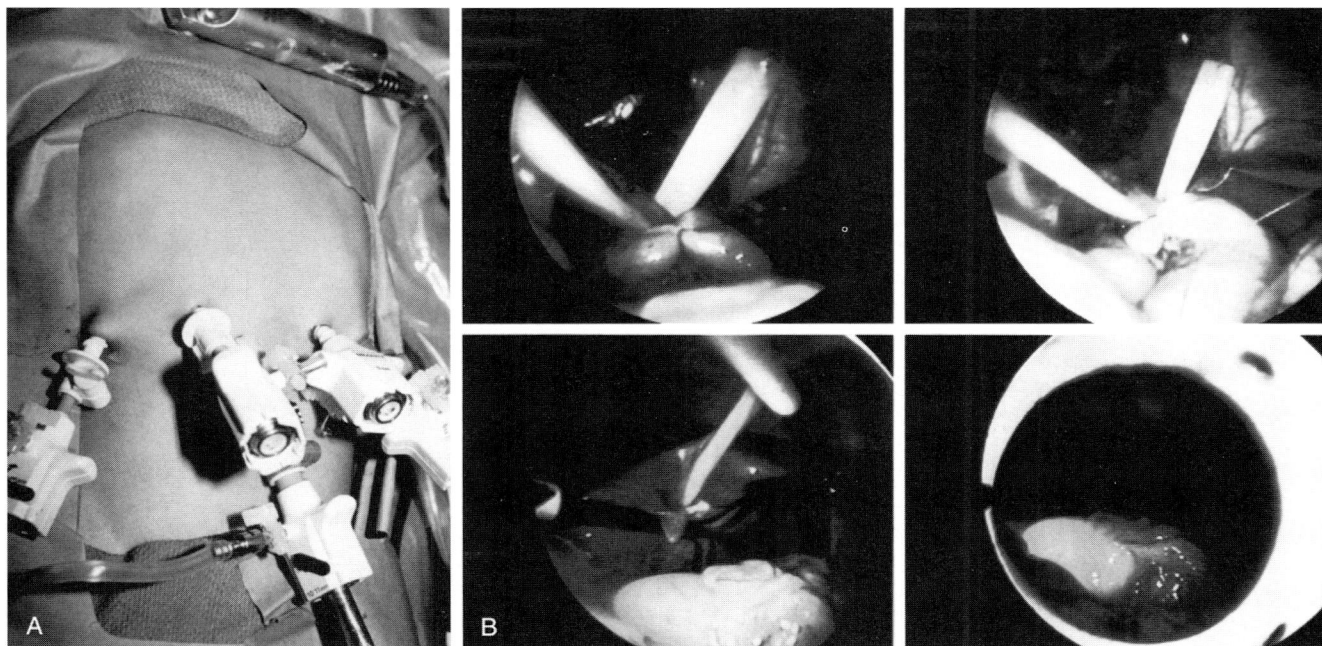

FIGURE 25–19. A, Operative photograph of "port" sites for a child undergoing laparascopic Nissen fundoplication. B, Operative endoscopic photograph demonstrating a completed Nissen procedure. A Penrose drain surrounds the esophagus. (A and B, From the slide collection of Dr. W. R. Thompson.)

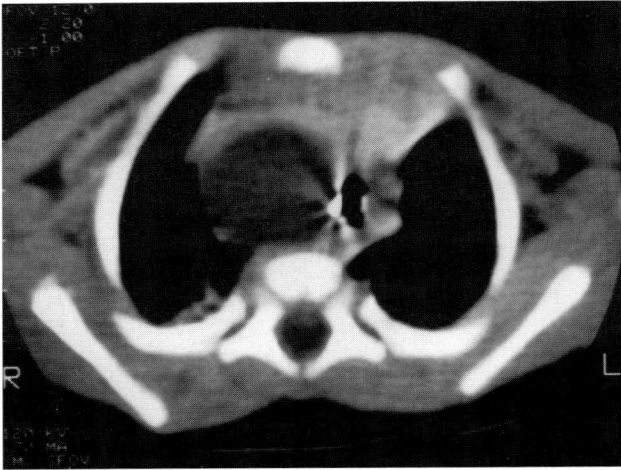

FIGURE 25–20. Chest computed tomography (CT) scan of an infant with an esophageal duplication. The mass is on the right side and is compressing the trachea and pushing it to the left. An operative approach via a right thoracotomy produced complete resection.

in the esophagus. The only evidence of a foreign body may be dysphagia and inability to swallow secretions, particularly in a child who is unable to give a history. Respiratory symptoms can be caused by tracheal compression or erosion of a long-standing foreign body into the esophageal wall. Coins and metal objects are readily seen on chest film, but a barium swallow may be necessary to display plastic or other nonopaque objects. The most common site of impaction is at the level of the cricopharyngeus, aortic arch, or esophageal hiatus. Many objects can be removed by using a Foley balloon and fluoroscopy (Campbell and Foley, 1983). Most esophageal foreign bodies in infants and children require prompt esophagoscopy, under anesthesia, for recovery.

Although most foreign objects can be retrieved without difficulty, perforation can occur. Open safety pins or other sharp objects that may have perforated the esophagus present special problems (Fig. 25–21) These, too, can be retrieved, but the children must be hospitalized and treated with antibiotics because erosion or perforation of the foreign bodies through the esophageal wall can cause serious mediastinal infection. Disk battery ingestion requires emergent endoscopy not only to remove the battery but also to inspect the esophageal mucosa (Temple and McNeese, 1983). Rarely, the trapping of a foreign body in the esophagus is the first clinical sign of the presence of a stricture of the esophagus, usually from reflux or a corrosive burn.

CORROSIVE BURNS OF THE ESOPHAGUS

Crawling unattended on the floor, small children are at risk for swallowing noxious substances because they instinctively reach for liquids in attractive containers. Frequently, these are corrosive cleaning fluids found under the kitchen sink. The potent alkalis con-

tained in the cleaning agents cause a devastating, full-thickness injury to the esophagus. Liquid lye causes more serious injury than granular preparations (Hawkins et al., 1980). In older children, ingestion of lye usually indicates a suicide attempt.

Acid ingestion is seen less often, primarily because acid is less available to young children. The accidental ingestion of acid causes mucosal injury more commonly than the full-thickness burn associated with alkali ingestion. Concentrated acid solutions may be extremely destructive, with extensive damage beginning in the mouth and extending through the length and full thickness of the esophagus. Even the stomach may be involved in severe acid injuries.

Diagnosis and Treatment

Pain, drooling, and inability to swallow are the chief symptoms. Respiratory symptoms may result from laryngeal injury. When a child is thought to have swallowed corrosive material, examination should commence with inspection of the lips, mouth, throat, and hypopharynx. Even if there are no obvious burns in these areas, the esophagus should be inspected. Observation of the child in the hospital for at least 24 hours is mandatory. Esophagoscopy within 48 hours of injury is useful in showing the extent of the injury. Endoscopy should be performed with the

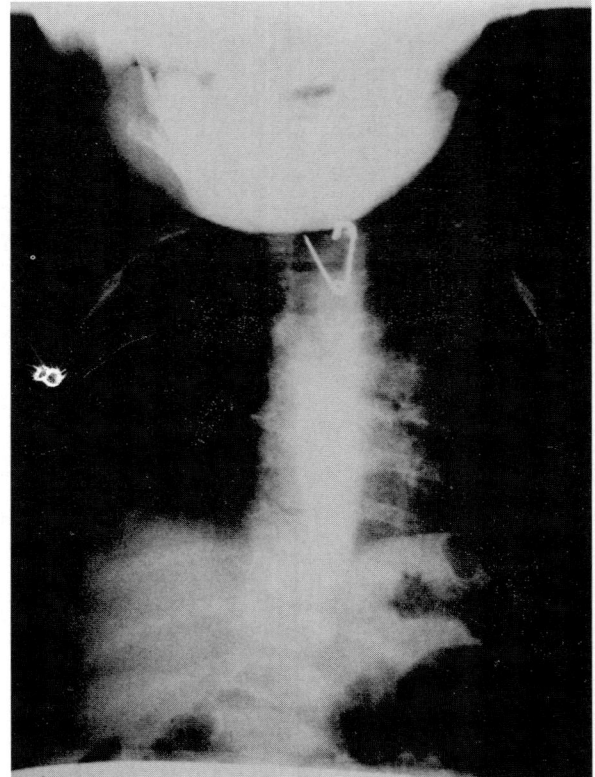

FIGURE 25–21. Chest radiograph demonstrating a swallowed safety pin that is lodged in the upper esophagus. Retrieval via an endoscope is possible, but care must be taken to avoid perforation of the esophagus.

patient under general anesthesia. With caustic burns, the esophagoscope should not be advanced beyond the first area of burn in the esophagus to prevent perforation. At this time, direct evaluation of the larynx and hypopharynx is important. If a significant burn of the esophagus is seen in the hypopharynx or upper esophagus, it is assumed that there is more extensive involvement distally. Cleveland and colleagues (1963) and Haller and associates (1971) recommended treatment with steroids and antibiotics if the esophagus was involved. These medications are continued for 4 to 6 weeks to minimize deposition of collagen and to control infection. The value of steroids remains controversial (Othersen et al., 1988). In a prospective trial, Anderson and co-workers (1990) showed "no benefit from the use of steroids to treat children who have ingested a caustic substance."

The healing esophagus is vulnerable to perforation, and follow-up endoscopy must be done with great care. Serial evaluation of the esophagus is best obtained by x-ray contrast study under fluoroscopic control (Kuhn and Tunell, 1983). When the burns are linear, or if there are multiple areas of involvement, the contour of the esophageal lumen is determined more accurately by using a silhouette technique with a barium-filled Penrose drain (Tunell et al., 1971) (Fig. 25–22). This technique affords a more exact status of the esophageal contour than does swallowed contrast material, which is subject to a streaming effect immediately below a stricture.

Dilatations are best delayed for 3 to 4 weeks after injury. Even in children with the most recalcitrant strictures, at least 6 months should be spent employing repeated dilatations in an attempt to restore an adequate lumen and permanently rehabilitate the esophagus (Dafoe and Ross, 1969; Wijburg et al., 1989). A gastrostomy may be necessary for feeding in severe cases and also as a route for retrograde bougienage. Use of lined Tucker's bougie dilators, drawn retrograde through the esophagus via a gastrostomy, represents a safe technique for esophageal dilatation in children (Tucker et al., 1974). A single short stricture may respond to direct installation of steroids through a fine needle adapted for use through the esophagoscope (Holder et al., 1969). Continued dilatations and repeated injections of steroids for several months have softened resistant strictures and preserved the esophagus in some patients. When multiple or extensive strictures develop that are not responsive to repeated dilatations, esophageal bypass must be considered. Other long-term complications include achalasia and carcinoma of the esophagus (Hopkins and Postlethwait, 1981).

ESOPHAGEAL REPLACEMENT

The primary indications for esophageal replacement in children are (1) severe caustic injuries in which the esophagus must be abandoned, despite

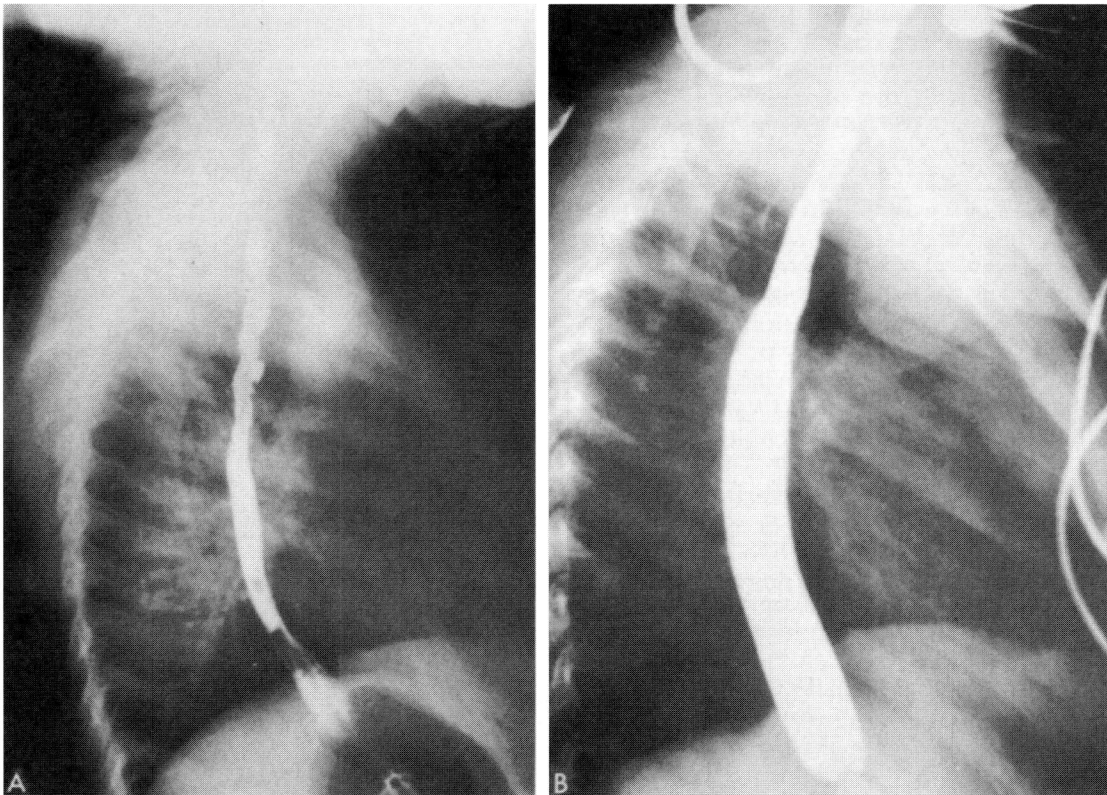

FIGURE 25–22. A, Barium swallow shows a long esophageal stricture from a caustic burn. B, In the same patient, the contour of the stricture is shown more accurately with a barium-filled Penrose drain, which has been drawn into the esophagus.

maximal dilatation therapy, and (2) esophageal atresia with or without tracheoesophageal fistula in which primary anastomosis is impossible or unsafe. Most operations for esophageal replacement are performed in children who have reached 1 year of age and weigh at least 10 kg. There are four major techniques of esophageal replacement: colon interposition, reversed gastric tube, total gastric transposition, and jejunal segment interposition.

Historical accounts of esophageal reconstruction begin with Czerny's description in 1877 of an operation to replace the cervical esophagus. Dale and Sherman (1955) established the colon as a safe and satisfactory esophageal substitute in children. In 1968, Burrington and Stephens showed that the reversed gastric tube was preferable to the colon in selected patients with a colon anomaly or an imperforate anus. Anderson and Randolph (1973) reported the adaptability of this gastric tube technique to infants with isolated esophageal atresia.

COLOESOPHAGOPLASTY

A variety of approaches may be employed, using either the right, the transverse, or the left colon and either a substernal or a retrohilar location of the conduit. The coloesophagoplasty (Fig. 25–23) is the most widely applied technique of esophageal replacement in children (Hendren and Hendren, 1985). Preopera-

tive studies include a barium enema to assess colon size, length, and anatomic configuration. Mechanical bowel preparation, supplemented with antibiotics, is advisable.

If the retrohilar intrathoracic route is planned for the colon position, the abdominal incision must be placed so that it can be extended easily into the left side of the chest in the fifth or sixth interspace. The decision as to which segment of colon is to be used is based on vascular anatomy. The middle colic artery usually provides reliable blood supply to the colon segment. When the right colon is used, its marginal artery is evaluated from the point of the ileocolic to the middle colic artery. If this portion of the marginal artery is well developed, the right colon can be used for bypass. Some surgeons prefer to use the left colon. Again, the marginal artery must be assessed along the mesenteric border to ensure that there are no gaps in the vessel. The blood supply to the proposed segment should be isolated and its adequacy tested by judicious placement of vascular clamps. If pulsations remain in the mesentery of the colon segment to be used, one may proceed with the appropriate ligations. Most of the transverse colon with either the hepatic or the splenic flexure and accompanying descending or ascending colon, respectively, is necessary to achieve appropriate length. It is preferable to isolate a segment of bowel of slightly greater length than needed rather than be hampered by inadequate length at the cervical anastomosis. Some surgeons recommend including the cecum and terminal ileum

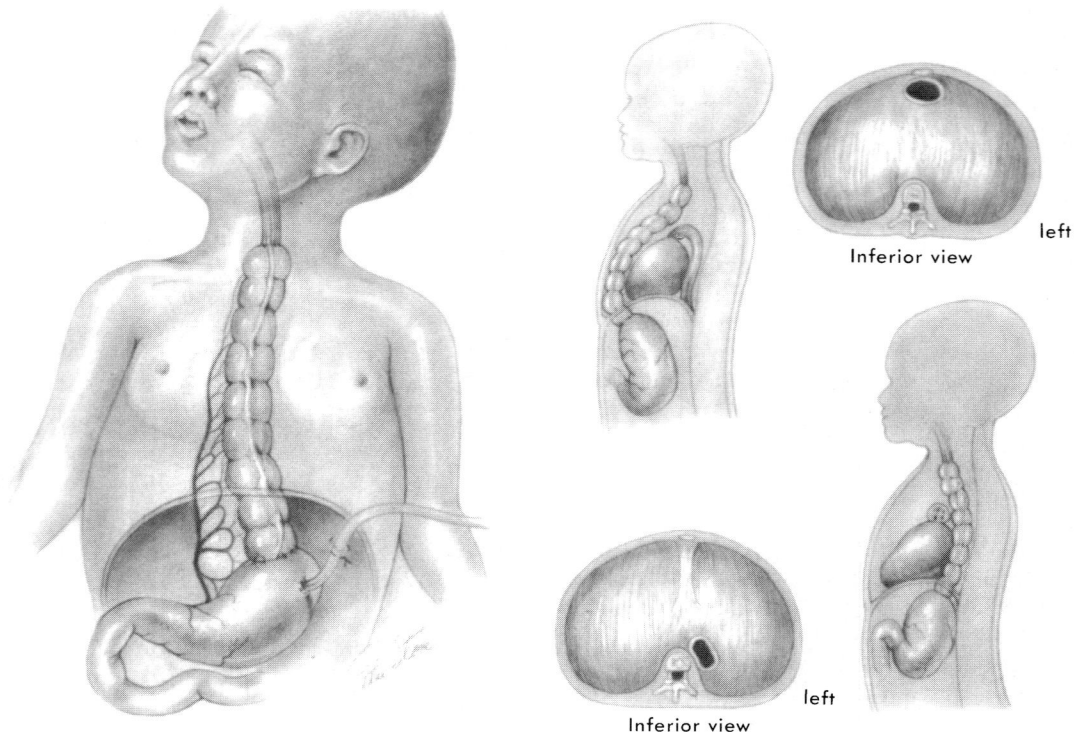

FIGURE 25–23. Coloesophagoplasty procedure. The colon may be placed in the substernal or the retrohilar position, depending on the surgeon's preference.

when the right colon is used and performing the appropriate trimming after the colon has been led into the neck.

The colon is divided between clamps and a colo-colic anastomosis creates continuity of the remaining abdominal colon. When the right colon is used, it is best to pass the colon segment behind the stomach through the gastrohepatic ligament, so that the vascular pedicle will lie behind the stomach. By this maneuver, subsequent traction on the vascular pedicle by a full stomach is avoided.

When the substernal position is selected, this space is developed by sharp and blunt dissection in the foramen of Morgagni immediately beneath the sternum (Fig. 25–24). The opening is enlarged until it can easily accommodate the colon without compression of its blood supply. An incision is made in the neck just above the jugular notch. With care to avoid the innominate vein, which lies immediately behind the upper sternum, the retrosternal space is entered just superficial to the thymus. In smaller children, the surgeon's fingers meet beneath the sternum and a channel can be created by blunt finger dissection. In older patients, a blunt instrument inserted beneath the sternum facilitates dissection. The dissection must be confined to the area immediately behind the central sternum to avoid tearing the pleura. When a tunnel of satisfactory size has been created, a long straight clamp is passed from above and the colon segment is drawn through the tunnel and out into the

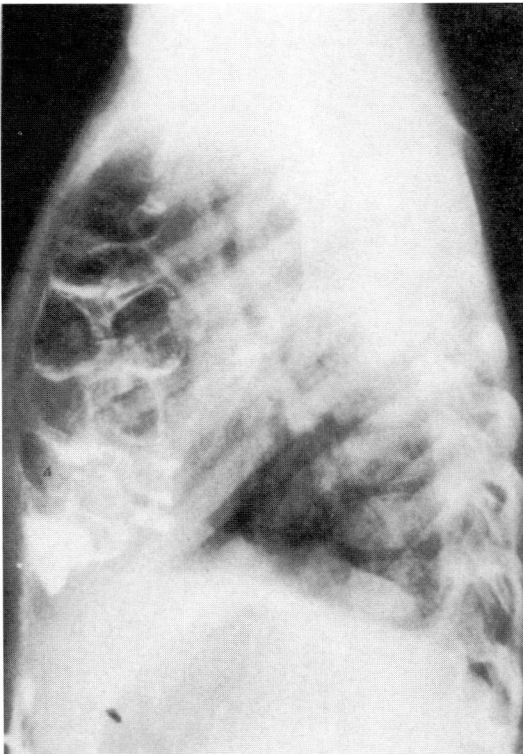

FIGURE 25–24. Barium swallow shows a retrosternal coloesophagoplasty in a 1-year-old patient with isolated esophageal atresia. Despite the colonic dilatation and the cascading of dye in the colonic folds, this child is eating normally and growing well.

cervical incision. The transit of swallowed material through the colon depends on gravity; therefore, it is not necessary to place the bowel in an isoperistaltic direction. At this time, the colon should be arranged at both ends to ensure that it is properly oriented and shows adequate pulsation in the small blood vessels.

The distal anastomosis between the lower end of the colon and the stomach is the next step. An incision is made in the presenting upper anterior stomach wall that conforms to the diameter of the colon, and the union is created with absorbable sutures to the inner row and interrupted nonabsorbable sutures on the outer layer. At this point, final refinements in the positioning of the colon are made, and any excess colon may be trimmed away. If the patient has had a previous esophagostomy, this is mobilized from the skin of the neck and brought into juxtaposition with the cervical colon for anastomosis. Two layers of nonabsorbable sutures are preferred. A small drain is led through the lateral corner of the wound, and the incision is closed. The drain is important because of the tendency of this anastomosis to leak.

Many surgeons advocate staging the operation by bringing the end of the colon out of the neck incision and delaying the esophagocolonic anastomosis. The determining factors with respect to delaying the cervical anastomosis are the general condition of the patient at this late stage in the procedure and the integrity of the blood supply to the distal portion of the conduit. A period of several days allows accurate assessment of the viability of the distal colon and permits the patient to stabilize.

A variant of coloesophagoplasty was introduced by Waterston (1964), who recommended placing the colon in the left hemithorax (Fig. 25–25). Exposure is obtained by extending the abdominal incision or using a separate thoracotomy. The colon segment is prepared as described earlier, but whenever possible, the left colon is selected. The segment is led from the abdomen into the chest through the esophageal hiatus or, preferably, through an incision in the diaphragm just lateral and slightly posterior to the hiatus. The colon and its vascular pedicle are drawn into the thorax and positioned behind the pulmonary hilus. By blunt and sharp dissection in the apex of the left side of the chest, a channel is created through Sibson's fascia into the neck. The opening created in the apical fascia must accommodate the colon and its mesentery without impinging on the blood supply. When the intrathoracic route is selected, the anastomosis to the stomach can be made as described previously. Alternatively, in patients whose distal esophagus is intact, an anastomosis may be made between the colon and the terminal portion of the esophagus above the diaphragm. This approach preserves the gastroesophageal junction and its diaphragmatic relations. Some surgeons consider pyloroplasty necessary for all colon interposition procedures, but this may not be required unless there has been vagal injury from an extensive esophageal burn. When the circulation of the distal colon is questionable, it is prudent to delay the cervi-

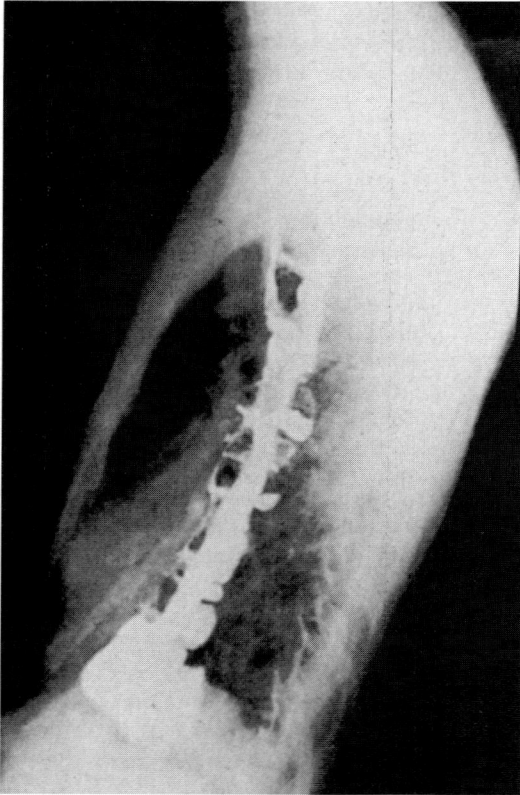

FIGURE 25–25. Barium swallow in a 14-year-old boy, 9 years after coloesophagoplasty for caustic stricture. The colon is in the retrohilar position advocated by Waterston.

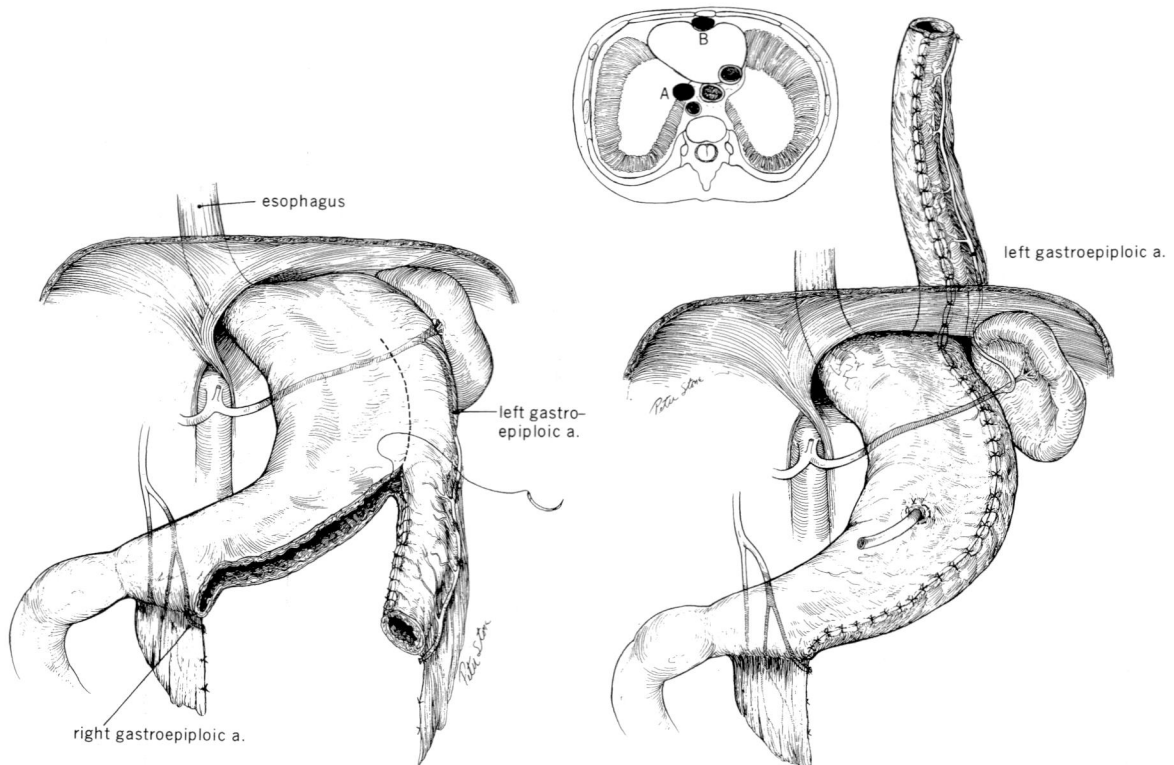

FIGURE 25–26. Important steps in the construction of a reversed tube gastric pedicle for esophageal reconstruction. A, The tube is started on the greater curvature, approximately 1 inch proximal to the pylorus. B, The gastric tube can be adapted to either the retrosternal or the retrohilar position.

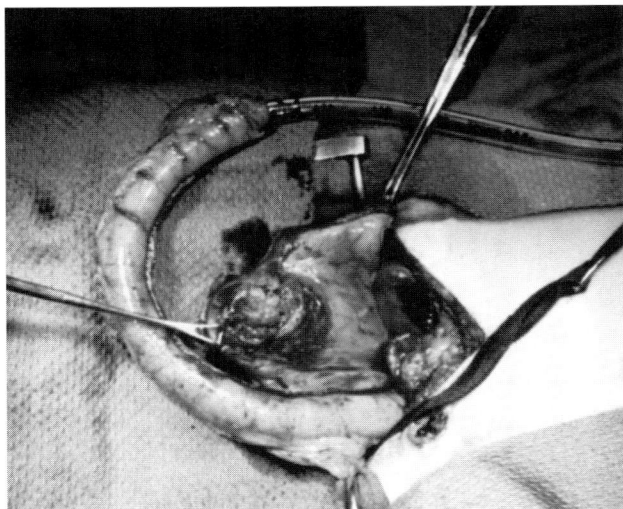

FIGURE 25–27. Operative photograph demonstrating the construction of a gastric tube over a chest tube.

cal anastomosis for several days until the viability of this bowel is determined.

Complications of colon interposition in the authors' experience include: (1) major colonic distention with serious compression of the lung (3 patients); (2) ulcer formation in the colon segment (1 patient); (3) leak at the cervical anastomosis (10 patients, of whom 5 healed spontaneously and 5 required surgical closure); (4) stenosis at the cervical anastomosis that required surgical revision (3 patients); (5) delayed gastric emptying that required separate pyloroplasty (2 patients); and (6) distal anastomotic stricture that required surgical revision (2 patients). Ischemic necrosis of the colon occurred once, and the transposed colon in this child was resected. Later a gastric tube interposition was performed, and the patient has since done well.

Despite the complications, these children have grown well and lead essentially normal lives. Colo-esophagoplasty has been a reliable method of reconstructing the esophagus with minimal complications in several large series of children (Ahmed and Spitz, 1986; Campbell et al., 1982; West et al., 1986).

ESOPHAGEAL RECONSTRUCTION BY USING THE TUBED GASTRIC PEDICLE

An esophageal conduit can be constructed from the greater curvature of the stomach (Fig. 25–26). The abdomen is entered through an upper transverse incision. Division of the gastrocolic omentum permits inspection of the left gastroepiploic artery at its origin from the splenic artery to determine its suitability to supply the tube.

The right gastroepiploic artery is divided approximately 2 cm proximal to the pylorus. An incision is then made in the wall of the stomach beginning 3 cm above the pylorus. A chest tube is inserted and pressed against the greater curvature to outline the

gastric tube. The size of the catheter varies with the size of the patient, but ranges from No. 18 to 24 French sizes (Fig. 25–27). The edges of the gastric tube are divided and stapled together using a stapling device. The final portion at the end of the tube that will lie in the neck is sutured in an interrupted manner. This allows subsequent trimming of the end of the tube to achieve proper length in the neck (Fig. 25–28). An incision is made in the left side of the neck just above the clavicle, and the cervical esophagus is dissected free.

As in colon bypass, the gastric tube may be placed in either the substernal or the intrathoracic position. Generally, the substernal tunnel can be made more quickly, because a thoracotomy is not required. However, the intrathoracic, retrohilar position of a substitute esophagus more nearly approaches normal anatomy. Occasionally, the native posterior mediastinal bed of the esophagus can be used.

For patients with esophageal atresia, the cervical esophagostomy created in the newborn period is dissected free and the edges are trimmed. In patients with caustic stricture without previous esophagostomy, the esophagus is divided at the level above the burned portion; the lower end of the esophagus is then removed. If the substernal location is chosen, the tunnel is prepared by blunt dissection from both the abdominal and the neck incisions. If the transthoracic route is elected, a posterolateral incision is made in the left side of the chest at the level of the sixth intercostal space, and a 2- to 3-cm opening is created in the diaphragm posterolateral to the esophageal hiatus. The tube is drawn through this new opening and positioned behind the left lung hilus. The opening in the diaphragm must be adequate to transmit the tube without obstructing the vascular pedicle. Next, a passage wide enough to admit the gastric tube is made at the apex of the thorax in Sibson's fascia. Care should be taken to protect the subclavian vessels that lie just anterior to the plane of dissection and to avoid the stellate ganglion that lies posteriorly. As the tube is brought into the neck, twisting must

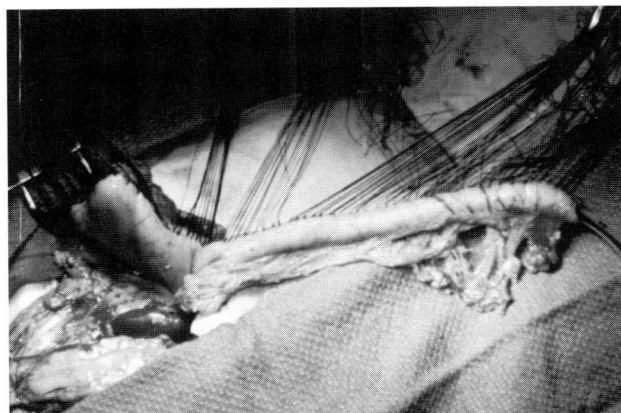

FIGURE 25–28. Operative photograph demonstrating the length that can be obtained with a reversed gastric tube so that it can reach into the neck. Multiple sutures are used to reinforce the staple lines.

be avoided, because it can impair the blood supply. As in coloesophagoplasty, the anastomosis between the gastric tube and the esophagus may be performed at this stage or may be delayed. The cervical anastomosis is made in two layers by means of interrupted sutures. Gastrostomy is performed routinely, as is pyloroplasty. The abdomen is closed without drainage, but the neck is drained.

Gastrostomy feedings are begun as soon as peristalsis returns. When the operation is completed in one stage, oral feedings are begun on the tenth day after a barium swallow has shown integrity of the gastric tube (Fig. 25–29). The thoracostomy tube is not removed until this time.

Complications of gastric tube interposition in 30 children at Children's Hospital have been major in 6 patients and minor in 7. The major complications are as follows: Three patients had intrathoracic leaks of the tube, 1 immediately postoperatively, which healed spontaneously, and 2 that were perforated during dilatation. One perforation was closed at operation; the other was unrecognized and the child died. Two cervical anastomoses required revision, and 1 patient had surgical closure of a fistula that persisted for 1 year. Gastric outlet obstruction due to a technical error required pyloroplasty in 1 patient. The minor complications included 5 cervical salivary leaks that closed spontaneously and 1 child with temporary stasis in a redundant gastric tube that produced an ulcer, which healed with antacids.

Children who have had esophageal reconstruction with a gastric tube have done well with regard to growth, nutrition, and overall adjustment. In a study comparing two large series of patients who had had either a reversed gastric tube or a colon interposition, the long-term outcome was equivalent (Anderson et al., 1992).

JEJUNAL ESOPHAGEAL REPLACEMENT

The jejunum has been used as an esophageal substitute for a variety of conditions in children (Ring et al., 1982). Saeki and co-workers (1988) reported good long-term results using jejunal interposition in infants with esophageal atresia. Advances in microvascular techniques have made possible free vascularized grafts of small bowel, principally in older children. A free jejunal graft is indicated mostly in situations where a standard interposition has failed (Fisher et al., 1984).

GASTRIC TRANSPOSITION

Use of a total gastric transposition with esophagogastric anastomosis has gained favor in some centers as the preferred method of esophageal replacement (Marujo et al., 1991; Valente et al., 1987). The entire stomach is mobilized and brought posteriorly in the

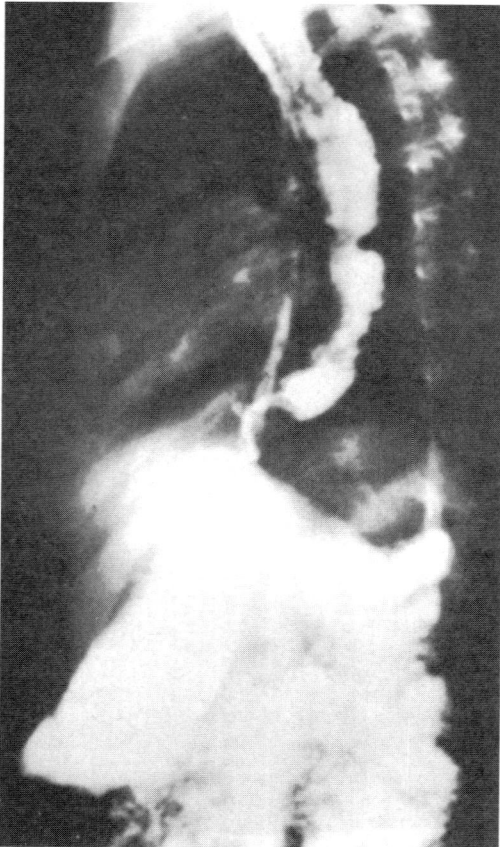

FIGURE 25–29. Barium swallow shows a gastric tube in the retrohilar position. There is mild reflux into the scarred esophageal remnant. Note the small but adequate gastric volume.

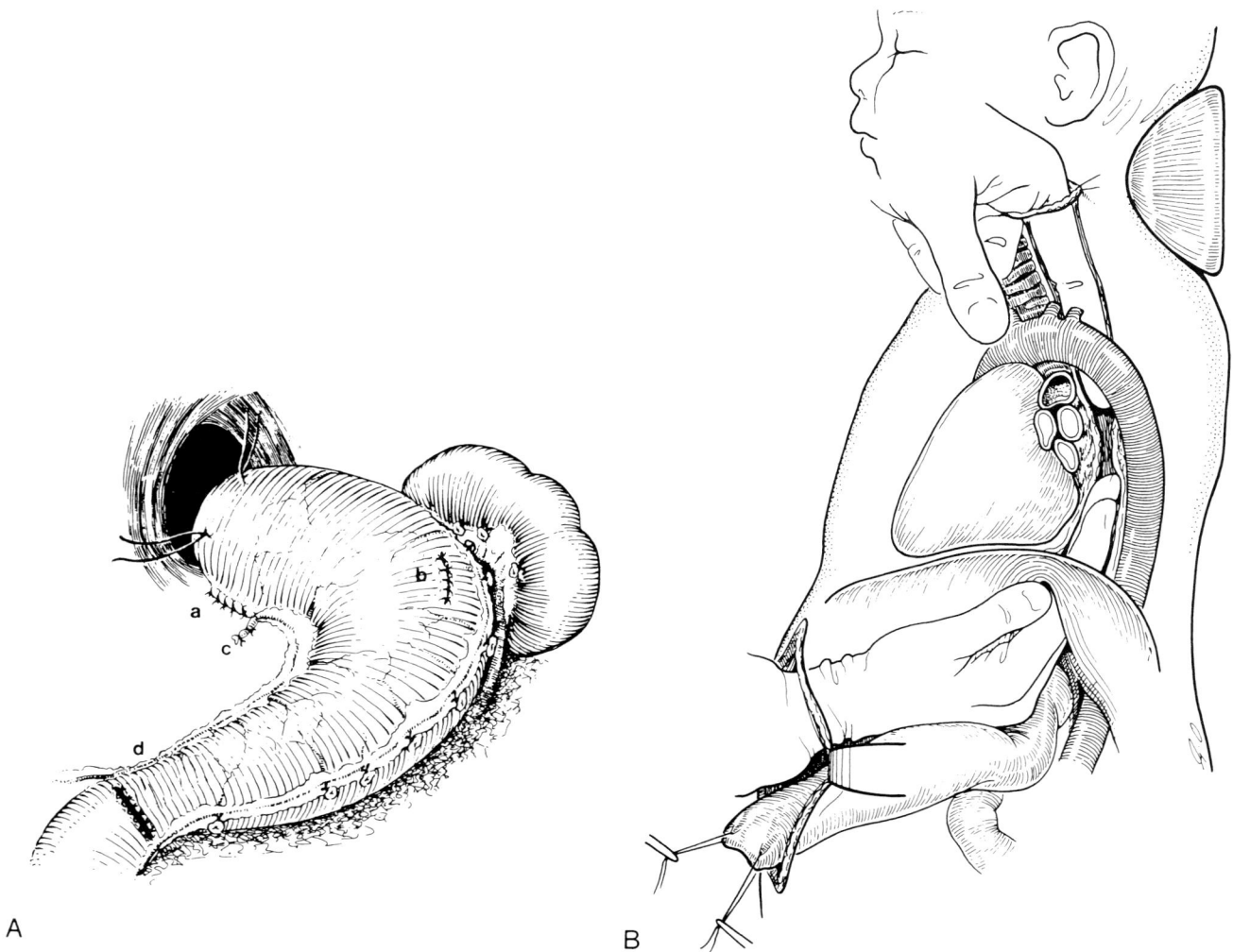

A

B

FIGURE 25–30. *A,* Diagram demonstrating the technique advocated by Spitz for mobilizing the stomach for total gastric transposition. A pyloroplasty has been performed and the sutures mark the site of the anastomosis on the apex of the stomach. a = Esophagogastric junction; b = gastrostomy site; c = left gastric artery; d = right gastric artery. *B,* The technique of creating a posterior mediastinal tunnel from above and below so that the stomach can be placed in the posterior mediastinum. (*A* and *B,* From Spitz, L.: Gastric transposition for esophageal substitution in children. J. Pediatr. Surg., 27:253, 1992.)

chest into the neck (Fig. 25–30). Complications of aspiration, reflux, and distention have been reported, although Spitz (1992) reported good results in extended follow-up. The chief advantage is the ease of construction with respect to the other modes of esophageal replacement.

SELECTED BIBLIOGRAPHY

Ashcraft, K. W., and Holder, T. M. (eds): Pediatric Esophageal Surgery. Orlando, FL, Grune & Stratton, 1986.

This monograph comprises contributions by outstanding workers in the fields of pediatric surgery and gastroenterology. The embryology, physiology, and surgical approaches to the manifestations of pediatric esophageal disease are illustrated.

Fonkalsrud, E. W., Foglia, R. W., Ament, M., et al.: Operative treatment for the gastroesophageal reflux syndrome in children. J. Pediatr. Surg., 24:525, 1989.

A careful analysis of a series of 420 infants and children over a 19-year period is described. The authors' stepwise diagnostic evaluation is presented. An algorithm for children with symptomatic reflux is described, which is useful in selecting patients for operation.

Hendren, W. H., and Hendren, W. G.: Interposition for esophagus in children. J. Pediatr. Surg., 20:829, 1985.

A series of 32 patients having esophageal substitution demonstrates the success of this operation. The operative technique for safe and successful construction of the colon interposition in children is beautifully illustrated.

Manning, P. B., Morgan, R. A., Coran, A. G., et al.: 50 years' experience with esophageal atresia and tracheoesophageal fistula. Ann. Surg., 204:446, 1986.

In this review of the experience at the University of Michigan, 426 patients with esophageal atresia and tracheoesophageal fistula were evaluated beginning with the first successful primary repair by Haight. Survival in the most recent group of 63 patients was 82.5%. The evolution and operative management, the incidence of associated anomalies, and the management of complications are detailed.

Randolph, J. G., Newman, K. D., and Anderson, K. D.: Current results in repair of esophageal atresia with tracheoesophageal fistula using physiologic status as a guide to therapy. Ann. Surg., 209:526, 1989.

The management of 118 infants with esophageal atresia is reviewed. A "modern" management plan was used in a series of 39 patients, with excellent results. The physiologic status of the infant, not arbitrary weight or x-ray findings, was the guide to the choice of management plan.

BIBLIOGRAPHY

Ahmed, A., and Spitz, L.: The outcome of colonic replacement of esophagus in children. Prog. Pediatr. Surg., 19:37, l986.

Anderson, K. D., Noblett, H., Belsey, R., and Randolph, J. G.: Long-term follow-up of children with colon and gastric tube interposition for esophageal atresia. Surgery 111:131, 1992.

Anderson, K. D., and Randolph, J. G.: The gastric tube for esophageal replacement in children. J. Thorac. Cardiovasc. Surg., 66:333, 1973.

Anderson, K. D., Rouse, T. M., and Randolph, J. G.: A controlled trial of corticosteroids in children with corrosive injury of the esophagus. N. Engl. J. Med., 323:637, 1990.

Ashcraft, K. W., Goodwin, C. D., Amoury, R. A., and Holder, T. M.: Early recognition and aggressive treatment of gastroesophageal reflux following repair of esophageal atresia. J. Pediatr. Surg., 12:317, 1977.

Ashcraft, K. W., Holder, T. M., and Amoury, R. A.: The Thal fundoplication for gastroesophageal reflux. J. Pediatr. Surg., 19:480, 1984.

Azizkhan, R. G., Tapper, D., and Eraklis, A.: Achalasia in childhood: A 20-year experience. J. Pediatr. Surg., 15:452, 1980.

Bettex, M., and Kuffer, F.: Long-term results of fundoplication in hiatus hernia and cardioesophageal chalasia in infants and children. Report of 112 consecutive cases. J. Pediatr. Surg., 4:526, 1969.

Bishop, P. J., Klein, M. D., Philippart, A. R., et al.: Transpleural repair of esophageal atresia without a primary gastrostomy: 240 patients treated between 1951 and 1983. J. Pediatr. Surg., 20:823, 1985.

Boix-Ochoa, J.: Diagnosis and management of gastroesophageal reflux in children. Surg. Annu., 13:123, 1981.

Bower, R. J., Sieber, W. K., and Kiesewetter, W. B.: Alimentary tract duplications in children. Ann. Surg., 188:669, 1978.

Buick, R. J., and Spitz, L.: Achalasia of the cardia in children. Br. J. Surg., 72:341, 1985.

Burrington, J. D., and Stephens, C. A.: Esophageal replacement with a gastric tube in infants and children. J. Pediatr. Surg., 3:246, 1968.

Campbell, J. B., and Foley, C.: A safe alternative to endoscopic removal of blunt esophageal foreign bodies. Arch. Otolaryngol., 109:323, 1983.

Campbell, J. R., Webber, B. R., Harrison, M. W., et al.: Esophageal replacement in infants and children by colon interposition. Ann. Surg., 144:29, 1982.

Canal, D. F., Vane, D. W., Goto, S., et al.: Reduction of lower esophageal sphincter pressure with Stamm gastrostomy. J. Pediatr. Surg., 22:54, 1987.

Carcassonne, M., Bensoussan, A., and Aubert, J.: The management of gastroesophageal reflux in infants. J. Pediatr. Surg., 8:575, 1973.

Cheu, H. W., Grosfeld, J., Heifetz, S. A., et al.: Persistence of Barrett's esophagus in children after antireflux surgery: Influence on follow-up care. J. Pediatr. Surg., 27:260, 1992.

Chittmittrapap, S., Spitz, L., Kiely, E. M., et al.: Anastomotic leakage following surgery for esophageal atresia. J. Pediatr. Surg., 27:29, 1992.

Cleveland, W. W., Chandler, M. D., and Lawson, R. B.: Treatment of caustic burns of the esophagus. J. A. M. A., 186:262, 1963.

Czerny, V.: Neue Opertionen. Zentralbl. Chir., 4:443, 1877.

Dafoe, C. X., and Ross, C. A.: Acute corrosive esophagitis. Thorax, 24:291, 1969.

Dale, W. A., and Sherman, C. D., Jr.: Late reconstruction of congenital esophageal atresia by intrathoracic colon transplantation. J. Thorac. Surg., 29:344, 1955.

DeLorimier, A. A., and Harrison, M. R.: Esophageal atresia: Embryogenesis and management. World J. Surg., 9:250, 1985.

DeLorimier, A. A., and Harrison, M. R.: Long gap esophageal atresia—Primary anastomosis after esophageal elongation by bougienage and esophagostomy. J. Thorac. Cardiovasc. Surg., 79:138, 1980.

Donahoe, P. K., and Gee, P. E.: Complete laryngotracheal cleft: Management and repair. J. Pediatr. Surg., 19:143, 1984.

Donahoe, P. K., and Hendren, W.: The surgical management of laryngotracheoesophageal cleft with tracheoesophageal fistula and esophageal atresia. Surgery, 71:363, 1972.

DuBois, J. J., Pokorny, W. J., Harberg, F. J., et al.: Current management of laryngeal and laryngotracheoesophageal clefts. J. Pediatr. Surg., 25:855, 1990.

Dudgeon, D. L., Morrison, C. W., and Woolley, M. M.: Congenital proximal tracheoesophageal fistula. J. Pediatr. Surg., 7:614, 1972.

Ein, S. H., Shandling, B., Wesson, D., et al.: Esophageal atresia with distal tracheoesophageal fistula: Associated anomalies and prognosis in the 1980s. J. Pediatr. Surg., 24:1055, 1989.

Euler, A. R., and Ament, M. E.: Detection of gastroesophageal reflux in the pediatric-age patient by esophageal intraluminal pH probe measurement (Tuttle test). Pediatrics, 60:65, 1977.

Euler, A. R., and Ament, M. E.: Value of esophageal manometric studies in the gastroesophageal reflux in infancy. Pediatrics, 59:58, 1977.

Filler, R. M., Randolph, J. G., and Gross, R. E.: Esophageal hiatus hernia in infants and children. J. Thorac. Surg., 47:551, 1964.

Filston, H. C., Rankin, J. S., and Grim, J. K.: Esophageal atresia: Prognostic features and contribution of preoperative telescopic endoscopy. Ann. Surg., 149:532, 1984.

Fisher, J., Payne, W. S., and Irans, G. B.: Salvage of a failed colon interposition in the esophagus with a free jejunal graft. Mayo Clin. Proc., 59:147, 1984.

Fonkalsrud, E. W., Foglia, R. P., Ament, M., et al.: Operative treatment for the gastroesophageal reflux syndrome in children. J. Pediatr. Surg., 24:525, 1989.

Forshall, I.: The cardioesophageal syndrome in childhood. Arch. Dis. Child., *30*:46, 1955.

Friesen, C. A., Holder, T. M., Ashcraft, K. W., et al.: Abbreviated esophageal pH monitoring as an indication for fundoplication in children. J. Pediatr. Surg., *27*:775, 1992.

Goh, D. W., and Brereton, R. J.: Success and failure with neonatal tracheoesophageal fistula. Br. J. Surg., *78*:834, 1991.

Haight, C., and Towsley, H. A.: Congenital atresia of the esophagus with tracheoesophageal fistula: Extrapleural ligation of fistula and end-to-end anastomosis of esophageal segments. Surg. Gynecol. Obstet., *76*:672, 1943.

Haller, J. A., Jr., Andrews, H. G., White, J. J., et al.: Pathophysiology and management of acute corrosive burns of the esophagus. Results of treatment in 285 children. J. Pediatr. Surg., *6*:578, 1971.

Hawkins, D. B., Demeter, M. J., and Burnett, T. E.: Caustic ingestion: Controversies in management. Laryngoscope, *90*:98, 1980.

Heller, E.: Extramukose Cardioplastik beim chronischem Cardiospasmus mit Dilatations des Oesophagus. Mitt. Grenzgeb. Med. Chir., *27*:141a, 1913.

Hendren, W. H., and Hendren, W. G.: Colon interposition for esophagus in children. J. Pediatr. Surg., *20*:829, 1985.

Herbst, J. J.: Medical treatment of gastroesophageal reflux. *In* Ashcraft, K. W., and Holder, T. M. (eds): Pediatric Esophageal Surgery. Orlando, FL, Grune & Stratton, 1986, pp. 181–191.

Hill, J. L.: Neuromotor esophageal disorders. *In* Welch, K. J., Randolph, J. G., Ravitch, M. M., et al. (eds): Pediatric Surgery. Chicago, Year Book Medical, 1986, pp. 720–725.

Holder, T. M.: Esophageal atresia and tracheoesophageal malformations. *In* Ashcraft, K. W., and Holder, T. M. (eds): Pediatric Surgery. Philadelphia, W. B. Saunders, 1993, pp. 249–270.

Holder, T. M., Ashcraft, K. W., and Leape, L.: The treatment of patients with esophageal strictures by local steroid injections. J. Pediatr. Surg., *4*:646, 1969.

Holder, T. M., McDonald, V. G., Jr., and Woolley, M. M.: The premature or critically ill infant with esophageal atresia. Increased success with a staged approach. J. Thorac. Cardiovasc. Surg., *44*:344, 1962.

Hollwarth, M., and Uray, E.: Physiology and pathophysiology of the esophagus in childhood. Prog. Pediatr. Surg., *18*:1, 1985.

Hopkins, R. A., and Postlethwait, R. W.: Caustic burns and carcinoma of the esophagus. Ann. Surg., *194*:146, 1981.

Hopkins, W. A.: The esophagus. *In* Gray, S. W., and Skandalakis, J. E. (eds): Embryology for Surgeons. Philadelphia, W. B. Saunders, 1972.

Howard, R., and Myers, N.: Esophageal atresia: A technique for elongating the upper pouch. Surgery, *58*:725, 1965.

Ibrahim, N. B., and Sandry, G. J.: Congenital oesophageal stenosis caused by tracheobronchial strictures in the oesophageal wall. Thorax, *36*:465, 1981.

Johnson, D. G.: The Nissen fundoplication. *In* Ashcraft, K. W., and Holder, T. M. (eds): Pediatric Esophageal Surgery. Orlando, FL, Grune & Stratton, 1986, pp. 193–208.

Jolley, S. G., Herbst, J. J., Johnson, D. G., et al.: Patterns of postcibal gastroesophageal reflux in symptomatic infants. Am. J. Surg., *138*:946, 1979.

Jolley, S. G., Johnson, D. G., Herbst, J. J., et al.: An assessment of gastroesophageal reflux in children by extended pH monitoring of the distal esophagus. Surgery, *84*:16, 1978.

Jolley, S. G., Tunell, W. P., Hoelzer, D. J., et al.: Postoperative small bowel obstruction in infants and children: A problem following Nissen fundoplication. J. Pediatr. Surg., *21*:407, 1986.

Jona, J. Z., Sty, J. R., and Glicklich, M.: Simplified radioisotope technique for assessing gastroesophageal reflux in children. J. Pediatr. Surg., *16*:114, 1981.

Kao, S. C., Smith, W. L., Sato, Y., et al.: Ultrafast CT of laryngeal and tracheobronchial obstruction in symptomatic postoperative infants with esophageal atresia and tracheoesophageal fistula. Am. J. Radiol., *154*:345, 1990.

Kimura, K., Soper, R. T., Kao, S. C., et al.: Aortosternopexy for tracheomalacia following repair of esophageal atresia: Evaluation by cine-CT and technical refinement. J. Pediatr. Surg., *25*:769, 1990.

Kluth, D.: Atlas of esophageal atresia. J. Pediatr. Surg., *11*:901, 1976.

Kuhn, J. R., and Tunell, W. P.: The role of cine-esophagography in caustic esophageal injury. Am. J. Surg., *146*:804, 1983.

Ladd, W. E.: The surgical treatment of esophageal atresia and tracheoesophageal fistula. N. Engl. J. Med., *230*:625, 1944.

Lanman, T. H.: Congenital atresia of the esophagus: A study of thirty-two cases. Arch. Surg., *41*:1060, 1940.

LaQuaglia, M. P., Gray, M., and Schuster, S. R.: Esophageal atresia and ante-thoracic skin tube esophageal conduits: Squamous cell cancer in the conduit 44 years following surgery. J. Pediatr. Surg., *22*:44, 1987.

Leape, L. L., Bhan, I., and Ramenofsky, M. L.: Esophageal biopsy in the diagnosis of reflux esophagitis. J. Pediatr. Surg., *16*:379, 1981.

Lemmer, J. H., Coran, A. G., Wesley, J. R., et al.: Achalasia in children: Treatment by anterior esophageal myotomy (modified Heller operation). J. Pediatr. Surg., *20*:333, 1985.

Leven, N. L.: Congenital atresia of the esophagus with tracheoesophageal fistula: Report of successful extrapleural ligation of fistulous communication and cervical esophagotomy. J. Thorac. Surg., *10*:648a, 1941.

Lilly, J. R., and Randolph, J. G.: Hiatal hernia and gastroesophageal reflux in infants and children. J. Thorac. Cardiovasc. Surg., *55*:42, 1968.

Lindahl, H., Rintala, R., and Louhimo, I.: Failure of the Nissen fundoplication to control gastroesophageal reflux in esophageal atresia patients. J. Pediatr. Surg., *24*:985, 1989.

Livaditis, A.: Esophageal atresia: A method of overbridging large segmental gaps. Z. Kinderchir., *13*:248, 1973.

Louhimo, I., and Lindahl, H.: Esophageal atresia: Primary results of 500 consecutively treated patients. J. Pediatr. Surg., *18*:217, 1983.

Mahour, G. H., Woolley, M. M., and Gwinn, J. L.: Elongation of the upper pouch and delayed reconstruction of the esophagus in esophageal atresia. J. Pediatr. Surg., *9*:373, 1974.

Malthaner, R. A., Newman, K. D., Parry, R., et al.: Alkaline gastroesophageal reflux in infants and children. J. Pediatr. Surg., 26:986, 1991.

Manning, P. B., Coran, A. G., Sloan, W. E., et al.: Fifty years' experience with esophageal atresia and tracheoesophageal fistula. Ann. Surg., *204*:446, 1986.

Martinez, D. A., Ginn-Pease, M. E., and Caniano, D. A.: Sequelae of antireflux surgery in profoundly disabled children. J. Pediatr. Surg., *27*:267, 1992.

Marujo, W. C., Tannuri, U., and Maksoud, J. G.: Total gastric transposition colon: An alternative to esophageal replacement in children. J. Pediatr. Surg., *26*:676, 1991.

McKinnon, L. J., and Kosloske, A. M.: Predictions and prevention of anastomotic complications of esophageal atresia at tracheoesophageal fistula. J. Pediatr. Surg., *25*:778, 1990.

Moncrief, J. A., and Randolph, J. G.: Congenital tracheoesophageal fistula without atresia of the esophagus: A method for diagnosis and surgical correction. J. Thorac. Cardiovasc. Surg., *51*:434, 1966.

Myer, C. M., Cotton, R. T., Holmes, D. K., et al.: Laryngeal and laryngotracheoesophageal clefts: Role of early surgical repair. Ann. Otol. Rhinol. Laryngol., *99*:98, 1990.

Myers, N. A.: Oesophageal atresia: The epitome of modern surgery. Ann. R. Coll. Surg. Engl., *54*:277, 1974.

Nakayama, D. K., Shorter, N. A., Boyle, J. T., et al.: Pneumatic dilatation and operative treatment of achalasia in children. J. Pediatr. Surg., *22*:619, 1987.

Neuhauser, B. D., and Berenberg, W.: Cardioesophageal relaxation as a cause of vomiting in infants. Radiology, *48*:480, 1947.

Newman, K. D.: The surgical management of laryngotracheoesophageal cleft. Woodbury, CT, Cine-med Video Library, 1988.

Nihoul-Fekete, C., Bawab, F., and Lortat-Jacob, S.: Achalasia of the esophagus in childhood. J. Pediatr. Surg., *24*:1060, 1989.

Nissen, R., and Rossettiu, M.: Die behandlung von Hiatushernien und Reflux-Oesophagitis mit Gastropexie und Fundoplication. Stuttgart, Geo. Thieme-Verlag, 1959.

Orringer, M. B., Kirsch, M. M., and Sloan, H.: Long-term esophageal function following repair of esophageal atresia. Ann. Surg., *186*:436, 1977.

Othersen, H. B., Parker, E. F., and Smith, C. D.: The surgical management of esophageal stricture in children: A century of progress. Ann. Surg., *207*:590, 1988.

Poenaru, D., Laberge, J. M., Neilson, I. R., et al.: A more than 25-

year experience with end-to-end versus end-to-side repair for esophageal atresia. J. Pediatr. Surg., *26*:472, 1991.

Pohlson, E. C., Schaller, R. T., and Tapper, D.: Improved survival with primary anastomosis in the low birth weight neonate with esophageal atresia and tracheoesophageal fistula. J. Pediatr. Surg., *23*:418, 1988.

Pretorius, D. H., Drose, J. A., Dennis, M. A., et al.: Tracheoesophageal fistula in utero, 22 cases. J. Ultrasound Med., *6*:509, 1987.

Puri, P., Ninan, G. K., Blake, N. S., et al.: Delayed primary anastomosis for esophageal atresia: 18 months to 11 years follow-up. J. Pediatr. Surg., *8*:1127, 1992.

Raffensperger, J. G.: Esophageal atresia and tracheoesophageal stenosis. *In* Raffensperger, J. G. (ed): Swenson's Pediatric Surgery. East Norwalk, CT, Appleton & Lange, 1990, pp. 697–717.

Randolph, J.: Experience with the Nissen fundoplication for correction of gastroesophageal reflux in infants. Ann. Surg., *198*:579, 1983.

Randolph, J. G., Lilly, J. R., and Anderson, K. D.: Surgical treatment of gastroesophageal reflux in infants. Ann. Surg., *180*:479, 1974.

Randolph, J. G., Newman, K. D., and Anderson, K. D.: Current results in repair of esophageal atresia with tracheoesophageal fistula using physiologic status as a guide to therapy. Ann. Surg., *209*:526, 1989.

Replogle, R. L.: Esophageal atresia: Plastic sump catheter for drainage of the proximal pouch. Surgery, *54*:657, 1963.

Ring, W. S., Varco, R. L., Heureux, R. R., et al.: Esophageal replacement with jejunum in children: An 18- to 30-year follow-up. J. Thorac. Cardiovasc. Surg., *83*:918, 1982.

Ryan, D. P., Muehrcke, D., Doody, D., et al.: Laryngotracheoesophageal cleft (type IV): Management and repair of lesions beyond the carina. J. Pediatr. Surg., *26*:962, 1991.

Saeki, M., Tsuchida, Y., Ogata, T., et al.: Long-term results of jejunal replacement of the esophagus. J. Pediatr. Surg., *23*:483, 1988.

Scherer, L. R., and Grosfeld, J. L.: Congenital esophageal stenosis, esophageal duplication, neurenteric cyst and esophageal diverticulum. *In* Ashcraft, K. W., and Holder, T. M. (eds): Pediatric Esophageal Surgery. Orlando, FL, Grune & Stratton, 1986, pp. 53–71.

Schropp, K. P., Lunsford, K., and Lobe, T. E.: Laparoscopic Nissen fundoplication in childhood. J. Pediatr. Surg., *28*:358, 1993.

Schwartz, M., and Filler, R. M.: Tracheocompression as a cause of apnea following repair of tracheoesophageal fistula: Treatment by aortopexy. J. Pediatr. Surg., *15*:842, 1980.

Shaul, D. B., Schwartz, M. Z., Marr, C., et al.: Primary repair without routine gastrostomy is the treatment of choice for neonates with esophageal atresia and tracheoesophageal fistula. Arch. Surg., *124*:1188, 1989.

Shono, T., Suita, S., Arima, T., et al.: Motility function of the esophagus before primary anastomosis and esophageal atresia. J. Pediatr. Surg., *28*:673, 1993.

Smith, C. D., Othersen, B., Gogan, N. J., et al.: Nissen fundoplication in children with profound neurologic disability: High risks and unmet goals. Ann. Surg., *215*:654, 1992.

Smith, E. I.: The early development of the trachea and the esophagus in relation to atresia of the esophagus and tracheoesophageal fistula. Contrib. Embryol. Carnegie Inst. Wash., No. 245, *36*:41, 1957.

Spitz, L.: Gastric transposition for esophageal substitution in children. J. Pediatr. Surg., *27*:252, 1992.

Spitz, L., Kiely, E., and Brereton, R. J.: Esophageal atresia: Five-year experience with 148 cases. J. Pediatr. Surg., *22*:103, 1987.

Spitz, L., and Kirtane, J.: Results and complications of surgery for gastroesophageal reflux. Arch. Dis. Child., *60*:743, 1985.

Stolar, C. J., Berdon, W. E., Dillon, P. W., et al.: Esophageal dilatation

and reflux in neonates supported by ECMO after diaphragmatic hernia repair. Am. J. Radiol., *151*:135, 1988.

Sulamaa, M., Gripenberg, L., and Ahvenainen, E. K.: Prognosis and treatment of congenital atresia of the esophagus. Acta Chir. Scand., *102*:141, 1951.

Superina, R. A., Ein, S. H., and Humphreys, R. P.: Cystic duplications of the esophagus and neurenteric cysts. J. Pediatr. Surg., *19*:527, 1984.

Temple, D. M., and McNeese, M. C.: Hazards of battery ingestion. Pediatrics, *71*:100, 1983.

Templeton, J. M., Templeton, J. J., Schneufer, L., et al.: Management of esophageal atresia and tracheoesophageal fistula in the neonate with severe respiratory distress syndrome. J. Pediatr. Surg., *20*:394, 1985.

Touloukian, R. J.: Reassessment of the end-to-side operation for esophageal atresia with distal tracheoesophageal fistula: A 22-year experience with 68 cases. J. Pediatr. Surg., *27*:562, 1992.

Tucker, J. A., Turtz, M. L., Silberman, H. D., et al.: Tucker retrograde esophageal dilatation, 1924–1974: A historical review. Ann. Otol. Rhinol. Laryngol. Suppl., *16*:1, 1974.

Tunell, W., Anderson, K. D., and Rosser S.: Esophagram with a barium-filled Penrose drain. J. Pediatr. Surg., *6*:567, 1971.

Turnage, R. H., Oldham, K. T., Coran, A. G., et al.: Late results of fundoplication for gastroesophageal reflux in infants and children. Surgery, *105*:457, 1989.

Ty, T. C., Burnet, C., and Beardmore, H. E.: A variation in the operative technique for the treatment of esophageal atresia with tracheoesophageal fistula. J. Pediatr. Surg., *2*:118, 1967.

Valente, A., Brereton, R. J., and Mackersie, A.: Esophageal replacement with whole stomach in infants and children. J. Pediatr. Surg., *22*:913, 1987.

Vane, D. W., Cosby, K., West, K., et al.: Late results following esophagomyotomy in children with achalasia. J. Pediatr. Surg., *23*:515, 1988.

Waterston, D. J.: Colonic replacement of the esophagus (intrathoracic). Surg. Clin. North Am., *44*:1441, 1964.

Waterston, D. J., Carter, R. E., and Aberdeen E.: Oesophageal atresia: Tracheoesophageal fistula. A study of survival in 218 infants. Lancet, *1*:819, 1962.

Weaver, D. D., Mapstone, C. L., and Uyu, P. L.: The VATER association. Analysis of 46 patients. Am. J. Dis. Child., *140*:225, 1986.

Wesley, J., Coran, A., and Sorahan T.: The need for evaluation of gastrointestinal reflux in brain-damaged children referred for feeding gastrostomy. J. Pediatr. Surg., *16*:866, 1981.

West, K. W., Vane, D. W., and Grosfeld, J.: Esophageal replacement in children: Experience with 31 cases. Surgery, *100*:751, 1986.

Wheatley, M. J., and Coran, A. G.: Pericardial flap interposition for the definitive management of recurrent tracheoesophageal fistula. J. Pediatr. Surg., *27*:1122, 1992.

Wheatley, M. J., Coran, A. G., and Wesley, J. R.: Efficacy of the Nissen fundoplication in the management of gastroesophageal reflux following esophageal atresia repair. J. Pediatr. Surg., *28*:53, 1993.

Wijburg, F. A., Heymans, H. S., and Urbanus, N. A.: Caustic esophageal lesions in childhood: Prevention of stricture formation. J. Pediatr. Surg., *24*:171, 1989.

Willich E.: Achalasia of the cardia in children. Pediatr. Radiol., *1*:229, 1973.

Wise, W. E., Caniano, D. A., and Harmel, R. P., Jr.: Tracheoesophageal anomalies in Waterston C neonates: A 30-year perspective. J. Pediatr. Surg., *22*:526, 1987.

Yazbeck, S., and Dubuck, S.: Fistules trachéo oesophagiennes congénitales sans atrésie de l'oesophage [English abstract]. Chir. Pediatr., *24*:113, 1983.

26

Pulmonary Arteriovenous Fistulas

H. Kim Lyerly and David C. Sabiston, Jr.

HISTORICAL ASPECTS

A pulmonary arteriovenous fistula was first described by Churton in 1897. The patient was a 12-year-old male whose multiple bilateral arteriovenous fistulas were found at postmortem examination. The primary clinical features of this malformation were distinguished 20 years later. These included epistaxis, telangiectasia, clubbing, cyanosis, and dyspnea (Wilkens, 1917). The chest film usually showed a radiopaque density in both lungs, and a massive hemothorax after rupture of one or more of the fistulas was a common cause of death. The classic triad of cyanosis, polycythemia, and clubbing of the fingers and toes was later described as characteristic of pulmonary arteriovenous fistulas (Reading, 1932). In 1940, Shenstone performed the first surgical excision of a pulmonary arteriovenous fistula, a pneumonectomy for a large, centrally located lesion (Hepburn and Dauphinee, 1942). Since that time, arteriovenous fistulas have been treated with increasingly conservative techniques, including lung-sparing procedures such as local excision and segmentectomy. More recently, nonoperative techniques have been advocated for the treatment of such fistulas. Angiographic embolization with metal coils was first performed in 1976 by Taylor (Taylor et al., 1978) but was first reported by Porstmann and associates in 1977 (Porstmann et al., 1977). Since that time, detachable balloons of either latex or silicone have been used to embolize pulmonary arteriovenous fistula, adding another therapeutic modality to the management of this condition.

ETIOLOGY

Pulmonary arteriovenous fistulas can be either acquired or congenital. Reports have shown acquired arteriovenous fistula after infection, metastatic carcinoma, trauma, and modified Fontan operations (Moore et al., 1989). However, the most common types are *congenital.* Approximately 40 to 50% of congenital fistulas are associated with hereditary hemorrhagic telangiectasia (Osler-Weber-Rendu disease). A review of pulmonary arteriovenous fistulas from the Mayo Clinic showed that hereditary telangiectasia was present in 47% of patients (Dines et al., 1983). Two patients (6%) had traumatic fistulas: One was due to a previous resection of a pulmonary neoplasm at the time of operation, and the other to an injury from shrapnel in the lung.

Several theories have been proposed concerning the pathogenesis of the congenital type of pulmonary arteriovenous fistula. Some experts believe that the problem is initiated by abnormalities in the septa that divide the primitive connection between the arterial and venous beds in the lung buds (Anabtawi et al., 1965). In this situation, incomplete degeneration of the vascular septa occurs in the second month of fetal life and produces an arteriovenous fistula. Other experts believe that the abnormality is caused by defects in the terminal capillary loops that permit dilatation and formation of vascular sacs (Hodgson et al., 1959; Stork, 1955). Some of these malformations involve the entire blood supply of a lobar segment; in addition, communications that join the pulmonary vessels with the systemic circulation in the chest wall have been reported (Robinson and Sabiston, 1981; Sammons, 1959; Steinberg et al., 1958). Most research has shown that the incidence is higher in men (60% of cases or more). An interesting observation is that pregnancy enhances the growth of pulmonary arteriovenous fistulas, perhaps because of hormonal and humoral responses (Hoffman and Rabens, 1974; Laroche, 1992).

PATHOLOGIC ASPECTS

Pulmonary arteriovenous fistulas are multiple in one-third to one-half of patients affected, and the lesions are bilateral in as many as 20% of patients. Of the 38 patients reviewed from the Mayo Clinic, 16 had single fistulas, and 16 had bilateral fistulas. In 5 patients, the fistulas were multiple in one lung, and in 4 patients, the fistulas were small and diffuse throughout both lungs. Of the single fistulas, 5 were in the left lower lobe, 5 were in the right lower lobe, 3 were in the left upper lobe, 2 were in the right upper lobe, and 1 was in the right middle lobe. Of the *multiple* and *bilateral* fistulas, all except 3 were in the lower lobes.

Pulmonary arteriovenous fistulas usually are supplied by several branches of the pulmonary artery. In addition, the systemic circulation may be involved through communications with the bronchial, intercostal, and internal mammary arteries or by direct branches of the thoracic aorta. The vascular channels within these fistulas are lined by endothelium. These spaces are usually thin-walled because of the low intraluminal pressure in most of these lesions. The veins that drain the fistulas become dilated and thin-walled, and they often show degenerative changes, including calcification. Thrombi may form within the fistulas (e.g., in systemic arteriovenous fistulas) and lead to bacterial endocarditis (Maier et al., 1948), or they may embolize to the brain, causing stroke or cerebral abscess. The tendency to form thrombi is increased by the polycythemia that affects many of these patients. When thrombi involve the bronchial wall, erosion may occur with ensuing hemoptysis that can be massive.

PHYSIOLOGIC ASPECTS

The obvious physiologic defect in a pulmonary arteriovenous fistula is a right-to-left shunt from the pulmonary artery directly into the pulmonary venous drainage. Significant and often undetected evidence of paradoxic embolization to the brain is an important feature of pulmonary arteriovenous fistula. Patients with pulmonary arteriovenous fistula with a feeding artery diameter as small as 3 mm are at risk of stroke (Hewes et al., 1985). In a series of patients with pulmonary arteriovenous fistula, 18% and 37% had clinical histories of stroke and transient ischemic attacks, respectively; 36% of patients who underwent screening computed tomography showed evidence of stroke (White et al., 1988). In addition to stroke, patients with pulmonary arteriovenous fistula are at risk for other major neurologic complications, including cerebral abscess. Most strokes are embolic and are thought to be caused by either paradoxic emboli or possibly thrombus formation in the pulmonary arteriovenous fistula.

Pennington and colleagues reported on eight patients who underwent detailed physiologic studies at rest and during exercise before therapeutic embolization (Pennington et al., 1992). Before treatment, six patients noted dyspnea on exertion, and three had symptoms suggesting paradoxic embolism. Resting studies showed hypoxemia, abnormally increased shunt fractions, chronic alveolar hyperventilation, mild decreases in diffusing capacity, and abnormal wasted ventilation. During exercise, oxygenation changed little from the resting values, but wasted ventilation increased markedly. Functional impairment was observed in most patients and was correlated with shunt fraction.

The right-to-left shunt can be small, but it may be appreciable with lesions that measure 2 cm or more in diameter. In the presence of a shunt of more than 20%, cyanosis, clubbing, and polycythemia with reduced oxygen saturation in the arterial blood, reticulocytosis, and an increase in the erythrocyte volume may occur.

In most patients with pulmonary arteriovenous fistulas, the cardiac index, intracardiac pressures, pulmonary and systemic arterial pressures, heart rate, and electrocardiographic results are within normal limits (Dines et al., 1974; Gomes et al., 1969; Mansour et al., 1971). The pulmonary vascular resistance usually is normal (Hultgren and Gerbode, 1954), and pulmonary hypertension is uncommon (Przybojewski and Maritz, 1980). With large fistulas, in which the shunt is great, the blood volume, cardiac output, central venous pressure, ventricular end-diastolic pressure, ventricular end-diastolic volume, ventricular volumes, and pulse pressure may increase. Congestive heart failure ensues when the shunt is severe. These changes revert to normal after the fistula is removed or occluded.

CLINICAL MANIFESTATIONS

Symptoms of arteriovenous fistula can occur at any time from infancy to later in life. In the review from the Mayo Clinic of 38 patients with this disorder, the mean age of onset of symptoms was 39 years (range of 3 to 73); nine patients were younger than 20 years old. In the classic form, cyanosis, clubbing of the digits, and dyspnea are present in patients with pulmonary arteriovenous fistulas. In this series, dyspnea was present in 47%, and epistaxis was present in 32%. Hereditary hemorrhagic telangiectasia was present in each of the latter groups. Ten patients (26%) had no pulmonary symptoms, and only five patients (13%) were completely asymptomatic.

A more recent review showed that of 76 patients with 276 pulmonary arteriovenous fistulas seen at the Johns Hopkins Hospital, epistaxis, dyspnea, hemoptysis, and hemothorax occurred in 79%, 71%, 13%, and 9%, respectively (White et al., 1988). Eighty-eight per cent had hereditary hemorrhagic telangiectasia, and 14% were diagnosed by family screening with measurement of arterial blood gases and chest radiography. Neurologic complications of right-to-left shunting were clearly associated with the presence of pulmonary arteriovenous fistula in this series of patients: Clinical histories showed strokes and transient ischemic attacks, and computed tomography demonstrated stroke in over one-third of patients.

In the Mayo Clinic series, 11 patients (29%) had a *bruit* that was audible over the lesion. These bruits are classically accentuated by inspiration and diminish with expiration. Abnormal laboratory findings included anemia in patients who had a history of bleeding; polycythemia related to a right-to-left shunt was present in 11 patients (29%). The highest hemoglobin count was 20.4 g/dl. In addition, blood gas measurements showed a degree of desaturation from which a figure for the degree of shunting can be derived.

IMAGING STUDIES

Because some patients with pulmonary arteriovenous fistulas are asymptomatic, lesions may be discovered on a routine chest film. Although the chest film findings are normal in some patients, they are abnormal in most patients and usually show either single or multiple densities. Most patients with pulmonary arteriovenous fistulas have a peripheral circumscribed noncalcified lesion connected by blood vessels to the hilus (Fig. 26–1). Tomograms sometimes can diagnose an arteriovenous fistula.

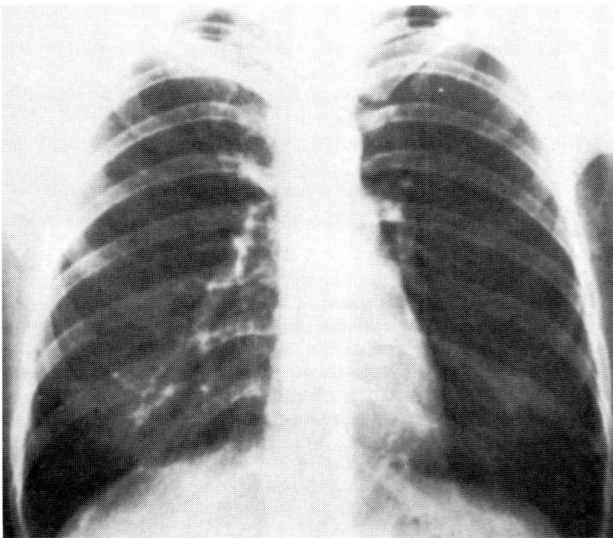

FIGURE 26–1. Chest film showing bilateral pulmonary fistulas in lower lobes. (From Dines, D. E., et al.: Pulmonary arteriovenous fistulas. Mayo Clin. Proc., *58:*176, 1983.)

Pulmonary angiography is the definitive test to document a suspected pulmonary arteriovenous fistula. It is also useful in determining the arterial source of the fistula, which may be the pulmonary artery or, less commonly, a systemic vessel. A pulmonary angiogram of a patient with multiple pulmonary arteriovenous fistulas is shown in Figure 26–2. Some fistulas are found at the capillary level, and angiography does not show *gross* lesions in these patients. In the authors' series, a systemic vessel was not involved in any of 28 patients who underwent pulmonary angiography. Other imaging studies that can document left-to-right shunting include isotope scanning using radiolabeled particles and rapid-sequence computed tomography.

Magnetic resonance imaging (MRI) has been valuable for distinguishing pulmonary vascular and nonvascular lesions. Rapid blood flow may be shown with little or no MRI signal. On MRI, the fistula is invisible because of rapid blood flow through the lumen. This technique shows promise as a noninvasive method of demonstrating and quantitating blood flow. Particularly in a large fistula, blood flows at a greater rate than the cut-off velocity. Moreover, the volume of blood flow through the fistula can be determined (Dinsmore et al., 1990; Webb et al., 1984).

Two-dimensional contrast echocardiography has been used for the detection and follow-up of pulmonary arteriovenous fistula. Left atrial appearance of microcavitations is significantly delayed in patients with pulmonary arteriovenous fistula compared with those with atrial left-to-right shunts. In 14 patients identified with pulmonary arteriovenous fistula by contrast echocardiography, abnormal blood gases were present in only 6 of 14, and chest film results were positive in 7 of 14. Successful balloon occlusion could be documented in 9 of 11 patients by contrast echocardiography, whereas 2 patients required repeat

embolotherapy. Thus, contrast echocardiography is sensitive for the identification of pulmonary arteriovenous fistulas (Barzilai et al., 1991).

MANAGEMENT

It is now known that even patients with asymptomatic pulmonary arteriovenous fistulas are at risk of stroke and other major neurologic complications. Less common complications include epistaxis, hemothorax, and severe hemoptysis. Although the reported morbidity and mortality rates for pulmonary arteriovenous fistulas vary, they are significant and usually necessitate treatment (Burke et al., 1986).

Although many patients diagnosed with pulmonary arteriovenous fistula have symptoms, some patients will be detected incidentally or by screening of relatives of patients with Osler-Weber-Rendu disease. Chest films and arterial blood gas determinations can be used to screen for pulmonary arteriovenous fistula, but other imaging modalities such as MRI and echocardiography, discussed earlier, may prove useful in screening high-risk individuals, even those with normal chest film results. Once pulmonary arteriovenous fistula is suspected through screening studies, a diagnostic pulmonary angiography should be performed.

Developments in percutaneous transcatheter embo-

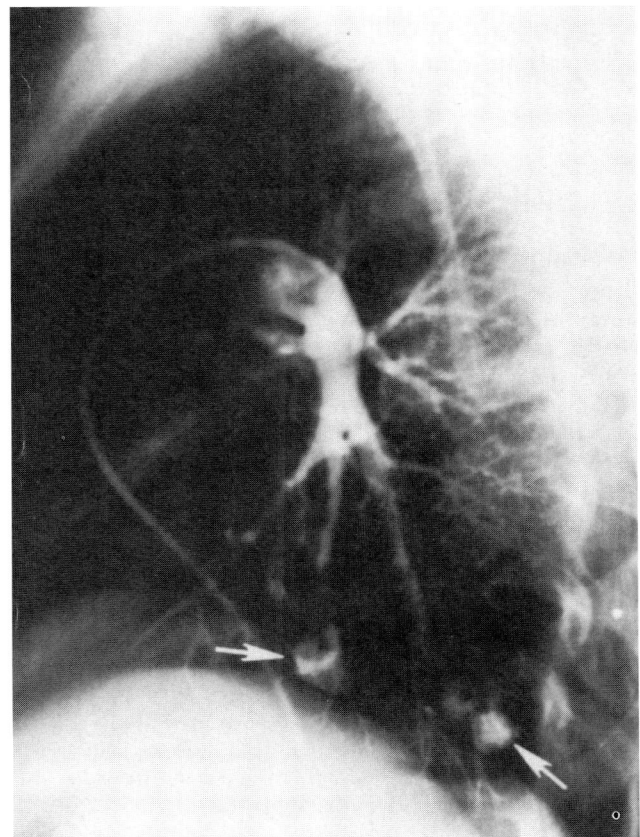

FIGURE 26–2. Pulmonary angiogram of an 11-year-old girl with multiple pulmonary arteriovenous fistulas in the lower lobes.

lization have facilitated treatment of patients with pulmonary arteriovenous fistula when surgery would have been hazardous or impossible. Embolization is now generally preferred to surgery because of its lower morbidity, lower mortality, reported efficacy, and patient acceptability. However, long-term outcomes have not been reported.

Percutaneous embolization of the pulmonary artery was first used by Taylor in attempts to close fistulas (Taylor et al., 1978). Percutaneous femoral vein puncture using Seldinger's technique allows embolization with large coils and may be particularly useful in controlling massive hemoptysis secondary to an acquired pulmonary arteriovenous fistula (Hoffman et al., 1980). Similarly, therapeutic balloon embolization for treatment of pulmonary arteriovenous fistulas has been accomplished (Hatfield and Fried, 1981; Terry et al., 1980). These authors believe that balloon occlusion is less hazardous than use of coils, because the risks of systemic embolization or occluding a branch to viable pulmonary tissue are decreased.

White and colleagues (1988) reported one of the largest series of embolization therapy of pulmonary arteriovenous fistula. Over a 10-year period, 276 pulmonary arteriovenous fistulas were occluded with balloon embolotherapy in 76 patients, 67 (88%) of whom had hereditary hemorrhagic telangiectasia. After embolotherapy, symptomatic hypoxemia was corrected, and serial values remained constant for 5 years. Complications were minimal, and patients did not require operation. Balloon embolotherapy is considered effective long-term therapy for pulmonary arteriovenous fistulas.

A more recent series was reported by Hartnell and colleagues (Hartnell et al., 1990). Forty-four pulmonary arteriovenous fistulas in 11 patients were occluded by transcatheter coil embolization with only one symptomatic complication, deep venous thrombosis, attributable to the procedure. Symptoms improved significantly and pulmonary arteriovenous shunting was reduced in the nine patients in whom embolization of all visible discrete lesions was successfully completed. Coil embolization is an effective alternative to other methods of treating pulmonary arteriovenous fistulas.

Although these reports documented excellent results with minimal complications, recent reports emphasize how important it is to be aware of the complications of the transcatheter occlusion techniques (Remy-Jardin et al., 1991). Failures and complications were analyzed retrospectively in 45 patients treated with embolotherapy or occlusion of pulmonary arterial circulation. Pulmonary arterial branches were occluded with steel coils in 19 patients with pulmonary arteriovenous malformations. Asymptomatic incidents included catheterization failures, vascular damage, partial occlusion, partial recanalization of the thrombus, ectopic deposition of a coil, and delayed bacterial contamination of the thrombus. A few cases of transient clinical and radiologic signs of pulmonary infarction were observed after complete occlusion of

the pulmonary artery and bronchial artery embolization.

To evaluate functional improvement after therapeutic embolization, Pennington and colleagues reported on eight patients who underwent detailed physiologic studies at rest and during exercise before and after therapeutic embolization (Pennington et al., 1992). Before treatment, six patients noted dyspnea on exertion, and three had symptoms suggesting paradoxic embolism. The arteriovenous fistulas were obliterated by therapeutic embolization with placement of coils or balloons in the feeder vessels. This treatment produced immediate relief of dyspnea and improved resting $P_{A_{O_2}}$ and shunt fraction. Exercise studies after embolization showed improved exercise capacity and gas exchange. However, chronic alveolar hyperventilation and reduced diffusing capacity remained unchanged. The abnormally decreased diffusing capacity suggests the presence of a diffuse pulmonary vascular abnormality.

Chilvers and colleagues assessed the effects of percutaneous transcatheter embolization on pulmonary function and exercise capacity in 15 patients with pulmonary arteriovenous fistula (Chilvers et al., 1990). Following steel coil embolization of all pulmonary arteriovenous fistulas with a feed vessel internal diameter greater than 3 mm (one to four sessions per patient), mean shunt fraction improved from 33% to 19% and resting $S_{A_{O_2}}$ from 86% to 92% with no change in vital capacity. Diffusing capacity was improved consistently only in patients with coexisting Osler-Weber-Rendu disease. Exercise capacity increased in the majority (unchanged in six) and $S_{A_{O_2}}$ during maximal exercise improved in all but one patient. The right-to-left shunts remaining following embolization may reflect the presence of numerous microscopic pulmonary arteriovenous fistulas in these patients.

Although several percutaneous therapeutic approaches are available, surgical excision remains indicated in some cases, particularly if the lesion is isolated. Surgical therapy is also indicated if there are no more than several fistulas, particularly if they are within the same lung. Whenever possible, the most conservative pulmonary resection is indicated, because it is unnecessary to remove normal tissue surrounding the lesion (Mansour et al., 1971). Prager and associates (1983) reported seven patients with pulmonary arteriovenous fistulas, each of whom was managed with surgical excision with no deaths, minimal morbidity, and excellent results with a follow-up of 1 to 27 years. Puskas and associates (1993) reported nine patients managed by conservative surgical excision; four underwent lobectomy, and five underwent segmentectomy or subsegmental excision. One patient underwent staged bilateral thoracotomies for multiple bilateral lesions.

In one patient with a large, solitary pulmonary arteriovenous fistula, it was possible to show and accurately correlate the preoperative decrease in shunt fraction and increase in room-air partial pressure of arterial oxygen with shunt occlusion by using a Swan-Ganz balloon catheter. Values were also ob-

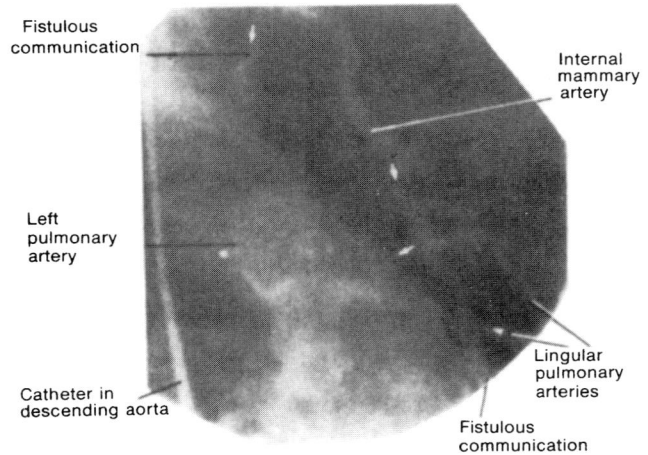

FIGURE 26–3. Cineangiogram of the middle of the left internal mammary artery in right anterior oblique projection. Filling of left pulmonary artery from fistula via lingular pulmonary arteries is shown. *Arrows* indicate fistulous communication. (From Robinson, L. A., and Sabiston, D. C., Jr.: Syndrome of congenital internal mammary-to-pulmonary arteriovenous fistula associated with mitral valve prolapse. Arch. Surg., Vol. 116, p. 1265. Copyright 1981, American Medical Association.)

tained 2 months after surgical excision; these results helped to determine the benefit of surgical excision of a large fistula in a high-risk patient who also had chronic obstructive pulmonary disease and a previous myocardial infarction (Harrow et al., 1978).

Surgical management is preferably by local or wedge resection, using a stapler to obtain maximal vascular and bronchial occlusion. For patients with multiple lesions, the decision to operate is more complicated. Among 36 of 63 patients who underwent operation and were monitored for a mean of 8 years, the operative approach was conservative, and there were no deaths. Morbidity was minimal, and only one fistula recurred. However, 6 of the 27 patients who were treated nonsurgically died (Dines et al., 1974). Generally, if the lesion is large, or if the patient is symptomatic or has an enlarging fistula or multiple, bilateral, well-localized fistulas, the fistula(s) should be excised. In addition, surgical excision is indicated for fistulas with a systemic arterial blood supply. In unusual cases with multiple and bilateral fistulas, simple *ligation* of the feeding vessels and local removal of the pulmonary arteriovenous fistula without resection of the parenchyma of the lung is indicated (Bjork, 1967). As reported, in patients with multiple bilateral lesions, staged bilateral thoracotomy can successfully resect lesions that are typically posterior in the lower lobes (Brown et al., 1982).

SYNDROME OF CONGENITAL INTERNAL MAMMARY ARTERY TO PULMONARY ARTERIOVENOUS FISTULAS

Congenital fistulas of the internal mammary artery to the pulmonary circulation are rare. Approximately 12 patients are described in the world literature. These lesions occasionally are associated with mitral valve prolapse (Robinson and Sabiston, 1981). The arteriovenous fistula provides a continuous murmur overlying its anatomic site; mitral valve prolapse can be

diagnosed by left ventricular angiography showing the ballooning mitral valve or by echocardiography. Definitive diagnosis of the arteriovenous fistula is best achieved by angiography of the internal mammary artery, which shows filling of the pulmonary artery through the fistula (Fig. 26–3). The arteriographic features of a right internal mammary artery fistulous communication in the right lower lobe are shown in Figure 26–4. The anatomic features of this fistula present at operation are shown in Figure 26–5. The diagnosis of congenital systemic pulmonary arteriovenous fistulas involving the internal mammary artery usually is made in the second or third decade of life (average age of 22 years, with a range of 9 to 32 years) (Robinson and Sabiston, 1981). As might be expected, the presentation depends on the size of the

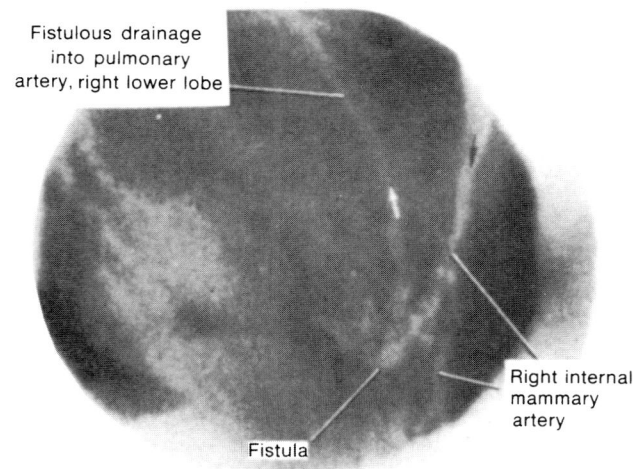

FIGURE 26–4. Cineangiogram in lateral projection of the distal right internal mammary artery shows fistulous communication (*arrows*) of the internal mammary artery with right lower lobe pulmonary artery branches. (From Robinson, L. A., and Sabiston, D. C., Jr.: Syndrome of congenital internal mammary-to-pulmonary arteriovenous fistula associated with mitral valve prolapse. Arch. Surg., Vol. 116, p. 1265. Copyright 1981, American Medical Association.)

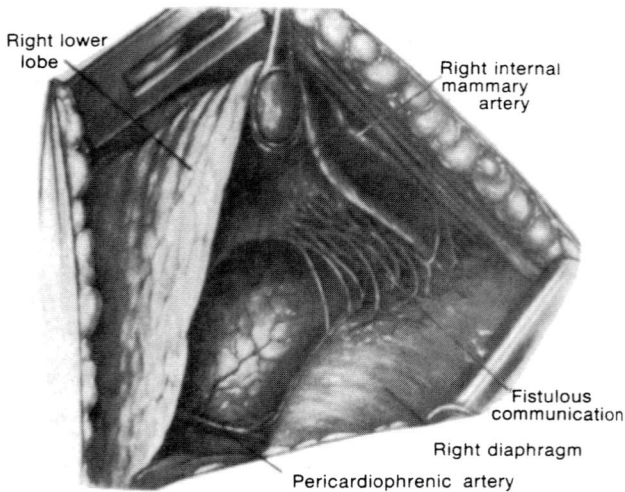

FIGURE 26–5. Operative findings seen through right anterolateral thoracotomy. Enlarged right internal mammary artery and pericardiophrenic artery form fistulous communication with pulmonary artery branches at the diaphragmatic aspect of the right lower lobe. (From Robinson, L. A., and Sabiston, D. C., Jr.: Syndrome of congenital internal mammary-to-pulmonary arteriovenous fistula associated with mitral valve prolapse. Arch. Surg., Vol. 116, p. 1265. Copyright 1981, American Medical Association.)

fistula and the shunt that is involved (Muenster et al., 1959; Thomas, 1959). Congenital arteriovenous fistulas usually enlarge with time and produce symptoms that include congestive heart failure and bacterial endocarditis. Therefore, surgical resection is generally indicated.

Detachable balloons also have been used to produce endovascular occlusion in several patients with multiple pulmonary arteriovenous fistulas; in one patient, this technique was used for a large peripheral aneurysm (Rankin et al., 1983). The preoperative and postoperative results are shown in Figures 26–6 and 26–7. However, the follow-up for the first patient was only 18 months and for the second patient 15 months at the time of the report. The role of this technique obviously depends on long-term follow-up.

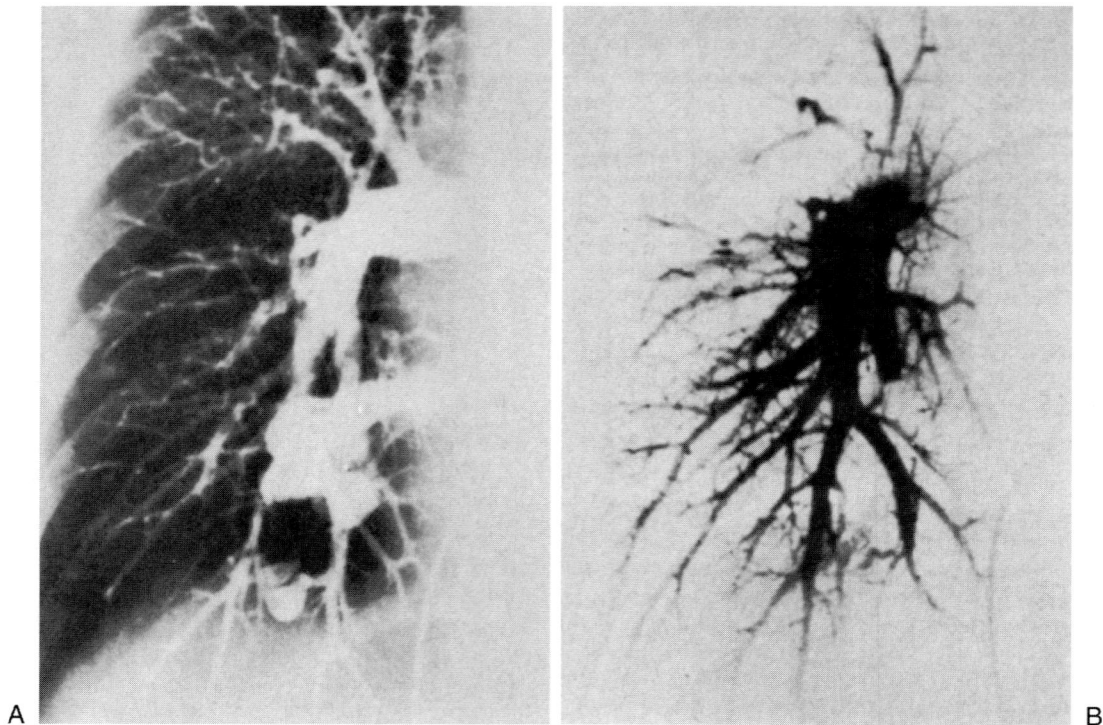

FIGURE 26–6. *A,* Anteroposterior right pulmonary arteriogram before treatment. A large pulmonary arteriovenous fistula is shown in the lower lobe with a small pulmonary arteriovenous fistula distal to it. *B,* Left pulmonary arteriogram shows two large fistulas in the lower lobe. All three large fistulas are large venous varices that are supplied by up to three fistulas per varix. (*A* and *B,* From Rankin, R. N., and Ahmad, D.: Embolization of arteriovenous fistulas and aneurysms with detachable balloons. Can. J. Surg., 26:317, 1983.)

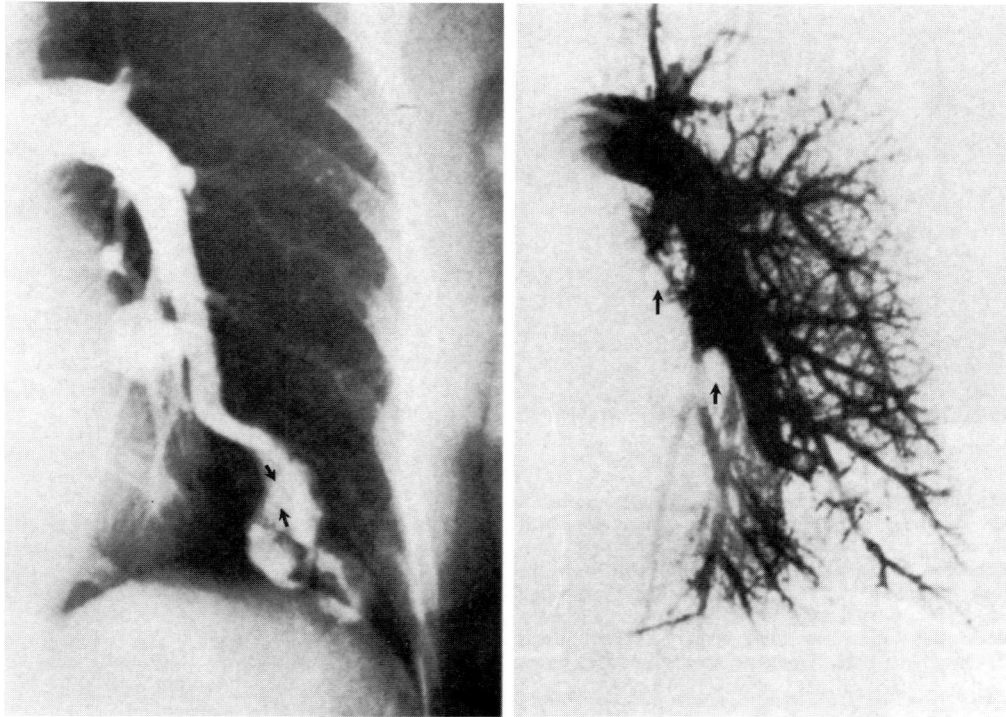

A

B

FIGURE 26–7. *A,* Right pulmonary arteriogram immediately after embolization. Large fistulas are no longer present. Occluding balloons are indicated by *arrows. B,* Left pulmonary arteriogram after embolization. Large fistulas are not visible. Occluding balloons are indicated by *arrows.* (*A* and *B,* From Rankin, R. N., and Ahmad, D.: Embolization of arteriovenous fistulas and aneurysms with detachable balloons. Can. J. Surg., *26:*317, 1983.)

SELECTED BIBLIOGRAPHY

Chilvers, E. R., Whyte, M. K., Jackson, J. E., et al.: Effect of percutaneous transcatheter embolization on pulmonary function, right-to-left shunt, and arterial oxygenation in patients with pulmonary arteriovenous malformations. Am. Rev. Respir. Dis., *142:*420, 1990.

The effects of percutaneous transcatheter embolization on pulmonary function and exercise capacity were assessed in patients with pulmonary arteriovenous fistula. Following steel coil embolization of all pulmonary arteriovenous fistulas with a feed vessel internal diameter greater than 3 mm (one to four sessions per patient), mean shunt fraction improved from 33 to 19% and resting SA_{O_2} from 86 to 92% with no change in VC. These findings indicate that embolization of all macroscopic pulmonary arteriovenous fistulas, undertaken primarily to reduce the risk of paradoxic embolization, is safe and substantially improves resting and exercise SA_{O_2} without evidence of loss of normal lung.

Peery, W. H.: Clinical spectrum of hereditary hemorrhagic telangiectasis (Osler-Weber-Rendu disease). Am. J. Med., *82:*989, 1987.

This authoritative and complete reference concerns hereditary hemorrhagic telangiectasis (Osler-Weber-Rendu disease). The disorder is autosomal dominant and occurs with systemic fibrovascular dysplasia in which telangiectases, arteriovenous malformations, and aneurysms may be distributed widely throughout the vascular structures of the body. Peery further emphasizes that major clinical manifestations include recurrent bleeding from mucosal telangiectases and arteriovenous malformations, hypoxemia, cerebral embolism, and brain abscess due to pulmonary arteriovenous fistulas. In addition, high-output congestive heart failure and portosystemic encephalopathy from hepatic arteriovenous malformations occur. Various additional neurologic symptoms due to central nervous system angiodysplasia have been reported. Therapy is primarily supportive and consists of iron supplementation and transfusion of blood. Septal dermoplasty and oral estrogens may allow prolonged remission of epistaxis, but permanent surgical cure is not often achieved, primarily because the angiodysplasia is diffused throughout the alimentary tract. For pulmonary arteriovenous fistulas, resection is preferred if possible, but ligation of major vessels and local excision or embolization may be indicated. The prognosis and survival rate of patients with this malformation are favorable if the complications are diagnosed adequately and treated appropriately.

Pennington, D. W., Gold, W. M., Gordon, R. L., et al.: Treatment of pulmonary arteriovenous malformations by therapeutic embolization. Rest and exercise physiology in eight patients. Am. Rev. Respir. Dis., *145:*1047, 1992.

Patients underwent detailed physiologic studies at rest and during exercise before and after therapeutic embolization. Functional impairment was observed in most patients and was correlated with shunt fraction. Obliteration of the pulmonary arteriovenous fistula resulted in immediate relief of dyspnea and improvement in resting PA_{O_2} and shunt fraction. Exercise studies after embolization showed improvement in exercise capacity and gas exchange. However, chronic alveolar hyperventilation and reduced diffusing capacity remained unchanged. Therapeutic embolization effectively reduces the degree of shunting, improving respiratory symptoms, exercise capacity, and gas exchange at rest and during exercise.

Puskas, J. D., Allen, M. S., Moncure, A. C., et al.: Pulmonary arteriovenous malformations: Therapeutic options. Ann. Thorac. Surg., *56:*253, 1993.

The authors report on the treatment of 21 patients (13 female, 8 male) with pulmonary arteriovenous fistula, presenting with dyspnea on exertion (67%), hereditary hemorrhagic telangiectasia (57%), and major neurologic events (33%). In the authors' early experience, eight patients had no specific treatment, and their case histories illustrate the major neurologic complications of untreated pulmonary arteriovenous fistulas. Nine patients (eight primarily, one after recurrence) underwent conservative surgical excision; four underwent lobectomy, and five underwent segmentectomy or subsegmental excision. One patient underwent staged bilateral thoracotomies for multiple bilateral lesions. The arterial oxygen tension was found to increase after excision of large or solitary pulmonary arteriovenous fistulas. All surgically treated patients were relieved of dyspnea, and none experienced postoperative recurrence of pulmonary arteriovenous fistulas or neurologic complications related to pulmonary arteriovenous fistulas. Five patients underwent balloon occlusion of pulmonary arteriovenous fistulas. Two patients chose to have solitary pulmonary arteriovenous fistulas occluded rather than undergo thoracotomy. One underwent surgical excision 5 years later, and the other required repeat balloon embolization 4 years later when recanalization of the pulmonary arteriovenous fistulas was documented. Three patients with numerous pulmonary arteriovenous fistulas received palliation with multiple balloon embolizations. The authors conclude that the high incidence of associated major neurologic complications mandates aggressive treatment of pulmonary arteriovenous fistulas whenever feasible, and they state that conservative surgical resection remains the treatment of choice. Balloon embolization is used as an alternative therapy for patients who are poor surgical risks or whose lesions are too numerous to resect.

Remy-Jardin, M., Wattinne, L., and Remy, J.: Transcatheter occlusion of pulmonary arterial circulation and collateral supply: Failures, incidents, and complications. Radiology, *180*:699, 1991.

Failures and complications were analyzed retrospectively in 45 patients treated with embolotherapy or occlusion of pulmonary arterial circulation. Pulmonary arterial branches were occluded with steel coils in 19 patients with pulmonary arteriovenous malformations. The management and prevention of complications, the role of bronchial arterial collateral pathways, and the importance of the site of pulmonary arterial occlusion in the development of pulmonary infarction are discussed.

Robinson, L. A., and Sabiston, D. C., Jr.: Syndrome of congenital internal mammary-to-pulmonary arteriovenous fistula associated with mitral valve prolapse. Arch. Surg., *116*:1265, 1981.

Congenital fistulas of the internal mammary artery to the pulmonary circulation are rare: only 12 patients are described in the world literature. Two additional patients are described who had an associated prolapse of the mitral valve, one of whom had mitral insufficiency. In most cases, the arteriovenous fistula is asymptomatic and is discovered when a continuous murmur is heard on routine chest examination. The definitive diagnosis is made best by selective arteriography. The embryologic origin of these fistulous communications may be the maldevelopment of accessory bronchial arteries arising from the internal mammary artery. Because of the potential risks of congestive heart failure as well as proximal dilation and degeneration of the parent artery, secondary hypertension, and endocarditis, operative closure of these arteriovenous fistulas is recommended.

White, R. I., Jr., Lynch Nyhan, A., Terry, P., et al.: Pulmonary arteriovenous malformations: Techniques and long-term outcome of embolotherapy. Radiology, *169*:663, 1988.

Over a 10-year period, 276 pulmonary arteriovenous fistulas were occluded with balloon embolotherapy in 76 patients, 67 (88%) of whom had hereditary hemorrhagic telangiectasia. After embolotherapy, symptomatic hypoxemia was corrected, and serial values have remained constant for 5 years. Complications were minimal, and no patient required surgery. Balloon embolotherapy is concluded to provide effective long-term therapy for pulmonary arteriovenous fistulas. Family screening should be recommended, because paradoxic embolization (stroke) may occur more often than has been recognized.

BIBLIOGRAPHY

Anabtawi, I. N., Ellison, R. G., and Ellison, L. T.: Pulmonary arteriovenous aneurysms and fistulas: Anatomical variations, embryology, and classification. Ann. Thorac. Surg., *1*:277, 1965.

Barzilai, B., Waggoner, A. D., Spessert, C., et al.: Two dimensional contrast echocardiography in the detection and follow up of congenital pulmonary arteriovenous malformations. Am. J. Cardiol., *68*:507, 1991.

Bjork, V. O.: Local extirpation of multiple bilateral pulmonary arteriovenous aneurysms. J. Thorac. Cardiovasc. Surg., *53*:293, 1967.

Brown, S. E., Wright, P. W., Renner, J. W., and Riker, J. B.: Staged bilateral thoracotomies for multiple pulmonary arteriovenous malformations complicating hereditary hemorrhagic telangiectasia. J. Thorac. Cardiovasc. Surg., *83*:285, 1982.

Burke, C. M., Safai, C., Nelson, D. P., and Raffin, T. A.: Pulmonary arteriovenous malformations: A critical update. Am. Rev. Respir. Dis., *134*:334, 1986.

Churton, T.: Multiple aneurysms of pulmonary artery. Br. Med. J., *1*:1223, 1897.

Dines, D. E., Arms, R. A., Bernatz, P. E., and Gomes, M. R.: Pulmonary arteriovenous fistulas. Mayo Clin. Proc., *49*:460, 1974.

Dines, D. E., Seward, J. B., and Bernatz, P. E.: Pulmonary arteriovenous fistulas. Mayo Clin. Proc., *58*:176, 1983.

Dinsmore, B. J., Gefter, W. B., Hatabu, H., and Kressel, H. Y.: Pulmonary arteriovenous malformations: Diagnosis by gradient-refocused MR imaging. J. Comput. Assist. Tomogr., *14*:918, 1990.

Gomes, M. R., Bernatz, P. E., and Dines, D. E.: Pulmonary arteriovenous fistulas. Ann. Thorac. Surg., *7*:582, 1969.

Harrow, E. M., Beach, P. M., Wise, J. R., et al.: Pulmonary arteriovenous fistula: Pre-operative evaluation with a Swan-Ganz catheter. Chest, *73*:92, 1978.

Hartnell, G. G., Jackson, J. E., and Allison, D. J.: Coil embolization

of pulmonary arteriovenous malformations. Cardiovasc. Intervent. Radiol., *13*:347, 1990.

Hatfield, D. R., and Fried, A. M.: Therapeutic embolization of diffuse pulmonary arteriovenous malformations. A. J. R., *137*:861, 1981.

Hepburn, J., and Dauphinee, J. A.: Successful removal of hemangioma of the lung followed by disappearance of polycythemia. Am. J. Med. Sci., *204*:681, 1942.

Hewes, R. C., Anster, M., and White, R. I., Jr.: Cerebral embolism—First manifestation of pulmonary arteriovenous malformation in patients with hereditary hemorrhagic telangiectasia. Cardiovasc. Intervent. Radiol., *8*:151, 1985.

Hodgson, C. H., Burchell, H. B., Good, C. A., and Clagett, O. T.: Hereditary hemorrhagic telangiectasia and pulmonary arteriovenous fistula. N. Engl. J. Med., *261*:625, 1959.

Hoffman, R., and Rabens, R.: Evolving pulmonary nodules: Multiple pulmonary arteriovenous fistulas. Am. J. Roentgenol. Radium Ther. Nucl. Med., *120*:861, 1974.

Hoffman, W. S., Weinburg, P. M., Ring, E., and Edmunds, L. H.: Massive hemoptysis secondary to pulmonary arteriovenous fistula: Treatment by a catheterization procedure. Chest, *77*:697, 1980.

Hultgren, H. N., and Gerbode, F.: Physiologic studies in a patient with pulmonary arteriovenous fistula. Am. J. Med., *17*:126, 1954.

Laroche, C. M., Wells, F., and Shneerson, J.: Massive hemothorax due to enlarging arteriovenous fistula in pregnancy. Chest, *101*:1452, 1992.

Maier, H. C., Himmelstein, A., Rilev, R. L., and Bunim, J. J.: Arteriovenous fistula of the lung. J. Thorac. Surg., *17*:13, 1948.

Mansour, K. A., Hatcher, C. R., Logan, W. D., and Abbott, O. A.: Pulmonary arteriovenous fistula. Am. Surg., *37*:203, 1971.

Moore, A. U., Kirby, W. C., Madden, W. A., and Gaither, N. S.: Development of pulmonary arteriovenous malformations after modified Fontan operations. J. Thorac. Cardiovasc. Surg., *98*:1045–1050, 1989.

Muenster, J. G., Graettinger, J. S., and Campkell, J. A.: Correlation of clinical and hemodynamic findings in patients with systemic arteriovenous fistulas. Circulation, *20*:1079, 1959.

Porstman, W., Munster, W., Futh, M., et al.: Preoperative embolization of the renal artery in kidney neoplasms. Z. Urol. Nephrol., *70*:165, 1977.

Prager, R. L., Laws, K. H., and Bender, H. W., Jr.: Arteriovenous fistula of the lung. Ann. Thorac. Surg., *36*:231, 1983.

Przybojewski, J. A., and Maritz, F.: Pulmonary arteriovenous fistula. S. Afr. Med. J., *57*:366, 1980.

Rankin, R. N., McKenzie, F. N., and Ahmad, D.: Embolization of arteriovenous fistulas and aneurysms with detachable balloons. Can. J. Surg., *26*:317, 1983.

Reading, B.: Case of congenital telangiectasia of lung, complicated by brain abscess. Tex. State J. Med., *28*:462, 1932.

Remy-Jardin, M., Wattinne, L., and Remy, J.: Transcatheter occlusion of pulmonary arterial circulation and collateral supply: Failures, incidents, and complications. Radiology, *180*:699, 1991.

Robinson, L. A., and Sabiston, D. C., Jr.: Syndrome of congenital internal mammary-to-pulmonary arteriovenous fistula associated with mitral valve prolapse. Arch. Surg., *116*:1265, 1981.

Sammons, B. P.: Arteriovenous fistula of the lung. Radiology, *72*:710, 1959.

Steinberg, I., Maisel, B., and Vogel, F. S.: Pulmonary arteriovenous fistula associated with capillary telangiectasia (Rendu-Osler-Weber disease). J. Thorac. Surg., *35*:517, 1958.

Stork, W. J.: Pulmonary arteriovenous fistulas. A. J. R., *74*:441, 1955.

Taylor, B. G., Cockerill, E. M., Maufredi, F., and Klatte, E. L.: Therapeutic embolization of the pulmonary artery in pulmonary arteriovenous fistula. Am. J. Med., *64*:360, 1978.

Terry, P. B., Barth, K. H., Kaufman, S. L., and White, R. I.: Balloon embolization for treatment of pulmonary artenovenous fistulas. N. Engl. J. Med., *302*:1189, 1980.

Thomas, G. I.: Arteriovenous fistula: Review of hemodynamic alterations and treatment. Q. Rev. Surg. Gynecol. Obstet., *16*:9, 1959.

Webb, W. R., Gamsu, G., Golden, J. A., and Crooks, L. E.: Nuclear magnetic resonance of pulmonary artenovenous fistula: Effects of flow. J. Comput. Assist. Tomogr., *8*:155, 1984.

Wilkens, G. D.: Ein Fall von multiplen pulmonalis Aneurysmen. Beitr. Klin. Tuberk., *38*:1, 1917.

27

Disorders of the Esophagus in the Adult

■ I Benign and Malignant Tumors of the Esophagus

Walter G. Wolfe and Mark W. Sebastian

HISTORICAL ASPECTS

The surgical management of esophageal cancer was addressed in the literature in anecdotal form only, until the advent of the cuffed endotracheal tube and positive-pressure anesthesia. Although esophageal surgery is therefore chiefly a 20th-century development, the contribution of esophagoscopy by Johann von Mikulicz in 1881 and his resection of the esophagus for carcinoma in 1886 deserve citation. Despite these advances and a belief that esophageal carcinoma was resectable, the esophagus maintained an unapproachable position in the thorax. Because the esophagus is surrounded on three sides by negative pressure and the vertebral column on the fourth, initial surgical management of esophageal neoplasm became possible only after the development of techniques that permitted safe access to intrathoracic structures. Subsequent advances in management required functional understanding of the esophageal physiology and its interaction with the proximal aerodigestive tract and distal stomach and gastrointestinal system. These advances were made possible by the development of techniques in esophageal manometry, cineradiography, flexible endoscopy, and computed tomography scanning.

Chief among these techniques is esophageal manometry, perfected in the laboratories of Ingelfinger (1958) in Boston and Code and associates (1958) at the Mayo Clinic. For the first time, the surgeon had the information necessary to direct operative management of esophageal problems along physiologic lines. Before this time, the esophagus was considered basically a conduit to permit ingested material to reach the stomach, and operations on it were based on anatomy.

Because the intrathoracic portion of the esophagus is so inaccessible, surgical therapy was first confined to the cervical and intra-abdominal portions of the esophagus. The first operations on the esophagus were probably performed to drain cervical abscesses caused by foreign-body perforation or to remove foreign bodies. The first recorded operation for removal of a foreign body from the cervical portion of the esophagus was performed by Goursaud of France in

1738, and this was followed by case reports of successful operations from the continent and Great Britain. David Cheever of Boston is said to have performed the first successful esophagotomy in the United States in 1864. A pharyngoesophageal diverticulum was resected successfully by Wheeler of Dublin in 1886. Billroth (1871) thought that localized carcinomas of the cervical esophagus were resectable, and his assistant Czerny successfully resected and reconstructed the cervical esophagus in a patient with carcinoma as early as 1877. Carcinoma of the cardia was first attacked surgically by von Mikulicz in 1898, but the patient died. Voelcker successfully resected a malignant lesion of the cardia in 1908.

Although the intrathoracic portion of the esophagus remained out of the surgeon's reach for many years, various reconstructive techniques were devised, primarily for the management of esophageal strictures secondary to ingestion of caustic materials. Some of these are used in modified form today. In 1905, Beck and Carrell, American surgeons, suggested a technique of antethoracic reconstruction of the esophagus by using a tube of the greater curvature of the stomach. This procedure was first used successfully by Jianu of Hungary in 1912. In 1907, Roux proposed the use of an isolated limb of jejunum for this purpose, and Lexer modified this procedure in 1908. His modification, an esophagodermatojejunogastric reconstruction, was the most common type of reconstructive procedure used at the time of Ochsner and Owens' review of the subject in 1934.

A transpleural esophagectomy was first performed in 1913 by Torek. In 1933, a successful one-stage esophagogastrectomy and esophagogastrostomy for carcinoma of the cardia was reported (Ohsawa, 1933). In 1937, Marshall (1938) of the Lahey Clinic was the first to perform this type of operation successfully in the United States. His technique was followed the next year by the frequently discussed operation of Adams and Phemister (1938). Later advances in surgical treatment have involved primarily modifications in technique born of a better understanding of the physiologic consequences of resection and anastomosis and the related but distinct surgical goals of palliation and resection with curative intent. Churchill and Sweet in

1942 described the left thoracic approach commonly employed, and Orringer and Sloan in 1978 introduced transhiatal esophagectomy without thoracotomy. Further refinements in treatment stem from the separation of squamous cell from adenocarcinoma in analyses, mobilization and use of the stomach for interposition and anastomosis, multimodal therapy, improved preoperative nutrition, and use of stapling devices to facilitate high intrathoracic anastomoses.

ANATOMY

Gross Anatomy

The esophagus is a tubular structure that extends from the pharynx at the level of C6 to the stomach, which it joins within the peritoneal cavity opposite the body of T11 (Fig. 27–1). It measures approximately 35 to 40 cm from the incisor teeth to the esophagogastric junction in the adult. At its upper end, the entrance to the esophagus is guarded by the upper esophageal sphincter, which is composed primarily of the cricopharyngeus muscle. This muscle runs trans-

versely across the posterior wall of the esophagus and connects the two lateral borders of the cricoid cartilage (Zaino et al., 1970). The muscle is bordered superiorly by the oblique fibers of the inferior pharyngeal constrictor muscle, which pass upward and backward from their origin on the thyroid cartilage and insert into a median raphe. Inferiorly, the cricopharyngeus muscle blends into the circular and longitudinal muscle fibers of the upper esophagus, which lies in the midline immediately posterior to the trachea before its entry into the thorax. There, the upper esophagus curves slightly to the left behind the great vessels and returns to the midline at the level of the aortic arch. It then inclines to the right as it continues in the posterior mediastinum. Ultimately, it crosses the thoracic aorta to the left of the midline and angles anteriorly to pass through the diaphragmatic hiatus, a noose of fibers made up predominantly of the right crus of the diaphragm, with varying contribution from the left crus. Other variations occur in the structure of the diaphragmatic hiatus; in the most common variation, the noose of muscular tissue receives equal contributions from both right and left diaphragmatic crura (Carey and Hollingshead, 1955).

An intra-abdominal esophageal segment of variable length is present before the organ joins the stomach. External identification of the esophagogastric junction may be difficult even at surgery. Although the stomach is covered with peritoneum and the esophagus is not, the gastric peritoneal reflection is variable and bare stomach may be present. Perhaps the best landmark is a sling of gastric muscle fibers (collar of Helvetius). Thus, macroscopic identification of the esophagogastric junction is difficult, if not impossible, except at autopsy. From a practical point of view, the esophagogastric junction can be described as that point where the esophageal tube meets the gastric pouch. Much emphasis has previously been placed in the cardiac incisura or the angle of His between the esophagus and the stomach. This emphasis is misleading, because the angle is not a constant finding and many patients do not exhibit it at all. The phrenoesophageal ligament or membrane, first described by Laimer in 1883, helps to hold the distal esophagus loosely in place. Composed of mature collagenous fibers, this structure is a continuation of the transverse fascia of the abdominal parietes. It receives contributions from the endothoracic fascia and pleura above and the peritoneum below, and the fibers fan out to insert into the lower 2 to 3 cm of the esophagus in the region of the lower esophageal sphincter.

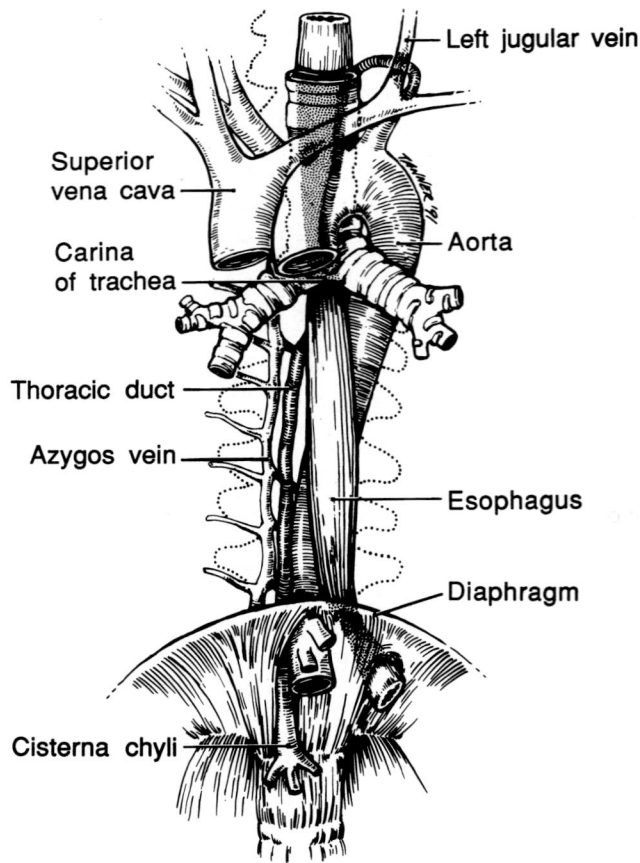

FIGURE 27–1. Anatomic figure demonstrating the relationship of the esophagus to other structures within the mediastinum. (From Wolfe, W. G., and Sebastian, M. W.: Complications in Thoracic Surgery. Chap. 22. St. Louis, C. V. Mosby, 1992, p. 245.)

Histology

Histologically, the esophageal wall consists of an inner circular layer of muscle and an outer longitudinal layer without a serosal covering (Higgs et al., 1965). The muscle layers consist of both striated and smooth muscle. The upper 5% of the esophagus consists solely of striated muscle, and the lower 54 to 62% consists of smooth muscle; a mixture constitutes the wall of the remaining esophagus in between (Meyer et al., 1986). Identification of a true anatomic sphincter has been difficult (Pera et al., 1975). Liebermann-Meffert and colleagues (1979), by using special techniques, identified a region of asymmetric muscle thickening in the esophageal wall below the diaphragm and above the angle of His that corresponds anatomically to the highest measurable pressures of the high-pressure zone. They pointed out that the inner circular layer is really semicircular. Stelzner (1971) emphasized the spiral nature of the "circular" muscle.

The mucous membrane of the esophageal lining consists of stratified squamous epithelium. Occasionally, ectopic islands of gastric mucosa have been identified, usually in the middle or upper portions of the esophagus. A prominent submucosa contains mucous glands, blood vessels, Meissner's plexus of nerves, and a rich network of lymphatic vessels. Transition from a squamous layer to a layer of junctional columnar epithelium occurs 1 to 2 cm cephalad to the esophagogastric junction. The squamocolumnar junction is not well defined because it is serrated. This junctional epithelium merges gradually with typical gastric mucosa distally in the stomach.

Vascular Supply

The blood supply is provided in the cervical portion of the esophagus by the inferior thyroid arteries and in the thoracic portion by branches from the aorta and by esophageal branches of the bronchial arteries (Swigert et al., 1950). Supplemental vessels come from arteries on the abdominal side of the diaphragm as well as from branches of the intercostal arteries. Important to the surgeon, particularly in mobilizing the esophagogastric junction, is the posterior gastric artery, a branch of the splenic artery, which is present 80 to 90% of the time and supplies the posterior wall of the stomach (Wald and Polk, 1983). A branch of the left inferior phrenic artery is often present and also supplies the esophagogastric junctional area of the stomach. The venous drainage is more complex (Butler, 1951). Venous channels course in both the lamina propria and the submucosa. In the region of the esophagogastric junction, they predominate in the lamina propria; elsewhere, they lie mainly in the submucosa (Spence, 1984). Subepithelial venous channels course longitudinally to empty above into the hypopharyngeal veins and below into the gastric veins. These channels also penetrate the esophageal muscle from which they receive branches. They leave the esophagus to form a periesophageal plexus; the longest trunks of this plexus accompany the vagus nerves. Venous drainage from the cervical portion of the esophagus is into the inferior thyroid and vertebral veins. Drainage from the thoracic portion is into the azygos and hemiazygos veins, and drainage from the abdominal portion is into the left gastric vein.

Lymphatic Drainage

The lymph vessels run longitudinally in the wall of the esophagus before penetrating the muscle layers to reach regional lymph nodes. After leaving the esophagus, these channels drain into the nearest group of nodes. Within the thorax, these nodes are identified by their location as tracheal, tracheobronchial, posterior mediastinal, and diaphragmatic. Lymphatic channels drain into the cervical nodes in the upper esophagus and into gastric and celiac nodes in the lower esophagus.

Innervation

The esophagus is innervated by both the parasympathetic and the sympathetic systems. In the neck, the parasympathetic supply is through branches of the recurrent laryngeal nerves and branches from the ninth and tenth cranial nerves and the cranial root of the eleventh nerve. The vagus nerves lie on either side of the esophagus for most of their course and form a plexus around it. As the hiatus is approached, two major trunks emerge; the left one comes to lie anteriorly and the right one posteriorly. The vagal plexus is joined by mediastinal branches of the thoracic sympathetic chain of the splanchnic nerves. The cervical esophagus receives its sympathetic supply from the pharyngeal plexus and lower down is supplied by fibers from the superior and inferior cervical sympathetic ganglia. Below the diaphragm, the esophagus receives fibers from the left greater splanchnic nerves, from the celiac plexus, and from plexuses around the left gastric and inferior phrenic arteries. The vagal trunk sends branches directly to the voluntary muscles of the esophagus and to the smooth muscle by parasympathetic preganglionic fibers. These branches synapse with the myenteric plexus of Auerbach (located between the inner circular and the outer longitudinal layers) and the plexuses of Meissner. Some unmyelinated fibers from the vagi pass directly to the muscular fibers of the muscularis mucosa. Afferent fibers are carried through both vagal and sympathetic nerves and do not synapse with the ganglion cells in the enteric plexuses. Terminal sensory nerve elements from widely branching filaments form a rich intramucosal network and communicate with the myenteric plexuses.

Benign Tumors and Cysts

Benign tumors of the esophagus are less common than their malignant counterparts; they constitute less than 10% of neoplasms of the esophagus. In general, they occur in patients at a younger age than carcinoma does, and their symptoms, if present, are usually of longer duration than when the organ contains malignancy.

Leiomyoma

Leiomyomas constitute two-thirds of the benign lesions of the esophagus. They occur more frequently in men than in women. The tumors may occur anywhere in the esophagus but are more commonly encountered in its lower third (Fountain, 1986) (Fig. 27–2). By 1978, 838 esophageal leiomyomas had been reported (Seremetis et al., 1973). Symptoms depend mainly on the size of the lesion; those smaller than 5 cm in diameter rarely produce symptoms. When symptoms occur, they consist primarily of dysphagia and a retrosternal feeling of pressure or of fullness. Esophageal leiomyomas are usually solitary, although rare instances of multiple tumors have been reported. Because the lesion is intramural with an overlying intact mucosa, bleeding is rare. Occasionally, a leiomyoma may grow to giant proportions and require esophagectomy (Kramer et al., 1986). Multiple leiomyomas are found in 2.4 to 4% of patients (Goddard and McCranie, 1973), and diffuse leiomyomatosis, in which the entire esophagus is studded with discrete confluent nodules, has been reported (Kabuto et al., 1980).

The radiographic appearance of a leiomyoma is typical and consists of a filling defect on esophagography with an intact esophageal mucosa (Schatzki and Hawes, 1950). The mass itself is usually ovoid with a sharply demarcated and smooth outline (see Fig. 27–2). Endoscopy may be deceiving because of the intact overlying mucosa. Usually, a filling defect in the esophageal wall is identifiable endoscopically. Only large encircling tumors, which are rare, cause obstruction to the passage of the endoscope. If a leiomyoma is suspected, the endoscopist should not perform a biopsy because it will complicate a subsequent surgical procedure. Histologically, the lesion consists of interlacing bundles of smooth muscle with eccentrically placed nuclei.

Patients with symptomatic leiomyomas are treated surgically. Depending on its location, the tumor is approached through either a right or a left thoracotomy, and can usually be enucleated through a longitudinal incision in the muscular wall of the esophagus without injuring the intact mucosa. A leiomyoma that involves the esophagogastric junction may pose a more complicated technical problem because these lesions often encircle the bowel, making enucleation of the tumor impossible. A limited esophagogastrectomy may be required for removal. Gastroesophageal competence should be restored by one of the plication procedures. Recently, reports of thoracoscopic removal of leiomyomata have appeared in the literature (Gossot et al., 1993). These reports are usually series of two to five patients involving upper-third lesions approached via right thoracoscopy with dual-lumen endotracheal tube, intraoperative esophagoscopy with transillumination, and opening of muscular layer perpendicular to the esophageal wall, with mucosal integrity assured via the esophagoscope.

Pedunculated Intraluminal Tumors

Various polypoid intraesophageal tumors have been described, including mucosal polyps, chondromas, lipomas, fibrolipomas, and myxofibromas. The most common histologic finding is a mixture of loose fibrous tissue with myxomatous fatty changes, best termed a *fibrolipoma* (Lolley et al., 1976). Dysphagia is the usual symptom and is sometimes associated with regurgitation and weight loss. The most dramatic presentation, but a rare one, involves regurgitation of the tumor through the mouth. Radiographic examination is not always diagnostic because the esophagus is sometimes so large that the tumor is obscured and the findings are confused with those of esophageal achalasia. Even esophagoscopy may be inconclusive because of the normal mucosal covering of the tumor.

Surgical removal is the treatment of choice for patients with pedunculated intraluminal tumors, although some tumors have been removed by means of a snare introduced through the esophagoscope. The site of origin of the tumor must be determined preoperatively to select the proper surgical approach. The approach may be through either a cervical incision or a high thoracic incision, and should be on the side opposite the origin of the tumor so that the pedicle can be seen readily after a longitudinal incision through the esophageal wall. The tumor is identified and removed from the esophagus, the pedicle is divided, and the defect in the esophageal wall is closed in two layers.

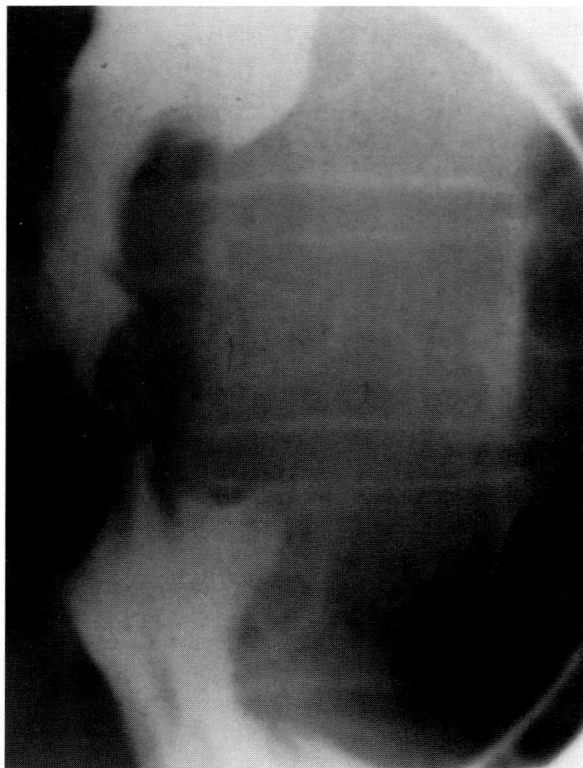

FIGURE 27–2. A large leiomyoma demonstrated on a barium swallow.

Cysts and Duplications of the Esophagus

Esophageal cysts are the second most common benign neoplasms of the esophageal wall. They represent an embryonal rest, are intramural, and may be lined with simple columnar ciliated epithelium or stratified squamous epithelium. The common location is in the wall of the upper thoracic esophagus in the region of the tracheal bifurcation. Radiographically, their appearance is identical to that of a leiomyoma, and surgical excision is conducted in the same manner as for a leiomyoma.

An esophageal duplication is a less common abnormality and consists of a tubular structure composed of muscular and submucosal layers with a squamous epithelial lining. It may extend the entire length of the normal esophagus parallel to it, and the muscular layers of the two may intermingle. Vertebral abnormalities are commonly associated with cysts and duplications, and the abnormality has been called the *split notochord syndrome* (Tarnay et al., 1970).

These lesions are surgically excised. The cystic lesions, like leiomyomas, can usually be enucleated easily. Excision of esophageal duplication is more difficult because of the intimate association with the esophageal wall and because some lesions may communicate with an intra-abdominal viscus (Fitzgibbons et al., 1980). Because the mucosa is not involved, esophageal duplications can usually be removed without esophageal resection.

Miscellaneous Benign Tumors

Several other benign tumors have been described and are mentioned here for completeness. These include squamous papilloma; granular cell myoblastoma, now reclassified as granular cell tumor (Sarma et al., 1986; Subramanyam et al., 1984); and hemangioma. Other benign lesions of the esophagus are lymphangiomas, neurofibromas, rhabdomyomas, osteochondromas, giant cell tumors, hamartomas, fibromas and lipomas, amyloid tumors, and eosinophilic granulomas.

Malignant Tumors

Incidence and Epidemiology

An estimated 10,000 Americans will have died from 11,000 diagnoses of esophageal cancer in 1992. The relatively uncommon nature of this condition in the United States is offset by a relatively higher incidence in France, Finland, Curacão, and Iceland and the high incidence found in the "esophageal cancer belt" extending from the Caspian Sea through Iran, Afghanistan, and Siberia to China. The distribution of esophageal cancer is 15% for the cervical esophagus, 50% for the middle esophagus, and 35% for the distal esophagus. Traditionally, 75% of esophageal cancer was of squamous histology. Recent data suggest a steady incidence of squamous cell and an increase in the incidence of adenocarcinoma since the early 1970s

(Silverberg and Lubera, 1988). Other patterns include a higher incidence of squamous cell cancer in black patients and a higher incidence of adenocarcinoma in white patients.

Carcinoma of the esophagus is predominantly a disease of men between the ages of 50 and 70 years. The incidence varies throughout the world; it is 3.5 per 100,000 among white men and 13.3 per 100,000 among black men in the United States (Garfinkel et al., 1980), and 130 per 100,000 in parts of the Honan province of North China (Day, 1975). The reason for the high incidence of esophageal carcinoma in China, Japan, Kazakhstan, Iran, and Brittany and among the native Bantu of South Africa is not clear (Doll et al., 1966).

Epidemiologic surveys show that two risk factors, smoking and high consumption of alcoholic beverages, predominate in patients with epidermoid cancer of the esophagus in Normandy and the United States (Wynder and Bross, 1961). Ingestion of nitrosamines is highly carcinogenic for the esophagus and may explain the high incidence of this condition among the South African Bantu and in some areas of China (McGlashan et al., 1968). Reference has been made to such predisposing lesions as esophageal achalasia, the columnar epithelium–lined lower esophagus, and corrosive lye strictures. An increased incidence has been reported in patients with the Patterson-Kelly syndrome (Wynder et al., 1957), which is discussed later, and in patients with tylosis (Shine and Allison, 1966).

Caustic Strictures

Strictures resulting from the ingestion of solid or liquid caustics are most frequently encountered in children who have swallowed the material accidentally or in adults who have ingested the material for suicidal purposes (Leape et al., 1971). The chemicals most commonly implicated in corrosive burns of the esophagus include alkaline caustics, acids or acid-like corrosives, and household bleaches. Lye, in the broad sense of the term, includes strong alkalis, most commonly sodium or potassium hydroxide. Most of the household cleaning agents, such as Dran-O, Liquid Plumr, and Easy-Off, contain one of these corrosive agents. Burns from the ingestion of such agents may involve the oral pharynx, larynx, esophagus, and stomach; 25 to 50% of patients with oral burns have an esophageal injury. Successful management requires prompt recognition and early treatment.

Caustic esophageal stricture is a precancerous lesion. In patients followed for at least 24 years, the risk of cancer of the esophagus developing was said to be increased a thousandfold (Kiviranta, 1952). Cancers engrafted on an esophagus injured by caustic agents are responsible for 1 to 4% of all cancers of the esophagus, and the average interval from injury to cancer development is about 40 years (Hopkins and Postlethwait, 1981).

Barrett's Esophagus (Columnar-Lined Esophagus)

Reflux of acid or alkaline secretions into the esophagus caused by esophagogastric incompetence as a result of a hypotensive lower esophageal sphincter is the most common cause of esophageal injury. Although reflux of acid peptic juices is more common, the sensitivity of the esophageal mucosa to the damaging effects of both acid and alkaline secretions has repeatedly been identified. The combination of acid and alkaline reflux is particularly deleterious to the esophageal mucosa (Gillison et al., 1972). Diagnosis and medical and surgical management of patients with gastroesophageal reflux disease are discussed in Chapter 28, part VI. Emphasis here is placed on Barrett's esophagus as a premalignant condition.

Barrett drew attention to a columnar epithelium–lined esophagus in 1950 and thought that it represented a congenitally short esophagus, with the stomach lying high within the thorax. Allison and Johnstone (1953) showed the distinction between the squamocolumnar mucosal junction and the functional junction between the esophagus and the stomach. This recognition that the intrathoracic structure was esophagus, not stomach, and description of the anomaly as "esophagus lined with gastric mucous membrane" began the current era of understanding of this disease. These authors also commented on the frequent association of a sliding esophageal hiatal hernia with this condition, and stated the belief that chronic peptic ulcer and adenocarcinoma could arise in a columnar-lined esophagus with peptic stricture. In 1957, Barrett changed his opinion and suggested, in a lecture given at the Mayo Clinic, that the entry be referred to as "the lower esophagus lined by columnar epithelium." This condition is referred to as *Barrett's esophagus.*

The condition was first considered to be congenital. Now, it is considered to be a response to the reflux of gastric acid into the lower esophagus, with ulceration and destruction of the squamous epithelium and replacement by the columnar epithelium. The universal association of a hypotensive lower esophageal sphincter and the almost constant association of a sliding esophageal hiatal hernia support this concept, as does documentation of the development of a lining of columnar epithelium in areas previously lined by squamous epithelium. Further support for this concept was provided by Bremmer and co-workers (1970), whose experimental studies showed that columnar cells form a new lining for an esophagus in which the squamous epithelium has been destroyed by acid gastric reflux.

Barrett's epithelium consists of a heterogeneous collection of cell types and patterns; some resemble gastric body and cardiac mucosa containing chief and parietal cells, and others appear similar to gastric mucosa that has undergone intestinal metaplasia. This specialized columnar epithelium is most often implicated in the development of dysplasia and adenocarcinoma (Paull et al., 1976).

The symptoms are those that characterize gastroesophageal reflux, which have been described earlier. The frequent association of a high-lying stricture accounts for the fact that dysphagia is a common symptom. The diagnosis is made radiographically in many patients, particularly when a stricture is present; a small sliding hernia with tubular esophagus intervening between the hernia and a high-lying stricture is characteristic. Endoscopy with biopsy confirms the diagnosis, which is further supported by the use of scintigraphy to identify the nature of the epithelium.

The prevalence of this condition in the general population is not known because many individuals with the disease are asymptomatic. Of patients with endoscopic evidence of esophagitis, 11% (Naef et al., 1975) to 27% (Winters et al., 1987) have Barrett's epithelium when biopsy is performed. Dysplastic changes may occur in Barrett's mucosa and precede the development of carcinoma in situ and invasive malignancy. The premalignant nature of Barrett's epithelium is recognized (Haggitt et al., 1978; Hawe et al., 1973), but its prevalence varies depending on the population of patients reviewed. Reported prevalence ranges from 8.6% (Naef et al., 1975) to 46% (Skinner et al., 1983). Prevalence rates may give a faulty impression of the risk of cancer developing in Barrett's esophagus. Cameron and associates in 1990 found a 20-fold greater prevalence of Barrett's esophagus by autopsy results. In follow-up studies of patients with this condition, the risk of cancer varied from 1 in 81 patient-years (Sprung et al., 1984) to 1 in 441 patient-years (Cameron et al., 1985). The report by Duhaylongsod and Wolfe in 1991 and Levine and colleagues in 1993 established the need for endoscopic surveillance. Endoscopic surveillance of patients with Barrett's esophagus is best performed with four quadrant biopsies at 1-cm intervals in the distal 3 cm of the esophagus, spanning from zero to 6 cm above the gastroesophageal junction and at 2-cm intervals to the squamocolumnar junction. Recent reports indicate p53 gene alterations in Barrett's esophagus (Moore et al., 1994).

Medical treatment has no beneficial effect on columnar (Barrett's) epithelium. Although antireflux operation occasionally results in regression of the abnormal epithelium, it never disappears entirely. Successful antireflux operation does not prevent the subsequent development of carcinoma. Therefore, it seems reasonable to adopt similar criteria for advising operation in these patients as in patients without the complication of Barrett's epithelium. Failure of medical management is the major indication, and the presence of severe dysplasia suggests the need for resection.

Patients who have been treated for Barrett's esophagus must be followed closely after the operation by radiography and endoscopy, because correction of reflux does not necessarily cause regression of the extent of the columnar epithelial lining and the patient is still at risk for developing cancer.

Pathology

Squamous cell carcinoma is the most common malignant tumor of the body of the esophagus and represents more than 95% of esophageal malignancies in some series (Figs. 27–3 and 27–4). Primary adenocarcinoma is rare, less than 1% (Raphael et al., 1966) to 7% of esophageal malignancies (Cederqvist et al., 1980) in earlier series, with an increasing incidence to as high as 25% noted in more recent series (Hesketh et al., 1989; Mayer, 1993). The most common glandular tumor of the esophagus is an adenocarcinoma that arises in the columnar epithelium of Barrett's esophagus (Hawe et al., 1973) (Fig. 27–5), which represented 86% of all adenocarcinomas of the esophagus in one series (Haggitt et al., 1978). Tumors similar in microscopic appearance to those arising in salivary glands represent less than one-fifth of all glandular tumors of the esophagus. These mucoepidermoid and adenoid cystic carcinomas arise from the ducts of the submu-

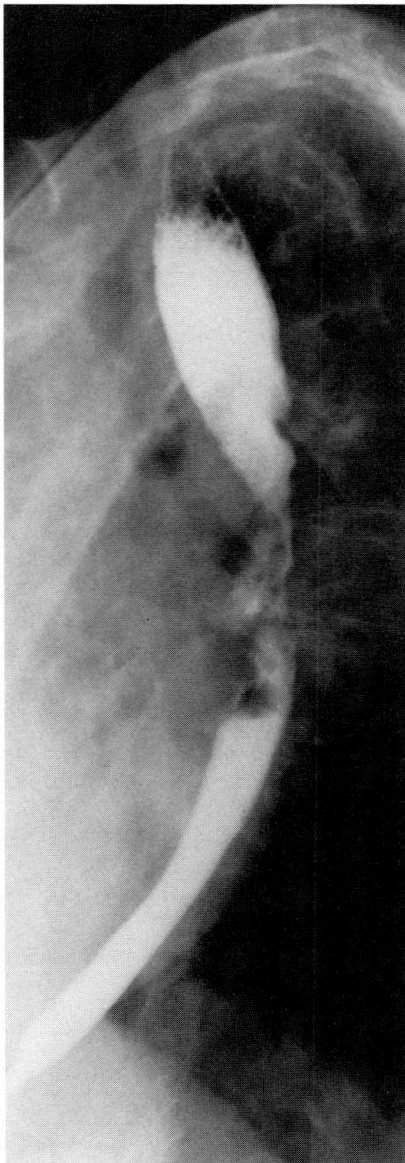

FIGURE 27–4. Pathologic specimen of a squamous cell carcinoma in the distal third of the esophagus from a patient with long-standing achalasia.

cosal glands. They are rare; only 27 cases were reported by 1980 (Bell-Thomson et al., 1980).

Most malignant lesions are ulcerating and encircle the esophageal lumen. These lesions are only rarely polypoid. The most common polypoid malignant lesion of the esophagus is a carcinosarcoma (Figs. 27–6 and 27–7), which has a slightly more favorable prognosis than squamous cell carcinoma (Stener et al., 1967). An even rarer polypoid lesion is a pseudosarcoma (Nichols et al., 1979). Another rare sarcomatous lesion of the esophagus is a leiomyosarcoma, which tends to ulcerate, in contrast to a benign leiomyoma. Primary malignant melanoma of the esophagus has been reported (Kreuser, 1979). An even more uncommon malignant esophageal tumor is a granular cell tumor (Sarma et al., 1986). Fibrosarcoma, rhabdomyosarcoma, plasmacytoma, and lymphosarcoma have also been reported.

The indolent biologic behavior of verrucous squamous cell carcinoma makes it more susceptible to cure than other esophageal malignancies (Meyerowitz and Shea, 1971). The oat-cell carcinoma is rare (Reid et al., 1980) and is considered a true apudoma arising from the argyrophilic Kulchitsky cells in the surface

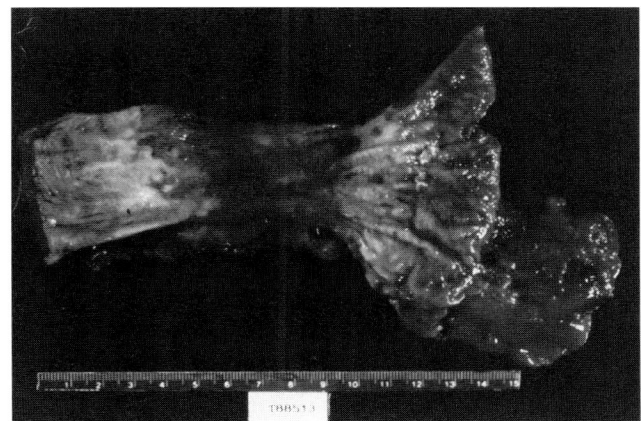

FIGURE 27–3. Typical squamous cell carcinoma in the middle third of the esophagus.

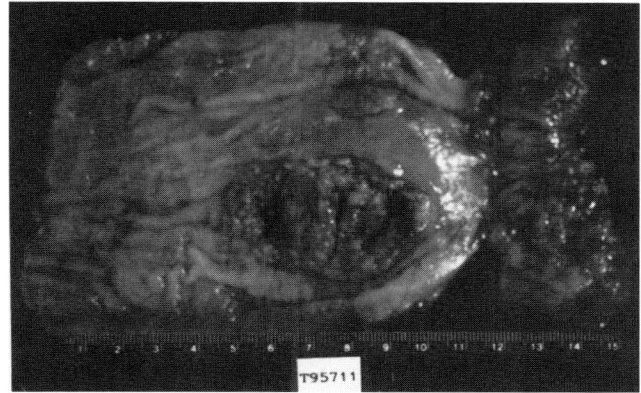

FIGURE 27–5. Resected specimen of a Barrett esophagus having adenocarcinoma in situ along with severe dysplasia.

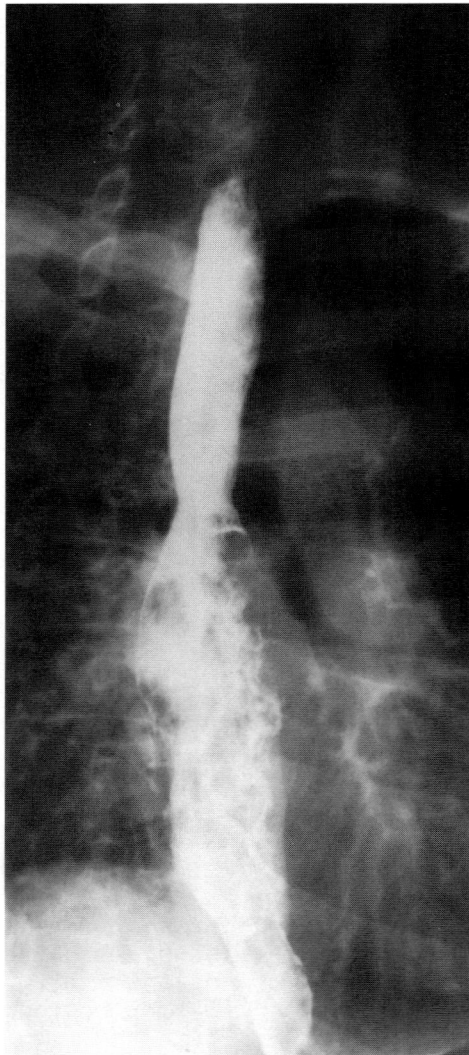

FIGURE 27–6. Barium swallow demonstrating a polypoid mass within the middle third of the esophagus, which is consistent with radiographic findings of a carcinosarcoma.

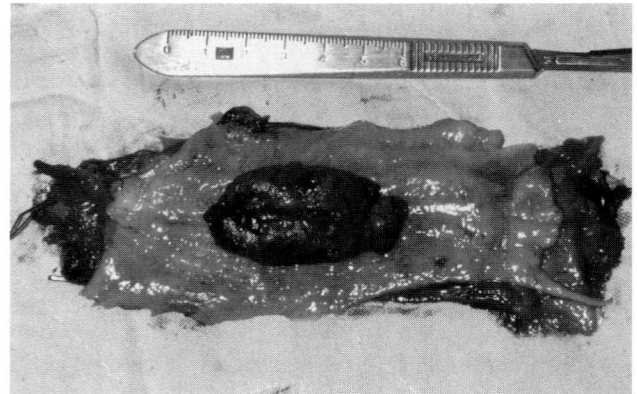

FIGURE 27–7. An esophageal specimen showing a polypoid carcinosarcoma after resection and esophagogastrectomy.

epithelium. Finally, the esophagus may be involved by primary tumors elsewhere in the body by direct extension or by blood-borne metastases.

Malignant lesions that involve the esophagogastric junction are almost invariably adenocarcinomas of gastric origin and constitute approximately half of the malignant tumors of the esophagus (Gunnlaugsson et al., 1970) The distinction between primary esophageal adenocarcinoma and adenocarcinoma of the gastric cardia with extension to the esophagus can be difficult (Figs. 27–8 and 27–9). Fewer than 15% of esophageal malignancies arise in the cervical region; all others arise in the intrathoracic body of the esophagus.

Although malignant tumors of the esophagus also spread by direct extension and by vascular invasion, the sites of nodal metastases are important in deciding therapy. Cervical esophageal carcinoma disseminates through the lymphatic vessels to cervical nodes, particularly the anterior jugular and supraclavicular nodes. Carcinomas arising in the thoracic esophagus

spread early to the local and mediastinal glands and to the supraclavicular nodes and, occasionally, to the subdiaphragmatic nodes. Those at the esophagogastric junction may involve local mediastinal and subdi-

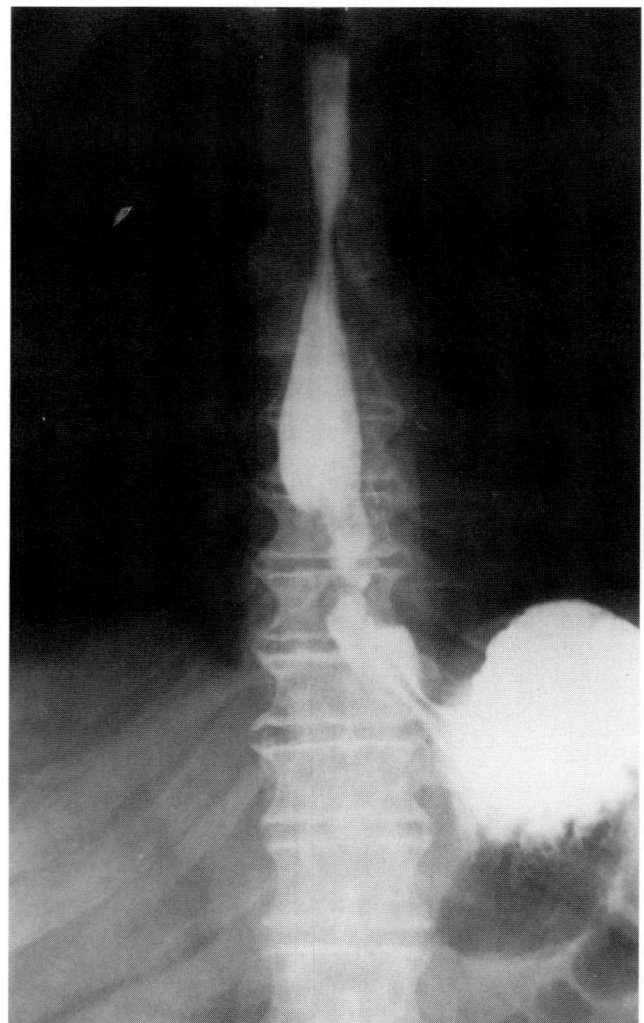

FIGURE 27–8. Adenocarcinoma associated with a hiatal hernia.

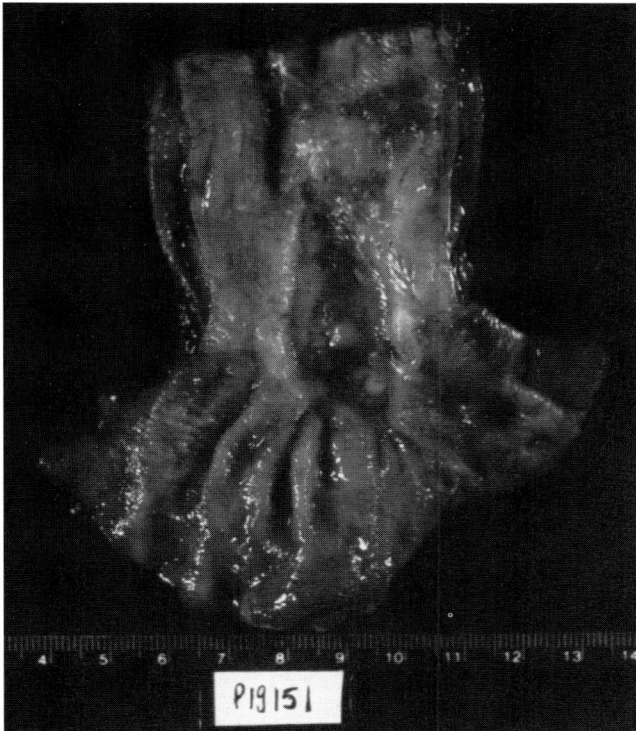

FIGURE 27–9. Adenocarcinoma of the distal third of the esophagus that is not associated with Barrett's epithelium.

aphragmatic nodes and nodes in the hilum of the spleen. Metastases through the bloodstream may produce liver, lung, brain, or bone implants. It is important to note that there is some increased use in the literature of the Japanese Society for Esophageal Diseases' classification of esophageal cancer. This classification differs from the *tumor-nodes-metastases* (TNM) staging in categorization of cervical or abdominal lymph node metastasis as distant metastasis (Shun'ichi et al., 1990).

Clinical Manifestations

The most common symptom of esophageal carcinoma is dysphagia. Initially, it is noted with the ingestion of solid foods, but ultimately swallowing even liquids and saliva becomes difficult. Weight loss and weakness are inevitable consequences. Aspiration pneumonitis is not infrequent as obstructive symptoms progress. Depending on the location of the tumor and the involvement of adjacent structures, recurrent nerve involvement or pulmonary symptoms may result from compression or invasion of the trachea or of the bronchi. Symptoms are rare until the tumor has totally encircled the esophagus, at which time the tumor may be relatively far advanced. Early diagnosis is important, and anyone over 40 years of age who complains of painful swallowing or of obstruction to swallowing should have diagnostic studies, including esophagoscopy, to exclude a malignant lesion.

Esophageal radiography provides the diagnosis with a high degree of accuracy. The usual finding is an irregular, ragged mucosal pattern with annular luminal narrowing. Unlike benign obstructive lesions, carcinoma is usually not associated with marked proximal dilatation of the esophagus.

The diagnosis should be confirmed by esophagoscopy not only to establish a tissue diagnosis but also to determine the anatomic limits of the lesion. Lesions that involve the upper portion of the esophagus in the region of the tracheal carina require bronchoscopy to determine the presence or absence of malignant involvement of the tracheobronchial tree. In addition to biopsies of the suspected lesion, cytologic study of smears from such a lesion is valuable. Other studies, such as esophageal motility, are rarely of use except to exclude one of the more common motility disturbances.

Treatment

Controversy persists concerning the proper management of patients with carcinoma of the esophagus. Some physicians consider surgical therapy unlikely to cure, and thus use irradiation for all patients. Other physicians prefer a combination of radiation therapy and resection or chemotherapy, radiation, and resection, and still other physicians use surgical therapy alone. Chemotherapy, used alone, has little role in the treatment of patients with esophageal cancer except when the lesion is nonresectable.

Radiation Therapy. Treatment of esophageal carcinoma by irradiation alone may be radical or palliative. If palliative, a dose in the range of 20 to 30 Gy (2000 to 3000 rads) during a 2-week period may provide temporary alleviation of pain, hemorrhage, and dysphagia with relatively little morbidity.

Radical treatment for cure necessitates a dose between 50 and 60 Gy (5000 to 6000 rads) delivered during 4 or more weeks. This form of treatment is not without risk because complications such as radiation pneumonitis and postradiation stricture are common. Unusual complications include tracheoesophageal fistula, radiation myelitis, hemorrhage, and constrictive pericarditis. Pearson (1977) is the strongest proponent for irradiation as the primary form of therapy, and his updated results in 288 patients with a 5-year survival rate of 17% are the best that radical radiotherapy has produced. It is not clear why others have not achieved comparable results, although selection of patients may have a role. In a review of the literature of the 25 years ending in 1979, Earlam and Cunha-Melo (1980b) reported an overall survival rate of only 6% after radiotherapy. If radiation alone has a role in the treatment of patients with esophageal malignancies, controversy would be least when it is applied to the cervical region of the esophagus.

Chemotherapy. Because systemic dissemination characterizes carcinoma of the esophagus, the use of chemotherapy in its management is logical, but its effectiveness in permanently controlling the disease has yet to be proved. Response rates vary from 5 to 50% and depend on the pharmacologic agent or operative chemotherapy coupled with preoperative radiation are increasingly common (Orringer, 1993; Wolfe et al., 1993). Resolution of dysphagia can be seen in 85% of patients. The most dramatic improvements in survival are seen in patients completing preoperative chemotherapy and radiation therapy and undergoing surgery, with histology showing no evidence of residual tumor. In these patients with a "sterile specimen," the most dramatic improvements in 5-year survival rates to 70% are seen. Combination therapy may increase the resectability rate in selected patients, although some reports suggest similar survival in patients undergoing preoperative chemotherapy and radiation therapy with surgery and those completing adjuvant therapy and not proceeding to resection (Naunheim, 1992).

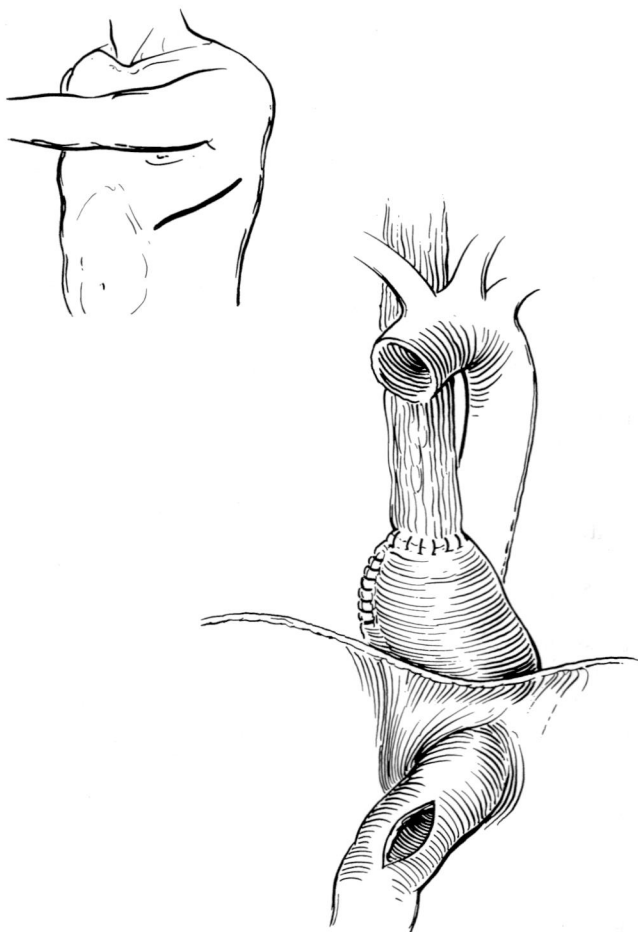

FIGURE 27–10. Diagram of incision for resection via a left thoracotomy.

combination of agents used, and the improvement is usually of brief duration (Coonley et al., 1984; Kelsen et al., 1983). Most of the agents found to be effective are accompanied by severe toxicity. The pulmonary complications of bleomycin are particularly worrisome when combined therapy is used. Intracavitary irradiation (brachytherapy) is being studied (Rowland and Pagliero, 1985).

Multimodal Therapy. Combined irradiation and surgical resection are preferred to resection alone by some physicians. Launois and associates (1981) reported a prospective randomized study that compared the results of preoperative irradiation with those after resection alone; the 5-year survival rates were not appreciably different.

The concept of combined therapy has been expanded to include chemotherapy in the hope of extending survival (Bains et al., 1982; Parker et al., 1985; Steiger et al., 1981). Commonly, one or more chemotherapeutic agents such as 5-fluorouracil and cisplatin and bleomycin combined with an irradiation dose of 30 to 36 Gy (3000 to 3600 rads) are administered before operation, followed by resection in 3 to 4 weeks. In some patients (up to 30% in some series) the local lesion completely disappears. Reports of pre-

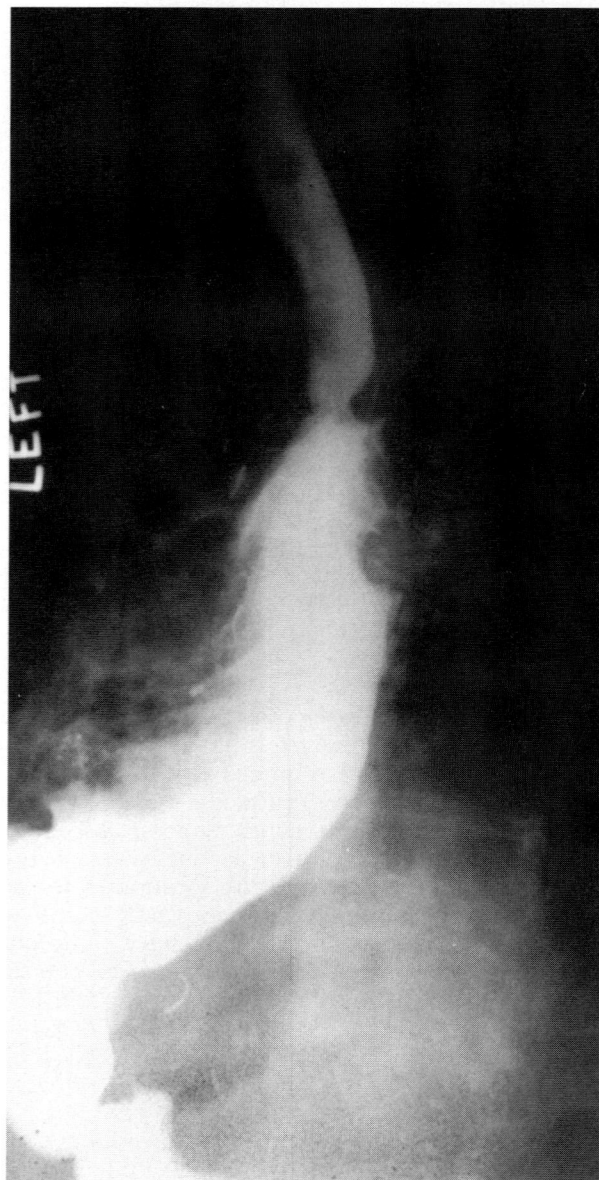

FIGURE 27–11. A reconstructed esophagogastrectomy through the left side of the chest using the Sweet procedure.

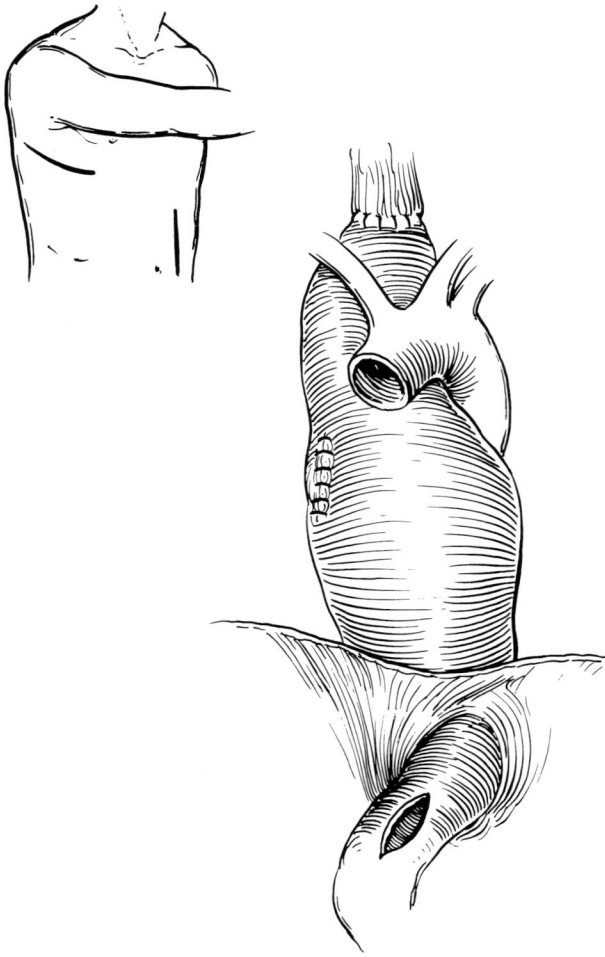

FIGURE 27–12. Diagram of the incision used for the Ivor-Lewis procedure.

Surgery. Various resective techniques have been used in the management of patients with carcinoma of the esophagus, both as staged operations and as definitive procedures. These techniques include esophagogastrectomy and esophagogastrostomy, or interposition of the small or large bowel or a revascularized intestinal autograft and the use of a Gavriliu gastric tube. Resection has also been combined with such staged reconstructive plastic procedures as the Wookey operation for cervical esophageal cancers and the formation of anterior thoracic skin tubes to reconstruct alimentary tract continuity. Many of these procedures have historical interest only. Emphasis here is placed on the operations that are most commonly used now.

Esophagogastrectomy with Esophagogastrostomy. Because it has a low hospital mortality and need not be staged, esophagogastrectomy with esophagogastrostomy is preferred in the surgical treatment of patients with lesions at all levels of the esophagus, as long as adequate stomach is available. The use of gastric substitution in 506 patients operated on for epidermoid cancer of the esophagus by Wang and colleagues, reported in 1992, showed use of the stom-

ach in 368 patients. For malignancies of the lower esophagus and esophagogastric junction, a left thoracotomy provides satisfactory exposure for resection and intrathoracic anastomosis (Figs. 27–10 and 27–11). For lesions that require an anastomosis at or proximal to the aortic arch, a combined abdominal and right thoracic approach is used (Figs. 27–12 and 27–13). When resection is performed for cervical esophageal cancer, a similar approach permits elevation of the freed stomach into the neck with primary cervical esophagogastrostomy, or a thoracotomy may be avoided by freeing the esophagus by blunt dissection from the neck and abdomen, resecting it, and elevating the freed stomach through the posterior mediastinum into the neck where an esophagogastrostomy is performed (Orringer and Sloan, 1978) (Figs. 27–14 and 27–15).

Regardless of the extent of the resection and the location of the anastomosis, careful mobilization of the stomach is essential to preserve its blood supply. The short gastric vessels are divided. The stomach is freed from the omentum and mesocolon, and care is taken to preserve the right gastroepiploic artery. When the local extension of the tumor demands, the spleen and part of the pancreas can be included in the resected specimen after division of the posterior gastric artery and usually also a branch of the left inferior phrenic artery. The left gastric artery is divided at its origin from the celiac axis and, if necessary, the duodenum is kocherized to permit further mobilization of the stomach. When feasible, an extramucosal pyloromyotomy is performed to minimize the postvagotomy effect. The stomach is divided at an appropriate level by a stapling device of proper

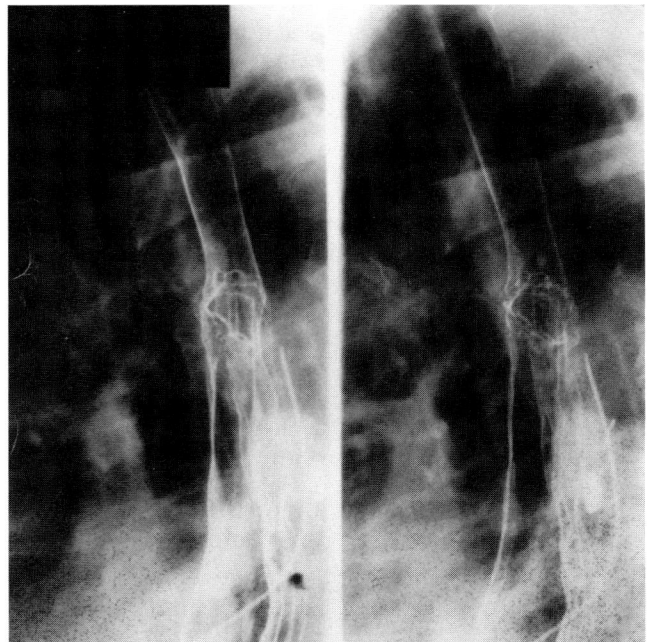

FIGURE 27–13. A stapled anastomosis after an Ivor-Lewis procedure with the stomach brought into the right side of the chest and the esophagogastrectomy completed just above the azygos vein.

A   **B**   **C**

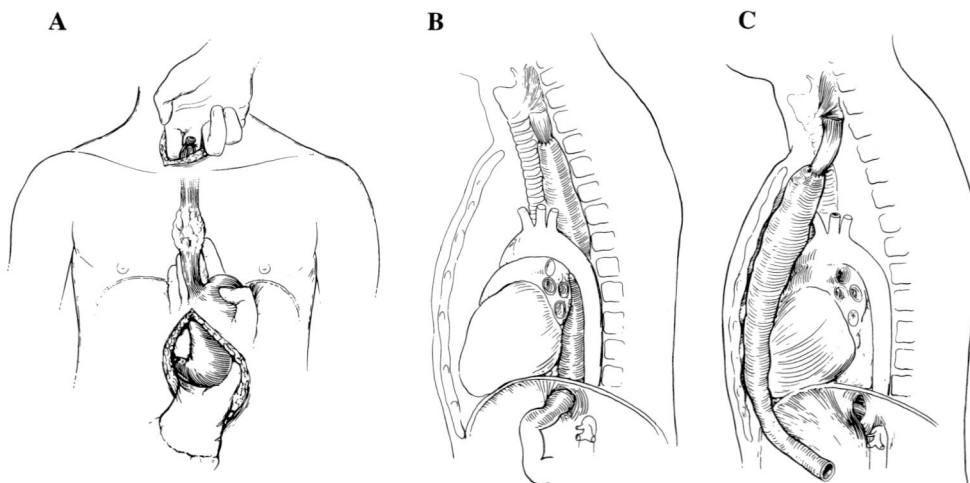

FIGURE 27–14. Diagram demonstrating transhiatal esophagogastrectomy *(A)* and placement of the stomach posteriorly *(B)* and substernally *(C)*.

size, and an end-to-side anastomosis between the stomach and the esophagus is performed without using clamps and while avoiding any tension. A number of anastomotic techniques can be used. A classic two-layer anastomosis with an inner layer of continuous catgut and an outer layer of interrupted silk sutures has proved to be satisfactory. Other techniques include single-layer sewn anastomoses and the use of the endoluminal enteric anastomosis (EEA) circular stapling device. The increasing use of the EEA stapling device has facilitated performance of high thoracic anastomoses (Fok et al., 1991).

Intercostal and nasogastric tube drainage are used to provide gastric decompression. The tubes are left in place for 4 or 5 days and removed after a contrast radiographic study confirms the integrity of the anastomosis, and oral feedings are begun.

Esophagogastrectomy with Colon or Jejunum Interposition. Of the other varieties of esophageal reconstruction, the interposed colon is perhaps most widely used as an alternative to esophagogastrostomy. For short distal segments, the jejunum and Roux-en-Y resection is usually preferred. If one needs to reconstruct in the neck, the colon is used. When insufficient stomach remains after resection, both are viable alternatives to esophagogastrostomy.

Results of Resection. The role of resection in treating patients with cancer of the esophagus has been challenged on the basis of low resectability and high mortality (Earlam and Cunha-Melo, 1980a). These views are based mostly on outdated information and do not reflect current practices. The report by Wu and Huang (1979) from the People's Republic of China more accurately reflects current practices. In a number of Chinese hospitals, the resectability was 80%, the hospital mortality was 3 to 5%, and the 5-year survival rate was almost 30%. The evolution of surgical treatment of esophageal cancer is reflected in a report from the Massachusetts General Hospital where 701 patients were reviewed. The mortality had fallen from 10.4% in the 1970s to 2.9% in the 1980s, with a 12.6% complication of anastomosis.

The best results have been obtained by the Chinese in asymptomatic patients diagnosed by screening techniques used in endemic areas. Resectability is 100% in these patients, the hospital mortality is 2.4%, and the 5-year survival rate is 90% (Huang et al., 1981).

Another recent development in the treatment strategy for esophageal cancer is in patient selection. The most extensive effort in the literature comes from Saito and co-workers, who have studied the impairment of host defense systems in patients with esophageal cancer. Since their initial report in 1991 of 21 serologic and immunologic markers in 32 patients and the relation of these markers to postoperative deaths, they have developed the *host defense index* (Saito et al., 1993). The HDI parameters that predict poor outcome after surgery include a depressed *cell-mediated immunity*, enhanced polyclonal immunoglobulin levels, enhanced neutrophil cytocidal activity, increased acute-phase protein concentrations, and altered nutritional status. The presence of these indicates reduction in cellular immunity and an elevation in chronic inflammatory response with a preoperative immunodeficiency-based predisposition to infection.

Palliative Procedures. Even with careful preoperative evaluation, some tumors cannot be removed successfully because of local extension to vital structures. In these patients, a palliative procedure is indicated. Various plastic tubes are available that can be passed through the lesion transorally and retrieved during operation through gastrotomy and firmly fixed in place. The Celestin tube is widely preferred (Fig. 27–16); it is associated with an operative mortality of approximately 10% but also with palliation of dysphagia in 75% of patients (Sanfelippo and Bernatz, 1973). For nonresectable lesions of the cardia, an alternative palliative procedure is a bypass technique. The fundus of the stomach is rotated into the thorax and anastomosed side-to-side to the proximal esophagus. For lesions higher in the thoracic esophagus, the stomach is mobilized, the esophagus is transected at the diaphragm and in the neck, and a cervical esophageal anastomosis to the substernally placed stomach is performed. The operation has limited applicability

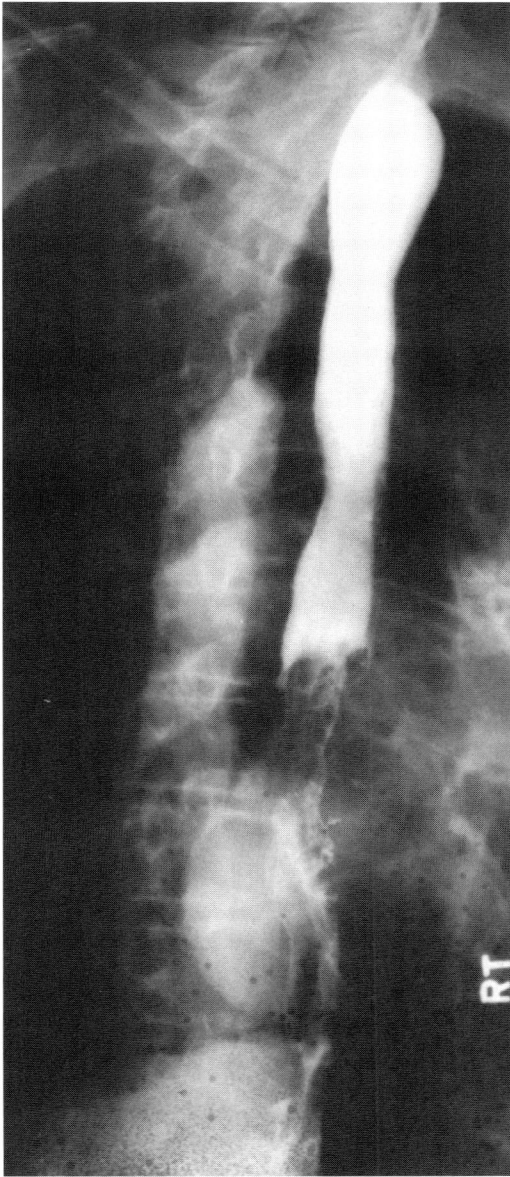

FIGURE 27–15. The stomach has been brought to the neck following a transhiatal esophagogastrectomy.

because of its high risk (Robinson et al., 1982). Although these procedures provide relief of dysphagia, longevity is unaffected; the average survival time is no more than 4 months, the same as it is for non-treated patients.

A technique with less risk is that of endoscopic intubation of nonresectable carcinoma of the esophagus. The Proctor-Livingston, Atkinson, Celestin, and Tytgat tubes are examples of such devices. A review of the experience in Great Britain with peroral intubation showed perforation in 9%, obstructed tubes in 8%, and dislodgment of the tube in 10% of patients; 4.5% of the patients died (Bennett, 1981).

Laser therapy for palliation of inoperable carcinoma of the esophagus is now being used, and the preliminary results are encouraging (Fleischer et al., 1982; Wolfe et al., 1987).

CONCLUSION

The literature shows wide variations in approaches to treatment of carcinoma of the esophagus. The subtleties inherent in analyzing the literature and determining a rational approach to this disease involve an intimate understanding of both the anatomy and physiology of the normal esophagus and the difference between the behavior of squamous cell carcinoma and that of adenocarcinoma that stems from the location of the tumors and from the aggressiveness of the tumors themselves. The dismal prognosis in the literature has added to the disparate approaches to treatment. There is a wide variance in operative approach, ranging from transhiatal esophagectomy without thoracotomy to laparotomy only. The degree

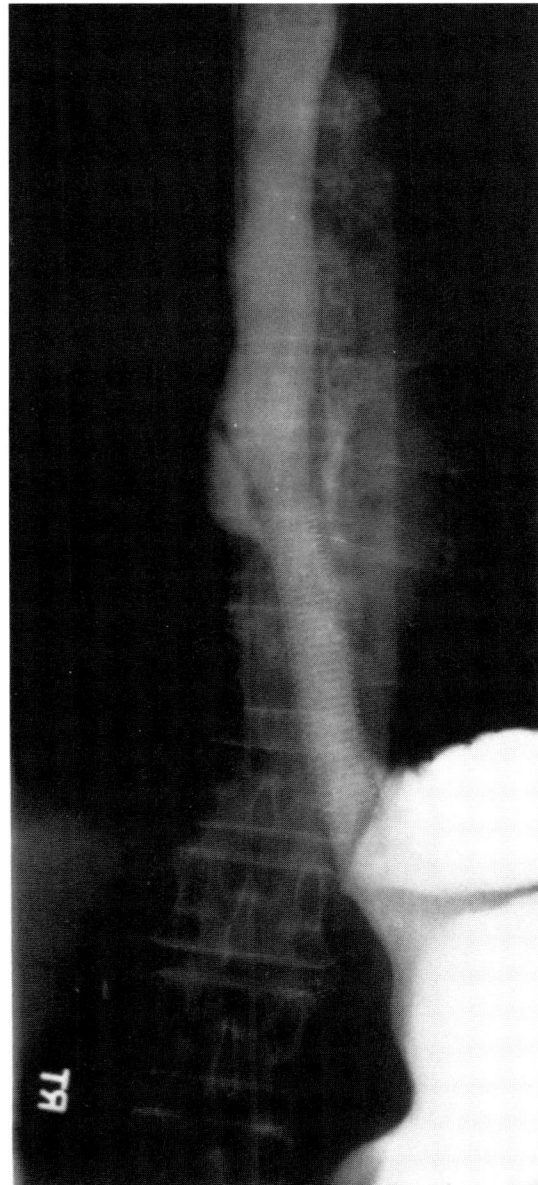

FIGURE 27–16. Placement of a Celestin tube in the distal third of the esophagus.

of excision ranges from local excision to wide local excision with extensive lymphadenectomy. The EEA stapling device has greatly facilitated use of mobilized stomach for intrathoracic anastomosis to the esophageal remnant in a simplified single anastomosis. Finally, the evolution of preoperative assessment of operative mortality to select proper candidates for curative resection, coupled with preoperative nutrition, chemotherapy, and radiation therapy with postoperative jejunal tube feeding, should allow selection of candidates who will benefit from aggressive management of this devastating disease.

SELECTED BIBLIOGRAPHY

DeMeester, T. R., and Matthews, H. R. (eds): Benign Esophageal Disease. Vol. 3 of the series International Trends in General Thoracic Surgery. St. Louis, C. V. Mosby, 1987.

Multiauthored, current, concise review of the subject.

Hacker, V., and Lotheissen, G.: Chirurgie der Speiseröhre. Band XXXIV. Neue Deutsche Chirurgie. Stuttgart, Enke, 1926.

This book is probably the best historical summary of early attempts to treat esophageal disease by surgical techniques. As so often happens in medicine, what now seems new and innovative was thought of and done before and unfortunately forgotten until modern advances permitted its reintroduction under more favorable circumstances.

Levine, Mark S.: Radiology of the Esophagus. Philadelphia, W. B. Saunders, 1989.

This is an excellent roentgenographic text of all esophageal disease.

Postlethwait, R. W.: Surgery of the Esophagus. 2nd ed. East Norwalk, CT, Appleton & Lange, 1986.

A new, updated, and totally rewritten edition of Postlethwait and Sealy's early esophageal monograph. The current edition has complete coverage of esophageal surgery and has an excellent bibliography.

Shahian, D. M, and Ellis, F. H., Jr.: Barrett's esophagus. In Shields, T. W. (ed): General Thoracic Surgery. 3rd ed. Philadelphia, Lea & Febiger, 1989, pp. 1024–1033.

Complete yet concise review of this poorly understood entity.

Siewart, J. R., and Hölscher, A. M. (eds): Diseases of the Esophagus. Berlin, Springer-Verlag, 1988.

Papers presented during International Esophageal Week in Munich summarize the state of the art concerning pathology, pathophysiology, diagnosis, and therapy of benign and malignant diseases of the esophagus.

Wolfe, W. G., Vaughn, A. L., Seigler, H. F., et al.: Survival of patients with carcinoma of the esophagus treated with combined-modality therapy. J. Thorac. Cardiovasc. Surg., 105:749, 1993.

This paper describes 5-year follow-up of chemotherapy, radiation therapy, and surgery in patients with both adenocarcinoma and squamous carcinoma of the esophagus.

BIBLIOGRAPHY

Adams, W. E., and Phemister, D. B.: Carcinoma of lower thoracic esophagus: Report of successful resection and esophagogastrostomy. J. Thorac. Cardiovasc. Surg., 7:621, 1938.

Allison, P. R., and Johnstone, A. S.: The oesophagus lined with gastric mucous membrane. Thorax, 8:87, 1953.

Bains, M. S., Kelsen, D. P., Beattie, E. J., Jr., et al.: Treatment of esophageal carcinoma by combined preoperative chemotherapy. Ann. Thorac. Surg., 34:512, 1982.

Barrett, N. R.: Chronic peptic ulcer of the oesophagus and "oesophagitis." Br. J. Surg., 38:175, 1950.

Barrett, N. R.: The lower esophagus lined by columnar epithelium. Surgery, 41:881, 1957.

Beck, C., and Carrell, A.: Demonstration of specimens illustrating a method of formation of prethoracic esophagus. Ill. Med. J., 7:463, 1905.

Bell-Thomson, J., Haggitt, R. C., and Ellis, F. H., Jr.: Mucoepidermoid and adenoid cystic carcinomas of the esophagus. J. Thorac. Cardiovasc. Surg., 79:438, 1980.

Bennett, J. R.: Intubation of gastro-oesophageal malignancies: A survey of current practice in Britain, 1980. Gut, 22:336, 1981.

Billroth, T.: Ueber die Resection des Oesophagus. Arch. Klin. Chir., 13:65, 1871.

Bremmer, C. G., Lynch, V. P., and Ellis, F. H., Jr.: Barrett's esophagus: Congenital or acquired? An experimental study of esophageal mucosal regeneration in the dog. Surgery, 68:209, 1970.

Butler, H.: Veins of oesophagus. Thorax, 6:276, 1951.

Cameron, A. J., Ott, B. J., and Payne, W. S.: The incidence of adenocarcinoma in columnar-lined (Barrett's) esophagus. N. Engl. J. Med., 313:857, 1985.

Cameron, A. J., Zinsmeister, A. R., Ballard, D. J., and Carney, J. A.: Prevalence of columnar-lined (Barrett's) esophagus. Comparison of population-based clinical and autopsy findings. Gastroenterology, 99:918, 1990.

Carey, J. M., and Hollingshead, W. H.: Anatomic study of esophageal hiatus. Surg. Gynecol. Obstet., 100:196, 1955.

Cederqvist, C., Nielsen, J., Berthelsen, A., et al.: Adenocarcinoma of the oesophagus. Acta Chir. Scand., 146:411, 1980.

Cheever, D. W.: Cited by Meade, R. H.: A History of Thoracic Surgery. Springfield, IL, Charles C. Thomas, 1961, p. 571.

Code, C. F., Creamer, B., Schlegel, J. F., et al.: An Atlas of Esophageal Motility in Health and Disease. Springfield, IL, Charles C. Thomas, 1958, pp. 1–134.

Coonley, C. J., Bains, M., Hilaris, B., et al.: Cisplatin and bleomycin in the treatment of esophagus carcinoma: A final report. Cancer, 54:2351, 1984.

Czerny, V.: Neue Operationen: Vorläufige Mittheilung. Zentrabl. Chir., 4:433, 1877.

Day, N. E.: Some aspects of the epidemiology of esophageal cancer. Cancer Res., 35:3304, 1975.

Doll, R., Payne, P., and Waterhouse, J. (eds): Cancer Incidence in Five Continents: A Technical Report. Vol. 1. New York, Springer-Verlag, 1966, pp. 1–241.

Duhaylongsod, F. G., and Wolfe, W. G.: Barrett's esophagus and adenocarcinoma of the esophagus and gastroesophageal junction. J. Thorac. Cardiovasc. Surg., 102:36, 1991.

Earlam, R., and Cunha-Melo, J. R.: Oesophageal squamous cell carcinoma. I: A critical review of surgery. Br. J. Surg., 67:381, 1980a.

Earlam, R., and Cunha-Melo, J. R.: Oesophageal squamous cell carcinoma. II: A critical review of radiotherapy. Br. J. Surg., 67:457, 1980b.

Fitzgibbons, R. J., Jr., Nugent, F. W., Ellis, F. H., Jr., and Braasch, J. W.: Unusual thoracoabdominal duplication associated with pancreaticopleural fistula. Gastroenterology, 79:344, 1980.

Fleischer, D., Kessler, F., and Haye, O.: Endoscopic Nd:YAG laser therapy for carcinoma of the esophagus: A new palliative approach. Am. J. Surg., 143:280, 1982.

Fok, M., Ah-Chong, A. K., Cheng, S. W. K., and Wong, J.: Comparison of a single-layer continuous hand-sewn method and circular stapling in 580 oesophageal anastomoses. Br. J. Surg., 78:342, 1991.

Fountain, S. W.: Leiomyoma of the esophagus. J. Thorac. Cardiovasc. Surg., 34:194, 1986.

Garfinkel, L., Poindexter, C. E., and Silverberg, E.: Cancer in black Americans. CA, 30:39, 1980.

Gillison, E. W., DeCastro, V. A., Nyhus, L. M., et al.: The significance of bile in reflux esophagitis. Surg. Gynecol. Obstet., 134:419, 1972.

Goddard, J. E., and McCranie, D.: Multiple leiomyomas of the esophagus. A. J. R., 259:117, 1973.

Gossot, D., Fourquier, P., el Meteini, M., and Celerier, M.: Technical aspects of endoscopic removal of benign tumors of the esophagus. Surg. Endosc., 7:102, 1993.

Goursaud, A. M.: Cited by Meade, R. H.: A History of Thoracic Surgery. Springfield, IL, Charles C. Thomas, 1961, p. 567.

Gunnlaugsson, G. H., Wychulis, A. R., Roland, C., et al.: Analysis of the records of 1657 patients with carcinoma of the esophagus and cardia of the stomach. Surg. Gynecol. Obstet., 130:997, 1970.

Haggitt, R. C., Tryzelaar, J., Ellis, F. H., Jr., et al.: Adenocarcinoma complicating columnar epithelium–lined (Barrett's) esophagus. Am. J. Clin. Pathol., 70:1, 1978.

Hawe, A., Payne, W. S., Weiland, L. H., et al.: Adenocarcinoma in the columnar epithelial–lined lower (Barrett) oesophagus. Thorax, 28:511, 1973.

Hesketh, P. J., Clapp, R. W., Doos, W. G., and Spechler, S. J.: The increasing frequency of adenocarcinoma of the esophagus. Cancer, 64:526, 1989.

Higgs, B., Shorter, R. G., and Ellis, F. H., Jr.: A study of the human esophagus with special reference to the gastroesophageal sphincter. J. Surg. Res., 5:503, 1965.

Hopkins, R. A., and Postlethwait, R. W.: Caustic burns and carcinoma of the esophagus. Ann. Surg., 194:146, 1981.

Huang, G. J., Zhang, D. W., Wang, G. Q., et al.: Surgical treatment of carcinoma of the esophagus: Report of 1647 cases. Chin. Med. J., 94:305, 1981.

Ingelfinger, F. J.: Esophageal motility. Physiol. Rev., 38:533, 1958.

Jainu, A.: Gastrotomie and Oesophagoplastik. Dtsch. Z. Chir., 118:383, 1912.

Kabuto, T., Taniguchi, K., Iwanaga, T., et al.: Diffuse leiomyomatosis of the esophagus. Dig. Dis. Sci., 25:388, 1980.

Kelsen, D., Hilaris, B., Coonley, C., et al.: Cisplatin, vindesine, and bleomycin chemotherapy of local-regional and advanced esophageal carcinoma. Am. J. Med., 75:645, 1983.

Kiviranta, U. K.: Corrosion carcinoma of esophagus: 381 cases of corrosion and 9 cases of corrosion carcinoma. Acta Otolaryngol., 42:89, 1952.

Kramer, M. D., Gibb, S. P., and Ellis, F. H., Jr.: Giant leiomyoma of the esophagus. J. Surg. Oncol., 33:166, 1986.

Kreuser, E. D.: Primary malignant melanoma of the esophagus. Virchows Arch. (Pathol. Anat.), 385:49, 1979.

Laimer, E.: Beitrag zur Anatomie des Oesophagus. Med. Jahrbücher, 1883, pp. 333–388.

Launois, B., Delarue, D., Campion, J. P., et al.: Preoperative radiotherapy for carcinoma of the esophagus. Surg. Gynecol. Obstet., 153:690, 1981.

Leape, L. L., Ashcraft, K. W., Scarpelli, D. G., et al.: Hazard to health—Liquid lye. N. Engl. J. Med., 284:578, 1971.

Levine, D. S., Haggitt, R. C., Blount, P. L., et al.: An endoscopic biopsy protocol can differentiate high-grade dysplasia from early adenocarcinoma in Barrett's esophagus. Gastroenterology, 105:40, 1993.

Lexer, E. B.: Oesophagoplastik: Verein für wissentschaftliche Heilkunde in Königsberg. Dtsch. Med. Wochenschr., 34:574, 1908.

Liebermann-Meffert, D., Allgöwer, M., Schmid, P., et al.: Muscular equivalent of the lower esophageal sphincter. Gastroenterology, 76:31, 1979.

Lolley, D., Razzuk, M. A., and Urschel, H. C., Jr.: Giant fibrovascular polyp of the esophagus. Ann. Thorac. Surg., 22:383, 1976.

Marshall, S. F.: Carcinoma of esophagus: Successful resection of lower end of esophagus with reestablishment of esophageal gastric continuity. Surg. Clin. North Am., 18:643, 1938.

Mayer, R. J.: Overview: The changing nature of esophageal cancer. Chest, 103:404S, 1993.

McGlashen, N. D., Walters, C. L., and McLean, A. E.: Nitrosamines in African alcoholic spirits and oesophageal cancer. Lancet, 2:1071, 1968.

Meyer, G. W., Austin, R. M., Brady, C. E., III, et al.: Muscle anatomy of the human esophagus. J. Clin. Gastroenterol., 8:131, 1986.

Meyerowitz, B. R., and Shea, L. T.: The natural history of squamous verrucose carcinoma of the esophagus. J. Thorac. Cardiovasc. Surg., 61:646, 1971.

Moore, J. H., Lesser, E. H., Erdody, D. H., et al.: Intestinal differentiation and p53 gene alterations in Barrett's esophagus and esophageal carcinoma. Int. J. Cancer, 56:487, 1994.

Naef, A. P., Savary, M., and Ozzella, L.: Columnar-lined lower esophagus: An acquired lesion with malignant predisposition. Report on 140 cases of Barrett's esophagus with 12 adenocarcinomas. J. Thorac. Cardiovasc. Surg., 70:826, 1975.

Naunheim, K. S.: Current status of preoperative treatment for carcinoma of the esophagus. Semin. Thorac. Cardiovasc. Surg., 4:270, 1992.

Nichols, T., Yokoo, H., Craig, R. M., et al.: Pseudosarcoma of the esophagus: Three new cases and review of the literature. Am. J. Gastroenterol., 72:615, 1979.

Ochsner, A., and Owens, N.: Anterothoracic oesophagoplasty for impermeable strictures of oesophagus. Ann. Surg., 100:1055, 1934.

Ohsawa, T.: The surgery of the esophagus. Arch. Jpn. Chir., 10:605, 1933.

Orringer, M. B.: Multimodality therapy for esophageal carcinoma—update. Chest, 103:4069, 1993.

Orringer, M. B., and Sloan, H.: Esophagectomy without thoracotomy. J. Thorac. Cardiovasc. Surg., 76:643, 1978.

Parker, E. F., Marks, R. D., Jr., Kratz, J. M., et al.: Chemoradiation therapy and resection for carcinoma of the esophagus: Short-term results. Ann. Thorac. Surg., 40:121, 1985.

Paull, A., Trier, J. D., Dalton, M. D., et al.: The histologic spectrum of Barrett's esophagus. N. Engl. J. Med., 295:476, 1976.

Pearson, J. G.: The present status and future potential of radiotherapy in the management of esophageal cancer. Cancer, 39(Suppl. 2):882, 1977.

Pera, C., Suner, M., and Capdevila, J.: Anatomical demonstration of the lower esophageal sphincter: A biometrical analysis of 300 specimens. Bull. Soc. Int. Chir., 34:285, 1975.

Raphael, H. A., Ellis, F. H., Jr., and Dockerty, M. B.: Primary adenocarcinoma of the esophagus: 18-year review and review of literature. Ann. Surg., 164:785, 1966.

Reid, H. A., Richardson, W. W., and Corrin, B.: Oat cell carcinoma of the esophagus. Cancer, 45:2342, 1980.

Robinson, J. C., Isa, S. S., Spees, E. K., et al.: Substernal gastric bypass for palliation of esophageal carcinoma: Rationale and technique. Surgery, 91:305, 1982.

Roux, C.: L'oesophago-jéjuno-gastrostomose, nouvelle opération pour rétrécissement infranchissable de l'oesophage. Sem. Méd., 27:37, 1907.

Rowland, C. G., and Pagliero, K. M.: Intracavitary irradiation in palliation of carcinoma of oesophagus and cardia. Lancet, 2:981, 1985.

Saito, T., Kinoshita, T., Shigemitsu, Y.: Risk factors associated with postoperative mortality in patients with esophageal cancer. Int. Surg., 78:93, 1993.

Sanfelippo, P. M., and Bernatz, P. E.: Celestin-tube palliation for malignant esophageal obstruction. Surg. Clin. North Am., 53:921, 1973.

Sarma, D. P., Rodriguez, F. H., Jr., Deiparine, E. M., and Weilbeacher, T. G.: Symptomatic granular cell tumor of the esophagus. J. Surg. Oncol., 33:246, 1986.

Schatzki, R., and Hawes, L. E.: Tumors of esophagus below mucosa and their roentgenological differential diagnosis. Rev. Gastroenterol., 17:991, 1950.

Seremetis, M. G., deGuzman, V. C., Lyons, W. S., et al.: Leiomyoma of the esophagus: A report of 19 surgical cases. Ann. Thorac. Surg., 16:308, 1973.

Shine, I., and Allison, P. R.: Carcinoma of the oesophagus with tylosis (keratosis palmaris et plantaris). Lancet, 1:951, 1966.

Shun'ichi, A., Tachibana, M., Shirasi, M., et al.: Lymph node metastasis in resectable esophageal cancer. J. Thorac. Cardiovasc. Surg., 100:287, 1990.

Silverberg, E., and Lubera, J. A.: Cancer statistics, 1988. CA, 38:5, 1988.

Skinner, D. B., Walther, B. C., Riddell, R. H., et al.: Barrett's esophagus: Comparison of benign and malignant cases. Ann. Surg., 198:554, 1983.

Spence, R. A. J.: The venous anatomy of the lower oesophagus in normal subjects and in patients with varices: An image analysis study. Br. J. Surg., 71:739, 1984.

Sprung, D. J., Ellis, F. H., Jr., and Gibb, S. P.: Incidence of adenocarcinoma in Barrett's esophagus [Abstract]. Am. J. Gastroenterol., 79:817, 1984.

Steiger, Z., Franklin, R., Wilson, R. F., et al.: Eradication and palliation of squamous cell carcinoma of the esophagus with chemotherapy, radiotherapy, and surgical therapy. J. Thorac. Cardiovasc. Surg., 82:713, 1981.

Stelzner, F.: Über den Dehnverschluss der terminalen Speiseröhre und seine Störunger. Dtsch. Med. Wochenschr., 96:1455, 1971.

Stener, B., Kock, N. G., Pettersson, S., et al.: Carcinosarcoma of the esophagus. J. Thorac. Cardiovasc. Surg., 54:746, 1967.

Subramanyam, K., Shannon, C. R., Patterson, M., et al.: Granular cell myoblastoma of the esophagus. J. Clin. Gastroenterol., 6:113, 1984.

Swigert, L. L., Siekert, R. G., Hanbley, W. C., et al.: Esophageal arteries: Anatomic study of 150 specimens. Surg. Gynecol. Obstet., 90:234, 1950.

Tarnay, T. J., Chang, C. H., Migert, R. G., et al.: Esophageal duplication (foregut cyst) with spinal malformation. J. Thorac. Cardiovasc. Surg., 59:293, 1970.

Torek, F.: The first successful case of resection of the thoracic portion of the oesophagus for carcinoma. Surg. Gynecol. Obstet., 16:614, 1913.

Voelcker, F.: Ueber Exstirpation der Cardia wegen Carcinoms. Verh. Dtsch. Ges. Chir., 37:126, 1908.

von Mikulicz, J.: Beiträge zur Technik der Operationen des Magencarcinoms. Arch. Klin. Chir., 57:524, 1898.

von Mikulicz, J.: Small contributions to the surgery of the intestinal tract. 1. Cardiospasm and its treatment. 2. Peptic ulcer of the jejunum. 3. Operative treatment of severe forms of invagination of the intestine. 4. Operation on malignant growths of the large intestine. Boston Med. Surg. J., 148:608, 1903.

Wald, H., and Polk, H. C., Jr.: Anatomical variations in hiatal and upper gastric areas and their relationship to difficulties experienced in operations for reflux esophagitis. Ann. Surg., 197:389, 1983.

Wang, L. S., Huang, M. H., Huang, B. S., and Chien, K. Y.: Gastric substitution for resectable carcinoma of the esophagus: An analysis of 368 cases. Ann. Thorac. Surg., 53:289, 1992.

Wheeler, W. I.: Pharyngocele and dilatation of pharynx, with existing diverticulum at lower portion of pharynx lying posterior to the oesophagus, cured by pharyngectomy, being the first case of the kind recorded. Dublin J. Med. Sci., 82:349, 1886.

Winters, C., Jr., Spurling, T. J., Chobanian, S. J., et al.: Barrett's esophagus: A prevalent, occult complication of gastroesophageal reflux disease. Gastroenterology, 92:118, 1987.

Wolfe, W. G., Burton, G. V., Seigler, H. F., et al.: Early results with combined modality therapy for carcinoma of the esophagus. Ann. Surg., 205:563, 1987.

Wolfe, W. G., Vaughn, A. L., Seigler, H. F., et al.: Survival of patients with carcinoma of the esophagus treated with combined-modality therapy. J. Thorac. Cardiovasc. Surg., 105:749, 1993.

Wu, Y. K., and Huang, K. C.: Chinese experience in the surgical treatment of carcinoma of the esophagus. Ann. Surg., 190:361, 1979.

Wynder, E. L., and Bross, I. J.: A study of etiological factors in cancer of the esophagus. Cancer, 14:389, 1961.

Wynder, E. L., Hultbert, S., Jacobson, F., et al.: Environmental factors in cancer of the upper alimentary tract: Swedish study with special reference to Plummer-Vinson (Paterson-Kelly) syndrome. Cancer, 10:470, 1957.

Zaino, C., Jacobsen, H. G., Lepow, H., et al.: The Pharyngoesophageal Sphincter. Springfield, IL, Charles C. Thomas, 1970, pp. 1–209.

■ II Disorders of the Esophagus in the Adult

André Duranceau

EMBRYOLOGY, ANATOMY, AND TISSUE ORGANIZATION OF THE ESOPHAGUS

Embryology of the Esophagus

Primitive Gut Formation

The primitive gut forms during the initial 4 weeks of development. During the second week, the embryo is a bilaminar disk formed by the ectoderm and the endoderm. When the mesoderm separates these two layers, the endoderm undergoes the changes necessary to become the primitive foregut (Gray and Skandalakis, 1972). The mesoderm then provides the material necessary for connective tissues, muscle coats of the gut, and serous coverings (Fig. 27–17).

Development of the larynx and of the tracheal diverticulum occurs during the seventh week. The larynx is seen as a protrusion of the anterior endodermal wall extending downward and surrounded by mesoderm. The elongating trachea develops alongside the esophagus without any fusion with it (Hamilton and Mossman, 1978; Moore, 1988) (Fig. 27–18). The esophagus at this point is very short, extending from the tracheal grove to the dilatation of the foregut, the future stomach. By the end of the seventh week, the esophagus reaches proportional relationships with its surrounding structures.

The gastroesophageal junction (GEJ) becomes better individualized as the greater curvature of the stomach grows larger. Following increased mitotic activity in this area, the height of the fundus and the acuteness of the angle of His become better defined and persist during subsequent development (Dankmeijer and Miète, 1961; Liebermann-Meffert, 1969) (Fig. 27–19). The supporting and anchoring structures of the esophagus result mostly from the mass of mesenchymal tissue that forms the early mediastinum. Around the distal esophagus, the septum transversum forms the diaphragm, and this is completed by the end of the sixth week.

The phrenoesophageal membrane, which holds the esophagus within the diaphragmatic hiatus, differentiates with the definitive formation of the diaphragmatic muscle.

Development of the Esophagus

Mucosa

When initially formed from the endoderm, the foregut shows a pseudostratified columnar epithelium surrounded by mesoderm (Fig. 27–20). With proliferation, the mucosa becomes multilayered and thicker

FIGURE 27–17. The endoderm becomes the primitive foregut. *a,* Endoderm over mesoderm. *b,* Endodermal rim. *c,* Formation of primitive intestinal tube. *d,* Primitive gut surrounded by mesoderm. (*a–d,* From Zuidema, G. D. [ed]: Shackelford's Surgery of the Alimentary Tract. Philadelphia, W. B. Saunders, 1996.)

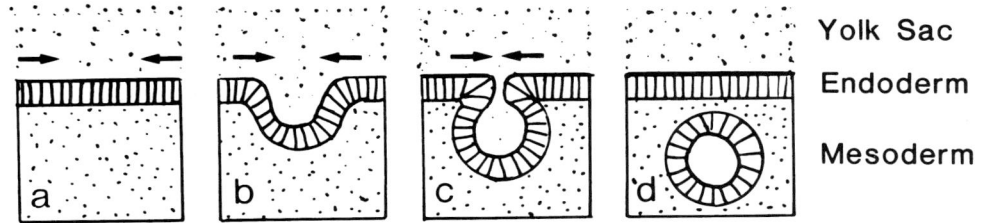

Yolk Sac
Endoderm
Mesoderm

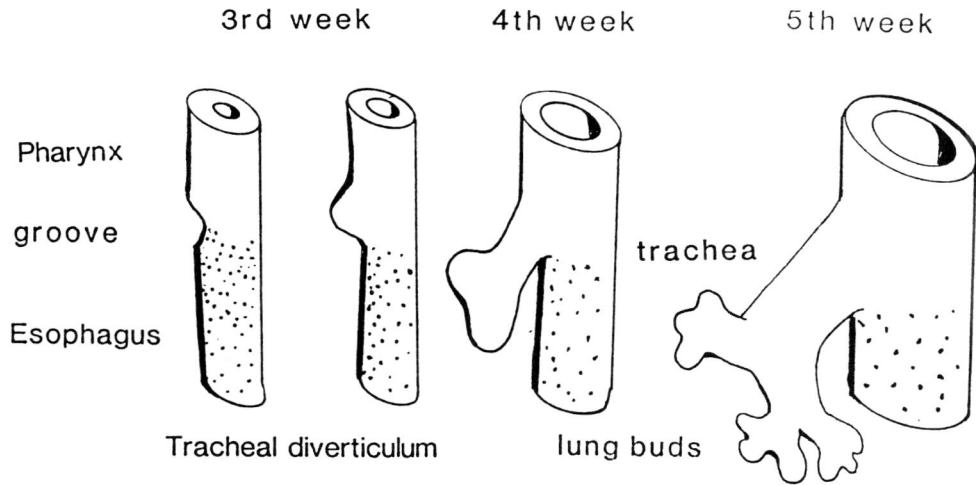

3rd week   4th week   5th week

Pharynx

groove

Esophagus

Tracheal diverticulum

trachea

lung buds

FIGURE 27–18. Appearance and downward elongation of trachea and lung bud. Both structures remain independent. (From Zuidema, G. D. [ed]: Shackelford's Surgery of the Alimentary Tract. Philadelphia, W. B. Saunders, 1996.)

FIGURE 27–19. Individualization of the gastroesophageal junction (GEJ). The cardia is held in place by its dorsal attachment while mitotic activity within the greater curvature of the stomach gives the gastric pouch its definitive configuration. (SSL = sagittal section length.) (From Zuidema, G. D. [ed]: Shackelford's Surgery of the Alimentary Tract. Philadelphia, W. B. Saunders, 1996.)

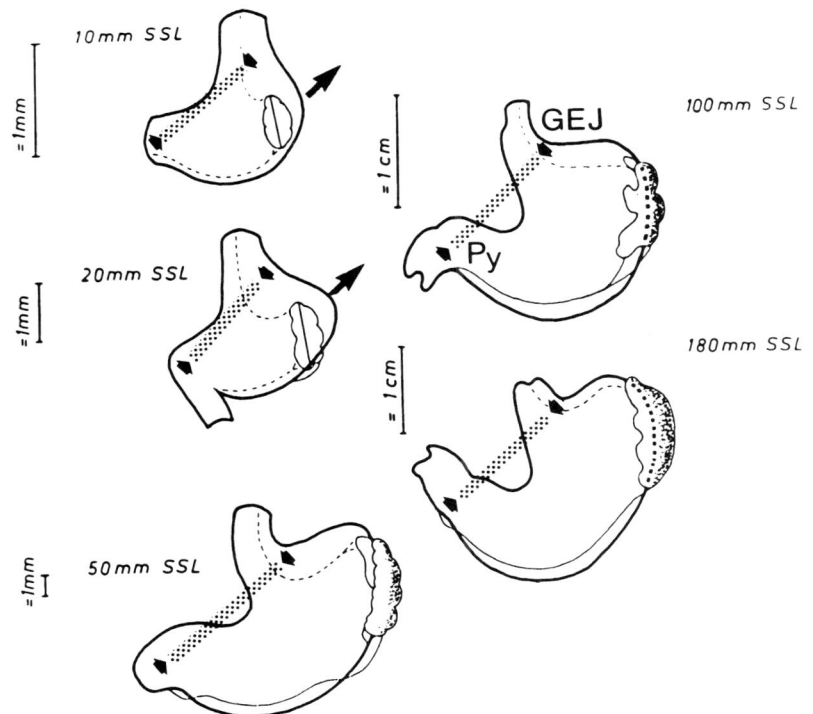

10mm SSL

20mm SSL

50mm SSL

GEJ

Py

100mm SSL

180mm SSL

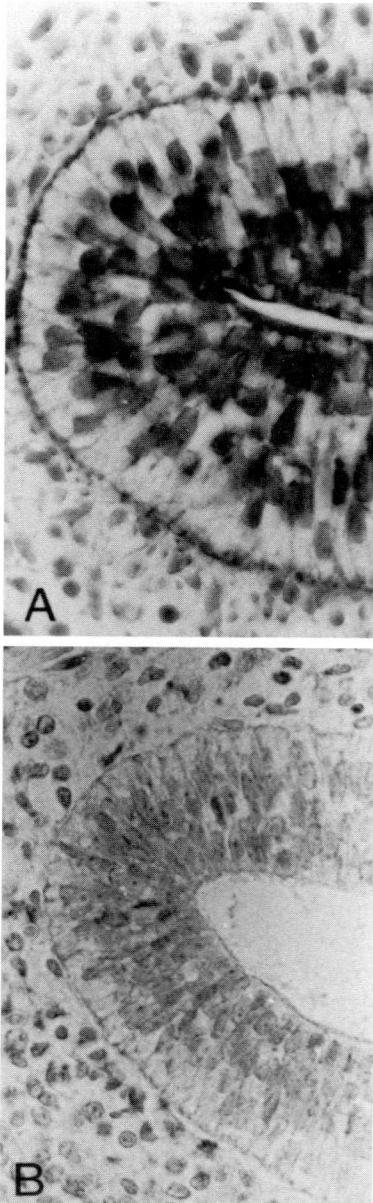

FIGURE 27–20. Esophageal epithelium *(A)* and gastric epithelium *(B)* in the embryo. The esophageal epithelium is stratified and columnar. (*A* and *B*, From Zuidema, G. D. [ed]: Shackelford's Surgery of the Alimentary Tract. Philadelphia, W. B. Saunders, 1996.)

(Johns, 1952). When the embryo grows from 12 to 25 mm, vacuoles will appear in the epithelium and increase progressively in number until the 29-mm stage (Fig. 27–21). This vacuolization of the epithelium then progressively decreases until the 75-mm stage. The overall significance of vacuolization remains unclear (Liebermann-Meffert, 1969).

At about the 40-mm stage, the basal layer gives rise to a ciliated columnar epithelium. These cells will cover the entire esophageal mucosa in the 60-mm embryo. These ciliated cells are progressively replaced by a stratified squamous epithelium migrating crani-

ally and caudally from the middle third of the esophagus. Some patches of the ciliated epithelium may remain at birth, usually in the proximal esophagus (Menard and Arsenault, 1987; Mueller-Botha, 1959) (Fig. 27–22).

Muscularis

The striated muscle is derived from the caudal branchial arches and is innervated by the motor branches of the vagi. Smooth musculature derives from the splanchnic mesoderm and receives innervation from the sympathetic nervous system. These cells originate from similar mesenchymal cells in the 10-mm embryo. The longitudinal and circular layers are complete at the 20-mm stage. In the 90-mm fetus, they show muscular arrangement comparable to that of the adult (Liebermann-Meffert, 1969; Liebermann-Meffert and Duranceau, 1994) (Fig. 27–23).

Vascular and Lymphatic Supply

Arterial venous and lymphatic flow follows a bidirectional pattern. Vessels originating from the branchial region irrigate distally, whereas the vascular supply (Fig. 27–24) of the celiac axis irrigates the esophagus in a cranial direction. Venous and lymphatic drainage follows the same flow pattern and appears 2 weeks after formation of the cardiovascular system (Hamilton and Mossman, 1978; Moore, 1988) (Fig. 27–25).

Innervation

Efferent fibers to the esophagus and foregut arise from the specialized dorsal motor nucleus. These nerves fuse in the last three branchial arches to form the vagi. Afferent fibers develop from the neuroblasts of the neural crest: They form the ganglions in the esophageal wall with a complete periesophageal neural network around the circular muscle layer before differentiation of the longitudinal muscle layer. Although the myenteric plexus can be identified in the fetus at 10 weeks (see Fig. 27–23B[3]), the innervation of the submucosa and muscularis mucosa becomes complete later, in the 90-mm fetus (Smith and Taylor, 1972).

Anatomy and Tissue Organization of the Esophagus

Macroscopic Features

The esophagus is a soft and flat muscular tube that opens at the cricopharyngeus level and ends at the junction with the stomach. It lies on the anterior aspect of the spine during most of its descent. Three natural narrowings also serve as identification landmarks during endoscopic procedures: the cricopharyngeus or upper esophageal sphincter, located between 14 and 16 cm from the incisors; the imprint of

PRENATAL DEVELOPMENT OF THE MUCOSA IN THE HUMAN ESOPHAGUS

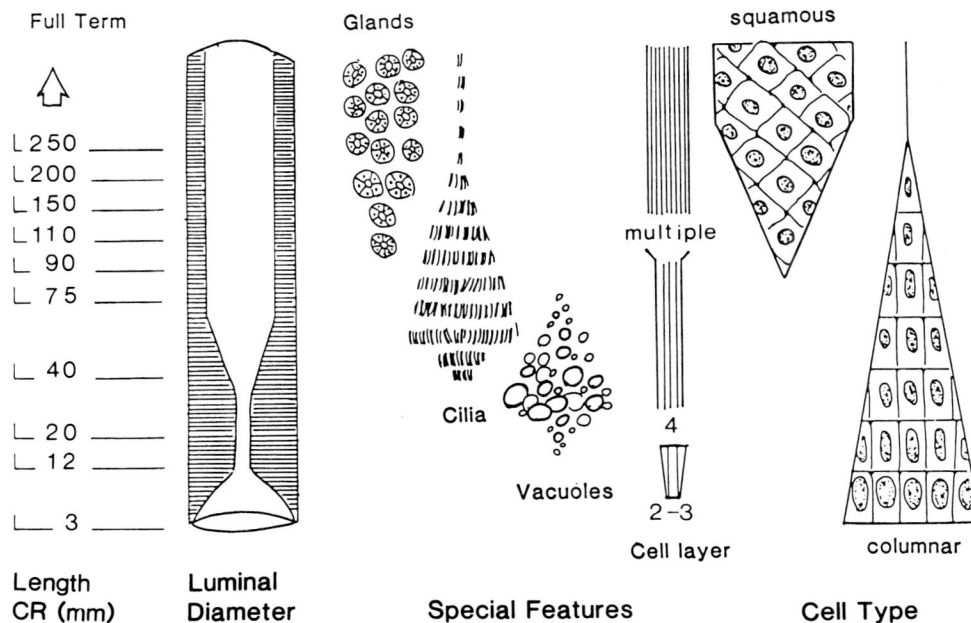

FIGURE 27–21. Development of the mucosa in the esophagus shows early changes in diameter related to changes in the type of epithelium. The vacuolization period occurs from 12- to 40-mm crown-rump length (CR) stage, with progressive disappearance of the vacuoles until the 75-mm stage. (From Zuidema, G. D. [ed]: Shackelford's Surgery of the Alimentary Tract. Philadelphia, W. B. Saunders, 1996.)

the aortic arch and left main bronchus, seen on the left anterior and lateral wall at 22 cm from the incisors; the third narrowing is at the lower end of the esophagus, between 40 and 45 cm from the incisors. This third narrowing may be explained by the function of the *lower esophageal sphincter* (LES), by the mechanical effect of the diaphragmatic hiatus, and by the angulation of the esophagus entering the stomach cavity (Savary and Miller, 1978) (Fig. 27–26).

The esophagus measures 22 to 28 cm in length, of which 2 to 6 cm may be intra-abdominal. The esophageal length is influenced by the subject's height (Liebermann-Meffert and Duranceau, 1994; Liebermann-Meffert and Siewert, 1992). The topographic anatomy of the esophagus is best described by computed tomography (CT) scan schematic views (Fig. 27–27). The relationship of the esophagus, with surrounding structures, within its mediastinal bed has been studied extensively by Lerche (1950) and described by Wegener (1983). Both the esophagus and the trachea are embedded between the pretracheal fascia anteriorly and the prevertebral fascia posteriorly. Posteriorly, this fascia extends from the base of the skull to the diaphragm. In the pretracheal space, the fascial plane surrounds the mediastinal vessels and fuses with the posterior fascia at the thoracic inlet to form the carotid sheaths (see Fig. 27–27B–F).

The esophagus has no serosa, but its location within these fascias gives a "mesentery effect" in which the supporting and the supplying structures to and from the esophagus are found. Anteriorly and laterally, the esophagus is anchored to the trachea by fibroelastic

tissues. Loose connective tissue keeps it attached to the posterior fascia. Anteriorly, the distal half of the esophagus is in close contact with subcarinal tissues and the posterior pericardium. The esophagus traverses the diaphragm through the hiatus at the level of the tenth dorsal vertebra. It is anchored in the hiatal orifice by the phrenoesophageal membrane, an extension of the subdiaphragmatic and endothoracic aponeurosis (see Fig. 27–41).

Supply to and from the Esophagus

ARTERIES

The arterial supply to the esophagus and its intramural organization has been studied extensively by Liebermann-Meffert and co-workers (1987, 1992). There are three principal sources of arterial blood for the esophagus (Fig. 27–28). In the neck, the superior and inferior thyroid arteries send small arteries to the cervical esophagus. In the chest, at the level of the aortic arch, three to five tracheobronchial arteries originate from under the aortic arch and one tracheobronchial artery arises from the anterior surface of the aorta just distal to the arch. One to two pairs of esophageal arteries may originate from the anterior surface of the descending aorta. At the GEJ, the left gastric artery supplies two to six arteries to the lower esophagus and to the anterior aspect of the cardia and proximal small curvature of the stomach. The splenic artery feeds the posterior esophageal wall and part of the posterior smaller and greater curvature of

Text continued on page 943

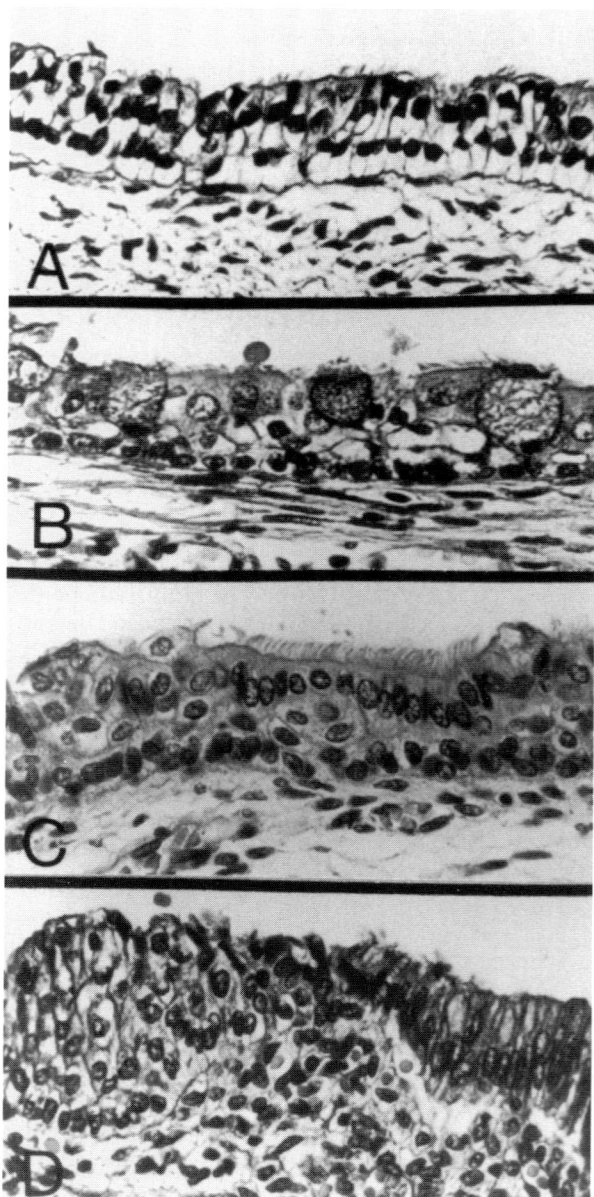

FIGURE 27–22. Development of the esophageal mucosa. *A*, Ciliated, pseudostratified columnar epithelium at 2 mm. *B*, Ciliated columnar cells and goblet cells at 190 mm. *C*, Squamous replacement process, with patches of remaining ciliated epithelium. *D*, Residual island of mucin-secreting cells in the esophagus of a newborn. (*A–D*, From Enterline, H., and Thompson, J.: Pathology of the Esophagus. Heidelberg, Springer-Verlag, 1984.)

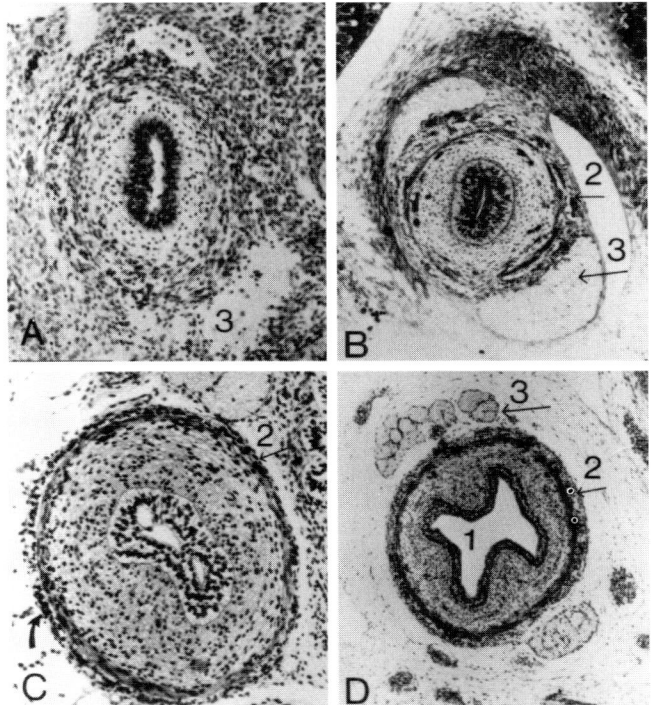

FIGURE 27–23. A–D, Development of esophageal muscle layers in the embryo. The inner muscle coat (2) is progressively covered by neural cells (3), precursors of the vagi. The longitudinal muscle appears over this early innervation at 40-mm CR. (A–D, From Enterline, H., and Thompson, J.: Pathology of the Esophagus. Heidelberg, Springer-Verlag, 1984.)

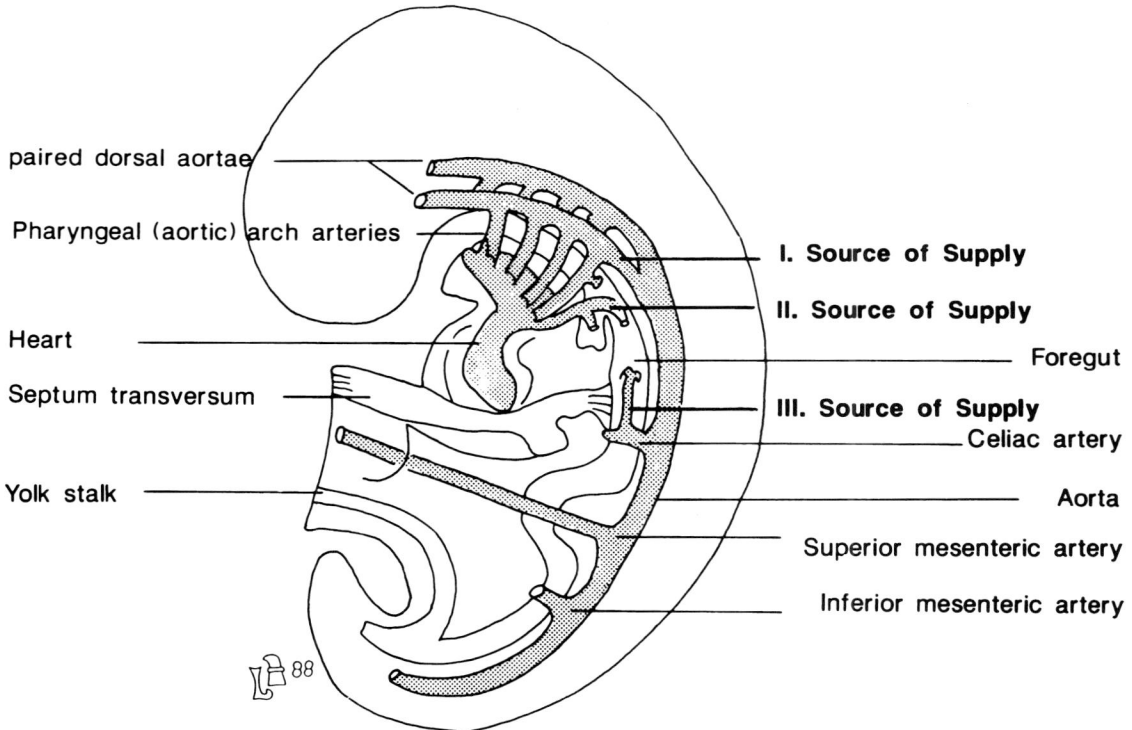

FIGURE 27–24. Development of the arterial blood supply for the foregut. Vessels from the branchial region irrigate distally. Vessels from the celiac axis irrigate cranially. (From Moore, K. L., and Persaud, T. V. N.: The Developing Human, 5th ed., Philadelphia, W. B. Saunders, 1993.)

DERIVATIVES OF

BRANCHIAL ARCHES

▸ Striated Muscle

▸ Vagus Nerve

▸ Aortic Arch

TRACHEAL BIFURCATION

SPLANCHNIC MESODERM

▸ Smooth Muscle

▸ Sympathetic Innervation

▸ Descending Aorta

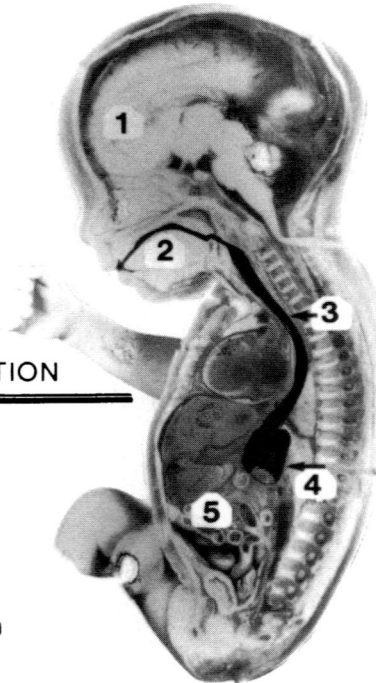

DIRECTION OF FLOW

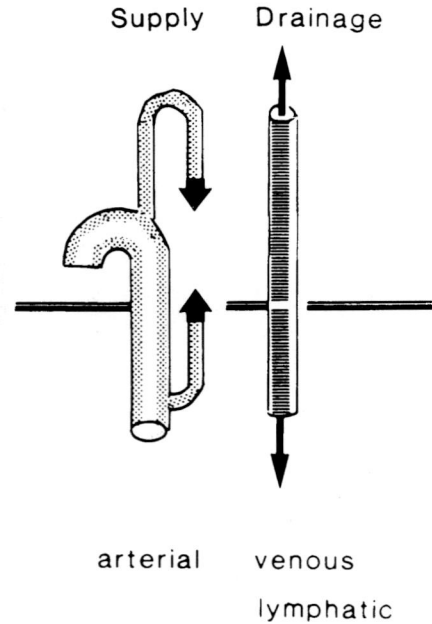

Supply   Drainage

arterial   venous

lymphatic

FIGURE 27–25. Bidirectional organization of vessels, lymphatics, and nerves above and below the tracheal bifurcation. (From Zuidema, G. D. [ed]: Shackelford's Surgery of the Alimentary Tract. Philadelphia, W. B. Saunders, 1995.)

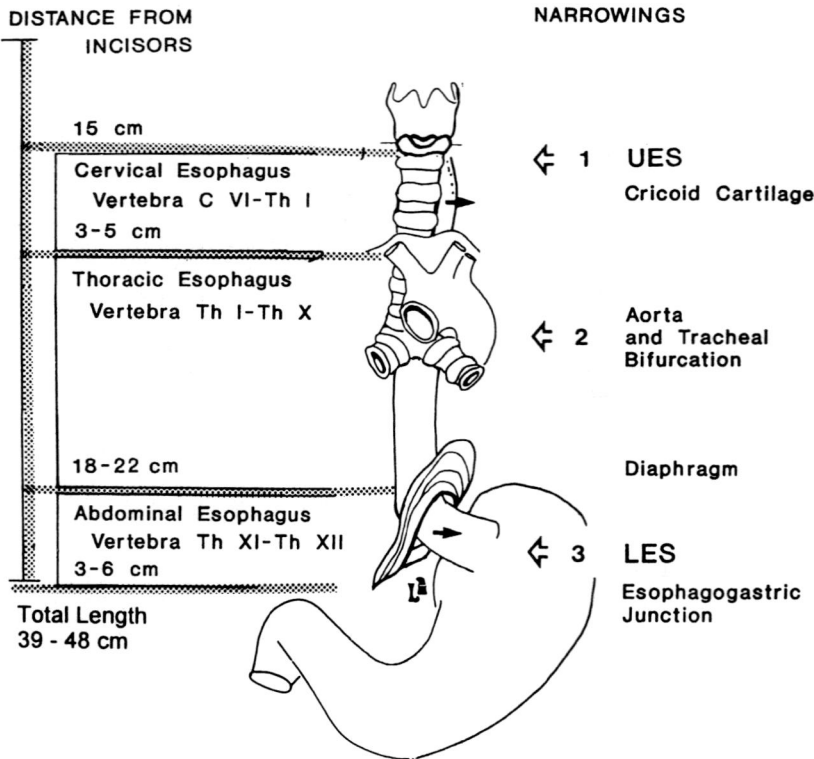

DISTANCE FROM
INCISORS

15 cm

Cervical Esophagus
Vertebra C VI–Th I
3–5 cm

Thoracic Esophagus
Vertebra Th I–Th X

18–22 cm

Abdominal Esophagus
Vertebra Th XI–Th XII
3–6 cm

Total Length
39 – 48 cm

NARROWINGS

⇐ 1   UES
Cricoid Cartilage

⇐ 2   Aorta
and Tracheal
Bifurcation

Diaphragm

⇐ 3   LES
Esophagogastric
Junction

FIGURE 27–26. Three narrowings can be identified at endoscopy: the pharyngoesophageal junction, the imprint of the aorta and left mainstem bronchus, and the esophagogastric junction. (UES = upper esophageal sphincter; LES = lower esophageal sphincter; C = cervical; Th = thoracic.) (From Zuidema, G. D. [ed]: Shackelford's Surgery of the Alimentary Tract. Philadelphia, W. B. Saunders, 1996.)

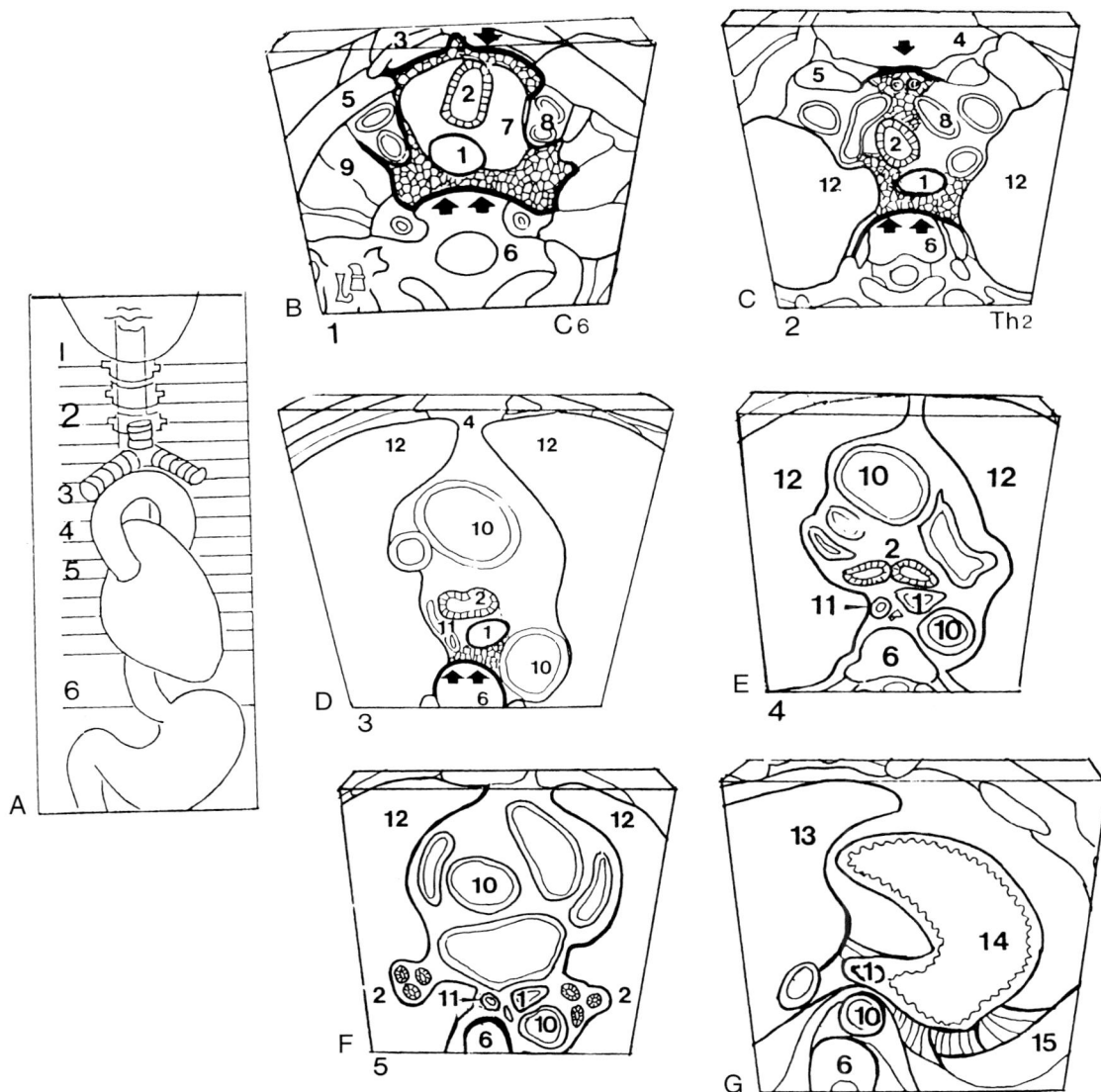

FIGURE 27–27. *A,* The topographic anatomy of the esophagus within its mediastinal bed. Anatomy of the esophagus in the neck and at the thoracic inlet *(B and C),* within the chest *(D–F),* and at the esophagogastric junction *(G).* (1 = esophagus; 2 = trachea; 3 = sternum; 4 = ribs; 5 = musculature; 6 = vertebra; 7 = thyroid gland; 8 = vessels; 9 = musculature; 10 = aorta and heart; 11 = azygos vein and thoracic duct; 12 = thoracic cavity; 13 = liver; 14 = stomach; 15 = spleen and ligaments.) *(A–G,* Adapted from Weisbrodt, N. W.: Neuromuscular organization of esophageal and pharyngeal motility. Arch. Intern. Med., *136:*524–531, 1976. Copyright 1976, American Medical Association.)

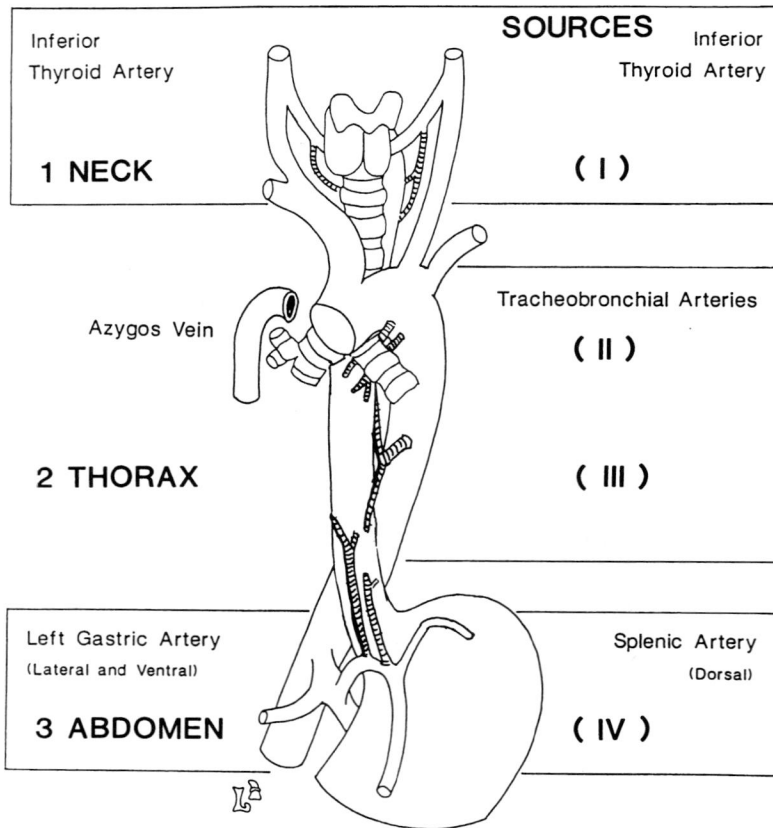

FIGURE 27–28. The arterial supply to the esophagus originates from three separate sources in the neck, chest, and upper abdomen. (From Zuidema, G. D. [ed]: Shackelford's Surgery of the Alimentary Tract. Philadelphia, W. B. Saunders, 1996.)

FIGURE 27–29. *A* and *B,* The arteries to the esophagus branch early to become a richly anastomosed intramural plexus. (*A* and *B,* From Zuidema, G. D. [ed]: Shackelford's Surgery of the Alimentary Tract. Philadelphia, W. B. Saunders, 1996.)

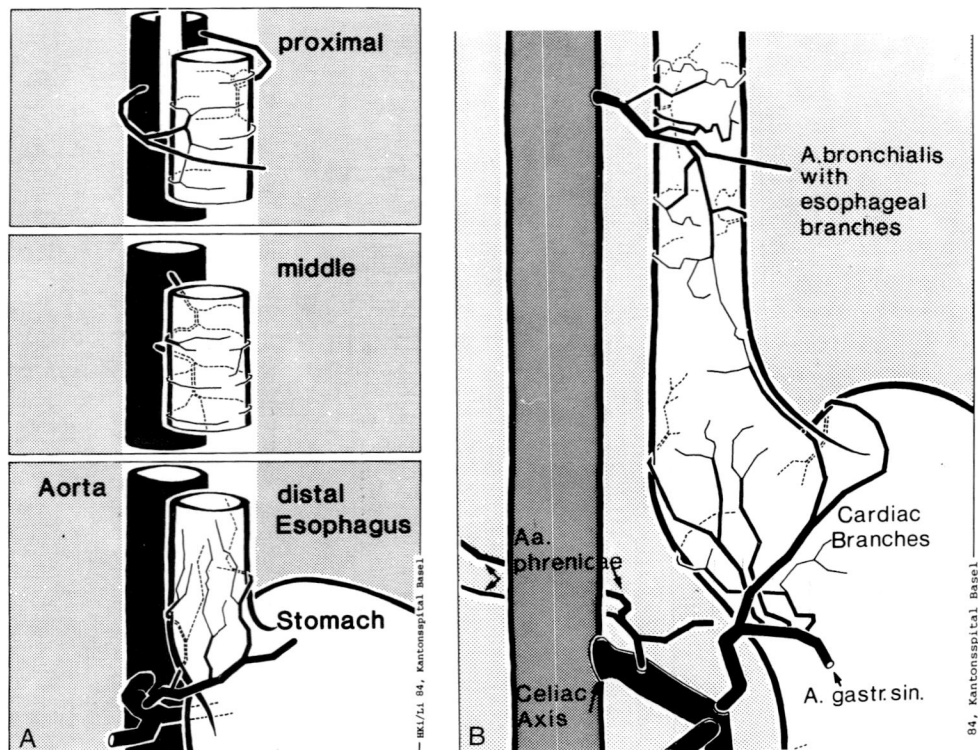

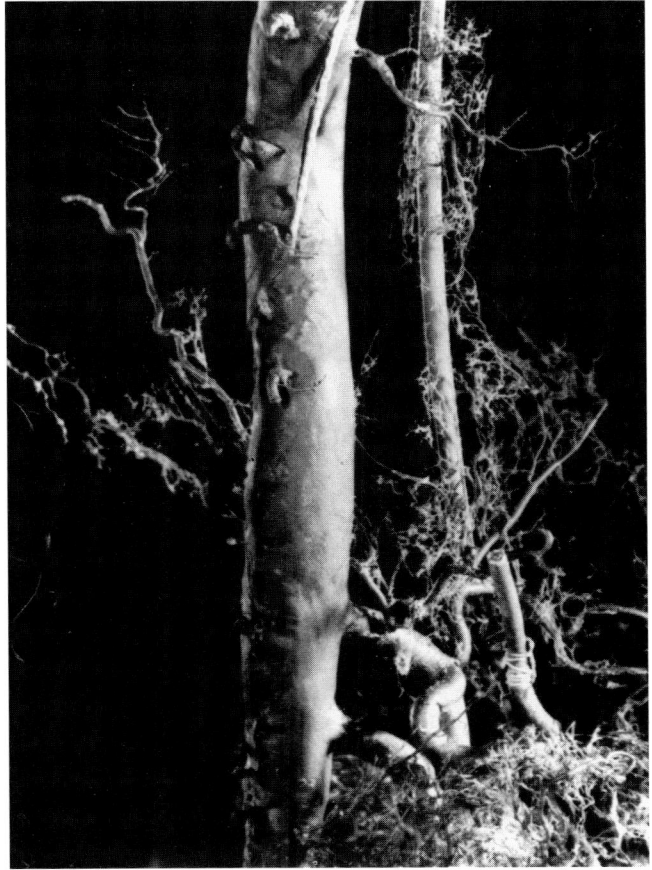

FIGURE 27–30. Arterial casts study showing the extensive connections of the arteries at the middle and lower esophageal levels. (From Zuidema, G. D. [ed]: Shackelford's Surgery of the Alimentary Tract. Philadelphia, W. B. Saunders, 1996.)

the stomach. At all levels, the esophageal arteries show early branching within the periesophageal tissues and within the wall, forming a richly anastomosed intramural plexus (Figs. 27–29 and 27–30).

VEINS

Intraesophageal veins follow a drainage pattern similar to that of the lymphatics from a subepithelial position. They drain in a submucous plexus to form communicating veins arranged longitudinally and perforating veins that pierce the muscularis, receiving contributing vessels from the muscle. They eventually form the extraesophageal veins, which drain into the inferior thyroid veins, the azygos and hemiazygos veins, the left gastric and the splenic veins, and the left gastroepiploic veins (Butler, 1951) (Figs. 27–31 to 27–33).

LYMPHATICS

Submucosal lymphatics form long channels that run parallel to the esophageal axis. These lymphatics may travel over a considerable distance in the mucosa and submucosa before passing through the muscularis into regional lymph nodes (see Fig. 27–32).

Once across the esophageal wall, lymphatics drain into subadventitial lymphatic trunks at the surface of the esophageal wall. These trunks have valves that

direct lymph flow toward regional lymph nodes in the neck and in the chest (see Figs. 27–31 and 27–33). In the abdomen, lymph drains toward the gastric superior, pericardial, and inferior diaphragmatic nodes. Lymph above the tracheal bifurcation drains mostly toward the neck. Lymph below the carina flows mostly toward the celiac nodes. Lymph flow at the bifurcation is bidirectional (Haagensen et al., 1972; Lehnert et al., 1947; Rouvière, 1932).

INNERVATION

Extraesophageal innervation is sympathetic and parasympathetic (Fig. 27–34). Sympathetic nerves enter the esophagus from the cervical and thoracic chains located along the dorsal vertebrae. The celiac plexus and ganglia send fibers to the distal esophagus and cardia. *Parasympathetic innervation* occurs through the vagus nerve. Both vagi originate from the dorsal vagal nucleus. They cross into the neck through the jugular foramina, where they innervate the pharynx, cervical esophagus, larynx, and trachea by their cervical plexus. Both nerves descend along the large vessels in the neck and are found along the posterior hilar structures in the chest. The recurrent laryngeal nerves originate from the vagi around the subclavian artery on the right and around the aortic arch on the left. Both recurrent nerves then ascend in their

From Lateral =
RIGHT THORACIC APPROACH

Thoracic Esophagus

Sup.Caval Vein

right Bronchi

Lung

Intercostal
Veins

Paratracheal
Lymph Nodes

Dorsal

Azygos Vein   right Vagus

MRIIC

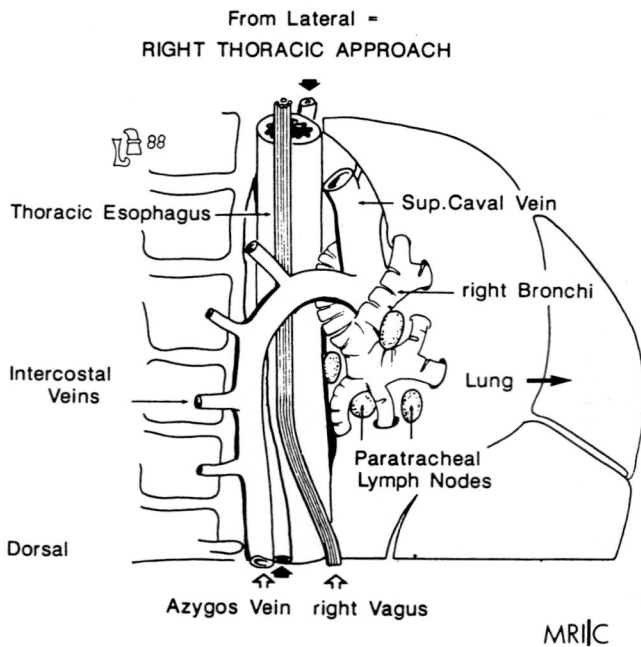

FIGURE 27–31. Venous drainage of the esophagus. In the right side of the chest, esophageal veins drain toward the azygos. Inferior thyroid veins, hemiazygos veins, and left gastric and gastroepiploic veins are the other tributaries from the esophagus. (*black arrow =* thoracic duct.) (From Zuidema, G. D. [ed]: Shackelford's Surgery of the Alimentary Tract. Philadelphia, W. B. Saunders, 1996.)

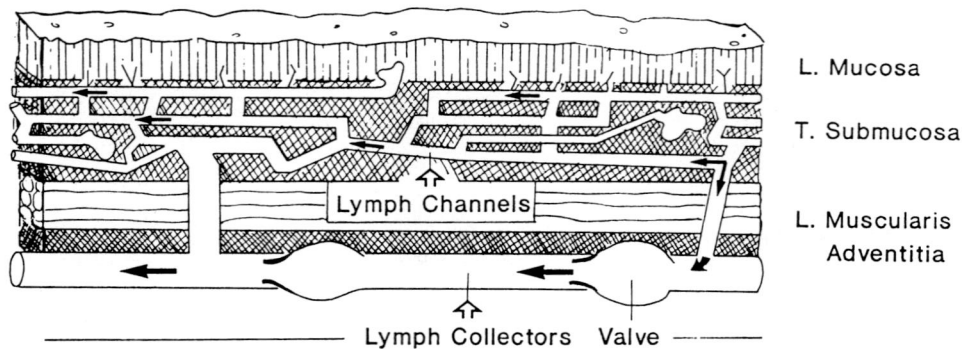

L. Mucosa

T. Submucosa

L. Muscularis
Adventitia

Lymph Channels

Lymph Collectors   Valve

FIGURE 27–32. Lymphatic drainage within the esophageal wall. (From Zuidema, G. D. [ed]: Shackelford's Surgery of the Alimentary Tract. Philadelphia, W. B. Saunders, 1996.)

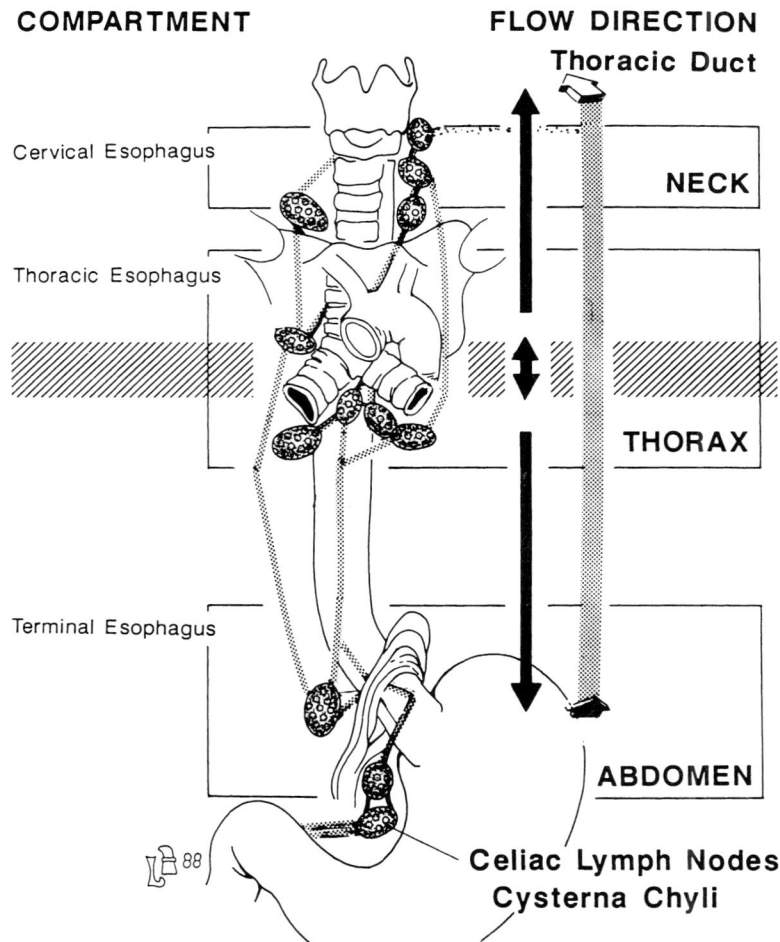

COMPARTMENT

Cervical Esophagus

Thoracic Esophagus

Terminal Esophagus

FLOW DIRECTION
Thoracic Duct

NECK

THORAX

ABDOMEN

Celiac Lymph Nodes
Cysterna Chyli

FIGURE 27–33. Bidirectional flow of lymph from the esophagus. Above the tracheal bifurcation, drainage is mostly toward the neck. Below the carina, lymph flows mostly toward the celiac nodes. Flow at the bifurcation is bidirectional and can be influenced by pathology. (From Zuidema, G. D. [ed]: Shackelford's Surgery of the Alimentary Tract. Philadelphia, W. B. Saunders, 1996.)

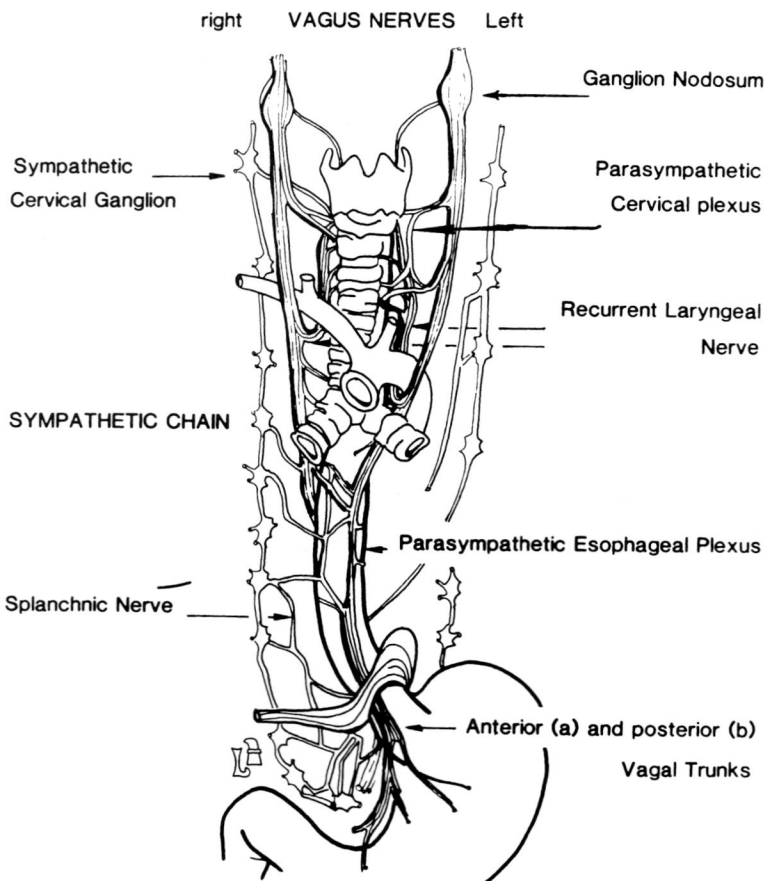

FIGURE 27–34. Innervation of the esophagus. (From Zuidema, G. D. [ed]: Shackelford's Surgery of the Alimentary Tract. Philadelphia, W. B. Saunders, 1996.)

respective tracheoesophageal grooves. After giving off branches to the lung, both vagi form a periesophageal plexus and then the right and left main trunks, identified above the hiatus just before crossing into the abdomen with the esophagus (see Fig. 27–34).

The intramural innervation shows a muscular plexus around the circular layer of the muscularis (Auerbach's plexus). Its cells are all along the esophagus, with maximal concentration around the terminal esophagus. Meissner's plexus is submucosal. Both are interconnected and are responsible for the fine-control mechanisms of esophageal function (Christensen, 1978; Cunningham and Sawchenko, 1990; Weisbrodt, 1976) (see Fig. 27–37B).

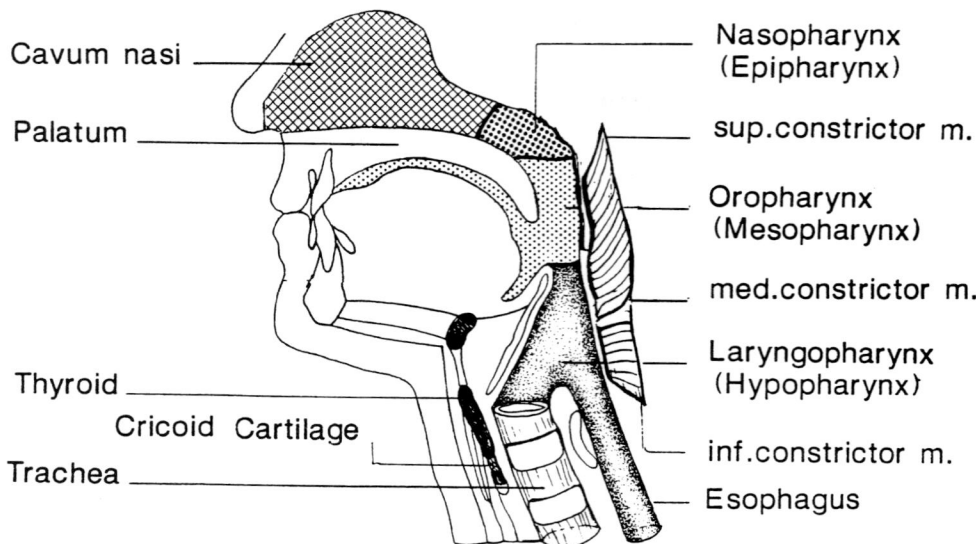

FIGURE 27–35. Anatomic division of the pharyngoesophageal junction. (From Zuidema, G. D. [ed]: Shackelford's Surgery of the Alimentary Tract. Philadelphia, W. B. Saunders, 1996.)

Tissue Organization

PHARYNGOESOPHAGEAL JUNCTION

The esophagus is limited proximally by the cricopharyngeus, a sling of striated muscle considered to be part of the inferior constrictor of the pharynx. It is inserted on both posterior laminae of the cricoid cartilage and exerts pressure at rest to close the proximal esophagus. The cricopharyngeus continues downward with the longitudinal and circular esophageal muscle (Zaino et al., 1978). The submucosa of the pharyngoesophageal junction may contain a large submucous venous plexus, possibly influenced by dysfunction in this region (Figs. 27–35 and 27–36A and B).

ESOPHAGEAL BODY

Adventitia. This represents loose connective tissue enveloping the esophagus. It contains nerves, lymphatics, and vessels.

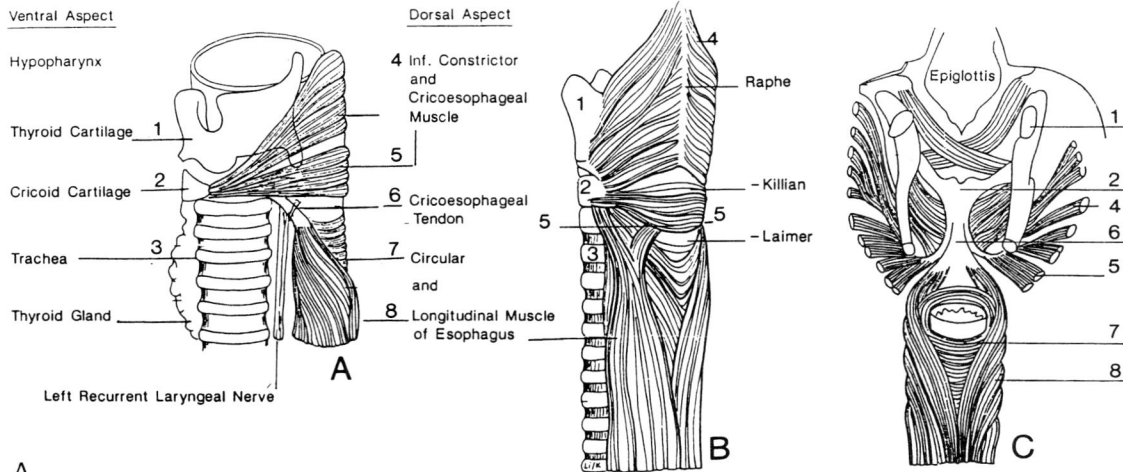

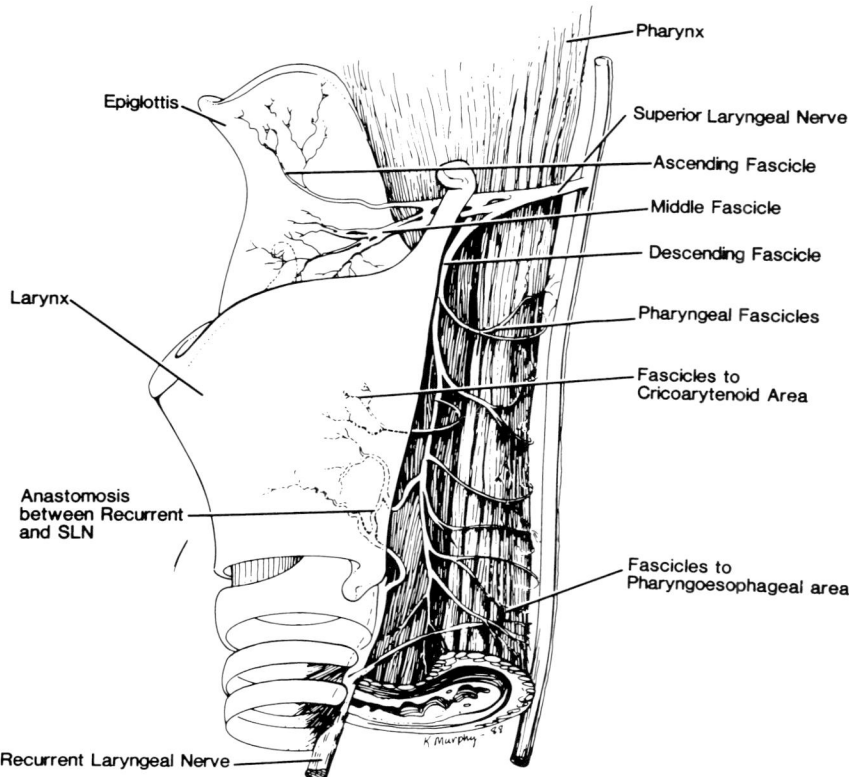

FIGURE 27–36. A (A–C), Muscular organization of the pharynx, UES, and cervical esophagus. B, Innervation of the pharyngoesophageal junction. (SLN = superior laryngeal nerve.) (A, From Zuidema, G. D. [ed]: Shackelford's Surgery of the Alimentary Tract. Philadelphia, W. B. Saunders, 1996; B, From The Esophagus, Castell D. O. Boston, Little, Brown, 1992. Published by Little, Brown and Company.)

Muscularis. The muscularis shows two muscle layers; the outer muscularis layer parallels the longitudinal axis of the esophagus (Fig. 27–37). Interconnecting fibers relate it to the inferior constrictor of the pharynx. At the GEJ, reorientation of the fibers is in continuity with longitudinal gastric muscle. The circular layer of the muscularis begins at the cricoid cartilage level, where the cricopharyngeus may blend to some degree with its fibers. Imperfect circles of muscle overlap and give the circular aspect to the layer along the esophageal body (Fig. 27–37A). There is progressive replacement of striated muscle fibers in the proximal esophagus by smooth muscle fibers over the distal two-thirds of the organ (Fig. 27–38). At the GEJ, the circular layer shows a special organization of its fibers. Asymmetric thickening occurs and accounts

for the elevated pressure zone recorded physiologically (Liebermann-Meffert et al., 1979, 1985) (Figs. 27–39 and 27–40).

Submucosa. The submucosa connects the muscularis and the mucosa. It is the strongest layer, containing elastic and collagenous fibers with a network of vessels and nerves. Deep esophageal glands penetrate the muscularis mucosa to enter the submucosa (see Fig. 27–39).

Mucosa. The muscularis mucosa is responsible for the rippling effect seen on the mucosa at endoscopy. The tunica propria projects into the epithelium, forming the papillae. The mucosa shows a multilayered squamous epithelium with a basal layer lying on the tunica propria. The junction of the squamous mucosa with the columnar epithelium of the stomach shows

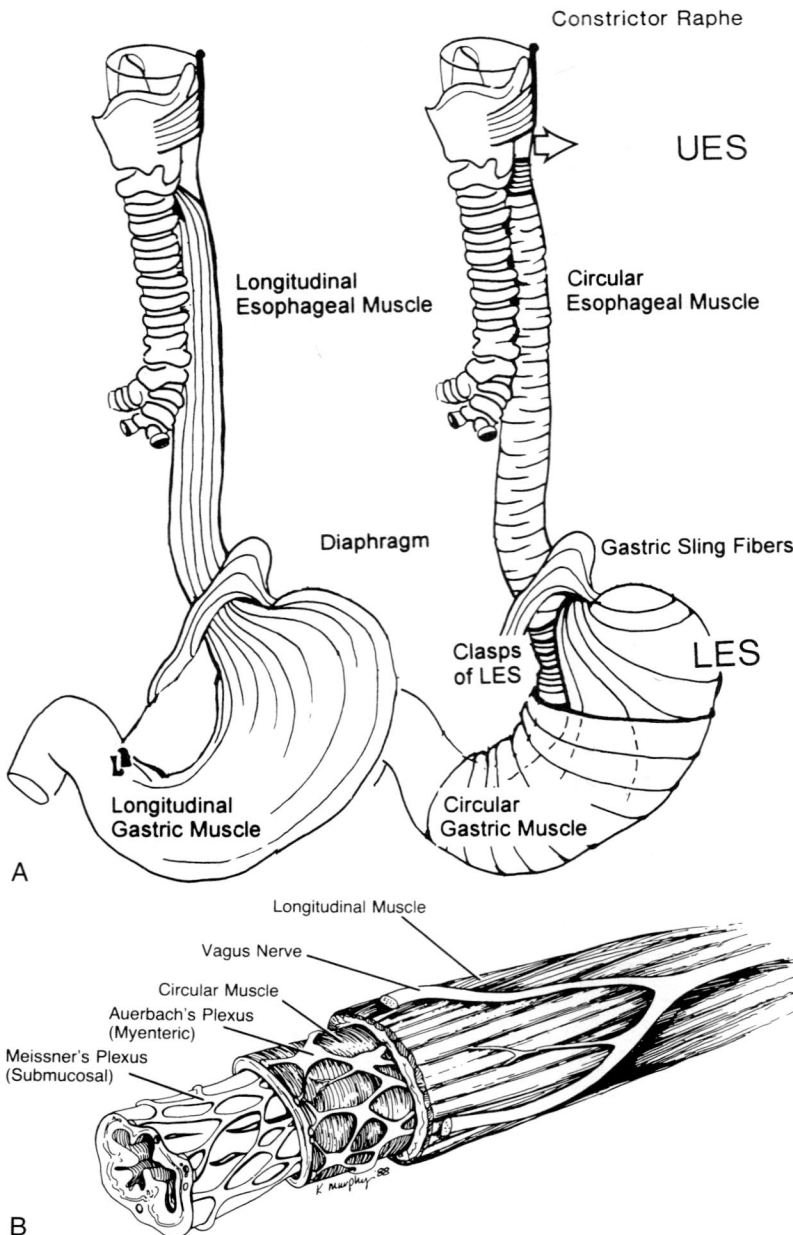

FIGURE 27–37. A and B, Architecture of the longitudinal and circular muscle layers in the esophagus. (UES = upper esophageal sphincter; LES = lower esophageal sphincter.) (A and B, From Zuidema, G. D. [ed]: Shackelford's Surgery of the Alimentary Tract. Philadelphia, W. B. Saunders, 1996.)

MUSCLE TYPE

Striated

HISTOLOGY

10

14

≈24 cm

Smooth

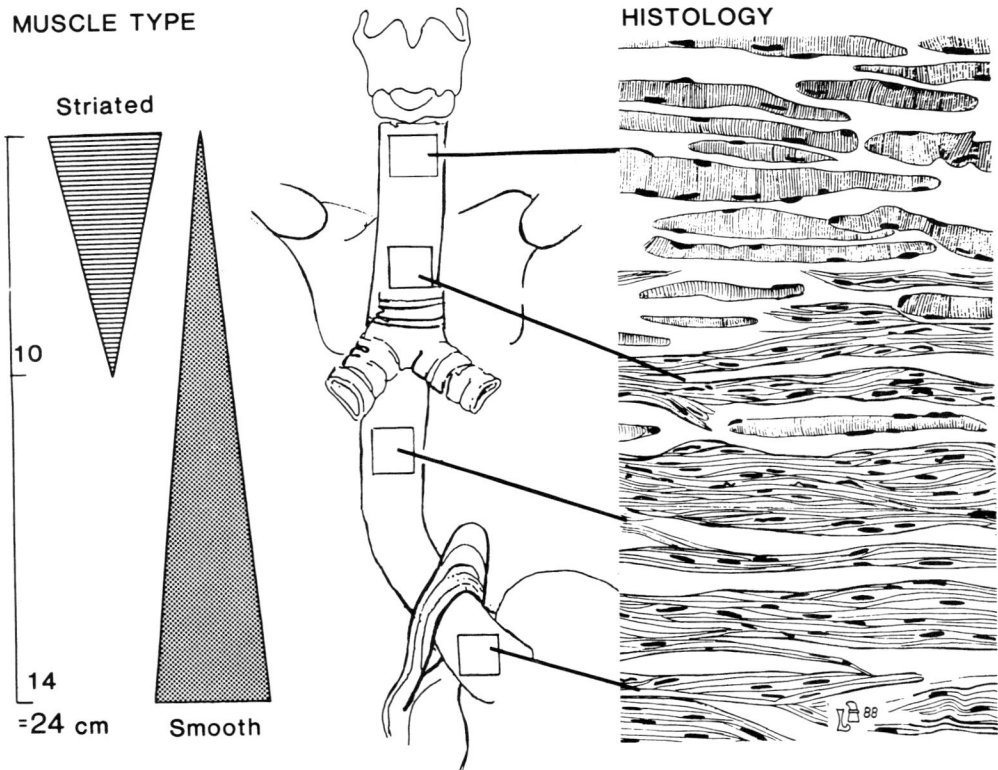

FIGURE 27–38. Progressive replacement of the striated muscle by smooth muscle in both layers of the esophagus. Below the tracheal bifurcation, only smooth muscle fibers persist. (From Zuidema, G. D. [ed]: Shackelford's Surgery of the Alimentary Tract. Philadelphia, W. B. Saunders, 1996.)

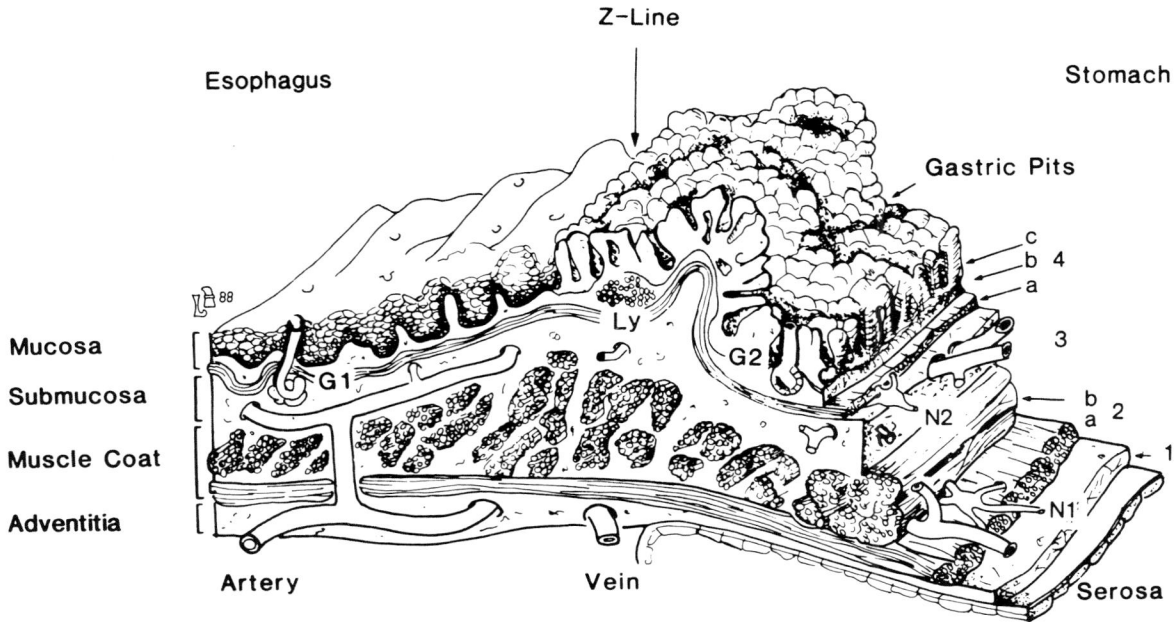

Z–Line

Esophagus

Stomach

Gastric Pits

c   4
b
a

3

Mucosa

Ly

G2

Submucosa

b   2
a

Muscle Coat

N2

1

Adventitia

N1

Artery

Vein

Serosa

FIGURE 27–39. Tissue organization at the esophagogastric junction. The Z line is usually a few centimeters above the anatomic junction. Thickening of the muscularis is identified at this level. (From Zuidema, G. D. [ed]: Shackelford's Surgery of the Alimentary Tract. Philadelphia, W. B. Saunders, 1996.)

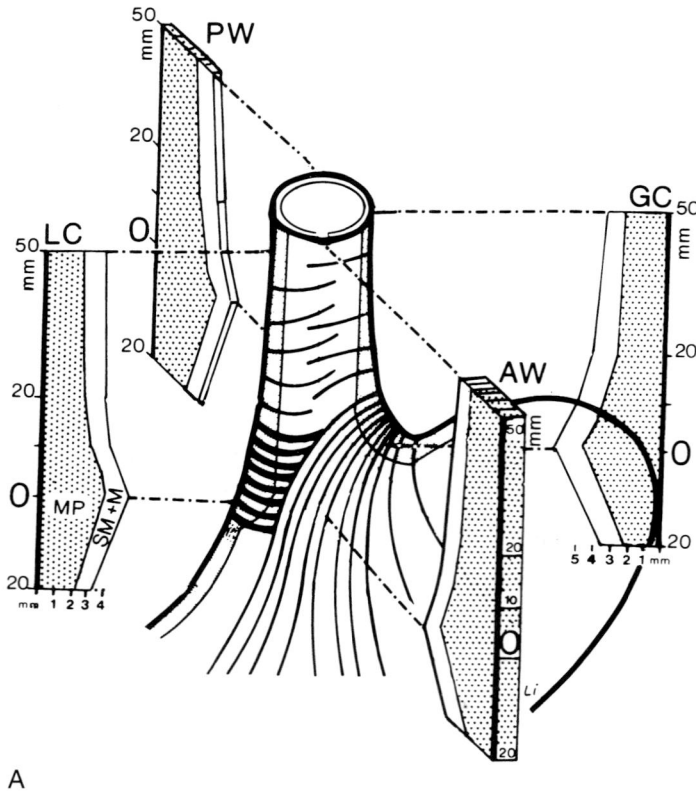

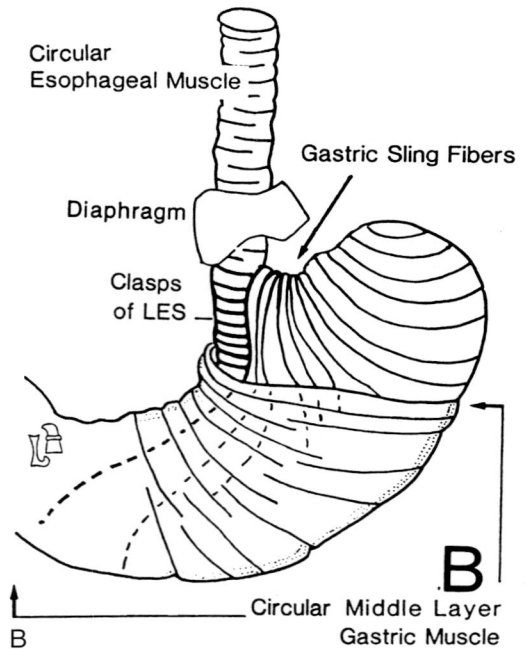

FIGURE 27–40. *A,* Muscular arrangement of the LES. Asymmetric thickening is described from serial measurements. (AW = anterior wall; PW = posterior wall; LC = lesser curvature; GC = greater curvature; MP = muscular layers; SM + M = submucosa and mucosa.) *B,* Structure and organization of the esophageal muscle in relation to the diaphragm. (*A* and *B,* From Zuidema, G. D. [ed]: Shackelford's Surgery of the Alimentary Tract. Philadelphia, W. B. Saunders, 1996.)

a serrated aspect, the Z line. This junction is usually a few centimeters above the anatomic junction (see Fig. 27–39).

GASTROESOPHAGEAL JUNCTION

The muscular organization is illustrated in Figure 27–40. The GEJ is held in place within the diaphragmatic hiatus by the phrenoesophageal membrane (Fig. 27–41). This membrane splits in two layers. The upper layer extends 2 to 4 cm above the hiatus and its elastic and collagenous fibers traverse the musculature to insert on the esophageal submucosa. The lower layer extends down on the cardia and fundus, where it blends with the gastric serosa, the gastrohepatic ligament, and the dorsal gastric mesentery. The precardial and pericardial "fat pad" is an accumulation of fatty tissue within the space between the two layers of the phrenoesophageal membrane.

PHYSIOLOGY OF THE ESOPHAGUS

Oral Phase of Swallowing

Following the formation of a bolus on the superior surface of the tongue, the mouth is first sealed by closing the lips. The tongue at this point contracts and, using the hard palate as support, pushes the bolus back toward the oropharynx. Tactile stimulation by the bolus at the anterior limits of the oropharynx elicits a pharyngeal response.

Pharyngeal Phase of Swallowing

Once stimulated, the pharyngeal phase involves several simultaneous events that, when coordinated, make swallowing comfortable. First, the velopharyngeal muscles of the soft palate effectively close the nasopharynx. Second, the larynx is pulled upward and anterior while the epiglottis folds over the additus of the larynx and while the false and true vocal cords are closed. The *upper esophageal sphincter* (UES) relaxes in an open position. Pharyngeal peristalsis is then initiated.

Motor Events

PHARYNX

The irregular configuration of the pharyngeal cavity makes it difficult to assess manometrically. Accurate recordings can be obtained with intraluminal strain gauge systems (Castell et al., 1990; Dodds et

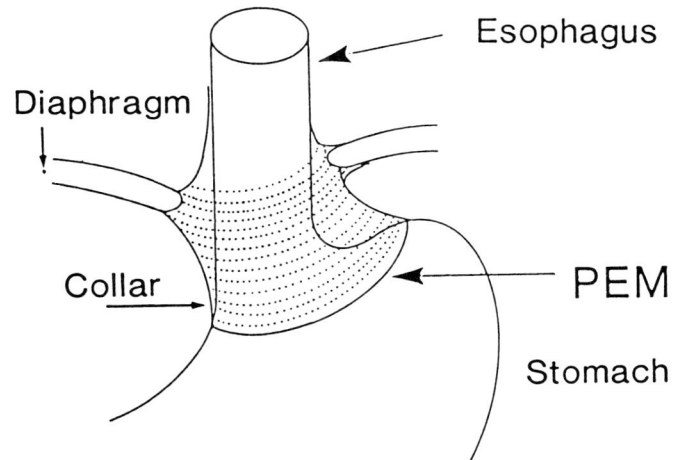

FIGURE 27–41. The phrenoesophageal membrane (PEM) supports and anchors the esophagogastric junction within the diaphragmatic hiatus. (From Zuidema, G. D. [ed]: Shackelford's Surgery of the Alimentary Tract. Philadelphia, W. B. Saunders, 1996.)

al., 1975). Maximal pharyngeal pressures are recorded just proximal to the UES, in the hypopharynx. Their pressures may range from 130 to 200 mm Hg. At oropharyngeal level, they average 100 mm Hg, and at the nasopharynx, mean pressures of 150 mm Hg are recorded. The peristaltic amplitude may be as high as 600 mm Hg. When progressing from the base of the skull toward the UES, the pharyngeal contraction advances very rapidly at a speed of 9 to 25 cm/sec. The contraction duration is very short at 0.55 sec or less. When the pharyngeal contraction is recorded using a perfused system, absolute contraction pressures are much lower (Fig. 27–42).

UPPER ESOPHAGEAL SPHINCTER

The cricopharyngeus muscle is mostly responsible for the high resting pressure zone at the junction of the pharynx with the esophagus (Fig. 27–43). Passive elastic forces are also responsible for some of the recorded pressures. The anatomic disposition of the cricopharyngeus with its bilateral insertion on both posterior and lateral laminae of the cricoid cartilage creates a sling effect. This gives an irregular configuration to the sphincter area, which Winans (1972) has documentated with a multilumen catheter. Besides this irregular configuration, the UES area moves upward with swallowing. These two factors led Kahrilas and colleagues (1987, 1988) and Cook and associates (1989) to propose the sleeve system to record UES pressures. Resting pressures in the UES result from continuous stimulation of the muscle fibers by branches of the ninth and eleventh nerves. These pressures averaged 32 to 101 mm Hg in Winans' study (1972). If a low-compliance system is used for recording, pressures range from 42 to 92 mm Hg (Knuff et al., 1982). Kahrilas and co-workers (1987) reported resting pressures in the awake individual of

FIGURE 27–42. The normal pharyngeal contraction travels at a speed of 9 to 25 cm/sec toward the upper esophagus. (DS = dry swallow.)

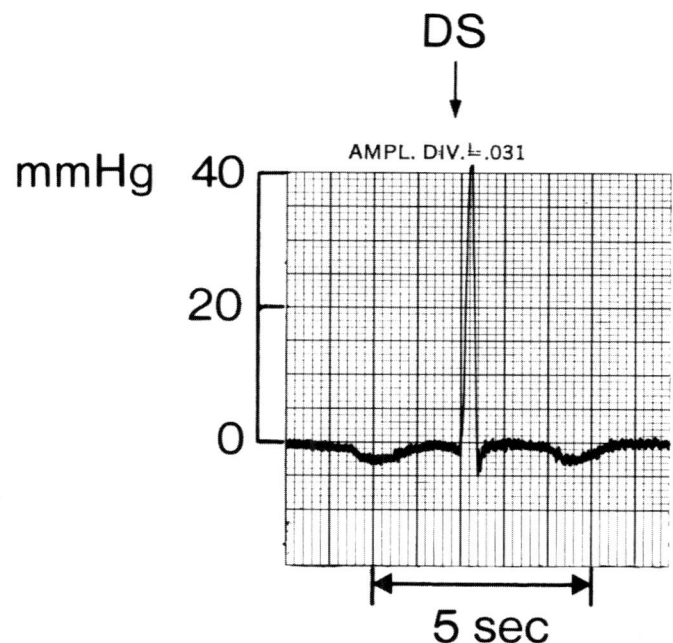

DS

mmHg 100

50

0

5 sec

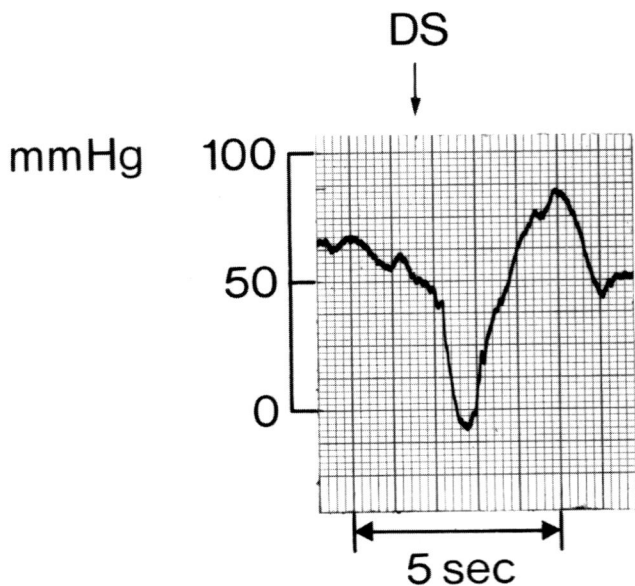

FIGURE 27–43. High-pressure zone of the UES. This area is difficult to record with precision.

FIGURE 27–44. Normal function at the pharyngoesophageal junction during pharyngeal contraction. UES relaxation is complete. The advancing pharyngeal contraction closes the UES and continues into the proximal esophagus as primary peristalsis.

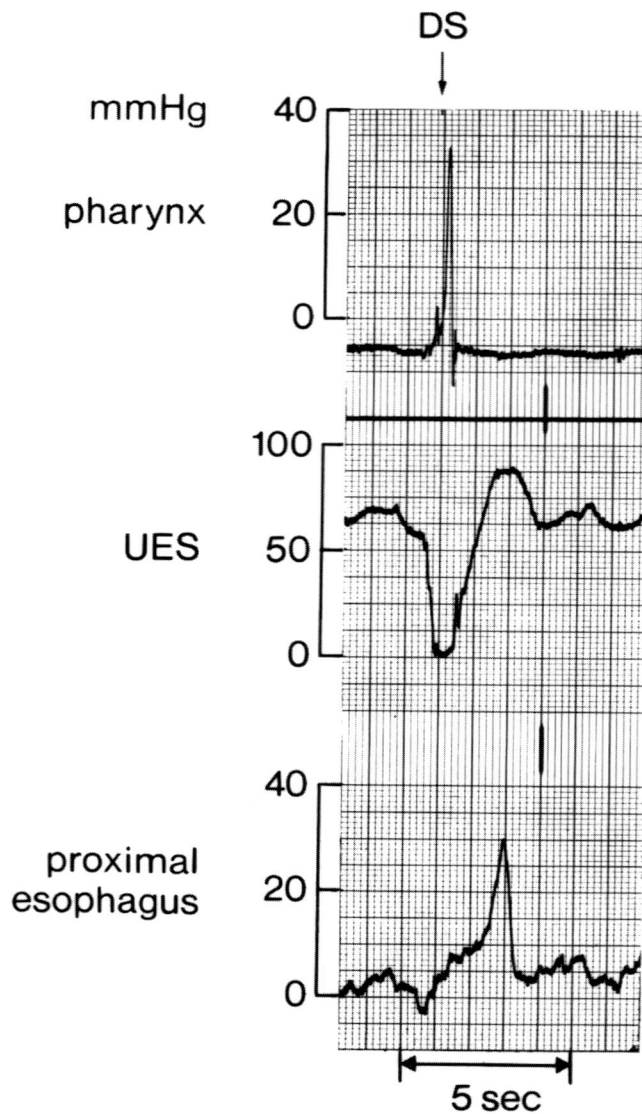

DS

mmHg 40

pharynx 20

0

100

UES 50

0

40

proximal
esophagus 20

0

5 sec

approximately 60 mm Hg. Castell and colleagues (1990) recorded mean pressures of 72 to 92 mm Hg using intraluminal strain gauges.

On swallowing, inhibition of all motor nerve stimulation to the UES occurs, causing the sphincter pressures to fall to ambient resting pressures at the pharyngoesophageal junction. This is recorded as sphincter relaxation. The sphincter remains open for 0.5 to 1.2 seconds, the duration of the pharyngeal contraction. The UES relaxes to cervical esophageal resting pressure in 93% of all swallows in normal volunteers. Coordination of sphincter opening during pharyngeal contraction is seen in almost all swallows. The sphincter is effectively closed by the sweeping wave of pharyngeal contraction that traverses the pharyngoesophageal junction, generating pressures that can triple the resting pressures of the sphincter (Dodds et al., 1975). Baseline pressures then return in the sphincter, and contraction continues into the cervical esophagus, starting the primary wave of peristalsis (Fig. 27–44).

Esophageal Body

In the proximal esophagus, the striated muscle receives direct innervation to its motor end plates from cells in the nucleus ambiguus. The smooth muscle receives indirect neural input from the dorsal motor nucleus of the vagus through the myenteric plexus. On innervation, the longitudinal muscle shortens while the circular muscle contracts sequentially in an aboral progression to generate peristalsis (Fig. 27–45).

Three distinct types of contractions are recorded in the esophagus (Fig. 27–46). *Primary peristalsis* is a normal propulsive wave in response to the stimulation of normal voluntary deglutition. *Secondary peristalsis* is a normal wave occurring without voluntary deglutition. This represents the best defense mechanism for the esophagus: When distended or irritated, this type of wave appears at the point of distention in an attempt to empty the esophagus of its content. *Tertiary waves* are usually abnormal if they occur following deglutition (Fig. 27–47A). They may also appear spontaneously between swallowings. Numerous stimulating factors are known to influence this spontaneous activity (Fig. 27–47B).

When the esophageal contraction appears in the proximal esophagus, it represents the continuation of the sweeping wave that started in the pharynx. Peak contraction pressures are weaker in the proximal esophagus (Fig. 27–48). Their strength increases progressively in the distal esophagus. Mean contraction pressures of 48 to 59 mm Hg were recorded in the proximal half of the esophagus with a mechanical perfusion system (Duranceau et al., 1983). If a non-compliant system is used for recording, values of 62 to 70 mm Hg are reported (Richter et al., 1987c). Contraction duration in the proximal half varied between 2.8 and 4.9 seconds.

In the distal half of the esophagus, mean contraction amplitude increases, reaching values of 55 to 74

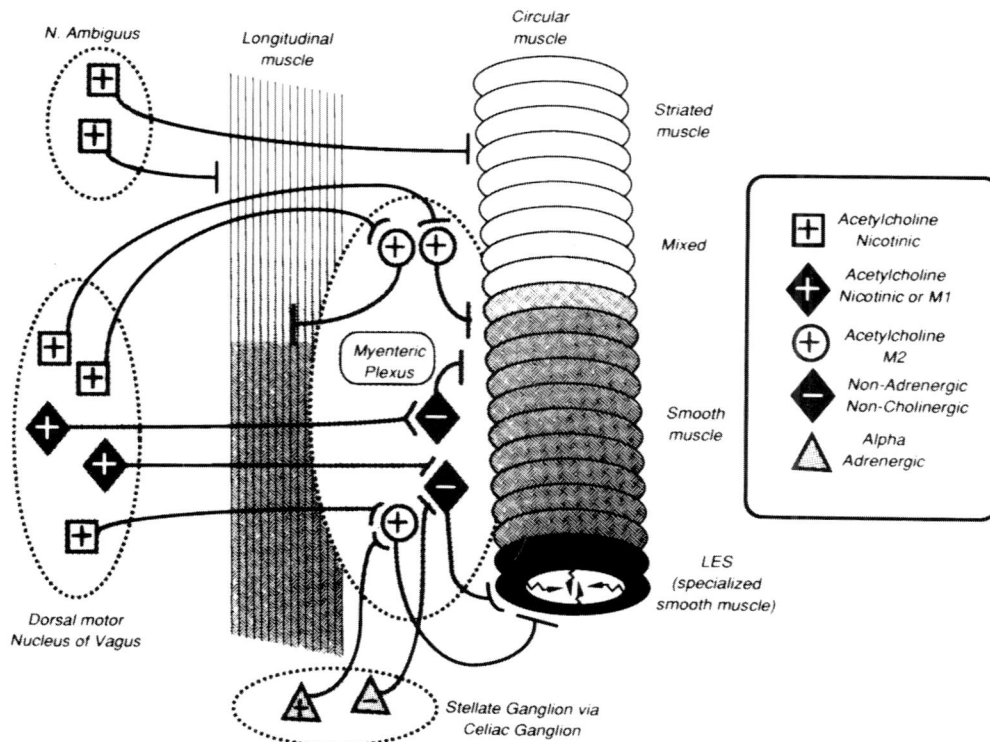

FIGURE 27–45. Schematic illustration of innervation to the striated and the smooth muscle of the esophagus. (From Kahrilas, P. J.: Functional anatomy and physiology of the esophagus. *In* The Esophagus, Castell, D. O. Boston, Little, Brown, 1992. Published by Little, Brown and Company.)

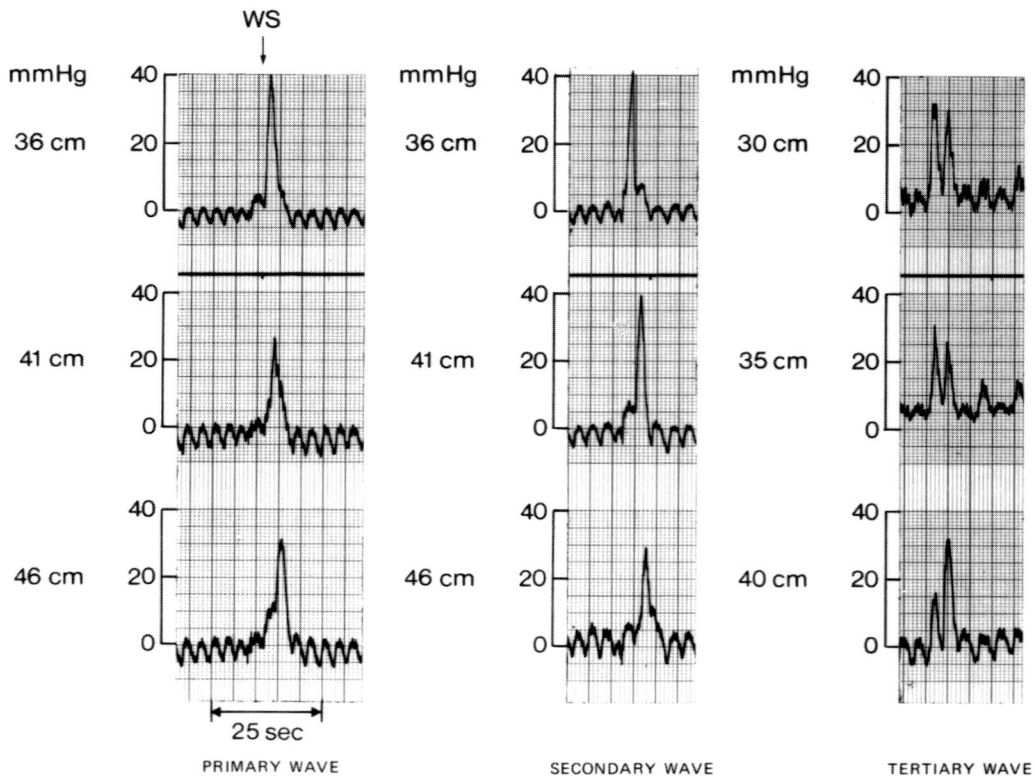

FIGURE 27–46. The primary contraction is a normal propulsive wave in response to deglutition. A secondary wave is normal peristalsis in response to distention or irritation. Tertiary waves are not propulsive and occur following deglutition or spontaneously. (WS = wet swallow.)

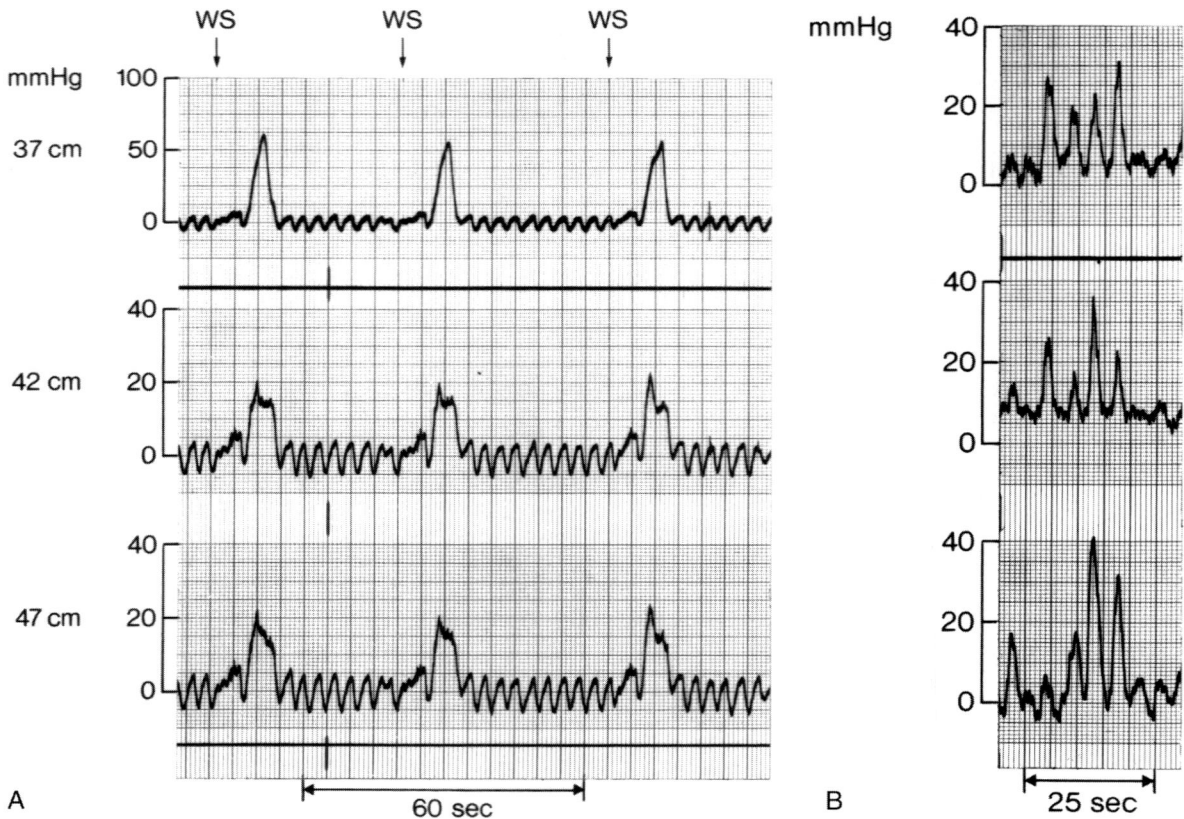

FIGURE 27–47. *A,* Tertiary waves in response to voluntary swallowing. *B,* Spontaneous, repetitive, and nonpropulsive contractions in the esophageal body.

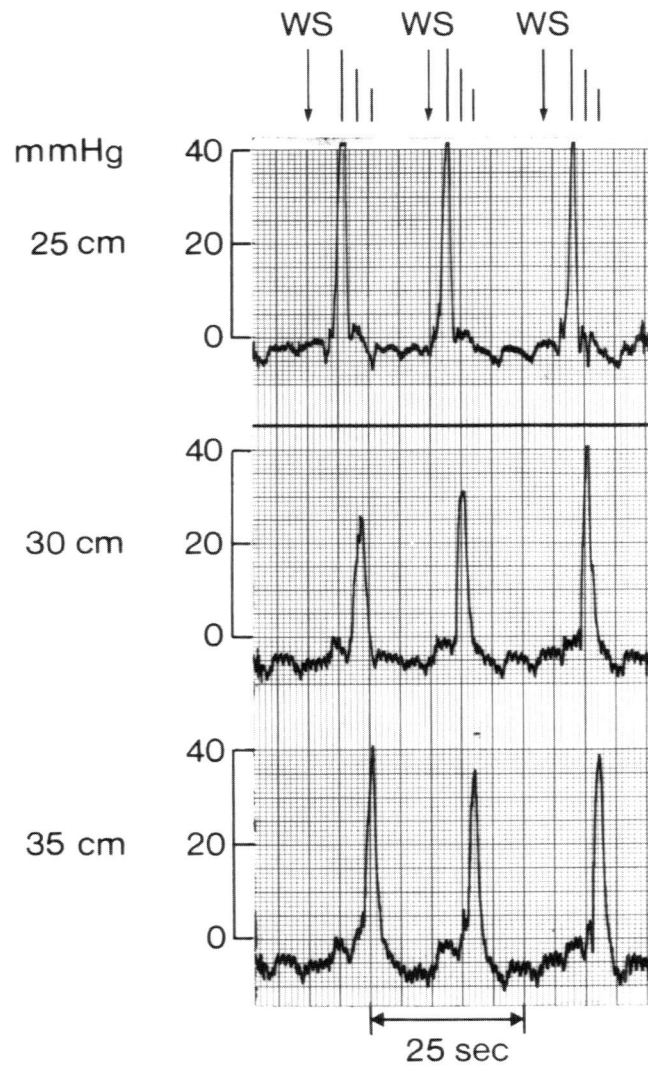

FIGURE 27–48. Normal peristalsis recorded in the proximal esophageal body.

mm Hg in the author's group (Fig. 27–49) and of 90 to 109 mm Hg in Richter's report. The duration of the contraction averaged 5 seconds.

The esophageal wave traverses the esophageal length at a speed of 3 cm/sec proximally. The velocity increases to 3.5 cm/sec in the distal esophagus to slow again immediately above the LES. Ninety-six per cent of all voluntary swallows show a peristaltic response.

A pressure-through is reported frequently at the junction of the proximal third and middle third, between 15 and 20 cm from the LES. The contraction pressures in this location are significantly lower, and this is possibly related to the transition zone from striated to smooth muscle.

Lower Esophageal Sphincter

The LES corresponds to a special muscle arrangement at the GEJ (see Fig. 27–40). Reorientation of the muscle fibers of the circular layer at this level coincides with an asymmetric thickening of the GEJ (Liebermann-Meffert et al., 1979). Manometrically, these muscle changes correspond to a high-pressure zone 3 to 4 cm in length and located just above the junction of the esophagus with the stomach. This muscle shows radial asymmetry (Winans, 1977), with highest pressures measured in the left posterior area (Fig. 27–50).

The smooth muscle of the LES high-pressure zone shows specialized features when compared with the esophageal muscle immediately above (Christensen, 1987). It remains in a contracted state mostly by myogenic activity influenced by a number of neural and hormonal factors (Table 27–1). LES relaxation is mediated by preganglionic cholinergic fibers and postganglionic nonadrenergic and noncholinergic nerves (see Fig. 27–45).

Absolute resting pressures in the LES of the author's control group was 24.8 mm Hg. The mean intragastric resting pressure in the same population was 7.3 mm Hg. Thus, a positive gradient of 17.5 mm Hg can be identified between esophagus and stomach at rest. Richter and colleagues (1987c) observed absolute resting LES pressure of 24.4 mm Hg when using a slow pull-through method. When using a rapid pull-through recording in the same group, pressures of 29 mm Hg were recorded during the Valsalva maneuver. The basal tone of the sphincter increases during gastric contractions (Dent et al., 1983) and in response to increases in intra-abdominal pressure.

The LES relaxes at the time of swallowing in order to allow esophageal peristalsis to push the bolus into the stomach cavity. Passage of the esophageal contraction through the sphincter area effectively closes the sphincter with pressures that double the resting val-

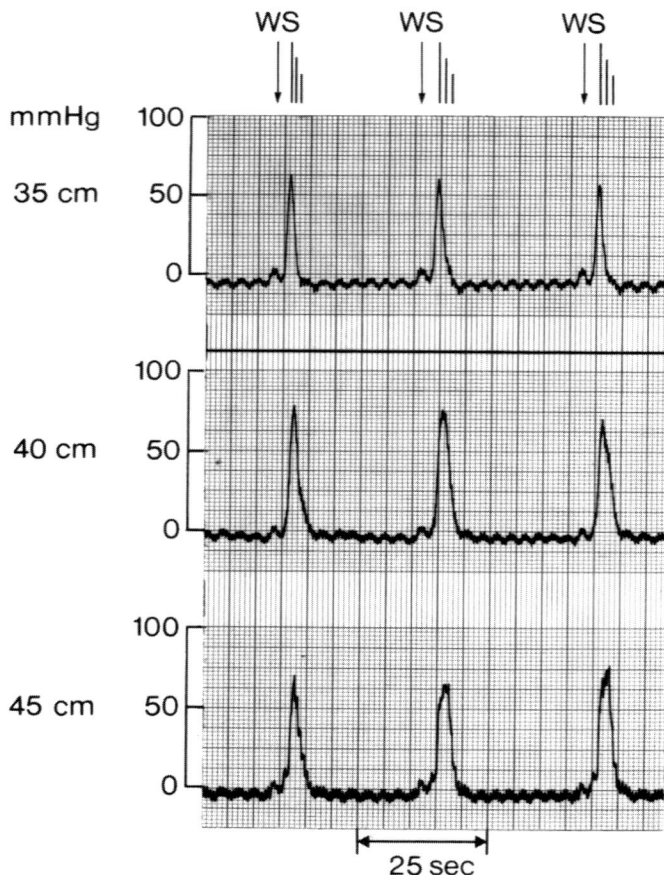

FIGURE 27–49. Normal peristalsis as seen in the distal half of the esophagus.

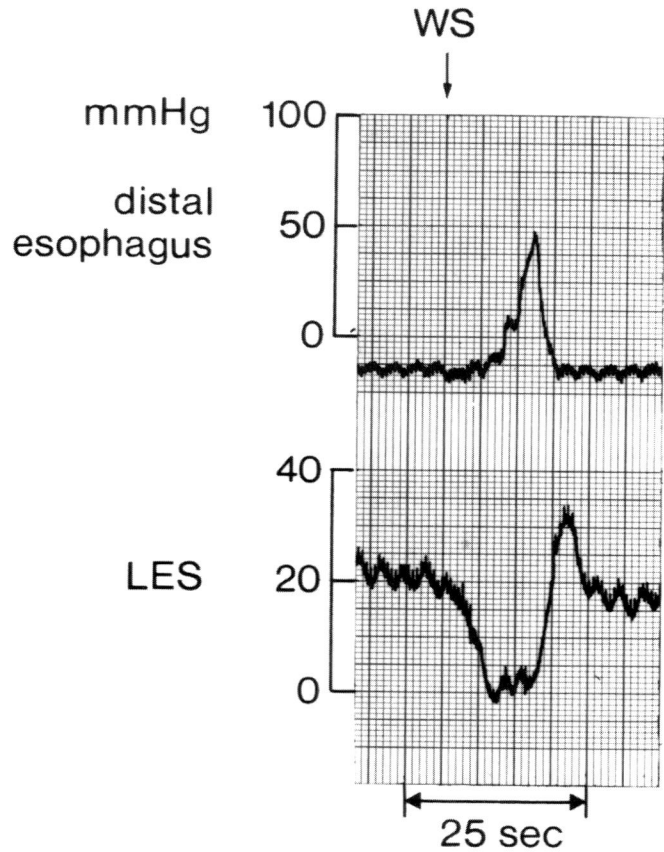

FIGURE 27–50. Normal LES. Relaxation is seen when deglutition (WS) occurs. The passing wave closes the sphincter, which then returns to normal baseline pressure. (WS = wet swallow.)

■ **Table 27–1.** LOWER ESOPHAGEAL SPHINCTER (LES) INFLUENCE FACTORS

Substance	Increase LES Pressure	Decrease LES Pressure
Hormones	Gastrin	Secretin
	Motilin	Cholecystokinin
	Substance P	Glucagon
		Somatostatin
		Gastric inhibitory polypeptide
		Vasoactive intestinal polypeptide
		Progesterone
Neural agents	Alpha-adrenergic antagonists	Alpha-adrenergic antagonists
	Beta-adrenergic antagonists	Beta-adrenergic antagonists
	Cholinergic antagonists	Cholinergic antagonists
	Protein	Fat
		Chocolate
		Ethanol
		Peppermint
Medication	Histamine	Barbiturates
	Antacids	Theophylline
	Metoclopramide	Prostaglandin $E_2 + I_1$
	Domperidone	Serotonin
	Prostaglandin F_{2a}	Meperidine
	Cisapride	Morphine
		Dopamine
		Calcium channel blockers

From Kahrilas, P. J.: Functional anatomy and physiology of the esophagus. *In* The Esophagus, Castell, D. O. Boston, Little, Brown, 1992. Published by Little, Brown and Company.

ues in the sphincter. Pressures then return to basal resting levels. The same type of relaxation is observed with secondary waves. Immediately after meals, usually on a distended stomach, *transient LES relaxations* (TLESR) occur, which last from 5 to 30 seconds (Dent et al., 1980). The spontaneous fall in LES resting pressures may play a role in belching and in the presence of physiologic as well as pathologic reflux (Dent et al., 1980).

DIAGNOSTIC TECHNIQUES

The Esophageal Laboratory and Its Role in Staging Reflux Esophagitis

The esophagus, in many of its diseases, remains a challenge to accurate diagnosis and management. Currently available techniques form the essential basis for a comprehensive esophageal laboratory: radiographic documentation of abnormalities; endoscopic assessment of mucosal damage; biopsy material for histologic documentation; motility studies of the esophagus and its sphincter; pH probe documentation of reflux events; radionuclide quantification of esophageal and gastric emptying; and potential difference measurements. These various investigative methods are all important to help quantify the abnormalities of esophageal disease, whether functional or caused by reflux disease or malignancies. These investigative methods can serve as a basis to accurately stage reflux disease and objectively document the results of treatment.

Radiology

Radiologic assessment of the esophagus remains the initial screening test in patients with esophageal symptoms. Standard examination techniques with full-column and double-contrast observations should document most mucosal and structural abnormalities when present (Ott, 1992).

Videoradiology is preferred in patients with oropharyngeal dysphagia. The rapidity of events dictates its use, since standard fluoroscopy and radiographic studies are considered inadequate to delineate the rapid movements taking place.

Standard radiographic techniques are important to classify diaphragmatic hernias into three types: Type I—sliding, Type II—paraesophageal, Type III—mixed with a sliding and paraesophageal component. However, radiology does not accurately assess mild reflux esophagitis. Ott and colleagues (1979) found that radiologic reflux could be observed in 25% of esophagitis patients, whereas it was seen in 20% of normal controls. Radiologic techniques do detect the anatomic abnormalities of reflux complications and stricture in 90 to 95% of studied patients (Ott et al., 1986). Radiographic evaluation of primary motor disorders may suggest the dysfunction. A good correlation with manometry is reported by Ott and associates (1989).

Motility studies remain essential to confirm and classify the dysfunction.

Virtually all benign and malignant neoplasms are detected by radiographic examinations. The noninvasive staging is completed by CT scan examination, which helps assess periesophageal and lymph node extension. Esophageal endoscopic ultrasound is superior for studying the depth of invasion, but is limited by the obstructive nature of the lesions.

Endoscopy

When only rigid instruments were available, the endoscopic assessment of both benign and malignant conditions of the esophagus was limited. The use of flexible instruments has simplified and improved the examination of the esophagus with a decreased morbidity.

REFLUX DISEASE

When minor degrees of inflammation exist in the mucosa, they are more difficult to classify because the endoscopic observation does not always correlate with the histologic diagnosis (Schuman and Rinaldo, 1966; Siegel and Hendrix, 1963; Ward et al., 1970). Siegel found a correlation in 72% of his observations, Ward and co-workers in 62.5% of their group, and Schuman and Rinaldo confirmed the endoscopic esophagitis in only 32% of their patients. The explanation given for this discrepancy between observation and histology was mostly sampling errors due to the patchy nature of reflux-induced mucosal inflammation or overinterpretation of esophageal mucosal damage. The method of biopsy may also have a role: Biopsies seem to show the minimal histologic changes better than the tiny pinch biopsies. When minimal damage exists, different endoscopists offer different interpretations. Endoscopy does not reliably detect lesser degrees of damage and chronic changes. Whenever severe esophagitis exists, the objectivity of observers is improved, producing a better correlation between observers and damage.

Therefore, the most recent classification proposed by Armstrong and colleagues (1991), the MUSE system, provides better visual information about the existing damage. Four categories of mucosal damage are reported: metaplasia, ulcers, stricture, and erosions (MUSE). Each has an objective damage level quantified on its own, and no place is given to minimal damage situations as viewed through the esophagoscope.

At present, a normal mucosa or a mucosa showing only erythema should be seen as offering very unreliable evidence of esophagitis. On the other hand, endoscopic documentation of erosions and ulcerations are unequivocal proof of mucosal damage, just as the presence of stricture and columnar-lined mucosa can be taken as evidence of severe reflux disease (Table 27–2).

■ **Table 27–2.** ENDOSCOPY

▲ E0 = Normal

▲ E1 = Erythema

EQUIVOCAL

——————— Evidence of esophagitis ———————

UNEQUIVOCAL

▲ E2 = Erosions and ulceration

▲ E3 = Stricture or columnar-lined esophagus

From Jamieson, G. G., and Duranceau, A.: Gastroesophageal Reflux. Philadelphia, W. B. Saunders, 1988.

ESOPHAGEAL MALIGNANCIES

When an esophageal malignancy is suspected, the purpose of endoscopy is to obtain a histologic diagnosis of the lesion while determining the proximal and, if possible, the distal limits of the tumor. The rigid endoscope may help assess fixation of the tumor in the mediastinum. It also provides larger biopsies with a higher diagnostic yield. When the flexible endoscope is used, multiple biopsies and brush cytologies will produce a similar diagnostic precision (Winawer et al., 1976).

ESOPHAGEAL BIOPSIES

The normal esophagus has a mucosa made up of an epithelial layer of squamous cells supported by a lamina propria and a muscularis mucosae. The squamous epithelium itself is not keratinized in its outer layer. Its middle layer shows plumper cells, and the basal layer shows cylindrical cells. The cells of the basal layer usually form less than 15% of the epithelium. The surface epithelium is supported by the lamina propria and the underlying muscularis mucosae. The lamina propria pushes papillae toward the surface of the epithelium, although these papillae usually do not extend over more than two-thirds of the thickness of the epithelium.

The initial events leading to early mucosal damage in reflux disease were studied by Ismail-Beigi and associates (1970), who believed that an increase in the basal layer thickness to form more than 15% of the total epithelium indicated reflux disease. Likewise, a penetration of the papillae over more than 66% of the epithelium thickness to come in close proximity to the esophageal lumen indicated reflux disease. These changes, however, were distributed at random over the 8 distal cm of the esophagus, and 20% of normal controls showed similar changes. Weinstein and coworkers (1975) found that over 50% of their controls showed these histologic changes in the distal 2.5 cm of the esophagus.

Acid or acid mixed with bile salts, pepsin, and trypsin affects the permeability of the mucosa, allowing diffusion of hydrogen ions. Damage results in the subepithelial and basal layers of the epithelium (Kiroff et al., 1987). This may stimulate a repair mechanism by directly damaging the basal layer of the epithelium, leading to an increased turnover of the basal layer and eventually to basal hyperplasia. This increased cellular activity leads to an increased blood supply, with more prominent papillae pushing toward the surface of the epithelium. The initial changes in the lamina propria considered to be the best indicator of reflux damage are the presence of neutrophils and eosinophils: They increase in proportion with the mucosal damage. Progression in the mucosal damage destroys the epithelium with erosions and ulcerations. These acute changes then allow chronic inflammatory changes to occur in the lamina propria and the submucosa. This inflammation rarely penetrates deeper than the submucosa.

If the ulceration, inflammation, granulation fibrosis, and the repair process continue over time, stricture and reepithelialization may occur, and the ulcerated part of the squamous mucosa will become progressively covered by a columnar mucosa that may grow in a cephalad direction (Bremner et al., 1970). This abnormal epithelium leads to the formation of a columnar-lined esophagus, with the columnar cells being gastric, junctional, or specialized in appearance. With persistent reflux, the mucosal junction between the squamous epithelium and the columnar epithelium tends to be damaged with the same repetition of early and progressive changes of mucosal insult. If esophageal biopsies show a normal epithelium or an epithelium with only basal cell hyperplasia, this only equivocally suggests esophageal reflux mucosal damage.

If, however, esophageal mucosal biopsies show acute inflammation with erosions or ulcerations, or if they reveal the fibrosis of a stricture or the columnar-lined epithelium of a Barrett mucosa, this can be considered unequivocal evidence of mucosal damage by reflux (Table 27–3).

Motility Studies

Documentation of esophageal function has evolved with the technical advances in esophageal manometry. Balloon recording, unperfused water columns, perfused catheters, noncompliant water-perfused systems, and intraluminal microtransducers are responsible for the progressive changes in observation and the improved precision in recording esophageal physiology.

Contraction pressures may vary significantly with

■ **Table 27–3.** HISTOLOGY

▲ H0 = Normal

▲ H1 = Basal cell hyperplasia

EQUIVOCAL

——————— Evidence of esophagitis ———————

UNEQUIVOCAL

▲ H2 = Acute epithelial or subepithelial inflammation and/or ulceration

▲ H3 = Fibrosis or columnar-lined esophagus

From Jamieson, G. G., and Duranceau, A.: Gastroesophageal Reflux. Philadelphia, W. B. Saunders, 1988.

recording methods and equipment. Moreover, changes with age, rate of swallowing, emotional state, posture, and body size and type can all modify esophageal motility tracings. For these reasons, a well-studied control population is necessary for any esophageal function laboratory.

Motor function studies of the esophagus provide the evidence for the physiologic abnormalities that are most commonly seen with motor disorders and with reflux disease. LES and esophageal body dysfunction can be quantified in reflux disease and help to stage the extent of dysfunction present with the mucosal abnormalities.

LOWER ESOPHAGEAL SPHINCTER ABNORMALITIES

The LES preserves the integrity of the esophagus. It was described as hypotensive in 9 out 10 reflux esophagitis patients first described by Atkinson and co-workers (1957). Winans and Harris (1967) and Pope (1967) suggested that motility systems could not offer reliable enough recordings of the LES. However, Haddad (1970) documented that patients with pH-documented free reflux had the lowest basal pressures in the LES. High LES pressures were not associated with reflux, whereas low LES pressures in the range of 0 to 10 mm Hg above gastric baseline pressure were seen with reflux. Behar and colleagues (1975) observed that the presence of endoscopic esophagitis was usually associated with poor LES tone. They also observed that when a very low tone existed in the LES, the chances of altering sphincter function by medical management alone were minimal over time. Kahrilas and associates (1986) showed that patients with increased reflux damage have significantly weaker LES resting pressures. Patients with a documented columnar-lined esophagus show the worst changes, with a virtually nonexistent LES tone (Iascone et al., 1983; Parilla et al., 1990, 1991; Stein et al., 1992). These patients have higher exposure to acid reflux.

Although an LES pressure below 10 suggests poor tone at the GEJ, much variation exists at this level and this is too imprecise to identify a potential for reflux. If the pressure in the LES is less than 6 mm Hg, this shows a reasonably high specificity compared with abnormal reflux on pH testing. A LES pressure that is extremely low or nonexistent identifies a more severe degree of reflux and a poorer prognosis for long-term medical therapy (Castell, 1991).

ESOPHAGEAL BODY DYSFUNCTION

Quantification of peristaltic activity and pressure amplitude is also of importance. Active esophagitis alters function. Esophageal body activity shows an increase in failed peristalsis and weaker contractions (Kahrilas, 1986). Patients with a columnar-lined esophagus also reveal the worst functional abnormalities in their esophageal body (Iascone et al., 1983; Parilla et al., 1990, 1991; Stein et al., 1992).

Motility studies offer objective and prognostic information on the physiologic damage present with reflux disease (Table 27–4). If motor function is normal in the esophageal body, with LES pressure values above 6 mm Hg, this is equivocal evidence of functional damage. If, however, esophageal contractions are intact, with an LES below 6 mm Hg, or if the esophageal contractions are aperistaltic and weak in conjunction with an nonexistent LES, this is considered strong evidence for physiologic abnormalities that cause damage.

24-Hour pH Monitoring

Twenty-four-hour pH monitoring has become the gold standard in establishing the presence of acid in the esophageal body. The amount, frequency, and time of acid exposure in the esophagus are measured by placing an electrode 5 cm above the manometric LES. Multiple pH probes can measure the esophageal exposure to acid reflux at different levels in the esophagus. This technique correlates reflux symptoms as well as oropharyngeal, pulmonary, or atypical chest pain symptoms with the presence or absence of reflux episodes.

When Johnson and DeMeester (1974) and DeMeester and co-workers (1976) looked at their normal population, total time of acid exposure in the normal group was always less than 4.2%. When Holscher and Weiser (1984) looked at their normal group, they suggested that 7% of total acid exposure was the normal acceptable level. Mattioli and colleagues (1989) showed over 12% of acid exposure in patients with nonconfluent erosive esophagitis. Kraus and associates (1990) suggested that the mean acid contact time measured during 24-hour pH monitoring better indicates possible reflux injury. The mucosal injury level also correlated to the period of acid exposure when Parilla and co-workers (1990, 1991) reported their reflux population and compared them with a normal group. The esophagitis group showed 15% of recording time exposure to an acid environment, whereas the columnar-lined esophagus patients showed a mean acid exposure of 26%. Stein and colleagues (1992) reported a higher acid exposure in their esophagitis group and an even more significant increase in patients with a columnar-lined esophagus.

■ **Table 27–4.** MANOMETRY

▲ M0 = Normal esophageal motility	LES >10 mm Hg
▲ M1 = Normal esophageal motility	LES 6–10 mm Hg
EQUIVOCAL		
———— Evidence of functional abnormality ———— associated with reflux		
UNEQUIVOCAL		
▲ M2 = Normal esophageal motility	LES <5 mm Hg
▲ M3 = Aperistaltic esophagus	LES <5 mm Hg

From Jamieson, G. G., and Duranceau, A.: Gastroesophageal Reflux. Philadelphia, W. B. Saunders, 1988.

■ **Table 27–5.** pH MONITORING

▲ R0 = No reflux

▲ R1 = <3 reflux episodes—SART or 4–7%—24-hr pH

EQUIVOCAL

——————— Evidence of reflux ———————

UNEQUIVOCAL

▲ R2 = >3 reflux episodes—SART or >7%—24-hr pH

▲ R3 = >12%—24-hr pH

From Jamieson, G. G., and Duranceau, A.: Gastroesophageal Reflux. Philadelphia, W. B. Saunders, 1988.
SART = standard acid reflux test.

They further suggested that alkaline exposure could also play a role in the increase in mucosal damage.

With the notion that there is good correlation between endoscopic esophagitis and pH parameters of acid reflux, objective documentation of reflux disease could be reported, as seen in Table 27–5, where mean acid contact time and percentage of acid exposure less than 7% represent equivocal proof of reflux disease. Exposure to acid between 8 and 12% or above 12% usually correlates with more damage to the esophageal mucosa and represents unequivocal evidence of reflux. Reflux esophagitis is quantified most objectively with endoscopy, histology, manometry, and 24-hour pH monitoring. With these four investigation methods, patients can be categorized according to the severity of their condition. As proposed by Jamieson and Duranceau (1988a), Table 27–6 summarizes a staging process for classification of reflux disease severity. This approach may promote a more uniform classification for better reporting and comparisons (Costantini et al., 1993; Feussner et al., 1991; Jamieson and Duranceau, 1988a).

ACID PERFUSION TESTING

The acid perfusion of Bernstein's test is used to reproduce and assess symptoms. It is qualitative and by itself does not reflect the severity of the reflux. The acid emptying test as employed by Booth and colleagues (1968) measures the emptying capacity of the esophagus when it is exposed to an acid bolus. This is a measure of one of the esophagus's defense mechanisms and may be abnormal in up to 50% of reflux esophagitis patients. Both the acid perfusion test and the acid clearance test are recorded in some way by the 24-hour pH recording, which measures both acid exposure over time and symptoms.

Radionuclide Emptying Studies

Both esophageal and gastric emptying studies, using liquid and solid radionuclide markers, should help to objectively quantify the end result of functional derangements that occur with reflux disease. Radionuclide esophagrams are not used to diagnose motor abnormalities or reflux disease. These provide objective information on esophageal emptying. The use of a bolus varying in consistency more precisely documents the emptying capacity. Peristaltic dysfunction, whether in reflux disease or motor disorders, causes poor bolus clearance in a significant proportion of patients (Richter et al., 1987a). Although not usually used for esophageal assessment, these studies add objectivity in measuring the results of various therapeutic options.

Potential Difference Measurements

In the esophagus, a higher potential difference exists with the esophageal mucosa when it is compared with the negative potential recorded at the level of the gastric mucosa. A reduction of potential difference appears when injury to the esophageal mucosa has occurred (Khamis et al., 1978). Although theoretically it can help detect columnar epithelium replacement in the esophagus, measurement of the potential difference in patients with this condition underestimates the extent of the pathologic epithelium. Orlando and associates (1982), Eckardt and co-workers (1983) and Herlihy and colleagues (1984) reported that the specificity of the method is 92 to 96% but that the sensitivity is only 50 to 70%.

ESOPHAGEAL MOTOR DISORDERS

Oropharyngeal Dysphagia

Oropharyngeal dysphagia refers to a symptom complex characterized by difficulty in propelling food or liquid from the oral cavity into the cervical esophagus. The causes of this special category of dysphagia are summarized in Table 27–7 and Figure 27–51.

■ **Table 27–6.** STAGING OF SEVERITY IN GASTROESOPHAGEAL REFLUX

	Endoscopy				Histology				Reflux				Manometry			
	0	1	2	3	0	1	2	3	0	1	2	3	0	1	2	3
Stage 0	○				○				○				○			
Stage 1		○				○				○				○		
Stage 2		○				○					○	○			○	○
Stage 3			○				○				○	○			○	○
Stage 4					Stricture formation or columnar-lined esophagus, or both											

From Jamieson, G. G., and Duranceau, A.: Gastroesophageal Reflux. Philadelphia, W. B. Saunders, 1988.

NEUROGENIC

. central

. peripheral

NEUROMUSCULAR

. end-plate diseases
. muscular

IATROGENIC

. surgery
. radiotherapy

MECHANICAL

. intraluminal
. extraluminal

STRUCTURAL

. idiopathic dysfunction
of UES

**GASTRO·ESOPHAGEAL
REFLUX**

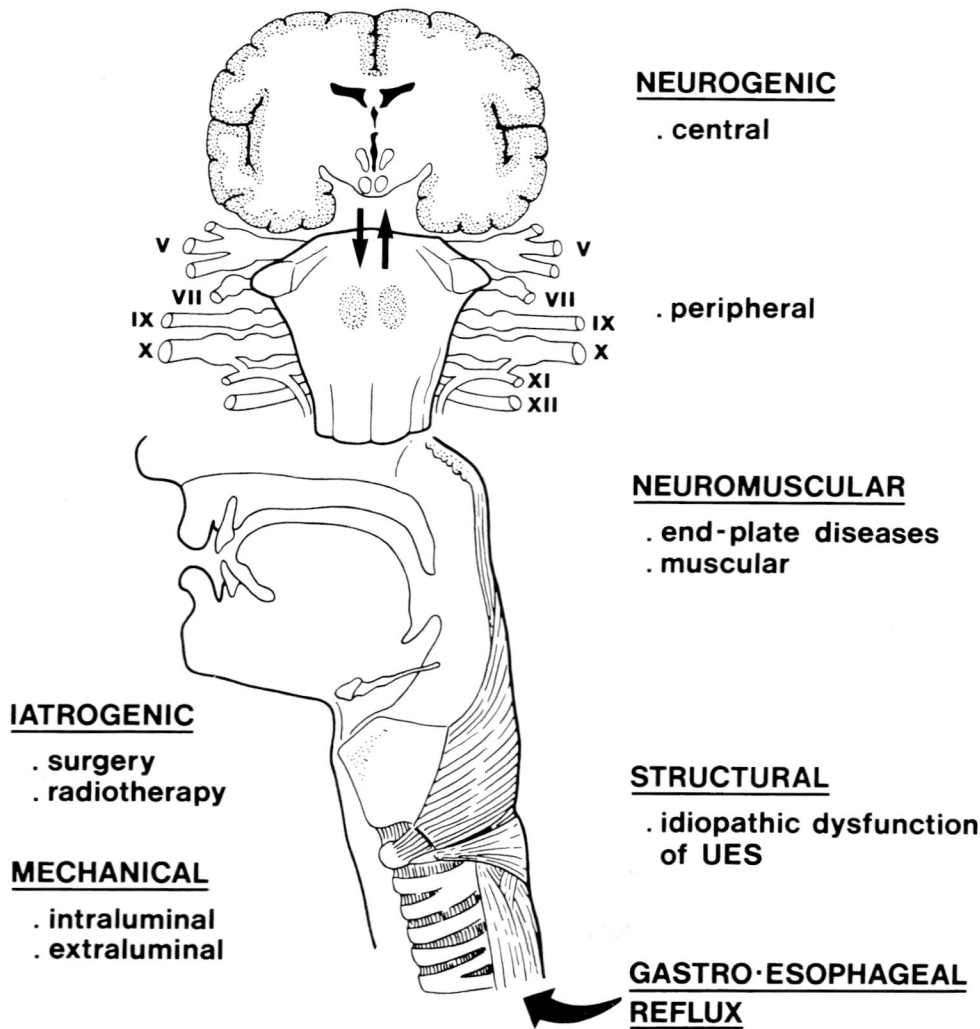

FIGURE 27–51. The causes of oropharyngeal dysphagia.

Assessment of Patients with Oropharyngeal Dysphagia

SYMPTOMS

Independently of the cause for the dysphagia, three categories of symptoms result from misdirection of an alimentary bolus: pharyngonasal or pharyngo-oral regurgitations and laryngotracheal aspiration. Thus, discomfort during meals and bronchopulmonary complications from aspiration are the main presenting patterns (Duranceau et al., 1988).

NEUROLOGIC DISEASE

Symptoms in the neurologic patient are most difficult to assess and to treat. Cerebrovascular disease may create difficulties of speech and expression. The dysarthric patient may show poor coordination of pharynx, larynx, and UES activity. The cerebrovascular accident victim often has difficulties in bolus formation and propulsion. Patients with Parkinson's disease show hesitancy in bolus preparation and in initiating swallows. Patients with amyotrophic lateral sclerosis, with their loss of motor neurons and control mechanisms, show absence of voluntary deglutition, dysarthria, and repetitive aspiration.

MUSCULAR DISEASE

Bilateral palpebral ptosis muscle weakness and repetitive efforts to swallow suggest muscular disease. Hoarseness, dysphonia, and nasal speech, when accompanying oropharyngeal dysphagia, suggest dystrophic disease with poor control of laryngeal and velopharyngeal muscles.

IDIOPATHIC DYSFUNCTION OF THE UPPER ESOPHAGEAL SPHINCTER

When oropharyngeal dysphagia cannot be explained by neurologic or muscular disease, intrinsic dysfunction of the UES must be suspected. These patients are often tense, although the underlying basis for a neuropsychogenic explanation of their condition is still lacking. Dysphagia at the oropharyngeal level, frequent food incarceration, and bouts of aspiration

■ Table 27–7. CAUSES OF OROPHARYNGEAL DYSPHAGIA

Neurologic

Central	Cerebrovascular disease
	Neurologic disorders
	Brain stem tumors
	Postsurgical and trauma
Peripheral	Neuropathy or invasion
	Botulism and tetanus

Myogenic

Motor end-plate disease	Myasthenia gravis
Skeletal muscle disease	Muscular dystrophy
	Myositis
	Metabolic myopathy

Cricopharyngeus Muscle Dysfunction

Idiopathic, without pharyngoesophageal diverticulum
With established pharyngoesophageal diverticulum

Iatrogenic

Head and neck surgery
Irradiation

Oropharyngeal Dysphagia from Lower Esophageal Disease

Reflux disease
Idiopathic motor dysfunction
Endoluminal or extraluminal obstructive causes

---

are the most frequent symptoms. When a pharyngoesophageal diverticulum is present, fresh food regurgitation frequently accompanies the oropharyngeal symptom complex.

IATROGENIC CAUSES

Ablative or explorative surgery in the neck may cause poor function at pharyngeal and UES level. Tracheostomy and thyroidectomy may limit normal laryngeal excursion. Irradiation causes dense ischemic fibrosis, with strictures often difficult to dilate.

FUNCTIONAL ABNORMALITIES OF THE LOWER ESOPHAGUS

Reflux disease presents as oropharyngeal dysphagia symptoms in 9 to 15% of patients with this condition. Idiopathic motor dysfunction as well as distal esophageal obstruction may also present in the same way. Only a complete esophageal investigation allows the proper diagnosis to be made.

RADIOLOGY

Radiologic assessment of the oropharyngeal dysphagia patient requires multiphasic multipositional studies using fluoroscopic and videorecording equipment (Curtis et al., 1984; Curtis and Hudson, 1983). Dysfunction of the pharynx, larynx, and UES, owing to the rapidity of events during the act of swallowing, can be accurately recorded only when using these techniques. They permit observation of the movements of the tongue and soft palate, the symmetry of pharyngeal contraction, the organization and activity of the larynx during its normal excursion, and the activity of the UES at rest and during swallowing. Even minute abnormalities in the function of these muscle groups can be documented. Hypopharyngeal pooling and stasis as well as pooling in the pyriform sinuses and in the valleculae suggest abnormal emptying (Figs. 27–52 to 27–54).

RADIONUCLIDE EMPTYING STUDIES

Emptying assessment of the oropharynx is easily obtained during esophageal radionuclide transit evaluation. In all categories of oropharyngeal dysphagia patients, it quantifies emptying with either a liquid or a solid bolus. Objective documentation of results are thus obtainable when using either medical or surgical treatment in these patients (Taillefer and Duranceau, 1988) (Figs. 27–55 and 27–56).

ENDOSCOPY

Direct laryngoscopy and the use of the short rigid esophagoscope are preferred to obtain detailed evaluation of the larynx, pharynx, hypopharynx, and UES area. This technique rules out any endoluminal lesion. The flexible endoscope subsequently allows complete

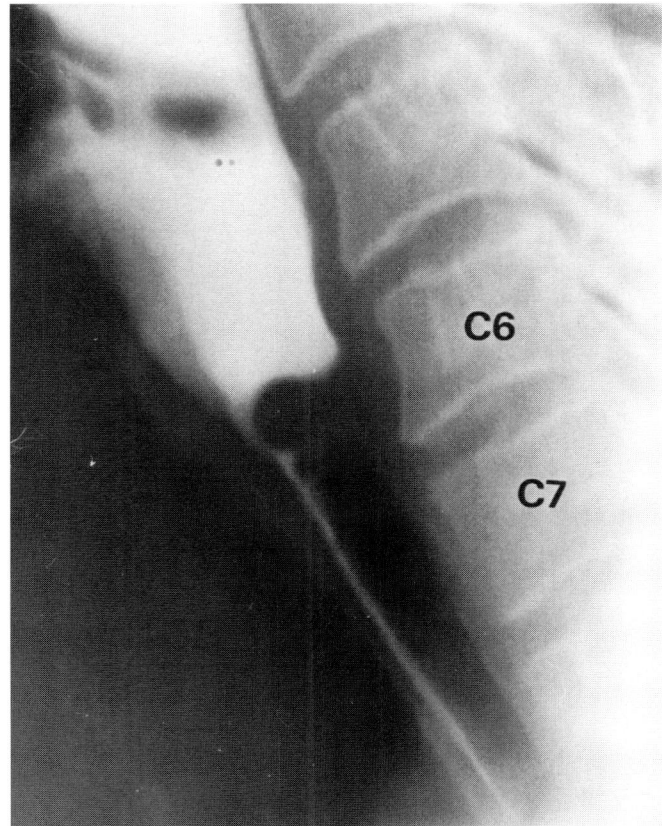

FIGURE 27–52. A cricopharyngeal bar suggests UES dysfunction when it is associated with symptoms of oropharyngeal dysphagia.

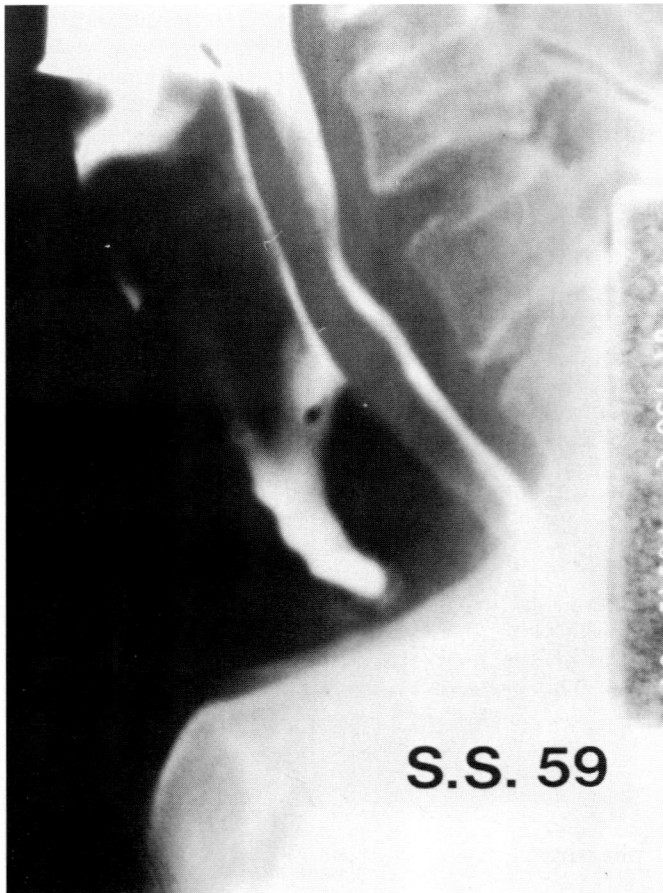

FIGURE 27–53. Hypopharyngeal stasis with tracheal aspiration in a patient with dysphagia from muscular disease.

FIGURE 27–54. Pseudotumor effect at UES level with hypopharyngeal stasis and tracheal aspiration.

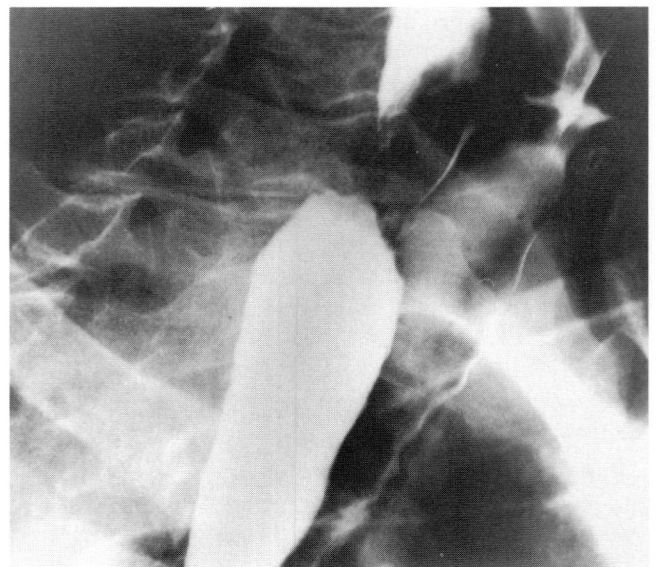

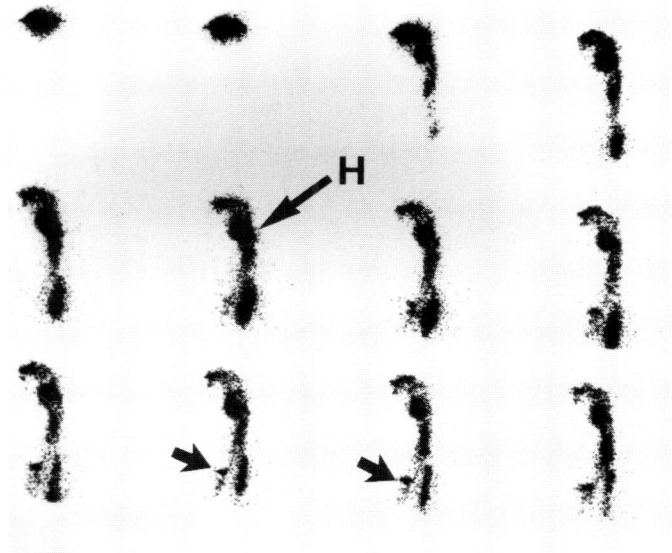

FIGURE 27-55. Hypopharyngeal stasis and tracheobronchial aspiration in a patient with oropharyngeal dysphagia. *Arrows* indicate tracheobronchial bifurcation. (H = hypopharynx.)

assessment of the distal esophagus. When a pharyngoesophageal diverticulum has been documented by radiographic studies, endoscopy is not considered a matter of urgency. Unless an underlying malignancy is suspected, the technique is considered dangerous. Its use can be delayed until the oropharyngeal problem has been corrected.

MOTILITY STUDIES

Manometric evaluation of the esophagus and its sphincters is essential to document both distal esophageal function and the physiologic abnormalities at the pharyngoesophageal junction. Physiologic evaluation of the UES must consider two important factors: the radial and axial asymmetry of the sphincter and the upward and anterior excursion of the sphincter during swallowing. Single-port recording catheters are not accurate to assess UES resting pressures. Multilumen recording catheters with port opening at the same level accurately assess the effects of the cricopharyngeus at rest (Winans, 1972). A circumferential pressure transducer probably provides the most accurate pressure values (Castell et al., 1990, 1992). The Dent sleeve catheter (Kahrilas et al., 1987) also has the advantage of recording sphincter pressures at any level along the sleeve membrane, even if sphincter movement occurs. A composite probe with a microtransducer at pharyngeal level and a sleeve catheter in the UES may be used. Assessment of relaxation and coordination in the sphincter is made difficult by the sphincter movement during deglutition. For that specific purpose, Castell and associates (1992) proposed positioning the recording sensor above the UES to study the opening phase of the sphincter. Actual methods of recording, even if they may provide accurate resting and closing pressures, certainly underestimate the true functional abnormalities present in patients with oropharyngeal dysphagia.

Treatment and Results

NEUROLOGIC DYSPHAGIA

Patients with oropharyngeal dysphagia of exclusive neurologic origin show functional abnormalities of resting pressures in the UES as well as incoordination and relaxation defects (Fig. 27-57). UES hypertension has been reported by Ellis and Crozier (1981), and Bonavina and co-workers (1985) reported incoordination and poor relaxation of the sphincter during the pharyngeal contraction. The author's group observed normal resting pressures, but relaxation was incomplete for 7 of 20 patients with neurogenic dysphagia. Poor coordination of sphincter opening during pharyngeal contraction was observed for 80% of all patients. Only neurologic oropharyngeal dysphagia patients have shown complete absence of relaxation or achalasia of their UES (Figs. 27-57B and C).

Cricopharyngeal myotomy is now reported for over 200 patients with dysphagia of exclusive neurologic origin. The operation aims to decrease the resistance to pharyngoesophageal transit by removing or lessening the sphincter effects of the cricopharyngeus (Figs. 27-58 to 27-60). The underlying motor abnormalities remain unchanged in the author's group's experience. Patients can be expected to improve if they retain an intact voluntary deglutition, if they show normal movements of the tongue, if they present with normal phonation, and if no dysarthria results from their central disease.

Results have been mixed and they vary with the disease category. Overall, 50% of treated patients report excellent results. The remaining patients may show initial improvement with subsequent deterioration (Duranceau et al., 1988).

Poor results are seen when the prognostic factors mentioned previously cannot be met. The mortality seen following this operation for neurologic condition may be as high as 12 to 20% (Duranceau et al., 1988),

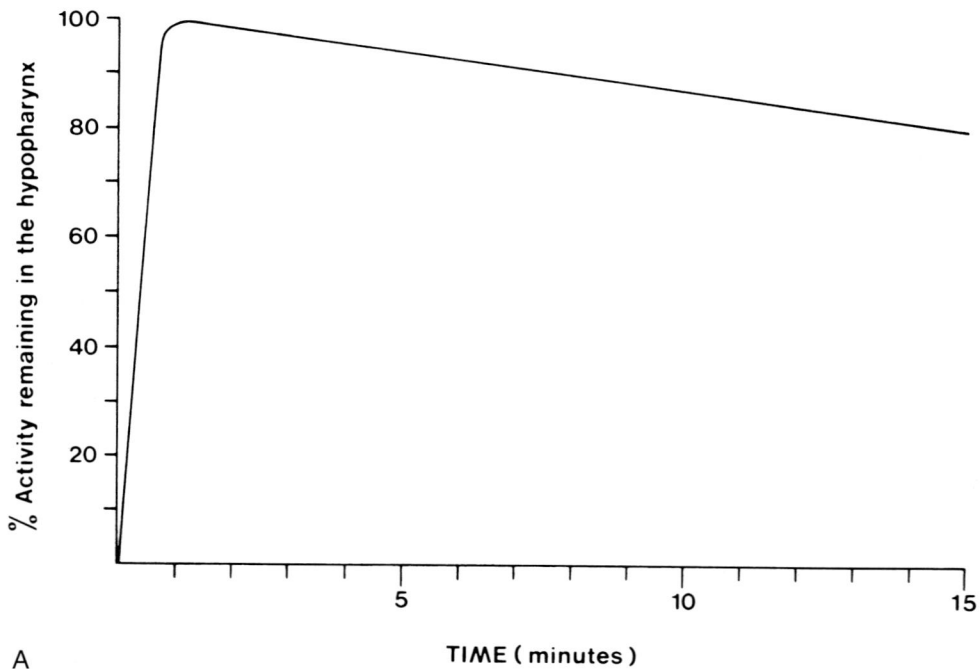

A

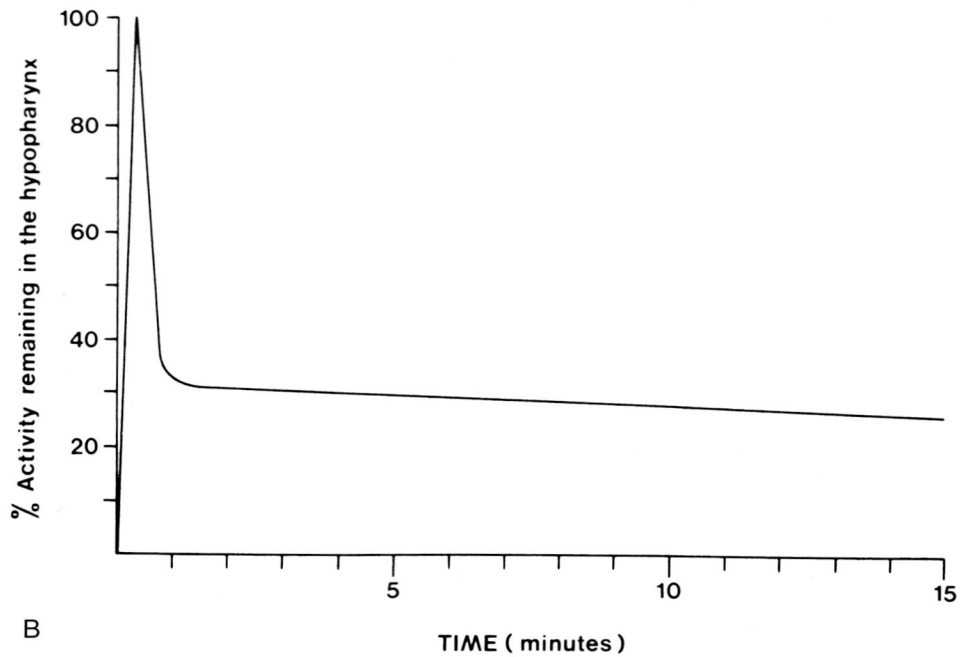

B

FIGURE 27–56. Quantification of hypopharyngeal emptying before *(A)* and after *(B)* cricopharyngeal myotomy in a patient with oropharyngeal dysphagia.

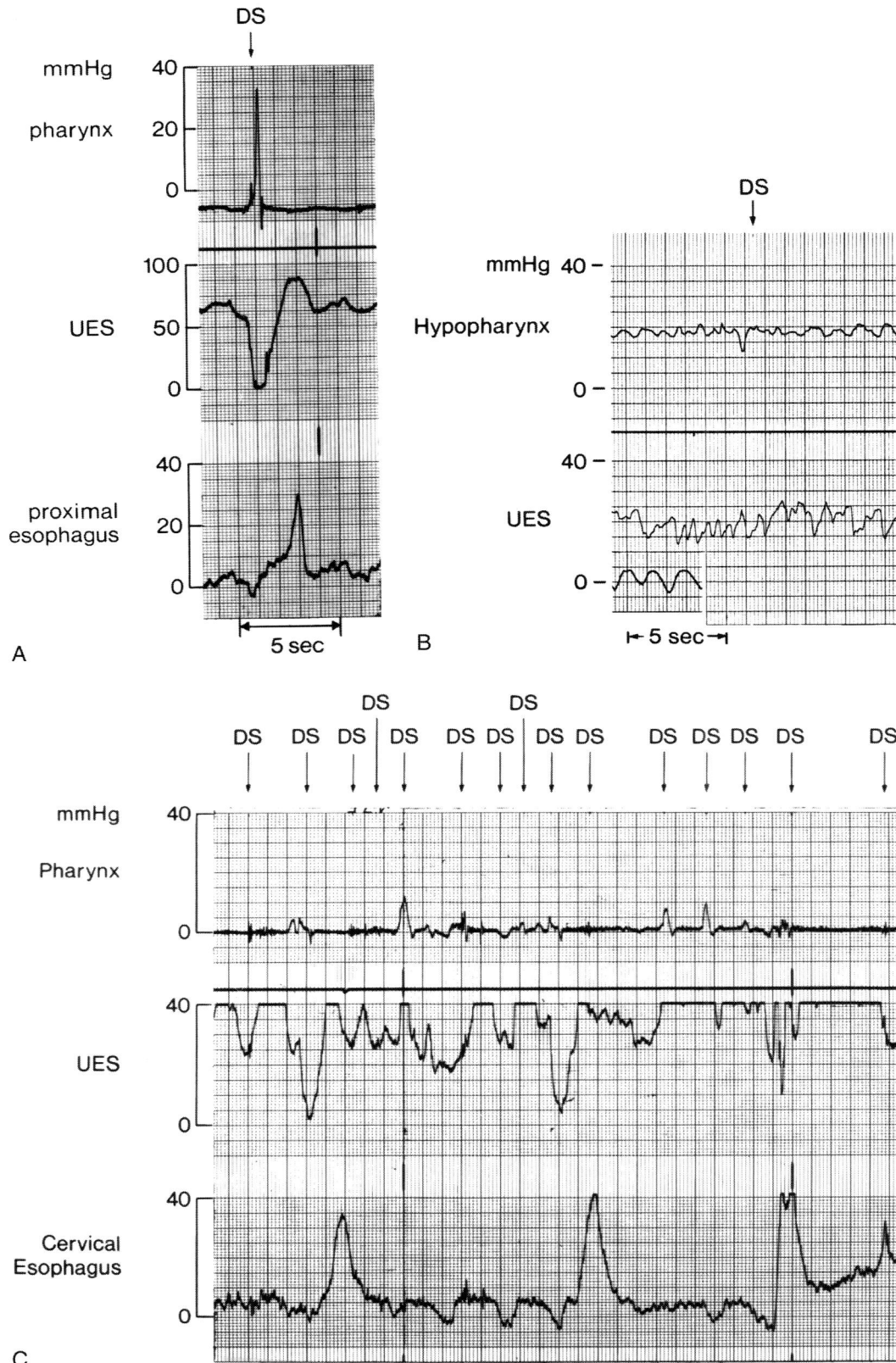

FIGURE 27–57. Oropharyngeal dysphagia of neurologic origin. *A,* Normal function of the pharyngoesophageal junction. *B,* Elevated resting pressures in the hypopharynx in a cerebrovascular accident victim. Dry swallow (DS) is followed by absent contraction in the hypopharynx and absent relaxation of the UES. *C,* Basilar artery thrombosis with repetitive DS followed by a powerless activity in the pharynx as well as absent, incomplete, and occasional complete opening of the UES.

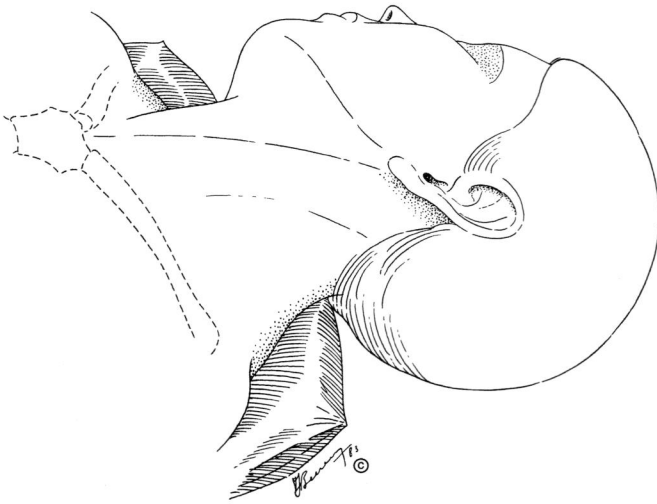

FIGURE 27–58. Cricopharyngeal myotomy for oropharyngeal dysphagia: cervical approach at the anterior border of the sternocleidomastoid muscle.

FIGURE 27–59. Cricopharyngeal myotomy: plane of dissection to reach the pharyngoesophageal junction.

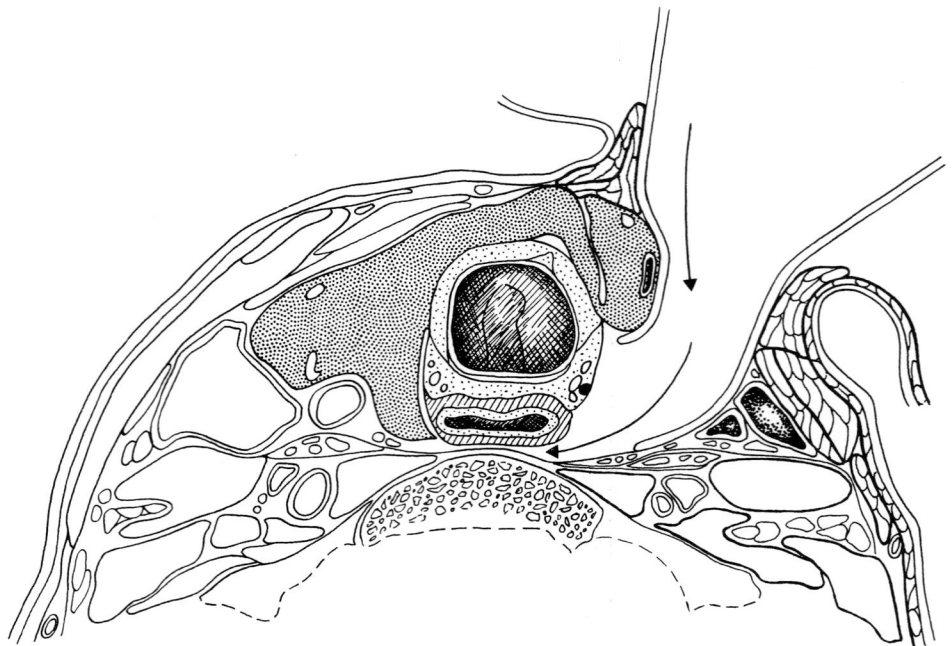

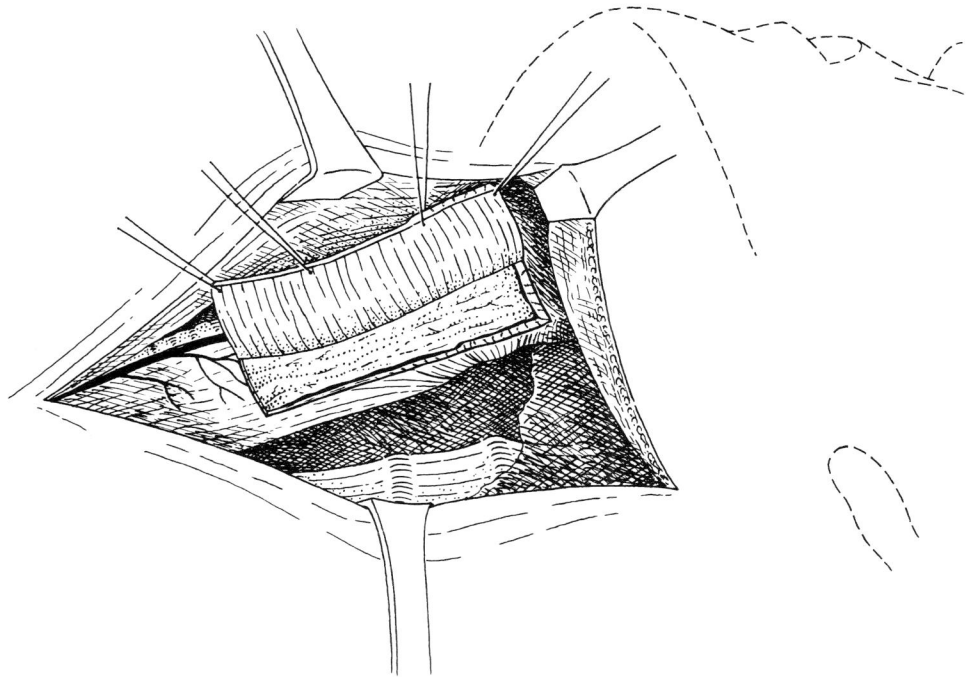

FIGURE 27–60. A 6-cm myotomy encompasses the musculature of the hypopharynx, the cricopharyngeus, and the proximal musculature of the cervical esophagus.

and stems from persistent aspiration with subsequent pulmonary and cardiovascular complications.

MUSCULAR DYSPHAGIA

Weaker and longer contractions in the pharynx of these patients are not powerful enough to propel the bolus past the cricopharyngeus area. The UES becomes a functional obstacle to food transit (Fig. 27–61; see also Figs. 27–52 to 27–54). Just as for neurologic patients, cricopharyngeal myotomy aims to abolish the resistance at the pharyngoesophageal junction (see Figs. 27–58 to 27–60). These patients, although they have a powerless pharynx, still improve in over 75% of cases (Duranceau et al., 1988; Taillefer and Duranceau, 1988). They retain adequate voluntary deglutition, and if they also retain appropriate muscular control of their larynx, comfortable swallowing is obtained following the myotomy with significant decrease in preoperative symptoms. Improvement in pharyngeal emptying is usually observed (see Figs. 27–55 and 27–56). Progression of the disease is the main factor controlling evolution following the myotomy. The appearance of dysphonia and hoarseness suggests deterioration of muscular function with potentially increased aspiration episodes. In these patients, laryngeal exclusion or excision is necessary to stop the aspiration problems (Fig. 27–62).

IDIOPATHIC DYSFUNCTION OF THE UPPER ESOPHAGEAL SPHINCTER

Dysfunction of the UES without any evidence of neurologic or muscular pathology to explain it is termed *idiopathic*. In these patients, no pharyngoesophageal diverticulum is present and the same type of cricopharyngeal myotomy is used as for patients with neurologic or muscular dysphagia (see Figs. 27–58 to 27–60). Over 80 patients operated for this condition have been reported, with seven-eighths showing excellent improvement following their operation.

The functional abnormalities present in the UES of patients when a pharyngoesophageal diverticulum is present have been assessed in a very meticulous study by Cook and colleagues (1992b) and by Jamieson and associates (1993). Using a sleeve sensor to assess the sphincter, these authors documented significantly higher intrabolus pressures in the hypopharynx during barium swallow studies (Figs. 27–63 to 27–66). At the same time, they measured the maximal luminal area of the open sphincter. The computed surface of the sphincter showed significantly less area than in controls. Documented histologic fibrosis and inflammation in the sphincter are responsible for a restrictive myopathy (Cook et al., 1992a). Thus, the decreased sphincter compliance and the high hypopharyngeal intrabolus pressures might eventually lead to diverticulum formation through repeated efforts of pharynx and hypopharynx.

The therapy for dysphagia secondary to UES dysfunction with an established pharyngoesophageal diverticulum is surgical. If the diverticulum is very small, an extensive cricopharyngeal myotomy over the pharyngoesophageal junction should allow the pouch to disappear with the symptoms (Duranceau and Jamieson, 1987; Ellis and Crozier, 1981; Jamieson et al., 1993; Lerut et al., 1987; Payne and King, 1983) (Fig. 27–67).

When the pouch is larger, section of the restrictive

Text continued on page 974

PHARYNX

NORMAL

OPMD

A

A.T. 74

B

C

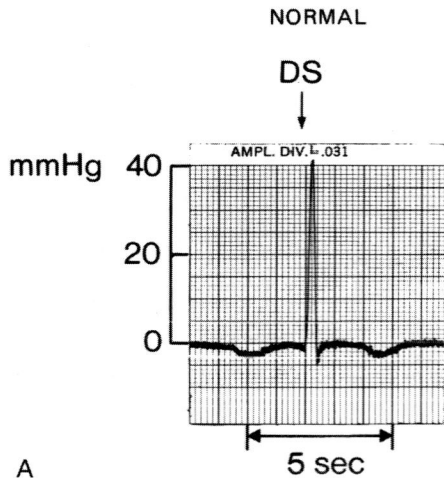

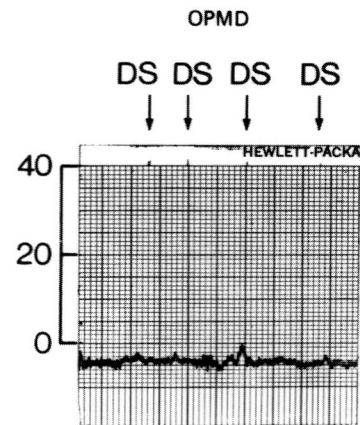

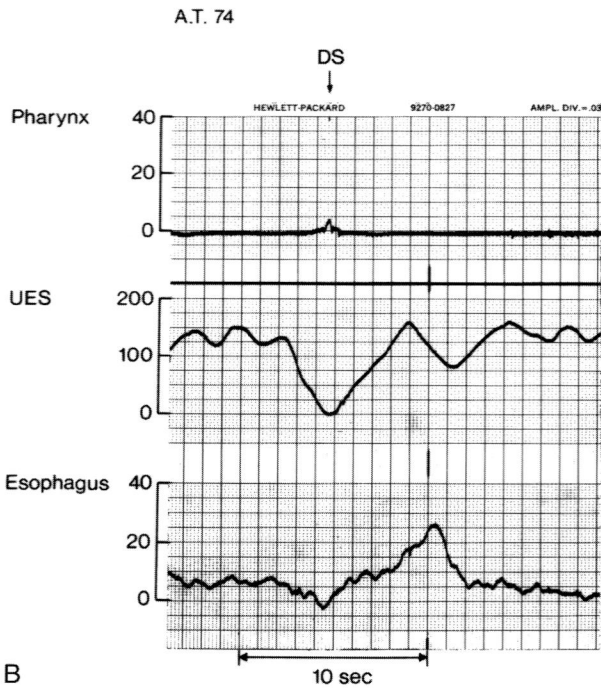

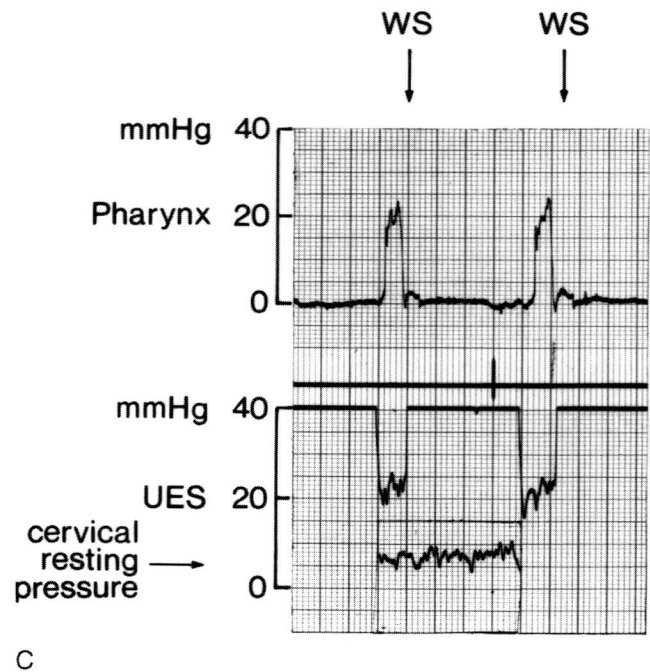

FIGURE 27–61. Oropharyngeal dysphagia in patients with oculopharyngeal muscular dystrophy (OPMD). *A,* When compared with a normal subject *(left),* the dystrophy patient shows repetitive and powerless contractions. *B,* The UES shows relaxation of increased duration when a hypotonic contraction of the pharynx is generated. *C,* Incomplete relaxation of the UES to cervical resting pressure.

FIGURE 27–62. Permanent tracheostomy with either laryngeal exclusion or laryngectomy may become the sole therapeutic option if tracheal aspirations cannot be improved by cricopharyngeal myotomy.

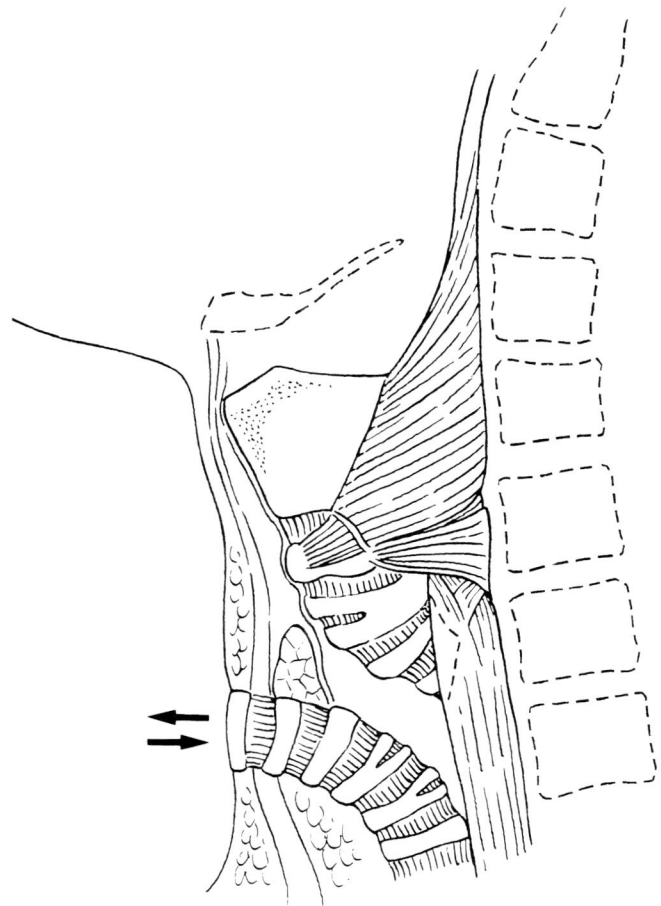

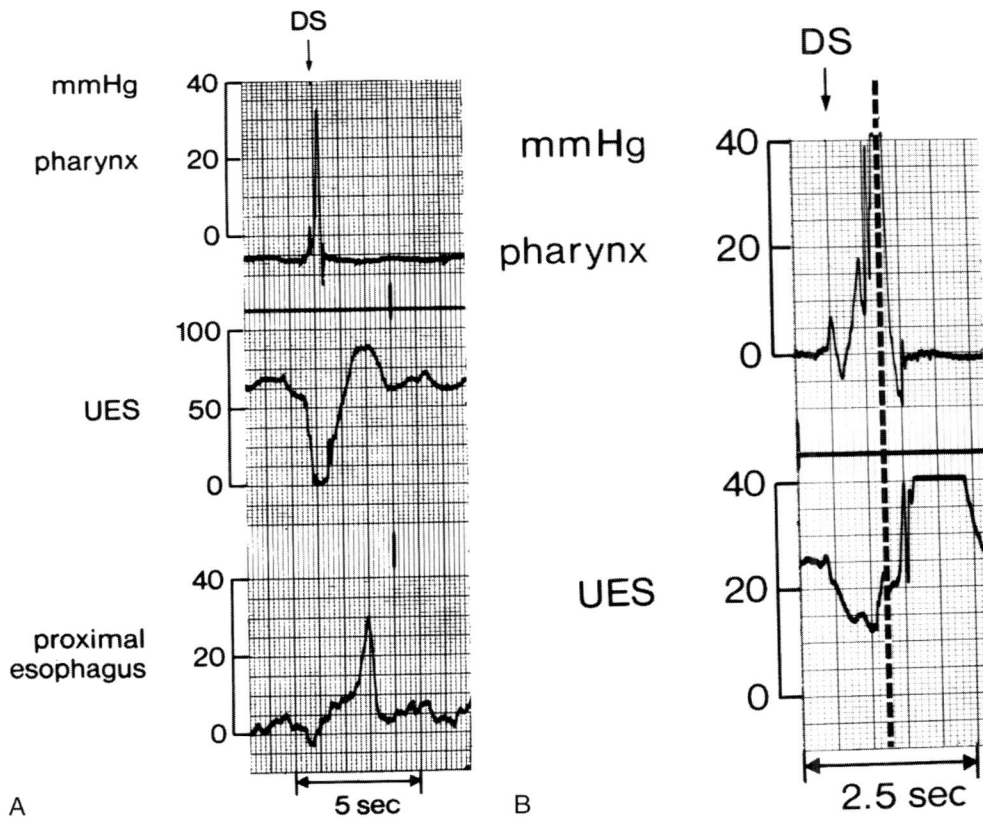

A

B

FIGURE 27–63. UES recording in a patient with a Zenker diverticulum, using standard manometry. When compared with normal function (A), premature closure of the sphincter against the persistent pharyngeal contraction can be observed and was interpreted as sphincter incoordination (B).

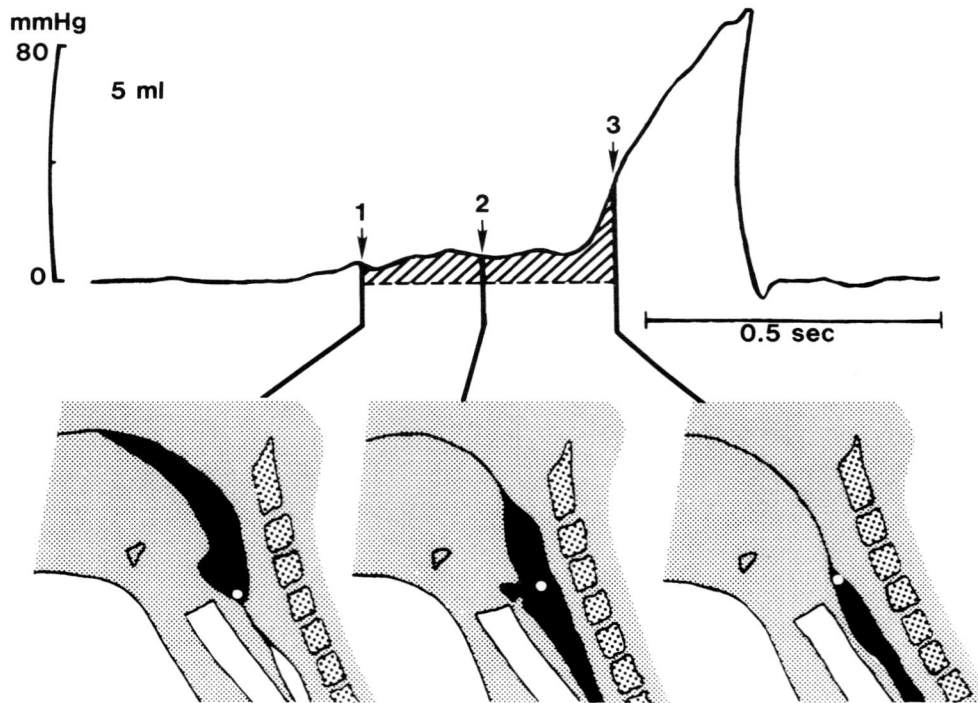

FIGURE 27–64. Sleeve recording and measurement of intrabolus pressure in a normal patient. (From Cook, I. J., Gabb, M., Panagopoulos, V., et al.: Pharyngeal [Zenker's] diverticulum is a disorder of upper esophageal sphincter opening. Gastroenterology, *103*:1229–1235, 1992.)

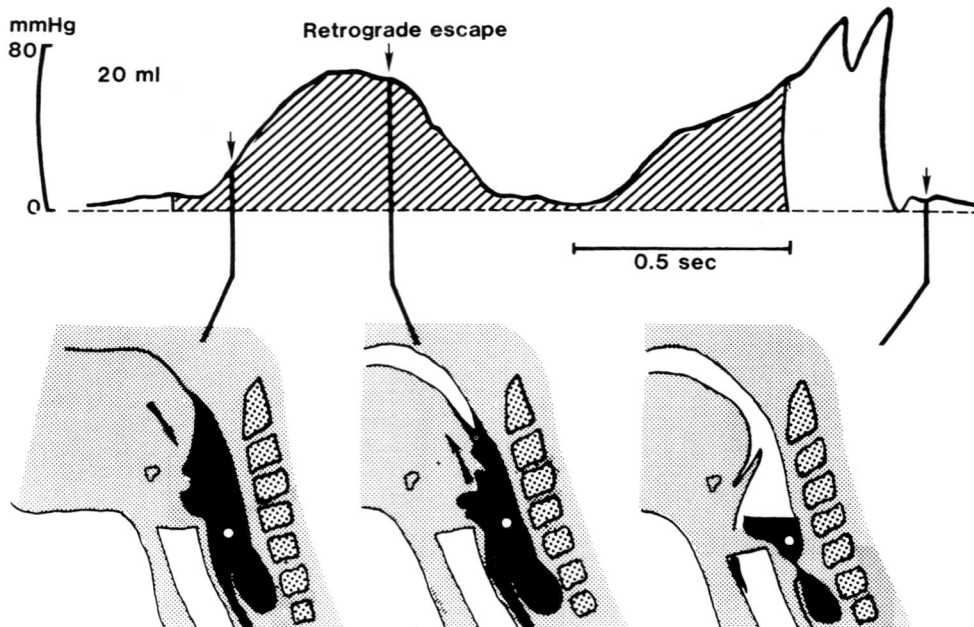

FIGURE 27–65. Manometric recording in a patient with Zenker's diverticulum. Hyperpressure is noted in the hypopharynx, whereas an incomplete relaxation of the sphincter is observed radiologically. This is due to restrictive disease in the sphincter. The end result over time probably will be diverticulum formation. (From Cook, I. J., Gabb, M., Panagopoulos, V., et al.: Pharyngeal [Zenker's] diverticulum is a disorder of upper esophageal sphincter opening. Gastroenterology, *103*:1229–1235, 1992.)

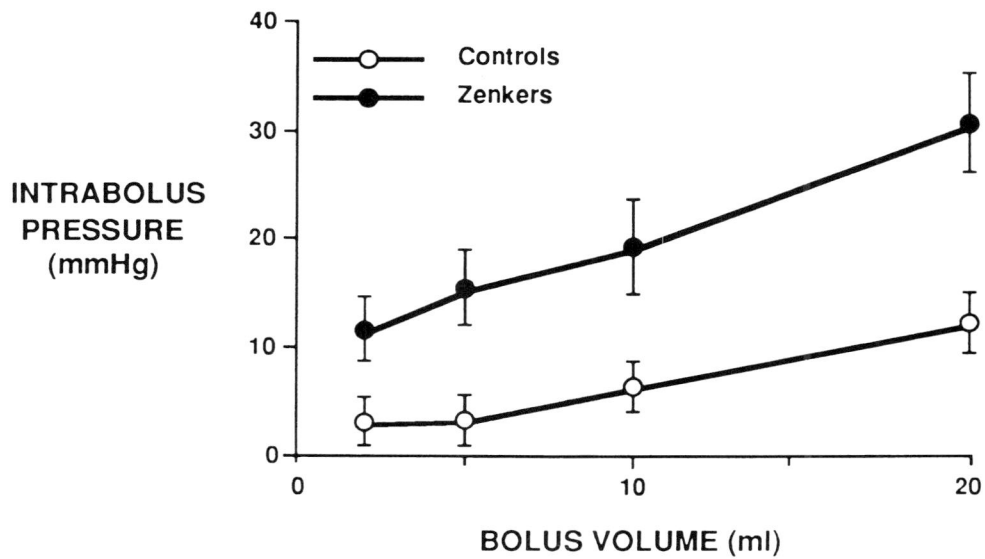

FIGURE 27–66. Significantly greater intrabolus pressures exist in the hypopharynx of Zenker's diverticulum patients when compared with normal subjects. (From Cook, I. J., Gabb, M., Panagopoulos, V., et al.: Pharyngeal [Zenker's] diverticulum is a disorder of upper esophageal sphincter opening. Gastroenterology, *103*:1229–1235, 1992.)

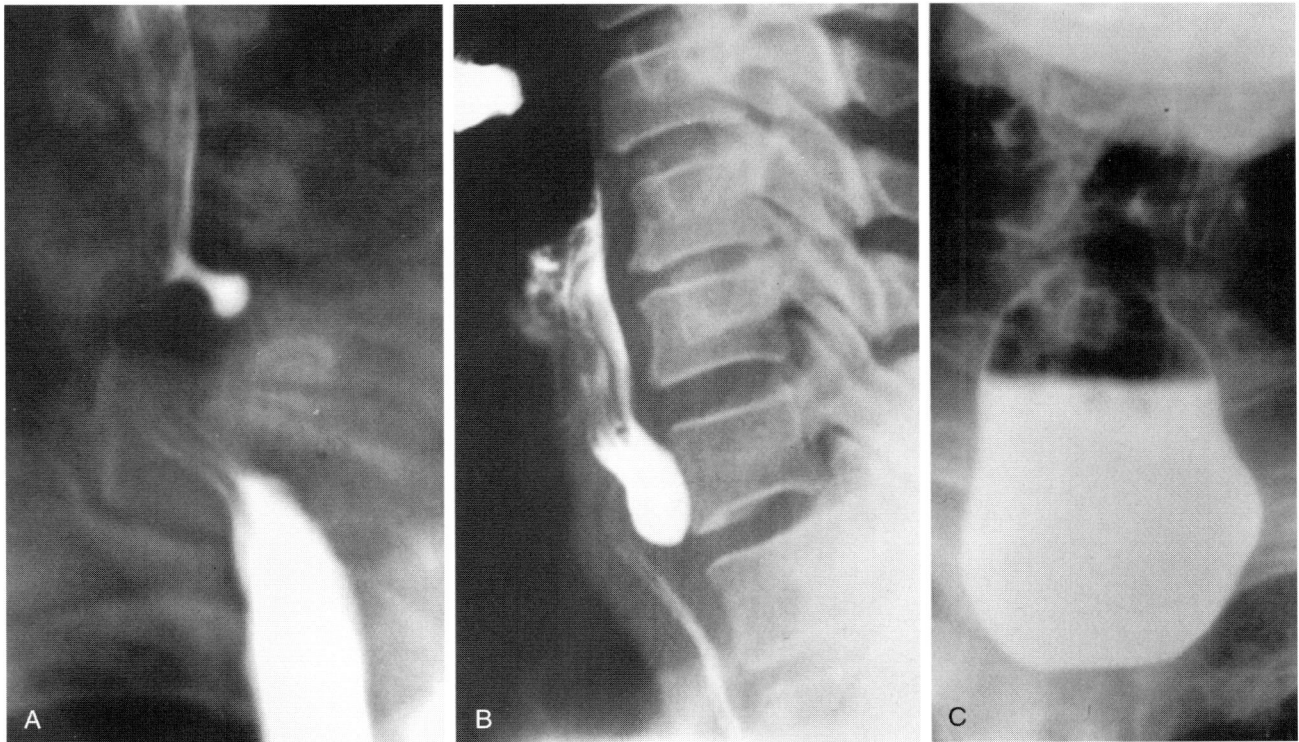

FIGURE 27–67. *A,* The very small diverticulum can be managed by cricopharyngeal myotomy of the pharyngoesophageal junction. *B,* The medium-sized diverticulum is managed by myotomy and suspension of the diverticulum. *C,* The large diverticulum requires resection and myotomy.

■ **Table 27–8.** DIAGNOSTIC CRITERIA OF PRIMARY IDIOPATHIC MOTOR DISORDERS

	Hypomotility	Hypermotility			
	Achalasia	*Diffuse Esophageal Spasm*	*Hyperperistalsis (Nutcracker Supersqueeze)*	*Hypertensive LES*	*Nonspecific Esophageal Motility Disorders*
Peristalsis	Totally absent in esophageal body High resting pressure	>30% Repetitive tertiary contraction (triphasic or more for at least 30% of swallows) Normal peristalsis between abnormal contractions	Normal	Normal	Spontaneous tertiary activity Occasional tertiary contractions in response to swallowing Peristalsis usually normal
Contraction amplitude	Weak, mirror-like organization at all recording levels	Duration and amplitude occasionally abnormal	Greater than 2 standard deviations above normal Increased amplitude in distal esophagus >180 mm Hg Increased duration of contractions >6 sec	Normal	Decreased or weak
Lower esophageal sphincter	Normal or increased resting pressures Incomplete or absent relaxation	LES occasionally hypertensive Occasional incomplete relaxation (30%)	Occasionally hypertensive	Hypertensive (>45 mm Hg) Normal or incomplete relaxation	Normal

cricopharyngeus and suspension of the diverticulum behind the pharynx (Fig. 27–68) aims to remove the abnormal muscle and allow a return to normal of hypopharyngeal pressures (Jamieson et al., 1993). If the diverticulum is too large to be suspended, resec-tion of the pouch while leaving the myotomy wide open is the treatment of choice (Fig. 27–69). Lerut and co-workers (1987) observed that the incidence of complications doubled if a diverticulectomy was performed without a myotomy. Moreover, long-term

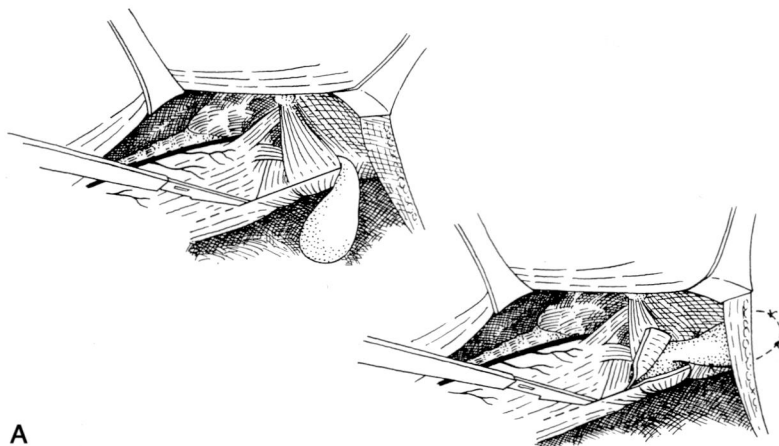

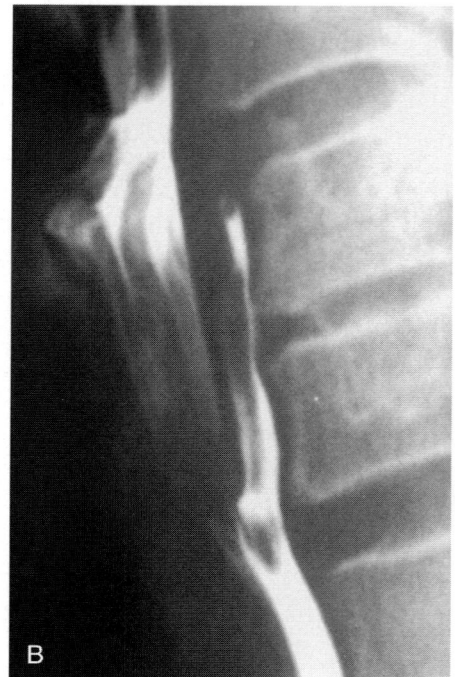

FIGURE 27–68. *A,* Cricopharyngeal myotomy and diverticulum suspension. *B,* Radiologic appearance of the suspended diverticulum.

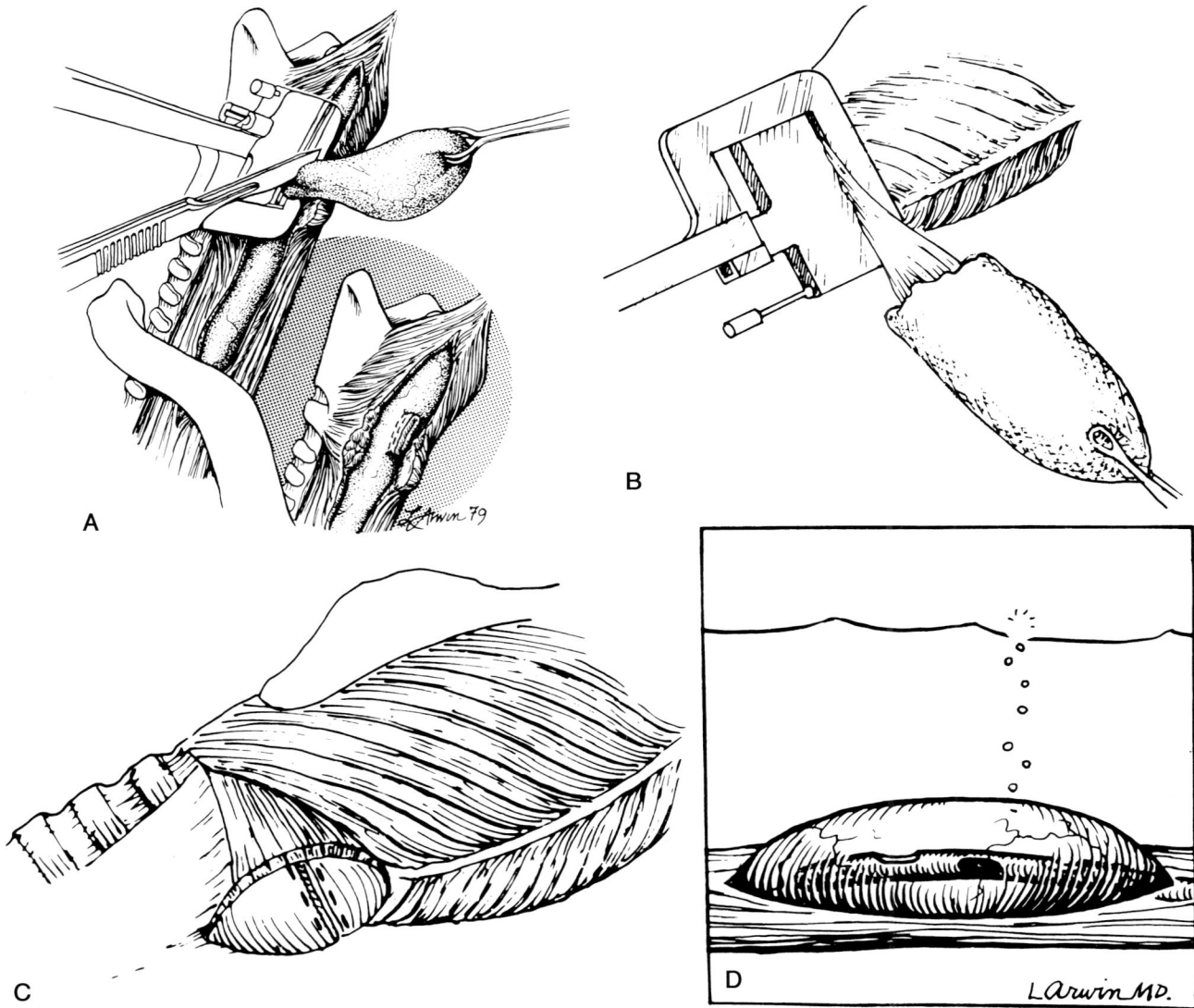

FIGURE 27–69. *A,* Resection of a larger diverticulum: The cricopharyngeal myotomy is completed, and vertical stapling is performed at the base of the diverticulum. An endoesophageal, mercury-filled bougie protects the integrity of the esophageal lumen. The myotomy is left open following the resection. *B,* Resection of a larger diverticulum using a transverse stapling technique. *C,* The myotomy is left wide open following the resection. *D,* As for other esophageal myotomies, testing for mucosal integrity is accomplished by air insufflation in the esophageal lumen while the myotomized esophagus is immersed. (*A,* From Orringer, M. B.: Extended cervical esophagotomy for cricopharyngeal dysfunction. J. Thorac. Cardiovasc. Surg., *80*:669, 1980; *B,* From Payne, W. S., and Reynolds, R. R.: Surgical treatment of pharyngoesophageal diverticulum [Zenker's diverticulum]. Surg. Rounds, 5:1, 1982. By permission of Mayo Foundation.)

follow-up reveals a high recurrence of the diverticulum following diverticulectomy alone. With the actual evidence at hand, solid justification exists to treat the pharyngoesophageal diverticulum as a complication of a restrictive myopathy, with myotomy followed by either diverticulum suspension or resection. Results are good to excellent in over 90% of reported cases.

Idiopathic Motor Disorders

The spectrum of esophageal motor disorders and their diagnostic criteria are given in Table 27–8. Dysfunction is associated with hypomotility and hypermotility abnormalities. Motor disorders that cause reflux disease are analyzed separately (Table 27–9).

Hypomotility Disorders

ACHALASIA

Achalasia is a more well known motor disorder because it is described better and responds to more precise diagnostic criteria. It is a condition seen frequently in young adults, with an incidence of 1 in 100,000 people (Earlam et al., 1969).

Cause. The cause of achalasia is still unknown. A

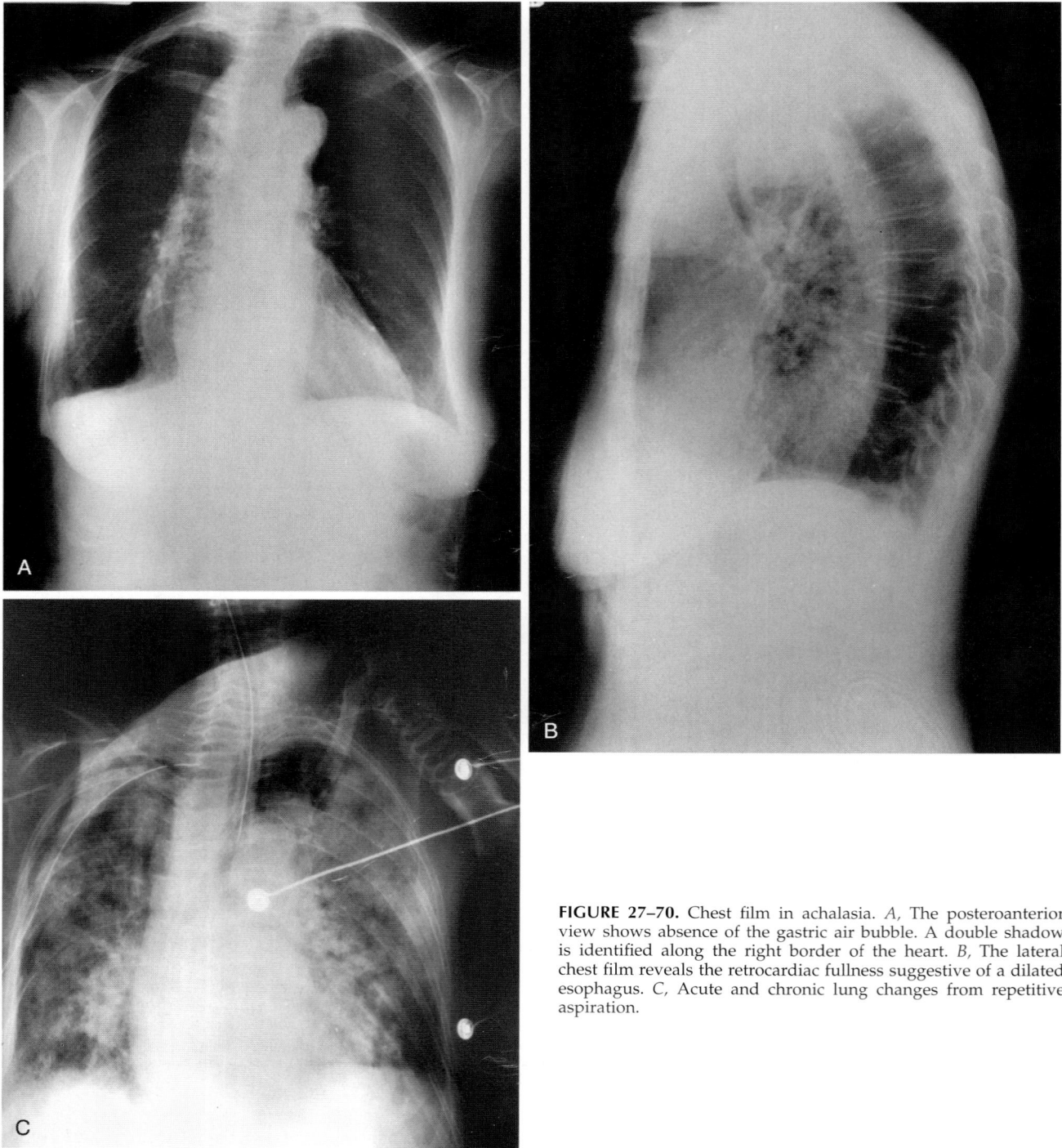

FIGURE 27–70. Chest film in achalasia. *A,* The posteroanterior view shows absence of the gastric air bubble. A double shadow is identified along the right border of the heart. *B,* The lateral chest film reveals the retrocardiac fullness suggestive of a dilated esophagus. *C,* Acute and chronic lung changes from repetitive aspiration.

loss of control at the postganglionic, nonadrenergic, and noncholinergic inhibitory nerves explains the dysfunction at the level of the LES and in the esophageal body (Wong and Maydonovitch, 1992) (see Fig. 27–45). Denervation has always been suggested as being responsible for this loss of control because of studies describing vagal injury at both the central and the peripheral levels (Cassella et al., 1964). The parasitic denervation seen in patients with Chagas' disease causes an achalasia-like condition in the

esophagus but with systemic manifestations. Severe physical and psychological stress can often be documented in achalasia patients, suggesting that a still undocumented mechanism causes the motor dysfunction.

Clinical Presentation. Clinically, most achalasia patients are seen when they are under 50 years of age, but older patients are not immune to the condition. Substernal dysphagia, the most frequent symptom, is accompanied by odynophagia, especially in the early

■ **Table 27–9.** ESOPHAGEAL MOTOR DISORDERS IN REFLUX DISEASE

| | Idiopathic Gastroesophageal Reflux | | Scleroderma and Reflux |
	Uncomplicated	*Complicated*	
Peristalsis	Normal	Normal or decreased (in proportion to wall damage)	Normal in striated esophagus Usually absent in smooth muscle esophagus
Contraction amplitude	Normal	Normal or decreased (in proportion to wall damage)	Adequate in striated esophagus Usually weak or absent in smooth muscle esophagus
Lower esophageal sphincter	Weak (gradient <6 mm Hg)	Weak or absent	Weak or absent

phases of the disease. Regurgitation of fresh food without any sour taste and loss of weight are also seen in most patients. Oropharyngeal dysphagia may occasionally be the sole presenting symptom of the disorder. Pulmonary complications from aspirations, namely pneumonitis, asthma-like syndrome, and pulmonary abscesses, are seen mostly in late-stage disease. Symptoms may be increased by cold liquids and are often influenced significantly by stressful situations. The most severe complication seen with achalasia is the development of a squamous cell carcinoma, which occurs in 1 to 10% of the achalasia population (Hankins and McLaughlin, 1975; Matthews and Pattison, 1988). These tumors are diagnosed late because they have a longer evolution without causing obstruction, and therefore carry a poorer prognosis.

Diagnosis

Radiology. Routine chest films may reveal the esophageal dilatation as well as acute or chronic sequelae of lung disease (Fig. 27–70). Esophageal dilatation seen with absent peristalsis and absent LES relaxation suggests the diagnosis (Fig. 27–71). The typical radiographic observation (Fig. 27–72) shows a smooth

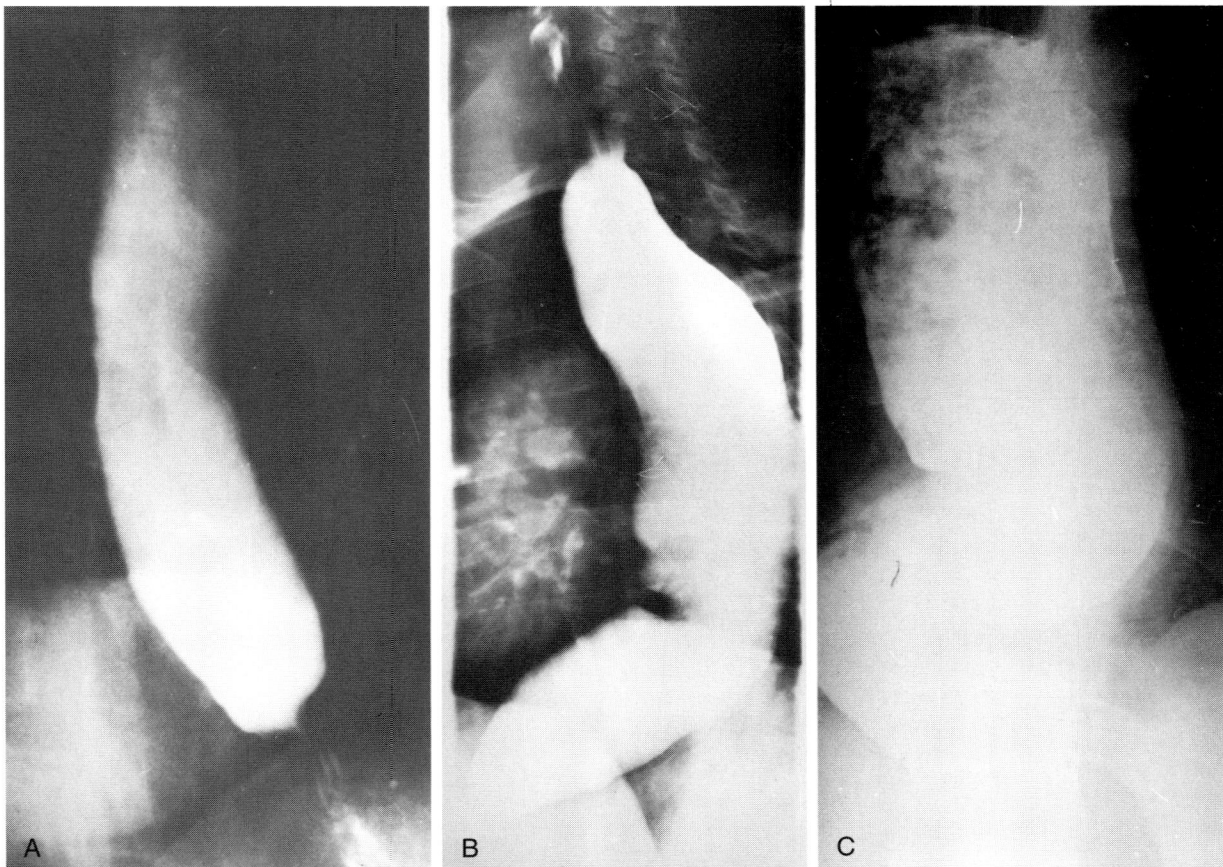

FIGURE 27–71. *A,* Moderate dilatation in achalasia. *B,* Intermediate esophageal widening with early angulation. *C,* Wide and tortuous megaesophagus.

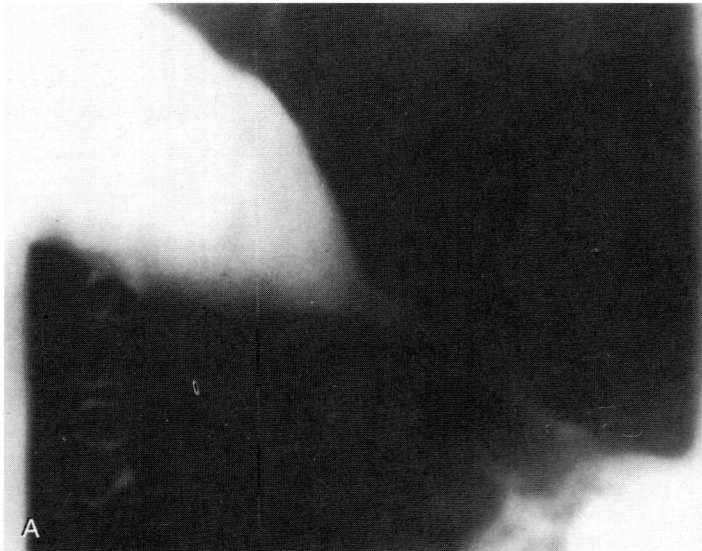

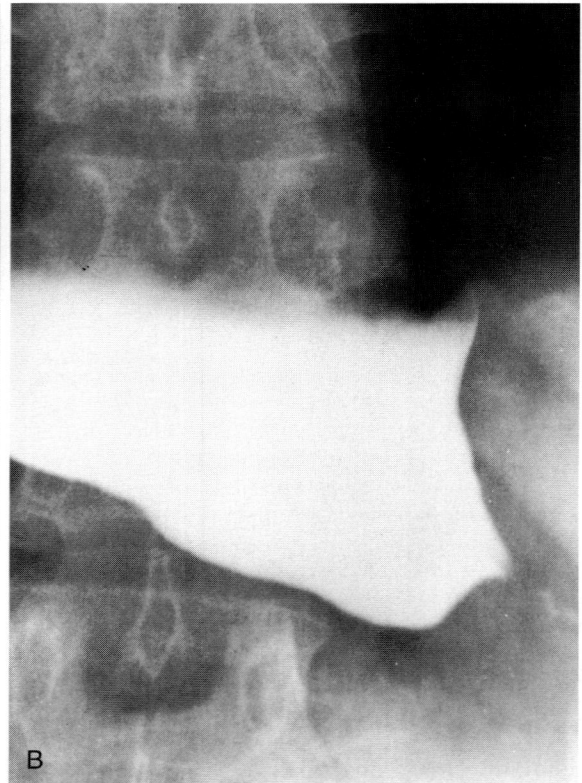

FIGURE 27–72. Detailed view of the LES region in achalasia. Tapering and bird's beak deformity in early achalasia *(A)* and in more advanced achalasia *(B)*.

tapered distal esophagus with a GEJ that opens poorly. However, radiologic findings do not always correlate with the length of evolution and with the symptoms. An achalasia esophagus smaller than 3 cm is considered to be in the early phase of evolution. Between 3 and 7 cm, it is considered to be at an intermediate stage, and over 7 cm, at a late stage (see Fig. 27–71). A small gastric cavity with no gastric air bubble may be seen with an absent LES relaxation (Orlando et al., 1978). Submucous infiltration by ade-

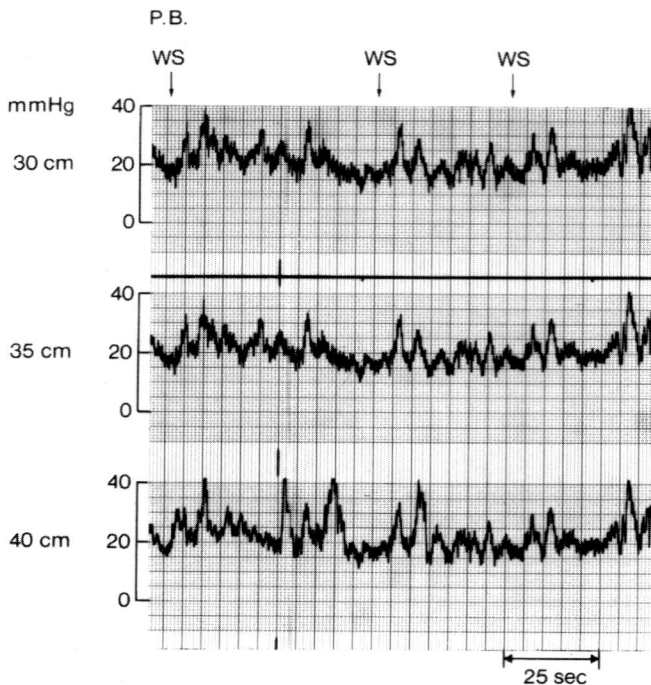

FIGURE 27–73. Esophageal body motor function in early achalasia. The resting pressure is elevated. Contractions in response to swallowing are stronger but without any peristalsis.

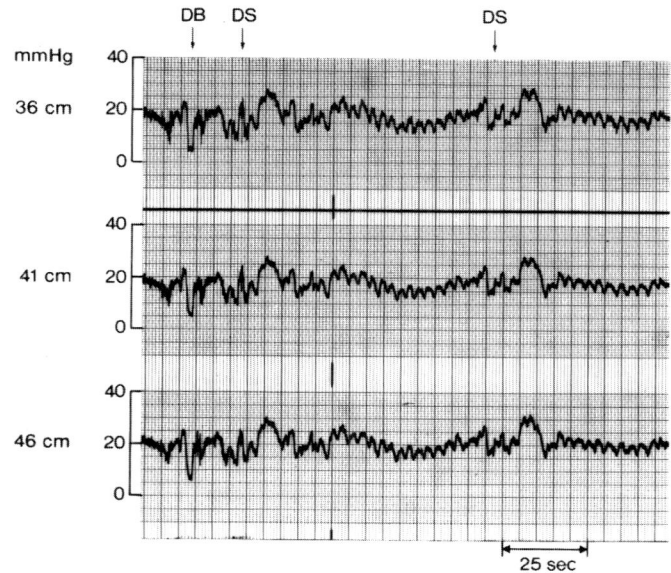

FIGURE 27–74. Esophageal body motor function in later achalasia: Flat nonperistaltic waves are seen in response to all swallows. The waves are identical at all recording levels. The resting pressures are increased. These changes are seen in the whole esophageal body, and no peristalsis is ever observed.

nocarcinoma of the cardia can give a similar picture and must be ruled out.

Endoscopy. The endoluminal aspect of the achalasic esophagus varies with the stage of evolution. In the early phase of achalasia, the esophagus may be perfectly normal. Resistance may be encountered at the GEJ owing to the hypertonic activity at the LES level. Progressive yielding of the junction without any evidence of mucosal lesion on the squamous epithelium or on the gastric epithelium of the subcardial region rules out carcinoma. In later stages, esophageal retention of liquids or solids is often encountered in a fasting patient. A thickened mucosa with wide folds and mild to moderate hyperhemia suggests stasis esophagitis.

Motility Studies. Evaluation of motor function is the only diagnostic study that can confirm achalasia (Castell, 1992; Hurwitz et al., 1979). The pharyngoesophageal junction shows normal activity. The esopha-

geal body reveals contraction abnormalities over its whole length, which are diagnostic. Elevated resting pressures are recorded and they remain constantly elevated with regard to atmospheric and intragastric pressures. All of the contractions seen in response to voluntary swallowing are nonpropulsive. They show mirror-like activity at all recording levels. During the early phase, when the esophagus is smaller, these contractions may seem stronger (Fig. 27–73). With progressive dilatation, weaker activity is recorded (Fig. 27–74). Denervation of the esophageal body is suggested when an administered cholinergic medication creates an exaggerated motor response of the esophagus. Bethanechol chloride (Urecholine) is currently used for this diagnosis, and when administered to achalasia patients, it progressively increases resting pressures as well as strength and duration of contractions (Fig. 27–75). This is frequently accompanied by

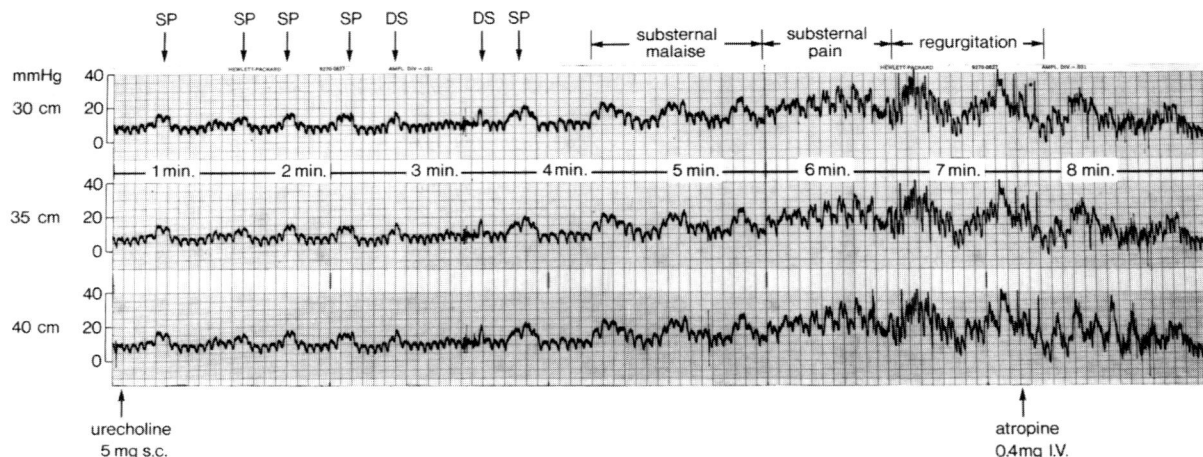

FIGURE 27–75. Esophageal body response to cholinergic stimulation with bethanechol chloride (Urecholine) in achalasia. The esophagus increases its spontaneous activity. Substernal malaise and pain are identified with the stronger contractions. Atropine abolishes the reaction.

chest pain and regurgitation. This reaction is abolished by the administration of atropine.

The LES in achalasia shows normal or elevated resting pressures. Instead of showing a proper opening on swallowing, incomplete or absent relaxation is the rule (Fig. 27–76). These functional abnormalities can be perfectly mimicked by an obstructive carcinoma of the GEJ.

Radionuclide Emptying Studies. Liquid and solid radionuclide emptying studies have been used to quantify results of treatment in achalasia patients (Gross et al., 1979; Holloway et al., 1983). The normal esophagus clears an ingested bolus within 15 seconds (Fig. 27–77A). In the achalasia patient, the esophagus shows significant retention at 2 minutes from ingestion (Fig. 27–77B). These studies add objectivity to symptoms, especially when assessing results of treatment (Fig. 27–77C and D).

Treatment. Management of achalasia is always palliative. It aims to improve dysphagia and poor esophageal emptying. Whatever methods are used to treat the condition, the abnormal motor function of achalasia does not return to normal.

Medication. Generally, nifedipine and diltiazem, as calcium channel blocking agents, are used to decrease the LES resting pressures. Traube and colleagues (1984, 1987) reported that this decrease in pressure reduces symptoms without improving the emptying.

Medication therapy is reserved for patients with early disease and minimal symptoms (Gelfond et al., 1982).

Dilatation. Forceful dilatation using pneumatic or hydrostatic dilators can improve symptoms and esophageal transit in achalasia patients. The dilator is placed fluoroscopically so that the bag is centered on the GEJ and remains in place during the procedure. Single or multiple high-pressure dilatations stretch or rupture the muscle of the LES. The immediate results are a decrease in LES pressures and an improved emptying curve (Gross et al., 1979). Good to excellent short-term results are reported in over 65% of patients. The main complication of dilatation is perforation, which has been reported in from 0 to 15% of patients, averaging around 4% in larger series. Gastroesophageal reflux is not mentioned as a frequent problem following forceful dilatation. However, Yon and Christensen (1975) reported a 7% incidence of reflux, and Bennett and Hendrix (1970) saw clinical and radiologic evidence of reflux in 17% of their dilatation group.

Esophageal Myotomy. Surgical esophagomyotomy for achalasia is more precise technically than dilatation, and it improves obstructive symptoms more effectively (Csendes et al., 1981). This operation can be performed through a left thoracotomy, by laparotomy, or using laparoscopic and thoracoscopic techniques (Pellegrini et al., 1992). The technical principles are

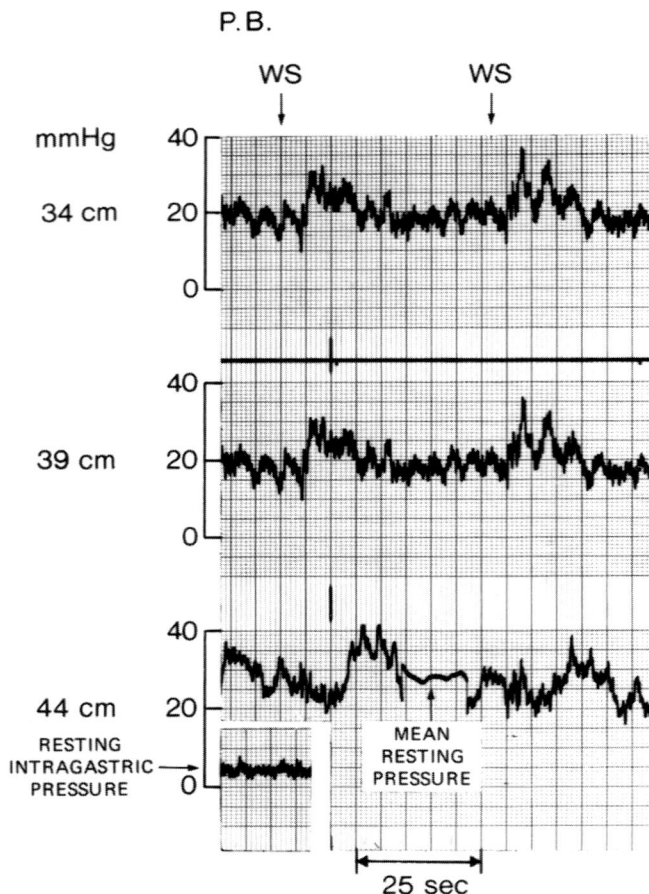

FIGURE 27–76. LES function in achalasia. Resting pressures are normal or above normal. LES relaxation to the level of intragastric pressure is incomplete or absent on swallowing.

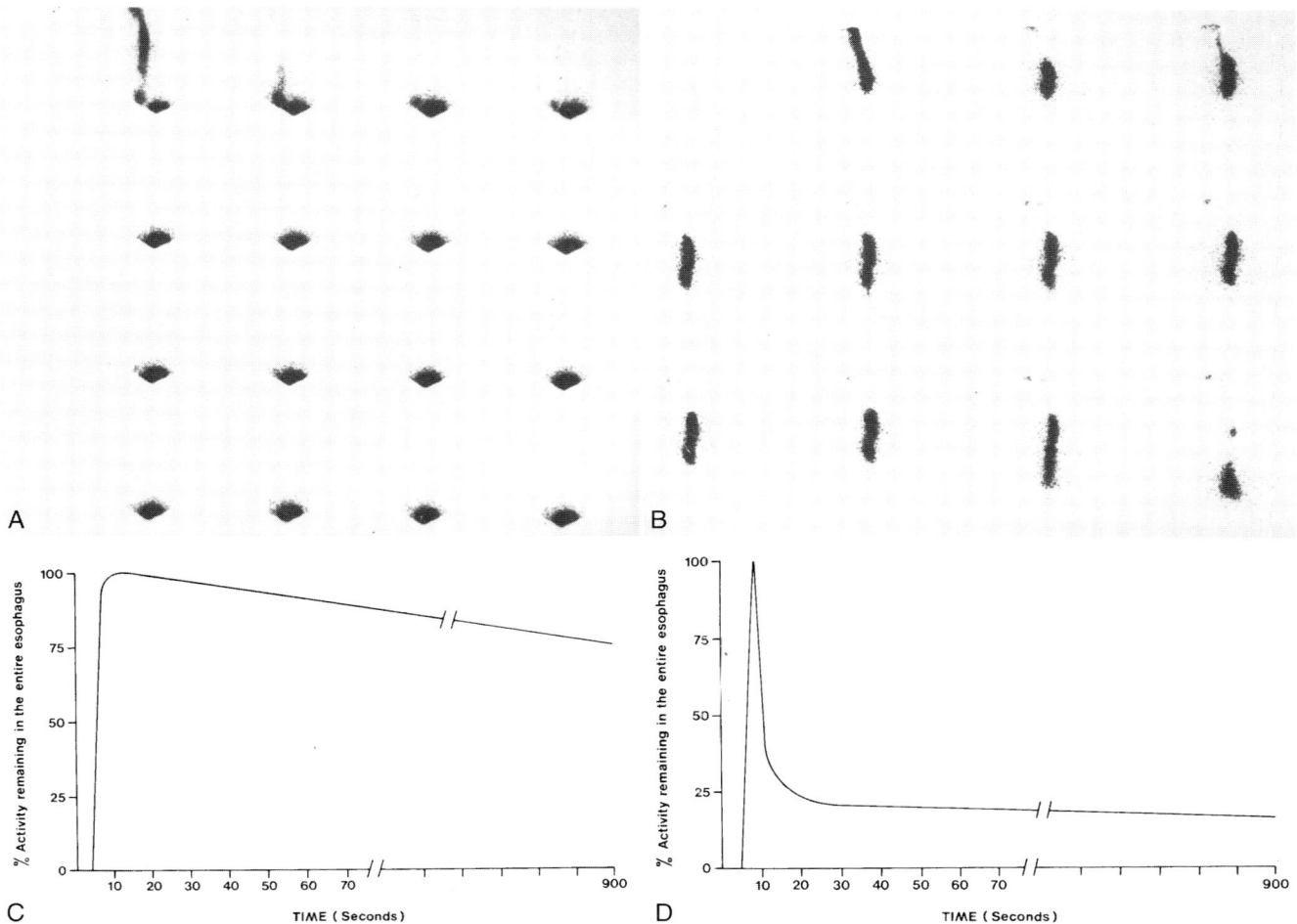

FIGURE 27–77. Esophageal emptying scintigram. *A,* The normal esophagus clears an ingested bolus rapidly. *B,* In achalasia, esophageal retention is significant over time. *C,* Emptying of the esophagus before esophageal myotomy. *D,* Emptying of the esophagus following esophageal myotomy.

identical whatever approach is used. Adequate exposure of the distal esophagus and GEJ is essential. A mercury bougie is passed and used as an intraesophageal stent for ease of manipulation during the myotomy.

A short 5- to 7-cm myotomy is completed on the distal esophagus (Fig. 27–78). It extends on the gastric wall for a distance of 1 cm. After the longitudinal and circular muscle layers are divided, the difference in vascular supply to the mucosa is observed at the junction between the esophageal and the gastric linings. The mucosa is dissected free from the muscularis over 50% of the esophageal circumference, allowing its protrusion between the cut muscle margins (Fig. 27–79).

Short-term and long-term results show the control of dysphagia in over 90% of operated patients. This corresponds to a decrease in resting pressures at LES level. The contraction amplitude is further weakened in the distal esophagus. The functional abnormalities usually remain unchanged following myotomy (see Fig. 27–78*B* and *C*). Return of some propulsive activity has been documented in the proximal esophagus following this operation (Topart et al., 1992).

Complications of surgical myotomy have been reviewed (Andreollo and Earlam, 1987; Moreno Gonzales et al., 1988). Mucosal perforations at operation occur in 1.1% of all patients and cause fistula formation and sepsis in 0.4%. Reflux disease is the feared long-term complication. Anatomic disruption and weakening of the LES are potentially responsible for its occurrence. It has been reported in from 0 to 52% of cases studied (Jamieson and Duranceau, 1988b), the incidence increasing with the passage of time and stabilizing at 13 years postmyotomy (Jara et al., 1979). These observations suggest that reflux disease may become troublesome over time. Many antireflux repairs have thus been suggested at the time of myotomy in order to prevent its complications. Adding an antireflux operation at the end of an atonic esophagus may lead to emptying problems. A total fundoplication has been shown to become too obstructive over time (Ellis and Gibb, 1975; Topart et al., 1992). A partial fundoplication offers satisfactory control of reflux symptoms without causing undue emptying problems (Fig. 27–80).

No treatment in achalasia returns a normal function. One aim prevails: Offering the best control of

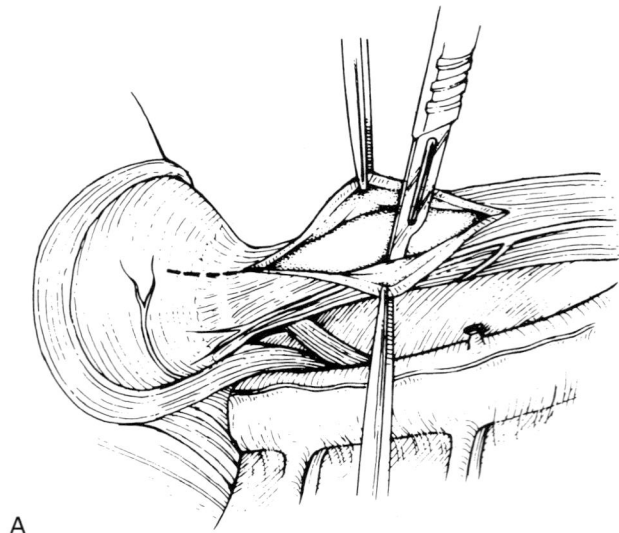

A

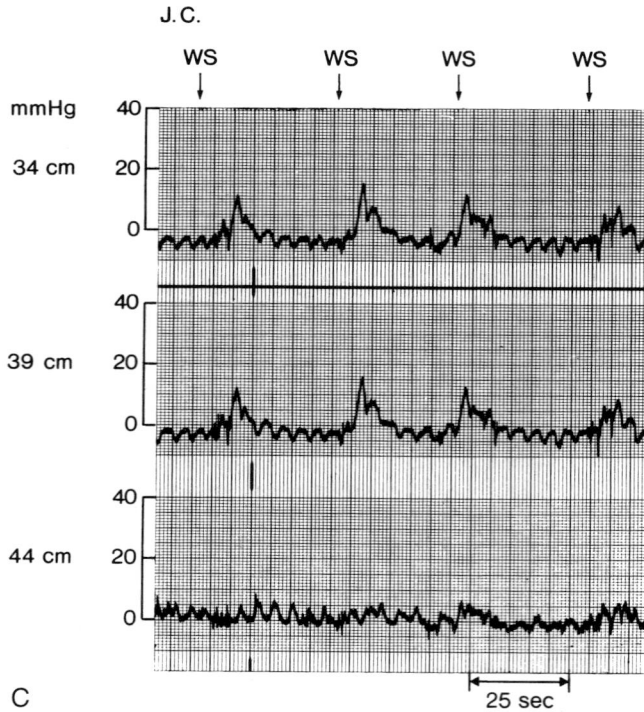

B

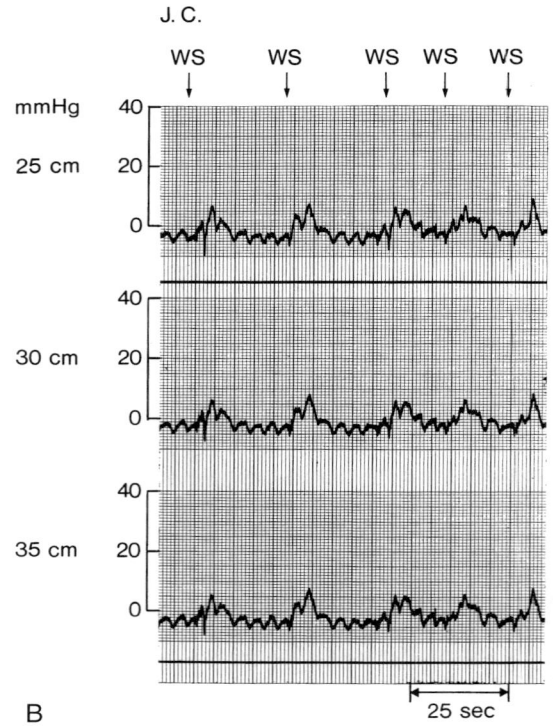

C

FIGURE 27-78. *A,* Short esophagomyotomy in achalasia. The distal esophagus and cardia are mobilized. The myotomy passes from the level of the inferior pulmonary vein down to the stomach, extending 1 cm on the gastric wall. *B,* Further weakening of esophageal body contractions following myotomy. *C,* Decrease in LES resting pressures following cardiomyotomy. (*A,* From Jamieson, G. G., and Debas, H. T. [eds]: Rob and Smith's Operative Surgery: Surgery of the Upper Gastrointestinal Tract. London, Chapman and Hall, 1994.)

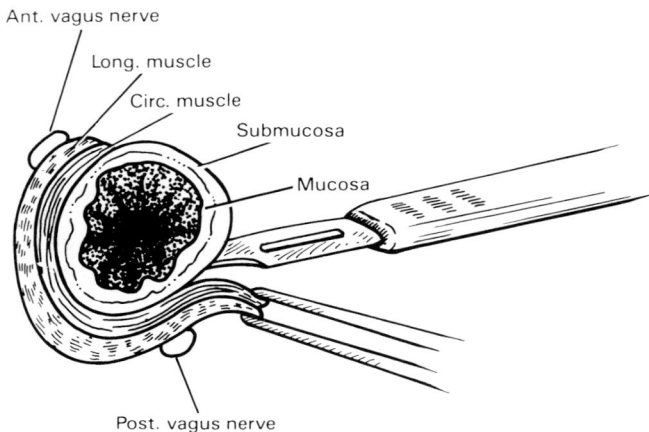

FIGURE 27-79. The muscularis is freed from the mucosa over approximately 50% of the esophageal circumference.

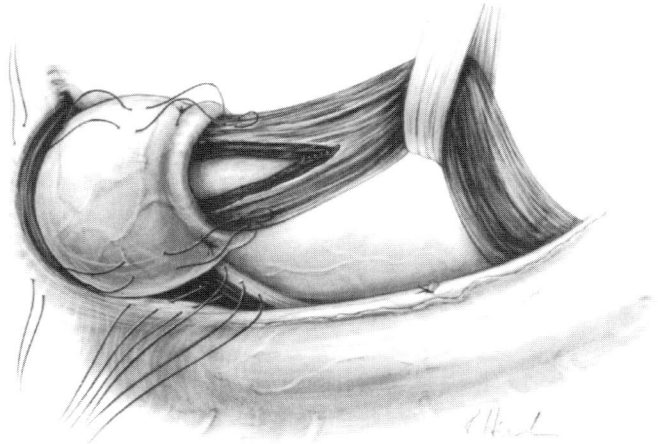

FIGURE 27–80. A partial fundoplication is added to prevent reflux. (From Skinner, D. B.: Atlas of Esophageal Surgery. Churchill Livingstone, New York, 1991.)

symptoms with the least chances of morbidity. Objective long-term follow-up is the only way to assess these results.

Hypermotility Disorders

Hypermotility disorders have been classified by Castell and associates according to manometric criteria. These dysfunction categories are: idiopathic diffuse esophageal spasm, hyperperistalsis (nutcracker or supersqueeze esophagus), and the hypertensive LES (Khan and Castell, 1988).

DIFFUSE ESOPHAGEAL SPASM

Cause. *Symptomatic idiopathic diffuse esophageal spasm* (SIDES) is a rare condition seen in 4% of all patients studied in an esophageal motility laboratory (Dalton et al., 1991). Its pathogenesis is unknown. Some reports have shown a muscle hypertrophy of longitudinal circular and muscularis mucosal layers (Gillies et al., 1967; Hurwitz et al., 1975). Cassella and associates (1965) observed no abnormalities of the smooth esophageal muscle itself, but saw possible degenerative changes in the peripheral branches of the vagus nerves. It remains unclear if all SIDES patients show the same macroscopic and microscopic changes.

It is possible that hyperdynamic disorders represent an evolutionary stage of a more diffuse disorder like achalasia. This remains speculative, since very few patients show this evolution over time (Fig. 27–81).

A relationship between emotional disturbances and esophageal contraction abnormalities has been suggested by Clouse and Lustman (1983; see also Clouse and Staiano, 1983). The fine mechanism leading to the dysfunction remains to be clarified.

Clinical Presentation. The association of dysphagia with odynophagia, especially with episodes of unexplained chest pain, usually leads to esophageal assessment and a correct diagnosis (Fig. 27–82). These symptoms are heard from particularly anxious individuals and they are worsened by stress. Substernal

chest pain irradiating to the back, the jaw, or the shoulders is often interpreted as angina or myocardial ischemia. For these reasons, patients with diffuse esophageal spasm are often referred to the esophageal

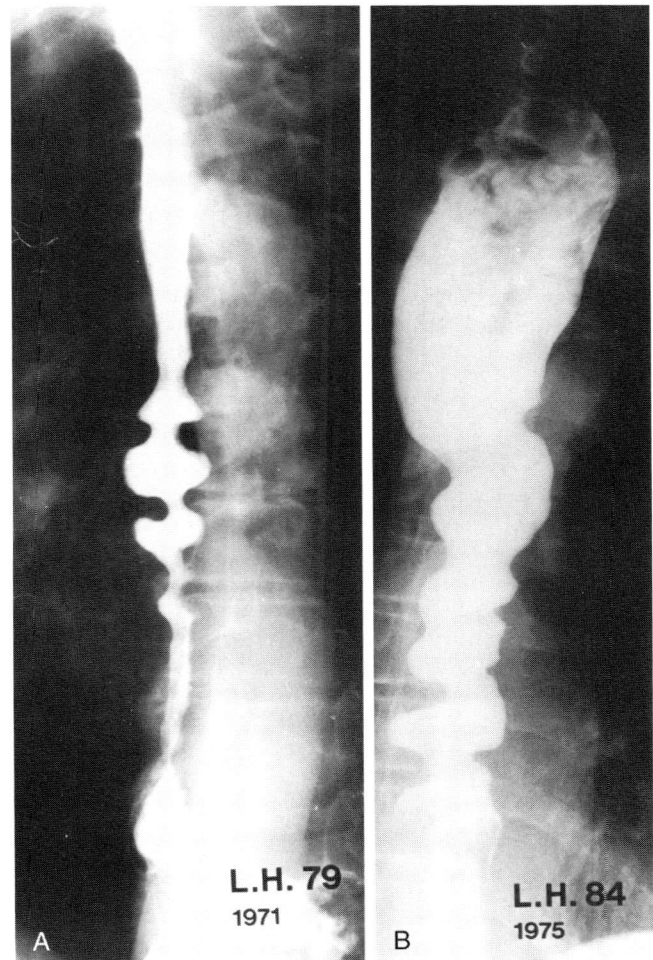

FIGURE 27–81. Hypermotility disorders. Symptomatic diffuse esophageal spasm in the same patient with a 5-year evolution. *A,* At age 79 years. *B,* At age 84 years.

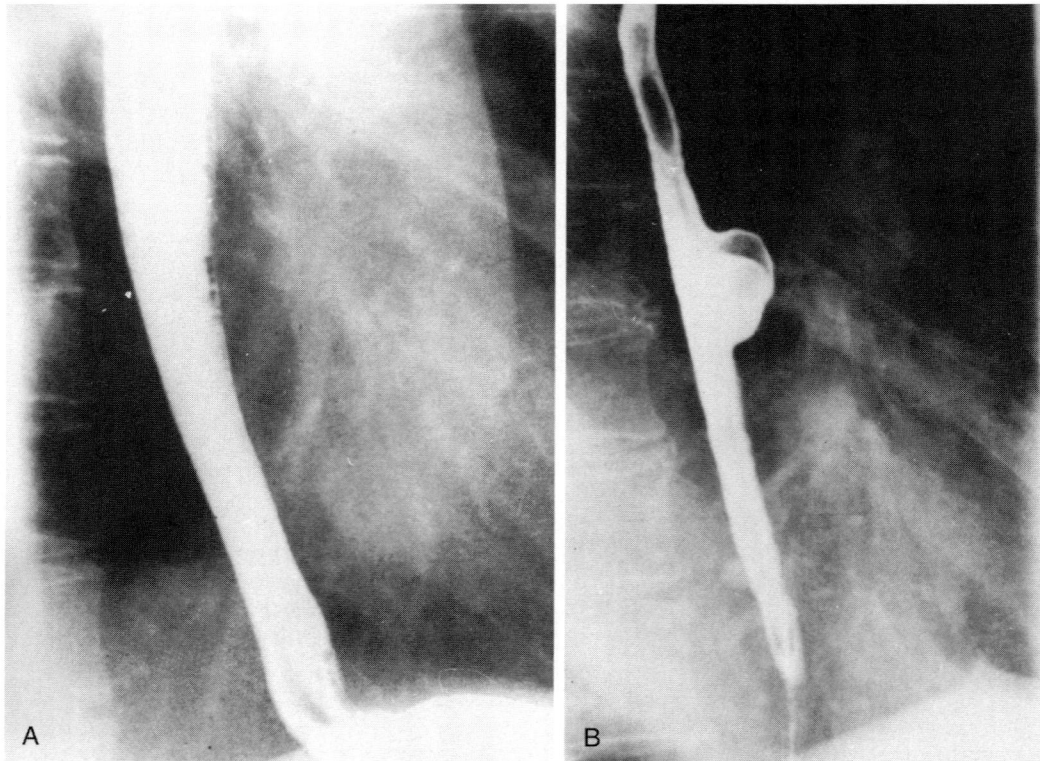

FIGURE 27–82. Hypermotility disorders. *A* and *B,* Intermittent appearance of a diverticulum in a patient repeatedly admitted to the intensive care unit for chest pain.

laboratory with a diagnosis of noncardiac chest pain, following assessment for coronary artery disease. Impaction and regurgitations of fresh food may occur, but not as steadily as in achalasia. Characterization of chest pain is particularly important, since identification of the triggering mechanisms is essential to classify the condition as secondary or idiopathic (Fig. 27–83).

Diagnosis

Radiology. The most suggestive presentation is the simultaneous segmental contractions observed in the smooth muscle section of the esophagus. Immediately below the UES, contractions appear normal. From the aortic arch level down to the GEJ, tertiary activity suggests the many visual aspects mentioned in the literature: a corkscrew, a rosary bead, or simple curling of the barium column (Fig. 27–84; see also Fig. 27–81). Intermittent appearance of a diverticulum may be observed (see Fig. 27–82) or an epiphrenic diverticulum may be present (Figs. 27–85 and 27–86). Chen and co-workers (1989) observed tertiary activity in 12 of 17 patients with a diffuse spasm diagnosis. They concluded that a normal radiographic study could not rule out a primary idiopathic motor disorder.

Endoscopy. Endoscopy may reveal contraction abnormalities during the examination. The mucosa is usually normal and the mouth of a diverticulum may be observed. A mucosal lesion at the GEJ must be ruled out.

Motility Studies. Esophageal motility studies are

the logical investigation in the diagnostic process (see Figs. 27–83, 27–84, and 27–86). The UES and the proximal third of the esophagus show normal function.

In the smooth muscle part of the esophagus, most voluntary swallows produce normal peristalsis. Tertiary contractions occur in more than 10% but less than 100% of voluntary swallows. These contractions must be of the triple-peak variety if they are to be considered abnormal (Castell, 1976; Richter et al., 1984, 1987c) (see Fig. 27–83). Although initially considered only with a pattern of repetitive multiphasic contractions of high amplitude and long duration (Code et al., 1958), the diagnosis of diffuse esophageal spasm may still be considered with contractions of normal amplitude (Dalton et al., 1991). The presence of spontaneous nonpropulsive activity between normal swallows must not be considered diffuse spasm; these contractions may be a variation of the normal. The LES is frequently mentioned as normal in patients with the diffuse spasm (DiMarino and Cohen, 1974). However, 10 patients in their study showed only a partial decrease in LES pressure with swallowing, and 9 showed an increase in basal LES pressure. Campo and Traube (1989) observed similar relaxation abnormalities. More recently, Dalton and colleagues (1991) observed incomplete relaxation in 13% of their studied patients and a hypertensive sphincter in 9% (see Fig. 27–84).

Treatment. The aim of therapy must be to remove symptoms. Triggering stimuli must be addressed and may require psychological assessment (Clouse and

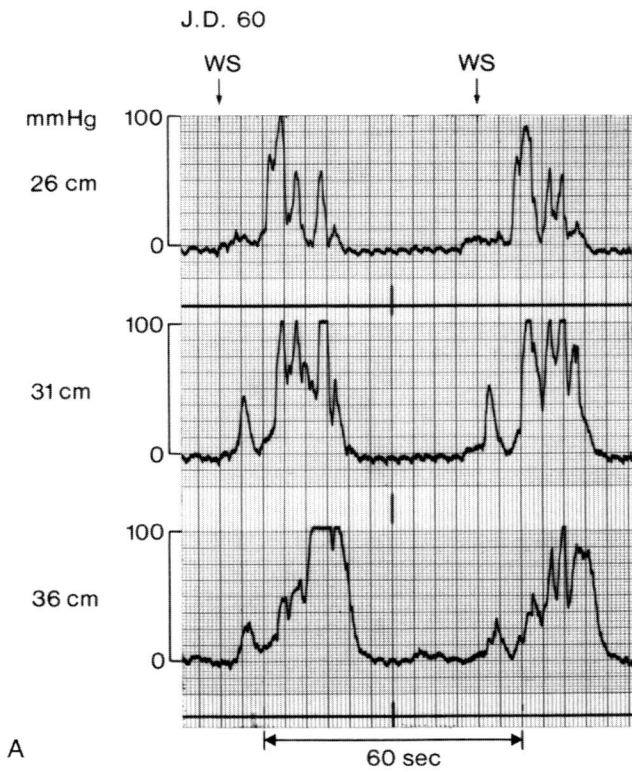

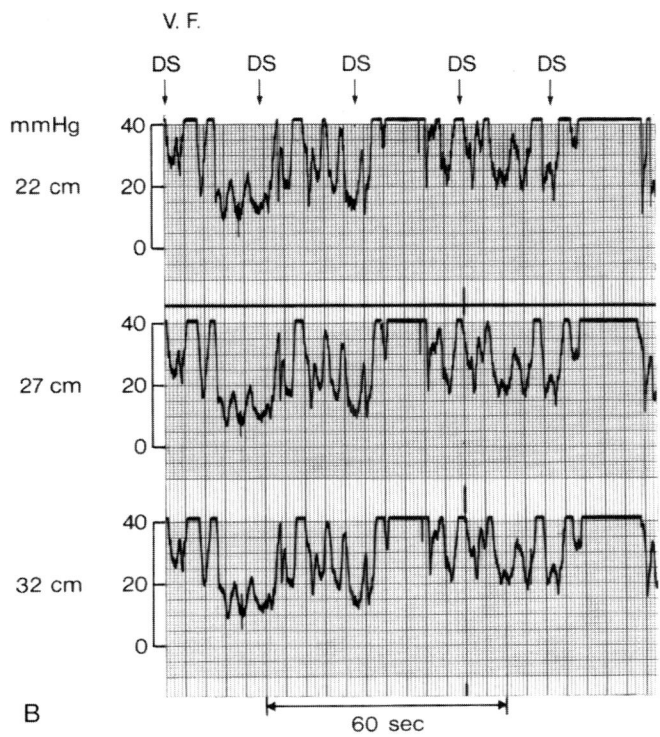

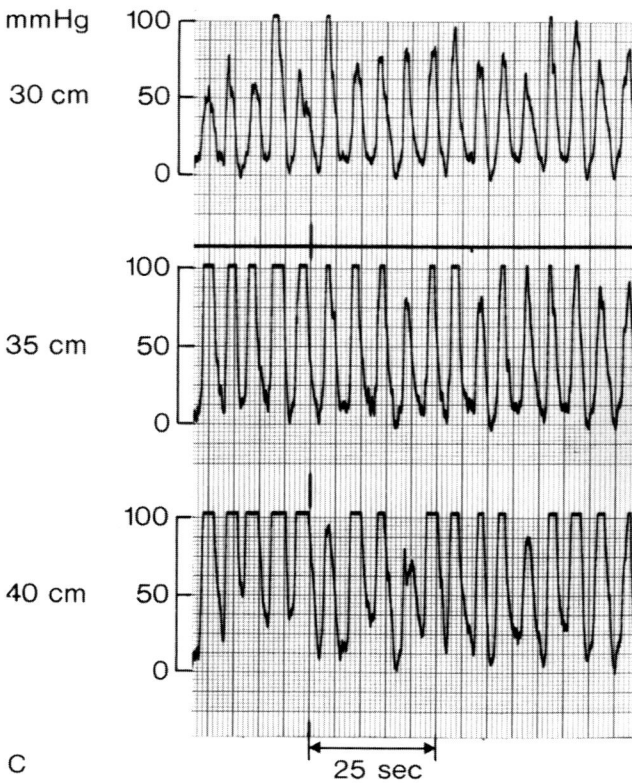

FIGURE 27–83. Hypermotility disorders: diffuse spasm. *A*, Multiphasic abnormal contractions of diffuse spasm seen in response to fewer than 100% of swallows. *B*, Repetitive long-duration contractions in a patient with idiopathic diffuse spasm. *C*, Chest pain and continuous hyperdynamic activity in a patient with spasm.

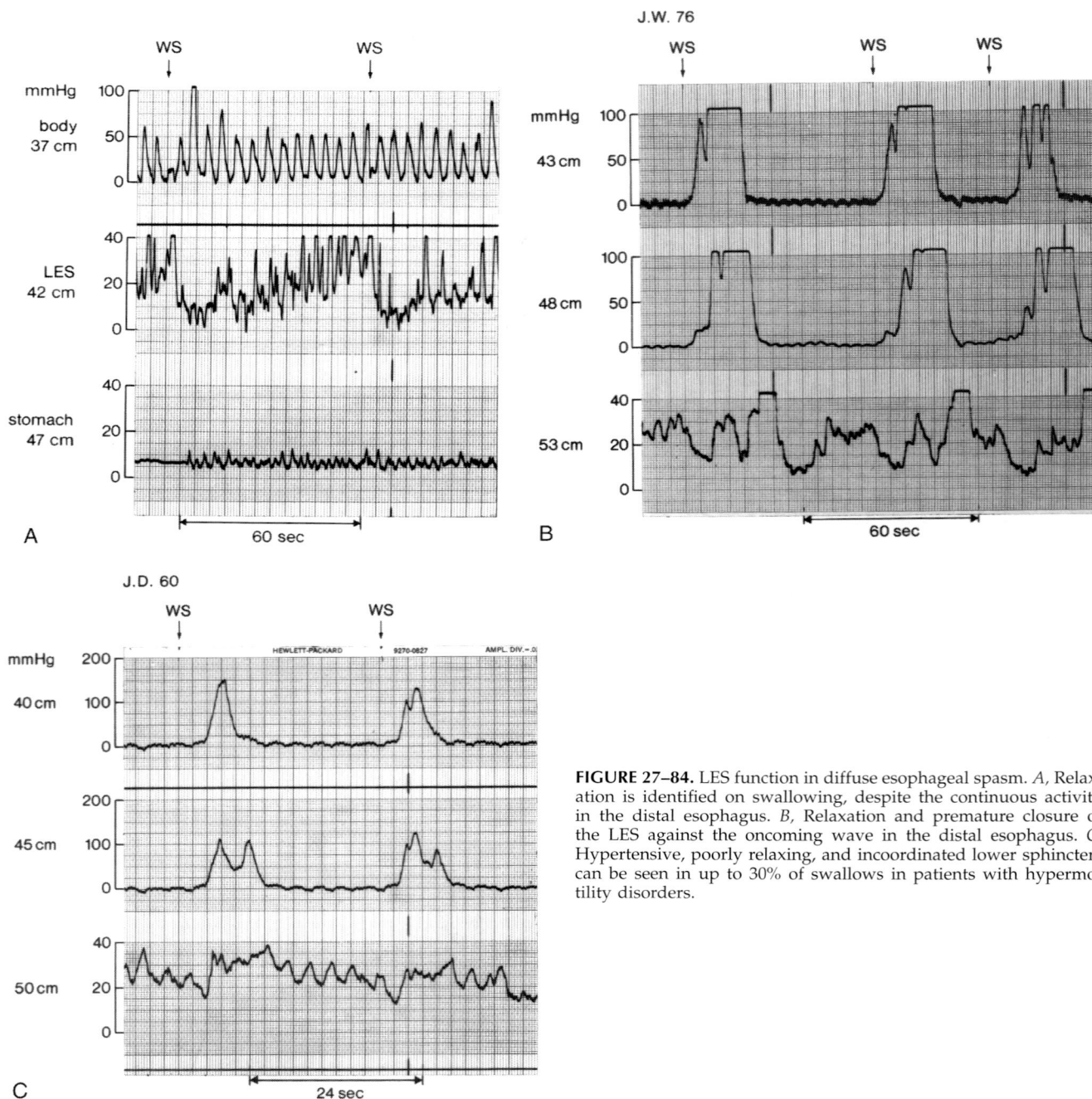

FIGURE 27–84. LES function in diffuse esophageal spasm. *A*, Relaxation is identified on swallowing, despite the continuous activity in the distal esophagus. *B*, Relaxation and premature closure of the LES against the oncoming wave in the distal esophagus. *C*, Hypertensive, poorly relaxing, and incoordinated lower sphincters can be seen in up to 30% of swallows in patients with hypermotility disorders.

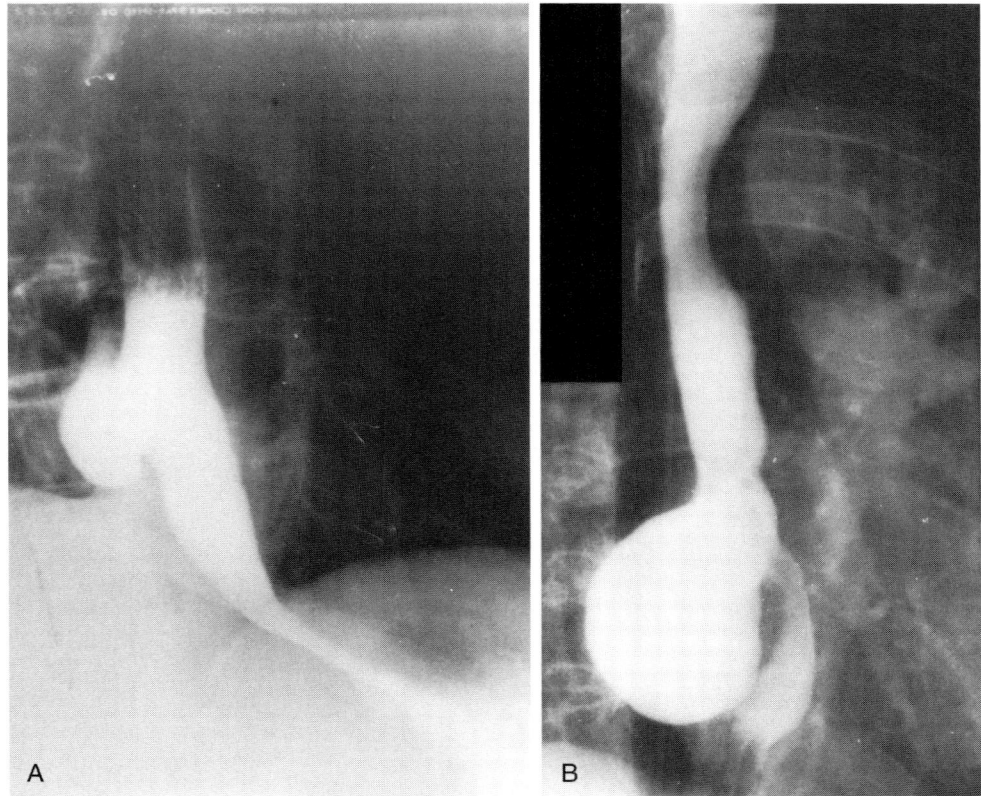

FIGURE 27–85. *A* and *B,* Progression of an epiphrenic diverticulum over a 6-year period in an asymptomatic patient.

Lustman, 1983). Since patients with hyperdynamic motor disorders frequently show a tense personality, control of the anxiety by the use of a mild sedative may decrease some symptoms while decreasing contraction pressures (Clouse et al., 1987).

When dysphagia and chest pain are closely related to meal time, patients should take sublingual nitroglycerin in order to decrease the effects of the abnormal contractions (Orlando and Bozymski, 1973) (Fig. 27–87). Calcium channel blocking agents may be used in patients with more frequent bouts of chest pain: They decrease the amplitude of contractions and reduce LES pressure (Richter et al., 1987b). Pneumatic dilatation of the GEJ can be suggested for diffuse spasm when a hypertensive LES or an incompletely relaxing sphincter is documented (Linsell et al., 1988). Very little data exist on this form of therapy.

Surgical treatment is considered only after full psychological assessment and a prolonged trial at medical control of symptoms. Significant incapacitation with adverse effects on normal life must be present. The results are not as good as for achalasia: Esophageal myotomy provides good to excellent results in 67 to 70% of operated patients (Ellis et al., 1964, 1988). A long esophageal myotomy extending to the aortic arch usually encompasses the whole area of abnormal function. The myotomy should extend on the proximal stomach, as in achalasia (Fig. 27–88). The mucosa is dissected free from the muscularis over 50% of the esophageal circumference (Fig. 27–89). The reason for this approach is the spectrum of sphincter dysfunction in diffuse esophageal spasm patients and its pres-

ence in up to 30% of studied patients. The effects of long myotomy in SIDES have been well documented: A decrease in esophageal resting and contraction pressures occurs, but the underlying motility disturbances are not affected (Leonardi et al., 1977; Paris et al., 1975). When the LES is transsected, a hypotensive sphincter must be expected and a partial fundoplication of the Belsey type should be added (Fig. 27–90). Conservative selection of patients with good correlation between radiologic symptoms and manometric abnormalities may improve results. The same treatment philosophy is followed when a distal esophageal diverticulum is present and symptomatic (Fig. 27–91). The functional alterations following diverticulectomy and myotomy create a hypotonic esophagus with a deficient LES (Fig. 27–92).

HYPERPERISTALSIS

Clinical Presentation. This condition is usually discovered in patients consulting for chest pain. Coronary disease is ruled out by appropriate investigation. Heartburn, regurgitations, and dysphagia are generally absent (Ferguson and Little, 1988). Hyperperistalsis is also described as the *nutcracker esophagus* or the *supersqueeze esophagus* (Clouse and Staiano, 1983). Patients with this condition show a strong emotional influence on their symptoms. They tend to be hypochondriacal and seek early medical attention with any symptom (Richter et al., 1986). Radiologic and endoscopic observations are usually normal. Radio-

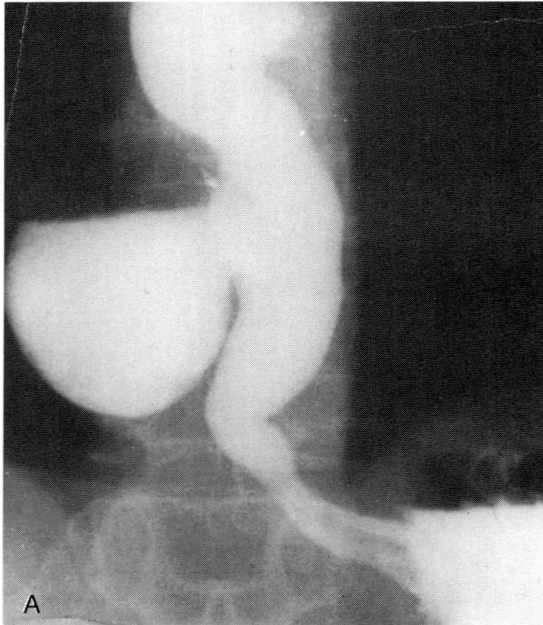

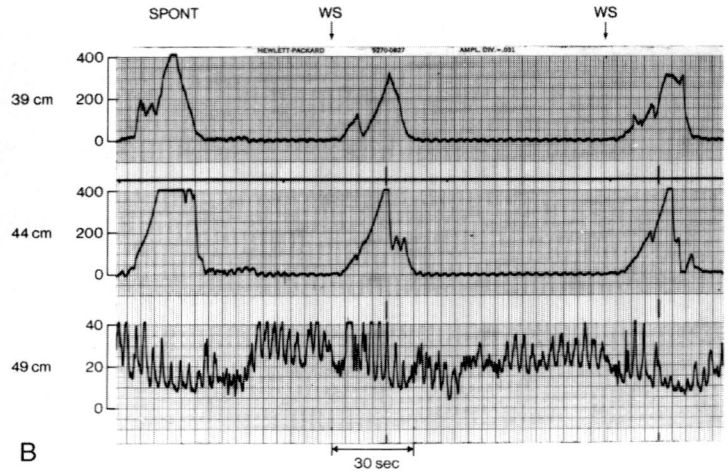

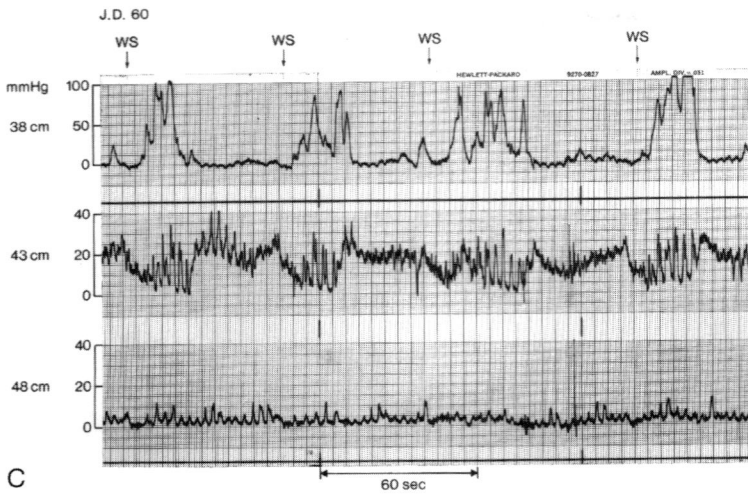

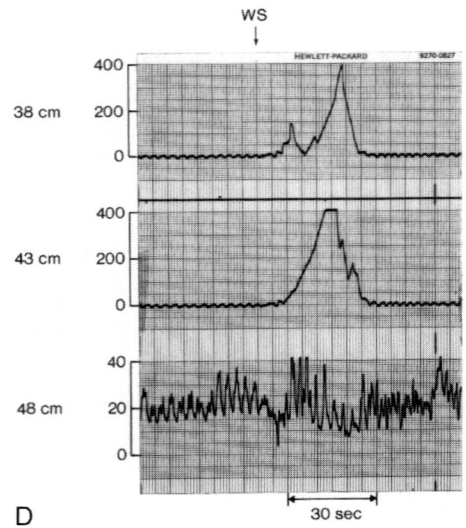

FIGURE 27–86. *A,* A large epiphrenic diverticulum. *B,* Strong spontaneous (SPONT) and antiperistaltic activity in the distal esophagus, with poor relaxation and coordination of the LES. *C* and *D,* Abnormal LES function in two patients with distal esophageal diverticula accompanied by hypermotility abnormalities.

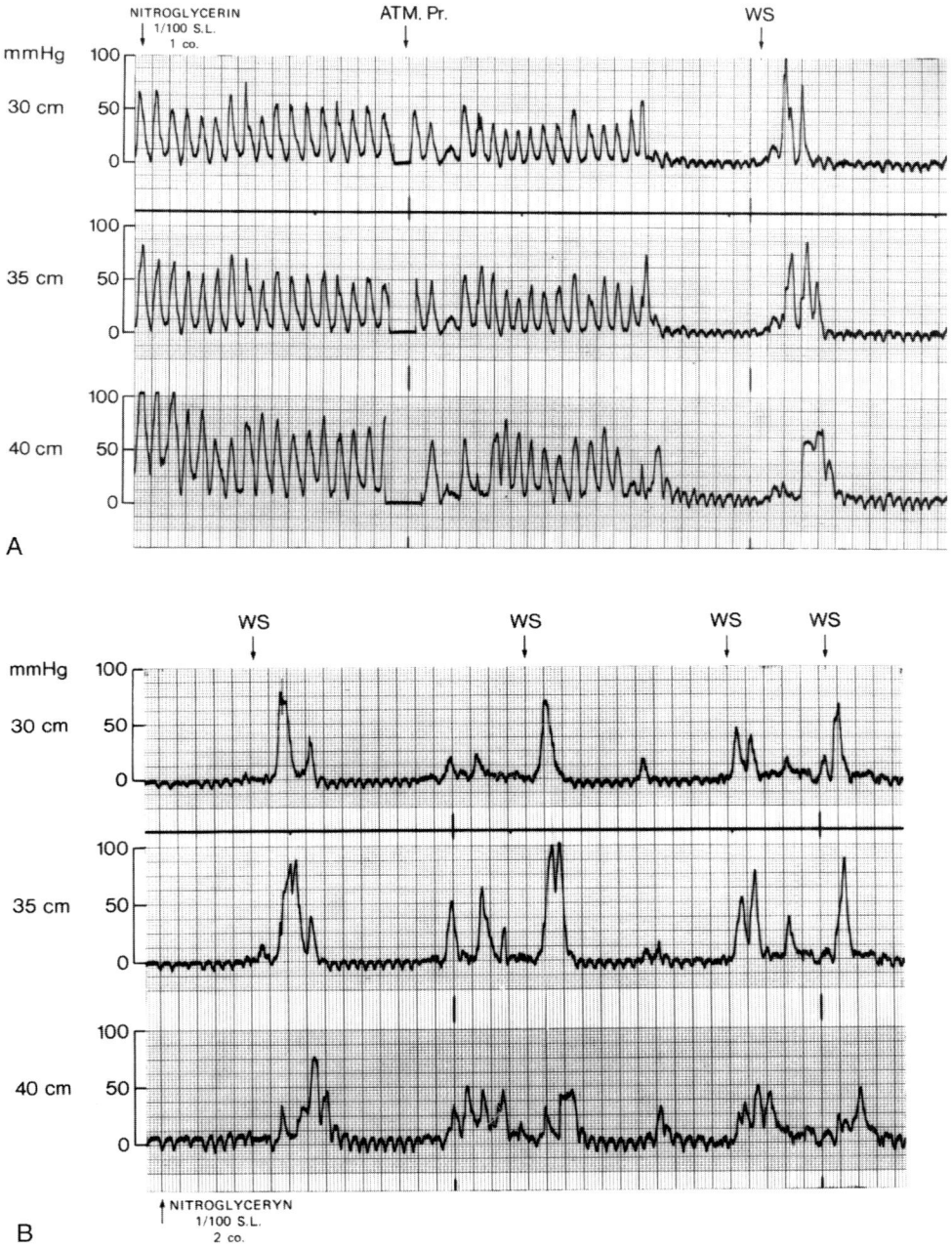

FIGURE 27–87. Medical management of hypermotility disorders. *A* and *B*, Nitroglycerin reduces the number of abnormal contractions in the esophageal body. Calcium channel blockers may also reduce smooth-muscle strength in the esophageal body and LES. (ATM. Pr. = atmospheric pressure.)

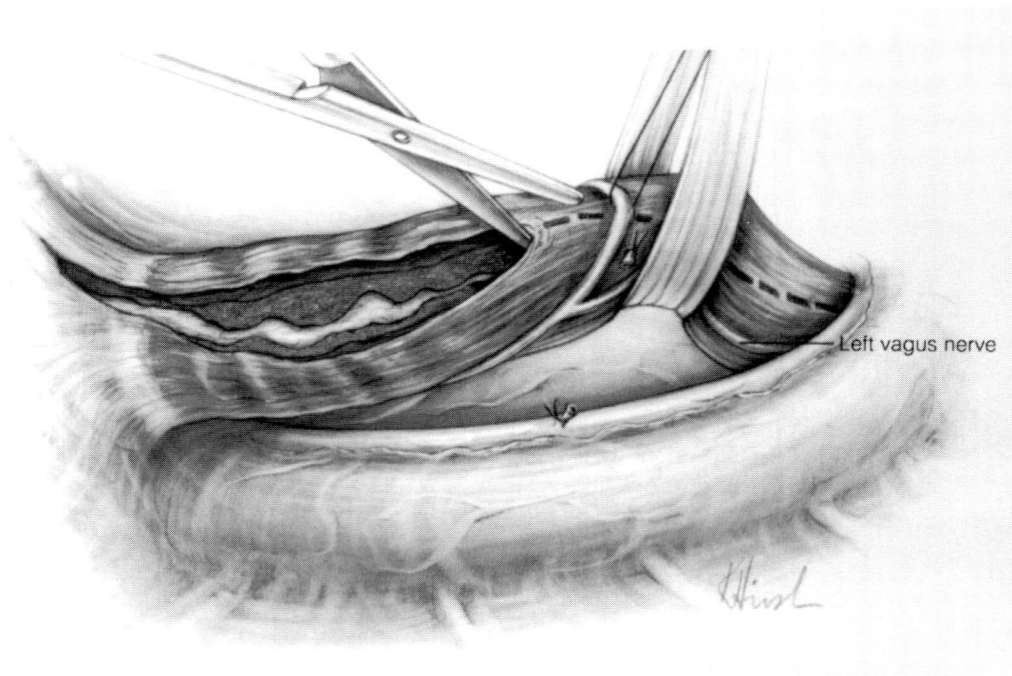

FIGURE 27–88. Surgical treatment for hypermotility disorders: long esophageal myotomy to the aortic arch, covering the abnormal motility area as documented at manometry. The LES area is included in the myotomy. (From Skinner, D. B.: Atlas of Esophageal Surgery. Churchill Livingstone, New York, 1991.)

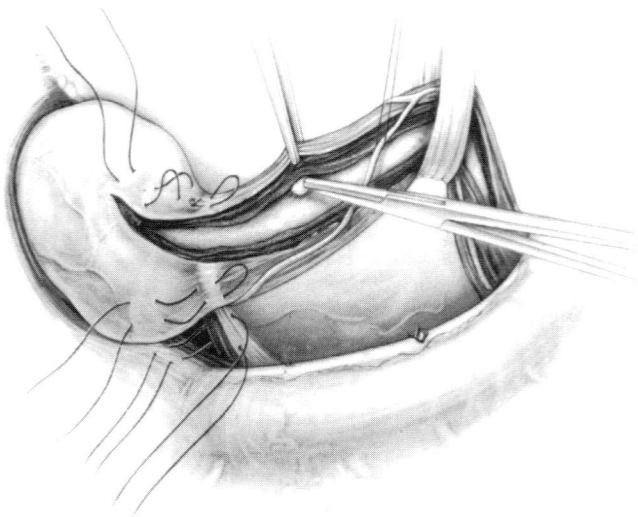

FIGURE 27–89. The mucosa is dissected free from the muscularis over 50% of the circumference. (From Skinner, D. B.: Atlas of Esophageal Surgery. Churchill Livingstone, New York, 1991.)

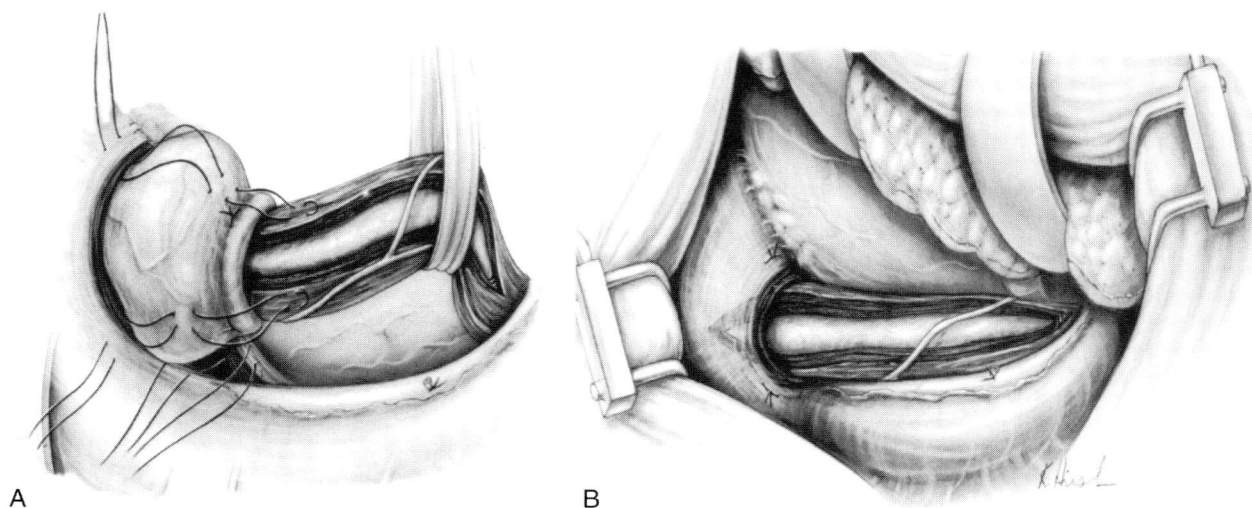

FIGURE 27–90. *A* and *B*, A partial fundoplication is added as a protection against reflux. (*A* and *B*, From Skinner, D. B.: Atlas of Esophageal Surgery. Churchill Livingstone, New York, 1991.)

nuclide transit studies reveal poor bolus transit in most of these patients (Benjamin et al., 1983).

Manometric Findings. The diagnosis is suggested when, on motility studies, swallowing is followed by peristaltic waves of increased amplitude. Peak contraction pressures are 2 to 3 standard deviations above normal (Castell, 1992). Mean values are reported above 180 mm Hg. LES may also show dysfunction with increased resting pressures.

Treatment. The primary approach is through medication with psychological assessment and support. Nifedipine (Richter et al., 1987b) and diltiazem (Richter and Castell, 1984) decrease symptoms of chest pain as well as the amplitude and duration of distal esophageal contractions. This medication also lowers the resting pressures of the distal sphincter.

Bougienage did not significantly change the amplitude of esophageal contractions or the resting pressures at LES level. Improvement in chest pain was recorded, but overall no objective benefit is obtained by bougienage (Winters et al., 1984).

Surgical myotomy was reported by Traube and associates (1987) in four patients for whom medical treatment was not satisfactory. Functional results 1 to 5 years after myotomy were a diminution in amplitude duration and percentage of bipeaked waves in the distal esophagus. Peristalsis was decreased. The LES was made hypotensive in all cases. Marked clinical improvement resulted. Ferguson and Little (1988) emphasized that operation offered poor results for most of these patients.

THE HYPERTENSIVE LOWER ESOPHAGEAL SPHINCTER

Isolated dysfunction of the LES with sphincter hypertension, hypercontraction, or poor relaxation was proposed as a separate entity by Garrett and Godwin (1969). It is diagnosed as a motor disorder when resting LES pressures are above 45 mm Hg, normal

relaxation is observed, and normal peristalsis is present in the esophageal body (Berger and McCallum, 1981; McCallum, 1991). Following the diagnosis, which is confirmed only through manometric studies, the therapeutic approach is that of other hyperdynamic disorders. Conservative management is in order, with smooth muscle relaxants, anxiety medication, and psychological investigation and support. Control of esophageal function must be reassessed over time to rule out further deterioration in function.

NONSPECIFIC MOTOR ABNORMALITIES

Despite efforts to improve the classification of motor disorders, functional abnormalities are often observed that cannot be classified. Decreased peristalsis, spontaneous tertiary activity, longer contractions, and repetitive contractions can all be considered abnormal. Still, when these are not part of a fixed pattern, their recording must not produce a wrong diagnosis and management.

Motor Disorders and Reflux Disease

Idiopathic Reflux Disease

The functional abnormalities of the esophagus in reflux disease patients are described in Table 27–9. Idiopathic gastroesophageal reflux disease is the most frequent condition assessed in the esophageal function laboratory. The motor dysfunction leading to this abnormal acid exposure has been initially documented by Atkinson and co-workers (1957), who observed that the LES was weak when reflux was present. Haddad (1970) emphasized later that if the LES pressure was constantly low, reflux episodes occurred more frequently. This was further established by Ahtaridis and colleagues (1981), who documented that

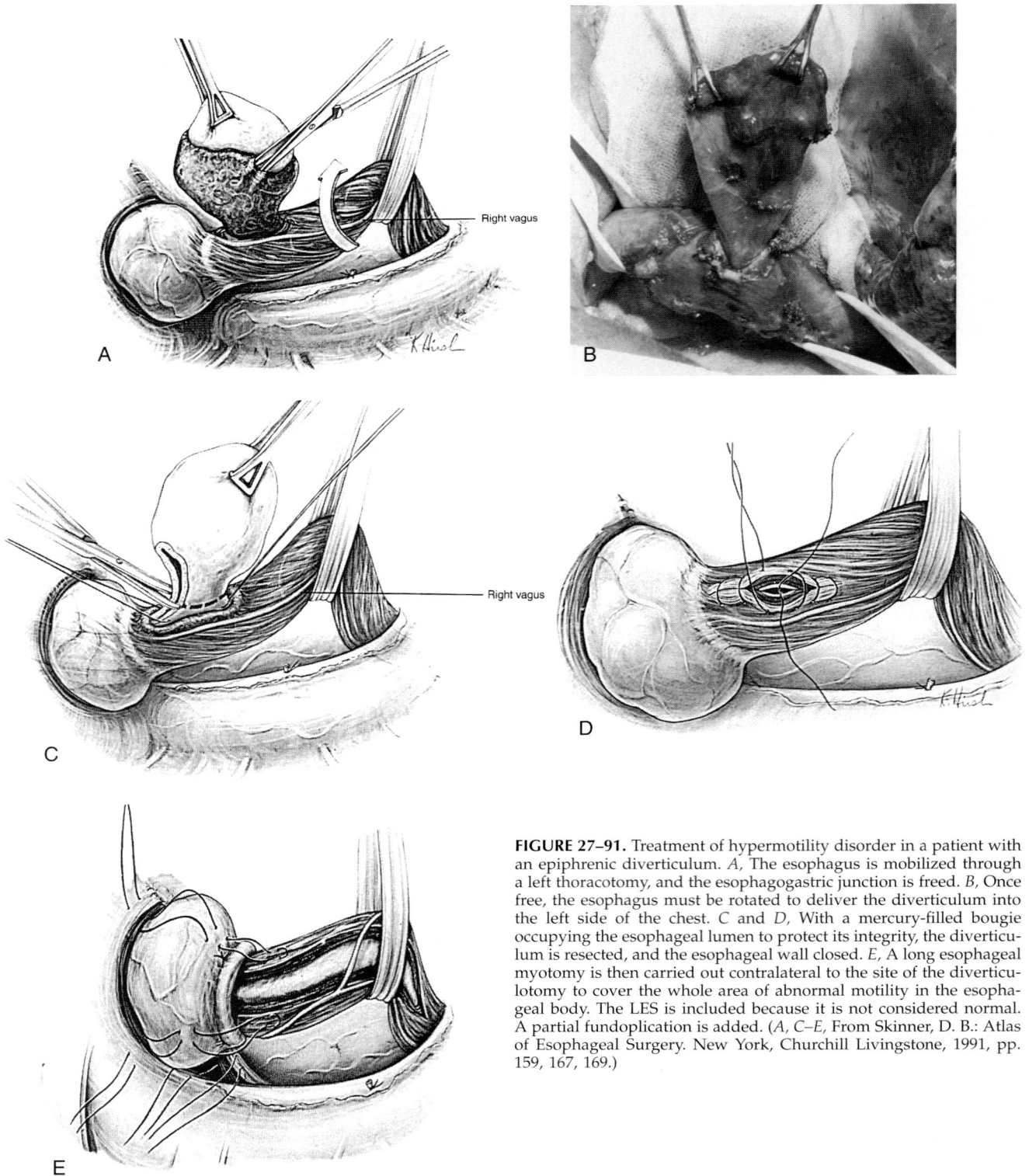

FIGURE 27–91. Treatment of hypermotility disorder in a patient with an epiphrenic diverticulum. *A,* The esophagus is mobilized through a left thoracotomy, and the esophagogastric junction is freed. *B,* Once free, the esophagus must be rotated to deliver the diverticulum into the left side of the chest. *C* and *D,* With a mercury-filled bougie occupying the esophageal lumen to protect its integrity, the diverticulum is resected, and the esophageal wall closed. *E,* A long esophageal myotomy is then carried out contralateral to the site of the diverticulotomy to cover the whole area of abnormal motility in the esophageal body. The LES is included because it is not considered normal. A partial fundoplication is added. (*A, C–E,* From Skinner, D. B.: Atlas of Esophageal Surgery. New York, Churchill Livingstone, 1991, pp. 159, 167, 169.)

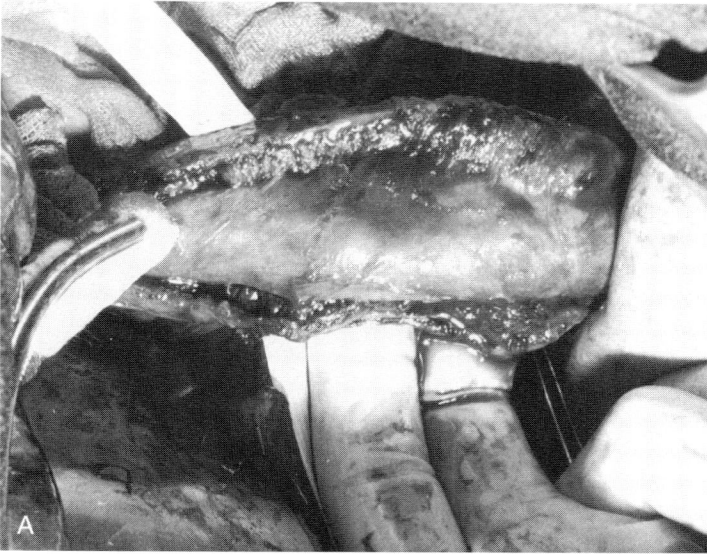

FIGURE 27–92. *A,* Completed diverticulectomy and long esophageal myotomy. *B,* The functional effects of myotomy are significant hypomotility and LES hypotension.

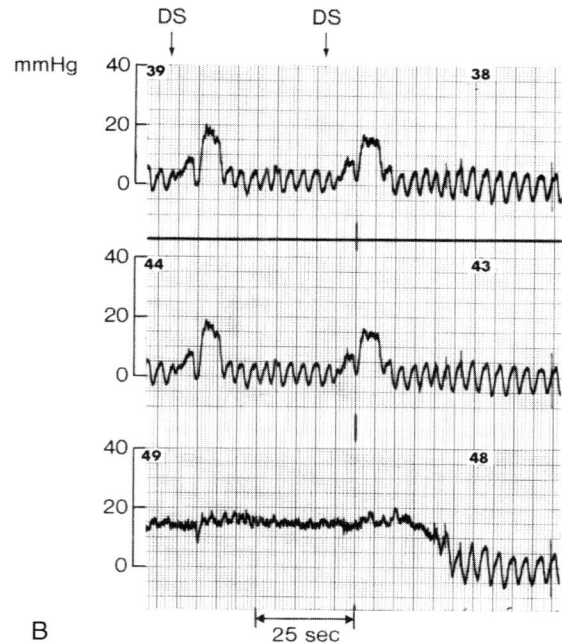

reflux was linearly related to LES pressures. Dent and associates (1980) reported that transient relaxation periods in the LES were responsible for reflux episodes in normal subjects. Dodds (1982), Dent (1988), and their co-workers reported later that in patients with reflux esophagitis, two-thirds of the reflux episodes occur initially with a normal sphincter. The LES becomes weaker with increasing esophagitis (Fig. 27–93).

The effects of repeat and prolonged reflux episodes on function of the esophagus have been suggested in a number of studies. Eastwood and co-workers (1975) reported that reflux episodes may cause LES hypotension, leading to further reflux and mucosal damage. Ransom and colleagues (1982) and Iascone and associates (1983) reported esophageal contraction abnormalities with poor amplitude and aperistalsis in patients with extensive reflux damage. Kahrilas and associates (1986), studying patients with normal noninflammatory reflux as well as those with mild and severe esophagitis, reported an increased incidence of failed peristalsis and decreased contraction amplitude occurring with increased mucosal damage. Parilla and co-workers (1990, 1991) and Mason and Bremner (1993) made similar observations. Stein and DeMeester (1993) suggested a correlation between the severity of sphincter hypotension and the extent of functional abnormalities in the esophageal body (Fig. 27–94).

It remains unclear whether correction of reflux disease leads to the disappearance of all these functional abnormalities.

Reflux Disease and Scleroderma

Ninety per cent of patients with scleroderma show abnormal function of the esophagus (Fig. 27–95). At-rophy of the smooth muscle portion of the esophagus with fibrous infiltration of its distal two-thirds produces total incompetence of the LES and disappearance of the normal propulsion and emptying mechanisms in the esophageal body. For 60% of these patients, this hypotony coupled with absent peristalsis and absent LES leads to a more severe form of reflux disease. A high percentage of reflux complications result (Duranceau et al., 1993; Henderson et al., 1988; Henderson and Pearson, 1973; Orringer, 1983). This is undoubtedly the most challenging form of reflux disease. Antireflux operations are not as successful in controlling reflux for these patients as for those with idiopathic reflux disease. Still, a decrease in acid exposure lessens the damage and improves patient comfort.

ESOPHAGEAL STRICTURES

Benign esophageal strictures are classified in Table 27–10. The most frequent cause (90%) of esophageal narrowing in North America is gastroesophageal reflux.

Peptic Strictures

Repeated mucosal insult by peptic juices causes ulcerations from destruction of the epithelium (Pollara, 1985). An attempt at repair may produce islets of regenerating epithelium underlined by inflammation and edema in the lamina propria. Inflammation and fibrosis are usually limited to the submucosa. In more severe cases, the reaction destroys the muscularis mu-

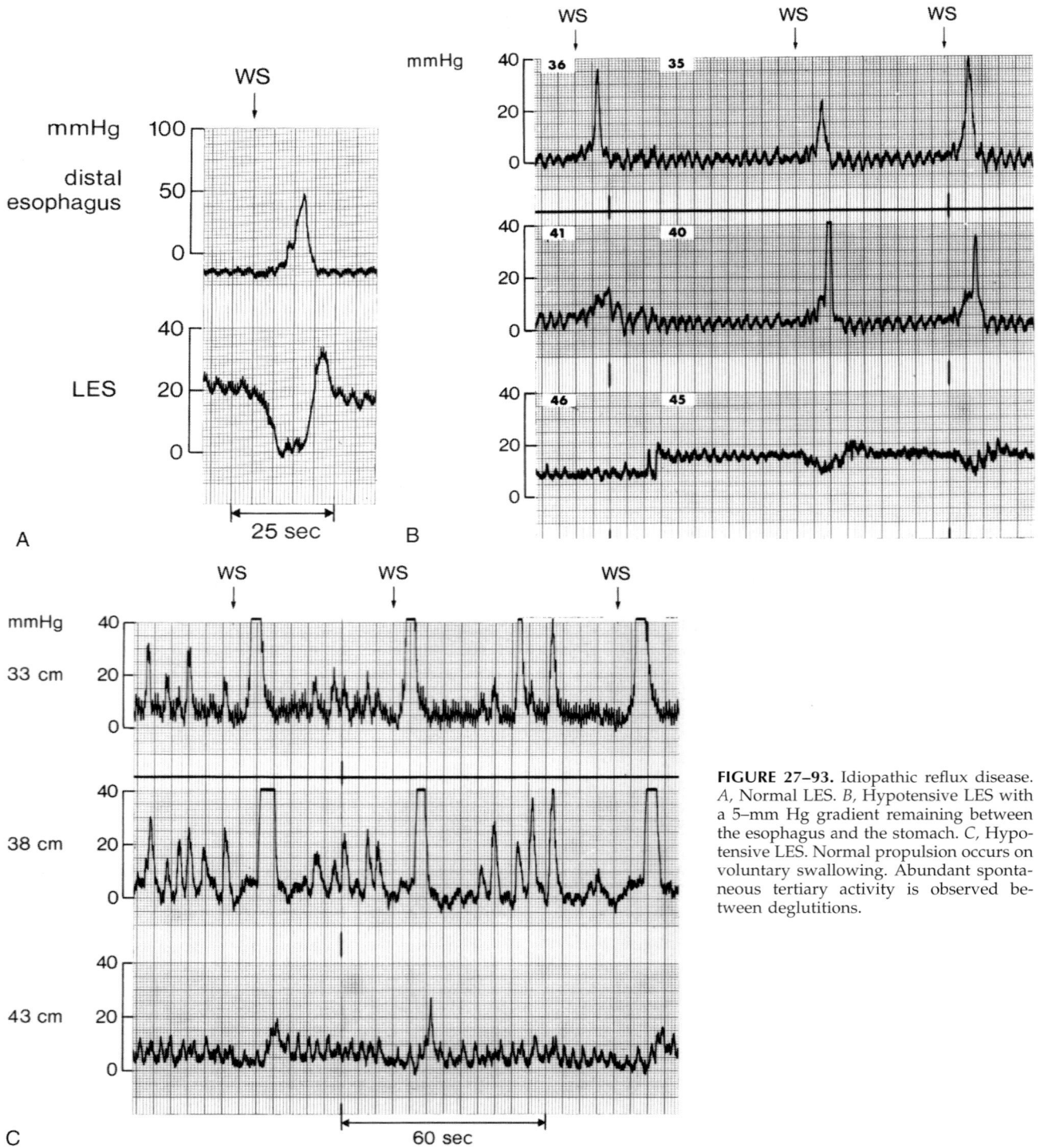

FIGURE 27–93. Idiopathic reflux disease. A, Normal LES. B, Hypotensive LES with a 5–mm Hg gradient remaining between the esophagus and the stomach. C, Hypotensive LES. Normal propulsion occurs on voluntary swallowing. Abundant spontaneous tertiary activity is observed between deglutitions.

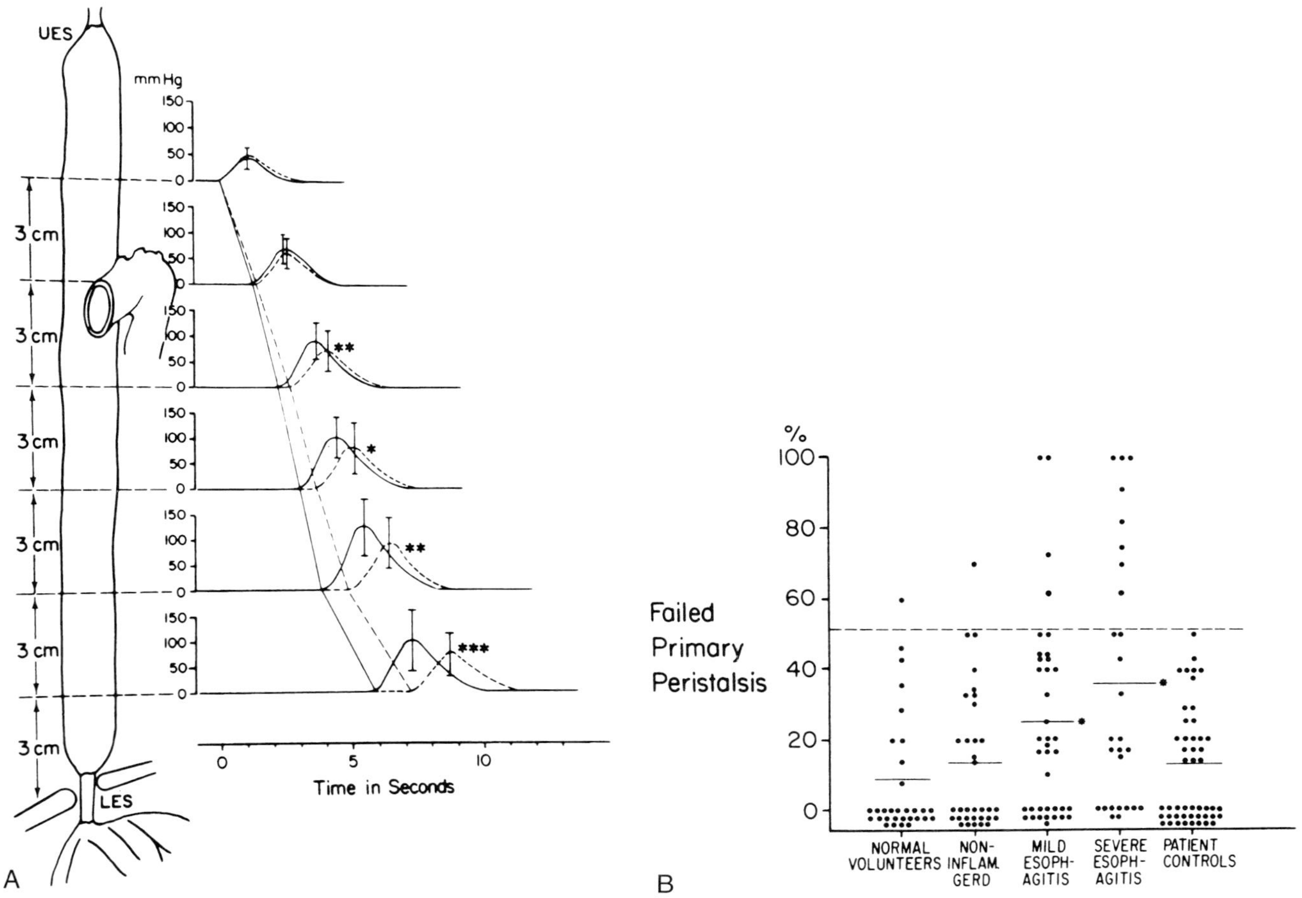

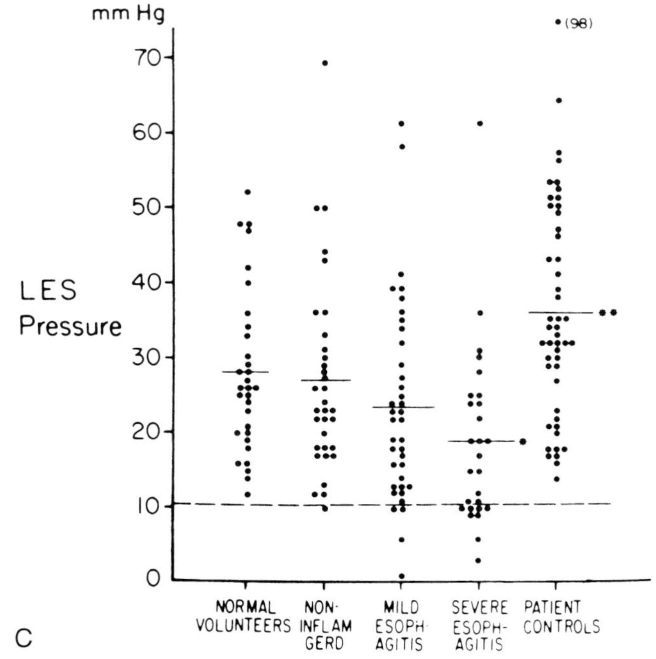

FIGURE 27–94. Peristalsis and LES function in esophagitis. *A*, With increasing reflux disease, the amplitude of peristaltic contraction decreases. *B*, Increased peristaltic failure with increasing severity of reflux esophagitis. *C*, Patients with severe esophagitis show the worst LES function. (*A–C*, From Kahrilas, P. J., Dodds, W. J., Hogan W. J., et al.: Esophageal peristaltic function in peptic esophagitis. Gastroenterology, *91*:897, 1986.)

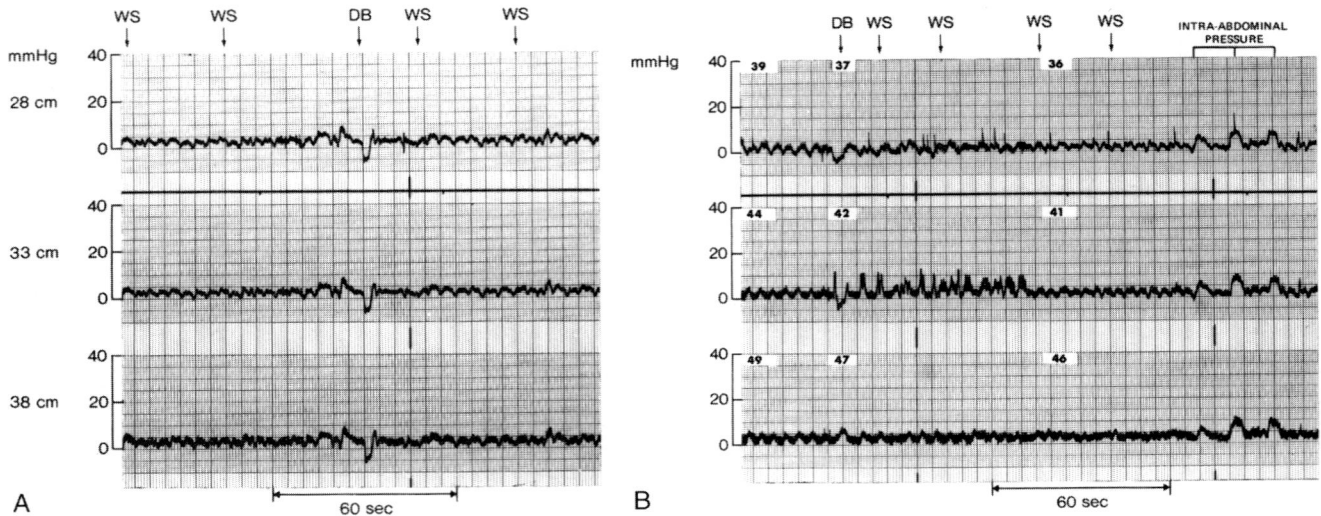

FIGURE 27–95. Reflux disease and scleroderma. *A,* Absent motor function in the middle and distal esophagus in a patient with CREST (calcinosis, Reynaud's phenomenon, esophageal motility disorders, sclerodactyly, and telangiectasia) syndrome. *B,* Absent LES high-pressure zone at esophagogastric junction. Transmission of pressure from the abdomen is recorded in the esophagus, revealing a common communicating cavity.

cosae and extends through the submucosa, depositing collagen and forming strictures in the circular muscle layer. Fibrosis and the inflammation of the longitudinal muscle layer may cause shortening (Fig. 27–96*A*). When stricture is found in association with a columnar-lined esophagus, it is located at the squamocolumnar junction and represents an epithelium-denuded area at the junction of both mucosa: Normal squamous epithelium is present above the stricture and the abnormal columnar epithelium is seen dis-

■ Table 27–10. BENIGN ESOPHAGEAL STRICTURES

Congenital
Tracheoesophageal remnant (choristoma)

Traumatic
Caustic
Foreign body
Surgical

Infection-related
Monilia
Pemphigus
Viral (Behçet)

Peptic
High strictures
Low strictures

Rings and Webs

Extraluminal Compression
Vascular
Mediastinal

tally. At the stricture level are connective tissue and granulation tissue, with a muscularis mucosa heavily infiltrated with inflammatory cells (Fig. 27–96*B*).

If penetrating ulcers are present, they are found either at the junction of the squamous mucosa and columnar-lined mucosa (Savary-Wolfe ulcers) or within the columnar-lined esophagus (Barrett's ulcer). Extension through the full thickness of the esophageal wall shows features similar to those of peptic ulcers of the stomach: Inflammation is often present in periesophageal tissues. In patients with chronic superficial esophagitis, even with a seemingly intact muscularis propria, gross periesophageal fibrosis may be present (Sandry, 1962).

Webs are thin, central, or eccentric narrowings of normal squamous epithelium without signs of inflammation, found mostly in the proximal esophagus. Rings are located at the level of the squamocolumnar junction in the distal esophagus. These concentric narrowings may significantly obstruct esophagogastric transit. They represent submucous connective tissue with chronic inflammatory cells covered by normal squamous epithelium above and normal gastric epithelium on the stomach side (Postlethwait and Sealy, 1967). This condition is always associated with a hiatal hernia. However, there is no solid evidence that it is caused by reflux disease (Fig. 27–96*C*).

Investigation

When an esophageal stricture is present, all efforts must be made to exclude a carcinoma. Subjective assessment followed by radiology and endoscopic examinations are the essential steps for this purpose. A decreased lumen with lack of distensibility of the esophageal wall and symmetric tapering proximally suggests a benign stricture. Asymmetry, marked ir-

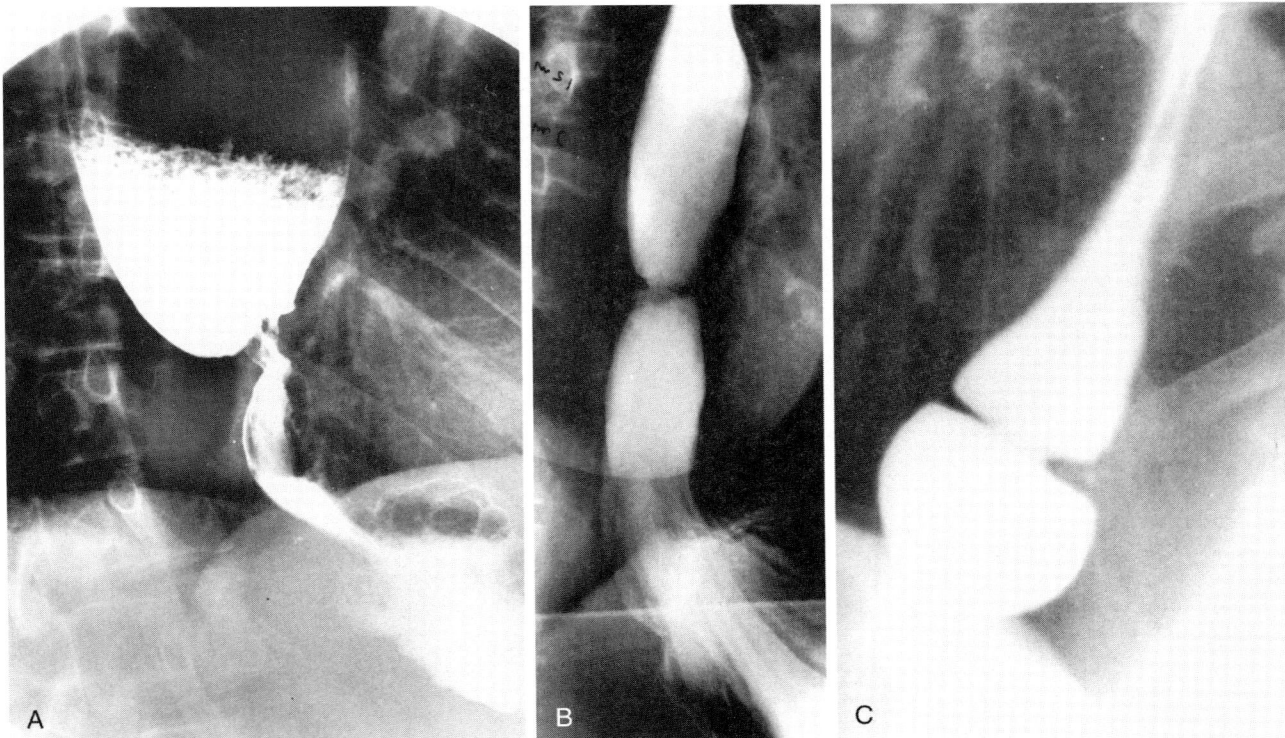

FIGURE 27–96. *A,* Severe stricture of the distal esophagus. *B,* The high stricture associated with a columnar cell–lined esophagus in the distal esophagus. *C,* A Schatzki ring at the squamocolumnar junction.

regularity, and deep ulceration suggest carcinoma. Guidewire dilatation may have to be performed in order to complete the examination and obtain tissue samplings of the narrowed segment.

Management

Table 27–11 summarizes the various steps in managing benign esophageal strictures of peptic origin.

Dilatation Therapy

Bougienage may improve swallowing, but it does not correct the underlying cause of the peptic stricture. For tight and long strictures, dilatation is gener-

■ **Table 27–11.** STEPS FOR MANAGING BENIGN ESOPHAGEAL STRICTURES OF PEPTIC ORIGIN

Dilatation
Dilatation and standard antireflux operation
Plastic procedures
   Intrathoracic
     Thal's repair
     Intrathoracic fundoplication
   Collis' gastroplasty
     Partial fundoplication
     Total fundoplication
   Bile diversion and acid reduction operation
Resection and reconstruction
   Stomach
   Jejunum
   Colon

---

ally started using a guidewire with rigid tapered plastic bougies of the Savary-Gilliard type. Balloon catheters have also been used to dilate irregular and tight strictures. When satisfactory permeability of the lumen has been obtained, antegrade bougienage using mercury-weighted Maloney bougies may be continued. The addition of appropriate antireflux medication can afford good symptomatic improvement in the elderly and in high-risk patients. For all patients with strictures due to reflux damage, consideration must be given to surgical correction of this severe complication, unless the medical condition contradicts such an approach.

Dilatations Followed by Standard Antireflux Operations

Dilatations followed by standard antireflux operations aim to correct dysphagia while preventing further damage from reflux disease. Naef and Savary (1972) and Safaie-Shirazi and colleagues (1975) reported excellent results using a total fundoplication following dilatation (Fig. 27–97A). However, standard antireflux operations fail in a larger proportion of patients when a stricture is present. Periesophagitis and shortening make it difficult to obtain a sufficient length of intra-abdominal esophagus. Even extensive esophageal mobilization to the aortic arch and freeing of the GEJ may not afford a comfortable 4 to 5 cm of esophagus under the diaphragm (Fig. 27–97B). Consequently, a tension-free repair is not possible. Belsey and Skinner (1972), Skinner and Belsey (1967), and

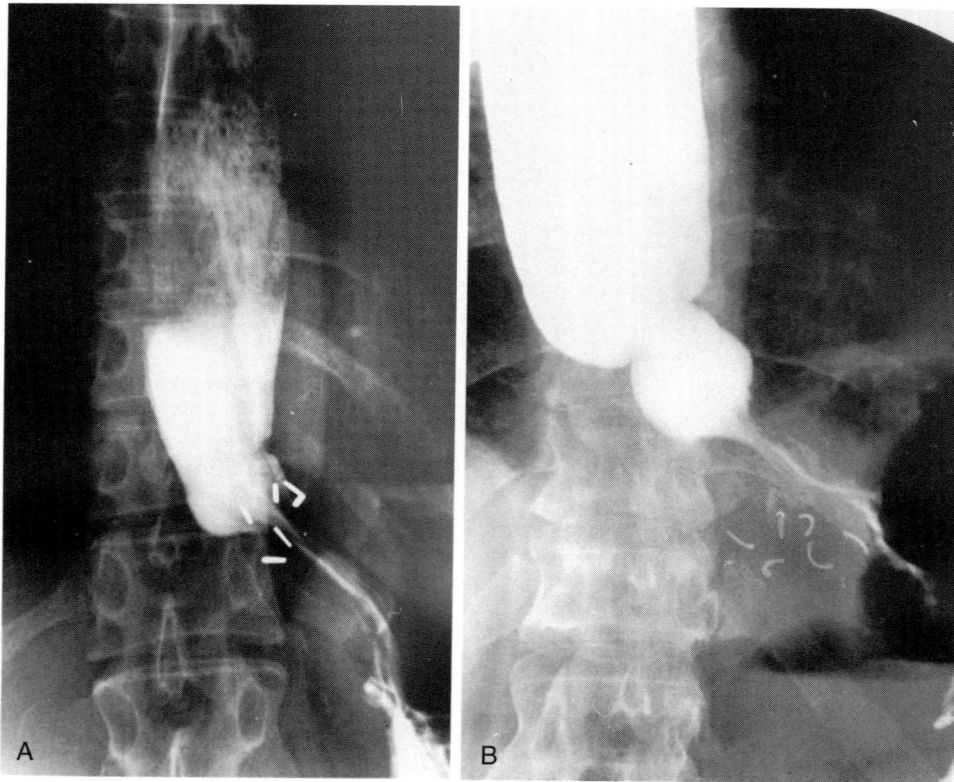

FIGURE 27–97. *A,* Total fundoplication in the management of reflux and stricture. *B,* A cut Collis gastroplasty associated to a total fundoplication when extensive esophageal dissection did not succeed in reducing the esophagogastric junction under the diaphragm.

Orringer and associates (1972) reported a 37% failure rate in patients at this stage of the disease. Results are often difficult to assess because the extent of damage in the esophageal wall and the degree of shortening are often impossible to clarify. Orringer and associates (1972) observed that a partial fundoplication of the Belsey type was not a proper antireflux operation when left in the chest. Hill and co-workers (1970) reported that the incidence of anatomic recurrences was minimal but that continued reflux was much higher.

Two attitudes have developed in regard to a shortened esophagus: Either create a functional antireflux operation that is left in the lower chest or elongate the esophagus in order to obtain a tension-free repair under the diaphragm.

Plastic Procedures

INTRATHORACIC FUNDOPLICATIONS AND STRICTUROPLASTY

When an antireflux operation cannot be reduced under the diaphragm without any tension on the repair, the repair may be left in the chest (Maher, 1988; Thal, 1968; Woodward, 1988). Thal (1968) proposed to split the esophageal stricture and to widen its lumen further by creating a fundic serosal patch. Later, in a modification of the initial operation, a skin graft had to be added to prevent restricturing of the repair over the serosa. These authors observed that even with the stomach serosa protected by a skin graft, a partial fundoplication repair suffered from free reflux and recurrent esophagitis. Total fundoplication added to

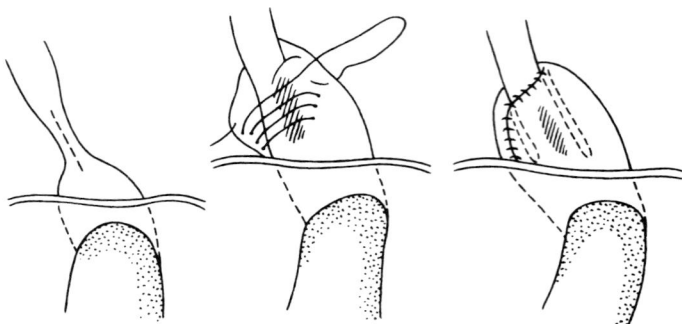

FIGURE 27–98. The Thal fundic patch repair.

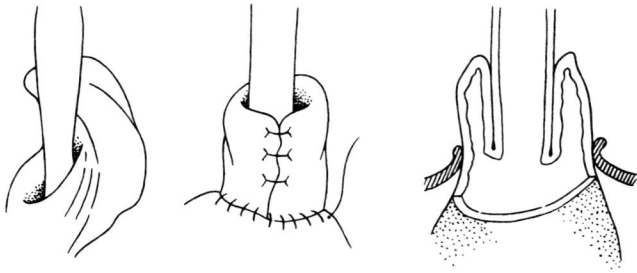

FIGURE 27–99. The intrathoracic fundoplication.

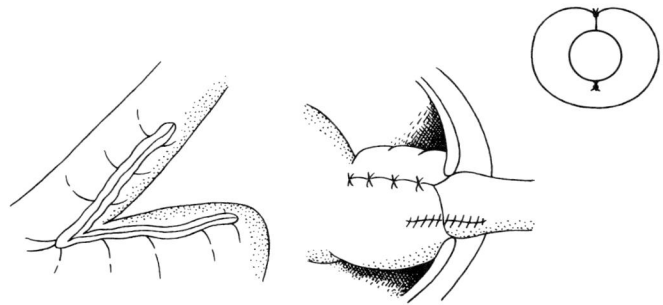

FIGURE 27–101. The cut Collis gastroplasty associated with a total fundoplication.

the patch gave satisfactory long-term results in 84% of patients (Woodward, 1988) (Fig. 27–98).

Krupp and Rosetti also suggested, in the mid-1960s, creating a total fundoplication to be left in the chest. This operation, as reevaluated by Maher (1988), offered good to excellent results in 82% of patients (Fig. 27–99). Both the Thal total fundoplication repair and the total intrathoracic fundoplication, although they are noted for their antireflux properties, suffer from their dangers—paragastric diaphragmatic hernias, gastric ulcerations in the supradiaphragmatic stomach, and gastric fistulization with mediastinal structures. Hugh and colleagues (1979) proposed the use of a vascularized antral patch esophagoplasty, arguing that it was acid-resistant and did not secrete acid. Permanent improvement and control of reflux damage with this operation still need to be documented over time.

ESOPHAGEAL ELONGATION GASTROPLASTY

Collis (1957) proposed a plastic repair for the short esophagus to lengthen the esophagus by creating a tube from the lesser curvature. This added intra-abdominal length to the repair but did not control reflux. A partial fundoplication was added to the gastroplasty by Pearson and Henderson (1976; see also Henderson, 1977; Orringer et al., 1976, 1977; Waters et al., 1988) (Fig. 27–100). However, the high incidence of persistent reflux stimulated a number of surgeons to propose a total fundoplication gastroplasty instead (Henderson, 1989; Henderson and Marryatt, 1983; Orringer, 1988; Orringer and Sloan, 1977) (Fig. 27–101). An uncut Collis gastroplasty with a stapled 3-cm gastroplasty tube created by mucosal apposition of

the anterior and posterior fundus was subsequently used extensively (Demos, 1984; Piehler et al., 1984) (Fig. 27–102).

ACID REDUCTION AND BILE DIVERSION OPERATIONS

Acid reduction and bile diversion operations have been used by Payne (1984) to manage untreatable strictures. These operations are proposed for repeat failures at reflux control as a last effort to preserve the esophagus. Stein and DeMeester (1993) reported that combined bile and acid reflux disease produced the worst mucosal damage in the esophagus. Acid reduction and bile diversion in these situations may help to control the extent of damage while preserving an intact esophagus. This is obtained at the cost of poor emptying in the stomach remnant.

Esophageal Resection

The undilatable stricture and the very long strictures caused by prolonged nasogastric tube drainage or by incoercible vomiting may have to be approached by resection. This treatment controls dysphagia and offers a replacement organ that will resist reflux damage while allowing proper reconstruction and minimal morbidity.

ESOPHAGECTOMY AND GASTRIC INTERPOSITION

This operation has become a first choice because it involves a single anastomosis either in the high chest or in the neck (Fig. 27–103). Reconstruction in the lower chest is contraindicated because it leads to a high proportion of restricturing from reflux. Orringer and co-workers (1977) reported minimal morbidity and mortality, with satisfying reconstruction comfort.

ESOPHAGECTOMY AND SMALL BOWEL INTERPOSITION

Resection of the strictured esophagus and replacement by small bowel has been proposed by Merendino and Dillard (1955) and reviewed by Polk (1980). Good results with decreased reflux symptoms have been reported.

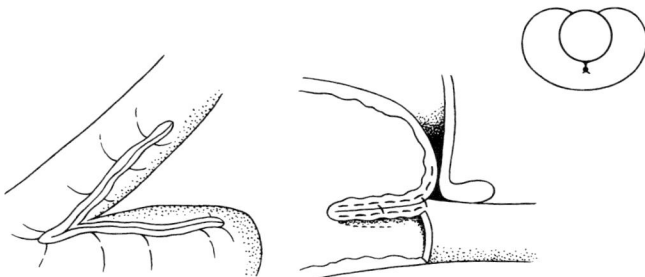

FIGURE 27–100. The cut Collis gastroplasty associated with a partial fundoplication.

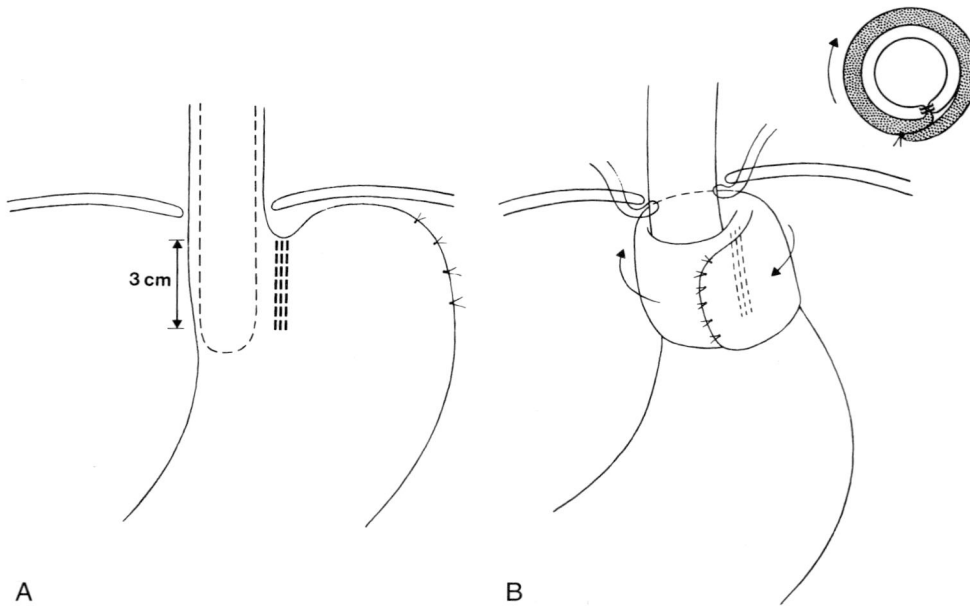

FIGURE 27–102. A, Uncut gastroplasty by the apposition of the anterior and posterior gastric walls using 3-cm staples along the proximal lesser curvature. B, Total wrap of the gastroplasty by the fundus.

ESOPHAGECTOMY WITH COLON INTERPOSITION

Until recently, colon interposition was the most commonly used reconstruction following resection for benign strictures (Fig. 27–104). In large series, morbidity and mortality were considered low enough for

this technique to be used. Good results were reported in 77% of all patients. Sixteen per cent of the patients show fair results, whereas 7% have a poor response. The mortality is 4.9% and necrosis of the colon occurs in 8% of all patients with long interpositions (Postlethwait, 1983b).

Corrosive Strictures

The damage to the esophageal wall resulting from exposure to chemical agents depends on the nature and the amount of the agent, the concentration of the substance, and the duration of the exposure. Accidental ingestion of lye is responsible for most of the lesions in children (Rothstein, 1986). In adolescents and young adults, suicide attempts are responsible for the resulting damage. Besides cleaning agents, alkali may be found in other forms: High-concentration potassium tablets, Clinitest tablets used for measuring sugar in the urine, vitamin C tablets, and doxycycline tablets may all be responsible for caustic damage. Small alkaline batteries ingested accidentally may cause similar lesions.

Pathophysiology

Caustic agents are alkaline or acid. Sixty per cent of esophageal injuries by caustics are the result of lye ingestion. Ingestion of strong acids is responsible for less than 10% of caustic damages (Postlethwait, 1986).

ALKALI

Experimentally, a 10% lye solution of sodium hydroxide causes transmural esophageal damage, and a 22% solution causes necrosis of the esophageal wall (Krey, 1952) (Fig. 27–105A). Common household

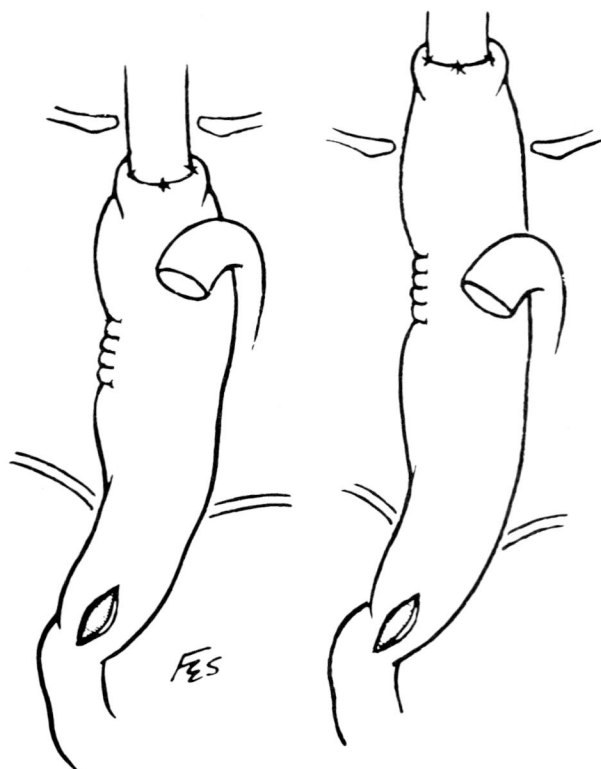

FIGURE 27–103. Gastric interposition with anastomosis in the apex of the chest or in the neck.

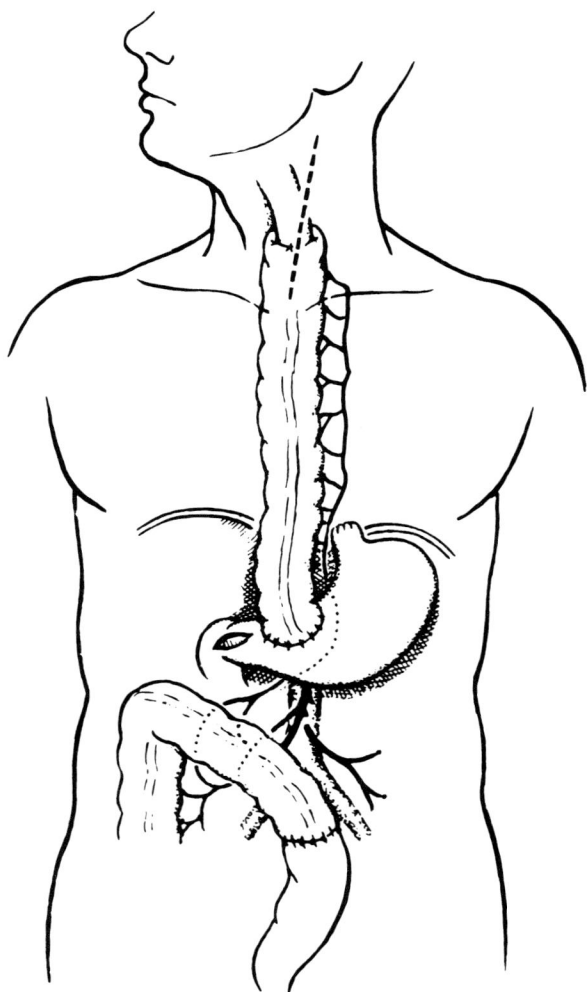

FIGURE 27–104. Colon interposition: The short segment is used for the distal esophagus, and the long segment is anastomosed to the cervical esophagus.

cleaners have a concentration of 25 to 36% in their liquid form and of 54 to 98% in their granular form. When in contact with the upper digestive tube, alkali damages the esophageal wall within 30 seconds after the exposure. An immediate liquefaction necrosis with diffusion of the agent through the layers of the esophagus causes this rapid damage. Immediate destruction of cells occurs with inflammation and subsequent vascular thrombosis. Secondary bacterial invasion supervenes. Sloughing of necrotic tissue with deposition of granulation tissue creates fibrotic strictures. Owing to the nature of the damage, chronic ulcerations may persist and encourage constant deposition of fibrous tissue. In its higher concentrations, lye induces transmural damage with involvement of periesophageal tissues.

ACID

Strong acids (sulfuric, nitric, hydrochloric) cause coagulation of the surface tissues. This initial reaction

may protect the esophageal wall. However, damage occurs to areas where exposure is prolonged. For these reasons, rapid esophageal passage with longer pooling in the gastric cavity causes acute lesions that may quickly progress to necrosis and perforation (Maull et al., 1979) (Fig. 27–105*B* and C).

Symptoms and Signs

ACUTE PHASE

Local pain and odynophagia may be present in the mouth and pharynx, and varies with the severity of injury. Ulcerations, edema, and hypersalivation may be observed.

Laryngeal burns cause respiratory difficulties with stridor and hoarseness. Esophageal damage causes dysphagia and odynophagia. Chest pain irradiating to the back with fever and tachycardia suggests deeper wall damage with developing infection. Progression of symptoms to chest and abdominal pain with a severe septic state suggest transmural damage and perforation.

CHRONIC PHASE

Proliferation of the granulation and fibrous tissues causes progressive dysphagia at the fifth or sixth week after injury. Stricture formation takes place in 10 to 25% of patients following solid alkali ingestion (Estrera et al., 1986). High-concentration liquid alkali causes increased damage, acutely and over time (Leape et al., 1971).

Clinical Assessment

RADIOLOGIC EXAMINATION

The initial radiologic assessment serves as a baseline for later examination. During the acute phase, spasm or atony may be observed. Ulcer narrowings from edema and inflammation may appear rapidly. Intramural retention of contrast material, air trapping in the esophageal cavity, and perforation indicate more severe burns (Fig. 27–105C).

Because symptoms do not always correlate with damage and because depth of injury is not always easy to assess, regular radiologic examination documents the development and extent of strictures.

Marchand (1955) suggested classifying esophageal strictures based on configuration and size of the lumen (Fig. 27–106).

ENDOSCOPIC EVALUATION

Endoscopic evaluation describes the areas and extent of the initial damage. Endoscopy is not accurate to indicate depth of injury. Assessment of pharynx and larynx by direct laryngoscopy may reveal proximal damage. Tracheoscopy and bronchoscopy must be completed if any aspiration damage may have occurred.

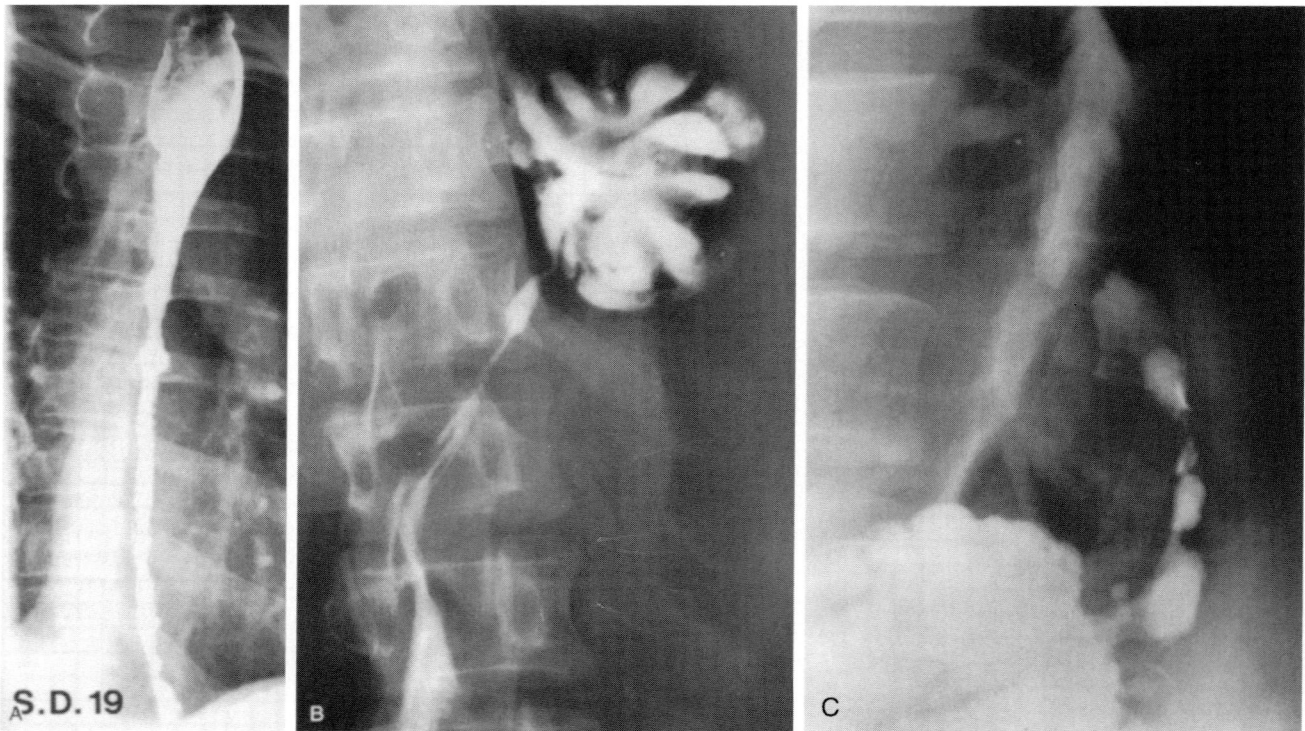

FIGURE 27–105. *A,* Severe damage to the esophagus from alkali ingestion. *B,* Transmural destruction and narrowing of the stomach by sulfuric acid ingestion. *C,* Intramural contrast, sacculation, ulceration, and fistulization indicate more severe burns.

Examination of the esophagus is undertaken with care and in a controlled situation. Erosions and exudates suggest second-degree burns. Circumferential discoloration, edema, and hematoma formation suggest deeper lesions. The endoscope is not inserted beyond areas of second- or third-degree burns to avoid the risks of perforation. The advantage of early endoscopy following caustic ingestion is to exclude patients without lesions from intensive immediate treatment. Long-term follow-up is still advised even if the initial assessment has not documented acute lesions: An upper digestive barium swallow at 1 month and 1 year after ingestion should rule out unexpected stricture formation.

Management

ACUTE PHASE

Cardona and Daly (1964) and Haller and colleagues (1971) have suggested, as general measures, that one identify the agent that has caused the damage and obtain within 12 to 24 hours a clear estimate of the severity and depth of the injury.

While respiratory and hemodynamics are being stabilized, antibiotics covering the mouth and esophageal flora are being started. Although some argue that steroids prevent stricture formation, strong evidence favoring their use is still lacking (Oakes et al., 1982).

No food or liquid should be given by mouth until endoscopic examination of pharynx, larynx, esophagus, and stomach has been completed.

Chest films and upper digestive barium examination should be obtained.

If no damage is found, all special measures are stopped. The patient is reassessed during the following year to rule out the appearance of undocumented damage.

If an esophageal burn is documented, treatment is continued for 3 weeks, when radiologic reassessment is obtained. The presence or absence of a stricture at this point determines subsequent treatment. Since full damage to the esophagus occurs within seconds of the contact, attempts at neutralization or gastric lavage are probably of little use.

When an alkaline battery has been ingested, it needs to be removed on an emergency basis because leakage can cause severe esophageal burns.

Complications to be looked for following ingestion of caustic substances include mediastinitis (20%), esophageal perforation (15%), and perforation of the stomach (10%). When esophageal ulcerations are present at endoscopy, 22% of these patients will develop a stricture (5.7% of total). Pulmonary complications may result from damage by the caustic, from aspiration, or by esophagotracheal fistulization. Mortality in recent decades is approximately 5% (Postlethwait, 1986). Major complications in the mediastinum and extensive necrosis may require total esophagectomy and gastrectomy (Brun et al., 1984; Estrera et al., 1986).

CHRONIC PHASE

Treatment of the caustic injury in the chronic phase is oriented toward the management of the established

Grade I

Grade II

Grade III

Grade IV

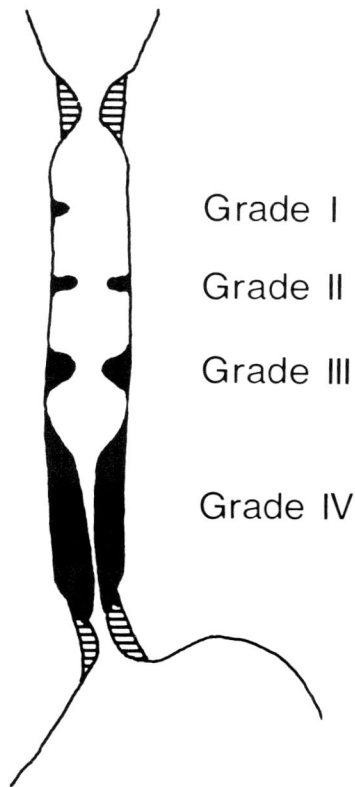

FIGURE 27–106. Classification of caustic injuries. Grade I: Short fibrous stricture involving less than the complete circumference; Grade II: string-like annular stricture of mucosa and submucosa; Grade III: dumbbell stricture with muscularis damage of less than 0.5 inch; Grade IV: long stricture of more than 0.5 inch.

stricture. Dilatations can be accomplished with Maloney bougies when the stricture is short. More extensive strictures require guidewire dilatations of the Savary-Gilliard type until proper lumen size is obtained. Gastric or colon bypass (see Figs. 27–103 and 17–104) of the strictured esophagus is indicated when complete stenosis is present or if marked irregularity and pocketing of the esophagus is evident. A tracheoesophageal fistula, the impossibility to reach a diameter larger than No. 40 French, or the impossibility to dilate without undue pain and mediastinal reaction are also indications for bypass. Subsequent esophagectomy may be considered, since a higher incidence of carcinoma is present in the damaged esophagus (Appelqvist and Salmo, 1980).

BENIGN TUMORS AND CYSTS

Benign tumors of the esophagus have been classified by Nemir and associates (1976) as epithelial, non-epithelial, and heterotopic (Table 27–12). Leiomyoma represent 36% of these benign lesions, and epithelial polyps, 25%. Cysts of the esophagus account for 10 to 20% of all benign esophageal lesions (Tapia and White, 1985).

Leiomyoma

Postlethwait and Musser (1974) and Postlethwait (1983a) observed these benign tumors in 51 of 1000 unselected esophagi examined at autopsy. It develops in men twice as often as in women, and the author estimates that approximately 80% of all tumor and cysts of the esophagus are leiomyomas. They are located mostly in the distal esophagus. The middle third is affected in 33% of reported cases and the proximal esophagus in 11% (Seremetis et al., 1976).

Pathology

Ninety-seven per cent of leiomyomas seem to originate in the circular muscle layer; the other 3% are polypoid and protrude outside the esophageal wall. Multiple lesions occur and some tumors may present with irregular shapes. Histologic examination reveals interlacing bundles of elongated cells with intracellular myofibrils. Interdigitation of fibrous tissue into the surrounding muscle may be seen, and there is usually no well-developed capsule around the tumor.

Symptoms

Half of the patients are asymptomatic. When present, symptoms are related to the size of the lesion. Dysphagia is present when the tumor is sufficiently large to cause obstruction. Chest pain may be present with substernal tightness or fullness. Hemorrhage is rare (3%) and presents when ulceration or transformation has occurred (Bruneton et al., 1981; Deverall, 1968).

Diagnosis

The esophagram shows a smooth, semilunar defect with intact mucosa and clear border (Fig. 27–107).

■ Table 27–12. BENIGN TUMORS AND CYSTS OF ESOPHAGUS

Epithelial	Heterotopic
Papillomas	Gastric mucosal
Polyps	Melanoblastic
Adenomas	Sebaceous gland
Cysts	Granular cell myoblastoma
	Pancreatic gland
	Thyroid nodule
Nonepithelial	
Myoma	
Leiomyoma	
Fibromyoma	
Lipomyoma	
Fibroma	
Vascular	
Hemangioma	
Lymphangioma	
Mesenchymal	
Reticuloendothelial	
Myxofibroma	
Giant cell	
Neurofibroma	
Osteochondroma	

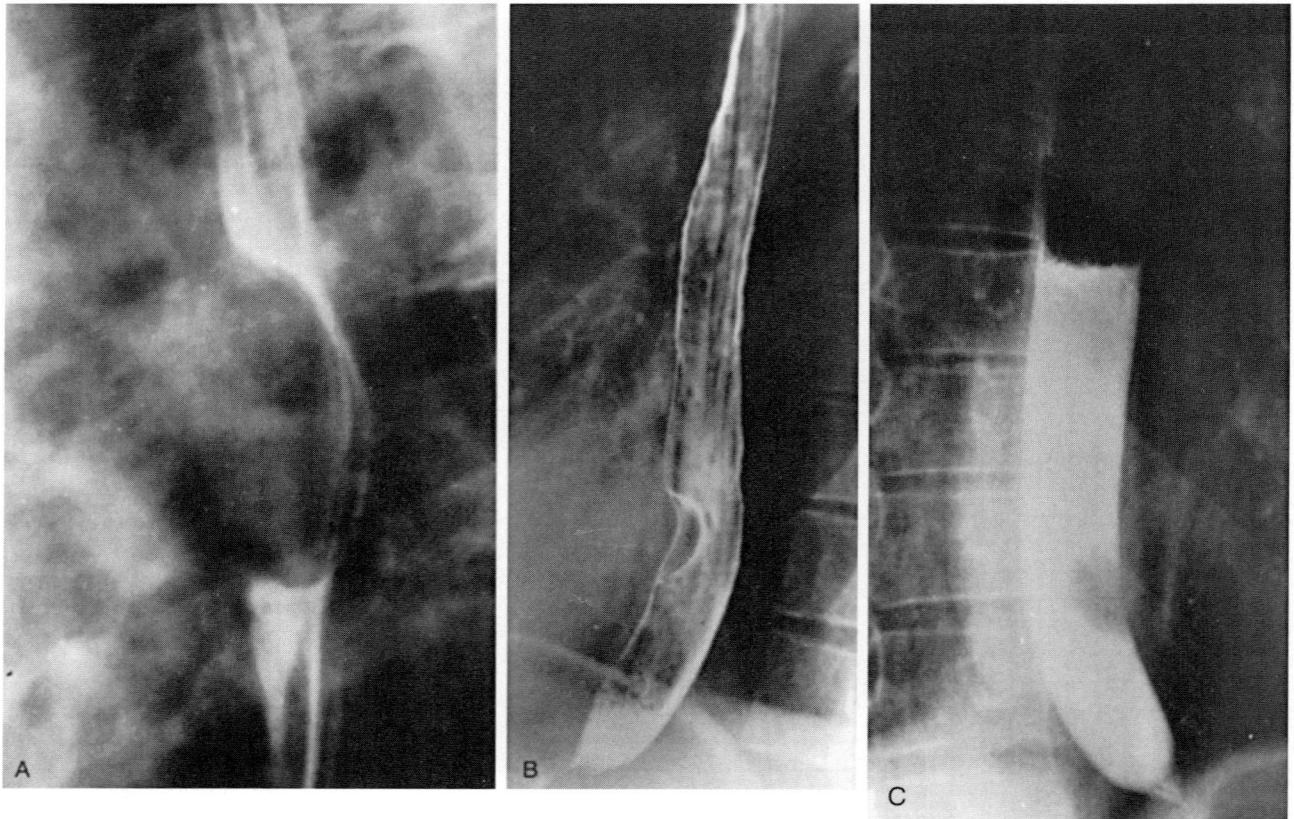

FIGURE 27–107. *A,* A large leiomyoma creating smooth mucosal compression. *B* and *C,* A small leiomyoma with intact mucosa and clear borders.

Esophageal opacification during CT scan examination (Fig. 27–108) may help locate the tumor within the esophageal wall. Larger tumors are seen near the cardia and may cause distortion of the GEJ.

Endoscopy confirms location and length of the tumor. The mucosa overlying the tumor is intact. It should not be biopsied because subsequent excision may be rendered more difficult. Similar imprints of tumors on the esophageal wall may result from bronchogenic cysts or large mediastinal lymph nodes.

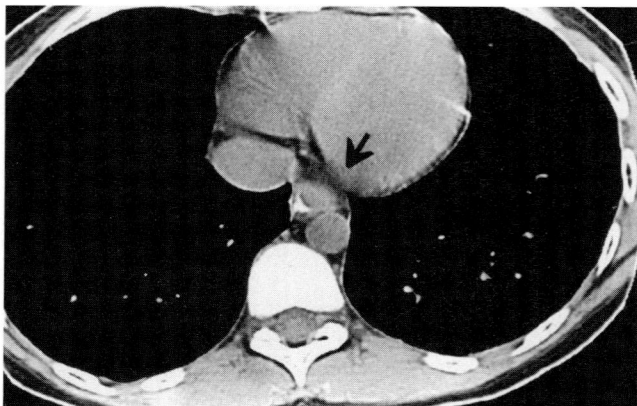

FIGURE 27–108. Esophageal opacification during CT scan of the chest locates the leiomyoma *(arrow)* within the esophageal wall.

Treatment

Indications for removal are the relief of symptoms and progression in size. It is important to obtain a clear tissue diagnosis in both indications. Symptoms eventually occur. Malignant transformation was documented in only two cases (Seremetis et al., 1976). Enucleation of the tumor is usually completed without problems following incision of the longitudinal muscle (Fig. 27–109). The mucosa should remain intact. If the tumor is large and circumferential and lies at the GEJ or if it is ulcerated and adherent to the mucosa, resection of the lesion with the esophagus is required.

■ **Table 27–13.** CYSTS OF THE MEDIASTINUM

Enterogenous	Mesothelial
Bronchogenic	Pleural
Esophageal	Pericardial
Gastroenteric	
	Lymphatic
Neuroenteric	
	Hygroma
Endodermal elements	Thoracic duct cyst
Ectodermal elements	
Vertebral defects	**Thymic**
	Nonspecific

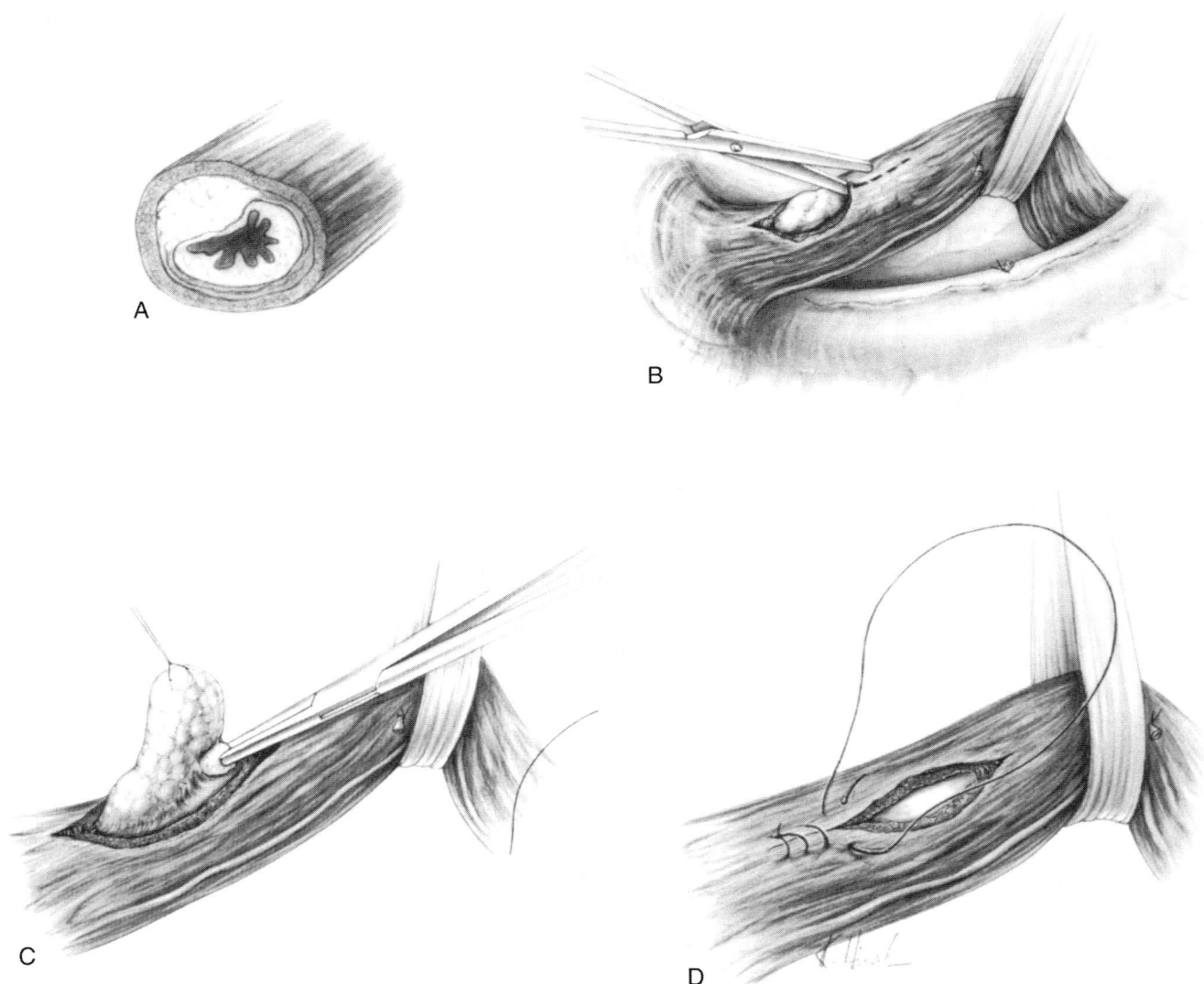

FIGURE 27–109. Enucleation of the tumor by thoracotomy. *A,* The tumor usually originates from the muscularis. *B,* Opening of the longitudinal musculature over the tumor. *C,* Progressive enucleation of the tumor; the mucosa is left intact. *D,* Closure of the muscularis. (*A–D,* From Skinner, D. B.: Atlas of Esophageal Surgery. Churchill Livingstone, New York, 1991.)

CYSTS AND DUPLICATION

A classification of mediastinal cysts is found in Table 27–13. Enterogenous or foregut cysts are usually divided into bronchogenic cysts and esophageal cysts. This division is based on the histologic findings in these lesions. Bronchogenic elements and islands of cartilage are found in bronchogenic cysts. A double layer of smooth muscle is the main histologic feature present in the walls of an esophageal cyst. Abnormal budding of the early bronchial tree causes these lesions to appear in the mediastinum. Most of these cystic tumors are then in anatomic contact with the esophagus or the tracheobronchial tree (Fig. 27–110).

Clinical Presentation

St-Georges and co-workers (1991) described symptoms in 86 patients with a cyst of the mediastinum. These lesions were closely adherent to the esophagus in 48% of patients and to the tracheobronchial tree in 32% of them. Forty-four patients (67%) were symptomatic with mostly chest pain (61%), cough, dyspnea, or fever. Nine patients had dysphagia.

Diagnosis

Standard posteroanterior and lateral chest films generally demonstrate the middle or posterior mediastinal location of the cyst and its relationship with adjacent structures. Barium swallows reveal an esophageal compression or displacement with an intact mucosa showing the smooth contour of benign intraparietal lesions (Fig. 27–111*A*). Endoscopy shows an intact mucosa. A CT scan usually suggests the cystic nature of the lesion (Fig. 27–111*B*).

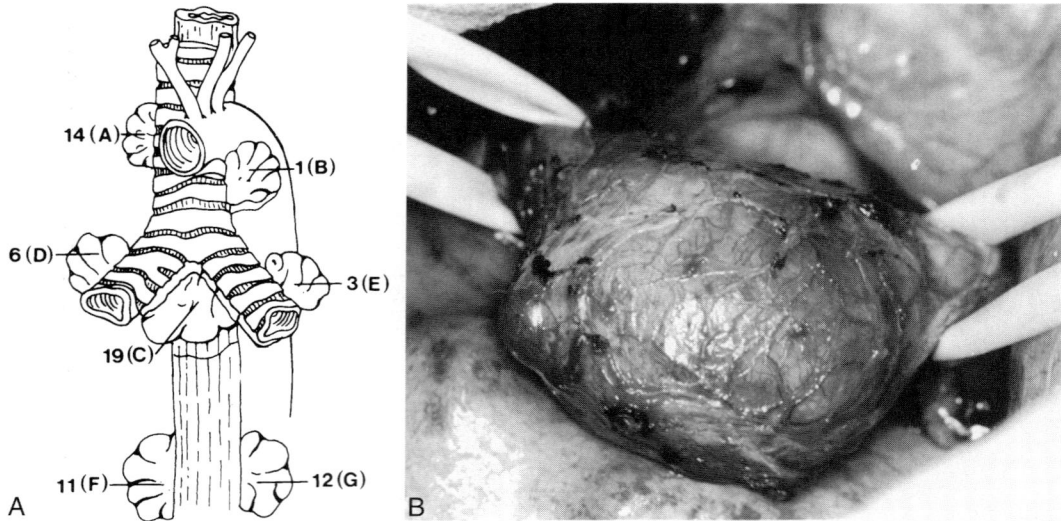

FIGURE 27–110. *A,* Most of the cystic tumors of the mediastinum may be in contact with the esophageal wall. *B,* Bronchogenic cyst of the mediastinum totally within the wall of the esophagus.

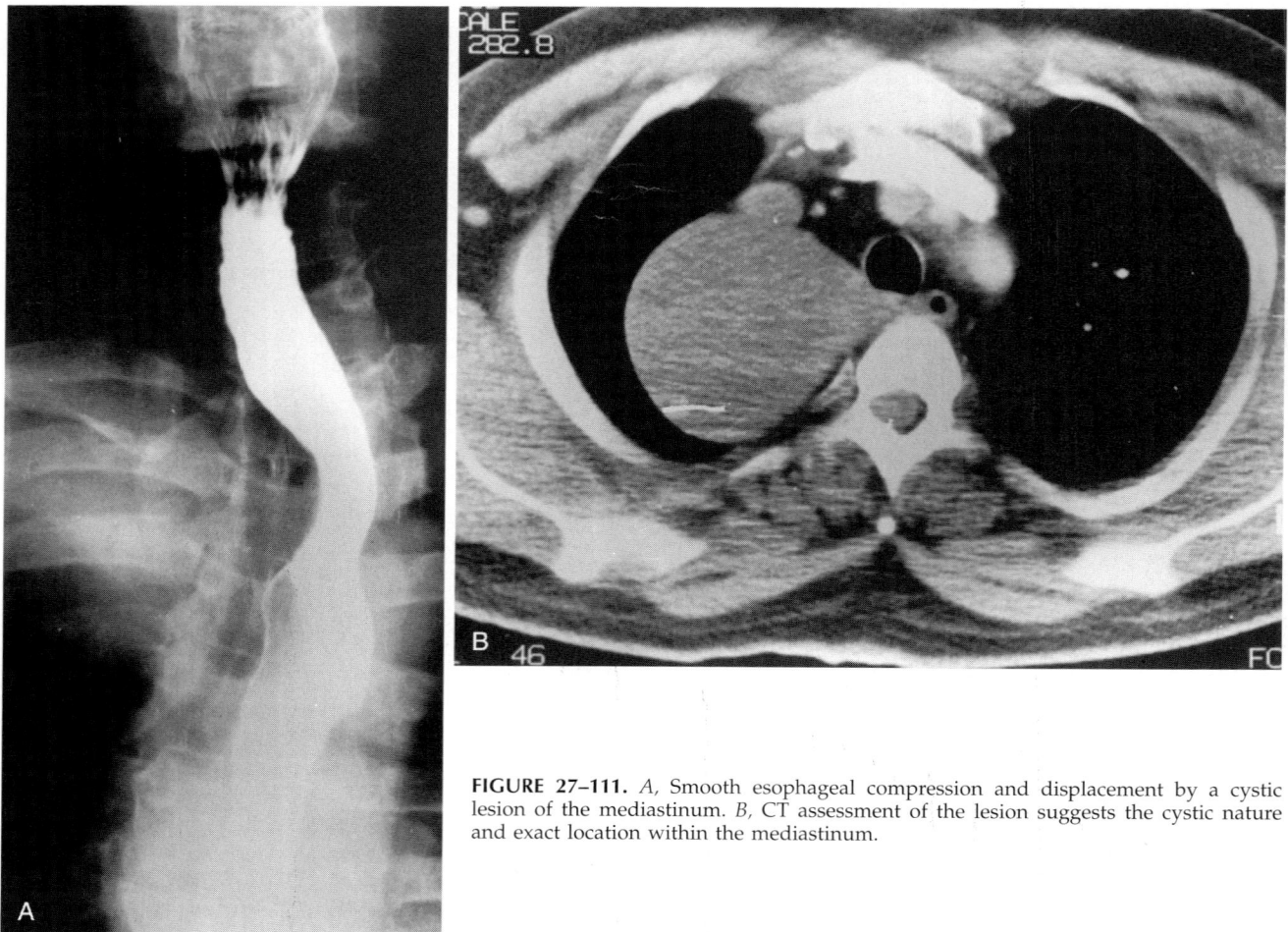

FIGURE 27–111. *A,* Smooth esophageal compression and displacement by a cystic lesion of the mediastinum. *B,* CT assessment of the lesion suggests the cystic nature and exact location within the mediastinum.

Treatment

Surgical excision is recommended for nearly all patients for two main reasons: to establish a definitive diagnosis and to prevent complications while alleviating the symptoms. Eighty-two per cent of the patients eventually become symptomatic from either compression or complications. Operation becomes more hazardous when complications have occurred, so early resection is recommended.

Like leiomyomas, these cysts are generally excised by enucleation, leaving the esophageal mucosa intact (see Fig. 27–109). Complete excision is necessary to obtain excellent results. Morbidity is minimal.

SELECTED BIBLIOGRAPHY

Jamieson, G. G. (ed): Surgery of the Oesophagus. London, Churchill Livingstone, 1988.

This is an encyclopedic work on surgery of the esophagus, undoubtedly the best referenced book on the subject.

Liebermann-Meffert, D.: Embryology and anatomy of the esophagus. In Zuidema, G. D. (ed): Shackelford's Surgery of the Alimentary Tract. Philadelphia, W. B. Saunders, 1994.

This concise but complete review of embryology, anatomy, and tissue organization of the esophagus helps illuminate not only developmental abnormalities and structural details but also the tridimensional organization of the esophagus within the chest.

REFERENCES

Ahtaridis, G., Snape, W. J., and Cohen, S.: Lower esophageal sphincter as an index of gastroesophageal acid reflux. Dig. Dis. Sci., 26:993, 1981.

Andreollo, N. A., and Earlam, R. J.: Heller's myotomy for achalasia: Is an added anti-reflux procedure necessary? Br. J. Surg., 74:765, 1987.

Appelqvist, P., and Salmo, M.: Lye corrosion carcinoma of the esophagus. A review of 63 cases. Cancer, 45:2655, 1980.

Armstrong, D., Monnier, P. H., Nicolet, M., et al.: Endoscopic assessment of oesophagitis. Gullet, 1:63, 1991.

Atkinson, M., Edwards, D. A. W., Honour, A. J., and Rowlands, E. N.: The oesophagogastric sphincter in hiatus hernia. Lancet, 2:1138, 1957.

Behar, J., Sheahan, D. G., Biancani, P., et al.: Medical and surgical management of reflux esophagitis. A 38-month report on a prospective clinical trial. N. Engl. J. Med., 293:263, 1975.

Belsey, R. H. R., and Skinner, D. B.: Management of esophageal stricture. In Skinner, D. B., Belsey, R. H. R., Hendrix, T. R., and Zuidema, G. D. (eds): Gastroesophageal Reflux and Hiatal Hernia. Boston, Little, Brown, 1972, pp. 173–196.

Benjamin, S. B., O'Donnell, J. K., Hancock, J., et al.: Prolonged radionuclide transit in nutcracker esophagus. Dig. Dis. Sci., 28:775, 1983.

Bennett, J. R., and Hendrix, T. R.: Treatment of achalasia with pneumatic dilatation. Mod. Treat., 7:1217, 1970.

Berger, K., and McCallum, R. W.: The hypertensive lower esophageal sphincter: A clinical and manometric entity. Gastroenterology, 80:1109, 1981.

Bonavina, L., Khan, N. A., and DeMeester, T. R.: Pharyngoesophageal dysfunctions: The role of cricopharyngeal myotomy. Arch. Surg., 120:541, 1985.

Booth, D. J., Kemmerer, W. T., and Skinner, D. B.: Acid clearing from distal esophagus. Arch. Surg., 96:731, 1968.

Bremner, C. G., Lynch, V. P., and Ellis, F. H., Jr.: Barrett's esophagus: Congenital or acquired? An experimental study of esophageal mucosal regeneration in the dog. Surgery, 68:209, 1970.

Brun, J. G., Celerier, M., Koskas, F., and Dubost, C.: Blunt thorax oesophageal stripping: An emergency procedure for caustic ingestion. Br. J. Surg., 71:698, 1984.

Bruneton, J. N., Drouillard, J., Roux, P., et al.: Leiomyoma and leiomyosarcoma of the digestive tract—A report of 45 cases and review of the literature. Eur. J. Radiol., 1:291, 1981.

Butler, H.: Veins of the esophagus. Thorax, 6:276, 1951.

Campo, S., and Traube, M.: Lower esophageal sphincter dysfunction in diffuse esophageal spasm. Am. J. Gastroenterol., 84:928, 1989.

Cardona, J. C., and Daly, J. F.: Management of corrosive esophagitis. Analysis of treatment, methods and results. N. Y. State J. Med., 64:2307, 1964.

Cassella, R. R., Brown, A. L., Jr., Sayre, G. P., and Ellis, F. H., Jr.: Achalasia of the esophagus: Pathologic and etiologic considerations. Ann. Surg., 160:474, 1964.

Cassella, R. R., Ellis, F. H., Jr., and Brown, A. L., Jr.: Diffuse spasm of the lower part of the esophagus. Fine structure of esophageal smooth muscle and nerve. J. A. M. A., 191:379, 1965.

Castell, D. O.: Achalasia and diffuse esophageal spasm. Arch. Intern. Med., 136:571, 1976.

Castell, D. O. (ed): The Esophagus. Boston, Little, Brown, 1992.

Castell, D. O.: pH monitoring versus other tests for gastroesophageal reflux disease: Is this the gold standard? In Richter, J. E. (ed): Ambulatory Esophageal pH Monitoring. New York, Igaku-Shoin, 1991, pp. 101–113.

Castell, J. A., and Dalton, C. B.: Esophageal manometry. In Castell, D. O. (ed.): The Esophagus. Boston, Little, Brown, 1992, pp. 143–160.

Castell, J. A., Dalton, C. B., and Castell, D. O.: Pharyngeal and upper esophageal sphincter manometry in humans. Am. J. Physiol., 258:G173, 1990.

Chen, Y. M., Ott, D. J., Hewson, E. G., et al.: Diffuse esophageal spasm: Radiographic and manometric correlation. Radiology, 170:807, 1989.

Christensen, J.: The innervation of motility of the esophagus. Front. Gastrointest. Res., 3:18, 1978.

Christensen, J.: Motor functions of the pharynx and esophagus. In Johnson, L. R. (ed): Physiology of the Gastrointestinal Tract. New York, Raven Press, 1987, pp. 595–612.

Clouse, R. E., and Lustman, P. J.: Psychiatric illness and contraction abnormalities of the esophagus. N. Engl. J. Med., 309:1337, 1983.

Clouse, R. E., Lustman, P. J., Eckert, T. C., et al.: Low-dose trazodone for symptomatic patients with esophageal contraction abnormalities. A double-blind, placebo-controlled trial. Gastroenterology, 92:1027, 1987.

Clouse, R. E., and Staiano, A.: Contraction abnormalities of the esophageal body in patients referred for manometry: A new approach to manometric classification. Dig. Dis. Sci., 28:784, 1983.

Code, C. F., Creamer, B., Schlegel, J. F., et al.: An Atlas of Esophageal Motility in Health and Disease. Springfield, IL, Charles C. Thomas, 1958.

Collis, J. L.: An operation for hiatus hernia with short esophagus. J. Thorac. Cardiovasc. Surg., 34:768, 1957.

Cook, I. J., Blumbergs, P., Cash, K., et al.: Structural abnormalities of the cricopharyngeus muscle in patients with pharyngeal (Zenker's) diverticulum. Gastroenterol. Hepatol., 7:556, 1992a.

Cook, I. J., Dodds, W. J., Dantas, R. O., et al.: Opening mechanisms of the human upper esophageal sphincter. Am. J. Physiol., 20:G748, 1989.

Cook, I. J., Gabb, M., Panagopoulos, V., et al.: Pharyngeal (Zenker's) diverticulum is a disorder of upper esophageal sphincter opening. Gastroenterology, 103:1229, 1992b.

Costantini, M., Crookes, P. F., Bremner, R. M., et al.: Value of physiologic assessment of foregut symptoms in a surgical practice. Surgery, 114:780, 1993.

Csendes, A., Velasco, N., Braghetto, I., and Henriquez, A.: A prospective randomized study comparing forceful dilatation and esophagomyotomy in patients with achalasia of the esophagus. Gastroenterology, 80:789, 1981.

Cunningham, E. T., Jr., and Sawchenko, P. E.: Central neural control of esophageal motility: A review. Dysphagia, 5:35, 1990.

Curtis, D. J., Cruess, D. F., and Berg, T.: The cricopharyngeal muscle: A videorecording review. A. J. R. Am. J. Roentgenol., 142:497, 1984.

Curtis, D. J., and Hudson, T.: Laryngotracheal aspiration: Analysis of specific neuromuscular factors. Radiology, *149*:517, 1983.

Dalton, C. B., Castell, D. O., Hewson, E. G., et al.: Diffuse esophageal spasm: A rare motility disorder not characterized by high-amplitude contractions. Dig. Dis. Sci., *36*:1025, 1991.

Dankmeijer, J., and Miète, M.: Sur le développement de l'estomac. Acta Anat., *47*:384, 1961.

DeMeester, T. R., Johnson, L. F., Joseph, G. J., et al.: Patterns of gastroesophageal reflux in health and disease. Ann. Surg., *184*:459, 1976.

Demos, N. J.: Stapled uncut gastroplasty for hiatal hernia: 12-year follow-up. Ann. Thorac. Surg., *38*:393, 1984.

Dent, J., Dodds, J., Friedman, R. H., et al.: Mechanism of gastroesophageal reflux in recumbent asymptomatic human subjects. J. Clin. Invest., *65*:256, 1980.

Dent, J., Dodds, W. J., Sekiguchi, T., et al.: Interdigestive phasic contractions of the human lower esophageal sphincter. Gastroenterology, *84*:453, 1983.

Dent, J., Holloway, R. H., Toouli, J., and Dodds, W. J.: Mechanisms of lower oesophageal sphincter incompetence in patients with symptomatic gastrooesophageal reflux. Gut, *29*:1020, 1988.

Deverall, P. B.: Smooth-muscle tumors of the oesophagus. Br. J. Surg., *55*:457, 1968.

DiMarino, A. J. Jr., and Cohen, S.: Characteristics of lower esophageal sphincter function in symptomatic diffuse esophageal spasm. Gastroenterology, *66*:1, 1974.

Dodds, W. J., Dent, J., Hogan, W. J., et al.: Mechanisms of gastroesophageal reflux in patients with reflux esophagitis. N. Engl. J. Med. *307*:1547, 1982.

Dodds, W. J., Hogan, W. J., Lydo, J. B., et al.: Quantitation of pharyngeal motor function in normal human subjects. J. Appl. Physiol., *39*:692, 1975.

Duranceau, A. C., Devroede, G., Lafontaine, E., and Jamieson, G. G.: Esophageal motility in asymptomatic volunteers. Surg. Clin. North Am., *63*:777, 1983.

Duranceau, A. C., and Jamieson, G. G.: Cricopharyngeal myotomy for pharyngoesophageal diverticula. *In* DeMeester, T. R., and Matthews, H. R. (eds): International Trends in General Thoracic Surgery: Benign Esophageal Disease. Vol. 3. St. Louis, C. V. Mosby, 1987, pp. 358–363.

Duranceau, A. C., Lafontaine, E., and Taillefer, R.: Oropharyngeal dysphagia. *In* Jamieson, G. G. (ed): Surgery of the Oesophagus. London, Churchill-Livingstone, 1988, pp. 413–434.

Duranceau, A. C., Topart, P., Deschamps, C., and Taillefer, R.: Gastroesophageal reflux control in operated scleroderma patients. *In* Nabeya, K., Hanaoka, T., and Nogami, H. (eds): Recent Advances in Diseases of the Esophagus. Tokyo, Springer-Verlag, 1993, pp. 115–121.

Earlam, R. J., Ellis, F. H., Jr., and Nobrega, F. T.: Achalasia of the esophagus in a small urban community. Mayo Clin. Proc., *44*:478, 1969.

Eastwood, G. L., Castell, D. O., and Higgs, R. H.: Experimental esophagitis in cats impairs lower esophageal sphincter pressure. Gastroenterology, *69*:146, 1975.

Eckhardt, V. F., Janisch, H. D., and Bettendorf, U.: Barrett's Syndrome: Correlation of oesophageal morphology with potential difference measurements. Z. Gastroenterol., *4*:296, 1983.

Ellis, F. H., Jr., and Crozier, R. E.: Cervical esophageal dysphagia: Indications for and results of cricopharyngeal myotomy. Ann. Surg., *194*:279, 1981.

Ellis, F. H., Jr., Crozier, R. E., and Shea, J. A.: Long esophagomyotomy for diffuse esophageal spasm and related disorders. *In* Siewert, J. R., and Holscher, A. H. (eds): Diseases of the Esophagus. New York, Springer-Verlag, 1988, pp. 913–917.

Ellis, F. H., Jr., and Gibb, S. P.: Reoperation after esophagomyotomy for achalasia of the esophagus. Am. J. Surg., *129*:407, 1975.

Ellis, F. H., Jr., Olsen, A. M., Schlegel, J. F., and Code, C. F.: Surgical treatment of esophageal hypermotility disturbances. J. A. M. A., *188*:862, 1964.

Estrera, A., Taylor, W., Mills, L. J., and Platt, M. R.: Corrosive burns of the esophagus and stomach: A recommendation for an aggressive surgical approach. Ann. Thorac. Surg., *41*:276, 1986.

Ferguson, M. K., and Little, A. G.: Angina-like chest pain associated with high-amplitude peristaltic contractions of the esophagus. Surgery, *104*:713, 1988.

Feussner, H., Petri, A., Walker, S., et al.: The modified AFP score: An attempt to make the results of antireflux surgery comparable. Br. J. Surg., *78*:942, 1991.

Garrett, J. M., and Godwin, D. H.: Gastroesophageal hypercontracting sphincter. Manometric and clinical characteristics. J. A. M. A., *208*:992, 1969.

Gelfond, M., Rozen, P., and Gilat, T.: Isosorbide dinitrate and nifedipine treatment of achalasia: A clinical, manometric and radionuclide evaluation. Gastroenterology, *83*:963, 1982.

Gillies, M., Nicks, R., and Skyring, A.: Clinical, manometric and pathological studies in diffuse esophageal spasm. Br. Med. J., *2*:527, 1967.

Gray, S. W., and Skandalakis, J. E. (eds): Embryology for Surgeons. The Embryological Basis for the Treatment of Congenital Defects. Philadelphia, W. B. Saunders, 1972.

Gross, R., Johnson, L. F., and Kaminski, R. J.: Esophageal emptying in achalasia quantitated by a radioisotope technique. Dig. Dis. Sci., *24*:945, 1979.

Haagensen, C. D., Feind, C. R., and Herter, F. P. (eds): The Lymphatics in Cancer. Philadelphia, W. B. Saunders, 1972.

Haddad, J. K.: Relation of gastroesophageal reflux to yield sphincter pressures. Gastroenterology, *58*:175, 1970.

Haller, J. A., Jr., Andrews, H. G., White, J. J., et al.: Pathophysiology and management of acute corrosive burns of the esophagus: Results of treatment in 285 children. J. Pediatr. Surg., *6*:578, 1971.

Hamilton, W. J., and Mossman, H. W. (eds): Human Embryology. Prenatal Development of Form and Function. 4th Ed. London, Macmillan, 1978.

Hankins, J. R., and McLaughlin, J. S.: The association of carcinoma of the esophagus with achalasia. J. Thorac. Cardiovasc. Surg., *69*:355, 1975.

Henderson, R. D.: Benign strictures of the esophagus. *In* Shields, T. W. (ed): General Thoracic Surgery. Philadelphia, Lea & Febiger, 1989, pp. 1012–1023.

Henderson, R. D.: Reflux control following gastroplasty. Ann. Thorac. Surg., *24*:206, 1977.

Henderson, R. D., and Marryatt, G.: Total fundoplication gastroplasty. Long-term follow-up of 500 patients. J. Thorac. Cardiovasc. Surg., *85*:81, 1983.

Henderson, R. D., Marryatt, G., and Henderson, R. F.: Surgical management of gastroesophageal reflux in patients with scleroderma. *In* Siewert, J. R., and Holscher, A. H. (eds): Diseases of the Esophagus. Berlin, Springer-Verlag, 1988.

Henderson, R. D., and Pearson, F. G.: Surgical management of esophageal scleroderma. J. Thorac. Cardiovasc. Surg., *66*:686, 1973.

Herlihy, K. J., Orlando, R. C., Bryson, J. C., et al.: Barrett's esophagus: Clinical, endoscopic, histologic, manometric and electrical potential difference characteristics. Gastroenterology, *86*:436, 1984.

Hill, L. D., Gelfand, M., and Bauermeister, D.: Simplified management of reflux esophagitis with stricture. Ann. Surg., *172*:638, 1970.

Holloway, R. H., Krosin, G., Lange, R. C., et al.: Radionuclide esophageal emptying of a solid meal to quantitate results of therapy in achalasia. Gastroenterology, *84*:771, 1983.

Holscher, A. H., and Weiser, H. F.: Reflux characteristics in health and disease. *In* Roman, C. (ed): Gastrointestinal Motility. Lancaster, England, M. T. P. Press, 1984, pp. 63–72.

Hugh, T. B., Lusby, R. J., and Coleman, M. J.: Antral patch esophagoplasty: A new procedure for acid-peptic esophageal stricture. Am. J. Surg., *137*:221, 1979.

Hurwitz, A. L., Duranceau, A., and Haddad, J. K.: Disorders of esophageal motility. Major Probl. Intern. Med., *16*:85, 1979.

Hurwitz, A. L., Way, L., and Haddad, J. K.: Epiphrenic diverticulum in association with an unusual motility disturbance: Report of surgical correction. Gastroenterology, *68*:795, 1975.

Iascone, C., DeMeester, T. R., Little, A. G., and Skinner, D. B.: Barrett's esophagus: Functional assessment, proposed pathogenesis, and surgical therapy. Arch. Surg., *118*:543, 1983.

Ismail-Beigi, F., Horton, P. F., and Pope, C. E., II: Histological consequences of gastroesophageal reflux in man. Gastroenterology, *58*:163, 1970.

Jamieson, G. G., Cook, I. J., and Shaw, D.: The pathogenesis of

Zenker's diverticulum and its normalisation by cricopharyngeal myotomy. ISDE Meeting Report, Kyoto, 1993.

Jamieson, G. G., and Duranceau, A.: Gastroesophageal Reflux. Philadelphia, W. B. Saunders, 1988a.

Jamieson, G. G., and Duranceau, A.: Reoperative surgery for problems after oesophagomyotomy. In Jamieson, G. G. (ed): Surgery of the Oesophagus. London, Churchill Livingstone, 1988b, pp. 797–802.

Jara, F. M., Toledo-Pereyra, L. H., Lewis, J. W., and Magilligan, D. J., Jr.: Long-term results of esophagomyotomy for achalasia of esophagus. Arch. Surg., 114:935, 1979.

Johns, B. A. E.: Developmental changes in the oesophageal epithelium in man. J. Anat., 86:431, 1952.

Johnson, L. F., and DeMeester, T. R.: Twenty-four-hour pH monitoring of the distal esophagus. A quantitative measure of gastroesophageal reflux. Am. J. Gastroenterol., 62:325, 1974.

Kahrilas, P. J.: Functional anatomy and physiology of the esophagus. In Castell, D. O. (ed): The Esophagus. Boston, Little, Brown, 1992.

Kahrilas, P. J., Dent, J., Dodds, W. J., et al.: A method for continuous monitoring of upper esophageal sphincter pressure. Dig. Dis. Sci., 32:121, 1987.

Kahrilas, P. J., Dodds, W. J., Dent, J., et al.: Upper esophageal sphincter function during deglutition. Gastroenterology, 95:52, 1988.

Kahrilas, P. J., Dodds, W. J., Hogan, W. J., et al.: Esophageal Peristaltic dysfunction in peptic esophagitis. Gastroenterology, 91:897, 1986.

Khamis, B., Kennedy, E., Finucane, J., and Doyle, J. S.: Transmucosal potential difference, diagnostic value in gastro-oesophageal reflux. Gut, 19:396, 1978.

Khan, A. A., and Castell, D. O.: Primary diffuse oesophageal spasm and related disorders. In Jamieson, G. G. (ed): Surgery of the Oesophagus. New York, Churchill Livingstone, 1988, pp. 484–488.

Kiroff, G. K., Mukerjhee, T. M., Dixon, B., et al.: Morphological changes caused by the exposure of rabbit oesophageal mucosa to hydrochloric acid and sodium taurocholate. Aust. N. Z. J. Surg., 57:119, 1987.

Knuff, T. F., Benjamin, S. B., and Castell, D. O.: Pharyngoesophageal (Zenker's) diverticulum: A reappraisal. Gastroenterology, 82:734, 1982.

Kraus, B. B., Wu, W. C., and Castell, D. O.: Comparison of lower esophageal sphincter manometrics and gastroesophageal reflux measured by 24-hour pH recording. Am. J. Gastroenterol., 85:692, 1990.

Krey, H.: On the treatment of corrosive lesions in the esophagus: An experimental study. Acta Otolaryngol. Suppl. 102:1,1952.

Krupp, S., and Rosetti, M.: Surgical treatment of hiatal hernias by fundoplication and gastropexy (Nissen repair). Ann. Surg., 164:927, 1966.

Leape, L. L., Ashcraft, K. W., Scarpelli, D. G., and Holder, T. M.: Hazard to health: Liquid lye. N. Engl. J. Med., 284:578, 1971.

Lehnert, T., Erlandson, A., and Decosse, J. J.: Lymph and blood capillaries of the human gastric mucosa. A morphologic basis for metastasis in early gastric carcinoma. Gastroenterology, 9:939, 1947.

Leonardi, H. K., Shea, J. A., Crozier, R. E., and Ellis, F. H., Jr.: Diffuse spasm of the esophagus. Clinical, manometric and surgical considerations. J. Thorac. Cardiovasc. Surg., 74:736, 1977.

Lerche, W.: The Esophagus and Pharynx in Action. A Study of Structure in Relation to Function. Springfield, IL, Charles C. Thomas, 1950.

Lerut, T., Vandekerkhof, J., Leman, G., et al.: Cricopharyngeal myotomy for pharyngoesophageal diverticula. In DeMeester, T. R., and Matthews, H. R. (eds): International Trends in General Thoracic Surgery: Benign Esophageal Disease. Vol. 3. St. Louis, C. V. Mosby, 1987, pp. 351–357.

Liebermann-Meffert, D.: Development of form and position of the human stomach and its mesenteries [German]. Acta Anat., 72:376, 1969.

Liebermann-Meffert, D., Allgower, M., Schmid, P., and Blum, A. L.: Muscular equivalent of the lower esophageal spincter. Gastroenterology, 76:31, 1979.

Liebermann-Meffert, D., and Duranceau, A.: Embryology of the esophagus. In Orringer, M. B. (ed): Shackelford's Surgery of the Alimentary Tract. Philadelphia, W. B. Saunders, 1994.

Liebermann-Meffert, D., Heberer, M., and Allgower, M.: The muscular counterpart of the lower esophageal sphincter. In DeMeester, T. R., and Skinner, D. B.: Esophageal Disorders: Pathology and Therapy. New York, Raven Press, 1985.

Liebermann-Meffert, D., Luescher, U., Neff, U., et al.: Esophagectomy without thoracotomy: Is there a risk of intramediastinal bleeding? A study on blood supply of the esophagus. Ann. Surg., 206:184, 1987.

Liebermann-Meffert, D., and Siewert, J. R.: Arterial anatomy of the esophagus. A review of the literature with brief comments on clinical aspects. Gullet, 2:3, 1992.

Linsell, J., Owen, W., and Anggiansa, H. A.: Management options for patients with diffuse esophageal spasm. In Siewert, J. R., and Holscher, A. H. (eds): Diseases of the Esophagus. New York, Springer-Verlag, 1988, pp. 909–912.

Maher, J. W.: Intrathoracic fundoplication for shortened esophagus. In Jamieson, G. G. (ed): Surgery of the Esophagus. London, Churchill Livingstone, 1988, pp. 321–326.

Marchand, P.: Caustic strictures of the oesophagus. Thorax, 10:171, 1955.

Mason, R. J., and Bremner, C. C.: Motility differences between long segment and short segment Barrett's esophagus. Am. J. Surg., 165:686, 1993.

Matthews, H. R., and Pattison, C. W.: Esophageal carcinoma as a complication of achalasia: The screening controversy. In Delarue, N. C., Wilkins, E. W., and Wong, J. (eds): International Trends in General Thoracic Surgery: Esophageal Cancer. Vol. 4. St. Louis, C. V. Mosby, 1988, pp. 11–15.

Mattioli, S., Pilotti, V., Spangaro, M., et al.: Reliability of 24-hour home esophageal pH monitoring in diagnosis of gastroesophageal reflux. Dig. Dis. Sci., 34:71, 1989.

Maull, K. I., Scher, L. A., and Greenfield, L. J.: Surgical implications of acid ingestion. Surg. Gynecol. Obstet., 148:895, 1979.

McCallum, R. W.: The hypertensive LES has quite special features. In Giuli, R., McCallum, R. W., and Skinner, D. B. (eds): Primary Motility Disorders of the Esophagus. London, J. Libbey Eurotext, 1991, pp. 825–829.

Menard, D., and Arsenault, P.: Maturation of human fetal esophagus maintained in organ culture. Anat. Rec., 217:348, 1987.

Merendino, K. A., and Dillard, D. H.: The concept of sphincter substitution by an interposed jejunal segment for anatomic and physiologic abnormalities at the esophagogastric junction, with special reference to reflux esophagitis, cardiospasm and esophageal varices. Ann. Surg., 142:486, 1955.

Moore, K. L.: The Developing Human: Clinically Orientated Embryology. 4th ed. Philadelphia, W. B. Saunders, 1988.

Moreno Gonzales, E., Garcia Alvarez, A., Landa Garcia, I., et al.: Results of surgical treatment of esophageal achalasia. Multicenter retrospective study of 1856 cases. GEEMO (Groupe Européen Etude Maladies Oesophagéennes) Multicentric Retrospective Study. Int. Surg., 73:69, 1988.

Mueller-Botha, G. S.: Organogenesis and growth of the gastroesophageal region in man. Anat. Rec., 133:219, 1959.

Naef, A. P., and Savary, M.: Conservative operation for peptic esophagitis with stenosis in columnar-lined lower esophagus. Ann. Thorac. Surg., 13:543, 1972.

Nemir, P., Wallace, H. W., and Fallahnejad, M.: Diagnosis and surgical management of benign diseases of the esophagus. Curr. Probl. Surg., 13:1, 1976.

Oakes, D. D., Sherck, J. P., and Mark, J. B. D.: Lye ingestion. Clinical patterns and therapeutic implications. J. Thorac. Cardiovasc. Surg., 83:194, 1982.

Orlando, R. C., and Bozymski, E. M.: Clinical and manometric effects of nitroglycerin in diffuse esophageal spasm. N. Engl. J. Med., 289:23, 1973.

Orlando, R. C., Call, D. L., and Bream, C. A.: Achalasia and absent gastric air bubble. Ann. Intern. Med., 88:60, 1978.

Orlando, R. C., Powell, D. W., Bryson, J. C., et al.: Esophageal potential difference measurements in esophageal disease. Gastroenterology, 83:1026, 1982.

Orringer, M. B.: The combined Collis-Nissen operation. In Jamieson, G. G. (ed): Surgery of the Oesophagus. London, Churchill Livingstone, 1988, pp. 327–335.

Orringer, M. B.: Surgical management of scleroderma reflux esophagitis. Surg. Clin. North Am., 63:859, 1983.

Orringer, M. B., Kirsh, M. M., and Sloan, H.: Esophageal reconstruction for benign disease. Technical considerations. J. Thorac. Cardiovasc. Surg., 73:807, 1977.

Orringer, M. B., Skinner, D. B., and Belsey, R. H.: Long-term results of the Mark IV operation for hiatal hernia and analyses of recurrences and their treatment. J. Thorac. Cardiovasc. Surg., 63:25, 1972.

Orringer, M. B., and Sloan, H.: Collis-Belsey reconstruction of the esophagogastric junction. Indications, physiology, and technical considerations. J. Thorac. Cardiovasc. Surg., 71:295, 1976.

Orringer, M. B., and Sloan, H.: Combined Collis-Nissen reconstruction of the esophagogastric junction. Ann. Thorac. Cardiovasc. Surg., 25:16, 1978.

Orringer, M. B., and Sloan, H.: Complications and failings of the combined Collis-Belsey operation. J. Thorac. Cardiovasc. Surg., 74:726, 1977.

Ott, D. J.: Radiology of the oropharynx and esophagus. In Castell, D. O. (ed): The Esophagus. Boston, Little, Brown, 1992.

Ott, D. J., Chen, Y. M., Hewson, E. G., et al.: Esophageal motility: Assessment with synchronous video tape fluoroscopy and manometry. Radiology, 173:419, 1989.

Ott, D. J., Cowan, R. J., Gelfand, D. W., et al.: The role of diagnostic imaging in evaluating gastroesophageal reflux disease. Postgrad. Radiol., 6:3, 1986.

Ott, D. J., Gelfand, D. W., and Wu, W. C.: Reflux esophagitis: Radiographic and endoscopic correlation. Radiology, 130:583, 1979.

Paris, F., Benages, A., Berenguer, J., et al.: Pre- and postoperative manometric studies in diffuse esophageal spasm. J. Thorac. Cardiovasc. Surg., 70:126, 1975.

Parrilla, P., Martinez De Haro, L. F., Ortiz, M. A., et al.: Correlation between endoscopic and pH-metric findings and motor oesophageal alterations in reflux oesophagitis. Dig. Surg., 8:210, 1991.

Parrilla, P., Ortiz, A., Martinez De Haro, L. F., et al.: Evaluation of the magnitude of gastro-oesophageal reflux in Barrett's oesophagus. Gut, 31:964, 1990.

Payne, W. S.: Surgical management of reflux-induced esophageal stenoses: Results in 101 patients. Br. J. Surg., 71:971, 1984.

Payne, W. S., and King, R. M.: Pharyngoesophageal (Zenker's) diverticulum. Surg. Clin. North Am., 63:815, 1983.

Pearson, F. G., and Henderson, R. D.: Long-term follow-up of peptic strictures managed by dilatation modified Collis gastroplasty, and Belsey hiatus hernia repair. Surgery, 80:396, 1976.

Pellegrini, C., Wetter, L. A., Patti, M., et al.: Thoracoscopic esophagomyotomy. Initial experience with a new approach for the treatment of achalasia. Ann. Surg., 216:291, 1992.

Piehler, J. M., Payne, W. F., Cameron, A. J., and Parolairo, C. T.: The uncut Collis-Nissen procedure for esophageal hiatus hernia and its complications. Probl. Gen. Surg., 1:1, 1984.

Polk, H.: Jejunal interposition for reflux esophagitis and esophageal stricture unresponsive to valvuloplasty. World J. Surg., 4:731, 1980.

Pollara, W. M., Zilberstein, B., Cecconello, I., et al.: Regeneration of esophageal epithelium in the presence of gastroesophageal reflux. In DeMeester, T. R., and Skinner, D. B.: Esophageal Disorders: Pathophysiology and Therapy. New York, Raven Press, 1985.

Pope, C. E., II: A dynamic test of sphincter strength: Its application to the lower esophageal sphincter. Gastroenterology, 52:779, 1967.

Postlethwait, R. W.: Benign tumors and cysts of the esophagus. Surg. Clin. North Am., 63:925, 1983a.

Postlethwait, R. W.: Chemical burns of the esophagus. In Postlethwait, R. W. (ed): Surgery of the Esophagus. East Norwalk, CT, Appleton & Lange, 1986, pp. 317–344.

Postlethwait, R. W.: Colonic interposition for esophageal substitution. Surg. Gynecol. Obstet., 156:377, 1983b.

Postlethwait, R. W., and Musser, A. W.: Changes in the esophagus in 1000 autopsy specimens. J. Thorac. Cardiovasc. Surg., 68:953, 1974.

Postlethwait, R. W., and Sealy, W. C.: Experiences with the treatment of 59 patients with lower esophageal web. Ann. Surg., 165:786, 1967.

Ransom, J. M., Patel, G. K., Clift, S. A., et al.: Extended and limited types of Barrett's esophagus in the adult. Ann. Thorac. Surg., 33:19, 1982.

Richter, J. E.: Diffuse esophageal spasm. In Castell, D. O., Richter, J. E., and Dalton, C. B. (eds): Esophageal Motility Testing. New York, Elsevier Science, 1987.

Richter, J. E., Blackwell, J. N., Wu, W. C., et al.: Relationship of radionuclide liquid bolus transport and esophageal manometry. J. Lab. Clin. Med., 109:217, 1987a.

Richter, J. E., and Castell, D. O.: Diffuse esophageal spasm: A reappraisal. Ann. Intern. Med., 100:242, 1984.

Richter, J. E., Dalton, C. B., Bradley, L. A., and Castell, D. O.: Oral nifedipine in the treatment of non-cardiac chest pain in patients with the nutcracker esophagus. Gastroenterology, 93:21, 1987b.

Richter, J..E., Obrecht, W. F., Bradley, L. A., et al.: Psychological comparison of patients with nutcracker esophagus and irritable bowel syndrome. Dig. Dis. Sci., 31:131, 1986.

Richter, J. E., Spurling, T. J., Cordova, C. M., and Castell, D. O.: Effects of oral calcium blocker diltiazem on esophageal contractions. Dig. Dis. Sci., 29:649, 1984.

Richter, J. E., Wu, W. C., Johns, D. N., et al.: Esophageal manometry in 95 healthy adult volunteers. Variability of pressures with age and frequency of "abnormal" contractions. Dig. Dis. Sci., 32:583, 1987c.

Rothstein, F. C.: Caustic injuries to the esophagus in children. Pediatr. Clin. North Am., 33:665, 1986.

Rouvière, H. C.: Anatomie des lymphatiques de l'homme. Paris, Masson, 1932.

Safaie-Shirazi, S., Zike, W. L., and Mason, E. E.: Esophageal stricture secondary to reflux esophagitis. Arch. Surg., 110:629, 1975.

St-Georges, R., Deslauriers, J., Duranceau, A., et al.: Clinical spectrum of bronchogenic cysts of the mediastinum and lung in the adult. Ann. Thorac. Surg., 52:6, 1991.

Sandry, R. J.: The pathology of chronic esophagitis. Gut, 3:189, 1962.

Sandry, R. J.: Pathology of reflux esophagitis. In Skinner, D. B., Belsey, R. H. R., Hendrix, T. R., and Zuidema, G. D. (eds): Gastroesophageal Reflux and Hiatal Hernia. Boston, Little, Brown, 1972, pp. 43–58.

Savary, M., and Miller, G.: The Esophagus. Handbook and Atlas of Endoscopy. Solothurn, Switzerland, Gossmann, 1978.

Schuman, B. M., and Rinaldo, J. A.: Relative frequency of esophagitis and gastritis in patients with symptomatic hiatus hernia. Gastrointest. Endosc., 12:14, 1966.

Seremetis, M. G., Lyons, W. S., De Guzman, V. C., and Peabody, J. W.: Leiomyomata of the esophagus. An analysis of 838 cases. Cancer, 38:2166, 1976.

Siegel, C. I., and Hendrix, T. R.: Esophageal motor abnormalities induced by acid perfusion in patients with heartburn. J. Clin. Invest., 42:686, 1963.

Skinner, D. B., and Belsey, R. H.: Surgical management of esophageal reflux and hiatus hernia. Long-term results with 1030 patients. J. Thorac. Cardiovasc. Surg., 53:33, 1967.

Smith, R. B., and Taylor, I. M.: Observations on the intrinsic innervation of the human fetal esophagus between the 10 mm and 140 mm crown-rump length stages. Acta Anat., 81:127, 1972.

Stein, H. J., and DeMeester, T. R.: Indications, technique and clinical use of ambulatory 24-hour esophageal motility monitoring in a surgical practice. Ann. Surg., 217:128, 1993.

Stein, H. J., Hoeft, S., and DeMeester, T. R.: Reflux and motility pattern in Barrett's esophagus. Dis. Esoph., 5:21, 1992.

Taillefer, R., and Duranceau, A. C.: Manometric and radionuclide assessment of pharyngeal emptying before and after cricopharyngeal myotomy in patients with oculopharyngeal muscular dystrophy. J. Thorac. Cardiovasc. Surg., 95:868, 1988.

Tapia, R. H., and White, V. A.: Squamous cell carcinoma arising in a duplication cyst of the esophagus. Am. J. Gastroenterol., 80:325, 1985.

Thal, A. P.: A unified approach to surgical problems of the esophagogastric junction. Ann. Surg., 168:542, 1968.

Topart, P., Deschamps, C., Taillefer, R., and Duranceau, A.: Long-term effect of total fundoplication on the myotomized esophagus. Ann. Thorac. Surg., *54*:1046, 1992.

Traube, M., Hongo, M., Magyar, L., and McCallum, R. W.: Effects of nifedipine in achalasia and in patients with high-amplitude peristaltic esophageal contractions. J. A. M. A., *252*:1733, 1984.

Traube, M., Tummala, V., Baue, A. E., and McCallum, R. W.: Surgical myotomy in patients with high-amplitude peristaltic esophageal contractions. Manometric and clinical effects. Dig. Dis. Sci., *32*:16, 1987.

Ward, A. S., Wright, D. H., and Collis, J. L.: The assessment of oesophagitis in hiatus hernia patients. Thorax, *25*:568, 1970.

Waters, P. F., Piazza, D., Cooper, J. D., et al.: Gastroplasty and partial fundoplication in patients with peptic esophagitis and acquired shortening: Results in long-term follow-up. *In* Siewert, J. R., and Holscher, A. H. (eds): Diseases of the Esophagus. Berlin, Springer-Verlag, 1988, pp. 1286–1290.

Wegener, O. H.: Whole-Body Computerized Tomography. Basel, S. Karger, 1983.

Weinstein, W. M., Bogoch, E. R., and Bowes, K. L.: The normal human esophageal mucosa: A histological reappraisal. Gastroenterology, *68*:40, 1975.

Weisbrodt, N. W.: Neuromuscular organisation of esophageal and pharyngeal motility. Arch. Intern. Med., *136*:524, 1976.

Winans, C. S.: Manometric asymmetry of the lower-esophageal high-pressure zone. Am. J. Dig. Dis., *22*:348, 1977.

Winans, C. S.: The pharyngoesophageal closure mechanism: A manometric study. Gastroenterology, *63*:768, 1972.

Winans, C. S., and Harris, L. D.: Quantitation of lower esophageal sphincter competence. Gastroenterology, *52*:773, 1967.

Winawer, S. J., Sherlock, P., and Hajdu, S. I.: The role of upper gastrointestinal endoscopy in patients with cancer. Cancer, *37*:440, 1976.

Winters, C., Artnak, E. J., Benjamin, S. B., and Castell, D. O.: Esophageal bougienage in symptomatic patients with the nutcracker esophagus. A primary esophageal motility disorder. J. A. M. A., *252*:363, 1984.

Wong, R. K. H., and Maydonovitch, C. L.: Achalasias. *In* Castell, D. O. (ed): The Esophagus. Boston, Little, Brown, 1992, pp. 233–260.

Woodward, E. R.: Fundic patch operation for peptic stricture. *In* Jamieson, G. G. (ed): Surgery of the Esophagus. London, Churchill Livingstone, 1988.

Yon, J., and Christensen, J.: An uncontrolled comparison of treatments for achalasia. Ann. Surg., *182*:672, 1975.

Zaino, C., Jacobson, H. G., Lepow, H., and Ozturk, C. H.: The Pharyngoesophageal Junction. Springfield, IL, Charles C. Thomas, 1978.

28
Esophageal Hiatal Hernia
■ I The Condition: Clinical Manifestations and Diagnosis

David B. Skinner

A small herniation of the gastric cardia upward through the esophageal hiatus of the diaphragm is a common finding on radiographic barium swallow examination and has no clinical significance at all unless accompanied by an abnormal degree of gastroesophageal reflux. Any discussion of esophageal hiatal hernia must distinguish between the inconsequential anatomic defect and the physiologic abnormality that can cause symptoms and severe complications. The two conditions, hiatal hernia and gastroesophageal reflux, may occur together, but each may occur in the absence of the other, and therefore they are discussed as separate entities (Hiebert and Belsey, 1961). The usual Type I axial or sliding hiatal hernia is very common and is estimated to occur in at least 10% of North American adults examined by barium swallow. Pathologic reflux is less common and is estimated to be present consistently in only 5% of those who have a hiatal hernia. Among patients with symptomatic reflux, approximately four-fifths have a coincidental Type I hiatal hernia, but one-fifth have no demonstrable radiographic abnormality at the hiatus.

NORMAL ANATOMY AND HIATAL HERNIA

The esophagus begins at the cricopharyngeal sphincter muscle (cricopharyngeus) at the level of the sixth cervical vertebral body. The sphincter muscle arises and inserts on the back of the cricoid cartilage of the larynx and superiorly blends into the inferior constrictor fibers of the hypopharynx. Anatomically, the cricopharyngeus is approximately 1 cm wide, but pressure recordings show a high-pressure zone that usually extends over several centimeters. The upper esophagus passes through the thoracic inlet constrained by adjacent anatomic structures, including the trachea anteriorly, the great vessels of the aortic arch laterally, and the vertebral bodies posteriorly. The aortic arch indents the esophagus approximately 8 cm below the cricopharyngeus and marks the junction of the upper and middle thirds of the esophagus. Below this, the esophagus normally dilates slightly, as determined by radiographic or endoscopic inspection. This occurs because the right lateral aspect of the esophagus is covered by the parietal pleura of the right hemithorax so that the esophagus is directly exposed to the less-than-atmospheric intrathoracic pressure. The midesophagus passes anteriorly from the tracheal bifurcation onto the surface of the pericardium. On the left lateral side the esophagus abuts the aorta and left pleura, and posteriorly, it contacts the azygos vein, the thoracic duct, and the vertebral bodies. In its lower third, the esophagus begins to deviate slightly toward the left and anterior to the aorta until it penetrates the diaphragm through the esophageal hiatus almost directly anterior to the aortic hiatus of the diaphragm. The average length of the esophagus in an adult is approximately 25 cm. The amount above the clavicles is approximately 4 cm in a young adult but decreases with age owing to anterior bowing of the skeleton. The aortic impulse on the esophagus is noted approximately 8 to 9 cm from the cricopharyngeus. The left atrial pulsation can be observed at the junction of the mid and lower esophagus, approximately 16 to 18 cm from the cricopharyngeus. The esophagus enters the hiatal tunnel, and the most distal 3 to 4 cm becomes intra-abdominal in a normal adult.

Throughout its length the esophagus consists of two muscular layers, an outer longitudinal layer and an inner zone of circular muscle fibers. The transition between longitudinal and circular fibers is not abrupt or anatomically distinct. "Bracket" longitudinal fibers appear to bind bands of circular muscle together. Some of these transitional fibers have an oblique orientation (Friedland et al., 1966; Higgs et al., 1965). In the adult, the esophagus has no true serosa or mesentery. However, in the embryo, there is a mesoesophagus during development of the foregut, and accordingly, the arterial and venous connections of the esophagus as well as lymphatic drainage proceed dorsally for the most part to the aorta, azygos vein, and thoracic duct, respectively. Although the esophagus does not have a true serosal layer, adjacent structures perform a serosa-like function by serving as points of origin and insertion for longitudinal muscle fibers. The serosa-like attachments include the membranous portion of the trachea and pericardium anteriorly and the pleural surfaces where these are adjacent to the esophagus.

The mucosa of the esophagus is separated from the muscle layers by a loose submucosa. This permits considerable mobility of the mucosa relative to the muscle layers and helps to explain the ability of the esophagus to make rapid changes in diameter and length during swallowing or vomiting. The submucosa includes a rich collateral blood supply that is sufficient to maintain the viability of the esophagus if the organ remains attached to nutrient arteries and veins at either its upper or lower end, even though all other segmental esophageal vessels are divided. The submucosa contains a rich lymphatic network. There is a well-developed layer of muscularis mucosae on which the mucosa itself rests. In humans, the esophagus is lined throughout its intrathoracic length by stratified squamous epithelium. The distal 2 to 3 cm of the esophagus is lined with the simple columnar epithelium of the gastric cardia type. Submocosal mucous glands may occur along the length of the esophagus but are noted particularly at the upper and lower ends. During fetal life, the esophagus is lined with glandular epithelium for a time. Rarely, in adults, rests of glandular epithelium may be found at various levels, most commonly in the cervical esophagus, surrounded by otherwise normal squamous epithelium.

The arterial blood supply reaches the esophagus from varying sources at different levels. The intra-abdominal segment of the esophagus is nourished by an ascending branch of the left gastric artery at the top of the gastrohepatic omentum. At approximately the level of the inferior pulmonary vein, a midesophageal artery passes directly from the aorta. There may be one or two additional direct aortic branches. Cephalad around the root of the lung, there are common arterial branches that provide both bronchial and esophageal arteries. The highest of these branches usually arises from the back of the aortic arch. The cervical esophagus receives blood supply from branches originating in the thyrocervical trunk of the subclavian arteries. As mentioned earlier, the submucosal network of arterial collaterals is sufficient to maintain viability of the esophagus even when all the segmental thoracic branches and the arterial supply at either the upper or lower end are divided, provided the blood supply at one end of the esophagus remains intact. Venous drainage of the esophagus enters the coronary vein and paracardial venous plexus below the diaphragm. Segmental veins join the azygos system from the thoracic esophagus and the high intercostal veins in its upper portion. The lymphatic drainage is mainly posterior toward the thoracic duct through most of the length of the esophagus, although there are anterior lymphatic connections to the subcarinal lymph nodes from the midportion and to the cervical lymph node from the upper esophagus.

The esophageal muscle is penetrated by the preganglionic fibers of the vagus nerve synapsing with the ganglion cells in the myenteric plexus of the esophagus. The upper esophagus receives this innervation from the recurrent branches of the vagus nerve after they have looped around the aortic arch or the subclavian artery. Sympathetic innervation occurs from the thoracic ganglion. Sensory innervation of the esophagus appears to be limited to fibers stimulated by muscular stretch or by temperature. These sensory fibers reach the central nervous system through the vagus nerves.

ANATOMY OF THE GASTROESOPHAGEAL JUNCTION

An understanding of the anatomy of the esophageal hiatus is essential to the understanding of mechanisms of reflux and its correction. Posteriorly, the diaphragm muscle arises from the lumbar vertebral bodies and the arcuate ligament and crosses over the aorta as it enters the abdomen. The diaphragm muscle rises initially in a cephalad direction. One vertebral body higher than the aortic hiatus, the muscle splits to form the aperture of the esophageal hiatus. The columns of diaphragm muscle rising off the vertebral body and arcuate ligament form two distinct pillars, the right and left crura. Although the esophageal hiatus lies slightly to the left of the midline, the margins of the hiatus in most dissections prove to arise from muscle of the right crus (Collis et al., 1954). There is, however, a great deal of variability and interdigitation of fibers from both crura. The looping of muscle fibers around the esophageal hiatus as the muscle passes toward its insertion in the central tendon of the diaphragm provides the diaphragmatic tunnel through which the esophagus passes as it enters the abdomen. This sling of muscle around the distal esophagus is approximately 2 cm in length. The muscle surrounding the esophagus in the diaphragmatic hiatus is innervated by the left phrenic nerve.

The hiatal aperture around the esophagus is closed by several layers that separate the thoracic and abdominal cavities. Of these the most important is the phrenoesophageal membrane, which anchors the esophagus within the hiatus. This membrane consists primarily of an extension of the endoabdominal fascia off the underside of the diaphragmatic muscle (Bombeck et al., 1966). This fascia extends slightly cephalad to form a cone-like structure as it approaches the esophagus. It is joined by fibroelastic tissue of the endothoracic fascia arising from the superior surface of the diaphragm, but the thoracic contribution to the membrane is less in amount and importance. The phrenoesophageal membrane formed by the fusion of the two fascial layers inserts in a series of fibrous attachments that penetrate the esophageal muscle and blend into the submucosa of the esophagus approximately 3 to 4 cm above the junction of the tubular esophagus with the stomach. The insertion of this membrane into the esophageal submucosa marks the point at which the esophagus becomes intra-abdominal. If one incises the layers of tissue anterior to the esophagus within the hiatus, the following layers are divided proceeding from the thoracic to abdominal direction: pleura, mediastinal fat, endothoracic fascia, endoabdominal fascia comprising the sheet of phrenoesophageal membrane, retroperitoneal fat, and peritoneum. In addition to the esophagus, the vagus nerves penetrate through the phrenoesophageal membrane on the wall of the esophagus. The hepatic branch of the right vagus nerve is given off just below the phrenoesophageal membrane, as is a major trunk of the left vagus nerve to the celiac plexus.

Discussion of the gastroesophageal junction requires precise definition of terms. A great deal of confusion has resulted from at least three different definitions that have been used to describe the esophagogastric junction (EGJ). To the endoscopist and radiologist, the mucosal junction of squamous and columnar epithelium is often called the EGJ. This junction is irregular, the ora serrata, and varies slightly in location. To define the esophagogastric junction as the mucosal junction ignores the fact that the most distal 2 to 3 cm of tubular, muscular esophagus is normally lined by columnar epithelium. A second and more realistic physiologic definition of the EGJ is the point at which esophageal muscular peristalsis stops. The peristaltic wave of the esophagus sweeps distally, ending with the closed distal esophageal segment, often referred to as the distal sphincter, at the junction where the muscular tube of esophagus joins the gastric pouch. This lowest portion of the muscular esophageal tube is lined with gastric-type columnar epithelium so that the muscular junction is distal to the mucosal junction. In normal individuals, this definition of the EGJ is most useful when discussing esophageal physiology and mechanisms of reflux.

In disease states such as achalasia or scleroderma, the esophageal peristaltic pattern is disrupted so that a third definition is necessary. In these cases, the EGJ is defined as the junction of the narrow-diameter esophageal swallowing tube with the large-diameter gastric pouch. This junction is usually 3 to 4 cm below the insertion of the phrenoesophageal membrane and coincides with the location of the most distal esophageal muscle contraction after peristalsis. Again, this definition places the junction slightly more caudal than the normal squamocolumnar mucosal junction. When the stomach is greatly distended, such as after a large meal, this segment of intra-abdominal tubular esophagus is shortened or effaced by the radial pull of the distended stomach wall. Thus, the length of the submerged segment of distal intra-abdominal esophagus seen by a radiologist during a barium swallow depends on the degree of gastric filling or retention. The theories concerning control of reflux focus on the role of the distal esophageal muscle and the length of intra-abdominal tubular esophagus. Accordingly, the most useful definitions for discussion of the EGJ are the latter two, rather than confusing the readily visible squamocolumnar junction with the EGJ.

HIATAL HERNIA

Hiatal hernias are divided into two main types. Each type involves a different anatomic defect and has different clinical significance (Fig. 28–1). The Type I axial or sliding hiatal hernia is common and is not significant unless it is accompanied by pathologic degrees of reflux. The abnormality is a slight dilatation in the diameter of the hiatal opening and a stretching or attenuation of the phrenoesophageal membrane, which permits a portion of the gastric cardia to slide upward into the hiatus. There is no defect or aperture in the endoabdominal fascia covering the hiatus and inserting into the esophagus so that there is no true peritoneal hernia sac. In most patients in whom this type of hernia is seen on barium swallow examination, the insertion of the phrenoesophageal membrane into the esophagus is at a normal location 3 to 4 cm above the junction, and there is no pathologic reflux. Another indication that the Type I hiatal hernia by itself is not a disease is the wide variation in incidence when this condition is seen by radiologists. Some radiologists boast that a Type I hiatal hernia can be shown with diligent effort,

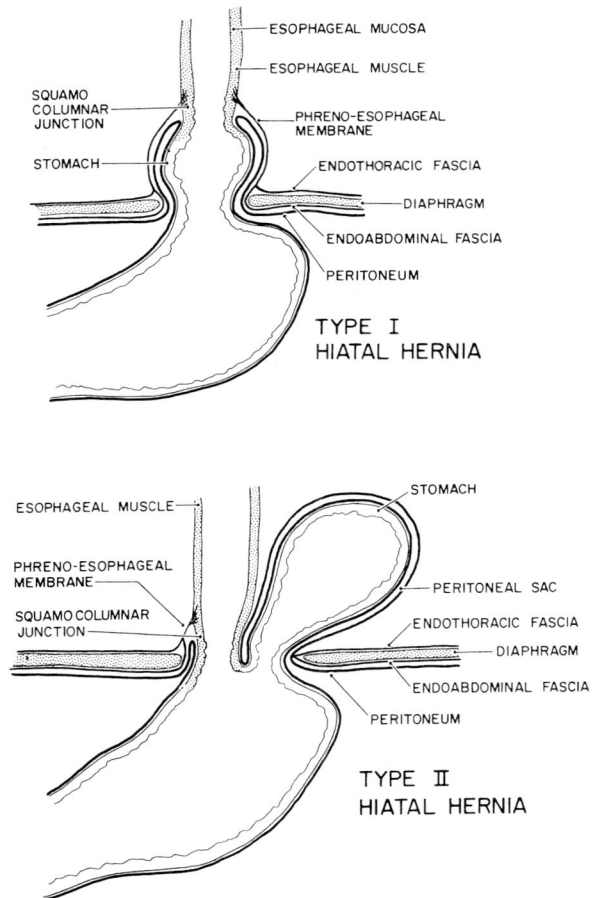

FIGURE 28–1. Diagrammatic representation of a Type I and Type II hiatal hernia. In the Type I hernia, the phrenoesophageal membrane is intact and there is no true peritoneal sac extending into the thorax. In the Type II hiatal hernia, there is a defect in the phrenoesophageal membrane, permitting a free peritoneal sac to enter the lower-pressure thoracic cavity. (From Skinner, D. B.: Hiatal hernia and gastroesophageal reflux. *In* Sabiston, D. C., Jr. [ed]: Davis-Christopher Textbook of Surgery. 12th ed. Philadelphia, W. B. Saunders, 1981.)

position, abdominal compression, and other maneuvers in up to 90% of barium swallow examinations. During the act of vomiting, the cardia of the stomach normally herniates slightly through the hiatus as the esophagus shortens and gastric and abdominal wall muscles contract violently. A Type I hiatal hernia can be shown by forceful maneuvers in normal individuals. The demonstration of this type of hiatal hernia under the artificial conditions of a stressful radiographic examination has no importance at all and should be disregarded unless clear evidence of spontaneous gastroesophageal reflux is seen.

In some patients, a larger Type I hiatal hernia is easily shown on radiographic study with the patient at rest. These patients who have a pouch of stomach greater than 3 cm that protrudes through the hiatus under resting conditions appear to have a higher association with abnormal degrees of gastroesophageal reflux (O'Sullivan et al., 1981). In these patients, the insertion of the phrenoesophageal membrane appears to be closer than normal to the gastroesophageal junction, as shown by both manometric evaluation and surgical dissection. Whether this low insertion of the phrenoesophageal membrane is congenital or acquired in an individual case is uncertain. Some of these patients give a history of regurgitation and reflux since childhood, which suggests a congenital problem. Other patients clearly acquire the symptoms and evidence of reflux later in life.

The presence of the Type I hiatal hernia itself does not indicate loss of the intra-abdominal segment of esophagus. The abdominal portion of esophagus is defined by the insertion of the phrenoesophageal membrane into the esophageal submucosa. As long as this insertion remains 3 to 4 cm above the junction of the tubular esophagus with the gastric pouch, the most distal esophagus remains within the abdominal pressure chamber, even when translocated cephalad through the hiatus. Increases in abdominal pressure are transmitted through the hiatus to compress the esophagus below the phrenoesophageal membrane. The high association of reflux with a larger Type I hiatal hernia suggests that the intra-abdominal esophagus may be lost in some of these patients. Mild degrees of esophagitis, which can be caused by overeating, alcoholic indulgence, and heavy smoking, may lead to periesophageal inflammation and adhesions between the oblique entrance of the phrenoesophageal membrane into the esophageal wall, with effective fusion of these structures and loss of the intra-abdominal esophagus. Another theory suggests that the buildup of fatty tissue at this critical junction may interfere with the transmission of abdominal pressures to the esophagus within a hiatal hernia pouch. However, a Type I hiatal hernia acquires clinical significance only when pathologic reflux is documented.

The second major type of hiatal hernia, the paraesophageal rolling or Type II hernia, is less common but is a significant clinical problem. In this type of hernia, there is a defect in the phrenoesophageal membrane, usually on the left ventral aspect of the hiatus, but also occasionally to the right and posteriorly. These defects allow protrusion of the peritoneum through the fascia in the manner of a true hernia sac. The adjacent stomach herniates through the defect in the fascia and enters the chest. Because the fascia no longer restrains the upward migration of the stomach and because intrathoracic pressure is less than abdominal pressure most of the time, the natural history of this defect is a progressive enlargement of the hernia. In advanced stages, the entire stomach may be herniated through the defect so that the cardia, still fixed by a portion of the phrenoesophageal membrane, and the pylorus come to lie close together. At this stage, there are almost always ventral and dorsal hernia sacs. This sets the stage for gastric volvulus, torsion, obstruction, strangulation, and intrathoracic gastric dilatation, any of which can be fatal (Fig. 28–2). Thus, the Type II hiatal hernia is considered a serious defect requiring surgical correction, even if the patient is asymptomatic.

With enlargement of the Type II hernia, the phrenoesophageal membrane frequently becomes attenuated, owing to the constant tension placed on it by the distortion of the stomach pulling on the cardia. When a patient has a herniation of the cardia well above the diaphragm in addition to a paraesophageal hernia sac, this type of hernia may be classified as a Type III or combined hiatal hernia with the clinical significance of the paraesophageal hernia as well as an increased incidence of reflux, which may accompany the larger Type I hernias. When other organs such as the colon or small intestine enter the paraesophageal hernia sac, the clinical implications are changed to reflect the possibility of obstruction or torsion of these other organs. This type can be classified as Type IV or multiorgan hiatal hernia.

NORMAL FUNCTION OF THE ESOPHAGUS AND CARDIA

The mechanisms by which the esophagus and cardia function normally to transport an ingested bolus and prevent reflux remain controversial despite an enormous amount of investigation. When two or more theories are supported by experimental and clinical evidence, both explanations are provided in this discussion.

The swallowing process is initiated with an upward and posterior thrust of the tongue and larynx so that the laryngeal orifice is covered by the epiglottis, and the solid, liquid, or gas bolus being ingested is thrust back into the hypopharynx. As the pharyngeal constrictors contract, there is a coordinated relaxation or opening of the cricopharyngeus muscle so that pharyngeal pressures exceed the cricopharyngeal sphincter pressure. The timing as well as amplitude of the contraction and relaxation of the constrictors and cricopharyngeus is important for smooth swallowing and can be disordered by neurologic damage in the brainstem or to the vagus and glossopharyngeal nerves, which suggests that the coordination is neurogenically controlled. As the cricopharyngeus re-

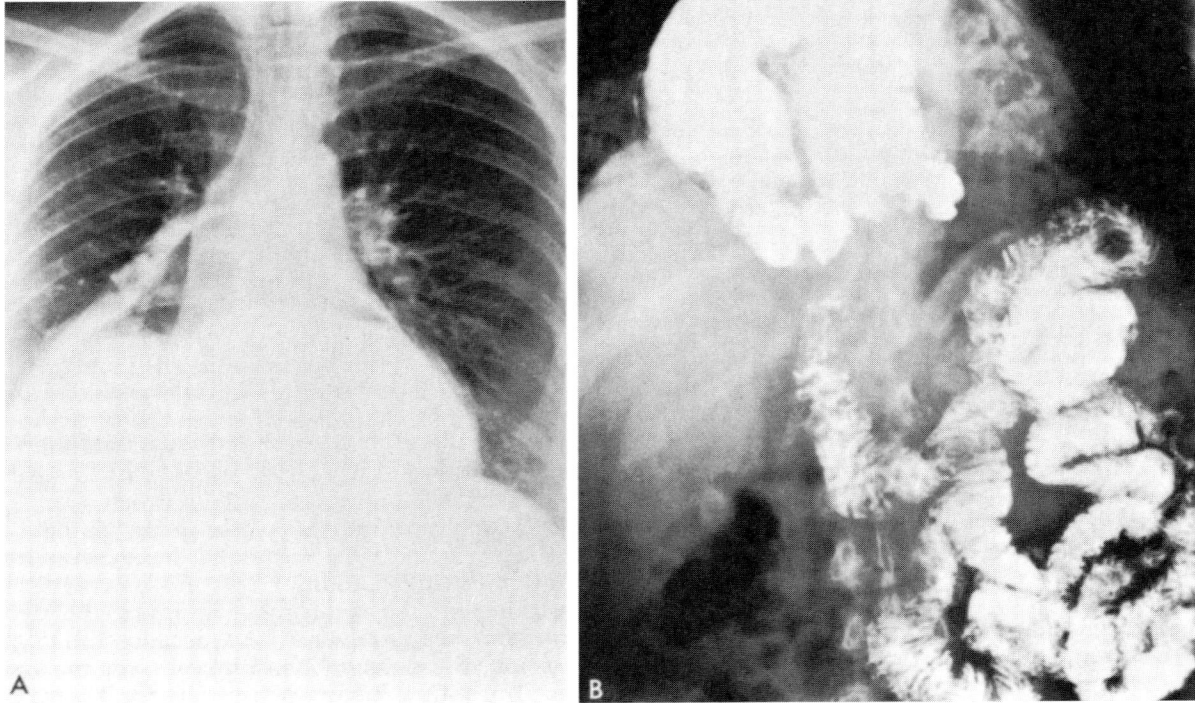

FIGURE 28–2. Typical radiographic appearance of a large Type II hiatal hernia. As in this case, there is often a loosening of the phrenoesophageal membrane as well, making it a combined sliding and paraesophageal, or Type III, hernia. *A,* Chest film. *B,* Barium swallow examination. (*A* and *B,* From Skinner, D. B.: Hiatal hernia and gastroesophageal reflux. *In* Sabiston, D. C., Jr. [ed]: Davis-Christopher Textbook of Surgery. 12th ed. Philadelphia, W. B. Saunders, 1981.)

laxes and then contracts again, a progressive peristaltic wave is initiated down the esophagus and is characterized by an initial phase of slight relaxation followed by a muscular contraction that normally is from 20 to 60 mm Hg in pressure. This pressure wave proceeds down the esophagus in a coordinated manner and travels caudally at the rate of 5 to 10 cm/sec. Intact innervation of the esophagus is essential for coordinated peristalsis, but it appears that the innervating fibers enter the esophageal wall much proximally to the level at which the contraction occurs, because a lower thoracic vagal transection has no effect on the peristalsis of the distal esophagus. Transection and reanastomosis of the esophagus do not interfere with the progression of the peristaltic wave across the anastomotic line if the innervation of the distal segment remains intact.

As the peristaltic wave reaches the distal esophagus, the high-pressure zone of the distal 3 to 4 cm of the esophagus relaxes to the level of resting gastric pressure. This segment contracts again as the bolus passes through the cardia, and the initial elevated resting pressure is restored. During the act of swallowing followed by primary peristalsis, the length of the esophagus shortens through longitudinal muscle contraction and is restored as the bolus passes distally in front of the contracting band of circular muscle.

Two theories regarding the relaxation of the distal segment should be considered. One explanation is that the distal esophageal muscle segment goes through an active phase of relaxation that is controlled by its innervation. The other explanation is that the resting pressure in the distal segment is reduced as the esophagus shortens through longitudinal muscle contraction and pulls upward on the phrenoesophageal membrane insertion. Because the membrane inserts from a lateral direction circumferentially, this action has the physical effect of tugging the lumen open and reducing pressure to that of the gastric cavity. The active phase would then be the contraction of the circular muscle as the bolus passes. Because there is anatomically no identifiable sphincter muscle in humans and subhuman primates and because the concept of one band of muscle maintaining a constant tonic contraction during rest without showing hypertrophy or different development from adjacent gastric or esophageal muscle appears to be improbable, the theory of passive relaxation and passive maintenance of tone in the distal esophagus because of its intra-abdominal location and small diameter relative to the stomach pouch is attractive. The explanation for failure of the distal segment to relax in achalasia can fit in with either theory. If active muscle relaxation is controlled by innervation, failure to relax would be expected in the denervated state of achalasia. Similarly, if the distal segment relaxation is passive and secondary to longitudinal muscle contraction against the phrenoesophageal membrane, the absence of peristalsis in achalasia could account for failure of the distal segment to relax.

Regardless of the precise mechanisms of peristalsis and distal segment relaxation, coordinated peristaltic clearing of the esophagus is an important aspect of protection against the noxious effects of gastroesophageal reflux (Booth et al., 1968). Distention of the esophagus or irritation of the mucosa can trigger a coordinated peristaltic contraction that is not initiated by an act of swallowing. This is called secondary peristalsis and may be a factor in the ability of the esophagus to clear regurgitated material without the patient's being aware of what is occurring.

The mechanism of the second function of the esophagus, the prevention of gastric reflux, is controversial (Skinner, 1985). The barrier preventing gastric reflux into the esophagus is identified by the resting high-pressure zone in the distal esophagus (Fyke et al., 1956). Many have accepted this as evidence for an active muscular sphincter, even though a distinct sphincter muscle cannot be identified anatomically. Discussion of the distal esophageal sphincter is widespread in publications. To understand the control of reflux, it is more useful to think of this high-pressure zone as a physiologic sphincter or barrier to reflux and to inquire into mechanisms by which it can be augmented.

The barrier to reflux can be described in several terms. It rests in the most distal 3 to 4 cm of the esophagus and is measured by a discrete zone of pressure elevated 8 to 20 mm Hg higher than resting intragastric pressure. In normal individuals, most of this high-pressure zone (HPZ) is caudal to the insertion of the phrenoesophageal membrane into the esophageal wall, or distal to the point of respiratory inversion on manometry studies. The HPZ corresponds to the submerged or compressed segment of esophagus seen on barium swallow examinations to remain closed after the peristaltic wave passes. Endoscopically, this barrier is seen as a segment of distal esophagus that remains closed even when air is insufflated into the thoracic esophagus. The ora serrata or gastroesophageal mucosal junction is often seen at the top of this closed segment.

Regardless of how the distal esophagus is described, this segment is responsible for the control of gastroesophageal reflux. At least two theories are supported by evidence concerning the function of the distal esophageal HPZ. The most widely accepted and classic theory is that the distal esophageal muscle is an intrinsic sphincter that maintains a closed tonic state of contraction during rest and actively relaxes during swallowing. This contraction is believed to be under neurologic and hormonal control (Cohen and Lipshutz, 1970). The second theory is that the distal esophageal HPZ is caused by the narrow-diameter distal esophageal tube entering abruptly into the larger digestive pouch within the common pressure chamber of the abdomen. According to the law of Laplace, it takes more force to distend the smaller-diameter tube than the larger-diameter pouch, and thus, the observed HPZ may represent these physical forces governing wall tension.

A number of hormones and chemicals influence foregut pressure, including that of the distal esophageal HPZ. Under the intrinsic muscle sphincter theory, these hormones work selectively on the sphincter muscle. Under the second theory, hormones that cause a general relaxation or tightening of foregut muscle would have a magnified effect, because the pressures governed by the law of Laplace are inversely related to the fourth power of the radius. A small change in radius of the narrow distal esophagus would have a greater effect on the force required to distend the wall than a similar percentage change in radius would have on the larger-diameter gastric pouch.

Although the behavior of the distal esophageal segment meets the physiologic definition of a muscular sphincter, several observations indicate that physical forces are important. No anatomically identifiable sphincter muscle has been found in primates. The first observations pointing toward physical forces accounting for the sphincter zone stem from the first antireflux repairs. Despite the trauma caused by the surgical dissection and suturing, the pressure in the distal esophageal segment is increased immediately postoperatively. If the pressure is generated by an intrinsic muscle tone, the surgical trauma should cause interference with muscular function rather than strengthening it in the early stages after operation. Additional observations indicate that a distal esophagus replaced by a small-diameter gastric tube can be effective in preventing reflux as long as there is a significant intra-abdominal segment of the gastric tube (Henderson, 1980). An HPZ in a small-diameter swallowing tube replacing the esophagus can be found when the replacement organ is a gastric tube, jejunal segment, or colon interposition segment (Skinner, 1985). When the distal esophagus is replaced by a gastric tube, this shows a similar pattern of increased or decreased pressure, depending on administration of specific hormones (Moossa et al., 1977). Finally, an in vitro model shows that competency of the cardia can be maintained when equalized intragastric and intra-abdominal pressures are applied to the outer surface of the esophagus, which is usual in the resting state. Under these circumstances, the control of reflux is directly proportional to the length of esophagus exposed to abdominal pressure, and a 3- to 4-cm segment of abdominal esophagus is sufficient to prevent reflux when there is a 10 cm H_2O abdominothoracic pressure difference (DeMeester et al., 1979). All these pieces of evidence point to the importance of the intra-abdominal segment of esophagus as a primary or at least important supplementary factor to whatever specific muscle function of the distal esophagus contributes to control of reflux. Thus, two measurable parameters of distal esophageal function are related to control of reflux: the pressure in the distal esophageal segment and the length of distal esophageal segment exposed to abdominal pressure.

GASTROESOPHAGEAL REFLUX AND ESOPHAGITIS

With this understanding of the anatomy and the physiologic components preventing reflux, some of the factors leading to reflux and esophagitis can be identified. The frequent association between pathologic reflux and a Type I hiatal hernia points to alterations in the anatomy of the hiatus that contribute to reflux in some cases. A widening of the hiatus tends to put some lateral tension on the distal esophageal segment, which increases its diameter and reduces the pressure required to distend the esophagus. The presence of an axial hiatal hernia itself, however, does not cause reflux in most patients. Presumably, this is because the phrenoesophageal membrane insertion still leaves an adequate segment of distal esophagus exposed to abdominal pressure transmitted into the hernia pouch from below. Under these circumstances, the extrinsic pressure on the stomach and abdominal portion of esophagus remains similar, even though the cardia and distal esophagus are seen radiographically to be above the diaphragm.

Factors that lead to recurrent or chronic elevation of gastric pressure contribute to reflux. Physiologic reflux normally occurs after meals, when the stomach is full and contracting (DeMeester et al., 1976). Failure of gastric emptying, as in pyloric stenosis, or a mass in the stomach, duodenum, pancreas, or gallbladder that delays gastric emptying can be a cause of secondary gastroesophageal reflux. Obliteration of the muscle tone in the esophageal wall, which occurs in scleroderma, can cause reflux. Dent and associates (1980) describe a phenomenon of spontaneous "inappropriate relaxation" of the HPZ preceding reflux. This appears to result from distention of the proximal stomach by air (aerophagea) of liquid gastric contents. Overdistention of the distal esophageal segment, which is created by Heller's esophagocardiomyotomy or forceful balloon dilatation, may lead to secondary reflux. A low insertion of the phrenoesophageal membrane into the distal esophagus, whether congenital or acquired, reduces the abdominal segment and its role in the control of reflux and encourages pathologic degrees of regurgitation. A congenitally low insertion of the phrenoesophageal membrane appears to be a common factor in severe reflux in children and young adults, who often recall that they had considerable regurgitation in early childhood. Obliteration of the angle of entry of the phrenoesophageal membrane into the esophagus with fusion of the membrane to the wall of the esophagus might occur in patients who have chronic low-grade esophagitis from heavy smoking or alcohol ingestion. Similarly, it can be envisioned that obese patients are more likely to have reflux because the cuff of extraperitoneal fatty tissue around the cardia prevents full transmission of intra-abdominal pressure to the abdominal segment of esophagus. Undoubtedly, there are unknown alterations in anatomy and control of foregut muscle tone that contribute to the problem.

From prolonged intraesophageal pH monitoring, it is known that reflux after meals is a normal event in healthy people. When reflux becomes prolonged or occurs throughout the day or at night, pathologic degrees of reflux are diagnosed. For esophagitis to develop as a complication of reflux, two factors must occur. The noxious gastric acid-peptic or pancreaticobiliary secretions must reach the esophagus with increased frequency, and the esophagus must be unable to clear the refluxed material back into the stomach. In normal individuals, acid in the esophagus is cleared by repeated peristaltic action, usually initiated by a swallow. Saliva has an important role in acid neutralization (Helm et al., 1982). In patients with esophagitis, delay in or lack of clearing acid and acid neutralization are frequently noted.

From prolonged pH monitoring, several patterns of reflux can be observed. In some patients, reflux occurs frequently during the day when they are in the upright position. These individuals often have the habit of snacking and of swallowing air to initiate the peristalsis required to clear the refluxed material. These habits, in turn, lead to persistent volume of air and food in the stomach, contributing to gastric distention and recurrent bouts of reflux. A recurrent cycle of ingestion, reflux, air swallowing, reflux, and so on is created. These patients are often highly aware of their reflux condition. However, the frequency of swallowing encourages acid clearing from the esophagus so that severe damage to the esophagus is not a great risk.

In other patients, reflux occurs at night while they are supine. Because swallowing is infrequent at night and absent during sound sleep, regurgitation during the night may lead to prolonged contact of the refluxed material with the esophageal mucosa, permitting injury to the mucosa to occur without the patient's awareness of the problem. A comparison of patterns of reflux with degrees of esophagitis shows a strong correlation between esophagitis and nocturnal reflux (Little et al., 1980). Patients with pure upright daytime reflux rarely have significant esophagitis. The most severe degrees of reflux, often requiring surgical management, usually occur both as daytime and nocturnal upright and supine reflux patterns.

When abnormal reflux occurs, the degree of damage to the esophagus may range from none, when the material is cleared rapidly, to a rapidly developing severe peptic stricture. It is useful to grade esophagitis by the degree of abnormality observed by the esophagoscopist. The absence of erythema or ulceration is graded as no esophagitis. Grade I is recorded when there is erythema of the mucosa without ulceration. In Grade 0 or Grade I, there may be microscopic changes of hypertrophy of the basal layer of the squamous epithelium and proximity of the rete pegs to the surface (Ismail-Beigi et al., 1970). However, these findings are nonspecific and may be caused by various stimulants to the esophagus, and therefore, they should not be interpreted as diagnostic of reflux esophagitis. Grade II esophagitis is noted when frank ulcerations are seen. Repeated chronic ulcerations lead to some fibrosis and stiffness of the wall of the esophagus, recorded as Grade III esophagitis. When a frank stricture occurs that prevents the passage of the esophagoscope, a Grade IV esophagitis or stricture is recorded. Progression from no esophagitis to a frank stricture may occur rapidly or may proceed slowly over a period of years. In some patients, the degree of esophagitis remains static for a long time. The earliest case of stricture that the author has seen was in a 5-day-old infant; postoperative severe reflux esophagitis in a debilitated patient with a nasogastric tube may lead to stricture formation within 5 to 10 days. It is because of the uncertainty of time sequence in progression to stricture that surgical correction of reflux esophagitis is advocated when the ulcerative phase is observed.

When chronic reflux esophagitis causes ulcerations, observations indicate that healing occurs by upward migration of the acid-resistant columnar cells of the gastric cardia into the ulcerated area. When this progression becomes marked and the columnar-type epithelium extends more than 3 cm into the tubular esophagus, the condition of Barrett's esophagus, or esophagus lined with columnar epithelium, occurs (Barrett, 1957). In many cases, this appears to be an acquired condition associated with chronic reflux. In others, the presence of rests or islands of gastric epithelium in the esophagus or the presence of normal-appearing gastric fundic mucosa, including parietal cells, suggests that there may be some cases in which gastric epithelium in the esophagus occurs congenitally as well. An important factor in Barrett's epithelium is the propensity of this stimulated mucosa to proceed toward neoplasia (Berenson et al., 1978; Skinner et al., 1983; Spechler et al., 1984). Thus, multiple biopsies must be taken at esophagoscopy, and the finding of dysplasia must be accepted as evidence of progression toward neoplasia.

In addition to esophagitis, stricture, and Barrett's esophagus, reflux may cause acute hemorrhage from the esophagus and aspiration of regurgitated contents into the lung. Cases of acute hemorrhage from esophagitis are rare. When seen, the entire lower esophageal mucosa is observed to be weeping blood as if a split-thickness skin graft had been taken and the bleeding was encouraged to persist by further washes of acid regurgitation over the raw mucosa. Although this type of frightening rapid bleeding from the surface is rare, chronic small amounts of bleeding sufficient to cause a guaiac-positive stool and mild anemia are a common problem with chronic ulcerative esophagitis. When the esophagus acquires a gastric mucosal lining, it is prone to deep penetrating ulcers on the gastric side of the squamocolumnar junction (Barrett, 1950; Sandry, 1962). These may erode into adjacent structures, including the aorta and heart, and lead to massive hemorrhage.

In patients with reflux, the possibility of regurgitation into the hypopharynx and aspiration into the larynx is always present. However, frank documented aspiration causing pulmonary symptoms is shown conclusively in only approximately 8% of patients who have documented pathologic reflux (Pellegrini et al., 1979; Skinner and Belsey, 1967). These patients also appear to share a disorder of esophageal motor function that inhibits clearing of regurgitated material into the esophagus. Because respiratory disease and reflux are both common problems in the population, a cause-and-effect relationship must be established by appropriate testing before assuming that one condition causes the other.

CLINICAL PRESENTATION

The Type I sliding hiatal hernia rarely causes symptoms severe enough for a patient to seek medical advice. Only when pathologic reflux is associated with the hiatal hernia are specific symptoms encountered. The Type II paraesophageal hernia may cause symptoms in the absence of reflux. These patients present with complaints of early satiety, vomiting after a large meal, epigastric distress, dysphagia, and gurgling noises within the chest. All of these symptoms relate to the intrathoracic pouch of herniated stomach filling up rapidly and reaching capacity. Dysphagia appears to be caused by lateral compression of the esophagus by the adjacent herniated viscus. With a large hernia, compression of the lung and occupation of a portion of the thoracic space may lead to cough after meals and occasionally dyspnea.

Symptoms caused by reflux are a more common clinical presentation. The classic symptoms are heartburn and regurgitation aggravated by postural changes such as stooping or lying flat. Heartburn is a term used by patients to mean different things and is a nonspecific symptom. The heartburn typically caused by reflux is a burning or hot sensation beneath the lower sternum and in the epigastrium. In severe cases, this may progress upward toward the neck and even into the shoulder and upper arm. This type of heartburn is usually relieved by ingestion of food or antacids. It occurs most commonly after meals but may almost be continuous in severe cases.

The regurgitation from reflux is of gastric contents. Patients note that the regurgitated material is sour, burns, or tastes bitter. If undigested food is regurgitated, this is not coming from the stomach and cannot be diagnosed as gastroesophageal reflux.

Dysphagia is a common symptom with reflux. It can also be caused by a carcinoma. For this reason, the symptom of dysphagia, or difficulty in swallowing, must be taken seriously, and every patient should have an evaluation of the esophagus, including at least a barium swallow or flexible fiberoptic esophagoscopy. Dysphagia may occur with reflux in the absence of esophagitis. In these cases, the difficulty in swallowing can be attributed to a degree of esophageal spasm or inefficient motor contraction of the esophagus. When the esophagitis has extended to a frank stricture, the difficulty in swallowing will be noted for solid food but not for liquids. The ingestion of hot or cold beverages or alcohol may cause an increase in burning. Heartburn usually diminishes as the stricture increases to protect the esophagus from regurgitated material. The dysphagia caused by diffuse esophageal spasm differs from the dysphagia of a stricture. The former occurs equally with liquids or solids, is episodic, and tends to improve as a meal progresses. There are other atypical symptoms caused by reflux. The pattern of angina pectoris may be mimicked by esophageal spasm triggered by reflux. In these cases, the chest pain may be severe and may cause a systemic reaction that mimics an acute myocardial infarction. In severe cases, a patient is often admitted directly to the coronary care unit for the esophageal spasm disorder.

Referral of symptoms to the neck may occur from reflux. In these cases, the patient has difficulty in initiating the swallow or complains of a persistent sensation of a lump in the neck. This may be misdiagnosed as globus hystericus. In these patients, reflux high into the cervical esophagus with a secondary irritation and spasm of the cricopharyngeus may be the cause.

Bleeding from reflux is rare, although occult blood in the stool is common with ulcerative esophagitis. When massive esophageal bleeding occurs, it is due either to unusual cases of diffuse hemorrhagic esophagitis or to a penetrating ulcer in the gastric mucosa lining the distal esophagus. These patients may have massive life-threatening hemorrhage.

Aspiration caused by reflux most commonly presents as nocturnal cough associated with regurgitation of food in the mouth, often awakening the patient. Morning hoarseness is another symptom suggesting nocturnal aspiration. Aspiration is particularly suspected in patients whose cough occurs mainly at night and not during the daytime. Severe aspiration from reflux can lead to lung abscess, recurrent pneumonia, or bronchiectasis. Asthma is occasionally suggested as being possibly caused by reflux. Cases in which this is truly documented are rare and controversial. However, a patient with an underlying asthmatic tendency may have more frequent attacks triggered by bouts of reflux. When any of these symptoms prompt a patient to see a physician, gastroesophageal reflux must be included in the differential diagnosis and objective tests must be used to confirm the correct diagnosis.

In children, reflux may be less apparent symptomatically, because young children are unable to describe their symptoms accurately and are not familiar with terms such as heartburn. Accordingly, in children, the disease may lead to complications such as failure to thrive, chronic anemia, and chronic aspiration without many complaints from the child. In these circumstances, objective means for diagnosing reflux are particularly important.

DIAGNOSIS OF REFLUX AND HIATAL HERNIA

In any patient suspected of having esophageal disease, a barium swallow is the first study indicated.

The radiologist should be informed of the suspicion of an esophageal disorder so that attention is paid to the important areas. Ordering an upper gastrointestinal radiograph frequently results in a cursory examination of the esophagus. The initial observation of the swallow should focus on the hypopharyngeal and cricopharyngeal swallowing mechanism and should exclude mechanical deformities above the aortic arch. The body of the esophagus is screened to exclude diverticula, extrinsic abnormalities, or mucosal abnormalities that might suggest neoplasia. The cardia is examined during and between swallows. During a swallow, the distal esophagus should open to permit passage of the bolus of barium. At the end of the swallow, the distal esophageal segment should remain closed. If free spontaneous gastroesophageal reflux is seen, this is highly significant, for the author has always been able to confirm this with quantitative tests for reflux. Of the maneuvers that may be used to stimulate reflux, Müller's maneuver, inhalation against a closed glottis, is most effective and significant. Some radiologists use a "water-sipping" test in which the patient is asked to swallow water with barium in the stomach and while the radiologist compresses the abdomen. This elicits physiologic reflux in most normal individuals and has no clinical significance. It is helpful to have the radiographic study recorded on videotape so that it may be inspected repeatedly, because swallowing disorders or a brief spurt of reflux may be difficult to interpret accurately in the course of the examination. If a mechanical deformity such as stricture is seen, multiple views of this should be obtained to help to decide whether it has the appearance of a neoplasm, an ulcerative benign stricture, or a motor disorder. However, the radiologist's opinion with regard to the etiology of the stricture cannot be considered diagnostic, and a tissue diagnosis is necessary in every case.

If the patient complains of dysphagia or the radiologist sees a mechanical abnormality in the esophagus, flexible fiberoptic endoscopy is done. A diagnosis may be obtained by biopsy or brushing. When the clinical problem is reflux, evidence for ulceration and erythema is recorded. The location of the squamocolumnar junction is noted relative to the aortic arch pulsation and relative to the entrance of the tubular esophagus into the gastric pouch. The number, depth, and arrangements of ulcerations should be reported. If a patulous cardia is seen throughout the respiratory cycle, this may confirm other evidence that reflux is present. If the complaint is dysphagia or if a hiatal hernia is present, a J maneuver during gastroscopy provides a look at the cardia from below. Early carcinoma in this area is difficult to visualize, and the retroflex maneuver with the gastroscope is most important. In every case, a full examination of the stomach and pylorus is made to exclude gastric factors that may contribute to increased reflux. If a stricture or severe esophagitis is encountered, or if Barrett's epithelium is suspected, multiple biopsies should be taken. If these do not give an exact diagnosis, deeper biopsies and brushings on a subsequent rigid esophagoscopy may be necessary to exclude carcinoma as a cause of the stricture and dysphagia.

In some patients with stricture, it is wise to do a series of dilatations after the initial endoscopy with balloon dilatation and then repeat the procedure later on to be certain of the diagnosis and the degree of improvement achieved by the dilatations. Bougienage is usually accomplished in these cases by using Maloney's mercury-filled tapered dilators, or the Savary graded dilator system passed over a guide (Monnier et al., 1985).

If reflux is suspected or a hiatal hernia is seen without reflux and if no free spontaneous reflux is seen by radiography, esophageal function tests may be necessary to make an exact diagnosis. A battery of esophageal function tests is commonly done on an outpatient basis and provides most of the information necessary for a diagnosis, except in the more confusing cases (Skinner and Booth, 1970). The esophageal function tests frequently used include esophageal manometry, a standardized acid reflux test using the pH electrode in the esophagus, an acid clearing test, and the acid perfusion test (Fig. 28–3). In more difficult cases in which the diagnosis is still uncertain, prolonged 24-hour pH monitoring and prolonged esophageal manometry may provide essential additional information. Each of these tests is done on an outpatient basis.

Esophageal manometry may be done with open-tip fluid-infused catheters that are bonded together with the openings at different levels. Alternatively, pressure-sensitive transducers in a chain of three or more may be used. Traditionally, manometry involves three recordings spaced 5 cm apart. The catheter is placed into the stomach and its position is confirmed by recording positive-pressure abdominal contractions with inspiration on all three channels. The catheter train is pulled back slowly across the gastroesophageal junction with recordings made at 0.5- or 1-cm intervals. A distal esophageal high-pressure zone is identified. Its amplitude, quality of relaxation, and portion reflecting intra-abdominal location are noted (Fig. 28–4). In the body of the esophagus, the proportion of progressive peristaltic contractions, amplitude of contractions, and presence of any tertiary contractions are noted. In the upper esophagus, the resting tone and timing of relaxation of the cricopharyngeus relative to hypopharyngeal contraction are recorded. Information obtained from this test describes the characteristics of the HPZ, including pressure and intra-abdominal length, and also reveals the presence of other esophageal motor abnormalities such as achalasia, spasm, or scleroderma.

After identification of the HPZ, an acid load is placed in the stomach for a standard acid-reflux test (Kantrowitz et al., 1969). In an adult, this is usually 300 ml of 0.1 normal HCl. The long intestinal pH electrode is positioned 5 cm above the HPZ in the lower esophagus. A standardized series of respiratory and postural maneuvers is done by the patient, in-

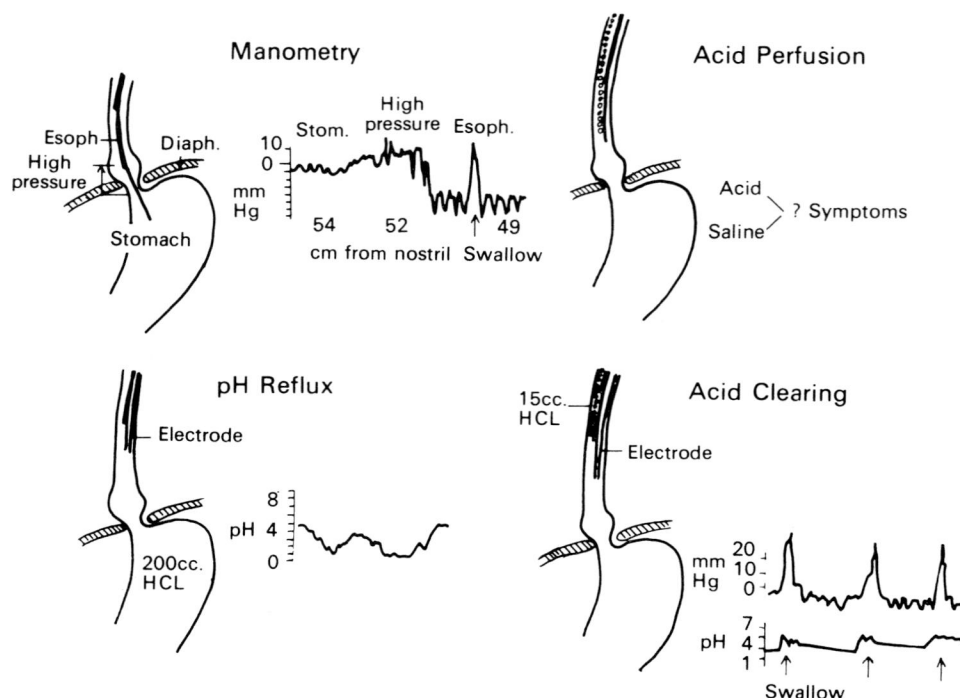

FIGURE 28–3. Placement for a triple-lumen manometric catheter and pH electrode during the performance of each of four esophageal function tests. Examples of the type of data obtained are shown (see text for details of technique and interpretation). (From Skinner, D. B., and Booth, D. J.: Assessment of distal esophageal function in patients with hiatal hernia and/or gastroesophageal reflux. Ann. Surg., 172:627, 1970.)

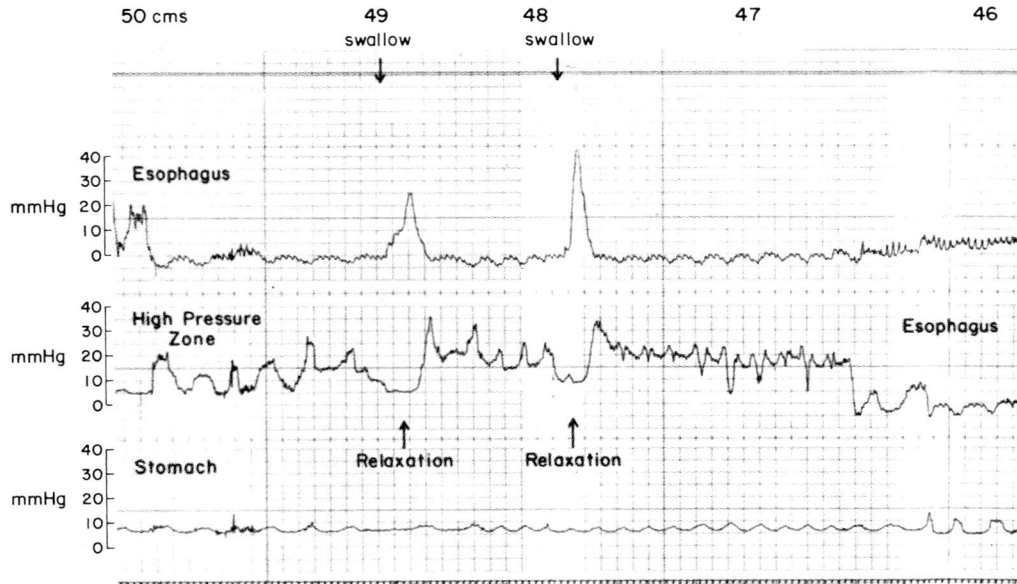

FIGURE 28–4. Manometric tracing showing the distal esophageal high-pressure zone. Recordings are made from catheter lumina spaced 5 cm apart. The catheter train is withdrawn from the stomach into the esophagus so that the proximal, middle, and distal recording channels pass sequentially through the high-pressure zone, which measures millimeters of mercury. Notice the relaxation with swallowing. (From Skinner, D. B.: Hiatal hernia and gastroesophageal reflux. *In* Sabiston, D. C., Jr. [ed]: Davis-Christopher Textbook of Surgery. 12th ed. Philadelphia, W. B. Saunders, 1981.)

cluding coughing, deep breathing, Valsalva's maneuver, and Müller's maneuver, in each of four body positions, supine, head down, right side down, and left side down. This test is standardized against results in a large number of normal volunteers. Three or more episodes of reflux measured by a drop of pH to less than 4 in the esophagus is an abnormal finding. In patients with severe reflux, it may not be possible to clear regurgitated acid from the esophagus.

With the pH probe still located 5 cm above the HPZ, a 15-ml bolus of 0.1 normal HCl is placed in the midesophagus through the proximal tip of the manometry catheter. After flushing this through with a small amount of water, the patient is asked to swallow at 30-second intervals. Normal individuals clear this amount of acid in 10 swallows or fewer and have a low incidence of esophagitis. Patients with reflux who cannot clear the acid have a high probability of esophagitis and require subsequent esophagoscopy for confirmation (Booth et al., 1968).

If symptoms are atypical, an acid perfusion test (Bernstein et al., 1962) is useful. The catheter remains positioned in the midesophagus, and the proximal end is led behind the patient. Two intravenous solution bottles joined by a Y connector are attached to the catheter. One bottle contains 0.1 normal HCl, and the other contains normal saline. One solution or the other is infused for approximately 10 minutes. The patient's spontaneous reaction to the infusion is recorded without coaching by the observer. If the infusion of the acid solution evokes the patient's own spontaneous symptoms, and these symptoms are not caused by saline, a positive acid perfusion test result

is recorded, indicating that the patient's symptoms can be reproduced by acid in the esophagus. This combined with a positive acid reflux test result provides a basis for diagnosing symptomatic reflux. Based on these tests, most cases of significant reflux, risk of esophagitis, and symptoms caused by reflux are diagnosed, and various complicating conditions such as the motor disorders of the esophagus can be eliminated.

In patients who have undergone previous esophageal therapy, in those whose symptoms are complicated or overlap with other known conditions, and in patients suspected of having reflux-induced aspiration or angina-like pain, prolonged 24-hour pH monitoring in the esophagus is invaluable (Johnson and DeMeester, 1974). After manometry, the pH probe is left 5 cm above the distal esophageal HPZ. The probe is connected to a portable pH meter and recorder for use at home (Falor et al., 1986). The patient is asked to record symptoms and activities during the ensuing 24 hours. During this time, the patient is instructed to eat normally but is restricted to a diet of fluids and food with a pH greater than 5. The number of bouts of reflux can be measured quantitatively based on their frequency and duration in both the supine and upright position. Alkaline reflux can be detected when the pH rises above 7. A scoring system is available based on known values in normal control subjects (Johnson and DeMeester, 1974). By this method, patients can be categorized as normal or abnormal for both upright and supine reflux, disorders of acid clearing can be identified, and correlation of unusual symptoms with reflux may be observed.

This test is the most sensitive and quantitative method for evaluating possible gastroesophageal reflux.

Radionuclide studies are being evaluated as new diagnostic techniques to investigate esophageal disorders. These techniques include imaging of the passage of a liquid or capsule containing a radioisotope through the esophagus (Ferguson et al., 1985) and observation by scintiscanning of reflux of radioactive liquids placed in the stomach (Dodds et al., 1981). The quantitative application of these studies is still being developed. At present, pH testing is still the basis for measuring reflux.

SUMMARY

With an understanding of the normal and abnormal anatomy and pathophysiology of hiatal hernia and reflux, knowledge of a range of symptom complexes, and availability of various tests of esophageal function, the clinician may quickly acquire all the information necessary to make a decision about treatment for reflux and hiatal hernia. As discussed in a later section, the principal indication for hiatal hernia repair is a paraesophageal Type II hiatal hernia, which should be repaired regardless of symptoms. There is no indication for the repair of a Type I axial hiatal hernia unless pathologic reflux causing symptoms and complications is present. When reflux is diagnosed as the cause of symptoms, medical therapy is initiated. Only in advanced cases with ulcerative esophagitis, stricture, bleeding observed to be coming from esophagitis, or documented aspiration shown to be caused by reflux on prolonged pH monitoring is antireflux therapy indicated. The several types of antireflux operations available and specific indications for each are discussed in later sections of this chapter.

SELECTED BIBLIOGRAPHY

DeMeester, T. R., Johnson, L. F., Joseph, G. J., et al.: Patterns of gastroesophageal reflux in health and disease. Ann. Surg., 184:459, 1976.

In this paper, the technique and interpretation for prolonged reflux monitoring are described. From analysis of a large number of patients studied, various patterns of abnormal reflux emerge. These, in turn, serve as the base for greater selectivity in treatment and identification of aberrant syndromes caused by reflux.

Skinner, D. B., and Belsey, R. H. R.: Management of Esophageal Disease. Philadelphia, W. B. Saunders, 1988.

Full-scale discussion of all aspects of diagnosis, complications, treatment, and outcome of hiatal hernia and gastroesophageal reflux. Extensive illustrations and references are provided.

BIBLIOGRAPHY

Barrett, N. R.: Chronic peptic ulcer of the esophagus and esophagitis. Br. J. Surg., 38:175, 1950.
Barrett, N. R.: The lower esophagus lined by columnar epithelium. Surgery, 41:881, 1957.
Berenson, M. M., Riddell, R. H., Skinner, D. B., and Freston, J. W.: Malignant transformation of esophageal columnar epithelium. Cancer, 41:544, 1978.

Bernstein, L. M., Fruin, R. C., and Pacini, R.: Differentiation of esophageal pain from angina pectoris: Role of the esophageal acid perfusion test. Medicine, 41:143, 1962.
Bombeck, C. T., Dillard, D. H., and Nyhus, L. M.: Muscular anatomy of the gastroesophageal junction and role of phrenoesophageal ligament: Autopsy study of sphincter mechanism. Ann. Surg., 164:643, 1966.
Booth, D. J., Kemmerer, W. T., and Skinner, D. B.: Acid clearing from the distal esophagus. Arch. Surg., 96:731, 1968.
Cohen, S., and Lipshutz, W.: Hormonal control of lower esophageal sphincter competence: Interaction of gastrin and secretin. Gastroenterology, 58:937, 1970.
Collis, J. L., Kelly, T. D., and Wiley, A. M.: Suturing of the crura of the diaphragm and the surgery of hiatus hernia. Thorax, 9:175, 1954.
DeMeester, T. R., Wernly, J. A., Bryant, G. H., et al.: Clinical and in vitro analysis of determinants of gastroesophageal competence. Am. J. Surg., 137:39, 1979.
DeMeester, T. R., Johnson, L. F., Joseph, G. J., et al.: Patterns of gastroesophageal reflux in health and disease. Ann. Surg., 184:459, 1976.
Dent, J., Dodds, W. J., Friedman, R. H., et al.: Mechanism of gastroesophageal reflux in recumbent asymptomatic human subjects. J. Clin. Invest., 65:256, 1980.
Dodds, W. J., Hogan, W. J., Helm, J. F., and Dent, J.: Pathogenesis of reflux esophagitis. Gastroenterology, 81:376, 1981.
Falor, W. H., Miller, J., Kraus, J., et al.: Twenty-four-hour monitoring of esophagopharyngeal pH in outpatients: Use of four-channel pH probe and computerized systems. J. Thorac. Cardiovasc. Surg., 91:716, 1986.
Ferguson, M. K., Ryan, J. W., Little, A. G., and Skinner, D. B.: Esophageal emptying and acid neutralization in patients with symptoms of esophageal reflux. Ann. Surg., 201:728, 1985.
Friedland, G. W., Melcher, D. H., Berridge, F. R., and Gresham, G. A.: Debatable points in the anatomy of the lower oesophagus. Thorax, 21:487, 1966.
Fyke, F. E., Jr., Code, D. F., and Schlegel, J. F.: The gastroesophageal sphincter in healthy human beings. Gastroenterologia (Basel), 86:135, 1956.
Helm, J. F., Dodds, W. J., and Hogan, W. J.: Acid neutralizing capacity of human saliva. Gastroenterology, 83:69, 1982.
Henderson, R. D.: The Esophagus: Reflux Primary Motor Disorders. Baltimore, Williams & Wilkins, 1980, p. 127.
Hiebert, C. A., and Belsey, R.: Incompetency of the gastric cardia without radiologic evidence of hiatus hernia. J. Thorac. Cardiovasc. Surg., 42:352, 1961.
Higgs, B., Shorter, R. G., and Ellis, F. H., Jr.: A study of the anatomy of the human esophagus with special reference to the gastroesophageal sphincter. J. Surg. Res., 5:503, 1965.
Ismail-Beigi, F., Horton, P. F., and Pope, C. E., II: Histological consequences of gastroesophageal reflux in man. Gastroenterology, 58:163, 1970.
Johnson, L. F., and DeMeester, T. R.: Twenty-four hour pH monitoring of the distal esophagus: A quantitative measure of gastroesophageal reflux. Am. J. Gastroenterol., 62:325, 1974.
Kantrowitz, P. A., Corson, J. G., Fleischli, D. L., and Skinner, D. B.: Measurement of gastroesophageal reflux. Gastroenterology, 56:666, 1969.
Little, A. G., DeMeester, T. R., Kirchner, P. T., et al.: Pathogenesis of esophagitis in patients with gastroesophageal reflux. Surgery, 88:101, 1980.
Monnier, V., Hsieh, V., and Savary, M.: Endoscopic treatment of esophageal stenosis using Savary-Gilliard bougies: Technical innovations. Acta Endoscopy, 15:119, 1985.
Moossa, A. R., Hall, A. W., Wood, R. A. B., et al.: Effect of pentagastrin infusion on gastroesophageal manometry and reflux status before and after esophagogastrectomy. Am. J. Surg., 133:23, 1977.
O'Sullivan, G. C., DeMeester, T. R., Smith, R. B., et al.: Twenty-four-hour pH monitoring of esophageal function. Arch. Surg., 116:581, 1981.
Pellegrini, C. A., DeMeester, T. R., Johnson, L. F., and Skinner, D. B.: Gastroesophageal reflux and pulmonary aspiration: Incidence, functional abnormality, and results of surgical therapy. Surgery, 36:110, 1979.

Sandry, R. J.: The pathology of chronic oesophagitis. Gut, 3:189, 1962.

Skinner, D. B.: Pathophysiology of gastroesophageal reflux. Ann. Surg., 101:546, 1985.

Skinner, D. B., and Belsey, R. H. R.: Surgical management of esophageal reflux and hiatus hernia: Long-term results with 1,030 patients. J. Thorac. Cardiovasc. Surg., 53:33, 1967.

Skinner, D. B., and Belsey, R. H. R.: Management of Esophageal Disease. Philadelphia, W. B. Saunders, 1988.

Skinner, D. B., and Booth, D. J.: Assessment of distal esophageal function in patients with hiatal hernia and/or gastroesophageal reflux. Ann. Surg., 172:627, 1970.

Skinner, D. B., Walther, B. C., Riddell, R. H., et al.: Barrett's esophagus: Comparison of benign and malignant cases. Ann. Surg., 198:554, 1983.

Spechler, S. J., Robbins, A. H., Rubins, H. B., et al.: Adenocarcinoma and Barrett's esophagus: An overrated risk? Gastroenterology, 87:927, 1984.

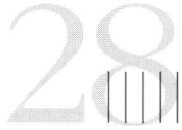

28 ■ II The Belsey Mark IV Antireflux Repair

David B. Skinner

In the early 1950s, gastroesophageal reflux and secondary esophagitis became recognized as a serious illness. Starting from methods for hiatal hernia repair, Belsey, in Bristol, England, developed by trial and error a specific antireflux operation that he called the Mark IV repair. This term recognized three preceding efforts to devise an antireflux repair that were unsuccessful. The first was similar to the repair described by Allison (1951), which was designed to correct reflux by shortening and reattaching the phrenoesophageal membrane. Allison's repair correctly recognized the importance of the intra-abdominal esophagus, but by circumferentially placing tension on the phrenoesophageal membrane, the esophageal diameter was widened and encouraged reflux. Allison recognized the high rate of persistent reflux after his repair in a long-term follow-up study.

The Mark IV repair remains an effective antireflux operation with a low incidence of complications and recurrences (Skinner and Belsey, 1967, 1988). It incorporates those principles deemed to be important in the control of reflux that are discussed in detail in the earlier section. Specifically, the Mark IV operation restores a 3- to 4-cm length of intra-abdominal esophagus, maintains a narrow diameter of the distal swallowing tube by compression from the adjacent gastric fundoplication, creates an abrupt change in diameter as the swallowing tube enters the gastric pouch, and leaves a portion of the circumference of the esophagus free posteriorly to dilate as necessary as a bolus of swallowed food passes (Fig. 28–5).

INDICATIONS FOR OPERATION

The Mark IV procedure, like all antireflux operations, is specifically designed to prevent gastrointestinal reflux and can be expected only to relieve symptoms and complications caused by this disturbance. The first step in choosing an antireflux operation is to be absolutely certain that the symptoms are caused by reflux or its complications. Because the complaints caused by reflux may be numerous and overlap with various other conditions, objective quantitation of reflux by esophageal function tests is essential. The next step is to ascertain the degree of esophagitis. Esophagoscopy to grade esophagitis is a prerequisite to a decision about the necessity for operative therapy and the type of operation that may prove most effective (see earlier section for esophageal function tests and grading of esophagitis).

Symptomatic gastroesophageal reflux (heartburn aggravated by postural change and postural regurgitation) in the absence of reflux complications is rarely, if ever, an indication for antireflux surgery. Symptomatic patients with no esophagitis, minimal Grade 1 esophagitis, or ulcerative Grade 2 esophagitis are initially treated medically. When acid reflux is the

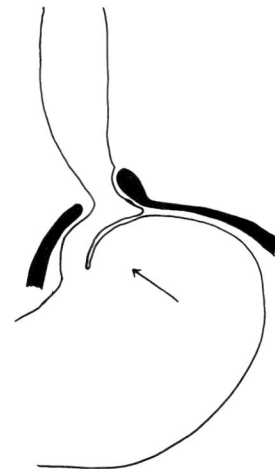

FIGURE 28–5. Principle of the Mark IV repair. The segment of lower esophagus restored to the abdomen is compressed by the positive intra-abdominal pressure against the posterior crural buttress.

cause of the symptoms and esophagitis, it is initially treated successfully by medication, including H_2 blockers in the great majority of patients. Occasionally, a proton pump inhibitor such as omeprozal must be prescribed for complete relief of symptoms and esophagitis. Failure of symptoms to respond to modern medical treatment reduces the possibility that reflux is the cause of the complaint. Therapy should be continued for at least 6 months to allow for temporary stresses in the life of the patient that may aggravate symptoms and to allow for seasonal variation in peptic acid disorders. Prompt relapse of troubling symptoms after medical therapy is stopped, particularly if omeprozal has been used, raises the issue of antireflux surgery as an alternative to prolonged, and perhaps lifelong, medical therapy. In young, otherwise healthy patients, antireflux surgery may be the preferred choice when severe symptoms recur after prolonged omeprozal treatment. The demands of certain occupations that require stooping, bending, or lifting may make postural therapy and medical treatment ineffective and make the surgical relief of symptoms inevitable.

The customary indication for antireflux operation is a complication of reflux, including ulcerative esophagitis, stricture, bleeding esophagitis, or repeated aspiration. When frank ulceration results from esophagitis and continues in spite of effective medical therapy, the virulence of the condition is established. The ulcer granulation tissue heals with the deposition of collagen in the submucosa. As the collagen contracts over time and the process of ulceration and healing is repeated or continuous, the outcome may be a stricture. This sequence of events is documented repeatedly and can occur with remarkable rapidity, for example, in a matter of days in some patients. Because ulcerative esophagitis is a known precursor of stricture and because stricture is more difficult to treat and has a poorer long-term prognosis, antireflux operation is recommended in patients with persistent ulcerative esophagitis who do not have overriding medical contraindications. Patients who present with a stricture are candidates for surgical relief. Repeated dilatation of the stricture with medical treatment for reflux is an alternative method of management, but it usually proves ineffective and unacceptable to most patients who are otherwise healthy and vigorous.

Rapid bleeding from esophagitis is occasionally seen and is an indication for antireflux operative intervention in approximately 1% of patients requiring operation. The bleeding is best handled acutely without operation by intravenous H_2 receptor blockers and an iced antacid drip through a nasoesophageal tube while the patient sits upright. After the bleeding ceases, which usually occurs within hours, the patient is evaluated and prepared for an elective antireflux operation to prevent a recurrence of this frightening complication.

Repeated aspiration of gastric contents into the lung is a serious complication of reflux and may occur in the absence of esophagitis or symptomatic heartburn. Any patient with morning hoarseness, chronic cough with recurrent episodes of acute bronchitis or pneumonia, and a history of nocturnal cough often associated with a sour or brackish taste in the mouth should be suspected of having reflux-induced aspiration. Respiratory symptoms and reflux are common in the general population. The coexistence of the two conditions does not establish a cause-and-effect relationship. In these patients, continuous long-term pH monitoring is essential to establish that reflux is the cause of the respiratory disorder.

In children, the indications for antireflux operation are less precise and more controversial. Frequent regurgitation and reflux are normal findings in children up to 12 to 18 months of age. After this time, almost all children acquire competency of the cardia, and the need for antireflux operation is rare during childhood and the teenage years. Because the natural history of frequent reflux in infancy and early childhood is progressive improvement, the decision with regard to whether to operate in a baby is difficult. Nevertheless, some young children do experience progression of complicated reflux to a stricture, with weight loss, failure to thrive, aspiration, and occult bleeding with anemia. When reflux is clearly interfering with the well-being of the child, which is documented by these complications, and the reflux does not respond readily to medical measures, including maintaining the child in a constant upright position with the so-called "chalasia chair," antireflux operation may yield dramatic results.

Another indication for antireflux operation is a complication of the condition called Barrett's esophagus (Allison and Johnstone, 1953; Barrett, 1953). It is normal for the distal 2 to 3 cm of the tubular esophagus to be lined with columnar epithelium as the transition between the acid-sensitive squamous epithelium of the esophagus and the acid-producing gastric mucosa. In some patients, this columnar epithelium may extend farther up the esophagus, may be associated with a zone of ulcerative esophagitis between the columnar epithelium and squamous mucosa, and may undergo degeneration to atypia, intestinalization, dysplasia, and neoplasia (Berenson et al., 1978). Deep, penetrating, gastric-type ulcers may occur in the esophagus lined with this aberrant gastric mucosa. When this condition is diagnosed, the patient is said to have Barrett's esophagus with or without Barrett's ulcer. The diagnosis is often suspected by radiographic findings and confirmed by endoscopy with multiple biopsies. Because the dysplasia and neoplasia are multicentric and interspersed among islands of more normal-appearing columnar and goblet cell mucosa, numerous biopsies are essential to exclude malignant degeneration. Whenever high-grade dysplasia or neoplasia is found in the biopsies, en-bloc esophagectomy for cure is recommended. In patients with no evidence of neoplastic degeneration or low-grade dysplasia, the indications for antireflux surgery in Barrett's esophagus are the same as for patients without the condition (i.e., persistent esophagitis, stricture, aspiration, or severe bleeding). Barrett's ulcer in the columnar mucosa is an indication for antireflux surgery, but a deep penetrating ulcer may require resection. Lifetime surveillance for neoplastic degeneration is necessary for all patients having Barrett's epithelium with metaplastic change. For those without low-grade dysplasia, a cytologic study or endoscopy with multiple biopsies at 2-year intervals appears adequate. For those with low-grade dysplasia, more frequent surveillance is necessary. It is not known whether and to what degree Barrett's epithelium may regress after a successful antireflux repair, and whether an antireflux repair eliminates the risk of future malignant degeneration in the abnormal epithelium.

PREOPERATIVE PREPARATION

When the diagnosis of reflux resistant to medical treatment is certain and ulcerative esophagitis is found, the indicated surgical procedure is done promptly. When a stricture or severe esophagitis is encountered or when the patient has had recent severe hemorrhage from esophagitis or a recent bout of aspiration pneumonia, time devoted to preoperative preparation increases the safety of the operation and the likelihood of a successful long-term outcome. A reflux-induced stricture consists of two components, true fibrosis from collagen deposition during the healing process and a degree of esophageal muscle spasm, edema, and inflammation from the acute ulceration. The latter is reversible, and persistent efforts to treat and heal the esophagitis medically before operation may convert a difficult stricture with a "short" esophagus into a straightforward problem that can be managed with an antireflux repair alone. When this course is followed, it is rare to find the indurated, edematous mediastinum that was commonly encountered in the past, making dissection difficult and producing a shortened esophageal tube that cannot be reduced beneath the diaphragm. Some patients with long-standing symptoms and a well-established stricture have too much fibrosis to enable the stricture to be reversed preoperatively. These patients often obtain a poor result from any type of antireflux procedure, including gastroplasty or fundic patch procedures, and require esophageal resection and reconstruction.

When the indication for operation is acute bleeding, the patient undergoes several days of intensive medical treatment to reverse the inflammation in the esophageal wall and mediastinum before the Mark IV operation is done. When aspiration is an indication for repair, several days of postural drainage, pulmonary physical therapy, and treatment with appropriate antibiotics are worthwhile before an antireflux repair.

CHOICE OF OPERATION

The surgeon who frequently operates for reflux and its complications has experience with several types of operations and chooses the one suited to the individual patient's requirements. Factors influencing the choice include whether a thoracic or abdominal approach is advantageous, whether the patient may be a candidate for a video-assisted procedure, whether the patient has had a previous antireflux repair, whether a resection or esophagomyotomy may be necessary, and the patient's body habitus. The Belsey Mark IV operation is done only through a thoracotomy incision.

In the author's practice, a thoracotomy approach is used for patients with extensive esophagitis in whom more than the usual mobilization of the esophagus is anticipated and when the possible need for a resection is anticipated. A thoracotomy approach is advantageous for repeated antireflux operations, because a primary cause of failure of the previous operation is likely to be insufficient esophageal mobilization. A thoracic approach provides better exposure and less difficult operating conditions in an obese patient. This approach is used when other pulmonary or mediastinal disease is noted.

Through the thoracic approach, the Belsey Mark IV or Nissen fundoplication is the usual antireflux repair. The degree of mobilization required for either is similar, and follow-up results offer little reason to choose one over the other. There are certain circumstances in which the Mark IV approach has advantages. These include patients with an esophageal motor disorder such as spasm, in whom the partial fundoplication is less likely to aggravate the esophageal obstruction than a full fundoplication. A modification of the Mark IV repair, in which the middle suture in each row is omitted, is combined with an esophagomyotomy in patients with standard or vigorous achalasia and after the resection and esophagomyotomy used for epiphrenic diverticulum (Belsey, 1966).

Although some surgeons use and advocate the Collis (1961) gastroplasty frequently, the author finds the need for this procedure to be rare if the patient is properly prepared for antireflux repair. When the Collis maneuver is used, it is combined with either a Mark IV or a Nissen type of fundoplication, and the residual fundus is wrapped around the newly created distal esophageal tube (Orringer and Sloan, 1978; Pearson and Henderson, 1973). Esophagectomy and reconstruction, preferably by an isoperistaltic segment of left colon or jejunum, are reserved for patients who have undergone multiple previous operations and in whom the esophagus is mainly an unyielding fibrous tube (Belsey, 1965). Occasionally, sufficient damage occurs to the esophagus in the course of a reoperation for stricture that a resection is preferable to attempts to repair the damage. All patients undergoing reoperation should be prepared for possible interposition.

MARK IV REPAIR

The Mark IV operation (Fig. 28–6) is a procedure of choice for the thoracic approach in antireflux repair and is used by many thoracic surgeons as their principal or best procedure for this condition. The operation

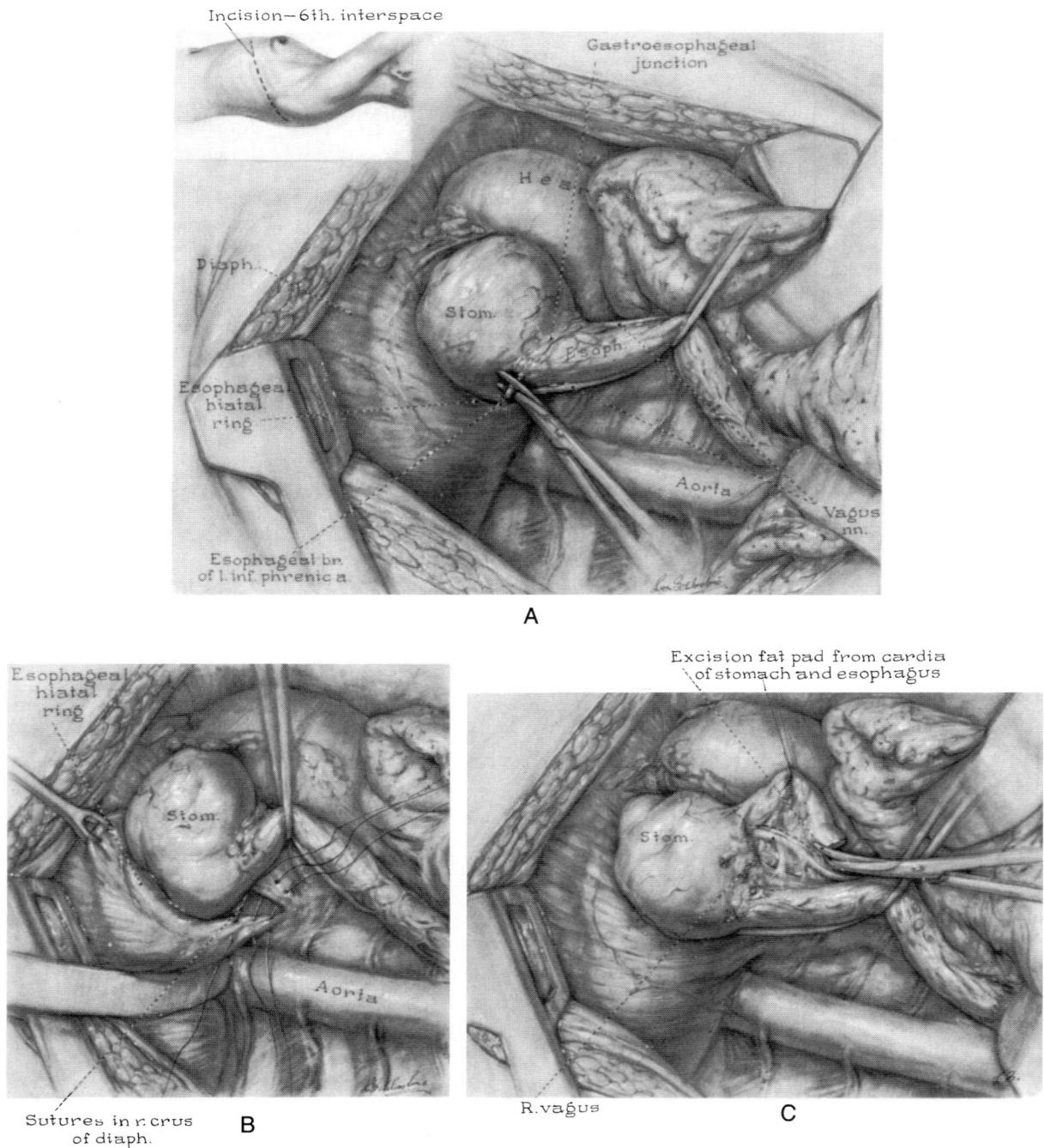

Incision—6th. interspace

Gastroesophageal junction

H.e.s.

Diaph.

Stom.

Esoph.

Esophageal hiatal ring

Aorta

Vagus nn.

Esophageal br. of l. inf. phrenic a.

A

Esophageal hiatal ring

Stom.

Aorta

Sutures in r. crus of diaph.   **B**

Excision fat pad from cardia of stomach and esophagus

Stom.

R. vagus   **C**

FIGURE 28–6. *A*, Mobilization of the distal esophagus and cardia is done through a left sixth interspace lateral thoracotomy. The esophagus with vagus nerves attached is completely freed up to the root of the lung. After the hernia sac is entered anteriorly, the entire circumference of the cardia is separated from its attachments. This requires division of branches from the left inferior phrenic artery laterally (illustrated) and left gastric artery posteriorly (not shown). *B*, At the start of the repair, sutures are placed in two limbs of the right crus posteriorly, but these are not tied until the completion of reconstruction. Tension on a clamp applied to the diaphragm anteriorly makes it easier to identify the strong tendinous tissue in the crus where the sutures should be placed. *C*, After complete mobilization of the esophagogastric junction, the pad of fibrofatty tissue at the cardia is excised anteriorly and laterally. The vagus nerves, which tend to be elevated off the esophagus during this dissection, are carefully preserved.

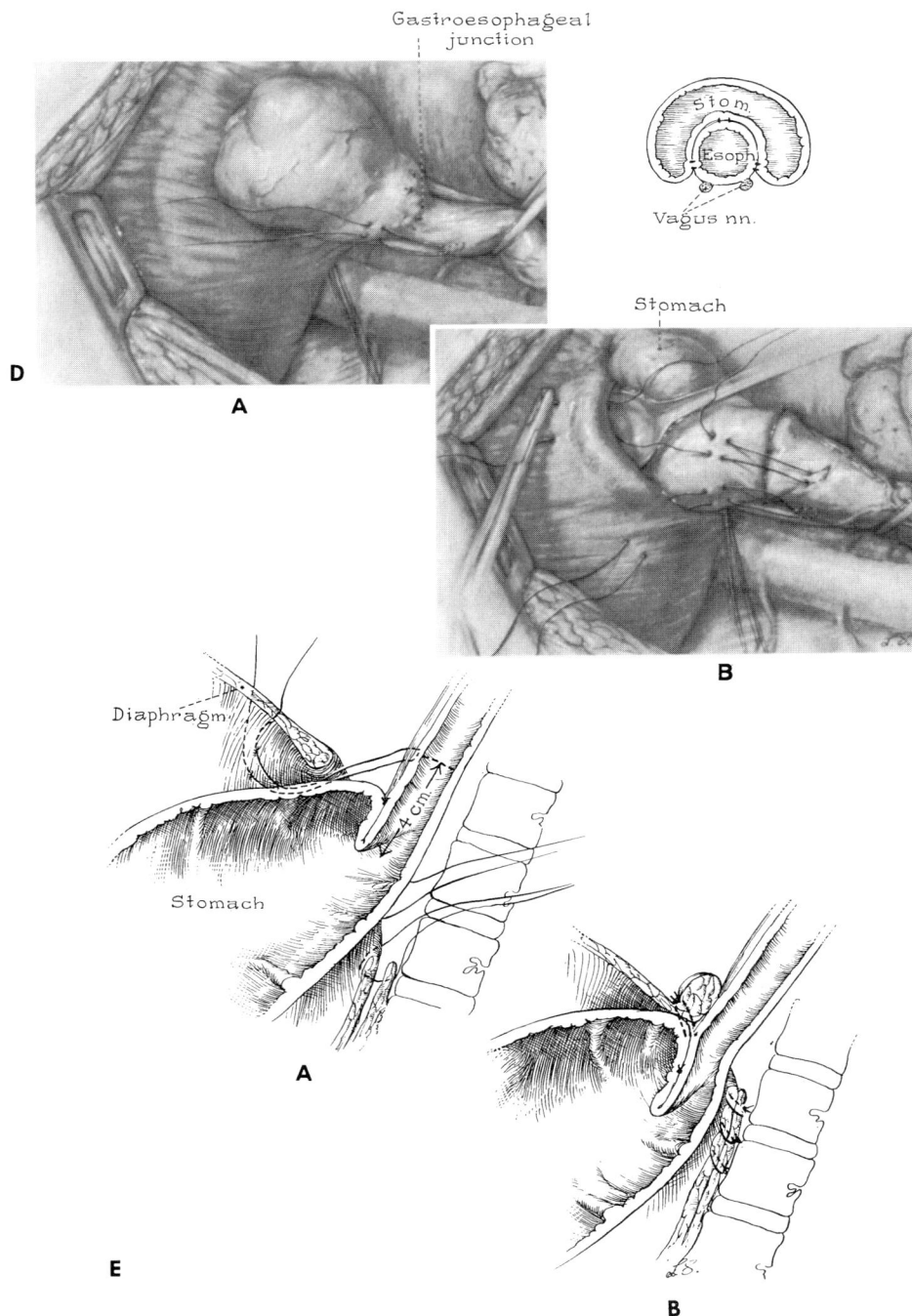

FIGURE 28–6 *Continued D,* **(A)** The reconstruction is started by placing the first of three mattress sutures between the fundus of the stomach and the esophagus 2 cm above the junction. The spacing of these sutures around the circumference of the esophagus is shown in the cross-sectional insert. **(B)** After completion of the first row of sutures, a second row of three mattress sutures is placed through the diaphragm, fundus, and esophagus. In the illustration, the first suture is in place, and the second is being passed through the diaphragm in the bowl of a spoon retractor, which is used to protect structures beneath the diaphragm. The posterior sutures in the crus are in place but have not been tied. *E,* Sagittal sections of the repair. **(A)** The sutures in the crus posteriorly have been placed but not yet tied. The first row of mattress sutures between the stomach and esophagus have been tied. One of the mattress sutures in the second row is illustrated. **(B)** The completed repair. The posterior sutures in the crus and second row of mattress sutures joining the diaphragm, stomach, and esophagus are tied after the reconstruction has been placed below the diaphragm. (*A–E,* From Belsey, R. H. R., and Skinner, D. B.: Surgical treatment: Thoracic approach. *In* Skinner, D. B., Belsey, R. H. R., Hendrix, T. R., and Zuidema, G. D. [eds]: Gastroesophageal Reflux and Hiatal Hernia. Boston, Little, Brown, 1972.)

is done through a left sixth interspace thoracotomy. For optimal long-term results, it is important to minimize post-thoracotomy discomfort. Thus, the surgeon should not fracture ribs or the costal margin or use an incision larger than necessary. Dividing the serratus anterior muscle is rarely necessary. In children and young adults, the rib cage is sufficiently pliable that an intercostal incision without dividing a rib provides satisfactory exposure. In older patients, postoperative discomfort is minimized if a short segment of the seventh rib is resected underneath the paraspinal muscle mass behind the posterior angle of the rib. The sixth interspace is chosen because it provides excellent exposure of the lower half of the esophagus and hiatus and causes less postoperative discomfort than does a lower interspace incision.

After the chest is opened, all adhesions to the lung are divided, and the pulmonary ligament is incised. The dissection of the esophagus is begun at the inferior pulmonary vein. The pleura overlying the esophagus is incised, and the esophagus is dissected free from the aorta. Normally, two or three esophagobronchial arteries from the aorta are clamped and ligated in mobilizing the esophagus. Anteriorly, the esophagus is freed from the pericardium. The vagal nerve plexus is left on the esophageal muscle. The right pleural reflection is carefully dissected off the esophagus to avoid entry into the opposite pleural cavity, where blood may accumulate unnoticed during the operation. Once the esophagus is freed circumferentially, a tape is passed around the organ and used to raise it. The dissection is extended cephalad well up under the arch of the aorta. The esophageal collateral blood supply in the submucosa is excellent, so there is no concern about causing esophageal ischemia by this mobilization. The thoracic approach for an antireflux repair is often chosen because of the advantage of extensive esophageal mobilization, so that failure to do this maneuver denies the patient the benefit of this approach.

After the proximal mobilization to the aortic arch is complete, the dissection is carried caudally. As the esophagus is raised from its bed, the vagus nerves are easily palpable as two taut strings behind the esophagus. Posteriorly, the dissection is carried down to the crura of the diaphragm. The right pleural reflection is bluntly dissected and the pericardium is mobilized off the right crus so that the tendinous origin of the crus is prepared for suturing. Anteriorly, the dissection is extended down until the cuff of diaphragmatic muscle is cleared circumferentially.

Upward retraction of the esophagus places tension on the phrenoesophageal membrane, which becomes visible inserting into the wall of the esophagus as it enters the hiatus. By using scissors, an incision is made in the phrenoesophageal membrane directly anteriorly and at a right angle to the axis of the esophagus. The incision passes through the endothoracic and endoabdominal fascia and retroperitoneal fat, and finally, the peritoneal sac is entered. The cardia is freed completely from the hiatus, preserving only the vagal nerve branches on the wall of the gastroesophageal

junction. The mobilization requires ligation and division of the ascending esophageal branch from the left gastric artery lying close to the right vagus nerve in the retroperitoneum. When the latter vessel is divided, the lesser peritoneal sac is opened, which completes the hiatal dissection. The fundus of the stomach is delivered up through the hiatus. The gastroesophageal junction anteriorly between the two vagus nerves is cleared of fibrofatty tissue to facilitate the repair. The stage is now set for the Mark IV reconstruction.

With the cardia retracted anteriorly, the decussation of the crura is visualized posteriorly. A 0 silk suture is placed through the tendinous portion of the right crus near its origin and through the left crus, catching a portion of the muscular cuff and piercing the endothoracic fascia immediately in front of the aorta. Two or three similar sutures are placed progressing anteriorly at 1-cm intervals. An average antireflux repair requires three such sutures, but as many as six or seven may be needed if the hiatus is large. These sutures are left in place and tied later, after the fundoplication is complete.

The first row of suturing for stomach plication to the esophagus is performed using 2-0 silk sutures placed first through the stomach and then obliquely through the esophageal wall 2 cm above the gastroesophageal junction. The suture is reversed and passed back obliquely through the esophagus and through the gastric fundus. Three of these mattress sutures are used. The first suture is placed near the left vagus nerve; the second (center) suture is placed anterior midway between the vagus nerves, and the third suture is placed adjacent to the right vagus nerve. An oblique suture catching a deep bite of both longitudinal and circular muscle is important to prevent the esophageal sutures from cutting through.

For the final row of sutures, 0 silk on a large, curved needle is used. A spoon inserted through the hiatus with the bowl on the underside of the diaphragm protects subdiaphragmatic organs. The needle is passed through the edge of the central tendon of the diaphragm into the bowl of the spoon and out through the hiatus. Next, the suture is passed through the fundus of the stomach and then an additional 2 cm cephalad on the esophagus, taking an oblique bite. The suture is then reversed, passing back through the esophagus and the fundus of the stomach and out through the tendinous portion of the diaphragm. Three sutures are placed in this row, corresponding in location to the sutures in the first row. After all three sutures are in place, the reconstructed cardia is set below the diaphragm manually before any tension is placed on the sutures. After pulling each suture up snugly to hold the reconstruction beneath the diaphragm, one ties the sutures gently. At this point, the repair should lie easily below the diaphragm without apparent tension. The posterior crural sutures are now tied, and care is taken to leave an orifice through the hiatus that is sufficient to admit the operator's index finger easily or to pass a No. 60 bougie without obstruction at the cardia. The thoracotomy is closed with chest tube drainage.

POSTOPERATIVE CARE

A nasogastric tube is not used routinely. The chest tube is removed after 48 hours or when drainage falls below 200 ml/day. Ambulation is started the evening of operation, and liquids may be taken by mouth on the next day. When the patient is eating well, a postoperative barium swallow examination is done to record the status of the repair. A satisfactory result should show the 4-cm segment of intra-abdominal esophagus and the adjacent fundoplication (Fig. 28–7). The lumen of the esophagus opens fully as the barium bolus passes, but remains closed otherwise.

At the time of discharge, usually the fifth postoperative day, the patient is advised to chew food carefully and avoid large boluses. Certain sticky foods such as soft bread and pithy vegetables tend to pass slowly through the reconstruction and should be avoided during the first month. Normal physical activity is encouraged. Depending on the patient's employment, work can usually be resumed within 3 to 6 weeks.

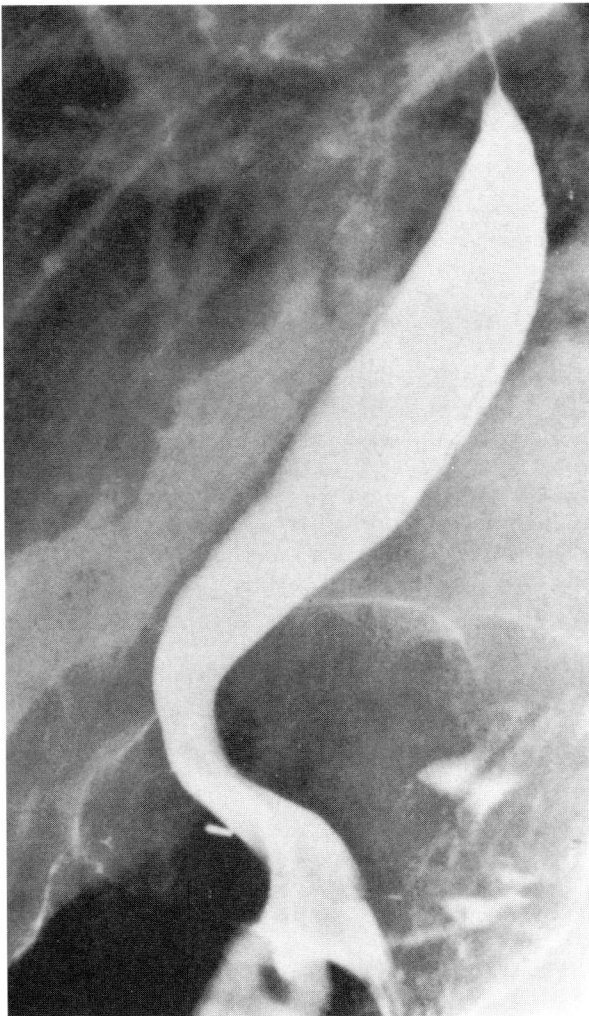

FIGURE 28–7. Postoperative barium swallow after Mark IV repair showing typical 4-cm segment of intra-abdominal esophagus compressed by adjacent gastric fundus.

FOLLOW-UP AND RESULTS

For the surgeon who is dedicated to perfecting the technique of antireflux repair and anxious to determine long-term results, an ongoing follow-up program is essential. After the first 6 months of check-ups, patients are asked to return at yearly intervals. Provided that the patient remains asymptomatic, a routine barium swallow and outpatient esophageal function tests should be repeated at 2 years and 5 years after operation. Any patient who returns complaining of symptoms remotely related to reflux should be evaluated promptly by a barium swallow, esophageal function tests, and if results of these are positive, esophagoscopy. In this way, objective evidence of the results of operation can be obtained in addition to assessing the patient's satisfaction with the operation. According to a systematic follow-up approach in which more than 97% of patients were accounted for, 85% of patients were asymptomatic and had a satisfactory barium swallow 5 or more years after a Mark IV repair (Skinner and Belsey, 1967). In a subsequent study, recurrence of specific symptoms of reflux or a recurrent hiatal hernia was found in 15% of 272 patients followed for more than 10 years, and 76% remained relieved of all preoperative symptoms (Orringer et al., 1972). In a separate independent evaluation of the operation, 71% of patients were completely free of symptoms after 10 years (Hiebert and O'Mara, 1979).

SELECTED BIBLIOGRAPHY

Hiebert, C. A., and O'Mara, C. S.: The Belsey operation for hiatal hernia: A twenty-year experience. Am. J. Surg., *137*:532, 1979.

  Long-term results (10-year follow-up) are given from another excellent series of Mark IV operations verifying the original Belsey experience.

Orringer, M. B., Skinner, D. B., and Belsey, R. H. R.: Long-term results of the Mark IV operation for hiatal hernia and analyses of recurrences and their treatment. J. Thorac. Cardiovasc. Surg., *63*:25, 1972.

  The long-term follow-up beyond 10 years for the Mark IV repair done in Belsey's clinic is reported along with an analysis of type and causes of recurrences.

Pearson, F. G., and Henderson, R. D.: Experimental and clinical studies of gastroplasty in the management of acquired short esophagus. Surg. Gynecol. Obstet., *136*:737, 1973.

  The rationale and use of the Collis gastroplasty combined with a Mark IV type of reconstruction is presented, and clinical results are given.

Skinner, D. B., and Belsey, R. H. R.: Surgical management of esophageal reflux and hiatus hernia: Long-term results with 1,030 patients. J. Thorac. Cardiovasc. Surg., *53*:33, 1967.

  This paper presents the first formal description of the Mark IV operation from Belsey's clinic, its indications, rationale, and results. Results from the early types of antireflux repairs are given. The uses of the operation in children, Type II hiatal hernia, and stricture cases are analyzed.

BIBLIOGRAPHY

Allison, P. R.: Reflux esophagitis, sliding hiatal hernia, and the anatomy of repair. Surg. Gynecol. Obstet., *92*:419, 1951.
Allison, P. R.: Hiatus hernia: A 20-year retrospective survey. Ann. Surg., *178*:273, 1973.
Allison, P. R., and Johnstone, A. S.: The esophagus lined with gastric mucous membrane. Thorax, *8*:87, 1953.

Barrett, N. R.: Chronic peptic ulcer of the oesophagus lined with gastric mucous membrane. Thorax, 8:87, 1953.

Belsey, R. H. R.: Functional disease of the esophagus. J. Thorac. Cardiovasc. Surg., 52:164, 1966.

Belsey, R. H. R.: Reconstruction of esophagus with left colon. J. Thorac. Cardiovasc. Surg., 49:33, 1965.

Belsey, R. H. R., and Skinner, D. B.: Surgical treatment: Thoracic approach. In Skinner, D. B., Belsey, R. H. R., Hendrix, T. R., and Zuidema, G. D.: Gastroesophageal Reflux and Hiatal Hernia. Boston, Little, Brown, 1972.

Berenson, M. M., Riddell, R. H., Skinner, D. B., and Freston, J. W.: Malignant transformation of esophageal columnar epithelium. Cancer, 41:544, 1978.

Collis, J. L.: Gastroplasty. Thorax, 16:197, 1961.

Henderson, R. D.: Reflux control following gastroplasty. Ann. Thorac. Surg., 24:206, 1977.

Hiebert, C. A., and O'Mara, C. S.: The Belsey operation for hiatal hernia: A twenty-year experience. Am. J. Surg., 137:532, 1979.

Orringer, M. B., Skinner, D. B., and Belsey, R. H. R.: Long-term results of the Mark IV operation for hiatal hernia and analyses of recurrences and their treatment. J. Thorac. Cardiovasc. Surg., 63:25, 1972.

Orringer, M. B., and Sloan, H.: Combined Collis-Nissen reconstruction of the esophagogastric junction. Ann. Thorac. Surg., 25:16, 1978.

Pearson, F. G., and Henderson, R. D.: Experimental and clinical studies of gastroplasty in the management of acquired short esophagus. Surg. Gynecol. Obstet., 136:737, 1973.

Skinner, D. B.: Atlas of Esophageal Surgery. New York, Churchill Livingstone, 1991.

Skinner, D. B.: Pathophysiology of gastroesophageal reflux. Ann. Surg., 202:546, 1985.

Skinner, D. B., and Belsey, R. H. R.: Management of Esophageal Disease. Philadelphia, W. B. Saunders, 1988.

Skinner, D. B., and Belsey, R. H. R.: Surgical management of esophageal reflux and hiatus hernia: Long-term results with 1,030 patients. J. Thorac. Cardiovasc. Surg., 53:33, 1967.

28 ▪ III The Nissen Fundoplication

Lucius D. Hill

The Nissen fundoplication was initially utilized by Rudolph Nissen in 1936 to protect the closure following resection of a benign lesion of the cardia. When he reviewed the progress of this patient 16 years later, Nissen was impressed with the lack of evidence of esophagitis. He first used the procedure for the primary indication of reflux control in 1955 and published his initial results the following year (Nissen, 1956). Owing to widespread dissatisfaction with the Allison repair, which was accompanied by recurrence rates as high as 50%, the new procedure was quickly adopted by many surgeons.

However, since its inception, the procedure has yielded an increasing number of reported complications worldwide. A MEDLARS search yielded over 50 reports in the last 15 years concerned specifically with serious complications of the Nissen procedure.

TECHNIQUE

The original procedure called for mobilization of the lower 5 to 8 cm of esophagus through an upper midline incision, and taking down the gastrohepatic omentum, including the hepatic branch of the vagus nerve. With the esophagus on tension with an encircling band, the gastrohepatic ligament was taken down. A large stomach tube was then passed down the esophagus with an accompanying nasogastric tube to prevent subsequent stenosis. The anterior and posterior walls of the fundus were wrapped with the right hand to encircle the newly reduced portion of intra-abdominal esophagus, and the posterior wall of the stomach was brought behind the esophagus, grasped, and stabilized with a Babcock clamp (Fig. 28–8A). The posterior wall of the fundus was brought to lie beside its anterior wall counterpart at approximately the level of the gastroesophageal (GE) junction, and these two serosal surfaces were sutured together starting as high on the esophagus as possible and including the esophagus in the first two stitches. Sutures were placed 1 to 1.5 cm apart for a distance ranging from 3 to 4 cm (Fig. 28–8B). If the patient had previously been identified as an acid hypersecretor, a left-sided truncal vagotomy was also added.

Since its first description, the procedure has undergone multiple modifications, both anatomic and technical, predominantly because of dissatisfaction with recurrence rates and complications. Many of the Nissen fundoplications done today have little in common with their 1956 predecessor.

MODIFICATIONS

Many surgeons complement the fundoplication with a posterior plication of the diaphragmatic crura, usually accomplished utilizing nonabsorbable sutures to narrow the hiatus such that one fingertip can still be inserted easily through the residual orifice alongside the esophagus. The degree of gastric mobilization can vary from Nissen's original description, in which no short gastric vessels are ligated, to the taking down of a portion or complete mobilization of the vaso-

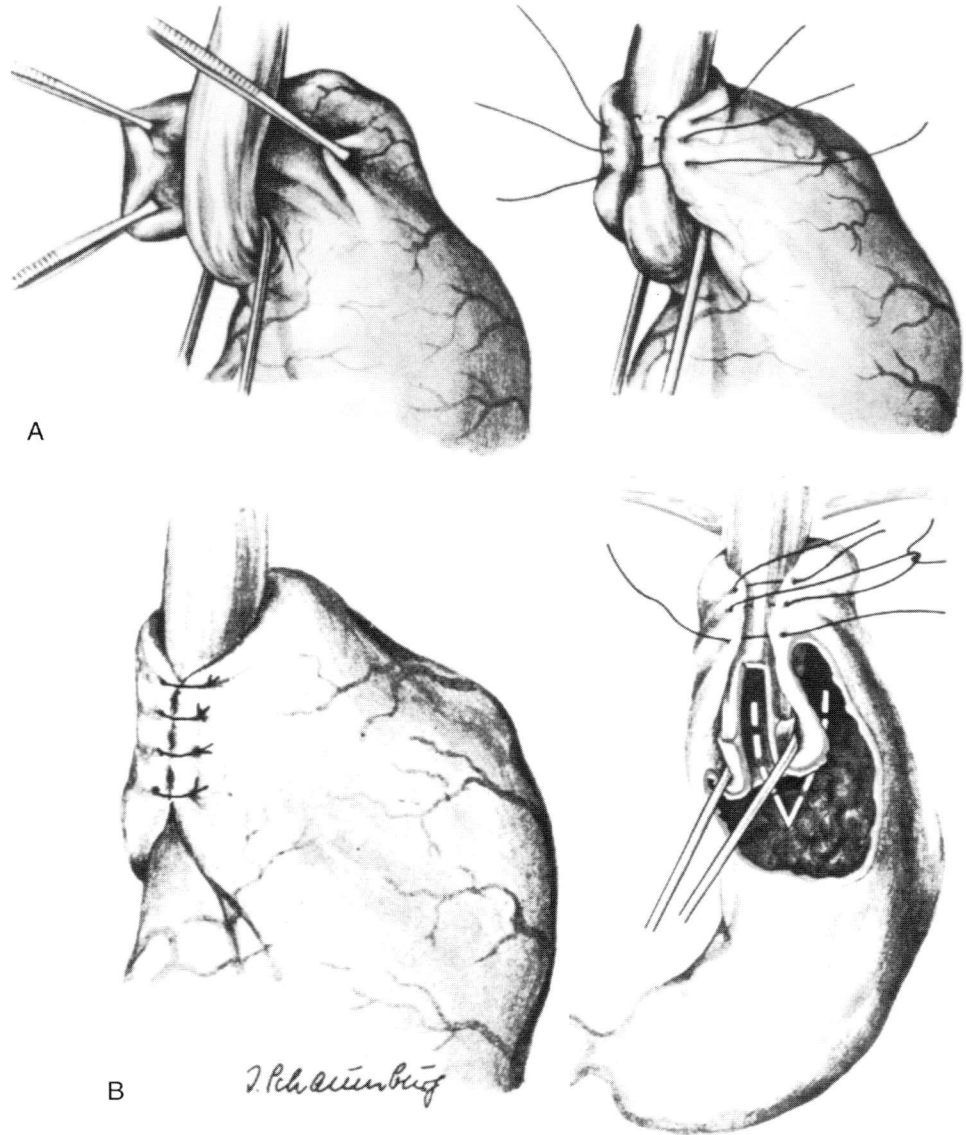

FIGURE 28–8. *A,* Basic technique of fundoplication. After the peritoneal attachment is freed, the cardia is drawn down in a caudad direction. The posterior wall is drawn forward medially to the esophagus, thus invaginating the terminal esophagus. *B,* Sutures are placed 1 to 1.5 cm apart to close the wrap. The two upper sutures include bites of the terminal esophagus as well as the gastric serosa of the anterior and posterior walls of the cardia. A cutaway of the anatomy also is shown. (*A* and *B,* From Nissen, R., and Rossetti, M.: Surgery of the Cardia Ventriculi. Basel, CIBA, 1963, p. 212.)

brevia. The recommendations for stenting the esophagus can vary anywhere from a No. 18 French nasogastric tube to a No. 50 mercury-filled bougie. Predominantly in response to recurrence and the postoperative problem of gas bloat, the fundoplication wrap itself has undergone multiple suggested modifications. Nissen suggested a method of tightening the wrap in the very obese patient by using the anterior rather than the posterior fundic wall to wrap the intra-abdominal esophagus. This is now known as the Rossetti modification of the Nissen fundoplication (Fig. 28–9). Other suggested revisions have included a double plication, an incomplete wrap, and a loose wrap or "floppy Nissen." The length of the fundoplication has varied significantly from 6 cm to studies in the cadaver that suggest that 4 cm is required to avoid reflux. More recently, animal laboratory studies have shown 2 to 3 cm to be adequate. In addition,

DeMeester (1984) recommended a 1.5 cm or single-stitch Nissen. In attempts to ensure the stability of the repair, thereby avoiding migration of the fundoplication, various authors have suggested fixation of the wrap to the right pillar of the diaphragm, the GE junction, and the median arcuate ligament. Both Kaminski and associates (1977) and Cordiano and co-workers (1976) noted improvement in esophageal function as determined by standard acid reflux test with anchoring of the GE junction to the preaortic fascia. Other reported modifications include the additions of vagotomy and pyloroplasty and parietal cell vagotomy in selected patients.

This multitude of operative innovations suggests a potential weakness in critically assessing the success of the procedure. With no gold standard or essential classic method of Nissen fundoplication, each clinical trial must be measured not only by a stated procedure

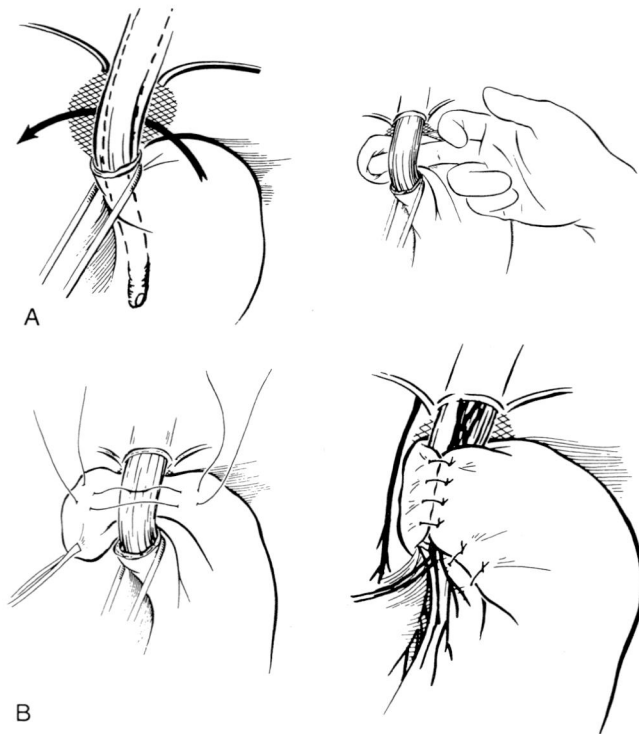

FIGURE 28–9. *A,* Technique of fundoplication. Four to 5 cm of distal esophagus is isolated and surrounded with a rubber tube for downward traction. A large-bore esophageal probe inserted by the anesthetist facilitates the identification of the cardia and prevents fundoplication from being too tight. The fundic wall is gently brought around the esophagus and grasped with an atraumatic clamp. *B,* Seromuscular, nonabsorbable, interrupted sutures are placed across the esophagus from fundic wall to fundic wall. The wall of the esophagus is not included in the sutures, which are tied to unite the gastric wall in front of the esophagus. The cuff of stomach should be loose, easily admitting one finger. (*A* and *B,* From Rossetti, M., and Hell, K.: Fundoplication for the treatment of gastroesophageal reflux in hiatal hernia. World J. Surg., *1*:440, 1977.)

but also by its descriptive account of actual technique.

CLINICAL EVALUATION

Many patients may respond to the newer proton pump inhibitors, but if reflux continues, particularly with respiratory complications, surgery should be considered. Indications for surgical intervention include failure to respond to medical management, stricture, ulcerative esophagitis with bleeding, pulmonary aspiration, and recurring pulmonary problems. The patient with these problems, if a reasonable risk, should be considered for surgical management. Severity of reflux should be assessed objectively with standard acid reflux test; for problem cases with upright reflux, 24-hour pH monitoring should be employed. Because reflux is a common disorder, the indications for operation should be strict. Paradoxically, however, Behar and associates (1975) conducted a prospective clinical trial that suggested that even those patients appropriate for initial medical management benefit

more from operative management. Patients with symptomatic reflux or low-grade esophagitis should be given a trial of medical management.

PATHOPHYSIOLOGY

Experimental and clinical studies have suggested that the Nissen fundoplication has potential for reflux control. The reestablishment of normal lower esophageal pressure is the most often cited mechanism for the Nissen procedure's success in reflux control. More recent investigations have shown that the presence of a musculomucosal flap valve mechanism is more likely responsible for withstanding the heavy pressures exerted against the GE junction than is the lower esophageal sphincter. The reestablishment of this flap valve is most likely responsible for bringing GE reflux under control, contradicting the hypothesis of a simple tightening effect on the lower esophageal sphincter. The presence of a more complicated flap valve mechanism is suggested by the success of various techniques of constructing the fundoplication itself. Most surgeons utilize the 360-degree wrap with variously sized intraesophageal stents in place. This technique is supported by experiments in cats using the repair with varying degrees of plication following a lower esophageal circular myotomy with pre- and postoperative comparison of lower esophageal sphincter (LES) manometry and pH testing. It was shown that a 2- to 3-cm 360-degree wrap was most effective at objectively controlling reflux. Subsequent concern over the postoperative problems of gas bloat and inability to belch and vomit led investigators to attempt repair with lesser degrees of fundoplication. These procedures were not only associated with a decrease in gas bloat but showed maintenance of a good level of reflux control.

The relatively new technique of the *floppy Nissen* involves purposely constructing a loose wrap with a relatively insignificant increase in LES pressure. This effectively controls reflux while limiting postoperative symptoms. This is another good technical demonstration of the importance of a valve mechanism over and above the LES pressure. The floppy Nissen is constructed not only with a No. 50 French dilator within the esophagus but also with a No. 15 Hager dilator external to the esophagus but within the plication. The problem with use of a bougie is that the surgeon has no way of knowing how tight or how loose the wrap is around the bougie. We have seen a number of cases in which the bougie was removed only to have the esophagus close tightly because it was constructed too tightly around the bougie. On the other hand, the wrap may remain wide open after the bougie is removed if it is constructed loosely about the bougie.

More recently, concern has been raised regarding the long-term results of the Nissen repair. Symptomatic and anatomic recurrence have varied from 3% in a small number of cases to 19% in the report of Negre and associates (1983). In the report of Rossetti and Hell (1977), which represents the continuance of the original Nissen procedure, the reported anatomic and symptomatic recurrence was 12.5% in 590 patients. These 590 patients were collected from a series of 1400 patients for a follow-up of less than 50% of patients who underwent surgery. Because over 50% of the patients were lost to follow-up, the validity of the study must be considered. None of the patients in the Rossetti and Hell follow-up underwent an objective test for reflux, and only a small number underwent an upper gastrointestinal (GI) series. An objective determination of the presence or absence of reflux in symptomatic patients is important in determining whether reflux has actually been curtailed.

BACKGROUND AND COMPLICATIONS

It has been suggested that even patients appropriate for initial medical management benefit more from surgery. More recently, a randomized trial of medical vs. surgical management by the Veterans Administration (VA) system in the United States showed that in men with complicated GE reflux disease, surgery is significantly more effective than medical therapy in improving the symptoms and endoscopic signs of esophagitis for up to 2 years, although medical treatment is also effective.

It is noteworthy that the two-stitch Nissen was employed in this study. The complication rate in the 67 patients undergoing surgery was high. The operative and postoperative complications are listed in Table 28–1, and the long-term complications, also very high, are listed in Table 28–2. The incidences of abdominal fullness of 56% and early satiety of 58% are indeed alarming. The fact that the total number of patients with more than one surgical symptom was 81% should be considered unacceptable for an elective surgical procedure.

The most common postoperative complication is the gas bloat syndrome with associated inability to belch or vomit. Reported incidences of some degree of gas bloat range up to 50%, even after 10 years of

■ **Table 28–1.** SURGICAL VS. MEDICAL THERAPY FOR GASTROESOPHAGEAL REFLUX: COMPLICATIONS FOLLOWING NISSEN REPAIR (67 PATIENTS)

Operative Complications (10 Patients: 15%)	Postoperative Complications (12 Patients: 18%)
Splenic injury: 5	Wound dehiscence: 1
Splenectomy: 1	Wound infection: 1
Esophageal perforation: 1	Pulmonary embolism: 1
Gastric perforation: 2	Pleural effusion: 1
Inadvertent vagotomy: 1	Prolonged ileus: 2
Reoperation (3 times): 1	Bleeding/transfusion: 2
	Mediastinal abscess: 1
	Intraperitoneal abcess: 1
Other: 4	

Data from Spechler, S. J., VA GERD Study Group, Department of Veterans Affairs: Comparison of medical and surgical therapy for complicated gastroesophageal reflux disease in veterans. N. Engl. J. Med., 326:786–792, 1992.

■ **Table 28–2.** SURGICAL VS. MEDICAL THERAPY FOR GASTROESOPHAGEAL REFLUX: LONG-TERM COMPLICATIONS FOLLOWING NISSEN REPAIR (67 PATIENTS)

Complication	Percentage of Patients
Abdominal fullness	56
Early satiety	58
Inability to belch	25
Inability to vomit	19
Total with more than 1 surgical symptom	81

Data from Spechler, S. J., VA GERD Study Group, Department of Veterans Affairs: Comparison of medical and surgical therapy for complicated gastroesophageal reflux disease in veterans. N. Engl. J. Med., 326:786–792, 1992.

follow-up. The associated symptoms of this syndrome are abdominal distention, subdiaphragmatic pressure sensations, and hiccups in 25% of patients. Ellis and Crozier (1984) cite dysphagia as the most common reason for reoperation. In many cases, this is secondary to an unidentified motility disorder, diffuse spasm, achalasia, or scleroderma. Immediate dysphagia can occur in up to 50% of patients and is usually transient, and most cases resolve or improve as postoperative edema subsides. A second group of patients, however, continues to have dysphagia over the long term. This complication could be avoided by using intraoperative pressure measurements at the time of surgery to determine how tight or how loose the wrap actually is.

REOPERATION FOR THE FAILED NISSEN OPERATION

The multi-institution study by the VA (Spechler et al., 1992) indicated that gas bloat, dysphagia, early satiety, and dumping syndrome are very common after the Nissen repair. An even more serious problem is the increasing number of reports of reoperation for the failed Nissen procedure: In 1988, the author reported 114 operations for failed Nissen repairs and indicated that this was simply the tip of the iceberg, in that many patients tolerate serious or debilitating postoperative problems before submitting to reoperation (Low et al., 1988). Since that publication, the series has increased to 190 cases. At reoperation, every attempt is made to determine why the operation has failed. The types of failure in the original 114 cases are listed in Table 28–3. An additional failure occurs in patients who hemorrhage. The author now has evaluated six patients who have hemorrhaged from ulcers in the lip of the wrap. Endoscopic appearance of the wrap in these patients suggests that the wrap is edematous and ischemic and subject to ulceration. Attempts to cauterize these ulcerations failed, and the patients developed exsanguinating bleeding.

With the slipped Nissen, the repair, which should be around the GE junction, slips down to the junction of the upper and middle third of the stomach, thereby obstructing the parietal cell mass. The parietal cell

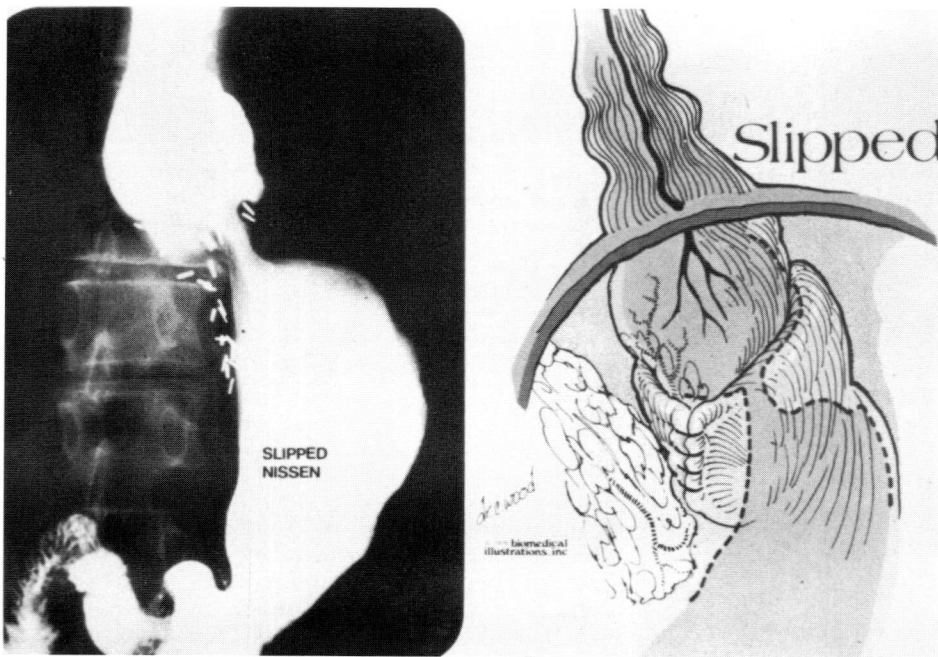

FIGURE 28–10. The slipped Nissen. The classic slipped Nissen shows the Nissen wrap having slipped from the gastroesophageal junction down to the junction of the upper and middle third of the stomach, thereby obstructing the parietal cell mass.

mass is the most potent acid-producing segment of the GI tract, and with obstruction, particularly at night with poor drainage and food retention, increased acid output may produce a variety of gastric ulcers that may go on to perforate and produce fistulas. The classic slipped Nissen is shown in Figure 28–10. The Nissen repair may disrupt partially or completely, producing the same symptom complex as the slipped Nissen. Gastric ulcers may form that penetrate the stomach, the diaphragm, and the lung, as illustrated in Figure 28–11. This patient developed a gastrobronchial fistula into the right lung. A patient with a transthoracic Nissen repair developed a gastric ulcer perforating the stomach and the diaphragm into the left lung. The transthoracic Nissen repair often produces an iatrogenic, thoracic, paraesophageal hernia with all of its complications.

Another serious complication is shown in Figure 28–12. The patient with a slipped Nissen developed a posterior penetrating gastric ulcer that bored into the aorta. A very alert surgeon, Dr. Edwin James, was able to get a clamp on the aorta, evacuate a huge clot, and sew up the aorta and the stomach. This patient is the only survivor of a gastroaortic fistula of whom the author is aware.

An even more serious complication is shown in

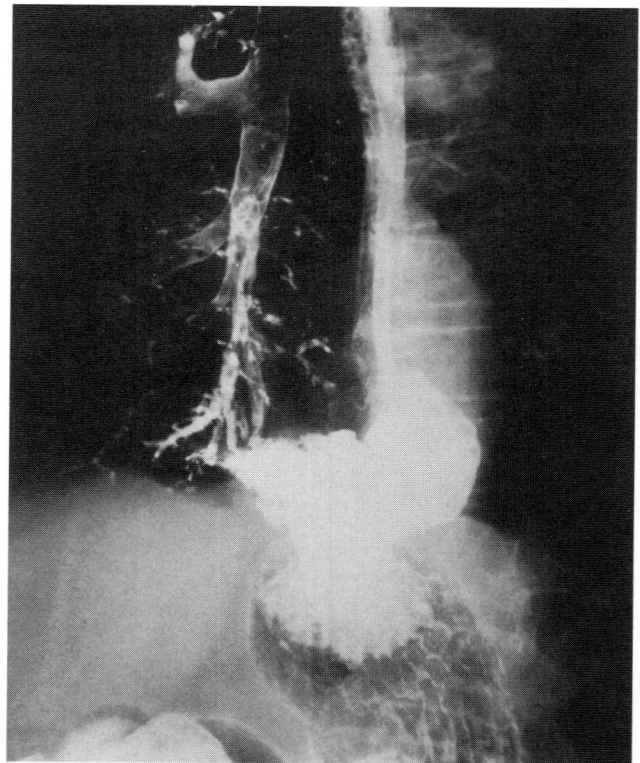

FIGURE 28–11. A gastric ulcer in a slipped Nissen has penetrated the stomach, the diaphragm, and the right lung, creating a gastrobronchial fistula.

■ **Table 28–3.** PREOPERATIVE AND INTRAOPERATIVE CAUSES OF FAILED NISSEN OPERATIONS

Cause of Failure	No. of Patients
Slipped Nissen	56
Patulous repair	24
Complete disruption	18
Partial disruption	15
Obstructed tight repair	2
Gastrobronchial fistula	2
Gastrocutaneous fistula	1
Gastropericardial fistula	1
Gastroaortic fistula	1
Multiple gastric perforations	1
Mucosal intussusception	1

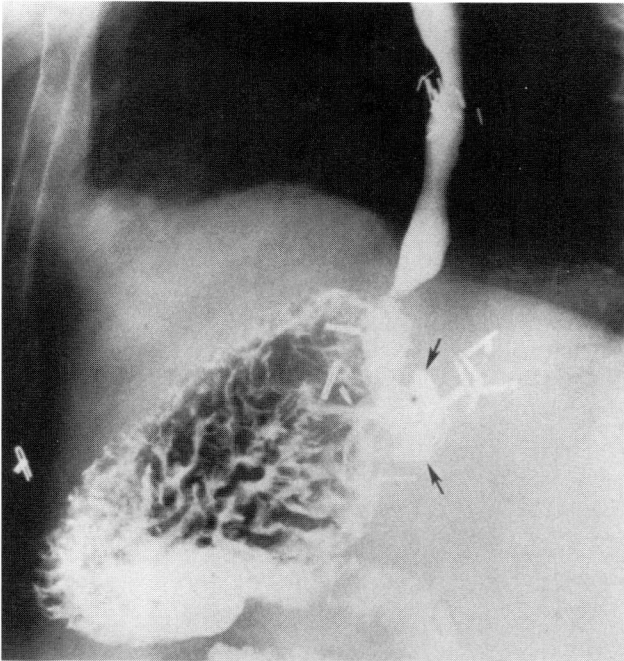

FIGURE 28–12. A slipped Nissen producing a large posterior gastric ulcer that perforated the aorta. Operative correction produced the only known survivor of a gastroaortic fistula.

SURGICAL REPAIR

Most patients underwent a takedown of the wrap with performance of a Hill repair. The fistulas were treated separately, and several cases required either jejunal interposition or resection of the GE junction. The results of reoperation over the long term showed an 83% good-to-excellent result. Some of these patients underwent surgery as many as 4 times and presented a serious technical challenge.

Another troublesome problem reported by several authors is the motility problem that occurs following the Nissen repair. Because the Nissen repair does not anchor the GE junction, the esophagus has no point of attachment or fulcrum from which to generate peristaltic waves to propel food and fluid aborally into the stomach. Consequently, the esophagus may lose its normal motility. Following takedown of the repair and anchoring of the GE junction, the motility returns to normal. Several authors, including Kaminski in the United States and Cordiano in Italy, have indicated that anchoring the Nissen repair to the pre-aortic fascia improved the motility postoperatively and precluded some of the dysphagia.

A MEDLARS search over the last 15 years shows

Figure 28–13. The operative photograph shows a patient who was admitted to the Coronary Care Unit with a diagnosis of myocardial infarction. The electrocardiogram showed diaphragmatic pericarditis. A barium swallow showed barium entering the pericardial sac. The patient was taken to surgery in very poor condition, and a huge gastric ulcer that had penetrated through the stomach, the diaphragm, and the pericardium was noted. The base of the ulcer was the myocardium. In this case of true "heartburn," the patient was in such poor condition that the diaphragm was closed as well as the ulcer, and the wrap was left in place. The patient developed an ulcer that bored along the left gastric pedicle into the liver, requiring reoperation. At reoperation, the left gastric pedicle was ligated in order to close the ulcer. The patient had undergone a *floppy Nissen,* which involves ligation of all of the short gastric vessels down to the antrum. Upon ligation of the left gastric artery, the entire stomach became gangrenous, requiring total gastrectomy. This patient is alive, but has serious GI complications. Another patient of the author's experienced a slipped Nissen, developed a gastropericardial fistula, and survived operation. These are the only two survivors of gastropericardial fistula of whom the author is aware.

Another serious complication is shown in Figure 28–14, which shows an exsanguinating hemorrhage that defied all attempts at curtailment of the bleeding. An ulcer was demonstrated in the edematous, ischemic wrap. In the author's study thus far, six patients have had serious bleeding from ulceration in the wrap.

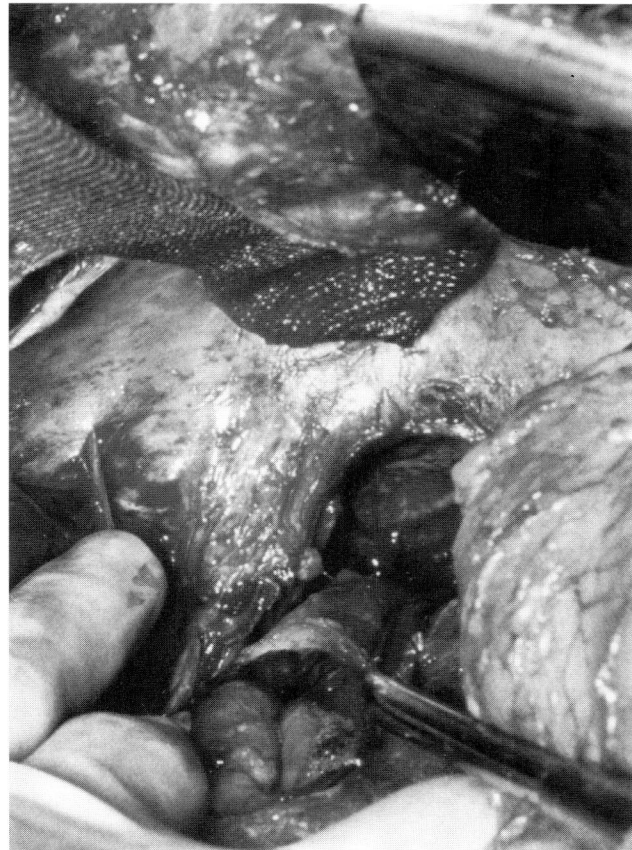

FIGURE 28–13. Surgical picture of a challenging complication of a gastropericardial fistula. A gastric ulcer from a slipped Nissen penetrated the stomach, the diaphragm, and the pericardium; the base of the ulcer was the myocardium. This represents a case of true "heartburn."

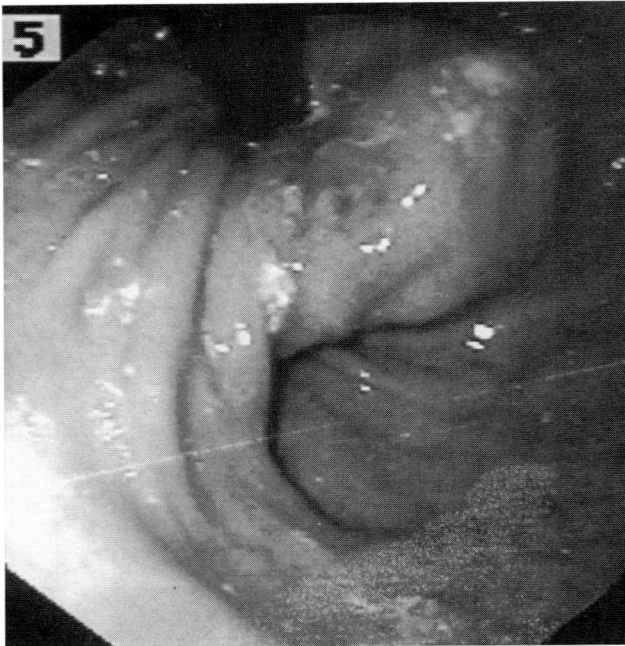

FIGURE 28–14. An ulcer in the edematous, ischemic wrap. This exsanguinating hemorrhage defied all attempts to curtail the bleeding.

an alarming number of serious complications with the Nissen repair, many of which required reoperation.

SUMMARY

The operation first performed by Rudolph Nissen in 1936 is widely used around the world and can effectively prevent reflux. Over the last 20 years, the large number of modifications of the original technique attest to dissatisfaction with the procedure. Despite these modifications, an increasing number of reports of complications and failures of the procedure have appeared. One basic problem with the technique is that it is a blind wrap of the stomach around the lower end of the esophagus with no objective determination of how tight or how loose the wrap might be. In addition, the placement of the wrap depends on sutures in the esophagus. The esophagus is the weakest portion of the GI tract, and the esophageal sutures, therefore, have little strength and may disrupt, leading to slippage. Further, when the wrap slips, it causes obstruction of the parietal cell mass, leading to overproduction of acid and gastric ulcers. These gastric ulcers may lead to bleeding, perforation, and fistula formation. These complications appear to be more common with the Nissen procedure than with any other technique. In fact, most of these complications have been reported only with the Nissen.

Furthermore, the Nissen fundoplication is not generally anchored. The stomach, therefore, may slip up and down and may reenter the thorax. Without a fulcrum, the esophagus cannot generate peristaltic waves strong enough to properly propel food ab-

orally. This accounts for the abnormal esophageal motility following a Nissen fundoplication, which accounts for a good deal of the dysphagia and gas bloat syndrome associated with the Nissen procedure.

In conclusion, the large number of complications and the failure rates with the Nissen repair are alarming. It is obvious that the first operation is the optimal time to do a definitive repair. With modern technology, it does not seem reasonable to use a blind wrap without objective determination of what is being done at operation. The surgeon has ample time to use proper techniques aided with modern technology, and with these newer techniques, the mortality, morbidity, and complication rates of reoperation should be avoidable.

BIBLIOGRAPHY

Alday, E. S., and Goldsmith, H. S.: Efficacy of fundoplication in preventing gastric reflux. Am. J. Surg., 126:322–324, 1973.

Allison, P. R.: Reflux esophagitis, sliding hiatal hernia and anatomy of repair. Surg. Gynecol. Obstet., 92:419–431, 1951.

Bahadorzadeh, K., and Jordan, P. H.: Evaluation of the Nissen fundoplication for treatment of hiatal hernia. Ann. Surg., 181:402–408, 1975.

Behar, J., Sheahan, D. G., Biancani, P., et al.: Medical and surgical management of reflux esophagitis. A 38-month report on a prospective clinical trial. N. Engl. J. Med., 293:263–268, 1975.

Bremner, C. G., and Rabin, M. R.: The Nissen fundoplication operation: Improved technique to prevent complications. In Stipa, S., Belsey, R. H. R., and Moraldi, A. (eds): Medical and Surgical Problems of the Esophagus. New York: Academic Press, 1981, pp. 71–74.

Cordiano, C., Rovere, G. Q. D., Agugiaro, S., and Mazzilli, G.: Technical modifications of the Nissen fundoplication procedure. Surg. Gynecol. Obstet., 143:977–978, 1976.

DeMeester, T. R. (Discussion of Ellis, F. H., and Crozier, R. E.): Reflux control by fundoplication: A clinical and manometric assessment of the Nissen operation. Ann. Thorac. Surg., 38:387–392, 1984.

Donahue, P. E., Samelson, S., Nyhus, L. M., and Bombeck, T.: The floppy Nissen fundoplication. Arch. Surg., 120:663–668, 1985.

Ellis, F. H.: Technique of fundoplication. In Stipa, S., Belsey, R. H. R., and Moraldi, A. (eds): Medical and Surgical Problems of the Esophagus. New York: Academic Press, 1981, p. 65.

Ellis, F. H., and Crozier, R. E.: Reflux control by fundoplication: A clinical and manometric assessment of the Nissen operation. Ann. Thorac. Surg., 38:387–392, 1984.

Guarner, V., Martinez, N., and Gavino, J. F.: Ten-year evaluation of posterior fundoplasty in the treatment of gastroesophageal reflux. Long-term and comparative study of 135 patients. Am. J. Surg., 139:200–203, 1980.

Hoffman, T. H., McDaniel, A., and Polk, H. C.: Slipped Nissen's fundoplication: A stitch in time [letter]. Arch. Surg., 116:1239, 1981.

Jordan, P. H.: Parietal cell vagotomy facilitates fundoplication in the treatment of reflux esophagitis. Surg. Gynecol. Obstet., 147:593–595, 1978.

Kaminski, D. L., Codd, J. E., and Sigmund, C. J.: Evaluation of the use of the median arcuate ligament in fundoplication for reflux esophagitis. Am. J. Surg., 134:724–729, 1977.

Leonardi, H. K., and Ellis, F. H.: Experimental fundoplication: Comparison of results of different techniques. Surgery, 82:514–520, 1977.

Low, D., Mercer, C. D., James, E. C., and Hill, L. D.: Post-Nissen syndrome. Surg. Gynecol. Obstet., 167:1, 1988.

Matikainen, M.: Nissen-Rossetti fundoplication for the treatment of gastroesophageal reflux. Acta Chir. Scand., 148:173–177, 1982.

Matikainen, M., and Kaukinen, L.: The mechanism of Nissen fundoplication. Acta Chir. Scand., 150:653–655, 1984.

Menguy, R.: A modified fundoplication which preserves the ability to belch. Surgery, 84:301–306, 1978.

Negre, J. B., Markkula, H. T., Keyrilainen, O., and Matikainen, M.: Nissen fundoplication: Results at 10 year follow-up. Am. J. Surg., *146*:635–637, 1983.

Nissen, R.: Eine einfache operation zur beeinflussung der refluxo-esophagitis. Schweiz. Med. Wochenschr., *86*:590, 1956.

Polk, H. C., and Zeppa, R.: Hiatal hernia and esophagitis: A survey of indications for operation and technique and results of fundoplication. Ann. Surg., *173*:775–781, 1971.

Rossetti, M., and Hell, K.: Fundoplication for the treatment of gastroesophageal reflux in hiatal hernia. W. J. Surg., *1*:439–444, 1977.

Spechler, S. J., VA GERD Study Group, Department of Veterans Affairs: Comparison of medical and surgical therapy for complicated gastroesophageal reflux disease in veterans. N. Engl. J. Med., *326*:786–792, 1992.

Thor, K., Hill, L. D., Mercer, C. D., and Kozarek, R. A.: Reappraisal of the flap valve mechanism. A study of a new valvuloplasty procedure in cadavers. Acta Chir. Scand., *153*:25–28, 1987.

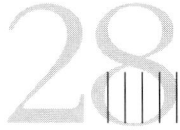

28

■ IV The Hill Repair

Lucius D. Hill and Peter Snopkowski

The Hill repair is an operation designed to restore the function of the antireflux barrier. The normal *gastroesophageal junction* (GEJ) is a highly competent barrier against reflux of gastric contents into the esophagus. With the development of a hiatal hernia, the GEJ slides into the posterior mediastinum and the barrier is lost, causing reflux. Gastroesophageal reflux, with its complications of esophagitis, heartburn, and pneumonitis, is the most common abnormality of the upper gastrointestinal (GI) tract. Despite the frequency of gastroesophageal reflux, the components of the antireflux barrier have been poorly understood until recently. For an antireflux procedure to be effective, the components of the antireflux barrier must be clearly understood.

ANTIREFLUX BARRIER

The antireflux barrier consists of the *gastroesophageal valve* (GEV), the *lower esophageal sphincter* (LES), the diaphragm, posterior fixation of the GEJ, and esophageal clearance. With our ability to measure the *lower esophageal sphincter pressure* (LESP), the GEV has been overlooked. The LES generates a pressure of around 15 to 18 mm Hg in the resting state and can generate pressures up to 100 mg Hg or more, but it is a weak sphincter and cannot alone withstand the large pressures exerted against the GEJ with heavy lifting, straining, and trauma.

The GEV can be viewed easily in the cadaver through a gastrostomy, and in patients through a retroflexed endoscope or a gastrostomy. The GEV has essentially the same structural appearance through a gastrostomy without an endoscope through the valve as it has through the retroflexed endoscope. The valve is created by the angle of entry of the esophagus into the stomach and is an intragastric musculomucosal fold that in the normal subject adheres to the endoscope through all phases of respiration. It opens with

swallowing, belching, and vomiting, and it closes promptly.

In our series using cadavers with no premorbid evidence of hiatal hernia or esophageal disease, we showed a measurable gradient of approximately 15 cm of water across the GEJ. This gradient can be eliminated effectively by depressing the fundus of the stomach 45 degrees. This maneuver causes the angle of His to become obtuse, which eliminates the gastroesophageal flap valve, converts the ostium of the esophagus into a funnel, and causes free reflux. Because there is no LES function in the cadaver, the presence of a gradient across the GEJ and the maneuver of depressing the cardia to eliminate the gradient help confirm the importance of the valve in an in situ preparation. The appearance of the valve through the retroflexed endoscope in 20 normal volunteers without reflux was studied to determine how the normal valve appears.

Thirty-two patients, with and without reflux, were examined with a retroflexed endoscope, and the valves were graded by a gastroenterologist blinded to the clinical status of the patient. From this study, we developed a grading system of the valve (Fig. 28–15).

In a separate gastric laboratory study of 33 patients who underwent both standard acid reflux testing and grading of the GEV, results were shown in terms of prediction of the clinical status of the patient (Table 28–4). It is noteworthy that grading of the GEV predicted the clinical picture in 32 of 33 patients, whereas measurement of the LESP correlated with the clinical picture in only 17. This study showed clearly that grading of the GEV portrays the clinical status more accurately than does measurement of the LESP.

The Grade I valve is a normal valve (Fig. 28–16). It consists of a musculomucosal fold adherent to the endoscope through all phases of respiration; it opens for swallowing and belching and closes promptly. The Grade II GEV is only slightly less well defined and shorter. It opens but closes promptly (Fig. 28–17). The

GRADING OF THE GEV

PATIENTS (N = 32)

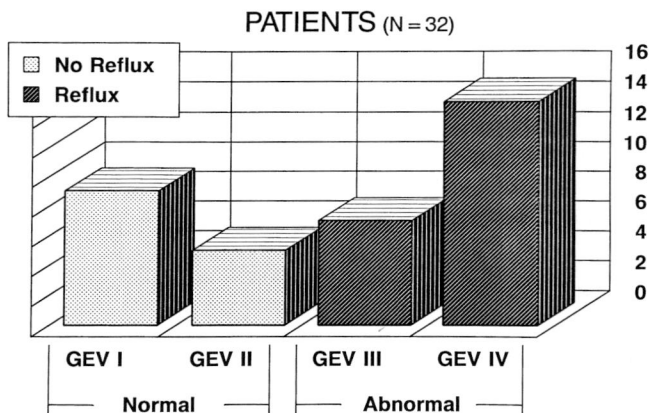

FIGURE 28–15. Grading system of the gastroesophageal valve (GEV) developed from retroflexed endoscopy in 32 patients with and without reflux.

Grade III valve opens frequently, remains open for varying periods, is poorly defined, and often is associated with a hiatal hernia (Fig. 28–18). The Grade IV valve shows no well-defined musculomucosal fold. The esophageal orifice is wide open and is invariably accompanied by a hiatal hernia (Fig. 28–19).

It is noteworthy that in 32 patients with or without a history of varying degrees of reflux, the GEV was graded by gastroenterologists blinded to the clinical status of the patient. No patient with Grade I or II GEV showed reflux, but all patients with Grade III and IV valves showed reflux (Fig. 28–15).

These studies show clearly that the GEV is an important component of the gastroesophageal barrier. The role of surgery, therefore, is to reestablish a normal Grade I, 180-degree valve in a patient who has lost the valve and is therefore suffering from reflux.

■ **Table 28–4.** PREDICTING THE CLINICAL STATUS OF THE GASTROESOPHAGEAL VALVE

No. of Patients	Accurate Prediction Using LESP*	Accurate Prediction Using Grading of GEV*
33	17	32

Key: GEV = gastroesophageal valve; LESP = lower esophageal sphincter pressure.
*Endoscopist was blinded to clinical picture.

In addition to re-creating the valve, calibrating of the LES is important, and it can be done with intraoperative measurement of the sphincter pressure. The relationship of the LES to the valve is shown in Figure 28–20. This computer-generated view shows that the sphincter resides inside the valve and aids the valve in discriminating among gas, liquids, and solids, and the sphincter does the discriminatory work while the valve does the heavy work in terms of preventing reflux. Increased intragastric pressure serves to close the valve against the lesser curve.

Posterior fixation of the GEJ is essential. This is lost when the patient develops a hiatal hernia and the GEJ ascends into the posterior mediastinum. The esophagus can no longer generate propulsive waves that are necessary for esophageal clearance, because the esophagus no longer has a fulcrum or point of fixation from which to work. It should be recalled that the entire GI tract, including the hollow as well as the solid viscera in humans and most vertebrate animals, is suspended by the dorsal mesentery to the posterior body wall. The esophagus is no exception to this rule. Extensive cadaver dissections demonstrate that the esophagus is primarily fixed posteriorly by a dense plate of fibroareolar tissue extending from the median arcuate ligament all the way to the aortic arch. The posterior attachment of the GEJ by the dorsal mesentery to the preaortic fascia is key to

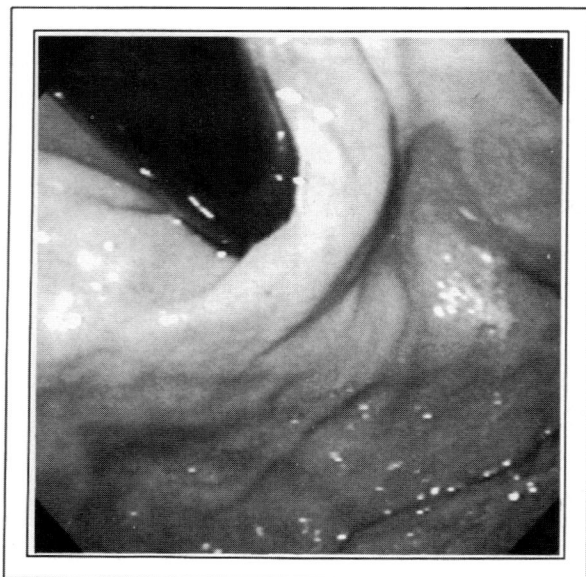

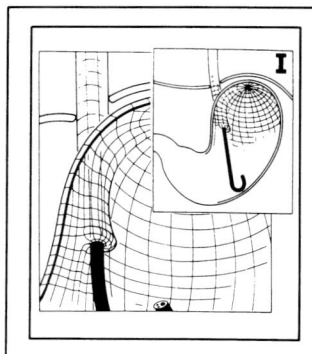

FIGURE 28–16. The Grade I valve is a normal valve. It is a musculomucosal fold that adheres to the retroflexed endoscope through all phases of respiration, and it opens for swallowing but closes promptly.

FIGURE 28–17. A Grade II GEV is slightly less well defined but still opens for swallowing, closes promptly, and does not allow reflux.

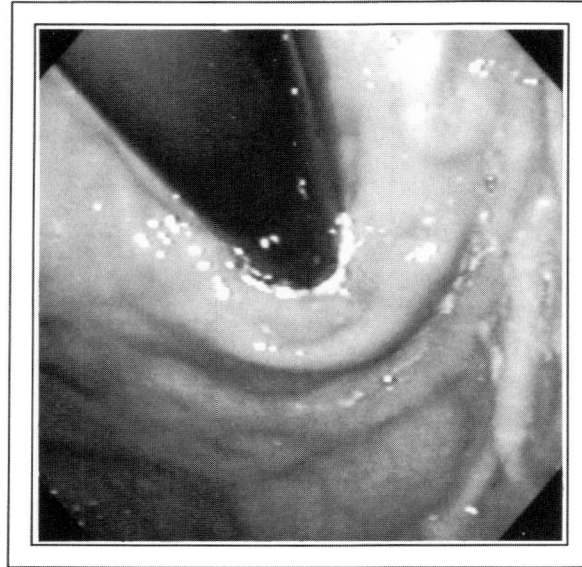

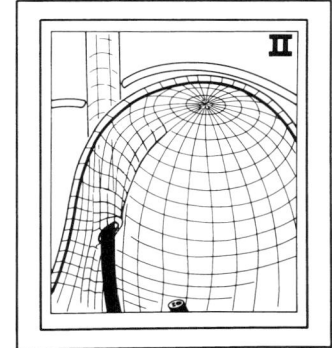

the integrity of the entire barrier to reflux. It has been demonstrated in the cadaver that with division of the posterior attachment, the GEJ slides into the chest, and the effect of the GEV is lost. This is also demonstrated with the retroflexed endoscope in humans. As the GEJ ascends into the posterior mediastinum, the valve is lost, and the sphincter is distracted. Reattachment of the GEJ is therefore important for restoration of esophageal function.

Closure of the enlarged diaphragmatic opening is important to prevent recurrence of hiatal hernia. The diaphragm should be closed loosely about the esophagus so that at least one finger can be placed alongside the esophagus with a nasogastric tube in the lumen. Fixation of the cardia to the rim of the diaphragm also is important to accentuate the valve and to close the opening into the posterior mediastinum

to prevent herniation of the cardia into the posterior mediastinum.

To summarize, the goals of operation are restoration of the GEV, calibration of the LES to the proper range, posterior fixation of the GEJ to restore esophageal peristalsis and clearance, reduction of the hiatal hernia, and closure of the diaphragm.

INDICATIONS FOR SURGICAL MANAGEMENT

Because the symptoms of esophagitis, including heartburn and dysphagia, are so common, it is important that the indications for surgical management remain strict. The important indications for operation are as follows:

FIGURE 28–18. The Grade III valve opens frequently, closes poorly, is poorly defined, and may be associated with a hiatal hernia.

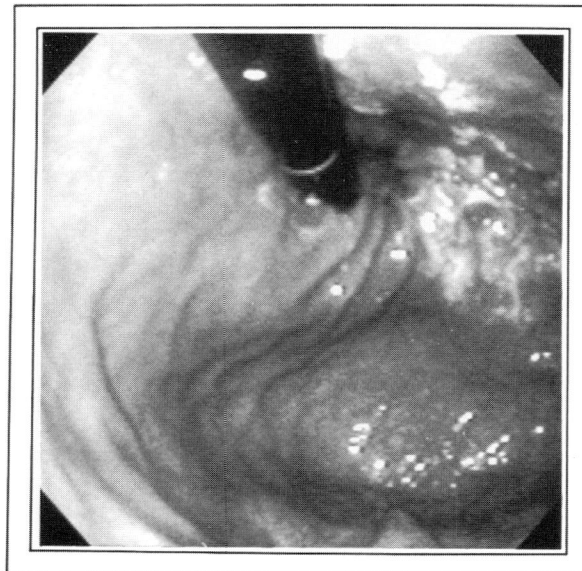

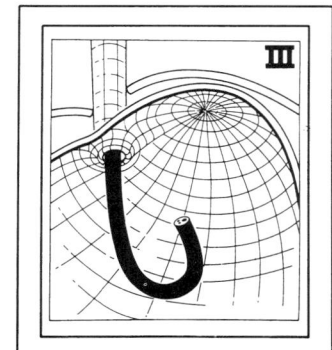

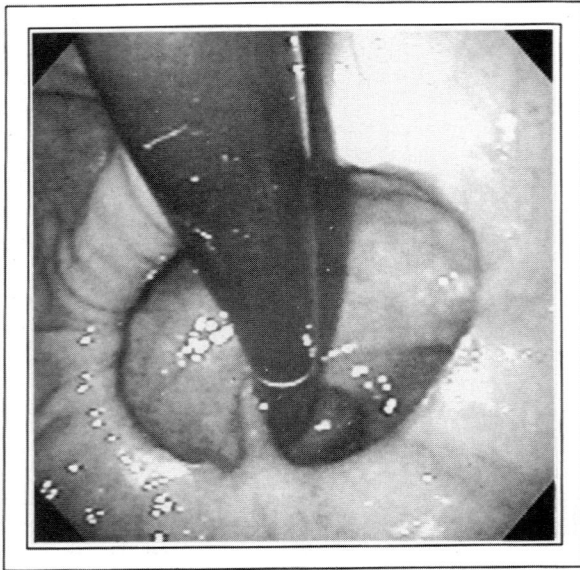

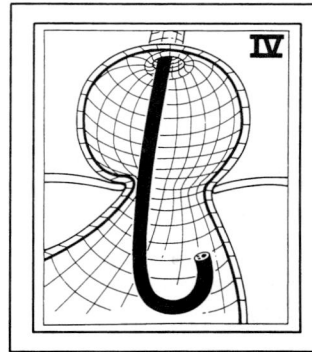

FIGURE 28–19. In patients with a Grade IV valve, there is no definable mucosal fold, the esophagus remains open most of the time it is viewed, and a hiatal hernia is invariably present.

Intractability. The most common indication for operation is failure to respond to medical management, called *intractability*. Medical management should be conducted by a gastroenterologist or internist interested in GI disorders. If this program is ineffective under the guidance of a competent physician, operation should be considered.

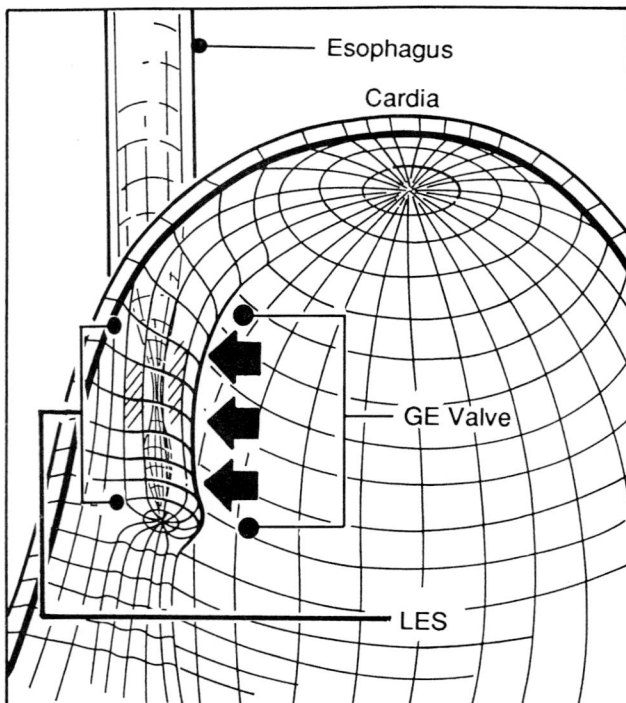

FIGURE 28–20. The relationship of the lower esophageal sphincter (LES) to the gastroesophageal valve (GE Valve). The sphincter resides inside the valve, aids the valve in discriminating among gas, liquid, and solids, and helps prevent reflux. The arrows are pressure vectors demonstrating that increased intragastric pressure closes the valve.

Esophagitis. The features of esophagitis have been outlined clearly by Pope and others, and may vary from edema and erythema of the mucosa accompanied by spasm to severe forms of ulcerative esophagitis with stricture.

Stricture and Ulceration. Approximately 14% of patients in our series have undergone surgery for stricture, and 2.5% have had discrete ulceration with or without stricture. The presence of a stricture usually indicates that refractory esophagitis has been allowed to proceed too long. Bleeding from these ulcers is usually slow and may produce chronic anemia. Perforations into the mediastinum and even into the pericardium have been reported. These complications are rare but indicate that large hiatal hernias are subject to a variety of problems. In addition to peptic ulceration, large hernias may produce pressure on the heart and lungs and create chest discomfort as well as limitation of cardiorespiratory reserve.

Bleeding. Bleeding from the esophagus is usually chronic, producing persistent anemia. Rarely, a tear in the esophagus from severe reflux or penetrating ulceration with submucosal bleeding leads to acute, serious bleeding. Approximately 10% of the patients in our series had chronic anemia.

Respiratory Complications. Larrain and Pope reported an excellent survey of the pulmonary complications of gastroesophageal reflux, which often are overlooked by physicians. A number of patients in our series had received long-term treatment for what was considered asthma. Careful questioning showed that the so-called asthma occurred when the patient was lying down or following episodes of reflux. Even with neutralization of the refluxed material with proton pump inhibitors such as omeprazole (Prilosec), the refluxed material is very damaging to the tracheobronchial tree and the vocal cords. In these individuals, surgical management is rewarding because it not only clears the symptoms of reflux but eliminates the symptoms related to aspiration or overflow into the tracheobronchial tree.

Large Hernias. In a small group of patients with sliding hiatal hernia, operation is required because the hernia is large enough to produce pressure symptoms in the chest with cardiorespiratory embarrassment. In these individuals, episodes of incarceration may cause pain so severe that it is interpreted as a myocardial infarction. In patients with large hernias, in addition to pressure symptoms, trauma to the stomach occurs where the diaphragm impinges on the displaced viscus and can lead to what is called a *callus ulceration* of the gastric mucosa, which may bleed either chronically or acutely.

Barrett's Esophagus. Patients with documented Barrett's esophagus who have progressive and increasing dysplastic changes in Barrett's epithelium while on intensive medical management are candidates for operative reflux control. Studies by Reid and associates, using flow cytometry to correlate genomic instability (diploidy/aneuploidy), have provided additional data to identify patients with Barrett's epithelium who are at increased risk for esophageal cancer. Esophageal reflux currently is the primary factor investigated in the evolution of Barrett's epithelium. Patients who have undergone a successful antireflux procedure have been shown to have regression of Barrett's esophagus after control of reflux. Patients with severe dysplasia should be evaluated by a competent pathologist, and if there is severe dysplasia, the patient may well have carcinoma in situ and is a candidate for resection of Barrett's epithelium.

PREOPERATIVE EVALUATION

Preoperative evaluation of the symptoms of *gastroesophageal reflux disease* (GERD) should identify the presence and severity of reflux and its potential complications while excluding or documenting co-existent problems. Upper gastrointestinal radiographs, although they are the most common initial examination, are somewhat insensitive to reflux. However, they do demonstrate stenosis with its level and length of extension and ulceration, as well as the type of hiatal hernia that is present. Other more objective tests include esophageal manometry with pH studies. These tests are important to establish the level of acid in the stomach, the volume of acid that is refluxing into the esophagus, and the LESP. These studies can be used postoperatively to test the success of the operation. In our laboratory, a sphincter pressure of less than 10 mm Hg suggests sphincter incompetence. A sphincter pressure in the range of 30 mm Hg or more suggests the possibility of a hypertensive sphincter or *super squeeze*. In addition, the standard acid reflux test can demonstrate the motility of the esophagus and the presence of high-pressure, simultaneous waves, which might reflect diffuse spasm.

In our experience, 24-hour pH monitoring is reserved for those patients in whom endoscopy and standard acid reflux testing have not clarified the problem. It can give an impression of the frequency as well as the severity of reflux. This has also enabled us to identify a subpopulation of patients with reflux who show an increased propensity to reflux in the upright position but with little or no reflux in the supine position. Preoperative endoscopy, with or without biopsy, provides valuable information regarding the presence of esophagitis, ulceration, and Barrett's esophagus, and it serves to rule out carcinoma.

Radionuclide studies are another valuable test for the detection of reflux, especially in patients who cannot tolerate or who refuse intubation for the pH and manometric studies. Russell and Velasco, in our laboratory, demonstrated very clearly that radionuclide studies not only can demonstrate reflux but can help discern early achalasia from diffuse spasm as well as other motility disorders and can detect delayed gastric emptying. The Hill repair is being done both by the conventional open technique and by the laparoscopic method.

OPEN TECHNIQUE

The conventional open technique is accomplished through an upper abdominal midline incision, and the abdomen is thoroughly explored. The pylorus in particular is examined carefully for any evidence of pyloric stenosis that might impede gastric emptying. The triangular ligament of the left lobe of the liver is divided so that the left lobe can be retracted to the patient's right. This exposes the esophageal hiatus with its covering phrenoesophageal membrane. An upperhand retractor with two blades is placed to facilitate exposure of the upper abdomen. The phrenoesophageal membrane is divided on the diaphragm (Fig. 28–21), while as much of the fibroareolar tissue that makes up the phrenoesophageal bundles as possible is kept with the GEJ. These bundles normally hold the GEJ in place in the diaphragm, and they are used to anchor the GEJ to the preaortic fascia. The lesser omentum is divided, and the esophageal hiatus is exposed. The esophagus is gently diverted to the patient's left, and the attachment of the cardia to the diaphragm is divided. We are able to accomplish the repair without dividing the short gastric vessels. Only rarely do we need to divide a short gastric vessel, and the dissection must be done with care so as not to damage the spleen. Capsular tears of the spleen may be repaired by cautery or by suturing and applying Avitene. Division of the phrenogastric and superior portions of the gastrosplenic ligament mobilizes the upper part of the gastric fundus, and the fundus can be rotated so that the posterior part of the stomach is visualized, allowing the GEJ to be retracted down and the hiatal hernia to be reduced. The bundles of tissue that constitute the anterior and posterior attachments of the GEJ to the diaphragm, the anterior and posterior phrenoesophageal bundles, can then be displayed. By retracting these caudally, an intra-abdominal segment of esophagus becomes

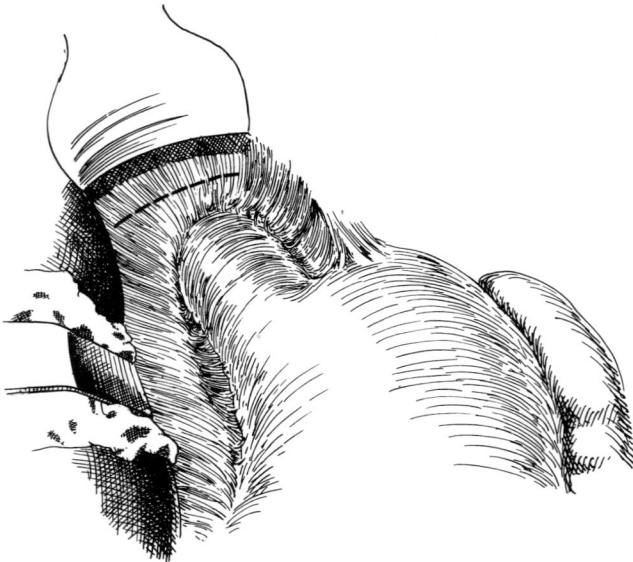

FIGURE 28–21. The phrenoesophageal membrane is divided on the diaphragm to retain the fibroareolar tissue on the stomach to be used in the repair.

visible. The anterior and posterior vagus nerves are visualized and kept in view so as not to be damaged.

Attention is again given to the pylorus. If the pylorus is scarred because the patient has had a duodenal ulcer or if there is a pyloric diaphragm obstructing the outlet of the stomach, a pyloromyotomy or pyloroplasty is planned. These findings should be interpreted in light of the patient's history. If the patient has a history of duodenal ulcer, not only should a pyloroplasty or pyloromyotomy be planned, but a vagotomy to decrease the gastric acid should be added. These findings should be anticipated by careful preoperative evaluation. Preoperative endoscopy should exclude pyloric stenosis or duodenal ulcer. Only if the duodenum is markedly scarred or if there is active ulceration should pyloroplasty and vagotomy be performed. We generally employ a highly selective vagotomy and Jaboulay pyloroplasty. If the pylorus is simply scarred and there is no active ulceration, the pylorus may be dilated and a pyloromyotomy performed. It is imperative to relieve any gastric outlet obstruction to obtain a good result from an antireflux procedure. However, it is unwise to add a vagotomy to a routine hiatal hernia repair; this might lead to complications without benefit to the patient.

Retracting the stomach to the patient's left exposes the preaortic fascia. The aorta and celiac axis are easily felt. The *median arcuate ligament* (MAL) is immediately above the celiac trunk. It can be exposed by careful blunt dissection at this point over the midpoint of the aorta. The celiac artery usually arises cephalad to the median arcuate ligament. When the free edge of the MAL has been exposed, the celiac artery can be compressed into the aorta and the fibroareolar tissue overlying the artery can be carefully divided. An instrument such as a Goodell dilator is passed beneath the MAL. If the instrument is in the correct plane, it should simply float beneath the preaortic fascia. If the instrument meets an obstruction, there may be a branch of the celiac artery in the midline, which may be damaged if force is used on insertion.

Dissection of the celiac axis has been the deterrent to performing this operation, in the opinion of other surgeons. If it is difficult to locate the MAL, and if the surgeon is not familiar with vascular surgery and is uncomfortable dissecting the celiac axis, a safer alternative procedure is recommended.

By retracting the esophagus to the patient's left, the esophageal hiatus can be exposed. The fibroareolar tissue overlying the aorta and the esophageal hiatus can be divided by sharp dissection, thereby exposing the aorta. A finger is passed gently beneath the preaortic fascia, down to the celiac artery, and the preaortic fascia can be lifted off the aorta. The fascia can be grasped with a Babcock clamp, and sutures are simply placed through the preaortic fascia. This is a much simpler and safer approach than dissecting out the celiac artery. In passing the finger behind the fascia, care must be taken not to damage short branches that pass from the aorta to the crura; if one stays in the midline, they can be avoided. This technique was described by Van Sant (Fig. 28–22) and is used by us quite frequently. We find it preferable, and we now rarely dissect the MAL.

The crura of the esophageal hiatus are loosely approximated behind the esophagus with nonabsorbable sutures. The crura are closed so that a finger can be placed alongside the esophagus to make certain that the closure is not too tight.

The stomach is rotated to expose the anterior and posterior phrenoesophageal bundles. The bundles are grasped with Babcock clamps well above the left gastric artery; care is taken not to traumatize the vagal nerves. Strong, nonabsorbable sutures are used for the repair. Sutures are taken through the anterior and posterior phrenoesophageal bundles and are passed through the preaortic fascia, which is lifted well off the aorta with a Babcock clamp. Usually, five sutures are placed in the anterior and posterior phrenoesophageal bundles and carried through the preaortic fascia (Fig. 28–23). These sutures are placed with the vagus nerves in full view so that they are not damaged. A single knot is placed in the top three sutures, which are clamped with long hemostats. Barrier pressure is measured by passing the side hole of the modified nasogastric tube attached to a monitor through the GEJ. If the pressure is above 40 mm Hg, the sutures are loosened, and if it is below 25 mm Hg, they are tightened. After the proper pressure is obtained, all five sutures are tied and a final pressure measurement is taken. The barrier is usually 34 cm in length. Additional cardiodiaphragmatic sutures are taken. The final appearance of the repair is shown in Figure 28–24. Besides the sphincter's being restored, the GEV is accentuated and can be readily palpated through the wall of the stomach. The valve measures from 34 cm along the lesser curve and is important

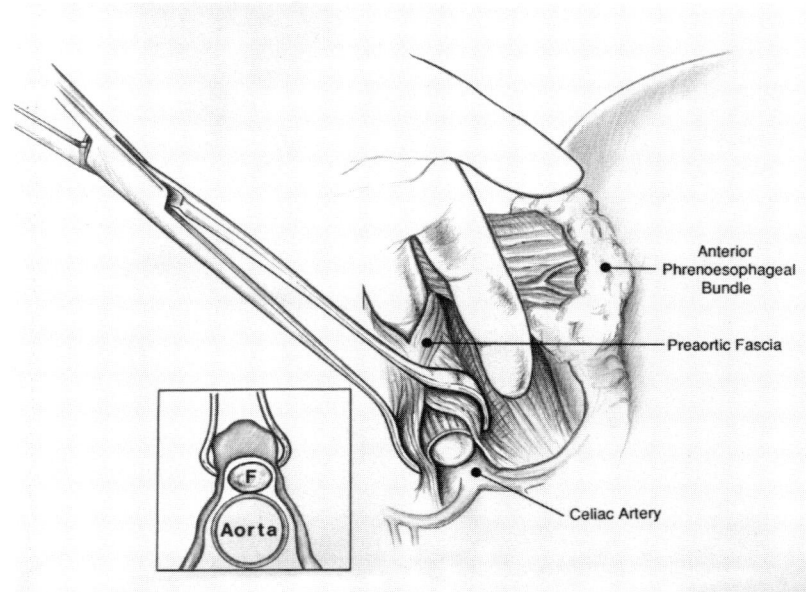

FIGURE 28–22. The fibroareolar tissue in the esophageal hiatus is divided, and a finger (F) is passed down posterior to the preaortic fascia, after which sutures may be placed in the preaortic fascia without dissecting out the median arcuate ligament. The preaortic fascia is lifted off the aorta with a Babcock stay suture.

in the prevention of reflux. In patients who have had previous operations with scarring and destruction of the GEJ, the valve may be destroyed or inadequate. In these cases, a gastrostomy is performed, and the valve is secured with sutures in the anterior and posterior edges of the valve, thereby lengthening the valve to 34 cm. Attempts to calibrate the cardia with a bougie are unsatisfactory, because it is impossible

to determine whether the wrap around the bougie is too tight or too loose.

INTRAOPERATIVE MANOMETRY

In 1977, our group first reported the use of a simplified method of measuring the pressure in the antire-

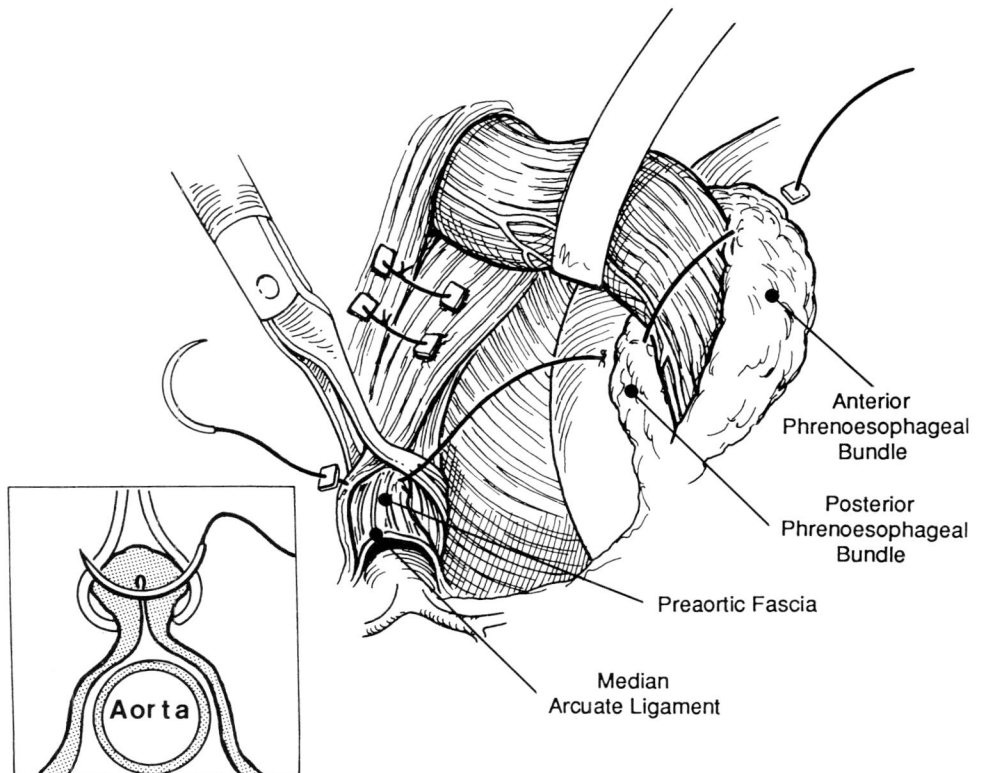

FIGURE 28–23. The hiatus is closed loosely around the esophagus, and sutures are commenced in the anterior and posterior phrenoesophageal bundles and carried through the preaortic fascia. The median arcuate ligament is not dissected out. Four such sutures are placed, and the top suture is tied with a single throw and a knot to allow for pressure measurements and alteration of the sutures according to the pressure obtained.

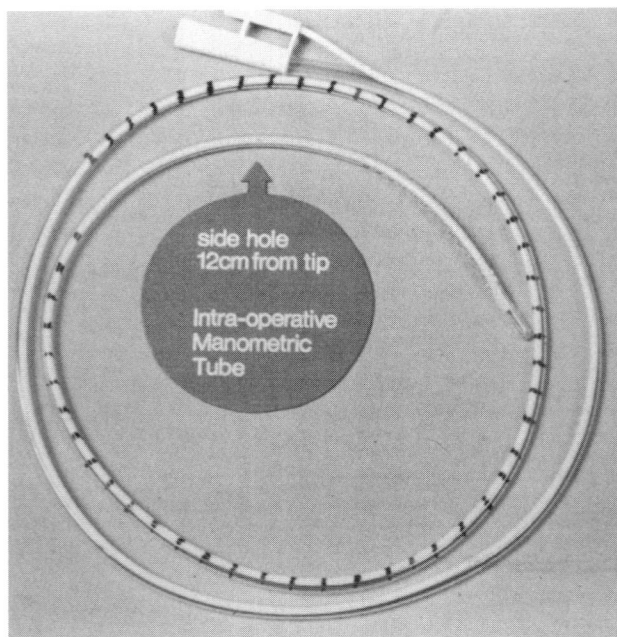

FIGURE 28–24. Modified nasogastric tube with a side hole that can be passed back and forth across the lower esophageal sphincter during surgery to determine the appropriate barrier pressure.

flux barrier during operation to objectively determine the pressure that has been created. This measurement is obtained by modifying the nasogastric tube that is routinely used in these patients. The tip of the smaller silastic sump portion of the tube is sealed at the end, and a 1-mm side hole is cut 18 cm from the tip of the tube (Fig. 28–25). This small silastic tube is attached to a strain gauge and to a manometer that produces a digital reading. If this manometer is not available, the pressure tube can simply be attached to the arterial line that the anesthesiologist has available. The tube is constantly perfused at a slow rate (0.7 ml/min). This apparatus is identical to the one that has been used in the gastric laboratory for over a decade and has been thoroughly standardized and used in over 19,000 patients at our institution. The side hole is passed across the GEJ at operation, and a baseline pressure is obtained prior to repair. Most often, there is no pressure whatever in the GEJ. As the side hole passes through the junction, both a tracing and a digital readout are obtained. After the repair, if the pressure is over 40 mm Hg, the sutures that have been placed are loosened. If the pressure is less than 20 mm Hg, the sutures are tightened. This process is continued until a pressure of between 25 and 35 mm Hg is obtained. The side hole must be pulled at a steady rate through the barrier. If it is pulled through too rapidly, a peak pressure may be missed.

In the repair of recurrent hernias, there is no doubt that intraoperative pressure measurement could prevent some of the disastrous complications of the Nissen procedure that occur when the wrap is either too loose or too tight. Further efforts to simplify intraoperative manometrics and to make the technique more

readily available are underway. The present technique is safe and simple, and it requires only a few minutes to obtain valuable information. It is our opinion that in a major antireflux operation so dependent on the construction of an adequate barrier, intraoperative assessment of the barrier should become a standard part of any technique.

It is important to point out that the Hill repair is not a fundoplication. The phrenoesophageal bundles are imbricated together, and there is no wrap of stomach around the lower esophagus. Very often this operation is described erroneously as partial fundoplication or a wrap. There is no intention on the part of the authors of this procedure to do a blind wraparound of the stomach, but rather a careful calibration of the antireflux barrier, restoration of the GEV, and posterior fixation of the GEJ. There is no wrap to slip. The basic differences between the gastroesophageal restoration repair and the Nissen repair are as follows:

1. The Hill procedure depends on augmentation of the intrinsic pressure and its special features. By placing tension on the collarsling musculature, the repair automatically restores the GEV, which has been shown to be important in the prevention of reflux. The Nissen repair depends on extrinsic pressure of a wrap around the lower esophagus with indirect pressure on the lower esophagus.

2. The Hill procedure anchors the GEJ posteriorly to its normal primary attachment, the preaortic fascia. The Nissen repair is allowed to float freely, and the

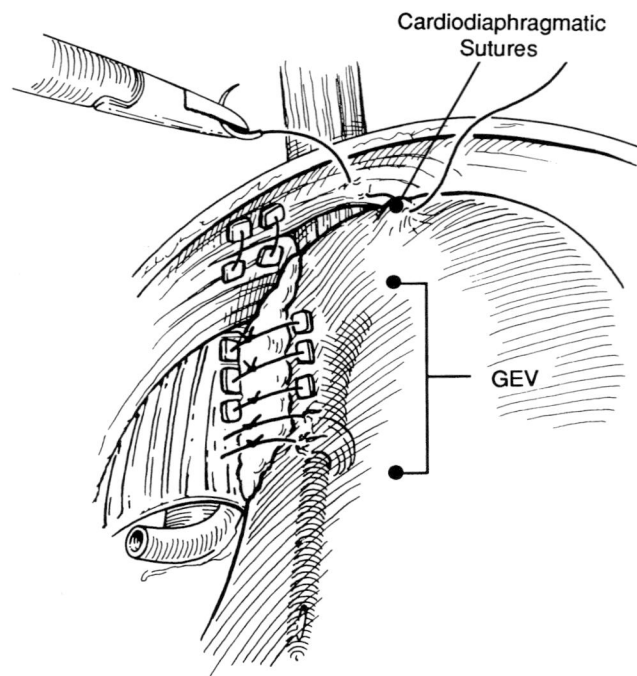

FIGURE 28–25. The final appearance of the repair. All four to five sutures are tied, anchoring the gastroesophageal junction to the preaortic fascia. If the procedure is done open, the gastroesophageal valve (*GEV*) can be palpated. If it is done closed, endoscopy is used to check the valve. Cardiodiaphragmatic sutures are placed to prevent herniation back into the posterior mediastinum.

GEJ is not anchored. The unanchored esophagus has no fulcrum from which to operate and almost always develops dysmotility, because the esophagus cannot generate propulsive waves.

3. In the Hill procedure, no sutures into the esophagus are used because the esophagus has no serosa and no strength. The Nissen procedure employs esophageal sutures to hold the wrap in place. The weakness of these sutures accounts for the frequency of the slipped Nissen. If these sutures are taken deeply, there is a risk of fistula formation from the esophagus.

4. In the Hill procedure, intraoperative pressure measurement is used to calibrate the barrier created at operation, giving an objective assessment of the competence of the reflux barrier. This should be used in all repairs—the Hill, the Belsey, or the Nissen. In the Nissen procedure, the surgeon relies on a bougie or a finger placed up into the esophageal lumen. We have seen a number of patients in whom a large bougie was used, and as soon as the bougie was removed, the wrap, which was made too tight, simply closed down, or the wrap that was made loosely remained open after removal of the bougie.

LAPAROSCOPIC TECHNIQUE

The laparoscopic technique is basically the same as the open technique except that an abdominal incision is not made, pneumoperitoneum is used, and the instruments are designed for working through trocars. The operation is performed through six 10-mm ports. Pneumoperitoneum is established, and the abdominal cavity is inflated with carbon dioxide to a pressure of 14 to 15 mm Hg. A 30-degree, 10-mm laparoscope (forward oblique) connected to a video camera is used. Trocars and retractors are introduced under direct vision (Fig. 28–26). The phrenoesophageal membrane is incised close to its diaphragmatic origin over the esophageal hiatus, thereby retaining the phrenoesophageal bundles on the stomach. These bundles of tissue represent the aggregate of fibroareolar tissue that normally holds the GEJ in the diaphragm, and they represent a strong aggregate of tissue suitable for holding the GEJ to the preaortic fascia. The diaphragm and the preaortic fascia are exposed, and the crura are closed loosely around the esophagus. Four repair sutures are placed through the anterior and posterior phrenoesophageal bundles and the preaortic fascia and tied with a single throw in the knot with a knot pusher. After all repair sutures have been placed, the first or uppermost suture is tied with a single throw in the knot, which is held in place by a knot pusher. This maneuver approximates the phrenoesophageal bundles to the preaortic fascia and places tension on the cardia. Intraoperative pressure measurements are then performed by adjusting suture tension, and an intraluminal pressure of about 25 to 30 mm Hg is developed. It should be remembered that the 15-mm pressure of the pneumoperitoneum should be added to the intraluminal pressure.

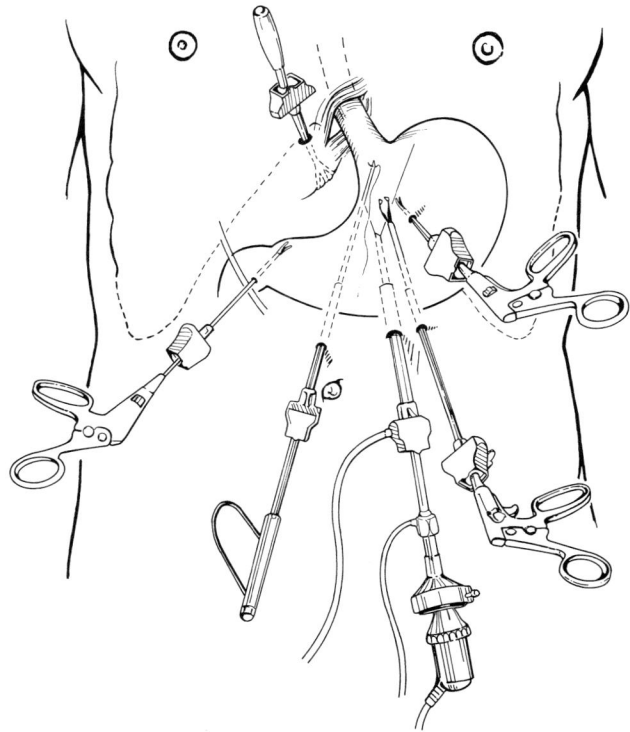

FIGURE 28–26. For the laparoscopic repair, six trocars are placed as shown. Five of these are 10-mm trocars; one is a 5-mm trocar.

This has been shown to produce a postoperative pressure of approximately 18 to 25 mm Hg, which is ideal. An intraoperative pressure of less than 12 mm Hg may be insufficient to prevent reflux. This method of measuring the barrier pressure is identical to that used daily in the GI laboratory. At this point, intraoperative endoscopy is performed to ensure the creation of a GEV Grade I. This type of valve shows a well-defined musculomucosal fold as viewed through the retroflexed endoscope. The musculomucosal fold is tightly apposed to the endoscope through all phases of respiration and measures 34 cm in length. When the desired suture tension is reached and the GEV Grade I has been achieved, all sutures are tied. The GEV is further accentuated by placing three or more additional sutures from the seromuscular layer of the gastric fundus to the edge of the crura of the esophageal hiatus. After final inspection, a second reading of the barrier pressure is obtained, which usually is very close to the first reading. The trocars are removed under direct visual control, and all wounds are closed.

PEPTIC ESOPHAGEAL STRICTURE

Surgical management of peptic strictures has been surrounded by controversy, much of which arose from a very unfortunate statement made by Norman Barrett in 1950 to the effect that "any portion of the gullet lined by columnar epithelium must be stomach." He presented the hypothesis that columnar epithelium above the diaphragm represented congenital shortening of the esophagus with an attenuated intrathoracic stomach. This concept persisted despite the fact that Allison and Johnstone, a short time later, described the columnar epithelium-lined esophagus and stated that the tubular portion of the gullet, even though lined with columnar epithelium above the diaphragm, was indeed esophagus. Motility studies have proved that the portion of the gullet between the stricture and the stomach has all of the manometric characteristics of the esophagus. This is an important concept, because the decision for or against resection of strictures rests on whether or not the esophagus is indeed shortened. In 1970, we reported our experience with 37 patients with advanced stricture treated with a simplified antireflux procedure. Following successful antireflux procedures, these strictures and ulcers opened up with surprising rapidity. Dilatation was done at operation and was required in less than half of the patients postoperatively. A representative patient in the reported series had a stricture of the midesophagus with a deep penetrating ulcer (Fig. 28–27). She had been unable to swallow solid food for 3 years and had been told she had an undilatable stricture with a short esophagus. At operation, the esophagus was straightened and the tortuousity eliminated, whereupon bougies could be passed and the stricture dilated. An antireflux procedure was performed, and 3 weeks post operation, a repeat upper gastrointestinal film showed the stricture to be open (Fig. 28–28). This procedure was done in 1970, and the patient remains well, swallows all solid food, and now has normal upper GI series results. A postoperative film of a 14-year-old patient who underwent surgery for a severe stricture is shown in Figure 28–29. A simplified antireflux procedure was performed, but the valve was not re-created and the sphincter pressure was not elevated sufficiently. At reoperation, the GEV was re-created and the LESP was raised to a level of 25 mm Hg, whereupon reflux was corrected and the stricture healed (Fig. 28–30). This case illustrates the very close relationship between correction of reflux and relief of stricture.

A later evaluation of strictures by Mercer and Hill (1986) reviewed a 20-year experience involving 160 patients undergoing antireflux operations with dilatation for peptic esophageal stricture. The mean follow-up was 47 months (range 6 to 240). One hundred seven patients who underwent surgery early in the course of the disease had the best results (90% good, 9% fair, 1% poor). The results of 31 patients who had undergone a previous failed operation were 52% good, 23% fair, and 26% poor. Twenty-two patients had multiple dilatations, and their antireflux procedures yielded 45% good, 23% fair, and 32% poor results. Intraoperative manometry improved results ($p < 0.05$), and postoperative reflux worsened the results. The postoperative LESP in patients without reflux was 17.7 ± 1.3 mm Hg, which was higher than the pressure in patients with reflux (8.9 ± 0.8 mm Hg). This review indicated that a conservative antire-

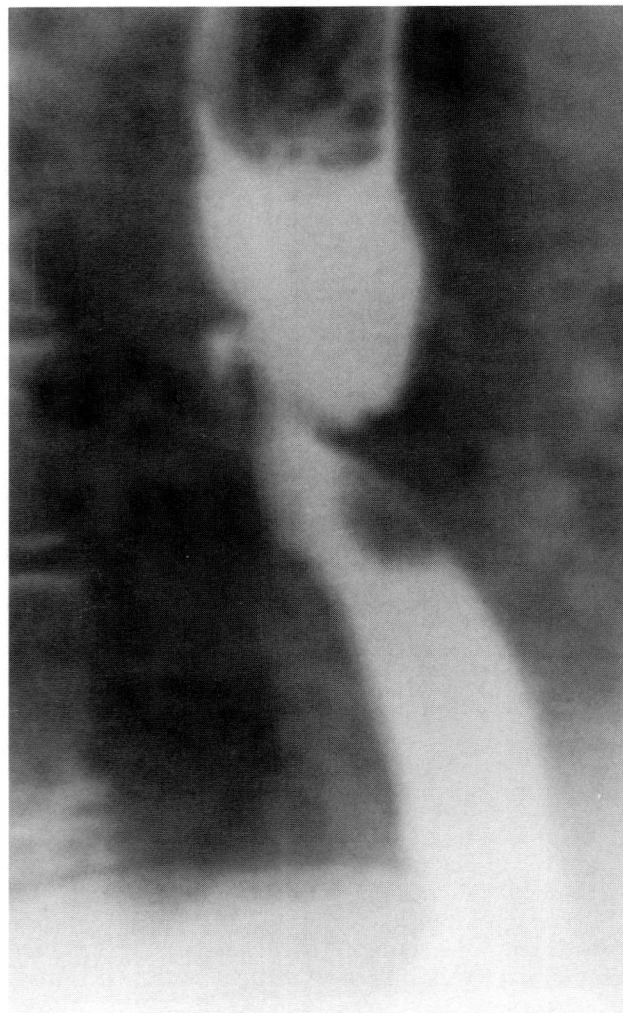

FIGURE 28–27. A stricture with a very narrow lumen and a deep penetrating ulcer. This was considered an undilatable stricture in a short esophagus. The patient was treated with a simplified antireflux procedure.

flux operation with dilatation is the treatment of choice in peptic esophageal strictures. Expansion of the series to over 200 patients has further confirmed these observations. In patients who have undergone multiple previous operations or multiple dilatations in whom transmural damage and fibrosis of the esophagus has destroyed the function of the esophagus, resection with either stomach or colon interposition is the only choice.

The manometric and pathologic composite studies show that strictures occur at the squamocolumnar junction, but the GEJ may be just above the diaphragm and can be reduced in these cases unless there have been multiple operations or multiple dilatations with perforations that have destroyed the esophagus.

When there is columnar lining of the esophagus, careful endoscopy with multiple biopsies must be done to make certain that neither Barrett's esophagus nor frank carcinoma is present. If Barrett's specialized

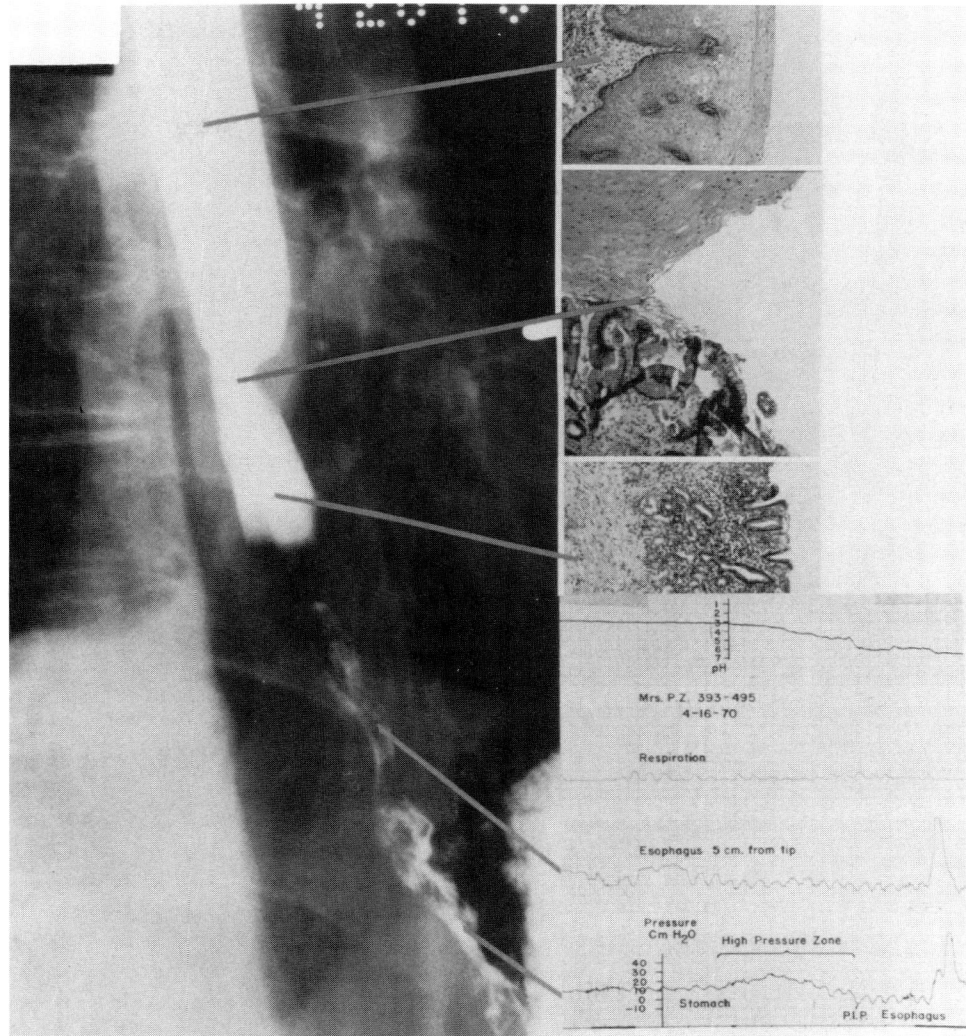

FIGURE 28–28. A composite postoperative study of the patient from Figure 28–26 3 weeks following surgery. The previous stricture has been dilated, and an antireflux procedure has been done. The reflux has been corrected as evidenced by the pH and pressure study, and the stricture has opened up. The patient remained well 18 years after operation.

metaplastic epithelium is present and if there is any doubt about whether a premalignant lesion is present, experienced pathologists are needed to make a careful analysis using flow cytometry. If specialized epithelium is accompanied by severe dysplasia with multiple sites of aneuploidy on flow cytometry, the patient should be considered for resection. As Haggitt and Reid have indicated, microinvasive carcinoma or frank carcinoma is already present in a number of these patients with severe dysplasia.

Following successful antireflux surgery, these strictures open up with surprising rapidity, and we are now seeing replacement of columnar epithelium by squamous epithelium in patients who have been followed for 3 to 5 years or more.

RESULTS

The most important criterion of success is patient satisfaction. If a patient is free of heartburn, can eat a full meal, can resume normal activity, and can be productive, the operation should be considered a suc-

cess. We also have employed a meticulous follow-up using pH and pressure studies 2 to 3 months after operation whenever possible.

Numerous series have appeared throughout the literature examining the relatively short-term success of the currently popular antireflux operations, the Nissen and the Belsey. We have performed three major retrospective studies of the long-term effect of surgical treatment with the Hill repair in more than 2000 patients undergoing surgery over a 25-year period. The results are summarized as follows: Excellent or good results have been obtained in over 94% with a recurrence rate of around 5%. The complication and mortality rates have been very low at 2.5% with one death in the last 600 operations for primary repair.

Our study of a 15- to 20-year follow-up of 167 patients, with an average follow-up of 17.8 years, is the only long-term study that includes evaluation of surgical therapy at an early stage and a general reassessment of the same population over a 20-year period. This study showed a good to excellent result in 88% of patients, and it is noteworthy that these procedures were done before intraoperative mano-

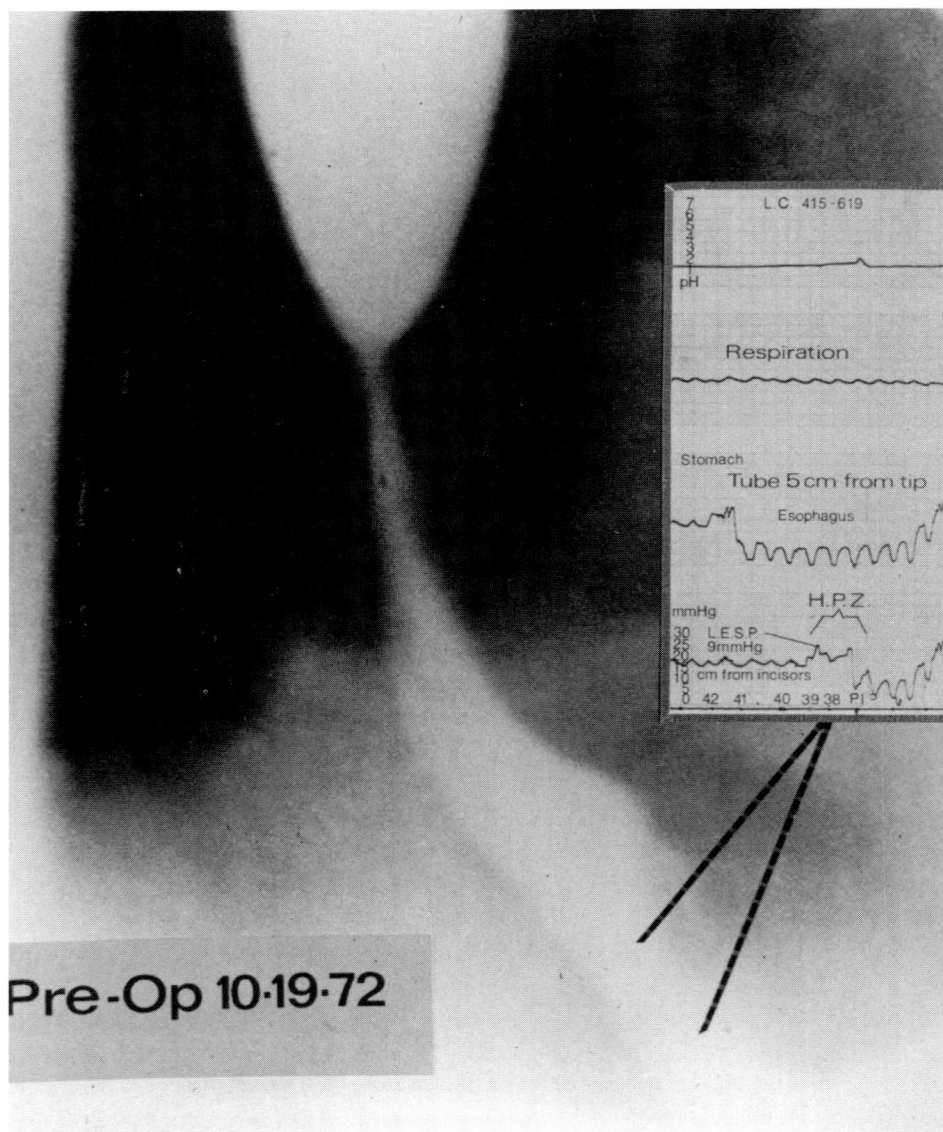

FIGURE 28–29. A 16-year-old male who underwent a simplified antireflux procedure for a very tight midesophageal stricture. The sphincter pressure was raised to only 9 mm Hg, which is inadequate, and reflux was not corrected. The stricture persisted.

metrics were in use. A more recent study of 115 patients followed up to 8 years while intraoperative pressure measurements and other technologic advances were available showed good to excellent results in 96% of patients. This study was conducted by an ophthalmologist who was far removed from GI surgery, so that the study might be unbiased.

The main complication in the last 500 patients has been dysphagia requiring esophageal dilatation. Adjustments in the intraoperative manometrics and, more recently, raising the level of the intraoperative pressure in the antireflux barrier to only 25 to 35 mm Hg have nearly eliminated the need for postoperative dilatation. Early in our experience, we encountered four fistulas that followed deep biopsy in the esophagus prior to operation. If a biopsy of the lower esophagus is required to exclude carcinoma or Barrett's esophagus, we wait at least 2 weeks to allow the biopsy to heal before performing an antireflux operation. Only one fistula occurred in a primary repair;

the others occurred in patients who had undergone previous operations. We have not encountered the devastating gastrobronchial, gastroaortic, gastropericardial, and gastrocutaneous fistulas, nor the severe gas bloat and other complications, that have been seen with the slipped Nissen procedure.

REPRODUCIBILITY

For an operation to be of value, it should be reproducible by others with good results. The Hill repair has been performed and reported by a number of surgeons around the world: Csendes and Larrain in Chile; Hermreck and Coates in the United States; Thomas, Van Sant, Warshaw, Ottinger, and Mercer in Canada; and Russell in Australia, to name a few. Csendes and Larrain achieved a 93% good result and no radiologic recurrence in 29 patients followed up to 16 months. Mercer has performed the Hill proce-

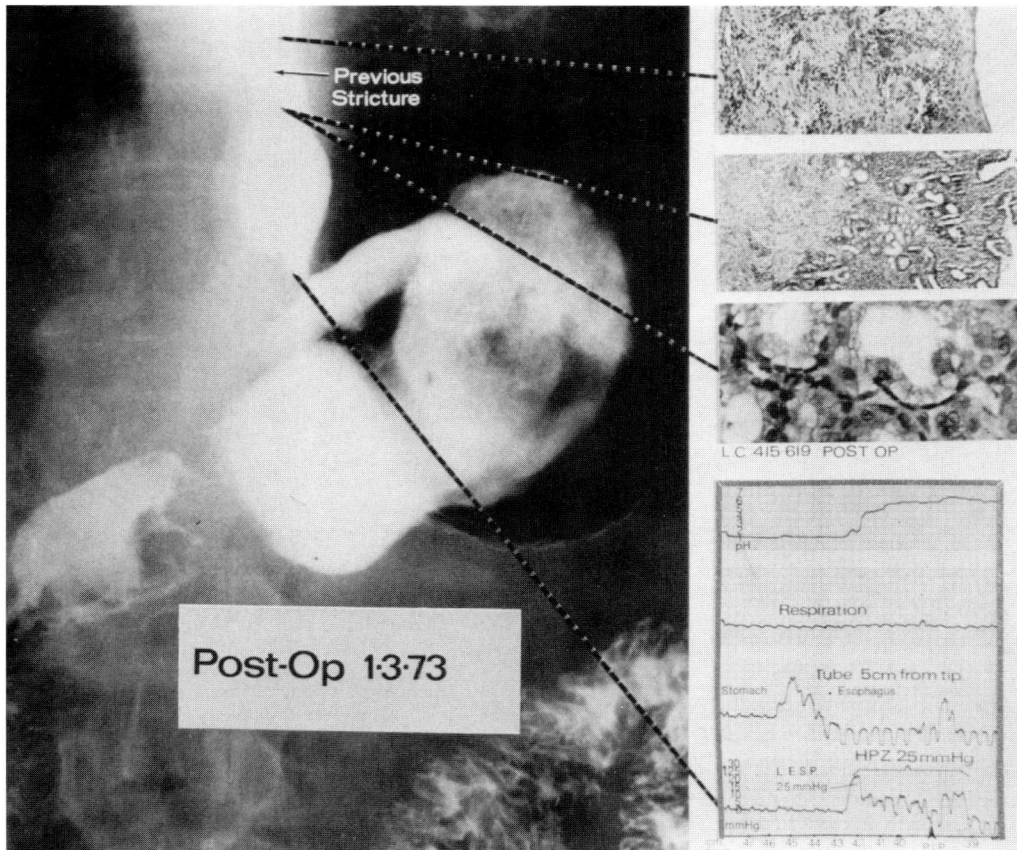

FIGURE 28–30. The patient from Figure 28–29 underwent reoperation, and the barrier pressure was raised to 25 mm Hg. Reflux was corrected as demonstrated on the pH tracing with the previous stricture healed. The patient remained well 15 years after the operation.

dure in 110 patients with 95% good results. Van Sant and associates have reported treating up to 400 patients with around 90% good results. A multi-institution study is underway that includes approximately 2500 patients, and the analysis thus far appears to yield a 90% good result over the long term without the complications reported with the Nissen procedure.

SUMMARY

In summary, the Hill procedure includes reconstruction of the normal GEJ and restoration of the GEV, restoring the esophagus to its normal point of attachment or fulcrum, and allowing it to generate forceful peristaltic waves to propel food aborally into the stomach. In short, esophageal motility is restored. The sphincter is calibrated and the pressure is measured so that a range of pressure is created that is high enough to prevent reflux but not so high as to create dysphagia. The GEV is restored, and the diaphragm is closed loosely about the esophagus. With careful selection of patients and careful performance of the procedure, good results can be obtained over the long term.

SELECTED BIBLIOGRAPHY

Hill, L. D., Aye, R. W., and Ramel, S.: Antireflux surgery: A surgeon's look. Gastroenterol. Clin. North Am., 19:745–775, 1990.

Excellent review of the present status of antireflux surgery.

Larrain, A., and Pope, C. E.: Respiratory complications of gastroesophageal reflux. In Hill, L. D., Kozarek, R., McCallum, R., and Mercer, C. D. (eds): The Esophagus: Medical and Surgical Management. Philadelphia, W. B. Saunders, 1988, pp. 70–77.

Respiratory complications account for a large portion of the gastroesophageal reflux problem. This is an important review of that complication.

Low, D. E., Anderson, R. P., Ilves, R., et al.: Fifteen- to twenty-year results after the Hill antireflux operation. J. Thorac. Cardiovasc. Surg., 98:444–450, 1989.

This study is the longest follow-up of antireflux surgery to be published. There was a mean follow-up of 17.5 years, and the results are excellent considering the fact that these patients were among the early patients to undergo this technique and surgeons were low on the learning curve, and the operations were done before the availability of new technology, including measurement of sphincter pressures.

Low, D. E., Mercer, C. D., James, E. C., and Hill, L. D.: Post Nissen syndrome. Surg. Gynecol. Obstet., 167:1–5, 1988.

This review presents the largest series of post-Nissen problems from any institution in the world. It is an excellent survey of the serious problems seen all too frequently with the Nissen procedure.

Mercer, C. D., and Hill, L. D.: Surgical management of peptic esophageal stricture. J. Thorac. Cardiovasc. Surg., 91:371–378, 1986.

This important article demonstrates clearly that a simplified antireflux procedure corrects most cases of peptic esophageal stricture. Resection is reserved only for those patients whose esophagus is destroyed.

Reid, B. J., Haggitt, R. C., and Rubin, C. E.: Barrett's esophagus and esophageal adenocarcinoma. *In* Hill, L. D., Kozarek, R., McCallum, R., and Mercer, C. D. (eds): The Esophagus: Medical and Surgical Management. Philadelphia, W. B. Saunders, 1988, pp. 157–166.

The Reid, Haggitt, and Rubin group has the largest collection of biopsies in Barrett's esophagus in the world. From this experience, they are able to show a direct relationship between Barrett's esophagus and adenocarcinoma.

Thor, K., Hill, L. D., Mercer, C. D., and Kozarek, R. A.: Reappraisal of the flap valve mechanism: A study of a new valvuloplasty procedure in cadavers. Acta Chir. Scand., *153*:25–28, 1987.

This paper represents publication of the cadaver work done to illustrate the importance of the gastroesophageal valve, which is the main component of the antireflux barrier. The valve, when visualized with the retroflexed endoscope, gives a better assessment of the clinical picture than measurement of the sphincter pressure does.

Spechler, S. J., VA GERD Study Group, Department of Veterans Affairs: Comparison of medical and surgical therapy for complicated gastroesophageal reflux disease in veterans. N. Engl. J. Med., *326*:786–792, 1992.

This important paper shows that surgery is more effective in the management of GERD than medical therapy is. The complications of the Nissen procedure used in the surgical group were unacceptably high.

BIBLIOGRAPHY

Allison, P. R., and Johnstone, A. S.: The oesophagus lined with gastric mucous membrane. Thorax, *8*:87–101, 1953.

Barrett, N. R.: The lower esophagus lined by columnar epithelium. Surgery, *41*:881–894, 1957.

Brand, D. L., Eastwood, I. R., Martin, D., et al.: Esophageal symptoms, manometry, and histology before and after antireflux surgery: A long-term follow-up study. Gastroenterology, *76*:1393–1401, 1979.

Cameron, A. J., Ott, B. J., and Payne, W. S.: The incidence of adenocarcinoma in columnar-lined (Barrett's) esophagus. N. Engl. J. Med., *313*:857–859, 1985.

Fyke, R. E., Code, C. F., and Schleggel, J. F.: The GE sphincter in healthy human beings. Gastroenterologia, *86*:135–150, 1956.

Hameeteman, W., Tytgat, G. N. J., Houthoff, H. F., et al.: Barrett's esophagus: Development of dysplasia and adenocarcinoma. Gastroenterology, *96*:1249–1256, 1989.

Hamilton, S. R., Smith, R. R. L., and Cameron, J. L.: Prevalence and characteristics of Barrett's esophagus in patients with adenocarcinoma of the esophagus or esophagogastric junction. Hum. Pathol., *19*:942–948, 1988.

Havelund, T., Laursen, L. S., Skoubo-Kristensen, E., et al.: Omeprazole and ranitidine in treatment of reflux oesophagitis: Double-blind comparative trial. Br. Med. J., *296*:89–92, 1988.

Hill, L. D.: Intraoperative measurement of lower esophageal sphincter pressure. J. Thorac. Cardiovasc. Surg., *75*:378–382, 1978.

Hill, L. D., Chapman, K. W., and Morgan, E. H.: Objective evaluation of surgery for hiatus hernia and esophagitis. J. Thorac. Cardiovasc. Surg., *41*:60, 1961.

Hill, L. D., Gelfand, M., and Bauermeister, D.: Simplified management of reflux esophagitis with stricture. Ann. Surg., *172*:639–651, 1970.

Hill, L. D., Morgan, E. H., and Kellogg, H. B.: Experimentation as an aid in management of esophageal disorders. Am. J. Surg., *102*:240–253, 1961.

Klinkenberg-Knol, E. C., Jansen, J. M. B., Festen, H. P. M., et al.: Double-blind multicentre comparison of omeprazole and ranitidine in the treatment of reflux oesophagitis. Lancet, *1*:349–351, 1987.

Leonardi, H. K., Crozier, R. E., and Ellis, F. H.: Reoperation for complications of the Nissen fundoplication. J. Thorac. Cardiovasc. Surg., *81*:50–56, 1981.

Little, A. G., Ferguson, M. K., and Skinner, D. B.: Reoperation for failed antireflux operations. Surgery, *91*:511–517, 1986.

Mittal, R. K., Dudley, F., Rochester, D. F., and McCallum, R.: Sphincteric action of the diaphragm during a relaxed lower esophageal sphincter in humans. J. Am. Physiol. Soc., G139, 1989.

Morgan, E. H., Hill, L. D., Siemsen, J. K., et al.: Studies of intraluminal esophageal and gastric pressure and pH. Bull. Mason Clin., *14*:53–89, 1960.

Negre, J. B.: Post fundoplication symptoms. Do they restrict the success of Nissen fundoplication? Ann. Surg., *198*:698–700, 1983.

Nissen, R.: Eine einfache operation zur beeinflussung der refluxoesophagitis. Schweiz. Med. Wochenschr., *86*:590, 1956.

Ovaska, J., Miettinen, M., and Kivilaakso, E.: Adenocarcinoma arising in Barrett's esophagus. Dig. Dis. Sci., *34*:1139–1336, 1989.

Patterson, D. J., Graham, D. Y., Smith, J. L., et al.: Natural history of benign esophageal stricture treated by dilatation. Gastroenterology, *85*:346–350, 1983.

Rabinovitch, P. S., Reid, B. J., Haggitt, R. C., et al.: Progression to cancer in Barrett's esophagus is associated with genomic instability. Lab. Invest., *60*:65–71, 1988.

Reid, B. J., et al.: Endoscopic biopsy can detect high-grade dysplasia or early adenocarcinoma in Barrett's esophagus without grossly recognizable neoplastic lesions. Gastroenterology, *94*:81–90, 1988.

Reid, B. J., Haggitt, R. C., Rubin, C. E., and Rabinovitch, P. S.: Barrett's esophagus. Correlation between flow cytometry and histology in detection of patients at risk for adenocarcinoma. Gastroenterology, *93*:1–11, 1987.

Rossetti, M., and Hell, K.: Fundoplication for the treatment of gastroesophageal reflux in hiatal hernia. World J. Surg., *1*:439–444, 1977.

Russell, C. O. H.: Control of reflux. *In* Hill, L. D., Kozarek, R., McCallum, R., and Mercer, C. D. (eds): The Esophagus: Medical and Surgical Management. Philadelphia, W. B. Saunders, 1988, pp. 45–46.

Skinner, D. B., Walther, B. C., Riddell, R. H., et al.: Barrett's esophagus. Comparison of benign and malignant cases. Ann. Surg., *198*:554–565, 1983.

Thor, K., and Silander, T.: Long-term randomized prospective trial of the Nissen procedure versus a modified Toupet technique. Ann. Surg., *210*:719–724, 1989.

Watson, A.: The role of antireflux surgery combined with fiberoptic endoscopic dilatation in peptic esophageal stricture. Am. J. Surg., *148*:346–349, 1984.

28

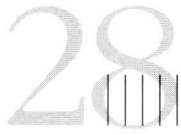

■ V Paraesophageal Hernia

Lucius D. Hill

Although it was originally estimated that paraesophageal hernia constituted approximately 3 to 4% of herniations through the esophageal hiatus, further data indicate that this disorder occurs in less than 2% of patients for whom surgical management is required for diaphragmatic hernias. In this condition, the esophageal hiatus is enlarged, and the stomach and, at times, even other viscera may herniate alongside the esophagus through the enlarged hiatus. The paraesophageal hernia is differentiated from the sliding hernia in that the *gastroesophageal junction* (GEJ), including the *lower esophageal sphincter* (LES) and *gastroesophageal valve* (GEV), is fixed in its normal intra-abdominal position by the posterior phrenoesophageal fascial complex, which is intact. The location of the GEJ below the diaphragm separates the true paraesophageal hernia from the other types of herniation through the esophageal hiatus. The other types include the sliding hernia, in which the GEJ slides into the posterior mediastinum with the GEJ at the cephalad or top end of the hernia. A third type of hernia is termed the *combined sliding and paraesophageal hernia,* in which the GEJ and the cardia slide up into the posterior mediastinum en masse so that the stomach is alongside the esophagus rather than below the esophagus. In the combined hernia, the angle of His may be preserved and the GEV may be intact, so that reflux is not a problem. In the sliding hernia, the GEV is lost and the sphincter may be distracted, so that reflux occurs.

Careful preoperative evaluation can separate these types of hernias. The standard acid reflux test can be used to determine the location of the sphincter and whether or not reflux is occurring. However, it may be difficult, if not impossible, in the true paraesophageal hernia to insert the pH and manometry tube into the stomach because of the acute angle that the stomach makes with the esophagus at the diaphragm. Endoscopy with the flexible scope usually can be accomplished and can determine whether or not the GEV is intact and located below the diaphragm.

Paraesophageal hernias are similar to other hernias in that they produce symptoms as a consequence of their size and because of the distortion of the viscera contained in them. The stomach may incarcerate or strangulate, or it may undergo torsion in the large hernial sac.

In the uncommon true paraesophageal hernia, the esophagus lies in its normal position fixed intra-abdominally by the firm posterior phrenoesophageal complex, a structure consisting of fibroelastic tissue extending from the esophageal wall into the hiatal rim of the diaphragm. Anteriorly and laterally, the components of the phrenoesophageal complex are markedly attenuated and, along with the peritoneum, form the sac of the herniation. In this form of hernia, the stomach rolls up into the posterior mediastinum anterior to the esophagus such that the greater curve lies superiorly in the thorax. However, the GEJ lies in its normal intra-abdominal position. This anatomic arrangement allows for competency of the cardia, as documented by normal pH and pressure study results and, therefore, the absence of gastroesophageal reflux (Fig. 28–31). As these hernias enlarge, more of the stomach may become incarcerated in the chest. Rarely, segments of small bowel and colon may be in the large intrathoracic sac. At times, the entire stomach and first portion of the duodenum may ascend into the thorax (Fig. 28–32). As more viscera become incarcerated in the chest, the esophageal hiatus widens. At this point, with incarceration in the chest, the posterior phrenoesophageal complex may become lax, allowing the GEJ to slide up into the chest, causing a combined paraesophageal and sliding hernia. It is imperative to define preoperatively whether there is a true paraesophageal hernia or a combined sliding and paraesophageal hernia. If the GEJ is incompetent and reflux is occurring, the hernia must be corrected as in a sliding hernia, and the repair must include an antireflux procedure.

NATURAL HISTORY

Paraesophageal hernias are benign until the hernia becomes large, usually when the patient is 30 to 40 years of age. At this time, symptoms of postprandial distress (retching and a sensation of nausea after eating) become common. With gastric distention, the patient experiences substernal pressure, particularly after eating, related to a dilated intrathoracic stomach. This pain can occasionally become so severe that the patient is admitted to the Emergency Room with a diagnosis of myocardial infarction. This pressure is often relieved with belching or vomiting. Patients do not complain of gastroesophageal reflux, and symptoms may be tolerated until complications occur, including ulceration in the herniated portion of the stomach, hemorrhage, volvulus, obstruction, or pulmonary complications such as aspiration.

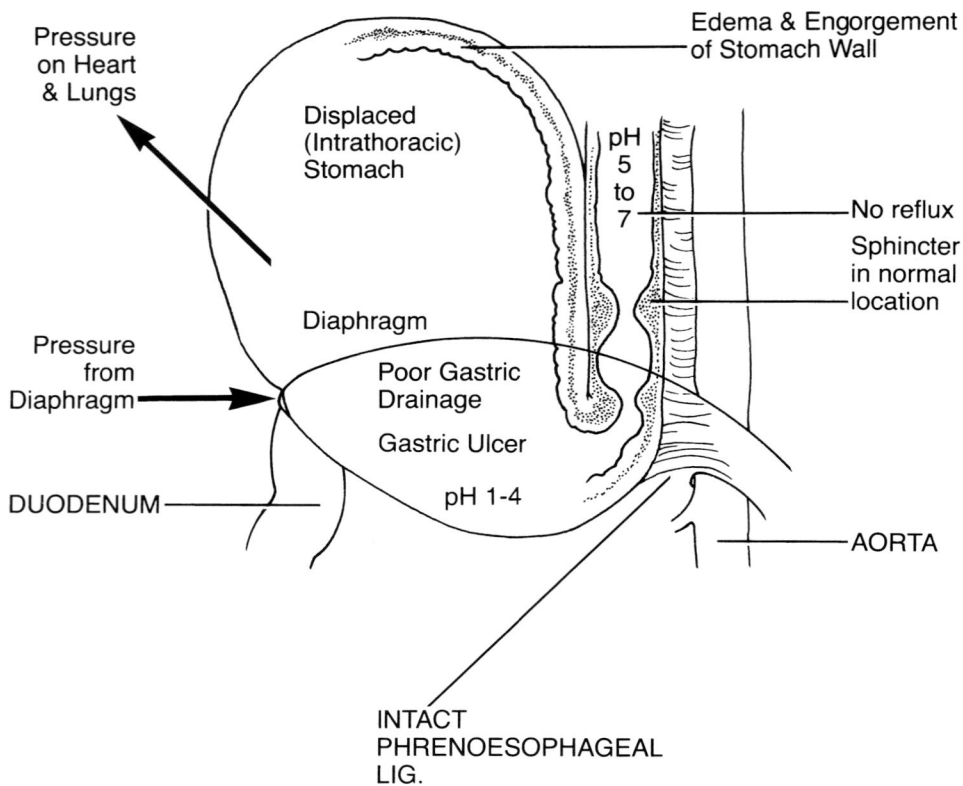

Pressure on Heart & Lungs

Displaced (Intrathoracic) Stomach

Edema & Engorgement of Stomach Wall

pH 5 to 7

No reflux

Sphincter in normal location

Diaphragm

Pressure from Diaphragm

Poor Gastric Drainage

Gastric Ulcer

pH 1-4

DUODENUM

AORTA

INTACT PHRENOESOPHAGEAL LIG.

FIGURE 28–31. The anatomic and physiologic appearance of a para-esophageal hernia. The stomach rolls up into the thorax anterior to the esophagus. The esophagus is fixed in its normal position by a plate of fibroareolar tissue and is functioning normally without allowing reflux. (LIG = ligament.)

Our reported series has seen a 30% incidence of chronic bleeding secondary to gastric ulceration within the intrathoracic segment of stomach. The ulceration is caused by poor gastric emptying with hypersecretion of acid and by trauma from torsion of the gastric wall and pressure from the diaphragm. Management of this ulceration mandates surgical correction of the problem, because the underlying pathophysiologic defect is mechanical. Antacid therapy will not allow healing of the ulcer, because the underlying problem is interference with gastric drainage and continued trauma to the gastric wall interfering with the blood supply to the stomach.

The most feared complication of paraesophageal hernia is volvulus and strangulation with infarction of the contained viscus and possible perforation into the mediastinum, causing mediastinitis. Other complications include pulmonary aspiration, varying from dyspnea to pneumonia.

It is of interest that most of our patients with mas-

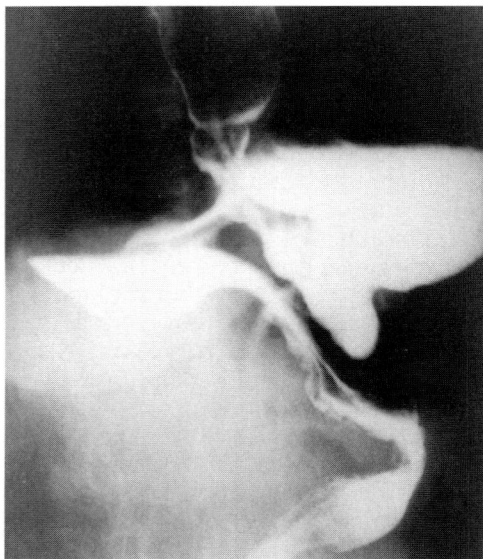

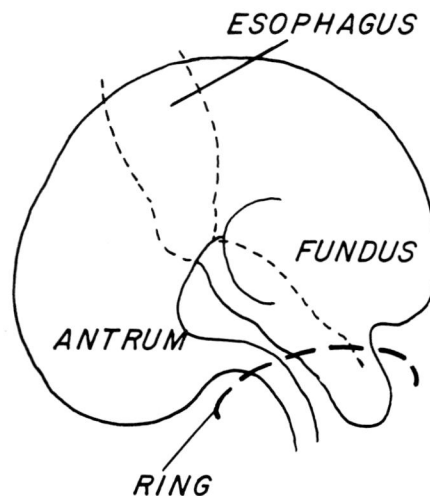

ESOPHAGUS

FUNDUS

ANTRUM

RING

FIGURE 28–32. The entire stomach and first portion of the duodenum may ascend into the thorax.

sive paraesophageal hiatus hernia were known to have had the hernia for many years before operation. Both physicians and surgeons caring for these patients often feel that the condition is harmless as long as the symptoms can be tolerated. These symptoms often are ignored despite the frequent reports of morbidity and even death associated with complicated hernia, and very often the striking radiologic changes are ignored. Unfortunately, once these complications develop, correcting the condition converts from a technically easy, elective operation with low morbidity and minimal mortality to a very complicated emergency operation with great risk.

Skinner and associates (1967) documented a series of 21 patients who were treated medically because of minimal symptoms. In this series, six patients died with complications such as strangulation, perforation, and hemorrhage.

DIAGNOSIS

The diagnosis of paraesophageal hernia is often made from a plain film of the chest in which the air fluid level posterior to the heart is seen (Fig. 28–33). An upper gastrointestinal (GI) series helps to evaluate the extent of the stomach involved in the hernia and provides information about gastric emptying. Rarely, barium enema examination may show part of the transverse colon included in the herniated viscus. Standard acid reflux testing should be done, although it may be difficult to insert the probe past the acutely angulated GEJ. However, with the probe just above

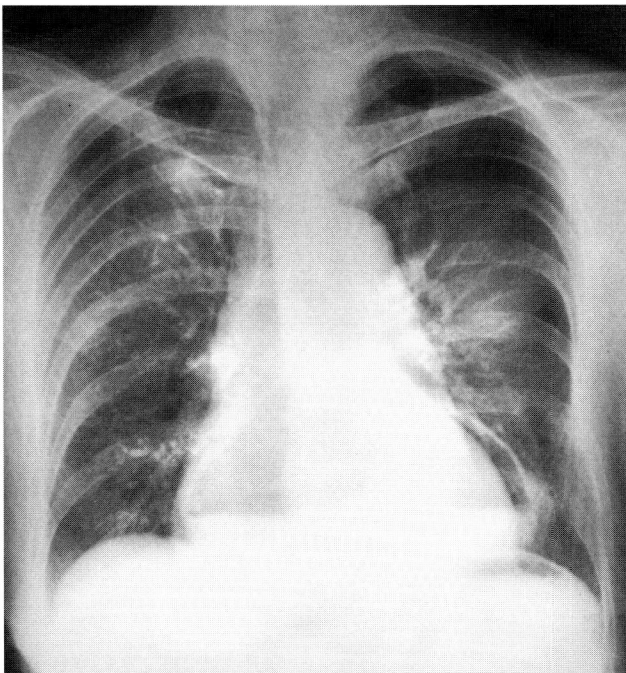

FIGURE 28–33. The diagnosis of paraesophageal hernia may be made by plain film of the chest showing an air fluid level behind the heart.

the GEJ, it can be determined whether the patient is refluxing.

TREATMENT

A paraesophageal hiatal hernia alone is a sufficient indication for operation, provided the risks of an elective surgical procedure are not prohibitive. Episodes of incarceration, bleeding, or obstruction are obvious indications for operations. Surgeons have been reluctant to operate in these cases, presumably because of previous poor results in patients who have undergone surgery for sliding hiatal hernias.

This lack of a clear understanding of the natural history of this condition by physicians who do not routinely deal with these patients has deterred clinicians from recommending surgical management for paraesophageal hernia. However, in contrast with the results of surgical intervention in sliding hiatal hernia, repair of esophageal hiatal hernia has met with almost complete success in elective cases. If the condition is accurately diagnosed and the operation is performed properly, there should be few, if any, recurrences.

SURGICAL TECHNIQUE

In the true paraesophageal hernia wherein the GEJ is anchored in its normal location and functioning properly, it is a technical mistake to free the esophagus circumferentially from the posterior part of the hiatus if the phrenoesophageal membrane is intact and maintaining the LES in its normal location within the abdominal cavity. Dissection posterior to the esophagus disrupts this attachment, allowing the GEJ to migrate into the chest with loss of the GEV, distraction of the sphincter, and creation of an iatrogenic sliding hiatus hernia.

The paraesophageal hernia may be approached either transthoracically or transabdominally. Using the transabdominal approach, the surgeon may be surprised to find that none of the stomach is within the abdomen (Fig. 28–34). The transthoracic approach would reveal the inverted stomach in the posterior mediastinum.

The hernial contents are carefully and usually reduced easily by slow manual traction. The sac of the hernia usually can be excised from the posterior mediastinum by a combination of blunt and sharp dissection. Reexpansion of the lungs with reduction of the hernia causes the hernia sac to collapse down into the abdomen, making the dissection easier. Dissection of this sac can be difficult if it has been present for a long time and firmly adheres to mediastinal tissue. In this situation, most of the sac should be excised and the hernial orifice should be closed, but dissection of the entire sac is not necessary. Once the hernia is reduced, the surgeon should reassess the problem.

If the GEJ is firmly fixed in the abdomen, as in true paraesophageal hernia, the attachments should

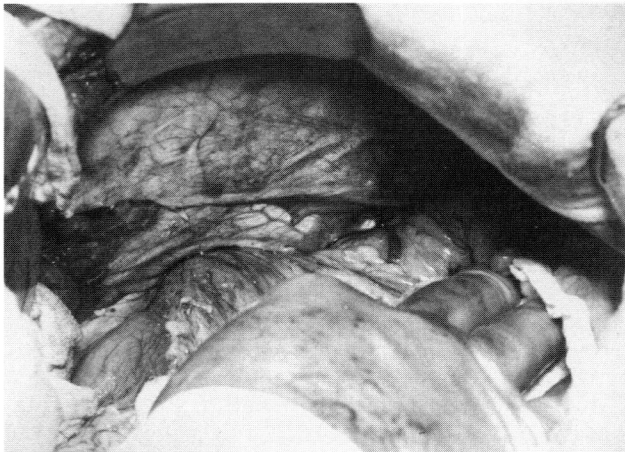

FIGURE 28–34. With the abdominal approach, the surgeon may be surprised to see none of the stomach in the abdomen. Only the pylorus is protruding through the enlarged esophageal hiatus.

remain intact (Fig. 28–35). If an intraoperative pressure study shows a good sphincter in its usual location and functioning normally, taking down the esophagus from its attachments is a technical mistake. It is interesting that the sphincter and the valve, which is held in place only by the posterior attachments and nowhere contacts the anterior or lateral portions of the diaphragm, can function normally, especially because the sharp angle of His at the GEJ, representing an accentuated valve mechanism, remains competent in these patients. Both the sphincter and the valve mechanism are preserved. If the GEJ can be seen to slide up into the posterior mediastinum, or if the sphincter pressure is too low, sutures along the lesser curvature, fixing the GEJ to the preaortic fascia, are important. In fact, in all cases, it is wise to add fixation sutures of the GEJ to the preaortic fascia to prevent subsequent development of a sliding hernia. The diaphragmatic opening, which may be

quite large, is then closed with interrupted, heavy, nonabsorbable sutures reinforced with Teflon pledgets. It has been our experience that the diaphragmatic tissues are strong enough to hold sutures well, even in the elderly patient in whom there is a huge hernial orifice. We have not used Marlex or other foreign material to close the opening because the diaphragmatic rim is lax enough to come together easily. This closure should be snug enough to allow the surgeon's index finger to be inserted alongside the esophagus, in which a nasogastric tube is present. In the completed repair, the large opening in the diaphragm is closed anterior to the esophagus (Fig. 28–36). Several fixation sutures are placed along the lesser curve to the preaortic fascia. With a mixed type of paraesophageal and sliding hernia, formal antireflux repair and sphincter calibration are necessary. If the patient is actively bleeding at the time of operation, a gastrostomy should be performed to locate the bleeding ulcer, which can then be repaired easily by simple suturing.

INCARCERATED PARAESOPHAGEAL HERNIA

In a previous report, we indicated that approximately 30% of patients with paraesophageal hernia develop incarceration. Incarceration is a surgical emergency that often is not appreciated. Review of the history of patients with incarcerated paraesophageal hernias shows they have had the hernia for many years. During this time, the patient may develop substernal pain and pressure so severe that myocardial infarction is diagnosed. In addition, gastric ulcer from poorly drained stomach may be present. It seems that as long as the entire stomach is in the chest, incarceration does not occur.

The first step in the development of incarcerated hernia is prolapse of the distended fundus into the

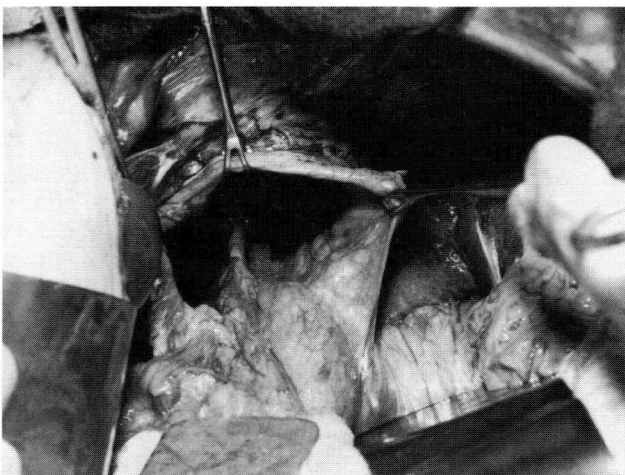

FIGURE 28–35. Following reduction of the hernia, the esophagus can be seen to be in its normal location fixed firmly posteriorly by a plate of fibroareolar tissue.

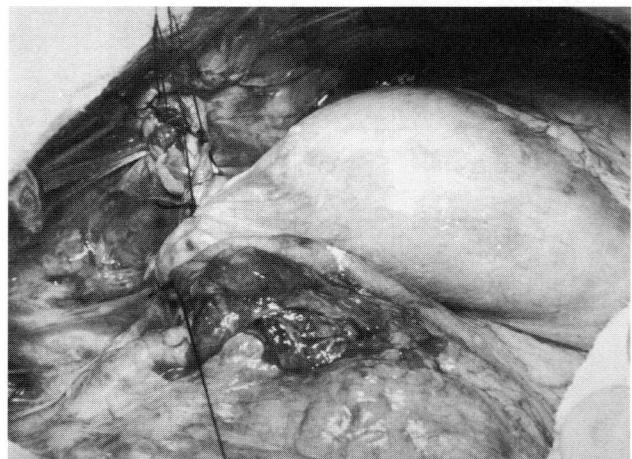

FIGURE 28–36. The completed repair shows the enlarged esophageal hiatus closed anterior to the esophagus, and fixation sutures have fixed the lesser curvature to the preaortic fascia. The posterior attachments of the esophagus are left intact.

FIGURE 28–37. Prolapse of the distended antrum into the abdomen is the first step in incarceration of a paraesophageal hernia.

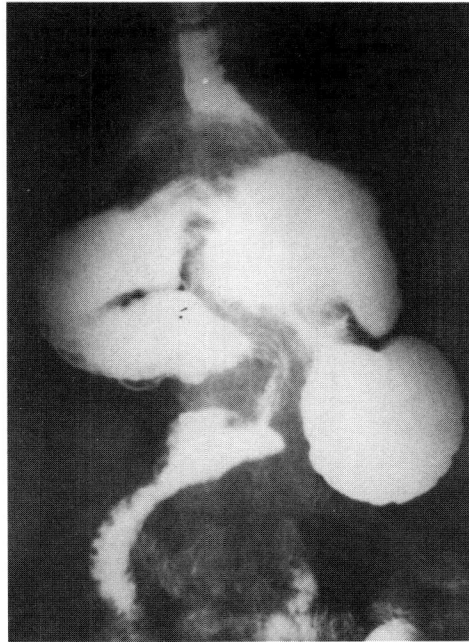

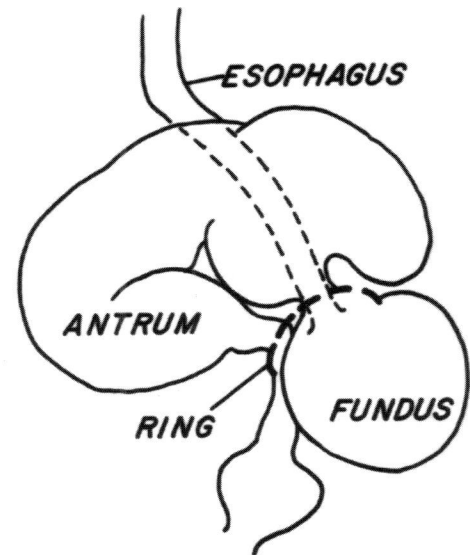

abdomen (Fig. 28–37). With further distention of the antrum and the fundus, the patient develops obstruction at multiple points. The midportion of the stomach, the terminal esophagus, and the first portion of the duodenum are all obstructed by the ring of the diaphragm. A flat plate of the abdomen would show the enormously dilated fundus filling the entire upper abdomen (Fig. 28–38). A concomitant chest film shows the enormously dilated antrum behind the heart displacing the thoracic viscera. Barium swallow clearly shows the dumbbell-shaped appearance of the stomach in both the chest and the abdomen. The pathophysiology of an incarcerated hernia is shown in Figure 28–39. In essence, there are two closed-loop obstructions as well as obstruction of the esophagus and the duodenum. At this point, the patient is in serious distress and the condition constitutes a surgical emergency. If this goes unrecognized, both the antrum and the fundus are subject to gangrene and perforation. If a nasogastric tube can be inserted past the GEJ into the fundus, the stomach can be decompressed. Following the rush of gas and gastric juice, the patient improves rapidly and can be prepared for an elective operation with very low risk of morbidity and mortality.

At operation, the enormously dilated gangrenous fundus is seen in the abdomen or, if the thoracic approach is used, the dilated antrum is noted in the chest. It may be necessary to divide the rim of the diaphragm and perform a gastrostomy to decompress the markedly distended stomach. Following reduction of the hernia, it is again important to determine whether the surgeon is dealing with a pure paraesophageal hernia, in which case the elective repair of paraesophageal hernia is indicated. If the GEJ is in the thorax and the surgeon is dealing with a sliding hernia, an antireflux procedure is indicated, along with closure of the large opening in the diaphragm. Analysis of 42 patients treated for paraesophageal hernia demonstrates the dramatic difference in outcome between patients who were diagnosed early and underwent an elective repair with no complications or recurrence and patients who were diagnosed

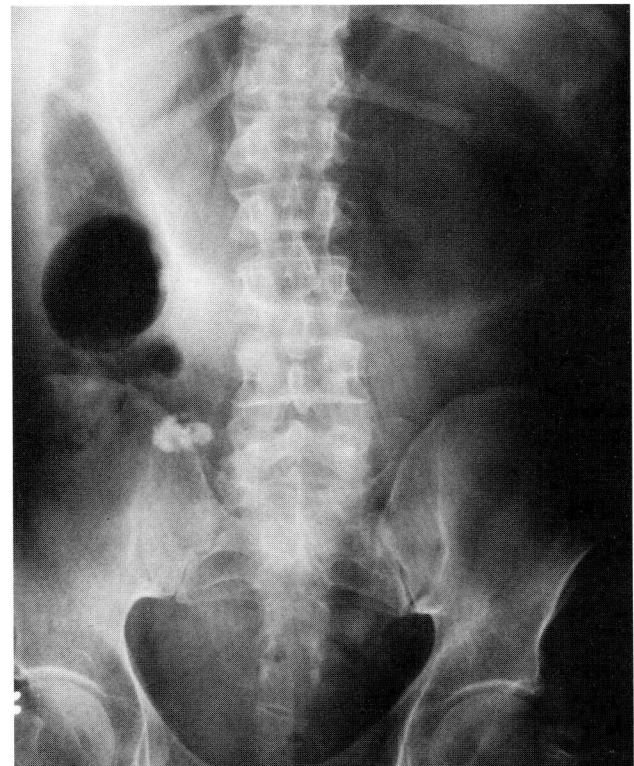

FIGURE 28–38. The enormously dilated prolapsed antrum fills the entire upper abdomen.

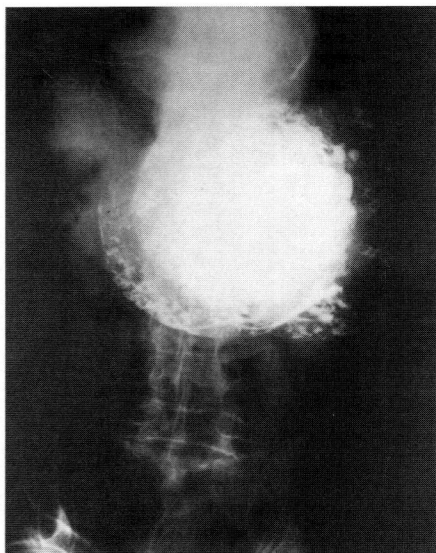

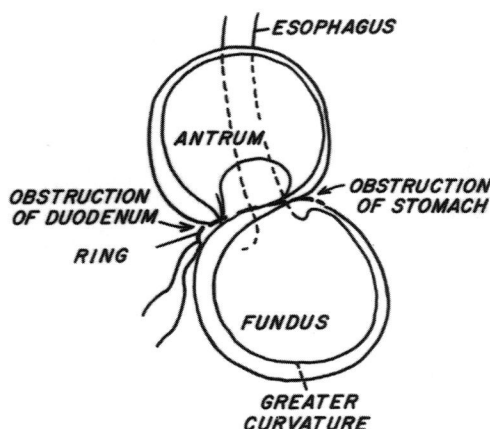

FIGURE 28–39. An incarcerated paraesophageal hernia presents two closed-loop obstructions as well as obstruction of the esophagus and duodenum. This is a surgical emergency.

late and developed serious complications (Table 28–5). Of the five patients in whom decompression was not possible, two died from cardiac arrest before reaching the operating room, two were salvaged by removal of the near-gangrenous stomach, and one was salvaged by reduction of a near-gangrenous stomach. This experience clearly underscores the fact that incarcerated paraesophageal hernia has a high mortality rate and is an indication for immediate operation. It follows that paraesophageal hernia is subject to serious complications, and if the patient is a reasonable risk for operation, elective repair of a paraesophageal hernia is indicated.

SUMMARY

True paraesophageal hernia is a rare condition and must be clearly differentiated from sliding hernia and a combined paraesophageal and sliding hernia. A true paraesophageal hernia presents the threat of incarceration and strangulation, and thus of considerable mortality and morbidity. In the good-risk patient, repair should result in very low risk and a long-term recurrence rate of less than 1%. Therefore, a paraesophageal hernia in a patient who is at reasonable risk for operation should be repaired.

■ **Table 28–5.** RESULTS OF TREATMENT OF COMPLICATED AND UNCOMPLICATED PARAESOPHAGEAL HERNIAS (42 PATIENTS)

Type of Hernia	Number	Results
Uncomplicated	28	Excellent: no mortality or recurrences
Complicated	14	
Decompressed	8	Good: no deaths
Not decompressed	6	3 preoperative deaths, 3 survived operation

SELECTED BIBLIOGRAPHY

Ellis, R. H., Crozier, R. E., and Shea, J. A.: Paraesophageal hiatus hernia. Arch. Surg., *121*:416, 1986.

This report summarizes extensive personal experience by the senior author managing 55 patients with paraesophageal hernia. These authors report that one-third of all the hiatal hernias encountered had a paraesophageal component. Emphasis is placed on the fact that "true" paraesophageal hernias have a normally situated gastroesophageal junction and, therefore, rarely are associated with reflux. When this has been manometrically verified, the authors emphasize that an antireflux operation is not necessary when the hernia is repaired. They do recommend routinely adding a gastrostomy to the anterior crural repair to prevent recurrence. Improvement was noted postoperatively in 88.49% of patients.

Ozdemir, I. A., Burke, W. A., and Ikins, P. M.: Paraesophageal hernia: A life-threatening disease. Ann. Thorac. Surg., *16*:547, 1973.

The authors reported 31 patients with paraesophageal hernia. Presentation of these patients was complicated by upper gastrointestinal hemorrhage in 10 patients, volvulus and obstruction in 9 patients, and gangrenous obstruction with perforation in 2 patients. Primary repair was accomplished in 28 patients with good results. The 2 patients who ultimately died were those whose course was complicated by obstruction, perforation, and mediastinitis. The authors note that the serious complications of paraesophageal hiatal hernia are life-threatening, and that therefore these hernias should be electively repaired when the diagnosis is made.

BIBLIOGRAPHY

Hill, L. D.: Incarcerated paraesophageal hernia. A surgical emergency. Am. J. Surg., *126*:286–291, 1973.
Hill, L. D., and Mercer, C. D.: Paraesophageal hernia. *In* Cameron, J. L. (ed): Current Surgical Therapy. Burlington, Ontario, B. C. Decker, 1984, pp. 22–24.
Hill, L. D., and Tobias, J. A.: Paraesophageal hernia. Arch. Surg., *96*:735, 1968.
MacDougall, J. T., Abbott, A. C., and Goodhard, T. K.: Herniation through congenital diaphragmatic defects in adults. Can. J. Surg., *6*:302, 1963.
Pearson, F. G., Cooper, J. D., Ilves, R., et al.: Massive hiatal hernia with incarceration: A report of 53 cases. Ann. Thorac. Surg., *35*:45–51, 1983.
Skinner, D. B., Belsey, R. H. R., and Russell, P. S.: Surgical management of esophageal reflux and hiatus hernia—Long-term results with 1030 patients. J. Thorac. Cardiovasc. Surg., *53*:33, 1967.
Sweet, R. H.: Thoracic Surgery. 2nd ed. Philadelphia, W. B. Saunders, 1954.

28

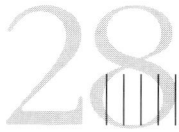

▪ VI Short Esophagus and Reflux Stricture

Mark B. Orringer

An esophageal reflux stricture is the end-result of the inflammatory reaction produced in the esophagus by regurgitation from the stomach of both acid and alkaline secretions through an incompetent lower esophageal sphincter mechanism. That gastroesophageal reflux can occur independently of a hiatal hernia has been emphasized (see part I of this chapter). Erosion of esophageal squamous epithelium by the chemical "burn" of gastric contents is associated with submucosal edema and inflammatory cellular infiltration, which may extend into the muscular layers of the esophageal wall and adjacent periesophageal tissues, producing edema and scarring of the mediastinal soft tissues and lymphadenopathy ("periesophagitis"). The healing process causes degrees of fibrosis. Because acute reflux esophagitis tends to be cyclical, with periods of quiescence followed by recrudescence, repetitive bouts of acute inflammation and then healing may produce progressive mural fibrous infiltration beginning in the submucosa and ultimately involving the muscle and periesophageal tissues. As fibrous deposition continues and collagen fibers within the stricture contract, not only does circumferential narrowing reduce the size of the lumen, but the esophagus shortens to various degrees during longitudinal contracture.

HISTORICAL ASPECTS

The surgical approach to esophageal reflux strictures has evolved progressively toward conservative and nonresective techniques. In earlier years, preoperative assessment of esophageal reflux strictures using radiographic studies, esophagoscopy, and biopsy, as well as the ease of dilatation, dictated the choice of operation. The more fibrous strictures that were difficult to dilate were considered "irreversible" and were treated by a variety of techniques of esophageal resection and reconstruction or esophagoplasties, including distal esophagectomy with esophagogastrostomy (Belsey, 1952; Dunlop, 1956; Tanner, 1955), jejunal interposition (Allison, 1948; Allison et al., 1943; Barnes and Redo, 1957; Merendino and Dillard, 1955), colonic interposition (Belsey, 1965; Neville and Clowes, 1963; Popov, 1961), the reversed gastric tube (Heimlich, 1962, 1972), plastic procedures on the distal esophageal stenosis with attempts at establishing valvular competence (Thal, 1968; Thal et al., 1965; Woodward,

1975), and resection of the stricture with esophagogastrostomy in combination with antrectomy, vagotomy, and Roux-en-Y gastroenterostomy (Ellis et al., 1958; Payne, 1970).

Hayward (1961), of Australia, was the first to suggest that most reflux strictures could be treated successfully with operative dilatation and an antireflux operation. Hill was the first to advocate this approach in the United States (Hill et al., 1970), and he emphasized the need to obtain adequate reflux control for this method to be successful. Surgical developments in this area have focused on techniques for obtaining the most reliable reflux control after dilatation of these strictures. These advances have come in part through greater insistence on objective evidence of reflux control, which has been permitted by refinements in techniques of esophageal manometry, as well as documentation of abnormal reflux with the intraesophageal pH probe. Since the pioneering work in esophageal manometry by Ingelfinger (1958) and Code and associates (1958) and the introduction of the long gastrointestinal pH electrode to assess competency of the distal esophageal sphincter mechanism by Tuttle and Grossman (1958), esophageal function laboratories have become essential to the practice of the modern esophageal surgeon. Esophageal mucosal exposure to refluxed gastric juice is now measured most directly with an intraesophageal pH electrode (DeMeester et al., 1976; Fuchs et al., 1982). Prolonged monitoring of distal esophageal pH is performed by positioning a pH probe 5 cm proximal to the upper end of the distal esophageal high-pressure zone as determined by prior manometry. Standardized scores expressing esophageal exposure to acid (total percentage of time pH <4, number of reflux episodes, number of episodes longer than 5 minutes, duration of the longest episode) have been developed for 24-hour pH monitoring, which has now emerged as the gold standard for diagnosing gastroesophageal reflux (DeMeester et al., 1980; Johnson and DeMeester, 1974). Just as the cardiac surgeon now relies on physiologic catheterization data and the pulmonary surgeon uses pulmonary function tests to predict the safety of a pulmonary resection, the esophageal surgeon now has a reliable, objective method for documenting not only the preoperative functional abnormality, but also the results of operations on the esophagus. The precision in both diagnosis and treatment that has come to characterize the cardiac surgeon should now be expected of the esophageal surgeon.

ANATOMIC CONSIDERATIONS

Three general varieties of esophageal reflux strictures are encountered clinically. The majority are short, 1 to 2 cm in length, and are localized to the esophagogastric junction (Fig. 28–40). At the other extreme are the more extensive strictures that involve the distal half or third of the esophagus (Fig. 28–41). This type of stricture most commonly occurs after prolonged nasogastric intubation in a critically ill patient who is supine for many days and, occasionally, after severe protracted vomiting, as in hyperemesis gravidarum or in association with gastric outlet obstruction. Finally, localized strictures occurring in the mid or upper thoracic esophagus should suggest the possibility of *Barrett's esophagus* (columnar epithelium–lined lower esophagus) (Figs. 28–42 and 28–43). In Barrett's esophagus, the stricture characteristically occurs at the squamocolumnar epithelial junction, which is in the mid or upper third of the organ in these patients. The esophagus distal to the stricture is lined by columnar or gastric-type epithelium, which may include acid-producing parietal cells, and a sliding hiatal hernia is generally present. Although originally thought to be a congenital abnormality, the columnar epithelium–lined esophagus is now viewed by most as an acquired condition that stems from reflux esophagitis and occurs through the process of

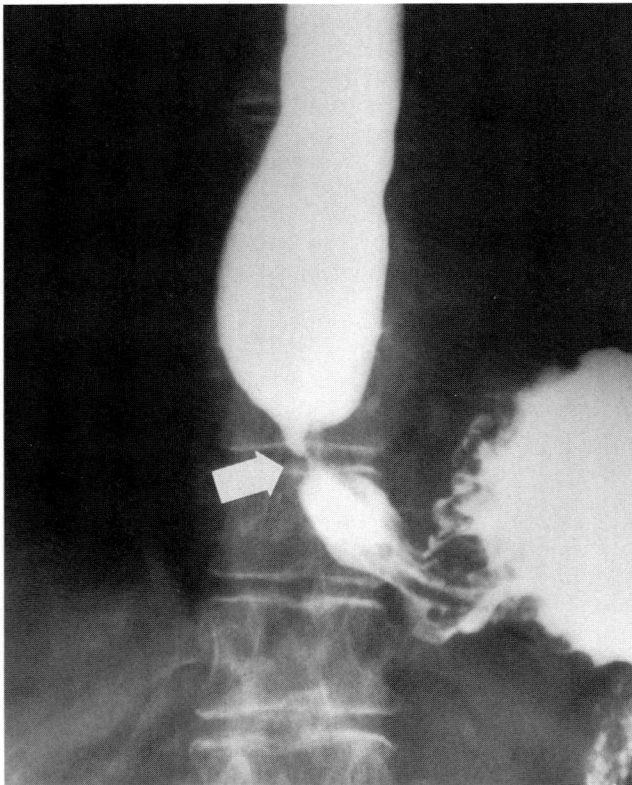

FIGURE 28–41. An 8-cm-long peptic esophageal stricture that followed severe protracted vomiting. There is an associated sliding hiatal hernia.

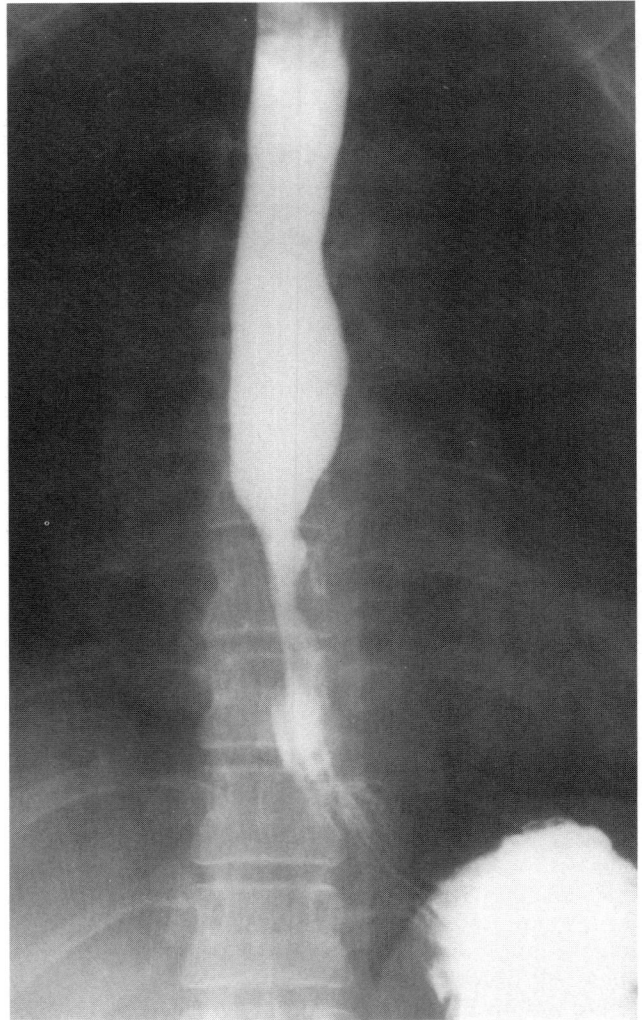

FIGURE 28–40. Esophagogram showing the most common type of peptic stricture. This high-grade stenosis *(arrow)* proximal to a small sliding hiatal hernia is less than 2 cm in length and is localized to the esophagogastric junction.

metaplasia. After the normal esophageal squamous epithelium is denuded by reflux esophagitis, the resulting ulcer is re-epithelialized by multipotential undifferentiated stem cells from the basal layers. These immature stem cells then differentiate into the columnar cells that characterize Barrett's mucosa (Spechler and Goyal, 1986). This pathologic entity is being reported with increasing frequency; its true incidence has undoubtedly been underestimated in the past, because barium esophagograms may not be diagnostic, and biopsies both above and below the stricture are a prerequisite for establishing the diagnosis. The premalignant nature of the columnar epithelium–lined esophagus is now well recognized: the reported prevalence of adenocarcinoma in this epithelium varies from 6 to 46% (Adler, 1963; Cameron et al., 1985; Harle et al., 1985; Hawe et al., 1973; Naef et al., 1972; Radigan et al., 1977; Skinner et al., 1983) (Fig. 28–44). Patients with Barrett's esophagus appear to have a 30- to 40-fold increase in the risk of developing esoph-

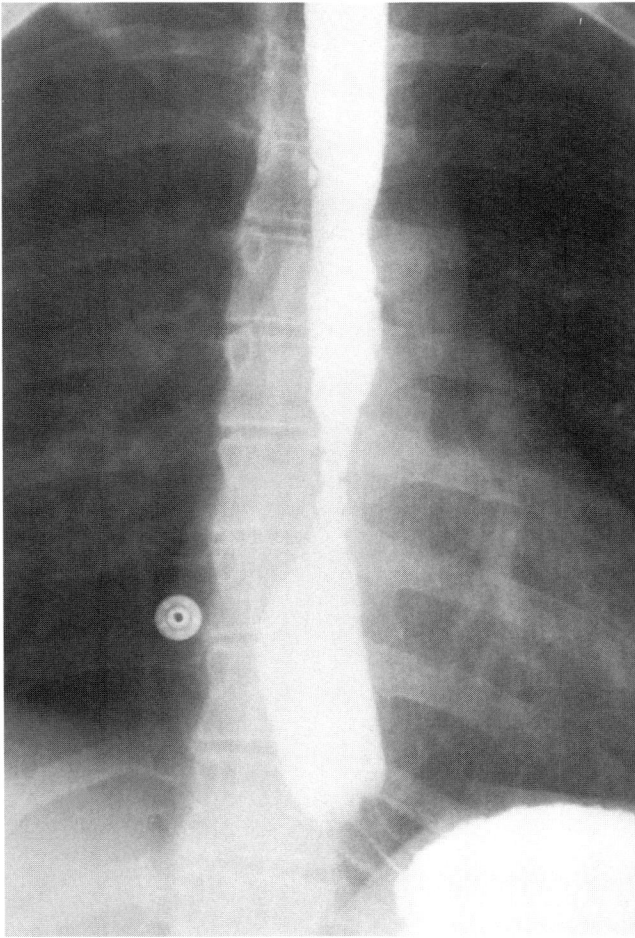

FIGURE 28–42. Esophagogram of a patient with long-standing dysphagia and Barrett's esophagus. The midesophageal stricture suggested Barrett's esophagus, and multiple biopsies distal to the stricture showed columnar epithelium. Normal squamous epithelium was found proximal to the stenosis. A sliding hiatal hernia was present.

ageal cancer over the general population (Cameron et al., 1985; Spechler et al., 1984).

The definition of the term *short esophagus* is controversial; some dispute that such an entity in association with gastroesophageal reflux even exists. According to Barrett (1950), peptic ulceration of the esophagus was first described by Albers in 1839, and Rokitansky later supported the existence of this pathologic entity. In a review of the literature, Tileston (1906) reported 44 patients with peptic ulceration of the esophagus and clearly described stenosis associated with this condition. As "reflux esophagitis" was popularized by Allison (1948), it became apparent that many of these patients with esophageal strictures had columnar epithelium distal to the stenosis. Erroneously, Barrett (1950) concluded that any portion of the swallowing passage lined by columnar epithelium is stomach. The term *short esophagus* thus arose because many regarded the columnar epithelium–lined length of the esophagus below the stricture as stomach. The result of this incorrect perception that strictures always occur at the anatomic esophagogastric junction was a policy of treating high strictures by resection and esophageal replacement with intestine to provide the "missing" length of esophagus. It has subsequently been recognized that columnar epithelium in the esophagus is generally an acquired lesion due to *reflux* esophagitis (Allison and Johnstone, 1953; Ellis et al., 1978; Mossberg, 1966; Naef et al., 1975). Furthermore, esophageal manometry has documented that there is a distal esophageal sphincter mechanism, although a weak one, at the *anatomic* esophagogastric junction, well below the squamocolumnar *epithelial* junction. This led Hill and associates (1970) to dispute the existence of the "short esophagus" and to argue that the esophagogastric junction can almost always be reduced below the diaphragmatic hiatus for their median arcuate ligament posterior gastropexy.

Most esophageal surgeons, however, believe that a true shortening of the distance between the esophageal introitus and the anatomic esophagogastric junction *does* occur as a result of the fibrous contracture associated with reflux esophagitis, similar to the well-recognized way that "shortening" may follow a caustic esophageal injury. In addition, clinical observation suggests that fibrosis need not be present for acquired esophageal shortening to occur, because some degree of contraction of both the circular and longitudinal esophageal musculature may be induced by reflux esophagitis, rendering it more difficult to reduce the esophagogastric junction below the diaphragm without tension. Therefore, although it may be a somewhat subtle and difficult concept to accept, the designation of "short esophagus" does not necessarily require that a stricture be present. It may follow an assessment of the anatomy at the time of hiatal hernia repair, with particular attention to the degree of stretch on the distal esophagus when the esophagogastric junction is reduced below the diaphragm. For practical purposes, the critical issue is not whether the esophagogastric junction can be reduced below the diaphragm, but rather the degree of residual tension on the distal esophagus when the reduction is complete, because tension associated with a hiatal hernia repair is just as undesirable as it is in repair of abdominal wall hernias at other sites, and the implications for subsequent recurrence are the same.

TREATMENT

The most important factor in the treatment of a benign esophageal reflux stricture is prevention—that is, controlling gastroesophageal reflux before mural fibrosis occurs. However, this requires that reflux esophagitis be diagnosed at a relatively early stage. Unfortunately, this diagnosis is hampered by two curious facets of the disease. First, there is a notoriously poor correlation between the patient's symptoms and the degree or extent of esophagitis. Some patients with severe heartburn and regurgitation with postural

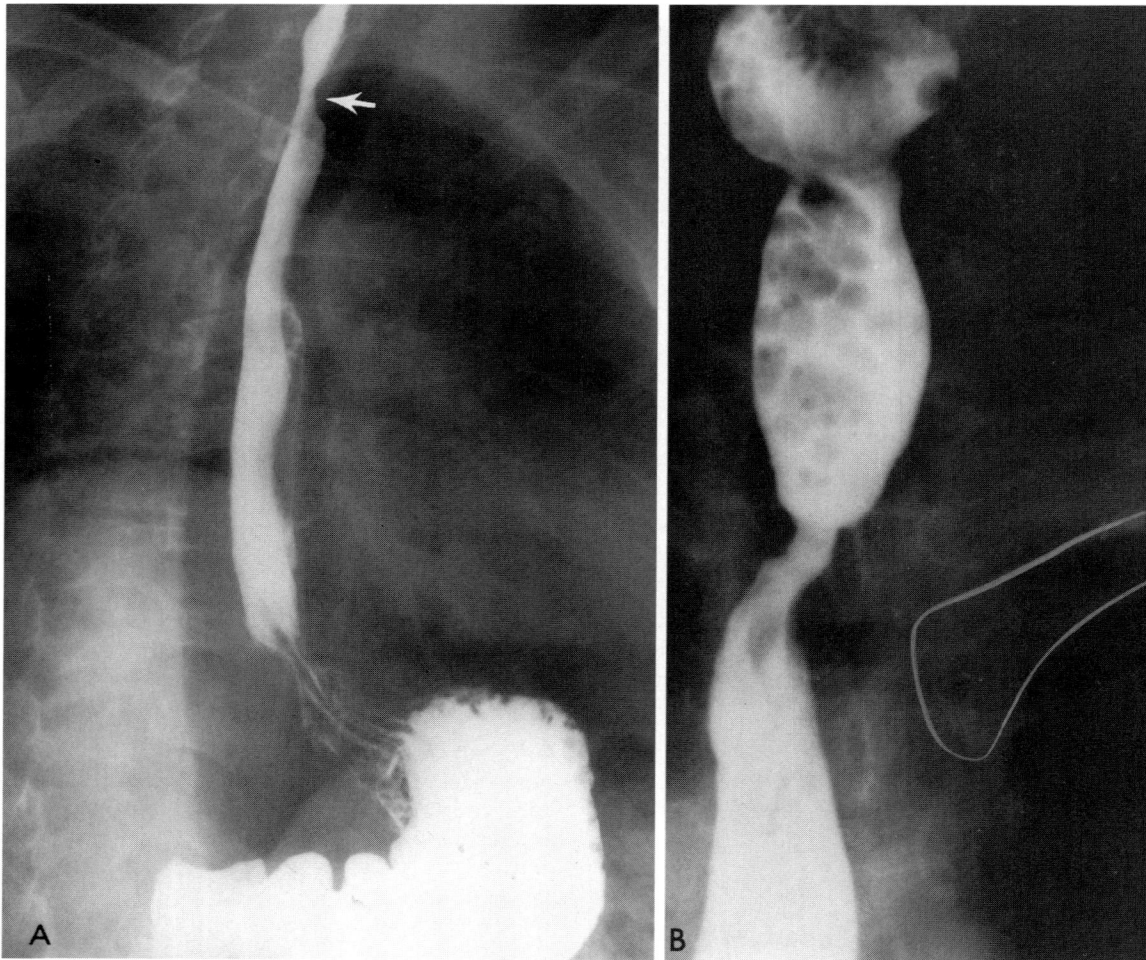

FIGURE 28–43. *A,* Cervicothoracic stricture *(arrow)* in a patient with a sliding hiatal hernia. *B,* Detail of the stricture, at the level of the clavicle *(highlighted),* initially thought to be secondary to carcinoma. Multiple esophageal biopsies at 5-cm intervals distal to the stricture revealed columnar epithelium. Squamous epithelium was found proximal to this unusually high stenosis that occurred in this case of Barrett's esophagus.

aggravation have little if any endoscopic evidence of esophagitis, whereas others have dysphagia from an established reflux stricture without a significant prior history of reflux symptoms. Second, one of the most widely used studies to evaluate the esophagus—the barium esophagogram—fails to detect esophagitis consistently and reliably before mural fibrosis has occurred. Although the radiologist may infer the presence of early esophagitis on the basis of distal spasm or at times demonstrate superficial mucosal irregularity with a carefully performed air-contrast study, he cannot consistently detect esophagitis until the barium swallow examination demonstrates some degree of esophageal narrowing. At this point, the report of a "mild" esophageal stricture may imply that the process has been detected at a sufficiently early stage that conservative therapy is adequate. As is evident from the endoscopic grades of esophagitis described below, however, a "mild" radiographic stricture is an advanced stage of esophagitis, and adequate therapy is long overdue.

Endoscopic Assessment

The degree and extent of esophagitis are important determinants of the type of therapy to be recommended. It is appropriate, therefore, that the evaluating surgeon use a consistent grading system for esophagitis to provide a more objective and meaningful description of the gross pathologic changes seen rather than the more traditional designations of "mild," "moderate," or "severe" esophagitis, which have inherent wide intraobserver variation. A number of endoscopic grading systems of esophagitis are used currently, but two of the most popular are those of Belsey (1967) and Savary and Monnier (Ollyo et al., 1992). The four grades of esophagitis proposed in the endoscopic grading system of Skinner and Belsey (1967) are as follows:

Grade I: Distal esophageal mucosal erythema (which may obscure the esophagogastric squamocolumnar epithelial junction)

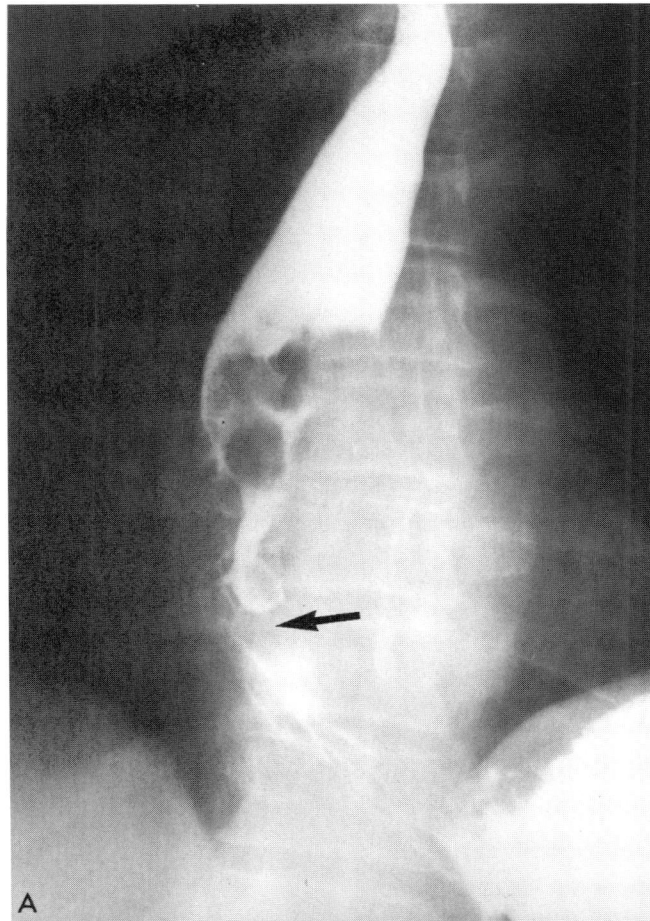

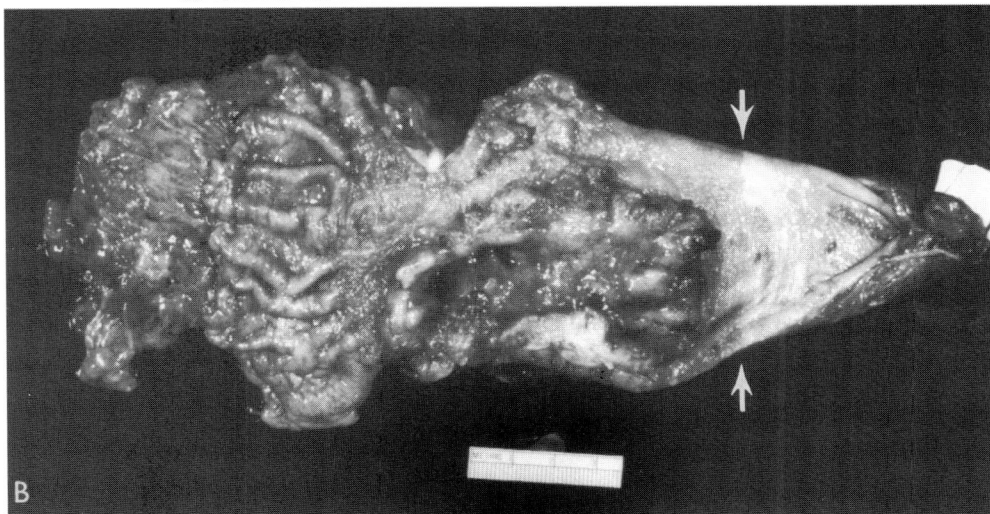

FIGURE 28–44. *A,* Adenocarcinoma arising in Barrett's esophagus. Esophagogram showing an extensive tumor proximal to a sliding hiatal hernia *(arrow* indicates the esophagogastric junction). *B,* Resected specimen showing the squamocolumnar epithelial junction *(arrows)* and the ulcerated adenocarcinoma arising in the columnar epithelium that lined the lower half of this case of Barrett's esophagus.

Grade II: Mucosal erythema with superficial
ulceration, typically linear and vertical and with
an overlying fibrinous membranous exudate
that is easily wiped away, leaving a bleeding
surface (which is often misinterpreted as "scope
trauma" by the inexperienced endoscopist)
Grade III: Mucosal erythema with superficial
ulceration and associated mural fibrosis (a
dilatable stricture)
Grade IV: Extensive ulceration and fibrous luminal
stenosis that is the result of irreversible
panmural fibrosis (an undilatable stricture)

The Savary-Monnier five-grade classification of reflux esophagitis is as follows (Ollyo et al., 1992):

Grade 1: Single or multiple erosions (may be
erythematous or covered by exudate) *on a single
mucosal fold*
Grade 2: Multiple erosions covering *several mucosal
folds;* may be confluent, but not circumferential
Grade 3: Multiple circumferential erosions
Grade 4: Ulcer, stenosis, or esophageal shortening
Grade 5: Barrett's epithelium: columnar mucosa reepithelialization that is circumferential or in the
form of an island or a strip

Dilatation

The surgeon confronted with a distal esophageal
stricture must answer two questions: Is the stricture
benign or malignant? If benign, can the stricture be
dilated? Both of these questions are answered by
esophagoscopy, which is a mandatory part of the
evaluation of *every* stricture. It cannot be overemphasized that dilatation of an esophageal stricture is
among the most dangerous of thoracic surgical operations performed; it requires patience and facility with
the variety of currently available techniques for in-
strumenting the esophagus. Regardless of the method
used, particularly for the initial endoscopic evaluation
of a distal esophageal stricture, which may be quite
uncomfortable for the patient, adequate sedation and
anesthesia are important so that the surgeon can de-
vote his complete attention to the endoscopic field
and not be distracted by a struggling, moving patient.
Modern advances in flexible fiberoptic esophagogastroscopy, video-transmitted optics, and instrumentation possible through the flexible esophagoscope have
made this the most readily available and widely used
technique for assessing esophageal stenoses. Complication is possible with passage of *any* instrument into
the esophagus, however, and a prior barium esophagogram to assess the level and length of the stricture,
the degree of obstruction it is causing, and any co-
existing esophageal pathology (e.g., tumor, diverticulum) should always be obtained and reviewed by the
endoscopist before proceeding with the operation.

The initial endoscopic assessment of the stricture
requires biopsies and brushings of the stenosis that
are adequate for cytologic evaluation. The combination of esophageal biopsy and brushings establishes

the diagnosis of esophageal cancer in more than 95%
of patients with carcinoma; if these studies yield no
evidence of neoplasm, the esophageal stricture can
generally be assumed to be benign with a high degree
of confidence. After biopsying the stricture, one performs dilatation. If the degree of stenosis is relatively
mild, as indicated by the esophagogram and the ability to pass the esophagoscope through the stenosis,
removal of the flexible esophagoscope and dilatation
of the stricture by "blind" passage of progressively
larger Hurst-Maloney mercury-filled tapered bougies
usually is possible. The standard flexible adult
esophagoscope is approximately the size of a No. 32
French bougie; therefore, if the esophagoscope can be
passed through the stricture, once it is removed from
the esophagus, dilatation with Hurst-Maloney bougies can be performed with a No. 32 French dilator,
progressing to sequentially larger sizes. In my experience, almost all strictures that can be dilated either
directly per os to the range of a No. 40 French bougie
can be further dilated *intraoperatively* to the No. 54
to No. 60 French range. Therefore, if the patient is
considered a likely candidate for antireflux surgery
(because of intractable esophagitis or dysphagia from
the stricture), aggressive dilatation all the way to the
No. 54 to No. 60 French range is not necessary at
the preoperative endoscopic assessment. However, in
patients in whom treatment of the reflux stricture
with periodic dilatations and a medical antireflux regimen is contemplated, dilatation to at least a No.
46 French size is necessary to restore comfortable
swallowing.

In patients with a high-grade esophageal stenosis
through which the flexible esophagoscope cannot be
advanced, there are two excellent options. Until the
availability of the Savary-Gilliard dilating system
(Monnier et al., 1985), patients with such "hard" reflux strictures were assessed routinely with the rigid
esophagoscope under general anesthesia. While the
stenosis is under direct vision, gum-tipped bougies
are passed under direct vision through the stricture
(Fig. 28–45). Gentle passage of these dilators allows
direct assessment of the pliability and length of the
stenosis. The largest gum-tipped dilator that will pass
through most rigid esophagoscopes is a No. 26
French. If an initially high-grade stenosis on barium
esophagogram is found to be pliable on probing with
the gum-tipped dilators, and minimal resistance is
encountered during dilatation, the esophagoscope may
be removed and the dilation continued with Hurst-
Maloney tapered dilators passed blindly through the
mouth. If, however, probing of the stricture reveals a
dense, rigid, "hard" stricture, blind passage of the
Hurst-Maloney dilator is not performed, because the
bougie may curl proximal to the nonyielding stenosis,
and perforation may occur. With such high-grade
hard stenoses, after removing the standard rigid
esophagoscope, I replace it with a special-order 45-
cm-long rigid esophagoscope (Pilling company) that
accommodates up to a No. 50 French size bougie (Fig.
28–46). This esophagoscope is introduced to the level
of the stricture; *under direct vision,* progressively larger

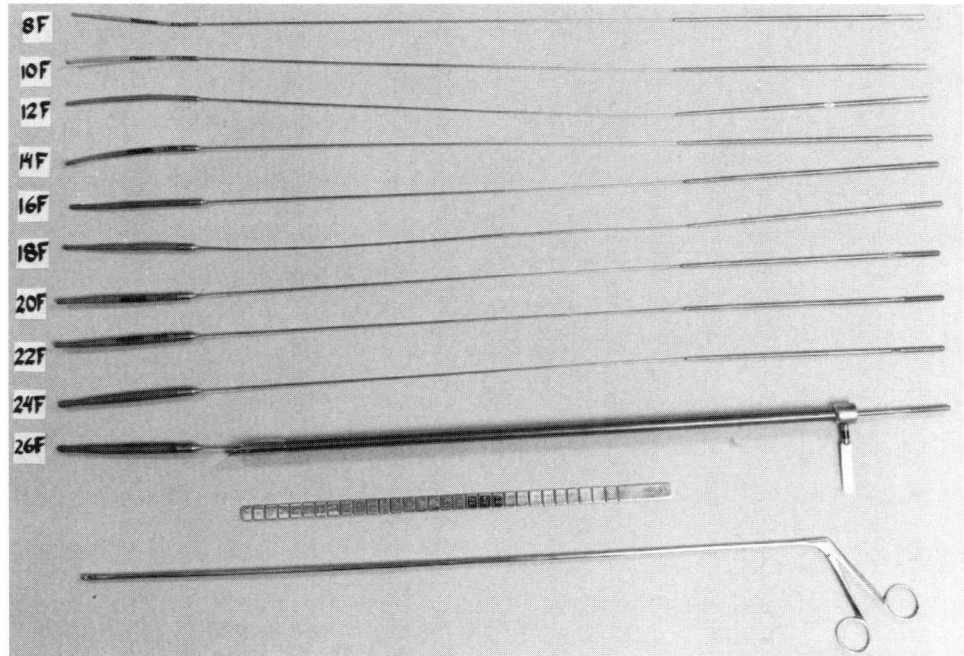

FIGURE 28–45. Required instruments for evaluation of peptic esophageal stricture. Precise, measured localization of the stricture in centimeters from the incisor teeth and adequate biopsies, as well as brushings from the stricture, are obtained. The gum-tipped Jackson dilators gently manipulated through the stenosis permit evaluation of the extent and pliability of the obstruction. The No. 26 French dilator is the largest size that will pass through the standard 45-cm rigid esophagoscope.

dilators, beginning with a No. 28 French and proceeding to a No. 50 French, are passed through the stenosis. After dilatation of the stricture, both esophageal biopsies and brushings for cytologic evaluation are performed to exclude carcinoma. Rigid esophagoscopy not only permits dilatation under direct vision, but also allows for a larger biopsy than is possible through the flexible fiberoptic instrument.

The Savary-Gilliard dilating system, however, has all but replaced the need for the large rigid esophagoscope for dilating difficult esophageal reflux strictures. For patients in whom the flexible esophagoscope cannot be insinuated through the stenosis, the Savary guidewire is negotiated through the stricture and into the stomach, the esophagoscope is removed, and the tapered polyvinyl bougies are passed progressively over the guidewire until the caliber of the lumen permits completion of the endoscopic assessment with multiple biopsies and brushings for cytologic assessment (Fig. 28–47).

As indicated earlier, symptoms may correlate poorly with the degree of esophagitis. In patients who

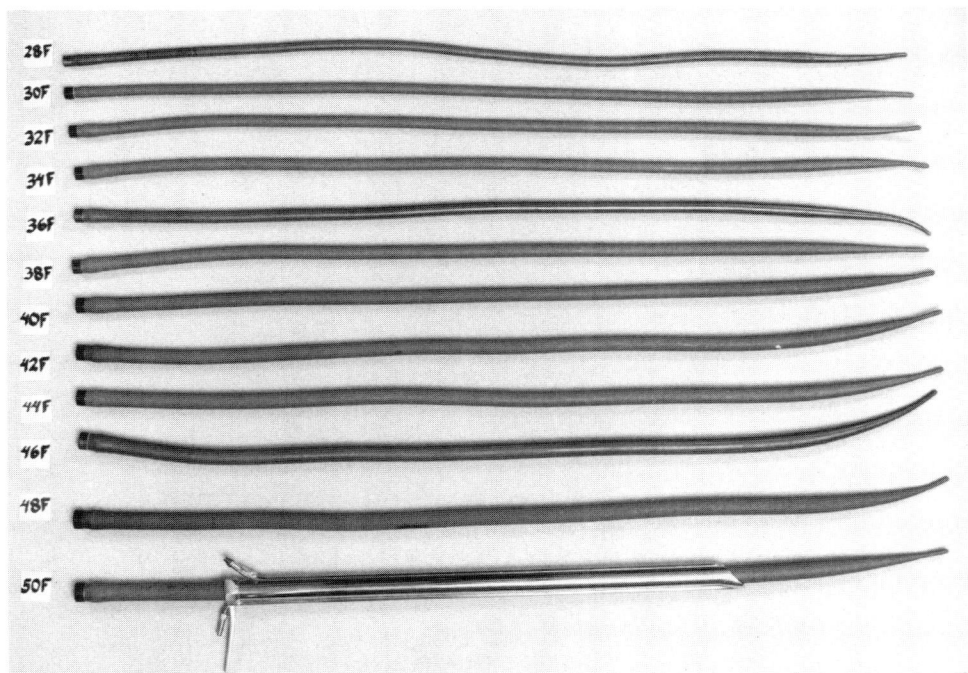

FIGURE 28–46. Tapered Hurst-Maloney esophageal dilators and 45-cm Pilling esophagoscope, which accommodates up to a No. 50 French bougie, thus permitting progressive dilatation of severe peptic strictures under direct vision.

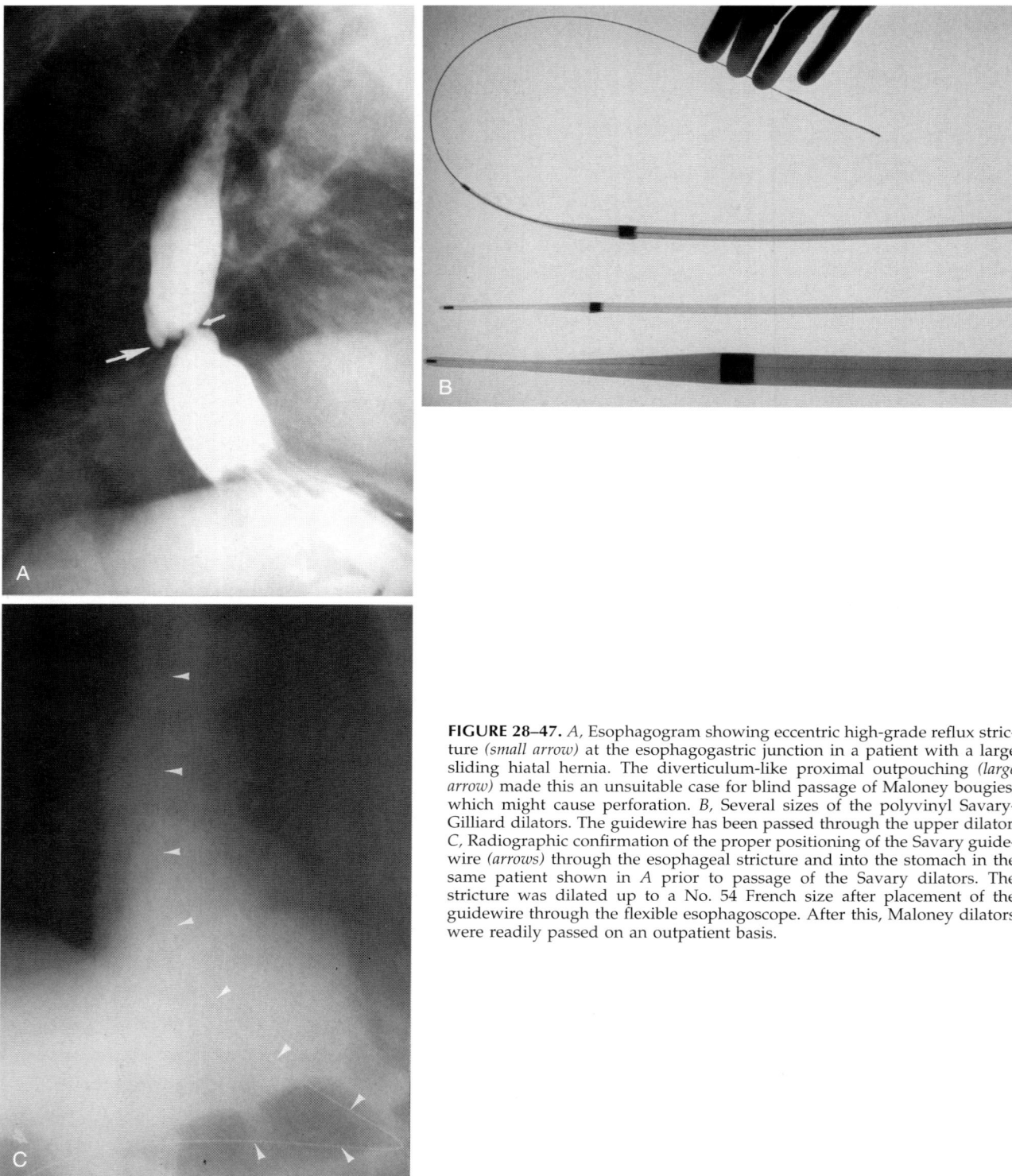

FIGURE 28–47. *A,* Esophagogram showing eccentric high-grade reflux stricture *(small arrow)* at the esophagogastric junction in a patient with a large sliding hiatal hernia. The diverticulum-like proximal outpouching *(large arrow)* made this an unsuitable case for blind passage of Maloney bougies, which might cause perforation. *B,* Several sizes of the polyvinyl Savary-Gilliard dilators. The guidewire has been passed through the upper dilator. *C,* Radiographic confirmation of the proper positioning of the Savary guidewire *(arrows)* through the esophageal stricture and into the stomach in the same patient shown in *A* prior to passage of the Savary dilators. The stricture was dilated up to a No. 54 French size after placement of the guidewire through the flexible esophagoscope. After this, Maloney dilators were readily passed on an outpatient basis.

have a reflux stricture and no significant heartburn or regurgitation, dilatation of the stricture relieves the dominant esophageal symptom—dysphagia—and the addition of a medical program for reflux control may constitute adequate therapy. These patients generally accept intermittent outpatient esophageal bougienage as a preferred alternative to impaired swallowing,

and between dilatations they are comfortable and satisfied with their ability to eat.

Some believe that the presence of Barrett's esophagus per se is an indication for an antireflux procedure to prevent the later development of malignancy (Skinner, 1985). However, careful long-term pathologic studies indicate that the presence of *dysplasia* in

Barrett's epithelium is the major risk factor for subsequent development of an adenocarcinoma, and that if there is no epithelial dysplasia on biopsy, the rate of malignant degeneration is probably in the range of 0.8% per year (Cameron et al., 1985). Therefore, for the patient with a reflux stricture with Barrett's epithelium that is not associated with endoscopic ulceration or microscopic dysplasia on biopsy, intermittent dilatations and medical therapy may still be reasonable treatment, particularly if the patient's only complaint is dysphagia. In contrast with such patients are those with high-grade peptic esophageal strictures who give a history of long-standing, severe reflux symptoms that gradually subsided as dysphagia occurred. Dilatation of the stricture in these patients relieves the dysphagia but also permits the return of significant regurgitation from the stomach into the esophagus. Thus, reflux symptoms again become prominent, and relief of the esophageal obstruction alone does not satisfy the patient.

Many physicians believe that esophageal bougienage in combination with a strict antireflux medical regimen is the treatment of choice for the patient with a peptic stricture (Wesdorp et al., 1982). The newest drug in the medical armamentarium against gastroesophageal reflux is the acid-pump inhibitor omeprazole, which is as effective as successful antireflux surgery in reducing pathologic esophageal acid exposure (Lundell, 1992). In the United States, there has been concern about the potential for induction of intestinal tumors by omeprazole because of a small reported incidence of small bowel tumors in rats exposed to high doses of this drug. The recommendation in the United States is to limit continuous omeprazole therapy to 8 weeks. In Europe, however, long-term omeprazole therapy has been used for several years in many patients without any reported small bowel tumors. Although this new drug therapy greatly benefits many patients with gastroesophageal reflux disease, other patients' persistent esophagitis, dysphagia, or intolerance of this medication warrants surgical intervention. Modern surgical advances have greatly changed the approach to esophageal reflux strictures, with the salvage of esophagi that were previously routinely resected (Toledo-Pereyra et al., 1976). Because of these developments and the fact that the patient with an esophageal reflux stricture, regardless of the severity of symptoms, has *advanced* reflux esophagitis, I still recommend surgical control of reflux in most patients who are relatively young and good candidates for operation.

Surgical Treatment

Peptic stricture and esophageal shortening interfere with the success of standard antireflux operations in these patients. The incidence of recurrent hiatal hernia or reflux in patients with strictures who undergo the standard Belsey Mark IV operation, for example, is between 45 and 75% (Donnelly et al., 1973; Orringer et al., 1972; Vollan et al., 1992). The mural inflammation, esophagitis, and esophageal shortening that characterize peptic esophageal strictures prevent the tension-free reduction of the prerequisite 3- to 5-cm segment of distal esophagus below the diaphragm, where the influence of positive intra-abdominal pressure transmitted to the esophagus by the partial fundoplication helps prevent reflux. Because the Belsey and Nissen fundoplications and the Hill median arcuate ligament repair all strive for an intra-abdominal location of the esophagogastric junction and all require sutures in the distal esophageal or periesophageal tissues, the long-term success of these antireflux procedures must be jeopardized if mural inflammation and esophageal shortening are present, because these factors necessitate not only suturing to inflamed tissues, but also fixing the esophagogastric junction below the diaphragm under tension. Mobilizing the short esophagus, if necessary to the level of the aortic arch, has been described as a way to better reduce the esophagogastric junction below the diaphragm (Little et al., 1988; Orringer et al., 1972). The necessity for such a maneuver, however, implies that the surgeon is concerned about the degree of tension on the repaired esophagus; I suggest that an alternative operation is needed.

The realization that peptic stricture and esophageal shortening adversely affected the results of the Mark IV operation led to Belsey's recommendation for resection rather than hernia repair in patients with reflux strictures requiring operation (Orringer et al., 1972). However, distal esophagectomy with an intrathoracic esophagogastric anastomosis is a poor operation for the patient with reflux esophagitis, because the lack of a lower esophageal sphincter combined with the iatrogenic hiatal hernia created are responsible for the development of reflux esophagitis in the residual esophagus in at least 40 to 60% of these patients. Various operations designed to prevent gastroesophageal reflux after an intrathoracic esophagogastric anastomosis have been reported (Bombeck et al., 1970; Demos and Biele, 1980; Okada et al., 1974), but none has been reliable or has gained widespread acceptance. The alternative techniques of distal esophagectomy and reconstruction with either a jejunal or a short-segment colonic interposition provide excellent relief of dysphagia and reflux symptoms in patients with peptic strictures. These are, of course, sizable and technically demanding operations, the need for which has been greatly diminished by the advent of newer, more conservative nonresective techniques.

In 1971, Pearson and associates reported success with the Collis gastroplasty operation (Collis, 1957, 1961) in combination with the Belsey hiatal hernia repair in patients with severe peptic esophagitis and secondary esophageal shortening. With elimination of reflux, the distal esophageal stenosis was resolved sufficiently to allow comfortable swallowing. The combined Collis-Belsey operation is performed through a left sixth or seventh intercostal space posterolateral thoracotomy rather than the thoracoabdominal incision described by Collis. As in the routine Belsey

Mark IV procedure, the fundus of the stomach is delivered into the chest through the hiatus without the routine use of a diaphragmatic counter-incision. This necessitates division and ligation of several of the short gastric vessels along the high greater curvature of the stomach. Progressively larger Hurst-Maloney tapered dilators, up to the range of No. 56 to 58 French size, are passed by the anesthetist per os and are guided across the esophagogastric junction by the surgeon, who supports the wall of the esophagus to avoid disruption. Satisfactory intraoperative dilatation may require considerable force. With a No. 54 French intraesophageal dilator in women or a No. 56 French dilator in men displaced against the lesser curvature of the stomach and with the fundus retracted in the opposite direction, the GIA surgical stapler is applied to the stomach adjacent to the dilator and parallel to the lesser curvature (Fig. 28–48). Use of the GIA surgical stapler to construct the gastroplasty tube, instead of the originally described gastric clamps, greatly simplifies this portion of the operation and prevents gastrointestinal contamination of the field (Orringer and Sloan, 1974). After advancing the knife assembly, a 5-cm-long gastric tube extension of the esophagus is created and is mechanically sutured closed by two staggered rows of stainless-steel staples. If there is a great deal of distal esophageal shortening and fibrosis, the stapler can be partially applied a second time to gain an additional 2 to 3 cm of "esophageal" length. The staple suture-line is then oversewn, and the dilator is removed. The standard

posterior crural sutures of No. 1 silk are placed and left untied for the present.

Pearson advocated a standard Belsey repair around the "new" distal esophagus (i.e., the gastroplasty tube) after intraoperative dilatation of the stricture and construction of the gastroplasty tube (Pearson et al., 1971) (Fig. 28–49). Two rows of sutures, each consisting of three horizontal mattress sutures of 2-0 silk, are placed in the newly created distal esophageal gastric tube. The first row is 2 cm above the new esophagogastric junction, and the second is 2 cm above the first and passes through the diaphragm. After the stomach is secured below the diaphragm and the posterior crural sutures have been tied, a 4-cm-long, tension-free segment of intra-abdominal "esophagus" is produced (Fig. 28–49C). Because the sutures of the Belsey reconstruction in this combined operation are taken in a resilient, healthy stomach (gastroplasty tube), the need to suture to inflamed distal esophagus is totally eliminated. The combined Collis-Belsey operation is conceptually sound, lengthening the functional distal esophageal tube to avoid tension on the repair and providing a resilient gastric tube, rather than the inflamed esophagus, around which to do the Belsey partial fundoplication. Pearson reported excellent relief of both dysphagia and reflux symptoms following dilatation of peptic strictures and the Collis-Belsey operation in 25 of 33 patients so treated and followed for 5 to 12 years (Pearson, 1977; Pearson and Henderson, 1976).

However, after initial enthusiasm for the combined

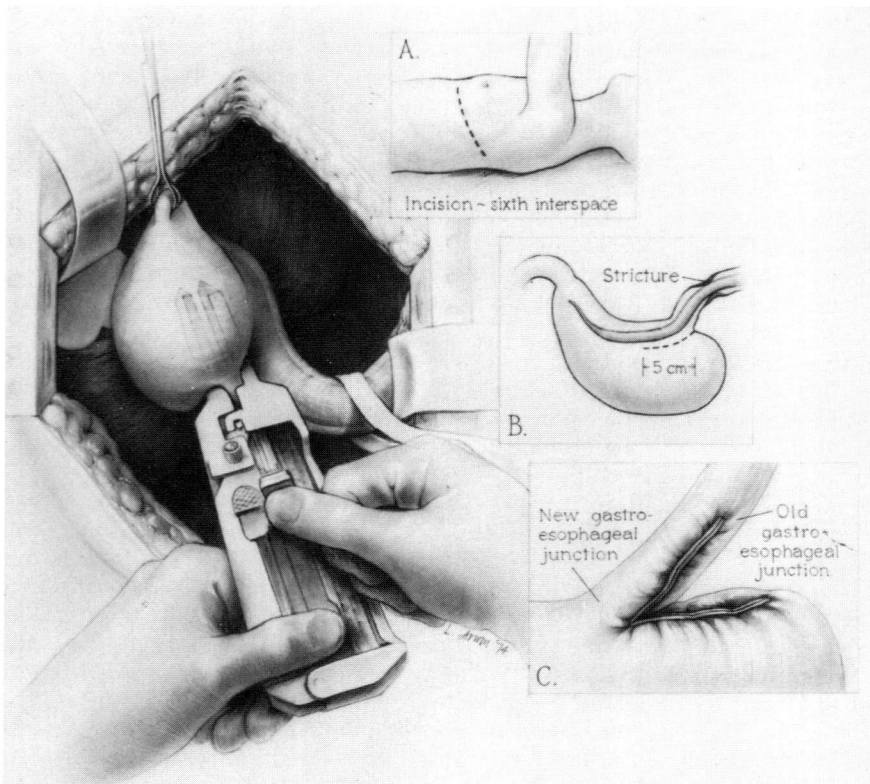

FIGURE 28–48. The Collis gastroplasty using the GIA stapler. *A,* The esophagus and fundus of the stomach are mobilized through a lateral thoracotomy in the sixth left intercostal space. *B,* A No. 54 French (in women) or No. 56 French (in men) Hurst-Maloney dilator is passed through the esophageal stricture and displaced against the lesser curvature of the stomach as the stapler is applied. The knife assembly is advanced *(main illustration),* and the stapler is removed. *C,* The result is a 3-cm-long gastric tube extension of the esophagus. An additional 2 to 3 cm of length can be gained by a second, partial application of the stapler, but this is seldom required. (*A–C,* From Orringer, M. B., and Sloan, H.: An improved technique for the combined Collis-Belsey approach to dilatable esophageal strictures. J. Thorac. Cardiovasc. Surg., *68:*298, 1974.)

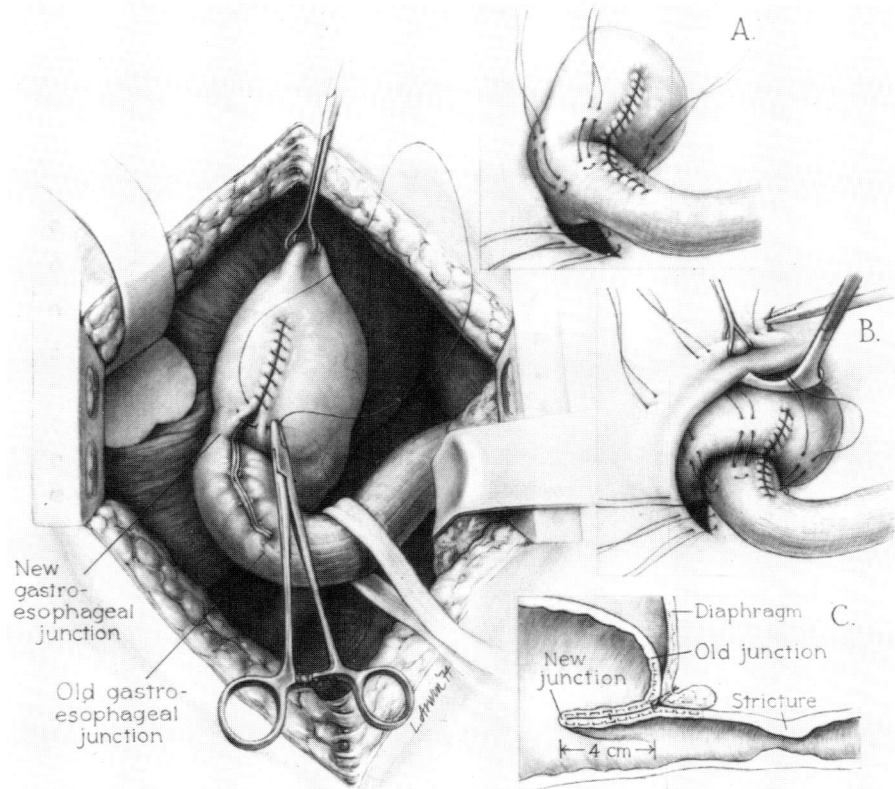

FIGURE 28–49. Belsey reconstruction of the esophagogastric junction after constructing the Collis gastroplasty tube. The *main illustration* depicts oversewing the staple suture line. *A,* Placement of standard posterior crural sutures and the first row of three mattress sutures between the fundus of the stomach and the new distal "esophagus," 2 cm above the new esophagogastric junction. *B,* Placement of the second row of mattress sutures through the diaphragm, fundus, and new distal "esophagus." *C,* The completed repair, showing a 4-cm segment of intra-abdominal distal "esophagus."

Collis-Belsey operation (Orringer and Sloan, 1976; Pearson and Henderson, 1973; Urschel et al., 1973), reports of unsatisfactory reflux control emerged from those who were assessing the objective results of the operation with the intraesophageal pH electrode. Orringer and Sloan (1977) suggested that construction of the gastroplasty tube reduces the amount of gastric fundus available for the fundoplication so much that an adequate 240-degree Belsey wrap around the new distal esophagus may not be possible (Fig. 28–50). Thus, even with a 3- to 7-cm intra-abdominal segment of functional distal esophagus, with an inadequate fundoplication, gastroesophageal reflux may not be prevented.

In an effort to improve reflux control after performance of the Collis gastroplasty, Henderson and associates (1977, 1985) and Orringer and associates (1978a, 1982) advocated the use of a 360-degree Nissen-type fundoplication. In my experience, if, at the initial endoscopic evaluation, it is ascertained that the stricture is benign and can be dilated per os to a No. 40 French bougie, treatment with dilatation and a combined gastroplasty-fundoplication operation most likely is possible. Almost every stricture that can be dilated to this size per os will be amenable to later forceful intraoperative dilation, done with the surgeon's hand supporting the mobilized esophagus from without, and resection can be avoided. Alternatively, if passage of a No. 40 French dilator through the stricture is not possible, a barium enema examination is done to evaluate the suitability of the colon as

an esophageal substitute, and the colon is prepared preoperatively in the event that intraoperative forceful dilatation of the stricture is unsuccessful and resection is required. The colon is also evaluated and prepared in patients with recurrent reflux esophagitis after multiple previous hiatal hernia repairs, because repetitive mobilization of the gastric fundus may not be viable and may contraindicate both construction of the Collis gastroplasty tube from the stomach and another fundoplication.

An average of five to six short gastric vessels are divided in the Collis-Nissen operation as the greater curvature of the stomach and gastric fundus are mobilized into the chest through the diaphragmatic hiatus. Great care must be taken to avoid undue tension on these vessels to prevent injury to the spleen. Moreover, gentle but precise ligation is required, because these vessels readily retract beneath the diaphragm and may be a source of subsequent intra-abdominal hemorrhage. If adhesions from previous operations at the hiatus require abdominal exposure, a 5- to 10-cm peripheral diaphragmatic counterincision is made 2 to 3 cm from the attachment of the diaphragm on the costal arch. Division of the costal arch is avoided if possible, because this is one of the most painful incisions, both in the early postoperative period and later. Thus, in my opinion, a separate abdominal incision, if necessary, is preferable to a thoracoabdominal one.

The stricture is dilated to the range of a No. 56 or 58 French bougie, and then the gastroplasty tube is constructed. It is seldom necessary to apply the GIA

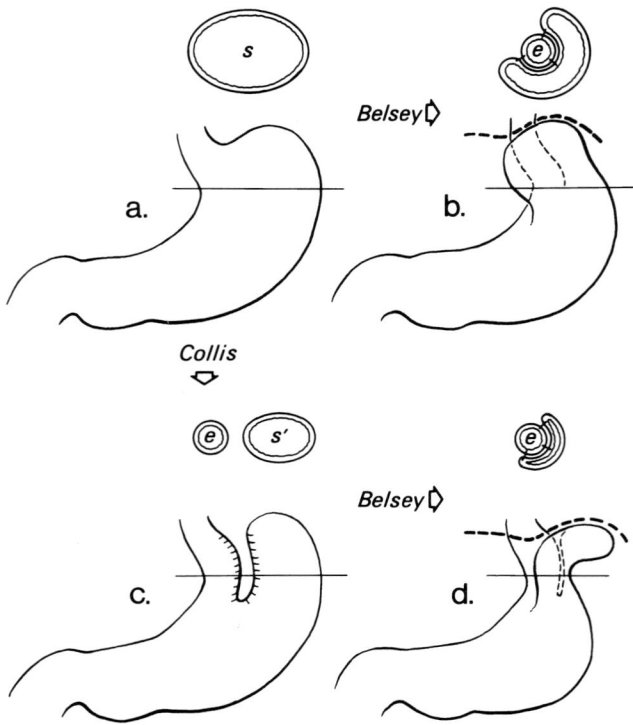

FIGURE 28–50. Limitation of fundoplication by Collis procedure. *a,* Cross-section through gastric fundus in the indicated plane shows the area of stomach (s) available for standard Belsey Mark IV repair, with 240-degree fundoplication shown in *b. c,* The use of stomach in the Collis procedure to form the new distal esophagus *(e)* results in a smaller area of gastric fundus *(s')* available for the Belsey fundoplication. *d,* Only a limited 180-degree fundoplication is possible after the Collis maneuver, and the elongated, narrowed gastric fundus is angulated beneath the diaphragm *(broken line)* as the second row of sutures of the Belsey repair are tied. *(a–d,* From Orringer, M. B., and Sloan, H.: Complications and failings of the combined Collis-Belsey operation. J. Thorac. Cardiovasc. Surg., 74:726, 1977.)

FIGURE 28–51. Nissen fundoplication after Collis gastroplasty. The main drawing illustrates the elongated, narrow gastric fundus available for the fundoplication after completion of the Collis procedure. *A,* Placement of the incision through the left sixth intercostal space. *B* and *C,* The gastric fundus is shown being wrapped around the gastroplasty tube and adjacent stomach. Note that the posterior crural sutures are left untied for the moment. *(A–C,* From Orringer, M. B., and Sloan, H.: Combined Collis-Nissen reconstruction of the esophagogastric junction. Ann. Thorac. Surg., 25:16, 1978.)

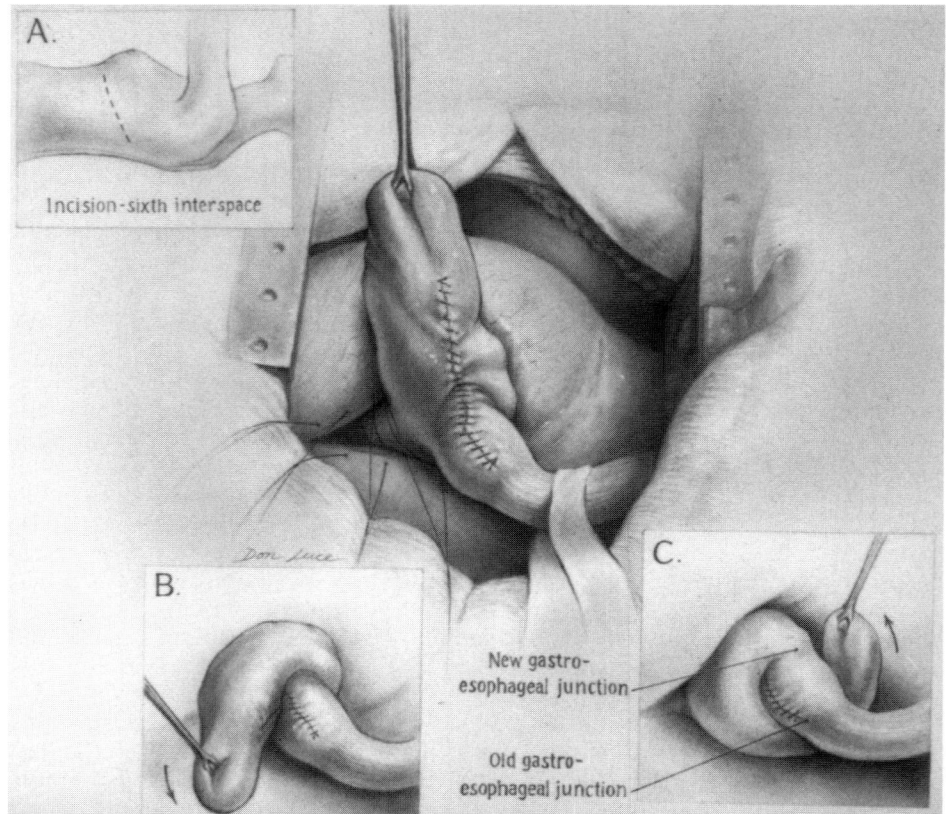

stapler more than once, because this "lengthens" the functional esophagus by approximately 5 cm. Earlier in my experience, after dilating strictures intraoperatively to the No. 54 to 60 French range and constructing the gastroplasty tube over these bougies, these large dilators were removed and replaced with a No. 46 French bougie around which the fundoplication was done. A relatively long 5- to 6-cm fundoplication was constructed, incorporating the proximal 3 to 4 cm of stomach and the distal 3 to 4 cm of the gastroplasty tube (Figs. 28–51 and 28–52). In more recent years, to minimize narrowing of the "neo-esophagus" and reduce the incidence of postoperative dysphagia, both the gastroplasty and fundoplication have been constructed over either a No. 54 French dilator (in women) or a No. 56 French dilator (in men) (Stirling and Orringer, 1988). In addition, the length of the fundoplication has been limited strictly to 3 cm, starting at the new esophagogastric junction and incorporating only the distal gastroplasty tube (Fig. 28–53). Four interrupted seromuscular 2-0 silk sutures are placed 1 cm apart. Each suture passes through the gastric fundus, then through the gastroplasty tube, and finally through the gastric fundus again. The sutures are tied with the No. 54 or 56 French dilator still within the gastroplasty tube, and

the silk suture line is then oversewn with a 4-0 running polypropylene Lembert stitch through the seromuscular layers on each side to prevent a subsequent leak from the fundoplication sutures.

The fundoplication is reduced beneath the diaphragm, and the posterior crural sutures are tied so that the hiatus admits one finger alongside the esophagus. Intraoperatively, silver clip markers are placed at the new esophagogastric junction (the apex of the gastroplasty tube) and at the edges of the diaphragmatic hiatus. On postoperative films, the distance between these two rows of markers represents the tension-free intra-abdominal segment of functional esophagus that is encircled completely by the gastric wrap (Fig. 28–54).

The severity of a reflux stricture is based intraoperatively on the degree of resistance encountered during dilatation, and it has important prognostic implications for resolution of the stricture, the need for subsequent dilatations, and the likelihood of long-term reflux control after operation. A *mild* stricture is one that is easily dilated during operation with minimal resistance; a *moderate* stricture requires some, but not excessive, forceful dilatation; and a *severe* stricture requires vigorous, forceful dilatation and is generally associated with marked periesophagitis, panmural

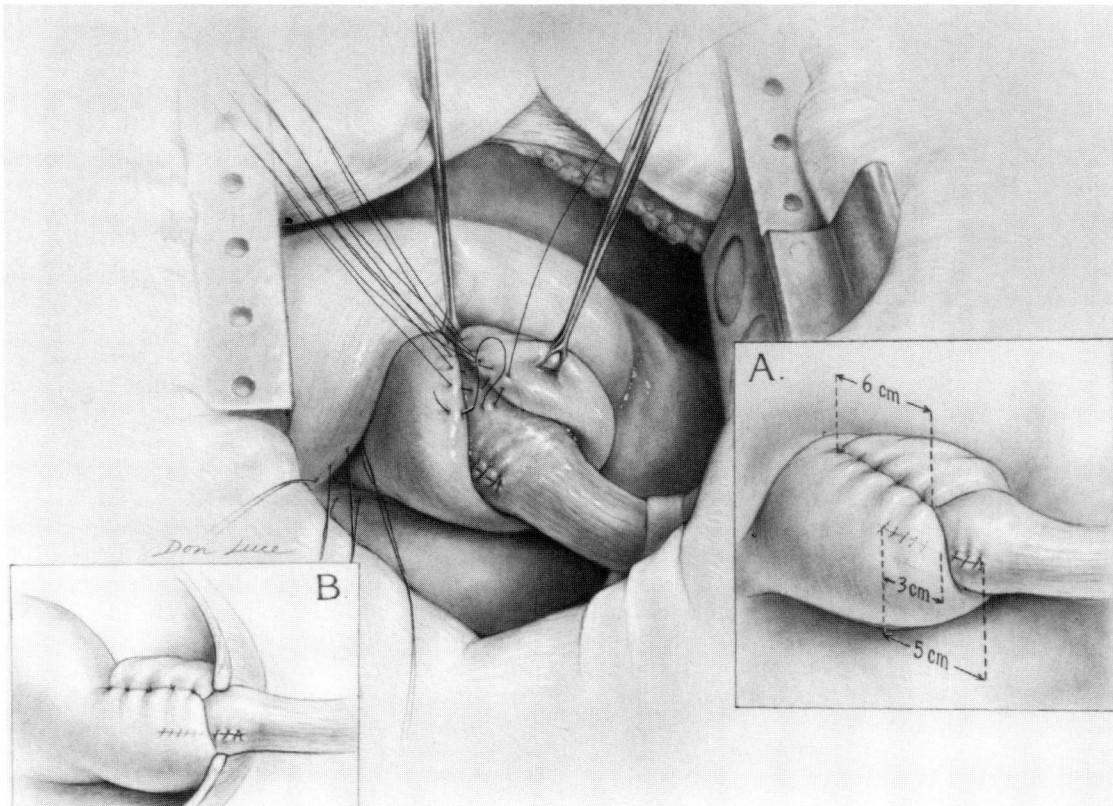

FIGURE 28–52. Originally advocated fundoplication length. Placement of the seromuscular sutures from the gastric fundus to the gastroplasty tube and back to the gastric fundus for the proximal three or four sutures and from the gastric fundus to the anterior stomach wall and then the gastric fundus for the distal three or four sutures. After these sutures are tied, the fundoplication includes the distal 3 to 4 cm of gastroplasty tube and the proximal 3 to 4 cm of stomach. *A,* The fundoplication, reduced in the abdomen, rests below the diaphragm without tension on the distal esophagus after the posterior crural sutures are tied *(B).* (*A* and *B,* From Orringer, M. B., and Sloan, H.: Combined Collis-Nissen reconstruction of the esophagogastric junction. Ann. Thorac. Surg., 25:16, 1978.)

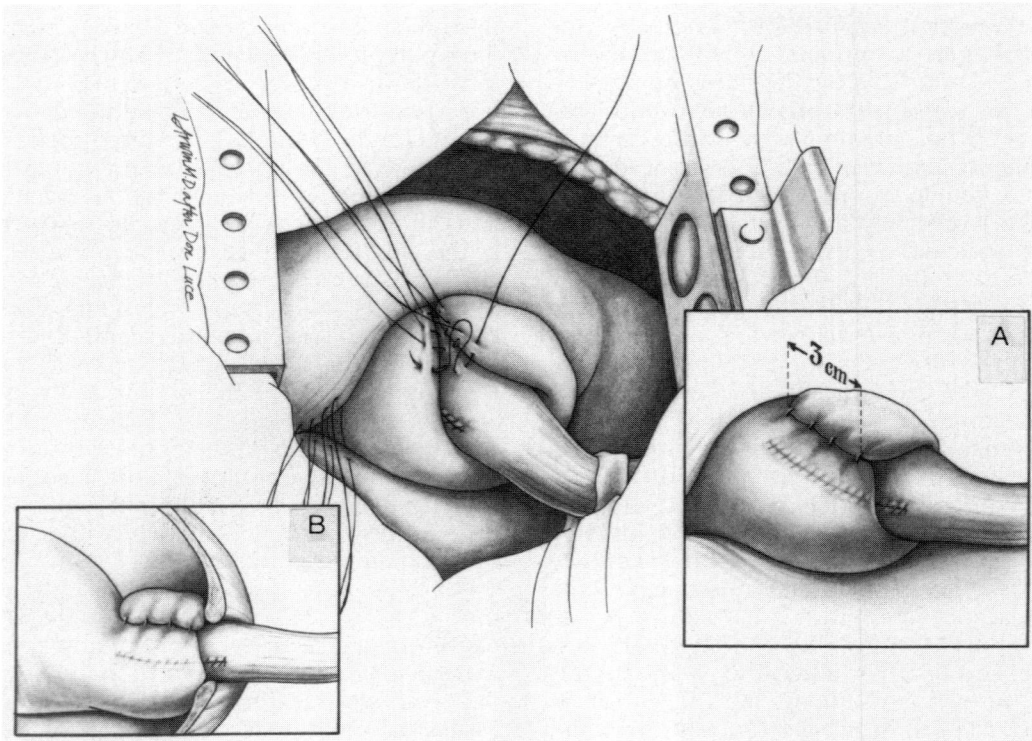

FIGURE 28–53. Currently advocated 3-cm-long fundoplication after Collis gastroplasty. Four seromuscular 2-0 silk sutures placed 1 cm apart *(main illustration)* are used to construct a 3-cm fundoplication around the gastroplasty tube *(A)*, not the proximal stomach, before reducing the wrap into the abdominal cavity *(B)*. *(A* and *B*, From Stirling, M. C., and Orringer, M. B.: The combined Collis-Nissen operation for esophageal reflux strictures. Ann. Thorac. Surg., *45*:148, 1988.)

fibrosis, and thickening of the esophagus. In this regard, I have been impressed that neither the severity of the stricture nor its ability to be dilated can be predicted accurately by its radiographic or endoscopic appearance, inasmuch as when the esophagus has been mobilized and is supported from without by the surgeon's hand, manipulation of Hurst-Maloney dilators through the stricture is almost always possible. In the rare case that antegrade dilatation is not possible, retrograde dilatation of severe strictures may be done using Hegar dilators passed through a high gastrotomy (Herrington et al., 1975).

Stirling and Orringer (1988) reported use of intraoperative dilatation and the combined Collis gastroplasty–Nissen fundoplication operation in 64 patients (average age of 51 years) with esophageal reflux strictures. During the same 12-year period in which these patients underwent surgery, the authors used intermittent outpatient esophageal dilatations and an aggressive antireflux medical regimen to successfully manage 30 patients (average age of 69 years) with reflux strictures and dysphagia, *without* significant reflux symptoms. Seventeen additional patients with reflux strictures required esophageal resection procedures because the strictures could not be dilated or because the stricture fractured during attempted dilatation (three patients). Additional associated esophageal pathology, such as a megaesophagus from achalasia, severe dysplasia in Barrett's epithelium, caustic

stricture, or inability to repeat fundoplication because of severe adhesions from previous antireflux repairs, necessitated resection in the other 14 patients.

In my experience, more than 95% of esophageal reflux strictures could be dilated. Among the 64 patients undergoing the Collis-Nissen operation, one died (1.6% mortality rate) from a pulmonary embolus 2 weeks after operation. Esophageal leaks occurred in two patients (3%), and both healed after drainage. Four patients were lost to follow-up; the remaining 59 patients were followed for an average of 43 months. At the time of most recent follow-up, reflux symptoms were eliminated or mild in 88% of the patients; 8% required an antireflux medical regimen to control symptoms; and 4% had uncontrolled reflux symptoms (Table 28–6). The preoperative severity of the stricture did not significantly influence the postoperative likelihood of unsatisfactory subjective reflux control. Reflux control was assessed objectively by routine preoperative and postoperative esophageal manometry and standard acid reflux testing with the intraesophageal pH electrode (Table 28–7). Although good reflux control was documented with the standard acid reflux test in 47 of 50 patients (94%) studied after 1 year, 10 of 29 patients (34%) who were studied 2 to 5 years postoperatively had abnormal reflux. Seven of these 10 patients, however, had no reflux symptoms at 2 to 5 years. Distal high-pressure zone pressure and length increased appreciably after the

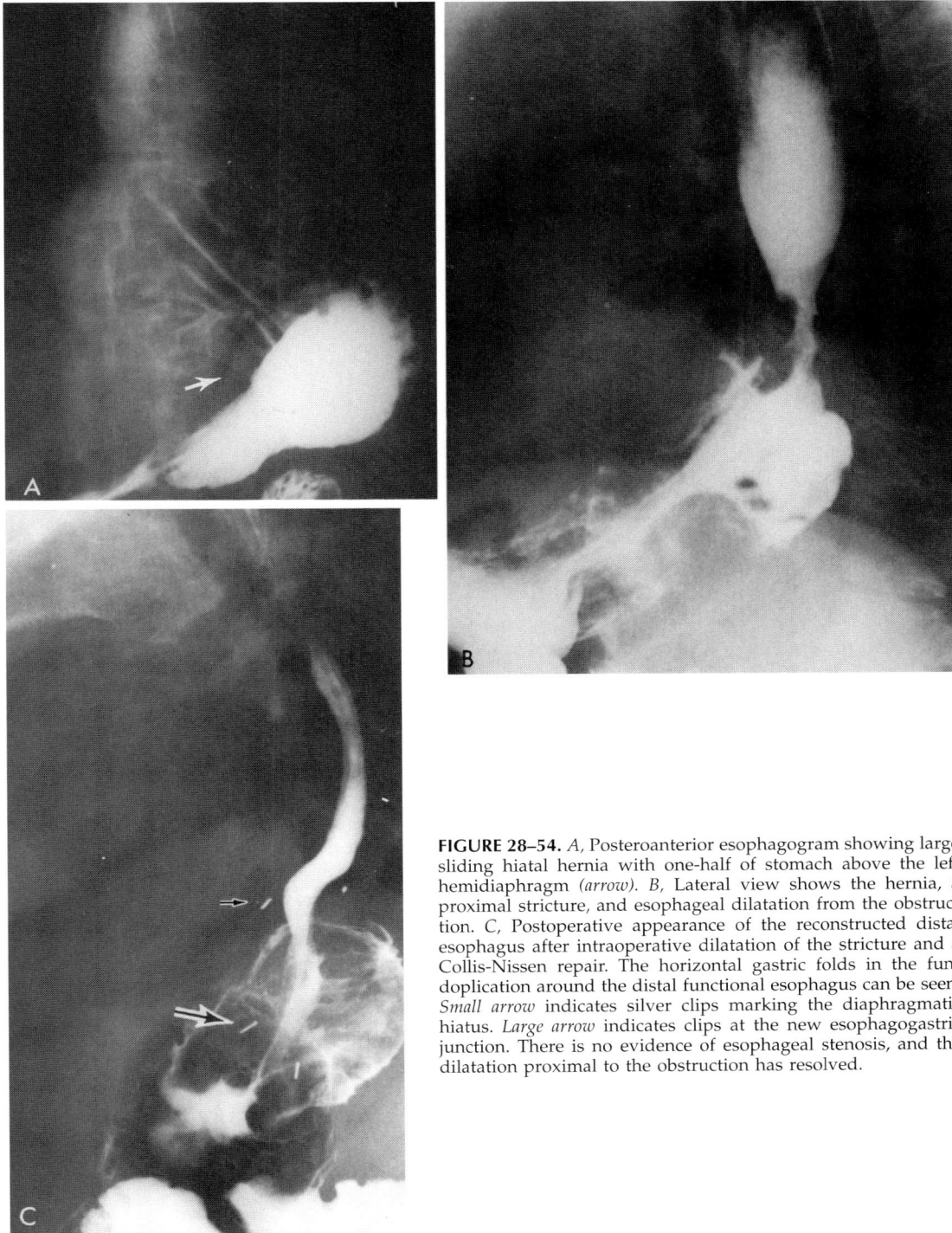

FIGURE 28–54. *A,* Posteroanterior esophagogram showing large sliding hiatal hernia with one-half of stomach above the left hemidiaphragm *(arrow). B,* Lateral view shows the hernia, a proximal stricture, and esophageal dilatation from the obstruction. *C,* Postoperative appearance of the reconstructed distal esophagus after intraoperative dilatation of the stricture and a Collis-Nissen repair. The horizontal gastric folds in the fundoplication around the distal functional esophagus can be seen. *Small arrow* indicates silver clips marking the diaphragmatic hiatus. *Large arrow* indicates clips at the new esophagogastric junction. There is no evidence of esophageal stenosis, and the dilatation proximal to the obstruction has resolved.

Collis-Nissen operation (see Table 28–7), and this increase was maintained over time. Patients with severe strictures were significantly ($p < .05$) more prone to objective reflux recurrence at a 2- to 5-year follow-up than were patients with less severe strictures.

In 81% of these patients, relief of dysphagia was satisfactory (no dysphagia or mild dysphagia not requiring dilatation) (see Table 28–6). Seven (12%) re-

quired occasional dilatations for dysphagia, and 4 (7%) required regular dilatations or reoperation. The need for early postoperative dilatations is significantly influenced by the severity of the stricture: 50% of those with mild strictures required at least one postoperative dilatation, compared with 73% of those with moderate strictures and 100% of those with severe strictures. Of the 38 patients (64%) who required

■ **Table 28–6.** SUBJECTIVE RESULTS OF COLLIS-NISSEN OPERATION FOR ESOPHAGEAL REFLUX STRICTURES (59 PATIENTS)

	Mild Stricture* (n = 34)		Moderate Stricture* (n = 15)		Severe Stricture* (n = 10)		Total (n = 59)	
	No.	*%*	*No.*	*%*	*No.*	*%*	*No.*	*%*
Reflux†								
None	28	82 } 91	12	80 } 87	8	80 } 80	48	81 } 52 (88%)
Mild	3	9	1	7	0		4	7
Moderate	2	6	2	13	1	10	5	8
Severe	1	3	0		1	10	2	4
Dysphagia‡								
None	26	76 } 85	9	60 } 73	7	70 } 80	42	71 } 48 (81%)
Mild	3	9	2	13	1	10	6	10
Moderate	3	9	3	20	1	10	7	12
Severe	2	6	1	7	1	10	4	7
Clinical status§								
Excellent	24	70 } 82	6	40 } 67	7	70 } 70	37	63 } 45 (77%)
Good	4	12	4	27	0		8	14
Fair	5	15	3	20	1	10	9	15
Poor	1	3	2	13	2	20	5	8

From Stirling, M. C., and Orringer, M. B.: The combined Collis-Nissen operation for esophageal reflux strictures. Ann. Thorac. Surg., 45:148, 1988.
Stricture: Mild = easily dilated; moderate = requiring some force to dilate; severe = requiring very forceful dilatation.
†*Reflux*: Mild = requires no treatment; moderate = controlled by medical therapy; severe = uncontrolled by medication or need for reoperation.
‡*Dysphagia*: Mild = requires no dilatation; moderate = requires occasional dilatation; severe = requires regular dilatations or reoperation.
§*Clinical status*: Excellent = asymptomatic; good = minimal reflux symptoms or mild dysphagia requiring no treatment; fair = symptoms controlled by medication or dilatation; poor = symptoms severe or reoperation required.

postoperative dilatations, 27 (72%) required early dilatation only (first 6 months) to achieve resolution of their dysphagia. Overall, comparing the degree of preoperative and postoperative dysphagia, dysphagia was improved postoperatively in 49 of the 59 patients (83%), was unchanged in 7 (12%), and was more severe in 3 (5%).

The overall *subjective* clinical status of these patients was defined as excellent (no symptoms) in 37 patients (63%), good (mild symptoms not requiring treatment) in 8 (14%), fair (reflux symptoms or dysphagia con-

trolled by medical therapy or dilatation) in 9 (15%), and poor (severe uncontrolled symptoms) in 5 (8%) (see Table 28–6). Therefore, the Collis-Nissen operation was successful (no symptoms or mild symptoms not requiring treatment) in 77% of these patients.

The effects of five variables on overall clinical status after the Collis-Nissen operation are cited in Table 28–8. Patients with scleroderma, severe preoperative dysphagia, follow-up longer than 48 months, and more severe strictures were less likely to obtain satisfactory clinical results than were their counterparts,

■ **Table 28–7.** OBJECTIVE RESULTS OF COLLIS-NISSEN OPERATION FOR ESOPHAGEAL REFLUX STRICTURES

Esophageal Function Tests	Mild Stricture*			Esophageal Function Tests	Severe Stricture*		
	Preop. (n = 36)	*1 Yr* (n = 27)	*2–5 Yr* (n = 17)		*Preop.* (n = 9)	*1 Yr* (n = 10)	*2–5 Yr* (n = 7)
Acid reflux test				Acid reflux test			
Normal (0–1 +)	2 (5%)	26 (96%)	12 (71%)	Normal (0–1 +)	1 (11%)	9 (90%)	2 (28%)
Abnormal (2–3 +)	34 (95%)	1 (4%)	5 (29%)	Abnormal (2–3 +)	8 (89%)	1 (10%)	5 (72%)
Distal HPZ				Distal HPZ			
Pressure (mm Hg)	3.5 ± 3.9	11.6 ± 3.5	10.8 ± 3.4	Pressure (mm Hg)	6.4 ± 4.5	10.8 ± 2.7	7.9 ± 3.7‡
Length (cm)	1.4 ± 1.6	4.4 ± 1.1	3.8 ± 1.2	Length (cm)	2.1 ± 1.7	4.1 ± 1.5	3.3 ± 1.6
	Moderate Stricture*				Total		
	Preop. (n = 16)	*1 Yr* (n = 13)	*2–5 Yr* (n = 5)		*Preop.* (n = 61)	*1 Yr* (n = 50)	*2–5 Yr* (n = 29)
Acid reflux test				Acid reflux test			
Normal (0–1 +)	2 (12%)	12 (92%)	5 (100%)	Normal (0–1 +)	5 (8%)	47 (94%)	19 (66%)
Abnormal (2–3 +)	14 (88%)	1 (8%)	0	Abnormal (2–3 +)	56 (92%)	3 (6%)	10 (34%)
Distal HPZ†				Distal HPZ			
Pressure (mm Hg)	1.4 ± 3.0	11.3 ± 3.8	11.2 ± 4.6	Pressure (mm Hg)	3.4 ± 4.1	11.4 ± 3.4	10.2 ± 3.8
Length (cm)	0.7 ± 1.5	3.8 ± 1.1	4.0 ± 1.2	Length (cm)	1.3 ± 1.6	4.2 ± 1.2	3.7 ± 1.2

From Stirling, M. C., and Orringer, M. B.: The combined Collis-Nissen operation for esophageal reflux strictures. Ann. Thorac. Surg., 45:148, 1988.
Stricture: Mild = easily dilated; moderate = requiring some force to dilate; severe = requiring forceful dilatation.
†HPZ = distal esophageal high pressure zone. HPZ pressure and length data are reported as mean ± standard deviation.
‡ < p 0.05 compared with mild and moderate strictures at 2–5 years.

■ **Table 28–8.** EFFECT OF VARIABLES ON CLINICAL OUTCOME (59 PATIENTS)

Variable	Satisfactory Results*		Unsatisfactory Results*	
	No.	*%*	*No.*	*%*
Scleroderma ($n = 11$)	6	55	5	45
No scleroderma ($n = 48$)	39	81	9	19
Mild-moderate preoperative dysphagia† ($n = 38$)	31	82	7	18
Severe preoperative dysphagia† ($n = 21$)	14	67	7	33
Follow-up 48 mo ($n = 25$)	16	64	9	36
Follow-up 48 mo ($n = 34$)	29	85	5	15
Mild stricture‡ ($n = 34$)	28	82	6	18
Moderate-severe stricture§ ($n = 25$)	17	68	8	32
Previous reflux operation ($n = 10$)	5	50§	5	50§
No previous reflux operation ($n = 49$)	40	82	9	18

From Stirling, M. C., and Orringer, M. B.: The combined Collis-Nissen operation for esophageal reflux strictures. Ann. Thorac. Surg., 45:148, 1988.

*Clinical results: Satisfactory = no symptoms or mild symptoms not requiring treatment; unsatisfactory = significant symptoms requiring treatment with antacids or dilatation.

†Preoperative dysphagia: Mild = no dilatations; moderate = requiring occasional dilatations; severe = requiring regular dilatations.

‡Stricture: Mild = easily dilated; moderate = requiring some force to dilate; severe = requiring forceful dilatation.

§$p < .05$ previous reflux operations compared with no previous reflux operations.

but these differences were not statistically significant. However, patients with reflux strictures for whom previous antireflux operations had failed were significantly ($p < .05$) less likely to have a satisfactory result than were those who had undergone no previous operation.

Four patients required reoperation. One patient with a mild stricture developed a paraesophageal hernia 3 years after the Collis-Nissen repair, and, despite reoperation, continued to have only a fair result. Two patients, one with a mild stricture and one with a moderate stricture, required transhiatal esophagectomy without thoracotomy for recurrent reflux esophagitis and had good results. One patient with a severe reflux stricture before an initial Collis-Nissen operation underwent pyloromyotomy and revision of the fundoplication for recurrent esophagitis 4 years later and had a subsequent good result.

Postoperative esophageal dilatations are performed liberally before discharge in patients with early complaints of dysphagia and to "calibrate" the esophagus postoperatively in patients with more severe strictures. One week after operation in those with moderate or severe strictures, a No. 50 French Maloney bougie is passed at the bedside before discharge. If resistance is encountered as this dilator is passed, subsequent outpatient dilatations are performed at 2-week intervals until there is no longer resistance. If no resistance is encountered when the dilator is initially passed, subsequent dilatations are performed only if dysphagia recurs during follow-up. Although the Collis-Nissen operation combined with intraoperative dilatation has successfully eliminated both reflux symptoms and dysphagia in 77% of patients with reflux strictures treated in this manner, a 23% failure rate for benign disease is still suboptimal. Careful long-term analysis of data is needed to predict which patients with dilatable strictures are likely to have a poor result from the Collis-Nissen operation and which patients are more likely to benefit from esophageal resection. As previously reported, patients with failed reflux operations had a 24% risk of recurrence

after an additional antireflux procedure (Stirling and Orringer, 1986). More recent data (Stirling and Orringer, 1988) indicate that patients with esophageal reflux strictures *in addition* to a failed previous repair are at an even higher risk for recurrence (50%), which is consistent with other reports (Mercer and Hill, 1986). On the basis of this information, esophageal resection in most patients with reflux strictures *and* a history of previous antireflux operation is recommended, because the failure rate is high with a more conservative operation. Bonavina and associates (1993) have reported a series of 65 patients with esophageal reflux strictures, 36 of whom were treated with fundoplication, 10 with a Collis gastroplasty and fundoplication, 4 with a duodenal diversion, and 15 with esophageal resection. Reflux control was poor in 9 (25%) of those patients who underwent a standard fundoplication, 6 of whom required reoperation. The authors advocate use of the Collis gastroplasty in patients with strictures when possible and employ resection for severe "hard" strictures (those associated with scleroderma, multiple previous operations, or severe dysplasia in Barrett's mucosa).

The combined Collis gastroplasty-fundoplication operation has also been used successfully in patients with scleroderma reflux esophagitis (Orringer et al., 1976; Orringer and Orringer, 1981; Pearson and Henderson, 1973). This population is particularly prone to peptic esophageal strictures, because the combination of lower esophageal sphincter incompetence and impaired motility causes prolonged contact between refluxed gastric acid and the esophageal mucosa. Despite systemic disease, severe dysphagia and reflux symptoms can be palliated by dilating the stricture and controlling reflux with a gastroplasty-fundoplication procedure. In my operative experience with scleroderma reflux esophagitis in 37 patients, 16 (43%) of whom have had peptic strictures, good to excellent relief from reflux symptoms was obtained in 89%. Ten of the 16 strictures totally regressed; 5 required intermittent dilatation. Because of the abnormal esophageal motility in these patients, however, significant problems can occur with esophageal emptying through the reconstructed distal esophagus. Therefore, in the scleroderma patient with a dilated, atonic esophagus and a reflux stricture, if medical therapy (including omeprazole) is ineffective, I am now more likely to recommend a transhiatal esophagectomy and cervical esophagogastric anastomosis than intraoperative dilatation and a Collis-Nissen repair.

Two additional nonresective operative techniques for managing peptic stricture and esophageal shortening should be mentioned. The fundic patch technique of Thal (Thal et al., 1965) originally was described for

use in patients with reflux strictures. Unfortunately, this procedure was subsequently applied to various problems of the esophagogastric junction (hiatal hernia with reflux esophagitis, achalasia, and perforation) (Thal, 1968) with the erroneous idea that it could prevent gastroesophageal reflux. It was soon recognized that addition of a Nissen fundoplication to the Thal operation was required for reflux control (Hollenbeck and Woodward, 1975; Maher et al., 1981; Thomas et al., 1972; Woodward, 1975) (Fig. 28–55). There are two primary objections to this approach: first, the need to intentionally incise and open the

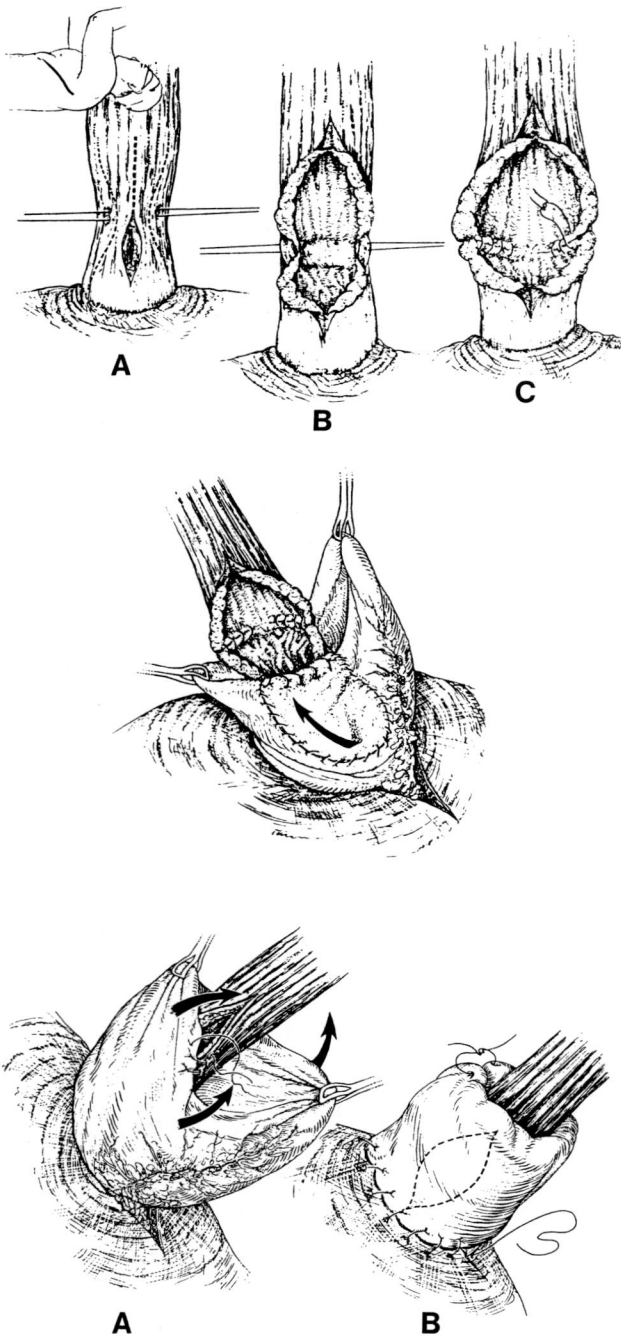

FIGURE 28–55. Combined Thal fundic patch operation and Nissen fundoplication for peptic esophageal stricture. *Upper panel: A,* Longitudinal incision of the stricture. *B,* The opened stricture. *C,* Transverse approximation of gastric fundus and esophagus, thus widening the stenotic area, but foreshortening the esophagus. *Middle panel:* The serosa of the gastric fundus is covered with a split-thickness skin graft and then rotated upward to fill the esophageal defect. *Lower panel: A,* The fundic patch is sutured into the esophageal defect. *B,* The fundus is wrapped around the lower esophagus and sutured to itself. (From Thomas, H. F., Clarke, J. M., Rayl, J. E., and Woodward, E. R.: Results of the combined fundic patch–fundoplication operation in the treatment of reflux esophagitis with stricture. Surg. Gynecol. Obstet., *135:*241, 1972. By permission of Surgery, Gynecology and Obstetrics.)

most inflamed and diseased portion of the esophagus, to which the gastric fundus is then sutured with the expectation that it will heal; and second, the need for an intrathoracic fundoplication—in effect, a man-made paraesophageal hiatal hernia. With this opera-

tion, not only have problems with suture-line disruption been appreciable (Strug et al., 1974), but also the mechanical complications of a paraesophageal hernia have been well documented (Polk, 1976; Richardson et al., 1982) (Fig. 28–56). For the same reasons, al-

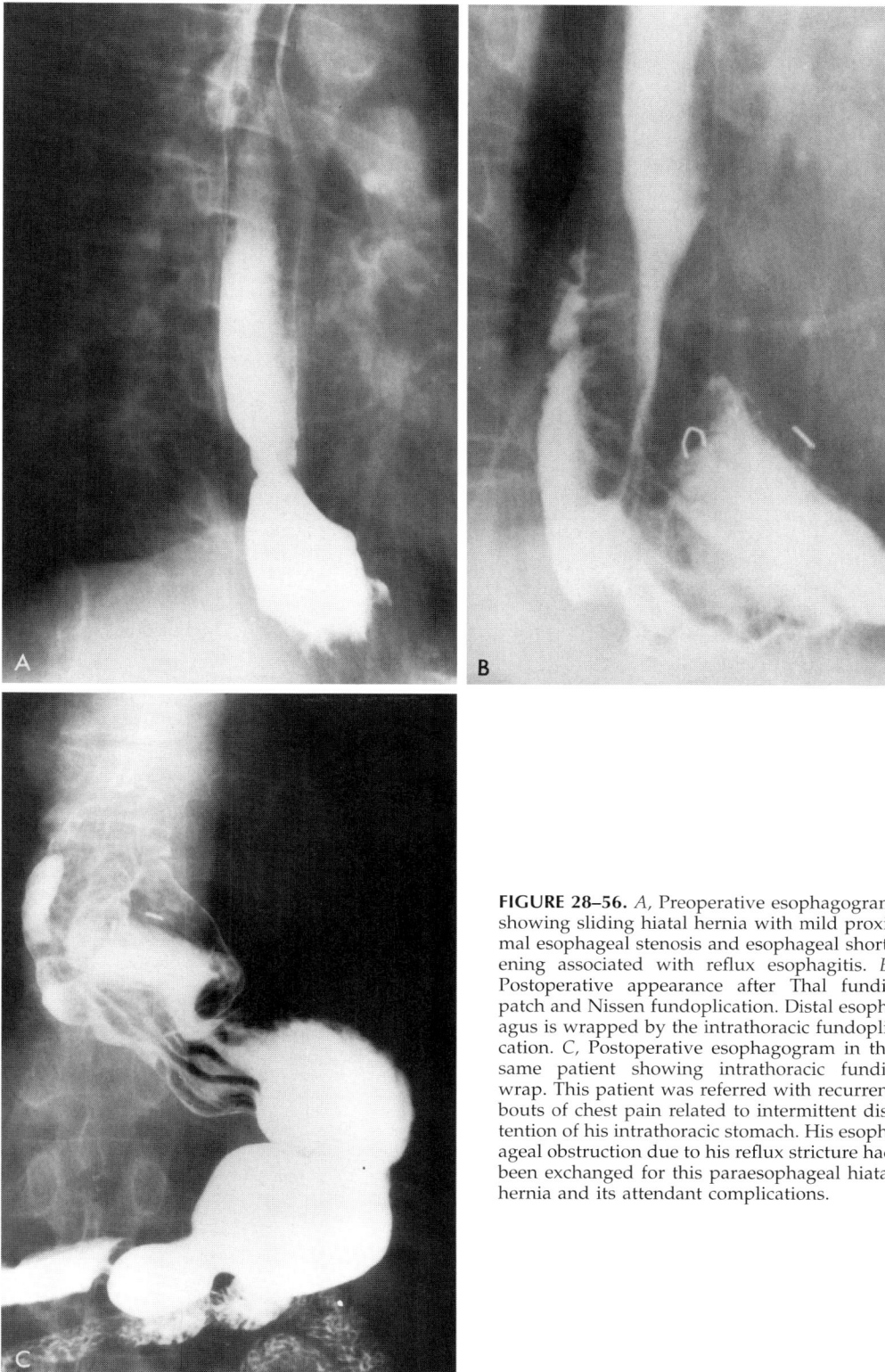

FIGURE 28–56. *A,* Preoperative esophagogram showing sliding hiatal hernia with mild proximal esophageal stenosis and esophageal shortening associated with reflux esophagitis. *B,* Postoperative appearance after Thal fundic patch and Nissen fundoplication. Distal esophagus is wrapped by the intrathoracic fundoplication. *C,* Postoperative esophagogram in the same patient showing intrathoracic fundic wrap. This patient was referred with recurrent bouts of chest pain related to intermittent distention of his intrathoracic stomach. His esophageal obstruction due to his reflux stricture had been exchanged for this paraesophageal hiatal hernia and its attendant complications.

though an intrathoracic fundoplication alone can provide a competent distal esophageal sphincter mechanism (Krupp and Rossetti, 1966; Safaie-Shirazi et al., 1974, 1975), the potential hazards of incarceration, strangulation, and bleeding from the intrathoracic stomach are real (Burnett et al., 1977; Rossman et al., 1979). I believe that it is always preferable to restore the fundoplication to the abdomen whenever possible to avoid these complications, and therefore the combined Collis gastroplasty-fundoplication technique is preferred in the event of a dilatable peptic stricture or short esophagus.

In the rare case in which a stricture proves to be nondilatable or attempts at dilatation produce esophageal disruption, resectional therapy and visceral esophageal substitution are required. Although jejunal interposition is an effective method of distal esophageal replacement (Polk, 1980), this technique has inherent difficulties with the delicate blood supply and length limitations of the jejunum. Colonic interposition with isoperistaltic left colon based on the ascending branch of the left colic artery is an excellent alternative that offers a more constant blood supply and greater length for esophageal reconstruction (Belsey, 1965; Keenan, 1984). The relative ease of mobilization of the left and transverse colon through a left thoracoabdominal incision permits one-stage esophageal resection and replacement of either the distal or the entire thoracic esophagus (Orringer et al., 1977). The naturally alkaline mucous secretions of the colon resist acid regurgitation from the stomach. Despite these advantages, colonic interposition is still a formidable operation in elderly or nutritionally depleted patients with esophageal obstruction. Increasing experience with *total* thoracic esophagectomy and esophageal replacement with the stomach anastomosed to the cervical esophagus indicates that this may be the best option in patients requiring esophageal resection for benign disease. Not only is the early postoperative danger from an intrathoracic anastomotic leak eliminated with this approach, but also the troublesome gastroesophageal reflux associated with an intrathoracic esophagogastric anastomosis is rarely of clinical significance (Orringer, 1985; Orringer and Stirling, 1988; Orringer and Sloan, 1978b). Among 55 patients who underwent a transhiatal esophagectomy and cervical esophagogastric anastomosis for benign disease and were followed beyond 5 years (average 101 months), 78% had no or mild dysphagia, 20% required an occasional outpatient dilatation, and 2% required dilatations. Regurgitation was denied in 56%, whereas 13% experienced occasional nocturnal regurgitation that required that they sleep elevated at night or on a wedge. None had experienced pulmonary complications of aspiration (Orringer et al., 1993).

SELECTED BIBLIOGRAPHY

Hayward, J.: The treatment of fibrous stricture of the oesophagus associated with hiatal hernia. Thorax, 16:45, 1961.

After his success with 14 patients with tough, fibrous strictures, this Australian surgeon was the first to express his view that resection of these stenoses is "seldom, if ever, needed and that good results can be obtained by repair of the hernia, dilatation of the stricture to the point of internal splitting at the time of operation, and postoperative dilatation by self bougienage." Although his contribution is seldom acknowledged, his conviction that fibrous tissue associated with reflux esophagitis will regress if the inflammatory stimulus can be eliminated is the foundation for the modern surgical approach to peptic esophageal strictures.

Henderson, R. D., and Marryatt, G. V.: Total fundoplication gastroplasty (Nissen) gastroplasty: Five-year review. Ann. Thorac. Surg., 39:74, 1985.

This report reviews the results of the combined Collis gastroplasty-"total" (Nissen) fundoplication in 351 patients followed for an average of 6.5 years. The series is exceptional in that 335 patients have 5 or more years of follow-up. The reported results are outstanding: 93% had excellent subjective and objective reflux control, 4% had mild residual symptoms, and 3% had persistent or recurrent symptoms. Only 10% of these patients had reflux strictures preoperatively, however. These authors have liberalized the use of the combined Collis-Nissen procedure in most patients requiring surgical control of reflux (not only those with strictures and esophageal shortening). Their unusually good results may therefore be "skewed" because patients with "uncomplicated" reflux might be expected to do well after the more standard repairs to the hiatal hernia. Nevertheless, this is an outstanding long-term follow-up study of the combined Collis-Nissen operation for control of gastroesophageal reflux and its complications.

Hill, L.D., Gelfand, M., and Bauermeister, D.: Simplified management of reflux esophagitis with stricture. Ann. Surg., 172:638, 1970.

This is a report of a group of 36 patients with esophageal strictures treated by dilatation of the stricture and Hill's median arcuate ligament (posterior gastropexy) repair. By using intraesophageal pH and manometric studies, the authors showed the existence of a lower esophageal sphincter well below the squamocolumnar epithelial junction in patients with Barrett's esophagus, thus proving that these strictures did not occur at the anatomic esophagogastric junction and that Barrett's concept of the "short esophagus" was incorrect. Good to excellent results were obtained in 85% of the reported patients for various periods of follow-up as long as 6 years. With this report, Hill became the first proponent in the United States of the nonresective operative approach to peptic esophageal strictures.

Mercer, C. D., and Hill, L. D.: Surgical management of peptic esophageal stricture: Twenty year experience. J. Thorac. Cardiovasc. Surg., 91:371, 1986.

A follow-up to Hill's 1970 publication, this report reviews the results of the authors' extensive experience in the surgical management of 160 patients with peptic stricture treated by dilatation and the Hill posterior gastropexy. Follow-up is from 6 to 240 months (average of 47 months). These authors emphasize the value of intraoperative manometry as a determinant of subsequent reflux control, a controversial concept. They also report that only 52% of patients who had undergone a previous failed antireflux operation had a good result, compared with 90% of those undergoing their first repair. They emphasize the merit of dilatation and conservative antireflux procedure in patients with peptic esophageal strictures.

Pearson, F. G., and Henderson, R. D.: Long-term follow-up of peptic strictures managed by dilatation, modified Collis gastroplasty, and Belsey hiatus hernia repair. Surgery, 80:396, 1976.

This report reviews results in 33 patients with peptic strictures who had undergone surgery more than 5 years earlier. Among 26 patients followed 5 to 12 years since operation, 25 had sustained excellent results, being able to eat a regular diet without dysphagia or reflux symptoms. There were no operative deaths in this series, and one esophageal perforation was sustained during dilatation. This experience provides convincing evidence that in patients with dilatable peptic strictures, dependable reflux control can be achieved with the combined Collis-Belsey procedure. However, although 24 of these patients underwent postoperative esophageal manometric studies, reflux control was not documented objectively with the intraesophageal pH probe.

Stirling, M. C., and Orringer, M. B.: The combined Collis-Nissen operation for esophageal reflux strictures. Ann. Thorac. Surg., 45:148, 1988.

This report reviews the results of esophageal dilatation and the Collis-Nissen operation in 59 patients with reflux strictures. The average follow-up was 43 months. *Subjectively*, reflux control was excellent or good (88%). *Objectively*, intraesophageal pH reflux testing showed good or excellent reflux control in 94% of patients at 1 year, but in only 66% at 2 to 5 years. Dysphagia was eliminated in 71%, was mild in 10%, was moderate (requiring occasional dilatation) in 12%, and was severe (requiring regular dilatations) in 7%. As reported by Mercer and Hill (1986), the combination of a reflux stricture and a previous failed antireflux operation greatly reduced the likelihood of a successful "redo" procedure; only 50% of these patients achieved a good result. It is suggested, therefore, that in this latter group of patients, resectional therapy may be a better option than a more conservative antireflux procedure.

BIBLIOGRAPHY

Adler, R. H.: The lower esophagus lined by columnar epithelium: Its association with hiatal hernia, ulcer, stricture, and tumor. J. Thorac. Cardiovasc. Surg., 45:13, 1963.

Allison, P. R.: Peptic ulcer of oesophagus. Thorax, 3:30, 1948.

Allison, P. R., and Johnstone, A. S.: The esophagus lined with gastric mucous membrane. Thorax, 8:87, 1953.

Allison, P. R., Johnstone, A. S., and Boyce, G. B.: Short esophagus with simple peptic ulceration. J. Thorac. Surg., 12:432, 1943.

Barnes, W. A., and Redo, S. F.: Evaluation of esophagojejunostomy in the treatment of lesions at the esophagogastric junction. Ann. Surg., 146:224, 1957.

Barrett, N. R.: Chronic peptic ulcer of the oesophagus and "oesophagitis." Br. J. Surg., 38:175, 1950.

Belsey, R.: Diaphragmatic hernia. In Modern Trends in Gastroenterology. New York, Hoeber, 1952, pp. 128–178.

Belsey, R. H.: Reconstruction of the esophagus with left colon. J. Thorac. Cardiovasc. Surg., 49:33, 1965.

Bombeck, C. T., Coelko, R. C. P., and Nyhus, L. M.: Prevention of gastroesophageal reflux after resection of the lower esophagus. Surg. Gynecol. Obstet., 130:1035, 1970.

Bonavina, L., Fontebasso, V., Bardini, R., et al.: Surgical treatment of reflux strictures of the oesophagus. Br. J. Surg., 80:317;320, 1993.

Burnett, H. F., Read, R. C., Morris, W. D., and Campbell, G. S.: Management of complications of fundoplication and Barrett's esophagus. Ann. Surg., 82:521, 1977.

Cameron, A. J., Ott, B. J., and Payne, W. S.: The incidence of adenocarcinoma in columnar-lined (Barrett's) esophagus. N. Engl. J. Med., 313:857, 1985.

Clarke, J. M., and Woodward, E. R.: Transthoracic fundoplication for hiatal hernia and short esophagus in a 3 year old child: Case report. Surgery, 64:858, 1968.

Code, C. F., Creamer, B., Schlegel, J. F., et al.: An Atlas of Esophageal Motility in Health and Disease. Springfield, IL, Charles C Thomas, 1958.

Collis, J. L.: An operation for hiatus hernia with short esophagus. Thorax, 12:181, 1957.

Collis, J. L.: Gastroplasty. Thorax, 16:197, 1961.

DeMeester, T. R., Johnson, L. F., Joseph, G. J., et al.: Patterns of gastroesophageal reflux in health and disease. Ann. Surg., 184:459, 1976.

DeMeester, T. R., Wang, C. I., Wernly, J. A., et al.: Technique, indications and clinical use of 24 hour esophageal pH monitoring. J. Thorac. Cardiovasc. Surg., 79:656, 1980.

Demos, N., and Biele, R. M.: Intercostal pedicle method for control of post-resection esophagitis. J. Thorac. Cardiovasc. Surg., 80:679, 1980.

Donnelly, R. J., Deverall, P. B., and Watson, D. A.: Hiatus hernia with and without stricture: Experience with the Belsey Mark IV repair. Ann. Thorac. Surg., 16:301, 1973.

Dunlop, E. E.: Problems in the treatment of reflux oesophagitis. Gastroenterologica, 86:287, 1956.

Ellis, F. H., Jr., Anderson, H. A., and Clagett, O. T.: Treatment of short esophagus with stricture by esophagogastrectomy and antral excision. Ann. Surg., 148:526, 1958.

Ellis, F. H., Jr., Leonardi, H. K., Dabuzhsky, L., et al.: Surgery for short esophagus with stricture: An experimental and clinical manometric study. Ann. Surg., 188:341, 1978.

Fuchs, K. H., DeMeester, T. R., and Albertucci, M.: Specificity and sensitivity of objective diagnosis of gastroesophageal reflux disease. Surgery, 102:575, 1987.

Harle, I. A., Finley, R. J., Belsheim, M., et al.: Management of adenocarcinoma in a columnar lined esophagus. Ann. Thorac. Surg., 40:330, 1985.

Hawe, A., Payne, W. S., Weiland, L. H., and Fontana, R. S.: Adenocarcinoma in the columnar epithelial lined lower (Barrett's) oesophagus. Thorax, 28:511, 1973.

Hayward, J.: The treatment of fibrous stricture of the esophagus associated with hiatus hernias. Thorax, 16:45, 1961.

Heimlich, H. J.: Esophagoplasty with reversed gastric tube. Am. J. Surg., 123:80, 1972.

Heimlich, H. J.: Peptic esophagitis with stricture treated by reconstruction of the esophagus with a reversed gastric tube. Surg. Gynecol. Obstet., 114:673, 1962.

Henderson, R. D.: Reflux control following gastroplasty. Ann. Thorac. Surg., 24:206, 1977.

Herrington, J. L., Jr., Wright, R. S., Edwards, W. H., et al.: Conservative surgical treatment of reflux esophagitis and esophageal stricture. Ann. Surg., 181:552, 1975.

Hill, L. D., Gelfand, M., and Bauermeister, D.: Simplified management of reflux esophagitis with stricture. Ann. Surg., 172:638, 1970.

Hollenbeck, J. I., and Woodward, E. R.: Treatment of peptic esophageal stricture with combined fundic patch fundoplication. Ann. Surg., 182:472, 1975.

Ingelfinger, F. J.: Esophageal motility. Physiol. Rev., 38:533, 1958.

Johnson, L. F., and DeMeester, T. R.: Development of 24 hour intraesophageal pH monitoring: A quantitative measure of gastroesophageal reflux. Am. J. Gastroenterol., 62:325, 1974.

Keenan, D. J. M., Hamilton, J. R. L., Gibbon, J., and Stevenson, H. M.: Surgery for benign esophageal stricture. J. Thorac. Cardiovasc. Surg., 88:182, 1984.

Krupp, S., and Rosetti, M.: Surgical treatment of hiatal hernia by fundoplication and gastropexy (Nissen repair). Ann. Surg., 164:927, 1966.

Little, A. G., Naunheim, K. S., Ferguson, M. K., and Skinner, D. B.: Surgical management of esophageal strictures. Ann. Thorac. Surg., 45:144, 1988.

Lundell, L.: Acid suppression in the long-term treatment of peptic stricture and Barrett's oesophagus. Digestion, 51(Suppl. 1):49–58, 1992.

Maher, J. W., Hocking, M. P., and Woodward, E. R.: Long-term follow-up of the combined fundic patch fundoplication for treatment of longitudinal peptic strictures of the esophagus. Ann. Surg., 194:64, 1981.

Mercer, C. D., and Hill, L. D.: Surgical management of peptic esophageal stricture. J. Thorac. Cardiovasc. Surg., 91:371, 1986.

Merendino, K. A., and Dillard, D. H.: The concept of sphincter substitution by an interposed jejunal segment for anatomic and physiologic abnormalities at the esophagogastric junction. Ann. Surg., 142:486, 1955.

Monnier, P., Hsieh, V., and Savary, M.: Endoscopic treatment of esophageal stenosis using Savary-Gilliard bougies: Technical innovations. Acta Endoscopia, 15:119, 1985

Mossberg, S. M.: The columnar lined esophagus (Barrett's syndrome): An acquired condition? Gastroenterology, 50:671, 1966.

Naef, A. P., and Savary, M.: Conservative operations for peptic esophagitis with stenosis in columnar-lined lower esophagus. Ann. Thorac. Surg., 13:543, 1972.

Naef, A. P., Savary, M., and Ozello, L.: Columnar-lined lower esophagus: An acquired lesion with malignant predisposition. J. Thorac. Cardiovasc. Surg., 70:826, 1975.

Neville, W. E., Clowes, G. H. A., Jr.: Surgical treatment of the complications resulting from cardioesophageal incompetence. Dis. Chest, 43:572, 1963.

Okada, N., Kuriyasma, T., Urmemoto, H., et al.: Esophageal surgery: A procedure for posterior invagination esophagogastrostomy in one stage without positional change. Ann. Surg., 179:27, 1974.

Ollyo, J.-B., Ch., Fontolliet, E., Brossard, F. L.: Savary's new endoscopic classification of reflux oesophagitis. Gullet, 22:307, 1992.

Orringer, M. B.: Transhiatal esophagectomy for benign disease. J. Thorac. Cardiovasc. Surg., 90:649, 1985.

Orringer, M. B., Dabich, L., Zarafonetis, C. J. D., and Sloan, H.: Gastroesophageal reflux in esophageal scleroderma: Diagnosis and implications. Ann. Thorac. Surg., 22:120, 1976.

Orringer, M. B., Kirsh, M. M., and Sloan, H.: Esophageal reconstruction for benign disease. J. Thorac. Cardiovasc. Surg., 73:807, 1977.

Orringer, M. B., Marshall, B., and Stirling, M. C.: Transhiatal esophagectomy for benign and malignant disease. J. Thorac. Cardiovasc. Surg., 105:265, 1993.

Orringer, M. B., and Orringer, J. S.: The combined Collis-Nissen operation: Early assessment of reflux control. Ann. Thorac. Surg., 33:534, 1982.

Orringer, M. B., and Orringer, J. S.: Combined Collis-gastroplasty-fundoplication for scleroderma reflux esophagitis. Surgery, 90:624, 1981.

Orringer, M. B., Skinner, D. B., and Belsey, R. H. R.: Long-term results of the Mark IV operation for hiatal hernia and analyses of recurrences and their treatment. J. Thorac. Cardiovasc. Surg., 63:25, 1972.

Orringer, M. B., and Sloan, H.: An improved technique for combined Collis-Belsey approach to dilatable esophageal strictures. J. Thorac. Cardiovasc. Surg., 68:298, 1974.

Orringer, M. B., and Sloan, H.: Collis-Belsey reconstruction of the esophagogastric junction. J. Thorac. Cardiovasc. Surg., 71:295, 1976.

Orringer, M. B., and Sloan, H.: Combined Collis-Nissen reconstruction of the esophagogastric junction. Ann. Thorac. Surg., 25:16, 1978a.

Orringer, M. B., and Sloan, H.: Complications and failings of the combined Collis-Belsey operation. J. Thorac. Cardiovasc. Surg., 74:726, 1977.

Orringer, M. B., and Sloan, H.: Esophagectomy without thoracotomy. J. Thorac. Cardiovasc. Surg., 76:643, 1978b.

Orringer, M. B., and Stirling, M. C.: Cervical esophagogastric anastomosis for benign disease functional results. J. Thorac. Cardiovasc. Surg., 96:887–893, 1988.

Payne, W. S.: Surgical treatment of reflux esophagitis and stricture associated with permanent incompetence of the cardia. Mayo Clin. Proc., 45:553, 1970.

Pearson, F. G.: Surgical management of acquired short esophagus with dilatable peptic stricture. World J. Surg., 1:463, 1977.

Pearson, F. G., and Henderson, R. D.: Experimental and clinical studies of gastroplasty in the management of acquired short esophagus. Surg. Gynecol. Obstet., 136:737, 1973.

Pearson, F. G., and Henderson, R. D.: Long-term follow-up of peptic strictures managed by dilatation, modified Collis gastroplasty, and Belsey hiatus hernia repair. Surgery, 80:396, 1976.

Pearson, F. G., Langer, B., and Henderson, R. D.: Gastroplasty and Belsey hiatal hernia repair. J. Thorac. Cardiovasc. Surg., 61:50, 1971.

Polk, H. C.: Jejunal interposition for reflux esophagitis and esophageal stricture unresponsive to valvuloplasty. World J. Surg., 4:731, 1980.

Polk, H. C., Jr.: Fundoplication for reflux esophagitis: Misadventures with the choice of operation. Ann. Surg., 183:645, 1976.

Popov, V. I.: Reconstruction of the esophagus in cases of stricture. Arch. Surg., 82:226, 1961.

Radigan, L. R., Glover, J. L., Shipley, F. E., and Shoemaker, R. E.: Barrett's esophagus. Arch. Surg., 112:486, 1977.

Richardson, J. D., Larson, G. M., Polk, H. C., Jr.: Intrathoracic fundoplication for shortened esophagus: A treacherous solution to a challenging problem. Am. J. Surg., 143:29, 1982.

Rossman, F., Brantigan, C. O., and Sawyer, R. B.: Obstructive complications of the Nissen fundoplication. Am. J. Surg., 138:860, 1979.

Safaie-Shirazi, S., Zike, W. L., and Masson, E. E.: Esophageal strictures secondary to reflux esophagitis. Arch. Surg., 110:629, 1975.

Safaie-Shirazi, S., Zike, W. L., Anuras, S., et al.: Nissen fundoplication without crural repair. Arch. Surg., 108:424, 1974.

Skinner, D. B.: The columnar-lined esophagus and adenocarcinoma [Editorial]. Ann. Thorac. Surg., 40:321, 1985.

Skinner, D. B., and Belsey, R. H. R.: Surgical management of esophageal reflux and hiatus hernia. J. Thorac. Cardiovasc. Surg., 53:33, 1967.

Skinner, D. B., Walther, B. C., Riddell, R. H., et al.: Barrett's esophagus: Comparison of benign and malignant cases. Ann. Surg., 198:554, 1983.

Spechler, S. J., and Goyal, R. K.: Barrett's esophagus. N. Engl. J. Med., 315:362, 1986.

Spechler, S. J., Robbins, A. H., Rubins, H. B., et al.: Adenocarcinoma and Barrett's esophagus: An overrated risk? Gastroenterology, 87:927, 1984.

Stirling, M. C., and Orringer, M. B.: Surgical treatment after the failed antireflux operation. J. Thorac. Cardiovasc. Surg., 92:667, 1986.

Stirling, M. C., and Orringer, M. B.: The combined Collis-Nissen operation for esophageal reflux strictures. Ann. Thorac. Surg., 45:148, 1988.

Strug, B. S., Jordan, P. H., Jr., and Jordan, G. L., Jr.: Surgical management of benign esophageal strictures. Surg. Gynecol. Obstet., 138:74, 1974.

Tanner, N. C.: Treatment of oesophageal hiatus hernia. Lancet, 2:1050, 1955.

Thal, A. P.: A unified approach to surgical problems of the esophagogastric junction. Ann. Surg., 168:542, 1968.

Thal, A. P., Hatafuko, T., and Kurtzman, R.: New operation for distal esophageal stricture. Arch. Surg., 90:464, 1965.

Thomas, H. G., Clarke, J. M., Rayl, J. E., and Woodward, E. R.: Results of the combined fundic patch fundoplication operation in the treatment of reflux esophagitis with stricture. Surg. Gynecol. Obstet., 135:241, 1972.

Tileston, W.: Peptic ulcer of the oesophagus. Am. J. Med. Sci., 132:240, 1906.

Toledo-Pereyra, L. H., Michel, H., Manifacio, G., and Humphrey, E. W.: Management of acid peptic esophageal strictures. J. Thorac. Cardiovasc. Surg., 72:518, 1976.

Tuttle, S. G., and Grossman, M. I.: Detection of gastroesophageal reflux by simultaneous measurement of intraluminal pressures and pH. Proc. Soc. Exp. Biol. Med., 98:225, 1958.

Urschel, H. C., Razzuk, M. A., Wood, R. E., et al.: An improved surgical technique for the complicated hiatal hernia with gastroesophageal reflux. Ann. Thorac. Surg., 15:443, 1973.

Vollan, G., Stangeland, L., Soreide, J. A., et al.: Long-term results after Nissen fundoplication and Belsey Mark IV operation in patients with reflux oesophagitis and stricture. Eur. J. Surg., 158:357–360, 1992.

Wesdorp, I. C. E., Bartelsman, J. F. W., Den Hartog Jager, F. C. A., et al.: Results of conservative treatment of benign esophageal strictures: A follow-up study in 100 patients. Gastroenterology, 82:487, 1982.

Woodward, E. R.: Sliding esophageal hiatal hernia and reflux peptic esophagitis. Mayo Clin. Proc., 50:523, 1975.

29 Diaphragm and Diaphragmatic Pacing

Peter Van Trigt III

DIAPHRAGM

Historical Aspects

The first traumatic diaphragmatic hernia was reported in 1579 by Paré, who described the post-mortem findings in two patients who died after a blunt injury and a gunshot wound, respectively (Sutton et al., 1967). In this report, Paré described an autopsy performed on an artillery captain who died of a strangulated intestinal obstruction after incarceration of the intestine through a traumatic laceration of the diaphragm sustained 8 months earlier. In 1853, Bowditch published the first account of traumatic diaphragmatic hernia diagnosed antemortem in the United States. He established five criteria for the physical diagnosis of the lesion: prominence and immobility of the left thorax, displacement to the right of the area of cardiac dullness, absent breath sounds over the left hemithorax, bowel sounds audible in the chest, and tympany to percussion over the left side of the chest. In 1886, Riolfi corrected a laceration of the diaphragm from a knife wound through which omentum had prolapsed (Grage et al., 1959). Naumann, in 1888, operated on a patient who had a traumatic diaphragmatic hernia and in whom the stomach had herniated into the left side of the chest (Grage et al., 1959). Before the 20th century, traumatic diaphragmatic hernia was a rarely reported condition.

Anatomy of the Diaphragm

The diaphragm consists of a central portion of a thin but strong aponeurosis and a peripheral muscular portion. The muscular components of the diaphragm are of sternal, costal, and lumbar origin. Embryologically, the middle leaflet of this central tendon develops from the transverse septum, which originates between the liver and the heart. It then grows caudad toward the dorsal mesentery of the foregut, with which it ultimately fuses. The transverse septum fuses with the pleuroperitoneal membrane from the lateral chest wall, joining the muscular components of the diaphragm and separating the pericardial, peritoneal, and pleural cavities. Thus, in an adult, the diaphragm is composed of two portions: the peripheral muscular portion and a central tendinous portion shaped like an inverted capital V. This central tendi-

nous portion is contiguous on its superior aspect with the pericardium (Fig. 29–1).

Three major openings in the diaphragm allow passage of structures from the chest to the abdomen: the aortic, esophageal, and vena caval openings. The aortic opening allows passage of the aorta, azygos vein, and thoracic duct. Through the esophageal hiatus pass the esophagus and vagus nerves, and the inferior vena cava passes alone through the caval opening.

Arterial supply to the diaphragm comes predominantly from the abdominal aorta and is composed of the right and left phrenic arteries. The anterior branch of the phrenic artery supplies the central most tendinous portion, which is contiguous with the pericardium. Additional arterial supply to the posterior portion of the diaphragm rises from the superior phrenic arteries, originating from the lower portion of the thoracic aorta, and the pericardiophrenic and musculophrenic arteries, originating from the internal mammary artery. Venous drainage of the diaphragm involves the right and left inferior phrenic veins, which drain medially into the inferior vena cava. On the left side, a venous arcade that connects the phrenic vein with the left renal vein provides additional drainage.

The right and left phrenic nerves provide both motor and sensory supply to the diaphragm. The right phrenic nerve enters the diaphragm just lateral to the opening of the inferior vena cava in the diaphragm; the left phrenic nerve enters lateral to the left border of the heart (see Fig. 29–1). Once these nerves enter the diaphragmatic muscle, they divide into four trunks: sternal, anterolateral, posterolateral, and crural. These trunks eventually course immediately below the peritoneal lining of the inferior surface of the diaphragm (see Fig. 29–1).

Disorders

Congenital Diaphragmatic Hernia

There are three types of congenital diaphragmatic hernias: posterolateral (Bochdalek's) hernia, subcostosternal (Morgagni's) hernia, and esophageal hiatal hernia.

The posterolateral (Bochdalek's) diaphragmatic hernia is the result of a congenital diaphragmatic defect in the posterior costal part of the diaphragm in the region of the tenth and eleventh ribs, which allows free communication between the thoracic and

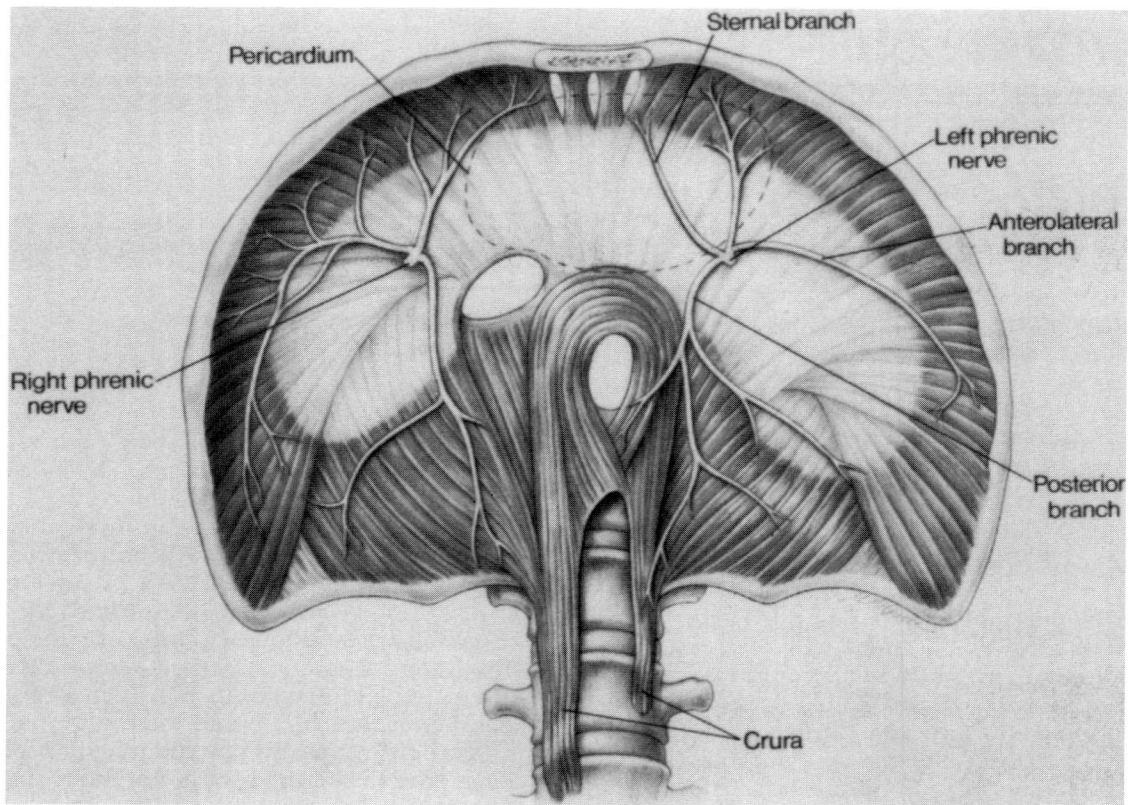

FIGURE 29–1. Anatomy of the diaphragm from the abdominal perspective, showing innervation.

the abdominal cavities. The defect is usually found on the left side (90% of patients) but may occur on the right side, where the liver often prevents detection (Gravier, 1974). The male-to-female ratio is 2 : 3, and this defect is associated with other congenital anomalies in 25% of patients. Because of the negative intrathoracic pressure, herniation of the abdominal contents occurs through left-sided defects, with resultant collapse of the left lung, shifting of the mediastinum to the right, and compression of the contralateral right lung. This type of congenital diaphragmatic hernia is usually manifested by acute respiratory distress in newborns (Symbas et al., 1977). Bochdalek's hernia in adults is usually detected as an asymptomatic posterior mediastinal mass on chest radiography. Studies using computed tomography (CT) have shown small asymptomatic Bochdalek's hernias present in 6% of otherwise normal patients (Tarver et al., 1989).

Chest films establish the diagnosis, displaying intestinal gas patterns within the thorax and the resultant shift of the relatively unstable and mobile neonatal mediastinum to the contralateral side. The clinical findings on examination include the presence of respiratory distress, the absence of breath sounds on the left side, and the presence of bowel sounds over the left side of the chest. Obstruction and strangulation of the bowel have been reported but are rare in the acute presentation of this entity. The usual cause of morbidity and mortality is progressive hypoxemia as a result of increased pulmonary vascular resistance

(PVR), decreased blood flow to the lungs, alveolar hypoxia, and further hypoxemia. Initial treatment consists of nasogastric decompression of the stomach and intestinal tract to reduce mediastinal shifting, replacement of fluids and electrolytes, correction of acid-base imbalance, positive-pressure respiratory support, and surgical correction of the diaphragmatic defect. For right-sided defects, repair is usually accomplished through a right-sided thoracotomy. For left-sided defects, an abdominal approach is preferred because of the malrotation and obstructing duodenal bands that can be present in this condition. Closure of the defect is accomplished by direct suture; chest tubes are placed in the involved hemithorax and are connected to underwater-seal drainage to assist expansion of the lung on the involved side.

TREATMENT

Treatment of newborn infants who have congenital diaphragmatic hernia and who develop severe respiratory distress requiring operative repair within the first 24 hours of life represents one of the most challenging problems in pediatric surgery. Postoperative mortality varies between 30 and 50% (Harrison and De Lorimier, 1981; Shochat et al., 1979). Pathologic examination of the lungs of infants who have died with congenital diaphragmatic hernia reveals a decrease in size and weight, with the ipsilateral lung being smaller and showing a distorted distribution of segmental airways. Total pulmonary volume is reduced owing to a smaller total number of alveoli as a result of a deficiency in bronchial generation. These pathologic findings led to an earlier assumption that the high mortality after repair of the diaphragmatic hernia is due to pulmonary hypoplasia. However, despite a reduction in total pulmonary volume, the contralateral lung in infants with congenital diaphragmatic hernia is usually able to maintain ventilation, and in surviving infants, the small hypoplastic ipsilateral lung eventually expands and fills the thoracic cavity (Wohl et al., 1977). In those survivors, total pulmonary volume becomes normal but there is an abnormal distribution; the ipsilateral lung contributes only 40% to total lung function (Hislop and Reid, 1976).

More recently, authors have emphasized the significance of an increase in PVR and a conversion to fetal circulation with increased pulmonary artery pressure as the primary abnormality responsible for the high postoperative morbidity and mortality (O'Callaghan et al., 1982). This hypothesis is supported by the clinical course of those neonates who die after repair of a diaphragmatic hernia. There is usually a great improvement in oxygenation in the immediate postoperative period, followed by deterioration 12 to 24 hours postoperatively, with progressive hypoxemia, acidosis, hypercarbia, and death despite all therapeutic manipulations to correct this progressive deterioration.

Cardiac catheterization studies that have been performed in children with a congenital diaphragmatic hernia show pulmonary arterial hypertension with a right-to-left shunt across the ductus, raised right ventricular end-diastolic pressure, and raised right atrial pressure with shunting across the foramen ovale. Pulmonary arteriography shows a decreased total pulmonary flow with shunting across the ductus and almost no perfusion of the lung on the side of the diaphragmatic hernia. The pulmonary vasculature of infants who have died with congenital diaphragmatic hernia has been investigated, and a significant increase in smooth muscle mass in the small pulmonary arteries has been documented (Naeye et al., 1976). Studies have established that this anatomically abnormal pulmonary vascular bed in infants with congenital diaphragmatic hernia (Levin, 1978) is capable of an exaggerated response to factors that produce pulmonary vasoconstriction in newborns (hypoxemia, hypercarbia, acidosis, hypothermia, increased transpulmonary pressure, and alveolar hypoxia) (Naeye et al., 1976). An exaggerated vasoconstrictive response of an abnormally hypertrophied pulmonary vascular bed leading to a rise of PVR appears to be the important mechanism leading to the often fatal hypoxemia in these neonates.

Pharmacologic interventions to break the vicious circle of hypoxia, increased PVR leading to decreased pulmonary flow, and shunting across the ductus and foramen ovale leading to further hypoxia have been attempted with the use of vasodilators such as tolazoline (Levy et al., 1977; Sumner and Frank, 1981) and,

more recently, prostaglandin E_1 (Cloutier et al., 1983; Ein et al., 1980). Earlier experience with tolazoline showed a significant incidence of complications associated with use of the drug, including hypotension, gastrointestinal bleeding, thrombocytopenia, seizures, and cardiac arrhythmias. Prostaglandin E_1 has been used clinically with significantly fewer complications, including fever, peripheral vasodilatation, and tremors.

In addition to pharmacologic interventions to alter PVR, *extracorporeal membrane oxygenation* (ECMO) has been used when more standard methods of support have failed to prevent progressive hypoxia and clinical deterioration (Hardesty et al., 1981; Redmond et al., 1987). ECMO is theoretically an ideal mode of support and therapy in this setting. It can immediately reduce or eliminate right-to-left shunting through the patent foramen ovale and ductus arteriosus and divert as much as 90% of the cardiac output from the right atrium into the extracorporeal circuit. Right atrial pressure and pulmonary blood flow are reduced, as is the volume of blood shunted across the atrium and through the ductus. Systemic hypoxemia and acidosis are reversed, and their vasoconstrictive effect on the pulmonary vasculature is eliminated. Transpulmonary pressures are reduced during ECMO, removing another potential pulmonary vasoconstricting factor. Reduction of PVR together with the improvement in systemic oxygenation and reduction in volume of ductal flow may lead to spontaneous closure of the ductus and resolution of the persistent fetal circulation that often occurs in the postoperative setting of these neonates. With this type of extracorporeal support, neonates can be supported for several days, and pulmonary function and PVR can return to normal (Sawyer et al., 1986; Trento et al., 1986). The impact of ECMO on survival in neonates with congenital diaphragmatic hernia was demonstrated by a review of 50 patients at the University of Michigan between 1974 and 1987 (Heiss et al., 1989). ECMO was introduced in 1981, defining a pre-ECMO cohort of 16 patients and a post-ECMO group of 34. Overall survival improved from 50 to 76% with the availability of ECMO.

Until recently, urgent repair was standard for congenital diaphragmatic hernia. Experience has shown, however, that delaying surgery in patients with severe cardiopulmonary compromise can correct acidosis, optimize oxygenation, reduce pulmonary hypertension, and stabilize the child to better tolerate the operation. For those patients not stabilized using ventilatory and pharmacologic means, *preoperative* ECMO has been advocated, repairing the defect while the patient is on bypass or after successfully weaning the patient from ECMO (Butler et al., 1993). In a review of an extremely high-risk group of neonates symptomatic of congenital diaphragmatic hernia at birth (mean PaO_2 of 33 mm Hg), 42 patients were repaired while on ECMO. Of the 42 patients, 18 (43%) survived; prematurity was a major risk factor, since no infants younger than 37 weeks of age survived (Lally et al., 1992). In another review, 7 of 9 babies placed on ECMO before repair of congenital diaphragmatic hernia due to failure of convential support died (West et al., 1992). Complications encountered in this high-risk group included hemorrhage requiring reexploration, recurrent hernia due to disruption of the suture line with growth when a prosthetic patch is used, and central nervous system hemorrhage. ECMO can profoundly affect survival in this high-risk group by reversing the effects of persistent pulmonary hypertension. Identification of the patient whose main problem is hypoplasia is a clinical difficulty, although several parameters measuring severity of illness have been prepared to aid in predicting outcome in the ECMO era (Wilson et al., 1991).

MORGAGNI'S HERNIA

In 1769, Morgagni first described the findings of substernal herniation of abdominal contents into the thoracic cavity (Morgagni, 1769). Since that time, this entity has frequently been called *Morgagni's hernia;* it has also been called *retrosternal hernia* or *Larrey's hernia.* Larrey, Surgeon General for Napoleon, described the surgical approach to the pericardial cavity through an anterior diaphragmatic defect (Thomas, 1972). The more appropriate descriptive name, *subcostosternal diaphragmatic hernia,* is attributed to Harrington (1948). This type of hernia is uncommon, representing approximately 3% of all surgically treated diaphragmatic hernias. It is rarely symptomatic, unlike its posterior counterpart, Bochdalek's hernia. With the increasing use of routine chest films and the need to exclude the possibility of a mediastinal neoplasm, most of these cases are brought to the attention of a thoracic surgeon. These hernias occur through a defect in the diaphragm just lateral to the xiphoid (usually to the right) and are associated with a well-formed hernia sac. They rarely produce symptoms in childhood, and most patients with Morgagni's hernia become symptomatic later in life, usually after age 40 years (Sinclair and Klein, 1993). Increased intra-abdominal pressure caused by obesity, trauma, or pregnancy may precipitate internal herniation through this part of the diaphragm. Most frequently, the transverse colon, either alone or in combination with some omentum, is most commonly involved in Morgagni's hernia (Fig. 29–2). Although most patients are not symptomatic and present with only an abnormal chest film, they may have symptoms of partial obstruction of the herniated viscus. Because the neck of the sac is usually small, the hernia may precipitate an acute or chronic colonic obstruction if it is left uncorrected, and this is an indication for surgical repair. Also indicated is an attempt to clearly define the hernia by preoperative diagnostic studies including contrast studies of the upper and lower intestine. An upper midline incision that extends into the subxiphoid area allows the best approach for repair. However, if the presence of a hernia is uncertain and there is a possibility of an anterior mediastinal mass causing the abnormal findings on the chest film, a right anterior thoracotomy

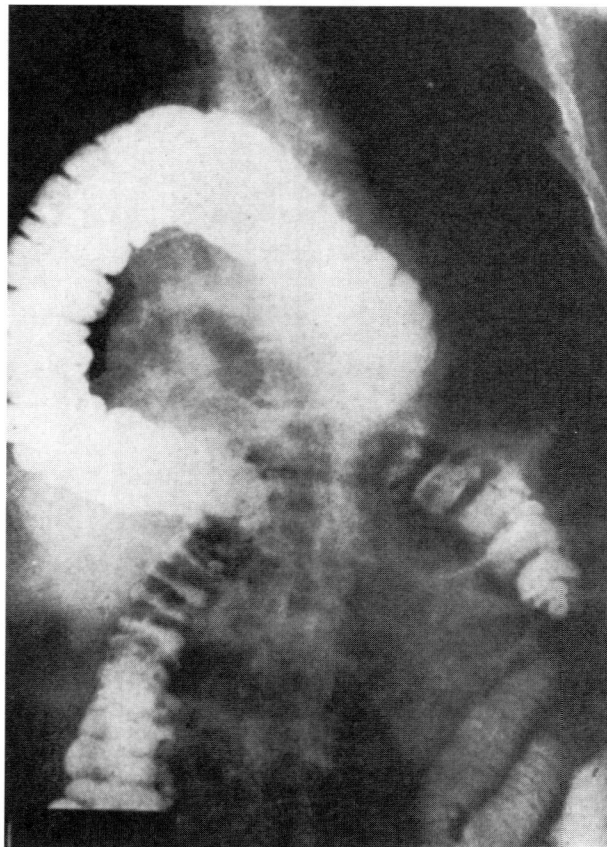

FIGURE 29–2. Subcostosternal (retrosternal, Morgagni's) hernia, showing most of the transverse colon displaced retrosternally.

incision allows good exposure of the area. The subcostal sternal defect can usually be repaired by direct suture after the contents of the hernia sac have been reduced. Laparoscopic repair of the defect has been reported (Kuster et al., 1992).

ESOPHAGEAL HIATAL HERNIA

Esophageal hiatal hernia is a common finding in adults. Less common is a congenital defect in the esophageal hiatus producing herniation of the stomach. It is common, however, for neonates and infants to have gastroesophageal reflux, which in some is associated with esophageal hiatal hernia. In symptomatic infants, gastroesophageal reflux is associated with a high degree of morbidity (Lilly and Randolph, 1968). Vomiting, respiratory complications, anemia, and failure to thrive are the four main diagnostic features of neonatal gastroesophageal reflux. The diagnosis is easily confirmed by esophagography together with fluoroscopy, which reveals free reflux of gastric contents into the esophagus, and by pH monitoring of the distal third of the esophagus. Esophagoscopy is not necessary for the diagnosis but is useful in evaluating the presence and severity of esophagitis. Conservative management involves maintaining the infant in an upright prone position, usually at an angle of 60 degrees for 24 hours a day until the baby outgrows the condition (Cahill et al., 1969; Lilly and Randolph, 1968). If medical management is unsuccessful, surgical repair is indicated. The type of repair is less important than the creation of a competent esophageal gastric sphincter, which prevents the reflux of gastric contents into the esophagus.

Tumors of the Diaphragm

Although primary tumors of the diaphragm are rare, the diaphragm is frequently involved with malignant tumors extending from contiguous structures, including the lungs, esophagus, stomach, liver, and retroperitoneum. Primary tumors of the diaphragm include cysts, inflammatory lesions, and benign or malignant neoplasms (Juvara and Priscu, 1966; Wiener and Chou, 1965).

In a review of 84 cases of primary tumor of the diaphragm (Olafsson et al., 1971), the male-to-female ratio was approximately equal (1:1.1). This ratio also applied to involvement of either the right or the left diaphragm, with the left side slightly predominating. The diagnosis is usually difficult to establish because these neoplasms are rare and the associated symptoms are nonspecific. The most common symptoms in order of frequency were epigastric or lower chest pain, cough, dyspnea, and gastrointestinal distress. Twenty per cent of the patients were asymptomatic, and in most the tumor was detected on the routine chest film. Routine chest films do not always provide a characteristic appearance, but CT has been helpful in localizing the exact site of the tumor.

In Olafsson's series, most primary tumors were benign (605), and the most frequently occurring benign tumors were cystic formations such as bronchial, mesothelial, or teratomal cysts. Most malignant tumors consisted of sarcomas, among which fibrosarcoma was the most common pathologic type. Trivedi (1958) reported three patients who had neurogenic diaphragmatic tumors and pulmonary osteoarthropathy and who were cured after resection. Radiographic manifestation of a diaphragmatic tumor consists of an enlarging mass on the diaphragmatic surface, which usually remains extrapleural (Anderson and Forrest, 1973).

Excision of the tumor is indicated whenever possible. Closure of the diaphragm by direct sutures is preferred, but when this is not possible, prosthetic material may serve as a replacement. In cases of inflammatory disease, such as hydatid disease or tuberculosis, treatment of the underlying condition is indicated.

Eventration and Unilateral Paralysis

Although previous authors have disagreed about the concept of the term, eventration is now generally recognized to be an abnormally high position of part or all of the diaphragm, usually associated with a sharp decrease in muscle fibers and a membranous appearance of the abnormal area. Eventrations of the diaphragm are divided etiologically into two groups: congenital or nonparalytic and acquired or paralytic (Thomas, 1968, 1970). Jean Louis Petit (1790) was the first to recognize this entity during autopsy studies in 1774. Beclard (1829) first used the term eventration. In 1923, Morrison did the first successful repair of an eventrated diaphragm and used one of the techniques of plication now applied to remove the redundancy associated with the eventration. Bisgard (1947) did the first successful repair of congenital eventration of the diaphragm and provided the current definition of eventration as "an abnormally high or elevated position of one leaf of the intact diaphragm as a result of paralysis, aplasia, or atrophy of varying degrees of the muscle fibers." He emphasized that the unbroken continuity of the diaphragm differentiates this entity from diaphragmatic hernia, which is sometimes difficult to establish on a clinical basis. Bilateral congenital eventration has been reported (Avnet, 1962).

Traumatic Perforation

Traumatic diaphragmatic hernias are produced by either blunt thoracoabdominal trauma or penetrating wounds of the diaphragm. Traumatic diaphragmatic hernia due to blunt trauma is thought to be produced by a sudden increase in the pleuroperitoneal pressure gradient that occurs at areas of potential weakness along the embryologic points of fusion (Childress and Grimes, 1961). Any patient with truncal penetrating trauma below the level of the nipples (fifth intercostal space) either anteriorly or posteriorly should be suspected of having diaphragmatic or intra-abdominal injuries. Automobile accidents are the most common cause of blunt traumatic diaphragmatic hernias, and in most series, approximately 90% involve the left hemidiaphragm (Brooks, 1978; McElwee et al., 1984; Pomerantz et al., 1968). Traumatic rupture of the right hemidiaphragm is thought to be less common because of the presence of the liver in the right upper quadrant to cushion the force applied against the diaphragm (Estrera et al., 1985). Defects due to blunt trauma are large, usually between 10 and 15 cm, and are generally located in the posterior aspect of the left hemidiaphragm (De la Rocha et al., 1982; Rodriguez-Morales et al., 1986). Through these defects, abdominal viscera can easily herniate into the thorax, and the stomach, spleen, colon, small intestine, and liver commonly enter the chest in that order of frequency (Orringer et al., 1975) (Fig. 29–3). Respiratory insufficiency due to compressed lung and a shift of the mediastinum to the contralateral side are common in the early phase of the injury, whereas symptoms of chronic intestinal obstruction are more common when the hernia has been present for a considerable period (Iuchtman et al., 1977).

Diagnosis of Traumatic Perforation

The diagnosis of diaphragmatic rupture can be elusive. Several centers have noted difficulty in diagnos-

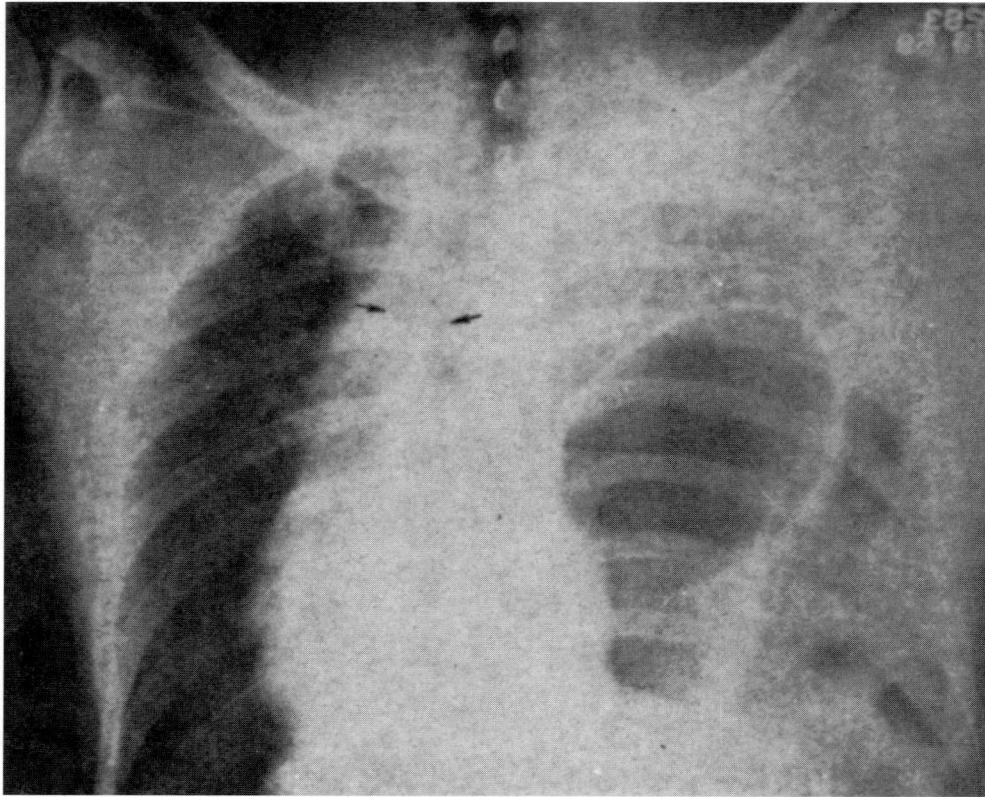

FIGURE 29–3. Blunt traumatic diaphragmatic hernia with stomach and bowel in left side of the chest. *Arrows* show lateral displacement of the tracheal shadow.

ing diaphragmatic injuries preoperatively because chest film findings and clinical signs lack specificity (Aronoff et al., 1982; Ebert et al., 1967; Miller et al., 1984). Of 68 patients with traumatic diaphragmatic hernia, in only 31% was the injury diagnosed preoperatively (Meyers and McCabe, 1993). Although not pathognomonic, the chest film is still the best initial screening examination, and absence of complete visualization of the entire hemidiaphragm should raise suspicion of injury (Carter et al., 1951; Ward et al., 1981). In patients sustaining blunt diaphragmatic hernias, the chest film in most series is diagnostic in approximately 50% of patients and is abnormal (hydropneumothorax, pneumothorax) but not diagnostic of the specific disorder in most of the remaining patients (Strug et al., 1974). Small tears due to perforating trauma are not often evident on the chest film, and the diagnosis of traumatic diaphragmatic hernia resulting from penetrating injuries to the abdomen or chest is usually made at the time of operation (Wiencek et al., 1986). Such tears in the diaphragm are not as large as those resulting from blunt trauma, and herniation of the abdominal contents into the thorax does not always occur immediately after the injury (Ebert et al., 1967).

Barium contrast studies are contraindicated in patients who are suspected of having diaphragmatic rupture with signs of obstruction because the air and contrast introduced into the bowel can become trapped and transform a partial obstruction in the herniated loop into a complete obstruction (Adamthwaite et al., 1983). A more recent case report describes the successful use of intraperitoneal technetium to diagnose a suspected right-sided diaphragmatic tear (Halldorsson et al., 1992).

Almost all series reviewing traumatic diaphragmatic hernia report a few patients with overlooked diaphragmatic injuries and delayed diagnosis, which often cause incarceration and strangulation of bowel (Brown and Richardson, 1985; Carter and Brewer, 1971). Some injuries can be overlooked even at operation, presumably because attention is diverted to the frequently encountered associated injuries (Table 29–1). Complete thoracotomy or exploratory laparotomy for trauma should always include careful inspection and palpation of both hemidiaphragms to avoid the morbidity of later intestinal obstruction and strangulation, which appear frequently (85%) within 3 to 5 years of the injury (Hood, 1971; Pomerantz et al., 1968). The expected yield of a careful search was documented in a report that found diaphragmatic injuries in 8.4% of 142 patients treated for blunt splenic trauma and in 8.8% of 102 patients with blunt hepatic rupture (Buckman et al., 1988).

Several cases of traumatic *intrapericardial* diaphragmatic hernias have been reported (Larrieu et al., 1980; Morrison and Mullens, 1978; van Loenhout et al., 1986). Most result from motor vehicle accidents. In these patients, chest films, CT scanning (Fagan et al., 1979), and echocardiography were helpful in estab-

■ Table 29–1. BLUNT DIAPHRAGMATIC
RUPTURE—ASSOCIATED INJURIES

Injury	No. of Injuries	Injury	No. of Injuries
Head	24	Femur fracture	5
Rib fracture	18	Pneumothorax	5
Pulmonary contusion	18	Humerus fracture	3
Spleen	18	Cervical spine fracture	2
Liver	18	Bladder rupture	2
Hemothorax	16	Myocardial contusion	2
Pelvic fracture	14	Lumbar spine fracture	1
Renal contusion	10	Pancreas	1
Hollow viscus	7	Shoulder dislocation	1
Pulmonary laceration	6	Clavicle fracture	1
Tibiofibular fracture	6	Aortic laceration	1

From Beal, S. L., and McKennan, M.: Blunt diaphragmatic rupture. Arch. Surg., Vol. 123, p. 82. Copyright 1988, American Medical Association.

lishing the diagnosis. Herniation of intra-abdominal organs into the pericardium results from a diaphragmatic tear in the transverse septum of the diaphragm. The most severe complication of intrapericardial diaphragmatic hernia is strangulation, which is more likely to develop in small tears than in larger hernias (Wetrich et al., 1969). The diagnosis can be made by means of barium swallow and barium enema to delineate stomach and bowel (Figs. 29–4 and 29–5).

Mortality of patients sustaining traumatic diaphragmatic hernia varies between 8 and 40%. Patients who sustain a blunt diaphragmatic hernia have the higher mortality because of the high incidence of associated injuries, which is almost 90% in most series (see Table 29–1).

Repair of Traumatic Hernia

Once the diagnosis of diaphragmatic hernia is made, repair should be made as soon as the patient is stabilized with regard to other significant injuries. Use of military antishock trousers that inflate the abdominal compartment is contraindicated in a patient with a suspected diaphragmatic hernia because this will further aggravate the pulmonary compromise caused by the herniated bowel. Because there is a high incidence of associated intra-abdominal injuries with blunt left diaphragmatic ruptures, patients whose injuries are diagnosed acutely after the injury should have transabdominal exploration so that associated injuries can be identified and corrected. If the diagnosis is delayed and there are no associated intra-abdominal injuries, repair is more easily accomplished by the transthoracic route. Right-sided herniations are often difficult to repair through an abdominal incision because of the presence of the liver, and a right-sided thoracotomy may be required to correct the defect. Whatever approach is chosen, the surgeon must be prepared to perform a combined thoracoabdominal operation through two different incisions (van Loenhout et al., 1986). Repair of the defect is accomplished by direct suture using a double layer of nonabsorbable suture and evacuation of the involved pleural cavity with a chest tube or with aspiration during the closure.

DIAPHRAGMATIC PACING

Historical Aspects

The fact that electricity could be used to stimulate movement of the diaphragm, the most important muscle of respiration, was first noted more than 200 years ago by Caldani, in 1786 (Schechter, 1970). In 1873, Hufeland proposed stimulating the phrenic nerve to treat asphyxia neonatorum. In 1818, Ure applied electricity from a voltaic battery to the phrenic nerve of a recently hung criminal. After observing "strong and laborious respirations," Ure proposed that if the spinal cord and blood vessels of the neck had not been damaged by the hangman's noose, resuscitation might have followed (Schechter, 1970). Duchenne (1872), an outstanding contributor to electrotherapy in the 19th century, clearly established phrenic nerve stimulation as the "best means of imitating natural respiration." Despite the early successes, electrophrenic stimulation did not become popular as a therapeutic technique, and when methods of negative-pressure and positive-pressure ventilation became available, stimulation of the phrenic nerves to activate the diaphragm disappeared from clinical practice.

In the 1940s, Sarnoff and associates (1948a, 1948b)

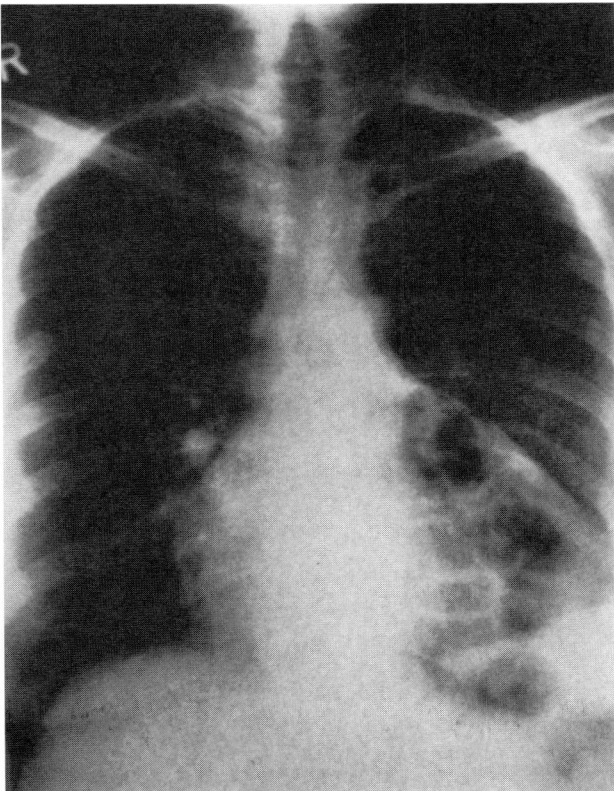

FIGURE 29–4. Chest film 1 year after blunt thoracoabdominal injury, showing bowel gas patterns within the cardiac silhouette.

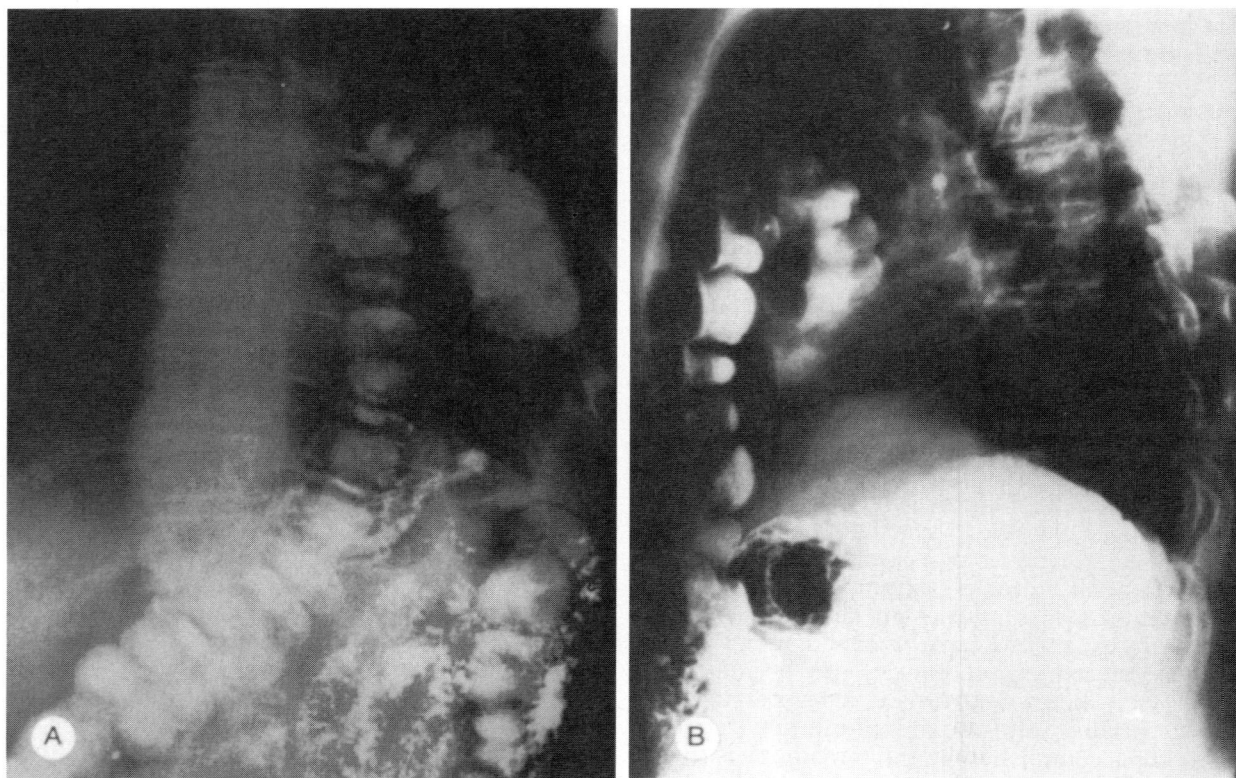

FIGURE 29–5. *A,* Contrast study showing barium-filled loops of colon intrapericardially (anteroposterior view). *B,* Lateral view locates the herniated colon to the anterior pericardial space.

became interested in electrical stimulation of the phrenic nerves as a method of aiding respiration in victims of bulbar poliomyelitis. In acute experiments, they showed the physiologic effects of electrical stimulation of the phrenic nerve and introduced the term *electrophrenic respiration.* Their experiments led to several important conclusions with regard to the technique, and these conclusions remain valid:

1. Artificial respiration by phrenic nerve stimulation can be performed in humans.
2. A smooth, gradual diaphragmatic contraction occurs when an increased voltage is applied to the phrenic nerve. The diaphragm thus performs a motion closely resembling that occurring during natural inspiration.
3. Respiratory minute volumes in excess of the patient's spontaneous minute volumes can be readily obtained with the submaximal stimulation of one phrenic nerve.
4. The depth of inspiration is proportional to the peak voltage applied to the phrenic nerve in humans, such as in the experimental model.
5. Adequate oxygenation of the blood can be maintained by electrophrenic respiration in the absence of spontaneous respiration.
6. The patient completely relinquishes spontaneous control of respiration when electrophrenic respiration is induced.

The development of an effective vaccine against poliomyelitis and the lack of the availability of implantable electrical stimulators probably discouraged the investigation of long-term phrenic nerve stimulation.

Beginning in the late 1950s and continuing until the present, Farmer and Glenn and their colleagues have been mainly responsible for the experimental development and clinical application of chronic diaphragmatic pacing by using radiofrequency signals to stimulate phrenic nerves through the intact skin (Farmer et al., 1978; Glenn et al., 1972). This group has acquired the greatest experience in using the technique and in doing so has defined the populations of patients in which chronic diaphragmatic pacing is efficacious. Moreover, their long-range interests and experience in this area have supplied information with regard to the safety of prolonged phrenic nerve stimulation and the mechanism of diaphragmatic fatigue by which effective pacing is usually limited to less than 24 consecutive hours (Kim et al., 1976).

Background

Through developing the technology of this field and applying those techniques to patients, Glenn defined the relative indications and contraindications for successful electrophrenic stimulation. Electroventilation by phrenic nerve stimulation is possible only with an intact peripheral nerve and muscle. Diaphragmatic pacing is indicated for patients who have chronic ventilatory insufficiency and in whom function of the phrenic nerves, lungs, and diaphragm is adequate to sustain ventilation by electrical stimulation. This includes some patients with paralysis of the respiratory muscles (quadriplegia) and with a central alveolar hypoventilation, also known as *sleep apnea* or *Ondine's curse*. Diaphragmatic pacing is not indicated in cases of ventilatory insufficiency that result from respiratory paralysis due to lower motor neuron lesions involving the phrenic nerve, from muscular dystrophy affecting the diaphragm, or from extensive parenchymal pulmonary disease. Muscle atrophy is not a contraindication, but it does increase the duration of the conditioning phase (Tibballs, 1991). With these careful indications for the procedure, properly chosen patients clearly benefit and can be freed from cumbersome ventilatory support systems (Brouillette et al., 1983; Glenn, 1987).

Electrical stimulation of motor nerves to achieve long-term contraction has been used successfully for diaphragm pacing only. The diaphragm can resist fatigue owing to its high oxidative capacity and high blood flow. Muscle fatigue has also been reduced by changing diaphragmatic muscle into a fatigue-resistant muscle through long-term application of slow stimulation frequencies. In normal diaphragmatic muscles, 55% of fibers are slow-twitch fatigue-resistant, 21% are fast-twitch fatigue-resistant, and 24% are fast-twitch fatigable (Lieberman et al., 1973). Fast-contracting muscles can be converted to slow-contracting muscles by electrical stimulation at low frequencies (10 Hz) over a period of months (Salmons and Henriksson, 1981). A fast-twitch muscle stimulated in this way will acquire the electrophysiologic and ultrastructural characteristics of a slow-twitch muscle. This strategy has been applied to diaphragmatic pacing in order to transform the diaphragmatic muscle to a new fatigue-resistant state (Talonen et al., 1990).

Apparatus

The diaphragmatic pacemaker commercially available, made by Avery Laboratory, located in Farmingdale, New York, consists of four components (Fig. 29–6). The receiver and electrode assembly are permanently implanted, and the transmitter and antenna remain external. The implanted radiofrequency receiver is inductively joined to the external transmitter and transforms the radiofrequency signals into an electrical impulse that is carried to the electrode placed behind the phrenic nerve (Fig. 29–7).

The transmitter-coded radiofrequency signals are generated by the external transmitter. Unlike the output signal of cardiac pacemakers, which produce a single impulse, the output signal of the diaphragmatic pacer is a train of pulses lasting between 1.2 and 1.45 seconds (shorter intervals in infants). The duration of the pulse train corresponds to the length of inspiration, and the number of pulse trains per minute estab-

lishes the respiratory rate (Nochomovitz et al., 1988). The pulse interval is usually preset at 50 msec, which allows effective contraction of the diaphragm muscle without producing rapid fatigue of diaphragmatic response (Bellemare and Bigland-Ritchie, 1987). Pulses have the same amplitude but differ in width, so that each successive pulse transmitted in each train is wider than its predecessor. The width of each radiofrequency pulse, after demodulation by the receiver, determines the amplitude of the current delivered to the phrenic nerve, which determines the depth of inspiration. The gradual increase in energy delivered during the pulse train is required to provide a smooth excursion of the diaphragm by progressively recruiting more and more nerve fibers (Bear and Talonen, 1987).

The usual settings of the transmitter for an adult are a respiratory rate of 12 breaths per minute with an inspiration time of 1.3 seconds and a pulse interval of 50 msec. The amplitude of the final signal is selected by gradually increasing the stimulus until diaphragmatic excursion is noted to be maximal, such as that recorded during fluoroscopy.

Antenna

The antenna transfers the radiofrequency signal from the transmitter across the intact skin to the subcutaneously implanted receiver. It is connected to a flexible wire lead that inserts into the transmitter. The antenna is placed directly over the implanted receiver and is secured in place with hypoallergenic tape. Because the intensity of the transmitted signal is determined by pulse width rather than by amplitude, the antenna can be displaced up to 2.5 cm from the center of the receiver without affecting operation.

Receiver

The implanted receiver (44 mm diameter, 15 mm thickness, 30.5 g weight) contains no batteries; an electronic integrated circuit obtains energy and stimulus information transcutaneously from the external transmitter by inductive electromagnetic coupling. The signal is demodulated into a unidirectional current, the amplitude of which varies directly with the width of the originally transmitted pulse. All components are hermetically sealed and encapsulated in an epoxy disk.

Electrodes

The electrodes contain a ribbon of platinum embedded in a silicone rubber cuff (Fig. 29–8). The surface area is calculated to be 11.5 mm^2. The cuff of the electrode is designed to fit loosely around a 1.5-cm segment of phrenic nerve and to permit firm fixation to the adjacent tissues without injuring the nerve. The ribbon electrode is available as bipolar or monopolar, but the monopolar electrode is preferred in all cases except when another electrical stimulation unit, such as a cardiac pacemaker, is in place. The advantage of

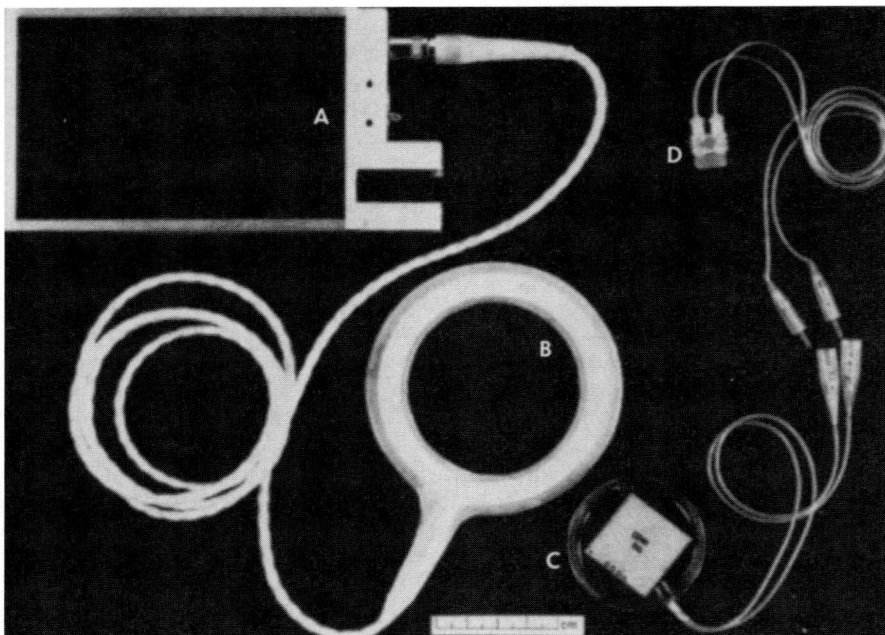

FIGURE 29–6. Components of the radio-frequency diaphragm pacemaker: *A*, transmitter; *B*, antenna; *C*, receiver; *D*, bipolar electrode.

the monopolar electrode is that it does not completely encircle the nerve and is therefore less likely to confine scar tissue that develops after implantation. The complete pacing system is shown in Figure 29–7.

Technique of Implantation

Although surgical techniques have been developed and used extensively for cervical implantation of the neuroelectrodes for diaphragmatic pacing, the thoracic approach is now preferred, except occasionally in the patient with extensive thoracic deformity or pleural disease, because accessory nerve fibers often join the phrenic nerve as it courses through the thoracic inlet. The usual approach for implantation of the platinum ribbon electrode on the phrenic nerve in the chest is through the second intercostal space anteri-

orly. If bilateral implants are indicated, the two operations are performed separately, at least 10 to 14 days apart, to avoid the greater danger of infection from the longer operation required for simultaneous implantation (Glenn and Phelps, 1985).

After sterile preparation, a transverse incision is made in the second intercostal space from the sternal border to the anterior axillary line (Fig. 29–9) The incision is extended in a muscle-splitting manner through the pectoralis major, and the internal mammary artery and vein are exposed, fully ligated, and divided. The pleura is opened, and the mediastinum is exposed. A segment of phrenic nerve presenting on a relatively flat surface between the base of the heart and the apex of the chest is selected as the site of implantation. On the right side, this is usually just above the junction of the azygos vein and the superior

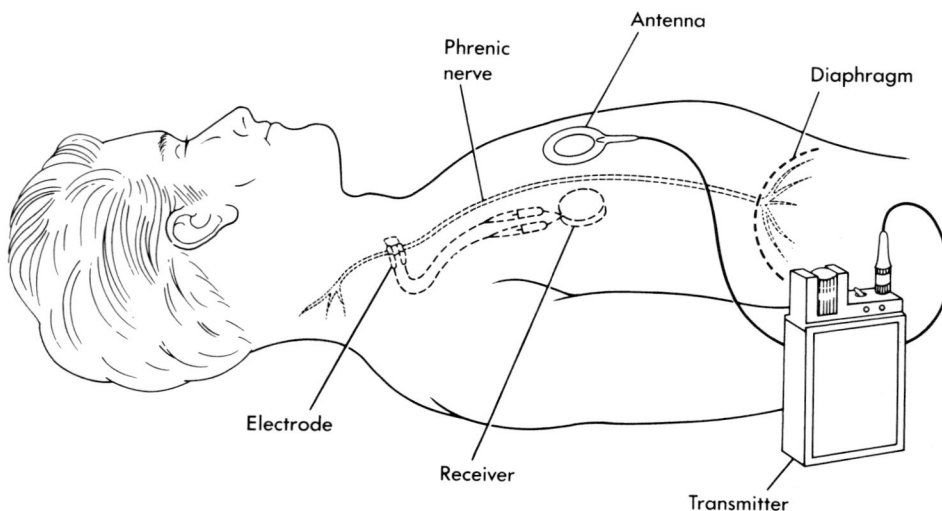

FIGURE 29–7. The relationship of the four components of the diaphragmatic pacer is shown, using a bipolar electrode. (From Avery Laboratories, Inc.: Diaphragm Pacer [product brochure 6011 B–5/79]. Farmingdale, NY, Avery Laboratories, Inc., May 1979.)

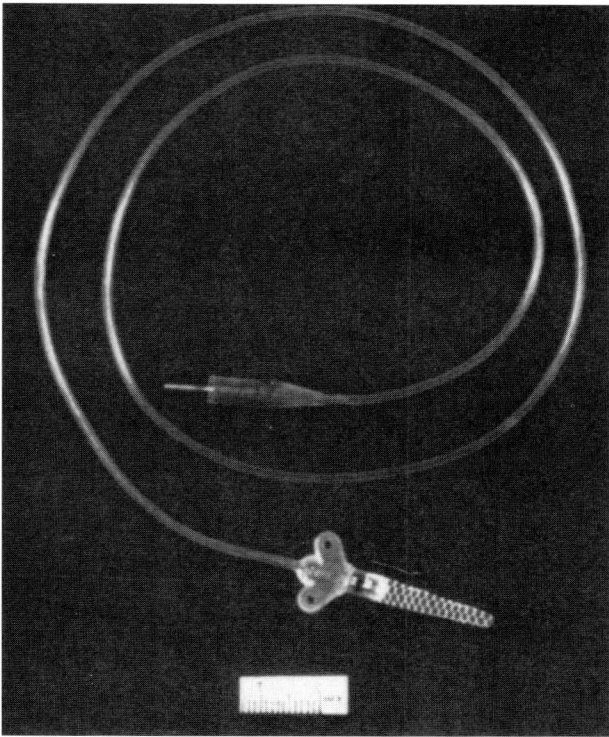

FIGURE 29–8. The newer platinum ribbon monopolar nerve electrode designed for phrenic nerve stimulation.

vena cava where the phrenic nerve passes across the middle of the superior vena cava (Wetstein, 1987). On the left side, the preferred site is where the phrenic nerve passes between the aortic arch and the left pulmonary artery.

The phrenic nerve is isolated by making 1.5-cm parallel incisions on each side of the phrenic nerve through the pleura and underlying areolar tissue. Care is taken to keep 2 to 3 mm from the nerve to preserve the perineural blood supply. The electrode cuff is then inserted carefully beneath the nerve (monopolar) and secured to the surrounding structures (see Fig. 29–9). Preparation must ensure that the surface of the platinum electrode lies directly in contact with the perineurium of the phrenic nerve. The lead wires are then passed through a subcutaneous tunnel to join those from the receiver. The receiver is placed in a subcutaneous pocket, which is either over the upper chest in the midclavicular line for quadriplegics or over the lower chest in the midaxillary line for patients with central alveolar hypoventilation. In infants and children, the receiver is implanted subcutaneously over the lateral abdomen. The subcutaneous pocket should be made so that no part of the apparatus lies directly under the incision. The copper coil of the receiver faces outward toward the undersurface of the skin. If bilateral units are implanted, the receivers must be separated by at least 15 cm to avoid cross-interference. Before the operation is terminated, the ability of the system to produce a diaphragmatic contraction should be shown by using a sterile antenna connected to an off-table transmitter,

which lies directly over the implanted radio receiver. If a good response is obtained, the threshold to stimulation is noted; it should be in the range of 0.1 to 2 ma. A higher threshold may signal displacement of the electrode or interposition of tissue between the electrode and the phrenic nerve. A pacing schedule is not begun until 12 to 14 days postoperatively to allow time for the wound to heal and for the perineural edema to resolve.

Preoperative Screening Tests

Proof that the phrenic nerve is viable is a prerequisite to implantation of a phrenic nerve electrode. To

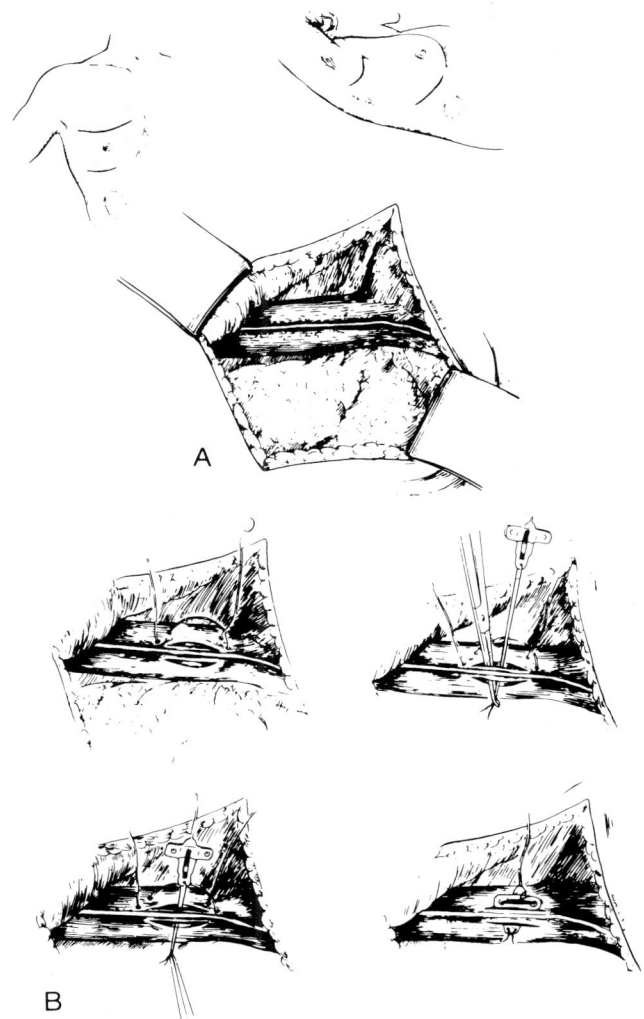

FIGURE 29–9. *A* and *B*, Transthoracic approach to the phrenic nerve. The mediastinum is exposed either through an incision in the second interspace anteriorly or through the third interspace in the axilla. The monopolar electrode is secured against the right phrenic nerve on the superior vena cava. If the nerve is isolated closer to the heart (within 5 cm), a bipolar electrode is required. (*A* and *B*, From Glenn, W. W. L., Hogan, J. F., and Phelps, M. L.: Ventilatory support to the quadriplegic patient with respiratory paralysis by diaphragm pacing. Surg. Clin. North Am., *60*:1055, 1980.)

determine that viable phrenic neurons exist, the nerve in the neck is electrically stimulated percutaneously. The usual response, when most neurons are viable, is a brisk contraction of the diaphragm of at least several centimeters. The absence of contraction when stimulating in the anatomic location of the nerve almost always means nonviability of the nerve. If there is doubt that the probe locates the nerve correctly, direct exploration is planned, together with preparation to apply the nerve electrode if a viable nerve is found. Phrenic nerve conduction time is also measured preoperatively. The normal conduction time from the neck to the diaphragm is generally between 7 and 10 msec in adults; the interval is shorter in infants and children. Prolongation over 12 msec may indicate serious local or systemic disease.

Pacing Schedule

The electrical parameters for phrenic nerve stimulation currently used by Glenn and colleagues have evolved after many years of extensive laboratory and clinical trials. Glenn initially used electrical parameters that included a frequency of 25 Hz (40 msec pulse interval), an inspiration duration of 1.35 seconds, and a pulse train repetition rate (respiratory rate) of 15 to 17 per minute.

The stimulus is pulse-width modulated with the current amplitude, increasing from the initial contraction (threshold stimulation) to the maximal contraction of the diaphragm, to obtain a smooth inspiratory diaphragmatic motion (Fig. 29–10). Clinical and experimental data acquired by Glenn show that when phrenic nerve stimulation is restricted to 12 hours daily, no harm is induced with respect to diaphragmatic fatigue. However, experiments in dogs with similar parameters have shown that if pacing is applied for several weeks or months without rest, diaphragmatic muscle function is reduced to less than 20% of normal and is accompanied by severe organic changes in the muscle that are irreversible (Ciesielski et al., 1983; Sato et al., 1970). The origination of fatigue after continuous electrophrenic stimulation in these investigations was studied by measuring end-plate potentials after continued repetitive electrical stimulation. The diaphragmatic fatigue was due to interference with transmission of impulses across the neuromuscular junction. Later, methods to reduce the electrical charge of the nerve and diaphragm were explored to reduce fatigue. Glenn and colleagues (1986) showed that pacing-induced fatigue of the diaphragm, such as that measured by the tidal volume during stimulation of the phrenic nerves, was significantly less when (1) the current applied to the nerve was just under that required for maximal tidal volume, (2) the respiratory rate was 10 per minute instead of 20, and (3) the frequency of stimulation was 10 Hz compared with a higher frequency. The type of waveform and whether the electrode was monopolar or bipolar made no significant difference to the onset or duration of fatigue. Muscle fatigue becomes a greater issue when bilateral pacing is required for full-time ventilatory support in infants, when unilateral pacing is often inadequate to accomplish adequate ventilation because of the instability of the mediastinum and the immaturity of the lungs and chest wall. As pacing is continued at a wide pulse interval (lower frequency) and the diaphragm muscle conditions to this lower stimulus frequency, there is fusion of the contractions. This causes muscle conditioning, which is due to conversion of the fast-contracting fibers of the diaphragm (high-glycolytic, white fibers) to slowly contracting fibers (low-glycolytic, red fibers) (Salmons and Henriksson, 1981). When nocturnal ventilatory support alone is indicated in central alveolar hypoventilation or sleep apnea, and only one hemidiaphragm is to be paced, the diaphragm must be paced more forcefully than for bilateral pacing. Because continuous pacing is not required and a period of several hours of rest is possible, this can be tolerated without inducing significant and irreversible muscle fatigue. The pulse interval is set at a relatively high frequency of approximately 50 msec (20 Hz) and a rate of 12 to 14 per minute. With these parameters, pacing for 10 to 12 hours followed by a similar period of rest is well tolerated, and fatigue of the diaphragm is minimal (Oda et al., 1981). Consequently, the patient with central alveolar hypoventilation without respiratory muscle paralysis can begin pacing for 8 to 10 hours nightly in the third week postoperatively.

Quadriplegic patients with respiratory muscle paralysis present a different problem in initiating a pacing schedule. These patients do not present for pacing until several months after the injury that caused the paralysis. During this time, they have had full-time mechanical ventilatory support, and the diaphragm has become weak from disuse and is easily fatigued by electrical stimulation (Nochomovitz et al., 1984). In these patients, the technique for achieving full-time

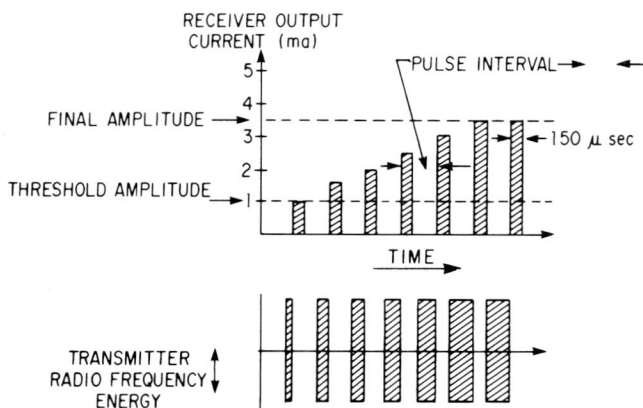

FIGURE 29–10. Schematic drawing of the electrical signals necessary to produce a single inspiration. The output of the transmitter is a train of biphasic pulses that vary progressively in width *(lower panel)*. The receiver modulates the signal and sends to the nerve-electrode a train of unidirectional impulses that vary in amplitude from 1 to 3.5 ma. The amplitude of the pulse is determined by the width of the corresponding biphasic signal. The first pulse is set at the threshold value and the final pulse at the current needed to produce a smooth diaphragmatic contraction.

pacing can be complex and prolonged. After pacing parameters have been selected and the initial threshold and maximal determination of diaphragm motion have been obtained, pacing is begun usually at 2 to 3 minutes an hour while the patient is awake. The duration of pacing can be advanced each day by several minutes hourly, as long as the minute volume is not decreased by more than 25% from the beginning to end of the pacing period (Harpin et al., 1986). It may take 6 weeks to 8 months to accomplish full-time ventilatory support to condition the diaphragm according to such a pacing schedule. If ventilation cannot be maintained except by bilateral simultaneous pacing, an attempt must be made to convert the diaphragm muscle fibers to nonfatiguing fibers. This is done by gradually decreasing the frequency of stimulation to 10 Hz, the respiratory rate to 8 per minute, and the current amplitude to submaximal. A considerably longer period is required to condition the diaphragm muscle in children because their respiratory components are immature. In addition, a permanent tracheostomy is needed with full-time pacing to keep the airway clear and unobstructed. Diaphragmatic pacing can actually exacerbate upper-airway obstruction because the usual coordinated pattern of simultaneous diaphragmatic and laryngeal muscle contraction during natural respiration is lost with artificial electrophrenic stimulation.

SELECTION OF PATIENTS FOR DIAPHRAGMATIC PACING

Successful diaphragmatic pacing is possible only in the presence of a viable phrenic nerve that can stimulate a normal diaphragm to contract and allow expansion of parenchyma of the lung that is capable of satisfactory ventilation and oxygenation. Malfunction of any of these structures significantly reduces the effectiveness of diaphragmatic pacing. Thus, a thorough evaluation of the components of respiration must precede a recommendation to pace the diaphragm (Mier et al., 1987). Diaphragmatic pacing is contraindicated in cases of diaphragmatic paralysis that result from (1) destruction of the anterior horn cells at the level of C3, C4, or C5; (2) damage to the peripheral axons of the phrenic nerve; (3) impaired diaphragmatic function secondary to atrophy, eventration, myositis, or muscular dystrophy; or (4) severe damage to pulmonary parenchyma (Glenn, 1978). Direct electrical stimulation of diaphragmatic muscle without using phrenic innervation has not been successful because of ineffective diaphragmatic contraction and early fatigability (Mugica et al., 1987). Thus, paralysis or paresis of the diaphragm, commonly encountered after coronary bypass grafting operations, is not amenable to electrophrenic pacing of the involved diaphragm. The cause of the phrenic nerve dysfunction is cold or stretching injury or ischemia (Estenne et al., 1985; Markland et al., 1985), and because of peripheral nerve involvement, electrophrenic pacing would not be effective.

Central Alveolar Hypoventilation

Central alveolar hypoventilation occurs when the respiratory center fails to respond to hypercapnia by increasing minute ventilation. Alternatively, the carotid body chemoreceptors may also not respond to hypoxemia. Periodic apnea can occur, especially during sleep. The clinical criteria for diagnosing central alveolar hypoventilation include (1) clinical features of hypoventilation, such as cyanosis, polycythemia, and cor pulmonale with right-sided heart failure; (2) hypoxemia and hypercapnia increasing during sleep; (3) hypoventilation during sleep, sometimes marked by periodic apnea; (4) almost normal results of ventilatory capacity tests; (5) reduced ventilatory response to induced hypoxemia and hypercapnia; and (6) absence of upper-airway obstruction during a sleep study or persistence of hypoventilation after relief of obstruction (Glenn, 1978). In the absence of an identifiable organic lesion of the respiratory centers, a cause of central alveolar hypoventilation may not be determined (Meisner et al., 1983). Frequently, there is a history of a previous attack of encephalitis or an undiagnosed febrile illness without an evident residual organic deficit. The presence of hypoventilation at birth or a history of apnea that suggests manifestations of the sudden infant death syndrome indicates the presence of a congenital defect in the respiratory center (Glenn, 1985).

Since 1966, Glenn and colleagues have used diaphragmatic pacing to treat 48 patients with defects in respiratory control secondary to the central alveolar hypoventilation syndrome. Since 1976, they have preferred the monopolar electrode to the bipolar electrode for both unilateral and bilateral stimulation. Three cases were categorized as being congenital; 11 were idiopathic as the cause of the central alveolar hypoventilation syndrome; and the remainder were due to organic lesions of the brain stem or above, usually due to vascular accidents. The mean age of the patients with idiopathic central alveolar hypoventilation was 55 years, with a range between 44 and 67 years. These patients were paced with a mean of 95 months and with a range of 17 to 168 months. Four patients died in this group; the mortality rate was 36%. Of 33 patients with central alveolar hypoventilation treated with diaphragmatic pacing because of lesions of the brain stem or above, 19 ultimately died (a mortality rate of 58%) (Glenn and Phelps, 1985).

Quadriplegia

The fact that diaphragmatic pacing could provide total ventilatory support in humans was shown by Glenn and colleagues in 1971 when they successfully transferred a ventilator-dependent quadriplegic patient to full-time electrophrenic respiration (Glenn et al., 1972). The patient was a 38-year-old man who sustained a spinal cord injury at the level of the first and second cervical segments. Five months after injury, he had a bipolar electrode placed around each phrenic nerve, using a cervical approach. Approximately 3 months after implantation, the patient was completely free of the mechanical respirator and was supported by radiofrequency electrophrenic respiration by alternating stimulation of the two phrenic nerves for 12 hours each. He was ultimately discharged from the hospital. Glenn and co-workers reported a series of 20 quadriplegic patients (Glenn et al., 1980) in whom full-time ventilatory support was achieved with diaphragmatic pacing in 8 patients and part-time support in an additional 8 patients. Similar results have been reported from other centers that specialize in the treatment of spinal cord injury (Oakes et al., 1980).

Use of the diaphragmatic pacing technique in quadriplegic patients requires special consideration of certain factors that have been well emphasized by Glenn and associates (1984):

1. The injury that produced quadriplegia must be localized to the first or second cervical segments of the spinal cord. If C3, C4, or C5 is involved, a portion of the anterior horn cells of the corresponding segments may be destroyed and the surviving neurons may become inadequate to achieve a satisfactory diaphragmatic function. Before permanent electrodes are implanted, nerve viability must be shown either by transcutaneous technique or by direct stimulation at the time of operation.

2. Some recovery of spontaneous ventilatory function may occur after spinal cord injury; therefore, the diaphragmatic pacing should be delayed until several months after injury to be certain it is really indicated.

3. Disuse atrophy of the diaphragm that is the result of the cervical spinal cord injury requires slow and gradual conditioning before diaphragmatic pacing can be expected to provide adequate ventilation.

4. Fatigue of the diaphragm requires that pacing be periodically interrupted to permit recovery of the neuromuscular junction. Fatigue that is not recognized can cause permanent damage to the neuromuscular junction, which can preclude successful electrophrenic respiration later.

5. Diaphragmatic pacing is indicated only in patients who are good candidates for long-term rehabilitation after they have been supported by conventional positive-pressure ventilation following the first few months after injury.

Sequential Stimulation

Baer and associates have proposed a new mode of phrenic nerve stimulation for diaphragmatic pacing that more clearly initiates natural muscle contractions, using the principle of sequential motor nerve stimulation (Baer et al., 1990). This allows individual nerve-muscle compartments to be stimulated at fairly low frequencies, thereby providing time for recovery even during muscle contractions, limiting muscle fatigue. This mode of stimulation provides smooth muscle contraction and shortens the conditioning phase after

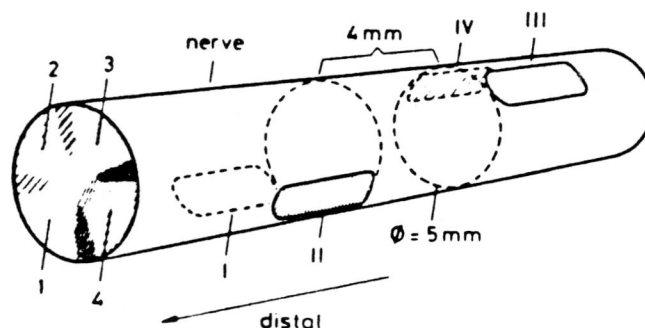

FIGURE 29–11. The quadripolar electrode configuration used for sequential stimulation. The electrode poles I–IV are placed around excitation compartments 1–4 in the cross surface of the phrenic nerve. The area of one electrode button is 6 mm. (From Talonen, P. P., Baer, G. A., Häkkinen, V., Ojala, J. K.: Neurophysiological and technical considerations for the design of an implantable phrenic nerve stimulator. Med. Biol. Eng. Comput., 28:31, 1990.)

the beginning of the long-term phrenic nerve stimulation from 2 to 3 months to 2 to 3 weeks.

The disadvantage of the unipolar electrode, used most often for clinical phrenic nerve stimulation, has been that the same part of the nerve is always stimulated, leaving no time for recovery. Alternate stimulation of the left and the right halves of the diaphragm has been used to allow time for recovery, until transformation of diaphragm muscle fibers from fast twitch to slow twitch occurs.

For sequential stimulation, the nerve is divided into four stimulating compartments with platinum electrode buttons positioned in two identical pairs

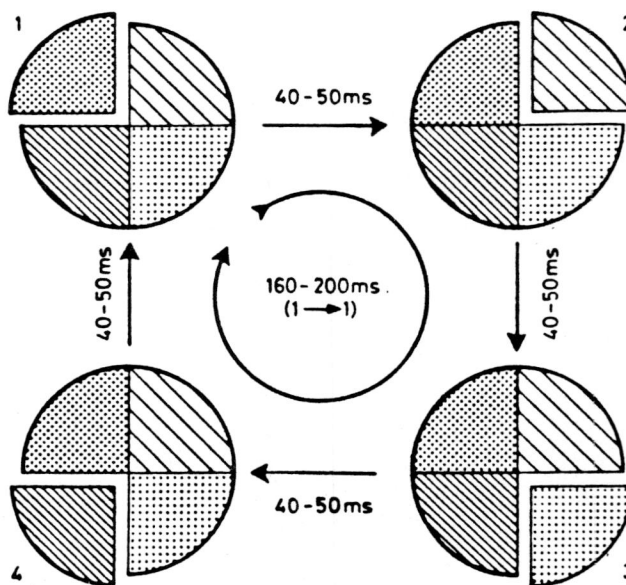

FIGURE 29–12. Principle of sequential nerve stimulation. Each of four nerve compartments controls a group of muscle fibers in a hemidiaphragm. When individual compartments are stimulated sequentially, the hemidiaphragm exerts a force similar to that of fused contraction. The pulse interval between each compartment is 40 to 50 ms *(outer diagram)* and the pulse interval of the same compartment is 160 to 200 ms *(inner circle).*

around the nerves, symmetric to the nerve axis but at some distance from each other in the longitudinal direction (quadripolar electrode). Stimulation occurs via longitudinal rather than transverse current flow, reducing the electrode charge needed for nerve activation (Fig. 29–11).

The principle of the sequential four-pole electrode stimulator is shown in Figure 29–12. Each of the compartments 1 to 4 is stimulated sequentially at a frequency of 5 to 6 Hz. This imitates natural activation of the nerve and allows most of the muscle fibers to rest during contraction of the muscle.

The quadipolar pacing system uses implanted receivers and a battery-operated control unit with outside antennas, similar to the Avery Laboratory system. The control unit allows adjustment of the stimulus intensity, frequency, and duration.

The four-pole system has been used in several patients (Talonen et al., 1990), with four patients having quadriplegia. The conditioning period for this group was significantly shortened compared with that for the unipolar pacing. The authors indicate that total independence from mechanical ventilation should be achieved within 2 months (Talonen et al., 1990).

Diaphragmatic Pacing in Infants

A series of phrenic nerve pacing in infants was reported by Ilbawi and associates (1985), who reviewed eight infants, ranging in age from 2.5 months to 8.5 months, who had central hypoventilation syndrome. Preoperative diagnosis was established by showing an inadequate ventilatory response to hypercapnia and hypoxia. Before placement of phrenic nerve electrodes, percutaneous measurements of phrenic nerve conduction time and diaphragmatic action potentials were performed to evaluate the feasibility of diaphragmatic pacing. Bilateral anterolateral inframammary thoracotomy incisions were made, entering the chest through the third intercostal space. Unipolar electrodes were passed around each phrenic nerve and connected to the receiver in a subcutaneous pocket created in the flank.

Patients were followed postoperatively for 6 months to 8 years. In all patients, bilateral phrenic nerve stimulation allowed either a sharp decrease in or a discontinuation of positive-pressure ventilation. Phrenic nerve conduction time and diaphragmatic action potential showed no evidence of nerve injury or muscle dysfunction after 8 years of pacing. This clinical experience confirms the previous work of Kim and colleagues (1976), who found that the histologic changes of phrenic nerves did not correlate with the duration of stimulation and that nerve injury was due to an inappropriate technique of electrode application (Fig. 29–13). The report by Ilbawi and co-workers (1985) suggested that diaphragmatic pacing in infants was safe, had no major side effects, and could be considered a viable long-term improvement over long-term positive-pressure ventilation. These conclusions were supported by other investigators (Cahill et al., 1983). The authors emphasized that tracheostomy is uniformly necessary in infants because pacing-related upper-airway obstruction is consistently observed as a result of failure to activate laryngeal and upper-airway muscles in synchrony with diaphragmatic contraction. This activation is necessary to counteract the negative pharyngeal pressure that is generated during inspiration. The authors also noted that it was uniformly necessary to use bilateral diaphragmatic pacing to sustain adequate ventilation in children, which precluded successful unilateral diaphragmatic pacing (Brouillette et al., 1983).

PACING FAILURES

Pacing failure causes a fall in oxygen saturation or a rise in P_{CO_2} as well as an increase in the threshold

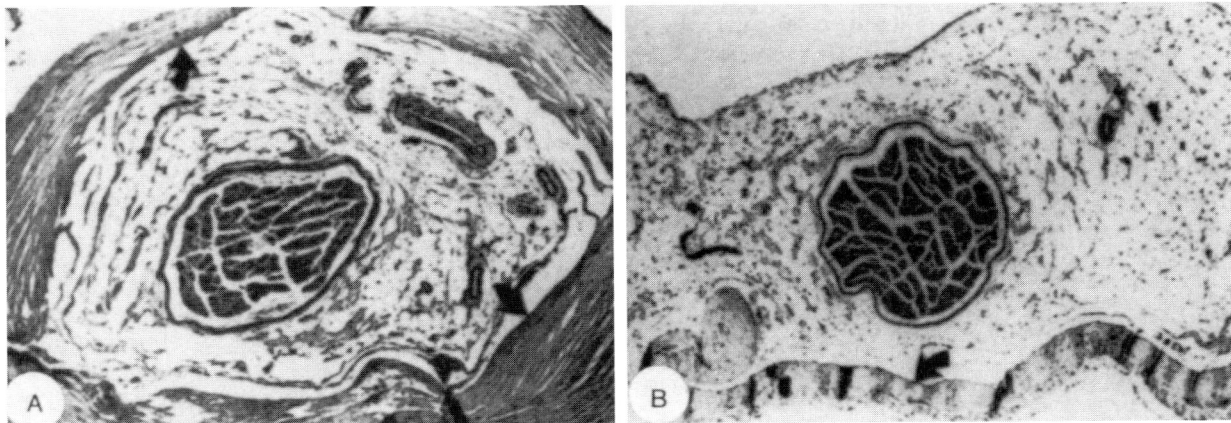

FIGURE 29–13. *A,* Section of the left phrenic nerve at the level of the electrode after bipolar stimulation for 126 days at 26 Hz. The epineural fibroadipose layer is surrounded completely by a thick fibrous capsule *(arrows),* but the nerve fascicle is histologically unremarkable. *B,* Section of the phrenic nerve at the electrode level after stimulation with a monopolar electrode for 154 days at 27 Hz. A band of fibrous tissue *(arrow)* has developed at the lower margin facing the electrode. The nerve fascicle is histologically unremarkable. (Hematoxylin and eosin stain, ×39.)

current required to initiate pacing. Causes of early failure include incorrect patient selection, surgical injury to the phrenic nerve at time of implantation, inappropriate pacing schedule, or upper-airway obstruction due to failure to activate stabilizing muscles of the upper airway synchronizing with diaphragmatic contraction (requiring a tracheostomy) (Moxham and Shneerson, 1993). Late pacing failure is usually due to reduced respiratory function from bronchospasm or pneumonia. Impaired diaphragmatic contractility from acidosis or hypophosphatemia will also impair pacing efficiency.

FUTURE GOALS

The perfection of a totally implantable, battery-powered diaphragmatic pacemaker that can be programmed and interrogated from an exterior device similar to current cardiac pacemaker technology is a goal (Glenn et al., 1986). An implanted energy source that could be developed from currently available technology would maintain an estimated battery life of 5 to 8 years for diaphragmatic pacing. Additionally, the development of a demand-type diaphragmatic pacemaker that would respond to ventilatory needs and act in synchrony with autonomic reflexes to maintain an open upper airway during respiration is the next goal in the evolution of artificial respiration by diaphragmatic pacing (Glenn, 1987). Perhaps the greatest contribution derived from the development of diaphragmatic pacing is the demonstration that peripheral nerves can be stimulated intermittently for extended periods by artificial pulses to achieve almost normal function of the neuromuscular unit without apparent damage. The development and application of diaphragmatic pacing represent a success story for neuroprosthetics and should serve as the basis for the application of similar techniques to other neurologically impaired but otherwise functional units of the body.

SELECTED BIBLIOGRAPHY

Anderson, L. S., and Forrest, J. V.: Tumors of the diaphragm. Am. J. Roentgenol. Radium Ther. Nucl. Med., 119:259, 1973.

The authors present a radiographic analysis of diaphragmatic tumors and a classification of those tumors into the following groups: primary benign neoplasms, primary malignant neoplasms, secondary malignant neoplasms, cysts, inflammatory lesions, and endometriosis.

Beal, S. L., and McKennan, M.: Blunt diaphragmatic rupture. Arch. Surg., 123:828, 1988.

The authors review 37 patients sustaining traumatic diaphragmatic hernia from blunt injury during a 12-month period. Because of a high incidence of associated injuries (36 of 37 patients) and a high incidence of shock on initial presentation (54%), the overall mortality was 40%. The difficulty in diagnosing traumatic diaphragmatic hernia was shown, in that the rupture was not initially recognized in 69% of patients, and the initial chest film was often nondiagnostic. The authors recommend a high index of suspicion for the injury in patients sustaining blunt trauma and also prompt exploratory laparotomy with complete inspection of both hemidiaphragms and primary repair of the diaphragmatic tear.

Glenn, W. W. L., Hogan, J. F., Loke, J. S. O., et al.: Ventilatory support by pacing of the conditioned diaphragm in quadriplegia. N. Engl. J. Med., 310:1150, 1984.

This report updates the Yale group's experience with diaphragmatic pacing in quadriplegic patients. The group reports changes in the method of pacing used in the 5 most recent patients, techniques that minimized fatigue of the diaphragm and permitted uninterrupted simultaneous pacing of both hemidiaphragms to produce a more physiologic form of respiration. The patients included in the study had continuous electrical pacing of both hemidiaphragms simultaneously for 11 to 33 months. The strength and endurance of the diaphragm muscle increased with diaphragmatic pacing. Biopsy specimens taken from 2 patients who had uninterrupted stimulation for 6 and 16 weeks showed changes that suggested the development of fatigue-resistant muscle fibers. When comparing the results of continuing bilateral diaphragmatic pacing in the current group with a previous group of 17 patients with respiratory paralysis, continuous bilateral pacing using low-frequency stimulation was superior because of more efficient ventilation of both lungs, less electrical energy required to effect the same ventilation, and absence of myopathic changes in the diaphragm muscle. The authors conclude that for patients with respiratory paralysis and intact phrenic nerves, continuous simultaneous pacing of both hemidiaphragms with low-frequency stimulation at a slow respiratory rate is a satisfactory method of providing full-time ventilatory support.

Glenn, W. W. L., and Phelps, M. L.: Diaphragm pacing by electrical stimulation of the phrenic nerve. Neurosurgery, 17:974, 1985.

In this review article, Glenn summarized his personal experience with diaphragmatic pacing in 77 patients. The indications and contraindications for the procedure are outlined, and the authors discuss the preoperative screening tests, which should be carefully completed before initiating this type of therapy. The operative technique is discussed and illustrated. The authors recommend that bilateral units be implanted at separate operations. A discussion of conduct of pacing as well as pacing schedules for diaphragmatic "conditioning" in quadriplegic patients is given. This is the most recent review of Glenn's experience in this area, which he has developed since the mid-1960s, and it provides his views of application of this technology to patients with chronic ventilatory insufficiency.

Ilbawi, M. N., Idriss, S. S., Hunt, C. E., et al.: Diaphragmatic pacing in infants: Techniques and results. Ann. Thorac. Surg., 40:323, 1985.

This report reviews eight infants with central hypoventilation syndrome who were treated with phrenic nerve pacing for periods between 6 months and 8 years. The ages of the patients ranged from 2½ to 8½ months at the time of phrenic nerve diaphragmatic pacing. The preoperative diagnosis was established by showing an inadequate ventilatory response to hypercapnia and hypoxia. Preoperative screening tests were performed on all patients and included measurement of phrenic nerve conduction time and diaphragmatic action potentials to assess the feasibility of diaphragmatic pacing. The electrodes were implanted through an anterior thoracotomy incision, with receiver implantation in the flank. There were no complications or deaths related to the procedure, and bilateral phrenic nerve stimulation allowed either sharp reduction in ventilatory requirement or discontinuation of positive-pressure ventilation. This report is encouraging in that it shows that prolonged phrenic nerve stimulation is safe in infants; in these selected patients, early initiation of diaphragmatic pacing can lead to an extended survival.

Meyers, B. F., and McCabe, C. J.: Traumatic diaphragmatic hernia—An occult marker of serious injury. Ann. Surg. 218:783, 1993.

Between 1982 and 1992, 68 patients were treated for traumatic diaphragmatic hernias at the Massachusetts General Hospital—25 from blunt injury and 43 from penetrating trauma. The authors emphasize the striking problem with making the diagnosis, because only 31% of the injuries were diagnosed prior to surgery. The mortality was 7.4%, with deaths due to coagulopathy, multisystem organ failure, and pulmonary embolism. Diaphragmatic injury is a predictor of serious associated injuries that, unfortunately, is also itself often occult.

Miller, L., Bennett, E. V., Root, H. D., et al.: Management of penetrating and blunt diaphragmatic injury. J. Trauma, 24:403, 1984.

The authors review a 5-year experience with 102 patients with diaphragmatic injury, mostly penetrating trauma (93 of 102). Chest films were normal in 40% of the patients, and a peritoneal lavage was not useful in the diagnosis. Most of the injuries were diagnosed at exploration, because the authors followed a policy of exploratory laparotomy for all penetrating wounds of the abdomen and lower thorax. Although associated injuries occurred in 87% of the patients, only 1 death occurred.

Moxham, J., and Shneerson, J. M.: Diaphragmatic pacing. Am. Rev. Respir. Dis., 148:533, 1993.

An up-to-date review article of the indications for diaphragmatic pacing. The authors discuss the choice of commercial systems available and principles of pacing schedules. About 1000 patients worldwide have now had diaphragmatic pacemakers implanted. The best results are obtained in this group, with 90% alive after 10 years. The significant limitations of the technique are also reviewed.

Sawyer, S. F., Falterman, K. W., Goldsmith, J. P., and Arensman, R. M.: Improving survival in the treatment of congenital diaphragmatic hernia. Ann. Thorac. Surg., 41:75, 1986.

This paper reviews 32 infants with congenital diaphragmatic hernia treated in the years 1979 to 1984. Twenty-four patients required immediate intubation and operative repair at less than 12 hours of age. The overall survival was 54% but this was significantly influenced by the date of treatment, because the survival in the last 3 years of the series was 82%, compared with 31% in the initial 3 years. The authors attribute the improved survival to more aggressive therapy to interrupt the vicious circle of persistent fetal circulation that accompanies the disorder. The authors describe the indications and use of both pharmacologic agents (pulmonary vasodilators, inotropic agents, buffering agents to prevent and treat acidosis) and mechanical interventions including high-frequency jet ventilation and extracorporeal membrane oxygenation (ECMO).

Thomas, T. V.: Congenital eventration of the diaphragm. Ann. Thorac. Surg., 10:180, 1970.

This collective review outlines the causes, symptoms, and indications for operative intervention for diaphragmatic eventration. A classification separating congenital (nonparalytic) from acquired (paralytic) eventration is established. The author carefully differentiates between diaphragmatic eventration and congenital diaphragmatic hernia in terms of the pathologic features and also the differences in therapy.

BIBLIOGRAPHY

Adamthwaite, D. N., Snijders, D. C., and Mirwis, J.: Traumatic pericardiophrenic hernia: A report of 3 cases. Br. J. Surg., 70:177, 1983.

Anderson, L. S., and Forrest, J. V.: Tumors of the diaphragm. Am. J. Roentgenol. Radium Ther. Nucl. Med., 119:259, 1973.

Aronoff, R. J., Reynolds, J., and Thal, E. R.: Evaluation of diaphragmatic injuries. Am. J. Surg., 144:671, 1982.

Avnet, N. L.: Roentgenologic features of congenital bilateral anterior diaphragmatic eventration. Am. J. Roentgenol., 88:743, 1962.

Baer, G. A., and Talonen, P. P.: International symposium on implanted phrenic nerve stimulators for respiratory insufficiency. Ann. Clin. Res., 19:399, 1987.

Baer, G. A., Talonen, P. P., Hakkinen, V., et al.: Phrenic nerve stimulation in tetraplegia. Scand. J. Rehab. Med., 22:107, 1990.

Beclard, E.: Cited by J. Cruveilhier in Atlas d'Anatomie Pathologique. Vol. 1, Book 17, Parte V. Paris, 1829, p. 2.

Bellemare, E., and Bigland-Ritchie, B.: Central components of diaphragmatic fatigue assessed by phrenic nerve stimulation. J. Appl. Physiol., 62:1307, 1987.

Bisgard, J. D.: Congenital eventration of the diaphragm. J. Thorac. Surg., 16:484, 1947.

Bowditch, H. L.: Diaphragmatic hernia. Buffalo Med. J., 9:1, 65, 94, 1853.

Brooks, J. W.: Blunt traumatic rupture of the diaphragm. Ann. Thorac. Surg., 26:199, 1978.

Brouillette, R. T., Ilbawi, M. N., and Hunt, C. E.: Phrenic nerve pacing in infants and children: A review of experience and report on the usefulness of phrenic nerve stimulation studies. J. Pediatr., 102:32, 1983.

Brown, G. L., and Richardson, J. D.: Traumatic diaphragmatic hernia: Continuing challenge. Ann. Thorac. Surg., 39:170, 1985.

Buckman, R. F., Piano, G., Durham, C. M., et al.: Major bowel and diaphragmatic injuries associated with blunt spleen or liver rupture. J. Trauma, 28:1317, 1988.

Butler, W. M., Stolar, C. J., and Altman, R. P.: Contemporary management of congenital diaphragmatic hernia. World J. Surg., 17:350, 1993.

Cahill, J. L., Aberdeen, E., and Waterston, D. J.: Results of surgical treatment of esophageal hiatal hernia in infancy and childhood. Surgery, 66:597, 1969.

Cahill, J. L., Okamoto, G. A., Higgins, T., and Davis, A.: Experiences with phrenic nerve pacing in children. J. Pediatr. Surg., 18:851, 1983.

Caldani, L. M. A.: Institutiones Physiologicae. Venice, Pezzana, 1786. In Schechter, D. C. (ed): Application of electrotherapy to

noncardiac thoracic disorders. Bull. N. Y. Acad. Med., 46:932, 1970.

Carter, B. N., Giuseffi, J., and Felson, B.: Traumatic diaphragmatic hernia. Am. J. Roentgenol., 65:56, 1951.

Carter, R., and Brewer, L. A., III: Strangulating diaphragmatic hernia. Ann. Thorac. Surg., 12:281, 1971.

Childress, M. E., and Grimes, O. F.: Immediate and remote sequelae in traumatic diaphragmatic hernia. Surg. Gynecol. Obstet., 113:573, 1961.

Ciesielski, T. E., Fukuda, Y., Glenn, W. W. L., et al.: Response of the diaphragm muscle to electrical stimulation of the phrenic nerve: A histochemical and ultrastructural study. J. Neurosurg., 58:92, 1983.

Cloutier, R., Fournier, L., and Levasseur, L.: Reversion to fetal circulation in congenital diaphragmatic hernia: A preventable postoperative complication. J. Pediatr. Surg., 18:551, 1983.

De la Rocha, A. G., Creel, R. J., Mulligan, G. W. N., et al: Diaphragmatic rupture due to blunt abdominal trauma. Surg. Gynecol. Obstet., 154:175, 1982.

Duchenne, G. B. A.: De l'electrisation localisée et de son application à la therapeutique par courants induits et par courants galvaniques interrompus et continus, par le dr. Duchenne. 3rd ed. Paris, Bailliere, 1872.

Ebert, P. A., Gaertner, R. A., and Zuidema, G. D.: Traumatic diaphragmatic hernia. Surg. Gynecol. Obstet., 125:59, 1967.

Ein, S. H., Barker, G., Olley, P., et al.: The pharmacologic treatment of newborn diaphragmatic hernia: A 2-year evaluation. J. Pediatr. Surg., 15:384, 1980.

Estenne, M., Yernault, J., De Smet, J., and De Troyer, A.: Phrenic and diaphragm function after coronary artery bypass grafting. Thorax, 40:293, 1985.

Estera, A. S., Landay, M. J., and McClelland, R. N.: Blunt traumatic rupture of the right hemidiaphragm: Experience in 12 patients. Ann. Thorac. Surg., 39:525, 1985.

Fagan, C. J., Schreiber, M. H., Amparo, E. G., et al.: Traumatic diaphragmatic hernia into pericardium: Verification of diagnosis by computed tomography. J. Comput. Assist. Tomogr., 3:405, 1979.

Farmer, W. C., Glenn, W. W. L., and Gee, J. B. L.: Alveolar hypoventilation syndrome: Studies of ventilatory control in patients selected for diaphragm pacing. Am.J. Med., 64:39, 1978.

Glenn, W. W. L.: Diaphragm pacing: Present status. PACE Pacing Clin. Electrophysiol., 1:357, 1978.

Glenn, W. W. L.: On diaphragm pacing. N. Engl. J. Med., 317:1477, 1987.

Glenn, W. W. L.: Pacing the diaphragm in infants. Ann. Thorac. Surg., 40:319, 1985.

Glenn, W. W. L., Hogan, J. F., Loke, J. S. O., et al.: Ventilatory support by pacing of the conditioned diaphragm in quadriplegia. N. Engl. J. Med., 310:1150, 1984.

Glenn, W. W. L., Hogan, J. F., and Phelps, M. L.: Ventilatory support of the quadriplegic patient with respiratory paralysis on diaphragm pacing. Surg. Clin. North Am., 60:1055, 1980.

Glenn, W. W. L., Holcomb, W. G., McLaughlin, A. J., et al.: Total ventilatory support in a quadriplegic patient with radiofrequency electrophrenic respiration. N. Engl. J. Med., 286:513, 1972.

Glenn, W. W. L., and Phelps, M. L.: Diaphragm pacing by electrical stimulation of the phrenic nerve. Neurosurgery, 17:974, 1985.

Glenn, W. W. L., Phelps, M. L., Elefteriades, J. A., et al.: Twenty years of experience in phrenic nerve stimulation to pace the diaphragm. PACE Pacing Clin. Electrophysiol., 9:780, 1986.

Grage, T. B., MacLean, L. D., and Campbell, G. S.: Traumatic rupture of the diaphragm: A report of 26 cases. Surgery, 46:669, 1959.

Gravier, L.: Congenital diaphragmatic hernias. South Med. J., 67:59, 1974.

Halldorsson, A., Esser, M. J., Rappaport, W., et al.: A new method of diagnosing diaphragmatic injury using intraperitoneal technectium—Case report. J. Trauma, 33:140, 1992.

Hardesty, R. L., Griffith, B. P., Debski, R. F., et al.: Extracorporeal membrane oxygenation: Successful treatment of persistent fetal circulation following repair of congenital diaphragmatic hernia. J. Thorac. Cardiovasc. Surg., 81:556, 1981.

Harpin, R. P., Gignac, S. P., Epstein, S. W., et al.: Diaphragm pacing and continous positive airway pressure. Am. Rev. Respir. Dis., 134:1321, 1986.

Harrington, S. W.: Various types of diaphragmatic hernias treated surgically: Report of 430 cases. Surg. Gynecol. Obstet., *86*:735, 1948.

Harrison, M. R., and De Lorimier, A. A.: Congenital diaphragmatic hernia. Surg. Clin. North Am., *61*:1023, 1981.

Heiss, K., Manning, P., Oldham, K. T., et al.: Reversal of mortality for congenital diaphragmatic hernia with ECMO. Ann. Surg., *209*:225, 1989.

Hislop, A., and Reid, L.: Persistent hypoplasia of the lung after repair of congenital diaphragmatic hernia. Thorax, *31*:452, 1976.

Hood, R. M.: Traumatic diaphragmatic hernia. Ann. Thorac. Surg., *12*:311, 1971.

Hufeland, C. W.: De usu vis electricae in asphyxia experimentis illustrato. Inaugural dissertation, Gottingae, 1873. *In* Schechter, D. C. (ed): Application of electrotherapy to noncardiac thoracic disorders. Bull. N. Y. Acad. Med., *46*:932, 1970.

Ilbawi, M. N., Idriss, F. S., Hunt, C. E., et al.: Diaphragmatic pacing in infants: Techniques and results. Ann. Thorac. Surg., *40*:323, 1985.

Iuchtman, M., Freire, E. C., and Jacob, E. R.: Acute diaphragmatic hernia caused by blunt trauma. Am. Surg., *43*:460, 1977.

Juvara, L., and Priscu, A.: Primary congenital diaphragmatic tumors. Surgery, *60*:255, 1966.

Kim, J. H., Manuelidis, E. E., Glenn, W. W. L., and Kaneyuki, T.: Diaphragmatic pacing: Histopathological changes in the phrenic nerve following long-term electrical stimulation. J. Thorac. Cardiovasc. Surg., *72*:602, 1976.

Kuster, G. R., Kline, L. E., and Garzo, G.: Diaphragmatic hernia through the foramen of Morgagni: Laparoscopic repair case report. J. Laparoendoscop. Surg., *2*:93, 1992.

Lally, K. P., Paranka, M. S., Roden, J., et al.: Congenital diaphragmatic hernia: Stabilization and repair on ECMO. Ann. Surg., *216*:569, 1992.

Larrieu, A. J., Wiener, L., Alexander, R., et al.: Pericardiodiaphragmatic hernia. Am. J. Surg., *139*:436, 1980.

Levin, D. L.: Morphologic analysis of the pulmonary vascular bed in congenital left-sided diaphragmatic hernia. J. Pediatr., *92*:805, 1978.

Levy, R. J., Rosenthal, A., Freed, M. D., et al.: Persistent pulmonary hypertension in a newborn with congenital diaphragmatic hernia: Successful management with tolazoline. Pediatrics, *60*:740, 1977.

Lieberman, D. A., Faulkner, J. A., Craig, A. B., and Maxwell, A. C.: Perfusion and histochemical composition of guinea pig and human diaphragm. J. Appl. Physiol., *34*:233, 1973.

Lilly, J. R., and Randolph, J. G.: Hiatal hernia and gastroesophageal reflux in infants and children. J. Thorac. Cardiovasc. Surg., *55*:42, 1968.

Markland, O. N., Moorthy, S. S., Mahomet, Y., et al.: Postoperative phrenic nerve palsy in patients with open-heart surgery. Ann. Surg., *39*:68, 1985.

McElwee, T. B., Myers, R. T., and Pennell, T. C.: Diaphragmatic rupture from blunt trauma. Am. Surg., *51*:143, 1984.

Meisner, H., Schober, J. G., Struck, E., et al.: Phrenic nerve pacing for the treatment of central hypoventilation syndrome—State of the art and case report. Thorac. Cardiovasc. Surg., *31*:21, 1983.

Meyers, B. F., and McCabe, C. J.: Traumatic diaphragmatic hernia—Occult marker of serious injury. Ann. Surg. *218*:783, 1993.

Mier, A., Brophy, C., Moxham, J., and Green, M.: Phrenic nerve stimulation in normal subjects and in patients with diaphragmatic weakness. Thorax, *42*:885, 1987.

Miller, L., Bennett, E. V., Jr., Root, H. D., et al.: Management of penetrating and blunt diaphragmatic injury. J. Trauma, *24*:403, 1984.

Morgagni, G. B.: Seats and causes of diseases. Zellts 54, Monograph on Hernia of the Diaphragm, 1769.

Morrison, J. A., and Mullens, J. E.: Traumatic intrapericardial rupture of the diaphragm. J. Trauma, *18*:744, 1978.

Morrison, J. M. W.: Elevation of one diaphragm unilateral phrenic paralysis: A radiological study with special reference to differential diagnosis. Arch. Radiol. Electrother., *27*:353, 1923.

Moxham, J., and Shneerson, J. M.: Diaphragmatic pacing. Am. Rev. Respir. Dis., *148*:533, 1993.

Mugica, J., Dejean, D., Smits, K., et al.: Direct diaphragm stimulation. PACE Pacing Clin. Electrophysiol., *10*:252, 1987.

Naeye, R. L., Shochat, S. J., Whitman, V., and Maisels, M. J.: Unsuspected pulmonary vascular abnormalities associated with diaphragmatic hernia. Pediatrics, *58*:902, 1976.

Nochomovitz, M. L., Hopkins, M., Brodkey, J., et al.: Conditioning of the diaphragm with phrenic nerve stimulation after prolonged disuse. Am. Rev. Respir. Dis., *130*:684, 1984.

Nochomovitz, M. L., Peterson, D. K., and Stellato, T. A.: Electrical activation of the diaphragm. Clin. Chest Med., *9*:349, 1988.

Oakes, D. D., Wilmot, C. B., Halverson, D., and Hamilton, R. D.: Neurogenic respiratory failure: A 5-year experience using implantable phrenic nerve stimulators. Ann. Thorac. Surg., *30*:188, 1980.

O'Callaghan, J. D., Saunders, N. R., Chatrath, R. R., and Walker, D. R.: The management of neonatal posterolateral diaphragmatic hernia. Ann. Thorac. Surg., *33*:174, 1982.

Oda, T., Glenn, W. W. L., Fukuda, Y., et al.: Evolution of electrical parameters for diaphragm pacing: An experimental study. J. Surg. Res., *30*:142, 1981.

Olafsson, G., Rausing, A., and Holen, O.: Primary tumors of the diaphragm. Chest, *59*:568, 1971.

Orringer, M. B., Kirsh, M. M., and Sloan, H.: Congenital and traumatic diaphragmatic hernia exclusive of the hiatus. Curr. Probl. Surg., *12*:33, 1975.

Petit, J. L.: Traite des Maladies Chirurgicales et des Operations Qui Leur Conviennent: Ouvrage Posthume de J. L. Petit. Vol. II. Rev. ed. Lesne, 1790, p. 233.

Pomerantz, M., Rodgers, B. M., and Sabiston, D. C., Jr.: Traumatic diaphragmatic hernia. Surgery, *64*:529, 1968.

Redmond, C. R., Graves, E. D., Falterman, K. W., et al.: Extracorporeal membrane oxygenation for respiratory and cardiac failure in infants and children. J. Thorac. Cardiovasc. Surg., *93*:199, 1987.

Rodriguez-Morales, G., Rodriguez, A., and Shatney, C. H.: Acute rupture of the diaphragm in blunt trauma: Analysis of 60 patients. J. Trauma, *26*:438, 1986.

Salmons, S., and Henriksson, J.: The adaptive response of skeletal muscle to increased use. Muscle Nerve, *4*:94, 1981.

Sarnoff, S. J., Hardenbergh, E., and Whittenberger, J. L.: Electrophrenic respiration. Am. J. Physiol., *155*:1, 1948a.

Sarnoff, S. J., Hardenbergh, E., and Whittenberger, J. L.: Electrophrenic respiration. Science, *108*:482, 1948b.

Sato, G., Glenn, W. W. L., Holcombe, W. G., and Wuench, D.: Further experience with electrical stimulation of the phrenic nerve: Electrically induced fatigue. Surgery, *68*:817, 1970.

Sawyer, S. F., Falterman, K. W., Goldsmith, J. P., and Arensman, R. M.: Improving survival in the treatment of congenital diaphragmatic hernia. Ann. Thorac. Surg., *41*:75, 1986.

Schechter, D. C.: Application of electrotherapy to noncardiac thoracic disorders. Bull. N. Y. Acad. Med., *46*:932, 1970.

Shochat, S. J., Naye, R. L, Frod, W. D. A., et al.: Congenital diaphragmatic hernia: New concept in management. Ann. Surg., *190*:332, 1979.

Sinclair, L., and Klein, B. L.: Congenital diaphragmatic hernia—Morgagni type. J. Emerg. Med., *11*:163, 1993.

Strug, B., Noon, G. P., and Beall, A. C., Jr.: Traumatic diaphragmatic hernia. Ann. Thorac. Surg., *17*:444, 1974.

Sumner, E., and Frank, J. D.: Tolazoline in the treatment of congenital diaphragmatic hernias. Arch. Dis. Child., *56*:350, 1981.

Sutton, J. P., Carlisle, R. B., and Stephenson, W. E.: Traumatic diaphragmatic hernia. Ann. Thorac. Surg., *3*:136, 1967.

Symbas, P. N., Hatcher, C. R., Jr., and Waldo, W.: Diaphragmatic eventration in infancy and childhood. Ann. Thorac. Surg., *24*:133, 1977.

Talonen, P. P., Baer, G. A., Hakkinen, V., and Ojala, J. K.: Neurophysiological and technical considerations for the design of an implantable phrenic nerve stimulator. Med. Biol. Eng. Comput., *28*:31, 1990.

Tarver, R. D., Conces, D. J., Cory, D. A., and Vix, V. A.: Imaging the diaphragm and its disorders. J. Thorac. Imag. *4*:1, 1989.

Thomas, T. V.: Congenital eventration of the diaphragm. Ann. Thorac. Surg., *10*:180, 1970.

Thomas, T. V.: Nonparalytic eventration of the diaphragm. J. Thorac. Cardiovasc. Surg., *55*:586, 1968.

Thomas, T. V.: Subcostosternal diaphragmatic hernia. J. Thorac. Cardiovasc. Surg., *63*:278, 1972.

Tiballs, J.: Diaphragmatic pacing: An alternative to long-term mechanical ventilation. Anaesth. Intensive Care, *19*:597, 1991.

Trento, A., Griffith, B. P., and Hardesty, R. L.: Extracorporeal membrane oxygenation experience (ECMO) at the University of Pittsburgh. Ann. Thorac. Surg., *42*:56, 1986.

Trivedi, S. A.: Neurolemmona of the diaphragm causing severe hypertrophic pulmonary osteoarthropathy. Br. J. Tuberc., *52*:214, 1958.

Ure, A.: Experiments made on the body of a criminal immediately after execution with physiological and philosophical observations. J. Sci. Arts, *12*:1, 1818. *In* Schechter, D. C. (ed): Application of Electrotherapy to Noncardiac Thoracic Disorders. Bull. N. Y. Acad. Med., *46*:932, 1970.

van Loenhout, R. M. M., Schiphorst, T. J. M. J., Wittens, C. H. A., and Pinackaers, J. A.: Traumatic intrapericardial diaphragmatic hernia. J. Trauma, *26*:271, 1986.

Ward, R. E., Flynn, T. C., and Clark, W. P.: Diaphragmatic disruption secondary to blunt abdominal trauma. J. Trauma, *21*:35, 1981.

West, K. W., Bengston, K., Rescorla, F. J., et al.: Delayed surgical repair and ECMO improves survival in congenital diaphragmatic hernia. Ann. Surg., *216*:454, 1992.

Wetrich, R. M., Sawyers, T. M. and Haug, C. A.: Diaphragmatic rupture with pericardial involvement. Ann. Thorac. Surg., *8*:361, 1969.

Wetstein, L.: Technique for implantation of phrenic nerve electrodes. Ann. Thorac. Surg., *43*:335, 1987.

Wiencek, R. G., Jr., Wilson, R. F., and Steiger, Z.: Acute injuries of the diaphragm. J. Thorac. Cardiovasc. Surg., *92*:989, 1986.

Wiener, M. F., and Chou, W. H.: Primary tumors of the diaphragm. Arch. Surg., *90*:143, 1965.

Wilson, J. M., Lund, D. P., Lillehei, C. W., and Vacanti, J. P.: Congenital diaphragmatic hernia: Predictors of severity in the ECMO era. J. Pediatr. Surg., *26*:1028, 1991.

Wohl, M. E. B., Griscom, N. T., Strieder, D. J., et al.: The lung following repair of a congenital diaphragmatic hernia. J. Pediatr., *90*:405, 1977.

Index

Note: Page numbers in *italics* refer to illustrations; page numbers followed by t refer to tables.

A

a waves, in pulse contour, 1368, *1368*
a/A P$_{O2}$ ratio, in respiratory support, 42
(A–a)D$_{O2}$. See *Alveolar-arterial oxygen gradient.*
Abdomen, compression of, in cardiac output maintenance, 1640–1641
  distention of, in tracheoesophageal fistula, 893–894
  injury of, with penetrating chest injury, 483, *484*
ABIOMED ventricular assist device, 2006, *2006*
Ablation, rotational, of coronary artery atheroma, 1176–1177
Abrasion, in pleurodesis, 2155, *2156*
Abscess, amebic, of pericardium, 1375
  lung. See *Lung abscess.*
  myocardial, 1707
  prosthetic valve, 1707
Absent pulmonary valve syndrome, in tetralogy of Fallot, 1470, *1470*
Absorption atelectasis, 51
  in pure oxygen therapy, 41, *42*
Academic credit, for computer application development, 397, *397*
Accessory pathways, concealed, 2047
  in paroxysmal supraventricular tachycardia, 2047
  in Wolff-Parkinson-White syndrome. See *Wolff-Parkinson-White syndrome.*
  Mahaim fibers and, 2048–2049
Accidents, chest injury in. See *Chest trauma, blunt.*
Acebutolol, in ventricular arrhythmias, 250t
Acetazolamide, in metabolic alkalosis, 259
Acetylcholine, in coronary spasm diagnosis, 1973
Acetylcholine receptors, antibodies to, in myasthenia gravis, 1101, *1105–1106*, 1105–1108
  in myasthenia gravis, 593
N-Acetylprocainamide, in ventricular arrhythmias, 250t
Achalasia, esophageal. See under *Esophagus.*
Acid, ingestion of. See *Corrosive substances, esophageal injury from.*
Acid citrate dextrose blood, metabolic alkalosis from, 49–50
Acid clearing test, in esophageal disorders, *1022,* 1023
Acid perfusion test, in esophageal disorders, 961, *1022,* 1025
Acid reduction procedures, in peptic stricture, 999
Acid-base balance, alterations in. See also *Acidosis; Alkalosis.*
  perioperative, 49–50
  evaluation of, 11–12
  Henderson-Hasselbalch equation in, 48
  historical aspects of, 48–49
  management of, after cardiac surgery, 259–260
    in cardiopulmonary bypass, *1261,* 1261–1262
  measurement of, 49–50

Acid-base balance *(Continued)*
  metabolism and, 48–49
  monitoring of, 49–50
  physiologic compensation in, 12
Acidosis, cardiopulmonary arrest in, 369
  causes of, 48–50
  in aortic stenosis, 1520
  in hypothermia, 1824
  in shock, 174
  lactic, in low cardiac output syndrome, 236
  metabolic, cardiopulmonary arrest in, 369
    compensation for, 12
    in cardioplegia, 1824
    in hypoplastic left heart syndrome, 1660
    in pediatric patients, 449
    in shock, 185
    in univentricular heart, 1617
    postoperative, 49, 259
  paradoxic intracellular, 50
    postoperative, oxygen therapy in, 44
  respiratory, compensation for, 12
    mechanical ventilation in, 57
    postoperative, 50, 259
Acid-reflux test, in esophageal disorders, *1022,* 1022–1023
Acquired immunodeficiency syndrome. See *Human immunodeficiency virus infection.*
Actinomyces israelii, 683, *684*
Actinomycosis, 683–684, *684*
Action potential, of conduction system, 1767, *1767,* 2033, *2033*
Activated clotting time, after cardiac surgery, 254, *254*
  in cardiopulmonary bypass, 139
Acute Physiology and Chronic Health Evaluation (APACHE), in shock, 173, 176, *177–178*
Acyclovir, in herpetic esophagitis, 741
  prophylactic, in immunodeficiency, 745, 746t
Acylated plasminogen-streptokinase activator complex, 1187
Adams-Oliver syndrome, Poland syndrome and, 507
Adenocarcinoma, of esophagus, 925–926, *925–927, 1063*
  of lung, 635
  of pleura, versus mesothelioma, 567
Adenoid cystic carcinoma, of bronchus, 663
  of esophagus, 925
  of trachea, 406, *407,* 437, 439, 663
Adenoma, bronchial. See under *Bronchus.*
  of parathyroid glands, 604
  of thyroid gland, 603
Adenomatous hamartoma of infancy, 662
Adenosine, in paroxysmal atrial tachycardia, 246
Adenosquamous carcinoma, of lung, pathology of, 635
Adhesions, in fibrothorax, 559–561

Esophagoplasty. See *Esophagus, reconstruction of.*
Esophagopulmonary fistula, 839
Esophagoscope, flexible, 86, *88*
  rigid, 85t, 85–86, *86–87*
Esophagoscopy, 84–95, 963, 965
  anesthesia for, 85
  complications of, 87, *88*
  contraindications for, 85
  cricopharyngeal muscle in, 86, *87*
  diagnostic, 84–90
    findings in, 87–89, 89t
    indications for, 84–85
    technique for, 85t, 85–86, *86–88*
    with ultrasonography, 89–90, *90*
  equipment for, 85, 85t, *86,* 90–91, *92,* 93–95, *94*
  in achalasia, 89, *94,* 94–95, 979
  in Barrett's esophagus, 88
  in biopsy, 959, 959t
  in brachytherapy, 92–93
  in carcinoma, 89, 91–92, *94,* 927
  in corrosive esophagitis, 88–89, 89t, 91, *93,* 900–901
  in diffuse spasm, 984
  in diverticulum, 89
  in foreign body removal, 90, *91*
  in gastroesophageal reflux, 897
  in hiatal hernia, 89, 1021–1022
  in malignancy, 959
  in neoplasms, 89, 91–92, *94*
  in pediatric patients, 85t, 85–86, *86–87*
  in peptic stricture dilatation, 1064–1065
  in peptic stricture evaluation, 1062, 1064
  in photodynamic therapy, 94
  in reflux, 87–88, 958, 959t
  in stenosis, 88
  in stricture dilatation, 90–91, *92*
  in tracheoesophageal fistula, 894
  in varices, 89, 94
  indications for, 84–85
  patient position for, 85–86, *87*
  procedure for, with flexible fibergastroscope, 86–87, *88*
    with rigid esophagoscope, 85t, 85–86, *86–87*
  pyriform sinus location in, 86, *87*
  therapeutic, 90–95, *91–94*
  ultrasonography with, 89–90, *90*
Esophagostomy, in esophageal atresia, 893
Esophagus, achalasia of, 974t, 975–983
    causes of, 975–976
    clinical features of, 976–977
    diagnosis of, 896, *897,* 976–981, *977–979, 980*
    esophagoscopy in, 89, *94,* 94–95
    etiology of, 896
    in pediatric patients, 896–897
    pathophysiology of, 1017–1018
    symptoms of, 896
    treatment of, 93–94, *94,* 896–897, 980–983, *982–983*
      thoracoscopic, 2160, *2161–2165,* 2162–2163, 2166
  acid perfusion test of, 961, *1022,* 1023
  acid-clearing test of, *1022,* 1023
  acid-reflux test of, *1022,* 1022–1023
  adenocarcinoma of, 925–926, *925–927, 1063*
  adenoid cystic carcinoma of, 925
  adventitia of, 947, *949*
  anastomosis of, 885, *885,* 888, *889–890,* 890–891
  anatomy of, *920,* 920–921, 937, *942–946, 943, 946, 948,* 1013–1015, *1015*
    developmental, 934, 936, *936–940*
    macroscopic, 936–937, *940–941*
    narrow sites, 84, *85,* 936–937, *940*
    topographic, 937, *941*
  anomalies of, *827*
  atresia of, *828,* 841, 885–893
    anatomy of, 886
    anomalies with, 885–886, *887*

Esophagus *(Continued)*
  clinical findings in, 886–887, *887–888,* 893, *893*
  embryology of, 885–886, *886*
  historical aspects of, 885, *885*
  incidence of, 886, *887*
  isolated, 892–893, *893*
  tracheoesophageal fistula with, 886–892, *887–892,* 895
  treatment of, 887–892
    bougienage in, 893
    complications of, 891–892, *892*
    delayed repair in, 890, *891*
    esophagostomy in, 893
    gastrostomy in, 890–891, *891,* 893
    nutritional support in, 887, 890–891
    primary repair technique in, 888, *889–890,* 890
    results of, 892
    risk categories in, 888
    staged repair in, 890–891
  types of, 886, *887*
  attachments of, 1040–1041
  Barrett's. See *Barrett's esophagus.*
  biopsy of, 959, 959t, 1021–1022, 1064
  blood supply of, *403,* 403–404, 921, 937, *942–943, 943,* 1014
    development of, 936, *939–940*
  body of, anatomy of, 947–948, *948–950,* 950
  bougienage of. See *Bougienage.*
  bronchogenic cyst of, 1005, *1006,* 1007
  burns of. See also *Corrosive substances; Esophagitis, reflux; Peptic stricture.*
    esophagoscopy in, 90, *91*
    in pediatric patients, 900–901, *901*
    treatment of, 90, *91*
  carcinoma of, Barrett's esophagus and. See *Barrett's esophagus.*
    caustic stricture transition to, 923
    clinical features of, 927
    diagnosis of, 927, 959
    endoscopy in, 959
    epidemiology of, 923
    esophagoscopy in, 89
    extension of, 926–927
    in achalasia, 977
    incidence of, 923
    metastasis of, 927
    pathology of, 924–927, *925–927*
    sites of, 923
    tracheal extension of, 408
    treatment of, 91–92, *94,* 927–932
      chemotherapy in, 927–928
      esophagogastrectomy in, *928–931,* 929–930
      historical aspects of, 919–920
      multimodal, 928
      palliative, 930–931, *931*
      radiation therapy in, 927–928
      surgical, *928–931,* 929–931
    versus peptic stricture, 996–997
  carcinosarcoma of, 925, *926*
  closure of, in airway obstruction relief, 291, *292*
  compression of, in aortic arch anomalies, 1300, 1302–1306
    in pulmonary artery sling, 1307, *1307*
  computed tomography of, 1195, *1196*
  congenital disorder(s) of, achalasia as, 896–897, *897*
    atresia as, 885–893, *885–893*
    developmental anomalies as, 826, *827–828*
    duplication as, 899, *900*
    gastroesophageal reflux in, 897–899, *898–899*
    laryngotracheal cleft with, 895
    neuromuscular, 896
    stenosis as, 895–896, *896*
    tracheoesophageal fistula as, 893–897, *894–895*
    webs as, 895–896, *896*
  corkscrew, in spasm, 896

Lymphoma *(Continued)*
  of mediastinum, 600–603
    benign giant, 606, *607*
    diagnosis of, 600
    Hodgkin's, 600, *601*
    non-Hodgkin's, 601–603, *602*
    symptoms of, 600
    treatment of, 600, 603
    ultrastructure of, 588t
  of myocardium, in HIV infection, 743
  of pericardium, 1375
  pleural effusion in, 544–545
  pseudolymphoma and, 662–663
Lymphoreticuloma, follicular, mediastinal, 606, *607*

M

MAC (minimum alveolar concentration), of
    anesthetics, 124
McGoon operation, in great artery transposition,
    1572–1573
  in mitral insufficiency, 1692
Machinery murmur, in patent ductus arteriosus,
    1276
MacIntosh blade, for laryngoscopy, 299, *299,* 301, *301*
Macleod's syndrome, hyperlucent lung in, 865, *866*
Macrophages, alveolar, elastase production in, 872
  in atherosclerosis formation, 2017, *2018*
  in multiple organ failure, 181
Magnesium, imbalance of, coronary artery spasm in,
    1982
  in cardioplegia solution, 1823–1824
  management of, after cardiac surgery, 259
Magnetic resonance angiography, in coronary artery
    disease, 1209, *1210–1211*
Magnetic resonance imaging, 1203–1223
  anatomic considerations in, *1204*
  cine, 1205, *1206,* 1207
  contraindications to, 1203
  contrast agents for, 1209
  echo planar imaging in, 1209
  gated imaging in, 1205
  gradient-recalled echo in, *1204,* 1205, *1206,* 1207
  in aortic disease, 1217–1220, *1218–1220*
  in aortic dissection, 1347, *1351*
  in bronchogenic cyst, 860
  in cardiac neoplasms, 1216–1217, *1216–1217,* 2075–
    2076, *2077*
  in cardiac thrombosis, 1216–1217
  in chest wall neoplasms, 516
  in congenital heart disease, 1211, 1213, *1213–1216,*
    1216
  in cor triatriatum, 1422–1423, *1423*
  in coronary artery disease, 1209, *1210–1211*
  in database, 392
  in ejection fraction measurement, 1207
  in left ventricular aneurysm, 1950
  in lung carcinoma, 638
  in mediastinal neoplasms, 586–587
  in myocardial infarction, 1207–1210, *1208*
  in myocardial ischemia, 1207–1210, *1208*
  in pericardial disease, 1217–1219, *1218–1219,* 1371
  in Poland syndrome, 507
  in pulmonary arteriovenous fistula, 913
  in pulmonary embolism, chronic, 807t
  in stroke volume measurement, 1207
  in thoracic aortic aneurysm, 1330, *1331*
  in tricuspid atresia, 1631–1632
  in valvular disease, 1209–1211, *1212–1213*
  principles of, 1203–1205, *1204, 1206,* 1207
  radiofrequency pulse in, 1205
  safety of, 1203
  spin-echo technique in, 1205, 1207
  transverse magnetization in, 1205
Magnetization, of cardioverter-defibrillator, 1807

Magnetization *(Continued)*
  transverse, in magnetic resonance imaging, 1205
Mahaim fibers, supraventricular arrhythmias and,
    2048–2049
Maintenance dose, in patient-controlled analgesia,
    154–155, 155t
Malignancy. See also specific disease, e.g., *Carcinoma;
    Mesothelioma.*
  pleural effusion in, 543–544
Malignant fibrous histiocytoma, of heart, 2083–2084
Malignant melanoma, metastasis of, to heart, *2084,*
    2084–2085
  to lung, 673–674
  of esophagus, 925
Mallampati's classification, of tongue versus
    pharyngeal size, 295, *296*
Mallinckrodt tracheal tubes, 335t, *336*
Malnutrition, in multisystem organ failure, treatment
    of, 199–201
Mammaplasty, in Poland's syndrome, 507
Mammary artery, internal, arteriovenous fistula of,
    915–916, *915–917*
  as coronary artery graft, 1909–1925
    angiography of, *1880,* 1881
    bilateral, 1898–1899
    disadvantages of, 1912
    free, 1915, *1915–1916*
    graft patency in, 1910–1911
    historical aspects of, 1885, 1910
    in Kawasaki's disease, 1994
    indications for, 1911
    left in-situ, 1914, *1914*
    multiple, 1918, 1920, *1921,* 1922t
    operative mortality and morbidity in, 1917–
      1918
    procurement of, 1896, 1912–1913, 1917
    right in-situ, 1914–1915, *1915*
    sequential grafting of, 1914, *1914*
    survival in, 1918, *1919–1921,* 1920, 1922t
    technique of, 1912–1917, *1913–1917*
  bypass of, with vertebral artery, in occlusive dis-
    ease of aortic arch branches, 1360t
  contractility of, along various segments, *1985*
  laceration of, 476
Mandatory minute ventilation, 58–59
Mandibular space, evaluation of, in tracheal
    intubation, 296, *296*
Mannitol, in renal failure prevention, 265
Manometry, of esophagus. See under *Esophagus.*
Manougiuan procedure, in aortic root enlargement,
    1753, *1754*
Mapping, electrophysiologic, in ventricular
    tachycardia, 2062–2064, *2064*
  intraoperative, in ischemic ventricular tachycar-
    dia, 2062–2064, *2064*
    in Wolff-Parkinson-White syndrome correc-
      tion, 2043
Marfan syndrome, aortic dissection in, 1345
  pectus excavatum correction in, 498
  thoracic aortic aneurysm in, 1327–1328, 1332–1334,
    1333–1337
Mark IV antireflux repair, 1025–1032
  alternatives to, 1027
  indications for, 1025–1027
  postoperative care in, 1031, *1031*
  preoperative preparation for, 1027
  results of, 1031
  technique of, 1027, *1028–1029,* 1030
Marshall, vein of, anatomy of, 1862, *1862*
  embryology of, *1408*
Martorell's syndrome. See *Aortic arch, branches of,
    occlusive disease of.*
Mask ventilation, airway difficulty and, *303*
  in cardiopulmonary resuscitation, 369–370
  technique of, 289–291
Massage, cardiac, in cardiopulmonary resuscitation,
    374–376, *376,* 2012

Mediastinum *(Continued)*
  subdivisions of, *576,* 576–577
    neoplasm location and, 583t, 583–584
  teratoma of, 595, *596*
  thymic cyst of, 610
  thymoma of. See *Thymoma.*
  widened, in great vessel injury, 468–469, *468–469*
  yolk-sac tumors of, 597–600, *599*
Medical history, in database, 386–387
  in tracheal intubation, 294–295
Medical literature services, 382–383, *385*
The Medical Record (TMR) database, 381
MEDLARS database, 383
MEDLINE database, 383
Medtronic Biomedicus pump, for ventricular assist
    devices, 2004, *2004*
Megaesophagus, in achalasia, *976–978,* 977–979
Meigs' syndrome, pleural effusion in, 544
Meissner's plexus, anatomy of, 946, *948*
Melanoma. See *Malignant melanoma.*
Membrane oxygenation, in cardiopulmonary bypass,
    1257
Meningitis, in coccidioidomycosis, 691
  in cryptococcosis, 695
Menstruation, pneumothorax during, 529–530
Meperidine, characteristics of, 154t
  dosage of, parenteral-oral conversions in, 158t
  in bronchoscopy, 73
  in epidural analgesia, 160t–161t
  in patient-controlled analgesia, 155t, 156
Mephentermine, action of, *143*
Mepivacaine, as local anesthetic, 127t
Mesenchymal patch, in tracheal reconstruction, 406
Mesenchymal tumor, mediastinal, 605
Mesenteric arteries, necrotizing arteritis of, after
    aortic coarctation repair, 1292
Mesocardia, in great artery transposition, 1558–1559
Mesoderm, in esophageal development, 934, *935*
Mesothelioma (cardiac), 2082
Mesothelioma (pleural), 566–570
  benign, 567–568, *568*
  clinical presentation of, 567, 569, *569*
  diffuse, 567–570, *569,* 569t–570t
  epithelial variant of, 567
  forms of, 567
  histology of, 566–567
  localized, 567–568, *568*
  malignant, diffuse, 568–570, *569*
    etiology of, 567
    localized, 568
    metastasis from, 569
    pathology of, 567
    staging of, 569, 569t
    treatment of, 569–570, 570t
  pathology of, 567
  pleural plaques and, 565
Message routes, in computer systems, 395
Metabolic acidosis. See under *Acidosis.*
Metabolic alkalosis. See under *Alkalosis.*
Metabolism, acids formed in, 48
  derangement of, cardiopulmonary arrest in, 369
    in blood transfusion, 256
    in low cardiac output syndrome, 236
    in multisystem organ failure, 199–201
    in septic shock, 194–195, 199–201
  in infants, thermoregulation and, 450, *450*
Metacholine, coronary artery spasm from, 1980
Metaproterenol, perioperative, 17
Metaraminol, action of, *143*
Metastasis, from germ-cell tumors, 598
  from heart, in myxoma, 2072
  from lung. See *Lung carcinoma, metastasis from.*
  from neuroblastoma, 590
  from seminoma, 597
  from thymoma, 595
  pathogenesis of, 669

Metastasis *(Continued)*
  to esophagus, 926–927
  to heart, *2084,* 2084–2085
    computed tomography of, 1197, *1197*
  to lung. See *Lung(s), metastasis to.*
  to mediastinum, 603
  to pericardium, 1375
  to pleura, 570–571
  to trachea, 408–409
Methadone, dosage of, parenteral-oral conversions
    in, 158t
Methicillin, 111
  bacteria resistant to, 108–109
Methotrexate, in lung carcinoma, 646
Methoxamine, action of, 143, *143,* 144t
Methyl methacrylate glue, in chest wall
    reconstruction, 219
Methylprednisolone, in heart-lung transplantation,
    2098–2099
Methylprednisone, in lung transplantation, 2129,
    2129
Metoclopramide, in aspiration prevention, 297
Metoprolol, in ventricular arrhythmias, 250t
  pharmacology of, 146t
Metronidazole, in amebiasis, 703
Mexiletine, in ventricular arrhythmias, 250t
Microatelectasis, postoperative, mechanical
    ventilation in, 316
Microbubbles, in echocardiography, 1240–1241, 1249
MicroMeSH literature search aid, 383
Midazolam, cardiovascular effects of, 123t
  in tracheal intubation, 302
    in cardiovascular disease, 297
Middle-lobe syndrome, in histoplasmosis, 689
  lobectomy in, 715, *716–719,* 720
Migraine headache, coronary artery spasm in, 1978
Miliary tuberculosis. See under *Tuberculosis.*
Military antishock trousers, in hypovolemic shock,
    186
Military injury, 456. See also *Chest trauma, blunt.*
Military position, in thoracic outlet syndrome, 617,
    619
Miller blade, for laryngoscopy, 299–300, *300*
Milrinone, after cardiac surgery, 242
Minimal effective analgesic concentration, 153–154,
    154t
Minimal inhibitory concentration, in antibiotic
    prophylaxis, 105
Minimum alveolar concentration, of anesthetics, 124
Minute oxygen consumption, pulmonary resection
    risk and, 16
Minute ventilation, calculation of, *24*
  spontaneous, in extubation success prediction, 326
Minute volume, in pediatric patients, 14t
  typical values of, 3t
Missile embolism, of pulmonary arteries, 780–781
Mitochondrial function, in septic shock, 195
Mitral arcade (hammock malformation), 1547–1548
Mitral insufficiency, 1688–1699. See also *Ebstein's
    anomaly; Mitral valve, prolapse of.*
  absent papillary muscles in, 1548
  acute, 1144, *1144*
  anatomic considerations in, postinfarction, 1958–
    1959
  anesthesia in, 129t, 132
  annular dilatation in, 1546–1547
  annuloplasty in, 1674, 1691–1692, 1696–1697
  aortic valve disease with, 1755
  asymptomatic, treatment of, 1690–1691
  atrial septal defect with, 1388
  chronic, 1144
  cleft leaflet in, 1551–1552, *1552*
  clinical features of, 132, 1549, 1689
    postinfarction, 1959t, 1959–1961, *1960*
  congenital, morphology of, 1546–1549, 1547t, *1548*
  diagnosis of, 1689–1690, *1690*

MVV. See *Maximal voluntary ventilation.*
Myasthenia gravis, 1100–1122
    acetylcholine receptor antibodies in, 1101, *1105–1106,* 1105–1108
    as autoimmune disorder, 1101–1102, 1105, 1107
    classification of, 1101, 1102t
    clinical features of, 1100–1103, *1101,* 1102t
    conditions associated with, 1102
    congenital, 1101
    definition of, 1100
    diagnosis of, 594, 1103–1105, *1104*
        algorithm for, 1119–1121, *1120*
    drugs interfering with, 1108, 1108t
    experimental allergic, 1107
    historical aspects of, 1100
    late-onset, thymus gland atrophy in, 1103
    medical treatment of, 1108–1110
        versus thymectomy, 1117, *1117*
    muscles affected by, 1100–1101, *1101,* 1101t
    neonatal, 1101
    pathogenesis of, *1105–1106,* 1105–1108
    plasmapheresis in, 1109
    prevalence of, 1100
    recurrence of, after thymectomy, *1117,* 1117–1119, 1118t, *1119*
    spontaneous remission in, 1101
    thymectomy in. See *Thymectomy.*
    thymoma and, 593–595, 1115–1116
    thymus gland and, 1102–1103, *1103,* 1107–1108
    treatment of, algorithm for, 1119–1121, *1120*
Myasthenic syndrome, 1101–1102
myc proto-oncogene, in lung cancer, 665
Mycobacteria, atypical, 754–755, 755t
    classification of, 754–755, 755t, 758, 760
Mycobacterial infections. See also *Tuberculosis.*
    in HIV infection, 739
    versus mycobacterial disease, 7–8, *759–761*
Mycobacterium avium-intracellulare infection, 755, 755t
    in HIV infection, 738–739
    lung resection in, 766, *767*
Mycobacterium bovis, 754–755
Mycobacterium kansasii, 755, 755t
Mycobacterium tuberculosis, 754–755, 755t. See also *Tuberculosis.*
Mycotic aneurysm, 1328
Mycotic infection(s). See *Fungal infection(s).*
Myoblastoma (granular cell tumor), of bronchus, 661
Myocardial depressant factor, in refractory hemorrhagic shock, 189
    in septic shock syndrome, 193
Myocardial infarction, acute, coronary artery bypass in, 1891–1892
    after coronary artery bypass, 231, *232,* 1901, 1928
    angiography in, 1190–1191
    angioplasty in, 1190–1191
    cardiogenic shock in, 201–205, 1892
        clinical manifestations of, 201–202
        diagnosis of, 201–202
        intra-aortic balloon pump in, 1999–2000
        mortality in, 201
        pathophysiology of, 201–202, *202*
        treatment of, 202–205, 204t
    cardiopulmonary arrest in, 368
    computed tomography in, 1197, *1197*
    coronary angioplasty in, 1172–1173
    coronary angioscopy in, 1178
    coronary artery bypass after, 1892
    echocardiography in, 1239–1240, *1241*
    fibrinolytic therapy in. See *Thrombolytic therapy.*
    healing in, 1822
    in cardiac catheterization, 1125–1126
    in coronary artery bypass, 1918
    in coronary atherosclerosis, 1887–1888
    in Kawasaki's disease, 1992
    in left ventricular aneurysm, 1943–1946, *1946*
    in Prinzmetal's angina, 1973, 1975

Myocardial infarction *(Continued)*
    infarct expansion in, 1187
    intra-aortic balloon pump in, refractory to medical therapy, 2001
        with cardiogenic shock, 1999–2000
        with mechanical complications, 2000
    intraoperative causes of, 244–245, *245*
    magnetic resonance imaging in, *1207,* 1207–1209
    mechanical complications of, intra-aortic balloon pump in, 2000
    mitral insufficiency in, 1688–1689, 1958–1968
        anatomic considerations in, 1958–1959
        clinical features of, 1959t, 1959–1961, *1960*
        diagnosis of, 1961–1962, *1961–1962*
        fixed, 1964–1966, *1964–1966*
        intra-aortic balloon pump in, 2000
        surgical treatment of, 1962–1966, *1963–1966*
        transient, 1963–1964
    monitoring in, 202–203
    pacing after, 1770–1771
    papillary muscle dysfunction in, clinical features of, 1960–1961
        surgical treatment of, 1964, *1965,* 1966
    papillary muscle rupture in, clinical features of, 1960, *1960*
        diagnosis of, 1961, *1961–1962*
        intra-aortic balloon pump in, 2000
        surgical treatment of, 1964, *1964–1965*
    pathology of, luminal narrowing in, 1849–1850, 1850t, *1851–1852,* 1852–1853
        plaque composition in, 1853, 1853t
    pathophysiology of, 1183–1184, *1183–1185,* 1816–1817, *1820–1822,* 1822
    perioperative, 128, 129t, *130,* 244–245, *245*
    pleural effusion after, 545
    prevention of, in coronary artery bypass, 1893–1894
    pulmonary embolism in, 781
    refractory to medical therapy, intra-aortic balloon pump in, 2001
    reperfusion treatment in, 202, 204
    resuscitation in, 1888
    risk reduction, lipid lowering in, 2023t
    stunned myocardium in, 202
    thrombolytic therapy for. See *Thrombolytic therapy.*
    treatment of, in cardiac surgery, 244
    ventricular septal defect in, 1968, 1970, *1970*
        intra-aortic balloon pump in, 2000
    ventricular tachycardia in, 2055–2056
Myocardial ischemia. See also *Ischemic heart disease; Myocardial infarction.*
    after pulmonary artery atresia with intact ventricular septum repair, 1503
    akinesia in, 1946
    anesthesia in, 128, 129t, *130*
    cardiac catheterization in, 1124
    diastolic creep in, 1816–1817, *1819*
    dyssynchrony in, 1946
    ejection fraction in, 1946
    end-diastolic volume in, 1997
    hypokinesia in, 1946
    in coronary artery hypoplasia, 1845
    in coronary atherosclerosis, 1886–1888
    in pulmonary atresia with intact ventricular septum, 1495, *1496,* 1606, *1606*
    in valvular disease, radionuclide imaging of, 1227–1228, *1228*
    intraoperative, treatment of, 128, *130*
    left ventricular aneurysm in, 1946
    magnetic resonance imaging in, *1207,* 1207–1209
    mitral insufficiency in. See *Myocardial infarction, mitral insufficiency in.*
    paradoxical motion in, 1946
    pathophysiology of, 1816–1817, *1818–1822,* 1822
    perioperative, mechanical ventilation in, 319
    repeated coronary artery bypass in. See *Coronary artery bypass, repeated.*

ISBN 0-7216-5757-5

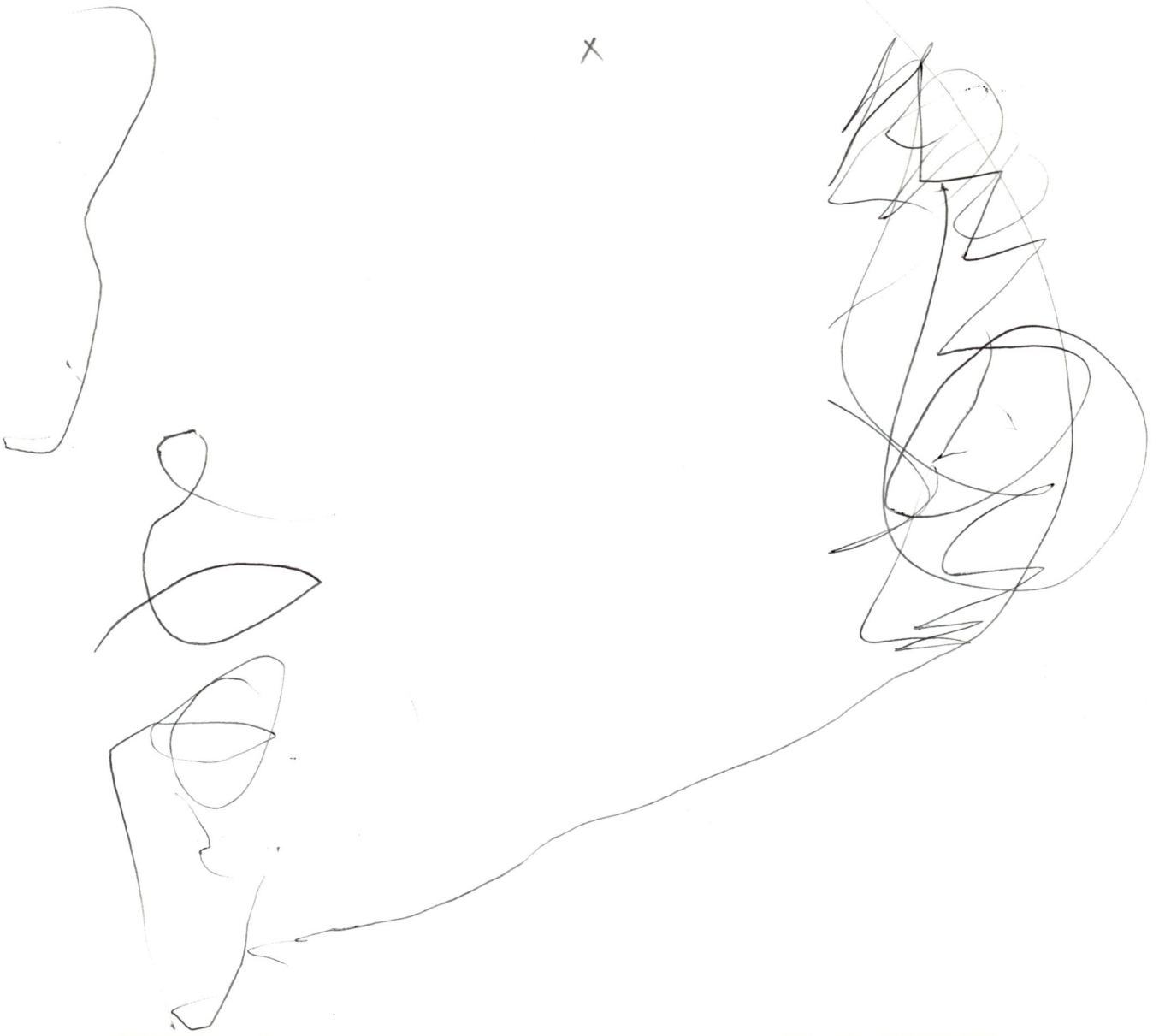